Textbook of the Neurogenic Bladder

2nd Edition

Edited by

Jacques Corcos MD
Professor of Urology
Director, Department of Urology
Jewish General Hospital
McGill University
Montréal, Québec
Canada

Erik Schick MD LMCC FRCSC
Emeritus Professor of Surgery (Urology)
University of Montréal
Former Chief and Honorary Member
Division of Urology
Maisonneuve-Rosemount Hospital
Montréal, Québec
Canada

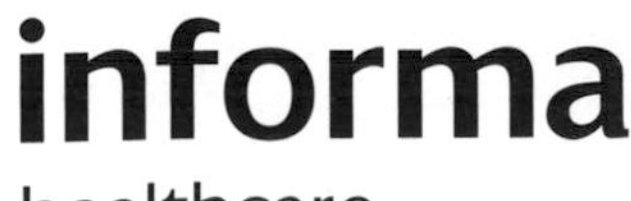

First published in the United Kingdom in 2004

Second edition published in the United Kingdom in 2008 by Informa Healthcare, Telephone House, 69-77 Paul Street, London, EC2A 4LQ. Informa Healthcare is a trading division of Informa UK Ltd. Registered Office: 37/41 Mortimer Street, London W1T 3JH. Registered in England and Wales number 1072954.

Tel: +44 (0)20 7017 5000
Fax: +44 (0)20 7017 6699
Website: www.informahealthcare.com

A CIP record for this book is available from the British Library.

Library of Congress Cataloging-in-Publication Data

Data available on application

ISBN-10: 0 415 42316 3
ISBN-13: 978 0 415 42316 8

Distributed in North and South America

Taylor & Francis
6000 Broken Sound Parkway, NW, (Suite 300)
Boca Raton, FL 33487, USA

Within Continental USA
Tel: 1 (800) 272 7737; Fax: 1 (800) 374 3401

Outside Continental USA
Tel: (561) 994 0555; Fax: (561) 361 6018
Email: orders@crcpress.com

Book orders in the rest of the world

Paul Abrahams
Tel: +44 207 017 4036
Email: bookorders@informa.com

Composition by C&M Digitals (P) Ltd, Chennai, India
Printed and bound in India by Replika Press Pvt. Ltd
Cover design by Catherine Schick

Contents

List of contributors

Mazen Abdelhady MD MSc Clinical Fellow, University of Western Ontario, London, Ontario, Canada.

Kate Abrahamsson MD Associate Professor, Pediatric Urology Section, The Queen Silvia Children's Hospital, Sahlgrenska Academy, University of Göteborg, Göteborg, Sweden.

Tala Al Afraa MD Research Fellow, University of Montréal, Division of Urology, Maisonneuve-Rosemont Hospital, Montréal, Québec, Canada.

Saad Aldousari MD Resident, Department of Urology, McGill University, Montréal, Québec, Canada.

Waleed Altaweel MD Resident, Department of Urology, McGill University, Montreal, Québec, Canada.

Karl-Erik Andersson MD PhD Professor, Wake Forest Institute for Regenerative Medicine, Wake Forest University Health Sciences, Winston Salem, NC, USA.

Gerard Apodaca PhD Professor of Medicine and Cell Biology and Physiology, Laboratory of Epithelial Cell Biology, University of Pittsburgh School of Medicine, Pittsburgh, PA, USA.

Walter Artibani MD Professor of Urology, Department of Oncological and Surgical Sciences, Urology Clinic, University of Padova, Padova, Italy.

Greg G Bailly MD FRCSC Assistant Professor, Department of Urology, Dalhousie University, Queen Elizabeth II Health Science Center, Halifax, NS, Canada.

Diego Barriéras MD FRCSC Assistant Clinical Professor, University of Montréal, Division of Urology, St-Justine Children's Hospital, Montréal, Québec, Canada.

Stuart B Bauer MD Senior Associate in Urology, Children's Hospital, Professor of Surgery (Urology), Harvard Medical School, Boston, MA, USA.

Djamel Bensmail MD Department of Physical Medicine and Rehabilitation, Neurourology and Andrology Unit, Raymond Poincaré Hospital, University of Versailles Saint Quentin en Yvelines, Garches, France.

Marianne Berényi MD PhD Director, Department of Developmental Neurology, Pediatric Institute, Budapest, Hungary.

Pierre E Bertrand MD FRCSC Assistant Professor of Urology, Division of Urology, University of Montréal, Maisonneuve-Rosemont Hospital, Montréal, Québec, Canada.

Fin Biering-Sørensen DrMedSci Head of Department, Clinic for Spinal Cord Injuries, The Neuroscience Centre, Rigshospitalet, Copenhagen University Hospital, Copenhagen, Denmark.

Lori A Birder PhD Associated Professor of Medicine and Pharmacology, Renal/Electrolyte Division, Department of Medicine, University of Pittsburgh School of Medicine, Pittsburgh, PA, USA.

Jerry G Blaivas MD Clinical Professor of Urology, Department of Urology, Weill College of Medicine, Cornell University, Institute for Bladder and Prostate Research, Lenox Hill Hospital, New York, NY, USA.

Bernard Boillot Division of Urology, Michallon University Hospital, Grenoble, France.

Timothy B Boone MD PhD Professor and Chair, Scott Department of Urology, Chairman, Department of Urology, Methodist Hospital, Baylor College of Medicine, Houston, TX, USA.

JLH Ruud Bosch MD PhD FEBU Professor and Chair, Department of Urology, University Medical Centre Utrecht, Utrecht, The Netherlands.

Nancy L Brackett PhD HCLD The Miami Project to Cure Paralysis, Department of Urology, University of Miami Miller School of Medicine, Miami, FL, USA.

Alison F Brading PhD Emeritus Professor, University Department of Pharmacology, Oxford University, Oxford, UK.

Guy Breault MD Resident, Department of Urology, McGill University, Montréal, Québec, Canada.

Homero Bruschini MD Professor of Urology, Division of Urology, University of São Paolo School of Medicine, São Paolo, Brazil.

Lysanne Campeau MD Resident, Department of Urology, McGill University, Montréal, Québec, Canada.

Steven Casha MD PhD FRCSC University of Calgary Spine Program and the Department of Clinical Neurosciences, Foothills Medical Centre, Calgary, Alberta, Canada.

Maria A Cerruto MD FEBU Assistant Professor of Urology, Department of Biomedical and Surgical Sciences, Urology Clinic, University of Verona, Verona, Italy.

Michael B Chancellor MD Professor of Urology and Obstetrics-Gynecology, Department of Urology and Obstetrics-Gynecology, McGowan Institute of Regenerative Medicine, University of Pittsburgh, Pittsburgh, PA, USA.

Emmanuel Chartier-Kastler MD PhD Professor of Urology, Department of Urology, Pitié-Salpetrière Hospital, Paris, France.

Pierre Clément PhD Pelvipharm Laboratories, Conseil National de la Recherche Scientifique, Gif-sur-Yvette, France.

Brian Cohen MD Fellow, Female Urology, Voiding Dysfunction and Reconstruction, Miller School of Medicine, Jackson Memorial Hospital, University of Miami, Miami, FL, USA.

Jacques Corcos MD Professor of Urology, Director of the Department of Urology, Jewish General Hospital, McGill University, Montréal, Québec, Canada.

Michael Craggs PhD CBiol Csci MIPEM Professor of Applied Neurophysiology, Division of Surgery and Interventional Sciences, University College London; Director of Spinal Research, Consultant Clinical Scientist, National Center for Spinal Research, Royal National Orthopaedic Hospital NHS Trust, Stanmore, Middlesex, UK.

Graham H Creasey MD FRCSD Professor of Neurosurgery, Department of Neurosurgery, Stanford University, Palo Alto, CA, USA.

G Willy Davila MD Chairman and Head, Department of Gynecology, Section of Urogyaecology and Reconstructive Pelvic Surgery, Cleveland Clinic Florida, Weston, FL, USA.

Dirk De Ridder MD PhD FEBU Head of Clinic, Urology and Neurourology Clinic, University Hospitals KU Leuven, National MS Hospital, Melsbroek, Belgium.

Gina A Defreitas MD Department of Surgery, Division of Urology, Humber River Regional Hospital, Toronto, Ontario, Canada.

Pierre Denys MD Department of Physical Medicine and Rehabilitation, Neurourology and Andrology Unit, Raymond Poincaré Hospital, University of Versailles Saint Quentin en Yvelines, Garches, France.

Angela DiGrande MSN APRN-BC Practioner Nurse, Northern California Urology Services, Shriners Hospital for Children, Saramento, CA, USA.

Ananias C Diokno MD FACS Executive Vice-President and Chief Medical Officer, William Beaumont Hospitals, Royal Oak, MI, USA.

Roger Dmochowski MD Professor of Urology, Vanderbilt Continence Center, Department of Urologic Surgery, Vanderbilt University Medical Center, Nashville, TN, USA.

John W Downie PhD Professor, Department of Pharmacology and Urology, Dalhousie University, Halifax, NS, Canada.

Marcus J Drake MA (Cantab) DM (Oxon) FRCS (Urol) Consultant Surgeon, Bristol Urological Institute, Southmead Hospital, University of The West of England, Bristol, United Kingdom.

Nader Elmayergi MD Bch Clinical Fellow, Department of Cardiology, University of Manitoba, Winnipeg, Manitoba, Canada.

Mostafa Elmissiry MbChBm Research Fellow, Section of Female Urology and Voiding Dysfunction, Cleveland Clinic Florida, Weston, FL, USA.

Magnus Fall MD PhD Professor, Deprtment of Urology, Institute of Clinical Sciences, Sahlgrenska University Hospital, University of Göteborg, Sweden.

Andrew Feifer MD Resident, Department of Urology, McGill University, Montréal, Québec, Canada.

Clare J Fowler MBBS MSc FRCP Reader and Consultant in Neuro-Urology, Department of Uro-Neurology, Institute of Neurology, University College of London, The National Hospital for Neurology and Neurosurgery, London, UK.

Jerzy B Gajewski MD FRCSC Professor of Urology and Pharmacology, Department of Urology, Dalhousie University, Queen Elizabeth II Health Science Centre, Halifax, Nova Scotia, Canada.

Hélène Gelez Pelvipharm Laboratories, Centre National de la Recherche Scientifique, Gif-sur-Yvette, France.

Gamal M Ghoniem MD FACS Head, Section of Female Urology, Voiding Dysfunction and Reconstruction, Clinical Professor of Surgery/Urology, NOVA Southeastern University, Ohio State University and University of South Florida and Cleveland Clinic Florida, Weston, FL, USA.

François Giuliano MD Assistance Publique-Hôpitaux de Paris, Neurourology and Andrology Unit, Department of Physical Medicine and Rehabilitation, Raymond Pointcaré Hospital, Garches, France.

Angelo E Gousse MD Associate Professor, Director of Urology Residency Program, Division of Female Urology, Voiding Dysfunction and Reconstruction, Miller School of Medicine, University of Miami, Miami, FL, USA.

Christian Gratzke MD Research Fellow, Wake Forest Institute for Regenerative Medicine, Wake Forest University Health Sciences, Winston Salem, NC, USA; and Department of Urology, Ludwig Maximilians University, Munich, Germany.

Derek J Griffiths MD Senior Visiting Fellow, Institute of Neurology, University College London, London, UK; and Consultant and Past Professor of Medicine, Division of Geriatric Medicine, University of Pittsburgh, Pittsburgh, PA, USA.

William C de Groat PhD Professor of Pharmacology, Division of Pharmacology, University of Pittsburgh School of Medicine, Pittsburgh, PA, USA.

Axel Haferkampl MD Professor of Urology, Department of Urology, University of Heidelberg, Germany.

Antal Hamvas MD PhD Associate Professor, Department of Urology, Semmelweis University, Budapest, Hungary.

Tomáš Hanuš MD PhD Professor of Urology, First Medical School, Charles University, Prague, Czech Republic.

Magdy Hassouna MD PhD FRCSC FACS Associate Professor of Surgery, Department of Surgery, University of Toronto, Toronto, Ontario, Canada.

Takamichi Hattori MD Professor, Department of Neurology, Chiba University, Chiba, Japan.

Sender Herschorn MD FRCSC Professor and Chair, Division of Urology, University of Toronto, Sunnybrook Health Science Center, Toronto, Ontorio, Canada.

Emad Ibrahim MD The Miami Project to Cure Paralysis, University of Miami Miller School of Medicine, Miami, FL, USA.

Ginger Isom-Batz MD Department of Urology, University of Texas, Southwestern Medical Center, Dallas, TX, USA.

Roman Jednak MD FRCSC Assistant Professor of Urology, Department of Urology, Director, Division of Pediatric Urology, The Montréal Children's Hospital, McGill University Health Centre, Montréal, Québec, Canada.

Ditlev Jensen MD PhD Assistant-Head, Department of Neurology, Rikshospitalet University Hospital, Oslo, Norway.

Yun Jeong Jeong MD PhD Department of Urology, Eulji University School of Medicine, Daejeon, Republic of Korea.

Martine Jolivet-Tremblay MD FRCSC Assistant Professor, Centre Hospitalier de l'Université de Montréal, Division of Urology, University of Montréal, Montréal, Québec, Canada.

Osamu Kamihira MD Chief, Department of Urology, Komaki Shimin Hospital, Komaki, Aishi, Japan.

Katona Ferenc MD PhD DSc Professor, Department of Developmental Neurology, Pediatric Institute, Budapest, Hungary.

Shinji Katsuragi MD Professor of Perinatology, National Cardiovascular Center, Suita, Osaka, Japan.

Mark Kellett BmedSci MD FRCP Greater Manchester Neurosciences Centre, Salford Royal Hospitals NHS Foundation Trust, Hope Hospital, Salford, Greater Manchester, UK.

Christopher E Kelly MD Assistant Professor, Department of Urology, New York University School of Medicine, New York, NY, USA.

Richard T Kershen MD Assistant Professor of Surgery, Director of Female Urology and Voiding Dysfunction, Division of Urology, Department of Surgery, The Continence Center, University of Vermont College of Medicine, Fletcher Allen Health Care, South Burlington, VT, USA.

Carlotte Kiekens MD Department of Physical Medicine and Rehabilitation, Rehabilitation Centre UZ Leuven, University Hospitals KU Leuven, Leuven, Belgium.

Dae Kyung Kim MD PhD Associate Professor, Department of Urology, Eulji University School of Medicine, Daejeon, Republic of Korea.

Bjorn Klevmark MD PhD Professor Emeritus, Department of Urology, Rikshospitalet University Hospital, Oslo, Norway.

Atsuo Kondo MD PhD President, Tsushima Rehabilitation Hospital, Tsushima, Aichi, Japan.

Jean-Jacques Labat MD Neurologist, Physical Medicine and Rehabilitation, Department of Urology, Hôtel-Dieu Hospital, University Hospital of Nantes, Nantes, France.

Steven P Lapointe MD FRCSC Urologist and Clinical Instructor, Department of Urology, University of Montréal, Cité de la Santé de Laval, Laval, Québec, Canada.

Marc Le Fort MD Physical Medicine and Rehabilitation, Department of Neurological Rehabilitation, Saint-Jacques Hospital, University Hospital of Nantes, Nantes, France.

Line Leboeuf MD FRCSC Assistant Professor of Urology, Division of Urology, University of Montréal, Maisonneuve-Rosemont Hospital, Montréal, Québec, Canada.

Ling K Lee MD FRCS Consultant Urological Surgeon, Department of Urology, Royal Bolton Hospital, Bolton, UK.

Gary E Lemack MD Associate Professor of Urology and Neurology, Department of Urology and Neurology, University of Texas Southwestern Medical Center, Dallas, TX, USA.

Patrick B Leu MD The Urology Center, Omaha, NE, USA.

Sivert Lindström MD PhD Professor, Department of Biomedicine and Surgery, University of Health Sciences, Linköping, Sweden.

Helmut G Madersbacher MD PhD Associate Professor of Urology, Neurourology Unit, Department of Neurology, Landeskrankenhaus, Medical University of Innsbruck, Innsbruck, Austria.

Attila Majoros MD PhD FEBU Assistant Professor, Department of Urology, Semmelweis University, Budapest, Hungary.

Anders Mattiasson MD PhD Professor of Urology, Department of Urology, Lund University Hospital, Lund, Sweden.

Paul Mitrofanoff MD Professor and Consultant, Division of Pediatric Surgery, Charles Nicolle University Hospital, Rouen, France.

John Morrison FB MB ChB PhD FRCSEd FIBiol Professor, Department of Physiology, Faculty of Medicine and Health Sciences, United Arab Emirates University, Al Ain, United Arab Emirates.

Hiep T Nguyen MD Assistant Professor of Surgery (Urology), Department of Urology, Harvard Medical School and Children's Hospital, Boston, MA, USA.

Osamu Nishizawa MD PhD Professor, Department of Urology, Shinshu University School of Medicine, Matsumoto-City, Nagano, Japan.

Victor W Nitti MD Professor and Vice-Chairman, Department of Urology, New York University School of Medicine, New York, NY, USA.

Reinier-Jacques Opsomer MD Associate Professor of Urology and Sexology, Centre de Pathologie Sexuelle Masculine (CPSM), Cliniques St-Luc, Université de Louvain, Brussels, Belgium.

Jürgen Pannek MD Professor and Chief of Neurourology, Department of Neurourology, Swiss Paraplegic Centre, Nottwil, Switzerland.

Inder Perkash MD FACS FRCS Professor of Urology, Stanford Consulting Staff Surgical Service, VA Palo Alto Health Care System, Palo Alto, CA, USA.

Brigitte Perrouin-Verbe MD Professor of Physical Medicine and Rehabilitation, Department of Neurological Rehabilitation, Saint-Jacques Hospital, University Hospital of Nantes, Nantes, France.

Joao Luiz Pippi-Salle MD PhD FRCSC FAAP Professor, Department of Surgery, Division of Urology, Hospital for Sick Children, University of Toronto, Toronto Ontario, Canada,

J Pindaro P Plese MD Professor of Neurosurgery, Department of Neurology, University of São Paolo School of Medicine, São Paolo, Brazil.

Simon Podnar MD DSc Neurologist and Neurophysiologist, Institute of Clinical Neurophysiology, Division of Neurology, University Medical Center Ljubljana, Ljubljana, Slovenia.

Imre Romics MD PhD DSc Professor and Chairman, Department of Urology, Semmelweis University, Budapest, Hungary.

Abdulrahman J Sabbagh MD FRCSC Consultant Neurosurgeon, Neuroscience Center, King Fahad Medical City, Ryad, Kingdom of Saudi Arabia.

Ryuji Sakakibara MD PhD Associate Professor, Neurology Division, Department of Internal Medicine, Sakura Medical Center, Toho University, Sakura, Japan.

Harriette Scarpero MD Assistant Professor, Department of Urology, Vanderbilt University Medical Center, Nashville, TN, USA.

Erik Schick MD (Louvain) LMCC FRCSC Emeritus Professor of Surgery (Urology), University of Montréal; Former Chief and Honorary Member, Division of Urology, Maisonneuve-Rosemont Hospital, Montréal, Québec, Canada.

Brigitte Schurch MD Professor of Neurology, Paraplegic Centre, University Hospital Balgrist, Zürich, Switzerland.

Satoshi Seki MD PhD Associate Professor, Shinshu University School of Medicine, Department of Clinical Urological and Pharmacological Research, Matsumoto-City, Nagano, Japan.

Ruhee Sidhu MD Research Associate, Institute for Bladder and Prostate Research, New York, NY, USA.

Ulla Sillén MD Professor, Pediatric Urology Section, The Queen Silvia Children's Hospital, Sahlgrenska Academy, University of Göteborg, Göteborg, Sweden.

Jean-Marc Soler MD Physical Medicine and Rehabilitation, Centre Bouffard Vercelli Cerbère, Cap Peyrefitte, France.

Miguel Srougi MD Professor and Chairman, Division of Urology, University of São Paolo School of Medicine, São Paolo, Brazil.

Manfred Stöhrer MD PhD Associate Professor, Department of Urology, University of Essen, Germany.

Anthony R Stone BSc MB FRCSEd Professor and Vice-Chair, Department of Urology, University of California Davis, Chief of Urology, Shriners Hospital of Northern California, Sacramento, CA, USA.

Emil A Tanagho MD Professor and Chairman Emeritus, Department of Urology, University of California, San Francisco, CA, USA.

Jocelyne Tessier MD FRCSC Assistant Clinical Professor of Urology, Division of Urology, University of Montréal, Maisonneuve-Rosemont Hospital, Montréal, Québec, Canada.

Vincent Tse WM MB BS FRACS (Urol) Assistant Professor, Department of Urology, Concord General Hospital, Concord, NSW, Australia.

William H Turner MD FRCSC (Urol) Consultant Urologist, Addenbrooke's Hospital, Cambridge University Hospitals, NHS Foundation NHS Trust, Cambridge, UK.

Philip Van Kerrebroeck MD PhD FEBU Professor of Urology, Chairman, Department of Urology, University Hospital, Maastricht, The Netherlands.

Paula J Wagner RN MSN C-FNP Family Nurse Practioner, Urology Clinic, University of California, Davis, Davis, CA, USA.

Christopher E Wolter MD Instructor in Urologic Surgery, Department of Urologic Surgery, Vanderbilt University Medical Center, Nashville, TN. USA.

Daniel J Won MD FACS FAAP Attending Pediatric Neurosurgeon. Department of Neurology, Kaiser Permanente Medical Centre, Fontana, CA, USA.

Jean-Jacques Wyndaele MD Dsci PhD Professor of Urology, Head, Laboratory for Urologic Animal Experiments; Head, Department of Urology, University of Antwerp, Antwerp, Belgium.

Brian S Yamada MD Attending Urological Surgeon, Capital Region Urological Surgeons, PLLC and St-Peter's Hospital, Albany, NY, USA.

Shokei Yamada MD PhD FACS Professor Emeritus, Former Chairman, Department of Neurosurgery, Loma Linda University School of Medicine, Loma Linda, CA; and Arrowhead Regional Medical Centre, Colton, CA; and, Kaiser Permanente Medical Centre, Fontana, CA, USA.

René Yiou MD PhD Division of Urology, Centre Hospitalier Universitaire Henri-Mondor, Créteil, France.

Tag Keun Yoo MD PhD Associate Professor, Department of Urology, Eulji University School of Medicine, Daejeon, Republic of Korea.

Naoki Yoshimura MD PhD Associate Professor, Department of Urology, University of Pittsburgh School of Medicine, Pittsburgh, PA, USA.

Philippe Zimmern MD Professor of Urology, Department of Urology, Bladder and Incontinence Center, UT Southwestern Medical Center, Dallas, TX, USA.

Introduction

Men who are occupied with the restoration of health of other men, by the joint exercise of skill and humanity are, above all, the noblest on earth. They even partake of divinity, since to preserve and renew is almost as noble as to create.

(Voltaire, 1694–1778)

As senior professors of urology, we noticed, for a long time, that students and residents are exceedingly interested in uro-oncology. Removing a prostate, or bladder, or kidney appears to be a noble task. They are happy because they 'kill the disease'! We noticed also that their interest declines when we speak to them about storage and voiding functions, physiology, neuropharmacology, and neurogenic bladders. There is possibly less glamour, fewer lives to save, less fear to assuage, and probably less money too in these 'neuro' fields. But we are probably right to say, at least from an epidemiologic point of view, that patients with voiding dysfunction, including those with neurogenic bladder dysfunction, are far more numerous than those suffering from urologic cancers. Neurourology and, more specifically, neurogenic bladder care are fascinating aspects of our speciality because they relate to function. Our surgeries do not produce large specimens, but, more interestingly, we reconstruct. The real challenge lies in functional results.

To share our passion with the reader, we have attempted to bring together some of the world's most distinguished experts in the field, assigning the difficult task of clear teaching to each of them. We asked them to summarize, synthesize, and simplify vast amounts of knowledge to make this book the reference source for students, residents, physicians, and health care professionals who want to have a precise, updated, well-documented, evidence-based, and authoritative opinion on all aspects of neurogenic bladders. We advised each author to try, according to our present level of comprehension, to explain all phenomena. We strongly believe that readers will better remember pathophysiologic events if they understand the nature of the underlying phenomena.

Since the first edition of this textbook in 2004, important new developments have occurred in relation to neurogenic bladder dysfunction. Consequently, this second edition is significantly expanded. We tried to incorporate these new aspects by updating all chapters. This, however, did not appear to be sufficient. We needed to add three new sections – special considerations on meningo-myelocele, sexual dysfunction in neurologic disorders, and ethical considerations – including a total of 19 new chapters to present a more comprehensive and complete view on the subject. More than 120 authors from five continents representing 21 countries agreed to participate with us in this exciting venture, ensuring a variety of approaches and allowing the expression of different opinions. Our deep gratitude goes to all of them.

This textbook will convey readers into several different aspects of the subspeciality. After reviewing the normal embryology, anatomy, and physiology of the lower urinary tract, complete with the physiology of normal sexual function in the first part, we devote a large segment of the second part to the epidemiology, pathology, and pathophysiology of different aspects of the neurogenic bladder. This essential part aims to clarify and explain the mechanisms underlying the different clinical entities developed in subsequent sections of the book.

One of the book's originalities is that it relates different neurologic pathologies to urethro-vesical dysfunction. We instructed the authors involved in the third part to briefly describe the pathophysiology of this neurologic disease and the way it alters lower urinary tract function.

All patients with vesico-urethral dysfunction – regardless of the nature of the neurologic process causing it – are investigated with the same diagnostic armamentarium. This constitutes the fourth part of the book. Clinical evaluation, imaging, electrophysiology, and, obviously, extensive urodynamic studies in adults as well as in infants and children are described in detail. A distinct chapter is devoted to cerebral representation of the voiding cycle, which opens up new avenues in our understanding of vesico-urethral function. Also, we found it useful to gather normal values from the literature – or at least what is believed to be normal – of different urodynamic parameters. This section ends with a practical guide to the diagnosis and follow-up of neurogenic bladders, a veritable handbook, on its own, for medical students and residents.

Different classifications of neurogenic bladder dysfunction, based on symptoms, site of neurologic lesions, and urodynamic findings, have been reported in the past. Recently, a new and highly original classification system has been proposed where structure and function are considered simultaneously. Professor Anders Mattiasson, former chairman of the Standardisation Committee of the International Continence Society, who presented this classification, accepted to develop it in the context of neurogenic bladder dysfunction. This chapter, on its own, constitutes the fifth part of the book.

Several new nonsurgical treatments, including new drugs and also new ways of administering them, have become standard in recent years. The electrical treatments mentioned a few years ago fill six chapters and represent new avenues in this field.

After the description of the surgical treatments available, which are still widely used and necessary, this sixth part ends with three fascinating chapters showing us what we believe will happen in neurogenic bladder management in the 21st century.

An entirely new section is devoted to meningo-myelocele patients. It deals not only with neonates, infants, and children, but also with adults, including recommendations for the follow-up of this special group of patients.

Part VII is a large synthesis, giving readers an overview of the different available treatments that depend on patient age and the main dysfunction presented, but keeping in mind the principle of vesico-urethral balance.

The eighth part describes the most frequent complications encountered and how to deal with them. A separate chapter is devoted to benign prostatic obstruction in neurogenic bladder patients, relatively frequent situations encountered in daily urologic practice.

Sexual problems were not considered in the previous edition of this book. We asked Professor Reinier-Jacques Opsomer to recruit a group of experts to explore these problems in this special group of patients. In the ninth part of our textbook, these different authors deal with the pathophysiology of sexual dysfunction in spinal cord injury and in neurologic diseases, such as multiple sclerosis and diabetes, available treatments for erectile dysfunction in neurologic patients in general, as well as fertility issues in men and problems related to pregnancy and delivery.

Follow-up, prognosis, and ethical considerations constitute parts X and XI.

Instead of reproducing *in extenso* some of the reports and guidelines published in the literature, we made a selection of the most pertinent ones for this book and indicated where they were published in printed form, and where they can be found on the Web. We consider it important to include such information because they represent a consensual view accepted by the international scientific community. In this way, readers can have access to the most recent versions of these reports and guidelines, which constitute the last part of the book.

Medicine in general and, more specifically, urology underwent tremendous evolution in recent decades. This radically modified our attitude toward neurogenic bladder dysfunction as well. We felt it was imperative to update our present-day knowledge of the subject in a practical, in-depth review of where we are today. We hope we have succeeded.

Once again, our deepest gratitude goes to each and every author who accepted our invitation to take part in this venture – for readily sharing their expertise with us, and for the time they took to write and/or update their respective chapters.

Last, but not least, our warmest gratitude goes to our wives, Sylvie and Micheline, who once again accepted to sacrifice part of our family life during the long months of intensive preparation of this book.

Jacques Corcos
Erik Schick
Montreal, 2008

Part I

The normal genito-urinary tract

1

Embryology of the lower urinary tract

Hiep T Nguyen and Emil A Tanagho

To better understand the diseases and congenital anomalies that affect the lower urinary tract, a thorough understanding of its embryology is essential. Our current understanding of lower urinary tract development is based upon observations derived from studies of fetal specimens and from clinical observations of congenital anomalies. However, these observations are only 'snap-shots' of a complex process that occurs during a brief period of time. Hence, much of what we know about the embryology of the lower urinary tract remains somewhat sketchy, and the exact details are filled by inferences and theories.

Development of germ layers

After fertilization of the ovum, the zygote undergoes cleavage and division to form a hollow sphere, the blastula. Some of the cells in the blastula aggregate to form an inner cell mass that will form the germ layers of the embryo (Figure 1.1). During the 2nd week of gestation, the inner cell mass flattens and forms two separate layers, the endoderm and ectoderm. A cleft develops within the ectoderm to form the amniotic cavity and within the endoderm to form the yolk sac. During the 3rd week of gestation, cells migrate from the endoderm and ectoderm to form a middle layer, the mesoderm. On the caudal end of the germ layers, the mesoderm does not develop, and the endoderm remains apposed to the ectoderm without an intervening layer of mesoderm.[1]

Development of the cloaca

At the caudal end where the endoderm and ectoderm remain apposed, the cloacal membrane is formed. Differential growth of the mesenchyme near the cloacal membrane causes the caudal end of the embryo to fold onto itself, forming a chamber, the cloaca (Figure 1.2). The cloaca is lined primarily by endoderm. Further growth causes the caudal end to flex further, placing the cloacal membrane on the ventral surface of the embryo. Around the 4th week of gestation, the urorectal septum, also known as Tourneux's fold, expands caudally toward the cloacal membrane (Figure 1.3). Concurrently, the two folds from the lateral aspect of the cloaca, Rathke's plicae, migrate medially.[2] As a result, the cloaca is divided into the urogenital sinus anteriorly and the rectum posteriorly. Similarly, the cloacal membrane is divided into the urogenital membrane and the anal membrane. Rupture of these membranes allows the urogenital sinus and anal canal to be in

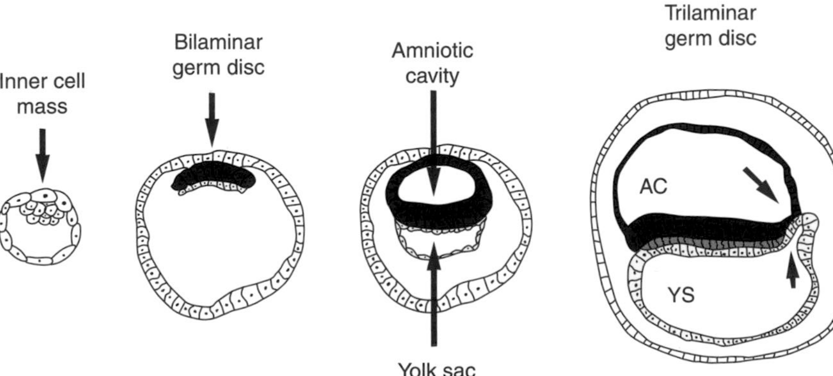

Figure 1.1
Development of the germ layers. An inner cell mass develops within the blastula. At the 2nd week of gestation, the cell mass differentiates to form two cell layers: ectoderm (blue) and endoderm (yellow). A cleft develops within each layer, forming the amniotic cavity (AC) and yolk sac (YS). During the 3rd week of gestation, a third layer, mesoderm (orange) develops in between the ectoderm and endoderm, except in the caudal region of the embryo (arrows).

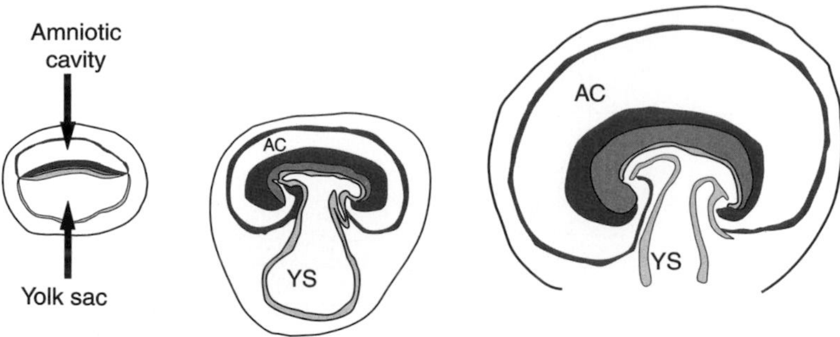

Figure 1.2
Creation of the cloaca. Differential growth of the mesenchyme in the cranial and caudal end of the embryo results in the infolding of yolk sac, creating the future GI and lower urinary tract. Rupture of the buccopharyngeal membrane (cranial) and the cloacal membrane (caudal) establishes communication between the amniotic cavity (AC) and the endoderm-lined yolk sac (YS, 3rd frame).

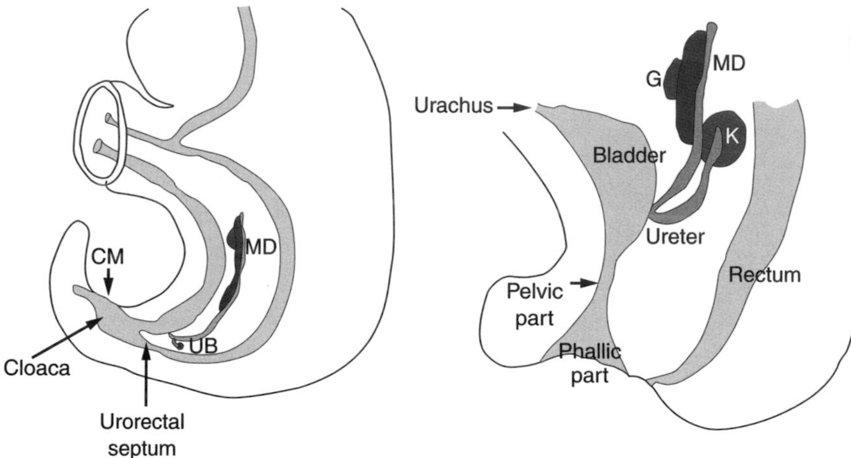

Figure 1.3
Differentiation of the cloaca. During the 4th week of gestation, the urorectal septum expands caudally to divide the cloaca into the urogenital sinus and the rectum. It also divides the cloacal membrane (CM) into the urogenital membrane and the anal membrane. The mesonephric duct (MD) develops adjacent to the primitive coelom. Cranially, it develops into the gonadal ductal system (G); caudally, it extends to join the urogenital sinus. A ureteric bud (UB) develops from each mesonephric duct and induces the surrounding mesenchyme to form the future kidney (K). After the 7th week of gestation, the urogenital sinus can be divided into three segments: the bladder, pelvic part, and phallic part.

communication with the amniotic cavity. This process of cloacal division is completed by the 7th week of gestation.

After this, the urogenital sinus can be morphologically divided into three segments (Figure 1.3). The largest and most cranial segment will give rise to the urinary bladder. The second segment, the pelvic part of the urogenital sinus, is the narrowest portion of the urogenital sinus and will give rise to the prostatic and membranous urethra in males. The third segment, the phallic part of the urogenital sinus, is separated from the amniotic cavity by the urogenital membrane and will give rise to the urethra and external genitalia.[1] The cranial portion of the urogenital sinus, the urachus, maintains its connection to the amniotic cavity.

Development of the trigone

Around the middle of the 3rd week of gestation, the mesonephric duct develops from the mesoderm adjacent to the coelom, the primitive peritoneum (Figure 1.3). The mesonephric duct extends caudally and by the 4th week of gestation reaches the urogenital sinus. The endodermal lining of the urogenital sinus fuses with the mesodermal epithelium of the mesonephric duct, allowing the mesonephric duct to drain into the cloaca. At this time, a diverticulum develops from the posteromedial aspect of the mesonephric duct, forming the ureteric bud. By the 5th week of gestation, the segment of mesonephric duct caudal to the ureteric bud dilates to form the common excretory duct (Figure 1.4). The right and left common excretory ducts are then absorbed into the urogenital sinus. They fuse together medially to form the primitive trigone.[3] As the common excretory ducts are absorbed, the openings to the ureters move cranially, while those to the mesonephric ducts move caudally.[4] Histologic evaluation of human fetuses demonstrated that, as early as the 12th week of gestation, myoblasts condensate mainly in the dorsal wall of the trigone and at the bladder outlet.[5] Expression of the androgen receptors is seen in the trigone of the bladder, indicating androgen involvement in the development of the vesico-ureteral junction.[6] The continuing muscle layers of the ureters cross the midline to form the interureteral fold. Muscle fibers forming the interureteral junction are demonstrable beginning at 14 weeks of gestation. The

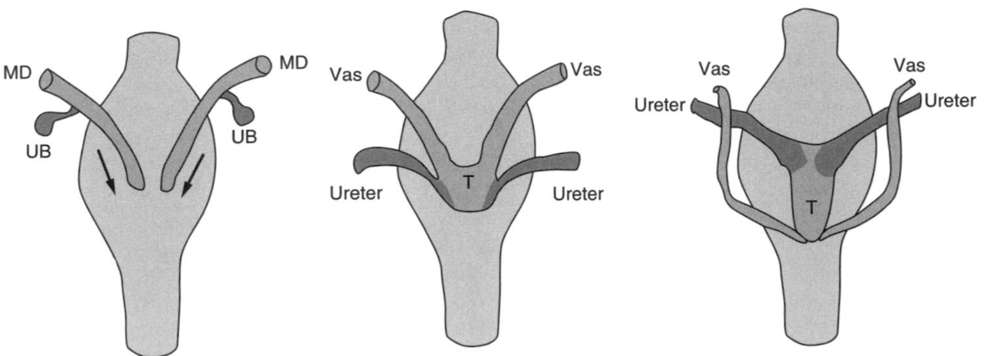

Figure 1.4
Development of the trigone. During the 5th week of gestation, the segment of the mesonephric duct (MD) caudal to the ureteric bud (UB) is absorbed into the urogenital sinus. The right and left side merge midline to form the trigone (T). In midline, growth of the trigone and vas continues caudally, pulling the orifice of vas distally. Laterally, growth occurs laterally and superiorly, pulling the ureteral orifice superiorly.

trigone develops continuously as a single, circular, muscular layer corresponding to the posterior part of the vesical sphincter muscle. The circular structure of this internal sphincter comes in close contact at its dorsal extension with the interureteral muscle, indicating a functional interaction and support of the distal uretero-vesical anchoring.[5] This pattern of development accounts for the contiguity of the musculature of the ureters with the trigone and the differential response of trigone musculature to pharmacologic agents compared to the bladder musculature.

Development of the bladder

By the 6th week of gestation, the cranial portion of the urogenital sinus dilates to form the primitive bladder, presumably due to the production of fluid/urine from the mesonephros and subsequently by the metanephros. At this stage the bladder wall is composed primarily of connective tissue. At the 7th week of gestation, mesenchyme at the dome of the primitive bladder begins to differentiate to form detrusor muscles. This process extends caudally and, by the 8th week of gestation, muscle development is seen diffusely throughout the bladder wall. However, the muscle is neither organized nor abundant. By the 12th week of gestation, the urachus closes, becoming a fibrous cord, the median umbilical ligament. The emptying of the bladder becomes primarily dependent on the urethra. Concurrently, the bladder muscle fibers begin to be organized into circular, interlacing, and longitudinal bundles. Muscle formation is especially abundant at the bladder base and in the trigone, where it is five times thicker than elsewhere in the bladder.[7]

By the 17th week of gestation, there are three muscle layers in the bladder: inner and outer longitudinal layers and a middle circular layer (Figure 1.5). Muscle bundles from the longitudinal layers interlace with the circular layer, making the distinction between the layers difficult except around the bladder neck.[8] The outer layer forms a complete sheet of muscle bundles around the bladder to the level of the bladder neck. In male fetuses, some of the muscle bundles from the outer layer extend into the prostate or loop around the proximal urethra. In female fetuses, these bundles end in the vesicovaginal septum. In contrast, the inner muscular layer is only present on the anterior bladder wall and is deficient posteriorly except in the region of the trigone. In the trigone, the inner longitudinal muscle layer extends caudally to become contiguous with the longitudinal muscle layer of the urethra. At the level of the bladder neck, the middle muscular layer is quiet prominent, since the muscle fibers in this area are quite closely packed together. The circularly oriented muscle bundles are complete anteriorly; they sweep through the sides of the bladder neck and fan outward as they travel posterior-cranially. The muscle bundles of the middle layer do not extend into the urethra but fuse to the lateral border of the trigone. As a result, by the 20th week of gestation, the bladder neck is bulky and pronounced. From the 20th week of gestation to term, there is continued increase in size of the muscles in the bladder, trigone, and urinary sphincter. Interestingly, while the bladder neck and trigone appear to develop in a gender specific manner, the bladder wall musculature develops uniformly, unrelated to gender. Its thickness and the mean profile area of smooth muscle bundles increase significantly with advancing gestation, mediated by linear growth patterns.[9]

The urothelium also undergoes extensive development during this time. The urothelium of the bladder is derived primarily from endoderm, while the urothelium of the upper urinary tract is derived from mesoderm. The presumed junction of the mesoderm and endoderm-derived urothelium occurs at the ureteral-vesical junction. However, the urothelium derived from mesoderm is histologically indistinguishable from that derived from endoderm.[10] The urothelium gradually differentiates from a simple cuboidal epithelium with smooth luminal surface to a stratified transitional epithelium of 3–7 cell layers with developed microridges.[11] Epithelial differentiation starts with the appearance

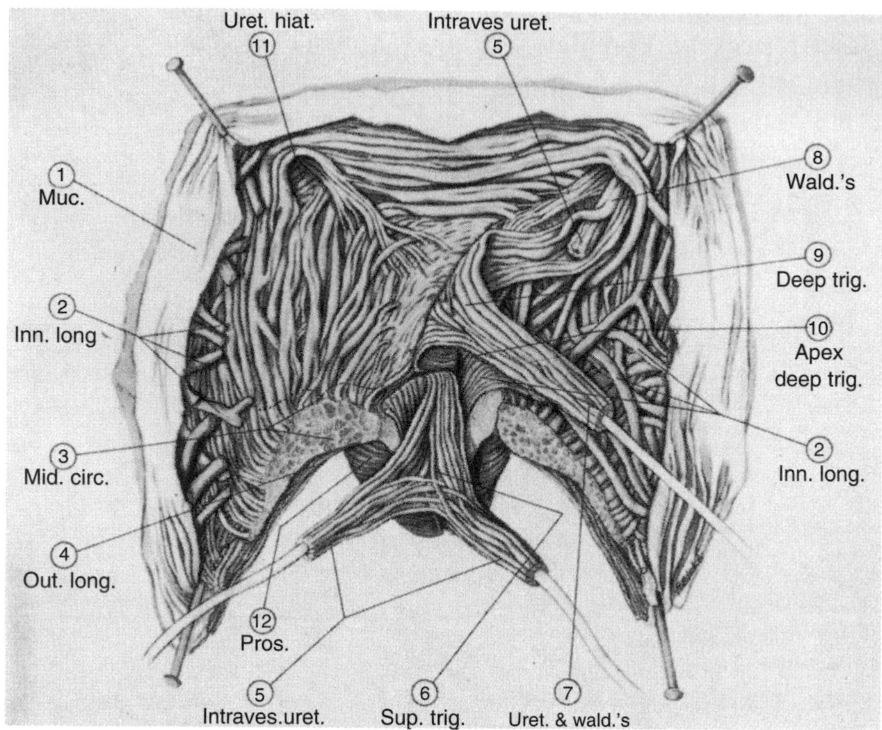

Figure 1.5
Muscle development of the bladder: (1) remaining edge of the bladder mucosa; (2) inner longitudinal muscle layer that extends toward the urethra (right side); (3) middle circular muscle layer that is most developed anteriorly; (4) outer longitudinal muscle layer; (5) intravesical ureter cut and reflected downward; (6) superficial trigone; (7) intramural ureter; (8) Waldeyer's sheath; (9) deep trigone; (10) apex of deep trigone extending toward the urethra; (11) ureteral hiatus; and (12) prostate. (From Tanagho and Smith.[8])

of microvilli and continues with the formation of both immature fusiform vesicles and ropy ridges. Differentiation continues with the formation of asymmetric unit membrane plaques and mature fusiform vesicles at the apical cytoplasm. Tight junctions, which are one of the cellular structures protecting the bladder from toxins in the urine, form early during urothelial differentiation.

Development of the urethra

The phallic segment of the urogenital sinus differentiates to form the urethra. During the 3rd week of gestation, mesenchymal cells from the region of the primitive streak migrate around the cloacal membrane, forming the cloacal folds. Cranial to the cloacal membrane, the cloacal folds fuse to form the genital tubercle. Concurrently, two protuberances, the genital swellings, develop lateral to the cloacal folds. During the 6th week of gestation, with the descent of the urorectal septum, the cloacal folds become subdivided into the anal and the urethral folds.

In male fetuses, the development of the penile urethra occurs in concert with the masculinization of the genitalia during the 8th week of gestation. Under the influence of androgens produced by the fetal testis, there is a rapid elongation of the genital tubercle, forming the phallus (Figure 1.6). During this process, the phallus pulls the urethral folds forward to form the lateral wall of the urethral groove.[1] By the 12th week of gestation, the penile urethra arises from the fusion of the urethral folds with primary luminization of the urethral groove.[12] Fusion of the urethral folds lined by endoderm results in a continuous mesodermal compartment around the penile urethra. Subsequent differentiation of this compartment forms the corpus spongiosum and cavernosum. During the 16th week of gestation, the glandular urethra develops. It is currently thought that in the glans, the fused urethral folds undergo endodermal to ectodermal transformation with secondary luminization of the urethral folds.[13]

The process of urethral development in female fetuses is less well understood. It is not known whether the development of the female urethra is dependent on sex hormones (such as estrogen or progesterone) or is simply a default pathway when androgens are not present. In female fetuses, the genital tubercle only elongates slightly and forms the clitoris (Figure 1.7). The urethral folds do not fuse as in male fetuses but rather differentiate into labia minora.[3] The urogenital groove remains open to the surface and forms the vestibule. Rupture of the urogenital membrane allows the bladder to drain into the amniotic cavity.[14]

Shortly after the formation of the urethra, the mesenchyme surrounding it begins to differentiate to form the two layers of the urethral musculature. They are present throughout the entire distance of the female urethra (Figure 1.8) and only in the proximal segment of the male urethra.[8] The inner layer is arranged longitudinally and is in continuity with the inner muscle layer of the bladder. This layer is relatively thick, since the muscle bundles are tightly packed and are held together by an abundance of collagen and elastic fibers. The outer layer consists of

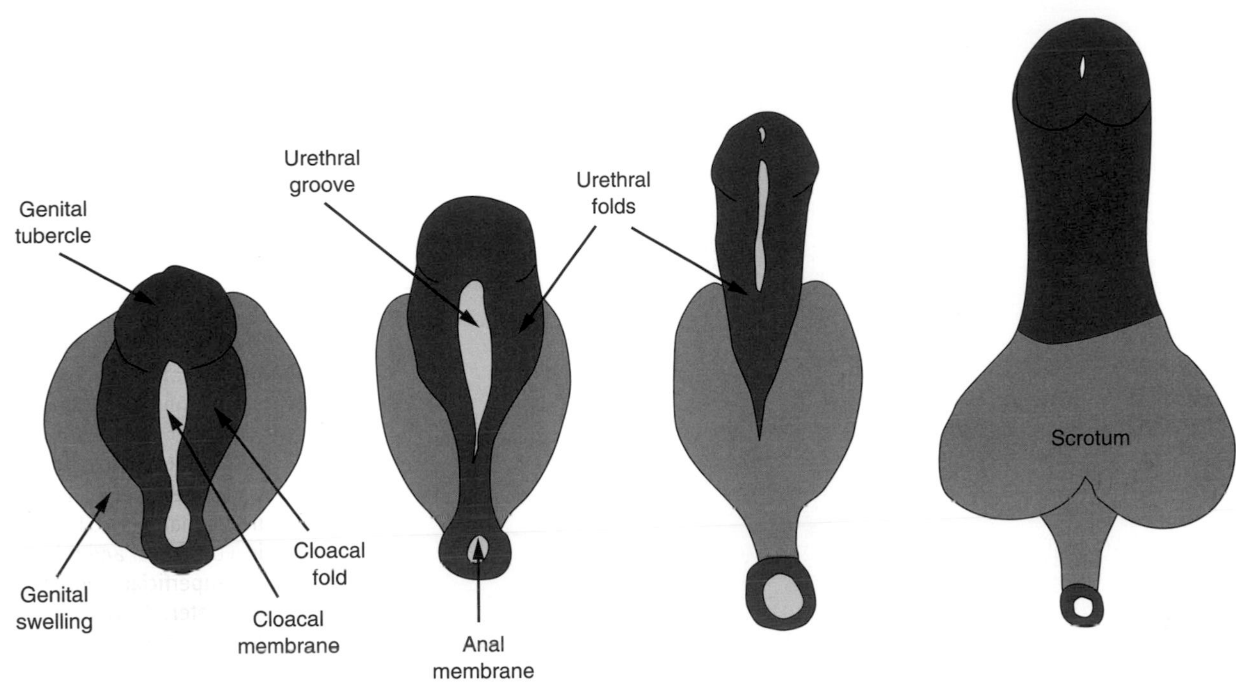

Figure 1.6
Development of the male urethra. Differentiation of the male urethra begins around the region of the cloacal membrane. Under the influence of androgens, the genital tubercle elongates and differentiates to form the glans and penis. Around the 12th week, the urethral folds fuse with primary luminization of the urethral groove. The genital swellings differentiate and fuse to form the scrotum.

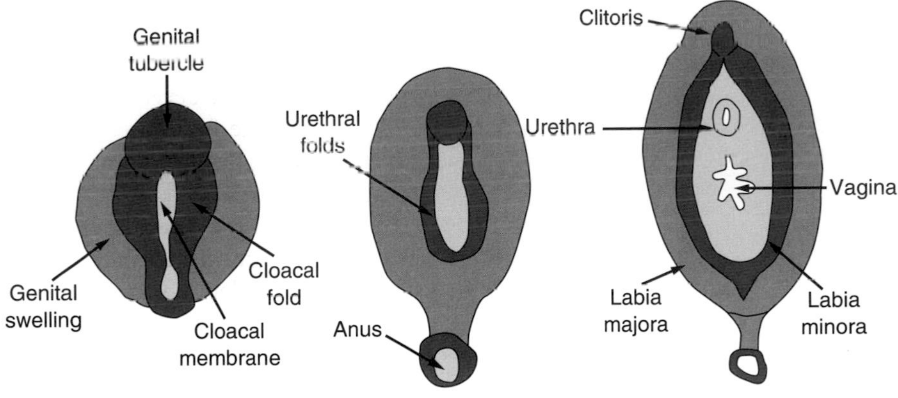

Figure 1.7
Development of the female urethra. The genital tubercle elongates slightly to form the clitoris. The urethral folds do not fuse and form the labia minora. The genital swellings differentiate to form the labia majora. Rupture of the urogenital membrane forms the opening of the female urethra.

semicircular fibers, looping around the urethra. This layer is thick proximally but tapers off distally.

Development of the external urinary sphincter

Around the 9th week of gestation, mesenchyme near the urogenital membrane condenses around the future urethra. In the male fetuses, this primarily occurs in the area of the future membranous urethra, and in the female fetuses, in the area of the mid-urethra. The mesenchyme develops into the external sphincter anteriorly and connective tissue with nerves and vessels posteriorly. By the 12th week of gestation, striated muscle fibers become apparent. A combination of detrusor, trigone, and urethral sphincter muscles provides the urinary continence mechanism. Recent studies indicate that the external sphincter has an omega-shaped configuration in both the male and female fetuses, most developed anteriorly and incomplete posteriorly.[15] In males the external urethral sphincter covers the ventral surface of the prostate as a crescent shape above the verumontanum, a horseshoe shape below the verumontanum, and a crescent

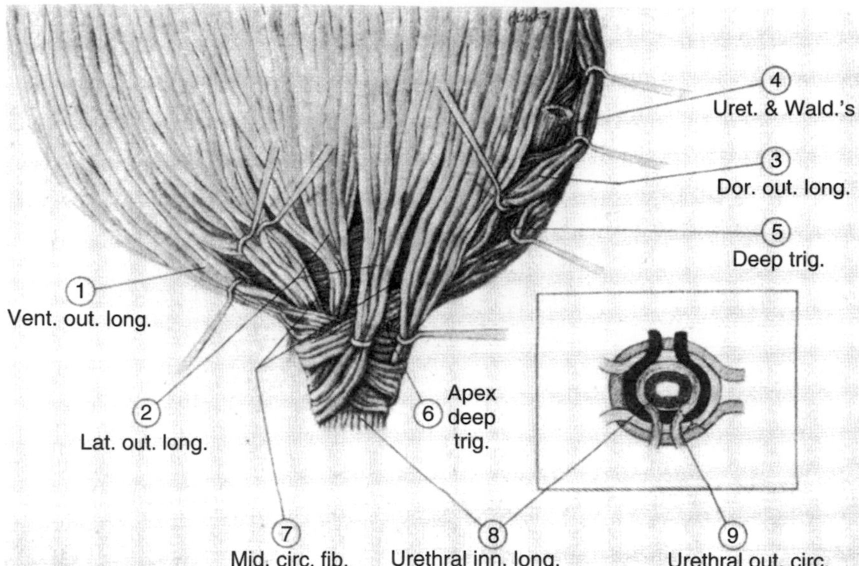

Figure 1.8
Arrangement of muscle around the female urethra: (1, 2, 3) the ventral, lateral, and dorsal outer longitudinal muscle layers of the bladder as they course downward to the urethra; (4) juxtavesical ureter surrounded by Waldeyer's sheath; (5) deep trigone; (6) apex of the deep trigone extending down toward the urethra; (7) middle circular muscle layer; (8) urethral inner longitudinal muscle layer; and (9) urethral outer circular layer. (From Tanagho and Smith.[8])

shape along the proximal bulbar urethra.[16] In females the external urethral sphincter covers the ventral surface of the urethra in a horseshoe shape. Caudally the same horseshoe-shaped external sphincter increases in size to envelop the distal vagina.

Development of the innervation to the lower urinary tract

At the 3rd week of gestation, the ectoderm begins to thicken in the mid-dorsal region in front of the primitive pit, forming the neural plate (Figure 1.9). The lateral edges of the neural plates rapidly grow to form the neural folds. The neural folds migrate toward the midline and fuse, forming a neural tube. In the wall of the recently closed neural tube there are neuroepithelial cells. These cells rapidly proliferate and differentiate to form the spinal cord.[17] Due to the rapid growth of the neuroepithelial cells, ventral and dorsal thickenings develop on each side of the neural tube. The ventral thickening contains the ventral motor horn cells and forms the motor area of the spinal cord, while the dorsal thickening contains sensory neurons and forms the sensory area of the spinal cord.

During subsequent stages of development, the axons of neurons in the ventral thickening begin to extend out into the spinal cord and migrate to their designated organs, providing motor innervation[1] (Figure 1.9). The bladder and urethra receive motor innervation from two areas of the spinal cord, the sympathetic and parasympathetic systems. Axons from neurons in the T11 to L2 region leave the spinal cord, forming the sympathetic nerve supply. These sympathetic fibers descend into the sympathetic trunk, then to the lumbar splanchnic nerves to reach the superior hypogastric plexus. This plexus then separates to form the right and left hypogastric nerves, which travel inferiorly to join the pelvic plexus (parasympathetic).[18] In the pelvic plexus, the axons from sympathetic nerves synapse, and postganglionic neurons are sent to the vesicle plexus. Axons from neurons in the S2–4 region form the parasympathetic system. They travel toward the bladder and form the pelvic plexus. After joining with the hypogastric nerves they form the vesical plexus, whose branches ramify in the adventitia and penetrate throughout the muscular bladder wall. The parasympathetic axons synapse with their respective postganglionic neurons within the bladder wall. It is believed that the parasympathetic cholinergic nerve fibers are in a 1:1 ratio with each muscle fiber, while the sympathetic nerve fibers are more richly distributed in the trigone, bladder base, and proximal urethra.[18]

In contrast to the axons of the neurons in the ventral thickening, those in the dorsal thickening descend or ascend to a lower or higher level within the spinal cord to form association neurons (Figure 1.9). Sensory innervation to the lower urinary tract develops from neurons arising outside of the neural tube.[19] During the invagination of the neural plate, a group of cells (neural crest cells) develops along each edge of the neural groove. They migrate on each side to the dorsolateral aspect of the neural tube. With growth and differentiation, these cells form dorsal root ganglia. Neurons in the dorsal root ganglia develop two processes. One penetrates the dorsal portion of the neural tube and synapses with association neurons or ascends to one of the higher brain centers. The second process extends

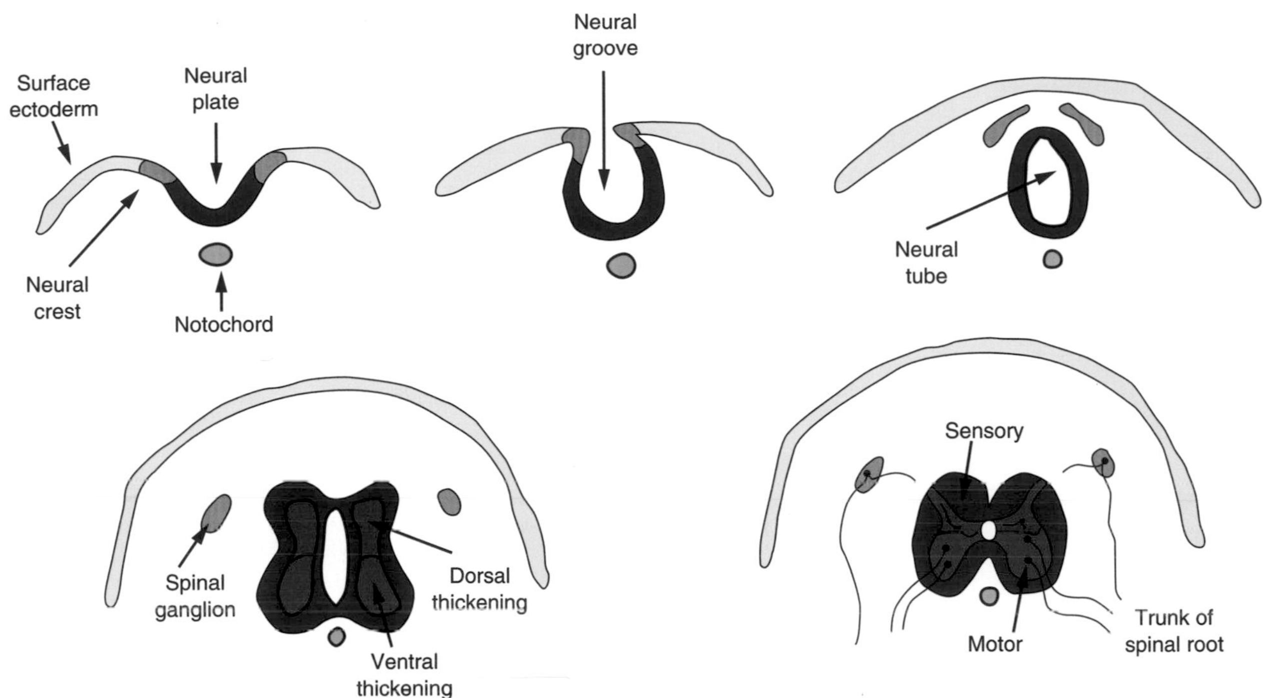

Figure 1.9
Development of motor and sensory innvervation to the lower urinary tract. Around the 3rd week of gestation, a pit is developed on the ectoderm, forming the neural plate (blue). The lateral edges fuse midline to form a neural tube. Ventral (red) and dorsal (pink) thickening develops around the neural tube to form the spinal cord. Axons from the ventral thickening extend toward the pelvis to provide innervation to the lower urinary tract. In contrast, sensory innervation develops from neural crest cells (brown). They aggregate to form a spinal ganglion. Neurons in the spinal ganglion develop two processes: one sent to the dorsal thickening to connect with the brain and spinal cord, and the second to the pelvic organs.

peripherally and terminates in sensory receptor organs. When combined with the ventral motor root, the peripherally growing axons form the trunk of the spinal nerves. The sensory pathways then parallel that of the motor pathways. The sensations of stretch and fullness in the bladder are believed to be mediated along the pelvic parasympathetic pathways, while the sensations of pain, touch, and temperature are along the sympathetic pathways.

Innervation to the external urethral sphincter is mediated primarily by motor somatic fibers. Axons from motor neurons in S2–3 exit the spinal cord and travel as part of the pelvic nerve or the pudendal nerve to reach the sphincter. Sensation from the striated musculature of the external sphincter is mediated via the pudendal nerve to S2 and to a lesser extent S3. Recent anatomic studies demonstrated that at the level of the bladder neck and the proximal part of the male urethra, unmyelinated nerve fibers destined for the smooth muscle fibers run alongside the myelinated nerve fibers destined for the striated muscle fibers. The majority of the unmyelinated nerve fibers approach the smooth muscular layers of the bladder neck and proximal urethra at the 5 and 7 o'clock positions, while the majority of the myelinated nerve fibers penetrate the sphincter at the 9 and 3 o'clock positions.[20]

The molecular biology of bladder development

While we are beginning to understand the morphologic events that occur during the development of the lower urinary tract, it remains largely unknown how this complex occurs. Recent studies have begun to elucidate the mechanism of cellular interaction that leads to the formation of muscle in the bladder. In a rat model, it has been observed that smooth muscle develops from undifferentiated mesenchyme. The process occurs in an orderly sequence of differentiation defined by the temporal expression of smooth muscle (alpha-actin, myosin, vinculin, desmin, vimentin, and laminin) markers.[21] Smooth muscle differentiation begins in the periphery of the bladder mesenchyme subjacent to the serosa and continues toward the epithelium. Concurrently, the epithelium lining the bladder also undergoes differentiation as defined by the temporal expression of epithelial (cytokeratins 5, 7, 8, 14, 18, and 19) protein markers.[21] Interestingly, without the bladder epithelium, the bladder mesenchyme does not differentiate into smooth muscle.[22] Consequently, it is believed that mesenchymal–epithelial interactions with bladder epithelium (urothelium) are necessary for the differentiation of bladder smooth muscle. Peptide growth factors such as keratinocyte growth factor (KGF) and transforming growth factors (TGF) alpha and beta are likely candidates as mediators of these mesenchymal–epithelial interactions.[23] The smooth muscle-inducing property is not unique to the fetal bladder epithelium but is also present in adult bladder epithelium and in epithelia of other organs such as the bowel, cornea, and uterus (although the amount of smooth muscle induction varies with the type of epithelium).[24] Similarly, there appear to be signals originating from the induced mesenchyme that affect the growth and differentiation of the bladder epithelium.[25] Consequently, reciprocal communication and induction between epithelium and mesenchyme are needed for the proper formation of the bladder.

In-vivo and in-vitro studies are beginning to provide insights into the process of bladder development. Unfortunately, much of the molecular mechanisms that govern the development of the lower urinary tract still remain to be defined.

References

1. Sadler TW. Langman's Medical Embryology, 5th edn. Baltimore: Williams & Wilkins, 1985: 410.
2. Stephens FD. In: Webser R, ed. Congenital Malformations of the Rectum, Anus and Genito-urinary tract. London: E & S Livingstone Ltd, 1963: 371.
3. Hamilton WJ, Mossman HW. The urogenital system. In: Human Embryology Prenatal Development of Form and Function. Hamilton WJ, ed. New York: Macmillan Press, 1976: 377.
4. Tejedo-Mateu A, Vilanova-Trias J, Ruano-Gil D. Contribution to the study of the development of the terminal portion of the Wolffian duct and the ureter. Eur Urol 1975; 1(1): 41–5.
5. Oswald J, Schwentner C, Lunacek A et al. Reevaluation of the fetal muscle development of the vesical trigone. J Urol 2006; 176(3): 1166–70.
6. Drews U, Sulak O, Oppitz M. Immunohistochemical localisation of androgen receptor during sex-specific morphogenesis in the fetal mouse. Histochem Cell Biol 2001; 116(5): 427–39.
7. Droes JT. Observations on the musculature of the urinary bladder and the urethra in the human foetus. Br J Urol 1974; 46(2): 179–85.
8. Tanagho EA, Smith DR. The anatomy and function of the bladder neck. Br J Urol 1966; 38: 54.
9. Koerner I, Peibl M, Oswald J et al. Gender specific chronological and morphometric assessment of fetal bladder wall development. J Urol 2006; 176(6 Pt 1): 2674–8.
10. Staack A, Hayward SW, Baskin LS et al. Molecular, cellular and developmental biology of urothelium as a basis of bladder regeneration. Differentiation 2005; 73(4): 121–33.
11. Ersoy Y, Ercan F, Cetinel S. A comparative ontogenic study of urinary bladder: impact of the epithelial differentiation in embryonic and newborn rats. Anat Histol Embryol 2006; 35(6): 365–74.
12. van der Werff JF, Nievelstein RA, Brands E et al. Normal development of the male anterior urethra. Teratology 2000; 61(3): 172–83.
13. Baskin LS. Hypospadias and urethral development. J Urol 2000; 163(3): 951–6.
14. Gosling JA. The structure of the female lower urinary tract and pelvic floor. Urol Clin North Am 1985; 12(2): 207–14.
15. Ludwikowski B, Brenner E, Fritsch H et al. The development of the external urethral sphincter in humans. BJU Int 2001; 87(6): 565–8.
16. Yucel S, Baskin LS. An anatomical description of the male and female urethral sphincter complex. J Urol 2004; 171(5): 1890–7.
17. Fujita H, Fujita S. Electron microscopic studies on neuroblast differentiation in the central nervous system of domestic fowl. Z Zellforsch Mikrosk, 1963; 60: 463.
18. Fletcher TF, Bradley WE. Neuroanatomy of the bladder-urethra. J Urol 1978; 119(2): 153–60.
19. Weston JA. The migration and differentiation of neural crest cells, in Advances in Morphogenesis, Abercrombie M, Brachet J, King TJ, eds. New York: Academic Press, 1970.
20. Karam I, Moudouni S, Droupy S et al. The structure and innervation of the male urethra: histological and immunohistochemical studies with three-dimensional reconstruction. J Anat 2005; 206(4): 395–403.
21. Baskin LS, Hayward SW, Young PF, Cunha GR. Ontogeny of the rat bladder: smooth muscle and epithelial differentiation. Acta Anat (Basel) 1996; 155(3): 163–71.
22. Baskin LS, Hayward SW, Young PF, Cunha GR. Role of mesenchymal–epithelial interactions in normal bladder development. J Urol 1996; 156(5): 1820–7.
23. Baskin LS, Sutherland RS, Thomson AA et al. Growth factors and receptors in bladder development and obstruction. Lab Invest 1996; 75(2): 157–66.
24. DiSandro MJ, Li Y, Baskin LS et al. Mesenchymal–epithelial interactions in bladder smooth muscle development: epithelial specificity. J Urol 1998; 160(3 Pt 2): 1040–6; discussion 1079.
25. Li Y, Lui W, Hayward SW et al. Plasticity of the urothelial phenotype: effects of gastro-intestinal mesenchyme/stroma and implications for urinary tract reconstruction. Differentiation 2000; 66(2–3): 126–35.

2

Simplified anatomy of the vesico–urethral functional unit

Saad Aldousari and Jacques Corcos

The bladder and urethra should necessarily be described together. Functionally speaking, these two organs cannot be dissociated and, anatomically, their connections are too imbricated to distinguish them as two different organs. The pelvic floor, with its muscles, fascia, and ligaments, is a separate anatomic entity, but, functionally, it is also an important component of urethra–vesical physiology.[1]

The bladder

The bladder (Figures 2.1a,b), located in the pelvis behind the pubic bone, can be divided into two portions. The dome, the upper part of the bladder is spherical, extensible, and mobile. The median umbilical ligament (urachus) ascends from its apex behind the anterior abdominal wall to the umbilicus, and the peritoneum behind it creates the median umbilical fold. In males, the superior surface of the dome is completely covered by the peritoneum extending slightly to the base. It is in close contact with the sigmoid colon and the terminal coils of the ileum. In females, the difference arises from the posterior reflection of the peritoneum on the anterior face of the uterus, forming the vesico–uterine pouch. In both sexes, the inferolateral part of the bladder is not covered by the peritoneum. In adults, the bladder is completely retropubic and can be palpated only if it is in overdistention. In contrast, at birth, it is relatively high and is an abdominal organ. It descends progressively, reaching its adult position at puberty.

The base of the bladder, i.e. the lower part, is fixed. The trigone, the post part of the base, is triangular between three orifices – two ureteral orifices and the urethral orifice or bladder neck.

At the level of the vesico–ureteral junction the ureters cross the bladder wall obliquely in a length of 1–2 cm. This type of path through the bladder wall creats a valve mechanism, preventing urine reflux toward the ureters when bladder pressure increases. This is achieved by the fact that the ureter pierces the bladder wall obliquely. As it passes through a hiatus in the detrusor (intramural ureter) compression and complete closure are completed by detrusor contraction. This intravesical portion of the ureter lies immediately beneath the bladder urothelium, and, therefore, it is backed by a strong plate of detrusor muscle. It is believed that with bladder filling, this results in passive occlusion of the ureter, like a flap valve.

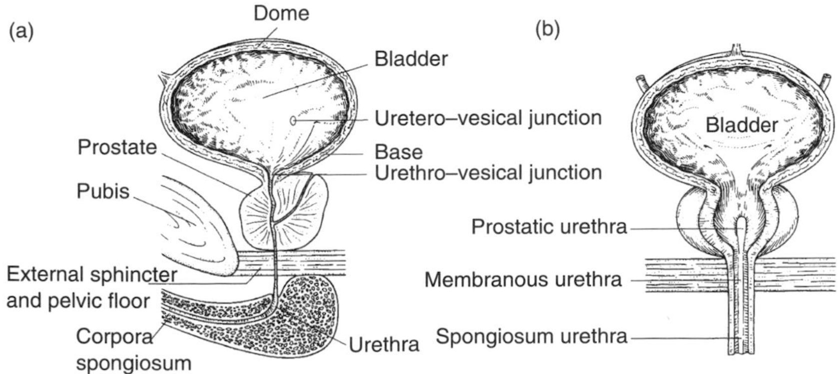

Figure 2.1
Anatomy of the vesicosphincteric unit in man. (a) Sagittal view; (b) Frontal view.

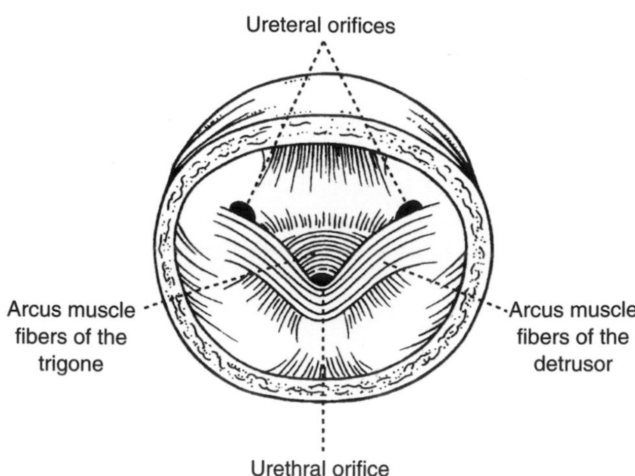

Figure 2.2
Trigone endovesical view.

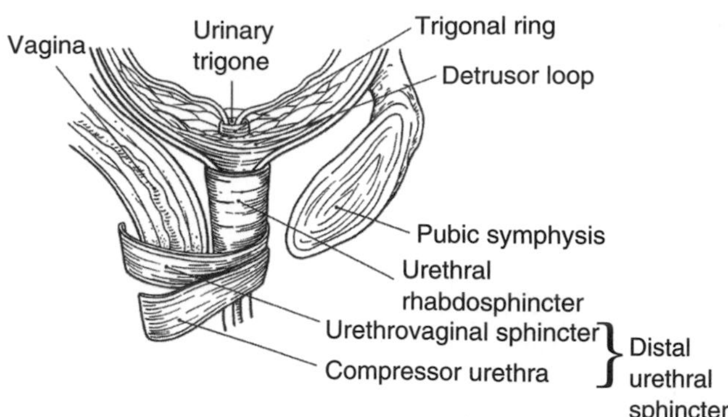

Figure 2.3
Architectural organization of the striated urethral sphincter. Location of its three components: the urethral rhabdosphincter, the compressor urethra, and the urethrovaginal sphincter.

At the level of the vesico–urethral junction or bladder neck, the original disposition of the muscle fibers allows closure during the bladder-filling phase (Figure 2.2).

The detrusor muscle

The detrusor muscle can be described as a sphere of smooth muscle bundles. It is a complex imbrication of smooth muscle fibers without a well-defined orientation, but is usually viewed as an external and internal longitudinal layer with a circular intermediate layer. These layers are inseparable in the upper aspect of the bladder. Near the bladder neck, on the other hand, they are clearly separable into the three layers mentioned earlier. In men and women, the muscle fibers of the inner longitudinal layer extend down into the urethra in a funnel-shaped structure, allowing continence and emptying of the bladder. In men, the middle circular layer forms a circular preprostatic sphincter, which is responsible for continence, as it forms a ring-like structure at the level of the bladder neck. The outer longitudinal layers are thickest posteriorly at the bladder base, providing a strong trigonal support. Laterally, fibers from this sheet pass anteriorly and fuse to form a loop around the bladder neck, participating in the continence mechanism.

The female bladder neck, on the other hand, differs from that of the male in the fact that its sphincteric function is limited. Some authors have denied its existence altogether.[2]

The bladder mucosa

The bladder mucosa, folded when the bladder is empty, is loosely adherent to the submucosal tissue and the detrusor. Over the trigone and all around the bladder neck it becomes much more adherent. The bladder mucosa is richly vascularized and very sensitive to pain, distention, temperature, etc.

Deep to this, the lamina propria forms a relatively thick layer of fibroelastic connective tissue that allows considerable distention. This layer is traversed by numerous blood vessels and contains smooth muscle fibers collected into a poorly defined muscularis mucosa. Beneath this layer lies the smooth muscle of the bladder wall.

The female urethra

The female urethra is 4 cm long and approximately 6 mm in diameter. It begins at the internal vesical orifice, extends downward and forward behind the symphysis pubis, and terminates at the external urethral meatus about 2 cm behind the glans clitoris. The urethral mucosa is surrounded by a rich, spongy, estrogen-dependent submucosal vascular plexus encased in fibroelastic and muscular tissue. The outer layer of the female urethra, covered two-thirds of its proximal length by a striated muscle, represents the external urinary sphincter. This sphincter has its largest diameter in the middle part of the urethra. The striated urogenital sphincter has two distinct portions: the upper sphincter portion, which is arranged circularly around the urethra, corresponds to the rhabdosphincter, whereas the lower portion comprises arch-like muscular bands (Figure 2.3). Many small mucous glands open into the urethra, forming what are called the paraurethral ducts, which are usually located on the lateral margin of the external urethral orifice.[2]

The male urethra

The male urethra (see Figures 2.1a,b) is 18–20 cm long and is usually divided into three portions: the proximal or prostatic urethra, the membranous urethra (both included in the posterior urethra), and the anterior urethra (composed of bulbar, pendulous urethra, and fossa navicularis).[3,4]

- The first segment (3–4 cm) is mainly a thin tube of smooth muscle lined by mucosa and extending through the prostate from the bladder neck to the apex of the prostate. At the origin of the prostatic urethra, the smooth muscle surrounding the bladder neck is arranged in a distinct circular collar, which becomes continuous distally with the capsule of the prostate. The internal sphincter extends from the internal vesical meatus through the prostatic urethra to the level of the veromontanum, providing passive continence via the sympathetic supply. The prostatic urethra ends distal to the veromuntanum.
- The second segment, erroneously called the membranous urethra (there is nothing membranous at that level), is also known as the sphincteric urethra. The external sphincter has an omega shape and surrounds the urethra with a fibrotic segment in its posterior midline. It is 2 cm long and 3–5 mm in thickness. It has an outer layer of striated muscle and an inner layer of smooth muscle, intrinsic to the urethral wall, making it both a voluntary and involuntary unit. Surrounding the external sphincter is a layer of periurethral striated muscle fibers, providing assistance in voluntary control (i.e. interruption of voiding).
- The last segment, the spongiose urethra, is contained in the corpus spongiosum of the penis and extends from the previous segment to the urethral meatus. Its diameter is 6 mm when passing urine. It is dilated at its commencement as the intrabulbar fossa and again within the glans penis, where it becomes the navicular fossa. All along the urethra, numerous small mucous glands (urethral glands) open into its lumen.

Vascular and lymphatic supply of the bladder and urethra

The superior and inferior vesical arteries are branches of the internal iliac arteries. The obturator and gluteal arteries also participate in the bladder arterial supply. In females, an additional branch is derived from the uterine and vaginal arteries. Venous drainage forms a complex, extensive network around the bladder and into a plexus on its inferolateral face, ending in the internal iliac veins.

Lymphatic drainage originates from all layers of the bladder and ends in the external iliac nodes. Most urethral lymphatic drainage terminates in the external iliac nodes, except for the spongiose urethra and the glans penis where it goes to the deep inguinal nodes and from there to the external iliac nodes.[3]

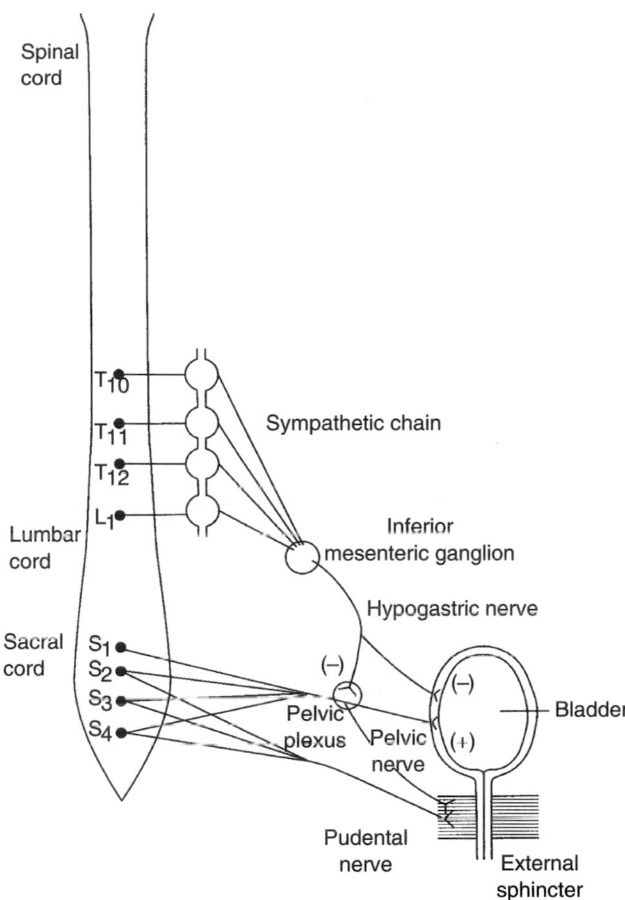

Figure 2.4
Spinal cord centers and nerves responsible for micturition.

Urethro–vesical unit innervation

Three nerves provide an anatomic and somatic innervation to the bladder (Figure 2.4).[5–7]

The hypogastric nerve

The hypogastric nerve has motor and sensitive fibers. It originates from preganglionic spinal neurons of the thoracolumbar intermediolateralis cord at the level of T10 to L1.[8]

Preganglionic axons reach the paravertebral sympathetic ganglionic chain, where they synapse with ganglionic neurons. Postganglionic axons cross the superior hypogastric plexus to reach the vesical or interior hypogastric plexus.

The adrenergic innervations delivered by these nerves are Β type at the level of the dome, and α_1 type at the level of the bladder base and neck (superficial trigone). The global effects of adrenergic bladder innervation are relaxation of the dome and contraction of the bladder neck. The hypogastric nerves are mainly adrenergic, but also have cholinergic as well as peptidergic contingents whose function is not well understood.

In contrast to the rich sympathetic innervation of the bladder neck in males, the bladder neck in females receives mainly cholinergic fibers and much less adrenergic innervation. This difference in nerve supply may relate to the main genital function attributed to the bladder neck in males and its lesser importance in females.

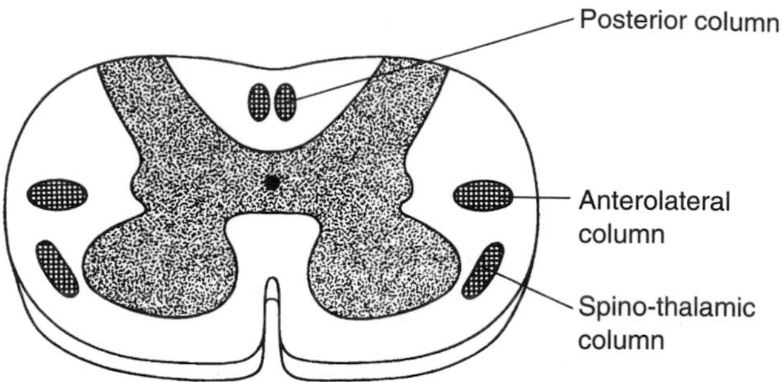

Figure 2.5
Transverse cut of the spinal cord showing the ascendent and descendent pathways of the vesico-sphincteric innervation.

The pelvic nerves

The pelvic nerves represent the parasympathetic component of bladder innervation. Their fibers arise from the 2nd to the 4th sacral segments of the spinal cord and merge at the level of the vesical plexus, from where branches reach the bladder. These fibers are cholinergic, but some noradrenergic fibers participate in the composition of the pelvic plexus.

The bladder, including the trigone, is profusely supplied by nerves from a dense plexus among the detrusor muscle fibers. The majority of these nerves are cholinergic and follow the vascular supply, only rarely extending among the nonstriated muscle components of the bladder and urethra.

Nonadrenergic noncholinergic innervation

Numerous neurotransmitters have been detected and studied in the intramural ganglia of the bladder: they include, among others, somatostatin, substance P, neurokinin, and bombesin. The anatomic and physiologic relationships between nonadrenergic/noncholinergic innervations and cholinergic/adrenergic innervations are still being debated.

The pudendal nerves

The pudendal nerves convey both notoriety and sensitivity, arising from the spinal motoneurones of Onuf's nucleus located at the base of the anterior horn of S2–S4. Their axons cross the pudendal plexus composed of the 2nd, 3rd, and 4th sacral nerves and merge to constitute the pudendal nerves that are responsible for innervation of all the striated muscles of the pelvic floor, including the urethral and anal sphincters.

A study carried out in the University Hospital Zurich by Reitz and colleague[9] has shown that somatosensory fibers of the pudendal nerve are projected onto sympathetic thoracolumbar neurons controling the bladder neck, a process called neuromodulation. It works on a spinal level and confers bladder neck competence and continence. The authors have also shown that involuntary detrusor contractions due to bladder overactivity or hyperreflexia can be suppressed by electrical pudendal nerve stimulation. This was explained by the fact that the stimulated pudendal afferents are directed in the spinal cord to influence both the inhibitory effects of the hypogastric or pelvic nerves on the bladder dome and the excitatory effects of the hypogastric nerve on the bladder neck by way of α-adrenergic receptors.

Afferent fibers

The origins of these sensory nerves incorporate different types of subepithelial receptors (simple or complex vesicles), capsulated or not, but with controversial distributions and functions (Figure 2.5). Present in sympathetic and adrenergic innervation, these sensory fibers transmit pain and awareness of distention to the central structures. Bladder afferents mainly follow the pelvic nerves. Urethral afferents follow the pelvic nerves for the proximal urethra, the hypogastric nerve for the mid-portion, and the pudendal nerves for the rest of the urethra and sphincter. However, their distribution is not clear-cut, and major overlapping exists.

The spinal sensory pathway (need to urinate, pain, temperature, urgency, sexual arousal) is found in the anterolateral white columns.

Fibers transmitting conscious sensitivity (bladder distention, ongoing micturition, tactile pressure) follow the posterior columns, synapsing in the gravelis nucleus and cuneatus of the brainstem before reaching the lateral ventral posterior nucleus of the thalamus and the cortex.

All these afferent pathways have important connections at the spinal cord and brainstem level with micturition

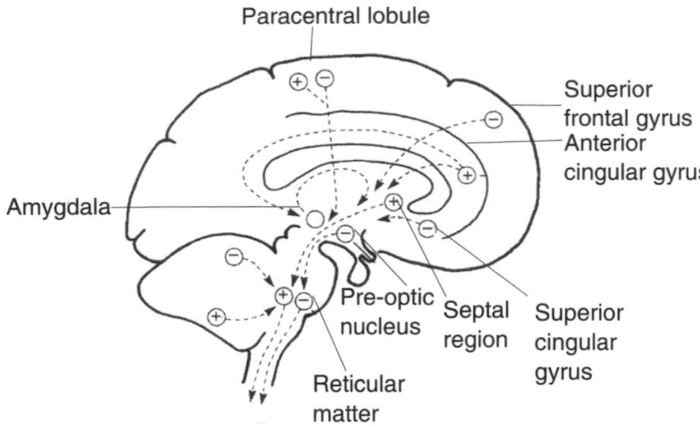

Figure 2.6
Micturition integration brain centers.

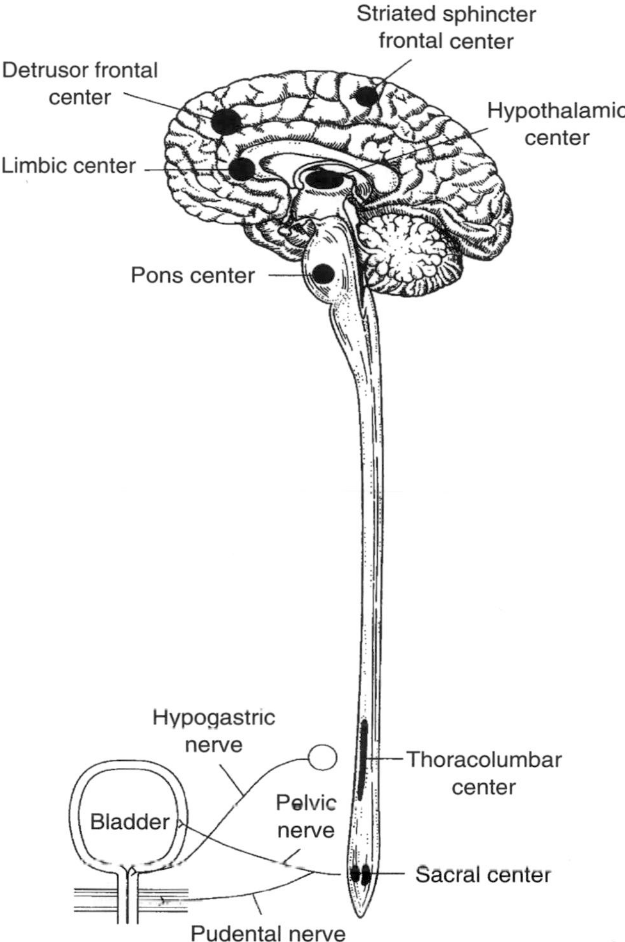

Figure 2.7
Micturition integration centers and nerves.

motor fibers and the limbic system that explain the affective component of micturition.

Micturition integration centers

Micturition is not only an autonomic function, but is also a voluntary and emotional function under upper central nervous system control (Figures 2.5, 2.6, and 2.7).

Micturition centers at the level of the brain

Micturition is regulated voluntarily by cortical centers at the level of the frontal lobe and diffusively in the premotrice area (paracentral lobule).

The emotional control of micturition is complex and involves the limbic system with participation of the hypothalamus, the hippocampus, the callosal gyrus, the supraorbitary cortex, the amygdala, and several nonspecific thalamic nuclei.

Locus caeruleus and subcaeruleus nucleus

At the level of the brainstem, particularly the pons and the medulla, stimulation of the locus caeruleus complex and subcaeruleus nucleus complex (LCC) provokes contraction or relaxation of the vesicosphincteric units located in the anterior and dorsal parts of the pons and being a component of the Barrington center. Neurons of the LCC are mainly nonadrenergic, but all kinds of neurotransmitters are involved (cholinergic, serotoninergic, enkephalinergic, etc.).

The LCC influences micturition through ascending and descending fibers. The ascending fibers regulate emotional and voluntary decision processes. Descending connections arise from the ventral part of the LCC and innervate most of the cord. Two catecholaminergic pathways follow the intermediolateral column and reach the sympathetic thoracolumbar and the parasympathetic sacral neurons.

References

1. Galeano C, Corcos J, Schick E. Anatomie simplifiée de l'unité fonctionnelle vesico-urethrale. In: Corcos J, Schick E, eds. Les Vessies Neurogènes de l'Adulte. Paris, France: Masson, 1996.
2. Haab F, Sebe P, Mondet F, Ciofu C. Functional anatomy of the bladder and urethra in females. In: Corcos J, Schick E, eds. The Urinary Sphincter. New York: Marcel Dekker, 2001.

3. Meyers RP. The male striated urethral sphincter. In: Corcos J, Schick E, eds. The Urinary Sphincter. New York: Marcel Dekker, 2001.
4. The urinary system. In: Gray's Anatomy. Edinburgh: Churchill Livingstone, 1995.
5. Thomson AS, Dabhoiwala NF, Verbeek FJ, Lamers WH. The functional anatomy of the ureterovesical junction. Br J Urol 1994; 73: 284–91.
6. Brooks JD, Chao W-M, Kerr J. Male pelvic anatomy reconstructed from the Visible Human data set J Urol 1998; 159: 868–72.
7. Williams PL, Warwick R, Dyson M, Bannister LH. Gray's Anatomy, 37th edn. New York: Churchill Livingstone, 1989.
8. Rosenstein DI, Alsikafi NF. Diagnosis and classification of urethral injuries. Urol Clin N Am 2006; 33: 73–85.
9. Reitz A, Schmid DM, Curt A, Knapp PA, Schurch B. Afferent fibers of the pudendal modulate sympathetic neurons controlling the bladder-neck. Neurourol Urodyn 2003; 22: 597–601.

3

Physiology of the urothelium

Lori A Birder, William C de Groat, and Gerard Apodaca

Introduction

The mucosal surface of the renal pelvis, ureters, and bladder is lined by the urothelium.[1] This specialized tissue forms a selective barrier that controls the passage of water, ions, solutes, and large macromolecules across the mucosal surface of the epithelium and prevents entry of pathogens into the underlying tissues. The barrier function of the urothelium depends, in part, on the presence of high resistance tight junctions, the unique lipid, protein, and carbohydrate composition of the apical membrane of the outermost umbrella cell layer, and changes in membrane turnover within the urothelium.[2–4] Beyond serving as a simple barrier, new investigation indicates that the urothelium performs a variety of additional functions including the ability to respond to chemical, mechanical, and thermal stimuli, as well as release of mediators such as ATP and nitric oxide (NO) that may communicate the state of the urothelial environment to the underlying nervous and muscular systems.[5] Study of urothelial sensory function is providing new therapeutic targets for bladder-associated diseases such as interstitial cystitis (IC), spinal cord injury, and detrusor overactivity that may result, in part, from urothelial responses to external stimuli or release of mediators.[5,6] This chapter will review the specialized anatomy of the urothelium and then explore new insights into the role of uroplakins (UPs), tight junctions, membrane turnover, urothelial-neuronal signaling, and, finally, the clinical implications of these recent findings.

Anatomy of the urothelium

Cellular composition of the urothelium

The urothelium forms the interface between the urinary space and the underlying vascular, connective, nervous, and muscular tissues.[1,7] It is a stratified epithelium, sometimes referred to as transitional epithelium, being somewhere in the continuum between nonkeratinizing stratified and pseudostratified epithelia. The urothelium is comprised of basal, intermediate, and umbrella cell layers (Figure 3.1a). The basal cell layer is one cell thick and is comprised of relatively small cells (~ 10 μm in diameter), which sit on a continuous basement membrane and form intimate contacts with the subjacent capillary bed. The basal cells are generally quiescent (the mitotic index is on the order of 0.1–0.5%) and have an estimated half-life of 3–6 months.[7,8] The intermediate cell layer is composed of one to several cell layers of pear-shaped cells (10–25 μm in diameter). The number of intermediate cell layers depends on the degree of bladder distention.[7] Like basal cells, intermediate cells are usually quiescent, but can rapidly differentiate when the outer umbrella cell layer is damaged.[7] The umbrella cell layer is composed of very large polyhedral cells with diameters of 25–250 μm (Figure 3.2). The long-lived umbrella cells can be multinucleate, although this is somewhat species dependent, and the generation of the multinucleate umbrella cells may result from intermediate cell–cell fusion.[7,9] A population of discoidal/fusiform vesicles is found under the apical membrane of the umbrella cell layer (Figure 3.1b). Although the shape of these vesicles is somewhat species dependent, their function is to deliver membrane and associated proteins to the apical surface of the umbrella cell.[1] Tight junctions are found at the apicolateral junction of the umbrella cells,[10] and form a tight seal between adjacent umbrella cells.

Specializations of the luminal membrane of umbrella cells

The apical surface of umbrella cells contains several specializations. It is covered by raised hinges (also called microplicae) and intervening areas called plaques (Figure 3.2). Plaques occupy approximately 70–90% of the surface of the umbrella cell.[7,11,12] The arrangement of hinges and plaques gives the apical surface its characteristic scalloped appearance, when viewed in cross-section (Figure 3.1b). The hinge

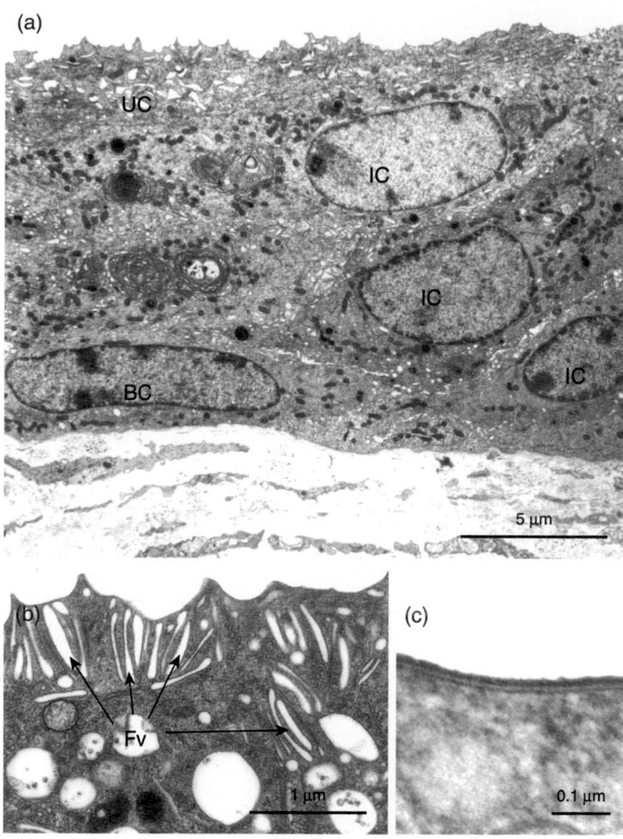

Figure 3.1
Ultrastructure of the urothelium. (a) Transmission electron micrograph of mouse urothelium showing umbrella cells (UC), intermediate cells (IC), and basal cells (BC). (b) Examples of fusiform vesicles (Fv) under the apical plasma membrane of the umbrella cells. (c) AUM of surface umbrella cells.

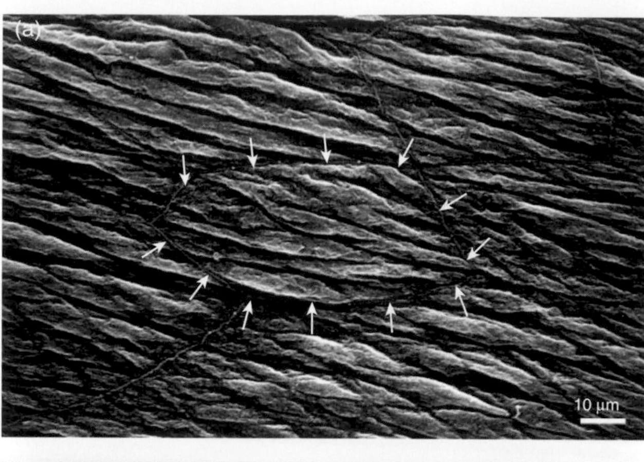

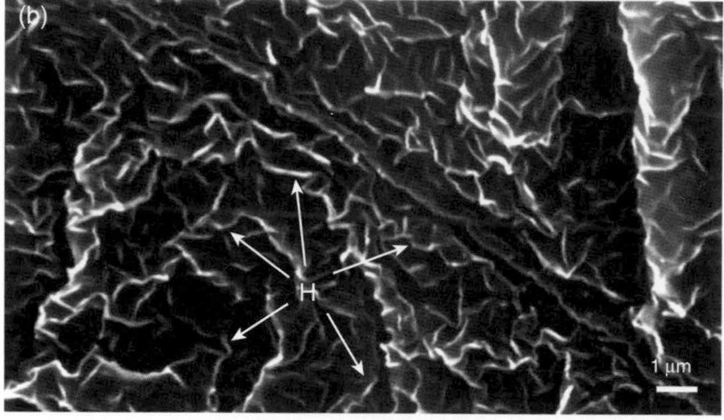

Figure 3.2
Scanning electron micrograph of mucosal surface of mouse umbrella cell layer. (a) The tight junction ring of an individual umbrella cell is demarcated by arrows. (b) High magnification view of apical surface of umbrella cell. Examples of hinges ('H') are marked with arrows.

areas are not well understood, but contain at least one unique protein called urohingin.[13] Because the plaque regions are crystalline in nature (see below), presumably all other apically distributed nonplaque proteins such as receptors and channels are localized to the hinge areas. The membrane associated with the hinge and plaque regions is highly detergent insoluble,[14] likely reflecting the unusual lipid composition of this membrane, which is rich in cholesterol, phosphatidyl choline, phosphatidyl ethanolamine, and cerebroside – a lipid profile similar to myelin.[15]

An additional characteristic of the membrane associated with the plaque regions is that the outer leaflet of the plasma membrane appears to be twice as thick as the inner leaflet, forming an asymmetric unit membrane (AUM; Figure 3.1c).[11,16,17] The AUM is composed of a paracrystalline array of 16-nm diameter AUM particles that are composed of six subunits, each of which occupies both the inner and outer ring of the AUM particle (Figure 3.3a).[17] A plaque contains approximately 1000–3000 AUM particles. Constituents of the AUM particles include the uroplakins (UPs), a family of five proteins including the tetraspanin family members UPIa and UPIb, and the type I single span proteins UPII, UPIIIa, and UPIIIb (Figure 3.3b).[18,19] In mammalian tissues, UPIa, UPII, UPIIIa, and UPIIIb are only expressed in the uroepithelium and are concentrated in the umbrella cell layer. UPIb is also expressed in the cornea and conjunctiva.[20] Recent genomic analysis indicates that UPs are likely formed by gene duplication and are absent in some vertebrates but are present in others including *Xenopus laevis* (frog), *Gallus gallus* (chicken), and *Denio rerio* (zebrafish).[21]

Both protein and structural studies are leading to a new understanding of how UPs interact to form AUM particles. Biochemical experiments using purified proteins have defined that UPIa forms heterodimers with UPII and UPIb pairs with UPIIIa or UPIIIb (Figure 3.3b).[19,22] Cryo-electron microscopy (EM) analysis indicates that the tetraspanins UP1a/UP1b form rod-shaped structures that interact with their UpII/UPIII bridging partner through interactions between the transmembrane and extracellular

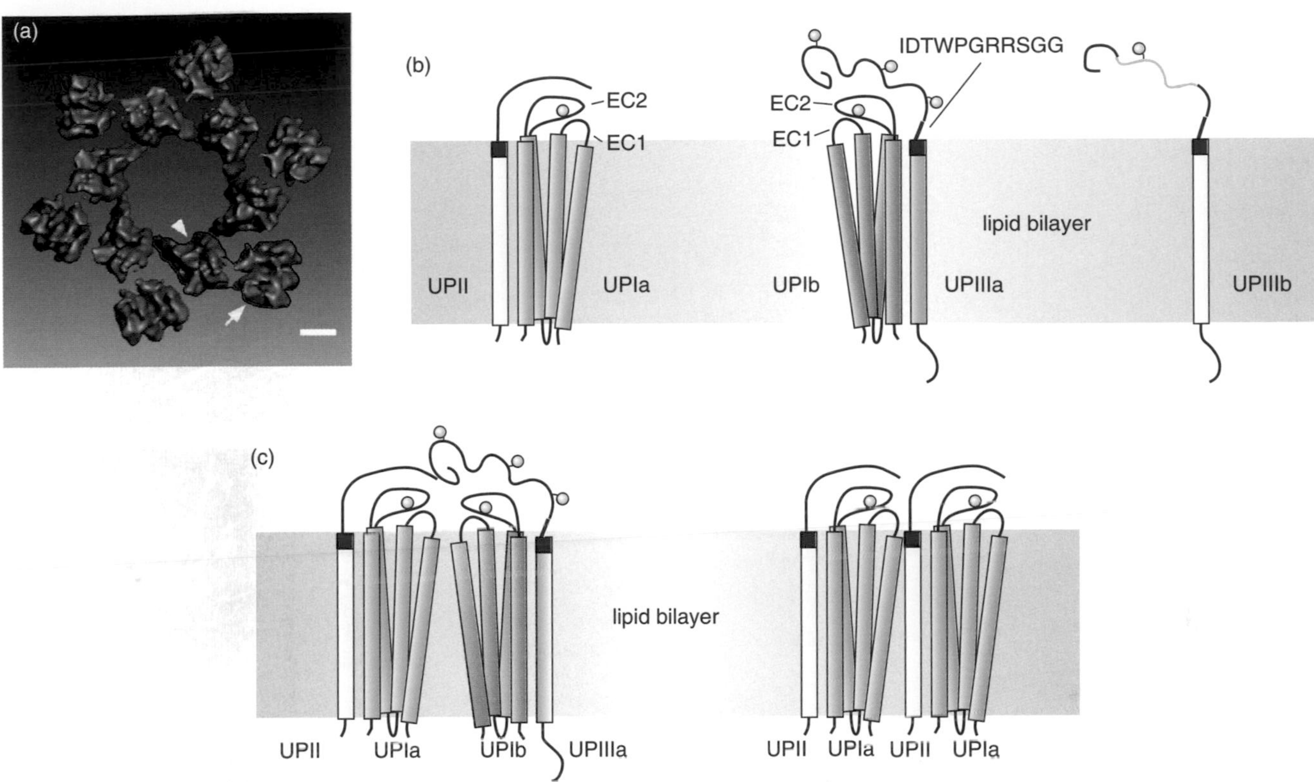

Figure 3.3
AUM particles. (a) 3D structure of the 16-nm AUM particle, which is composed of 6 subunits (the perimeter of one subunit is marked in blue) that occupy the inner and outer ring of the particle. A UPIa/UPII heterodimer is indicated by an arrowhead and a UPIb/UPIII heterodimer is indicated by an arrow. Bar = 2 nm. (Reprinted with permission Min et al.[23]) (b) Interactions between UPIa/UPII and UPIb/UPIIIa. UPIa and UPIb are members of the tetraspanin family of proteins and have four transmembrane domains. UPII, UPIIIa, and UPIIIb cross the membrane once and are type I membrane proteins. They share a 'conserved domain' (shown in red), which includes the N-terminal portion of the transmembrane region and, in UPIIIa and UPIIIb, extends towards the extracellular domain. The sequence of the extracellular region of the conserved domain of UPIIIa is shown in single amino acid code. The region of the extracellular domain of UPIIIb colored in yellow is > 90% identical to a portion of the human DNA mismatch repair enzyme-related PMSR6 protein. The small green circles represent potential sites for N-linked glycan addition. (c) The left-most heterotetrameric interaction that occurs between UPIa/UPII in the inner ring and UPIb/UPIIIa in the outer ring is primarily mediated by the extracellular domains of UPII and UPIIIa. The right-most interaction between adjacent UPIa/UPII heterodimers occurs in the inner ring and involves pairings between the transmembrane domains of UPIa and UPII.

domains of the two molecules.[23] The extracellular 'head' domain of UPII or UPIIIa extends over the second extracellular domain of the tetraspanin protein (Figure 3.3b,c). The UPIa/UPII pairs are localized to the inner ring of the AUM particle, while the UPIb/UPIIIa pairs are localized to the outer ring. Interactions between adjacent UPIa/UPII pairs in the inner ring are mediated through association between UPIa with the neighboring UPII of the adjacent UPIA/UPII pair, whereas interactions between UPIa/UPII in the inner ring and UPIb/UPIIIa in the outer ring occur through attachments between the extracellular head regions of UPII and UPIIIa (Figure 3.3c). Further study is sure to give a finer resolution and understanding of how UPs assemble to form AUM particles, and how the latter coalesce to form plaques. Discussion below will examine UP function and the role these proteins may play in urinary tract diseases.

Urothelial barrier function: role of claudins and disruption by antiproliferative factor (APF)

An important function of the umbrella cells that line the mucosal surface of the urinary bladder is to form a barrier between the constituents of the urinary space (including toxic metabolites and pathogens) and the underlying

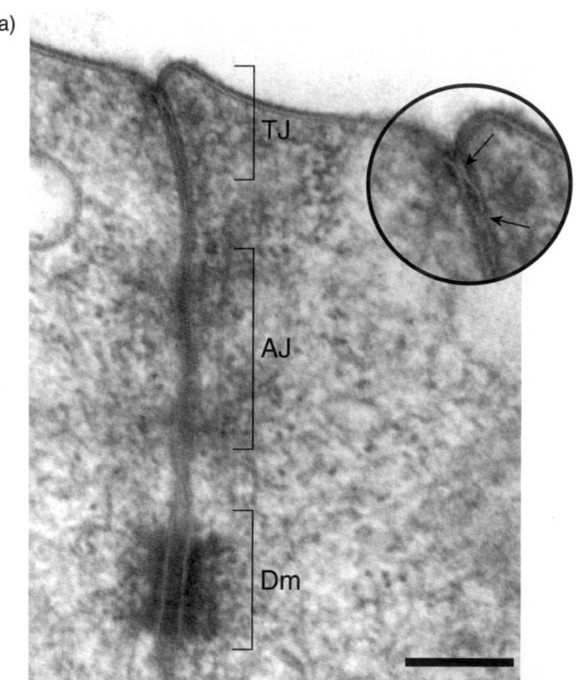

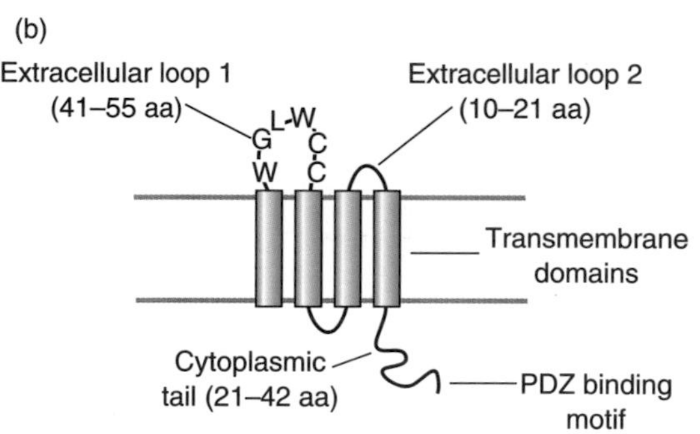

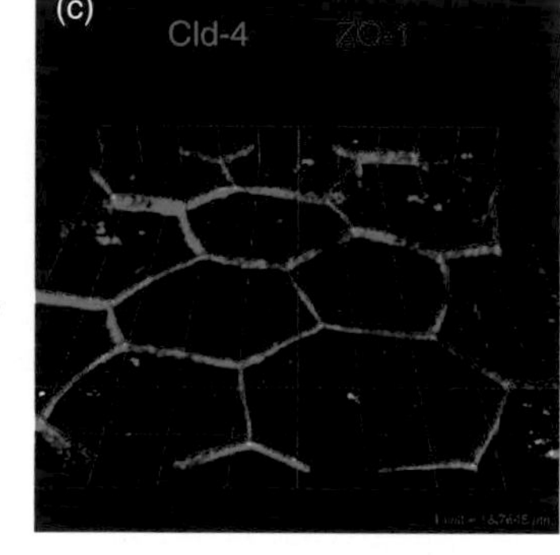

Figure 3.4
Tight junctions and claudins in urothelium. (a) TEM analysis of the junctional complex between adjacent rat umbrella cells showing the tight junction (TJ), adherens junction (AJ), and desmosome (Dm). The region of the tight junction is magnified in the inset. 'Kissing points' are marked with arrows. Bar = 0.5 μm. (b) Topology of the claudins. The approximate length of the extracellular loops and cytoplasmic domains is variable and depends on the claudin species involved. The location of the WGLWCC signature motif in the first extracellular loop of all claudin family members is shown. (c) Localization of claudin-4 (Cld-4) and the tight junction associated protein ZO-1 in the umbrella cell layer. Scale, one unit is ~ 16.8 μm. (Figure 3.4c is reprinted with permission from Acharya et al.[10])

muscular, neuronal, and vascular tissues. Several factors contribute to this barrier function. The first is a mucin/glycosaminoglycan layer that closely apposes the apical surface of the umbrella cell and may prevent bacterial attachment and diffusion of urine components across the epithelium.[24,25] The second is an apical plasma membrane rich in cholesterol and glycosphingolipids with an inherently low permeability to urea and water.[3] Third, and the subject of the following two subsections, a high-resistance paracellular barrier that is formed by the umbrella cell-associated tight junctions[2] and is disrupted by APF released from interstitial cystitis (IC) urothelial cells. The fourth factor is the plaque proteins described above that may play an important role in forming the apical membrane barrier to solutes (see discussion below). Finally, and also discussed below, is membrane turnover at the apical plasma membrane of the umbrella cell, which allows for surface area expansion during filling and recovery of membrane during voiding.[1]

Role of claudins

The tight junction is located at the apico-lateral junction of a polarized epithelial cell and forms a continuous belt that functions as a regulated seal between neighboring epithelial cells.[26] Tight junctions regulate paracellular transport (gate function) and restrict movement of lipids and membrane proteins between the apical and basolateral plasma membrane domains (fence function). The tight junctions of all epithelial cells, including those of umbrella cells, show characteristic regions where the membrane of apposing cells comes in close proximity to form so-called 'kissing points' (Figure 3.4a).[27] When examined by freeze fracture techniques, the kissing points appear as multiple anastamosing filamentous 'strands' that surround the apico-lateral junction of the epithelial cells.[28] Tight junctions are composed of multiple proteins including the claudins, a family of 24 membrane proteins that share the following common features: a molecular mass of 20–25 kDa, four transmembrane domains, two extracellular loops, the presence of a conserved WGLWCC 'signature motif' in the first extracellular loop, and a C-terminal PDZ (PSD-95, discs large, ZO-1)-binding motif that allows for interactions with PDZ domains of tight junction-associated cytoplasmic proteins such as ZO-1 (Figure 3.4b).[29]

Claudins are localized to junctional strands, and when claudins are expressed ectopically in nonpolarized L-cell fibroblasts they induce cell–cell interactions and formation of strands.[30] The expression pattern of claudins is tissue and segment specific,[31,32] and can be developmentally regulated.[32,33] A significant body of recent work indicates that claudins regulate paracellular ion transport, and the current model is that the extracellular loops of claudins present on apposing cell surfaces combine to form pores that allow selective transport of ions.[26–28] Presumably, the specific claudins expressed by the epithelium, and their ability to form homomeric and heteromeric claudin–claudin interactions, are the molecular basis of the distinct paracellular transport properties associated with each epithelium. Hereditary loss of claudin-14 leads to deafness[34] and loss of claudin-16 expression results in hypomagnesemia and hypercalciuria.[35] In addition, a growing literature indicates that changes in claudin expression may alter the metastic potential of numerous tumor types,[36] and tight junctions are likely to play an important, albeit ill-defined role in bladder cancer.[37] Claudins are also targets for bacterial and fungal toxins including *Clostridium perfringens* enterotoxin[38] and ochratoxin A.[39]

Our knowledge of the claudin family members expressed in the urothelium and the role they play in forming this high-resistance barrier ($> 75\,000\ \Omega \cdot cm^2$) is incomplete but growing. Claudins-4, -8, -12, and possibly -13 are expressed by the uroepithelium of rat, mouse, and rabbit bladder.[10] Claudins-8 and -12 are localized to the tight junction of the umbrella cell layer, whereas claudin-4 is associated with the tight junctions as well as the basolateral surface of the umbrella cells and the plasma membrane of the underlying cell layers (Figure 3.4c). The localization of claudin-4 to basolateral membranes is consistent with the possibility that it may play an additional role in cell–cell adhesion. Other studies indicate that additional claudin species are expressed by human uroepithelium including claudins-3, -4, -5, and -7.[40] Claudin-3 is found in the umbrella cell tight junction, claudin-5 is expressed at the basolateral surface of the umbrella cell layer, while claudins-4 and -7 are localized at the intercellular borders of all urothelial cell layers. RT-PCR data indicate that claudins-1, -2, -8, and -10 may also be expressed. Further analysis using cultured human urothelial cells indicates that expression of claudin isoforms is dependent on the time in culture and modulators of signaling by the epidermal growth factor (EGF) receptor and the nuclear hormone receptor peroxisome proliferator activated receptor.[40] Activation of the latter, in the presence of EGF receptor antagonists, promotes terminal differentiation of the cultured urothelium. In addition to regulating claudin expression, this treatment also promotes localization of claudins to the tight junctions and intercellular borders of the cultured urothelium.

Further study will increase our understanding of how claudins contribute to the high-resistance phenotype-associated urothelium, and how disruptions of tight junctions contribute to bladder diseases such as outlet obstruction, bacterial cystitis, IC, and experimentally-induced spinal cord injury, all of which are characterized by alterations of the urothelium and umbrella cell junctional complex.[41–48]

Antiproliferative factor and urothelial barrier function

IC is a painful bladder syndrome that affects predominantly women.[49] It is of unknown etiology and is often characterized by pain in the bladder or surrounding pelvic region and may be accompanied by urgency and frequency. Cytoscopic examination can reveal petechial hemorrhages and ulcers that extend into the lamina propria (Hunner's ulcers), while at the cellular level there is a loss and/or thinning of the urothelium. Intriguingly, isolated urothelial cells from patients with IC, but not those of control patients, release antiproliferative factor (APF), which, as the name implies, slows urothelial cell growth.[50]

APF has been isolated and purified and is a nonapeptide (T-V-P-A-A-V-V-V-A, in single amino acid code) that is identical to residues 541–549 of the 6th transmembrane domain of the Wnt ligand receptor Frizzled 8.[50] The peptide is glycosylated by a sialic acid α-2,3 linked to galactose β1-3-*N*-acetylgalactosamine, which in turn is α-O-linked to the N-terminal T_{541} residue of the APF peptide. The sialic acid moiety is not required for APF activity, but the *N*-acetylgalactosamine is. The putative receptor for APF was recently identified and is the cytoskeleton-associated protein 4/p63, which is expressed by isolated urothelial cells.[51] Addition of function-blocking antibodies to the receptor, or downregulation of the receptor by siRNA technology, diminishes the ability of APF to decrease urothelial proliferation. The pathways that are modulated downstream of receptor activation and regulate cell proliferation remain to be identified.

In addition to its role in regulating proliferation, APF may also regulate urothelial tight junction barrier function. Cultured urothelium from IC patients shows increased paracellular flux of tracers such as mannitol and inulin.[52] Furthermore, expression of two tight junction-associated proteins, ZO-1 and occludin, is decreased. Significantly, treatment of urothelial cells derived from normal tissues with purified APF results in increased paracellular flux and decreased expression of ZO-1 and occludin.[52] These studies indicate that the leaky urothelium observed in patients with IC may result, in part, from APF-induced defects in the umbrella cell-associated tight junction. It is not known if APF acts through the cytoskeleton-associated protein 4/p63 receptor to induce these changes, nor is there any information about the pathways that occur downstream of receptor activation are not known.

Functions of plaque-associated proteins

Analysis of knockout mice lacking UPIIIa or UPII indicates that plaques may play a role in barrier function. UPIIIa knockout mice show few plaques, likely reflecting the ability of the minor amounts of UPIIIb to form heterodimers with UPIb.[53] In contrast, UPII knockout mice form no plaques, stressing the importance of this UP in plaque formation.[54] Intriguingly, the apical membranes of umbrella cells from UPIIIa knockout animals show increased permeability to the normally membrane impermeant dye methylene blue.[53] Biophysical analysis confirms these findings and demonstrates that bladders from UPIIIa knockout animals have a significant increase in water and urea permeability across the umbrella cell layer; however, junctional permeability appears to be unchanged.[4] These results are the first indication that integral membrane proteins may contribute to the apical membrane permeability barrier of the uroepithelium. It has not been reported whether UPII knockout mice share a similar phenotype, but it is likely to be the case.

In addition to defects in permeability, lack of UPII and UPIIIa expression has other dramatic consequences including formation of a hyperplastic uroepithelium with small umbrella cells, perhaps a result of increased turnover of the epithelium or lack of normal apical membrane traffic, and enlarged obstructed ureters (a result of urothelial hyperplasia).[53,54] The latter leads to vesicoureteral reflux, resulting in hydronephrosis and, eventually, death in some animals.[53] Although vesicoureteral reflux is a hereditary disease that affects ~ 0.5–1.0% of the human population, the mode of inheritance is not well understood.[55] The knockout animals indicate that deficiencies in plaque subunits or plaque formation may account for some of these genetic abnormalities. However, two groups have examined patients with primary vesicoureteral reflux and observed no genetic linkage between the disease and defects in the UPIIIa locus.[56,57] In contrast, mutations in the UPIIIa gene are associated with renal hypodysplasia,[58,59] a disease characterized by small kidneys with decreased numbers of nephrons and other developmental defects. In one study, de novo mutations in the gene encoding UPIIIa were found in 4 of 17 children with renal hypodysplasia,[58] while a separate analysis showed a much lower rate of de novo mutations (approaching 0.4%).[59] Mutations observed included conversion of glycine at position 202 to an aspartate in the so-called 'conserved domain' (I-D-T-W-P-G_{202}-R-R-S-G-G-M-I-V-I-T-S-I-L-G-S-L-P-F-F) of the UPIIIa gene[59] (Figure 3.3b). The possible significance of this mutation is described below.

Why UPII/UPIIIa deficiency or mutations in UPIIIa leads to growth and developmental defects is unknown. It could simply reflect the altered permeability barrier, or there may be other causes. One possibility is that UPIIIa may be involved in downstream signaling events that are important for proper growth and differentiation. Intriguingly, a *Xenopus* ortholog of UPIIIa (called xUPIIIa) is expressed in the kidney, urinary tract, ovary, and eggs of the frog along with xUP1b.[60,61] xUP1a, xUPII, and xUPIIIb mRNA are also expressed in frog tissues.[21] Antibodies to the extracellular domain of xUPIIIa block egg fertilization, implicating xUPIIIa in this process.[60] The data thus far indicate that xUPIIIa and xUP1b form a complex at the plasma membrane with the ganglioside GM-1, at least when expressed in HEK293 cells (Figure 3.5).[61] At the cell surface the xUPIIIa/xUP1b complex interacts with the *Src* kinase, modulating *Src* localization and negatively regulating its activity.[61] Upon interaction with the oocyte, the sperm releases a proteinase(s) that likely acts upon the G-R-R_{188} motif present in the conserved domain of xUPIIIa.[62] The cleavage of xUPIIIa relieves the inhibitory action of xUPIIIa/xUP1b on *Src*, which then phosphorylates tyrosine residue 249 in the cytoplasmic domain of xUPIIIa.[62] Exogenously added cathepsin-B (which recognizes and cleaves peptides containing G-R-R residues) can also promote xUPIIIa cleavage, *Src* activation, and xUPIIIa phosphorylation. While the function of the cleaved, phosphorylated fragment of xUPIIIa remains to be defined, activated *Src* stimulates downstream Ca^{2+} release by activating xPLCγ, eventually resulting in resumption of meiosis II. Although it is unknown whether UPIIIa plays a related function in regulating signaling within mammalian urinary tract-associated tissues, such a requirement could explain the significant abnormalities associated with loss of UPs in mammalian systems.[6] It is intriguing to note that G_{186} in xUPIIIa is equivalent to G_{202} in the conserved domain of hUPIIIa, mutation of which results in renal hypodysplasia.

Membrane turnover at the apical surface of umbrella cells

Coordinated exocytosis/endocytosis in response to stretch

A crucial aspect of the barrier function of the uroepithelium is that it must be maintained in the face of cyclical changes in hydrostatic pressure as the bladder fills and empties. At the organ level, this is accomplished by

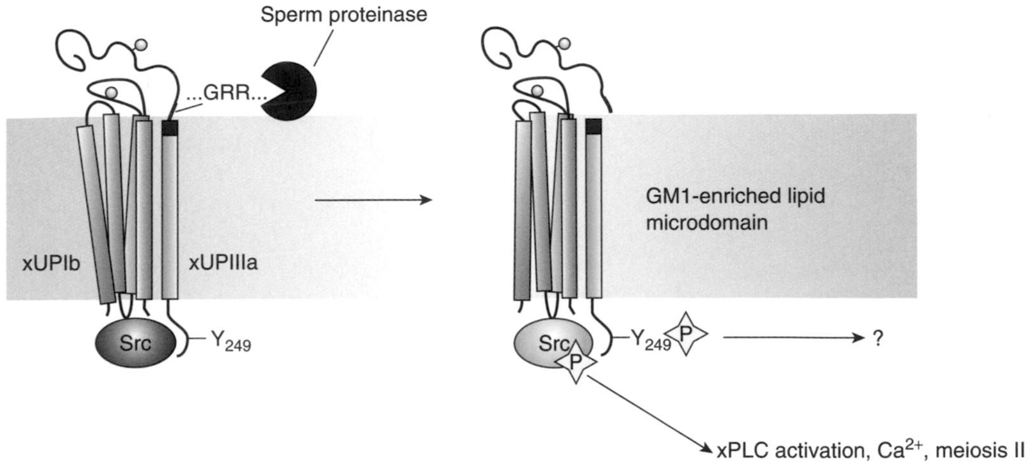

Figure 3.5
Function of xUP1b/xUPIIIa in *Xenopus* sperm-egg fertilization. xUPI1/xUPIIIa are found in cholesterol- and GM1-enriched lipid microdomains at the surface of eggs. Src is associated with this complex in an inactive state. Cathepsin-B-like enzymes released from sperm proteolyze xUPIIIa, possibly at the G-R-R motif found in the conserved domain. The cleavage of xUPIIIa results in the autophosphorylation of Src Y_{415} (not shown) as well as Src-dependent phosphorylation of Y_{239} in the cytoplasmic domain of xUPIIIa. Activated Src phosphorylates xPLC (not shown) and stimulates increased cytoplasmic Ca^{2+} and entry into meiosis II. The function of phosphorylated cleaved xUPIIIa is unknown.

unfolding of the highly wrinkled mucosal surface during bladder filling and refolding upon voiding. At the cellular level this accommodation involves both changes in the morphology and membrane dynamics of the uroepithelium. As the bladder fills the uroepithelium becomes thinner, apparently the result of intermediate and basal cells spreading laterally to accommodate the increased urine volume.[7,9] The umbrella cells undergo a large shape change that involves progression from a roughly cuboidal morphology in the empty bladder to one that is flat and squamous in the filled bladder.[7,9] The umbrella cell shape transformation is accompanied by discoidal/fusiform vesicle exocytosis that increases the apical surface area of the umbrella cell and the overall surface area of the bladder, allowing the bladder to accommodate additional urine volume (Figure 3.6).[63,64]

Surprisingly, stretch not only stimulates exocytosis, but it also stimulates rapid endocytosis.[63] The endocytosed membrane components including UPs are likely transported to lysosomes where they are degraded,[63] as the amount of endocytosed membrane proteins and UPs decreases with increasing exposure to stretch. Recycling of internalized membrane may also occur, but this has not been examined. Apparently, the rates of endocytosis and exocytosis are such that the net effect is to add membrane to the apical surface of the cell. At first glance it seems counterintuitive that hydrostatic pressure would simultaneously induce exocytosis and endocytosis; however, hydrostatic pressure-induced endocytosis would modulate the increase in apical surface area brought about by exocytosis, and it would ensure turnover of membrane components.

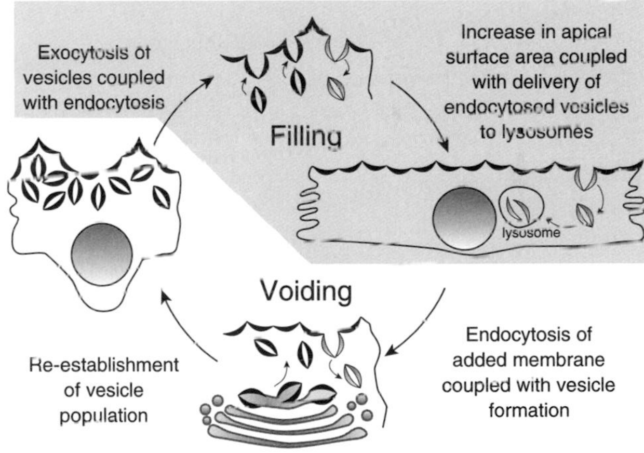

Figure 3.6
Model for vesicle dynamics in umbrella cells. Filling stimulates both exocytosis and endocytosis. The net rates of these processes are such that membrane is added to the apical surface. Endocytosed membrane is delivered to lysosomes where contents are degraded. Upon voiding the added membrane is internalized and re-establishment of the vesicle pool may result from both endocytosis and de novo synthesis along the biosynthetic pathway. (Reprinted with permission from Apodaca.[1])

Beyond serving as a system to modulate surface area expansion in response to filling, exocytosis and endocytosis are likely to play a crucial role in modulating the release of mediators and regulating the surface density of the increasingly large number of channels, receptors, and other proteins localized to the plasma membranes of the urothelial cells.[65] In doing so, these membrane trafficking pathways can modulate the sensory and transducer functions of the epithelium described below. Exocytosis and endocytosis may also play important roles in bladder disease processes. For example, the uroepithelium of patients with IC releases increased amounts of ATP and expresses increased levels of $P2X_2$ and $P2X_3$ receptors,[66–70] both the likely consequence of increased exocytosis. Furthermore, binding of uropathogenic *Escherichia coli* to the umbrella cell surface is dependent on surface expression of uroplakin Ia.[71,72] Following binding, bacteria can be internalized by the umbrella cell, where they serve as a source of recurrent infection.[73] By blocking bacterial association and internalization, recurrent bacterial infections may be prevented.

Events following voiding

In cells such as neurons or mast cells, exocytosed membrane is recovered in a process termed compensatory endocytosis.[74] In the case of the umbrella cell, apical membrane added during bladder filling needs to be recovered upon voiding (Figure 3.6); however, there is little understanding of this process. Early studies instilled fluid-phase endocytic markers into the bladder just after urination.[16,75] However, filling the bladder increases stretch and stimulates the stretch-induced endocytosis described above.[63] Other studies placed urothelial tissue in hypotonic buffer, which increases cell volume and surface area, and subsequently in isotonic buffer, which stimulates endocytosis.[76] Although the physiologic significance of this experimental manipulation is unclear, endocytosis was rapid and dependent on the actin and microtubule cytoskeletons.[77] Finally, there is evidence that apical membrane added during short-term or extended stretch is rapidly recovered when the stretch stimulus is removed.[77] The intracellular fate of internalized membrane is not known. One possibility is that it serves to re-establish the population of discoidal vesicles.[16,75] However, endocytosed marker proteins (including fluid-phase and membrane-bound lectins) only label a small fraction of the total discoidal vesicle pool,[16,75,78] indicating that the majority of discoidal vesicles may be formed de novo from newly synthesized proteins (Figure 3.6).

Modulation of exocytosis by second messengers, Rab GTPases, ATP, adenosine, and EGF receptor signaling

Role of second messengers

Exocytosis in the umbrella cells requires metabolic energy (in the form of ATP) and the actin, intermediate filament, and microtubule cytoskeletons.[77,79,80] In addition, discoidal/fusiform vesicle exocytosis is regulated by Ca^{2+} and cAMP. Raising cytoplasmic Ca^{2+}, either by treating the epithelium with the Ca^{2+} ionophore A23187 or with the ER Ca^{2+} uptake inhibitor thapsigargin, stimulates exocytosis in the umbrella cell layer.[64] Conversely, exocytosis is blocked when tissue is bathed in a nominally Ca^{2+}-free solution or if cells are treated with inhibitors of inositol 1,4,5-trisphosphate (IP3)-dependent Ca^{2+} release pathways.[64] Thus both extracellular and intracellular Ca^{2+} may play a role in this process. An additional secondary messenger that is produced when the urothelium is exposed to hydrostatic pressure is cAMP.[63] Artificially raising cAMP in umbrella cells, by treating tissue in the absence of pressure with forskolin, causes a dramatic increase in exocytic activity, but not endocytic activity.[63] Unopposed by endocytosis, forskolin induces change in the apical surface area of umbrella cells of greater than 120%. Forskolin also stimulates exocytosis in isolated uroepithelial cells.[81] Treatment with H-89, an inhibitor of the downstream cAMP effector protein kinase A, partially inhibits (by ~ 50%) stretch-induced changes in the apical surface area of umbrella cells.[63] These data indicate that cAMP, possibly acting through protein kinase A, modulates stretch-induced exocytic traffic in umbrella cells.

Role of Rab27b

The majority of, if not all, membrane trafficking events are regulated by Rab GTPases, which regulate cargo selection, vesicle budding, organelle motility, and vesicle fusion.[82] Which ones regulate discoidal vesicle exocytosis remains an open question, although Rab27b is expressed in the bladder and is localized to discoidal vesicles.[83] The other isoform of Rab27, Rab27a, has been implicated in melanosome traffic and exocytosis of lytic granules in cytotoxic T-cells.[84] Rab27a links melanosomes, through melanophilin, to the unconventional myosin Va, which interacts with the actin cytoskeleton and serves to retain melanosomes at the cell periphery.[84] In a similar manner, Rab27b could interact with myosin motor proteins to tether discoidal/fusiform vesicles to the actin cytoskeleton, ultimately promoting vesicle exocytosis. In fact, discoidal/fusiform vesicles are scattered throughout the umbrella cell cytoplasm of unstretched tissue, but accumulate under the apical membrane as the bladder fills.[11,63,85]

ATP release and exocytosis

Isolated urothelium releases ATP from both mucosal and serosal surfaces when exposed to hydrostatic pressure,[86–89] and it is hypothesized that ATP released from the serosal surface of the urothelium during bladder filling stimulates $P2X_3$-containing receptors on suburothelial sensory nerve fibers, thus signaling information about urinary bladder filling.[90] ATP release may occur, in part, by vesicular release as it is inhibited by the secretory inhibitor brefeldin A (BFA), and potential stores of ATP are observed in tissue stained with the ATP-binding dye quinacrine.[91] However, pharmacologic analysis indicates that release of ATP may also occur through other mechanisms including connexin hemichannels, ABC proteins, and nucleoside transporters.[91] Other studies indicate that ATP release may depend on the activity of the amiloride-sensitive epithelial sodium channel, which is proposed to act as a mechanosensor in this system.[87] ATP release may also require expression of the transient receptor potential channel, vanilloid subfamily member (TRPV1), an ion channel expressed by nociceptive (pain sensing) afferent neurons and the urothelium.[92] Isolated bladders from TRPV1 knockout animals fail to release ATP in response to pressure and do not increase umbrella cell apical surface area in response to pressure.[92] The link between TRPV1 and ATP release is unknown, but could reflect TRPV1 conductance of extracellular Ca^{2+} into the cell.

In addition to playing a role in transmitting information to the nervous system, ATP may also play a role in regulating exocytosis in the umbrella cell layer. $P2X_2$, $P2X_3$, $P2X_4$, and $P2X_5$ receptor subunits are expressed on the serosal surfaces of urothelial cells.[93–95] Intriguingly, addition of apyrase (a membrane-impermeant exonucleotidase) to the serosal, but not mucosal, side of isolated urothelial tissue prevents stretch-induced exocytosis in umbrella cells, indicating that extracellular ATP release acts as an upstream signal for exocytosis.[91] Furthermore, the P2 receptor inhibitor PPADS blocks stretch-induced exocytosis, pointing to P2 receptor involvement in this process. Significantly, stretch-regulated exocytosis is inhibited in knockout mice lacking expression of $P2X_2$, $P2X_3$, or both subunits, implicating these particular purinergic receptors in discoidal/fusiform vesicle exocytosis. ATP-stimulated exocytosis is blocked by treatments that remove extracellular Ca^{2+} or prevent release of Ca^{2+} from intracellular stores, indicating that Ca^{2+} is an important second messenger in this process.[91] In addition to the previously described role for urothelially released ATP as a signal for bladder filling,[90] these observations establish ATP as a physiologically relevant upstream signal for regulating membrane turnover in umbrella cells.

Adenosine receptor expression and function

Adenosine receptors are expressed in all tissues and play important roles in regulating cellular functions such as neurotransmission, cell polarization, regulation of ion transport, and exocytosis.[96,97] Surprisingly little is known about how adenosine modulates bladder function in general, and uroepithelial biology in particular. Western blot analysis confirms expression of all four receptors in the urothelium, and immunofluorescence staining shows that A_1, A_{2a}, A_{2b}, and A_3 receptors are expressed in urothelium/submucosa, with A_1 being found on the apical surface of the umbrella cell layer.[98] The other receptors are expressed along the basolateral surfaces of the umbrella cell layer and the plasma membranes of the underlying urothelial cell layers. Stretching the epithelium stimulates release of adenosine from both surfaces of the tissue, and when adenosine is added to the serosal or mucosal surface of urothelium there is an increase in exocytosis.[98] Deaminase (which converts adenosine into inosine) abolishes these adenosine-induced capacitance increases. While A_1-, A_{2a}-, and A_3-, selective agonists all increase membrane capacitance after being administrated serosally, only an A_1-selective agonist increases membrane capacitance significantly after being administrated mucosally.[98] Antagonists of adenosine receptors, as well as deaminase, have no effect on stretch-induced capacitance increases. However, adenosine potentiates the effects of stretch when added to the mucosal surface of pressure-stimulated epithelium.[98] These results indicate that the urothelium is a site of adenosine biosynthesis, and that adenosine receptor signaling may contribute to the modulation of umbrella cell exocytosis.

Role of EGF receptor in exocytosis

EGF/EGF-receptor is known to play an important role in urothelial proliferation during regeneration and during neoplastic transformation.[99–101] Surprisingly, new work indicates that apical EGF-receptor signaling may play a central role regulating umbrella cell exocytosis.[102] When isolated urothelium is stretched the ensuing increase in exocytosis is marked by two phases: a rapid phase that occurs during the first 30 minutes of stretch, followed by an extended slow phase that occurs over the next several hours. The slow phase depends on protein synthesis and is inhibited by cyclohexamide and BFA. The early phase is not inhibited by these agents, indicating that it may involve exocytosis of preformed vesicles. Slow-phase exocytosis is inhibited by EGF receptor antagonists, and the exogenous addition of EGF stimulates exocytosis in the absence of stretch after a lag of 30–60 minutes. Although urine is known to contain EGF, undiluted urine does not stimulate exocytosis in this system. Stretch stimulates EGF receptor activation and this activation appears to depend on upstream cleavage of the heparin-binding (HB)-EGF transmembrane precursor at the apical surface of the umbrella cell, releasing HB-EGF to bind to apically localized EGF receptors (Figure 3.7). Once activated, the EGF receptor stimulates activation of downstream ERK/p38 MAP kinase signaling cascades. The latter are known to regulate transcription and could explain the protein synthesis dependence of late-phase exocytosis. The protein products that are synthesized upon stretch and required for exocytosis are not known.

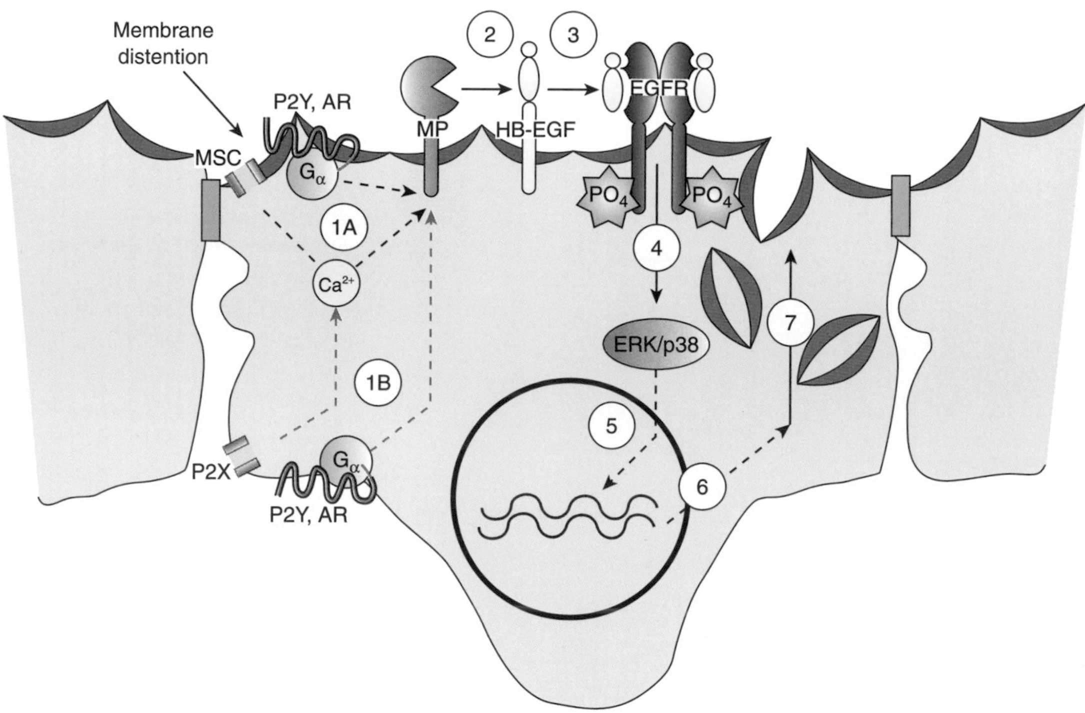

Figure 3.7
Regulation of exocytosis by transactivation of EGF receptor and downstream MAPK-dependent protein synthesis. Bladder filling may activate mechanosensitive ion channels (MSC) and/or stimulate release of mediators such as ATP and adenosine (not shown), which bind to P2X, P2Y, or adenosine receptors (AR). The increased intracellular Ca^{2+} that results from P2X or MSC activation or stimulation of heterotrimeric G proteins downstream of ligand binding to P2Y receptors or ARs initiates at the mucosal (step 1A) or possibly serosal (step 1B) surfaces of the cell. Either pathway activates metalloproteinase activity through an uncharacterized mechanism. The metalloproteinase (possibly a member of the disintegrin and metalloproteinase family or matrix-associated metalloproteinase family) cleaves apical pro-HB-EGF (step 2) to liberate soluble HB-EGF, which stimulates EGF receptor dimerization and cytoplasmic autophosphorylation (step 3). The activated EGF receptor stimulates signaling molecules including those that may activate p38 and ERK1/2 MAPK signaling pathways (step 4). MAPK signaling pathways may regulate the transcription of gene products (step 5), which encode unknown proteins (step 6) that facilitate exocytosis of discoidal vesicles that mediate the late-phase expansion of apical surface area (step 7). (Reprinted with permission from Balestreine and Apodaca.[102])

Autocrine activation of EGFR by mechanical stimuli such as stretch may occur as a result of receptor transactivation. In this process upstream stimuli such as elevated intracellular Ca^{2+} and activation of G-protein-coupled receptors promotes proteolytic processing and release of ErbB family ligands, typically HB-EGF, that bind to and activate the EGF receptor.[103] In addition to P2X receptors the umbrella cells also likely express G-protein coupled P2Y receptors at their mucosal surface.[91] One plausible model is that ATP binds to P2Y receptors, which in turn stimulate a heterotrimeric G-protein to activate proteolytic cleavage and release of ligand(s) such as HB-EGF. Alternatively, the increased Ca^{2+} stimulated by ATP binding to P2X receptors could result in EGFR transactivation.[91] It is equally plausible that many of the mediators previously found to stimulate exocytosis, such as adenosine and agents that increase intracellular Ca^{2+} and cAMP,[63,64,91,98] may act, in part, by EGFR transactivation. Thus EGF receptor transactivation and signaling may be a common pathway to stimulate exocytosis in the umbrella cell layer.

Urothelial-neuronal signaling

Innervation of the urothelium

Recent studies have shown that both afferent and autonomic efferent nerves are located in close proximity to the urothelium (Figure 3.8). Peptidergic (substance P, calcitonin-gene-related peptide, CGRP), P2X-, and TRPV1-immunoreactive nerve fibers presumed to arise from afferent neurons in the lumbosacral dorsal root ganglia are distributed throughout the urinary bladder musculature as well as in a plexus beneath and extending into the urothelium.[92,104–106] In humans with neurogenic detrusor overactivity intravesical administration of resiniferatoxin, a C-fiber afferent neurotoxin, reduces the density of TRPV1 and $P2X_3$ immunoreactive suburothelial nerves, indicating that these are sensory nerves.[107]

Immunohistochemical markers for cholinergic (choline acetyltransferase (ChAT)) and adrenergic nerves (tyrosine hydroxylase) are also detected in the

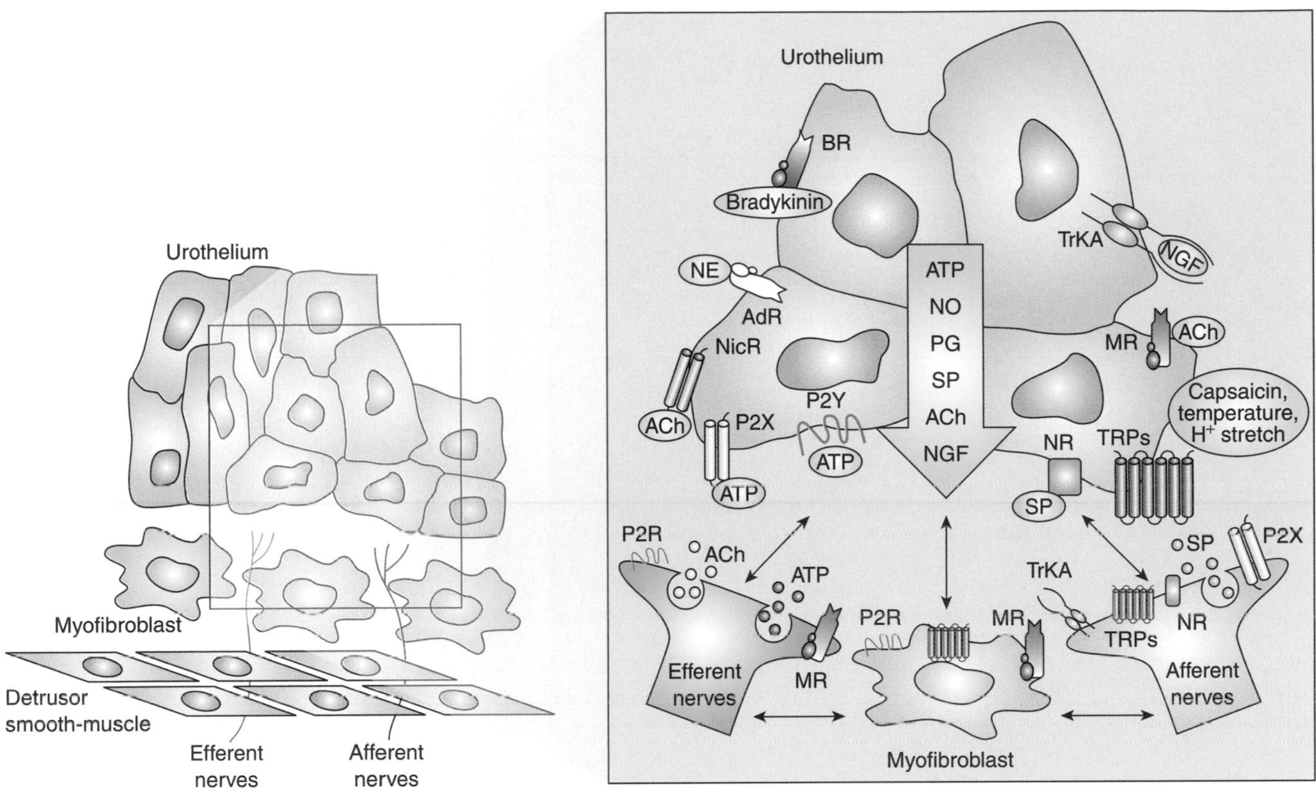

Figure 3.8
Hypothetical model that depicts possible interactions between bladder afferent and efferent nerves, urothelial cells, smooth muscle, and myofibroblasts. Stimulation of receptors and channels on urothelial cells can release mediators that target bladder nerves and other cell types; urothelial cells can also be targets for neurotransmitters released from nerves or other cell types. Urothelial cells can be activated by either autocrine (i.e. autoregulation) or paracrine (release from nearby nerves or other cells) mechanisms. Abbreviations: ACh, acetylcholine; AdR, adrenergic receptor; BR, bradykinin receptor; H^+, proton; MR, muscarinic receptor; NE, norepinephrine; NGF, nerve growth factor; NR, neurokinin receptor; NicR, nicotinic receptor; NO, nitric oxide; P2R, purinergic 2 receptor unidentified subtype; P2X and P2Y, purinergic receptors; PG, prostaglandin; SP, substance P; Trk A, receptor tyrosine kinase A, high affinity receptor for nerve growth factor; TRPs, transient receptor potential channels.

suburothelial regions of the bladder.[105,108] While this would commonly indicate the presence of efferent autonomic nerves, in the guinea pig bladder some ChAT immunoreactivity near the urothelium may be present in sensory rather than efferent nerves.[108] This conclusion is based on the finding that the ChAT-positive nerves do not exhibit neurofilament-200 staining. Because intramural autonomic efferent neurons in both the cat and guinea pig bladder express neurofilament-200 immunoreactivity,[108,109] it is proposed that the neurofilament-200 negative/ChAT-positive staining represents cholinergic sensory nerves.[108]

A network of cells with morphologic characteristics similar to those of myofibroblasts or interstitial cells is also detected in the suburothelial space of the bladder in both humans and animals (Figure 3.8).[110–112] These cells, which are extensively linked by gap junctions and have close contact with nerves, can respond to neurotransmitters, such as ATP released from nerves or urothelial cells, suggesting that they could act as intermediaries in urothelial–nerve interactions.[111,112] Thus the anatomic substrates for bidirectional urothelial–neural communication exist in the urinary bladder.

Involvement of the urothelium in 'sensing' chemical and mechanical stimuli

The urothelium is becoming increasingly appreciated as a responsive structure capable of detecting physiologic and chemical stimuli, and releasing a number of signaling molecules. Examples of neuronal 'sensor molecules' (i.e. receptors/ion channels) that have been identified in urothelium include receptors for bradykinin, neurotropins (trkA and p75), purines (P2X and P2Y), adenosine (A_1, A_{2a}, A_{2b}, and A_3), norepinephrine (α and β), acetylcholine (nicotinic and muscarinic), protease-activated receptors (PARs), amiloride/

Table 3.1 *Comparison of sensor properties of urinary bladder urothelial cells and primary afferent nerves*

Sensor function/Stimuli	Urothelial sensor molecules	Primary afferent sensor molecules
ATP	P2X/P2Y	P2X/P2Y
Capsaicin/Resiniferatoxin	TRPV1	TRPV1
Heat	TRPV1; TRPV2; TRPV4	TRPV1; TRPV2; TRPV3; TRPV4
Cold	TRPM8; TRPA1	TRPM8; TRPA1
H^+	TRPV1	TRPV1; ASIC; DRASIC
Osmolarity	In part TRPV4	In part TRPV4
Bradykinin	B1; B2	B1; B2
Acetylcholine	Nicotinic/muscarinic	Nicotinic/muscarinic
Norepinephrine	α/β subtypes	α/β subtypes
Nerve growth factor	p75/trkA	p75/trkA
Mechanosensitivity	Amilioride sensitive Na^+ channels	Amilioride sensitive Na^+ channels

mechanosensitive Na^+ channels and a number of TRP channels (TRPV1, TRPV2, TRPV4, TRPM8) (Table 3.1).[69,92,113–121] Examples of factors released from urothelial cells following physical and chemical stimulation include ATP, NO, acetylcholine, adenosine, APF, cytokines, prostanoids, and various trophic factors.[50,67,87,113–115,121–123] These and other data accumulated over the last several years indicate that urothelial cells display a number of properties similar to sensory neurons (nociceptors/mechanoreceptors), and that both types of cells use diverse signal-transduction mechanisms to detect physiologic stimuli.

Urothelium-associated purinergic receptors: role in bladder pathology

Since the first report in 1997 of distention-evoked ATP release from bladder urothelium,[87] and the subsequent demonstration that distention of the ureter evokes ATP release into the ureteral lumen,[86] there is abundant evidence that supports a role for urothelial-derived ATP release in both autocrine and paracrine signaling in the urinary tract. The expression of P2X and P2Y purinergic receptor subtypes in cells (urothelium, nerves, myofibroblasts) located at or near the luminal surface of the bladder [69,111,112] and the sensitivity of these cells to ATP (indicated by an ATP-induced increase in $[Ca^{2+}]_i$ [115] raises the possibility that basolateral ATP release from urothelial cells could influence not only adjacent urothelial cells, but also myofibroblasts and nerves (Figure 3.8). In addition, intercellular coupling mediated by gap junctions in myofibroblasts could provide a mechanism for long-distance spread of signals from the urothelium to the detrusor muscle.[112]

A role of purinergic sensory mechanisms in normal bladder function was first demonstrated in studies in anesthetized $P2X_3$ null mice that exhibit abnormal reflex bladder activity.[88,90] In these animals ATP release from the urothelium is normal but the excitatory effect of exogenous ATP on bladder afferent nerves is blocked. Immunohistochemistry, which shows abundant $P2X_3$ immunoreactive nerves in the suburothelial plexus in wild type animals, reveals a complete absence of these fibers in null mice, whereas staining for CGRP and TRPV1 receptors is unaffected, indicating that the afferent innervation is still intact. Afferent nerve activity, which increases progressively during gradual bladder distention in wild-type animals, is attenuated in the $P2X_3$ null mice. In addition, the bladder volume for inducing a micturition reflex was increased in the null mice. Subsequent studies in $P2X_2$ null and $P2X_2$/$P2X_3$ null mice (i.e., double knockouts) revealed reduced urinary bladder reflexes and decreased afferent nerve activity upon bladder distention.[124] These experiments indicate an important contribution of heteromeric $P2X_{2/3}$ receptors to mechanosensory transduction in the urinary bladder. Although it is likely that a major factor underlying the defect in bladder function in $P2X_{2/3}$ receptor null mice is the change in afferent excitability, it should be noted as mentioned earlier that stretch-evoked exocytosis in cultured urothelial cells is inhibited in mice lacking expression of either $P2X_2$, $P2X_3$, or both subunits,[91] raising the possibility that the function of the urothelium as well as that of afferent nerves is abnormal in these animals.

Immunohistochemical studies in patients exhibiting neurogenic detrusor overactivity reveal an increased density of suburothelial $P2X_3$ immunoreactive nerves.[125] In some patients who respond clinically to intravesical administration of the C-fiber neurotoxin resiniferatoxin, $P2X_3$ staining is reduced.[125] The staining is also reduced in patients responding to intravesical administration of botulinum toxin A.[126] These data indicate that neurogenic detrusor overactivity is associated with an increased expression of $P2X_3$ receptors in afferent nerves or increased density of these nerves.

Changes in the expression of purinergic receptors in the urothelium and changes in the urothelial release of ATP are also detected in pathologic conditions. In cats with feline interstitial cystitis (FIC), a painful bladder disorder, $P2X_1$ and $P2Y_2$ immunoreactivity in the urothelium is decreased.[69] Urothelial cells isolated from FIC cats also exhibit greater stretch-evoked release of ATP.[67] A similar enhancement of ATP release is detected in urothelial cells from patients with IC.[70] ATP can also act in an autocrine manner to enhance its own release from urothelial cells.[70] This autofeedback mechanism may be more important in pathologic conditions. Enhanced release of ATP into the bladder lumen in response to bladder distention is also observed in chronic spinal cord injured rats and in rats with chemically irritated bladders.[127,128] ATP released from the urothelium can directly depolarize and initiate firing in sensory nerves by activating P2X channels[124] or by activating P2Y receptors on afferent nerves to stimulate intracellular second messenger pathways that, in turn, modulate other ion channels. For example, it has been shown recently in sensory neurons that ATP enhances TRPV1 currents by lowering the threshold for protons, capsaicin, and heat.[129] This response, which is presumably mediated by activation of intracellular protein kinases and phosphorylation of the TRPV1 channel,[130] represents a novel mechanism by which large amounts of ATP released from damaged or sensitized cells in response to injury or inflammation may trigger the sensation of pain.

TRPV1 and involvement in hypersensitivity disorders

The ability of capsaicin to evoke NO release from rat urothelium, reported in 1998, provided the first, albeit indirect, demonstration that TRPV channels are expressed in urothelial cells and that urothelial cells and afferent neurons may share some common properties.[113] TRPV1 is a member of a TRPV subfamily, consisting of six mammalian members (TRPV1–TRPV6), which are in turn part of a TRP superfamily that consists of several subfamilies (TRPC, TRPM, TRPA, TRPML, TRPP) that can regulate intracellular Ca^{2+} concentrations, either by modulating or acting as Ca^{2+} entry pathways in the plasma membrane or by activating intracellular signaling pathways for intracellular Ca^{2+} release from several types of organelles.[121,131,132] Many members of the TRPV subfamily (TRPV1–TRPV4) are heat-activated channels that are non-selectively permeable for cations and modestly permeable to Ca^{2+}.[121] In addition, TRPV1–TRPV4 also function as chemosensors for a broad array of endogenous and synthetic ligands.

TRPV1, previously known as the capsaicin receptor or the vanilloid receptor type 1, is a ligand-gated ion channel activated by capsaicin, heat, acidosis, and endogenous agonists (such as anandamide, 12-hydroxyeicosatetranoic acid).[121,133,134] Interest in this channel was stimulated by early studies of the pungent actions of agents such as capsaicin and resiniferatoxin (RTX).[131,135] Capsaicin (first isolated from chili peppers in 1919) became a 'hot' topic when it was found to have specific binding sites in a number of tissues including sensory nerves.[136–138] This culminated in the cloning of TRPV1, using capsaicin as a ligand.[133]

Both the upper and lower urinary tract are densely innervated by capsaicin-sensitive primary afferent neurons in a number of species including man.[136] Early functional studies revealed that capsaicin-sensitive C-type bladder afferent nerves play a role in micturition.[136,139] The capsaicin-sensitive nerves exhibit both a sensory and also an 'efferent' function that is mediated by release of peptides such as substance P and CGRP that can affect bladder smooth muscle and participate in sensory transmission in the spinal cord.[135,140] Capsaicin selectively activates unmyelinated (C-fiber type) bladder afferent nerves but does not affect myelinated (A-δ) afferent nerves. Stimulation of C-fiber bladder afferents with capsaicin or resiniferatoxin reduces the volume threshold for inducing micturition, increases voiding frequency, induces bladder hyperactivity, produces a burning sensation in the bladder or pain behavior in animals, and elicits bladder contractions and plasma protein extravasation.[136–140]

The expression of capsaicin-sensitive nerve fibers in the lower urinary tract was first demonstrated following binding of radiolabeled resiniferatoxin in the bladder and urethra of the rat.[138] Subsequently the use of antibodies to TRPV1 revealed TRPV1 immunoreactivity in a subpopulation of bladder afferent (C-fiber) nerves.[104,141] These fibers are localized near and within the bladder mucosa, as well as in close proximity to blood vessels and smooth muscle cells.

TRPV1 is expressed not only by afferent nerves that form a close contact with the bladder epithelium but also by non-neuronal cells such as urothelial cells and myofibroblasts.[104,110] The first indication of this broader distribution of TRPV1 in the bladder was the demonstration that capsaicin could evoke the release of NO in the bladder and that this effect persisted after complete denervation.[113] Subsequently it was shown that TRPV1 is expressed in urothelial cells (Figure 3.9) and that capsaicin evokes the release of NO from cultured urothelial cells as well as from sensory neurons.[104] In addition, activation of urothelial TRPV1 receptors with capsaicin or resiniferatoxin increases intracellular calcium and can evoke the release of other transmitters such as ATP.[92,104] As noted in sensory neurons, these responses are enhanced by low pH, blocked

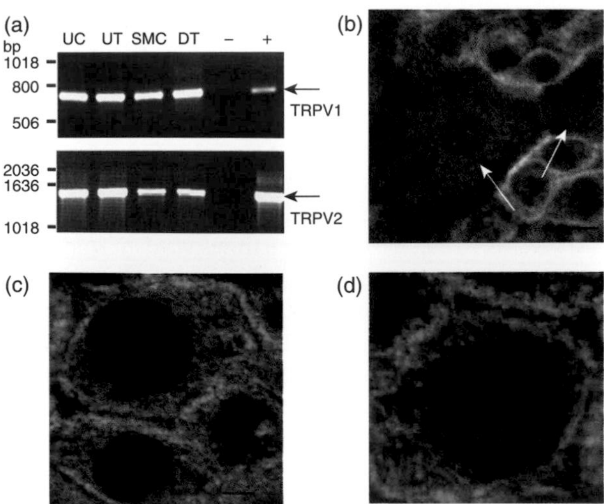

Figure 3.9
TRPV1 and TRPV2 expression was detected in urothelial and smooth muscle cells of the urinary bladder from the rat. (a) Reverse transcription-PCR analysis of TRPV1 and TRPV2 mRNA expression in dissociated bladder urothelial cells (UC), bladder urothelium (UT), dissociated bladder smooth muscle cells (SMC), and de-epithelialized bladder tissue (DT, smooth muscle following removal of the urothelium). Control lanes indicate input of no template (–), dorsal root ganglion cDNA (+ for TRPV1), or brain cDNA (+ for TRPV2). Arrows indicate predicted product sizes (TRPV1, 704 bp; TRPV2, 1436 bp). (b) Confocal image of bladder urothelium in bladder whole mounts stained for TRPV1 (cy3, red) and cytokeratin 17 (FITC, green), a marker for basal urothelial cells. A diffuse cytoplasmic pattern of TRPV1 staining can be seen in the apical and underlying urothelial layers (nuclei are unstained). Arrows indicate apical cells within the field from a single plane of focus. (c) Enlarged image of basal cells depicting TRPV1 (cy3, red) and cytokeratin (FITC, green) immunoreactivity. (d) Elimination of TRPV1 staining with the antibody preabsorbed with antigenic peptide. (Scale bars: b, 15 μm; c, 5 μm; d, 4 μm).

by TRPV1 antagonists, and eliminated in TRPV1 null mice.[104] In afferent neurons, TRPV1 is thought to integrate/amplify the response to various stimuli and to play an essential role in the development of inflammation-induced hyperalgesia. Thus, it seems likely that urothelial TRPV1 might participate in a similar manner, in the detection of irritant stimuli following bladder inflammation or infection.

Cultured urothelial cells from TRPV1 null mice also exhibit a reduction in stretch-evoked and hypotonic-evoked ATP release and a stretch-evoked increase in membrane capacitance.[92] In addition, TRPV1 knockout mice have a higher frequency of low-amplitude, nonvoiding bladder contractions, suggesting the possibility of a small but ongoing role for TRPV1 in normal micturition or urine storage. TRPV1 null mice also exhibit a reduction in bladder distention-evoked c-fos expression in the spinal cord and reflex voiding.[92] These changes may result from loss of TRPV1 expression not only in afferent nerves that form close contacts with bladder urothelial cells but also in urothelial cells themselves. Thus the function of TRPV1 in the bladder extends beyond pain sensation to include participation in normal voiding function, and is essential for mechanically-evoked purinergic signaling by the urothelium.

TRPV1 immunoreactivity is also present in a population of cells located in the suburothelial space.[110] These cells have morphologic characteristics of myofibroblasts and stain intensively for vimentin and the gap junction protein connexin 43. It is proposed that these 'myofibroblast' or 'interstitial' type cells function as 'pacemaker' cells in the bladder and have the capacity to modulate bladder sensations.[110–112] This hypothesis is given added support by the fact that many nerve fibers terminate on these cells, thus providing a means to modulate the sensitivity of bladder filling sensations. An understanding of the mechanisms underlying these cell–cell interactions may lead to the identification of novel targets for pharmacologic management of various bladder disorders.

TRPV1 has attracted considerable attention as a potential contributor to bladder diseases. TRPV1 knockout mice display differences in the response to chemically-induced irritation or inflammation of the bladder as compared to their wild-type counterparts.[142,143] Furthermore, patients suffering from neurogenic detrusor overactivity exhibit significant increases in the number of TRPV1-expressing nerves as well as increased TRPV1 expression within the urothelium.[107,144] Intravesical administration of vanilloid compounds produces beneficial effects in patients with bladder disorders such as neurogenic detrusor overactivity or hypersensitivity disorders such as IC.[145–155] However, intravesical vanilloids also reduce the number of bladder sensory fibers immunoreactive for TRPV1 or $P2X_3$ and therefore the clinical efficacy of these agents may be due largely to depletion of afferent transmitters or degeneration of the peripheral afferent nerves in the wall of the urinary bladder rather than desensitization of TRPV1 receptors in nerves or urothelium.[107,144] Thus it will not be possible to determine the contribution of TRPV1 receptors to lower urinary tract dysfunction in patients until the development and clinical testing of selective TRPV1 antagonists.

Additional TRP channels

Much less is known about the involvement of other TRPs in bladder function or disease. TRPV4, which is a non-selective cation channel activated by heat, shear stress, changes in osmolarity, and lipid ligands, is expressed within the epithelium of the lower urinary tract (see Table 3.1).[156–158] A definitive role for TRPV4 in bladder function has not been established. However, at other sites in the body, TRPV4 seems to play a role in bronchial hyper-responsiveness, hypo-osmotic induced hyperalgesia, and in the development of neuropathic pain.[121,159]

While little is known about the involvement of the cold-sensing TRP channels (TRPM8 and TRPA1) in bladder function, the effect of cold temperature on lower urinary tract function has long been of interest.[160,161] The instillation of cold solutions (known as the ice water test) elicits involuntary detrusor contractions in patients with either chronic spinal cord lesions or following bladder outlet obstruction.[161–164] This reflex is believed to be mediated by activation of C-type bladder afferent nerves sensitive to cold temperatures. The finding that intravesical instillation of menthol facilitates the bladder cooling reflex in both the cat and human suggests that TRPM8, a cold- and menthol-sensing channel, may be involved in triggering the reflex.[165–167] In the urinary bladder, TRPM8-positive immunoreactivity is found in nerves as well as in the urothelium.[168,169]

TRPA1 (formerly named ANKTM1) has been characterized as a thermoreceptor activated by noxious cold. Recent studies have shown that this channel is localized within the bladder urothelium and in sensory nerves that innervate the urinary bladder.[169,170] TRPA1 channels are activated by isothiocyanates or thiosulfinite compounds, which are the pungent ingredients in mustard oil and garlic, respectively, and by cinnamaldehyde and acrolein, the latter compound being the active metabolite of cyclophosphamide, an anticancer drug that produces hemorrhagic cystitis. Both mustard oil and cyclophosphamide have been used extensively to produce animal models of bladder irritation. Activation of TRPA1 channels with various agonists elicits contractions of bladder smooth muscle, which are due to release of tachykinins and cyclooxygenase metabolites.[170] The effect on smooth muscle contractility of agents capable of stimulating TRPA1 is comparable in potency to capsaicin, supporting the speculation that this channel may play a role in bladder function.

Cholinergic receptors: role in overactive bladder

The presence of muscarinic and nicotinic receptors in the urothelium is attracting interest in the role of acetylcholine as a chemical mediator of neural–urothelial interactions.[118,123,171–173] These receptors could be stimulated by acetylcholine released from urothelial cells as well as by cholinergic nerves that are detected in close proximity to the urothelial cells in the rat bladder (Figure 3.8).[123,174] Exogenous muscarinic and nicotinic cholinergic agonists applied to cultured urothelial cells elicit an increase in intracellular Ca^{2+} concentration and evoke the release of NO and ATP.[67,118] In bladder strips or whole bladder preparations muscarinic agonists also stimulate the release of a smooth muscle inhibitory factor from the urothelium.[171,172] Electrical stimulation of the pelvic nerve or reflex activation of the autonomic nervous system by spinal cord injury[41,175] can elicit changes in urothelial permeability as well as changes in the morphology of the urothelium in the rat, raising the possibility that autonomic or sensory nerves make 'synaptic connections' with the urothelial cells. Further studies are needed to determine if acetylcholine is involved in these connections.

The clinical effect of antimuscarinic agents in decreasing sensory symptoms in the overactive bladder may be related in part to blocking of muscarinic receptors in the urothelium or afferent nerves. These agents prevent stimulation of postjunctional muscarinic receptors by acetylcholine released from bladder efferent nerves and result in increased bladder capacity. Evidence that the urothelium expresses a complement of muscarinic receptors (M1–M5) along with recent studies that reveal a difference in muscarinic receptor density between normal, aging, and pathologic bladder urothelium has sparked an interest in the role of the urothelium in these disorders.[116,176–178]

Since antimuscarinic agents effectively enhance the storage phase of micturition, when parasympathetic nerves are silent, it has been postulated that the release of acetylcholine from the urothelium may contribute to detrusor overactivity.[179] Recent studies show that urothelial cells express the acetylcholine-synthesizing enzymes ChAT and carnitine acetyltransferase and can release acetylcholine following both mechanical and chemical stimulation.[123,180] Once released, there are a number of sites where urothelial-derived acetylcholine could exert an effect, including smooth muscle, nerves, and urothelial-muscarinic and/or nicotinic receptors, thereby participating in feedback mechanisms to modify urothelial function. Because stimulation of cholinergic receptors in urothelial cells elicits the release of ATP, cholinergic mechanisms in the urothelium could alter bladder sensation indirectly by triggering purinergic stimulation of nearby afferent nerves.

The functions of cholinoceptors in the urothelium have been evaluated by testing the effects of intravesically administered cholinergic agonists and antagonists on urine storage and voiding in cats and rats.[118,173,181,182] In chronic spinal cord injured cats intravesical infusion of carbachol, a muscarinic-nicotinic agonist, as well as oxotremorine methiodide, a quaternary muscarinic agonist that should have a relatively low ability to penetrate the urothelial barrier, decreases bladder capacity and enhances the number of premicturition contractions[182] during cystometrograms, but does not alter the amplitude of micturition contractions. These effects are blocked by intravesical administration of atropine sulfate or the quaternary analog, atropine methylnitrate. Intravesical administration of neostigmine methylsulfate, a quaternary anticholinesterase agent, mimicks the facilitatory effects of muscarinic agonists. The effects of neostigmine are blocked by atropine. These results indicate that activation of muscarinic receptors in the urothelium or in suburothelial afferent nerves facilitates the spinal micturition reflex mediated by C-fiber afferent nerves.[183] In the rat a similar facilitation of bladder activity induced by intravesically-administered muscarinic agonists is reported.[173,182]

Intravesical application of nicotine in the rat elicits two effects: a decrease in the frequency of reflex micturition in low concentrations and an increase in frequency in high concentrations.[118] The inhibitory effect is blocked by methyllycaconitine, an antagonist of $\alpha 7$ nicotinic receptors, whereas the facilitatory effect is blocked by hexamethonium, an antagonist of $\alpha 3$ type nicotinic receptors. Methyllyaconitine alone does not alter reflex bladder activity, whereas hexamethonium alone decreases reflex bladder activity, suggesting the existence of a tonically active nicotinic facilitatory mechanism. Nicotine also increases intracellular Ca^{2+} in cultured urothelial cells by activating hexamethonium-sensitive receptors.[118] These data coupled with the results of RT-PCR experiments that revealed the expression of multiple subtypes of nicotinic receptors in rat urothelial cells ($\alpha 3$, $\alpha 5$, $\alpha 7$, $\beta 3$, and $\beta 4$) raise the possibility that sensory mechanisms in the urothelium are modulated by complex nicotinic mechanisms.[118]

Urothelial cells express the various proteins necessary for the synthesis and storage of acetylcholine including the plasma membrane choline transporter ChAT, as well as the enzyme responsible for the metabolism of acetylcholine (acetylcholinesterase).[123,180] Acetylcholine is released from the bladder urothelium in rats[123,180] and humans.[178,184] Synthesis and release of acetylcholine has also been reported in epithelial cells in the lung.[185] However, the mechanism of release is uncertain. Recently botulinum toxin has been used to evaluate the release mechanism. Botulinum toxin, which is used clinically to treat a number of bladder disorders including neurogenic detrusor overactivity, detrusor–sphincter dyssynergia, as well as IC, inhibits detrusor muscle contractions by suppressing the release of transmitters such as ATP and Ach from bladder nerves by blocking exocytosis.[186–188] However, besides targeting bladder nerves, botulinum toxins also target the urothelium. Botulinum toxin type A significantly reduces stretch-evoked ATP release from bladder mucosa and also blocks intravesical ATP-induced bladder overactivity.[127,128,189] On the other hand, acetylcholine release from urothelial cells seems to be mediated by different mechanisms than those such as vesicular storage and exocytosis that underlie the release of ATP and ACh from nerves and the release of ATP from the urothelium.[123] These results suggest that it is unlikely that botulinum toxin therapy is targeting urothelial-derived Ach release to produce symptomatic relief of bladder overactivity.

Adrenergic receptors: role in bladder outlet obstruction

The urothelium expresses both alpha and beta subtypes of adrenergic receptors (see Table 3.1) which, when stimulated, trigger an increase in intracellular Ca^{2+} leading to the release of a number of mediators including ATP and NO.[113,114] Because of the close proximity of adrenergic nerves to the urothelium, it is possible that neurally-released norepinephrine may have an effect on the urothelial cells and thereby influence bladder function. Patients with a variety of lower urinary tract symptoms due to benign prostatic hyperplasia and even IC are often treated with selective α_1-adrenergic receptor antagonists.[190,191] Studies utilizing adrenergic receptor subtype null mice suggest an important role for adrenergic receptors, in particular α_{1D}, in regulation of bladder function.[192] The α_{1D} receptor is expressed within the bladder urothelium and tonic activation of these receptors by catecholamines may modulate bladder sensory mechanisms.

Nitric oxide

NO is involved in many functions of the lower urinary tract, ranging from inhibitory transmission in the urethra to modulation of bladder afferent nerves and bladder reflex pathways in the spinal cord.[193] The localization of neuronal nitric oxide synthase (nNOS) and/or NADPH-diaphorase (a marker for NOS) in efferent and afferent nerve fibers in addition to NOS isoforms (n, e, and i) in the urothelium suggest a role for NO in the micturition reflex pathway.[114,193] The release of NO from urothelium or other cells is thought to either facilitate or inhibit activity of bladder afferent nerves. For example, intravesical administration of oxyhemoglobin results in a bladder hyperactivity, demonstrating an inhibitory role for NO in the control of bladder reflexes.[194] Spinal cord injury or chronic bladder inflammation alters the expression of NOS, which raises the possibility that the neurotransmitter function of NO is plastic and can be altered by chronic pathologic conditions.[195,196] For example, it is reported that in cats with FIC, baseline levels of NO released from mucosal or bladder smooth muscle strips are increased.[197] Pharmacologic experiments revealed that the NO is produced by an iNOS-mediated Ca^{2+}-independent mechanism. High levels of NO in bladder or intestinal epithelia increase permeability to hydrophilic macromolecules.[198] This action might contribute to the loss of urothelial barrier function occurring in many disease states. High levels of NO also suppress the activity of ion channels in bladder afferent neurons, consistent with the inhibitory effect of intravesical administration of NO donors on the urinary bladder hyperactivity occurring in animals treated with cyclophosphamide.[199–201] It is reported that NO levels in the urine are decreased in some patients with interstitial cystitis.[202] This decrease could be linked with increased pain responses due to reduced NO inhibitory modulation of sensory nerves in the urinary bladder.

Future directions/clinical significance

Research during the last several years has markedly changed how we view the function of the urothelium. This tissue not only acts as a highly efficient barrier, but also exhibits properties similar to those of nociceptive and mechanoceptive afferent neurons. Activation of urothelial cells by chemical, thermal, or mechanical stimuli can evoke the release of various mediators or neurotransmitters that impact neural activity and ultimately bladder function. Thus urothelial cells exhibit specialized sensory and signaling properties that allow them to respond to their chemical and physical environment and to engage in reciprocal communication with neighboring cells in the bladder wall. It is conceivable that the effectiveness of some agents currently used in the treatment of bladder disorders may involve an action on urothelial receptors and/or release mechanisms. For example, botulinum neurotoxin type A (BoNT/A), which has been used to treat lower urinary tract symptoms such as frequency and urgency incontinence due to neurogenic or idiopathic detrusor overactivity, may act in part by suppressing the release of mediators (ATP and neuropeptides) from both neural and urothelial cells. Suppression of neurotransmitter release from urothelium could blunt afferent activity driven by urothelial-derived mediators. Thus pharmacologic interventions aimed at targeting urothelial receptor/ion channel expression or release mechanisms may provide a new strategy for the clinical management of bladder disorders.

Acknowledgments

I thank Dr Elena Hawryluk and Dr Puneet Khandelwal for their constructive and helpful comments while preparing this manuscript. The transmission and scanning electron micrographs were prepared by M von Bodungen and W Giovanni Ruiz. This work was supported by grants from the NIH to GA (R37DK54425), LB (DK54824), and WCD (DK49430).

References

1. Apodaca G. The uroepithelium: not just a passive barrier. Traffic 2004; 5: 1–12.
2. Lewis SA. Everything you wanted to know about the bladder epithelium but were afraid to ask. Am J Physiol 2000; 278: F867–74.
3. Negrete HO, Lavelle JP, Berg J, Lewis SA, Zeidel ML. Permeability properties of the intact mammalian bladder epithelium. Am J Physiol 1996; 271: F886–94.
4. Hu P, Meyers S, Liang F-X et al. Role of membrane proteins in permeability barrier function: uroplakin ablation elevates urothelial permeability. Am J Physiol 2002; 283: F1200–7.
5. Birder LA, de Groat WC. Mechanisms of disease: involvement of the urothelium in bladder dysfunction. Nature Clin Pract Urol 2007; 4: 46–54.
6. Jenkins D, Woolf AS. Uroplakins: new molecular players in the biology of urinary tract malformations. Kidney Int 2007; 71: 195–200.
7. Hicks M. The mammalian urinary bladder: an accommodating organ. Biol Rev 1975; 50: 215–46.
8. Martin BF. Cell replacement and differentiation in transitional epithelium: a histological and autoradiographic study of the guinea-pig bladder and ureter. J Anat 1972; 112: 433–55.
9. Petry G, Amon H. Licht- und elecktronenmikroskopiche Studien über Struktur und Dynamik des Übergangsepithels. Zeitschrift für Zellforschung 1966; 69: 587–612.
10. Acharya P, Beckel J, Wang E et al. Distribution of the tight junction proteins ZO-1, occludin, and claudin-4, -8, and -12 in bladder epithelium. Am J Physiol 2004; 287: F305–18.
11. Hicks RM. The fine structure of the transitional epithelium of rat ureter. J Cell Biol 1965; 26: 25–48.
12. Kachar B, Liang F, Lins U et al. Three-dimensional analysis of the 16 nm urothelial plaque particle: luminal surface exposure, preferential head-to head interaction, and hinge formation. J Mol Biol 1999; 285: 595–608.
13. Yu J, Manabe M, Sun TT. Identification of an 85–100 kDa glycoprotein as a cell surface marker for an advanced stage of urothelial differentiation: association with the interplaque ('hinge') area. Epithel Cell Biol 1992; 1: 4–12.
14. Liang F, Kachar B, Ding M et al. Urothelial hinge as a highly specialized membrane: detergent-insolubility, urohingin association, and in vitro formation. Differentiation 1999; 65: 59–69.
15. Hicks M, Ketterer B, Warren R. The ultrastructure and chemistry of the luminal plasma membrane of the mammalian urinary bladder: a structure with low permeability to water and ions. Phil Trans Royal Soc London Series B: Biol Sci 1974; 268: 23–38.
16. Porter K, Kenyon K, Badenhausen S. Specializations of the unit membrane. Protoplasma 1967; 63: 262–74.
17. Walz T, Häner M, Wu X-R et al. Towards the molecular architecture of the asymmetric unit membrane of the mammalian urinary bladder epithelium: a closed 'twisted ribbon' structure. J Mol Biol 1995; 248: 887–900.
18. Wu X-R, Lin J-H, Walz T et al. Mammalian uroplakins. A group of highly conserved urothelial differentiation-related membrane proteins. J Biol Chem 1994; 269: 13716–24.
19. Deng F-M, Liang F-X, Tu L et al. Uroplakin IIIb, a urothelial differentiation marker, dimerizes with uroplakin Ib as an early step of urothelial plaque assembly. J Cell Biol 2002; 159: 685–94.
20. Adachi W, Okubo K, Kinoshita S. Human uroplakin Ib in ocular surface epithelium. Invest Ophthalmol Vis Sci 2000; 41: 2900–5.
21. Garcia-España A, Chung P-J, Zhao X et al. Origin of the tetraspanin urolakins and their co-evolution with associated proteins: implications for uroplakin structure and function. Mol Phylo Evol 2006; 41: 355–67.
22. Wu X-R, Medina JJ, Sun TT. Selective interactions of UPIa and UPIb, two members of the transmembrane 4 superfamily, with distinct single transmembrane-domained proteins in differentiated urothelial cells. J Biol Chem 1995; 270: 29752–9.
23. Min G, Wang H, Sun T-T, Kong X-P. Structural basis for tetraspanin functions as revealed by the cryo-EM structure of uroplakin complexes at 6-angstrom resolution. J Cell Biol 2006; 173: 975–83.
24. Parsons CL, Boychuk D, Jones S, Hurst R, Callahan H. Bladder surface glycosaminoglycans: an epithelial permeability barrier. J Urol 1990; 143: 139–42.

25. Parsons CL, Greenspan C, Moore SW, Mulholland SG. Role of surface mucin in primary antibacterial defense of bladder. Urology 1977; 9: 48–52.
26. Van Itallie C, Anderson JM. The molecular physiology of tight junction pores. Physiology 2004; 19: 331–8.
27. Tsukita S, Furuse M. Pores in the wall: claudins constitute tight junction strands containing aqueous pores. J Cell Biol 2000; 149: 13–16.
28. Tsukita S, Furuse M, Itoh M. Multifunctional strands in tight junctions. Nature Rev Mol Cell Biol 2001; 2: 285–93.
29. González-Mariscal L, Betanzos A, Nava P, Jaramillo BE. Tight junction proteins. Progress Biophys Mol Biol 2003; 81: 1–44.
30. Furuse K, Sasaki H, Fujimoto K, Tsukita S. A single gene product, claudin-1 or -2, reconstitutes tight junction strands and recruits occludin in fibroblasts. J Cell Biol 1998; 143: 391–401.
31. Rahner C, Mitic LL, Anderson JM. Heterogeneity in expression and subcellular localization of claudins 2, 3, 4, and 5 in the rat liver, pancreas, and gut. Gastroenterology 2001; 120: 411–22.
32. Kiuchi-Saishin Y, Gotoh S, Furuse M et al. Differential expression patterns of claudins, tight junction membrane proteins, in mouse nephron segments. J Am Soc Nephrol 2002; 13: 875–86.
33. Pummi KP, Heape AM, Grénman RA, Peltonen JTK, Peltonen SA. Tight junction proteins ZO-1, occludin, and claudins in developing and adult human perineurium. J Histochem Cytochem 2004; 52: 1037–46.
34. Wilcox ER, Burton QL, Naz S et al. Mutations in the gene encoding tight junction claudin-14 cause autosomal recessive deafness DFNB29. Cell 2001; 104: 165–72.
35. Simon DB, Lu Y, Choate KA et al. Paracellin-1, a renal tight junction protein required for paracellular Mg^{2+} resorption. Science 1999; 285: 103–6.
36. Swisshelm K, Macek R, Kubbies M. Role of claudins in tumorogenesis. Adv Drug Deliv Rev 2005; 57: 919–28.
37. Haynes MD, Martin TA, Jenkins SA et al. Tight junctions and bladder cancer (review). Int J Mol Med 2005; 16: 3–9.
38. McClane BA. The complex interactions between *Clostridium perfringens* enterotoxin and epithelial tight junctions. Toxicon 2001; 39: 1781–91.
39. McLaughlin J, Padfield PJ, Burt JPH, O'Neill CA. Ochratoxin A increases permeability through tight junctions by removal of specific claudin isoforms. Am J Physiol 2004; 287: C1412–17.
40. Varley C, Hill G, Pellegrin S et al. Autocrine regulation of human urothelial cell proliferation and migration during regenerative responses in vitro. Exp Cell Res 2005; 306: 216–29.
41. Apodaca G, Kiss S, Ruiz WG et al. Disruption of bladder epithelium barrier function after spinal cord injury. Am J Physiol 2003; 284: F966–76.
42. Kreft ME, Romih R, Sterle M. Antigenic and ultrastructural markers associated with urothelial cytodifferentiation in primary explant outgrowths of mouse bladder. Cell Biol Int 2002; 26: 63–74.
43. Kreft ME, Sterle M, Veranic P, Jezernik K. Urothelial injuries and the early wound healing response: tight junctions and urothelial cytodifferentiation. Histochem Cell Biol 2005; 123: 529–39.
44. Lavelle J, Meyers S, Ramage R et al. Bladder permeability barrier: recovery from selective injury of surface epithelial cells. Am J Physiol 2002; 283: F242–53.
45. Leppilahti M, Hirvonen J, Tammela TL. Influence of transient overdistension on bladder wall morphology and enzyme histochemistry. Scand J Urol Nephrol 1997; 31: 517–22.
46. Leppilahti M, Kallioinen M, Tammela TL. Duration of increased mucosal permeability of the urinary bladder after acute overdistension: an experimental study in rats. Urol Res 1999; 27: 272–6.
47. Mulvey MA, Lopez-Boado YS, Wilson CL et al. Induction and evasion of host defenses by type 1-piliated uropathogenic *Escherichia coli*. Science 1998; 282: 1494–7.
48. Veranic P, Jezernik K. The response of junctional complexes to induced desquamation in mouse bladder urothelium. Biol Cell 2000; 92: 105–13.
49. Chai TC, Keay S. New theories in interstitial cystitis. Nature Clin Pract Urol 2004; 1: 85–9.
50. Keay SK, Szekely Z, Conrads TP et al. An antiproliferative factor from interstitial cystitis patients is a frizzled 8 protein-related sialoglycopeptide. Proc Natl Acad Sci USA 2004; 101: 11803–8.
51. Conrads TP, Tocci GM, Hood BL et al. CKAP64/p63 is a receptor for the Frizzled-8 protein-related antiproliferative factor from interstitial cystitis patients. J Biol Chem 2006; 281: 37836–43.
52. Zhang C-O, Wang J-Y, Koch KR, Keay S. Regulation of tight junction proteins and bladder epithelial paracellular permeability by an antiproliferative factor from interstiitial cystitis patients. J Urol 2005; 174: 2382–7.
53. Hu P, Deng F-M, Liang F-X et al. Ablation of uroplakin III gene results in small urothelial plaques, urothelial leakage, and vesicoureteral reflux. J Cell Biol 2000; 151: 961–71.
54. Kong XT, Deng FM, Hu P et al. Roles of uroplakins in plaque formation, umbrella cell enlargement, and urinary tract diseases. J Cell Biol 2004; 167: 1195–204.
55. Dillon MJ, Goonasekara CD. Reflux nephropathy. J Am Soc Nephrol 1998; 9: 2377–83.
56. Giltay JC, van de Meerakker J, van Amstel HK, de Jong TP. No pathogenic mutations in the uroplakin III gene of 25 patients with primary vesicoureteral reflux. J Urol 2004; 171: 931–2.
57. Kelly H, Ennis S, Yoneda A et al. Uroplakin III is not a major candidate gene for primary vesicoureteral reflux. Eur J Human Gen 2005; 13: 500–2.
58. Jenkins D, Bitner-Blindzicz M, Malcolm S et al. De novo uroplakin IIIa heterozygous mutations cause human renal dysplasia leading to severe kidney failure. J Am Soc Nephrol 2005; 16: 2141–9.
59. Schönfelder E-M, Knüppel T, Tasic V et al. Mutations in uroplakin IIIA are a rare cause of renal hypodysplasia in humans. Am J Kidney Dis 2006; 47: 1004–12.
60. Sakakibara K, Sato K-i, Yoshino K-i et al. Molecular identification and characterization of *Xenopus* egg uroplakin III, and egg raft-associated transmembrane protein that is tyrosine-phosphorylated upon fertilization. J Biol Chem 2005; 280: 15029–37.
61. Hasan AKMM, Ou Z, Sakakibara K et al. Characterization of *Xenopus* egg membrane microdomains containing uroplakin Ib/III complex: roles of their molecular interactions for subcellular localization and signal transduction. Genes Cells 2007; 12: 251–67.
62. Hasan AKMM, Sato K-i, Sakakibara K et al. Uroplakin III, a novel Src substrate in *Xenopus* egg rafts, is a target for sperm protease essential for fertilization. Dev Biol 2005; 286: 483–92.
63. Truschel ST, Wang E, Ruiz WG et al. Stretch-regulated exocytosis/endocytosis in bladder umbrella cells. Mol Biol Cell 2002; 13: 830–46.
64. Wang E, Truschel ST, Apodaca G. Analysis of hydrostatic pressure-induced changes in umbrella cell surface area. Methods 2003; 30: 207–17.
65. Birder LA. More than just a barrier: urothelium as a drug target for urinary bladder pain. Am J Physiol 2005; 289: F489–95.
66. Tempest HV, Dixon AK, Turner WH et al. $P2X_2$ and $P2X_3$ receptor expression in human bladder urothelium and changes in interstitial cystitis. BUJ Int 2004; 93: 1344–8.
67. Birder LA, Barrick SR, Roppolo JR et al. Feline interstitial cystitis results in mechanical hypersensitivity and altered ATP release from bladder urothelium. Am J Physiol 2003; 285: F423–9.
68. Sun Y, Chai TC. Up-regulation of $P2X_3$ receptor during stretch of bladder urothelial cells from patients with interstitial cystitis. J Urol 2004; 171: 448–52.
69. Birder LA, Ruan HZ, Chopra B et al. Alterations in P2X and P2Y purinergic receptor expression in urinary bladder from normal cats and cats with interstitial cystitis. Am J Physiol 2004; 287: F1084–91.
70. Sun Y, Keay S, DeDeyne P, Chai TC. Augmented stretch activated adenosine triphosphate release from bladder uroepithelial cells in patients with interstititial cystitis. J Urol 2001; 166: 1951–6.
71. Min G, Stolz M, Zhou G et al. Localization of uroplakin Ia, the urothelial receptor for bacterial adhesin FimH, on the six inner

domains of the 16 nm urothelial plaque particle. J Mol Biol 2002; 317: 697–706.

72. Kau AL, Hunstad DA, Hultgren SJ. Interaction of uropathogenic *Escherichia coli* with host uroepithelium. Curr Opin Microbiol 2005; 8: 54–9.
73. Anderson GG, Palermo JJ, Schilling JD et al. Intracellular bacterial biofilm-like pods in urinary tract infections. Science 2003; 301: 105–7.
74. Gundelfinger ED, Kessels MM, Qualmann B. Temporal and spatial coordination of exocytosis and endocytosis. Nat Rev Mol Cell Biol 2003; 4: 127–39.
75. Hicks R. The function of the Golgi complex in transitional epithelium. J Cell Biol 1966; 30: 623–44.
76. Chang A, Hammond T, Sun T, Zeidel M. Permeability properties of the mammalian bladder apical membrane. Am J Physiol 1994; 267: C1483–92.
77. Lewis S, de Moura J. Incorporation of cytoplasmic vesicles into apical membrane of mammalian urinary bladder epithelium. Nature 1982; 297: 685–8.
78. Amano O, Kataoka S, Yamamoto T. Turnover of asymmetric unit membranes in the transitional epithelial superficial cells of the rat urinary bladder. Anat Rec 1991; 229: 9–15.
79. Sarikas S, Chlapowski F. Effect of ATP inhibitors on the translocation of luminal membrane between cytoplasm and cell surface of transitional epithelial cells during the expansion-contraction cycle of the rat urinary bladder. Cell Tiss Res 1986; 246: 109–17.
80. Sarikas SN, Chlapowski F. The effect of thioglycolate on intermediate filaments and membrane translocation in rat urothelium during the expansion-contraction cycle. Cell Tiss Res 1989; 258: 393–401.
81. Deng F-M, Ding M, Lavker RM, Sun TT. Urothelial function reconsidered: a role in urinary protein secretion. Proc Natl Acad Sci USA 2001; 98: 154–9.
82. Zerial M, McBride H. Rab proteins as membrane organizers, Nature Rev Mol Cell Biol 2001; 2: 107–17.
83. Chen Y, Samaraweera P, Sun TT, Kreibich G, Orlow SJ. Rab27b association with melanosomes: dominant negative mutants disrupt melanosomal movement. J Invest Dermatol 2002; 118: 933–40.
84. Seabra MC, Mules EH, Hume AN. Rab GTPases, intracellular traffic and disease. Trends Mol Med 2002; 8: 23–30
85. Lewis S, de Moura J. Apical membrane area of rabbit urinary bladder increases by fusion of intracellular vesicle: an electrophysiological study. J Membr Biol 1984; 82: 123–36.
86. Knight GE, Bodin P, de Groat WC, Burnstock G. ATP is released from guinea pig ureter epithelium on distention. Am J Physiol 2002; 282: F281–8.
87. Ferguson DR, Kennedy I, Burton TJ. ATP is released from rabbit urinary bladder epithelial cells by hydrostatic pressure changes – a possible sensory mechanism? J Physiol (Lond) 1997; 505(Pt 2): 503–11.
88. Vlaskovska M, Kasakov L, Rong W et al. P2X3 knock-out mice reveal a major sensory role for urothelially released ATP. J Neurosci 2001; 21: 5670–7.
89. Lewis SA, Lewis JR. Kinetics of urothelial ATP release. Am J Physiol 2006; 291: F332–40.
90. Cockayne DA, Hamilton SG, Zhu Q-M et al. Urinary bladder hyporeflexia and reduced pain-related behaviour in $P2X_3$-deficient mice. Nature 2000; 407: 1011–15.
91. Wang ECY, Lee J-M, Ruiz WG et al. ATP and purinergic receptor-dependent membrane traffic in bladder umbrella cells. J Clin Invest 2005; 115: 2412–22.
92. Birder LA, Nakamura Y, Kiss S et al. Altered urinary bladder function in mice lacking the vanilloid receptor TRPV1. Nature Neurosci 2002; 5: 856–60.
93. Elneil S, Skepper JN, Kidd EJ, Williamson JG, Ferguson DR. Distribution of $P2X_1$ and $P2X_3$ receptors in the rat and human urinary bladder. Pharmacology 2001; 63: 120–8.
94. Lee HY, Bardini M, Burnstock G. Distribution of P2X receptors in the urinary bladder and the ureter of the rat. J Urol 2000; 163: 2002–7.
95. Ferguson DR. Urothelial function. BJU Int 1999; 84: 235–42.
96. Fredholm BB, Ijzerman AP, Jacobson KA, Klotz K-N, Linden J. International union of pharmacology. XXV. Nomenclature and classification of adenosine receptors. Pharmacol Rev 2001; 53: 527–52.
97. Jacobson KA, Gao Z-G. Adenosine receptors as therapeutic targets. Nature Rev Drug Discov 2006; 5: 247–64.
98. Yu W, Zacharia LC, Jackson EK, Apodaca G. Adenosine receptor expression and function in bladder uroepithelium. Am J Physiol 2006; 291: C254–65.
99. Cheng J, Huang H, Zhang ZT et al. Overexpression of epidermal growth factor receptor in urothelium elicits urothelial hyperplasia and promotes bladder tumor growth. Cancer Res 2002; 62: 4157–63.
100. Baskin LS, Sutherland RS, Thomson AA, Hayward SW, Cunha GR. Growth factors and receptors in bladder development and obstruction. Lab Invest 1996; 75: 157–66.
101. Bindels EM, van der Kwast TH, Izadifar V, Chopin DK, de Boer WI. Functions of epidermal growth factor-like growth factors during human urothelial reepithelialization in vitro and the role of erbB2. Urol Res 2002; 30: 240–7.
102. Balestreire EM, Apodaca G. Apical EGF receptor signaling: regulation of stretch-dependent exocytosis in bladder umbrella cells. Mol Biol Cell 2007; 18: 1312–23.
103. Daub H, Weiss FU, Wallasch C, Ullrich A. Role of transactivation of the EGF receptor in signalling by G-protein-coupled receptors. Nature 1996; 379: 557–60.
104. Birder LA, Kanai AJ, de Groat WC et al. Vanilloid receptor expression suggests a sensory role for urinary bladder epithelial cells. Proc Natl Acad Sci USA 2001; 98: 13396–401.
105. Dickson A, Avelino A, Cruz F, Ribeiro-da-Silva A. Peptidergic sensory and parasympathetic fiber sprouting in the mucosa of the rat urinary bladder in a chronic model of cyclophosphamide-induced cystitis. Neuroscience 2006; 141: 1633–47.
106. Jen PY, Dixon JS, Gosling JA. Immunohistochemical localization of neuromarkers and neuropeptides in human fetal and neonatal urinary bladder. Br J Pharmacol 1995; 75: 230–5.
107. Brady CM, Apostolidis AN, Harper M et al. Parallel changes in bladder suburothelial vanilloid receptor TRPV1 and pan-neuronal marker PGP9.5 immunoreactivity in patients with neurogenic detrusor overactivity after intravesical resiniferatoxin treatment. BJU Int 2004; 93: 770–6.
108. Gillespie JI, Markerink-van Ittersum M, de Vente J. Sensory collaterals, intramural ganglia and motor nerves in the guinea-pig bladder: evidence for intramural neural circuits. Cell Tissue Res 2006; 235: 33–45.
109. Ruan HZ, Birder LA, Xiang Z et al. Expression of P2X and P2Y receptors in the intramural parasympathetic ganglia of the cat urinary bladder. Am J Physiol 2006; 290: F1143–52.
110. Ost D, Roskams T, Van der Aa F, De Ridder D. Topography of the vanilloid receptor in the human bladder: more than just the nerve fibers. J Urol 2002; 168: 293–7.
111. Sui GP, Wu C, Fry CH. Electrical characteristics of suburothelial cells isolated from the human bladder. J Urol 2004; 171: 938–43.
112. Brading AF, McCloskey KD. Mechanisms of disease: specialized interstitial cells of the urothelium: an assessment of current knowledge. Nat Clin Pract Urol 2005; 2: 546–54.
113. Birder LA, Apodaca G, de Groat WC, Kanai AJ. Adrenergic and capsaicin-evoked nitric oxide release from urothelium and afferent nerves in urinary bladder. Am J Physiol 1998; 275: F226–9.
114. Birder LA, Nealen ML, Kiss S et al. Beta-adrenoceptor agonists stimulate endothelial nitric oxide synthase in rat urinary bladder urothelial cells. J Neurosci 2002; 22: 8063–70.
115. Burnstock G. Purine-mediated signaling in pain and visceral perception. Trends Pharmacol Sci 2001; 22: 182–8.

116. Chess-Williams R. Muscarinic receptors of the urinary bladder: detrusor, urothelial and prejunctional. Auton Autocoid Pharmacol 2002; 22: 133–45.
117. Chopra B, Barrick SR, Meyers S et al. Expression and function of bradykinin B1 and B2 receptors in normal and inflamed rat urinary bladder urothelium. J Physiol 2005; 562: 859–71.
118. Beckel JM, Kanai A, Lee SJ, de Groat WC, Birder LA. Expression of functional nicotinic acetylcholine receptors in rat bladder epithelial cells. Am J Physiol 2006; 290: F103–10.
119. Wolf-Johnston AS, Buffington CA, Roppolo JR et al. Increased NGF expression in urinary bladder and sensory neurons from cats with feline interstitial cystitis. Soc Neurosci Abstr 2003; 608: 4.
120. Ossovskaya VS, Bunnett NW. Protease-activated receptors: contribution to physiology and disease. Physiol Rev 2005; 84: 579–621.
121. Nilius B, Owsianik G, Voets T, Peters JA. Transient receptor potential cation channels in disease. Physiol Rev 2007; 87: 165–217.
122. Birder LA, Wolf-Johnston A, Griffiths D, Resnick NM. Role of urothelial nerve growth factor in human bladder function. Neurourol Urodyn 2007; 26: 405–9.
123. Hanna-Mitchell AT, Beckel JM, Barbadora S et al. Non-neuronal acetylcholine and the urothelium. Life Sci 2007; 80: 2298–302.
124. Cockayne DA, Dunn PM, Zhong Y et al. P2X2 knockout mice and P2X2/P2X4 double knockout mice reveal a role for the P2X2 receptor subunit in mediating multiple sensory effects of ATP. J Physiol 2005; 567: 621–39.
125. Brady CM, Apostolidis A, Yiangou Y et al. P2X3-immunoreactive nerve fibres in neurogenic detrusor overactivity and the effect of intravesical resiniferatoxin. Eur Urol 2004; 46: 247–53.
126. Apostolidis A, Popat R, Yiangou Y et al. Decreased sensory receptors P2X3 and TRPV1 in suburothelial nerve fibers following intradetrusor injections of botulinum toxin for human detrusor overactivity. J Urol 2005; 174: 977–82.
127. Khera M, Somogyi GT, Kiss S, Boone TB, Smith CP. Botulinum toxin A inhibits ATP release from bladder urothelium after chronic spinal cord injury. Neurochem Int 2005; 45: 987–93.
128. Smith CP, Vemulkonda VM, Kiss S, Boone TB, Somogyi GT. Enhanced ATP release from bladder urothelium during chronic inflammation: effect of botulinum toxin A. Neurochem Int 2005; 47: 291–7.
129. Tominaga M, Wada M, Masu M. Potentiation of capsaicin receptor activity by metabotropic ATP receptors as a possible mechanism for ATP-evoked pain and hypersensitivity. Proc Natl Acad Sci 2001; 98: 6951–6.
130. Sculptoreanu A, de Groat WC, Buffington CA, Birder LA. Protein kinase C contributes to abnormal capsaicin responses in DRG neurons from cats with feline interstitial cystitis. Neurosci Lett 2005; 381: 42–6.
131. Hicks GA. TRP channels as therapeutic targets: hot property, or time to cool down? Neurogastroenterol Motil 2006; 18: 590–4.
132. Levine JD, Alessandri-Haber N. TRP channels: targets for the relief of pain. Biochimi Biophys Acta 2007; 1772: 989–1003.
133. Caterina MJ, Schumacher MA, Tominaga M et al. The capsaicin receptor: a heat-activated ion channel in pain pathway. Nature 1997; 89: 816–24.
134. Hwang SW, Cho H, Kwak J et al. Direct activation of capsaicin receptors by products of lipoxygenases: endogenous capsaicin-like substances. Proc Natl Acad Sci 2000; 97: 6155–60.
135. Szallasi A, Blumberg PM. Vanilloid (capsaicin) receptors and mechanisms. Pharmacol Rev 1999; 51: 150–221.
136. Maggi CA. The dual sensory and efferent functions of the capsaicin-sensitive primary sensory neurons in the urinary bladder and urethra. In: Maggi CA, ed. The Autonomic Nervous System, Vol. 3. London: Harwood, 1993: 383–422.
137. Dasgupta P, Fowler CJ. Chillies from antiquity to urology. Br J Urol 1997; 80: 845–52.
138. Szallasi A, Conte B, Goso C, Blumberg PM, Manzini S. Characterization of a peripheral vanilloid (capsaicin) receptor in the rat urinary bladder. Life Sci 1993; 52: PL221–6.
139. Maggi CA, Barbanti G, Santicioli P et al. Cystometric evidence that capsaicin-sensitive nerves modulate the afferent branch of micturition reflex in humans. J Urol 1989; 142: 150–4.
140. Maggi CA. The dual function of capsaicin-sensitive sensory nerves in the bladder and urethra. Ciba Found Symp 1990; 151: 77–83.
141. Avelino A, Cruz C, Nagy I, Cruz F. Vanilloid receptor 1 expression in the rat urinary tract. Neuroscience 2002; 109: 787–97.
142. Silva C, Charrua A, Dinis P, Cruz F. TRPV1 knockout mice do not develop bladder overactivity during acute chemical bladder inflammation. Soc Neurosci Abstr 2004; 288: 16.
143. Szallasi A, Cruz F, Geppetti P. TRPV1: a therapeutic target for novel analgesic drugs? Trends Molec Med 2006; 12: 545–54.
144. Apostolidis A, Brady CM, Yiangou Y et al. Capsaicin receptor TRPV1 in urothelium of neurogenic human bladders and effect of intravesical resiniferatoxin. Urology 2005; 65: 400–5.
145. Chancellor MB, de Groat WC. Intravesical capsaicin and resiniferatoxin therapy: spicing up the ways to treat the overactive bladder. J Urol 1999; 162: 3–11.
146. Lazzeri M, Spinelli M, Zanollo A, Turini D. Intravesical vanilloids and neurogenic incontinence: 10 years experience. Urol Int 2004; 72: 145–9.
147. Payne CK, Mosbaugh PG, Forrest JB. Intravesical resiniferatoxin for the treatment of interstitial cystitis: a randomized, double-blind, placebo controlled trial. J Urol 2005; 173: 1590–4.
148. Cruz F, Guimaraes M, Silva C et al. Desensitization of bladder sensory fibers by intravesical capsaicin has long lasting clinical and urodynamic effects in patients with hyperactive or hypersensitive bladder dysfunction. J Urol 1997; 157: 585–9.
149. de Seze M, Wiart L, Joseph PA et al. Capsaicin and neurogenic detrusor hyperreflexia, a double blind placebo controlled study in 20 patients with spinal cord lesions. Neurourol Urodyn 1998; 17: 513–23.
150. Dinis P, Silva J, Ribeiro MJ et al. Bladder C-fiber desensitization induces a long-lasting improvement of BPH-associated storage. LUTS: a pilot study. Eur Urol 2004; 46: 88–93.
151. Fowler CJ, Jewkes D, McDonald WI, Lynn B, de Groat WC. Intravesical capsaicin for neurogenic bladder dysfunction. Lancet 1992; 339: 1239.
152. Geirsson G, Fall M, Sullivan L. Clinical and urodynamic effects of intravesical capsaicin treatment in patients with chronic traumatic spinal detrusor hyperreflexia. J Urol 1995; 154: 1825–9.
153. Apostolidis A, Gonzales GE, Fowler CJ. Effect of intravesical resiniferatoxin (RTX) on lower urinary tract symptoms, urodynamic parameters, and quality of life of patients with urodynamic increased bladder sensation. Eur Urol 2006; 50: 1299–305.
154. Mukerji G, Yiangou Y, Agarwal SK, Anand P. Transient receptor potential vanilloid receptor subtype 1 in painful bladder syndrome and its correlation with pain. J Urol 2006; 176: 797–801.
155. Kalsi V, Fowler CJ. Therapy insight: bladder dysfunction associated with multiple sclerosis. Nat Clin Prac Urol 2005; 2: 492–501.
156. Liedtke W. TRPV4 plays an evolutionary conserved role in the transduction of osmotic and mechanical stimuli in live animals. Pflugers Arch 2005; 451: 176–80.
157. Gevaert T, Vriens J, Everaerts W, Nilius B, De Ridder D. TRPV4 is localized on urothelium: does it play a role in afferent bladder signaling? Eur Urol Suppl 2007; 6: 38.
158. Barrick S, Lee H, Caterina M et al. Expression and function of TRPV4 in urinary bladder urothelium. Soc Neurosci Abstr 2003; 608: 6.
159. Alessandri-Haber N, Dina OA, Joseph EK, Reichling D, Levine JD. A transient receptor potential vanilloid 4-dependent mechanism of hyperalgesia is engaged by concerted action of inflammatory mediators. J Neurosci 2006; 26: 3864–74.
160. Cheng C-L, Chai CY, de Groat WC. Detrusor-sphincter dyssynergia induced by cold stimulation of the urinary bladder of rats. Am J Physiol 1997; 41: R1271–82.

161. Wein AJ. Neuromuscular dysfunction of the lower urinary tract. In: Walsh PC, Retik AB, Stamey TA, Vaughn ED, eds. Campbell's Urology. Saunders, Philadelphia, 1992: 573–642.
162. Chai TC, Gray J, Steers W. The incidence of a positive ice water test in bladder outlet obstructed patients: evidence for bladder neural plasticity. J Urol 1998; 160: 34–8.
163. Gotoh M, Yoshikawa Y, Kondo AS et al. Positive bladder cooling reflex in patients with bladder outlet obstruction due to benign prostatic hyperplasia. World J Urol 1999; 17: 126–30.
164. Hirayama A, Fujimoto K, Matumoto Y, Ozono S, Hirao Y. Positive response to ice water test associated with high-grade bladder outlet obstruction in patients with benign prostatic hyperplasia. Urology 2003; 62: 909–13.
165. Peier AM, Moqrich A, Hergarden AC et al. A TRP channel that senses cold stimuli and menthol. Cell 2002; 108: 705–15.
166. Jiang CH, Mazieres L, Lindstrom S. Cold and menthol-sensitive C afferents of cat urinary bladder. J Physiol 2002; 543: 211–20.
167. Geirsson G, Lindstrom S, Fall M. The bladder cooling reflex and the use of cooling as stimulus to the lower urinary tract. J Urol 1999; 162: 1890–6.
168. Stein RJ, Santos S, Nagatomi J et al. Cool (TRPM8) and hot (TRPV1) receptors in the bladder and male genital tract. J Urol 2004; 172: 1175–8.
169. Barrick S, Chopra B, Caterina M et al. Expression and function of the cold channels in urinary bladder urothelium: TRPM8 and TRPA1. 24th Annual American Pain Society Meeting, Banff, Canada, 2005.
170. Andrade EL, Ferreira J, Andre E, Calixto J. Contractile mechanisms coupled to TRPA1 receptor activation in rat urinary bladder. Biochem Pharmacol 2006; 72: 104–14.
171. Hawthorn MH, Chapple CR, Cock M, Chess-Williams R. Urothelium-derived inhibitory factor(s) influences on detrusor muscle contractility in vitro. Br J Pharmacol 2000; 129: 416–9.
172. Templeman L, Chapple CR. Chess-Williams R. Urothelium derived inhibitory factor and cross-talk among receptors in the trigone of the bladder of the pig. J Urol 202; 167: 742–5.
173. De Groat WC. The urothelium in overactive bladder: passive bystander or active participant? Urology 2004; 64: 7–11.
174. Beckel JM, Barrick SR, Keast JR et al. Expression and function of urothelial muscarinic receptors and interactions with bladder nerves. Soc Neurosci Abstr 2004; 846: 23.
175. Birder LA. Role of the bladder epithelium in urinary bladder dysfunction after spinal cord injury. In: Weaver LC, Polosa C, eds. Autonomic Dysfunction after Spinal Cord Injury: The Problems and Underlying Mechanisms. Progress in Brain Research. Amsterdam: Holland: Elsevier, 2004.
176. Tong YC, Cheng JT, Hsu CT. Alterations of M(2)-muscarinic receptor protein and mRNA expression in the urothelium and muscle layer of the streptozotocin-induced diabetic rat urinary bladder. Neurosci Lett 2006; 406: 216–21.
177. Mansfield KJ, Liu L, Mitchelson FJ et al. Muscarinic receptor subtypes in human bladder detrusor and mucosa, studied by radioligand binding and quantitative competitive RT-PCR: changes in ageing. Br J Pharmacol 2005; 144: 1089–99.
178. Braverman AS, Lebed B, Linder M, Ruggieri MR. M2 mediated contractions of human bladder from organ donors is associated with an increase in urothelial muscarinic receptors. Neurourol Urodyn 2007; 26: 63–70.
179. Yoshida M, Inadome A, Maeda Y et al. Non-neuronal cholinergic system in human bladder urothelium. Urology 2006; 67: 425–30.
180. Lips KS, Wunsch J, Zarghooni S et al. Acetylcholine and molecular components of its synthesis and release machinery in the urothelium. Eur Urol 2007; 51: 1047–53.
181. Kim YT, Yoshimura N, Masuda H, De Miguel F, Chancellor MB. Antimuscarinic agents exhibit local inhibitory effects on muscarinic receptors in bladder afferent pathways. Urology 2004; 65: 238–42.
182. de Groat WC. Integrative control of the lower urinary tract: preclinical perspective. Br J Pharmacol 2006; 147: S25–40.
183. Cheng CL, Liu JC, Chang SY, Ma CP, de Groat WC. Effect of capsaicin on the micturition reflex in normal and chronic spinal cord-injured cats. Am J Physiol 1999; 277: R786–94.
184. Yoshida M, Miyamae K, Iwashita H, Otani M, Inadome A. Management of detrusor dysfunction in the elderly: changes in acetylcholine and adenosine triphosphate release during aging. Urology 2004; 63: 17–23.
185. Proskocil BJ, Sekhon SS, Jia Y et al. Acetylcholine is an autocrine or paracrine hormone synthesized and secreted by airway bronchial epithelial cells. Endocrinol 2004; 145: 2498–506.
186. Tiwari A, Naruganahalli KS. Current and emerging investigational medical therapies for the treatment of overactive bladder. Expert Opin Investig Drugs 2006; 15: 1017–37.
187. Chancellor MB. Urgency, botulinum toxin and how botulinum toxin can help urgency. J Urol 2005; 174: 818.
188. Toft BR, Nordling J. Recent developments of intravesical therapy of painful bladder syndrome/interstitial cystitis: a review. Current Opin Urol 2006; 16: 268–72.
189. Atiemo H, Wynes J, Chuo J et al. Effect of botulinum toxin on detrusor overactivity induced by intravesical adenosine triphosphate and capsaicin in a rat model. Urology 2005; 65: 622–6.
190. Toh KL, Ng CK. Urodynamic studies in the evaluation of young men presenting with lower urinary tract symptoms. Int J Urol 2006; 13: 520–3.
191. Yassin A, Saad F, Hoesl CE et al. Alpha-adrenoceptors are a common denominator in the pathophysiology of erectile function and BPH/LUTS – implications for clinical practice. Andrologia 2006; 38: 1–12.
192. Ishihama H, Momota Y, Yanase H et al. Activation of alpha1D adrenergic receptors in the rat urothelium facilitates the micturition reflex. J Urol 2006; 175: 358–64.
193. Andersson KE, Persson K. Nitric oxide synthase and the lower urinary tract: possible implications for physiology and pathophysiology. Scand J Urol Nephrol Suppl 1995; 175: 43–53.
194. Pandita RK, Mizusawa H, Andersson KE. Intravesical oxyhemoglobin initiates bladder overactivity in conscious, normal rats. J Urol 2000; 164: 545–50.
195. de Groat WC, Kruse MN, Vizzard MA et al. Modification of urinary bladder function after spinal cord injury. Adv Neurol 1997; 72: 347–64.
196. Vizzard MA. Neurochemical plasticity and the role of neurotrophic factors in the bladder reflex pathways after spinal cord injury. Prog Br Res 2006; 152: 97–115.
197. Birder LA, Wolf-Johnston A, Buffington CA et al. Altered inducible nitric oxide synthase expression and nitric oxide production in the bladder of cats with feline interstitial cystitis. J Urol 2005; 172: 625–9.
198. Kolios G, Valata V, Ward SG. Nitric oxide in inflammatory bowel disease: a universal messenger in an unsolved puzzle. Immunology 2004; 113: 427–37.
199. Yoshimura N, Seki S, de Groat WC. Nitric oxide modulates Ca^{2+} channels in dorsal root ganglion neurons innervating rat urinary bladder. J Neurophysiol 2001; 86: 304–11.
200. Ozawa H, Chancellor MB, Jung SY et al. Effect of intravesical nitric oxide therapy on cyclophosphamide-induced cystitis, J Urol 1999; 162: 2211–16.
201. Korkmaz A, Oter S, Sadir S et al. Peroxynitrite may be involved in bladder damage caused by cyclophosphamide in rats. J Urol 2005; 173: 1793–6.
202. Hosseini A, Ehren I, Wiklund NP. Nitric oxide as objective marker for evaluation of treatment response in patients with classic interstitial cystitis. J Urol 2004; 172: 2261–5.

4

Physiology of the smooth muscles of the bladder and urethra

Marcus J Drake and William H Turner

Introduction

The lower urinary tract is a complex entity, whose function remains incompletely understood. The muscles of the bladder and urethra are crucial in normal urinary function, and smooth muscle dysfunction is important in the pathophysiology of storage and voiding disorders.[1] In recent decades there has been a substantial increase in the knowledge base of LUT function, from the whole organ to the molecular level, acquired through the application of increasingly sophisticated experimental tools (reviewed in reference 1). This chapter outlines salient points in current understanding of detrusor and urethral smooth muscle physiology.

Molecular cell biology of the detrusor

The biologic behavior of a cell is determined by the proteins present in the cellular membrane, particularly the receptors and the ion channels, along with the components of the intracellular second messenger systems.

Receptors

Cellular response to hormones and neurotransmitters is determined by binding of ligands to specific membrane-bound receptors. This can result in either direct modification of ionic permeability of cell membranes (ionotropic action), or synthesis of intermediary substances known as second messengers (metabotropic action). Many different receptor types have been identified, reflecting the diverse array of endogenous ligands.

Adrenergic receptors

Adrenergic receptors mediate responses to the circulating hormone epinephrine and the neurotransmitter norepinephrine. They are classified as α-adrenoceptors or β-adrenoceptors, with further subclassification on the basis of structure and response to pharmacologic agonists and antagonists into α_1 (α_{1A-D} and α_{1L}), α_2 (α_{2A-C}), and β_{1-3}. Beta-adrenoceptors are distributed throughout the urethra and bladder,[2–4] and induce relaxation in precontracted detrusor muscle by complex mechanisms.[5] Subtype-selective ligand studies show the presence of β_2 and β_3 receptors.[6] The latter elicit relaxation of human detrusor strips and reduce spontaneous activity,[7] and have been proposed as a possible therapeutic target in detrusor overactivity.

Cholinergic receptors

Tissue response to the neurotransmitter acetylcholine is mediated by muscarinic and nicotinic receptors. Nicotinic receptors are predominantly in the central nervous system, peripheral ganglia of the autonomic nervous system, and on skeletal muscle, but functional non-neuronal nicotinic receptors are present in the lower urinary tract.[8] Muscarinic receptors are classified on the basis of specific response to pharmacologic agents (M_{1-5}) and molecular structure (m_{1-5}).[9] M_3 receptors predominate on receptor-binding studies, although a 3:1 predominance of m_2 over m_3 has been reported using subtype-specific immunoprecipitation.[10] Functionally, the M_3 is the predominant mediator of acetylcholine response in the bladder, as indicated by observations in numerous situations including specific antagonists and receptor knockout mouse models.[11,12] The role of the M_2 receptor is unclear. In pathologic circumstances, a change in the receptor subtype mediating contraction more towards the M_2 receptor is apparent, which appears to be due to detrusor hypertrophy.[13] With aging, fewer muscarinic receptors may be expressed, but the relative preponderance of M_2 and M_3 receptors is largely unaltered.[14]

The response to cholinergic stimulation in the isolated whole organ is more complex than might be anticipated from observations made on isolated strips of muscle. Several components of the intravesical pressure change in response to cholinergic stimulation have been described.[15–17] An initial tonic peak response increases with bladder distention and is inhibited by M_2 and M_3 muscarinic receptor antagonists; this settles to a steady-state response which is not affected by bladder volume. In addition, phasic contractions are superimposed on the steady-state activity. The phasic contractions are not an obvious feature at low bladder volume, but become disproportionately apparent at high volumes. Indeed the fluid volume which elicits a prominent phasic component of the cholinergic response can be used to define bladder capacity, a concept which is otherwise difficult to standardize in the isolated organ.[18]

Purinergic receptors

Purinoceptors are present in the lower urinary tract, the agonists for which are extracellular adenosine, adenosine diphosphate (ADP), and adenosine triphosphate (ATP). The purinoceptors are classified as P_1 or P_2; they show differing affinity for the endogenous agonists. P_1 is further subclassified into A_1 and A_{2A-2B}, and P_2 into P_{2t}, P_{2u}, and P_{2x-z}. Several subtypes of the P_{2x} receptor are present in rat and human bladder.[19,20] The contractile response of the rat bladder to ATP is mediated mainly through P_{2x}-purinoceptors and A_1-purinergic receptors.[21] The P_{2x1} receptor appears to predominate on smooth muscle cells,[22] but there is considerable plasticity in P_{2x} receptors according to physiologic circumstances.

Other receptors

Histamine H_1 receptors are present on smooth muscle cells.[23,24] Detrusor cells also express the vanilloid receptor VR_1.[25]

Ion channels

The lipid bilayer of the cell membrane is relatively impermeable to the passage of charged ions. The presence of transmembrane protein channels allows ionic transfer into and out of the cytoplasm, the properties of the channels enabling tight control of the intracellular composition and membrane potentials.

Potassium channels

Several types of potassium (K^+) channels are recognized, falling into two main groups: voltage-sensitive channels, and inward rectifying channels, which conduct inward K^+ current much more readily than outward. There is substantial functional overlap between the two groups. Calcium-activated K^+ channels include the SK, BK, and maxi-K^+ channels. K_{ATP} channels are inward rectifying channels whose configuration is determined by the metabolic state of the cell. They are linked to sulfonylurea receptors and are sensitive to the action of glibenclamide. K^+ channel opening drugs, such as cromakalim, probably act by reducing the sensitivity of K^+ channels to inhibition by ATP.

The ion channels present in the bladder are complex (reviewed in reference 26). Currents characteristic of several types of K^+ channel have been identified in detrusor myocytes, including voltage-sensitive delayed rectifier current, Ca^{2+}-activated maxi K^+ channels, SK and BK channels, and glibenclamide-sensitive K^+ channels. K^+ channels appear to be fundamental both in determining the membrane potential and in repolarization following the action potential. K_{ATP} channels strongly influence the membrane potential in the bladder, since activation of only a small proportion of the channels present significantly inhibits action potentials.[27] Potassium channel blocking drugs have varying effects on the membrane potential and they tend to increase spontaneous mechanical activity in isolated detrusor strips. Different K^+ channel blocking drugs affect the action potential in various ways, some blocking after-hyperpolarization, some slowing depolarization. Activation of K^+ channels, in particular the large-conductance calcium-activated K^+ (BK) channels, reduces excitability and contractility of detrusor muscle.[28] BK channels are involved in the β-adrenoceptor agonist-induced relaxation in precontracted detrusor muscle.[5]

Overall, the high sensitivity of BK channels to both intracellular calcium and voltage may make them negative feedback regulators,[29] modulating human detrusor smooth muscle phasic contractility.[30]

Calcium channels

Several types of membrane channels allow the influx of Ca^{2+}, both specific and nonselective, but voltage-operated Ca^{2+} channels appear to predominate in smooth muscle.[31] Voltage-operated Ca^{2+} channels are classified according to the properties of the currents passing through them, comprising L-type (long lasting), T-type (transient), or N-type (neither L nor T).

L-type Ca^{2+} channels are numerous in detrusor muscle, permitting high ion flux rates, which can result in a rapid rise in cytoplasmic Ca^{2+} levels. They only allow current flow in one of three possible channel states (open state), which is strongly regulated by the membrane potential. In guinea pig bladder they are inactivated by a rise in intracellular free Ca^{2+} ions, but also show the unusual property of being switched into a long open state by depolarization, and having two open states, features that may have important implications for contractile function. In detrusor strips from most animals studied, L-type Ca^{2+} channel blockers, such as nifedipine, reduce spontaneous contractile activity. Furthermore, the upstroke of the action potential is produced by current flowing through these channels.

T-type channels are also present in the bladder, which possibly have a role in replenishment of intracellular calcium stores. Activity of these channels may underlie depolarizations that lead to action potentials. They may also couple functionally to SK channels, contributing to the stability of the resting membrane potential in detrusor smooth muscle.[32] Detrusor myocytes from overactive human bladders have a higher T-type current density.[33] T-type Ca^{2+} channel activity increases in partial bladder outlet obstruction.[34] Antibodies affecting the function of this channel have been suggested to underlie alterations in bladder behavior in diabetics.[35]

Nonspecific cation channels

Exogenously-applied ATP elicits large inward currents in dispersed bladder smooth muscle cells from human and pig.[36] P_{2x} channels are ionotropic and, following binding of ATP, they permit Ca^{2+} flux, although Ca^{2+} may only carry 10% of the nonselective cation current.[31] In many smooth muscles, activation of M_2 receptors results in G-protein-mediated, nonselective, depolarizing cation current, facilitated by M_3 receptor-mediated release of Ca^{2+} from intracellular stores.[31] This acetylcholine response is biphasic in some smooth muscles, with a Ca^{2+}-activated inward chloride current preceding a sustained nonselective cation current. Oscillation of inward currents has been observed as a result of exposure to endothelin-1, probably as a consequence of periodic activation of Ca^{2+}-activated chloride channels.[37]

Detrusor cells possess stretch-activated nonselective cation channels, which cause cell membrane depolarization. The degree of depolarization is modulated by secondary activation of Ca^{2+}-activated K^+ channels, which allow potassium to leave the cell.[38] As a result, the cellular response to stretch depends on the rate at which it is applied. Strips of detrusor muscle respond to rapid stretch with a rapid depolarization and increase in action potential frequency, leading to a nonsustained contraction. Slowly-applied stretch does not activate this contractile response, presumably because K^+ channel activation keeps up with opening of the stretch-activated channels, preventing depolarization.

A further conductance mediated by the influx of sodium, with a smaller inward calcium current, has been identified in mouse detrusor cells,[39] while the presence of a sodium-calcium exchanger has also been surmised.[40]

Sodium channels

A family of sodium (Na^+) channels has been cloned and characterized pharmacologically, using Na^+ channel antagonists such as tetrodotoxin (TTX). Although many smooth muscles express Na^+ channels, their physiologic role is uncertain.[41]

Chloride channels

Chloride channels permit passive transfer of Cl^- across the cell membrane and may regulate cell volume and membrane excitability in smooth muscles. The calculated Cl^- equilibrium potential is −35 to −20 mV, while the measured intracellular Cl^- concentration is typically 40–50 mM, indicating that an active transport system contributes to the accumulation of Cl^-.[41] Patch clamp studies have also revealed Ca^{2+}-dependent Cl^- currents in smooth muscle.

Second messenger systems

G-proteins form a vast family of related proteins, each comprising several subunits. The binding of ligands to some cell surface receptors alters the subunit interactions within specific G-protein complexes, the precise nature of the response being determined by the type of G-proteins related to the receptor. The G-proteins in turn activate or inhibit enzymes such as phospholipase C (PLC), adenylate cyclase, or guanylate cyclase, changing the levels of soluble second messengers. Adenylate and guanylate cyclase synthesize cyclic adenosine monophosphate (cAMP) and cyclic guanine monophosphate (cGMP), respectively. PLC cleaves a membrane-bound phospholipid, phosphatidyl inositol diphosphate (PIP_2) into diacylglycerol (DAG) and inositol triphosphate (IP_3). As a consequence, the phosphorylation state of diverse proteins throughout the cell is altered, affecting multiple aspects of cellular function. The effects of the cyclic nucleotides are altered by phosphodiesterases (PDEs).[42] A selective PDE4 inhibitor reduces overactive bladder contractions in rats with bladder outlet obstruction, at doses that have no effect on voiding bladder contractions.[43] Similar effects on phasic activity in human detrusor strips have been described.[44]

The subtypes of muscarinic receptors have differing second messenger effects. M_1, M_3, and M_5 receptors link to the $G_{q/11}$ family of G-proteins, which activate PLC. M_2 and M_4 receptors couple with the $G_{i/o}$ family and influence cAMP levels, along with K^+ and Ca^{2+} channel activity. M_3 receptors mediate contraction by activation of PLC and protein kinase A, whereas the M_2 signal transduction cascade may include activation of rho kinase, protein kinase C (PKC), and possibly further mechanisms yet to be identified.[45, 46] The rho kinase pathways make a greater contribution in the denervated bladder[45,46] and in spontaneously hypertensive rats.[47]

Second messenger effects of α_1-adrenoceptors are mediated by $G_{q/11}$, whereas β-adrenoceptors are linked to a G_s which activates adenylate cyclase.[41] The Ca^{2+} ion can be considered a second messenger, as it forms a complex with the cytoplasmic protein calmodulin, resulting in accelerated breakdown of cAMP and activation of the contractile apparatus. Muscarinic receptor activation induces calcium sensitization in detrusor smooth muscles.[48]

Cellular physiology of the detrusor

Functionally, muscle cells alternate between states of active shortening and quiescence, determined by various stimuli, which serve to impose control over shortening and to maintain cell functionality.

Passive membrane properties and cell coupling

The degree to which the smooth muscle membrane will allow ions to pass between the intracellular and extracellular compartments varies, as the channels through which the ions pass change permeability according to various factors. At rest, the tendency of the ion to move down its concentration gradient is balanced by an electrical membrane potential (equilibrium potential). The overall membrane potential approximates to the membrane potential of the most permeant ion; at rest this is K^+, due to BK channels. Resting membrane potential in detrusor is −40 to −45 mV in the guinea pig and −60 mV in the human.[49–51]

Electrical activity spreads between cells through specialized intercellular connections, characterized by the presence of proteins of the connexin family. Only a very small number of gap junctions is required to achieve effective coupling and a small increase in gap junction density could significantly influence tissue properties. The passive electrical behavior of nerve and smooth muscle cell membranes is quantified using two constants, derived from analysis of the spread of injections of subexcitation threshold current through microelectrodes. The space constant (λ) is an index of the decay of the injected current with distance, whilst the time constant (τ) describes the decay of current spread with time. Large values of λ indicate good intercellular coupling, exemplified by pregnant myometrium or cardiac muscle, while large values of τ indicate resistance to membrane charging. Measurement of current spread in guinea pig detrusor suggests that cells are coupled to their close neighbors, but that the tissue as a whole is poorly coupled,[50,52] and electrical coupling between cells more than 40 μm apart axially only occurs rarely. The detrusor also shows higher tissue impedance than other smooth muscles.[52,53] Furthermore, although double sucrose-gap recordings can be made in some small mammal detrusor strips, the electrical activity is not often resolved into clear spikes, and in the normal pig detrusor the technique does not work, probably because of insufficient electrical coupling. This may explain the technical difficulties encountered during attempts to record electromyogram activity in the bladder.[54]

Poor coupling is consistent with the observation that gap junctions are infrequent in detrusor smooth muscle,[55] though recent evidence has emerged to indicate some communication across gap junctions between detrusor muscle cells in the guinea pig.[56] From a functional point of view, these features match well with the requirements that adjustments in the length of the smooth muscles can take place without the activity spreading to produce synchronous activation of the whole bladder wall. Thus both connexin 43 and connexin 45 are expressed at low levels in normal human detrusor, but the former can be upregulated in patients with urge incontinence.[57]

Active membrane properties

Some smooth muscles show the facility to develop 'action potentials', which are a transient change in the membrane potential as a result of temporary alterations in ionic fluxes across the cell membrane (Figure 4.1).[58] Action potentials in detrusor muscle can be precipitated by various neuromuscular transmitters and by stretch. The phases of the action potential are the result of coordinated action of distinct membrane conductances and have been assessed using patch clamp studies on isolated myocytes from several species. The upstroke results from Ca^{2+} entry through voltage-dependent Ca^{2+} channels, while the repolarization phase is attributed to voltage-dependent K^+ channels and Ca^{2+}-dependent K^+ channels. Subsequently, the cell shows a prolonged after-hyperpolarization during which the membrane potential is more negative than the resting potential.

Cell shortening

Contractile proteins

In both striated and smooth muscle, the contractile apparatus is made up of structural proteins arranged as thick

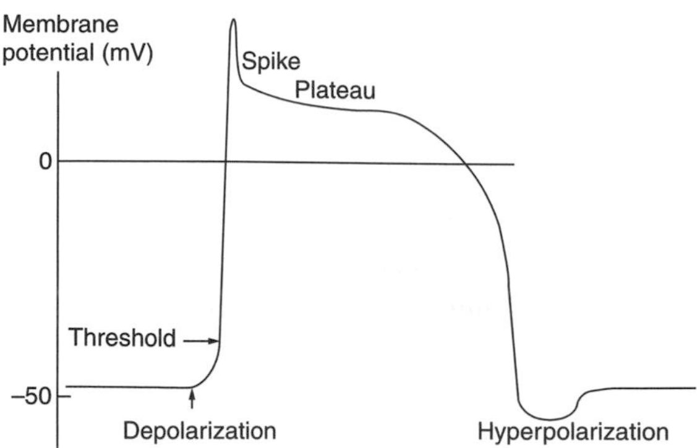

Figure 4.1
Phases of the action potential. A schematic representation of the phases of the action potential in the detrusor muscle cell. From the resting membrane potential, an extrinsic stimulus causes a slight depolarization. If this is sufficient to reach a threshold level, a transient reversal of the cell membrane potential occurs as a result of a rapid increase in the membrane permeability to calcium. This is followed by a plateau phase, before the cell repolarizes due to restoration of potassium as the most permeant ion. For a brief period, the membrane potential may become even more negative, 'after-hyperpolarization', rendering the cell less excitable, as a greater extrinsic stimulus will be required to bring the cell to its threshold potential.

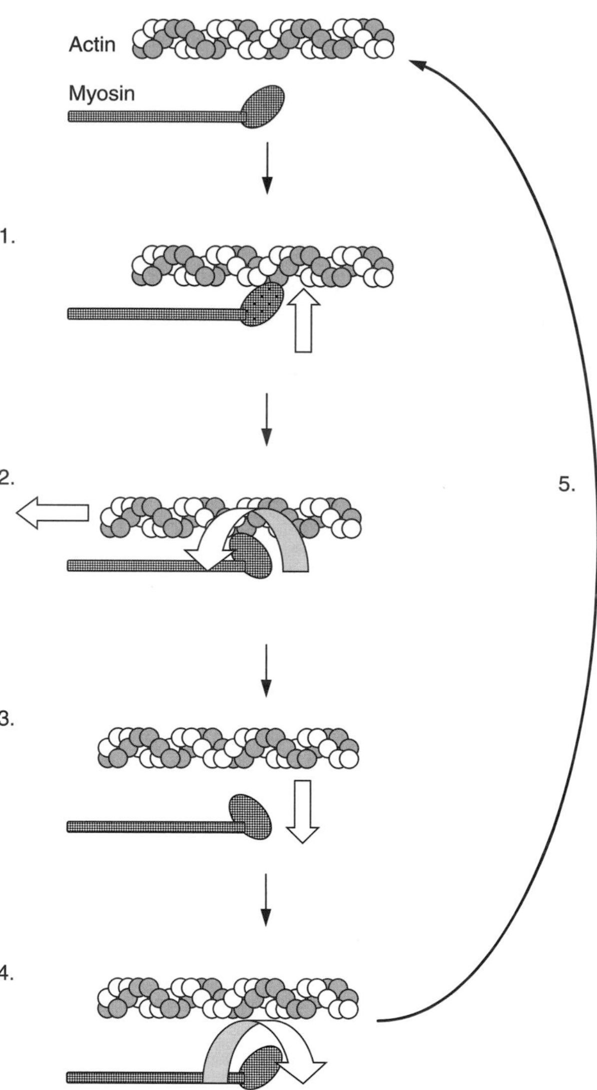

Figure 4.2
The phases in the sliding filament hypothesis of muscle contraction: (1) attachment of the myosin heads to actin filaments; (2) angulation of the attachment within the myosin molecule; (3) release of the binding; (4) straightening of the myosin angulation; and (5) repetition.

(myosin) and thin (actin) filaments. The sliding filament theory of contraction, developed in skeletal muscle, suggests that muscle shortening occurs because overlapping fibers of fixed length (the thick and thin filaments) slide past each other in an energy-consuming process. Figure 4.2 illustrates the phases involved to achieve this. The configuration of the cytoskeleton is such that actin from all parts of the cell is drawn inwards towards the center, resulting in overall cell shortening. The process is powered by hydrolysis of ATP and regulated by the concentration of free calcium in the cytoplasm.

Myosin is the major component of the thick filaments in all tissues, smooth muscle myosin consisting of a heavy chain pair (MHC) and a light chain pair (MLC) (Figure 4.3). It has a globular head formed by folding of the N′-terminus of the MHC pair, while the C′-terminal parts intertwine to form an α-helix, which constitutes the thick filament. Smooth muscle myosin *in vivo* occurs in various isoforms, which influence assembly and function of the contractile apparatus, the types of MHC present in the muscle determining its biomechanical behavior. Two isoforms, SM1 and 2, differing in the C′-terminal portions, are generated by alternative splicing of the mRNA encoded by a single smooth muscle MHC gene.[59] The relative expression of these isoforms is influenced by acute spinal cord injury.[60] Further isoforms are generated by alternative splicing at the 5′-end of the MHC mRNA, determining an insert that encodes seven amino acids in the N′-region, near the ATP-binding site. Noninserted MHC (SM-A) predominates in tonically active muscle, while the majority of MHC is inserted (SM-B) in phasic tissues, such as the bladder and visceral muscle in general.[61] SM-B has higher actin-induced ATPase activity and can move actin faster in an *in vitro* motility assay. MLCs are sited at the head–rod junction of the MHCs. They occur as a pair of 20 kDa chains (MLC20), and a 17 kDa pair (MLC17). The MLC20 is also known as the regulatory light chain because it regulates smooth muscle contraction according to its degree of

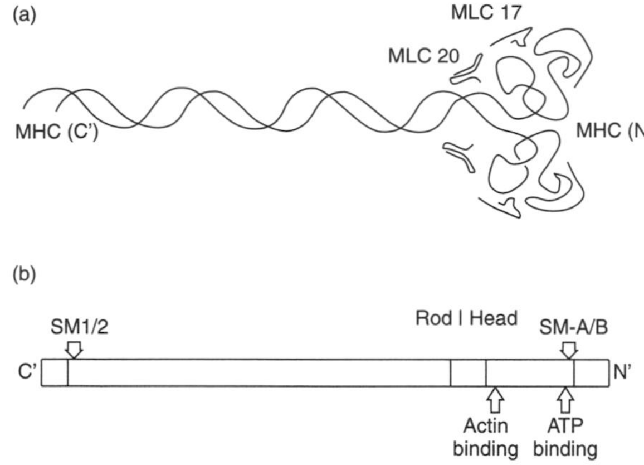

Figure 4.3
Smooth muscle myosin. (a) Schematic drawing of smooth muscle myosin, showing the relationship between the two myosin heavy chain molecules (MHC) and the myosin light chains (MLC 20 and 17). (b) Schematic representation of the MHC, showing regions of actin and ATP binding and sites of isoform variation for SM1/2 and SM-A/B.

phosphorylation. MLC17 extends close to the MHC ATP-binding site and is termed the essential light chain because its removal leads to loss of ATPase activity. MLC isoforms are recognized which can influence shortening velocity in some smooth muscle types.[62,63] Obstruction in the mouse bladder induces increased expression of C-terminal (SM1) and N-terminal (SM-A) myosin heavy chain isoforms.[64]

Regulation of the contractile apparatus

The key event determining activation of smooth muscle cell contractile proteins is a sufficient rise in cytosolic Ca^{2+} concentration. Increased Ca^{2+} leads to the formation of a complex with the cytoplasmic protein calmodulin, resulting in activation of myosin light chain kinase (MLCK). Following phosphorylation of a specific site on the regulatory light chain by MLCK, using ATP as the phosphate donor, crossbridges form between myosin and actin. Angulation in the myosin molecule results in relative movement between the two types of fiber, which is the basis of cellular shortening. Once phosphorylated, repetitive cycles of attachment and angulation continue until MLC20 is dephosphorylated by myosin light chain phosphatase, which is usually bound tightly to myosin. This entire process can be modulated by intracellular factors. For example, MLCK is subject to phosphorylation by various kinases,[65] which influence its affinity for Ca^{2+}–calmodulin. One enzyme that can achieve this is phosphokinase A, which is activated by cAMP.[66] A rho kinase inhibitor suppresses myosin regulatory light chain phosphorylation.[67] The composition of thin filament-associated proteins, particularly tropomyosin, actin, and calponin, changes in bladder hypertrophy due to partial outlet obstruction.[68] The relationship between MLC phosphorylation and force generation is nonlinear.[69]

Two sources of Ca^{2+} can generate the elevation in cytoplasmic levels determining contraction:

1. Release of Ca^{2+} stored intracellularly in the sarcoplasmic reticulum (SR) through pharmacomechanical coupling, mediated by IP_3 and ryanodine receptors. Ryanodine receptors trigger release of Ca^{2+} stores in response to an initial rise in intracellular Ca^{2+}, hence the term 'calcium-induced calcium release' (CICR). IP_3 receptors are also regulated by intracellular Ca^{2+}, with a marked increase in channel opening as the levels start to rise, followed by a reduction in activity at higher levels. Local calcium transients occur in discrete subsarcolemmal hot spots, which subsequently spread to CICR over wider areas, and can be attenuated by uncoupling of voltage-dependent calcium channels from ryanodine receptors in the hot spots.[70] Muscarinic receptor activation appears primarily to work through generation of IP_3, but it can also cause a small degree of direct extracellular Ca^{2+} entry by activating nonselective cation channels and increasing the action potential frequency.
2. Influx of extracellular Ca^{2+} across the surface membrane, associated with altered cell membrane potential, through electromechanical coupling. The depolarization phase of the action potentials is associated with rapid entry of Ca^{2+} into the intracellular compartment, which is further enhanced as a consequence of CICR from intracellular stores.

The central role of Ca^{2+} in smooth muscle contraction is summarized in Figure 4.4.

At this stage, the relative importance of electromechanical and pharmacomechanical coupling, and of intracellular or extracellular Ca^{2+} sources in detrusor contraction, remains unclear[71] and may vary with the magnitude of stimulation. The situation is highly complicated, as several further factors influence the ability of smooth muscle to generate phasic or tonic contraction. Shortening velocity is higher when intracellular Ca^{2+} and phosphorylation are high, while fairly low Ca^{2+} and phosphorylation support high levels of force generation. Myosin light chain dephosphorylation does not necessarily lead to relaxation: myosin may remain attached to actin for a period of time in what is known as a latch state, by mechanisms which are not fully understood. This allows maintenance of tension with minimal consumption of ATP. Some smooth muscles can maintain tone at low levels of LC_{20} phosphorylation, implying a different mechanism of regulation of contraction, directed at actin rather than myosin. Caldesmon inhibits actomyosin ATPase activity.

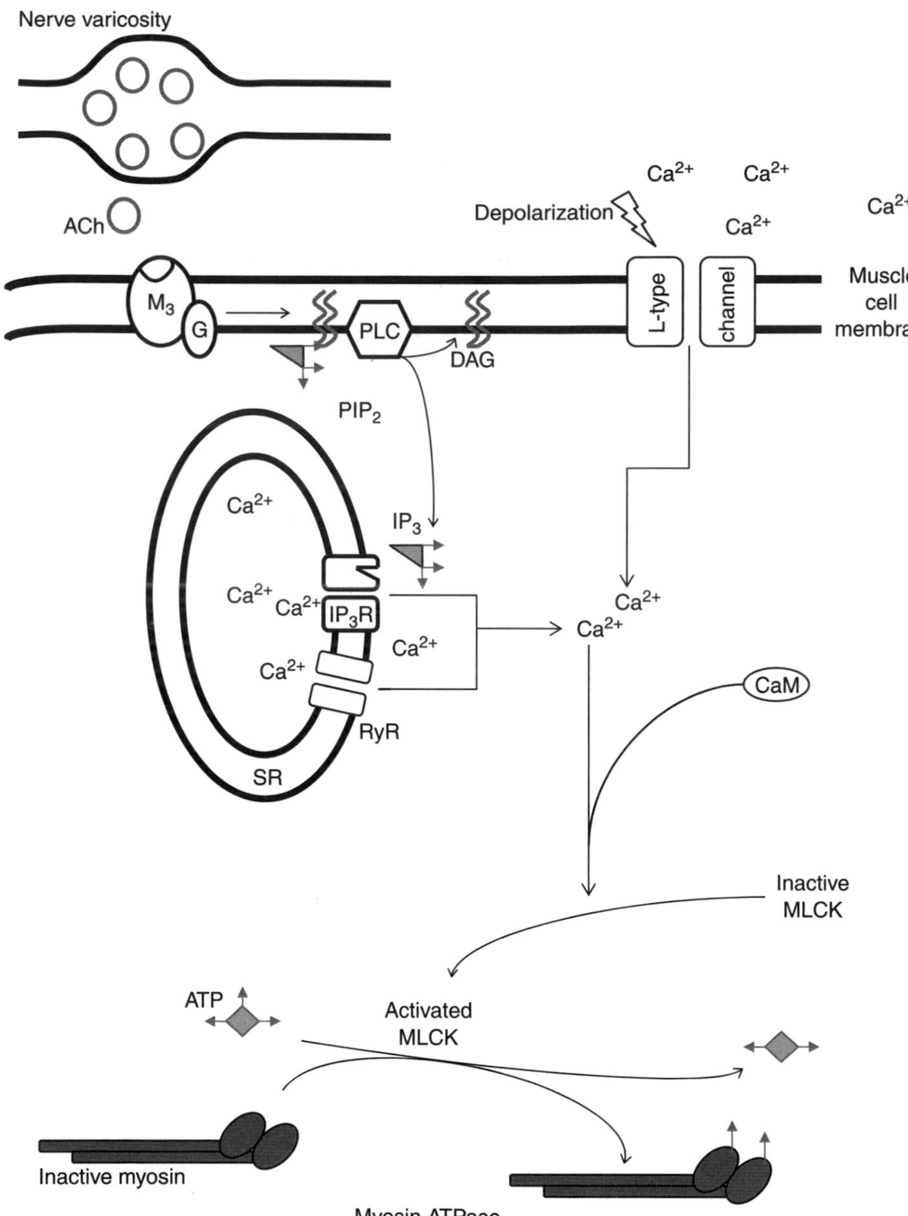

Figure 4.4
The role of calcium in detrusor muscle contraction. Cytosolic calcium increases rapidly as a result of release of intracellular stores, mainly in the sarcoplasmic reticulum, in response to second messenger signaling through the inositol triphosphate pathway and calcium-induced calcium release through ryanodine receptors. Extracellular calcium can also enter the cytoplasm through L-type calcium channels in the cell membrane in response to depolarization. The resulting generation of a calcium calmodulin complex activates myosin light chain kinase, leading to binding of actin by myosin and cell shortening. ACh, acetyl choline; G, G protein; PLC, phospholipase C; PIP2, phosphatidyl inositol diphosphate; IP3(R), inositol triphosphate (receptor); DAG, diacyl glycerol; SR, sarcoplasmic reticulum; RyR, ryanodine receptor; CaM, calmodulin; MLCK, myosin light chain kinase.

When phosphorylated, caldesmon releases actin, allowing it to interact with myosin. PKC, activated by DAG, is also believed to play an important role in the regulation of sustained smooth muscle contraction in general, though its role in the detrusor is not known.[72] Related to the PKC activation pathway may be other proteins, such as mitogen-activated protein kinase, caldesmon, small GTP-binding proteins, calponin, and others.[65]

Detrusor relaxation

The Ca^{2+} stores in the bladder are relatively labile: they can be readily depleted in Ca^{2+}-free solution, and rapidly filled from the extracellular source. Relaxation occurs when Ca^{2+} is taken back into the intracellular stores through the sarcoplasmic/endoplasmic reticulum Ca^{2+} ATPase (SERCA) pump. Some Ca^{2+} is also lost across the cell membrane and has to be replenished between contractions to ensure a steady state for calcium balance. Mechanisms by which stores are replenished are uncertain, but could include action of a cellular membrane Ca^{2+}–Na^{+} antiport, or a Ca^{2+}–ATPase.[72] A proportion of the calcium channels in the detrusor cell membrane are T-type,[33] which are active at a more negative membrane potential than L-type channels. Thus, at resting membrane potential, they may permit Ca^{2+} entry at a rate which will allow replenishment of stores, but not fast enough to precipitate contraction.

CICR does not only lead to contraction, but may also promote activation of membrane-bound Ca^{2+}-activated channels. For example, CICR from ryanodine receptors appears to have a strong functional influence on BK channels in the surface membrane. This may have a protective effect, as excessive accumulation of calcium activates Ca^{2+}-dependent enzymes such as proteases and lipases and can trigger apoptosis. Detailed discussion of the regulation of Ca^{2+} is given by Horowitz and colleagues.[65]

Detrusor strips show adjustable passive stiffness characterized by strain softening: a loss of stiffness on stretch to a new length distinct from viscoelastic behavior. At the molecular level, strain softening appears to be caused by cross-link breakage. Potassium- or carbachol-induced contraction rapidly restores the passive stiffness lost to strain softening, but this can be prevented by the rhoA kinase inhibition.[73]

Metabolism

Relatively little is known about metabolic processes in normal detrusor muscle. The response of the bladder to various stimuli is biphasic, comprising a rapid phasic rise in tension, followed by a prolonged period of force generation, the latter ensuring contraction is maintained until completion of voiding. The sustained phase is sensitive to depletion of glucose,[74] since glycogen stores in the detrusor are relatively small.[75] It is also acutely affected by removal of oxygen from the bathing medium, even though intracellular levels of ATP may be high.[76] This suggests that sustained tension is supported by high energy phosphates derived directly from oxidative phosphorylation, rather than cytosolic ATP. However, the basal metabolic rate is high[74] and oxygen-consuming energy production accounts for only 60% of heat generated during contraction, so that bladder muscle produces lactate under aerobic conditions (aerobic glycolysis).[77]

Tissue physiology of the bladder

Spontaneous activity

Spontaneous contractions occur in isolated detrusor strips, although the proportion of strips showing activity and the frequency of the contractions show marked species variation.[78,79] Individual contractions in isolated detrusor strips generally occur on a baseline of nearly zero tension, rising briefly to a variable amplitude and then falling back to baseline (Figure 4.5). This contrasts with intestinal smooth muscle, where contractions often fuse into a sustained high-tension tetanus. Fused tetanic contractions occur very infrequently in normal detrusor strips, a further indicator that electrical coupling is relatively poor.

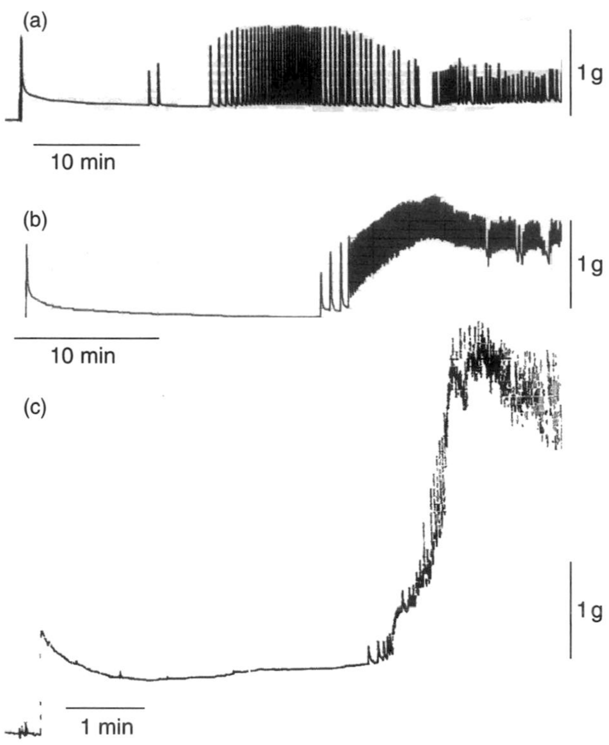

Figure 4.5
Spontaneous contractile activity. Patterns of contractile activity shown by isolated human detrusor muscle strips. (a) Phasic: repetitive contractions of about 30 s duration, each returning to baseline. (b) Tonic: a sustained rise in tension, often with superimposed phasic activity. (c) Fused tetanic contraction: rarely exhibited by muscle strips from normal bladders.

Spontaneous activity appears to have a myogenic basis, as it is not abolished by various receptor antagonists or nerve blockade. In most species, L-type Ca^{2+} channel blockers reduce spontaneous mechanical activity, while K^+ channel blocking drugs have the opposite effect. Some smooth muscles show spontaneous changes in membrane potential, in the form of action potentials or oscillations ('slow waves'). Quantal release of neurotransmitter from nearby nerve fibers also leads to fluctuations in the membrane potential, manifesting as excitatory junction potentials (EJPs) or inhibitory junction potentials (IJPs). EJPs are depolarizations below the threshold, but if enough transmitter reaches a muscle cell in a limited time period, summation of the EJPs may depolarize sufficiently to initiate an action potential, resulting in contraction of the cell. The extent to which the action potential will be propagated through the tissue depends on the degree of intercellular coupling. In poorly coupled tissues, the rate of EJPs greatly exceeds the level of spontaneous mechanical activity. Spontaneous action potentials can be recorded in individual

intravesical volumes, ranging from 0 to 500 ml or more. The range of intravesical volumes necessitates substantial adjustments within the detrusor and urothelium, such that individual smooth muscle cells elongate many times their resting length without increased tension.[115] Several investigators have proposed that the ability of the bladder to stretch with minimal increase in intravesical pressure might be achieved through action of a relaxant factor. Nerve-induced detrusor relaxation involving nitric oxide (NO) has been reported,[116] but other investigators have been unable to find detrusor relaxation in response to nerve stimulation.[117] Detrusor cells express some receptors which can mediate relaxation. Studies in the rat have suggested the presence of an unidentified relaxant factor released by muscarinic receptor activation.[118] The significance of these observations in normal bladder function has yet to be established.

Because the bladder is able to expel urine regardless of the volume contained, ergonomic considerations require that the ratio of the surface area to the volume is kept to its minimum, optimizing the bladder configuration for voiding if required. The ability to maintain tone without generalized contraction despite considerable stretch may arise in part from spontaneous action potentials unrelated to the innervation,[119] resulting in localized contractile activity. This will tend to maintain tone in the organ as a whole and allow adjustment to the increase in volume, without synchronous mass contraction of the entire bladder.

During bladder filling, several species show transient rises in intravesical pressure unrelated to micturition,[120] particularly when the bladder is filled at physiologic rates.[121,122] The mechanisms responsible for these nonmicturition contractions (NMCs) are not understood, but phasic fluctuations in intravesical pressure have been reported in several preparations where pathways of the micturition reflex have been interrupted.[122–125] Intramural contractile activity with minimal pressure rise has been also been reported during bladder filling, taking the form of localized shortenings, termed 'micromotions',[126] or propagating waves.[125] These observations indicate that peripheral mechanisms can generate bladder activity independent of the CNS and that NMCs are based on different mechanisms from micturition. Some understanding of these phenomena may be gained by comparison with the upper urinary tract, where autonomous areas of localized contractility ('pacemakers') synchronize and initiate peristalsis in response to distention.[127] A corresponding arrangement into peripheral autonomous modules has been proposed in the bladder.[128] In this model, modules are proposed as functional contractile units within the detrusor, analogous to the motor unit arrangement of skeletal muscle (Figure 4.7). Each module would be capable of contracting in isolation, perhaps consequent upon pacemaker activity, resulting in a localized contraction. The coordination of activity in neighboring modules would lead to organized contraction of a greater proportion of the bladder wall. Coordination of separate modules might occur through either ICC-like cell networks, or through direct myogenic transmission.[129] The existence of localized contractions in whole organ contractility has been described in rodents[16,18,130,131] and humans[132,133] (Figure 4.8). This results in a complex relationship between the intramural contractility and intravesical pressure.[134]

Voiding

Voiding is initiated by the CNS, which activates the parasympathetic efferents, resulting in widespread synchronous detrusor contraction and consequent increase in intravesical pressure. Simultaneously, a complex series of reflexes ensures appropriate configuration of the bladder outlet and relaxation of the continence mechanisms, resulting in urine flow. In order to ensure complete emptying, force of contraction has to be sustained throughout the voiding phase. A particular feature of the detrusor is the ability to sustain near-maximal force generation in the face of significant length changes. This is influenced both by ergonomic considerations as alluded to above and also the maintenance of the stimulus to contract until complete emptying has been achieved. Implicitly, sustained efferent activity will achieve the latter, but conceivably peripheral mechanisms underlying NMC activity could make an important contribution.

Regionalization in the bladder

Functional distinctions can be drawn between various regions of the bladder musculature. The body of the detrusor serves to store and expel urine periodically. The bladder base, particularly the trigone, differs in terms of the microanatomic arrangement of the muscle, the profile of receptors expressed, and the predominantly sympathetic innervation. This region may have a role in sensory return, and anatomic configuration of the bladder outlet and vesicoureteric junctions during voiding.

The bladder neck in men provides a sphincter function to ensure prograde propulsion on ejaculation. Some differences in neuromuscular transmission compared with the rest of the bladder may be present at the bladder neck. Pituitary adenylate cyclase activating protein (PACAP) 38 and VIP relax the pig urinary bladder neck.[135] PACAP 38 is involved in inhibitory neurotransmission.[136] In addition, presynaptic modulation influences transmitter release.[137]

Urothelium and suburothelial region

The urothelium maintains a barrier function, but it also appears to exhibit sensory and signaling properties that

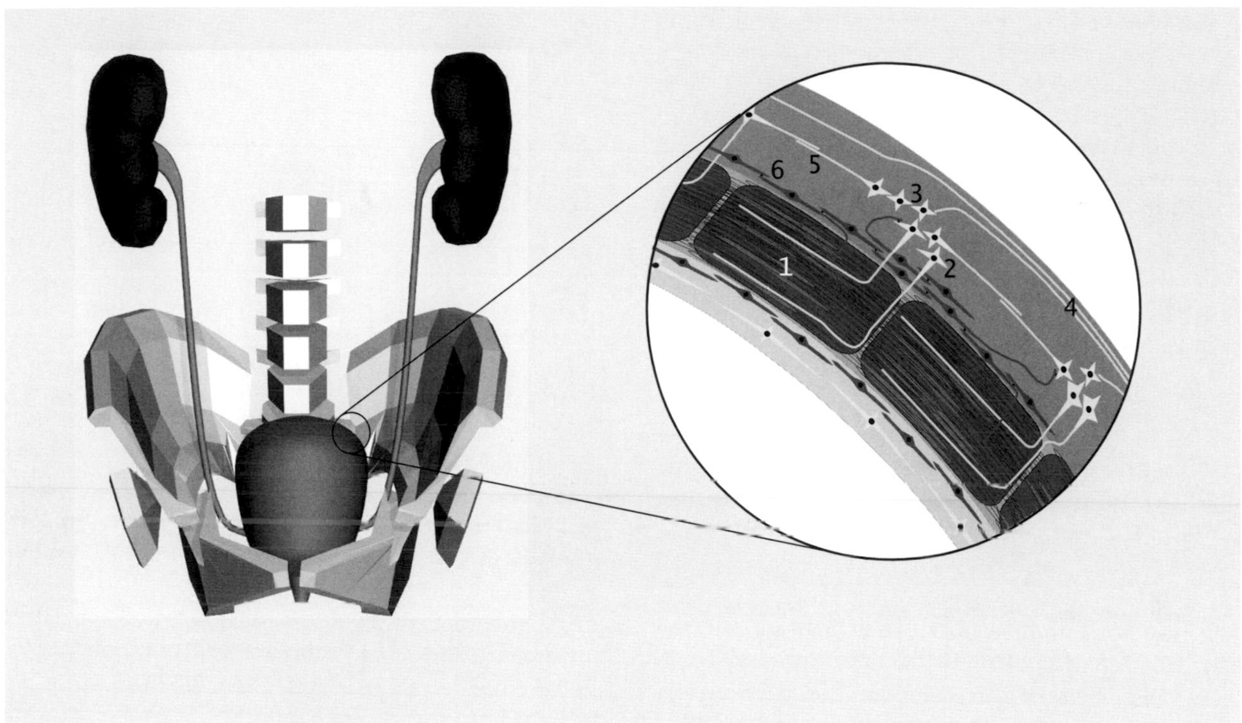

Figure 4.7
The peripheral autonomous module hypothesis of the detrusor. A schematic representation of the bladder wall, showing muscle blocks (1) defined by the region of distribution of axons of dominant motor neurons within intramural ganglia (2). These cells are influenced by a circuit made up of other neurons in the ganglion (3), which integrate information from diverse inputs, such as collaterals from suburothelial afferents (4) and axons from neighboring modules (5). Once a dominant motor neuron reaches a threshold of excitation, it fires action potentials, resulting in autonomous contraction localized to the muscle block supplied. Communications between modules across a hypothetical 'myovesical plexus', in the form of axons connecting the integrative circuitry of neighboring modules (5), or myofibroblast processes passing between muscle blocks (6), result in coordinated activity in a greater proportion of the bladder wall. This physiologic proposal has implications in the comprehension of pathophysiologic processes underlying conditions such as detrusor overactivity, since pathologically enhanced activity within modules or enhanced coordination of neighboring modules could facilitate uninhibited detrusor contraction outwith volitional control.

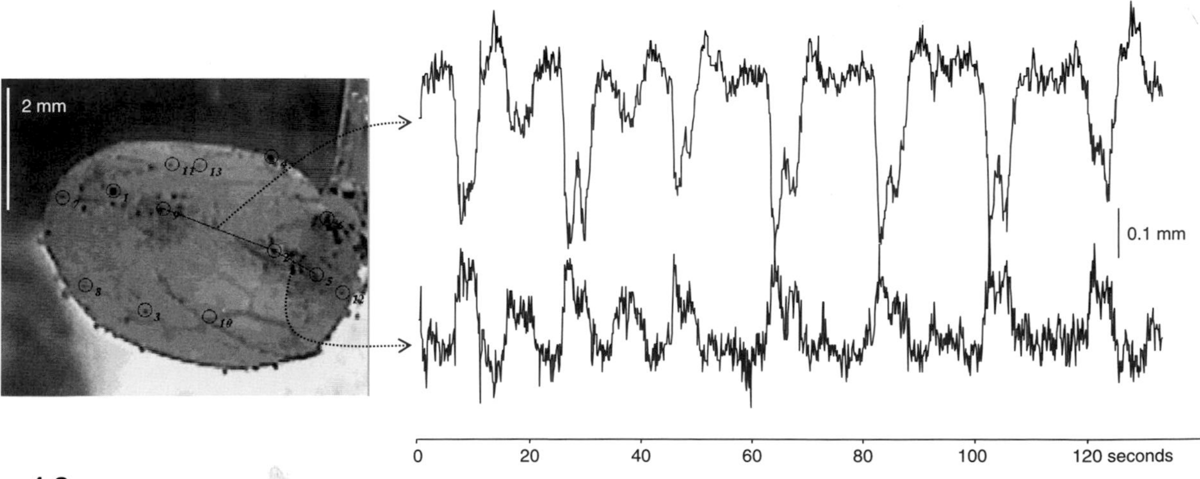

Figure 4.8
Activity in an autonomous module. Localized activity arising spontaneously in an isolated mouse bladder. Separation of multiple markers on the bladder surface was assessed, indicated on the photograph in the left panel. On the right are plotted marker separations in two regions. In one, spontaneous localized shortenings were observed, with concurrent elongations in the neighboring region, indicating autonomous behavior in discrete areas, i.e. functional modularity. Markers outside these regions maintained a constant separation.

allow response to the chemical and physical surroundings and reciprocal communication with subjacent structures. The urothelium secretes factors that can influence muscle contractility.[138] Substances released by the urothelium significantly alter the contractile response to carbachol[139] and electrical field stimulation,[140] while a diffusible inhibitory substance can reduce detrusor contractility.[139] The mechanisms involved have yet to be clarified, but the urothelium does release ATP[141] and other substances in response to stretch, proportionate to the degree of intravesical distention. The stretch response could result from the presence of mechanosensitive sodium channels, the density of which varies according to changes in the local conditions.[142] Urothelial cells express a range of receptors and release substances that can regulate the activity of underlying nerves.[143,144] This may have clinical significance: for example, urothelial expression of bradykinin receptors alters in models of bladder pathophysiology.[145] The suburothelial region is densely innervated and a wide range of putative neurotransmitters is present,[83] which may be released locally ('sensory efferents').[146] In addition, there is an extensive suburothelial network of myofibroblastic interstitial cells.[55] The urothelium synthesizes and releases transmitters, including ATP[147,148] and acetylcholine.[149] Their release may be modulated by the epithelial sodium channels on the apical surface of the urothelial cells, resulting in responsiveness to stretch.[142] Hormonal influences mediated by aldosterone have also been described.[150]

The physiology of the urethra

Bladder outlet function is derived from a complex integration of skeletal muscle in the pelvic floor and urethral wall, urethral smooth muscle, lamina propria, and urothelium. There are clear species variations, and the behavior of the skeletal component of the outlet has been shown by electromyography to differ in the rat and the guinea pig, with the suggestion that the rat urethra is therefore a less good model of the human urethra.[151] There are also marked regional variations, even in just the smooth muscle component. Whereas the female pig urethra is arranged in three smooth muscle layers, an inner longitudinal, a mid circular, and an outer longitudinal layer, the female human urethra has a smooth muscle bilayer consisting of an inner longitudinal and an outer circular layer.[152] The longitudinal muscle is anatomically continuous with the detrusor, implying a possible role in bladder neck opening and urethral shortening at the onset of voiding.[152] The circular layer is not continuous with the detrusor and is arranged in a disposition typical of a muscular sphincter, so it may be important for maintaining urethral closure. These anatomic distinctions may contribute to the functional attributes of the urethra in preventing leakage during storage, yet allowing urine flow during voiding. At this stage, however, understanding of the underlying processes is patchy.

Molecular cell biology of the urethra

Receptors

Adrenergic receptors are important in maintenance of urethral closure, and in the circular smooth muscle of the urethra there is evidence for the α_{1A} subtype,[153] and also the α_{1L} subtype.[154]

Muscarinic receptors show regional and interspecies variation. Cholinergic contraction of the normal pig urethra appears to be mediated via M_2 and, to a lesser extent, M_3 receptors in circular muscle, but only by M_3 receptors in longitudinal muscle.[155] M_1, M_2, and M_3 receptors may be involved in carbachol-induced contraction of the circular muscle of the rabbit urethra. The circular muscles have been reported to show a minimum or no response to muscarinic stimulation *in vitro*.[156]

Ion channels

Potassium channels

Exposure to the potassium channel opener levcromakalim causes relaxation of strips of proximal urethral smooth muscle from the female pig, associated with hyperpolarization and an outward K^+ current, both of which are blocked by glibenclamide.[157] The channel responsible is inhibited by intracellular ATP, reactivated by nucleoside diphosphates, and may be regulated by intracellular magnesium levels.[158] The channel was felt to differ from the ATP-sensitive channel in the guinea pig bladder, because of different conductance and reactivation properties. Sulfonylurea receptor subtypes have been shown to regulate ATP-sensitive potassium channel activity in the pig urethra.[159] The diversity of potassium channels in urethral smooth muscle is also shown by drug effects; another potassium channel opener, nicorandil, appears to induce relaxation in proximal pig urethra through two independent mechanisms,[160] and the action of mefenamic acid on the smooth muscle of proximal pig urethra shows three effects, on different potassium channels.[161] Further components of the outward K^+ current are a Ca^{2+}- and voltage-sensitive BK current and a voltage-activated, Ca^{2+}-insensitive DK current. The resting membrane potential in proximal urethral smooth muscle cells varies according to species and gender, with spontaneous hyperpolarizations and depolarizations apparent in a minority of cells.[162]

Other channels

In urethral smooth muscle of the human, sheep, guinea pig, and rabbit, both L-type and T-type Ca^{2+} channels and Ca^{2+}-dependent Cl^- currents have been identified.[163,164] The former seem to be responsible for the upstroke of the action potential. Drug effects have also shown diversity in the behavior of Ca^{2+} channels.[165]

Cell and tissue physiology of the urethra

Innervation

The bladder outlet receives neuronal inputs from several sources, both somatic and autonomic, mediating voluntary and involuntary mechanisms. Nerve-mediated contractions and relaxations occur in urethral smooth muscle, depending on the stimulation parameters, and the urethra appears to have both excitatory and inhibitory innervation, differing from the detrusor where direct innervation appears to be solely excitatory.[162] The predominant excitatory innervation is noradrenergic. Tamsulosin has been shown *in vivo* to reduce urethral resting pressure [166] and to be a potent urethral α_1 adrenoceptor blocker *in vitro*.[167] In addition, a parasympathetic cholinergic excitatory input to the urethra has been identified in male rats, but not in females,[168] and there may also be a purinergic component.[169] Evidence is now also available for the role of glutamatergic and serotonergic mechanisms in the regulation of urethral function, possibly at the spinal level,[170,171] and this stimulated the development of duloxetine as a clinical therapy for stress urinary incontinence.[172]

Nitrergic innervation from nerves with cell bodies in the major pelvic ganglia is also present and is primarily inhibitory. There is evidence for the presence of nitric oxide synthase in the striated muscle of the female urethra in the human[173] and in the guinea pig.[174] Nitric oxide donors have also been shown *in vivo* to reduce urethral resting pressure.[175] The constitutive carbon monoxide-producing enzyme heme oxygenase-2 coexists with neuronal nitric oxide synthase in nerve trunks of the human urethra.[176]

Generation of tonic contraction

Smooth muscle tension is one of the factors contributing to the maintenance of intraurethral pressure at a level exceeding the intravesical pressure, thereby ensuring continence. *In-vivo* studies of the effects of cholinergic and adrenergic agonists and antagonists on urethral pressure in humans have had variable results, but suggest that there is a tonic activity in the sympathetic innervation, with minimal contribution from cholinergic stimulation. Overall, sympathetic nervous activity is crucial to the maintenance of urethral closure.

Urethral smooth muscle generates spontaneous tone, which is greater in strips from the proximal urethra than the distal urethra *in vitro*.[177] This may be dependent on electrical membrane events, the force of contraction depending on the amplitude and duration of the plateau of electrical 'slow waves', and also on Ca^{2+} release from intracellular stores.[178] L-type Ca^{2+} current and Ca^{2+}-activated Cl^- current both seem to contribute to the generation of slow waves, whereas BK and DK currents appear to oppose depolarization during the plateau phase of the slow wave and may therefore modulate Ca^{2+} entry.

Rabbit urethra appears to contain interstitial cells, acting as specialized pacemaking cells that may be responsible for initiating slow waves in smooth muscle cells.[179–181] Partial tissue dissection with collagenase reveals a small population of branched cells, which may be myofibroblasts. These cells exhibit regular spontaneous depolarizations, which increase in frequency when exposed to norepinephrine (nonadrenaline) and are blocked by perfusion with calcium-free solution. They show Ca^{2+}-activated Cl^- current and spontaneous transient inward currents, which can be blocked by Cl^- channel blockers.[182] Calcium oscillations in these cells, related to ryanodine-sensitive intracellular stores, and the role of a Na^{+}-Ca^{2+} mechanism in the regulation of their spontaneous activity, have been demonstrated.[183,184] Accordingly, generation of tone may result from pacemaker activity of a small group of cells in the urethra, rather than intrinsic properties of the smooth muscle cells themselves. Electrical activity in these cells may also be modulated by nitrergic mechanisms.[185]

Urethral relaxation

The urethral pressure drops during micturition, prior to increase in intravesical pressure. When cholinergic and adrenergic responses are blocked, intrinsic nerve stimulation relaxes the tone of urethral muscle strips. Nerve-mediated relaxation is at least partly nitrergic,[169] acting by activating soluble guanylate cyclase.[186] Phosphodiesterase 5 inhibitors can modulate this relaxation.[187] The urothelium in the proximal urethra may enhance nerve-mediated smooth muscle relaxation by releasing NO.[188] Carbon monoxide may also act as an inhibitory transmitter, although with significantly lower potency than NO.[189,190]

Several other mediators may influence urethral tone. Relaxation can be mediated through β-adrenoceptors, via β_2 and β_3 subtypes.[3] Prostaglandins could increase or decrease both longitudinal and circular smooth muscle layer tension.[191] Prostaglandin synthesis inhibitors increase tension and spontaneous activity in pig urethral smooth muscle, whereas E series prostaglandins and VIP have the opposite effect. Serotonin produces substantial relaxation, partly inhibited by specific 5-HT receptor antagonists. ATP and adenosine can also elicit relaxation of urethral smooth muscle, in a manner similar to nerve-mediated relaxation, although the role of P2Y receptors is unclear.[192, 193]

Presynaptic modulation

Activation of α_2 adrenoceptors and muscarinic receptors can inhibit both the release of norepinephrine from adrenergic nerve terminals and the release of acetylcholine from cholinergic nerve terminals. This was interpreted as negative feedback control, indicating that the components of the urethral dual innervation may cross-regulate. The release of NO from nitrergic nerves in the rabbit urethra is reduced and increased by stimulation of prejunctional α_1 and α_2 adrenergic receptors, respectively,[194] whereas NO inhibits release of norepinephrine from adrenergic nerves,[195] and it may modulate the release of acetylcholine from the neuromuscular junction in urethral skeletal muscle.[196] Neuropeptide Y (NPY) has an inhibitory effect on the adrenergic component of electrically induced contractions in the urethra.[197]

Conclusion

The physiology of smooth muscles of the detrusor and urethra is complex and must be viewed in the context of the integrative function of the entire lower urinary tract and the functional requirements to achieve storage, voiding, and voluntary control. There are several levels of control and integration, including the brainstem, sacral spinal cord, peripheral ganglia, and intramural mechanisms, with a substantial voluntary input. This makes the study of smooth muscle physiology fascinating, but intellectually demanding. We remain far from a complete understanding of how the substantial number of pieces of the jigsaw gathered so far fit together, though substantial progress has been made.

References

1. Turner WH, Brading AF. Smooth muscle of the bladder in the normal and the diseased state: pathophysiology, diagnosis and treatment. Pharmacol Ther 1997; 75: 77.
2. Yamanishi T, Chapple CR, Yasuda K et al. Identification of beta-adrenoceptor subtypes in lower urinary tract of the female pig. J Urol 2002; 168: 2706.
3. Yamanishi T, Chapple CR, Yasuda K et al. The functional role of beta-adrenoceptor subtypes in mediating relaxation of pig urethral smooth muscle. J Urol 2003; 170: 2508.
4. Yamanishi T, Chapple CR, Yasuda K et al. Role of beta-adrenoceptor subtypes in mediating relaxation of the pig bladder trigonal muscle in vitro. Neurourol Urodyn 2003; 22: 338.
5. Uchida H, Shishido K, Nomiya M et al. Involvement of cyclic AMP-dependent and -independent mechanisms in the relaxation of rat detrusor muscle via beta-adrenoceptors. Eur J Pharmacol 2005; 518: 195.
6. Igawa Y, Yamazaki Y, Takeda H et al. Relaxant effects of isoproterenol and selective beta3-adrenoceptor agonists on normal, low compliant and hyperreflexic human bladders. J Urol 2001; 165: 240.
7. Biers SM, Reynard JM, Brading AF. The effects of a new selective beta3-adrenoceptor agonist (GW427353) on spontaneous activity and detrusor relaxation in human bladder. BJU Int 2006; 98: 1310.
8. Beckel JM, Kanai A, Lee SJ et al. Expression of functional nicotinic acetylcholine receptors in rat urinary bladder epithelial cells. Am J Physiol Renal Physiol 2006; 290: F103.
9. Eglen RM. Muscarinic receptor subtypes in neuronal and non-neuronal cholinergic function. Auton Autacoid Pharmacol 2006; 26: 219.
10. Wang P, Luthin GR, Ruggieri MR. Muscarinic acetylcholine receptor subtypes mediating urinary bladder contractility and coupling to GTP binding proteins. J Pharmacol Exp Ther 1995; 273: 959.
11. Tran JA, Matsui M, Ehlert FJ. Differential coupling of muscarinic M1, M2, and M3 receptors to phosphoinositide hydrolysis in urinary bladder and longitudinal muscle of the ileum of the mouse. J Pharmacol Exp Ther 2006; 318: 649.
12. Morimura K, Ohi Y, Yamamura H et al. Two-step Ca^{2+} intracellular release underlies excitation–contraction coupling in mouse urinary bladder myocytes. Am J Physiol Cell Physiol 2006; 290: C388.
13. Ruggieri MR Sr, Braverman AS. Regulation of bladder muscarinic receptor subtypes by experimental pathologies. Auton Autacoid Pharmacol 2006; 26: 311.
14. Schneider T, Hein P, Michel-Reher MB et al. Effects of ageing on muscarinic receptor subtypes and function in rat urinary bladder. Naunyn Schmiedebergs Arch Pharmacol 2005; 372: 71.
15. Lagou M, Gillespie JI, Andersson K-E et al. Bladder volume alters cholinergic responses of the isolated whole mouse bladder. J Urol 2006; 175: 771.
16. Lagou M, Gillespie JI, Kirkwood TBL et al. Muscarinic stimulation of the isolated whole mouse bladder; physiological responses in young and ageing mice. Auton Autacoid Pharmacol 2006; 26: 253.
17. Lagou M, Gillespie JI, Andersson KE et al. Bladder volume alters cholinergic responses of the isolated whole mouse bladder. J Urol 2006; 175: 771.
18. Drake MJ, Hedlund P, Harvey IJ et al. Partial outlet obstruction enhances modular autonomous activity in the isolated rat bladder. J Urol 2003; 170: 276.
19. Moore KH, Ray FR, Barden JA. Loss of purinergic P2X(3) and P2X(5) receptor innervation in human detrusor from adults with urge incontinence. J Neurosci 2001; 21: RC166.
20. Lee HY, Bardini M, Burnstock G. Distribution of P2X receptors in the urinary bladder and the ureter of the rat. J Urol 2000; 2002: 163.
21. Khattab MM, Al-Hrasen MN, El-Hadiyah TM. Contractile activity of ATP and diadenosine tetraphosphate on urinary bladder in the rat: role of A1- and P2X-purinoceptors and nitric oxide. Auton Autacoid Pharmacol 2007; 27: 55.
22. O'Reilly BA, Kosaka AH, Chang TK et al. A quantitative analysis of purinoceptor expression in the bladders of patients with symptomatic outlet obstruction. BJU Int 2001; 87: 617.
23. Neuhaus J, Weimann A, Stolzenburg JU et al. Histamine receptors in human detrusor smooth muscle cells: physiological properties and immunohistochemical representation of subtypes. World J Urol 2006; 24: 202.

24. Khanna OP, DeGregorio GJ, Sample RC et al. Histamine receptors in urethrovesical smooth muscle. Urology 1997; 10: 375.
25. Ost D, Roskams T, van der Aa F et al. Topography of the vanilloid receptor in the human bladder: more than just the nerve fibers. J Urol 2002; 168: 293.
26. Brading AF. Spontaneous activity of lower urinary tract smooth muscles: correlation between ion channels and tissue function. J Physiol 2006; 570: 13.
27. Petkov GV, Heppner TJ, Bonev AD et al. Low levels of K(ATP) channel activation decrease excitability and contractility of urinary bladder. Am J Physiol Regul Integr Comp Physiol 2001; 280: R1427.
28. Werner ME, Knorn AM, Meredith AL et al. Frequency encoding of cholinergic- and purinergic-mediated signaling to mouse urinary bladder smooth muscle: modulation by BK channels. Am J Physiol Regul Integr Comp Physiol 2007; 292: R616.
29. Ghatta S, Nimmagadda D, Xu X et al. Large-conductance, calcium-activated potassium channels: structural and functional implications. Pharmacol Ther 2006; 110: 103.
30. Darblade B, Behr-Roussel D, Oger S et al. Effects of potassium channel modulators on human detrusor smooth muscle myogenic phasic contractile activity: potential therapeutic targets for overactive bladder. Urology 2006; 68: 442.
31. Kotlikoff MI, Herrera G, Nelson MT. Calcium permeant ion channels in smooth muscle. Rev Physiol Biochem Pharmacol 1999; 134: 147.
32. Yanai Y, Hashitani H, Kubota Y et al. The role of Ni^{2+}-sensitive T-type Ca^{2+} channels in the regulation of spontaneous excitation in detrusor smooth muscles of the guinea-pig bladder. BJU Int 2006; 97: 182.
33. Sui GP, Wu C, Severs N et al. The association between t-type Ca^{2+}-current and outward current in isolated human detrusor cells from stable and overactive bladders. BJU Int 2007; 99(2): 436–41.
34. Li L, Jiang C, Hao P et al. Changes in T-type calcium channel and its subtypes in overactive detrusor of the rats with partial bladder outflow obstruction. Neurourol Urodyn 2007; 26(6): 870-8.
35. Wan EC, Gordon TP, Jackson MW. Autoantibody-mediated bladder dysfunction in type 1 diabetes. Scand J Immunol 2007; 65: 70.
36. Inoue R, Brading AF. Human, pig and guinea-pig bladder smooth muscle cells generate similar inward currents in response to purinoceptor activation. Br J Pharmacol 1991; 103: 1840.
37. Kajioka S, Nakayama S, McCoy R et al. Inward current oscillation underlying tonic contraction caused via ETA receptors in pig detrusor smooth muscle. Am J Physiol Renal Physiol 2004; 286: F77.
38. Wellner M-C, Isenberg G. Properties of stretch-activated channels in myocytes from the guinea-pig urinary bladder. J Physiol (Lond) 1993; 466: 213.
39. Thorneloe KS, Nelson MT. Properties of a tonically active, sodium-permeable current in mouse urinary bladder smooth muscle. Am J Physiol Cell Physiol 2004; 286: C1246.
40. Besarani D, Wu C, Fry CH. The influence of changes in extracellular and intracellular sodium concentration on detrusor contractility. BJU Int 2006; 97: 1083.
41. Kuriyama H, Kitamura K, Itoh T et al. Physiological features of visceral smooth muscle cells, with special reference to receptors and ion channels. Physiol Rev 1998; 78: 811.
42. Uckert S, Stief CG, Mayer M et al. Distribution and functional significance of phosphodiesterase isoenzymes in the human lower urinary tract. World J Urol 2005; 23: 368.
43. Nishiguchi J, Kwon DD, Kaiho Y et al. Suppression of detrusor overactivity in rats with bladder outlet obstruction by a type 4 phosphodiesterase inhibitor. BJU Int 2007; 99(3): 680–6.
44. Oger S, Behr-Roussel D, Gorny D et al. Relaxation of phasic contractile activity of human detrusor strips by cyclic nucleotide phosphodiesterase type 4 inhibition. Eur Urol 2007; 51: 772.
45. Braverman AS, Tibb AS, Ruggieri MR, Sr. M2 and M3 muscarinic receptor activation of urinary bladder contractile signal transduction. I. Normal rat bladder. J Pharmacol Exp Ther 2006; 316: 869.
46. Braverman AS, Doumanian LR, Ruggieri MR, Sr. M2 and M3 muscarinic receptor activation of urinary bladder contractile signal transduction. II. Denervated rat bladder. J Pharmacol Exp Ther 2006; 316: 875.
47. Rajasekaran M, Wilkes N, Kuntz S et al. Rho-kinase inhibition suppresses bladder hyperactivity in spontaneously hypertensive rats. Neurourol Urodyn 2005; 24: 295.
48. Durlu-Kandilci NT, Brading AF. Involvement of Rho kinase and protein kinase C in carbachol-induced calcium sensitization in beta-escin skinned rat and guinea-pig bladders. Br J Pharmacol 2006; 148: 376.
49. Fry CH, Wu C, Sui GP. Electrophysiological properties of the bladder. Int Urogynecol J Pelvic Floor Dysfunct 1998; 9: 291.
50. Bramich NJ, Brading AF. Electrical properties of smooth muscle in the guinea-pig urinary bladder. J Physiol 1996; 492: 185.
51. Mostwin JL, Karim NS, van Koeveringe G. Electrical properties of obstructed guinea pig bladder. Adv Exp Med Biol 1995; 385: 21.
52. Fry CH, Cooklin M, Birns J et al. Measurement of intercellular electrical coupling in guinea-pig detrusor smooth muscle. J Urol 1999; 161: 660.
53. Parekh AB, Brading AF, Tomita T. Studies of longitudinal tissue impedance in various smooth muscles. Prog Clin Biol Res 1990; 327: 375.
54. Ballaro A, Mundy AR, Fry CH et al. A new approach to recording electromyographic activity of detrusor smooth muscle. J Urol 2001; 166: 1957.
55. Sui GP, Rothery S, Dupont E et al. Gap junctions and connexin expression in human suburothelial interstitial cells. BJU Int 2002; 90: 118.
56. Neuhaus J, Wolburg H, Hermsdorf T et al. Detrusor smooth muscle cells of the guinea-pig are functionally coupled via gap junctions in situ and in cell culture. Cell Tissue Res 2002; 309: 301.
57. Neuhaus J, Pfeiffer F, Wolburg H et al. Alterations in connexin expression in the bladder of patients with urge symptoms. BJU Int 2005; 96: 670.
58. Mostwin JL. The action potential of guinea pig bladder smooth muscle. J Urol 1986; 135: 1299.
59. Nagai R, Kuro-o M, Babij P et al. Identification of two types of smooth muscle myosin heavy chain isoforms by cDNA cloning and immunoblot analysis. J Biol Chem 1989; 264: 9734.
60. Wilson TS, Aziz KA, Vazques D et al. Changes in detrusor smooth muscle myosin heavy chain mRNA expression following spinal cord injury in the mouse. Neurourol Urodyn 2005; 24: 89.
61. Chacko S, DiSanto M, Menon C et al. Contractile protein changes in urinary bladder smooth muscle following outlet obstruction. In: Advances in Bladder Research. Edited by L. Baskin and Hayward. New York: Kluwer Academic/Plenum, 1999.
62. Malmqvist U, Arner A, Uvelius B. Contractile and cytoskeletal proteins in smooth muscle during hypertrophy and its reversal. Am J Physiol 1991; 260: C1085.
63. Malmqvist U, Amer A. Correlation between isoform composition of the 17 kDa myosin light chain and maximal shortening velocity in smooth muscle. Pflugers Arch Eur J Physiol 1991; 418: 523.
64. Austin JC, Chacko SK, DiSanto M et al. A male murine model of partial bladder outlet obstruction reveals changes in detrusor morphology, contractility and myosin isoform expression. J Urol 2004; 172: 1524.
65. Horowitz A, Menice CB, Laporte R et al. Mechanisms of smooth muscle contraction. Physiol Rev 1996; 76: 967.
66. Conti MA, Adelstein RS. The relationship between calmodulin binding and phosphorylation of smooth muscle myosin kinase by the catalytic subunit of 3':5' cAMP-dependent protein kinase. J Biol Chem 1981; 256: 3178.
67. Isotani E, Zhi G, Lau KS et al. Real-time evaluation of myosin light chain kinase activation in smooth muscle tissues from a transgenic calmodulin-biosensor mouse. Proc Natl Acad Sci USA 2004; 101: 6279.
68. Mannikarottu AS, Disanto ME, Zderic SA et al. Altered expression of thin filament-associated proteins in hypertrophied urinary bladder smooth muscle. Neurourol Urodyn 2006; 25: 78.

69. Rembold CM, Wardle RL, Wingard CJ et al. Cooperative attachment of cross bridges predicts regulation of smooth muscle force by myosin phosphorylation. Am J Physiol Cell Physiol 2004; 287: C594.
70. Hotta S, Yamamura H, Ohya S et al. Methyl-beta-cyclodextrin prevents Ca^{2+}-induced Ca^{2+} release in smooth muscle cells of mouse urinary bladder. J Pharmacol Sci 2007; 103: 121.
71. Andersson K-E. Pharmacology of lower urinary tract smooth muscle and penile erectile tissue. Pharm Rev 1993; 45: 253.
72. Fry CH, Skennerton D, Wood D et al. The cellular basis of contraction in human detrusor smooth muscle from patients with stable and unstable bladders. Urology 2002; 59: 3.
73. Speich JE, Borgsmiller L, Call C et al. ROK-induced cross-link formation stiffens passive muscle: reversible strain-induced stress softening in rabbit detrusor. Am J Physiol Cell Physiol 2005; 289: C12.
74. Uvelius B, Arner A. Changed metabolism of detrusor muscle cells from obstructed rat urinary bladder. Scand J Urol Nephrol Suppl 1997; 184: 59.
75. Haugaard N, Wein AJ, Levin RM. In vitro studies of glucose metabolism of the rabbit urinary bladder. J Urol 1987; 137: 782.
76. Zhao Y, Wein AJ, Bilgen A et al. Effect of anoxia on in vitro bladder function. Pharmacology 1991; 43: 337.
77. Wendt IR, Gibbs CL. Energy expenditure of longitudinal smooth muscle of rabbit urinary bladder. Am J Physiol Cell Physiol 1987; 252: C88.
78. Brading AF, Williams JH. Contractile responses of smooth muscle strips from rat and guinea-pig urinary bladder to transmural stimulation: effects of atropine and alpha,beta-methylene ATP. Br J Pharmacol 1990; 99: 493.
79. Sibley GN. A comparison of spontaneous and nerve-mediated activity in bladder muscle from man, pig and rabbit. J Physiol Lond 1984; 354: 431.
80. Daniel EE, Cowan W, Daniel VP. Structural bases for neural and myogenic control of human detrusor muscle. Can J Physiol Pharmacol 1983; 61: 1247.
81. Gabella G. The structural relations between nerve fibres and muscle cells in the urinary bladder of the rat. J Neurocytol 1995; 24: 159.
82. Hirst GDS, Chaote JK, Cousins HM et al. Transmission by postganglionic axons of the autonomic nervous system: the importance of the specialised neuroeffector junction. Neuroscience 1996; 73: 7.
83. Drake MJ, Hedlund P, Mills IW et al. Structural and functional denervation of human detrusor after spinal cord injury. Lab Invest 2000; 80: 1491.
84. Mills IW, Greenland JE, McMurray G et al. Studies of the pathophysiology of idiopathic detrusor instability: the physiological properties of the detrusor smooth muscle and its pattern of innervation. J Urol 2000; 163: 646.
85. Kinder RB, Mundy AR. Atropine blockade of nerve-mediated stimulation of the human detrusor. Br J Urol 1985; 57: 418.
86. Lundberg JM. Pharmacology of cotransmission in the autonomic nervous system: integrative aspects on amines, neuropeptides, adenosine triphosphate, amino acids and nitric oxide. Pharmacol Rev 1996; 48: 113.
87. Brading AF, Inoue R. Ion channels and excitatory transmission in the smooth muscle of the urinary bladder. Z Kardiol 1991; 7: 47.
88. Luheshi GN, Zar MA. Presence of non-cholinergic motor transmission in human isolated bladder. J Pharm Pharmacol, 1990; 42: 223.
89. Westfall TD, Kennedy C, Sneddon P. The ecto-ATPase inhibitor ARL 67156 enhances parasympathetic neurotransmission in the guinea pig urinary bladder. Eur J Pharmacol 1997; 329: 167.
90. Gosling JA, Gilpin SA, Dixon JS et al. Decrease in the autonomic innervation of human detrusor muscle in outflow obstruction. J Urol 1986; 136: 501.
91. Persson K, Andersson K-E. Non-adrenergic, non-cholinergic relaxation and levels of cyclic nucleotides in rabbit lower urinary tract. Eur J Pharmacol 1994; 268: 159.
92. Zagorodnyuk VP, Costa M, Brookes SJ. Major classes of sensory neurons to the urinary bladder. Auton Neurosci 2006; 390: 126–7.
93. Clapham DE. TRP channels as cellular sensors. Nature 2003; 426: 517.
94. Mukerji G, Yiangou Y, Corcoran SL et al. Cool and menthol receptor TRPM8 in human urinary bladder disorders and clinical correlations. BMC Urol 2006; 6: 6.
95. Andrade EL, Ferreira J, Andre E et al. Contractile mechanisms coupled to TRPA1 receptor activation in rat urinary bladder. Biochem Pharmacol 2006; 72: 104.
96. Powell DW, Mifflin RC, Valentich JD et al. Myofibroblasts. I. Paracrine cells important in health and disease. Am J Physiol 1999; 277: C1.
97. Klemm MF, Exintaris B, Lang RJ. Identification of the cells underlying pacemaker activity in the guinea-pig upper urinary tract. J Physiol 1999; 519: 867.
98. Drake MJ, Fry CH, Eyden B. The structural characterisation of myofibroblasts in the bladder. BJU Int, 2006; 97(1): 29–32.
99. Faussone-Pellegrini MS, Thuneberg L. Guide to the identification of interstitial cells of Cajal. Microsc Res Tech 1999; 47: 248.
100. Drake MJ, Hedlund P, Andersson K-E et al. Morphology, phenotype and ultrastructure of fibroblastic cells from normal and neuropathic human detrusor: lack of myofibroblastic characteristics. J Urol 2003; 169: 1573.
101. Smet PJ, Jonavicius J, Marshall VR et al. Distribution of nitric oxide synthase-immunoreactive nerves and identification of the cellular targets of nitric oxide in guinea-pig and human urinary bladder by cGMP immunohistochemistry. Neuroscience 1996; 71: 337.
102. McCloskey KD, Gurney AM. Kit positive cells in the guinea pig bladder. J Urol 2002; 168: 832.
103. Popescu LM, Gherghiceanu M, Cretoiu D et al. The connective connection: interstitial cells of Cajal (ICC) and ICC-like cells establish synapses with immunoreactive cells. Electron microscope study in situ. J Cell Mol Med 2005; 9: 714.
104. McCloskey KD. Characterization of outward currents in interstitial cells from the guinea pig bladder. J Urol 2005; 173: 296.
105. McCloskey KD. Calcium currents in interstitial cells from the guinea-pig bladder. BJU Int 2006; 97: 1338.
106. Kuijpers KA, Heesakkers JP, Jansen CF et al. Cadherin-11 is expressed in detrusor smooth muscle cells and myofibroblasts of normal human bladder. Eur Urol 2007; 52(4): 1213–21.
107. Hashitani H, Yanai Y, Suzuki H. Role of interstitial cells and gap junctions in the transmission of spontaneous Ca signals in detrusor smooth muscles of the guinea-pig urinary bladder. J Physiol 2004; 559: 567.
108. Hashitani H. Interaction between interstitial cells and smooth muscles in the lower urinary tract and penis. J Physiol 2006; 576: 707.
109. Lagou M, Drake MJ, Markerink-van Inttersum M et al. Interstitial cells and phasic activity in the isolated mouse bladder. BJU Int 2006; 98: 643.
110. Lagou M, de Vente J, Kirkwood TB et al. Location and innervation of interstitial cells in the mouse bladder. BJU Int 2006; 97: 1332.
111. Biers SM, Reynard JM, Doore T et al. The functional effects of a c-kit tyrosine inhibitor on guinea-pig and human detrusor. BJU Int 2006; 97: 612.
112. Kubota Y, Kajioka S, Biers SM et al. Investigation of the effect of the c-kit inhibitor Glivec on isolated guinea-pig detrusor preparations. Auton Neurosci 2004; 115: 64.
113. Gillespie JI, Harvey IJ, Drake MJ. Agonist and nerve induced phasic activity in the isolated whole bladder of the guinea pig. Exp Physio 2003; 88: 343.
114. Mukerji G, Yiangou Y, Grogono J et al. Localization of M2 and M3 muscarinic receptors in human bladder disorders and their clinical correlations. J Urol 2006; 176: 367.
115. Uvelius B. Isometric and isotonic length–tension relations and variations in longitudinal smooth muscle from rabbit urinary bladder. Acta Physiol Scand 1976; 92: 1.
116. James MJ, Birmingham AT, Hill SJ. Partial mediation by nitric oxide of the relaxation of human isolated detrusor strips in response to electrical field stimulation. Br J Clin Pharmacol 1993; 35: 366.

117. Triguero D, Prieto D, Garcia Pascual A. NADPH-diaphorase and NANC relaxations are correlated in the sheep urinary tract. Neurosci Lett 1993; 163: 93.
118. Fovaeus M, Fujiwara M, Hogestatt ED et al. A non-nitrergic smooth muscle relaxant factor released from rat urinary bladder by muscarinic receptor stimulation. J Urol 1999; 161: 649.
119. Brading AF, Turner WH. The unstable bladder: towards a common mechanism. Br J Urol 1994; 73: 3.
120. Vaughan CW, Satchell PM. Urine storage mechanisms. Prog Neurobiol 1995; 46: 215.
121. Igawa Y, Mattiasson A, Andersson KE. Micturition and premicturition contractions in unanesthetized rats with bladder outlet obstruction. J Urol 1994; 151: 244.
122. Klevmark B. Motility of the urinary bladder in cats during filling at physiological rates. II. Effects of extrinsic bladder denervation on intramural tension and on intravesical pressure patterns. Acta Physiol Scand 1977; 101: 176.
123. Mills IW, Drake MJ, Noble JG et al. Are unstable detrusor contractions dependent on efferent excitatory innervation? Neurourol Urodyn 1998; 17: 352.
124. Sethia KK, Brading AF, Smith JC. An animal model of non-obstructive bladder instability. J Urol 1990; 143: 1243.
125. Sugaya K, de Groat WC. Influence of temperature on activity of the isolated whole bladder preparation of neonatal and adult rats. Am J Physiol Regul Integr Comp Physiol 2000; 278: R238.
126. Coolsaet BL, Van Duyl WA, Van Os-Bossagh P et al. New concepts in relation to urge and detrusor activity. Neurourol Urodyn 1993; 12: 463.
127. Constantinou CE, Yamaguchi O. Multiple-coupled pacemaker system in renal pelvis of the unicalyceal kidney. Am J Physiol 1981; 241: R412.
128. Drake MJ, Mills IW, Gillespie JI. Model of peripheral autonomous modules and a myovesical plexus in normal and overactive bladder function. Lancet 2001; 358: 401.
129. Hashitani H, Fukuta H, Takano H et al. Origin and propagation of spontaneous excitation in smooth muscle of the guinea-pig urinary bladder. J Physiol 2001; 530: 273.
130. Drake MJ, Harvey IJ, Gillespie JI. Autonomous activity in the isolated guinea pig bladder. Exp Physiol 2003; 88: 19.
131. Drake MJ, Gillespie JI, Hedlund P et al. Muscarinic stimulation of the isolated whole rat bladder; pathophysiological models of detrusor overactivity. Auton Autacoid Pharmacol 2006; 26: 261.
132. Van Os-Bossagh P, Kosterman LM, Hop WC et al. Micromotions of bladder wall in chronic pelvic pain (CPP): a pilot study. Int Urogynecol J Pelvic Floor Dysfunct 2001; 12: 89.
133. Drake MJ, Harvey IJ, Gillespie JI et al. Localised modular contractions in the normal human bladder and in urinary urgency. BJU Int 2005; 95: 1002.
134. Gevaert T, Ost D, de Ridder D. Comparing study of autonomous activity in bladders from normal and paraplegic rats. Neurourol Urodyn 2006; 25(4): 368–78.
135. Hernandez M, Barahona MV, Recio P et al. Neuronal and smooth muscle receptors involved in the PACAP- and VIP-induced relaxations of the pig urinary bladder neck. Br J Pharmacol 2006; 149: 100.
136. Hernandez M, Barahona MV, Recio P et al. PACAP 38 is involved in the non-adrenergic non-cholinergic inhibitory neurotransmission in the pig urinary bladder neck. Neurourol Urodyn 2006; 25: 490.
137. Hernandez M, Recio P, Victoria Barahona M et al. Pre-junctional α_2-adrenoceptors modulation of the nitrergic transmission in the pig urinary bladder neck. Neurourol Urodyn 2007; 26(4): 578–83.
138. Maggi CA, Santicioli P, Parlani M et al. The presence of mucosa reduces the contractile response of the guinea-pig urinary bladder to substance P. J Pharm Pharmacol 1987; 39: 653.
139. Hawthorn MH, Chapple CR, Cock M et al. Urothelium-derived inhibitory factor(s) influences on detrusor muscle contractility in vitro. Br J Pharmacol 2000; 129: 416.
140. Levin RM, Wein AJ, Krasnopolsky L et al. Effect of mucosal removal on the response of the feline bladder to pharmacological stimulation. J Urol 1995; 153: 1291.
141. Ferguson DR, Kennedy I, Burton TJ. ATP is released from rabbit urinary bladder epithelial cells by hydrostatic pressure changes – a possible sensory mechanism? J Physiol 1997; 505: 503.
142. Burton TJ, Edwardson JM, Ingham J et al. Regulation of Na^+ channel density at the apical surface of rabbit urinary bladder epithelium. Eur J Pharmacol 2002; 448: 215.
143. Birder LA, Nakamura Y, Kiss S et al. Altered urinary bladder function in mice lacking the vanilloid receptor TRPV1. Nat Neurosci 2002; 5: 856.
144. Birder LA, Kanai AJ, de Groat WC et al. Vanilloid receptor expression suggests a sensory role for urinary bladder epithelial cells. Proc Natl Acad Sci USA 2001; 98: 13396–401.
145. Chopra B, Barrick SR, Meyers S et al. Expression and function of bradykinin B1 and B2 receptors in normal and inflamed rat urinary bladder urothelium. J Physiol 2005; 562: 859.
146. Maggi CA, Meli A. The sensory-efferent function of capsaicin-sensitive sensory neurons. Gen Pharmacol 1988; 19: 1.
147. Salas NA, Somogyi GT, Gangitano DA et al. Receptor activated bladder and spinal ATP release in neurally intact and chronic spinal cord injured rats. Neurochem Int 2007; 50: 345.
148. Khera M, Somogyi GT, Kiss S et al. Botulinum toxin A inhibits ATP release from bladder urothelium after chronic spinal cord injury. Neurochem Int 2004; 45: 987.
149. Lips KS, Wunsch J, Zarghooni S et al. Acetylcholine and molecular components of its synthesis and release machinery in the urothelium. Eur Urol 2006; 51(4): 1042–53.
150. Burton TJ, Cooper DM, Dunning-Davies B et al. Aldosterone stimulates active Na^+ transport in rabbit urinary bladder by both genomic and non-genomic processes. Eur J Pharmacol 2005; 510: 181.
151. Walters RD, McMurray G, Brading AF. Comparison of the urethral properties of the female guinea pig and rat. Neurourol Urodyn 2006; 25: 62.
152. Dass N, McMurray G, Greenland JE et al. Morphological aspects of the female pig bladder neck and urethra: quantitative analysis using computer assisted 3-dimensional reconstructions. J Urol 2001; 165: 1294.
153. Nasu K, Moriyama N, Fukasawa R et al. Quantification and distribution of alpha1 adrenoceptor subtype mRNAs in human proximal urethra. Br J Pharmacol 1998; 123: 1289.
154. Bagot K, Chess-Williams R. Alpha(1A/L)-adrenoceptors mediate contraction of the circular smooth muscle of the pig urethra. Auton Autacoid Pharmacol 2006; 26: 345.
155. Yamanishi T, Chapple CR, Yasuda K et al. The role of M2 muscarinic receptor subtypes mediating contraction of the circular and longitudinal smooth muscle of the pig proximal urethra. J Urol 2002; 168: 308.
156. Ek A, Alm P, Andersson KE et al. Adrenergic and cholinergic nerves of the human urethra and urinary bladder. A histochemical study. Acta Physiol Scand 1977; 99: 345.
157. Teramoto N, Creed KE, Brading AF. Activity of glibenclamide-sensitive K^+ channels under unstimulated conditions in smooth muscle cells of pig proximal urethra. Naunyn Schmiedebergs Arch Pharmacol 1997; 356: 418.
158. Teramoto N, McMurray G, Brading AF. Effects of levcromakalim and nucleoside diphosphates on glibenclamide-sensitive K^+ channels in pig urethral myocytes. Br J Pharmacol 1997; 120: 1229.
159. Yunoki T, Teramoto N, Ito Y. Functional involvement of sulphonylurea receptor (SUR) type 1 and 2B in the activity of pig urethral ATP-sensitive K^+ channels. Br J Pharmacol 2003; 139: 652.
160. Teramoto N, Brading AF. Nicorandil activates glibenclamide-sensitive K^+ channels in smooth muscle cells of pig proximal urethra. J Pharmacol Exp Ther 1997; 280: 483.
161. Teramoto N, Brading AF, Ito Y. Multiple effects of mefenamic acid on K^+ currents in smooth muscle cells from pig proximal urethra. Br J Pharmacol 2003; 140: 1341.

162. Creed KE, Oike M, Ito Y. The electrical properties and responses to nerve stimulation of the proximal urethra of the male rabbit. Br J Urol 1997; 79: 543.
163. Hollywood MA, Woolsey S, Walsh IK et al. T- and L-type Ca^{2+} currents in freshly dispersed smooth muscle cells from the human proximal urethra. J Physiol 2003; 550: 753.
164. Bradley JE, Anderson UA, Woolsey SM et al. Characterization of T-type calcium current and its contribution to electrical activity in rabbit urethra. Am J Physiol Cell Physiol 2004; 286: C1078.
165. Teramoto N, Tomoda T, Ito Y. Mefenamic acid as a novel activator of L-type voltage-dependent Ca^{2+} channels in smooth muscle cells from pig proximal urethra. Br J Pharmacol 2005; 144: 919.
166. Reitz A, Haferkamp A, Kyburz T et al. The effect of tamsulosin on the resting tone and the contractile behaviour of the female urethra: a functional urodynamic study in healthy women. Eur Urol 2004; 46: 235.
167. Yamaguchi T, Nagano M, Osada Y. Effects of different alpha-1 adrenoceptor blockers on proximal urethral function using in vivo isovolumetric pressure changes. J Smooth Muscle Res 2005; 41: 247.
168. Kakizaki H, Fraser MO, De Groat WC. Reflex pathways controlling urethral striated and smooth muscle function in the male rat. Am J Physiol 1997; 272: R1647.
169. Bridgewater M, MacNeil HF, Brading AF. Regulation of tone in pig urethral smooth muscle. J Urol 1993; 150: 223.
170. Chang HY, Cheng CL, Chen JJ et al. Roles of glutamatergic and serotonergic mechanisms in reflex control of the external urethral sphincter in urethane-anesthetized female rats. Am J Physiol Regul Integr Comp Physiol 2006; 291: R224.
171. Boy S, Reitz A, Wirth B et al. Facilitatory neuromodulative effect of duloxetine on pudendal motor neurons controlling the urethral pressure: a functional urodynamic study in healthy women. Eur Urol 2006; 50: 119.
172. Thor KB. Serotonin and norepinephrine involvement in efferent pathways to the urethral rhabdosphincter: implications for treating stress urinary incontinence. Urology 2003; 62: 3.
173. Ho KM, Borja MC, Persson K et al. Expression of nitric oxide synthase immunoreactivity in the human female intramural striated urethral sphincter. J Urol 2003; 169: 2407.
174. Walters RD, McMurray G, Brading AF. Pudendal nerve stimulation of a preparation of isolated guinea-pig urethra. BJU Int 2006; 98: 1302.
175. Reitz A, Bretscher S, Knapp PA et al. The effect of nitric oxide on the resting tone and the contractile behaviour of the external urethral sphincter: a functional urodynamic study in healthy humans. Eur Urol 2004; 45: 367.
176. Ho KM, Ny L, McMurray G et al. Co-localization of carbon monoxide and nitric oxide synthesizing enzymes in the human urethral sphincter. J Urol 1999; 161: 1968.
177. Bridgewater M, Davies JR, Brading AF. Regional variations in the neural control of the female pig urethra. Br J Urol 1995; 76: 730.
178. Hashitani H, Yanai Y, Kohri K et al. Heterogeneous CPA sensitivity of spontaneous excitation in smooth muscle of the rabbit urethra. Br J Pharmacol 2006; 148: 340.
179. Seki N, Karim OM, Mostwin JL. The effect of experimental urethral obstruction and its reversal on changes in passive electrical properties of detrusor muscle. J Urol 1992; 148: 1957.
180. Sergeant GP, Hollywood MA, McHale NG et al. Ca^{2+} signalling in urethral interstitial cells of Cajal. J Physiol 2006; 576: 715.
181. Sergeant GP, Thornbury KD, McHale NG et al. Interstitial cells of Cajal in the urethra. J Cell Mol Med 2006; 10: 280.
182. Sergeant GP, Thornbury KD, McHale NG et al. Characterization of norepinephrine-evoked inward currents in interstitial cells isolated from the rabbit urethra. Am J Physiol Cell Physiol 2002; 283: C885.
183. Johnston L, Sergeant GP, Hollywood MA et al. Calcium oscillations in interstitial cells of the rabbit urethra. J Physiol 2005; 565: 449.
184. Bradley E, Hollywood MA, Johnston L et al. Contribution of reverse Na^+–Ca^{2+} exchange to spontaneous activity in interstitial cells of Cajal in the rabbit urethra. J Physiol 2006; 574: 651.
185. Sergeant GP, Johnston L, McHale NG et al. Activation of the cGMP/PKG pathway inhibits electrical activity in rabbit urethral interstitial cells of Cajal by reducing the spatial spread of Ca^{2+} waves. J Physiol 2006; 574: 167.
186. Dokita S, Smith SD, Nishimoto T et al. Involvement of nitric oxide and cyclic GMP in rabbit urethral relaxation. Eur J Pharmacol 1994; 266: 269.
187. Werkstrom V, Svensson A, Andersson KE et al. Phosphodiesterase 5 in the female pig and human urethra: morphological and functional aspects. BJU Int 2006; 98: 414.
188. Pinna C, Eberini I, Puglisi L et al. Presence of constitutive endothelial nitric oxide synthase immunoreactivity in urothelial cells of hamster proximal urethra. Eur J Pharmacol 1999; 367: 85.
189. Werkstrom V, Alm P, Persson K et al. Inhibitory innervation of the guinea-pig urethra; roles of CO, NO and VIP. J Auton Nerv Syst 1998; 74: 33.
190. Werkstrom V, Ny L, Persson K et al. Carbon monoxide-induced relaxation and distribution of heme oxygenase isoenzymes in the pig urethra and lower esophagogastric junction. Br J Pharmacol 1997; 120: 312.
191. Andersson KE, Ek A, Persson CG. Effects of prostaglandins on the isolated human bladder and urethra. Acta Physiol Scand 1997; 100: 165.
192. Werkstrom V, Andersson KE. ATP- and adenosine-induced relaxation of the smooth muscle of the pig urethra. BJU Int 2005; 96: 1386.
193. Pinna C, Glass R, Knight GE et al. Purine- and pyrimidine-induced responses and P2Y receptor characterization in the hamster proximal urethra. Br J Pharmacol 2005; 144: 510.
194. Seshita H, Yoshida M, Takahashi W et al. Prejunctional alpha-adrenoceptors regulate nitrergic neurotransmission in the rabbit urethra. Eur J Pharmacol 2000; 400: 271.
195. Yoshida M, Akaike T, Inadome A et al. The possible effect of nitric oxide on relaxation and noradrenaline release in the isolated rabbit urethra. Eur J Pharmacol 1998; 357: 213.
196. Garcia-Pascual A, Costa G, Labadia A et al. Partial nicotinic receptor blockade unmasks a modulatory role of nitric oxide on urethral striated neuromuscular transmission. Nitric Oxide 2005; 13: 98.
197. Zoubek J, Somogyi GT, De Groat WC. A comparison of inhibitory effects of neuropeptide Y on rat urinary bladder, urethra, and vas deferens. Am J Physiol 1993; 265: R537.

5

Physiology of the striated muscles

John FB Morrison

INTRODUCTION

This chapter is concerned with the physiologic control of the external urethral sphincter, the pelvic floor muscles, and other striated muscles functionally associated with the pelvic diaphragm in the set of conditions described collectively as the 'neurogenic bladder' or 'overactive bladder (OAB)'. Following spinal cord lesions, striated muscles generally develop spasticity, for example following a cervical or thoracic spinal cord transection, and a corresponding increase in tone is seen in the striated muscle of the external urethral sphincter and pelvic floor. Alternatively, muscle tone can be flaccid, if there is a lower motoneurone lesion affecting the cauda equina. Partial and mixed lesions also occur and reflex activities can be modified in the remodeling of the neural networks that regulate these muscles, or by the denervation and reinnervation of neurones or skeletal muscle. The muscles themselves also respond to these changes in activity, and, for example, hypoplastic changes and replacement by fibrous tissue can also occur as a result of denervation.

There have been a number of reviews and books on the subject[1–9] during the last couple of decades, and recently there has been a substantial body of genetic and molecular data concerning the mechanisms that operate in muscles of different types, and the mechanisms that operate to maintain the stability of the link between motoneurone and muscle at the nerve–muscle junction. The striated muscles of the lower urinary tract are specialized in function, and are subject to neural coordination that causes them to work together as a functional group. Within this overall concept there remain areas of muscle that are specialized for different tasks related to the visceral systems with which they are principally associated. Examples include the pubo-rectalis or the fibers of levator ani that loop behind the urethra, and there are also differences between the mechanisms controlling the urethral sphincter, the associated paraurethral muscles, and the muscle fibers that compose the bulk of levator ani. These differences extend to the histologic and biochemical properties of the muscle fibers, the pattern and source of innervation, the reflex behavior, and the role in voluntary control of the lower urinary tract.

NORMAL STRUCTURE AND FUNCTION

Morphology of the striated muscle of the lower urinary tract

Gross anatomy

Striated muscle occurs in the pelvic floor and within the urethra, and both of these contribute to continence mechanisms; smooth muscle as well as skeletal muscle occurs within the urethra, and the roles of these are sometimes difficult to separate. *In-vivo* recordings of intraurethral pressure have been made following blockade of the nicotinic receptors in various mammals,[10–14] and all suggest that the somatic innervation of the striated muscle of this region plays a part in generating the resting urethral pressure.

Striated muscle of the rhabdosphincter

The external urethral sphincter consists of circular striated muscle concentrated over about 40% of the length of the urethra (from 20 to 60% of its length in humans). In the rat, the distribution of striated muscle in the urethra is similar, but there is also a mass of muscle that forms an arch at the perineal membrane that can compress the urethra from above in the lower third.[12]

Various recent studies have focused on the mechanisms that operate in the human and animal rhabdosphincter.[15–20] In the human female the striated muscle is said to form an outer sleeve (the external urethral sphincter or

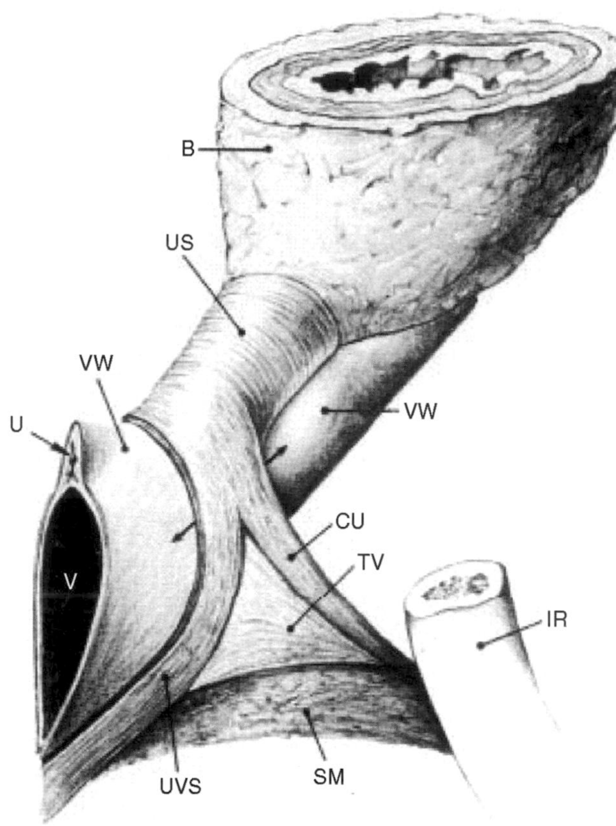

Figure 5.1
Striated urogenital sphincter muscle showing its urethral sphincter (US), compressor urethrae (CU), and urethrovaginal sphincter (UVS). Also shown, B, bladder; IR, ischiopubic ramus; SM, smooth muscle; TV transverse vaginal muscle; U, urethra; V, vagina; VW, vaginal wall.[48]

rhabdosphincter), and this surrounds the inner smooth muscle (Figure 5.1). This female rhabdosphincter is separate from the muscle of the anterior pelvic floor. The fibers are oriented in a circular direction and are thickest in the middle third of the urethra, but the posterior segment, adjacent to the vaginal wall, is thinner than elsewhere. These striated muscle cells are smaller than in the pelvic floor and exert tone upon the urethral lumen for long periods of time, and this muscle also aids closure. In the human male, the striated muscle also encircles the urethra, and unlike the female these small fibers merge with larger diameter fibers of adjacent muscles. One possibility is that these larger fibers are a proximal extension of striated muscle from the bulb of the penis.[6] Other views relate to observations on the striated muscle of the prostatic capsule, where fast and slow fibers are present.[7] In tissues taken from transplant donors it was found that the male rhabdosphincter consists of 35% fast and 65% slow fibers, while in the female only 13% of fibers are fast-twitch fibers (see later).

It has previously been speculated that a morphologic abnormality in this sphincter might be found in some women who present with urinary retention. It was hypothesized that these women have urethral sphincter overactivity and work hyperplasia of urethral rhabdosphincter fibers. However, in a recent investigation it was shown by electron microscopy that excessive peripheral sarcoplasm with lipid and glycogen deposition occurred in these cells together with sarcoplasmic accumulation of normal mitochondria, which were absent from the control.[21] Clearly other cellular pathology is present in these patients.

Levator ani

The levator ani is a sling of muscle in the shape of a thin broad sheet attached to the pubis anteriorly and laterally as far as the ischial spine; anteriorly the muscle is absent in the midline and a fat-filled space lies immediately behind the pubic symphysis.[22] In the human male a few fibers attach to the perineal body behind the prostate to form the levator prostatae. In the female these fibers attach to the lateral vaginal wall to form the pubo-vaginalis or sphincter vaginae. Other fibers attach to the anorectal flexure and fuse with the deep part of the external anal sphincter to form pubo-rectalis; other components are called pubococcygeus and iliococcygeus, which tend to merge into one. Levator ani plays an important role in maintaining the position of the pelvic viscera. On contraction of the pelvic floor, the anterior movement of the vagina produces some compressive action on the urethra against the pubis near the location of the urethral sphincter, reinforcing its action, e.g. during coughing.[6]

In the human female, the paraurethral tissues are joined with muscle fibers of the most medial portion of the levator ani in the region of the proximal urethra. At this site, the medial fibers of levator ani insert into the vaginal wall and provide an arching mechanism that can constrict the urethra.[23] It has also been suggested that the medial fibers of the levator ani muscle have a specific role in controling vesical neck position and in urinary continence mechanisms.[24] The role of the levator ani appears to be to support the proximal urethra and to pull the bladder neck in an anterior direction, such that the lumen is constricted between arching fibers and connective tissue of the levator ani and a connective tissue band (endopelvic fascia) anteriorly. When the levator ani relaxes, the bladder neck can descend, and the lumen can open because the external compression is reduced; at this stage support is provided by the connective tissue of the arcus tendineus fasciae.[7,25] Acute spinal anesthesia has been used to block nerve impulses to the pelvic floor and its effect is to disrupt the active muscular mechanism that supports the bladder neck in healthy continent women.[26] A significant loss of support was demonstrable during spinal anesthesia, indicating that activity originating in the spinal cord and pelvic floor muscles was a major factor responsible for support of the bladder neck.

A recent gross anatomic study of the human female levator ani suggests that the innervation of this muscle is separate from the pudendal nerve; the levator ani nerve in humans runs along the superior surface of the pelvic floor and is innervated by S3–5.[27] Animal studies using neuroanatomic tracing techniques confirm that, in the rat, the origin of the levator ani nerve differs from that of the pudendal nerve within the spinal cord.[9,28,29]

The distribution and properties of different types of striated muscle fibers

Functional properties of fast and slow muscle

Striated muscle fibers can be divided into different types depending on their speed of contraction and their susceptibility to fatigue. Ranvier's classic observations[30] on slowly-contracting 'red' and fast-contracting 'white' muscle indicated that there were at least two types of striated muscle fibers, and studies of the mechanical properties indicated human muscles contain slow twitch and fast twitch fibers (Figure 5.2) which take about 100 ms and 30 ms to reach the peak of their contractions, respectively. The fast units often develop much larger forces, and those that produce the greatest force are fatiguable (the force generated declines on repetitive stimulation); this is the basis of the subdivision of the fast fibers into two subgroups: fatiguable and fatigue resistant. In contrast, the slow units tend to produce smaller forces, and are resistant to fatigue. The proportions of these vary between different muscles.[31]

The fast fibers are innervated by larger alpha motoneurones while the slow fibers are innervated by alphamotoneurones of smaller diameter and lower conduction velocity. The latter are generally tonically active, whereas the former are only activated in a phasic or transient manner; this is known as the 'size principle'.[32] One consequence of the size principle is that the smaller, type I, slow fibers are tonically active and the tonic activity is a result of the regular firing of action potentials along the motoneurones: thus the tonic activity of the striated muscle of the urethral sphincter is generated within the spinal cord and dependent upon the temporal pattern of impulses in different pudendal motoneurones. It is only relatively recently that the relationship between function and histochemical properties has been intensively investigated.

Histochemistry

The dominance of oxidative enzymes, such as succinate dehydrogenase, in slow twitch (type I) fibers and the lack of these in fast fatiguable (type II) fibers is an important histochemical correlate. In the human urethral sphincter, the presence of small diameter fibers containing oxidative enzymes suggests that these are slow fibers, which are adapted to produce a steady tension. There is some evidence that there may also be a few larger fibers that have less ATPase reactivity, and these may be involved less with tonic activity and more with squeezing the urethra at times of transient stresses, such as during coughing. The blood supply of the slow (fibers type I) is rich, whereas the capillary supply in fast fibers is less so. This correlation may be due to the production and release of angiogenic factors – factors that cause the growth of blood vessels – and this will be discussed briefly below. The development of slow and fast contractile properties in striated muscle fibers may be related to the levels of certain transcription factors that are involved in myogenesis. One such factor is MyoD; the mRNA levels of this factor differ between slow and fast muscle, and it is associated particularly with the nuclei of the fastest muscle fibers.[33]

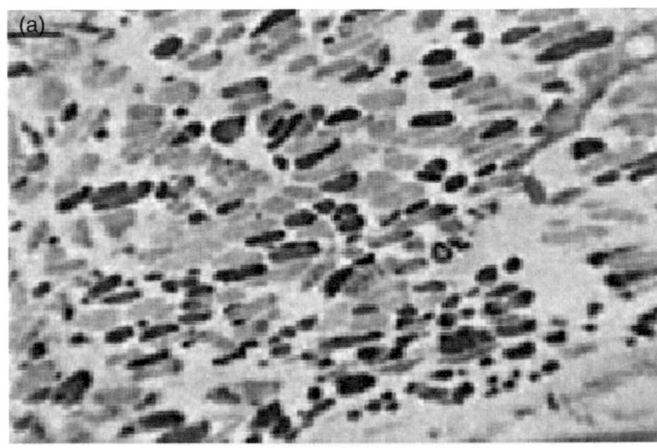

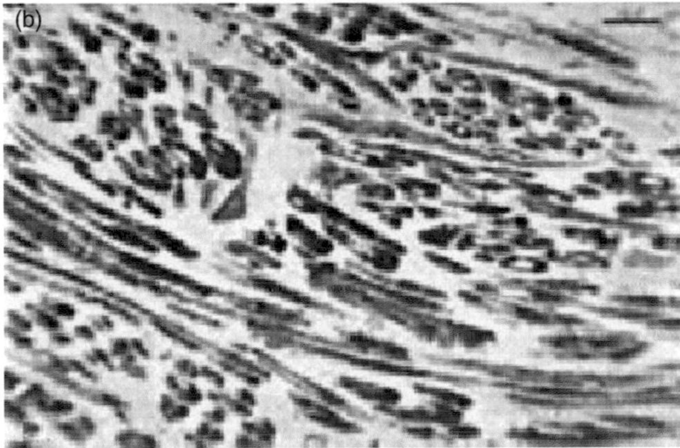

Figure 5.2
Sections from the proximal third of the human male urethra (a) and the female membranous urethra (b) stained for ATPase at pH 4.3, in which the slow-twitch fibers appear darkly stained. Note that most of the female striated muscle is slow twitch, whereas a significant proportion of the male fibers are fast twitch.[6]

The periurethral fibers of the levator ani contains both type I and larger, type II (fast twitch) fibers, which are more concerned with rapid motor responses such as voluntary squeeze;[34] in contrast, the striated fibers of the external urethral sphincter consist mainly of type I (slow twitch) fibers, which are associated with the generation of tone. However, as stated previously, there are sex differences and in the male rhabdosphincter approximately one-third of striated muscle fibers are fast fibers, while in the female only about one-eighth of fibers are fast twitch. Fast and slow muscle fibers differ in their content of oxidative enzymes, creatine kinase, and myoglobin, have different forms of myosin, differences in the expression of transcription factors, and differences in the distribution of nitric oxide synthase in the sarcolemma. The following sections contain some details on these differences.

Creatine kinase Fast and slow muscle contractions are both dependent on ATP availability, and the enzyme creatine kinase, which is normally responsible for energy storage and catalyzes the exchange of high-energy phosphate between creatine phosphate and ATP, is present in highest concentration in the fast fibers. Dahlstedt et al[35] used a mutant animal that was deficient in creatine kinase and showed that the fast fibers fatigued more quickly and this may be related to changes in phosphate concentration on cross-bridge function and the handling of ionized calcium by the sarcoplasmic reticulum. A reduction in maximum tetanic force production has also been observed in CK-deficient animals.[36]

Myoglobin An oxygen storage protein, myoglobin occurs in striated muscle fibers, and is present in higher concentrations in the type I slow muscles of the sort that predominate in the urethral sphincter.[35] Myoglobin is present in oxidative skeletal muscle fibers and facilitates oxygen delivery during periods of high metabolic demand. Its role in muscle performance has been studied in animals that are genetically deficient in myoglobin. Myoglobin-deficient mice have striated muscle fibers that have adapted to the deficiency by converting type I to type II in the soleus muscle as well as other changes, including the expression of angiogenic and endothelial growth factors, which may account for the preserved exercise capacity of these models.[36]

Myosin Biochemical analysis of the myosin chains in different muscles has indicated that the muscle of the rabbit external urethral sphincter has a type of myosin more closely associated with fast red muscles than slow white ones.[37,38] Biochemical analysis of the human external urethral sphincter suggested that there is a degree of diversity in the proportions of fast and slow myosin molecules in different specimens, and this is not related to age.[39,40] In rabbits, fast type myosin exceeded slow type in amount. The ratio of fast to slow myosins in the female was different from that in the male external urethral sphincter, and there appears to be a selective decrease in the volume of type 2 (fast) muscle fibers and/or conversion of type 2 to type 1 (slow) muscle fibers with age and multiparity.[39,40] In male rabbits, the urethral striated muscle appeared to have mainly fast myosin but slow myosin occurred in higher amounts in the proximal region and tended to decrease toward the distal end of the urethra.[40,41] As mentioned earlier, the presence of fast myosin may correlate with the existence of fast muscle extending downwards from the prostatic capsule.

Nitric oxide synthase The essential enzyme in the formation of nitric oxide, nitric oxide synthase, is a mediator in smooth muscle and the nervous system. However, it has been found recently that nitric oxide synthase, which generates the neuromodulator nitric oxide, is present in the sarcolemma of urethral striated muscle fibers.[13,42] Generally speaking, it is found in fast fibers, but there are reports of it also in the larger, slow twitch fibers in the human membranous urethra. In somatic muscles, the presence of nitric oxide synthase in some sarcolemmal membranes appears to be associated with the syntrophin group of proteins that contain multiple protein interaction motifs, and are associated closely with dystrophin. Alpha-syntrophin also has an important role in synapse formation and in the organization of utrophin, the acetylcholine receptor, and acetylcholinesterase at the neuromuscular synapse.[43] Recent studies suggest that there may be a significant role for nitric oxide in the striated muscle of the urethral sphincter.[13,15,44]

Relationship between muscle contractile properties and innervation

Fast fibers are innervated by faster-conducting alpha-motoneurones, and the slow twitch fibers are innervated by the slower alpha-motoneurones. The fast fatiguable fibers also have larger diameters than the fast, fatigue-resistant fibers, which, in turn, are larger than the slow fibers. The nature of the motor innervation of muscle appears to play an important role in determining the contractile properties of the muscle fibers they innervate. Buller et al[45] transected the nerves to the fast flexor digitorum longus and the slow soleus, and reconnected them so that the motoneurones that originally innervated one of these now grew back to reinnervate the other. Their findings were that fast muscle becomes slower and slow muscle becomes faster after cross-innervation. These results have been confirmed by others; however, it is suggested that only about 50% of the cross-reinnervated fibers undergo a change in histochemical type.

The results above indicate that there is a gradation in the properties of striated muscles in the pelvic floor and associated structures, and structures that are specialized for production of tone usually contain a majority of slow twitch fibers. These smaller diameter muscle fibers are innervated by smaller diameter alpha-motoneurones, which also conduct more slowly than those that innervate the fast striated muscle fibers. However, there is increasing evidence of a spectrum of properties, which is not surprising given that the striated muscle of the lower urinary tract must maintain tone, but also respond to transient needs, such as during coughing.

Development of the striated muscle of the urethral sphincter and its innervation

In humans, the urethral sphincter first develops as a condensation of mesenchyme around the urethra after the division of the cloaca, and pubo-rectalis appears soon after, following the opening of the anal membrane. Striated muscle fibers can be clearly differentiated at 15 weeks.[16] At this time, the smooth muscle layer also becomes thicker at the level of the bladder neck and forms the inner part of the urethral musculature. The urethral sphincter is a functional unit composed of central smooth muscle fibers and peripheral striated muscle fibers, which develops mainly in the anterior wall of the urethra. It appears to have an omega-shaped configuration that is recognizable after 10 weeks of gestation in both sexes.[47] The rectovesical septum was found to be well developed in neonates, and studies of various markers suggested that this membrane was unlikely to lead to apoptosis of muscle cells in the posterior part of the external sphincter in males after birth. These authors also concluded that the function of the muscle may change during development because of neuronal maturation. Oelrich[48] described the male urethral sphincter as a striated muscle in contact with the urethra from the base of the bladder to the perineal membrane. This muscle develops before the prostate, which develops as a growth from the urethra through the striated muscle sphincter. The muscle fibers of the urethral sphincter are 25–30% smaller than those in adjacent muscles.

Borirakchanyavat et al[49] studied the sequential expression of smooth and striated muscle proteins in the intrinsic urethral sphincter, where smooth and striated muscle are in adjacent positions, in embryos of 14, 16, and 18 days' gestation, neonates on postnatal day 1, and in adult rats. Sections of the urethra and adjacent levator ani muscles were studied histologically with hematoxylin and eosin, anti-alpha-smooth muscle actin, anti-alpha-sarcomeric actin, and anti-striated muscle myosin heavy chain antibodies. Striated muscle myosin heavy chain protein was absent in the urethral sphincter of the embryo and neonate, and was expressed only in the mature myotubule of adults. Alpha-smooth muscle actin was expressed throughout the urethral sphincter of embryonic and neonatal animals. In adults, alpha-smooth muscle actin was confined to the smooth muscle component of the urethra. Coexpression of alpha-smooth and alpha-sarcomeric muscle actin by the striated sphincter myotubule was noted only in neonates. These authors concluded that the development of the intrinsic urethral sphincter is characterized by sequential expression of well characterized muscle marker proteins. Given the coexpression of smooth and striated muscle markers by developing sphincter myotubule, the authors were tempted to suggest the possibility that transdifferentiation of smooth to striated muscle occurs in the developing genitourinary tract.

Many of the details of these processes have been worked out on animal models, but a paper has been published in which the expression of a protein (p27kip1) has been studied in the muscle fibers of levator ani muscle from aging women and has been related to cell differentiation and degeneration in aging.[50] This protein shows changing expression in differentiating skeletal muscle cells during development, and relatively high levels of p27 RNA were detected in the normal human skeletal muscles. These authors indicated that pelvic floor disorders are associated with an appearance of moderate cytoplasmic p27 expression in perimenopausal patients, and are accompanied by hypertrophy and transition of type II into type I fibers. Elderly patients show shrinking and fragmentation of muscle fibers associated with strong cytoplasmic p27 expression relative to a control group of premenopausal patients.

Innervation of the pelvic floor musculature

During the course of development, each muscle fiber is normally innervated by more than one motoneurone, and these are progressively withdrawn so that in the adult each muscle fiber is innervated by only one alpha-motoneurone. The process of synapse elimination in rats appears to be dependent on the removal of factors that tend to favor polyneuronal innervation, including basic fibroblast growth factor and ciliary neurotrophic factor.[51] Some of these factors are considered in more detail in the section on the cell biology of muscle. In the child and the adult human the following details apply.

Peripheral motor nerves

The peripheral innervation of the striated muscle has been described in a number of reviews,[4,5,9] and there has been recent interest in the innervation of the striated muscle by nitrergic axons.[13,44] Onuf's nucleus is a group of cell bodies of motoneurones that innervate the striated muscle of the anal, urethral, and vaginal sphincters, the pelvic floor, and bulbocavernosus, and is situated in the ventral horn of the sacral cord. While the striated muscle of the external urethral sphincter appears to be innervated mainly by the pudendal nerve, there is also evidence of a minor innervation that reaches the muscle via a pathway traversing the pelvis or using the pelvic nerve.[52–54] This appears to be the case in the rat, dog, and human, although some authors believe that the pelvic pathway is absent in the dog.[55] The innervation of the skeletal muscle of the distal urethra appears to be essentially unilateral,[56] as is the innervation of the pelvic floor.[53] Some of the innervation of the urethral sphincter, probably sensory in nature, arises from branches of the dorsal nerve of the penis.[54] The role of the pudendal innervation of the striated muscles in generating resistance has been studied and the conclusion made that the pudendal nerve was of major importance in maintaining urethral resistance in healthy human females;[56] the influence of vaginal delivery on the pudendal nerve has long been recognized, and several recent studies exist concerning this mechanism.[57,58] However, there are some rat studies that suggest that the pudendal nerve can also play a role in urethral relaxation.[59] It has been generally assumed that the innervation of striated muscle in this region is akin to that found in other parts of the somatic musculature. However, studies suggest that the innervation of levator ani originates outside Onuf's nucleus, and more work is needed to understand fully the complex innervation of this region.[9,27–29,60,61]

Pudendal motoneurones are smaller in diameter than many somatic neurones, in keeping with the size of the muscle fibers they innervate, and they also have a spontaneous repetitive discharge. This tonic activity gives rise to the periurethral skeletal muscle tone and about one-third of the intraurethral pressure at rest is attributable to the tonic activity in the motoneurones that innervate these striated muscles.[62] Not only are these motoneurones smaller in size, their conduction velocities are also less,[63] and there are few synaptic contacts on their surface,[64] which possibly reflects the lack of muscle spindle afferents in urethral muscle, and the lack of Ia afferent input to these motoneurones.[65] There were relatively few monosynaptic inputs from primary afferents in sphincteric motoneurones.[64,66] In addition, Renshaw cell inhibition and crossed disynaptic inhibition are absent.[65,67] Morphologic and functional studies have provided greater insight into the mechanism whereby these cells are activated, and there has been considerable interest in the role of 5-HT in their control.[68–71]

In humans the tonic activity of the pudendal nerves has been studied by infiltration of local nerve block,[72] during which the rate of urine flow during voluntary micturition fell to about 50% of the control values. Pudendal nerve degeneration during childbirth has been offered as a reason for denervation of both the anal and the urethral sphincter in women.[73–75] In contrast, electromyographic (EMG) studies on the urethral sphincter have shown that in some women who experience urinary retention there is an altered activity of the EUS, which was described as bizarre repetitive discharges (Figure 5.3).[75–77]

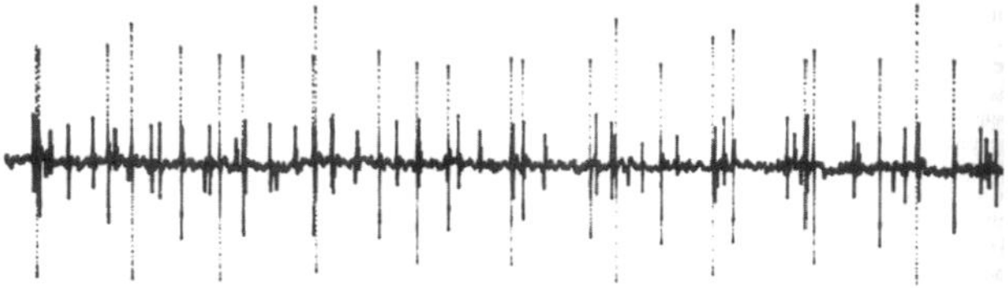

Figure 5.3
Recording of the EMG of the urethral striated muscle in a normal woman during the filling phase of the micturition cycle. The recording was made with a concentric needle electrode. The electrode is picking up signals from at least four different motor units, distinguishable by the amplitude of the spikes. A large increase in the number of units firing is seen during maneuvers that increase intra-abdominal pressure.[75]

Reflex control

One of the unique features of the pelvic floor muscles is that they react to afferent stimuli originating from the skin and muscle of the lower limbs as well as to the state of distention of the bladder and colon: if the bladder is relaxed and filling slowly, then one particular response may occur; however, if the bladder is full and contracting, the behavior of the pelvic floor may be completely different. Reflex control has been considered previously,[4,9,78,79] and the following is a short summary of the conclusions.

Somatic reflexes

Cutaneous stimulation of sacral dermatomes is particularly effective in modulating the activity of the pelvic floor and external urinary sphincter. Light touch of the perineal area is known to cause reflex contraction of the pelvic floor muscles and external anal sphincter, and has been used as a clinical test of segmental nerves to this region. Mechanical stimulation of the urethra in both sexes elicits a complex urethrogenital reflex which includes activation of all of the perineal muscles and clonic activity in some. These reflexes show a coordinated pattern of reflex activity involving the somatic, sympathetic, and parasympathetic systems innervating reproductive organs, dependent on a central motor pattern generator within the spinal cord.[80,81] Painful stimuli in the perineal skin induce a marked increase in EMG activity in periurethral striated muscle; cooling the perineal skin caused a smaller excitation.[80]

Contraction or relaxation of the pelvic floor can also occur in response to proprioceptive stimuli that arise during movement or postural change. Convergence of such afferent inputs from different sources on the activity of pelvic floor and sphincteric muscles is the potential role of afferent impulses from muscles or joints as an adjunct in bladder training and pelvic floor exercises. A variety of maneuvers can cause changes in pelvic floor/sphincteric tone, including attempts to relax and contract the pelvic floor, the Valsalva maneuver, coughing, hip adduction, gluteal contraction, backward tilting of the pelvis, and sit-ups. During hip adduction and gluteal muscle contraction, the urethra contracts concomitantly with the pelvic floor muscles, but not during contraction of the abdominal muscles.

Viscerosomatic reflexes

A guarding reflex that maintains continence by causing urethral sphincter contraction during flow has been described.[82] However, when urethral flow is associated with a bladder contraction, this guarding reflex is overpowered by another reflex that promotes voiding, when relaxation of the sphincter accompanies a rise in bladder pressure or a micturition contraction.[79]

Passive increments in intravesical pressure in spinal rats have been found to elicit contractile activity in the middle region of the urethra mediated by pelvic nerve afferents and sympathetic and somatic nerve efferents.[83,84] It is thought that these reflexes may significantly contribute to the maintenance of continence, for example in patients with stress incontinence.

Micturition has a major inhibitory influence on the pelvic floor activity in humans. Relaxation of the external anal sphincter occurs at the start of the rise in bladder pressure, and precedes the start of urine flow;[85] it is thought to occur concomitantly with the relaxation of the pelvic floor that allows descent of the bladder.[86] The inhibition extends not only to a depression of tonic activity at rest, but causes a reduction in the excitability of pudendal motoneurones involved in reflex functions.[87] In animal models, colonic distention and stimulation of anal afferents also suppress periurethral muscle EMG activity.[80,88–90]

However, this simple explanation becomes more complicated by studies of the periurethral muscle EMG using fine-wire electrodes directly inserted into the region of the urethral sphincter in anesthetized animals. In some animal models, for example the rat, bladder contractions were accompanied by an alternating oscillatory pattern of on–off bursting in EMG activity during the period when the bladder pressure was rising most rapidly. These periods of oscillatory firing in the periurethral EMG during the rising phase of micturition contraction were never seen in spinal animals, and some authors believe that they are generated by supraspinal mechanisms.[91] Recent work on the guinea pig has suggested that this model is closer to the human, and several recent papers have focused on the striated muscle of the urethra in this species and its mechanisms of control.[13,14,68,70,92]

Role of central pathways in the control of the pelvic floor musculature

Anatomy

Spinal cord

The spinal innervation of the striated muscle and the central spinal origins of these have already been described; there are also several recent reviews.[8,9,93,94]

Brainstem and hypothalamus

The central nervous control over the pelvic floor muscles and associated sphincters depends on important descending pathways from regions of the brainstem (particularly the pons and medulla) and the hypothalamus. The dorsolateral pons contains two regions, one of which excites, and the other inhibits tonic activity in the pelvic floor muscles. These regions are close to Barrington's micturition center of the cat and the dorsolateral pontine tegmentum of the rat.[9,95–99] These projections are fairly specific in that they target pudendal motoneurones innervating the urethral sphincter, but not those supplying the anal sphincter. In animals, descending pathways from the pontine micturition center appear to be involved directly in inhibiting the pudendal motoneurones in Onuf's nucleus (Figure 5.4) while those from the L-region facilitate and excite the sphincteric motoneurones. Interneurones that utilize γ-amino butyric acid (GABA) appear to be responsible for the reciprocal inhibition of the sphincteric motoneurones during micturition mediated within the sacral cord[5,9,100,101] (see Figure 4.6).

The paraventricular nuclei of the hypothalamus (which contain oxytocin), and nuclei in the brainstem, including the ipsilateral caudal pontine lateral reticular formation, and the contralateral caudal nucleus retroambiguus also project to the pudendal motoneurones in Onuf's nucleus[97] via the ipsilateral anterior and contralateral white matter in the spinal cord.

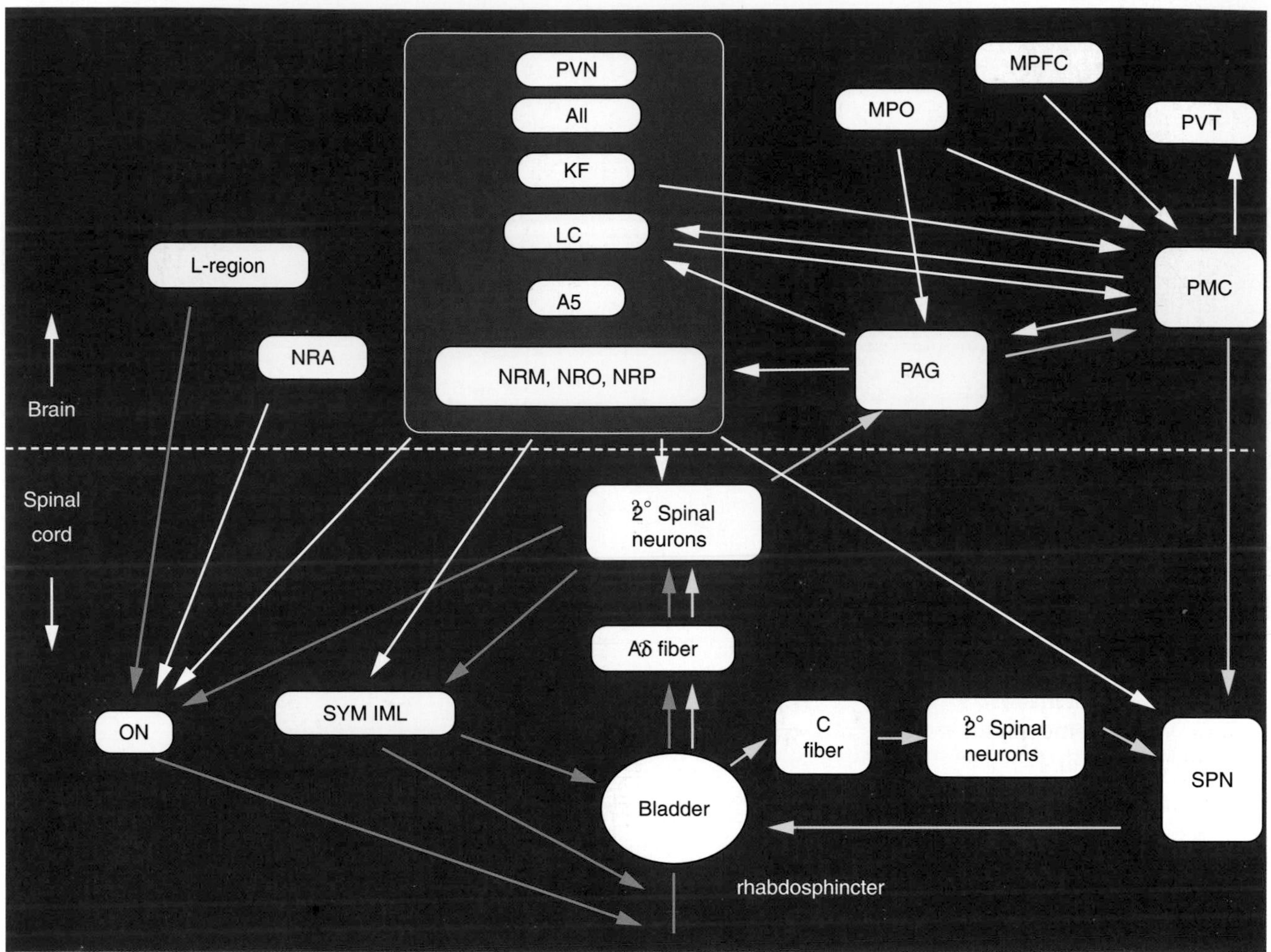

Figure 5.4

Diagram of documented neuroanatomic connections of the primary and secondary components of storage and micturition reflexes. The connections of the primary components of the storage reflexes are shown in red, whereas the connections of the primary components of the micturition reflexes are shown in gold. The connections of the secondary (or modulatory) components of the reflexes are shown in white. Abbreviations: All, All group of dopaminergic neurons; A5, A5 group of noradrenergic neurons; KF, Kollicke–Fuse nucleus; LC, locus coeruleus; MPFC, medial prefrontal cortex; MPO, medial preoptic nucleus of the hypothalamus; NRA, nucleus retroambiguus; NRM, nucleus raphe magnus; NRO, nucleus raphe obscuris; NRP, nucleus raphe pallidus; ON, Onuf's nucleus; PAG, periaqueductal gray; PMC, pontine micturition center; PVN, paraventricular nucleus; PVT, periventricular thalamic nucleus; SPN, sacral parasympathetic nucleus; SYM IML, sympathetic intermediolateral nucleus.[5]

The medullary raphe nuclei and nucleus gigantocellularis reticularis also have a predominantly inhibitory action on bladder motility and sphincteric reflexes.[102–104] We now have results from positron emission tomography (PET) studies and transcortical stimulation that indicate that in humans there are mechanisms that correlate well with what was found in previous animal studies.

The nucleus retroambiguus, located in the caudal ventrolateral medulla, contains motoneurons involved in respiration and control of abdominal musculature. In addition, this nucleus has a prominent projection to Onuf's nucleus.[95,105] It has been speculated that this projection activates sphincter motoneurones coincident with activation of the abdominal muscles during forceful expiration such as coughing, laughing, and sneezing.

Dopaminergic contributions to the control of the urethral sphincter have recently been examined,[106] and this group concluded that activation of D2-like dopamine receptors at a supraspinal site can suppress activity of the striated muscle urethral sphincter.

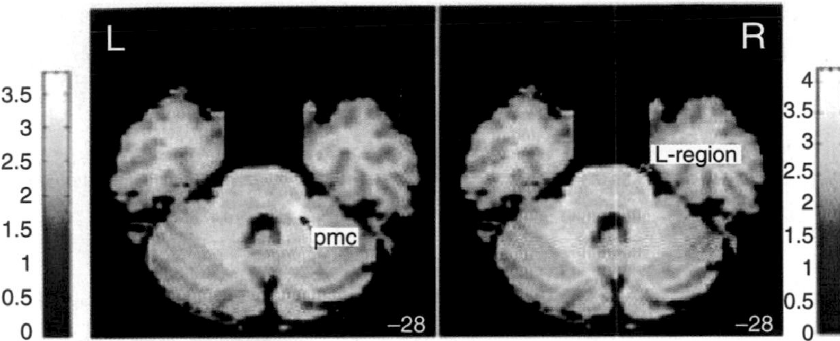

Figure 5.5
PET scan of brainstem with increased activity in vicinity of pontine micturition center (pmc) during voiding. Alternatively, increased activity in L-region association with holding of urine.[5]

Studies on the human CNS during micturition

Spinal cord

The advent of magnetic and electrical stimulators has changed our ability to study the spinal mechanisms of control in the urethral sphincter.[94,107–111] There have also been recent advances in therapy using drugs that interfere with serotonin or noradrenaline metabolism and handling that show promise in some conditions and which act within the spinal cord.[112,113]

Brainstem

Several PET studies have provided evidence that the brainstem is involved in the control of micturition and the external sphincters: men and women were studied during micturition and showed an increased blood flow in the dorsal part of the pons close to the fourth ventricle, an area analogous to the pontine micturition center in the cat (Figure 5.5).[9,99,114,115] A second group of volunteers was asked to micturate during scanning, but were unable to do so. These individuals showed no activation in the dorsal, but did have an area of high blood flow in the ventral pons, similar to the location of the L-region – the pontine storage center in cats. It would appear that these subjects contracted their urethral sphincters and withheld their urine, although they had a full bladder and tried to urinate. There is therefore a reasonable correlation between the information in cats and humans concerning the brainstem regulation of voiding and urine storage (Figure 5.6).[115]

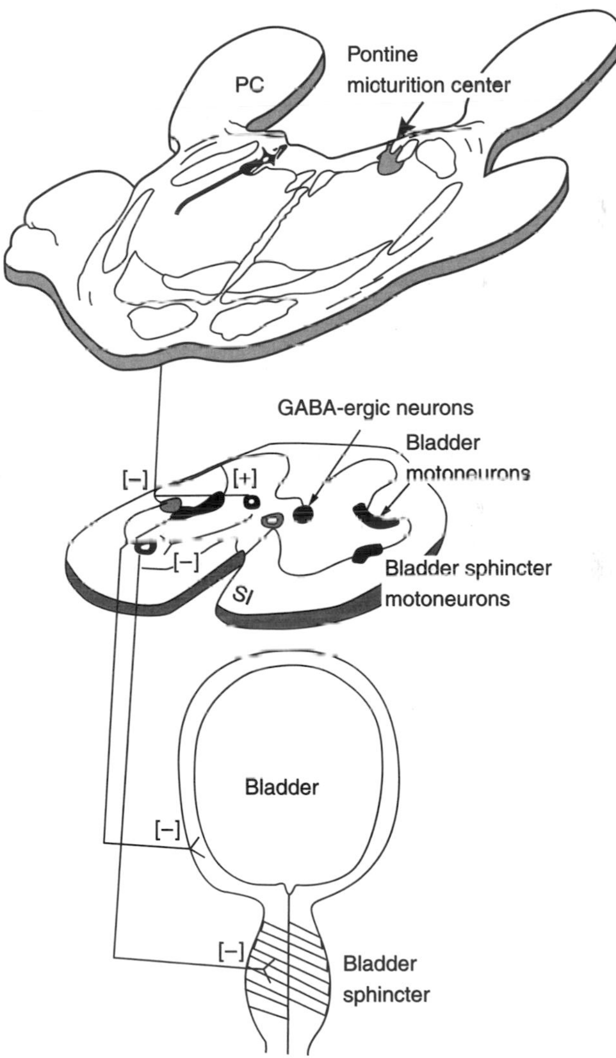

Figure 5.6
Coordination of voiding with external urethral sphincter. Descending glutamatergic input to sacral spinal cord excites bladder neurons in sacral parasympathetic neurons. Simultaneous activation of GABA neurons inhibits sphincter neurons in Onuf's nucleus. Conversely, during attempts at urine storage activation of GABA neurons provides input to bladder neurons while providing excitatory input to sphincter neurons.[5] Cerebellar Peduncle, PC; S1, first sacral spinal segment.

Cortex and hypothalamus: the voluntary control of micturition

PET scanning studies in humans have shown that two cortical areas, the cingulate gyrus and the prefrontal cortex, and the hypothalamus, including the preoptic area, are activated during micturition.[115–117] Cerebral blood flow in the cingulate gyrus was significantly decreased during voluntary withholding of urine and during the urge to void. The prefrontal cortex is active when micturition takes place and during involuntary urine withholding. Possibly, activation of the prefrontal cortex and the anterior cingulate gyrus do not reflect specific involvement in micturition, but more in general mechanisms, such as attention and response selection. The prefrontal cortex plays a role in making the decision whether or not micturition should take place at that particular time and place. Forebrain lesions including the anterior cingulate gyrus are known to cause urge incontinence.[118] The cingulate gyrus influences strongly descending pathways involved in the facilitation of motoneurons and interneurons.

Another PET study on adult female volunteers identified brain structures involved in the voluntary motor control of the pelvic floor. Concomitant activations of the cerebellum, supplementary motor cortex, and thalamus were also commonly present, and the anterior cingulate gyrus was also activated during sustained pelvic floor straining. A recent fMRI study also concluded that the inhibitory control of the micturition reflex requires activity of many structures including the basal ganglia, parietal cortex, limbic system, and cerebellum.[119] There is a also recent review of this area.[9]

In humans, electrophysiologic studies by Hansen[120] also support the view that cortical centers are involved in the descending control of pelvic floor muscles. He provided evidence that the state of the bladder has a significant influence on sphincteric reflex function. Voluntary influences on the pelvic floor, anal sphincter, urethral sphincter and bulbocavernosus muscles of man were studied by transcranial cortical stimulation using either high voltages or short-duration magnetic pulses.[120–122] In contrast to the effects of a small stimulus to the cortex, which causes a short burst of activity in leg muscles, the responses of the anal and urethral sphincters were maintained for 1–2 s, despite the short latency. Voluntary contraction of the external anal sphincter could cause facilitation of the response to cortical stimulation in a number of other muscles, such as tibialis anterior. In humans it had been believed that pelvic floor muscles increase their activity during bladder filling. Hansen[120] also showed that the excitability of pudendal motoneurones could be altered by bladder filling: initially, when bladder volume is low, there appears to be some inhibition of pudendal motoneurones, but when the bladder is full, the motoneurones are facilitated. This facilitation may have been voluntary, as a consequence of sensory information from the bladder. Changes in the excitability of pudendal motoneurones have been reported in humans and in cats.[87,104,123] In humans these techniques have been used during spinal surgery in patients where bowel or bladder function is at risk; the most effective site of stimulation is C4/C3.[124,125]

STRUCTURE AND FUNCTION FOLLOWING NEUROLOGIC LESIONS AND DURING DEVELOPMENT AND AGING

Cell biology of striated muscle and the peripheral nerve–muscle junction

The amount of specific knowledge on the striated muscle of the lower urinary tract is relatively sparse compared with that on other somatic muscles; however, there is a large and increasing body of information derived from somatic muscles that is relevant to the maintenance and regeneration/reinnervation of the muscles of the lower urinary tract. This information, if applied to the muscles of the lower urinary tract, will provide a tremendous impetus to investigate the potential of the new molecules that are being recognized as playing a part in some of the cellular responses associated with stress and strain in pelvic tissues. For example, we are now beginning to understand the molecular basis of the muscle response to stress and the replacement of muscle with fibrous tissue; similarly, we are beginning to understand the factors that operate when stretch of nerves results in partial muscle denervation, and, more importantly, the functional reinnervation of the tissues. The following section aims to highlight some of the mechanisms that operate in the maintenance of the mechanical properties of muscles and the nerves that innervate them, the nerve–muscle junction, the factors that are essential for new functional connections following stress and strain injuries, and the factors that operate during development. Some of the molecules and genes that regulate these processes will be considered individually and in greater detail towards the end of this section.

Effects of denervation on striated muscle

Denervation-induced atrophy is a common clinical observation that is used in diagnosis of disorders of the lower motoneurone, and there should be no surprise that changes in various muscle proteins occur in this condition. For example, Boudriau et al[126] showed that the cytoskeletal lattice in rat fast- and slow-twitch skeletal muscle atrophied following denervation. However, the relative contents of dystrophin and desmin were reduced in the slow-twitch muscle (soleus), while significant increases were shown in the fast-twitch gastrocnemius muscle. In both muscles, a major increase in alpha-tubulin levels were observed, associated with a distinct rearrangement of the microtubule network toward a predominantly longitudinal alignment. It was concluded that fast-twitch muscles are relatively more resistant to denervation-induced atrophy and that the relative increase of the structural proteins in gastrocnemius may be related to this.

Concomitant changes occur in the sarcoplasmic reticulum, where the activity of the calcium pump appears to be decreased in both fast- and slow-twitch muscles following denervation, and these changes were associated with prolongation of twitch contraction times and slowed rates of tension development.[127] These results, however, contrast with some of the earlier findings[128] that suggested that denervation resulted in decreases in calcium pump activity in fast-, but not slow-twitch muscle. Other calcium-binding proteins, such as calsequestrin and parvalbumin, were present in higher concentrations in fast-twitch muscles following denervation. Neuromuscular activity has a modulatory effect, and the expression of parvalbumin is greatly enhanced by phasic, and drastically decreased by tonic, motor neuron activity.

Effects of axotomy on motoneurones: reinnervation following axotomy

Following axotomy, changes occur in the distal portion of the nerve (fragmentation of the axons and degeneration of the Schwann cells), in the morphology of the dendritic fields and in other parameters of the cell bodies within the spinal cord. As the cut neurone terminals begin to grow back toward the peripheral tissues, dramatic changes can be seen, including upregulation of ciliary neurotrophic factor alpha (CNTF alpha) observed in denervated rat muscle[129] and other neurotrophins as well as their receptors.[130] These neurotrophins are produced endogenously by the lesioned nerve and are capable of significantly accelerating the regeneration of both sensory and motor axons after peripheral nerve damage.

Schwann cells also play a role in guiding growing or regenerating nerve terminals back into paralyzed and partially denervated muscles. Trachtenberg and Thompson[131] found that application of a soluble neuregulin isoform, glial growth factor II (GGF2), to developing rat muscles alters the morphology of the Schwann cells at the motoneurone terminal, the nerve terminals themselves, and the postjunctional region of the muscle fibers. The Schwann cells put out processes and migrate away from the synapse, and the nerve terminals retract from acetylcholine receptor-rich synaptic sites, and their axons grow, in association with Schwann cells, to the ends of the muscle. These axons make effective synapses only after withdrawal of the GGF2.

Our understanding of the basic events underlying synapse formation, maintenance, and plasticity has progressed considerably over the last few years, primarily because of the numerous studies that have focused on the nerve–muscle junction and the use of electrophysiologic, morphologic, pharmacologic, and recombinant DNA technology. We will consider two scenarios, first that occurring during development, and second, that pertinent to reinnervation following injury.

Molecular factors involved in stability of synapses

Synapse formation and maintenance at the somatic nerve–muscle junction depends upon the expression of a number of molecules, some of which are considered essential: agrin, muscle-specific kinase (MuSK) and rapsyn;[132] and others, including the neuregulins and neurotrophins, that have important actions. These molecules work together to ensure the development of the complex arrangement seen in the adult skeletal nerve–muscle junction, and are also involved in the maintenance of these structures and the processes necessary for reinnervation and reinstatement of a functional synapse between motoneurones and skeletal muscle.

Agrin

Agrin was originally isolated from the basal lamina of the synaptic cleft, and has been found to be synthesized and secreted by motoneurons. It triggers formation of acetylcholine receptor (AChR) clusters on cultured myotubes,[133] and when deficient, the postsynaptic AChR aggregates are markedly reduced in number, size, and density in muscles of agrin-deficient mutant mice. These results support the hypothesis that agrin is a critical organizer of postsynaptic differentiation.[134] Animals deficient in this factor show abnormal intramuscular nerve branching and presynaptic differentiation.

The same group[135] found that differentiation of the postsynaptic membrane at the neuromuscular junction requires (a) agrin (derived from the presynaptic nerve), (b) MuSK, a component of the agrin receptor in muscle, and (c) rapsyn, a protein that interacts with AChRs. From a functional viewpoint, it appears that agrin, arising from the motor nerve, works through MuSK in the postsynaptic membrane to determine a synaptogenic region within which synaptic differentiation occurs.[135] The process reinforces developing clusters of nicotinic receptors, but also seems to have effects on the neural growth cone so that it differentiates into a stable nerve terminal in contact with the muscle endplate region. There is also evidence that the specialized presynaptic mechanisms that enable release of neurotransmitter are also stabilized by this system.[136]

Muscle-specific kinase (MuSK)

During development, MuSK (and agrin) enable the clustering of nicotinic receptors in the postsynaptic membrane at the endplate, which occurs as a result of gene transcription in the muscle nuclei immediately below the endplate. Similar aggregations of acetylcholinesterase (AChE) also develop because of the complex actions of these molecules.

The role of MuSK in adults appears to be a continuation of this process – it seems to stabilize the nerve–muscle junction, maintaining levels of the nicotinic receptor at the endplate as well as the functional integrity of the junction and inhibition of axonal growth and remodeling.[137] Mutations of MuSK give rise to certain myesthenic syndromes.[138,139]

AChE is associated with the basal lamina within the nerve–muscle junction, and its localization to this position appears to depend on complexes of AChE with a type of collagen (collagen Q) present in the basal lamina and with MuSK. This is further evidence that the MuSK complex may be involved in the regulation of synaptic gene expression at the nerve–muscle junction.[140,141]

Rapsyn

The role of rapsyn was studied by Bartlett et al,[142] who found that its absence resulted in pre- and postsynaptic defects, including failure to cluster AChRs. The mRNA level for ciliary neurotrophic factor (CNTF) was decreased in the rapsyn-deficient muscles compared with those of controls, although those for NGF, BDNF, NT-3, and TGF-beta$_2$ were not affected. These authors suggested that failure to form postsynaptic specializations in rapsyn-deficient mice caused an alteration in the CNTF cytokine signaling pathway within skeletal muscle, which may, in turn, account for the increased muscle–nerve branching and motoneuron survival seen in rapsyn-deficient mice. This conclusion is supported by the observations of English and Schwartz,[51] who found that the postnatal elimination of polyneuronal innervation can be inhibited by basic fibroblast growth factor and ciliary neurotrophic factor.

Neuregulins

Neuregulins (NRGs) are a subfamily of molecules similar to endothelial growth factor and play a part in the development of Schwann cells and the formation of the nerve–muscle junction. They activate a Ras/MAP kinase signaling cascade, which ultimately induces nAChR epsilon-subunit gene expression in the subendplate nuclei.[143] Neuregulin appears to act on the postsynaptic erbB family of receptor tyrosine kinases, and acts at synaptic sites.[134,144] Curare, which blocks nicotinic receptors, reduces synaptic neuregulin expression in a dose-dependent manner, yet has little effect on synaptic agrin or a muscle-derived heparan sulfate proteoglycan. This modulation of postsynaptic structures by alterations of synaptic activity and changes in the expression of synaptic regulatory factors is part of the mechanism by which nerves influence the function of muscle. A number of factors change as a result of such blockade of electrical activity, including an increase in the number and a decrease in the size of AChR aggregates, and reductions in brain-derived neurotrophic factor and NT-3, and these were thought to indicate the existence of a local, positive feedback loop between synaptic regulatory factors that translates activity into structural changes at neuromuscular synapses.[145] This loop was targeted in some studies in which the neuroregulin-1 gene was disrupted: knockouts showed peripheral neuronal projections defasciculated and displayed aberrant branching patterns within their targets. Motor nerve terminals were transiently associated with broad bands of postsynaptic AChR clusters. Initially, Schwann cell precursors accompanied peripheral projections, but later, Schwann cells were absent from axons in the periphery. Following the initial stages of synapse formation, sensory and motor nerves withdrew and degenerated. These studies suggest that NRG-1-mediated signaling is involved in the normal maintenance of synapses; however, the interactions are more complex, involving the motoneuron terminal, muscle, and the Schwann cells at the nerve–muscle junction. It appears that NRG-1 plays a central role in the normal maintenance of peripheral synapses, and ultimately in the survival of CRD-NRG-1-expressing neurons.[146] The role of neuregulin in the development and maintenance of the nerve–muscle junction has recently been questioned,[147] but there is increasing evidence for its involvement in signaling between axons and Schwann cells,[148] and in the differentiation of muscle spindles.[149]

Neurotrophins and other trophic factors

Neurotrophins are a family of protein growth factors structurally related to the nerve growth factor (NGF) and include neurotrophin-1 (nerve growth factor; NGF), neurotrophin-2 (NT-2), neurotrophin-3 (NT-3), and neurotrophin-4/5 (NT-4). Other growth factors include basic fibroblast growth factor (bFGF), brain-derived neurotrophic factor (BDNF), glial-derived neurotrophic factor (GNDF), and ciliary neurotrophic factor (CNTF).

A variety of neurotrophins and growth factors are expressed in the skeletal muscle during the critical period of synapse formation.[150] The relationship between neurotrophins and the development of the nerve–muscle junction during development is not completely worked out, but it is known that during fetal life the molecular nature of the nicotinic receptor differs from the adult: the gamma subunit of the AChR in the fetus is replaced by the epsilon subunit in the adult. It has been shown that this changeover in postsynaptic molecular organization could be interfered with by genetic manipulation that prevented the normal development of the receptor.[151] The result was that the structural development of the endplate was compromised and there was a severely reduced AChR density and a profound reorganization of AChR-associated components of the postsynaptic membrane and cytoskeleton. The development of the motor endplate appears to depend on the activity of muscle cell nuclei that are located in the vicinity of the postsynaptic membrane. NT-3 appears to be involved in this process.[150] Jasmin et al[152] proposed that transcription processes in these nuclei are functionally different to those of nuclei of the extrasynaptic sarcoplasm. Thus, renewal of proteins concerned with neuromuscular transmission in the postsynaptic membrane appears to occur via a mechanism involving the activation of genes in nuclei adjacent to the nerve–muscle junction using chemical signals originating from motoneurons. Such interaction between presynaptic nerve terminals and the postsynaptic sarcoplasm indicates that the entire signal transduction pathway is compartmentalized at the level of the neuromuscular junction. Such chemical signals are discussed later and include neuregulin and agrin, and there is evidence that these are involved during both development and recovery from injury.

NT-4 and BDNF occur in motoneurons and muscle fibers, and the latter can release them during contractions. They both enhance synaptic transmission at neuromuscular junctions by activating tyrosine kinase receptor B (TrkB). Some of their actions are presynaptic – BDNF can increase the release of synaptic vesicles – and NT-4 can increase local levels of neuregulin or other nerve-derived modulators.[153] Thus NT-4 influences the development of presynaptic neuronal terminals, and such regulation is specific to the axonal branch that innervates that specific myocyte within the motor unit;[154] a consequence of this is that neurotrophin-induced synaptic changes can be spatially restricted to the site of neurotrophin secretion and appear not to spread to neighboring synapses, i.e. the part of the motor unit subjected to NT-4 is targeted individually, and the effects do not spread to other terminals of the motoneurone. CNTF is a member of the neurotrophin family that, amongst other things, regulates agrin-induced postsynaptic differentiation,[155] induces axons and their nerve terminals to sprout within adult skeletal muscles,[156] has trophic actions on denervated skeletal muscle,[157] and is highly correlated with the reinnervation activity of Schwann cells.[158]

Regeneration of striated muscle; satellite cells; fibrosis

Regeneration and repair of skeletal muscle

Skeletal muscle satellite cells are situated between the sarcolemma and the basement membrane and have the potential to develop into skeletal muscle. Normally they are quiescent and differ from skeletal muscle in that they have only one nucleus, and appear to be a reserve population of cells that can differentiate into skeletal muscle, particularly following muscle injury, when they proliferate extensively.[159] Some of these dividing satellite cells can fuse with each other to form a multinucleate cell and produce myofibrils. It has been estimated that each human being has around 10^{10} satellite cells and that these normally form a relatively static population, except in injury or disease, when they proliferate.[160,161] Satellite cells appear to undergo self-renewal such that they may participate in repeated episodes of injury-induced regeneration.[162,163]

These cells possess a number of molecular markers, such as Pax-7, that are used to monitor their activities. It seems likely that these cells do not form a homogeneous population and at least three varieties probably exist,[164] one of which may have a hemopoietic origin. Other workers have also provided evidence for a progenitor cell coming from the bone marrow via the myeloid line.[165–168] IGF-1 has been identified as a mediator that enhances the recruitment of hemopoietic cells to sites of tissue damage.[169,170] There is some doubt as to the quantitative aspects of this transformation normally,[171] and some authors argue that the hemopoietic stem cells, while migrating to muscle tissue, do not take part in intrinsic myogenicity.[172] It is possible that only a minority of satellite cells is responsible for adult muscle regeneration and that these stem cells survive the effects of aging to retain their intrinsic potential throughout life.[173]

Different types of muscle fibers (types 1 and 2) in limb muscles appear to regenerate using intrinsically different precursor cells, and this may be relevant to the regeneration of the tonic muscle variety found in the rhabdosphincter.[174] Several attempts have been made to provide damaged muscle tissue with stem cells. One study suggests that implantation of cellularized scaffolds is better than direct injection for delivering myogenic cells into regenerating skeletal muscle.[175,176]

Molecular changes during denervation and reinnervation

Following denervation of a muscle, nerve terminal withdrawal is accompanied by a loss of AChRs at corresponding postsynaptic sites during the process of synapse elimination in developing and in adult neuromuscular junctions. The dismantling of the postsynaptic specialization involves rapid dissolution of some structures and slower loss of others.[177] MuSK, normally restricted to the motor endplate, starts to appear outside the endplate region on the muscle fibers within a few days, and takes about two weeks to disappear from the endplate itself; the distribution of MuSK is precisely coordinated with that of the nicotinic receptors[178,179] and other factors that influence the distribution are muscle activity, and agrin. After reimplantation of a nerve into the denervated rat soleus muscle, ectopic neuromuscular junctions develop outside the junctional region, and neural-derived agrin is able to cause protein aggregation in the early stages of new endplate formation, and also to initiate the distribution of organelles which appear as the apparatus reaches maturity.[180]

Another feature of muscle that is affected by innervation and denervation is the arrangement of the costameres: normal innervated skeletal muscle fibers contain dystrophin and beta-dystroglycan in an arrangement referred to as a costamere. These molecules are arranged in a transverse direction in a rib-like pattern with stripes over the Z and M lines, but the orientation of these molecules becomes longitudinal rather than transverse after denervation. Electrical stimulation of denervated muscle causes these costameres to revert to the normal transverse orientation, and neural agrin also simulates this change.[181]

Regeneration and repair in the urethral rhabdosphincter and levator ani

The presence of satellite cells in the rhadsosphincter has been demonstrated, and their proliferation can be enhanced through both the endogenous and exogenous actions of hepatocyte growth factor (HGF) and insulin-like growth factor-1 (IGF-1) via extracellular signal–related kinase 1 and 2 (ERK1/2) and – akt murine thymoma viral oncogene homolog–1 (Akt).[182] The question of whether the urethral rhabdosphincter can regenerate using satellite cells has been approached recently using the same mechanisms as occur in skeletal muscles. Satellite cells were shown to proliferate and form multinucleated myotubes *in vitro*, and this was associated with complete recovery of the striated urethral sphincter *in vivo*, as assessed by normalization of muscle strength and of myofiber number and diameter.[183] Local injections of stem cells into the urethral rhabdosphincter were able to improve the pressure at which urine leakage occurred.[184] The rhabdosphincter appears to change its proportion of different muscle fiber types with age,[185] and it has already been noted that these two fiber types appear to derive from different precursor cells,[174] but this specific question with respect to the urethral sphincter is unresolved at the present time.

The rat levator ani muscle is susceptible to age, treatment with androgens, and to denervation.[186–188] It has been found that the satellite cell pool is unaffected by aging, and does not respond mitotically following denervation. However, it appears to be susceptible to androgen treatment or withdrawal.[189,190]

The therapeutic implications of this knowledge and the possible origin of the sphincteric satellite cells are exciting, and several lines of activity in relation to sphincteric regeneration have been followed.[191,192] Implantation of extrinsic muscle precursor cells into the rhabdosphincter has been shown to result in selective incorporation into striated myofibers,[191] and can recapitulate a myogenic program when injected into an irreversibly injured sphincter. Furthermore, there is evidence that the maturation of these cells activates nerve regeneration and restores functional motor units.[193,194] A recent review, however, points to some of the difficulties of this new technology;[193] however, there remains hope that cell therapy may provide some therapeutic benefit for the treatment of urinary incontinence in humans.

Development of fibrosis in skeletal muscle

The recovery of muscle function following injury is a challenging problem if techniques are to be developed to improve striated muscle function when it is weakened by injury. Kasemkijwattana et al[195,196] and Menetrey et al[197] observed a massive muscle regeneration occurring in the first two weeks following injury that was subsequently followed by the development of muscle fibrosis. The possibility of enhancement of muscle growth and regeneration, as well as the prevention of fibrotic development, was considered, and three growth factors capable of enhancing myoblast proliferation and differentiation *in vitro* and of improving the healing of the injured muscle *in vivo* were identified. The three growth factors capable of improving muscle regeneration and improving muscle force in an injured muscle were bFGF, IGF, and NGF. The same group considered the use of gene transfer using an adenovirus to deliver an efficient and persistent expression of these growth factors to the injured muscle. These studies may indicate a new strategy to aid efficient muscle healing with complete functional recovery following muscle contusion and strain injury.

The process of fibrosis may be associated with the activities of another family of membrane proteins, the integrins, which are responsible for the regulation of interactions between the myocytes and the extracellular matrix.[198] Integrin beta1D provides a strong link between the cytoskeleton and extracellular matrix, necessary to support mechanical tension during muscle contraction. It is expressed in the cell membranes of striated muscle tissues, and binds to both cytoskeletal and extracellular matrix proteins.

Angiogenesis and capillary density

IGF-1 also appears to be involved in the regulation of the size of myocytes and the capillary density.[198] Muscle hypoplasia results from disruption of the IGF-1 gene and its effects are seen on cell proliferation, differentiation, and apoptosis during development; the concomitant reduction in capillary density may result from both direct and indirect influences on angiogenesis. It appears that the sympathetic innervation may influence angiogenesis through the release of the cotransmitter neuropeptide Y (NPY). NPY mediates neurogenic ischemic angiogenesis at physiologic concentrations by activating Y2/Y5 receptors and eNOS, in part due to the release of vascular endothelial growth factor (VEGF).[199] A review indicates the range of mediators that may be involved in the formation of new blood vessels.[200]

Reflex control of the striated muscle of the lower urinary tract following spinal injury

It has been known for over 50 years that somatic events influence the bladder of paraplegic patients,[201] and recently there is increasing evidence for a role of viscero or somatic convergence in the control of the human pelvic floor. Such interactions are particularly true in patients with overactive bladders. Another feature of human paraplegia is that some patients develop automatic bladders and achieve some degree of sphincter inhibition during micturition, whereas others have a hypertonic sphincter and require regular catheterization. In experimental studies for the last 30 years, scientists have reported that the motor pathway to the external sphincters and pelvic floor is subject to control from events in viscera and the segmental innervation of somatic structures. The pathways that control the striated muscle of the external sphincter as well as the detrusor smooth muscle are summarized in Figures 5.4 and 5.6. Figure 5.4 indicates that certain nuclei in the brainstem are of particular importance in the regulation of the external sphincter, including the L-region and the nucleus retroambiguus, which have major projections to Onuf's nucleus, and are of particular importance in maintaining continence and facilitating urine storage.[5,9] This topic has been reviewed recently.[9,202,203]

In a study of chronic spinal cats, Sasaki[63] found detrusor–sphincteric dyssynergia in about 50% of chronic spinal cats, while the other 50% achieved some sphincter inhibition during bladder contractions. Sphincteric responses to stimuli were affected by the state of bladder filling, and when the bladder was empty, tactile stimulation of the perineal skin caused an increase in EUS activity and detrusor contractions in spinal animals, the opposite of what occurs in animals with a normal intact neuroaxis. In contrast, when the bladder was full, rhythmic detrusor contractions were present, and tactile stimulation caused EUS activity and bladder contractions, and noxious stimulation of the skin resulted in an immediate contraction of the bladder, followed by some depression of ongoing rhythmic contractions. The effects on the sphincter depended on the state of the sphincter, and when dyssynergia was present, innocuous tactile stimulation was accompanied by a prolonged increase in EUS activity that was not inhibited during micturition contractions. Reflex responses of the sphincter induced by electrical stimulation of afferents in the pudendal nerve were inhibited in spinal animals with a normal synergic relationship between the bladder and urethra, but in dyssynergia, relaxation of the sphincter and inhibition of pudendal nerve reflex responses during bladder contractions were absent. There has been recent interest in the role of 5-hydroxytryptamine (5-HT) in the injured spinal cord; it was shown that the disruption of phasic activity in the external urethral sphincter in spinal cord injury could be improved to some extent by treatment with 8-OH-DPAT.[204]

The clinical literature clearly distinguishes between lesions of the spinal cord in which the peripheral innervation of the striated muscle of the pelvic floor and sphincters is intact, and lesions in which there is peripheral denervation. There may also be a small group where there is a mix of a high lesion and some peripheral denervation. Perlow and Diokno[205] found that a neurogenic bladder developed in spinal patients with lesions at T7 and above, whereas peripheral denervation was common in lesions at vertebral T11 and below. Vesicosphincteric dyssynergia developed in about two-thirds of their patients with neurogenic bladders; the increased excitability of pudendal motoneurones was associated with increased excitability of the bulbocavernosus reflex.[206] During the phase of spinal shock following spinal cord injury in humans, bladder filling was found to be accompanied by an increased urethral resistance in the bladder neck region, not associated with an increased EMG activity of the pelvic floor,[207] presumably associated with smooth muscle activity. Areflexia could also be present. In some patients with spinal cord injuries, bladder contraction and distention of the rectum resulted in inhibition of EMG activity in the external urethral and anal sphincters, whereas in the levator ani, there was sometimes an initial excitation of the muscle.[208]

Rossier et al,[209] using pudendal nerve blockade and injections of phentoamine to dissociate the effects of striated and smooth muscle, found that the dyssynergia was due to the passage of impulses along the pudendal nerves, and that about two-thirds of the urethral pressure was due to striated muscle tone developed by this impulse activity – rather more than in normal subjects.[72] Rossier et al[209] commented that there was no evidence of a sympathetic innervation of striated muscle. However, more recent experiments on cats have suggested that the cholinergic preganglionic fibers of the sympathetic system can grow and form functional contacts with denervated striated muscle following the experimental section of spinal roots.[210] Possibly a more detailed study of reinnervation of the striated muscle of the lower urinary tract in humans would support this possibility.

Investigation of the neural connectivity can now be performed using a variety of neurophysiologic and radiologic techniques. Thiry and Deltenre[211] found that electrical stimulation of the head can be used to assess the volitional as well as segmental and suprasegmental influences on the behavior of the external urethral sphincter; however, subjects were not tolerant of the electrical stimuli. Magnetic stimulation of the brain, spinal cord, and peripheral nerves, however, has been pioneered in the last decade or so and appears to be tolerated better; its use has had considerable impact on the study of the neural control of the striated muscle of the anal sphincter.[95,212–221] It has most recently enabled the study of the control of different parts of the sphincteric apparatus around the anus, and has allowed the effects of birth trauma on different parts of the external anal sphincter to be defined.[222–224] In the lower urinary tract there were early demonstrations of the usefulness of the technique in studying the central and peripheral pathways to the external urethral sphincter,[225,226] perineum,[227] pelvic floor,[228] and bulbocavernosus.[217,229,230] Magnetic stimulation has also been used to confirm the presence of complete or partial lesion of the spinal cord and functional characteristics of the latter.[231] The potential therapeutic use of magnetic stimulation has been pioneered by Craggs in hyperreflexic states.[232,233]

An alternative approach to the hypertonic sphincter has been used by Phelan et al,[234] who reported the results following injection of botulinus toxin into the spastic urethral sphincter. Botulinus toxin (Botox) acts presynaptically to prevent the release of acetylcholine at the nerve–muscle junction. It is a very powerful lethal neurotoxin and is delivered in very small doses in these studies, and acts to dissociate the link between high frequencies of impulses in the pudendal motoneurones and the contractile response. These authors claimed that this could be a useful treatment for some patients' sphincter dyssynergia.

In a study of the lower urinary tract in patients with neurologic disorders, Sakakibara et al[235] studied patients with detrusor–sphincteric dyssynergia, and found that one group had uninhibited external sphincter relaxation. In these patients there was an abnormal reduction of external urethral sphincter pressure (by 64 ± 27 cmH_2O (mean ± standard deviation)) and variation in both the sphincteric pressure and EMG. Fluoroscopy showed that bladder neck opening was commonly associated with extreme urge sensation. This appears possibly to be the normal reflex response to bladder contraction involving a major reduction in efferent activity to the striated muscle. However, other patients with detrusor–external sphincter dyssynergia failed to relax their sphincters during attempted voiding, and fluoroscopic imaging showed an incomplete or absent urethral opening at the external sphincter. The mean reduction of urethral pressure during attempted voiding in this group was only 6.4 ± 6.7 cmH_2O and 5.0 ± 9.5 cmH_2O (females and males, respectively). Possibly this group were unable to inhibit the pudendal motoneuron activity. These results correlate reasonably well with the study on cats by Sasaki et al.[236]

Reflex control of the striated muscle of the lower urinary tract following other neurologic lesions

Parkinson's disease

Chemical or surgical lesions of dopamine-containing neurons in the basal ganglia in the rat cause changes in motor activity akin to those seen in Parkinson's disease, and the urodynamic results suggest that the bladder of these animals is overactive. The dopaminergic nerves that are affected in Parkinson's disease projections of dopamine-containing fibers from the substantia nigra have opposing effects on the bladder depending on whether the D1 or D2 receptors are activated. Activation of D2 receptors is excitatory to micturition, whereas D1 receptors are inhibitory. However, these receptors can also suppress activity of the striated muscle urethral sphincter, and the urge incontinence symptoms often seen in patients with Parkinson's disease may be aggravated because of the decreased urethral resistance induced by D2 dopamine receptor activation.[106]

In humans, Pavlakis et al[237] described detrusor dyssynergia in the majority of Parkinson's disease patients studied, and the EMG investigations showed that a few patients had a voluntary contraction of the perineal floor in an attempt to prevent leakage, while others had sphincter bradykinesia, which was associated with the generalized skeletal muscle hypertonicity found in Parkinsonism. This was reinvestigated by Stocchi et al,[238] who found that incomplete pelvic floor relaxation was present in about one-quarter of patients, while another quarter had hyperreflexia associated with vesicosphincteric synergy; a further 10% had hyperreflexia with vesicosphincteric synergy associated with incomplete pelvic floor relaxation. Urologic manifestations of Parkinson's disease tend to be associated with the severity and duration of the condition.

Stroke

A commonly used experimental model of stroke involves ligation of the middle cerebral artery of the rat, which results in cerebral ischemia and infarction. The urodynamic status of this model is characterized by bladder overactivity consistent with the loss of cerebral inhibition of the lower urinary tract.[105,239] Urodynamic studies on incontinent patients following a stroke showed a disturbance in the function of the striated muscle of the lower urinary tract including detrusor–sphincter dyssynergia.[240] Sakakibara et al[241] reported bladder hyper-reflexia, detrusor–sphincter dyssynergia, and uninhibited sphincter relaxation in patients with stroke. The same group[242] subsequently demonstrated that frontal lobe disease may cause disorders of storage as well as of voiding; they observed uninhibited sphincter relaxation and unrelaxing sphincter on voiding and disturbances of bladder function in these patients.

References

1. Torrens M, Morrison JFB. The Physiology of the Lower Urinary Tract. Berlin: Springer-Verlag, 1987.
2. Morrison J. Central nervous control of the bladder. In: Jordan D, ed. Central Nervous Control of Autonomic Function, Vol 11. London: Harwood, 1997: 129–50.
3. de Groat W, Downie J, Levin R et al. Basic neurophysiology and neuropharmacology. In: Abrams P, Khoury S, Wein A eds. Incontinence. UK: Health Publication, 1999: 105–54.
4. Morrison JFB. Physiology of the striated muscles of the pelvic floor. In: Corcos J, Schick E, eds. The Urinary Sphincter. New York: Marcel Dekker, 2001: 43–70.
5. Morrison J, Steers W, Brading AF et al. Neurophysiology and neuropharmacology. In: Abrams P, Cardozo L, Khoury S, Wein A eds. Incontinence. UK: Health Publication, 2002: 83–164.
6. Gosling J, Alm P, Bartsch G, Bubaker L, Creed K, Delmas V et al. Gross anatomy of the urinary tract. In: Abrams P, Khoury S, Wein A eds. Incontinence. UK: Health Publications, 1999: 21–56.
7. Delancey J, Gosling JA, Creed K et al. Gross anatomy and cellular biology of the lower urinary tract. In: Abrams P, Cardozo L, Khoury S, Wein A eds. Incontinence. Health Publication, 2002: 17–82.
8. de Groat WC. Integrative control of the lower urinary tract: pre-clinical perspective. Br J Pharmacol 2006; 147(Suppl 2): S25–40.
9. Morrison J, Birder L, Craggs M et al. Neural control. In: Abrams P, Cardozo L, Khoury S, Wein A eds. Incontinence. Health Publication, 2005: 367–422.
10. Greenland JE, Brading AF. Urinary bladder blood flow changes during the micturition cycle in a conscious pig model. J Urol 1996; 156(5): 1858–61.
11. Thind P. The significance of smooth and striated muscles in the sphincter function of the urethra in healthy women. Neurourol Urodyn 1995; 14(6): 585–618.
12. Andersson PO, Malmgren A, Uvelius B. Functional responses of different muscle types of the female rat urethra in vitro. Acta Physiol Scand 1990; 140(3): 365–72.
13. Walters RD, McMurray G, Brading AF. Pudendal nerve stimulation of a preparation of isolated guinea-pig urethra. BJU Int 2006; 98(6): 1302–9.
14. Walters RD, McMurray G, Brading AF. Comparison of the urethral properties of the female guinea pig and rat. Neurourol Urodyn 2006; 25(1): 62–9.
15. Yucel S, De SA Jr, Baskin LS. Neuroanatomy of the human female lower urogenital tract. J Urol 2004; 172(1): 191–5.
16. Yucel S, Baskin LS. An anatomical description of the male and female urethral sphincter complex. J Urol 2004; 171(5): 1890–7.
17. Tunn R, Goldammer K, Neymeyer J et al. MRI morphology of the levator ani muscle, endopelvic fascia, and urethra in women with stress urinary incontinence. Eur J Obstet Gynecol Reprod Biol 2006; 126(2): 239–45.
18. Stolzenburg JU, Neuhaus J, Liatsikos EN et al. Histomorphology of canine urethral sphincter systems, including three-dimensional reconstruction and magnetic resonance imaging. Urology 2006; 67(3): 624–30.
19. Karam I, Droupy S, Abd-Alsamad I et al. Innervation of the female human urethral sphincter: 3D reconstruction of immunohistochemical studies in the fetus. Eur Urol 2005; 47(5): 627–33.
20. Karam I, Moudouni S, Droupy S et al. The structure and innervation of the male urethra: histological and immunohistochemical studies with three-dimensional reconstruction. J Anat 2005; 206(4): 395–403.
21. Andrich DE, Rickards D, Landon DN, Fowler CJ, Mundy AR. Structural assessment of the urethral sphincter in women with urinary retention. J Urol 2005; 173(4): 1246–51.
22. Fritsch H, Lienemann A, Brenner E, Ludwikowski B. Clinical anatomy of the pelvic floor. Adv Anat Embryol Cell Biol 2004; 175: III–64.
23. DeLancey JO. Functional anatomy of the female lower urinary tract and pelvic floor. Ciba Found Symp 1990; 151: 57–69.
24. DeLancey JO, Starr RA. Histology of the connection between the vagina and levator ani muscles. Implications for urinary tract function. J Reprod Med 1990; 35(8): 765–71.
25. DeLancey JO. The pathophysiology of stress urinary incontinence in women and its implications for surgical treatment. World J Urol 1997; 15(5): 268–74.
26. Haeusler G, Sam C, Chiari A et al. Effect of spinal anaesthesia on the lower urinary tract in continent women. Br J Obstet Gynaecol 1998; 105(1): 103–6.
27. Barber MD, Bremer RE, Thor KB et al. Innervation of female levator ani muscles. Am J Obstet Gynecol 2002; 187: 64–71.
28. Bremer RE, Barber MD, Coates KW, Dolber PC, Thor KB. Innervation of intrapelvic skeletal muscles in the female rat. Anat Rec 2003; 275A: 1031–41.
29. Bremer RE, Barber MD, Coates KW, Dolber PC, Thor KB. Innervation of the levator ani and coccygeus muscles of the female rat. Anat Rec A Discov Mol Cell Evol Biol 2003; 275(1): 1031–41.
30. Ranvier L. De quelques faits relatifs a l'histologie et a la physiologie des muscles stries. Arch Physiol Norm Pathol 1874; 1: 5–18.
31. Burke R. Motor units: anatomy, physiology and functional organisation. Handbook of Physiology Section 1: The Nervous System Volume 2, Part 1. Washington, American Physiological Society, 1981: 335–442.
32. Henneman E, Olson CB. Relations between structure and function in the design of skeletal muscles. J Neurophysiol 1965; 28: 581–98.

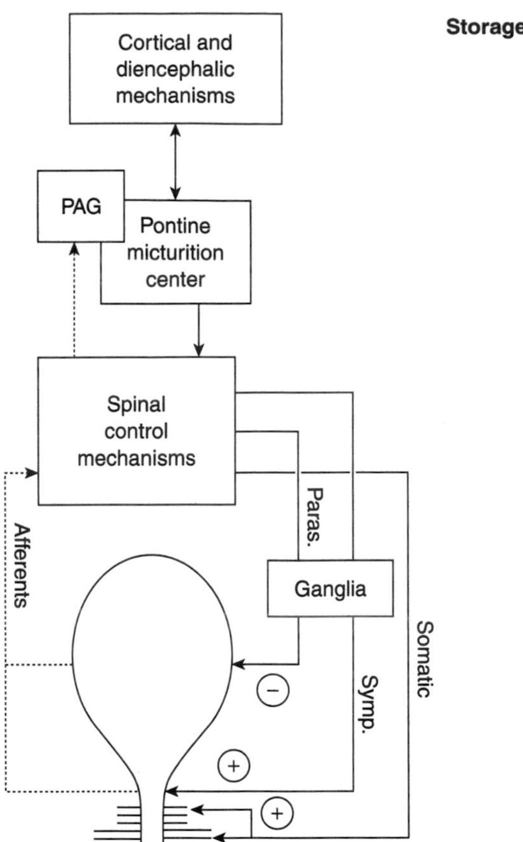

Figure 6.2
During storage, there is continuous and increasing afferent activity from the bladder. There is no spinal parasympathetic (paras.) outflow that can contract the bladder. The sympathetic (symp.) outflow to urethral smooth muscle, and the somatic outflow to urethral and pelvic floor striated muscles keep the outflow region closed. Whether or not the sympathetic innervation to the bladder (not indicated) contributes to bladder relaxation during filling in humans has not been established. PAG = periaqueductal gray.

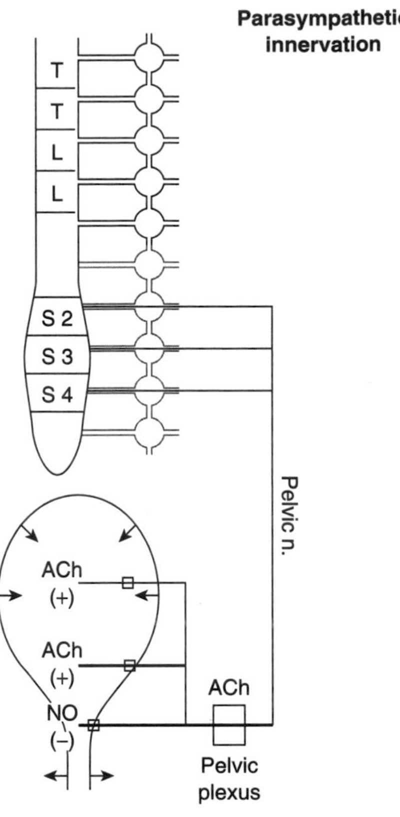

Figure 6.3
The parasympathetic (pelvic nerve) innervation mediates contraction of the bladder (acetylcholine=ACh, muscarinic receptors) and relaxation of the urethra (NO = nitric oxide). T = thoracic, L = lumbar, S = sacral segments.

while the outflow region is contracted, enabling urine storage at low intravesical pressure, or they initiate micturition by relaxing the outflow region and contracting the bladder smooth muscle. Parasympathetic activation excites the bladder and relaxes the outflow region (Figure 6.3), and sympathetic activation inhibits the bladder body and excites the bladder outlet and urethra (Figure 6.4). Somatic nerves activate the striated urethral sphincter (rhabdosphincter; Figure 6.5).

The *sensory* (afferent) innervation, which anatomically can be found in the parasympathetic, sympathetic, and somatic nerves, transmits information about bladder filling and contractile bladder activity to the CNS.

Parasympathetic neurons, mediating contraction of the detrusor smooth muscle and relaxation of the outflow region, are located in the sacral parasympathetic nucleus in the spinal cord at the level of S2–S4.[4] The axons pass through the pelvic nerve and synapse with the postganglionic nerves in either the pelvic plexus, in ganglia on the surface of the bladder (vesical ganglia), or within the walls of the bladder and urethra (intramural ganglia).[5] The preganglionic neurotransmission is mediated by acetylcholine (ACh) acting on nicotinic receptors. This transmission can be modulated by adrenergic, muscarinic, purinergic, and peptidergic presynaptic receptors.[4] The postganglionic neurons in the pelvic nerve mediate the excitatory input to the human detrusor smooth muscle by releasing ACh acting on muscarinic receptors. However, an atropine-resistant component has been demonstrated, particularly in functionally and morphologically altered human bladder tissue (see below). The pelvic nerve also conveys parasympathetic fibers to the outflow region and the urethra. These fibers exert an inhibitory effect and thereby relax the outflow region. This is mediated partly by nitric oxide, although other transmitters might be involved.[6,7]

Most of the *sympathetic* innervation of the bladder and urethra originates from the intermediolateral nuclei in the

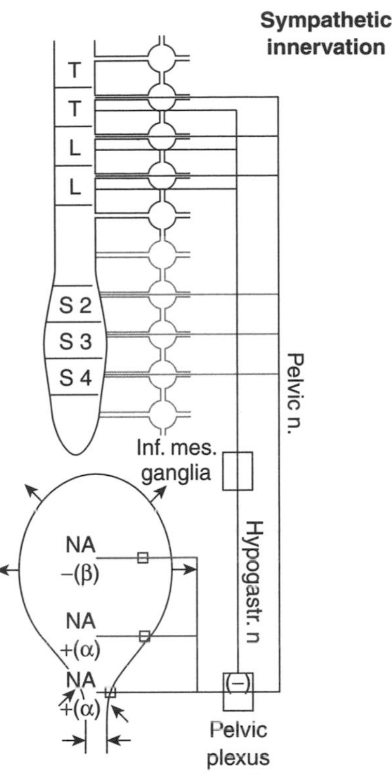

Figure 6.4
Sympathetic innervation (hypogastric nerve) mediates contraction of the bladder outlet and urethral smooth muscle (NA = noradrenaline, α-adrenoceptors) and relaxes the bladder (NA = noradrenaline, β-adrenoceptors). T = thoracic, L = lumbar, S = sacral segments.

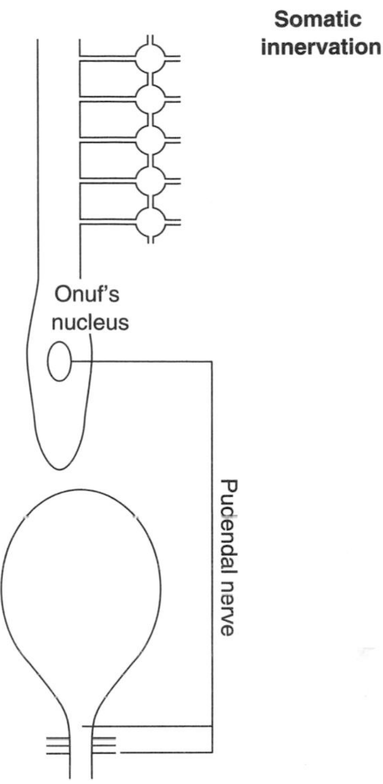

Figure 6.5
During storage, activity in somatic nerves (pudendal nerve) keeps the striated urethral sphincter (rhabdosphincter) closed. During micturition, this activity is suppressed.

thoracolumbar region (T10–L2) of the spinal cord. The axons travel either through the inferior mesenteric ganglia and the hypogastric nerve, or pass through the paravertebral chain and enter the pelvic nerve. Thus, sympathetic signals are conveyed in both the hypogastric and pelvic nerves.

The predominant effects of the sympathetic innervation of the lower urinary tract in man are inhibition of the parasympathetic pathways at spinal and ganglion levels, and mediation of contraction of the bladder base and the urethra. However, in several animals, the adrenergic innervation of the detrusor is believed to relax the detrusor directly. Noradrenaline is released in response to electrical stimulation of detrusor tissues *in vitro*, and the normal response of detrusor tissues to released noradrenaline is relaxation.

Somatic motoneurons, activating the external urethral sphincter (EUS), are located in the Onuf's nucleus, a circumscribed region of the sacral ventral horn at the level of S2–S4. EUS motoneurons send axons to the ventral roots and into the pudendal nerves.[8]

The *sensory* (afferent) nerves monitor the urine volume and pressure during urine storage, transmitting the information to the CNS.[9] Most of the sensory innervation of the bladder and urethra reaches the spinal cord via the pelvic nerve and dorsal root ganglia. In addition, some afferents travel in the hypogastric nerve. The afferent nerves of the EUS travel in the pudendal nerve to the sacral region of the spinal cord.[5] There are several populations of afferents in the bladder. The most important for the micturition process are myelinated Aδ fibers and unmyelinated C fibers. The Aδ fibers respond to passive distention and active contraction (low threshold afferents), thus conveying information about bladder filling.[10] The activation threshold for Aδ fibers is 5–15 mm H_2O, which is the intravesical pressure at which humans report the first sensation of bladder filling.[4] C fibers have a high mechanical threshold and respond primarily to chemical irritation of the bladder mucosa or cold.[11,12] Following chemical irritation, the C-fiber afferents exhibit spontaneous firing when the bladder is empty and increased firing during bladder distention.[11] These fibers are normally inactive and are therefore termed 'silent fibers'.

Local control of the bladder

The cholinergic and adrenergic mechanisms involved in bladder storage and emptying functions have been extensively investigated.[13–16] Non-adrenergic, non-cholinergic (NANC) bladder mechanisms, on the other hand, have been studied mainly in research animals, and their relevance in humans has not been established.[16]

Cholinergic mechanisms

Cholinergic nerves

Although histochemical methods that stain for acetylcholine esterase (AChE) are not specific for ACh-containing nerves, AChE staining has been used as an indirect marker of cholinergic nerves.[5] The vesicular ACh transporter (VACht) is a marker specific for cholinergic nerve terminals.[17] In rats, for example, bladder smooth muscle bundles are supplied with a very rich number of VAChT-positive terminals also containing neuropeptide Y (NPY), nitric oxide synthase (NOS), and vasoactive intestinal polypeptide (VIP).[18] Similar findings have been made in human bladders of neonates and children.[19] The muscle coat of the bladder showed a rich cholinergic innervation and small VAChT-immunoreactive neurons were found scattered throughout the detrusor muscle. VAChT-immunoreactive nerves were also observed in a suburothelial location in the bladder. The function of these nerves is unclear, but a sensory function or a neurotrophic role with respect to the urothelium cannot be excluded.[19]

Muscarinic receptors

Acetylcholine, acting on muscarinic receptors on the detrusor myocytes, is a main contractile transmitter in the mammalian bladder. Muscarinic receptors comprise five subtypes, encoded by five distinct genes.[20] In the human bladder, the mRNAs for all muscarinic receptor subtypes have been demonstrated.[21,22] The M_2 predominates over the M_3 receptor subtype (3:1 ratio).[21–24] These receptors have been located not only on the detrusor myocytes, but also on other structures, including urothelium, interstitial cells, and suburothelial nerves.[25] Detrusor smooth muscle contains muscarinic receptors mainly of the M_2 and M_3 subtypes.[26–29] The receptors are functionally coupled to G-proteins, but the signal transduction systems are different.[26–28]

The M_3 receptors in the human detrusor are believed to be the most important for detrusor contraction.[30] In bladder strips from M_3 knockout mice, 95% of the contraction induced by carbachol was mediated by M_3 receptors.[31] However, these mice had an almost normal cystometric pattern owing to the remaining purinergic activation mechanism.[32]

Stimulation of M_3 receptors has previously been considered to cause contraction through phosphoinositide hydrolysis.[33,34] However, several studies have suggested that other signaling pathways can be involved.[35–37] There may be species differences in the signaling pathways used by the different muscarinic receptor subtypes.[38] However, taken together available evidence suggests that the main pathways for M_3 receptor activation of the human detrusor are calcium influx via L-type calcium channels and inhibition of myosin light chain phosphatase through activation of Rho-kinase and protein kinase C, leading to increased sensitivity to calcium of the contractile machinery.[37,39,40]

The functional role for the M_2 receptors has not been clarified, but it has been suggested that M_2 receptors may oppose sympathetically mediated smooth muscle relaxation through β-ARs.[41] M_2 receptor stimulation may also activate nonspecific cation channels,[42] inhibit K_{ATP} channels through activation of protein kinase C,[43,44] and use other signaling pathways.[38] An investigation using M_2, M_3, and M_2/M_3 double knockout mice revealed that the M_2 receptor may have a role in indirectly mediating bladder contractions by enhancing the contractile response to M_3 receptor activation, and that minor M_2 receptor-mediated contractions may also occur.[45]

On the other hand, in certain disease states, the contribution of M_2 receptors to detrusor contraction may increase. Thus, in the denervated rat bladder, M_2 receptors, or a combination of M_2 and M_3, mediated contractile responses.[38,46–48] In obstructed, hypertrophied rat bladders, there was an increase in total and M_2 receptor density, whereas there was a reduction in M_3 receptor density.[49] The functional significance of this change for voiding function has not been established, and preliminary experiments on the human detrusor could not confirm these observations.[50,51] Pontari et al[52] analyzed bladder muscle specimens from patients with neurogenic bladder dysfunction to determine whether the muscarinic receptor subtype mediating contraction shifts from M_3 to the M_2 receptor subtype, as found in the denervated, hypertrophied rat bladder. They concluded that whereas normal detrusor contractions are mediated by the M_3 receptor subtype, in patients with neurogenic bladder dysfunction, contractions can be mediated by the M_2 receptors.

Muscarinic receptors may also be located on the presynaptic nerve terminals and participate in the regulation of transmitter release. The inhibitory prejunctional muscarinic receptors have been classified as M_2 in the rabbit[53,54] and rat,[55] and M_4 in the guinea-pig,[56] rat,[57] and human[58] bladder. Prejunctional facilitatory muscarinic receptors appear to be of the M_1 subtype in the rat and rabbit urinary bladder.[53–55] Prejunctional muscarinic facilitation has also been detected in human bladders.[59] The muscarinic facilitatory mechanism seems to be upregulated in overactive bladders from chronic spinal cord transected rats. The facilitation in these preparations is primarily mediated by M_3 muscarinic receptors.[59]

Muscarinic receptors have also been demonstrated on the urothelium/suburothelium,[25,28,60] but their functional importance has not been clarified. It has also been suggested that muscarinic receptors on structures other than the myocyte (urothelium/suburothelium) may be involved in the release of an unknown inhibitory factor.[28,61,62]

Several studies have suggested that muscarinic receptors mediate activation of bladder afferent nerves.[63,64] De Laet et al[65] demonstrated an inhibitory effect of systemically given oxybutynin on the afferent part of the micturition effect in rats by recording afferent activity in the pelvic nerve. Boy et al,[66] who studied the effect of tolterodine on sensations evoked by intravesical electrical stimulation and during bladder filling in healthy female subjects, found that the drug had a significant effect on afferent fibers, probably located in the suburothelium. These findings are in line with the clinical observations that antimuscarinics at clinically recommended doses have little effect on voiding contractions and may act mainly during the bladder storage phase, increasing bladder capacity.[30,67,68]

The muscarinic receptor functions may be changed in different urologic disorders, such as outflow obstruction, neurogenic bladders, idiopathic detrusor overactivity, and diabetes.[69]

Adrenergic mechanisms

Adrenergic nerves

Fluorescence histochemical studies have shown that the body of the detrusor receives a relatively sparse innervation by noradrenergic nerves. The density of noradrenergic nerves increases markedly towards the bladder neck, where the smooth muscle receives a dense noradrenergic nerve supply, particularly in the male. The importance of the noradrenergic innervation of the bladder body has been questioned since patients with a deficiency in dopamine β-hydroxylase, the enzyme that converts dopamine to noradrenaline, void normally.[70] Noradrenergic nerves also occur in the lamina propria of the bladder, only some of which are related to the vascular supply. Their functional significance remains to be shown.

α-Adrenoceptors

In the human detrusor, β-ARs dominate over α-ARs, and the normal response to noradrenaline is relaxation.[13] The number of α-ARs in the human detrusor was found to be low,[71] in some studies too low for a reliable quantification.[72] Malloy et al[73] reported that even if the total α_1-AR expression was low, it was reproducible. Among the high affinity receptors for prazosin, only α_{1A} and α_{1D}-mRNAs were expressed in the human bladder. The relation between the different subtypes was α_{1D}: 66% and α_{1A}: 34%, with no expression of α_{1B}.

Even if the α-ARs have no significant role in normal bladder contraction, there is evidence that there may be changes after, for example, bladder outlet obstruction.[74] However, Nomiya and Yamaguchi[75] concluded that neither an upregulation of α_1-ARs, nor a downregulation of β-ARs, occurs in human obstructed bladder, and that it was not likely that detrusor α_1-ARs are responsible for the overactivity observed in patients with bladder outflow obstruction.

It has been shown that α_1-ARs are located *prejunctionally* on cholinergic nerve terminals in the rat urinary bladder.[76] Activation of these receptors facilitates ACh release and enhances neurogenic contractions. Terazosin inhibited phenylephrine-induced facilitation of the neurally-evoked contractions and facilitation of ACh release.[77] Szell et al[78] found that the α_{1A}-AR subtype on the cholinergic nerve terminals mediated the prejunctional facilitation.

In a recent study, Trevisani and coworkers[79] examined the influence of α_1-ARs on neuropeptide release from primary sensory neurons of the lower urinary tract in rats. The α_1-agonist, phenylephrine, caused an intracellular Ca^{2+} mobilization in cultured lumbar and sacral dorsal root ganglion neurons, as well as a release of substance P from terminals of capsaicin-sensitive sensory neurons from the lumbar enlargement of the dorsal spinal cord and urinary bladder, and increased plasma protein extravasation in the urinary bladder. These effects were abolished by alfuzosin. The authors concluded that α_1-ARs are functionally expressed by capsaicin-sensitive, nociceptive, primary sensory neurons of the rat lower urinary tract, and their activation may contribute to signal irritative and nociceptive responses arising from this region. Parts of the beneficial effects of α_1-adrenoceptor antagonists in the amelioration of storage symptoms in the lower urinary tract could be derived from their inhibitory effect on neurogenic inflammatory responses.

β-Adrenoceptors

The β-ARs of the human bladder were shown to have functional characteristics typical of neither β_1- nor β_2-ARs.[80,81] Normal as well as neurogenic human detrusors are able to express β_1-, β_2-, and β_3-AR mRNA, and selective β_3-AR agonists effectively relaxed both types of detrusor muscle.[82,83] An investigation comparing the subpopulations of β-ARs in research animals revealed significant differences amongst species.[84] Studies in human detrusor tissue revealed an expression of β_3-AR mRNA of 97% over β_1- (1.5%) and β_2- (1.4%) AR mRNA, concluding that if the amount of mRNA reflects the population of receptor protein, β_3-ARs mediate bladder relaxation.[85] This is in accordance with several *in-vitro* studies, and it seems that atypical β-AR-mediated responses reported in early studies of β-AR antagonists are mediated by β_3-ARs.[82,83] It can also partly explain why the clinical effects of selective β_2-AR agonists in bladder overactivity have been controversial and largely inconclusive.[86] It has been speculated that, in detrusor overactivity associated with outflow obstruction, there is a lack of an inhibitory β-AR-mediated noradrenaline response, but this has never been verified in humans.[75,87,88] Several β3-AR agonists have shown effect profiles *in vitro* and in animal models that should be promising for treatment of detrusor overactivity and the overactive bladder (OAB) syndrome.[82,83,89–91] Whether or not β3-AR stimulation will be an effective way of treating these conditions has to await proof of concept studies.

Afferent signaling from the urothelium/suburothelium

Recent evidence suggests that the urothelium/suburothelium may serve not only as a passive barrier, but also as a specialized sensory and signaling unit, which, by producing nitric oxide, ATP, and other mediators, can control the activity in afferent nerves, and thereby the initiation of the micturition reflex.[92–94] Both afferent and autonomic efferent nerves are located in close proximity to the urothelium.[95–98] The urothelium has been shown to express, for example, nicotinic, muscarinic, tachykinin, adrenergic, bradykinin, and transient receptor potential (TRP) receptors.[93,95,96,99]

While antimuscarinics were traditionally considered to develop their beneficial effects via muscarinic receptors located on detrusor smooth muscle, there is increasing evidence that additional effects involve muscarinic receptors within the urothelium and bladder afferent (sensory) nerves.[100,101] Intravesical oxybutynin has been shown to have a direct anesthetic effect within the bladder wall by temporarily desensitizing C-fiber afferents without affecting Aδ fibers.[102] Systemic oxybutynin also influences bladder sensory nerves by inhibiting the afferent part of the micturition reflex.[65] Similar results were found for intravesical and intravenous application of tolterodine.[63] Very recently, Iijima et al[103] analyzed the effects of the M_3 receptor-selective muscarinic antagonist darifenacin on bladder afferent activity of the rat pelvic nerve. Darifenacin significantly reduced bladder afferent activity, which might be an additional factor in the treatment of OAB.

Lips and coworkers directly analyzed the ACh content in the urothelium and characterized the molecular component of its synthesis and release machinery.[104] They found ACh to be present in the urothelium in a nanomolar range per gram of wet weight. RT-PCR data supported the presence of carnitine acetyltransferase (CarAT) but not choline acetyltransferase (CHAT). Vesicular ACh transporter (VAChT), used by neurons to shuffle ACh into synaptic vesicles, was detected in subepithelial cholinergic nerve fibers, but not by RT-PCR or immunohistochemistry in the urothelium. The authors concluded that this urothelial non-neuronal cholinergic system differs widely from that of neurons with respect to molecular components of the ACh synthesis and release machinery. Consequently, these two systems might be differentially targeted by pharmacologic approaches.

Low pH, high K, increased osmolality, and low temperatures can influence afferent nerves, possibly via effects on the vanilloid receptor (capsaicin-gated ion channel, TRPV1), which is expressed both in afferent nerve terminals and in the urothelial cells.[96] TRPV1 is expressed throughout the afferent limb of the micturition reflex pathway, including in urinary bladder unmyelinated (C-fiber) nerves that detect bladder distention or the presence of irritant chemicals.[105,106] TRPV1 is expressed by urothelial cells as well as by afferent nerves in proximity to urothelial cells in the urinary bladder.[95,96] Birder et al showed that TRPV1-null mice are anatomically normal.[96] However, bladder function seems to be altered, including a reduction of *in-vitro*, stretch-evoked ATP release and membrane capacitance. Urothelial cells from TRPV1-null mice were also shown to exhibit a decrease in hypotonic-evoked ATP release.[96]

A network of interstitial cells (ICs), extensively linked by Cx43-containing gap junctions, was found to be located beneath the urothelium in the human bladder.[107–109] This interstitial cellular network was suggested to operate as a functional syncytium, integrating signals and responses in the bladder wall. The firing of suburothelial afferent nerves, conveying sensations and regulating the threshold for bladder activation, may be modified by both inhibitory (e.g., nitric oxide) and stimulatory (e.g., ATP, tachykinins, prostanoids) mediators. There may be several types of ICs within the bladder wall. These NO/cGMP-positive cells can be separated into two main groups:[110] cells in the suburothelial space (suburothelial ICs) and cells associated with an outer layer of muscle. Three subtypes of muscle ICs have been identified:[111] cells on the outer surface of the bladder wall (muscle-coat ICs), cells on the surface of muscle bundles (surface muscle ICs), and cells within the muscle bundles (intramuscular ICs).

ATP, generated by the urothelium, has been suggested as an important mediator of urothelial signaling.[92,112] P2X and P2Y purinergic receptor subtypes are expressed in cells (urothelium, nerves, and myofibroblasts) that are situated near the luminal surface of the bladder. ATP was shown to potentiate the response of vanilloids in sensory neurons by lowering the threshold for protons, capsaicin, and heat.[113] Thus, ATP possibly triggers pain when released from injured or damaged cells.[94] Supporting such a view, intravesical ATP induces detrusor overactivity in conscious rats.[114] Furthermore, mice lacking the P2X3 receptor were shown to have hypoactive bladders.[115,116]

There seem to be other, thus far unidentified, factors in the urothelium that could influence bladder function.[16]

Even if these mechanisms can be involved in, for example, the pathophysiology of OAB, their functional importance remains to be established.

Nonadrenergic, noncholinergic mechanisms

In most animal species, the bladder contraction induced by stimulation of nerves consists of at least two components, one atropine-resistant and one mediated by NANC mechanisms.[13] NANC contractions have been reported to occur in normal human detrusor, even if not representing more than a few percent of the total contraction in response to nerve stimulation.[117–119] However, a significant degree of NANC-mediated contraction may exist in morphologically and/or functionally changed human bladders, and has been reported to occur in hypertrophic bladders, idiopathic detrusor instability, interstitial cystitis bladder, neurogenic bladders, and in the aging bladder.[118,120–125] The NANC component of the nerve-induced response may be responsible for up to 40–50% of the total bladder contraction (see below).

NANC neurotransmission: ATP There is good evidence that the transmitter responsible for the NANC component is ATP, acting on P2X receptors found in the detrusor smooth muscle membranes of rats and humans.[112,127,128] The receptor subtype predominating in both species seemed to be the $P2X_1$ subtype. Moore et al[129] reported that detrusor from patients with idiopathic detrusor instability had a selective absence of $P2X_3$ and $P2X_5$ receptors, and suggested that this specific lack might impair control of detrusor contractility and contribute to the pathophysiology of urge incontinence. On the other hand, O'Reilly et al[123] found that, in patients with idiopathic detrusor instability, $P2X_2$ receptors were significantly elevated, whereas other P2X receptor subtypes were significantly decreased. They were unable to detect a purinergic component of nerve-mediated contractions in control (normal) bladder specimens, but there was a significant purinergic component of approximately 50% in unstable bladder specimens. They concluded that this abnormal purinergic transmission in the bladder might explain symptoms in these patients. The same group confirmed that the $P2X_1$ receptor was the predominant purinoceptor subtype also in the human male bladder.[128] They found that the amount of $P2X_1$ receptor per smooth muscle cell was larger in obstructed than in control bladders. This suggests an increase in purinergic function in the overactive bladder arising from bladder outlet obstruction.

NANC neurotransmission: neuropeptides Various bioactive peptides have been demonstrated to be synthesized, stored, and released in the human lower urinary tract, including atrial natriuretic peptide (ANP), bradykinin, calcitonin gene-related peptide (CGRP), endothelin, enkephalins, galanin, neuropeptide Y, somatostatin, substance P (SP), and vasoactive intestinal polypeptide (VIP).[13] However, their functional roles have not been established.[130–132] In human bladder, Uckert et al[132] found contractant effects of SP and ET-1, a relaxant effect of VIP, and very little effects of ANP and CGRP.

As discussed by Maggi, neuropeptide-containing, capsaicin-sensitive primary afferents in the bladder and urethra may not only have a sensory function ('sensory neuropeptides'), but also a local effector or efferent function.[4,130] In addition, they may play a role as neurotransmitters and/or neuromodulators in the bladder ganglia and at the neuromuscular junctions. As a result, the peptides may be involved in the mediation of various effects, including micturition reflex activation, smooth muscle contraction, potentiation of efferent neurotransmission, and changes in vascular tone and permeability. Evidence for this is based mainly on experiments in animals. Studies on isolated human bladder muscle strips have failed to reveal any specific local motor response attributable to a capsaicin-sensitive innervation.[131] However, cystometric evidence that capsaicin-sensitive nerves may modulate the afferent branch of the micturition reflex in humans has been presented.[133] In a small number of patients suffering from bladder hypersensitivity disorders, intravesical capsaicin produced a long-lasting, symptomatic improvement. It has been discussed whether peptides are involved in the pathogenesis of detrusor overactivity. Results from immunohistochemical studies have provided evidence that outflow obstruction, which is commonly associated with detrusor overactivity, causes a reduction in the density of peptide-containing nerves.[134]

Tachykinins Endogenous tachykinins, substance P (SP), neurokinin A (NKA), and neurokinin B (NKB), are widely distributed in the central and peripheral nervous system. They are found in afferent pathways of the bladder and urethra, and there is considerable evidence that they act as transmitters in sensory nerves.[4] In addition, these peptides have been shown to produce diverse biologic effects, such as smooth muscle contraction, facilitation of transmitter release from nerves, vasodilatation, and increased plasma permeability. Their actions are mediated by activation of three distinct receptor types termed NK-1, NK-2, and NK-3. Rat and guinea pig detrusors contain both NK-1 and NK-2 receptors, whereas the NK-2 receptor seems to be the only mediator of contractile responses to tachykinins in human bladder smooth muscle, where the potency of neurokinins was shown to be NKA > NKB >> SP.[135] Nociceptive transmission is mainly mediated through NK_1-receptors.

The potential role of tachykinins, particularly SP, in the atropine-resistant component of the contractile response induced by electrical stimulation, has been studied by several investigators.[13,132] With few exceptions, these studies did not favor the view that SP, released from postganglionic nerve terminals, has an excitatory transmitter role. However, evidence has been presented that SP may play a role in the afferent branch of the micturition reflex.[13,15] Green et al[136] tested the hypothesis that aprepitant, an NK-1 receptor antagonist, may be efficacious in the treatment of urge urinary incontinence. In a double-blind, randomized, placebo-controlled, parallel group pilot study on postmenopausal women with a history of urge urinary incontinence or mixed incontinence, they found that aprepitant significantly decreased the average daily number of micturitions and urgency episodes compared with placebo, and concluded that NK-1 receptor antagonism may represent a novel therapeutic approach to treating OAB.

Endothelins Endothelins (ET-1, ET-2, ET-3) and ET (ET_A, ET_B) receptors have been demonstrated in the bladder. Via their receptors, ETs can initiate both short-term (contraction) and long-term (mitogenesis) events in targets cells in the bladder and urethra. Saenz de Tejada et al[137] demonstrated ET-like immunoreactivity in the transitional epithelium, serosal mesothelium, vascular endothelium, smooth muscles of the detrusor (nonvascular) and vessels, and in fibroblasts of the human bladder. This cellular distribution was confirmed in *in-situ* hybridization experiments. The authors suggested that ET may act as an autocrine hormone in the regulation of the bladder wall structure and smooth muscle tone, and that it may regulate cholinergic neurotransmission by a paracrine mechanism. In patients with benign prostatic hypertrophy (BPH), the density of ET receptors in the bladder was significantly lower than in men without this disorder.[138] ET-1 is known to induce contraction in animal as well as human detrusor muscle.[13,132] The contractile effect of ETs seems to be mediated mainly by the ET_A receptor, and the ET_B receptor could not be linked to contraction.[139] However, in human bladder smooth muscle, ETs may not only have a contractile action, but could also be linked to proliferative effects. Supporting this view, Khan et al[140] found that ET_A and ET_B receptor antagonists inhibited rabbit detrusor and bladder neck smooth muscle cell proliferation, and they suggested that ET-1 antagonists may prevent smooth muscle cell hyperplasia associated with partial bladder outflow obstruction.

Many authors have suggested that ET may play a pathophysiologic role in bladder outlet obstruction associated with BPH.[16] In the bladder, ETs may be implicated in detrusor hypertrophy and its functional consequences. Thus, Schröder et al[141] studied the effect of an orally administered endothelin converting enzyme (ECE) inhibitor by cystometry in conscious rats with and without bladder outflow obstruction (BOO). They concluded that ECE inhibition did not prevent an increase in bladder weight after BOO, but it appeared to have a beneficial effect on detrusor function and decrease detrusor overactivity in conscious rats.

Vasoactive intestinal polypeptide Vasoactive intestinal polypeptide (VIP) was shown to inhibit spontaneous contractile activity in isolated detrusor muscle from several animal species, and from humans, but to have little effect on contractions induced by muscarinic receptor stimulation or by electrical stimulation of nerves.[13] Uckert et al[132] found a moderate relaxant effect of VIP on isolated, carbachol-contracted human detrusor and a less than twofold increase in intracellular cyclic AMP concentration. In isolated rat bladder, VIP had no effect, and in isolated guinea pig bladder, VIP produced contraction. Stimulation of the pelvic nerves in cats increased the VIP output from the bladder, and increased bladder blood flow, although moderately.[142] VIP injected iv induced bladder relaxation in dogs.[143] On the other hand, VIP given iv to patients in a dose causing increases in heart rate had no effect on cystometric parameters.[144] Plasma concentrations of VIP were obtained, which, in other clinical investigations, had been sufficient to cause relaxation of smooth muscle.[144] Even if a decrease in VIP concentrations has been found in bladders from patients with idiopathic detrusor overactivity, the role of this peptide in bladder function has not been established.[145]

Calcitonin gene-related peptide Calcitonin gene-related peptide (CGRP) is widely distributed in nerve endings in the bladder, and considered a sensory neuromodulator.[131] However, whether CGRP has a role in the control of bladder motility is controversial. In pig detrusor, CGRP did not alter the response to potassium, carbachol, substance P, or electrical field stimulation (EFS).[146] In hamsters, CGRP caused dose-dependent inhibition of the response to EFS, but about 20% of the preparations did not respond.[147] In human detrusor strips, the relaxing effect of CGRP on carbachol-induced contraction was negligible, despite a slight increase in cGMP levels.[132] Most probably, the main role of CGRP is that of a sensory neuromodulator.

Neuropeptide Y Neuropeptide Y (NPY) and noradrenaline are stored in separate vesicles at sympathetic nerve terminals, and NPY is preferentially released at high frequencies of stimulation.[148] In rat bladders, abundant NPY-containing nerves were found, and exogenously added NPY contracted detrusor strips and potentiated the noncholinergic motor transmission. A possible motor transmitter function of the peptide in the rat bladder was suggested.[13,149] However, other investigators studying rat and guinea pig bladders found no contractile response to exogenous NPY, but inhibitory effects on cholinergic and

NANC-induced contractions.[150,151] The human bladder is richly endowed with NPY containing nerves.[152–155] In neonates and children, small ganglia scattered throughout the detrusor muscle of urinary bladder were found, of which approximately 95% contained NPY.[19] It seems as if NPY can be found in adrenergic as well as cholinergic nerves. However, in the human bladder only very few if any functional NPY receptors were found.[156] Thus a role for NPY in bladder function remains to be established.

Prostanoids Prostanoids are synthesized from a common precursor, arachidonic acid, a process catalyzed by the enzyme cyclooxygenase (COX). This process occurs locally in both bladder muscle and mucosa, and is initiated by various physiologic stimuli such as stretch of the detrusor muscle, but also by injuries of the vesical mucosa, nerve stimulation, and by agents such as ATP and mediators of inflammation.[105,157–159] There seem to be species variations in the spectrum of prostanoids and the relative amounts synthesized and released by the urinary bladder. Biopsies from the human bladder were shown to release prostanoids in the following quantitative order: $PGI_2 > PGE_2 > PGF_{2\alpha} > TXA_2$.[160]

$PGF_{2\alpha}$, PGE_1, and PGE_2 contract isolated detrusor muscle, whereas PGE_1 and $PGF_{2\alpha}$ relax or have no effect on urethral smooth muscle.[13] Even if prostaglandins have contractile effects on the human bladder, it is still unclear whether they contribute to the pathogenesis of detrusor overactivity. Prostanoids may affect the bladder in two ways: directly by effects on the smooth muscle and/or indirectly via effects on the neurotransmission.[105] Probably, prostanoids do not act as true effector messengers along the efferent arm of the micturition reflex, but rather as a neuromodulator of the efferent and afferent neurotransmission.[105,161] An important physiologic role might be sensitization of sensory nerves. Evidence for a sensitizing effect of PGE_2 has also been demonstrated *in vivo*. It was shown in the rat urinary bladder that intravesical instillation of PGE_2 lowered the threshold for reflex micturition, an effect which was blocked by systemic capsaicin desensitization. Indomethacin pretreatment and systemic capsaicin increased the micturition threshold without affecting the amplitude of the micturition contraction.[105] Since intravesical PGE_2 did not reduce the residual volume in capsaicin-pretreated animals, it was suggested that endogenous prostanoids enhance the voiding efficiency through an effect, direct or indirect, on sensory nerves.

Prostanoids may also be involved in the pathophysiology of different bladder disorders. As pointed out by Maggi, in cystitis there may be an exaggerated prostanoid production leading to intense activation of sensory nerves, increasing the afferent input.[105]

Schröder et al[141] investigated whether the PGE_2 receptor EP1 was involved in the regulation of normal micturition, the response to intravesical PGE_2 administration, and the development of bladder hypertrophy and overactivity due to BOO. Moderate BOO was created in EP1 receptor knockout (EP1KO) mice and their wild-type (WT) counterparts. After 1 week cystometry was performed in conscious animals before and after PGE_2 instillation. Findings were compared to those in unobstructed control animals. There was no difference between unobstructed EP1KO and WT mice in urodynamic parameters, but EP1KO mice did not respond to intravesical PGE_2 instillation, while WT mice showed detrusor overactivity. The lack of EP1 receptor did not prevent bladder hypertrophy due to BOO. After BOO, WT mice had pronounced detrusor overactivity, while this was negligible in EP1KO mice. It was concluded that the EP1 receptor appears not to be essential for normal micturition or the mediation of bladder hypertrophy due to BOO, but to have a role in the development of detrusor overactivity caused by PGE_2 and outlet obstruction.

COX is the pivotal enzyme in prostaglandin synthesis. It has been established that this enzyme exists in two isoforms, one constitutive (COX-1) and one inducible (COX-2).[162] The constitutive form is responsible for the normal physiologic biosynthesis, whereas the inducible COX-2 is activated during inflammation.[163,164] Park et al[165] demonstrated that the expression of COX-2 was increased as a consequence of bladder outflow obstruction. If prostaglandins generated by COX-2 contribute to bladder overactivity, selective inhibitors of COX-2 would, theoretically, be one possible target for pharmacologic therapy. Whether or not available selective COX-2 inhibitors would be useful as treatment for bladder overactivity remains to be established.

Lee et al[166] investigated whether a new PE_1 receptor antagonist, PF-2907617-02, would influence the regulation of normal micturition in rats, if it affected bladder function in animals with partial BOO. They found PF-2907617-02 to have a significantly increased bladder capacity, micturition volume, and micturition interval, but no effect on other urodynamic parameters. Intravesical PGE_2 induced detrusor overactivity. The antagonist significantly reduced the stimulatory effects of PGE_2. In obstructed animals, PF-2907617-02 significantly increased micturition interval, but not bladder capacity and residual volume. The drug also decreased the frequency and amplitude of nonvoiding contractions. The authors concluded that the EP_1 receptor was involved in the initiation of the micturition reflex, both in normal rats and in animals with BOO. It may also contribute to the generation of detrusor overactivity after BOO, thus EP_1 antagonists may have potential as a treatment of detrusor overactivity in humans.

Nitric oxide Evidence has accumulated that L-arginine-derived NO is responsible for the main part of the inhibitory NANC responses in the lower urinary tract.[13] However, NO may have different roles in the bladder and the urethra.

Nitrergic nerves: In biopsies taken from the lateral wall and trigone regions of the human bladder, a plexus of NADPH-diaphorase-containing nerve fibers was found.[167] Samples from the lateral bladder wall contained many NADPH-reactive nerve terminals, particularly in the subepithelial region immediately beneath the urothelium; occasionally they penetrated into the epithelial layer. Immunohistochemical investigations of pig bladder revealed that the density of NO synthase (NOS) immunoreactivity was higher in trigonal and urethral tissue than in the detrusor.[168]

Functional effects of NO: Relaxations to electrical stimulation were found in small biopsy preparations of the human detrusor.[169] The relaxations were sensitive to the NOS-inhibitor nitro L-arginine (L-NOARG), but insensitive to tetrodotoxin, and it was suggested that NO, generated from the detrusor, was important for bladder relaxation during the filling phase. However, Elliott and Castleden[170] were unable to demonstrate a nerve-mediated relaxation in human detrusor. In the pig detrusor, the NO donor SIN-1, and exogenous NO relaxed muscle preparations, which were precontracted by carbachol and endothelin-1, by approximately 60%. However, isoprenaline was about 1000 times more potent than SIN-1 and NO and caused complete relaxation. Nitroprusside, SIN-1, and NO were only moderately effective in relaxing isolated rat, pig, and rabbit detrusor muscle, compared to their effects on the urethral muscle.[168,171,172]

It appears to be unlikely that NO has a major role as a neurotransmitter causing direct relaxation of the detrusor smooth muscle, since the detrusor sensitivity to NO and agents acting via the cyclic GMP system is low.[173] This is also reflected by the finding in rabbits that cyclic GMP is mainly related to urethral relaxation, and cyclic AMP to urinary bladder relaxation.[174] However, this does not exclude that NO may modulate the effects of other transmitters, or that it has a role in afferent neurotransmission.

Phosphodiesterases LUT smooth muscle can be relaxed by drugs increasing the intracellular concentrations of cyclic AMP (cAMP) or cyclic GMP (cGMP).[16,173,175] Multiple types of adenylyl cyclases exist, which catalyze the formation of cAMP.[176,177] In LUT smooth muscles, increases in cAMP seem to have a main role in bladder relaxation, whereas cGMP is important for urethral relaxation.[16,172,174,175,178] Several agents, acting through different receptors linked to adenylyl cyclase, or directly stimulating the enzyme, have been shown to relax the bladder and simultaneously to increase the intracellular concentrations of cAMP. Many endogenous agents as well as drugs have cGMP as their common mediator in eliciting different physiologic responses. There are multiple types of soluble and particulate guanylyl cyclases which catalyze cGMP synthesis.[179] Soluble guanylyl cyclase is the target of NO, which binds to its heme moiety and activates the enzyme, with resulting increase in cGMP. cGMP, in turn, regulates protein phosphorylation, ion channel conductivity, and phosphodiesterase (PDE) activity.

Both cAMP and cGMP are degraded by PDEs, a heterogenous group of hydrolytic enzymes.[180–183] Since cAMP seems to be more important than cGMP for detrusor function, the cAMP pathway in this tissue has been the most extensively investigated. Truss et al[184–188] demonstrated the presence of five PDE isoenzymes (PDE1–5) in human and porcine detrusor and suggested that the cAMP pathway and the calcium/calmodulin-stimulated PDE (PDE1) could be of functional importance in the regulation of detrusor tone. The same enzymes were demonstrated in the rat[189] and rabbit bladder.[190] Further studies revealed messenger RNA for PDEs 1A, 1B, 2A, 4A, 4B, 5A, 7A, 8A, and 9A in human bladder tissue.[132] PDE1 was shown to be localized to the epithelium of the human urinary tract, including ureteral and bladder urothelium.[191]

Significant relaxation of human detrusor muscle *in vitro*, paralleled by increases in cyclic nucleotide levels, was induced by papaverine, vinpocetine (nonselective inhibitor of PDE1), and forskolin, suggesting that the cAMP pathway and PDE1 may be important in regulation of smooth muscle tone.[185] *In vitro*, human detrusor muscle was relatively inert to sodium nitroprusside, and to agents acting via the cGMP system.[185] However, animal studies indicated that the NOS pathway involves not only the detrusor but also the urothelium/suburothelium, and the urothelium expresses nNOS and produces GMP.[110,111,192] This would mean that also inhibitors of cGMP degradation could influence bladder function via these structures. However, it has not been established which PDE enzymes are located to these tissues. PDE4 has been implicated in the control of bladder smooth muscle tone. PDE4 inhibitors reduced the *in-vitro* control response of guinea pig,[193] rat,[194] and non-human primate bladder strips,[194] and also suppressed rhythmic bladder contractions of the isolated guinea pig bladder.[111] PDE inhibition (PDE4 and 5), alone or in combination, for treatment of LUTS seems to deserve further exploration.

Based on these findings, it was speculated that some PDE1 inhibitors might be beneficial in the treatment of OAB and low-compliance bladder through relaxation of bladder smooth muscle.[184] Truss et al[184] presented preliminary clinical data with the PDE1 inhibitor vinpocetine in OAB patients not responding to standard antimuscarinic therapy, which suggested a possible role for vinpocetine in the treatment of urgency, frequency, and urge incontinence. The results of a larger randomized, double-blind, placebo-controlled, multicenter trial with vinpocetine showed a tendency in favour of vinpocetine over placebo; however, statistically significant results were documented for one parameter only.[185]

Summary

There is abundant evidence that cholinergic neurotransmission is predominant in the activation of the human detrusor. This may not be the case in animals, which should be considered when animal models are used for study of bladder function. Release of ACh, which stimulates M_3 and M_2 receptors on the detrusor smooth muscle cells, will lead to bladder contraction. Other neurotransmitters/modulators (e.g. ATP) have been demonstrated in the bladder of both animals and humans, but their roles in the human bladder remain to be established.

Urethra

Sufficient contraction of the urethral smooth muscle is an important function to provide continence during the storage phase of the micturition cycle. Equally important is a coordinated and complete relaxation during the voiding phase. The normal pattern of voiding in humans is characterized by an initial drop in urethral pressure followed by an increase in intravesical pressure.[13,195] The mechanism of this relaxant effect has not been definitely established, but several factors may contribute. One possibility is that the drop in intraurethral pressure is caused by stimulation of muscarinic receptors on noradrenergic nerves, diminishing NA release and thereby tone in the proximal urethra. Another is that contraction of longitudinal urethral smooth muscle in the proximal urethra, produced by released ACh, causes shortening and widening of the urethra, with a concomitant decrease in intraurethral pressure. A third possibility is that a NANC mechanism mediates this response.[13]

Cholinergic mechanisms

Cholinergic nerves The urethral smooth muscle receives a rich cholinergic innervation, of which the functional role is largely unknown. Most probably, the cholinergic nerves cause relaxation of the outflow region at the start of micturition by releasing NO and other relaxant transmitters, based on the principle of cotransmission, as multiple transmitters were found to be colocalized in cholinergic nerves. In pig urethra, colocalization studies revealed that AChE-positive and some NOS-containing nerves had profiles that were similar. These nerves also contained NPY and VIP. NO-containing nerves were present in a density lower than that of the AChE positive nerves, but higher than the density of any peptidergic nerves.[196] Coexistence of ACh and NOS in the rat major pelvic ganglion was demonstrated by double immunohistochemistry.[197] In the rat urethra, colocalization studies confirmed that NOS and VIP are contained within a population of cholinergic nerves.[17]

Muscarinic receptors In rabbits, there are fewer muscarinic receptor binding sites in the urethra than in the bladder.[198] Muscarinic receptor agonists contract isolated urethral smooth muscle from several species, including humans, but these responses seem to be mediated mainly by the longitudinal muscle layer.[13] Investigating the whole length of the female human urethra, it was found that ACh contracted only the proximal part and the bladder neck.[199] If this contractile activation is exerted in the longitudinal direction, it should be expected that the urethra is shortened and that the urethral pressure decreases. Experimentally, *in-vitro* resistance to flow in the urethra was only increased by high concentrations of ACh.[200,201] However, in humans, tolerable doses of bethanechol and emeprone had little effect on intraurethral pressure.[202,203]

Prejunctional muscarinic receptors may influence the release of both noradrenaline (NA) and ACh in the bladder neck/urethra. In urethral tissue from both rabbit and humans, carbachol decreased and scopolamine increased concentration-dependently the release of [^{3}H] NA from adrenergic, and of [^{3}H] choline from cholinergic nerve terminals.[202] This would mean that released ACh could inhibit NA release, thereby decreasing urethral tone and intraurethral pressure.

Studies in the pig urethra show that M_2 receptors are predominant over M_3. Additionally, contraction of the circular muscle appears to be mediated by M_2 and M_3, while the longitudinal response is mainly mediated by M_3 receptors.[205] This may have clinical interest since subtype-selective antimuscarinic drugs (M_3) are being introduced as a treatment of bladder overactivity.

Adrenergic mechanisms

Adrenergic nerves The well-known anatomic differences between the male and female urethra are also reflected in the innervation. In the human male, the smooth muscle surrounding the preprostatic part of the urethra is richly innervated by both cholinergic and adrenergic nerves, and considered a 'sexual sphincter', contracting during ejaculation and thus preventing retrograde transport of sperm.[206] The role of this structure in maintaining continence is unclear, but probably not essential.

In the human female, the muscle bundles run obliquely or longitudinally along the length of the urethra, and in the whole human female urethra, as well as in the human male urethra below the preprostatic part, there is only a scarce supply of adrenergic nerves.[5,207] Fine varicose nerve terminals can be seen along the bundles of smooth muscle cells, running both longitudinally and transversely. Adrenergic terminals can also be found around blood vessels. Colocalization studies in animals have revealed that adrenergic nerves, identified by immunohistochemistry using tyrosine hydroxylase (TH), also contain NPY.[208] Chemical sympathectomy in rats resulted in a complete disappearance of the adrenergic nerves, while NOS-containing nerve fibers were not affected by the treatment.[209] This suggests that NOS is not contained within adrenergic nerves.

Both α- and β-ARs have been found in isolated urethral smooth muscle from animals as well as humans.[200,210–212]

α-Adrenoceptors In humans, up to about 50% of the intraurethral pressure is maintained by stimulation of α-ARs, as judged from results obtained with α-AR antagonists and epidural anesthesia in urodynamic studies.[213,214] In human urethral smooth muscle, both functional and receptor binding studies have suggested that the α_1-AR subtype is the predominating postjunctional α-AR.[13,215] However, most *in-vitro* investigations of human urethral α-ARs were done in males, and the results support the existence of a sphincter structure in the male proximal urethra, which cannot be found in the female. Other marked differences between sexes in the distribution of α_1- and α_2-ARs (as found in, for example, rabbits), or in the distribution of α_1-AR subtypes, do not seem to occur.[216]

Separating the entire length of the isolated female human urethra into seven parts, from the external meatus to the bladder neck, it was found that NA (α_1 and α_2), but not clonidine (α_2), produced concentration-dependent contractions in all parts, with a peak in the middle to proximal urethra.[199] Also a similarity in patterns between NA-induced contraction and the urethral pressure profile in the human urethra was demonstrated.

Among the three high affinity α_1-AR subtypes (α_{1A}, α_{1B}, α_{1D}) identified in molecular cloning and functional studies, α_{1A} seems to predominate in the human lower urinary tract. However, a receptor with low affinity for prazosin (the α_{1L}-AR) was found to be prominent in the human male urethra and may represent a functional phenotype of the α_{1A}-AR.[217,218] In the human female urethra, the expression and distribution of α_1-AR subtypes were determined and mRNA for the α_{1A} subtype was predominant. Autoradiography confirmed the predominance of the α_{1A}-AR.[216]

The studies cited above suggest that the sympathetic innervation helps to maintain urethral smooth muscle tone through α_1-AR receptor stimulation. If urethral α_1-ARs are contributing to the lower urinary tract symptoms, which can also occur in women, an effect of α_1-AR antagonists should be expected in women with these symptoms.[219,220] This was found to be the case in some studies, but was not confirmed in a randomized, placebo-controlled pilot study, which showed that terazosin was not effective for the treatment of 'prostatism-like' symptoms in aging women.[221]

Urethral α_2-ARs are able to control the release of NA from adrenergic nerves, as shown in *in-vitro* studies. In the rabbit urethra, incubated with [^{3}H]NA, electrical stimulation of nerves caused a release of [^{3}H], which was decreased by NA and clonidine and increased by the α_2-AR antagonist rauwolscine.[204] Clonidine was shown to reduce intraurethral pressure in humans, an effect that may be attributed partly to a peripheral effect on adrenergic nerve terminals.[222] More probably, however, this effect is exerted on the central nervous system with a resulting decrease in peripheral sympathetic nervous activity. The subtype of prejunctional α_2-AR involved in [^{3}H]NA secretion in the isolated guinea pig urethra was suggested to be of the α_{2A} subtype.[56]

Prejunctional α_2-AR regulation of transmitter release is not confined to adrenergic nerves.[13] Electrical field stimulation (EFS; frequencies above 12 Hz) of spontaneously contracted smooth muscle strips from the female pig urethra evoked long-lasting, frequency-dependent relaxations in the presence of prazosin, scopolamine, and the NOS inhibitor L-NOARG, suggesting the release of an unknown relaxation-producing mediator. Treatment with a selective α_2-AR agonist markedly reduced the relaxations evoked by EFS at all frequencies tested (16–30 Hz). This inhibitory effect was completely antagonized by the α_2-AR antagonist rauwolscine, and the results suggested that the release of the unknown mediator in the female pig urethra can be modulated via α_2-ARs.[223]

β-Adrenoceptors In humans, the β-ARs in the bladder neck were suggested to be of the β_2 subtype, as shown by receptor binding studies using subtype selective antagonists.[224] However, β_3-ARs can be found in the striated urethral sphincter.[225]

Although the functional importance of urethral β-ARs has not been established, they have been targets for therapeutic intervention. Selective β_2-AR agonists have been shown to reduce intraurethral pressure, while β-AR antagonists did not influence intraurethral pressure in acute studies.[226–229] The theoretic basis for the use of β-AR antagonists in the treatment of stress incontinence is that blockade of urethral β-ARs may enhance the effects of NA on urethral α-ARs. Even if propranolol has been reported to have beneficial effects in the treatment of stress incontinence, this does not seem to be an effective treatment.[13]

After selective β_2-AR antagonists have been used as a treatment of stress incontinence, it seems paradoxical that the selective β_2-AR agonist clenbuterol was found to cause significant clinical improvement in women with stress incontinence.[230] The positive effects were suggested to be a result of an action on urethral striated muscle and/or the pelvic floor muscles.[225,231]

Nonadrenergic, noncholinergic mechanisms

The mechanical response to autonomic nerve stimulation and to intra-arterial ACh injection on resistance to flow in the proximal urethra was tested in male cats. It was found that sacral ventral root stimulation produced an atropine-sensitive constriction when basal urethral resistance was low, but dilatation when resistance was high.[232] The latter response was reduced, but not abolished, by atropine. When urethral constriction had been produced by phenylephrine, injection of ACh produced a consistent decrease in urethral resistance, which was then not reduced by atropine. It was suggested that parasympathetic dilatation of the urethra may be mediated by an unknown NANC transmitter released from postganglionic neurons. The predominant transmitter is believed to be NO.

Nitric oxide NO has been shown to be an important inhibitory neurotransmitter in the lower urinary tract.[13,233] NO-mediated responses in smooth muscle preparations are found to be linked to an increase in cGMP formation, which has been demonstrated in several urethra preparations.[172,174,178,234] Subsequent activation of a cGMP-dependent protein kinase (cGK) has been suggested to hyperpolarize the cell membrane, probably by causing a leftward shift of the activation curve for the K^+-channels, thereby increasing their open probability.[235,236] There have also been reports suggesting that NO in some smooth muscles might act directly on the K^+ channels.[237,238] Other mechanisms for NO-induced relaxations, mediated by cGMP, might involve reduced intracellular Ca^{2+} levels by intracellular sequestration, or reduced sensitivity of the contractile machinery to Ca^{2+}, both mechanisms acting without changing the membrane potential.[239] Electrophysiologic registrations from urethral smooth muscle are scarce; however, following NANC stimulation in some preparations of urethral smooth muscle from male rabbits, a hyperpolarization was found.[240]

Persson et al[241] investigated the cGMP pathway in mice lacking cGK type 1 (cGKI). In the wild type controls, EFS elicited frequency-dependent relaxations in urethral preparations. The relaxations were abolished by L-NOARG, and instead a contractile response occurred. In cGKI –/– urethral strips, the response to EFS was practically absent, but a small relaxation generally appeared at high stimulation frequencies (16–32 Hz). This relaxant response was not inhibited by L-NOARG, suggesting the occurrence of additional relaxant transmitter(s).[241]

The abundant occurrence of NOS-immunoreactive (IR) nerve fibers in the rabbit urethra also supports the present view of NO as the main inhibitory NANC mediator.[172] Using cGMP antibodies, target cells for NO were localized in rabbit urethra. Spindle-shaped cGMP-IR cells, distinct from the smooth muscle cells, formed a network around and between the urethral smooth muscle bundles.[242] Similar cGMP-IR interstitial cells were found in guinea pig and human bladder/urethra, but in contrast to the findings in rabbits, smooth muscle cells with cGMP immunoreactivity were found in the urethral tissues, following stimulation with sodium nitroprusside.[243] The occurrence of cyclic GMP immunoreactivity in smooth muscle cells seems logical, since NO is believed to stimulate guanylyl cyclase with subsequent cGMP formation in the cells.

The function of the interstitial cells has not been established, but since they have morphologic similarities to the interstitial cells of Cajal (ICC) in the gut, which are considered pacemaker cells, it has been speculated that they also may have a similar function in the lower urinary tract. Studies performed in rabbit urethral tissue showed regular spontaneous depolarization of these interstitial cells, suggesting that they indeed may have pacemaker function.[244] The specific marker for ICC, c-kit, was used to demonstrate these cells also in the guinea pig bladder, further suggesting the existence of this mechanism in the lower urinary tract.[245]

Role of phosphodiesterases NO has been demonstrated to be an important inhibitory neurotransmitter in the smooth muscle of the urethra and its relaxant effect is associated with increased levels of cGMP.[16] However, few investigations have addressed the cAMP- and cGMP-mediated signal transduction pathways and their key enzymes in the mammalian urethra. Morita et al[138] examined the effects of isoproterenol, prostaglandin E1 and E2, and SNP on the contractile force and tissue content of cAMP and cGMP in the rabbit urethra. They concluded that both cyclic nucleotides can produce relaxation of the urethra. Werkstrom et al[246] demonstrated the significance of NO and cGMP in the control of urethral relaxation. Using female pig urethral smooth muscle, they studied NANC relaxations induced by means of electrical field stimulation, and observed that the NOS inhibitor nitro-L-arginine (L-NOARG) inhibited relaxations registered at low frequencies of stimulation. Measurement of cyclic nucleotides in preparations subjected to continuous nerve stimulation revealed an increase in cGMP. In the presence of L-NOARG, there was a significant decrease in cGMP content in comparison to the control tissue. Werkstrom et al also characterized the distribution of PDE-5, cGMP, and PKG1 in female pig and human urethra, and evaluated the effect of pharmacologic inhibition of PDE-5 in isolated smooth muscle preparations. After stimulation with the NO donor, DETA NONO-ate, the cGMP immunoreactivity in urethral and vascular smooth muscles increased. There was a wide distribution of cGMP- and vimentin-positive interstitial cells between pig urethral smooth muscle bundles. PDE-5 immunoreactivity could be demonstrated within the urethral and vascular smooth muscle cells, but also in vascular endothelial cells that expressed cGMP-IR. Nerve-induced relaxations of urethral preparations were enhanced at low concentrations of sildenafil, vardenafil, and tadalafil, whereas there were direct smooth muscle relaxant actions of the PDE-5 inhibitors at high concentrations. The occurrence of other cGMP-degrading PDEs in the male urethral structures does not seem to have been studied.

Randomized-controlled studies (RCTs) on sildenafil[248] and tadalafil,[249] respectively, analyzed the impact of PDE-5 inhibitors on lower urinary tract symptoms. Both studies found significant improvements in symptom scores (International Prostate Symptom Score), but there was interestingly no change in maximum flow rate. Thus, the mechanism and site(s) of action for these positive effects of the PDE-5 inhibitors have not been established. The lack of effect on flow rate suggests that the site action may be different from that of α_1-AR antagonists. Considering preclinical experimental evidence, a relaxant effect on urethral smooth muscle could be expected, and may not be completely excluded.

Carbon monoxide The role of CO in urethral function is still controversial. It has been assumed that CO causes relaxation through the cGMP pathway. A weak relaxant effect of exogenous CO, compared to NO, was found in the rabbit urethra, suggesting that CO is not an important mediator of relaxation in this tissue.[242] However, there are known interspecies differences of urethral relaxant responses to CO. In guinea pig urethras the maximal relaxant response to CO did not exceed 15 ± 3%, compared to 40 ± 7% in pigs.[234,246] The distribution of the CO-producing enzymes heme oxygenases HO-1 and HO-2 was investigated in urethral smooth muscle of several species. In guinea pigs, HO-2 immunoreactivity was found in all nerve cell bodies of intramural ganglia, localized between smooth muscle bundles in the detrusor, bladder base, and proximal urethra.[246] In the pig urethra, HO-2 immunoreactivity was found in coarse nerve trunks, and HO-1 immunoreactivity in nerve cells, coarse nerve trunks, and varicose nerve fibers within urethral smooth muscle. In strip preparations, exogenously applied CO evoked a small relaxation associated with a small increase in cyclic GMP, but not cyclic AMP, content.[250] However, HO-2 and the NO-producing enzyme neuronal NO synthase (nNOS) were found coexisting in nerve trunks of human male and female urethras, suggesting the possibility of interaction between both systems.[251]

Naseem et al[252] found that, in the presence of hydrogen peroxide, the relaxation responses to both CO and NO in the rabbit urethra were significantly increased, and it was suggested that hydrogen peroxide may amplify NO- and CO-mediated responses. In pigs, an even more pronounced increase in relaxant response to CO in female pig urethra, using YC-1, a stimulator of sGC, suggested a possible role for CO as potential messenger function for urethral relaxation.[234]

Vasoactive intestinal peptide In various species, VIP-containing urethral ganglion cells have been demonstrated, and numerous VIP immunoreactive nerve fibers have been observed around ganglion cells, in the bladder neck, in the urethral smooth muscle layers, in lamina propria, and in association with blood vessels.[5] However, whether the findings have relevance in man is not proven.

In the pig urethra, VIP and NOS seem to be partly colocalized within nerve fibers.[196] In the rabbit urethra VIP-IR nerve fibers occurred throughout the smooth muscle layer, although the number of nerves was lower than that of NOS-IR structures and a marked relaxation of the isolated rabbit urethral muscle to VIP was reported.[242] Both pelvic and hypogastric nerve stimulation in dogs increased the bladder venous effluent VIP concentration, supporting the view that VIP can be released also from urethral nerves.[143] VIP had a marked inhibitory effect on the isolated female rabbit urethra contracted by NA or EFS, without affecting NA release, but in human urethral smooth muscle, relaxant responses were less consistent. However, a modulatory role in neurotransmission could not be excluded.[253] Infusion of VIP in humans, in amounts that caused circulatory side-effects, had no effects on urethral resistance, despite the fact that plasma concentrations of VIP were obtained which, in other clinical investigations, had been sufficient to cause relaxation of the lower esophageal sphincter and to depress uterine contractions.[144] Therefore, the physiologic importance of VIP for the lower urinary tract function in humans was questioned, and it is still unclear whether or not VIP contributes to NANC-mediated relaxation of the human urethra.[144]

NANC neurotransmission: ATP ATP has been found to cause smooth muscle relaxation via G-protein coupled P2Y receptors.[254] ATP may also induce relaxation via breakdown to adenosine. In strips of precontracted guinea pig urethra, it was found that ATP caused relaxation and inhibited spontaneous electrical activity.[255] In precontracted preparations ATP had almost no effect on EFS-induced relaxation in isolated male rabbit circular urethral smooth muscle; however, suramin, a nonselective P2Y-purinoceptor antagonist, and L-NOARG, both concentration-dependently attenuated the relaxation. ATP and related purine compounds (adenosine, AMP, and ADP) each reduced induced tonic contractions in a concentration-dependent manner. The outflow of ATP, measured using the luciferase technique, was markedly increased by EFS.[256] The findings suggested that P2Y purinoceptors exist in the male rabbit urethra, and that ATP and related purine compounds may play a role in NANC neurotransmission. This conclusion was further supported in studies on circular strips of hamster proximal urethra precontracted with arginine vasopressin. EFS caused frequency-dependent relaxations, which were attenuated by suramin and reactive blue. Exogenous ATP produced concentration-related relaxations, which were also attenuated by suramin and reactive blue.[257] The relevance of this system in man remains to be established.

Summary

Available information supports the idea that sympathetic activity, via release of NA and stimulation of urethral smooth muscle α_1-ARs, is a main factor in the maintenance of intraurethral pressure and thus of continence. NO, produced by NOS within cholinergic nerves, seems to be the predominant inhibitory neurotransmitter in the urethra, even if there is good evidence for the existence of other, as yet unidentified, inhibitory transmitters.

References

1. Morrison JF, Birder L, Craggs M et al. Incontinence. In: Abrams CL, Khoury S, Wein A eds. 3rd International Consultation on Incontinence, Vol 21. France: Health Publication, 2005: 363–422.
2. Griffiths D, Holstege G, Dalm E, de Wall H. Control and coordination of bladder and urethral function in the brainstem of the cat. Neurourol Urodyn 1990; 9: 63–82.
3. Blok BF, Holstege G. Two pontine micturition centers in the cat are not interconnected directly: implications for the central organization of micturition. J Comp Neurol 1999; 403: 209–18.
4. de Groat WC, Boot AM, Yoshimura N. Neurophysiology of micturition and its modification in animal models of human diseases. In: Maggi CA, ed. Nervous Control of the Urogenital System, Vol 3. London: Harwood Publishers, 1993; 3: 227–90.
5. Lincoln J, Burnstock G. Autonomic innervation of the urinary bladder and urethra. In: Maggi CA, ed. Nervous Control of the Urogenital System, Vol 3. London: Harwood Academic Publishers, 1993 1993: 33–68.
6. Werkstrom V, Persson K, Ny L et al. Factors involved in the relaxation of female pig urethra evoked by electrical field stimulation. Br J Pharmacol 1995; 116: 1599–604.
7. Hashimoto S, Kigoshi S, Maramatsu I. Nitric oxide-dependent and -independent neurogenic relaxation of isolated dog urethra. Eur J Pharmacol 1993; 231: 209–14.
8. Thor KB, Donatucci C. Central nervous system control of the lower urinary tract: new pharmacological approaches to stress urinary incontinence in women. J Urol 2004; 172: 27–33.
9. Yoshimura N, de Groat WC. Neural control of the lower urinary tract. Int J Urol 1997; 4: 111–25.
10. Janig W, Morrison JF. Functional properties of spinal visceral afferents supplying abdominal and pelvic organs, with special emphasis on visceral nociception. Progr Brain Res 1986; 67: 87–114.
11. Habler HJ, Jonig W, Koltzentburg M. Activation of unmyelinated afferent fibres by mechanical stimuli and inflammation of the urinary bladder in the cat. J Physiol 1990; 425: 545–62.
12. Fall M, Lindstrom S, Mazieres L. A bladder-to-bladder cooling reflex in the cat. J Physiol 1990; 427: 281–300.
13. Andersson K. Pharmacology of lower urinary tract smooth muscles and penile erectile tissues. Pharmacol Rev 1993; 45: 253–308.
14. de Groat WC, Yoshimura N. Pharmacology of the lower urinary tract. Annu Rev Pharmacol Toxicol 2001; 41: 691–721.
15. Morrison JF, Steers W, Brading AF et al. Neurophysiology and neuropharmacology. In: Abrams P, Cardozo L, Khoury S, Wein A, eds. Incontinence. Plymbridge: Plymbridge Distributors, 2002: 83–163.
16. Andersson KE, Arner A. Urinary bladder contraction and relaxation: physiology and pathophysiology. Physiol Rev 2004; 84: 935–86.
17. Arvidsson U, Riedl M, Elde R, Meister B. Vesicular acetylcholine transporter (VAChT) protein: a novel and unique marker for cholinergic neurons in the central and peripheral nervous systems. J Comp Neurol 1997; 378: 454–67.
18. Persson K, Andersson KE, Alm P. Choline acetyltransferase and vesicular acetylcholine transporter protein in neurons innervating the rat lower urinary tract. Proc Soc Neurosci 1997; 596.
19. Dixon JS, Jen PY, Gosling JA. The distribution of vesicular acetylcholine transporter in the human male genitourinary organs and its co-localization with neuropeptide Y and nitric oxide synthase. Neurourol Urodyn 2000; 19: 185–94.
20. Caulfield MP, Birdsall NJ. International Union of Pharmacology. XVII. Classification of muscarinic acetylcholine receptors. Pharmacol Rev 1998; 50: 279–90.
21. Sigala S, Mirabella G, Peroni A et al. Differential gene expression of cholinergic muscarinic receptor subtypes in male and female normal human urinary bladder. Urology 2002; 60: 719–25.
22. Hinata N, Shirakawa T, Okada H et al. Quantitative analysis of the levels of expression of muscarinic receptor subtype RNA in the detrusor muscle of patients with overactive bladder. Mol Diagn 2004; 8: 17–22.
23. Wang P, Luthin GR, Ruggieri MR. Muscarinic acetylcholine receptor subtypes mediating urinary bladder contractility and coupling to GTP binding proteins. J Pharmacol Exp Ther 1995; 273: 959–66.
24. Yamaguchi O, Shishido K, Tamura K. Evaluation of mRNAs encoding muscarinic receptor subtypes in human detrusor muscle. J Urol 1996; 156: 1208–13.
25. Mukerji G, Yiangou Y, Grogono J et al. Localization of M2 and M3 muscarinic receptors in human bladder disorders and their clinical correlations. J Urol 2006; 176: 367–73.
26. Eglen RM, Hegde SS, Watson N et al. Muscarinic receptor subtypes and smooth muscle function. Pharmacol Rev 1996; 48: 531–65.
27. Hegde SS, Eglen RM. Muscarinic receptor subtypes modulating smooth muscle contractility in the urinary bladder. Life Sci 1999; 64: 419–28.
28. Chess-Williams R. Muscarinic receptors of the urinary bladder: detrusor, urothelial and prejunctional. Auton Autacoid Pharmacol 2002; 22: 133–45.
29. Eglen RM. Muscarinic receptor subtypes in neuronal and non-neuronal cholinergic function. Auton Autacoid Pharmacol 2006; 26: 219–33.
30. Andersson KE, Wein AJ. Pharmacology of the lower urinary tract: basis for current and future treatments of urinary incontinence. Pharmacol Rev 2004; 56: 581–631.
31. Matsui M, Noromura D, Karasawa H. Multiple functional defects in peripheral autonomic organs in mice lacking muscarinic acetylcholine receptor gene for the M3 subtype. Proc Natl Acad Sci USA 2000; 97: 9579–84.
32. Igawa Y, Zhang X, Nishizawa O et al. Cystometric findings in mice lacking muscarinic M2 or M3 receptors. J Urol 2004; 172: 2460–4.
33. Andersson KE, Holmquist F, Fovaeus M et al. Muscarinic receptor stimulation of phosphoinositide hydrolysis in the human isolated urinary bladder. J Urol 1991; 146: 1156–9.
34. Harriss DR, Marsh KA, Birmingham AT, Hill SJ. Expression of muscarinic M3-receptors coupled to inositol phospholipid hydrolysis in human detrusor cultured smooth muscle cells. J Urol 1995; 154: 1241–5.
35. Jezior JR, Brady JD, Rosenstein DI et al. Dependency of detrusor contractions on calcium sensitization and calcium entry through LOE-908-sensitive channels. Br J Pharmacol 2001; 134: 78–87.
36. Wibberley A, Chen Z, Hu E et al. Expression and functional role of Rho-kinase in rat urinary bladder smooth muscle. Br J Pharmacol 2003; 138: 757–66.
37. Schneider T, Hein P, Michel MC. Signal transduction underlying carbachol-induced contraction of rat urinary bladder. I. Phospholipases and Ca^{2+} sources. J Pharmacol Exp Ther 2004; 308: 47–53.
38. Braverman AS, Ruggieri MR Sr. Muscarinic receptor transcript and protein density in hypertrophied and atrophied rat urinary bladder. Neurourol Urodyn 2006; 25: 55–61.
39. Takahashi R, Nishimura J, Hirano K et al. Ca^{2+} sensitization in contraction of human bladder smooth muscle. J Urol 2004; 172: 748–52.
40. Peters SL, Schmidt M, Michel MC. Rho kinase: a target for treating urinary bladder dysfunction? Trends Pharmacol Sci 2006; 27: 492–7.

41. Hegde SS, Choppin A, Bonhaus D et al. Functional role of M2 and M3 muscarinic receptors in the urinary bladder of rats in vitro and in vivo. Br J Pharmacol 1997; 120: 1409–18.
42. Kotlikoff MI, Dhulipala P, Wang YX. M2 signaling in smooth muscle cells. Life Sci 1999; 64: 437–42.
43. Bonev AD, Nelson MT. Muscarinic inhibition of ATP-sensitive K^+ channels by protein kinase C in urinary bladder smooth muscle. Am J Physiol 1993; 265: C1723–8.
44. Nakamura K, Hirano J, Itazawa S et al. Protein kinase G activates inwardly rectifying K(+) channel in cultured human proximal tubule cells. Am J Physiol Renal Physiol 2002; 283: F784–91.
45. Ehlert FJ, Griffin MT, Abe DM et al. The M2 muscarinic receptor mediates contraction through indirect mechanisms in mouse urinary bladder. J Pharmacol Exp Ther 2005; 313: 368–78.
46. Braverman A, Legos J, Young W et al. M2 receptors in genito-urinary smooth muscle pathology. Life Sci 1999; 64: 429–36.
47. Braverman AS, Luthin GR, Ruggieri MR. M2 muscarinic receptor contributes to contraction of the denervated rat urinary bladder. Am J Physiol 1998; 275: R1654–60.
48. Braverman AS, Luthin GR, Ruggieri MR. Interaction between muscarinic receptor subtype signal transduction pathways mediating bladder contraction. Am J Physiol Regul Integr Comp Physiol 2002; 283: R663–8.
49. Braverman AS, Ruggieri MR Sr. Hypertrophy changes the muscarinic receptor subtype mediating bladder contraction from M3 toward M2. Am J Physiol Regul Integr Comp Physiol 2003; 285: R701–8.
50. Stevens L, Tophill P, Chess-Williams R. A comparison of muscarinic receptor-mediated function in the normal and the neurogenic overactive bladder. J Urol (Suppl) 2004; 171: 143 (abstract 535).
51. Stevens L, Chess-Williams R, Chapple C. Muscarinic receptor function in the idiopathic overactive bladder. J Urol (Suppl) 2004; 171: 140–1 (abstract 527).
52. Pontari MA, Braverman AS, Ruggieri MR. The M2 muscarinic receptor mediates in vitro bladder contractions from patients with neurogenic bladder dysfunction. Am J Physiol Regul Integr Comp Physiol 2004; 286: R874–80.
53. Tobin G, Sjogren C. In vivo and in vitro effects of muscarinic receptor antagonists on contractions and release of [3H]acetylcholine in the rabbit urinary bladder. Eur J Pharmacol 1995; 281: 1–8.
54. Inadome A, Yoshida M, Takahashi W et al. Prejunctional muscarinic receptors modulating acetylcholine release in rabbit detrusor smooth muscles. Urol Int 1998; 61: 135–41.
55. Somogyi GT, de Groat WC. Evidence for inhibitory nicotinic and facilitatory muscarinic receptors in cholinergic nerve terminals of the rat urinary bladder. J Auton Nerv Syst 1992; 37: 89–97.
56. Alberts P. Classification of the presynaptic muscarinic receptor subtype that regulates 3H-acetylcholine secretion in the guinea pig urinary bladder in vitro. J Pharmacol Exp Ther 1995; 274: 458–68.
57. D'Agostino G, Barbieri A, Chiossa E et al. M4 muscarinic autoreceptor-mediated inhibition of 3H-acetylcholine release in the rat isolated urinary bladder. J Pharmacol Exp Ther 1997; 283: 750–6.
58. D'Agostino G, Bolognesi ML, Lucchelli A et al. Prejunctional muscarinic inhibitory control of acetylcholine release in the human isolated detrusor: involvement of the M4 receptor subtype. Br J Pharmacol 2000; 129: 493–500.
59. Somogyi GT, de Groat WC. Function, signal transduction mechanisms and plasticity of presynaptic muscarinic receptors in the urinary bladder. Life Sci 1999; 64: 411–18.
60. Mansfield KJ, Lui L, Mitchelson FJ et al. Muscarinic receptor subtypes in human bladder detrusor and mucosa, studied by radioligand binding and quantitative competitive RT-PCR: changes in ageing. Br J Pharmacol 2005; 144: 1089–99.
61. Fovaeus M, Fujiwara M, Hogestatt ED et al. A non-nitrergic smooth muscle relaxant factor released from rat urinary bladder by muscarinic receptor stimulation. J Urol 1999; 161: 649–53.
62. Hawthorn MH, Chapple CR, Cock M et al. Urothelium-derived inhibitory factor(s) influences on detrusor muscle contractility in vitro. Br J Pharmacol 2000; 129: 416–19.
63. Yokoyama O, Yusup A, Miwa Y et al. Effects of tolterodine on an overactive bladder depend on suppression of C-fiber bladder afferent activity in rats. J Urol 2005; 174: 2032–6.
64. Hedlund P ST, Lee T, Andersson K-E. Effects of tolterodine on afferent neurotransmission in normal and resiniferatoxin-treated conscious rats. J Urol 2007; 178: 326–31.
65. De Laet K, De Wachter S, Wydaele JJ. Systemic oxybutynin decreases afferent activity of the pelvic nerve of the rat: new insights into the working mechanism of antimuscarinics. Neurourol Urodyn 2006; 25: 156–61.
66. Boy S, Schurch B, Nehring G et al. The effect of tolterodine on sensations evoked by electrical stimulation and bladder filling sensations. Eur Urol Suppl 2006; 5: 223 (abstract 804).
67. Finney SM, Andersson CE, Gillespie JI et al. Antimuscarinic drugs in detrusor overactivity and the overactive bladder syndrome: motor or sensory actions? BJU Int 2006; 98: 503–7.
68. Blake-James BT, Rashidian A, Ikeda Y et al. The role of anticholinergics in men with lower urinary tract symptoms suggestive of benign prostatic hyperplasia: a systematic review and meta-analysis. BJU Int 2007; 99: 85–96.
69. Andersson KE. New roles for muscarinic receptors in the pathophysiology of lower urinary tract symptoms. BJU Int 2000; 86(Suppl 2): 36–42; discussion 42–3.
70. Gary T, Robertson D. Lessons learned from dopamine beta-hydroxylase deficiency in humans. News Physiol Sci 1994; 9: 35–9.
71. Michel MC, Vrydag W. Alpha1-, alpha2- and beta-adrenoceptors in the urinary bladder, urethra and prostate. Br J Pharmacol 2006; 147(Suppl 2): S88–119.
72. Goepel M, Wittmann A, Rubben H, Michel MC. Comparison of adrenoceptor subtype expression in porcine and human bladder and prostate. Urol Res 1997; 25: 199–206.
73. Malloy BJ, Price DT, Price RR et al. Alpha1-adrenergic receptor subtypes in human detrusor. J Urol 1998; 160: 937–43.
74. Hampel C, Dolber PC, Smith MP et al. Modulation of bladder alpha1-adrenergic receptor subtype expression by bladder outlet obstruction. J Urol 2002; 167: 1513–21.
75. Nomiya M, Yamaguchi O. A quantitative analysis of mRNA expression of alpha 1 and beta-adrenoceptor subtypes and their functional roles in human normal and obstructed bladders. J Urol 2003; 170: 649–53.
76. Persson K, Pandita RK, Spitsbergen JM et al. Spinal and peripheral mechanisms contributing to hyperactive voiding in spontaneously hypertensive rats. Am J Physiol 1998; 275: R1366–73.
77. Somogyi GT, Tanowitz M, de Groat WC. Prejunctional facilitatory alpha 1-adrenoceptors in the rat urinary bladder. Br J Pharmacol 1995; 114: 1710–16.
78. Szell EA, Yamamoto T, de Groat WC et al. Smooth muscle and parasympathetic nerve terminals in the rat urinary bladder have different subtypes of alpha(1) adrenoceptors. Br J Pharmacol 2000; 130: 1685–91.
79. Trevisani M, Campi B, Gatti F et al. The influence of alpha(1)-adrenoreceptors on neuropeptide release from primary sensory neurons of the lower urinary tract. Eur Urol 2007; 52: 901–8.
80. Nergardh A, Boreus LO, Naglo AS. Characterization of the adrenergic beta-receptor in the urinary bladder of man and cat. Acta Pharmacol Toxicol (Copenh) 1977; 40: 14–21.
81. Larsen JJ. Alpha and beta-adrenoceptors in the detrusor muscle and bladder base of the pig and beta-adrenoceptors in the detrusor muscle of man. Br J Pharmacol 1979; 65: 215–22.
82. Igawa Y, Yamazaki Y, Takeda H et al. Functional and molecular biological evidence for a possible beta3-adrenoceptor in the human detrusor muscle. Br J Pharmacol 1999; 126: 819–25.
83. Takeda M, Obara K, Mizusawa T et al. Evidence for beta3-adrenoceptor subtypes in relaxation of the human urinary bladder detrusor:

analysis by molecular biological and pharmacological methods. J Pharmacol Exp Ther 1999; 288: 1367–73.
84. Yamazaki Y, Takeda H, Akahane M et al. Species differences in the distribution of beta-adrenoceptor subtypes in bladder smooth muscle. Br J Pharmacol 1998; 124: 593–9.
85. Yamaguchi O. Beta3-adrenoceptors in human detrusor muscle. Urology 2002; 59: 25–9.
86. Andersson KE, Chapple C, Wein A. The basis for drug treatment of the overactive bladder. World J Urol 2001; 19: 294–8.
87. Rohner TJ, Hannigan JD, Sanford EJ. Altered in vitro adrenergic responses of dog detrusor msucle after chronic bladder outlet obstruction. Urology 1978; 11: 357–61.
88. Tsujii T, Azuma H, Yamaguchi T, Oshima H. A possible role of decreased relaxation mediated by beta-adrenoceptors in bladder outlet obstruction by benign prostatic hyperplasia. Br J Pharmacol 1992; 107: 803–7.
89. Igawa Y, Yamazaki Y, Takeda H et al. Relaxant effects of isoproterenol and selective beta3-adrenoceptor agonists on normal, low compliant and hyperreflexic human bladders. J Urol 2001; 165: 240–4.
90. Tanaka N, Tomai T, Mukaiyama H et al. Beta(3)-adrenoceptor agonists for the treatment of frequent urination and urinary incontinence: 2-[4-(2-[[(1S,2R)-2-hydroxy-2-(4-hydroxyphenyl)-1-methylethyl]amino]ethyl) phenoxy]-2-methylpropionic acid. Bioorg Med Chem 2001; 9: 3265–71.
91. Woods M, Carson N, Norton NW et al. Efficacy of the beta3-adrenergic receptor agonist CL-316243 on experimental bladder hyperreflexia and detrusor instability in the rat. J Urol 2001; 166: 1142–7.
92. Andersson KE. Bladder activation: afferent mechanisms. Urology 2002; 59: 43–50.
93. de Groat WC. The urothelium in overactive bladder: passive bystander or active participant? Urology 2004; 64: 7–11.
94. Birder LA, de Groat WC. Mechanisms of disease: involvement of the urothelium in bladder dysfunction. Nat Clin Pract Urol 2007; 4: 46–54.
95. Birder LA. Involvement of the urinary bladder urothelium in signaling in the lower urinary tract. Proc West Pharmacol Soc 2001; 44: 85–6.
96. Birder LA, Nakamura Y, Kiss S et al. Altered urinary bladder function in mice lacking the vanilloid receptor TRPV1. Nat Neurosci 2002; 5: 856–60.
97. Dickson A, Avelino A, Cruz F et al. Peptidergic sensory and parasympathetic fiber sprouting in the mucosa of the rat urinary bladder in a chronic model of cyclophosphamide-induced cystitis. Neuroscience 2006; 139: 671–85.
98. Jen PY, Dixon JS, Gosling JA. Immunohistochemical localization of neuromarkers and neuropeptides in human fetal and neonatal urinary bladder. Br J Urol 1995; 75: 230–5.
99. de Groat WC. Integrative control of the lower urinary tract: preclinical perspective. Br J Pharmacol 2006; 147(Suppl 2): S25–40.
100. Andersson KE. New pharmacologic targets for the treatment of the overactive bladder: an update. Urology 2004; 63: 32–41.
101. Andersson KE. Antimuscarinics for treatment of overactive bladder. Lancet Neurol 2004; 3: 46–53.
102. De Wachter S, Wyndaele JJ. Intravesical oxybutynin: a local anesthetic effect on bladder C afferents. J Urol 2003; 169: 1892–5.
103. Iijima K, De Wachter S, Wyndaele J-J. Effects of the M3 receptor selective muscarinic receptor antagonist darifenacin on bladder afferent activity of the rat pelvic nerve. Eur Urol 2007; 52: 842–7.
104. Lips KS, Wunsch J, Zarghooni S et al. Acetylcholine and molecular components of its synthesis and release machinery in the urothelium. Eur Urol 2007; 51: 1042–53.
105. Maggi CA. Prostanoids as local modulators of reflex micturition. Pharmacol Res 1992; 25: 13–20.
106. Chancellor MB, de Groat WC. Intravesical capsaicin and resiniferatoxin therapy: spicing up the ways to treat the overactive bladder. J Urol 1999; 162: 3–11.
107. Sui GP, Rothery S, Dupont E et al. Gap junctions and connexin expression in human suburothelial interstitial cells. BJU Int 2002; 90: 118–29.
108. Sui GP, Wu C, Fry CH. Electrical characteristics of suburothelial cells isolated from the human bladder. J Urol 2004; 171: 938–43.
109. Brading AF, McCloskey KD. Mechanisms of disease: specialized interstitial cells of the urinary tract – an assessment of current knowledge. Nat Clin Pract Urol 2005; 2: 546–54.
110. Gillespie JI, Markerink K, van Ittersum M, de Vente J. Endogenous nitric oxide/cGMP signalling in the guinea pig bladder: evidence for distinct populations of sub-urothelial interstitial cells. Cell Tissue Res 2006; 325: 325–32.
111. Gillespie JI, Markerink K, van Ittersum M, de Vente J. cGMP-generating cells in the bladder wall: identification of distinct networks of interstitial cells. BJU Int 2004; 94: 1114–24.
112. Burnstock G. Purine-mediated signalling in pain and visceral perception. Trends Pharmacol Sci 2001; 22: 182–8.
113. Tominaga M, Wada M, Masu M. Potentiation of capsaicin receptor activity by metabotropic ATP receptors as a possible mechanism for ATP-evoked pain and hyperalgesia. Proc Natl Acad Sci USA 2001; 98: 6951–6.
114. Pandita RK, Andersson KE. Intravesical adenosine triphosphate stimulates the micturition reflex in awake, freely moving rats. J Urol 2002; 168: 1230–4.
115. Cockayne DA, Hamilton SG, Zhu QM et al. Urinary bladder hyporeflexia and reduced pain-related behaviour in P2X3-deficient mice. Nature 2000; 407: 1011–5.
116. Vlaskovska M, Kasakov L, Rong W et al. P2X3 knock-out mice reveal a major sensory role for urothelially released ATP. J Neurosci 2001; 21: 5670–7.
117. Luheshi GN, Zar MA. Presence of non-cholinergic motor transmission in human isolated bladder. J Pharm Pharmacol 1990; 42: 223–4.
118. Sjogren C, Andersson KE, Husted S et al. Atropine resistance of transmurally stimulated isolated human bladder muscle. J Urol 1982; 128: 1368–71.
119. Sibley GN. A comparison of spontaneous and nerve-mediated activity in bladder muscle from man, pig and rabbit. J Physiol 1984; 354: 431–43.
120. Smith CC. In vitro response of human bladder smooth muscle in unstable obstructed male bladders: a study of pathophysiological causes. Neurourol Urodyn 1994; 134: 14–15.
121. Bayliss M, Wu C, Newgreen D et al. A quantitative study of atropine-resistant contractile responses in human detrusor smooth muscle, from stable, unstable and obstructed bladders. J Urol 1999; 162: 1833–9.
122. Saito M, Kondo A, Kato T, Miyake K. [Response of the human neurogenic bladder induced by intramural nerve stimulation]. Nippon Hinyokika Gakkai Zasshi 1993; 84: 507–13.
123. O'Reilly BA, Kosaka AH, Knight GF et al. P2X receptors and their role in female idiopathic detrusor instability. J Urol 2002; 167: 157–64.
124. Palea S, Artibani W, Ostardo E et al. Evidence for purinergic neurotransmission in human urinary bladder affected by interstitial cystitis. J Urol 1993; 150: 2007–12.
125. Wammack R, Wiebe E, Dienes HP, Hohenfellner R. Die Neurogene Blase in vitro. Akt Urol 1995; 26: 16–18.
126. Yoshida M, Homma Y, Inadome A et al. Age-related changes in cholinergic and purinergic neurotransmission in human isolated bladder smooth muscles. Exp Gerontol 2001; 36: 99–109.
127. Lee HY, Bardini M, Burnstock G. Distribution of P2X receptors in the urinary bladder and the ureter of the rat. J Urol 2000; 163: 2002–7.
128. O'Reilly BA, Kosaka AH, Chang TK et al. A quantitative analysis of purinoceptor expression in the bladders of patients with symptomatic outlet obstruction. BJU Int 2001; 87: 617–22.

129. Moore KH, Ray FR, Barden JA. Loss of purinergic P2X(3) and P2X(5) receptor innervation in human detrusor from adults with urge incontinence. J Neurosci 2001; 21: RC166.
130. Maggi CA. The mammalian tachykinin receptors. Gen Pharmacol 1995; 26: 911–44.
131. Maggi CA. The dual, sensory and 'efferent' function of the capsaicin-sensitive primary sensory neurons in the urinary bladder and urethra. In: Maggi CA, ed. Nervous Control of the Urogenital System, Vol 3. London: Harwood Publishers 1993; 3: 348–422.
132. Uckert S, Stief CG, Lietz B et al. Possible role of bioactive peptides in the regulation of human detrusor smooth muscle – functional effects in vitro and immunohistochemical presence. World J Urol 2002; 20: 244–9.
133. Maggi CA, Barbanti G, Santicioli P et al. Cystometric evidence that capsaicin-sensitive nerves modulate the afferent branch of micturition reflex in humans. J Urol 1989; 142: 150–4.
134. Chapple CR, Milner P, Moss HE, Burnstock G. Loss of sensory neuropeptides in the obstructed human bladder. Br J Urol 1992; 70: 373–81.
135. Giuliani S, Patacchini R, Barbanti G et al. Characterization of the tachykinin neurokinin-2 receptor in the human urinary bladder by means of selective receptor antagonists and peptidase inhibitors. J Pharmacol Exp Ther 1993; 267: 590–5.
136. Green SA, Alon A, Ianas J et al. Efficacy and safety of a neurokinin-2 receptor antagonist in postmenopausal women. J Urol 2006; 176: 2523.
137. Saenz de Tejada I, Mueller JD, de Las Morenas A et al. Endothelin in the urinary bladder. I. Synthesis of endothelin-1 by epithelia, muscle and fibroblasts suggests autocrine and paracrine cellular regulation. J Urol 1992; 148: 1290–8.
138. Kondo S, Morita T, Tashima Y. Benign prostatic hypertrophy affects the endothelin receptor density in the human urinary bladder and prostate. Urol Int 1995; 54: 198–203.
139. Okamoto-Koizumi T, Takeda M, Komeyama T et al. Pharmacological and molecular biological evidence for ETA endothelin receptor subtype mediating mechanical responses in the detrusor smooth muscle of the human urinary bladder. Clin Sci (Lond) 1999; 96: 397–402.
140. Khan MA, Shukla N, Auld J et al. Possible role of endothelin-1 in the rabbit urinary bladder hyperplasia secondary to partial bladder outlet obstruction. Scand J Urol Nephrol 2000; 34: 15–20.
141. Schroder A et al. Detrusor responses to prostaglandin E2 and bladder outlet obstruction in wild-type and Ep1 receptor knockout mice. J Urol 2004; 172: 1166–70.
142. Andersson PO, Bloom SR, Mattiasson A, U'velius B. Bladder vasodilatation and release of vasoactive intestinal polypeptide from the urinary bladder of the cat in response to pelvic nerve stimulation. J Urol 1987; 138: 671–3.
143. Andersson PO, Sjogren C, Urnas B, Uvnas-Moberg K. Urinary bladder and urethral responses to pelvic and hypogastric nerve stimulation and their relation to vasoactive intestinal polypeptide in the anaesthetized dog. Acta Physiol Scand 1990; 138: 409–16.
144. Klarskov P, Holm-Bentzen M, Norgaard T et al. Vasoactive intestinal polypeptide concentration in human bladder neck smooth muscle and its influence on urodynamic parameters. Br J Urol 1987; 60: 113–18.
145. Gu J, Restarick JM, Blank MA et al. Vasoactive intestinal polypeptide in the normal and unstable bladder. Br J Urol 1983; 55: 645–7.
146. Persson K, Garcia-Pusual A, Andersson KE. Difference in the actions of calcitonin gene-related peptide on pig detrusor and vesical arterial smooth muscle. Acta Physiol Scand 1991; 143: 45–53.
147. Giuliani S, Santicioli P, Lippi A et al. The role of sensory neuropeptides in motor innervation of the hamster isolated urinary bladder. Naun Schmiedebergs Arch Pharmacol 2001; 364: 242–8.
148. Lacroix JS, Stjarne P, Anggard A, Lundberg JM. Sympathetic vascular control of the pig nasal mucosa (III): Co-release of noradrenaline and neuropeptide Y. Acta Physiol Scand 1989; 135: 17–28.
149. Iravani MM, Zar MA. Neuropeptide Y in rat detrusor and its effect on nerve-mediated and acetylcholine-evoked contractions. Br J Pharmacol 1994; 113: 95–102.
150. Zoubek J, Somagyi GT, de Groat WC. A comparison of inhibitory effects of neuropeptide Y on rat urinary bladder, urethra, and vas deferens. Am J Physiol 1993; 265: R537–43.
151. Lundberg JM, Hua XY, Franco-Cereceda A. Effects of neuropeptide Y (NPY) on mechanical activity and neurotransmission in the heart, vas deferens and urinary bladder of the guinea-pig. Acta Physiol Scand 1984; 121: 325–32.
152. Crowe R, Noble J, Robson T et al. An increase of neuropeptide Y but not nitric oxide synthase-immunoreactive nerves in the bladder neck from male patients with bladder neck dyssynergia. J Urol 1995; 154: 1231–6.
153 Dixon JS, Jen PY, Gosling JA. A double-label immunohistochemical study of intramural ganglia from the human male urinary bladder neck. J Anat 1997; 190 (Pt 1): 125–34.
154. Gu J, Blank MA, Huang WM et al. Peptide-containing nerves in human urinary bladder. Urology 1984; 24: 353–7.
155. Iwasa A. [Distribution of neuropeptide Y (NPY) and its binding sites in human lower urinary tract. Histological analysis]. Nippon Hinyokika Gakkai Zasshi 1993; 84: 1000–6.
156. Davis B, Goepel M, Bein S et al. Lack of neuropeptide Y receptor detection in human bladder and prostate. BJU Int 2000; 85: 918–24.
157. Brown WW, Zenser TV, Davis BB. Prostaglandin E2 production by rabbit urinary bladder. Am J Physiol 1980; 239: F452–8.
158. Downie JW, Karmazyn M. Mechanical trauma to bladder epithelium liberates prostanoids which modulate neurotransmission in rabbit detrusor muscle. J Pharmacol Exp Ther 1984; 230: 445–9.
159. Jeremy JY, Dandona P. Fluoride but not phorbol esters stimulate rat urinary bladder prostanoid synthesis: investigations into the roles of G proteins and protein kinase C. Prostaglandins Leukot Med 1987; 29: 129–39.
160. Jeremy JY, Tsang V, Mikhailidis DP et al. Eicosanoid synthesis by human urinary bladder mucosa: pathological implications. Br J Urol 1987; 59: 36–9.
161. Andersson KE, Sjogren C. Aspects on the physiology and pharmacology of the bladder and urethra. Prog Neurobiol 1982; 19: 71–89.
162. Feng L, Sun W, Xia Y et al. Cloning two isoforms of rat cyclooxygenase: differential regulation of their expression. Arch Biochem Biophys 1993; 307: 361–8.
163. Pairet M, Engelhardt G. Distinct isoforms (COX-1 and COX-2) of cyclooxygenase: possible physiological and therapeutic implications. Fundam Clin Pharmacol 1996; 10: 1–17.
164. Vane JR, Botting RM. Mechanism of action of anti-inflammatory drugs. Scand J Rheumatol Suppl 1996; 102: 9–21.
165. Park JM, Yang T, Arend LJ et al. Cyclooxygenase-2 is expressed in bladder during fetal development and stimulated by outlet obstruction. Am J Physiol 1997; 273: F538–44.
166. Lee T, Hedlund P, Newgreen D, Andersson KE. Urodynamic effects of a novel EP1-receptor antagonist in normal rats and rats with bladder outlet obstruction. J Urol 2007; 177: 1562–7.
167. Smet PJ, Edyvane KA, Jonavicius J, Marshall VR. Distribution of NADPH-diaphorase-positive nerves supplying the human urinary bladder. J Auton Nerv Syst 1994; 47: 109–13.
168. Persson K, Alm P, Johansson K et al. Nitric oxide synthase in pig lower urinary tract: immunohistochemistry, NADPH diaphorase histochemistry and functional effects. Br J Pharmacol 1993; 110: 521–30.
169. James MJ, Birmingham AT, Hill SJ. Partial mediation by nitric oxide of the relaxation of human isolated detrusor strips in response to electrical field stimulation. Br J Clin Pharmacol 1993; 35: 366–72.
170. Elliott RA, Castleden CM. Nerve mediated relaxation in human detrusor muscle. Br J Clin Pharmacol 1993; 36: 479; author reply 80–1.
171. Persson K, Igawa Y, Mattiasson A, Andersson KE. Effects of inhibition of the L-arginine/nitric oxide pathway in the rat lower urinary tract in vivo and in vitro. Br J Pharmacol 1992; 107: 178–84.

172. Persson K, Andersson KE. Non-adrenergic, non-cholinergic relaxation and levels of cyclic nucleotides in rabbit lower urinary tract. Eur J Pharmacol 1994; 268: 159–67.
173. Andersson KE. Pathways for relaxation of detrusor smooth muscle. Adv Exp Med Biol 1999; 462: 241–52.
174. Morita T, Tsujii T, Dokita S. Regional difference in functional roles of cAMP and cGMP in lower urinary tract smooth muscle contractility. Urol Int 1992; 49: 191–5.
175. Wheeler MA, Ayyagari RR, Wheeler GL et al. Regulation of cyclic nucleotides in the urinary tract. J Smooth Muscle Res 2005; 41: 1–21.
176. Sunahara RK, Dessauer CW, Gilman AG. Complexity and diversity of mammalian adenylyl cyclases. Annu Rev Pharmacol Toxicol 1996; 36: 461–80.
177. Cooper DM, Crossthwaite AJ. Higher-order organization and regulation of adenylyl cyclases. Trends Pharmacol Sci 2006; 27: 426–31.
178. Dokita S, Smith SD, Nishimoto T et al. Involvement of nitric oxide and cyclic GMP in rabbit urethral relaxation. Eur J Pharmacol 1994; 266: 269–75.
179. Lucas KA, Pitari GM, Kazerounian S et al. Guanylyl cyclases and signaling by cyclic GMP. Pharmacol Rev 2000; 52: 375–414.
180. Conti M, Jin SL. The molecular biology of cyclic nucleotide phosphodiesterases. Progr Nucleic Acid Res Mol Biol 1999; 63: 1–38.
181. Francis SH, Jurko IV, Corbin JD. Cyclic nucleotide phosphodiesterases: relating structure and function. Progr Nucleic Acid Res Mol Biol 2001; 65: 1–52.
182. Beavo JA, Brunton LL. Cyclic nucleotide research – still expanding after half a century. Nat Rev Mol Cell Biol 2002; 3: 710–18.
183. Rybalkin SD, Yan C, Bornfeldt KE et al. Cyclic GMP phosphodiesterases and regulation of smooth muscle function. Circ Res 2003; 93: 280–91.
184. Truss MC, Steif CG, Uckert S et al. Initial clinical experience with the selective phosphodiesterase-I isoenzyme inhibitor vinpocetine in the treatment of urge incontinence and low compliance bladder. World J Urol 2000; 18: 439–43.
185. Truss MC, Steif CG, Uckert S et al. Phosphodiesterase 1 inhibition in the treatment of lower urinary tract dysfunction: from bench to bedside. World J Urol 2001; 19: 344–50.
186. Truss MC, Uckert S, Steif CG et al. Cyclic nucleotide phosphodiesterase (PDE) isoenzymes in the human detrusor smooth muscle. II. Effect of various PDE inhibitors on smooth muscle tone and cyclic nucleotide levels in vitro. Urol Res 1996; 24: 129–34.
187. Truss MC, Uckert S, Steif CG et al. Cyclic nucleotide phosphodiesterase (PDE) isoenzymes in the human detrusor smooth muscle. I. Identification and characterization. Urol Res 1996; 24: 123–8.
188. Truss MC, Uckert S, Steif CG et al. Effects of various phosphodiesterase-inhibitors, forskolin, and sodium nitroprusside on porcine detrusor smooth muscle tonic responses to muscarinergic stimulation and cyclic nucleotide levels in vitro. Neurourol Urodyn 1996; 15: 59–70.
189. Qiu Y, Kraft P, Graig EC et al. Identification and functional study of phosphodiesterases in rat urinary bladder. Urol Res 2001; 29: 388–92.
190. Qiu Y, Kraft P, Graig EC et al. Cyclic nucleotide phosphodiesterases in rabbit detrusor smooth muscle. Urology 2002; 59: 145–9.
191. Morley DJ, Hawley DM, Ulbright TM et al. Distribution of phosphodiesterase I in normal human tissues. J Histochem Cytochem 1987; 35: 75–82.
192. Gillespie JI, Markerink K, van Ittersum M, de Vente J et al. Expression of neuronal nitric oxide synthase (nNOS) and nitric oxide-induced changes in cGMP in the urothelial layer of the guinea pig bladder. Cell Tissue Res 2005; 321: 341–51.
193. Longhurst PA, Briscoe JA, Rosenberg DJ et al. The role of cyclic nucleotides in guinea-pig bladder contractility. Br J Pharmacol 1997; 121: 1665–72.
194. Snyder PB, Esselstyn JM, Loughney K et al. The role of cyclic nucleotide phosphodiesterases in the regulation of adipocyte lipolysis. J Lipid Res 2005; 46: 494–503.
195. Tanagho EA, Miller ER. Initiation of voiding. Br J Urol 1970; 42: 175–83.
196. Persson K, Alm P, Johansson K et al. Co-existence of nitrergic, peptidergic and acetylcholine esterase-positive nerves in the pig lower urinary tract. J Auton Nerv Syst 1995; 52: 225–36.
197. Persson K, Alm P, Uvelius B, Andersson KE. Nitrergic and cholinergic innervation of the rat lower urinary tract after pelvic ganglionectomy. Am J Physiol 1998; 274: R389–97.
198. Johns A. Alpha- and beta-adrenergic and muscarinic cholinergic binding sites in the bladder and urethra of the rabbit. Can J Physiol Pharmacol 1983; 61: 61–6.
199. Taki N, Taniguchi T, Okada K et al. Evidence for predominant mediation of alpha1-adrenoceptor in the tonus of entire urethra of women. J Urol 1999; 162: 1829–32.
200. Persson CG, Andersson KE. Adrenoceptor and cholinoceptor mediated effects in the isolated urethra of cat and guinea-pig. Clin Exp Pharmacol Physiol 1976; 3: 415–26.
201. Andersson KE, Persson CG, Alm P et al. Effects of acetylcholine, noradrenaline, and prostaglandins on the isolated, perfused human fetal urethra. Acta Physiol Scand 1978; 104: 394–401.
202. Ek A, Andersson KE, Ulmsten U. The effects of norephedrine and bethanechol on the human urethral closure pressure profile. Scand J Urol Nephrol 1978; 12: 97–104.
203. Ulmsten U, Andersson KE. The effects of emeprone on intravesical and intraurethral pressure in women with urgency incontinence. Scand J Urol Nephrol 1977; 11: 103–9.
204. Mattiasson A, Andersson KE, Sjogren C. Adrenoceptors and cholinoceptors controlling noradrenaline release from adrenergic nerves in the urethra of rabbit and man. J Urol 1984; 131: 1190–5.
205. Yamanishi T, Chapple CR, Yasuda K et al. The role of M2 muscarinic receptor subtypes mediating contraction of the circular and longitudinal smooth muscle of the pig proximal urethra. J Urol 2002; 168: 308–14.
206. Gosling JA, Dixon JS, Lendon RG. The autonomic innervation of the human male and female bladder neck and proximal urethra. J Urol 1977; 118: 302–5.
207. Ek A, Alm P, Andersson KE, Persson CG. Adrenergic and cholinergic nerves of the human urethra and urinary bladder. A histochemical study. Acta Physiol Scand 1977; 99: 345–52.
208. Alm P, Zygmunt PK, Iselin C et al. Nitric oxide synthase-immunoreactive, adrenergic, cholinergic, and peptidergic nerves of the female rat urinary tract: a comparative study. J Auton Nerv Syst 1995; 56: 105–14.
209. Persson K, Johansson K, Alm P et al. Morphological and functional evidence against a sensory and sympathetic origin of nitric oxide synthase-containing nerves in the rat lower urinary tract. Neuroscience 1997; 77: 271–81.
210. Levin RM, Wein AJ. Quantitative analysis of alpha and beta adrenergic receptor densities in the lower urinary tract of the dog and the rabbit. Invest Urol 1979; 17: 75–7.
211. Latifpour J, Kondo S, O'Hollaren B et al. Autonomic receptors in urinary tract: sex and age differences. J Pharmacol Exp Ther 1990; 253: 661–7.
212. Ek A, Alm P, Andersson KE, Persson CG. Adrenoceptor and cholinoceptor mediated responses of the isolated human urethra. Scand J Urol Nephrol 1977; 11: 97–102.
213. Appell RA, England HR, Hussell HR, McGuire EJ. The effects of epidural anesthesia on the urethral closure pressure profile in patients with prostatic enlargement. J Urol 1980; 124: 410–11.
214. Furuya S, Kumamoto Y, Yokoyama E et al. Alpha-adrenergic activity and urethral pressure in prostatic zone in benign prostatic hypertrophy. J Urol 1982; 128: 836–9.
215. Brading AF, McCoy R, Dass N. Alpha1-adrenoceptors in urethral function. Eur Urol 1999; 36(Suppl 1): 74–9.
216. Nasu K, Moriyama N, Fukasawa R et al. Quantification and distribution of alpha1-adrenoceptor subtype mRNAs in human proximal urethra. Br J Pharmacol 1998; 123: 1289–93.

217. Daniels DV, Gever JR, Jaspar JR et al. Human cloned alpha1A-adrenoceptor isoforms display alpha1L-adrenoceptor pharmacology in functional studies. Eur J Pharmacol 1999; 370: 337–43.
218. Fukasawa R, Tamiguchi N, Moriyama N et al. The alpha1L-adrenoceptor subtype in the lower urinary tract: a comparison of human urethra and prostate. Br J Urol 1998; 82: 733–7.
219. Chai TC, Belville WD, McGuire EJ, Nyquist L. Specificity of the American Urological Association voiding symptom index: comparison of unselected and selected samples of both sexes. J Urol 1993; 150: 1710–13.
220. Lepor H, Machi G. Comparison of AUA symptom index in unselected males and females between fifty-five and seventy-nine years of age. Urology 1993; 42: 36–40; discussion 40–1.
221. Lepor H, Theune C. Randomized double-blind study comparing the efficacy of terazosin versus placebo in women with prostatism-like symptoms. J Urol 1995; 154: 116–8.
222. Nordling J, Meyhoff HH, Christensen NJ. Effects of clonidine (Catapresan) on urethral pressure. Invest Urol 1979; 16: 289–91.
223. Werkstrom V, Persson K, Andersson KE. NANC transmitters in the female pig urethra – localization and modulation of release via alpha 2-adrenoceptors and potassium channels. Br J Pharmacol 1997; 121: 1605–12.
224. Levin RM, Ruggieri MR, Wein AJ. Identification of receptor subtypes in the rabbit and human urinary bladder by selective radioligand binding. J Urol 1988; 139: 844–8.
225. Morita T, Iizuka H, Iwara T, Kondo S. Function and distribution of beta3-adrenoceptors in rat, rabbit and human urinary bladder and external urethral sphincter. J Smooth Muscle Res 2000; 36: 21–32.
226. Laval KU, Hannappel J, Lutzeyer W. Effects of beta-adrenergic stimulating and blocking agents on the dynamics of the human bladder outlet. Urol Int 1978; 33: 366–9.
227. Rao MS, Bapna BC, Sharma PL et al. Clinical import of beta-adrenergic activity in the proximal urethra. J Urol 1980; 124: 254–5.
228. Vaidyanathan S, Rao MS, Bapna BC et al. Beta-adrenergic activity in human proximal urethra: a study with terbutaline. J Urol 1980; 124: 869–71.
229. Thind P, Lose G, Colstrup H, Andersson KE. The influence of beta-adrenoceptor and muscarinic receptor agonists and antagonists on the static urethral closure function in healthy females. Scand J Urol Nephrol 1993; 27: 31–8.
230. Ishiko O, Ushiroyama T, Saji F et al. Beta(2)-adrenergic agonists and pelvic floor exercises for female stress incontinence. Int J Gynaecol Obstet 2000; 71: 39–44.
231. Morita T, Kihara K, Nagamatsu H et al. Effects of clenbuterol on rabbit vesicourethral muscle contractility. J Smooth Muscle Res 1995; 31: 119–27.
232. Slack BE, Downie JW. Pharmacological analysis of the responses of the feline urethra to autonomic nerve stimulation. J Auton Nerv Syst 1983; 8: 141–60.
233. Burnett AL. Nitric oxide control of lower genitourinary tract functions: a review. Urology 1995; 45: 1071–83.
234. Schroder A, Hedlund P, Andersson KE. Carbon monoxide relaxes the female pig urethra as effectively as nitric oxide in the presence of YC-1. J Urol 2002; 167: 1892–6.
235. Peng W, Hoidal JR, Farrukh IS. Regulation of Ca(2+)-activated K+ channels in pulmonary vascular smooth muscle cells: role of nitric oxide. J Appl Physiol 1996; 81: 1264–72.
236. Robertson BE, Schubert R, Hescheler J, Nelson MT. cGMP-dependent protein kinase activates Ca-activated K channels in cerebral artery smooth muscle cells. Am J Physiol 1993; 265: C299–303.
237. Bolotina VM, Najibi S, Palacino JJ et al. Nitric oxide directly activates calcium-dependent potassium channels in vascular smooth muscle. Nature 1994; 368: 850–3.
238. Koh SD, Campbell JD, Carl A, Sanders KM. Nitric oxide activates multiple potassium channels in canine colonic smooth muscle. J Physiol 1995; 489 (Pt 3): 735–43.
239. Warner TD, Mitchell JA, Sheng H, Murad F. Effects of cyclic GMP on smooth muscle relaxation. Adv Pharmacol 1994; 26: 171–94.
240. Ito Y, Kimoto Y. The neural and non-neural mechanisms involved in urethral activity in rabbits. J Physiol 1985; 367: 57–72.
241. Persson K, Pandita RK, Aszadi A et al. Functional characteristics of urinary tract smooth muscles in mice lacking cGMP protein kinase type I. Am J Physiol Regul Integr Comp Physiol 2000; 279: R1112–20.
242. Waldeck K, Ny L, Persson K, Andersson KE. Mediators and mechanisms of relaxation in rabbit urethral smooth muscle. Br J Pharmacol 1998; 123: 617–24.
243. Smet PJ, Jonavicius J, Marshall VR, de Vente J. Distribution of nitric oxide synthase-immunoreactive nerves and identification of the cellular targets of nitric oxide in guinea-pig and human urinary bladder by cGMP immunohistochemistry. Neuroscience 1996; 71: 337–48.
244. Sergeant GP, Hollywood MA, McCloskey KD et al. Role of IP(3) in modulation of spontaneous activity in pacemaker cells of rabbit urethra. Am J Physiol Cell Physiol 2001; 280: C1349–56.
245. McCloskey KD, Gurney AM. Kit positive cells in the guinea pig bladder. J Urol 2002; 168: 832–6.
246. Werkstrom V, Alm P, Persson K, Andersson KE. Inhibitory innervation of the guinea-pig urethra; roles of CO, NO and VIP. J Auton Nerv Syst 1998; 74: 33–42.
247. Werkstrom V, Alm P, Persson K et al. Inhibitory innervation of the guinea-pig urethra: roles of CO, NO, and VIP. J Auton Nerv Syst 1998; 74: 33.
248. McVary KT, Monnig W, Camps JL et al. Sildenafil citrate improves erectile function and urinary symptoms in men with erectile dysfunction and lower urinary tract symptoms associated with benign prostatic hyperplasia: a randomized, double-blind trial. J Urol 2007; 177: 1071–7.
249. Roehrborn C, Kaminetsky JC et al. The efficacy and safety of tadalafil administered once a day for lower urinary tract symptoms (LUTS) in men with benign prostatic hyperplasia. J Urol (Suppl) 2006; 175: 527 (abstract 1636).
250. Werkstrom V, Ny L, Persson K, Andersson KE. Carbon monoxide-induced relaxation and distribution of haem oxygenase isoenzymes in the pig urethra and lower oesophagogastric junction. Br J Pharmacol 1997; 120: 312–18.
251. Ho KM, Vy L, McMurray G et al. Co-localization of carbon monoxide and nitric oxide synthesizing enzymes in the human urethral sphincter. J Urol 1999; 161: 1968–72.
252. Naseem KM, Mumtaz FH, Thompson CS et al. Relaxation of rabbit lower urinary tract smooth muscle by nitric oxide and carbon monoxide: modulation by hydrogen peroxide. Eur J Pharmacol 2000; 387: 329–35.
253. Sjogren C, Andersson KE, Mattiasson A. Effects of vasoactive intestinal polypeptide on isolated urethral and urinary bladder smooth muscle from rabbit and man. J Urol 1985; 133: 136–40.
254. Dalziel HH, Westfall DP. Receptors for adenine nucleotides and nucleosides: subclassification, distribution, and molecular characterization. Pharmacol Rev 1994; 46: 449–66.
255. Callahan SM, Creed KE. Electrical and mechanical activity of the isolated lower urinary tract of the guinea-pig. Br J Pharmacol 1981; 74: 353–8.
256. Ohnishi N, Park YC, Karita T, Kajimoto N. Role of ATP and related purine compounds on urethral relaxation in male rabbits. Int J Urol 1997; 4: 191–7.
257. Pinna C, Puglisi L, Burnstock G. ATP and vasoactive intestinal polypeptide relaxant responses in hamster isolated proximal urethra. Br J Pharmacol 1998; 124: 1069–74.

7

Integrated physiology of the lower urinary tract

Naoki Yoshimura, Jeong Yun Jeong, Dae Kyung Kim, and Michael B Chancellor

Introduction

The urinary bladder and its outlet, the urethra, serve two main functions: (1) storage of urine without leakage and (2) periodic release of urine. These two functions are dependent on central as well as peripheral autonomic and somatic neural pathways.[1–6] Since the lower urinary tract switches in an all-or-none manner between storage and elimination of urine, many of the neural circuits controling voiding exhibit phasic patterns of activity rather than tonic patterns occurring in autonomic pathways to other viscera. Micturition is also a special visceral mechanism because it is dependent on voluntary control, which requires the participation of higher centers in the brain, whereas many other visceral functions are regulated involuntarily. Because of these complex neural regulations, the central and peripheral nervous control of the lower urinary tract is susceptible to a variety of neurologic disorders. This chapter will summarize clinical and experimental data to describe the complexity of the peripheral and central nervous systems controling urine storage and elimination in the lower urinary tract.

Peripheral nervous system

Efferent pathways of the lower urinary tract

During urine storage, the bladder outlet is closed and detrusor (bladder smooth muscle) is quiescent, allowing intravesical pressure to remain low over a wide range of bladder volumes. On the other hand, during voluntary voiding, the initial event is a relaxation of striated urethral muscles, followed by a detrusor muscle contraction. These two different activities are mediated by three sets of peripheral nerves: parasympathetic (pelvic), sympathetic (hypogastric), and somatic (pudendal) nerves (Figure 7.1):[7]

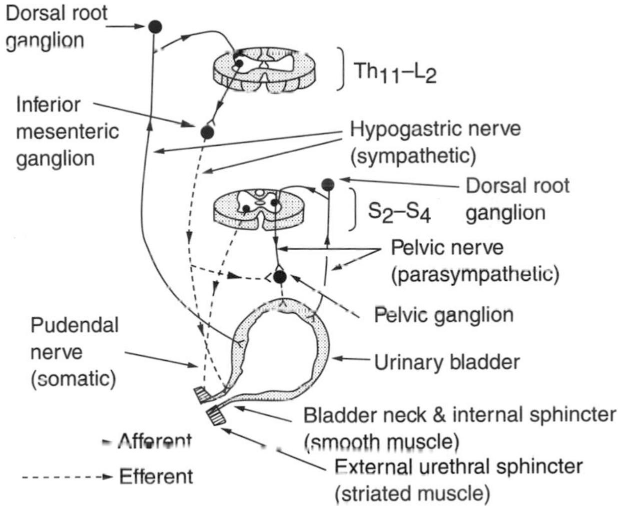

Figure 7.1
Sympathetic, parasympathetic, and somatic innervation of the lower urinary tract. Sympathetic preganglionic pathways emerge from the thoracolumbar cord (Th_{11}–L_2) and pass to the inferior mesenteric ganglia. Preganglionic and postganglionic sympathetic axons then travel in the hypogastric nerve to the pelvic ganglia and lower urinary tract. Parasympathetic preganglionic axons which originate in the sacral cord (S_2–S_4) pass in the pelvic nerve to ganglion cells in the pelvic ganglia and postganglionic axons innervate the bladder and urethral smooth muscle. Sacral somatic pathways are contained in the pudendal nerve, which provides an innervation to the external urethral sphincter striated muscles. Afferent axons from the lower urinary tract are carried in these three nerves. (Reproduced from Yoshimura and de Groat with permission.)[7]

1. Pelvic parasympathetic nerves, which arise at the sacral level of the spinal cord, provide an excitatory input to the bladder and an inhibitory input to the urethral smooth muscle to eliminate urine.
2. Hypogastric sympathetic nerves, which arise at the upper lumbar level of the spinal cord, excite the

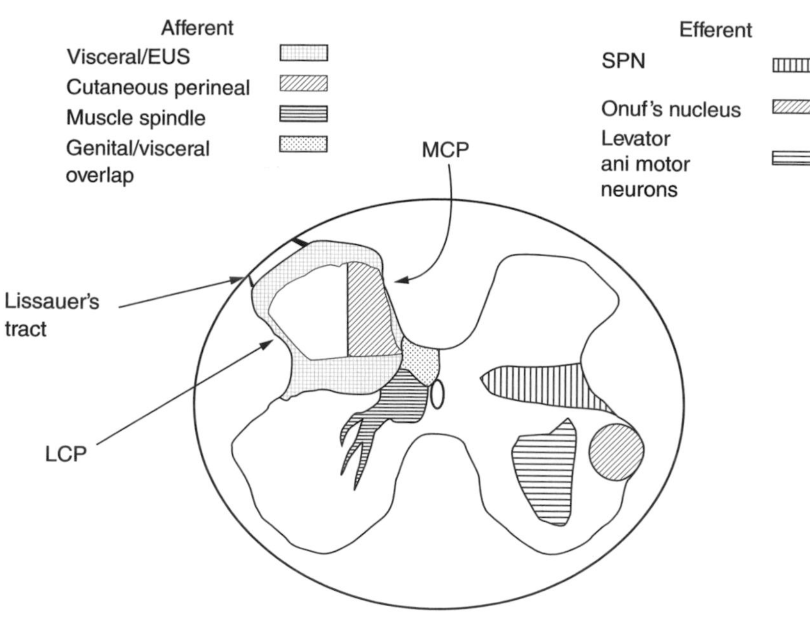

Figure 7.2
Neuroanatomic distribution of primary afferent and efferent components of storage and micturition reflexes within the sacral spinal cord. Afferent components are shown on the left side, whereas efferent components are shown on the right side. Both components are distributed bilaterally and thus overlap extensively. Visceral afferent components represent bladder and urethral afferents contained in the pelvic nerve. External urethral sphincter (EUS) afferents have the same distribution as visceral afferents. Genital (glans penis/clitoris) afferent fibers are contained in the pudendal nerves. Cutaneous perineal afferent components represent afferent fibers that innervate the perineal skin and that are contained in the pudendal nerve. Muscle spindle afferent components represent 1α/β afferent fibers contained in the levator ani nerve that innervate muscle spindles in the levator ani muscle. SPN, sacral parasympathetic nucleus; LCP, lateral collateral afferent projection; MCP, medial collateral afferent projection. (Reproduced from de Groat et al with permission.)[80]

internal sphincter smooth muscle and inhibit the detrusor to store urine.

3. Pudendal somatic nerves, which arise at the sacral level of the spinal cord, elicit excitatory effects to the external sphincter striated muscle to facilitate urine storage in the bladder.

Parasympathetic pathways

Parasympathetic preganglionic neurons (PGNs) innervating the lower urinary tract are located in the lateral part of the sacral intermediate gray matter in a region termed the sacral parasympathetic nucleus (SPN).[1,8–11] Parasympathetic PGNs send axons through the ventral roots to peripheral ganglia, where they release the excitatory transmitter acetylcholine (ACh) which activates postsynaptic ganglionic-type nicotinic receptors.[2,6,7] Parasympathetic postganglionic neurons in humans are located in the detrusor wall layer and not as an independent ganglion, which is known as the major pelvic ganglion in the rodent. Parasympathetic postganglionic nerve terminals release ACh, which can excite various muscarinic receptors in bladder smooth muscles.[12–15] Both M2 and M3 muscarinic subtypes are found in bladder smooth muscle. Studies of subtype-selective receptor knockout mice revealed that the M3 subtype is the major receptor in bladder contractions.[16,17]

The postganglionic parasympathetic input to the urethra elicits inhibitory effects mediated at least in part via the release of nitric oxide (NO), which directly relaxes the urethral smooth muscle.[18–24] Several neuropeptides, including vasoactive intestinal polypeptide (VIP) and neuropeptide Y (NPY), are also released at postganglionic neurons, which may function as modulators of neural transmission.[25,26] Thus, the excitation of sacral parasympathetic efferent pathways induces a bladder contraction and urethral relaxation to promote bladder emptying during voiding (Figure 7.2).

Sympathetic pathways

Sympathetic outflow from the rostral lumbar spinal cord provides a noradrenergic excitatory and inhibitory input to the bladder and urethra[18] to facilitate urine storage. The peripheral sympathetic pathways follow a complex route which passes through the sympathetic chain ganglia to the interior mesenteric ganglia and then via the hypogastric nerves to the pelvic ganglia (see Figure 7.1).[27] Sympathetic PGNs make synaptic connections with postganglionic neurons in the inferior mesenteric ganglion as well as with postganglionic neurons in the paravertebral ganglia and pelvic ganglia.[1,2,28,29] Ganglionic transmission in sympathetic pathways is also mediated by ACh acting on ganglionic-type nicotinic receptors. Sympathetic postganglionic terminals which release norepinephrine elicit contractions of bladder base and urethral smooth muscle and relaxation of the bladder body to facilitate urine storage.[1,2,18,30]

Somatic pathways

Somatic efferent motoneurons which innervate the external striated urethral sphincter muscle and the pelvic floor musculature are located along the lateral border of the ventral horn in the sacral spinal cord, commonly referred to as the Onuf's nucleus (see Figure 7.2).[31] Sphincter motor neurons also exhibit transversely oriented dendritic bundles that project laterally into the lateral funiculus, dorsally into the intermediate gray matter, and dorsomedially toward the central canal. Somatic nerve terminals release ACh, which acts on skeletal muscle type nicotinic receptors to induce a muscle contraction (see Figure 7.1).

Combined activation of sympathetic and somatic pathways elevates bladder outlet resistance and contributes to urinary continence. This condition is usually found when one feels a 'strong desire to void' in the storage phase, being evident with increased external sphincteric EMG activity in the urodynamic study.

Afferent pathways of the lower urinary tract

The pelvic, hypogastric, and pudendal nerves also contain afferent axons that transmit information from the lower urinary tract to the lumbosacral spinal cord.[7,32,33] The primary afferent neurons of the pelvic and pudendal nerves are contained in sacral dorsal root ganglia, whereas afferent innervation in the hypogastric nerves arises in the rostral lumbar dorsal root ganglia (see Figure 7.1). The central axons of the dorsal root ganglion neurons carry the sensory information from the lower urinary tract to second-order neurons in the spinal cord.[10,11,31,32] Visceral afferent fibers of the pelvic[11] and pudendal[31] nerves enter the cord and travel rostrocaudally within Lissauer's tract (see Figure 7.2).

Sensory information, including the feeling of bladder fullness or bladder pain, is conveyed to the spinal cord via afferent axons in the pelvic and hypogastric nerves.[33,34] Pelvic nerve afferents, which monitor the volume of the bladder and the amplitude of the bladder contractions, consist of small myelinated Aδ and unmyelinated C axons. Electrophysiologic studies in cats and rats have revealed that the normal micturition reflex is mediated by myelinated Aδ-fiber afferents, which respond to bladder distention (Figure 7.3).[4,33,35]

While sensing bladder volume is of particular relevance during urine storage, afferent discharges that occur during a bladder contraction have an important reflex function and appear to reinforce the central drive that maintains bladder contractions.[36] Afferent nerves that respond both to distention and contraction, i.e. 'in series tension receptors', have been identified in the pelvic and hypogastric nerves of cats and rats.[37–40] Afferents that respond only to bladder filling have been identified in the rat bladder,[41] and appear to be volume receptors, possibly sensitive to stretch of the mucosa. In the cat bladder, some 'in series tension receptors' may also respond to bladder stretch.[42] In the rat there is now evidence that many C-bladder afferents are volume receptors that do not respond to bladder contractions, a property that distinguishes them from 'in series tension receptors'.[41]

During inflammation and neuropathic conditions there is recruitment of C-fiber bladder afferents, which form a new functional afferent pathway that can cause bladder overactivity and bladder pain (Figure 7.3).[43] In cats, C-fiber afferents have high thresholds and are usually

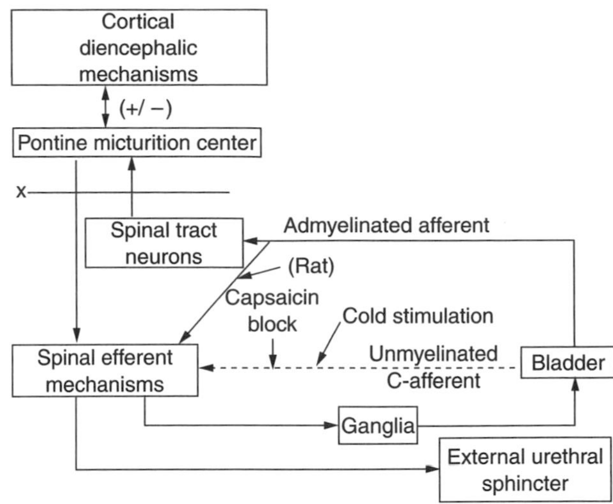

Figure 7.3
The central reflex pathways that regulate micturition in the cat and rat. In animals such as cats and rats with an intact neuraxis, micturition is initiated by a supraspinal reflex pathway passing through the pontine micturition center (PMC) in the brainstem. The pathway is triggered by myelinated afferents (Aδ) connected to tension receptors in the bladder wall (Bladder). Spinal tract neurons carry information to the brain. PMC is controlled by excitatory and inhibitory pathways (+/–) in cortical and diencephalic mechanisms. In spinalized animals, connection of the brainstem and the sacral spinal cord is interrupted (X) and micturition is initially blocked. In animals with chronic spinal cord injuries (SCI), a spinal reflex mechanism emerges which is triggered by unmyelinated (C-fiber) bladder afferents. The C-fiber reflex pathway is usually weak or undetectable in animals with an intact nervous system. Capsaicin blocks the C-fiber reflex in chronic SCI animals. Cold stimulation also activates the C fiber-mediated micturition reflex. However, following SCI voiding, reflex in the rat is still triggered by myelinated Aδ afferents connecting to spinal efferent mechanisms (Rat), whereas voiding reflex in the cat is totally abolished by capsaicin treatment.

unresponsive to mechanical stimuli such as bladder distention and therefore have been termed 'silent C fibers'. However, many of these fibers do respond to chemical, noxious, or cold stimuli.[34,44,45] Previous studies in the rat using patch clamp techniques revealed that C-fiber afferent neurons are relatively unexcitable due to the presence of high-threshold, tetrodotoxin-resistant sodium channels and low-threshold A-type potassium channels.[46] Activation of C-fiber afferents by chemical irritation induces detrusor overactivity, which is blocked by administration of capsaicin, a neurotoxin of C-fiber afferents.[1,47,48] However, since capsaicin does not block normal micturition in cats as well as rats, it appears that C-fiber afferents are not essential for normal conscious voiding (Figure 7.3).[1,47,49–51]

Afferent fibers innervating the urethra are also important to modulate lower urinary tract function (Figure 7.4). Talaat[52] has reported in dogs that urethral afferent fibers in the pelvic and pudendal nerves are sensitive to the passage of urine and that, during saline flow through the urethra, pudendal nerve afferents were activated at a much lower pressure in comparison to pelvic nerve afferents, discharges of which were induced by high-pressure flow that caused a distention of the urethra. High thresholds (over 60 cmH_2O) for activation of urethral afferents in the pelvic nerves were also identified in rats.[53] It has also been documented that conduction velocities of cat pudendal nerve afferent fibers responding to electrical stimulation of the urethra are approximately twice as fast (45 m/s) as pelvic nerve afferent fibers responding to the same stimulation (20 m/s).[54] In addition, urethral afferents in the pudendal and pelvic nerves of the cat seem to have different receptor properties. Pudendal nerve afferents responding to urine flow, some of which may be connected to Pacinian corpuscle-like structures in the muscle layers and the deeper parts of urethral mucosa, exhibited a slowly adapting firing pattern,[55] whereas small myelinated or unmyelinated urethral afferents in the hypogastric nerves and myelinated urethral afferents in the pelvic nerves responding to urine flow or urethral distention are reportedly connected to rapidly adapting receptors.[39,56]

Nociceptive C fibers are also present in pelvic and pudendal nerves innervating the urethra.[57,58] Previous studies have demonstrated that C-fiber afferent fibers identified with positive staining of calcitonin gene-related peptide (CGRP) or substance P were found in the subepithelium, the submucosa, and the muscular layer in all portions of the urethra.[59,60] Moreover, the activation of these urethral C fibers induced by urethral capsaicin application elicited nociceptive behavioral responses, which disappeared after pudendal nerve transection,[61] and increased electromyographic (EMG) activity of pelvic floor striated muscle, including the external urethral sphincter (EUS).[57,58] It is also known that urethral C-fiber activation by capsaicin suppressed reflex bladder contractions.[62]

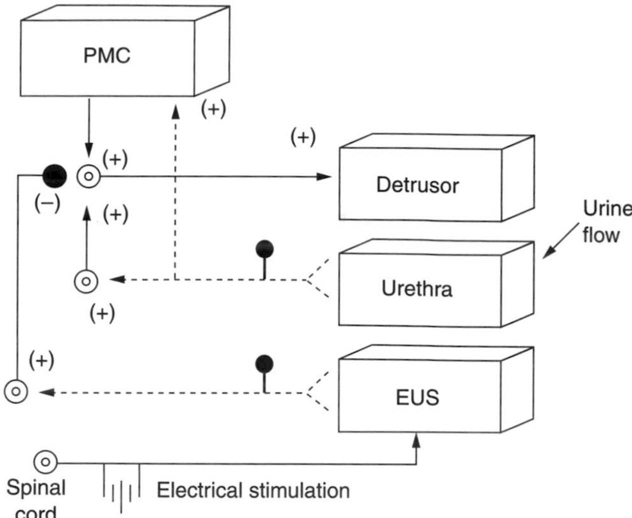

Figure 7.4
Urethra-to-bladder reflexes. Activity in afferent nerves (dashed lines) from the urethra can facilitate parasympathetic efferent outflow to the detrusor via a supraspinal pathway passing through the pontine micturition center (PMC) as well as by a spinal reflex pathway. Afferent input from the external urethral sphincter (EUS) can inhibit parasympathetic outflow to the detrusor via a spinal reflex circuit. Electrical stimulation of motor axons in the S1 ventral root elicits EUS contractions and EUS afferent firing, which in turn inhibits reflex bladder activity; (+) excitatory and (–) inhibitory mechanisms. (Reproduced from de Groat et al with permission.)[80]

Interaction between urothelium and afferent nerves

There is increasing evidence that bladder epithelial cells play an important role in modulation of bladder activity by responding to local chemical and mechanical stimuli and then sending chemical signals to the bladder afferent nerves, which then convey information to the central nervous system (Figure 7.5).[63] It has been shown that urothelial cells express nicotinic, muscarinic, tachykinin, and adrenergic receptors,[1,14] as well as vanilloid receptors,[64] and can respond to mechanical as well as chemical stimuli and in turn release chemicals such as adenosine triphosphate (ATP), prostaglandins, and NO (Figure 7.5).[63,65–67] These agents are known to have excitatory and inhibitory actions on afferent neurons, which are located close to or in the urothelium.[7,68,69] Studies using $P2X_3$, an ATP receptor, in knockout mice have revealed that urothelially released ATP during bladder distention can interact with $P2X_3$ receptors in bladder afferent fibers to modulate bladder activity, and that a loss of $P2X_3$ receptors resulted in bladder hypoactivity.[65,70] It has also been demonstrated that vanilloid

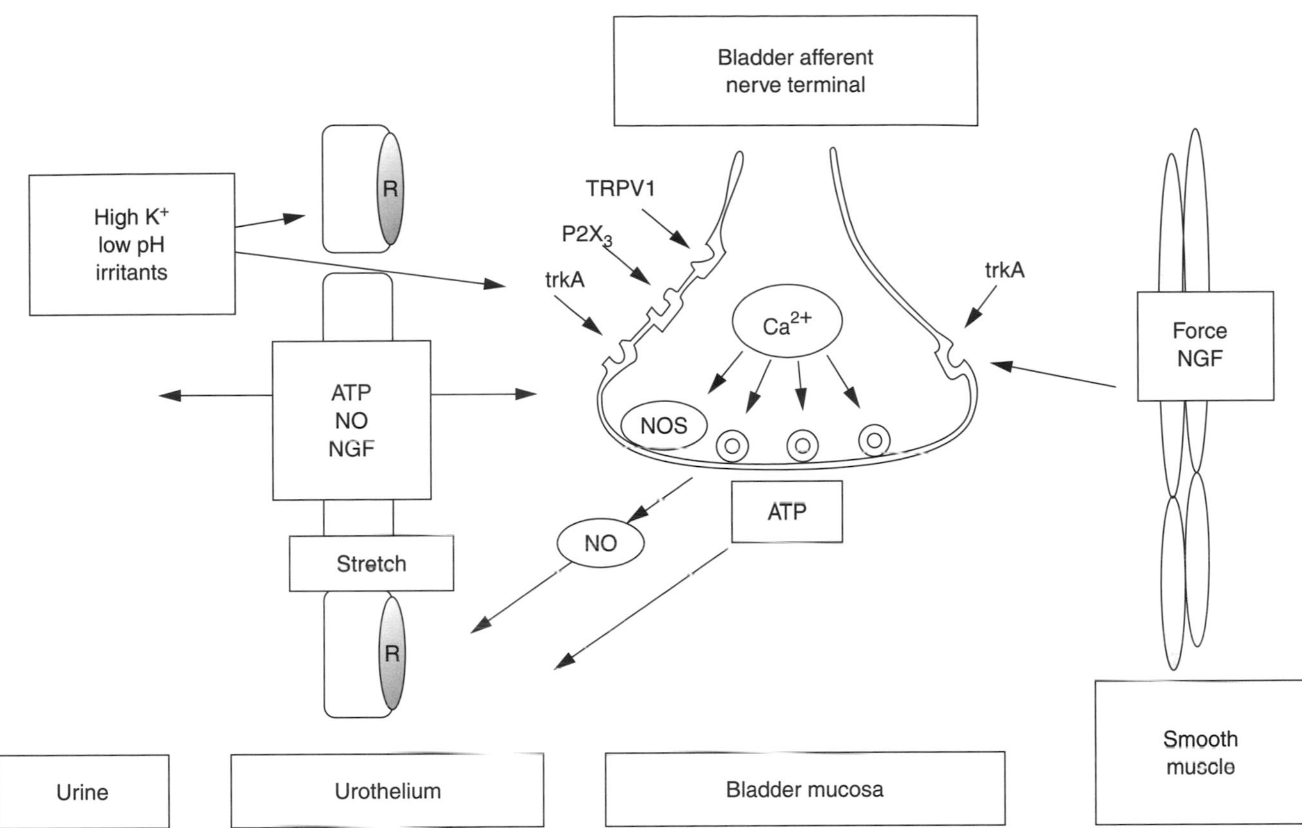

Figure 7.5
Interactions between chemical mediators released from bladder epithelial cells and smooth muscles and afferent nerve endings in the bladder mucosa. ATP and NO can be released from the urothelium and may sensitize the mechanoreceptors via an activation of $P2X_3$ and TRPV1 receptors, respectively, which respond to stretch of the mucosa during bladder distention. This mechanism can be induced by the presence of high urinary potassium concentrations, and possibly by other sensitizing solutions within the bladder lumen, such as those with high osmolality or low pH; the presence in the tissues of inflammatory mediators may also sensitize the endings. The smooth muscle can generate force that may influence some mucosal endings, and the production of nerve growth factor (NGF) is another mechanism that can influence the mechanosensitivity of the sensory ending, via the trkA receptor. NOS, nitric oxide synthase.

receptor (TRPV1)-knockout mice exhibited reduced NO and ATP release from urothelial cells, as well as alterations in bladder function.[71]

The urothelium also appears to modulate contractile responses of the detrusor smooth muscle to muscarinic and other stimulation. Hawthorn and associates[72] demonstrated in the pig bladder that there is a greater muscarinic receptor density in the urothelium than in the detrusor smooth muscle. Contractions of urothelium denuded muscle strip were inhibited in the presence of a second bladder strip with an intact urothelium, but not if the second strip was denuded. Thus, the detrusor smooth muscle is sensitive to a diffusible inhibitory factor released from the urothelium.

Overall, it seems likely that urothelial cells exhibit specific signaling properties that allow them to respond to their chemical and physical environments and engage in reciprocal communication with neighboring nerves and smooth muscles in the bladder wall.

Reflex circuitry controling micturition

Coordinated activities of the peripheral nervous system innervating the bladder and urethra during urine storage and voiding depend upon multiple reflex pathways organized in the brain and spinal cord. The central pathways controling lower urinary tract function are organized as on-off switching circuits that maintain a reciprocal relationship between the urinary bladder and urethral outlet.[1,69,73] The principal reflex components of these switching circuits are listed in Table 7.1 and illustrated in Figure 7.6.

Table 7.1 *Reflexes to the lower urinary tract*

Afferent pathways	Efferent pathways	Central pathways
Urine storage Low-level vesical afferent activity (pelvic nerve)	1. External sphincter contraction (somatic nerves) 2. Internal sphincter contraction (sympathetic nerves) 3. Detrusor inhibition (sympathetic nerves) 4. Ganglionic inhibition (sympathetic nerves) 5. Sacral parasympathetic outflow inactive	Spinal reflexes
Micturition High-level vesical afferent activity (pelvic nerve)	1. Inhibition of external sphincter activity 2. Inhibition of sympathetic outflow 3. Activation of parasympathetic outflow to the bladder	Spinobulbospinal Reflexes
	4. Activation of parasympathetic outflow to the urethra	Spinal reflex

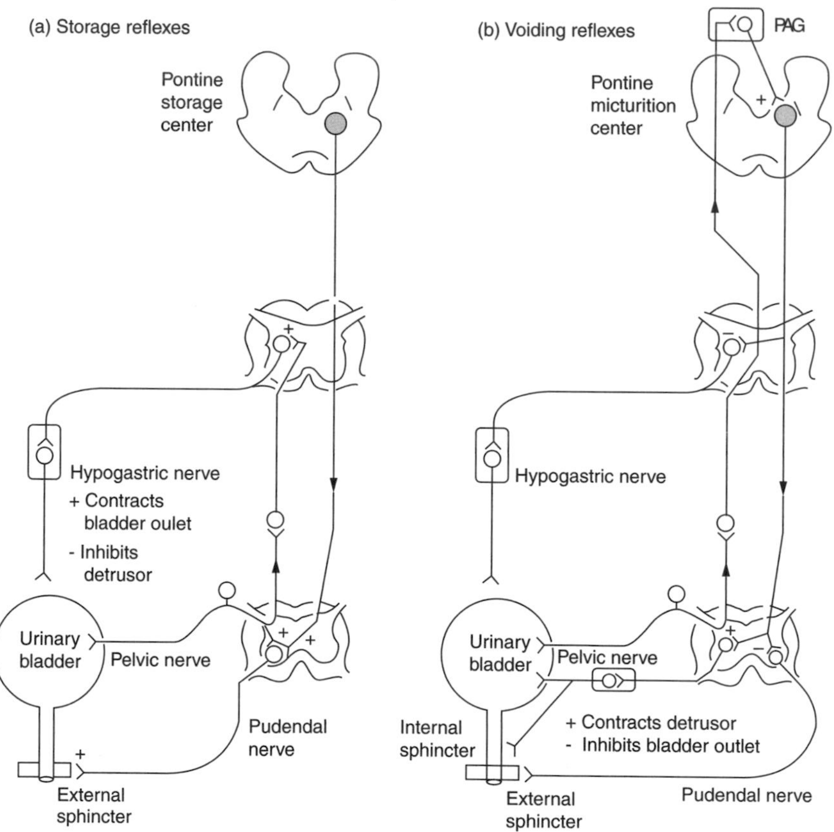

Figure 7.6
Neural circuits controling continence and micturition. (A) Storage reflexes. During urine storage, bladder distention produces low-level firing in bladder afferent pathways, which in turn stimulates (1) the sympathetic outflow to the bladder outlet (bladder base and urethra) and (2) pudendal outflow to the external sphincter muscle. These responses are elicited by spinal reflex pathways. Sympathetic firing also inhibits detrusor muscle and transmission in bladder ganglia. A region in the rostral pons (the pontine storage center) increases external urethral sphincter activity. (B) Voiding reflexes. During elimination of urine, intense bladder afferent firing activates spinobulbospinal reflex pathways passing through the pontine micturition center, which stimulate the parasympathetic outflow to the bladder and internal sphincter smooth muscle and inhibit the sympathetic and pudendal outflow to the bladder outlet. Ascending afferent input from the spinal cord may pass through relay neurons in the periaqueductal gray (PAG) before reaching the pontine micturition center. (Reproduced from Yoshimura and de Groat with permission.)[7]

The storage phase of the bladder

The bladder functions as a low-pressure reservoir during urine storage. In both humans and animals, bladder pressures remain low and relatively constant when bladder volume is below the threshold for inducing voiding (Figure 7.7). The accommodation of the bladder to increasing volumes of urine is primarily a passive phenomenon dependent on the intrinsic properties of the vesical smooth muscle and the quiescence of the parasympathetic efferent pathway.[1,4,7] The bladder-to-sympathetic reflex also contributes as a negative feedback or urine storage mechanism that promotes closure of the urethral outlet and inhibits neurally mediated contractions of the bladder during bladder filling (Table 7.1).[74] Reflex activation of the sympathetic outflow to the lower urinary tract can be triggered

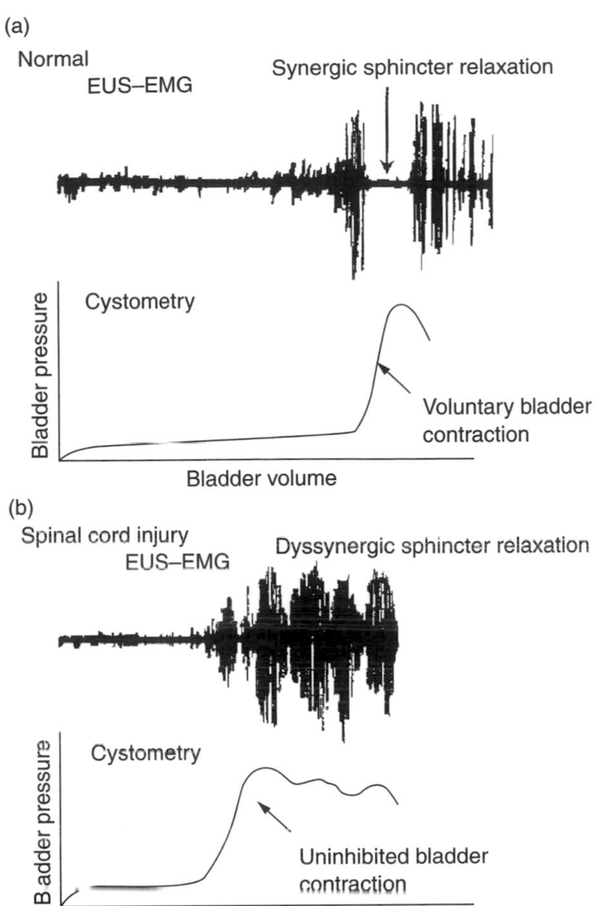

Figure 7.7
Combined cystometry and external urethral sphincter electromyography (EUS–EMG) recordings comparing reflex voiding responses in a normal adult (A, Normal) and in a spinal cord injury (SCI) patient (B, SCI). The abscissas represent bladder volume and the ordinates in cystometrograms represent bladder pressure. In panel A, a slow infusion of fluid into the bladder induces a gradual increase of EMG activity, but no apparent changes in bladder pressure. When a voluntary voiding starts, an increase of bladder pressure (voluntary bladder contraction) is associated with a cessation of EUS–EMG activity (synergic sphincter relaxation). On the other hand, in an SCI patient (B), the reciprocal relationship between bladder and sphincter is abolished. During bladder filling, uninhibited bladder contraction occurs in association with an increase in sphincter activity (detrusor-sphincter dyssynergia). Loss of the reciprocal relationship between bladder and sphincter in SCI patients interferes with bladder emptying. (Reproduced from Yoshimura with permission.)[75]

by afferent activity induced by distention of the urinary bladder.[1,74] This reflex response is organized in the lumbosacral spinal cord and persists after transection of the spinal cord at the thoracic levels (Figure 7.7).[75]

During bladder filling the activity of the sphincter electromyogram also increases (see Figure 7.7), reflecting an increase in efferent firing in the pudendal nerve and an increase in outlet resistance that contributes to the maintenance of urinary continence. Pudendal motoneurons are activated by bladder afferent input (the guarding reflex).[76] External urethral sphincter (EUS) motoneurons are also activated by urethral/perineal afferents in the pudendal nerve.[77] This reflex may represent, in part, a continence mechanism that is activated by proprioceptive afferent input from the urethra/pelvic floor and which induces closure of the urethral outlet. These excitatory sphincter reflexes are organized in the spinal cord. It is also reported that a supraspinal urine storage center is located in the dorsolateral pons. Descending inputs from this region activate the pudendal motoneurons to increase urethral resistance (see Figure 7.6).[78,79]

Sphincter-to-bladder reflexes

During the urine storage phase the bladder-to-external urethral sphincter guarding reflex which triggers sphincter contractions during bladder filling could in turn activate sphincter muscle afferents, which initiate an inhibition of the parasympathetic excitatory pathway to the bladder.[80] Previous studies in cats and monkeys have demonstrated that contractions of the EUS stimulate firing in muscle proprioceptive afferents in the pudendal nerve, which then activate central inhibitory mechanisms to suppress the micturition reflex (see Figure 7.4).[80] It is also known that stimulation of somatic afferent pathways projecting in the pudendal nerve to the caudal lumbosacral spinal cord can inhibit voiding function. The inhibition can be induced by activation of afferent input from various sites, including the penis, vagina, rectum, perineum, urethral sphincter, and anal sphincter.[1,81] Electrophysiologic studies in cats showed that the inhibition was mediated by suppression of interneuronal pathways in the sacral spinal cord and also by direct inhibitory input to the parasympathetic preganglionic neurons.[82] A similar inhibitory mechanism has been identified in monkeys by directly stimulating the anal sphincter muscle.[83] In monkeys at least part of the inhibitory mechanism is localized in the spinal cord because it persisted after chronic spinal cord injury.

The emptying phase of the bladder

The storage phase of the bladder can be switched to the voiding phase either involuntarily (reflexly) or voluntarily (Figure 7.7). The former is readily demonstrated in the human infant or in patients with neuropathic bladder. When bladder volume reaches the micturition threshold, afferent activity originating in bladder mechanoceptors triggers micturition reflexes. The afferent fibers which trigger micturition in the rat and cat are small myelinated Aδ fibers (see Figure 7.3).[35,84,85] These bladder afferents in the pelvic nerve synapse on neurons in the sacral spinal cord, which then send their axons rostrally to a micturition center (the pontine micturition center) in the dorsolateral pons (see Figure 7.6).[84–89]

Activation of this center reverses the pattern of efferent outflow to the lower urinary tract, producing firing in the sacral parasympathetic pathways and inhibition of sympathetic and somatic pathways (see Figure 7.6). The expulsion phase consists of an initial relaxation of the urethral sphincter followed in a few seconds by a contraction of the bladder, resulting in the flow of urine through the urethra. Relaxation of the urethral smooth muscle during micturition is mediated by activation of a parasympathetic pathway to the urethra that triggers the release of nitric oxide[18,21] and by removal of excitatory inputs to the urethra (see Figure 7.6). Studies in the rat and cat indicate that activity ascending from the spinal cord may pass through a relay center in the periaqueductal gray before reaching the pontine micturition center (see Figure 7.6).[90–94] Thus, voiding reflexes depend on a spinobulbospinal pathway which passes through an integrative center in the brain (see Figure 7.6B). Secondary reflexes elicited by flow of urine through the urethra also facilitate bladder emptying.[1,4,62] Inhibition of EUS reflex activity during micturition is dependent, in part, on supraspinal mechanisms because it is weak or absent in chronic spinal cord injured animals and humans, resulting in simultaneous contractions of bladder and urethral sphincter (i.e. detrusor sphincter dyssynergia) (see Figure 7.7).[75,95,96]

Urethra-to-bladder reflexes

It has been reported that myelinated afferents innervating the urethra could contribute to bladder emptying during the voiding phase. Barrington[97,98] reported that urine flow or mechanical stimulation of the urethra with a catheter could excite afferent nerves that, in turn, facilitated reflex bladder contractions in the anesthetized cat (see Figure 7.4). He proposed that this facilitatory urethra-to-bladder reflex could promote complete bladder emptying. A study in the anesthetized rat has provided additional support for Barrington's findings.[62] Measurements of reflex bladder contractions under isovolumetric conditions during continuous urethral perfusion (0.075 ml/min) revealed that the frequency of micturition reflexes was significantly reduced when urethral perfusion was stopped or following infusion of 1% lidocaine into the urethra. Intraurethral infusion of nitric oxide donors (*S*-nitroso-*N*-acetylpenicillamine, SNAP, or nitroprusside, 1–2 mmol) markedly decreased urethral perfusion pressure (approximately 30%) and decreased the frequency of reflex bladder contractions (45–75%), but did not change the amplitude of bladder contractions. It was thus concluded that activation of urethral afferents during urethral perfusion could modulate the micturition reflex.

Barrington also identified two components of this facilitatory urethra-to-bladder reflex during voiding. One component was activated by a somatic afferent pathway in the pudendal nerve and produced facilitation by a supraspinal mechanism involving the pontine micturition center.[97] The other component was activated by a visceral afferent pathway in the pelvic nerve and produced facilitation by a spinal reflex mechanism.[98] Afferent fibers which respond to urine flow in the urethra were found in the pelvic, hypogastric, and pudendal nerves, although it has been reported that the properties of urethral afferents in pelvic/hypogastric and pudendal nerves are different, as described above.

Spinal and supraspinal pathways involved in the micturition reflex

Spinal cord

In the spinal cord, afferent pathways terminate on second-order interneurons that relay information to the brain or to other regions of the spinal cord. Since spinal reflex pathways controling bladder and urethral activities are mediated by disynaptic or polysynaptic pathways, interneuronal mechanisms play an essential role in the regulation of lower urinary tract function. Electrophysiologic[10,84,99,100] and neuroanatomic techniques[101–104] have identified interneurons in the same regions of the spinal cord that receive afferent input from the bladder. As shown in Figure 7.2, horseradish peroxidase (HRP) labeling techniques in the cat revealed that afferent projections from the EUS and levator ani muscles (i.e. pelvic floor) project into different regions of the sacral spinal cord. The EUS afferent terminals are located in the superficial layers of the dorsal horn and at the base of the dorsal horn, whereas the levator ani afferents project into a region just lateral to the central canal and extending into the medial ventral horn. The EUS afferents overlap very closely with the central projections of visceral afferents in the pelvic nerve that innervate the bladder and urethra (Figure 7.2). Intracellular labeling experiments also showed that the dendritic patterns of EUS motoneurons[105] and parasympathetic PGN[9] are similar. Pharmacologic experiments revealed that glutamic acid is the excitatory transmitter in these pathways. In addition, approximately 15% of interneurons located medial to the sacral parasympathetic nucleus in laminae V–VII make inhibitory synaptic connections with the PGN.[10,106] These inhibitory neurons release γ-aminobutyric acid (GABA) and glycine. Reflex pathways which control the external sphincter muscles also utilize glutamatergic

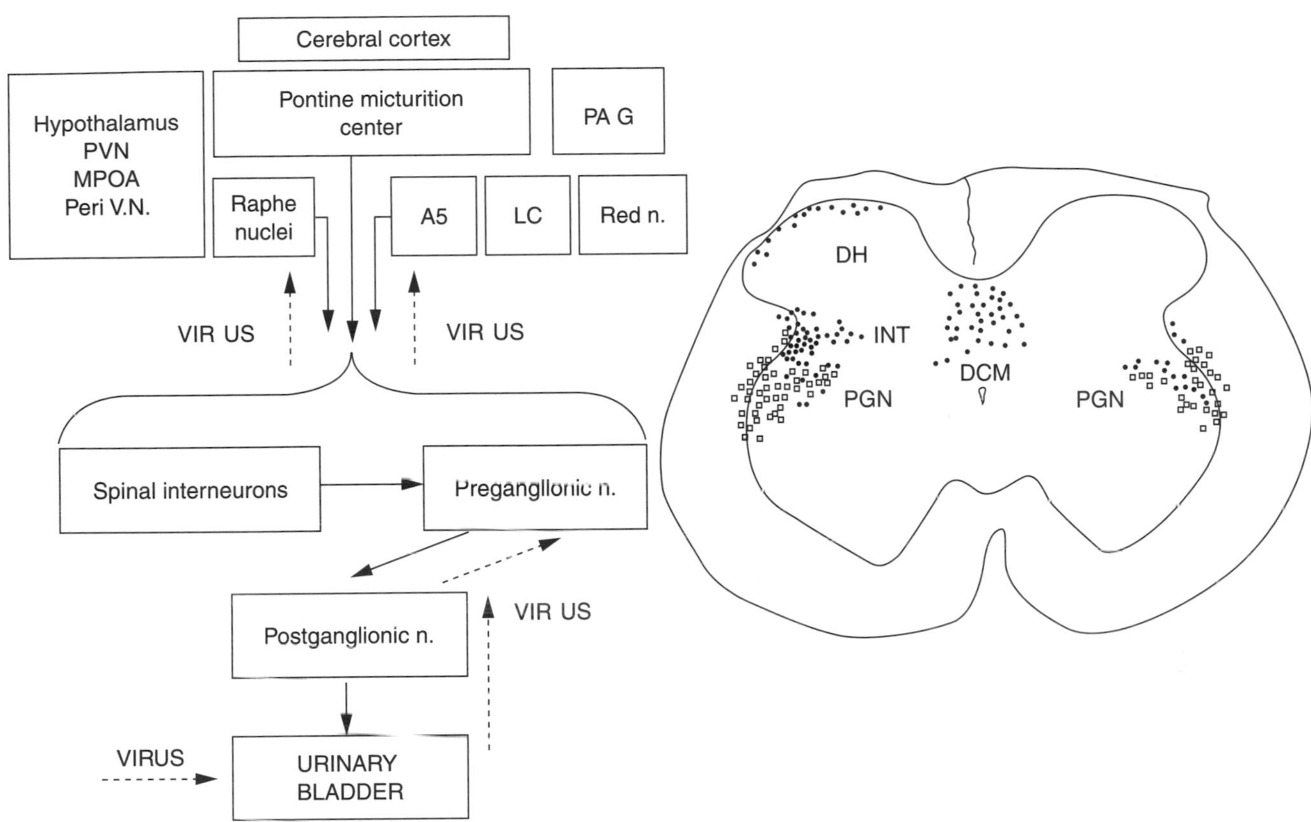

Figure 7.8
Transneuronal virus tracing of the central pathways controling the urinary bladder of the rat. Injection of pseudorabies virus into the wall of the urinary bladder leads to retrograde transport of virus (dashed arrows) and sequential infection of postganglionic neurons, preganglionic neurons, and then various central neural circuits synaptically linked to the preganglionic neurons. At long survival times, virus can be detected with immunocytochemical techniques in neurons at specific sites throughout the spinal cord and brain, extending to the pontine micturition center in the pons (i.e. Barrington's nucleus or the laterodorsal tegmental nucleus) and to the cerebral cortex. Other sites in the brain labeled by virus are (1) the paraventricular nucleus (PVN), medial preoptic area (MPOA), and periventricular nucleus (Peri V.N.) of the hypothalamus; (2) periaqueductal gray (PAG); (3) locus coeruleus (LC) and subcoeruleus; (4) red nucleus (Red n.); (5) medullary raphe nucleus; and (6) the noradrenergic cell group designated A5. L6 spinal cord section showing the distribution of virus labeled parasympathetic preganglionic neurons (□) and interneurons (•) in the region of the parasympathetic nucleus 72 h after injection of the virus into the bladder. Interneurons (INT) in the dorsal commissure and the superficial laminae of the dorsal horn (DH) are also shown. The left side shows the entire population of preganglionic neurons (PGN) labeled by axonal tracing with fluorogold injected into the pelvic ganglia. The right side shows the distribution of PRV-labeled bladder PGN (□) among the entire population of FG-labeled PGN (□). Bladder PGN were labeled with PRV and FG. Composite diagram of neurons in 12 spinal sections (42 μm). (Reproduced from de Groat et al with permission.)[99]

excitatory and GABAergic/glycinergic inhibitory interneuronal mechanisms.

Central and spinal neural pathways controling lower urinary tract function have also been identified by transneuronal tracing studies using neurotropic viruses such as pseudorabies virus (PRV) (Figure 7.8). PRV can be injected into a target organ and then move intra-axonally from the periphery to the central nervous system. Because PRV can be transported across many synapses it could sequentially infect all the neurons that connect directly or indirectly to the lower urinary tract.[102–104] Interneurons identified by retrograde transport of PRV injected into the urinary bladder are located in the region of the sacral parasympathetic nucleus (SPN), the dorsal commissure (DCM), and the superficial laminae of the dorsal horn (see Figure 7.8).[10,102,104] A similar distribution of labeled interneurons has been noted after injection of virus into the urethra[9] or the EUS,[102] indicating a prominent overlap of the interneuronal pathways controling the various target organs of the lower urinary tract.

The micturition reflex can be modulated at the level of the spinal cord by interneuronal mechanisms activated by afferent input from cutaneous and striated muscle targets. The micturition reflex can also be modulated by inputs from other visceral organs.[1,4,7,73,84,107–110] Stimulation of afferent fibers from various regions (anus, colon/rectum, vagina, uterine cervix, penis, perineum, pudendal nerve) can inhibit the firing of sacral interneurons evoked by bladder distention.[83] This inhibition may occur as a result of presynaptic inhibition at primary afferent terminals or due to direct postsynaptic inhibition of the second-order neurons. Direct postsynaptic inhibition of bladder PGN can also be elicited by stimulation of somatic afferent axons in the pudendal nerve or by visceral afferents from the distal bowel.[108,111]

Pontine micturition center

The dorsal pontine tegmentum has been firmly established as an essential control center for micturition in normal subjects. First described by Barrington,[112] it has subsequently been called 'Barrington's nucleus', the 'pontine micturition center' (PMC),[113] or the 'M region'[78,92,114] due to its medial location.

Studies in animals using brain-lesioning techniques revealed that neurons in the brainstem at the level of the inferior colliculus have an essential role in the control of the parasympathetic component of micturition.[1,4,7] Removal of areas of brain above the colliculus by intercollicular decerebration usually facilitates micturition by elimination of inhibitory inputs from more rostral centers, whereas transections at any point below the colliculi abolish micturition.[115] In addition, bilateral lesions in the region of the locus coeruleus in the cat or the dorsolateral tegmental nucleus in the rat abolish micturition, whereas electrical or chemical stimulation of this region induces a bladder contraction and a reciprocal relaxation of the urethra, leading to bladder emptying.[78,86–89,116]

In addition to providing axonal inputs to the locus coeruleus and the sacral spinal cord,[117–119] neurons in the PMC also send axon collaterals to the paraventricular thalamic nucleus, which is thought to be involved in the limbic system modulation of visceral behavior.[119] Some neurons in the PMC also project to the periaqueductal gray region,[120] which regulates many visceral activities as well as pain pathways.[121] Thus, neurons in the PMC communicate with multiple supraspinal neuronal populations that may coordinate micturition with other functions. Although the circuitry in humans is uncertain, brain imaging studies have revealed increases in blood flow in this region of the pons during micturition.[122] In addition, it has been reported that in a case study of a multiple sclerosis patient, coordinated bladder contraction and urethral relaxation was induced by ectopic activation of a region in the dorsolateral pontine tegmentum.[123] Thus the PMC appears critical for the normal micturition reflex across species.

Neurons in the PMC provide direct synaptic inputs to sacral PGN, as well as to GABAergic neurons in the sacral DCM.[113] The former neurons carry the excitatory outflow to the bladder, whereas the latter neurons are thought to be important in mediating an inhibitory influence on EUS motoneurons during voiding.[120] As a result of these reciprocal connections, the PMC can promote coordination between the bladder and urethral sphincter.

Central pathways modulating the micturition reflex

Transneuronal tracing studies using PRV injected into the lower urinary tract also identified various areas in the brain (see Figure 7.8).[102–104,124] Thus, central control of voiding is likely to be complex. Injection of PRV into the rat bladder labeled many areas of the brainstem, including the laterodorsal tegmental nucleus (the PMC); the medullary raphe nucleus, which contains serotonergic neurons; the locus coeruleus, which contains noradrenergic neurons; periaqueductal gray; and noradrenergic cell group A5. Several regions in the hypothalamus and the cerebral cortex also exhibited virus-infected cells (see Figure 7.8). Neurons in the cortex were located primarily in the medial frontal cortex. Similar brain areas were labeled after injection of virus into the urethra and urethral sphincter, suggesting that coordination between different parts of the lower urinary tract is mediated by a similar population of neurons in the brain.[102–104,124]

Studies in humans indicate that voluntary control of voiding is dependent on connections between the frontal cortex and the septal/preoptic region of the hypothalamus as well as connections between the paracentral lobule and the brainstem.[1] Lesions to these areas of cortex appear to directly increase bladder activity by removing cortical inhibitory control. Brain imaging studies in human volunteers have implicated both the frontal cortex and the anterior cingulate gyrus in control of micturition and have indicated that micturition is controlled predominately by the right side of the brain.[113,125]

Positron emission tomography (PET) scans were also used to examine which brain areas are involved in human micturition.[126] In their study, when 17 right-handed male volunteers were scanned, 10 volunteers were able to micturate during scanning. Micturition was associated with increased blood flow in the right dorsomedial pontine tegmentum, the periaqueductal gray (PAG), the hypothalamus, and the right inferior frontal gyrus. Decreased blood flow was found in the right anterior cingurlate gyrus when urine was withheld. The other seven volunteers were not able to micturate during scanning, although they had a full bladder and tried vigorously to micturate. In this group, during these unsuccessful attempts to micturate, increased blood flow was detected in the right ventral pontine tegmentum. It has been reported that descending inputs from this area can activate the pudendal motoneurons to increase urethral resistance during urine storage in cats.[80,114,127]

Another study using PET scans in 11 healthy male subjects also revealed that increased brain activity related to increasing bladder volume was seen in the PAG, in the midline pons, in the mid-cingulate cortex, and bilaterally in the frontal lobe area, suggesting that the PAG receives information about bladder fullness and relays this information to areas involved in the control of bladder storage.[128] The PAG has multiple connections with higher centers such as the thalamus, insula, cingulate, and prefrontal cortices. It seems that the influences from these higher centers have a role in determining when and where one may void safely.

Increased blood flow also occurred in the right inferior frontal gyrus during unsuccessful attempts to micturate, and decreased blood flow occurred in the right anterior cingulate gyrus during the withholding of urine. The results suggest that the human brainstem contains specific nuclei responsible for the control of micturition, and that the cortical and pontine regions for micturition are predominantly on the right side.

A PET study was also conducted in adult female volunteers to identify brain structures involved in the voluntary motor control of the pelvic floor.[129] The results revealed that the superomedial precentral gyrus and the most medial portion of the motor cortex are activated during pelvic floor contraction, and the superolateral precentral gyrus is activated during contraction of the abdominal musculature. In these conditions, significant activations were also found in the cerebellum, supplementary motor cortex, and thalamus. The right anterior cingulate gyrus was activated during sustained pelvic floor straining.

Recently, functional MRI (fMRI) has been popular in the study of brain activities. In the neurourologic applications, fMRI has been especially useful in studying functional brain changes associated with pelvic floor muscle contraction owing to its improved resolution compared to PET. Several fMRI studies reported strong activities of the supplementary motor area (SMA) in the motor cortex during repetitive pelvic muscle contractions in a full-bladder condition, while previous studies with PET were unable to record this in detail.[130–132] SMA is known to be involved in motor timing and inhibition of motor control. An fMRI study combined with the MMPI (Minnesota Multiphasic Personality Inventory) reported that self-control, including self-inhibition, is related to the activity of SMA.[133] In a recent series of 30 healthy volunteers (15 women, 15 men), Kuhtz-Buschbeck et al[132] reported a strong and consistent recruitment of the SMA, with foci of peak activity located in the posterior portion of the SMA, suggesting involvement of this region in involuntary pelvic floor muscle control. They also found significant activation bilaterally in the frontal opercula, the right insular cortex, and the right supramarginal gyrus, and weaker signals in the primary motor cortex and dorsal pontine tegmentum. However, no significant gender-related difference was found.

Overall, these results in animals and humans indicate that various regions in the central nervous system are necessary for voluntary control of lower urinary tract function.

Developmental changes of bladder reflexes

The neural mechanisms involved in storage and elimination of urine undergo marked changes during postnatal development.[134] In a postnatal period in humans, as well as animals, supraspinal neural pathways controling lower urinary tract function are immature, and voiding is regulated by primitive reflex pathways organized in the spinal cord (Figure 7.9). In neonate animals such as rats and cats, voiding is dependent on an exteroceptive somato-bladder reflex mechanism triggered when the mother licks the genital or perineal region of the young animal. This exteroceptive perineal-to-bladder reflex is regulated by primitive reflex pathways organized in the sacral spinal cord (see Figure 7.9). In humans, the neonatal bladder is more of a conduit of urine than a storage organ and, without control from the central nervous system, the bladder will reflexively empty into a diaper when it reaches functional capacity. Primitive reflex activities organized in the spinal cord such as perineal-to-bladder reflexes are also observed in infants.[99]

Previous studies have also reported that bladder-cooling reflexes are positive in neurologically normal infants and children about age 4 years.[135] The bladder ice water cooling test is performed by quickly instilling up to 100 ml of 4°C sterile saline. The normal adult can maintain a stable bladder without uninhibited bladder contractions. The bladder cooling response is triggered by activation of cold receptors within the bladder wall supplied by unmyelinated C-fiber afferents, and organized by segmental spinal reflex pathways.[45,136] Overall, it appears that during a postnatal period, primitive reflex activities organized in the spinal cord such as perineal-bladder reflexes or C-fiber-mediated cooling reflexes are dominant, due to immature control of the central nervous system (Figure 7.9).

However, transneuronal tracing studies using PRV have demonstrated that micturition reflex pathways in the spinal cord and brain are already connected anatomically at birth, despite the fact that voiding in neonatal rats does not depend on neural mechanisms in the brain.[104] When PRV was injected into the bladder of 2- and 10-day-old rat pups, the labeled neurons were found in various sites in the brain, such as the PMC, the nucleus raphe magnus, A5 and A7 regions, parapyramidal reticular formation, the periaqueductal gray, locus coeruleus, the lateral hypothalamus, medial preoptic area, and the frontal cortex (see Figure 7.8).[104] Thus, even in neonatal animals, supraspinal pathways may already be connected, but may either be nonfunctioning or functioning in an inhibitory manner to suppress

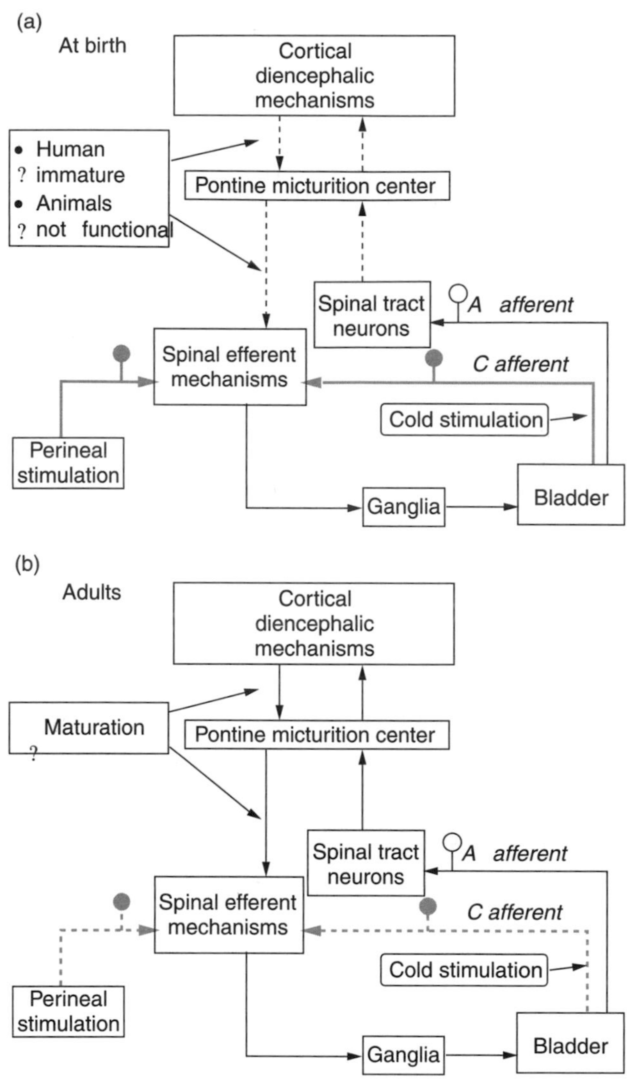

Figure 7.9
Organization of micturition reflex pathways in postnatal (A) and adult periods (B). A, Since in a postnatal period in humans, as well as animals, supraspinal neural pathways controling lower urinary tract function are immature, voiding is regulated by primitive reflex pathways organized in the spinal cord. In neonate animals such as rats and cats, voiding is dependent on an exteroceptive somato-bladder reflex mechanism triggered when the mother licks the genital or perineal region of the young animal (perineal stimulation). Similar reflexes are also observed in infants. Bladder cooling reflexes mediated by C-fiber bladder afferents are positive in neurologically normal infants (Cold stimulation). B, When the central nervous system matures in adults (Maturation), reflex voiding is brought under voluntary control, which originates in the higher center of the brain and, at the same time, primitive spinal reflex activities such as perineal-bladder reflexes or C-fiber-mediated cooling reflexes are masked. However, the primitive neonatal micturition reflexes could be unmasked by pathologic processes that disturb the descending neuronal control of normal voiding, such as spinal cord injury (also see Figure 7.3).

the spinobulbospinal micturition reflex, allowing micturition to be induced by primitive spinal reflex mechanisms.[134]

As the central nervous system matures during the postnatal period, reflex voiding is brought under voluntary control, which originates in the higher center of the brain and, at the same time, primitive spinal reflex activities such as perineal-to-bladder reflexes or C-fiber-mediated cooling reflexes are masked (see Figure 7.9).[134] Electrophysiologic studies using patch-clamp recording techniques in rat spinal cord slice preparations indicate that developmental changes in sacral parasympathetic pathways are due in part to alterations in excitatory synaptic transmission between interneurons and preganglionic neurons.[100] However, the primitive neonatal micturition reflexes such as positive bladder cooling responses and/or spinal perineal-to-bladder reflexes could be unmasked by pathologic processes that disturb the descending neuronal control of normal voiding, such as spinal cord injury (see Figures 7.3 and 7.9).[99,134]

References

1. de Groat WC, Booth AM, Yoshimura N. Neurophysiology of micturition and its modification in animal models of human disease. In: Maggi CA, ed. The Autonomic Nervous System, Vol. 3, Nervous Control of the Urogenital System. London: Harwood Academic Publishers, 1993: 227–90.
2. de Groat WC, Booth AM. Synaptic transmission in pelvic ganglia. In: Maggi CA, ed. The Autonomic Nervous System, Vol. 3, Nervous Control of the Urogenital System. London: Harwood Academic Publishers, 1993: 291–347.
3. Van Arsdalen K, Wein AJ. Physiology of micturition and continence. In: Krane RJ, Siroky M, eds. Clinical Neurourology. New York: Little Brown & Company, 1991: 25–82.
4. Torrens M, Morrison JFB. The Physiology of the Lower Urinary Tract. Berlin: Springer-Verlag, 1987.
5. Chai TC, Steers WD. Neurophysiology of micturition and continence. Urol Clin North Am 1996; 23: 221–36.
6. Chancellor MB, Yoshimura N. Physiology and pharmacology of the bladder and urethra. In: Walsh PC, Retik AB, Vaughan C, Wein A, eds. Campbell's urology, Vol. 2. Philadelphia: Saunders, 2002: 831–86.
7. Yoshimura N, de Groat WC. Neural control of the lower urinary tract. Int J Urol 1997; 4: 111–25.
8. Nadelhaft I, de Groat WC, Morgan C. Location and morphology of parasympathetic preganglionic neurons in the sacral spinal cord of the cat revealed by retrograde axonal transport of horseradish peroxidase. J Comp Neurol 1980; 193: 265–81.
9. Morgan CW, de Groat WC, Felkins LA, Zhang SJ. Intracellular injection of neurobiotin or horseradish peroxidase reveals separate types of preganglionic neurons in the sacral parasympathetic nucleus of the cat. J Comp Neurol 1993; 331: 161–82.
10. de Groat WC, Vizzard MA, Araki I, Roppolo JR. Spinal interneurons and preganglionic neurons in sacral autonomic reflex pathways. In: Holstege G, Bandler R, Saper C, eds. The emotional motor system, Progress in brain research. Amsterdam: Elsevier Science Publishers, 1996: 97–111.
11. Morgan C, Nadelhaft I, de Groat WC. The distribution of visceral primary afferents from the pelvic nerve to Lissauer's tract and the spinal gray matter and its relationship to the sacral parasympathetic nucleus. J Comp Neurol 1981; 201: 415–40.

12. Eglen RM, Hegde SS, Watson N. Muscarinic receptor subtypes and smooth muscle function. Pharmacol Rev 1996; 48: 531–65.
13. Maeda A, Kubo T, Mishina M, Numa S. Tissue distribution of mRNAs encoding muscarinic acetylcholine receptor subtypes. FEBS Lett 1988; 239: 339–42.
14. Kondo S, Morita T, Tashima Y. Muscarinic cholinergic receptor subtypes in human detrusor muscle studied by labeled and nonlabeled pirenzepine, AFDX–116 and 4DAMP. Urol Int 1995; 54: 150–3.
15. Yamaguchi O, Shishido K, Tamura K et al. Evaluation of mRNAs encoding muscarinic receptor subtypes in human detrusor muscle. J Urol 1996; 156: 1208–13.
16. Matsui M, Motomura D, Karasawa H et al. Multiple functional defects in peripheral autonomic organs in mice lacking muscarinic acetylcholine receptor gene for the M3 subtype. Proc Natl Acad Sci USA 2000; 97: 9579–84.
17. Matsui M, Motomura D, Fujikawa T et al. Mice lacking M2 and M3 muscarinic acetylcholine receptors are devoid of cholinergic smooth muscle contraction but still viable. J Neurosci 2002; 22: 10623–7.
18. Andersson K-E. Pharmacology of lower urinary tract smooth muscles and penile erectile tissues. Pharmacol Rev 1993; 45: 253–308.
19. Lundberg JM. Pharmacology of cotransmission in the autonomic nervous system: integrative aspects on amines, neuropeptides, adenosine triphosphate, amino acids and nitric oxide. Pharmacol Rev 1996; 48: 113–78.
20. Fraser MO, Flood HD, de Groat WC. Urethral smooth muscle relaxation is mediated by nitric oxide (NO) released from parasympathetic postganglionic neurons. J Urol 1995; 153: 461A.
21. Bennett BC, Kruse MN, Roppolo JR et al. Neural control of urethral outlet activity in vivo: role of nitric oxide. J Urol 1995; 153: 2004–9.
22. Persson K, Igawa Y, Mattiasson A, Andersson K-E. Effects of inhibition of the L-arginine/nitric oxide pathway in the rat lower urinary tract in vivo and in vitro. Br J Pharmacol 1992; 107: 178–84.
23. Thornbury KD, Hollywood MA, McHale NG. Mediation by nitric oxide of neurogenic relaxation of the urinary bladder neck muscle in sheep. J Physiol 1992; 451: 133–44.
24. Takeda M, Lepor H. Nitric oxide synthase in dog urethra: a histochemical and pharmacological analysis. Br J Pharmacol 1995; 116: 2517–23.
25. Keast JR, de Groat WC. Immunohistochemical characterization of pelvic neurons which project to the bladder, colon or penis in rats. J Comp Neurol 1989; 288: 387–400.
26. Tran LV, Somogyi GT, de Groat WC. Inhibitory effects of neuropeptide Y on cholinergic and adrenergic transmission in the rat urinary bladder and urethra. Am J Physiol 1994; 266: R1411–17.
27. Kihara K, de Groat WC. Sympathetic efferent pathways projecting to the bladder neck and proximal urethra in the rat. J Auton Nerv Syst 1997; 62: 134–42.
28. Janig W, McLachlan EM. Organization of lumbar spinal outflow to distal colon and pelvic organs. Physiol Rev 1987; 67: 1332–404.
29. Lincoln J, Burnstock G. Autonomic innervation of the urinary bladder and urethra. In: Maggi CA, ed. The autonomic nervous system, Vol. 3, Nervous control of the urogenital system. London: Harwood Academic Publishers, 1993: 33–68.
30. Levin RM, Ruggieri MR, Wein AJ. Identification of receptor subtypes in the rabbit and human urinary bladder by selective radioligand binding. J Urol 1988; 139: 844–8.
31. Thor KB, Morgan C, Nadelhaft I et al. Organization of afferent and efferent pathways in the pudendal nerve of the female cat. J Comp Neurol 1989; 288: 263–79.
32. de Groat WC. Spinal cord projections and neuropeptides in visceral afferent neurons. Progr Brain Res 1986; 67: 165–87.
33. Janig W, Morrison JFB. Functional properties of spinal visceral afferents supplying abdominal and pelvic organs, with special emphasis on visceral nociception. Progr Brain Res 1986; 67: 87–114.
34. Habler HJ, Janig W, Koltzenburg M. Activation of unmyelinated afferent fibres by mechanical stimuli and inflammation of the urinary bladder in the cat. J Physiol 1990; 425: 545–62.
35. Mallory B, Steers WD, de Groat WC. Electrophysiological study of micturition reflexes in rats. Am J Physiol 1989; 257: R410–21.
36. Kruse MN, Mallory BS, Noto H et al. Properties of the descending limb of the spinobulbospinal micturition reflex pathway in the cat. Brain Res 1991; 556: 6–12.
37. Iggo A. Tension receptors in the stomach and the urinary bladder. J Physiol 1955; 128: 593–607.
38. Floyd K, Hick VE, Morrison JF. Mechanosensitive afferent units in the hypogastric nerve of the cat. J Physiol 1976; 259: 457–71.
39. Bahns E, Ernsberger U, Janig W, Nelke A. Functional characteristics of lumbar visceral afferent fibres from the urinary bladder and the urethra in the cat. Pflugers Archiv 1986; 407: 510–18.
40. Morrison JF. The physiological mechanisms involved in bladder emptying. Scand J Urol Nephrol Suppl 1997; 184: 15–18.
41. Morrison JFB. ATP may be a natural modulator of the sensitivity of bladder mechanoreceptors during slow distensions. First International Consultation on Incontinence, Monaco, 1998.
42. Downie JW, Armour JA. Mechanoreceptor afferent activity compared with receptor field dimensions and pressure changes in feline urinary bladder. Can J Physiol Pharmacol 1992; 70: 1457–67.
43. Yoshimura N, Seki S, Chancellor MB et al. Targeting afferent hyperexcitability for therapy of the painful bladder syndrome. Urology 2002; 59: 61–7.
44. Janig W, Koltzenburg M. Pain arising from the urogenital tract. In: Maggi CA, ed. The autonomic nervous system, Vol. 3, Nervous control of the urogenital system. London: Harwood Academic Publishers, 1993: 525–78.
45. Fall M, Lindström S, Mazieres L. A bladder-to-bladder cooling reflex in the cat. J Physiol 1990; 427: 281–300.
46. Yoshimura N, White G, Weight FF, de Groat WC. Different types of NA^+ and A-type K^+ currents in dorsal root ganglion neurons innervating the rat urinary bladder. J Physiol 1996; 494: 1–16.
47. Maggi CA. The dual, sensory and efferent function of the capsaicin-sensitive primary sensory nerves in the bladder and urethra. In: Maggi CA, ed. The autonomic nervous system, Vol. 3, Nervous control of the urogenital system. London: Harwood Academic Publishers, 1993: 383–422.
48. Birder LA, Roppolo JR, Erickson VE, de Groat WC. Increased *c-fos* expression in lumbosacral projection neurons and preganglionic neurons after irritation of the lower urinary tract in the rat. Brain Res 1999; 834: 55–65.
49. Cheng C-L, Ma C-P, de Groat WC. Effects of capsaicin on micturition and associated reflexes in the rat. Am J Physiol 1993; 265: R132–8.
50. de Groat WC, Kawatani M, Hisamitsu T et al. Mechanisms underlying the recovery of urinary bladder function following spinal cord injury. J Auton Nerv Syst 1990; 30(Suppl): S71–7.
51. Cheng C-L, Ma C-P, de Groat WC. Effect of capsaicin on micturition and associated reflexes in chronic spinal rats. Brain Res 1995; 678: 40–8.
52. Talaat M. Afferent impulses in the nerves supplying the urinary bladder. J Physiol (Lond) 1937; 89: 1–13.
53. Feber JL, van Asselt E, van Mastrigt R. Neurophysiological modeling of voiding in rats: urethral nerve response to urethral pressure and flow. Am J Physiol 1998; 274: R1473–81.
54. Bradley W, Griffin D, Teague C, Timm G. Sensory innervation of the mammalian urethra. Invest Urol 1973; 10: 287–9.
55. Todd JK. Afferent impulses in the pudendal nerves of the cat. Q J Exp Physiol 1964; 49: 258–67.
56. Bahns E, Halsband U, Janig W. Responses of sacral visceral afferents from the lower urinary tract, colon and anus to mechanical stimulation. Pflugers Arch 1987; 410: 296–303.

57. Conte B, Maggi CA, Giachetti A et al. Intraurethral capsaicin produces reflex activation of the striated urethral sphincter in urethane-anesthetized male rats. J Urol 1993; 150: 1271–7.
58. Thor KB, Muhlhauser MA. Vesicoanal, urethroanal, and urethrovesical reflexes initiated by lower urinary tract irritation in the rat. Am J Physiol 1999; 277: R1002–12.
59. Hokfelt T, Schultzberg M, Elde R et al. Peptide neurons in peripheral tissues including the urinary tract: immunohistochemical studies. Acta Pharmacol Toxicol (Copenh) 1978; 43: 79–89.
60. Warburton AL, Santer RM. Sympathetic and sensory innervation of the urinary tract in young adult and aged rats: a semi-quantitative histochemical and immunohistochemical study. Histochem J 1994; 26: 127–33.
61. Lecci A, Giuliani S, Lazzeri M et al. The behavioral response induced by intravesical instillation of capsaicin in rats is mediated by pudendal urethral sensory fibers. Life Sci 1994; 55: 429–36.
62. Jung SY, Fraser MO, Ozawa H et al. Urethral afferent nerve activity affects the micturition reflex; implication for the relationship between stress incontinence and detrusor instability. J Urol 1999; 162: 204–12.
63. Ferguson DR, Kennedy I, Burton TJ. ATP is released from rabbit urinary bladder epithelial cells by hydrostatic pressure changes – a possible sensory mechanism? J Physiol 1997; 505: 503–11.
64. Birder LA, Kanai AJ, de Groat WC et al. Vanilloid receptor expression suggests a sensory role for urinary bladder epithelial cells. Proc Natl Acad Sci USA 2001; 98: 13396–401.
65. Vlaskovska M, Kasakov L, Rong W et al. P2X3 knock-out mice reveal a major sensory role for urothelially released ATP. J Neurosci 2001; 21: 5670–7.
66. Birder LA, Apodaca G, De Groat WC, Kanai AJ. Adrenergic- and capsaicin-evoked nitric oxide release from urothelium and afferent nerves in urinary bladder. Am J Physiol 1998; 275: F226–9.
67. Birder LA, Nealen ML, Kiss S et al. Beta-adrenoceptor agonists stimulate endothelial nitric oxide synthase in rat urinary bladder urothelial cells. J Neurosci 2002; 22: 8063–70.
68. Bean BP, Williams CA, Ceelen PW. ATP-activated channels in rat and bullfrog sensory neurons: current–voltage relation and single-channel behavior. J Neurosci 1990; 10: 11–19.
69. Dmitrieva N, Burnstock G, McMahon SB. ATP and 2-methyl thioATP activate bladder reflexes and induce discharge of bladder sensory neurons. Soc Neurosci Abstr 1998; 24: 2088.
70. Cockayne DA, Hamilton SG, Zhu QM et al. Urinary bladder hyporeflexia and reduced pain-related behaviour in P2X3-deficient mice. Nature 2000; 407: 1011–15.
71. Birder LA, Nakamura Y, Kiss S et al. Altered urinary bladder function in mice lacking the vanilloid receptor TRPV1. Nat Neurosci 2002; 5: 856–60.
72. Hawthorn MH, Chapple CR, Cock M, Chess-Williams R. Urothelium-derived inhibitory factor(s) influences on detrusor muscle contractility in vitro. Br J Pharmacol 2000; 129: 416–19.
73. de Groat WC. Nervous control of the urinary bladder of the cat. Brain Res 1975; 87: 201–11.
74. de Groat WC, Theobald RJ. Reflex activation of sympathetic pathways to vesical smooth muscle and parasympathetic ganglia by electrical stimulation of vesical afferents. J Physiol 1976; 259: 223–37.
75. Yoshimura N. Bladder afferent pathway and spinal cord injury: possible mechanisms inducing hyperreflexia of the urinary bladder. Progr Neurobiol 1999; 57: 583–606.
76. Park JM, Bloom DA, McGuire EJ. The guarding reflex revisited. Br J Urol 1997; 80: 940–5.
77. Fedirchuk B, Hochman S, Shefchyk SJ. An intracellular study of perineal and hindlimb afferent inputs onto sphincter motoneurons in the decerebrate cat. Exp Brain Res 1992; 89: 511–16.
78. Holstege G, Griffiths D, De Wall H, Dalm E. Anatomical and physiological observations on supraspinal control of bladder and urethral sphincter muscles in the cat. J Comp Neurol 1986; 250: 449–61.
79. Kohama T. [Neuroanatomical studies on the urine storage facilitatory areas in the cat brain. Part I. Input neuronal structures to the nucleus locus subcoeruleus and the nucleus radicularis pontis oralis.] Nippon Hinyokika Gakkai Zasshi 1992; 83: 1469–77.
80. de Groat WC, Fraser MO, Yoshiyama M et al. Neural control of the urethra. Scand J Urol Nephrol Suppl 2001: 35–43; discussion 106–25.
81. de Groat WC, Booth AM, Krier J et al. Neural control of the urinary bladder and large intestine. In: Brooks CM, Koizumi K, Sato A, eds. Integrative functions of the autonomic nervous system. Tokyo: Tokyo University Press, 1979: 50–67.
82. de Groat WC, Booth AM, Milne RJ, Roppolo JR. Parasympathetic preganglionic neurons in the sacral spinal cord. J Auton Nerv Syst 1982; 5: 23–43.
83. McGuire EJ, Morrissey SG, Schichun Z, Horwinsk E. Control of reflex detrusor activity in normal and spinal injured non-human primates. J Urol 1983; 129: 197–9.
84. de Groat WC, Nadelhaft I, Milne RJ et al. Organization of the sacral parasympathetic reflex pathways to the urinary bladder and large intestine. J Auton Nerv Syst 1981; 3: 135–60.
85. Vera PL, Nadelhaft I. Conduction velocity distribution of afferent fibers innervating the rat urinary bladder. Brain Res 1990; 520: 83–9.
86. Kuru M. Nervous control of micturition. Physiol Rev 1965; 45: 425–94.
87. Nishizawa O, Sugaya K, No to H et al. Pontine micturition center in the dog. J Urol 1988; 140: 872–4.
88. Mallory BS, Roppolo JR, de Groat WC. Pharmacological modulation of the pontine micturition center. Brain Res 1991; 546: 310–20.
89. Noto H, Roppolo JR, Steers WD, de Groat WC. Excitatory and inhibitory influences on bladder activity elicited by electrical stimulation in the pontine micturition center in rat. Brain Res 1989; 492: 99–115.
90. Noto H, Roppolo JR, Steers WD, de Groat WC. Electrophysiological analysis of the ascending and descending components of the micturition reflex pathway in the rat. Brain Res 1991; 549: 95–105.
91. Blok BF, Holstege G. Direct projections from the periaqueductal gray to the pontine micturition center (M-region). An anterograde and retrograde tracing study in the cat. Neurosci Lett 1994; 166: 93–6.
92. Blok BF, De Weerd H, Holstege G. Ultrastructural evidence for a paucity of projections from the lumbosacral cord to the pontine micturition center or M-region in the cat: a new concept for the organization of the micturition reflex with the periaqueductal gray as central relay. J Comp Neurol 1995; 359: 300–9.
93. Matsuura S, Allen GV, Downie JW. Volume-evoked micturition reflex is mediated by the ventrolateral periaqueductal gray in anesthetized rats. Am J Physiol 1998; 275: R2049–55.
94. Matsuura S, Downie JW, Allen GV. Micturition evoked by glutamate microinjection in the ventrolateral periaqueductal gray is mediated through Barrington's nucleus in the rat. Neuroscience 2000; 101: 1053–61.
95. Blaivas JG. The neurophysiology of micturition: a clinical study of 550 patients. J Urol 1982; 127: 958.
96. Rossier AB, Ott R. Bladder and urethral recordings in acute and chronic spinal cord injury patients. Int J Urol 1976; 31: 49–59.
97. Barrington FJF. The component reflexes of micturition in the cat. Parts I and II. Brain 1931; 54: 177–88.
98. Barrington FJF. The component reflexes of micturition in the cat. Part III. Brain 1941; 64: 239–43.
99. de Groat WC, Araki I, Vizzard MA et al. Developmental and injury induced plasticity in the micturition reflex pathway. Behav Brain Res 1998; 92: 127–40.
100. Araki I, de Groat WC. Developmental synaptic depression underlying reorganization of visceral reflex pathways in the spinal cord. J Neurosci 1997; 17: 8402–7.

101. Birder LA, de Groat WC. Induction of *c-fos* gene expression of spinal neurons in the rat by nociceptive and non-nociceptive stimulation of the lower urinary tract. Am J Physiol 1993; 265: R643–8.
102. Nadelhaft I, Vera PL. Neurons in the rat brain and spinal cord labeled after pseudorabies virus injected into the external urethral sphincter. J Comp Neurol 1996; 375: 502–17.
103. Vizzard MA, Erickson VL, Card JP et al. Transneuronal labeling of neurons in the adult rat brainstem and spinal cord after injection of pseudorabies virus into the urethra. J Comp Neurol 1995; 355: 629–40.
104. Sugaya K, Roppolo JR, Yoshimura N et al. The central neural pathways involved in micturition in the neonatal rat as revealed by the injection of pseudorabies virus into the urinary bladder. Neurosci Lett 1997; 223: 197–200.
105. Sasaki M. Morphological analysis of external urethral and external anal sphincter motoneurones of cat. J Comp Neurol 1994; 349: 269–87.
106. Araki I. Inhibitory postsynaptic currents and the effects of GABA on visually identified sacral parasympathetic preganglionic neurons in neonatal rats. J Neurophysiol 1994; 72: 2903–10.
107. de Groat WC. Excitation and inhibition of sacral parasympathetic neurons by visceral and cutaneous stimuli in the cat. Brain Res 1971; 33: 499–503.
108. de Groat WC. Inhibitory mechanisms in the sacral reflex pathways to the urinary bladder. In: Ryall RW, Kelly JS, eds. Iontophoresis and transmitter mechanisms in the mammalian central nervous system. Amsterdam: Elsevier, 1978: 366–8.
109. Morrison JF, Sato A, Sato Y, Yamanishi T. The influence of afferent inputs from skin and viscera on the activity of the bladder and the skeletal muscle surrounding the urethra in the rat. Neurosci Res 1995; 23: 195–205.
110. McGuire EJ. Experimental observations on the integration of bladder and urethral function. Trans Am Assoc Genitourin Surg 1976; 68: 38–42.
111. de Groat WC, Ryall RW. Reflexes to sacral parasympathetic neurones concerned with micturition in the cat. J Physiol 1969; 200: 87–108.
112. Barrington FJF. The relation of the hind-brain to micturition. Brain 1921; 4: 23–53.
113. Blok BFM, DeWeerd H, Holstege G. The pontine micturition center projects to sacral cord GABA immunoreactive neurons in the cat. Neurosci Lett 1997; 233: 109–12.
114. Blok BFM, Holstege G. Neuronal control of micturition and its relation to the emotional motor system. Progr Brain Res 1996; 107: 113–26.
115. Tang PC, Ruch TC. Localization of brain stem and diencephalic areas controlling the micturition reflex. J Comp Neurol 1956; 106: 213–45.
116. Sugaya K, Matsuyama K, Takakusaki K, Mori S. Electrical and chemical stimulations of the pontine micturition center. Neurosci Lett 1987; 80: 197–201.
117. Valentino RJ, Chen S, Zhu Y, Aston-Jones G. Evidence for divergent projections to the brain noradrenergic system and the spinal parasympathetic system from Barrington's nucleus. Brain Res 1996; 732: 1–15.
118. Ding YQ, Takada M, Tokuno H, Mizuno N. Direct projections from the dorsolateral pontine tegmentum to pudendal motoneurons innervating the external urethral sphincter muscle in the rat. J Comp Neurol 1995; 357: 318–30.
119. Otake K, Nakamura Y. Single neurons in Barrington's nucleus projecting to both the paraventricular thalamic nucleus and the spinal cord by way of axon collaterals: a double labeling study in the rat. Neurosci Lett 1996; 209: 97–100.
120. Blok BF, van Maarseveen JT, Holstege G. Electrical stimulation of the sacral dorsal gray commissure evokes relaxation of the external urethral sphincter in the cat. Neurosci Lett 1998; 249: 68–70.
121. Valentino RJ, Pavcovich LA, Hirata H. Evidence for corticotropin releasing hormone projections from Barrington's nucleus to the periaqueductal gray and dorsal motor nucleus of the vagus in the rat. J Comp Neurol 1995; 363: 402–22.
122. Blok BFM, Willemsen ATM, Holstege G. A PET study on the brain control of micturition in humans. Brain 1997: 111–21.
123. Yoshimura N, Nagahama Y, Ueda T, Yoshida O. Paroxysmal urinary incontinence associated with multiple sclerosis. Urol Int 1997; 59: 197–9.
124. Marson L. Identification of central nervous system neurons that innervate the bladder body, bladder base, or external urethral sphincter of female rats: a transneuronal tracing study using pseudorabies virus. J Comp Neurol 1997; 389: 584–602.
125. Fukuyama H, Matsuzaki S, Ouchi Y et al. Neural control of micturition in man examined with single photon emission computed tomography using 99mTc-HMPAO. Neuroreport 1996; 7: 3009–12.
126. Blok BF, Willemsen TM, Holstege G. A PET study on brain control of micturition in humans. Brain 1997; 120: 111–21.
127. Holstege JC, Van Dijken H, Buijs RM et al. Distribution of dopamine immunoreactivity in the rat, cat and monkey spinal cord. J Comp Neurol 1996; 376: 631–52.
128. Athwal BS, Berkley KJ, Hussain I et al. Brain responses to changes in bladder volume and urge to void in healthy men. Brain 2001; 124: 369–77.
129. Blok BF, Sturms LM, Holstege G. A PET study on cortical and subcortical control of pelvic floor musculature in women. J Comp Neurol 1997; 389: 535–44.
130. Zhang H, Reitz A, Kollias S et al. An fMRI study of the role of suprapontine brain structures in the voluntary voiding control induced by pelvic floor contraction. Neuroimage 2005; 24: 174–80.
131. Seseke S, Baudewig J, Kallenberg K et al. Voluntary pelvic floor muscle control – an fMRI study. Neuroimage 2006; 31: 1399–407.
132. Kuhtz-Buschbeck JP, van der Horst C, Wolff S et al. Activation of the supplementary motor area (SMA) during voluntary pelvic floor muscle contractions – an fMRI study. Neuroimage 2007; 35: 449–57.
133. Matsui M, Yoneyama E, Sumiyoshi T et al. Lack of self-control as assessed by a personality inventory is related to reduced volume of supplementary motor area. Psychiatry Res 2002; 116: 53–61.
134. de Groat WC, Araki I. Maturation of bladder reflex pathways during postnatal development. Adv Exp Med Biol 1999; 462: 253–63.
135. Geirsson G, Lindstrom S, Fall M. The bladder cooling reflex and the use of cooling as stimulus to the lower urinary tract. J Urol 1999; 162: 1890–6.
136. Chancellor MB, de Groat WC. Intravesical capsaicin and resiniferatoxin therapy: spicing up the ways to treat the overactive bladder. J Urol 1999; 162: 3–11.

8

Physiology of normal sexual function

Hélène Gelez, Pierre Clément, and François Giuliano

Introduction

The lifting of the Victorian veil, which covered the Western world with prudishness and sexual taboos until the first half of the twentieth century, was followed by profound changes in social attitudes producing a so-called sexual revolution in the 1960s. As a result, a rational approach to sexual physiology and sexual dysfunctions, developed by researchers from multiple scientific fields, progressively emerged and led to a better knowledge of human sexuality, even if there is still significant progress to be made, especially for female sexual physiology. In both genders, sexual behavior is divided in appetitive and consummatory components.[1] Appetitive behaviors are associated with sexual desire, excitement, and arousal, whereas consummatory behaviors consist of genital stimulation leading to orgasm. Initially, the human sexual response was described by Masters and Johnson[2] as including four interactive phases: excitation, plateau, orgasm, and resolution. This definition has subsequently been revised by Kaplan[3] and Levin[3,4] to lead to a commonly accepted model, consisting of desire, excitation, orgasm, and resolution. Each of these phases is controlled by a complex and coordinated interplay of multiple components of the brain, spinal cord, and relevant peripheral organs. Many of the mechanisms of control of the different aspects of sexual function are not fully delineated, although homologies and, most often analogies, with mammalian animal models have allowed the improvement of our understanding of the physiology of human sexual function.

Female sexual function

The female sexual life phases consist of puberty, adulthood, pregnancy, and menopause. Puberty is defined as sexual maturation and refers to the process of physical and physiologic changes by which a child's body becomes an adult body capable of reproduction. Then, adult females experience menstrual cycles consisting of different phases: menstruation, follicular phase, ovulation, and luteal phase. The ovarian cycle's duration varies across species (4 days in rats, 17 days in sheep, 28 days in women), but in all species they are tightly controlled by steroid hormones. Women are able to express sexual desire and to engage in sexual intercourse at any time, contrary to females in most animal species which display sexual activity only during a precise period of the ovarian cycle, around ovulation. Female sexual behavior consists of proceptive components associated with sexual desire, excitement and arousal, and receptivity, commonly reflected by the lordosis reflex in female rodents.[1,3,4] Each of these phases is controlled by both the autonomic and somatic nervous systems, and their interconnections with different spinal and supraspinal centers.

Neuroanatomy

Female genitalia

The female genital sexual anatomy consists of the perineum, the external genitalia, and the vagina. The perineum is the short stretch of skin situated between the anus and the bottom of the vulva, extending from the inferior boundary of the pelvis to the symphysis pubis and the inferior edges of the pubic bone. The urogenital diaphragm, also known as the triangular ligament, is part of the perineum and consists of a sheet of tissue stretching across the pubic arch, formed by the deep transverse perineal and the sphincter urethrae muscles.

The vagina is a muscular canal extending from the cervix to the exterior of the body. The vaginal opening is at the caudal end of the vulva, behind the opening of the urethra. The vaginal mucosa, which lines the vaginal walls, is thick and has a protective layer of stratified squamous, nonkeratinized epithelium. The lumen of the vagina is usually small, with the walls that surround it generally in

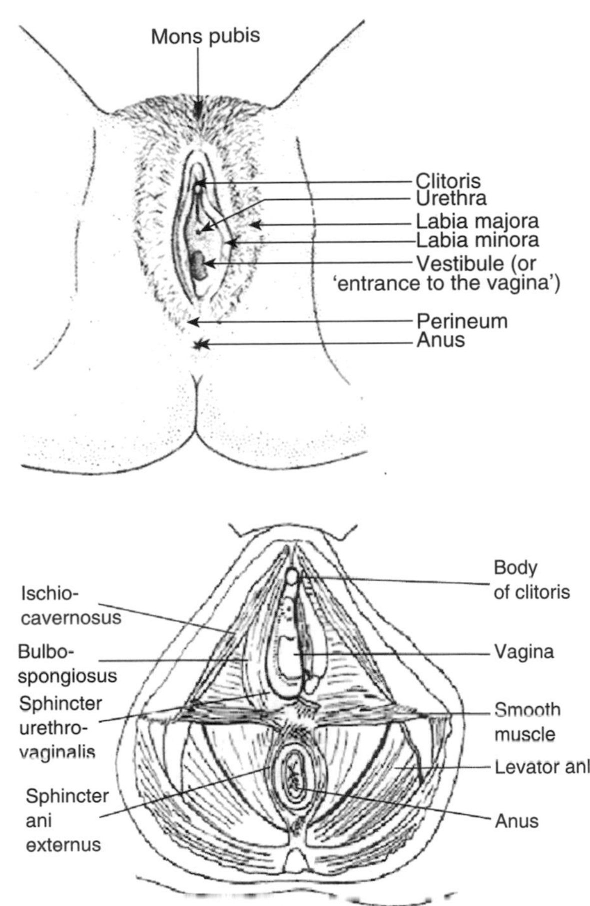

Figure 8.1
(a) Anatomy of female genitalia. (b) Muscular support of the female pelvic floor.

contact with each other. The vaginal canal is capable of stretching during sexual intercourse as well as childbirth.

The external genitalia of the female are collectively referred to as the vulva and include the mons veneris, labia majora, labia minora, clitoris, vulvovaginal glands (also called Bartholin's glands), and the vestibule of the vagina (Figure 8.1A). The mons pubis, also called the mons veneris in females, is the soft tissue present in both genders just above the genitals (above the vulva in females), raised above the surrounding area due to a pad of fat lying just beneath it which protects the pubic bone. It is anterior to the symphysis pubis. The labia majora are two prominent longitudinal cutaneous folds which extend downward and backward from the mons pubis to the perineum. Each labium has two surfaces, an outer, pigmented and covered with hairs, and an inner, smooth and containing sebaceous glands which render it moist. The labia minora are two smaller folds located medial to the labia majora and anteriorly surrounding the clitoris. Anteriorly, each labium divides into two portions: the upper division passes above the clitoris, forming a fold extending beyond the clitoral glans clitoridis, and named the preputium clitoridis; the lower division passes under the clitoral glans and forms the frenulum clitoridis. The labia minora surround a space, called the vestibule, into which the vagina and urethra open. These labia lack hair but have a large supply of venous sinuses, sebaceous glands, and nerves.

The anatomy of the clitoris has recently been clarified in a series of dissections of fresh and fixed cadaver tissue.[5–7] The clitoris is a multiplanar structure located near the anterior junction of the labia minora, above the opening of the urethra and vagina, and consists of the glans, the body, and erectile bodies (the paired bulbs, crura, and corpora). The glans is the only visible external part of the clitoris and is entirely or partially protected by the clitoral hood or prepuce, a covering of tissue similar to the foreskin of the male penis. The clitoral body contains a pair of corpora cavernosa and extends several centimeters upwards and to the back, before splitting into two arms, the clitoral crura. These crura extend around and to the interior of the labia majora.

The pelvic floor is composed of muscles having their origin on the interior of the bony pelvis and inserting onto the caudal coccygeal vertebrae.[8] The levator ani is composed of two major muscles, the pubococcygeus and iliococcygeus, and the coccygeus muscles form the pelvic diaphragm.[9,10] The striated perineal muscles consist of the sexually dimorphic bulbospongiosus and ischiocavernosus muscles, and the external anal and urethral sphincters (Figure 8.1B).[7,11,12] In addition, the vagina is surrounded by a circular layer of smooth muscles, as well as an important longitudinal smooth muscle layer (Figure 8.1B).

Peripheral innervation

Peripheral innervation of the female genital organs has been described in humans,[13,14] as well as in different rodent species. Neuroanatomic studies show that female genital organs are innervated by the autonomic nervous system, but also by somatic and sensory fibers.

Afferent innervation Sensory fibers from the pelvic, pudendal, and hypogastric nerves innervate the female genital organs and relay information to the spinal cord (in the thoracolumbar and lumbosacral segments) (Figure 8.2).[13–16]

Pelvic nerve sensory fibers innervate the vagina, the cervix, and the body of the uterus, with the greatest concentration in the fornix of the vagina.[17] The sensory fibers conveyed by the pelvic nerve enter the spinal cord via the S2–S3 dorsal roots in women, and the L6–S1 dorsal roots in female rats, essentially in the Lissauer's tract from which collaterals extend to the dorsal horn, the sacral parasympathetic nucleus (SPN), and the dorsal gray commissure (DGC).[18,19]

The pudendal nerve provides sensory innervation to the clitoris, perineum, and urethra; the major branch of the sensory pudendal nerve gives rise to the dorsal nerve of

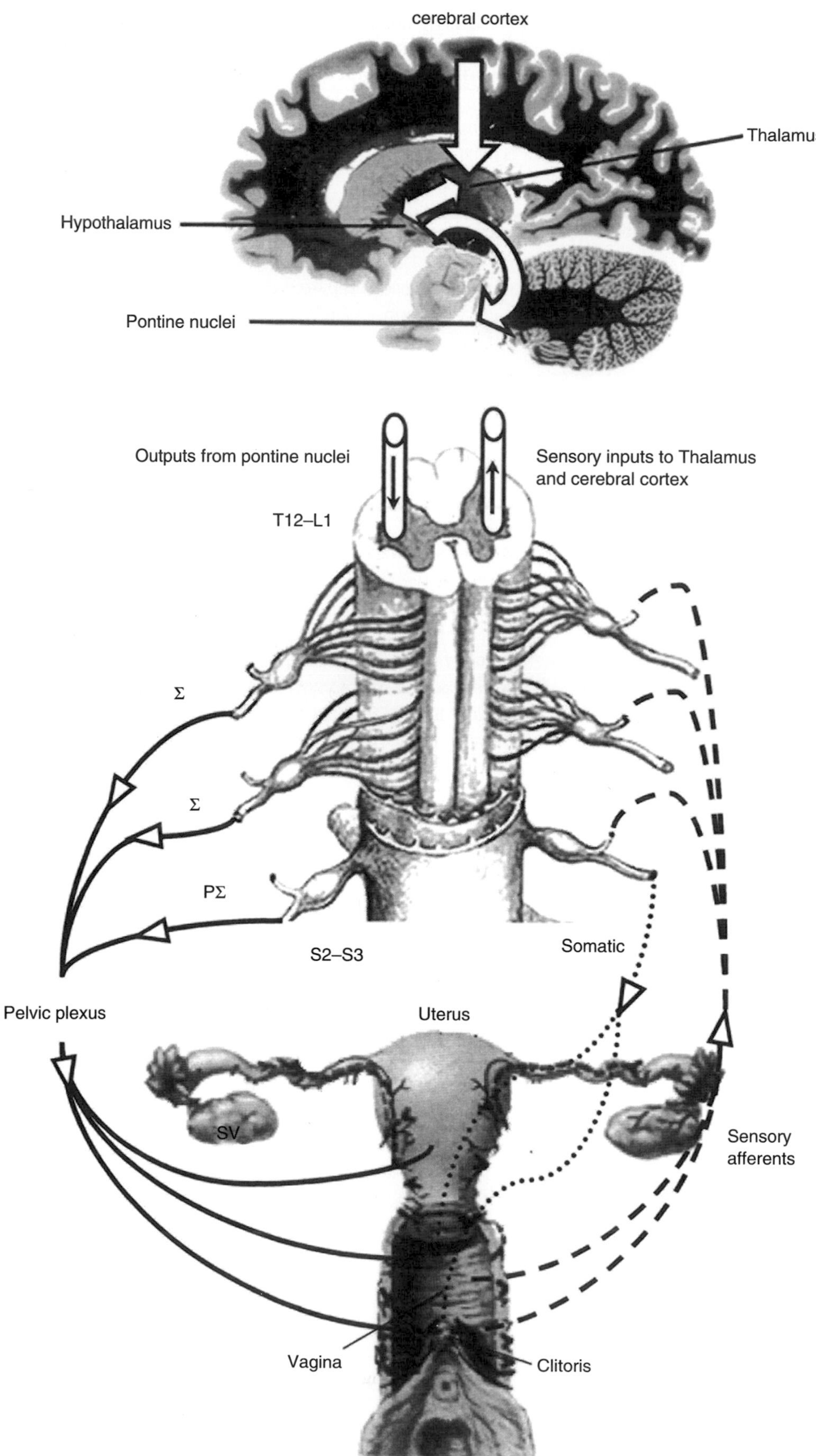

Figure 8.2
Neural pathways controlling female sexual response. Sympathetic (Σ), parasympathetic (PΣ), and somatic nerves originating in lumbosacral spinal nuclei command the peripheral anatomical structures that control female sexual responses. Sensory afferents originating in genital areas are integrated at the spinal and brain levels. Activity of spinal preganglionic and motor neurons is under the influence of peripheral and supraspinal inputs.

the clitoris, while other branches innervate the perineal skin and urethra. The pudendal afferent fiber terminations are located in the dorsal column, the medial half of Lissauer's tract, the extreme edge of the dorsal horn, and in the DGC in the lumbosacral segments L6–S1.[20,21] The dorsal nerves of the clitoris originate below the pubic bone and form two bundles that fan out laterally on the clitoral bodies, where they join to form the single clitoral body.[7]

The hypogastric nerve also contains some axons of afferent neurons originating in the uterus and the cervix and reaches the thoracolumbar segments of the spinal cord.[22]

There is also evidence that vagal afferent fibers likely convey sensory information from the female genital organs directly to the nucleus of the tractus solitaris (NTS), bypassing the spinal cord. Indeed, it is noteworthy that women with complete upper spinal cord injury are still able to perceive genital sensation.[23] Furthermore, in the rat, it has been shown that afferent fibers in the vagus nerve are implicated in the responses to vagino-cervical stimulation (VCS).[24]

Efferent innervation The female genital organs receive parasympathetic, sympathetic, and somatic innervation via three nerves: the pelvic, hypogastric, and pudendal (Figure 8.2).

Parasympathetic fibers to the vagina and the clitoris are conveyed by the pelvic nerve originating from the sacral segments (S2–S4) of the spinal cord from the SPN.[18] The neural fibers of the pelvic nerve travel in the pelvic plexus and send branches in the cavernous nerves, which originate from the autonomic nerve plexus around the vagina and extend to the proximal urethra and the clitoral body. In the rat, preganglionic neurons of the SPN are located almost exclusively (98%) within the L6–S1 spinal cord segment,[19] corresponding to the sacral S2–S4 segments in humans.

Autonomic sympathetic fibers destined to the vagina and the clitoris are conveyed by the paravertebral sympathetic chain and the hypogastric nerve. Sympathetic preganglionic neurons originate from the thoracolumbar segments of the spinal cord (T13–L2 in rats) from two separate nuclei, the DGC and the intermediolateral cell column, and represent the main sympathetic outflow to the genital tract.[25]

The pudendal nerve originates from the splanchnic branches of the sacral plexus and provides innervation to the pelvic floor, and anal and urethral sphincters.[11,20] The pudendal motoneurons are located in the the ventral cord of the sacral spinal segments in the Onufrowicz's (Onuf's) nucleus. In rats, the Onuf's nucleus is anatomically divided into the dorsomedial and the dorsolateral nuclei.[20,26]

Spinal and supraspinal centers: neuroanatomic consideration

In this section details of the neuroanatomic connections between the spinal and brain centers involved in the control of female sexual responses are provided, while their functional role will be addressed in the following paragraphs.

Spinal centers The pseudorabies virus (PRV), a transneuronal retrograde tracer, has been used to identify the spinal neurons destined to the clitoris, vagina, cervix, and uterus in rats. The major input to the clitoris originates from the lumbosacral segments of the spinal cord (L5–S1), in the SPN where the preganglionic neurons of the pelvic nerve are located, and in the DGC.[27] Fewer PRV-labeled neurons were found in other areas of the spinal cord, including the T13–L2 segments where the sympathetic preganglionic neurons of the hypogastric nerve and the lumbosacral paravertebral sympathetic chain are located. PRV injection in both the clitoris and vagina labeled neurons in similar regions of the spinal cord, with numerous PRV-labeled neurons in the L6–S1 segments in the superficial, medial, and lateral regions of the dorsal horn, the SPN, the DGC and intermediomedial nucleus, the intermediate gray, and ventral horn.[28]

The spinal neurons destined to the uterus and cervix have also been identified. When PRV was injected in the uterus and cervix, preganglionic neurons and putative interneurons were labeled in the lumbosacral spinal cord (L6–S1) and the lower segments of the thoracic cord (T11–T13), mainly in the lateral horn area (SPN and intermediolateral nucleus), lateral aspect of the dorsal horn, intermediate gray, and the DGC.[29]

Sensory projections from the pelvic area and spinal neurons involved in different aspects of the female sexual response have also been examined by quantifying the Fos protein, a marker of neuronal activation. Electrical stimulation of the pelvic nerve in anesthetized rats activated primarily neurons in the L6–S1 segments of the spinal cord, in the superficial dorsal horn, the DGC, and lateral laminae V–VII in the region of the SPN.[30] VCS elicited by copulation with a sexually vigorous male or by manual stimulation with a lubricated glass rod increased the expression of Fos protein immunoreactivity primarily in the L6–S1 segments throughout the dorsal horn and in the dorsal and medial gray commissure.[31–33] These results confirm the neuroanatomic data obtained from tracing studies showing that afferent information from the female genital organs is received by neurons in specific areas of the dorsal horn, especially in the lumbosacral segments.

Brain centers Similar neuroanatomic studies using PRV have been conducted to investigate the brain centers involved in the multisynaptic circuitry controling female sexual responses. Tracing techniques have evidenced two major ascending pathways: the spinothalamic and the spinoreticular pathways, which relay sensory information to the brain.[34] The spinothalamic pathway travels in the dorsal columns and dorsal lateral quadrant, crosses the brainstem, passes through the medial lemniscus, and reaches the specific nuclei of the thalamus (nucleus ventralis posterolateralis and nucleus ventralis posteromedialis). A last relay sends information to the somatosensory cortex. Most of the spinoreticular fibers cross to the opposite side of the cord (below T8) and travel in the lateral spinal columns, terminating in brainstem reticular formation and the nonspecific nuclei of the thalamus.

The descending pathways from the brain to the female genital organs have been identified by examining the distribution of PRV in different spinal and supraspinal centers.[27,28,35] Four days after PRV injection in the clitoris and the vagina, PRV-positive neurons were found in the nucleus paragigantocellularis (nPGi), Barrington's nucleus, raphe magnus, A5 region, and in the hypothalamus primarily in the paraventricular nucleus (PVN). PRV-positive cells were occasionally localized in the raphe pallidus, caudal ventrolateral periaqueductal gray (PAG), and lateral hypothalamus (LH). After a 5-day survival period, more PRV-positive neurons were observed in the areas described above and in additional brain regions including the dorsal, lateral, and ventrolateral PAG, nucleus of the tractus solitarius (NTS), the medial preoptic area (MPOA), and the ventral part of the ventromedial hypothalamic nucleus (VMNvl), with few PRV cells in the bed nucleus of the stria terminalis (BNST), zona incerta, and medial amygdala (MeA).

Physiology of the female sexual response

The female sexual response consists of sexual desire, arousal, and orgasm. This includes genital and behavioral responses characterized by peripheral physiologic events occurring mainly in the genital organs, and a central drive originating from the spinal and supraspinal centers.

It has always been difficult to define sexual desire and to dissociate sexual desire from sexual arousal. It is now commonly accepted that sexual arousal generally reflects an increase in blood flow to the genital organs and clitoral erectile tissues, whereas sexual desire refers to a psychologic state characterizing sexual interest and motivation to engage in sexual contact.[36] In women, the central drive is crucial and constitutes the key element of the mechanisms controlling libido. Accordingly, it is crucial to emphasize that an increase of vaginal blood flow is not necessarily associated with the subjective feeling of sexual arousal.[37]

Peripheral physiologic changes during the female sexual response

Genital arousal Physiologic sexual arousal in both humans and animals can be defined as an increase in autonomic activation that prepares the body for sexual activity and decreases the amount of sexual stimulation necessary to induce orgasm. In women, the first studies focused on extragenital measures such as heart rate, respiration, blood pressure, sweat production, and body temperature, considered as indexes of sexual arousal.[2] Other methods were subsequently developed to measure vaginal temperature[38] and monitor changes in clitoral and vaginal blood flow: for example photoplethysmography measuring vaginal pulse amplitude,[39] the oxygenation-temperature method,[40] and clitoral color doppler ultrasonography.[41] It has been shown that genital arousal results in an increase in blood flow to the vagina, clitoris, and labia mediated by the parasympathetic nervous system. The erectile tissue of the clitoris shows vasocongestion and tumescence, in the same way as does the penis. Sexual arousal is also associated with vaginal lubrication resulting from blood engorgement and increased permeability of epithelial capillary tufts, also mediated by the parasympathetic nervous system.

Some data suggested that female genital arousal is controlled, as in males, by a balance between the facilitatory parasympathetic and inhibitory sympathetic inputs. However, a facilitatory effect of the sympathetic nervous system resulting in an increase in blood flow to striated and smooth muscles that participate in different sexual responses, such as increased heart and breathing rates, has been proposed.[42]

Electrical stimulation of the sacral roots in women increases vaginal blood flow.[43] Analogous models have been developed in rats, rabbits, and dogs. In *in-vivo* experiments performed in various animal species, electrical stimulation of the pelvic nerve mimicks the type of stimulation normally received by females during intromissive copulation and results in vaginal response and clitoral tumescence characterized by an increase in vaginal blood flow, vaginal wall pressure, vaginal length, clitoral and intracavernosal pressure, and blood flow, and a decrease in vaginal luminal pressure.[44–46] It is interesting to note that, in the rat, stimulation of the paravertebral sympathetic chain reverses the effect of pelvic nerve stimulation.[44]

Orgasm Orgasm is the third and probably the shortest phase of the human sexual response cycle; it is the most reinforcing component of sexual behavior and is followed by a feeling of euphoria and satisfaction during the resolution phase. In women, orgasm is usually obtained by stimulation of the clitoris and/or the vagina, although cervical stimulation may also be perceived as pleasurable during orgasm.[47] Orgasm results in rhythmic contractions of the vagina, uterus, and anal sphincter and changes in vaginal and clitoral blood flow.[48–51] Increases in heart rate, blood pressure, and respiration are associated.[2,52] Orgasmic responses are regulated by both the autonomic and somatic nervous systems. The pudendal nerve that conveys sensory information from the vulva and the striated pelvic perineal muscles plays a critical role in the occurrence of clitoral orgasm. The pelvic and hypogastric nerves conveying sensory information from the internal pelvic organs may be involved in 'coital orgasm'. Nevertheless, it must be emphasized that the exact physiologic support for orgasm remains unknown. An experimental model attempting to mimick sexual climax in humans has been developed in the rat. The urethrogenital (UG) reflex is induced by mechanical stimulation of the distal urethra and consists in the female of rhythmic contractions of the vagina, uterus, and striated perineal muscles, i.e. the external urethral and anal sphincters.[53] Examination of spinal neuronal Fos activation suggests that the UG reflex is mediated by the pudendal sensory nerve and comprises activation of the hypogastric, pelvic, and pudendal motor nerves.[54] The UG reflex is not dependent on vagal pathways since this reflex can still be evoked after vagal nerve cuts in female rat.[54]

Some women have reported a dramatic increase in secretions during orgasm, described as female ejaculation by some authors. When female ejaculation occurs, it involves, as in males, the ejection of significant amounts of fluid in gushes through the urethra at the moment of sexual climax.[55] However, it remains unclear whether ejaculation in women consistently occurs and is associated with orgasm, and whether these secretions are different from urine.[56]

Orgasm is also associated with hormonal changes: in particular, an increase in circulating levels of prolactin, oxytocin (OT), vasopressin (AVP), adrenaline, and vasointestinal polypeptide (VIP) has been reported.[56,57]

Central control of female sexual response

Spinal network Functional approaches have demonstrated that local physiologic changes associated with sexual arousal result mainly from spinal reflex mechanisms. Two main spinal sexual reflexes have been evidenced: the bulbocavernous reflex involving sacral segments S2–S4 and another reflex involving vaginal and clitoral cavernosal autonomic nerve stimulation and producing clitoral, labial, and vaginal engorgement.[58] Different data demonstrated that the spinal cord is sufficient to generate female sexual responses, without functional connections to supraspinal centers. Women diagnosed with complete spinal cord injury retain the capacity of increased blood flow and/or lubrication upon masturbation.[56,59,60] Orgasm is also a reflex mediated by the spinal cord: women with complete spinal cord injury are still able to achieve orgasm during audiovisual erotic combined with manual genital stimulation.[60] However, women with injury of the lower motoneurons and S2–S5 dermatomes are less likely to reach orgasm compared to women with injury at or above T11.[61] This suggests that orgasmic responses require intact reflexes that relay in the sacral spinal cord.

In male rats, recent studies have identified a group of lumbar spinothalamic (LSt) neurons, which likely represent a spinal generator for ejaculation.[62] An increased *c-fos* expression has been evidenced in these neurons after ejaculation in male rats, but not after VCS applied to females. However, a similar neuronal subpopulation conveying copulatory stimuli to the spinal cord and regulating genital arousal and orgasm can also exist in females, but, so far, has not been evidenced.

In the animal model mimicking human climax, the UG reflex induced by urethral stimulation can be elicited only in acutely spinalized females.[53] Indeed, in spinally intact anesthetized females, this reflex is tonically inhibited by neurons in the nPGi of the ventral medulla.

In fact, the spinal centers involved in the control of female sexual responses are under descending excitatory and inhibitory control from supraspinal brain sites.

Brain network It now commonly accepted that sexual desire is mainly controlled by brain mechanisms. Any individual, in order to engage in sexual intercourse, must be able to respond to hormonal and neurochemical changes that signal sexual desire. Sexual arousal also includes a central component that increases neural 'tone' or awareness to respond to sexual incentives, defined as 'arousability' by Whalen.[63] Contrary to the peripheral physiologic changes which have been well identified in both humans and animals, the neural pathways involved in the control of female sexual desire and central arousal remain largely unknown. The majority of the data available have been obtained from animal studies, and there is an abundant literature regarding the central control of lordosis in female rodents. However, it remains difficult to extrapolate these data to human sexual behavior since there is no human counterpart of lordosis.

Brain imaging studies have been conducted in humans to identify the brain centers activated during female sexual responses, but most of them focus on orgasmic reflexes. Positron emission tomography studies have evidenced that orgasm, compared to pre-orgasm arousal, enhances activation in the PVN, PAG, amygdala, hippocampus, striatum, cerebellum, and different cortical areas.[64] During self-masturbation, the NTS, thalamus, somatosensory and motor cortices, and sensory areas of the spinal medulla are activated. However, further studies are needed to identify the brain areas specifically activated during orgasm and to discriminate with those specifically activated during sexual arousal.

This functional dissociation can be evaluated in animal models, by examining and comparing the neural pathways controling appetitive and consummatory sexual responses. In female rats, mating with males results in increased *c-fos* expression in different hypothalamic nuclei, such as the MPOA, VMN, PVN, arcuate nucleus, and in the structures belonging to the mesolimbic dopaminergic pathway: the ventral tegmental area (VTA), MeA, nucleus accumbens (Nac), but also in the lateral septum, striatum, BNST, and the medial central gray.[65–67] A similar Fos staining was elicited by manual VCS.[68, 69]

However, a neuronal activation detected in a brain area in response to sexual stimulation does not necessarily imply the involvement of this structure in the control of sexual response. Functional approaches have confirmed the role of some of these brain structures. In female rats, lesion of the MPOA, Nac, or striatum abolishes proceptive behaviors,[70–74] whereas lesion of the VMN, VTA, PAG, or nPGi blocked the stereotyped reflex of lordosis.[75–77] Many of these structures have been labeled after PRV injection in the clitoris and the vagina.[28]

The MPOA plays a critical role in the control of female sexual desire. Neurochemical changes occurring in the MPOA have been measured in close association with sexual desire. Many neurotransmitters, neuropeptides, and pharmacologic agents (dopamine (DA), OT, melanocortin, and opioids agonists) have been reported to exert facilitatory effects on proceptive behaviors, when microinfused into the MPOA. Furthermore, in anesthetized female rats, electrical stimulation of the MPOA resulted in an increase in vaginal blood flow and wall tension.[44] The MPOA does not directly innervate the spinal cord and neuroanatomic data suggest that the major MPOA output relays in the PAG and nPGi before reaching the spinal circuits regulating female genital reflexes (Figure 8.3).[78] Female sexual drive may also be controlled by other neural pathways. The mesolimbic dopaminergic pathway is involved in rewarding and motivational processes, including sexual motivation. In this pathway, neurons of the VTA project to the Nac and the MeA, two critical structures for the display of sexual desire. The MPOA, which sends direct outputs to the VTA and the NAc, and receives neuronal inputs from the MeA, may modulate sexual responses through these central interconnections.

Multiple evidence from lesion, electrical stimulation, and neurochemical experiments indicates that the ventromedial hypothalamus (VMH) contains neural mechanisms that facilitate female sexual behavior.[79] The VMN is critical for lordosis and is the main site of action for steroid hormones.[79–81] However, the role of the VMH in the control of genital responses has not been investigated yet.

The PVN could also be involved in the control of female sexual response. The PVN is an important integrative site for the sympathetic nervous system and supplies OT to the peripheral circulation. Both copulation with a male and VCS result in *c-fos* activation within the OT neurons of the PVN in female rats.[82] Furthermore, neurons of the PVN are labeled after PRV injection in the clitoris and the vagina and directly project to the lumbosacral segments of the spinal cord (Figure 8.3).[28,83] However, the exact role of the PVN in the control of female sexual function remains to be determined.

The nPGi and the PAG are two other areas labeled with PRV after injection in the clitoris and the vagina, and have direct connections with the MPOA (Figure 8.3).[28] The nPGi regulates a variety of autonomic and somatic functions and could be involved in female sexual function, as a tonic inhibitory center. The PAG is known to be an important relay for sexually relevant stimuli and has extensive connections with brainstem and hypothalamic nuclei involved in female sexual function.[78] The PAG receives and integrates autonomic input from the MPOA and the PVN and appears to inhibit the nPGi, thereby desinhibiting sexual reflexes.

Hormonal control of female sexual response

Role of sex steroids on physiologic genital changes Androgens, acting directly or through their conversion to estrogens in the central nervous system (CNS) and in the periphery, are essential for the development of reproductive function and play a critical role in maintaining the structural and functional integrity of vaginal tissues, and modulating physiologic changes occurring during sexual arousal.[84,85] Ovariectomy caused vaginal atrophy and reduced vaginal epithelial cell maturation.[86] In addition, clinical and experimental studies have suggested a role for estrogens in modulating genital blood flow. In women, the decline in circulating estrogen associated with the menopause affects vaginal lubrication and can be responsible for clitoral fibrosis and diminished thinning of the vagina wall.[87]

Likewise, ovariectomized or estrogen-deprived female rats show a low increase in vaginal and clitoral blood flow following pelvic nerve stimulation and a significantly reduced vaginal lubrication in comparison to controls.[84] In these females, normal physiologic responses associated with sexual arousal can be restored by estrogen treatment. Vaginal smooth muscle contractility seems also to be regulated by estrogens.[88] It has been suggested that estrogens may modulate blood flow by regulating the local levels of NO and VIP.[89,90]

In contrast, the physiologic changes that accompany orgasmic responses have been shown to be present even in the absence of steroid hormones.[47] Furthermore, ovariectomy does not affect the UG reflex.[53]

Role of steroid hormones in sexual behavior In women both estrogens and androgens are critical for sexual desire, arousal, and orgasm. The fluctuations of circulating hormones across the ovarian cycle are often associated with libido changes.[91] The strong motivation for sexual activity at the time of ovulation may be due to the peak of steroid hormones. Furthermore, administration of androgens seems to enhance sexual interest.[92]

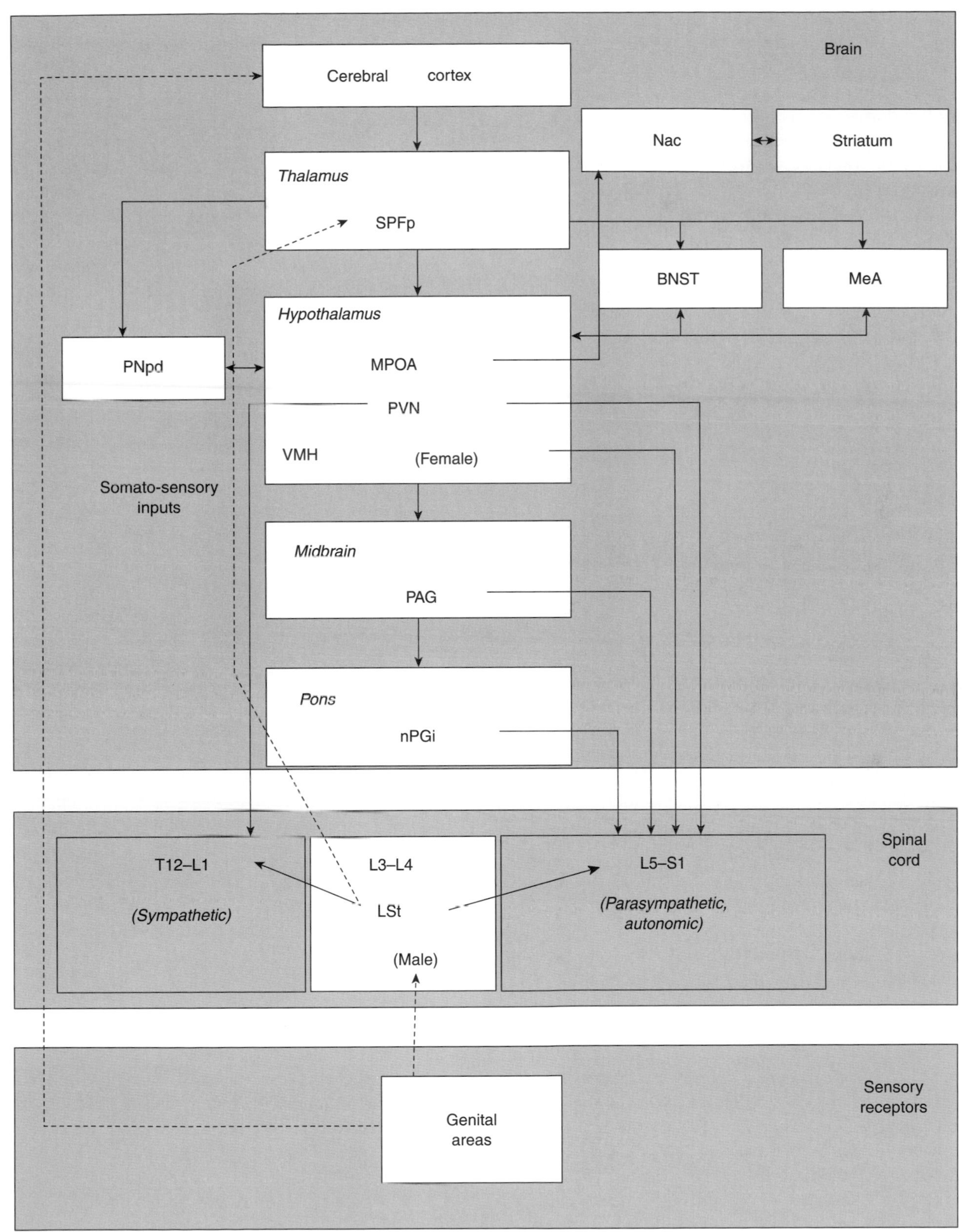

Figure 8.3
Diagram of brain structures and putative central pathways involved in sexual responses. Hatched lines indicate sensory afferents. Abbreviations: BNST, bed nucleus of stria terminalis; LSt, lumbar spinothalamic; MeA, medial amygdaloid nucleus; MPOA, medial preoptic area; Nac, nucleus accumbens; PAG, periaqueductal gray; nPGi, paragigantocellular nucleus; PNpd, posterodorsal preoptic nucleus; PVN, paraventricular hypothalamic nucleus; SPFp, parvicellular part of the subparafascicular thalamus; VMH, ventromedial hypothalamus.

In animals also, both appetitive and consummatory sexual behaviors are tightly regulated by sex steroids. Estradiol and progesterone regulate different aspects of female sexual behavior and must be present in a precise temporal sequence that varies across species.[80] Ovariectomized females do not display any trait of sexual activity and treatment with estradiol alone restores only receptive behaviors whereas both sex steroids are necessary to induce proceptivity. The VMH plays a critical role in the hormonal regulation of lordosis. Neurons in the VMH, and particularly the ventrolateral region, concentrate both estradiol and progesterone receptors.[79]

Neurotransmitters and neuropeptides regulating female sexual response

The presence of a variety of neurotransmitters has been demonstrated in the vagina and the clitoris, but their physiologic role at the peripheral level remains largely unknown. However, numerous animal studies have evidenced central mechanisms of action of different neurotransmitters and neuropeptides in the control of female sexual responses.

Acetylcholine and noradrenaline The respective role of the sympathetic (classic neurotransmitter noradrenaline, NA) and parasympathetic (classic neurotransmitter acetylcholine, Ach) systems in the control of female sexual response remain unclear. At the peripheral level, NA exerts an inhibitory effect on female sexual genital responses.[45] Despite the rich cholinergic vaginal innervation, Ach appears to play a minor role in the control of vaginal blood flow, sexual arousal, and orgasm. In women, atropine delivered intravenously does not affect the vaginal blood increase elicited by masturbation, nor subjective sexual arousal.[93] In female rats, intravenous injection of atropine only slightly decreased vaginal blood engorgement and vaginal smooth muscle contractions induced by pelvic nerve stimulation.[44]

Nonadrenergic noncholinergic neurotransmitters Several nonadrenergic noncholinergic (NANC) neurotransmitters/mediators have been identified in the female animal genital tract including vasoactive intestinal polypeptide (VIP), nitric oxide (NO), neuropeptide Y (NPY), calcitonin gene-related peptide (CGRP), and substance P (SP). At the peripheral level, VIP and NO are generally considered as the most important facilitatory neurotransmitters of the genital arousal response, whereas NPY seems to produce inhibitory effects. In women, intravenous injection of VIP increases vaginal blood flow and elicits vaginal lubrication.[94,95] *In-vivo* experimental models have shown that NO can play a role in the control of vaginal blood flow, vaginal smooth muscle contraction, and clitoral erection.[96–98] Clinically, sildenafil enhances vaginal vasocongestion during erotic stimulus in healthy premenopausal women, but improves sexual arousal and orgasm in a minority of women suffering from sexual disorders.[99–101]

Dopamine The effects of dopaminergic drugs in humans parallel those reported in animals. In rats, several studies monitored dopamine (DA) release during different phases of sexual behavior. DA increases in the MPOA, Nac, and dorsal striatum during copulation, but is also associated with anticipatory aspects of sexual activity.[102–104] Pharmacologic studies showed that the effects of dopaminergic agonists or antagonists on female lordosis are variable and can have both facilitatory and inhibitory effects, according to the hormonal status of the females.[105] Overall, the D1-like receptors, especially D5, play a critical role in the control of lordosis.[106,107] However, which DA receptor subtypes control female appetitive behaviors remain unclear. A recent study conducted in humans showed an association between the D4 receptor gene and scores in scales measuring human sexual behavior including desire, arousal, and function.[108]

Serotonin Selective serotonin (5-HT) reuptake inhibitors (SSRIs) are noted for their inhibitory effects on female sexual behavior. Decreased libido, arousal difficulties, and delayed orgasm or anorgasmia are often reported by patients treated with antidepressant and antipsychotic drugs which directly or indirectly act on 5-HT receptors.[47,109] However, inhibitory side-effects vary from one antidepressant to another. Fewer adverse sexual effects may be observed when the antidepressant drug interacts with dopaminergic or noradrenergic systems, known to induce facilitatory effects on sexual behavior.[110–112]

In rats, the descending serotoninergic pathway originating in the nPGi inhibits the UG reflex.[113,114] However, in the female rat, sexual behavior can be both facilitated and inhibited by 5-HT, depending on which subtypes of 5-HT receptors are activated.[115,116] 5-HT1A receptors mediate inhibitory effects on female lordosis, whereas activation of 5-HT2A/2C receptors facilitates not only female receptivity but also appetitive behaviors.[117–119]

Gamma-aminobutyric acid (GABA) and glutamate The presence of gabaergic and glutamatergic interneurons in the spinal cord leads to the hypothesis that these neurons, through their respective inhibitory and excitatory properties, can be involved in the intraspinal integration of information from the periphery. Furthermore, GABA and glutamate receptors in the VMH have been reported to mediate, respectively, facilitatory and inhibitory effects on female lordosis.[120–122]

Melanocortin The melanocortin system is involved in the control of both appetitive and consummatory components of female sexual behavior. Administration of α-melanocyte stimulating hormone (α-MSH) in the lateral ventricle, MPOA, VMN, median eminence, or zona incerta enhances female lordosis.[123–128] Melanotan-II and bremelanotide (PT-141), two peptides analog of α-MSH, selectively increase proceptive behaviors, such as solicitation and hops and darts, without affecting lordosis.[129,130] The facilitatory effect of these peptides on female sexual desire is located within the MPOA, whereas their injection in the VMN has no effect.[131]

A recent clinical study reported a positive effect of bremelanotide, a nonselective agonist of MC receptors, on sexual desire in premenopausal women with sexual arousal disorder.[132]

Oxytocin and vasopressin Data from humans and animal studies suggested that oxytocin (OT) might be involved in the control of sexual desire, arousal, and orgasm. In female rats, OT and arginine vasopressin (AVP) have opposite effects on female sexual behavior. Administration of an OT agonist in the MPOA enhances proceptivity, whereas injection of an OT antagonist decreases proceptive behaviors and increases male-directed agonistic behavior.[133–136] Conversely, intracerebroventricular injection of AVP decreases not only lordosis but also hops and darts,[137,138] whereas injection of an antagonist of 1a subtype vasopressin receptors (V1a) administered the MPOA stimulates sexual receptivity[139] and tends to increase hops and darts.[137] Both OT and V1a antagonist effects are localized in the MPOA, suggesting that endogenous OT and AVP can act synergistically between the MPOA, PVN, and the VMH, to contribute to the regulation of female sexual behavior. OT may also be involved in the control of orgasm, and could act synergistically with sex hormones to facilitate muscle contractions.

Opioids In women, long-term opioid use has been associated with anorgasmia, absence of menstrual periods, elimination of sexual dreams, and infertility in some cases.[140] The effects of acute opioid administration on sexual behavior are very different from long-term opioid use. For example, opioid users describe the acute administration of heroin as producing an instantaneous, orgasm-like 'rush' of euphoria.[141] Endogenous opioids appear to be released during genital stimulation and orgasm, and may play an important role in the euphoric feeling of orgasm by binding to opioid receptors in the amygdala, the MPOA, the PVN, the NST, and/or the cingulate cortex, and by mediating the activation of other brain structures that receive projections from these areas.

Opioid receptors are involved to a varying degree in the control of female sexual behavior. In female rats, selective μ-opioid receptor agonists administered in the lateral ventricle, MPOA, or VMN inhibit the lordosis reflex, whereas δ-opioid receptor agonists, when injected in the lateral ventricle but not in the MPOA, have a facilitatory effect on both proceptive and receptive behaviors.[142–144]

Male sexual function

The different aspects of male sexual function include sexual desire, erection, ejaculation, and orgasm. The knowledge of the central nervous system control of male sexual function appears to lag far behind the understanding of local physiologic processes. The variety of transmitters that affect sexual behavior indicate that several neuronal systems are involved in the control of the different aspects of sexual function.

Little is known about the physiology of male sexual desire and this issue will not deserve a detailed paragraph in the present review. Sexual desire, also termed libido in humans, is defined as the biologic need for sexual activity. It encompasses detection of a suitable mate, approach to it, and establishment of initial contact. Behaviors associated with sexual desire are highly variable and dependent on the context. Amongst the different factors that have been shown to be involved in the regulation of male sexual desire, dopaminergic and serotonergic systems, and gonadal hormones seem to play a key role. In both laboratory animal and human males, experimental and clinical data indicate that activation of central dopaminergic neurotransmission stimulates sexual behavior.[145,146] However, results in favor of the participation of DA are ambiguous and further investigations are necessary to clarify the role of this neurotransmitter. Conversely, increased central serotonergic neurotransmission can be associated with decreased libido in humans[147] and decreased sexual motivation in animals.[148] The importance of androgens, and more particularly testosterone, in enhancing libido is well known and has been reviewed elsewhere.[149]

Penile erection

Neuroanatomy of the penis

The penis is composed of three cylindrical spongy bodies, the paired corpora cavernosa and the corpus spongiosum, which surround the urethra (Figure 8.4). The corpora cavernosa lie side by side on the dorsal aspect of the penis, while the corpus spongiosum stands ventrally. At the level of the perineum, the corpora cavernosa split bilaterally to form the penile crura; each crus is attached to the pelvis via the ischiopubic ramus. The distal part of the corpus spongiosum expands and covers the distal part of the corpora cavernosa to form the penile glans. The penile skin is continuous with that of the abdominal wall and covers the

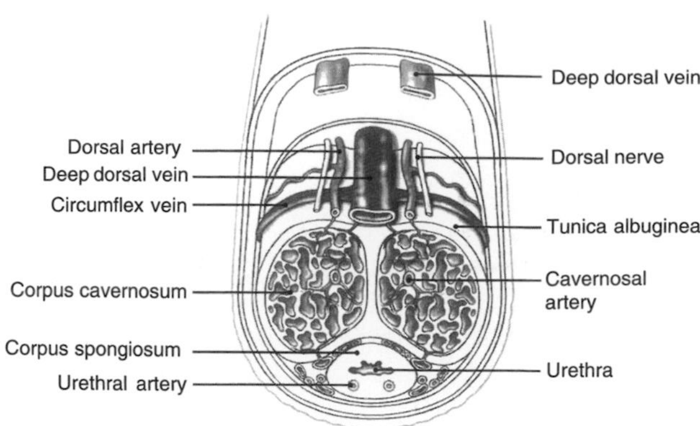

Figure 8.4
Transversal section of the penis.

glans of the penis as the prepuce to reattach at the coronal sulcus. The corpora cavernosa and corpus spongiosum share common miscroscopic features. These formations consist of sinuses (trabeculae) lined by endothelium and separated by connective tissue septa. Surrounding the corpora cavernosa is the tunica albuginea. This multilayered structure of inner circular and outer longitudinal layers of connective tissue affords great flexibility, rigidity, and tissue strength to the penis. The inner coat contains the cavernous tissue and supports it by radiating throughout the cavernosum bodies. The outer coat extends from the penile glans to the proximal crura and provides strength to the tunica albuginea. The tunica albuginea is composed of fibrillar collagen in organized arrays interlaced with elastin fibers.

The vascular components of the penis are of particular importance in erectile function (Figure 8.4). The blood supply to the penis is primarily provided by the internal pudendal artery, a branch of the internal iliac artery. Alternatively, the main blood supply to the erectile tissue can be provided by accessory internal pudendal arteries. After passing through the Alcock's canal, the internal pudendal artery becomes the common penile artery which, at the level of the perineum, gives off the bulbourethral, cavernosum, and dorsal penile arteries. The bulbourethral artery supplies the urethra and the glans. The cavernosal arteries, which run in the corpora cavernosa, give rise to the helicine resistance arteries furnishing the trabecular erectile tissue with blood. The dorsal penile artery proceeds down the penis on its dorsal aspect to supply superficial components of the penis, and possibly the erectile bodies via circumflex arteries. The venous drainage system of the penis occurs at three levels. Superficially, on the dorsal aspect of the penis, the superficial dorsal vein drains the skin into the saphenous vein via the external pudendal veins. The intermediate system consists of the deep dorsal and circumflex veins. The deep dorsal vein receives blood from emissary veins, which arise from subtunical venules draining trabeculae and passing through the tunica albuginea, and circumflex veins. In the infrapubic region, the deep dorsal vein drains into the pelvic preprostatic venous plexus or the internal pudendal veins. The deep drainage system includes the crural and cavernosal veins that drain the deeper cavernous tissue and empty into the internal iliac veins via the internal pudendal veins.

The innervation of the penis is provided by sympathetic, parasympathetic, and somatic (motor and sensory) systems. Sympathetic preganglionic fibers arise from preganglionic neurons located from the 11th thoracic to the 2nd lumbar spinal cord segments (T11–L2) in humans. The sympathetic preganglionic fibers travel throughout the thoracic paravertebral sympathetic chain and then via the lumbar splanchnic nerves to the prevertebral ganglia in the inferior mesenteric and superior hypogastric plexi. From there, fibers reach the pelvic plexus via the hypogastric nerves. In addition, sympathetic preganglionic axons synapse with ganglion cells in the sacral and caudal lumbar ganglia of the paravertebral sympathetic chain and then postganglionic fibers reach the pelvic plexus via the pelvic nerves. The parasympathetic preganglionic fibers originate in neurons located in the second, third, and fourth sacral spinal cord segments (S2–S4) in humans. The parasympathetic preganglionic fibers traveling via the pelvic nerve join sympathetic nerves to form the pelvic plexus. One branch of the pelvic plexus that innervates the penis is the cavernous nerve. Autonomic fibers passing in the cavernous nerve provide innervation to cavernosal smooth muscle cells as well as to the arterial supply of the penis. Sacral motoneurons (S2–S4) also send projections, via the pudendal nerves, to the ischiocavernosus muscles. Their rhythmic contractions reinforce penile erection by compression of the engorged corpora cavernosa. The somatic sensory pathway consists of the dorsal nerve of the penis, a sensory branch of the pudendal nerve. The dorsal nerve of the penis carries impulses to the upper sacral and, in rats, lower lumbar segments of the spinal cord from sensory receptors harbored in the penile skin, prepuce, and glans. Encapsulated receptors (Krause–Finger corpuscles) have been found in the glans, but the majority of afferent terminals are represented by free nerve endings.[150]

Local control of erection

Penile erection takes place when dilation of the penile arteries, mechanical occlusion of veins draining erectile tissue because of the rigidity of the tunica albuginea, and relaxation of the smooth cells of the erectile tissue occur. Penile artery dilation results in increased arterial blood flow to the penis, constriction of emissary veins which drain the corpora cavernosa results in decreased outflow from the penis, and erectile tissue relaxation results in

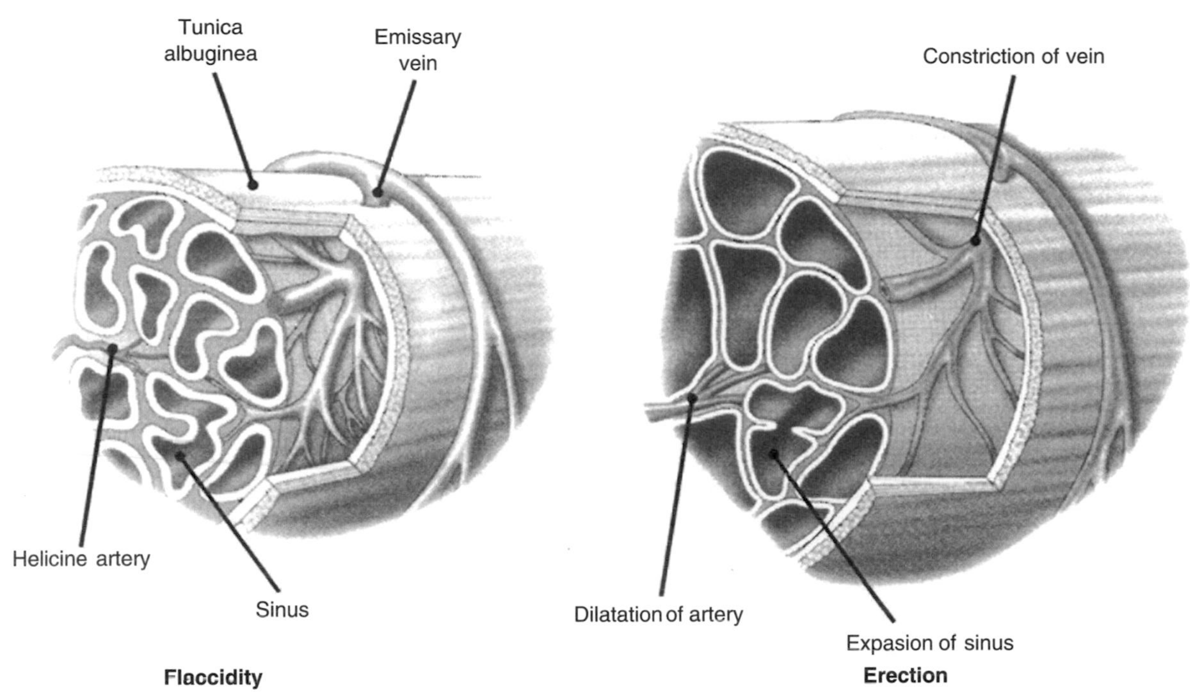

Figure 8.5
Vascular events occurring during erection. Vasodilatation of helicine arteries increase blood inflow in corpus cavernosum sinuses which, by expanding, press emissary veins against the rigid tunica albuginea resulting in decreased blood outflow. The final outcome is blood engorgement of the corpora cavernosa and resulting increase in volume and rigidity of the penis.

engorgement of the penis with blood (Figure 8.5). Both arterial and erectile tissue relaxations rely upon a change in the tone of the arterial wall smooth muscle fibers and of that of the erectile tissue (trabeculae of the corpora cavernosa). It is the amount of intracellular, cytoplasmic calcium that controls the tone of smooth muscle fibers. Increasing this amount, through the release of calcium from intracellular stores (sarcoplasmic reticulum) and/or facilitating its entry from the extracellular milieu, leads to contraction. In the flaccid state, smooth muscle fibers of the penis and penile arteries are contracted. Decreasing the amount of intracellular calcium, through pumping it back into the sarcoplasmic reticulum or expelling it out of the cell, leads to relaxation. During erection, the smooth muscle fibers of the penis and penile arteries are relaxed. Depending on the smooth muscle fibers involved, intracellular calcium movements are either spontaneous or controlled by information from the extracellular milieu. With regard to the penis, this information is carried by a variety of chemical messengers that are released by endothelial cells and autonomic nerve terminals. Both endothelial cells and nerve terminals are present in the penis and penile arteries. Chemical messengers either interact with specific receptors present at the surface of the smooth muscle fiber membrane, or cross the membrane to reach intracellular targets. Interaction of the messengers with their receptors activates the first step of cascades of intracellular mechanisms. Erection is mainly due to the increased synthesis of two intracellular second messengers, the cyclic nucleotides guanosine monophosphate (cGMP) and adenosine monophosphate (cAMP). cGMP and cAMP are degraded by phosphodiesterases. The pro-erectile chemicals facilitate the synthesis or the accumulation, or prevent the degradation of cGMP and/or cAMP. Increasing the amounts of intracellular cGMP and cAMP leads to relaxation. Because smooth muscle fibers of the penis are connected with gap junctions, it is not required that chemical messengers reach all of the cells to elicit an effect. Indeed, gap junctions allow for a rapid spread of electro-tonic current and intercellular diffusion of second messengers and ions.[151]

The neurotransmitters released by the postganglionic nerve terminals of the sympathetic and parasympathetic pathways in the penis are of particular importance in the local control of erection. NA and NPY are released in the erectile tissue by the terminals of sympathetic fibers. NA is the major contractile agent of the cavernosal as well as penile artery smooth muscle cells, and NPY enhances its effects. NA plays a role in flaccidity and detumescence.[152] The terminals of parasympathetic fibers release Ach, VIP, and NO. Ach contracts cavernosal smooth muscle *in vitro*, and erection is rather resistant to the cholinergic antagonist atropine. Therefore Ach cannot be the candidate to exert a direct relaxant effect on cavernosal smooth muscle. In fact, it activates the synthesis of NO by NO synthase in endothelial cells through muscarinic receptors located on endothelial cells. The relaxant effects of VIP[153] and NO[154,155] released by nerve terminals in the penis have been demonstrated. NO increases the production of cGMP in smooth muscle fibers, and it is recognized as the most important factor in the local relaxation of erectile tissue smooth muscle. The importance of this mechanism in humans is supported by the successful development of phosphodiesterase type-5 inhibitors, which prevent catabolism of cGMP, in the treatment of erectile dysfunction, regardless of whether the cause is due to psychogenic, organic, or mixed factors.[156] In addition to the release of transmitters by the endings of autonomic postganglionic motor fibers, there exists a release of neuropeptides by the peripheral endings of autonomic sensory fibers. Although some of these peptides (e.g. substance P (SP) and calcitonin gene-related peptide (CGRP)) display vasorelaxant effects *in vitro*, their physiologic role in the control of erection remains to be demonstrated. Endothelin, one of the most powerful endogenous vasoconstricting peptides, is synthesized in the endothelial cells of the erectile tissue and has been suggested to contribute to the maintenance of corpora cavernosa smooth muscle tone.[152] The role of prostanoids, which can be produced locally in human corpus cavernosum, is unclear. Some of them (e.g. prostaglandin F_2 and thromboxane A_2) may exert a contractile effect on erectile tissue, whereas others (prostaglandins E_1 and E_2) cause relaxation. Local administration (intracavernosal or transurethral) of prostaglandin E_1 has been found effective for the treatment of erectile dysfunction in humans, although the route of administration can cause mild penile pain.[157]

In contrast with other visceral tissues (e.g. gut, uterus) which possess smooth muscle cells that contract spontaneously and rhythmically (pacemaker cells), and intrinsic innervation (autonomic ganglion cells present in the wall or at the outer surface of the organ), the erectile tissue is devoid of such an autonomy. Therefore its activity is dependent on the autonomic innervation that originates in the spinal cord.

Spinal control of erection

The spinal cord contains the three sets of motoneurons (thoracolumbar sympathetic, sacral parasympathetic, and sacral somatic) that are anatomically linked with the penis and functionally involved in the erectile response elicited by any kind of sexual stimulation, i.e. peripheral and/or central. The majority of the sympathetic preganglionic cell bodies whose axons run in the paravertebral sympathetic chain are located in the intermediolateral cell column of T11–L2 spinal segments. Other sympathetic preganglionic neurons, which send axons into the hypogastric nerve, originate in the DGC.[158] The cell bodies of the preganglionic parasympathetic neurons are located in the intermediolateral cell column of the S2–S4 segments of the spinal cord in an area referred to as the SPN. In humans, the sacral motoneurons are located in the ventral cord of the S2–S4 spinal segments in the Onuf's nucleus. In rats, two distinct nuclei (dorsomedial and dorsolateral) constitute the Onuf's nucleus; the somatic motoneurons innervating the ischiocavernosus muscles are found in the dorsolateral nucleus.[12] The different spinal centers involved in the control of erection are reciprocally connected, allowing synchronization of the peripheral events leading to erection. The intraspinal network extending over the thoracolumbar and sacral spinal segments has been revealed by neuroanatomic tract tracing techniques using the transsynaptic retrograde transport of PRV injected in the penis of rats.[12]

The spinal cord represents a key structure integrating excitatory and inhibitory information from the periphery and from supraspinal nuclei. Erection likely occurs when the convergence of peripheral and supraspinal information onto the spinal cord elicits a lowering of the activity of the thoracolumbar sympathetic 'anti-erectile' pathway and an increase in the activity of both the sacral parasympathetic and somatic pro-erectile pathways. There may also be a pro-erectile role for a component of the sympathetic innervation which is responsible for vasoconstriction of nonpenile areas to divert blood to the penis.[159]

The primary role of afferent signals from the genitalia in the induction of erection (i.e. reflexive erection) is well documented. In anesthetized rats, electrical stimulation of the dorsal nerve of the penis elicits evoked potentials on the cavernous nerve,[160] intracavernosal pressure rises, and contraction of the perineal striated muscles.[160,161] In humans too, genital stimulation elicits penile erection, an increased blood flow to the penis, and contraction of the perineal striated muscles.[162,163] These data indicate that stimulation of penile sensory pathways is able to recruit the different autonomic and somatic nuclei of the spinal cord that control erection. Several lines of evidence indicate that the spinal cord contains the necessary circuitry for producing penile erection. In animals with a complete section of the spinal cord at the thoracic level, genital stimulation can elicit reflexive erection as well as secretion of seminal fluid from the accessory sex glands, contraction of the perineal striated muscles, and movements of the hindlimbs, that are mediated by spinal segments lower than the lesioned ones.[164,165] Reflexive erections are also observed in patients with a lesion of the spinal segments higher than the sacral ones.[166,167]

Not only has the spinal cord to manage with the circuits of erection, it is also responsible for the coordination of erection with other sexual responses such as ejaculation, and the inhibition of the activity of other pelvic functions such as micturition and defecation. The hyperreflexia, dyssynergia, altered erection, and/or ejaculation observed in patients with a lesion of the spinal cord reflect the important role of supraspinal structures in this coordination.

Supraspinal control of erection

In humans and animals, penile erection occurs in several contexts, some of which are not related to the sexual context (*in utero* or during paradoxical sleep). It is possible that several different areas of the brain contribute to the occurrence of erection in the different contexts.[168] Each context may reflect the contribution of a unique combination of several brain nuclei, and one brain nucleus may participate in the occurrence of erection in several contexts. The participation of each nucleus in erection depends on the amount of excitatory and inhibitory information that it receives from the periphery and from other central nuclei, and to a lesser extent on its hormonal environment.

The first candidates for a role in the supraspinal control of erection are those nuclei containing neurons that project directly onto the sacral spinal cord. With regard to penile erection in rats, these neurons have been localized using detection of PRV injected in the corpus cavernosum and retrogradely transported to the CNS.[169] Neurons containing PRV were found in a variety of areas of the medulla oblongata (raphe nuclei, nPGi, locus coeruleus, and Barrington's nucleus), pons (A5 noradrenergic cell group and PAG), and hypothalamus (PVN). Expression of the transcription factor encoded by the immediate early gene *c-fos* has also been used to identify populations of neurons activated following sexual behavior in male rats.[65,170,171] In addition, investigation of the *c-fos* pattern of expression showed neuronal activation in forebrain regions (MPOA, BNST, and MeA) integrating higher sensory inputs with hormonal ones and sending information to brainstem sites. Attempts to demonstrate the role of these brain structures in the control of erection have used, among other, selective central stimulation or lesions in animal models. MPOA is a key structure in the central control of male sexual behavior. Electrostimulation of this brain area induces erection,[172] and lesions at this site limit copulation[173,174] although they do not impair either erection in the presence of an inaccessible female on heat (noncontact erection) or erection induced by mechanical stimulation of the penis (reflexive erection).[175] MPOA is not a source of direct projections to the spinal cord, instead it integrates sensory and hormonal signals and projects to brain nuclei in direct connection with the spinal centers involved in the control of erection. One of these brain nuclei of particular importance is the PVN, more particularly the parvocellular part. It contains neurons that send direct oxytocinergic and vasopressinergic projections to the lumbosacral cord.[83] Lesions in the PVN increase the latency of noncontact erections and diminish their number, but are devoid of effect upon erection during copulation, and facilitate reflexive erections.[176,177] Conversely, stimulation of PVN induces erection in anesthetized rats.[178] The nPGi provides descending serotoninergic fibers to the lumbosacral cord. Its bilateral lesion releases inhibition exerted upon reflexive erections and erections during copulation.[176,179,180] Finally, lesions of the MeA, that have no effect upon erections during copulation, facilitate reflexive erections but depress noncontact erections.[181]

Among the supraspinal neurologic conditions that can cause erectile dysfunction through alteration of central pathways are brain tumor, stroke, encephalitis, Parkinson's disease, dementias, the olivopontocerebellar degeneration (Shy–Drager syndrome), and epilepsy of the temporal lobe.[182] In contrast, erections occur after lesions of the pyriform cortex and amygdaloid complex (the Kluver–Bucy syndrome).

Central neurochemical regulation of erection

The precise role of endogenous substances in the regulation of one sexual aspect is difficult to define because of the wide range of sexual parameters affected, species differences, conflicting results depending on the site in the CNS where the substance acts, and the existence of receptor subtypes. An extensive review of the studies dealing with the central neurochemical regulation of sexual behavior is beyond the scope of the present review and has been proposed elsewhere.[145,183,184] Here, we attempted to present briefly the data directly related to erectile and ejaculatory (later in the text) functions. Erection is an integrated and coordinated process involving different brain structures and a variety of centrally acting neurotransmitters and hormones.

Depending on the site of action and the 5-HT receptor subtype activated, 5-HT enhances or inhibits erection. Activation of spinal 5-HT1A receptors inhibits reflexive erection,[185] whereas spinal 5-HT2C receptors are thought to enhance erectile activity.[186] The involvement of DA in penile erection was first suggested by the observation of enhanced erection in Parkinson's patients treated with DA agonists.[187] Later, it was demonstrated in rats that stimulation of D1 receptors in PVN[188] and D1 or D2/3 receptors in the spinal cord[189] can produce erection. In addition, it was found that the microinjection of a D4 agonist into the PVN elicited penile erection in rats.[190] The D1/D2-like agonist apomorphine has been registered in Europe for the treatment of erectile dysfunction, although its use is limited because of frequently occurring side-effects as well as limited efficacy.[191] Conversely, to the periphery where it has been found that adrenaline and NA can exert anti-erectile activity by acting on α1 adrenoreceptors,[192] brain α2 adrenergic receptor stimulation was found to inhibit erections.[193] OT can trigger erection in rats when injected into the PVN and hippocampus[194] as well as by acting on OT receptors located in the lumbosacral spinal cord.[195] Morphine, a preferential agonist for μ opioid receptor subtypes, when injected into the PVN prevents noncontact penile erections that occur in male rats in the presence of an inaccessible sexually receptive female.[196] In addition to the primary pro-erectile role of NO locally produced in erectile tissue, this substance has been involved as an important pro-erectile messenger in the CNS, and especially within the PVN.[197,198] NO seems to play a pivotal role since DA and OT induce NO release in PVN, and NO synthase inhibitors delivered within the PVN reverse the proerectile effect of DA and OT.[199] Adrenocorticotropic hormone (ACTH) and α-MSH are peptides derived from a common precursor, pro-opiomelanocortin. Both ACTH and α-MSH can trigger penile erection when injected in cerebral ventricles of rats [200,201] by acting on melanocortin receptors.[201] In erectile dysfunction patients, the use of the melanocortin 3/4 receptor subtype agonist PT-141 (bremelanotide) has proven effective in restoring erectile function.[202] Prolactin has been shown to decrease the frequency of reflexive erections in rats by acting at a supraspinal site.[203,204] In addition, prolactin may have a direct effect on the penis through a contractile effect on the cavernous smooth muscle.[205]

Ejaculation

Spermatozoa transported from the epididymis and secretions of the bulbourethral glands, prostate, and seminal vesicles compose the sperm. In human males, the fluid is released from the glands in a specific sequence during ejaculation. The first portion of the ejaculate consists of a small amount of fluid from the bulbourethral glands. This is followed by a low-viscosity opalescent fluid from the prostate containing a few spermatozoa. Then the principal portion of the ejaculate is secreted which contains the highest concentration of spermatozoa, along with secretions from the epididymis, and vas deferens, as well as prostatic and seminal vesicle fluids. The last fraction of the ejaculate consists of seminal vesicle secretions.

Anatomic organization of sexual organs involved in ejaculation

The importance of the autonomic nervous system in regulating the ejaculatory response is well documented. All of these organs receive a dense autonomic innervation composed of sympathetic and parasympathetic axons mainly coming from the pelvic plexus. The ganglia of the pelvic plexus, that are dispersed in amongst the pelvic organs in most animal species, contain fibers from both pelvic and hypogastric nerves and from the caudal paravertebral sympathetic chain.[206] In addition to adrenergic and cholinergic mechanisms of regulation of ejaculation, NANC factors including ATP,[207–209] NPY,[210,211] VIP,[212,213] and NO[154,213] have been shown to have a direct participation in the peripheral control of ejaculation.

Two main categories of anatomic structures involved in ejaculation can be distinguished depending on the phase they participate in.

Organs of emission

Epididymis: The epididymis, the organ in which spermatozoa undergo final maturation and storage prior to ejaculation, receives fibers originating in the superior and inferior spermatic plexi. Both adrenergic and cholinergic axons have been found to contact smooth muscle cells of the epididymis.[214] The presence of VIP,[215] NPY (colocalized with NA in the sympathetic fibers),[216] CGRP,[217] SP,[218] and NO synthase[215] immunoreactive fibers has also been reported in the cauda epididymis.

Ductus deferens: Neuroanatomic studies have identified a limited number of categories of nerve endings in the ductus (or vas) deferens. It is widely accepted that the ductus deferens is dually innervated in the sense that both adrenergic and cholinergic nerves, arising from the pelvic plexus, exist. VIP and NPY are the most common peptides found in the nerve endings in the ductus deferens in various animal species. Other peptides including enkephalin, SP, somatostatin, and CGRP have also been detected in the ductus deferens, although to a lesser extent.[218,219] As an additional autonomic pathway of importance, the nitrergic network can be cited since its fibers have been shown to terminate in the ductus deferens.[220]

Seminal vesicles: They are a pair of tubular glands whose stroma is composed of smooth muscle layers. Seminal vesicles, responsible for the secretion of 50–80% of the entire ejaculatory volume, receive a dual sympathetic and parasympathetic innervation from the hypogastric and pelvic nerves via the pelvic plexus. The adrenergic innervation is distributed in both inner and outer smooth muscle layers. In contrast, the cholinergic nerve endings are located at the level of the epithelium. The distribution of fibers immunoreactive for VIP and NPY has been shown to share some similarities with that of parasympathetic and sympathetic nerve endings, suggesting the colocalization of VIP and NPY with Ach and NA, respectively.[221,222] Finally, NO synthase has also been found to be expressed in nerve fibers branching within the seminal vesicle.[223]

Prostate gland: Roughly considered, the prostate gland is a tangle of fibromuscular tissue and alveolar epithelium that secretes 15–30% of the sperm. Anatomic, neurochemical, and functional studies have pointed out the interspecies heterogeneity of the structure of the prostate. Despite this, some common features concerning the autonomic control of contractile and secretory functions of the prostate can be underlined. As in other genital organs, i.e. the ductus deferens and seminal vesicle, the prostate is dually innervated by the sympathetic and parasympathetic systems. The distribution of the adrenergic fibers driven by the pelvic nerve is restrained to blood vessels supplying the prostate.[224] The neural inputs reaching the prostatic parenchyma appear to originate from adrenergic and cholinergic postganglionic neurons that are under the influence of sympathetic tone conducted by the hypogastric nerve.[219] A study using a transneuronal tracing technique has demonstrated the presence of adrenergic and cholinergic axon terminals in the outer muscle layer and inner secretory layer of the prostatic acini, respectively.[225] Autoradiographic investigations carried out in rats and humans indicate that muscarinic receptors and α1 adrenoreceptors are predominant in the nonpathologic prostate, although α2 and β adrenoreceptors have also been detected.[226,227] VIP is the most common peptidergic neurotransmitter in the prostate.[222] The second most abundant neuropeptide in the prostate is NPY.[228] In addition, axon terminals immunoreactive for enkephalin have been detected in the smooth muscle layers of the prostate.[222, 229] Lastly, immunohistochemical data have reported the existence of a dense nitrinergic innervation of glandular epithelium, fibromuscular stroma, and blood vessels.[230]

Bulbourethral glands: Typically, the bulbourethral or Cowper's glands, that empty their secretions into the urethra, are closely invested by a layer of striated muscle, namely the bulboglandularis. The autonomic innervation of the bulbourethral glands has received little attention. Whereas no adrenergic elements have been detected in the bulbourethral glands of rats, cholinergic fibers were found around acini.[219] Retrograde tracing experiments suggest that these cholinergic fibers may constitute a sacral parasympathetic innervation of the bulbourethral glands.[231]

Anatomic structures participating in expulsion

Bladder neck and urethra: The bladder neck and the urethra, both containing smooth muscle layers, play an important role in the ejaculatory reflex. These structures receive a dual innervation from the sympathetic and parasympathetic systems, the axons of which travel along the hypogastric and pelvic nerves that join in the pelvic plexus. The urethral distribution of adrenergic and cholinergic axon terminals exhibits a similar pattern, both branching within the smooth muscle layers.[232] Both α1 and α2 adrenoreceptors have been identified in the urethra of various species, with the first being mainly located in smooth muscle cells and the second in the submucosa.[233] Another cholinergic extrinsic efferent is composed of somatic fibers that proceed via the pudendal nerve to the striated muscle layer, namely the rhabdosphincter, at the distal part of the urethra.[232] The existence of ganglion cells located in the smooth muscle layers of the urethra has been reported.[234] These cells have been shown to be immunoreactive for NPY and NO synthase.[235,236] Histochemical studies performed in several species have revealed the presence of VIP-containing nerve endings that synapse with smooth muscle cells of the bladder neck and the urethra.[234] Depending on the animal tested, enkephalin and somatostatin have also been detected in ganglion cells and/or axon terminals.[237,238] Finally, urethral afferents, reaching the lumbosacral spinal cord via pelvic, hypogastric and pudendal nerves, have been found to contain SP and CGRP.[237,239]

Perineal striated muscles: The pelvic floor striated muscles, including the ischiocavernosus, bulbospongiosus, and levator ani, have a preponderant role in the expulsion of semen from the urethra. They appear to be solely innervated by motoneurons whose fibers travel in the motor branch of the pudendal nerve.

Peripheral neural pathways

Afferents The dorsal nerve of the penis, a sensory branch of the pudendal nerve, carries impulses to the lower lumbar and upper sacral segments (sacral in human) of the spinal cord from sensory receptors harbored in the penile skin, prepuce, and glans (Figure 8.6).[240,241] Encapsulated receptors (Krause–Finger corpuscles) have been found in the glans, but the majority of afferent terminals are represented by free nerve endings.[150] Stimulation of the Krause–Finger corpuscles, which can be potentiated by sensory information coming from various peripheral areas such as the penile shaft, perineum, and testes, facilitates the ejaculatory reflex. In various mammalian species, a relatively sparse sensory innervation of the ductus deferens, prostate, and urethra has been evidenced, which reaches the lumbosacral spinal cord via the pudendal nerve.[242,243] A second afferent pathway comprises fibers traveling along the hypogastric nerve and, after passing through the paravertebral lumbosacral sympathetic chain, it enters the spinal cord via the thoracolumbar dorsal roots.[244] Sensory afferents terminate in the medial dorsal horn and the DGC of the spinal cord.[20, 21]

Efferents The soma of the preganglionic sympathetic neurons are located in the intermediolateral cell column and in the central autonomic region of the thoracolumbar segments of the spinal cord.[245,246] The sympathetic fibers,

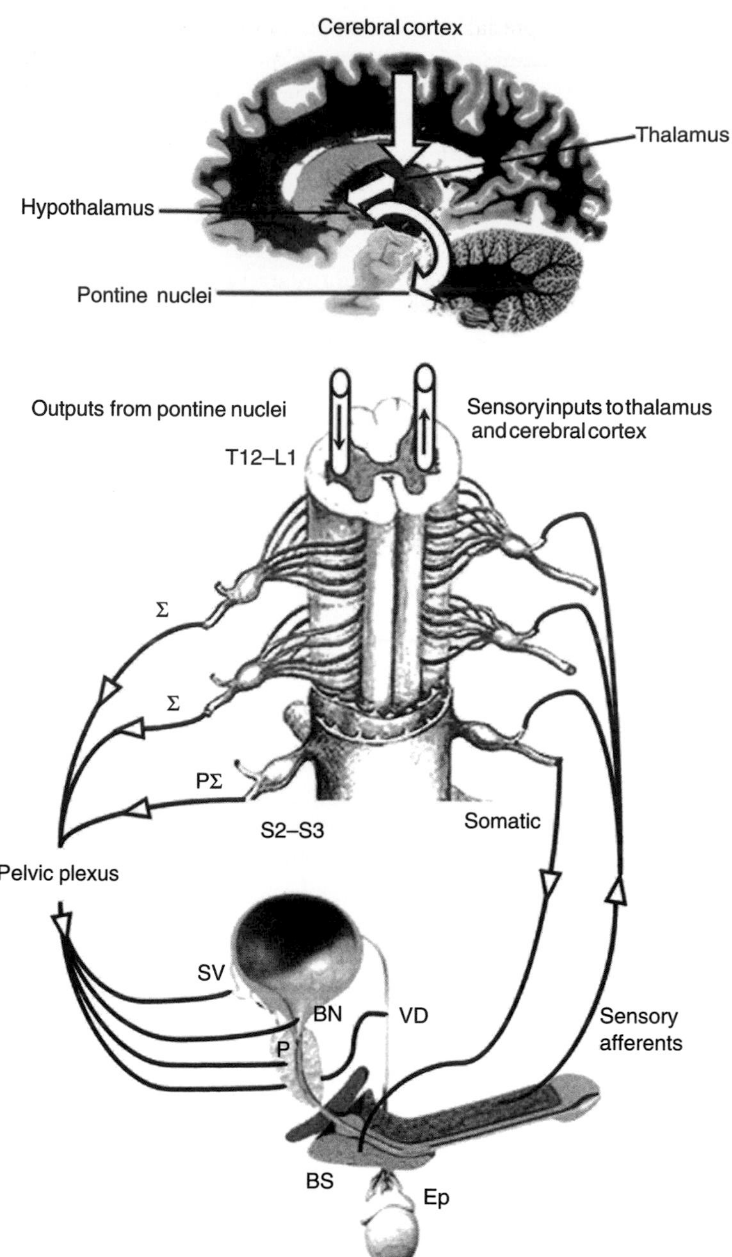

Figure 8.6
Neural pathways controlling ejaculation. Sympathetic (Σ), parasympathetic (PΣ), and somatic nerves originating in lumbosacral spinal nuclei command the peripheral anatomical structures responsible for ejaculation. Sensory afferents originating in genital areas are integrated at the spinal and brain levels. Activity of spinal preganglionic and motor neurons is under the influence of peripheral and supraspinal inputs. Abbreviations: BN, bladder neck; BS, bulbospongiosus muscle; Ep, epididymis; P, prostate; SV, seminal vesicle; VD, vas deferens.

emerging from the spinal column via the ventral roots, relay in the paravertebral sympathetic chain. In the majority of mammalian species, the fibers then proceed to the inferior mesenteric ganglia, whether directly via the splanchnic nerves or after relaying in the celiac superior mesenteric ganglia via the intermesenteric nerves.[247] Emanating from the inferior mesenteric ganglia are the hypogastric nerves that, after joining the parasympathetic pelvic nerve, form the pelvic plexus from which arise fibers innervating the anatomic structures involved in ejaculation (Figure 8.6). The cell bodies of the preganglionic parasympathetic neurons are located in the intermediolateral cell column of the lumbosacral segments of the spinal cord, i.e. SPN.[19] The SPN neurons send projections, traveling in the pelvic nerve, to the postganglionic cells located in the pelvic plexus.

Efferents of somatic motoneurons, whose cell bodies are found at the lumbosacral spinal level (sacral level in man) in the Onuf's nucleus, exit the ventral horn of the medulla and proceed via the motor branch of the pudendal nerve to the pelvic floor striated muscles, including the bulbospongiosus and ischiocavernosus muscles (Figure 8.6).[248]

Functional considerations

Sensory nervous system Sensory inputs have been shown sufficient to provoke an expulsion reflex or even a complete ejaculatory response (forceful expulsion of semen).

In an experimental paradigm developed in anesthetized rat with complete transection of the spinal cord at the T8 level, urethral distention by accumulating liquid infused into the urethra elicited rhythmic contractions of bulbospongiosus muscles.[53] In the anesthetized and intact rat, pudendal nerve (the motor branch innervating the bulbospongiosus and ischiocavernosus muscles) firing was elicited in response to electrical stimulation of the dorsal nerve of the penis and pelvic nerve, which convey sensory information from the penis and urethrogenital tract, respectively.[249]

In humans also, contractions of the bulbospongiosus muscles identified with electromyographic electrodes were evidenced following electrostimulation of the penile dorsal nerve, mechanical distention of the posterior urethra, and magnetostimulation of the sacral root.[250–252] These procedures are currently used routinely to evaluate the integrity of neural pathways controling ejaculation, and have also served as a basis for developing a method that produces ejaculation in patients with neurogenic anejaculation. This method, namely penile vibratory stimulation, consists of placing a vibration-delivering device on the glans of the penis, either the dorsum or frenulum, and applying 2.5 mm amplitude vibrations for 5–15 minutes in 1–3 series.[253,254] Penile vibratory stimulation facilitated a complete ejaculatory response in a significant number of men with spinal cord injury.[253]

Autonomic nervous system Both sympathetic and parasympathetic tones act in a synergistic fashion to initiate seminal emission by activating smooth muscle contraction and epithelial secretion, respectively, throughout the seminal tract.

From experimental studies carried out in different animal species, it has been demonstrated that activation of the sympathetic nervous system, whether stimulation of sympathetic nerves (hypogastric or splanchnic) or by the use of sympathomimetic agents, elicited a strong contractile response in the ducti deferens,[255,256] seminal vesicles,[257,258] prostate,[259,260] and urethra.[259] Contractions induced by sympathetic stimulation were blocked, only partially in ducti deferens and seminal vesicles,[261] by α_1-adrenergic antagonists.[256] The functional role of parasympathetic cholinergic fibers conveyed by the pelvic nerves is still not fully defined, likely because of the differences in gross and microscopic anatomy of the prostate among species that do not allow straightforward extrapolation between animals. Contractions of the ductus deferens in rodents,[256,262] and of the prostate[260] and urethra[263] in dogs, were elicited by electrical stimulation of the pelvic nerves, although no appreciable emission of fluid was observed.[260] Pharmacologic evidence relating to a cholinergic mechanism for both contraction and secretion of prostate and seminal vesicles exists.[258,264,265] Essentially, these glands were activated by cholinomimetic compounds acting on muscarinic receptors.[266] Altogether, the results of pelvic nerve stimulation and pharmacologic cholinergic activation led to the suggestion that sympathetic innervation to the prostate includes both adrenergic and cholinergic components, in contrast to the conventional view of the organization of pelvic autonomic pathways.

In addition, peptidergic and purinergic systems are involved in the peripheral control of ejaculation although the precise mechanism remains to be clarified. Several lines of evidence have shown that VIP and NPY participate in contraction and secretion of prostate and seminal vesicles,[261,264,267] by apparently modulating NA release.[221] The same regulatory role has been reported for NPY in ductus deferens contractions.[221] Finally, evidence has been marshaled that ATP, the main endogenous purine, acts as a cotransmitter with NA to produce prostatic, seminal vesicle, and ductus deferens contractions.[268–270]

In humans, disruption of sympathetic pathways supplying the bladder neck, ductus deferens, and prostate is widely accepted to be the cause of postoperative anejaculation or retrograde ejaculation.[271,272] The essential role of sympathetic innervation is best illustrated by surgical strategies that, by sparing sympathetic efferents, successfully preserve normal ejaculatory function in patients who have undergone retroperitoneal lymphadenectomy for testicular cancer or resection for rectal cancer.[273,274] In addition, in paraplegic men whose ability to ejaculate is commonly severely impaired, semen was obtained upon electrical stimulation of the hypogastric plexus.[275] As far as we know, there is no clear clinical evidence for a functional role of parasympathetic innervation in the ejaculatory process.

Somatic nervous system The expulsion phase of ejaculation is under the sole control of the somatic nervous system. Forceful propulsion of semen out of the urethra via the glans meatus is caused by rhythmic contractions of perineal muscles and smooth muscles of the urethra. Owing to the fact that relatively noninvasive measurement of perineal muscle activity is possible in man, the expulsion phase has been shown to be characterized by synchronous activation of the ischiocavernosus, bulbospongiosus, and levator ani muscles, and the anal and urethral external sphincters.[276,277] The contractions are regular, with an interburst interval starting at approximately 0.6 s and increasing by about 100 ms for each subsequent interburst interval. The typical number of bursts of contractions varies from 10 to 15, depending on the subject, although each subject's pattern of contractions is reproducible.[276] In the case of lesion of the pudendal nerves, as may occur after trauma[278] or neuropathy related to diabetes,[279] retrograde and/or dribbling ejaculation is observed.

Central physiology of ejaculation

As described previously, the sympathetic and parasympathetic nervous systems, closely interconnected in the pelvic plexus which represents an integrative peripheral crossroad site, act in synergy to command physiologic events occurring during ejaculation. Both sympathetic and parasympathetic tones are under the influence of sensory genital and/or cerebral erotic stimuli integrated and processed at the spinal cord level.

Spinal network The thoracolumbar sympathetic and lumbosacral parasympathetic spinal ejaculatory nuclei, specifically the SPN, play a pivotal role in ejaculation as they integrate peripheral and cerebral signals and send coordinated outputs to pelvic organs that allow a normal ejaculation to occur. Integrity of these spinal nuclei is necessary and sufficient for the expression of ejaculation as demonstrated by the induction of the ejaculatory reflex after peripheral stimulation in animals with spinal cord transection and in humans after spinal cord lesion.[53,253] The conversion of sensory information into secretory and motor outputs involves spinal interneurons which have been identified in rats.[62] The presence of these cells, named lumbar spinothalamic (LSt) cells, has been demonstrated in laminae X and VII of spinal lumbar segments 3 and 4. Immunohistochemical investigations have shown that LSt cells contain galanin, cholecystokinin, and enkephalin. In rat, spinal cord fibers of the sensory branch of the pudendal nerve terminate close to LSt cells,[20] although a direct connection has not yet been proved. LSt neurons project to the sympathetic and parasympathetic preganglionic neurons innervating the pelvis as well as the motoneurons of the dorsomedial nucleus innervating the bulbospongiosus muscles (Figure 8.3).[280] In addition, LSt cells send direct projections to the parvocellular subparafascicular nucleus of the thalamus.[281] All these data support a crucial role for LSt in coordinating the spinal control of ejaculation, although descending pathways that terminate on LSt have not yet been identified.

A critical issue that is under increasing debate is the identification of the ejaculation trigger. A theory, proposed by Marberger,[282] stipulates the triggering event as the build-up of a prostatic pressure chamber created by seminal secretions entering the posterior (bulbous) urethra with concomitant closure of the bladder neck. The resulting distention of the bulbous urethra, communicated through sensory pathways to spinal ejaculatory centers, causes a series of rhythmic reflex contractions of the pelvic striated muscles responsible for forceful propeling of urethral content. Experimental and clinical data exist that support this description, although several lines of evidence, recently discussed in greater detail,[283] actually contradict it. Indeed, it has been demonstrated that:

(1) Anesthesia of the urethra by infusion with lidocaine did not prevent bulbospongiosus muscle contractions elicited by urethral distention in the rat.[284]
(2) Pharmacologic inhibition of seminal emission by α-adrenergic receptor antagonists did not prevent the occurrence of pelvic striated muscle contractions resulting in dry ejaculation, nor did it alter the related orgasmic sensation.[277]
(3) Endorectal ultrasonography studies undertaken in healthy volunteers did not evidence the formation of a prostatic pressure chamber before semen expulsion.[285, 286]
(4) Distention of the urethra with a small volume of saline is unable to provoke bulbospongiosus muscle contractions,[252] suggesting that, in the case of dry ejaculation, another mechanism triggers the expulsion phase.

Altogether these findings indicate that the expulsion phase of ejaculation can occur in the absence of urethral stimulation, and that the prostatic pressure chamber concept does not provide a definitive answer to the identity of the ejaculation trigger. Our purpose is not to reject the fact that stimulation of the urethra can initiate contractions of pelvic striated muscles – there is clear evidence in favor of this phenomenon – but rather we postulate this expulsion reflex as a secondary mechanism which may take place, in the absence of any sexual cue, to prevent possibly deleterious accumulation of seminal fluid within the urethrogenital tract. The search for another possible site triggering ejaculation has given rise to interesting studies. The relatively recent identification in the rat of a potential spinal ejaculatory generator in an ideal position for integrating peripheral and supraspinal inputs and commanding autonomic and motor outputs responsible for ejaculation seems promising,[62] although the evidence for such an integrative spinal site in man remains to be provided.

Brain network As a centrally integrated and highly coordinated process, ejaculation involves cerebral sensory areas and motor centers which are tightly interconnected (Figure 8.3). Recent findings, based on studies investigating *c-fos* pattern of expression, have revealed, in distinct species, brain structures specifically activated when the animals ejaculate.[171,287] This was further confirmed by investigators using a 5-HT1A subtype receptor agonist (8-OH-DPAT) as a pro-ejaculatory pharmacologic agent.[288] As a whole, these data strongly suggest the existence of a cerebral network specifically related to ejaculation that is activated whatever the preceding sexual activity, i.e. mounts and intromissions in rats. The brain structures belonging to this cerebral network comprise discrete regions lying within the posteromedial bed nucleus of stria terminalis (BNSTpm), the posterodorsal medial amygdaloid nucleus (MeApd), the posterodorsal preoptic nucleus (PNpd), and the parvicellular part of the subparafascicular thalamus (SPFp). Reciprocal connections between those substructures and the MPOA of the hypothalamus, a brain area known as essential in controling sexual behavior,[289] has been reported in anatomic and functional studies.[287,290]

The pivotal role of MPOA in ejaculation has been documented in several experiments where both phases of ejaculation were abolished after MPOA lesion[291] or elicited after chemical[292,293] or electrical[114,294] stimulations of this brain area. Neuroanatomic studies failed to reveal the existence of direct connections between the MPOA and the spinal ejaculatory centers. However, it was shown that MPOA projects to other brain regions involved in ejaculation such as the PVN,[295] the PAG,[296] and the nPGi.[297] The PVN has long been known as a key site for neuroendocrine and autonomic integration.[298] Parvocellular neurons of the PVN directly innervate autonomic preganglionic neurons in the lumbosacral spinal cord[83,299] and pudendal motoneurons located in the L5–L6 spinal segment in rats.[20] The PVN also sends direct projections to nPGi in the brainstem.[300] Bilateral chemical lesion of the PVN with N-methyl-D (NMDA) was associated with a one-third reduction in the weight of the seminal material ejaculated.[301] Retrograde and antegrade tracing studies have shown that the SPFp sends projections to the BNST, MeA, and MPOA[240,302] and receives inputs from LSt cells.[201] These data suggest a pivotal role for the SPFp, although functional investigations are lacking. The other forebrain structures which have been proposed, based on *c-fos* pattern of expression, to take part in regulation of the ejaculatory process in rat are the MeA, BNST, and PNpd.[171,290] Their precise roles remain unclear but they may be involved in the relay of genital sensory signals to the MPOA.

In the brainstem, the nPGi and PAG have received increasing attention. A strong inhibitory role for the nPGi, which projects to pelvic efferents and interneurons in the lumbosacral spinal cord,[113,303] on ejaculation in rats has been suggested from investigations using an experimental model, namely urethrogenital reflex, mimicking the expulsion reflex.[113,304] The same experimental paradigm was used to demonstrate the important role of the PAG[305] in controling expulsion reflex. In addition, as established in neuroanatomic studies, the PAG constitutes a relay between the MPOA and nPGi.[290,306] Clearly, midbrain structures exert a regulating function on ejaculation, but further investigations are required for revealing the details of the mechanism.

A study using positron emission tomography (PET) to investigate increases in regional cerebral blood flow in man during ejaculation showed that the strongest activation occurs in the mesodiencephalic transition zone, including the VTA, medial and ventral thalamus, and SPFp.[307] Regarding the role of the neocortex in ejaculation, several studies have shown the intense activation of the parietal cortex during ejaculation by PET and functional magnetic resonance imaging (fMRI) techniques.[307,308] This brain area is considered as a site which receives sensory information from pudendal sensory nerve fibers.[309]

Neurochemical regulation Similarly to the erectile function, various neurotransmitters and neurohormones participate in the control of ejaculation. However, less is known about the neurochemical regulation of ejaculation despite the recent progress in this field. Several lines of experimental evidence support the involvement of DA in ejaculation. It was shown that D2/D3 receptor stimulation promotes seminal emission and ejaculation in conscious rats and triggers ejaculation in anesthetized rats, likely by acting in the MPOA.[310–312] A great body of evidence supports the inhibitory role of cerebral 5-HT on ejaculation in the rat model. The stimulation of somatodendritic 5-HT1A autoreceptors regulating 5-HT neuron firing has been demonstrated to shorten the ejaculatory latency time.[313,314] However, as suggested by Rehman and coworkers, 5-HT1A receptors at different locations (brain, raphe nuclei, spinal cord, and autonomic ganglia) may modulate ejaculation in opposing ways.[315] Stimulation of postsynaptic 5-HT2C receptors was responsible for inhibition of male rat ejaculatory behavior.[316] Selective serotonin reuptake inhibitors, which are prescribed for the treatment of depression, often delay ejaculation in humans and are currently used 'off-label' for treatment of premature ejaculation.[148] Activation of the cholinergic muscarinic receptors in MPOA has been shown to reduce the ejaculatory threshold in copulating male rats.[317] Delivered either systemically or centrally, OT decreases ejaculation latency and postejaculatory interval (i.e. the refractory period) in copulating male rats.[318]

Orgasm The orgasm is undoubtedly one of the most pleasurable sensations known to mankind and has been associated with reward in rats,[319] although very little is known about the underlying physiologic mechanisms that control orgasmic responses. Orgasm is a cerebral process that usually follows a series of peripheral physical events comprising contraction of accessory sexual organs and the urethral bulb, and build-up and release of pressure in the distal urethra.

It is noteworthy that orgasm is reported by patients who do no longer have ejaculation, for example after radical prostatectomy.[320,321] Furthermore, orgasmic sensations generated cerebrally without input from genitals or without ejaculation have been reported in humans.[322] These clinical data indicate that the emission of sperm as well as its expulsion are not mandatory for orgasm to occur and support a distinction between ejaculation and orgasm from a physiologic perspective.

Table 8.1 *Comparison of genital peripheral physiological changes, neuroanatomical pathways and neurotransmitters involved in the control of sexual responses in male and female*

	Female	Male
Neuroanatomy		
Genital organs	Vagina, clitoris, pelvic striated muscles	Penis, organs of emission (epididymis, ductus deferens, seminal vesicles, prostate, and bulbourethral glands), organs of expulsion (bladder neck, urethra, pelvic striated muscles)
Peripheral innervation		
Afferent	Pelvic, hypogastric, pudendal (dorsal nerve of the clitoris), vagal	Pelvic, hypogastric, pudendal (dorsal nerve of the penis)
Efferent	Pelvic (parasympathetic), hypogastric (sympathetic), pudendal (somatic)	Pelvic (parasympathetic), hypogastric (sympathetic), pudendal (somatic)
Peripheral physiologic changes		
Genital arousal	Increased blood flow to vagina and clitoris Clitoral erection Vaginal lubrication	Erection: Increased blood flow to the penis Decreased outflow from the penis Erectile tissue relaxation
Orgasm	Rhythmic contractions of vagina, uterus and anal sphincter	Ejaculation: Emission: contraction of ductus deferens, seminal vesicles, prostate, urethra Expulsion: rhythmic contractions of perineal muscles and smooth muscles of the urethra
Spinal and supraspinal centers involved in sexual responses *(identified by PRV injection in genital organs or Fos activation after copulation)*		
Spinal	L5–S1: medial and lateral dorsal horn, SPN, DGC, Onuf's nucleus	T12–L1: IML, DGC L3–L4: LSt cells L5–S1: dorsal horn, SPN, Onuf's nucleus
Brain	MPOA, VMN, PVN, LH, arcuate nucleus, MeA, Nac, VTA, BNST, lateral septum, PAG, nPGi, Barrington's nucleus, raphe magnus, raphe pallidus, A5 region	MPOA, VMN, PVN, LH, MeA, Nac, VTA, BNST, lateral septum, PAG, nPGi, SPFp, Barrington's nucleus, raphe magnus, raphe pallidus, A5 region
Neurochemical control of sexual responses		
Sexual desire (central drive)	**DA** **5-HT** **OT** **Melanocortin** **Estradiol, progesterone**	**DA** **5-HT** **Androgens**
Genital arousal	**DA** (central) **5-HT** (central) **OT** (central) **Opioids** (central) **NO** (central and peripheral) **Melanocortin** (central) **Estrogens**	**DA** (central) **5-HT** (central) **NA** (central and peripheral) **OT** (central) **Opioids** (central) **NO** (central and peripheral) **Melanocortin** (central) **Androgens** (central and peripheral)

Table 8.1 *(Continued)*

	Female	Male
Ejaculation/orgasm	**DA** (central) **5-HT** (central) **OT** (central) **Opioids** (central)	**DA** (central) **5-HT** (central) **NA** (peripheral) **OT** (central) **Androgens** (central and peripheral)

CONCLUSION

Although individuals may differ in their experience of pleasure and subjective feeling during sexual intercourse, a common human sexual response, consisting of four interactive phases (excitement, arousal, orgasm, resolution), has been defined and refers to both men and women. Indeed, in both sexes, sexual behavior occurs as a sequence of behavioral events including appetitive and consummatory components which are, according to the incentive sequence model,[323] the same for both sexes. Interestingly, the physiologic correlates and the neural mechanisms controling these sexual responses also share numerous commonalities between males and females (reviewed by McKenna[324]) (Table 8.1):

1. Male and female genitalia are anatomically very different, but the clitoris can be viewed as somewhat analogous to the penis, with comparable neuroanatomic organization and similar vasocongestion during sexual arousal
2. Peripheral innervation of the genital organs is comparable between male and female, with sensory afferents conveyed by the pudendal, pelvic, and hypogastric nerves, and efferent outflows arising from multiple segments of the spinal cord.
3. The multisynaptic circuitry controling sexual responses is remarkably similar between males and females, with the likely exception of the vagus nerve for females. Neuronal activation induced by copulation or PRV injection in the vagina and clitoris or in the penis results in a very comparable labeling in the lumbosacral segments of the spinal cord and neurons within the hypothalamus, midbrain, and brainstem.
4. In both genders, genital sexual arousal and orgasm are controlled by a coordinated regulation between the sympathetic, parasympathetic, and somatic systems, and are mainly the product of spinal reflexes. Studies in spinal cord injured patients or animals with spinal cord transection have shown that, with adequate genital stimulation, the spinal cord can generate sexual responses.
5. In both sexes, spinal centers involved in the control of sexual responses are under excitatory and inhibitory inputs from the brain.
6. The MPOA and PVN play a critical role in the control of sexual responses and regulate both male and female sexual desire and genital arousal. These structures have numerous interconnections with the PAG and MeA, which probably participate in sexual function. In females, the VMN is clearly involved in the control of consummatory sexual behaviors, while its role in males remains to be investigated.
7. In males, descending serotonergic pathways from the brainstem, especially from the nPGi, exert an inhibitory control on spinal sexual reflexes. It seems probable that the same mechanism also occurs in females, although it has not been clearly evidenced.
8. Among the diversity of neurotransmitters and neuropeptides which can affect sexual responses, DA, 5-HT, and OT are believed to play a major role in both male and female sexual function.

This chapter reviewed numerous similarities in the mechanisms controling normal sexual function in males and females, and in particular a similar neural and neurochemical organization. However, there is a significant difference between the genders arising from the mechanisms of the central drive. In men, physiologic performance, such as obtaining and maintaining a good erection, is sufficient for them to consider themselves a good sexual partner and to enjoy sexual intercourse. In contrast, in women, the feeling of subjective arousal results more from central mechanisms, cognitive processes, and psychologic changes than from peripheral vasocongestive feedback.[37] Further investigations and major advances are needed in order to help patients from both genders complaining about sexual dysfunction.

References

1. Beach FA. Sexual attractivity, proceptivity, and receptivity in female mammals. Horm Behav 1976; 7: 105–38.
2. Masters W, Johnson V. Human Sexual Response. Boston: Little Brown, 1966.
3. Kaplan H. Disorders of Sexual Desire. New York: Simon and Schuster, 1979.

4. Levin RJ. Normal sexual function. In: Gelder MG, Lopez-Ibor JJ, Andreasen N, eds. New Oxford Textbook of Psychiatry. Oxford: Oxford University Press, 2000: 875–82.
5. O'Connell HE, Hutson JM, Anderson CR, Plenter RJ. Anatomical relationship between urethra and clitoris. J Urol 1998; 159(6): 1892–97.
6. O'Connell HE, Sanjeevan KV, Hutson JM. Anatomy of the clitoris. J Urol 2005; 174(4 Pt 1): 1189–95.
7. Yucel S, De SA Jr, Baskin LS. Neuroanatomy of the human female lower urogenital tract. J Urol 2004; 172(1): 191–5.
8. Barber MD, Bremer RE, Thor KB, Dolber PC, Kuehl TJ, Coates KW. Innervation of the female levator ani muscles. Am J Obstet Gynecol 2002; 187(1): 64–71.
9. Shafik A. The role of the levator ani muscle in evacuation, sexual performance and pelvic floor disorders. Int Urogynecol J Pelvic Floor Dysfunct 2000; 11(6): 361–76.
10. Shafik A, Doss S, Asaad S. Etiology of the resting myoelectric activity of the levator ani muscle: physioanatomic study with a new theory. World J Surg 2003; 27(3): 309–14.
11. Breedlove SM, Arnold AP. Hormone accumulation in a sexually dimorphic motor nucleus of the rat spinal cord. Science 1980; 210(4469): 564–6.
12. Schroder HD. Organization of the motoneurons innervating the pelvic muscles of the male rat. J Comp Neurol 1980; 192(3): 567–87.
13. Bell C. Autonomic nervous control of reproduction: circulatory and other factors. Pharmacol Rev 1972; 24(4): 657–736.
14. Janig W, McLachlan EM. Organization of lumbar spinal outflow to distal colon and pelvic organs. Physiol Rev 1987; 67(4): 1332–404.
15. Berkley KJ, Robbins A, Sato Y. Functional differences between afferent fibers in the hypogastric and pelvic nerves innervating female reproductive organs in the rat. J Neurophysiol 1993; 69(2): 533–44.
16. Peters LC, Kristal MB, Komisaruk BR. Sensory innervation of the external and internal genitalia of the female rat. Brain Res 1987; 408(1–2): 199–204.
17. Langworthy OR. Innervation of the pelvic organs of the rat. Invest Urol 1965; 2: 491–511.
18. Morgan C, Nadelhaft I, de Groat WC. The distribution of visceral primary afferents from the pelvic nerve to Lissauer's tract and the spinal gray matter and its relationship to the sacral parasympathetic nucleus. J Comp Neurol 1981; 201(3): 415–40.
19. Nadelhaft I, Booth AM. The location and morphology of preganglionic neurons and the distribution of visceral afferents from the rat pelvic nerve: a horseradish peroxidase study. J Comp Neurol 1984; 226(2): 238–45.
20. McKenna KE, Nadelhaft I. The organization of the pudendal nerve in the male and female rat. J Comp Neurol 1986; 248(4): 532–49.
21. Ueyama T, Arakawa H, Mizuno N. Central distribution of efferent and afferent components of the pudendal nerve in rat. Anat Embryol (Berl) 1987; 177(1): 37–49.
22. Berkley KJ, Robbins A, Sato Y. Afferent fibers supplying the uterus in the rat. J Neurophysiol 1988; 59(1): 142–63.
23. Komisaruk BR, Gerdes CA, Whipple B. 'Complete' spinal cord injury does not block perceptual responses to genital self-stimulation in women. Arch Neurol 1997; 54(12): 1513–20.
24. Cueva-Rolon R, Sansone G, Bianca R et al. Vagotomy blocks responses to vaginocervical stimulation after genitospinal neurectomy in rats. Physiol Behav 1996; 60(1): 19–24.
25. Nadelhaft I, Roppolo J, Morgan C, de Groat WC. Parasympathetic preganglionic neurons and visceral primary afferents in monkey sacral spinal cord revealed following application of horseradish peroxidase to pelvic nerve. J Comp Neurol 1983; 216(1): 36–52.
26. Schroder HD. Onuf's nucleus X: a morphological study of a human spinal nucleus. Anat Embryol (Berl) 1981; 162(4): 443–53.
27. Marson L. Central nervous system neurons identified after injection of pseudorabies virus into the rat clitoris. Neurosci Lett 1995; 190(1): 41–4.
28. Marson L, Murphy AZ. Identification of neural circuits involved in female genital responses in the rat: a dual virus and anterograde tracing study. Am J Physiol Regul Integr Comp Physiol 2006; 291(2): R419–28.
29. Papka RE, Williams S, Miller KE, Copelin T, Puri P. CNS location of uterine-related neurons revealed by trans-synaptic tracing with pseudorabies virus and their relation to estrogen receptor-immunoreactive neurons. Neuroscience 1998; 84(3): 935–52.
30. Birder LA, Roppolo JR, Iadarola MJ, de Groat WC. Electrical stimulation of visceral afferent pathways in the pelvic nerve increases c-fos in the rat lumbosacral spinal cord. Neurosci Lett 1991; 129(2): 193–6.
31. Chinapen S, Swann JM, Steinman JL, Komisaruk BR. Expression of c-fos protein in lumbosacral spinal cord in response to vaginocervical stimulation in rats. Neurosci Lett 1992; 145(1): 93–6.
32. Ghanima A, Bennis M, Rampin O. c-fos expression as endogenous marker of lumbosacral spinal neuron activity in response to vaginocervical-stimulation. Brain Res Brain Res Protoc 2002; 9(1): 1–8.
33. Lee JW, Erskine MS. Vaginocervical stimulation suppresses the expression of c-fos induced by mating in thoracic, lumbar and sacral segments of the female rat. Neuroscience 1996; 74(1): 237–49.
34. Cliffer KD, Burstein R, Giesler GJ Jr. Distributions of spinothalamic, spinohypothalamic, and spinotelencephalic fibers revealed by anterograde transport of PHA-L in rats. J Neurosci 1991; 11(3): 852–68.
35. Marson L. Identification of central nervous system neurons that innervate the bladder body, bladder base, or external urethral sphincter of female rats: a transneuronal tracing study using pseudorabies virus. J Comp Neurol 1997; 389(4): 584–602.
36. Goldstein I, Giraldi A, Kodigliu A et al. Physiology of female sexual function and pathophysiology of female sexual dysfunction. In: Lue TF, Basson R, Rosen R, Giuliano F, Khoury S, Montorsi F, editors. Sexual Medicine. Sexual dysfunctions in men and women. Paris: Health Edition; 2004: p. 683–748.
37. Laan E, Everaerd W, van d, V, Geer JH. Determinants of subjective experience of sexual arousal in women: feedback from genital arousal and erotic stimulus content. Psychophysiology 1995; 32(5): 444–51.
38. Fisher S, Osofsky H. Sexual responsiveness in women. Psychological correlates. Arch Gen Psychiatry 1967; 17(2): 214–26.
39. Sintchak G, Geer JH. A vaginal plethysmograph system. Psychophysiology 1975; 12(1): 113–15.
40. Levin RJ, Wagner G. Human vaginal fluid – ionic composition and modification by sexual arousal [proceedings]. J Physiol 1977; 266(1): 62–3P.
41. Goldstein I, Berman JR. Vasculogenic female sexual dysfunction: vaginal engorgement and clitoral erectile insufficiency syndromes. Int J Impot Res 1998; 10(Suppl 2): S84–90.
42. Meston CM, Gorzalka BB. The effects of sympathetic activation on physiological and subjective sexual arousal in women. Behav Res Ther 1995; 33(6): 651–64.
43. Levin RJ, Macdonagh RP. Increased vaginal blood flow induced by implant electrical stimulation of sacral anterior roots in the conscious woman: a case study. Arch Sex Behav 1993; 22(5): 471–5.
44. Giuliano F, Allard J, Compagnie S et al. Vaginal physiological changes in a model of sexual arousal in anesthetized rats. Am J Physiol Regul Integr Comp Physiol 2001; 281(1): R140–9.
45. Park K, Goldstein I, Andry C et al. Vasculogenic female sexual dysfunction: the hemodynamic basis for vaginal engorgement insufficiency and clitoral erectile insufficiency. Int J Impot Res 1997; 9(1): 27–37.
46. Vachon P, Simmerman N, Zahran AR, Carrier S. Increases in clitoral and vaginal blood flow following clitoral and pelvic plexus nerve stimulations in the female rat. Int J Impot Res 2000; 12(1): 53–7.

47. Meston CM, Levin RJ, Sipski ML, Hull EM, Heiman JR. Women's orgasm. Annu Rev Sex Res 2004; 15: 173–257.
48. Bohlen JG, Held JP, Sanderson MO, Ahlgren A. The female orgasm: pelvic contractions. Arch Sex Behav 1982; 11(5): 367–86.
49. Gillan P, Brindley GS. Vaginal and pelvic floor responses to sexual stimulation. Psychophysiology 1979; 16(5): 471–81.
50. Levin RJ. Sex and the human female reproductive tract – what really happens during and after coitus. Int J Impot Res 1998; 10(Suppl 1): S14–21.
51. Kratochvil S. [Vaginal contractions in female orgasm]. Cesk Psychiatr 1994; 90(1): 28–33.
52. Bohlen JG, Held JP, Sanderson MO, Patterson RP. Heart rate, rate–pressure product, and oxygen uptake during four sexual activities. Arch Intern Med 1984; 144(9): 1745–8.
53. McKenna KE, Chung SK, McVary KT. A model for the study of sexual function in anesthetized male and female rats. Am J Physiol 1991; 261(5 Pt 2): R1276–85.
54. Marson L, Cai R, Makhanova N. Identification of spinal neurons involved in the urethrogenital reflex in the female rat. J Comp Neurol 2003; 462(4): 355–70.
55. Kratochvil S. [Orgasmic expulsions in women]. Cesk Psychiatr 1994; 90(2): 71–7.
56. Hines TM. The G-spot: a modern gynecologic myth. Am J Obstet Gynecol 2001; 185(2): 359–62.
57. Carmichael MS, Warburton VL, Dixen J, Davidson JM. Relationships among cardiovascular, muscular, and oxytocin responses during human sexual activity. Arch Sex Behav 1994; 23(1): 59–79.
58. Munarriz R, Kim NN, Goldstein I, Traish AM. Biology of female sexual function. Urol Clin North Am 2002; 29(3): 685–93.
59. Sipski ML, Alexander CJ, Rosen RC. Physiologic parameters associated with sexual arousal in women with incomplete spinal cord injuries. Arch Phys Med Rehabil 1997; 78(3): 305–13.
60. Sipski ML, Alexander CJ, Rosen RC. Sexual response in women with spinal cord injuries: implications for our understanding of the able bodied. J Sex Marital Ther 1999; 25(1): 11–22.
61. Sipski ML, Alexander CJ, Gomez-Marin O, Grossbard M, Rosen R. Effects of vibratory stimulation on sexual response in women with spinal cord injury. J Rehabil Res Dev 2005; 42(5): 609–16.
62. Truitt WA, Coolen LM. Identification of a potential ejaculation generator in the spinal cord. Science 2002; 297(5586): 1566–9.
63. Whalen RE. Sexual motivation. Psychol Rev 1966; 73(2): 151–63.
64. Whipple B, Komisaruk BR. Brain (PET) responses to vaginal–cervical self-stimulation in women with complete spinal cord injury: preliminary findings. J Sex Marital Ther 2002; 28(1): 79–86.
65. Coolen LM, Peters HJ, Veening JG. Fos immunoreactivity in the rat brain following consummatory elements of sexual behavior: a sex comparison. Brain Res 1996; 738(1): 67–82.
66. Erskine MS, Hanrahan SB. Effects of paced mating on c-fos gene expression in the female rat brain. J Neuroendocrinol 1997; 9(12): 903–12.
67. Pfaus JG, Heeb MM. Implications of immediate–early gene induction in the brain following sexual stimulation of female and male rodents. Brain Res Bull 1997; 44(4): 397–407.
68. Pfaus JG, Marcangione C, Smith WJ, Manitt C, Abillamaa H. Differential induction of Fos in the female rat brain following different amounts of vaginocervical stimulation: modulation by steroid hormones. Brain Res 1996; 741(1–2): 314–30.
69. Tetel MJ, Getzinger MJ, Blaustein JD. Fos expression in the rat brain following vaginal-cervical stimulation by mating and manual probing. J Neuroendocrinol 1993; 5(4): 397–404.
70. Guarraci FA, Megroz AB, Clark AS. Effects of ibotenic acid lesions of the nucleus accumbens on paced mating behavior in the female rat. Behav Neurosci 2002; 116(4): 568–76.
71. Hoshina Y, Takeo T, Nakano K, Sato T, Sakuma Y. Axon-sparing lesion of the preoptic area enhances receptivity and diminishes proceptivity among components of female rat sexual behavior. Behav Brain Res 1994; 61(2): 197–204.
72. Jenkins WJ, Becker JB. Role of the striatum and nucleus accumbens in paced copulatory behavior in the female rat. Behav Brain Res 2001; 121(1–2): 119–28.
73. Whitney JF. Effect of medial preoptic lesions on sexual behavior of female rats is determined by test situation. Behav Neurosci 1986; 100(2): 230–5.
74. Yang LY, Clemens LG. Function of intromissions on intromission-return latency of female rats during paced sexual behavior. Physiol Behav 1997; 61(6): 889–94.
75. Lonstein JS, Stern JM. Site and behavioral specificity of periaqueductal gray lesions on postpartum sexual, maternal, and aggressive behaviors in rats. Brain Res 1998; 804(1): 21–35.
76. Mathews D, Edwards DA. Involvement of the ventromedial and anterior hypothalamic nuclei in the hormonal induction of receptivity in the female rat. Physiol Behav 1977; 19(2): 319–26.
77. Zemlan FP, Kow LM, Pfaff DW. Effect of interruption of bulbospinal pathways on lordosis, posture, and locomotion. Exp Neurol 1983; 81(1): 177–94.
78. Marson L, Foley KA. Identification of neural pathways involved in genital reflexes in the female: a combined anterograde and retrograde tracing study. Neuroscience 2004; 127(3): 723–36.
79. Pfaff DW. Estrogens and Brain Function. New York: Springer, 1980.
80. Rubin BS, Barfield RJ. Induction of estrous behavior in ovariectomized rats by sequential replacement of estrogen and progesterone to the ventromedial hypothalamus. Neuroendocrinology 1983; 37(3): 218–24.
81. Rubin BS, Barfield RJ. Progesterone in the ventromedial hypothalamus facilitates estrous behavior in ovariectomized, estrogen-primed rats. Endocrinology 1983; 113(2): 797–804.
82. Flanagan LM, Pfaus JG, Pfaff DW, McEwen BS. Induction of FOS immunoreactivity in oxytocin neurons after sexual activity in female rats. Neuroendocrinology 1993; 58(3): 352–0.
83. Luiten PG, Ter Horst GJ, Karst H, Steffens AB. The course of paraventricular hypothalamic efferents to autonomic structures in medulla and spinal cord. Brain Res 1985; 329(1–2): 374–8.
84. Min K, Munarriz R, Kim NN et al. Effects of ovariectomy and estrogen replacement on basal and pelvic nerve stimulated vaginal lubrication in an animal model. J Sex Marital Ther 2003; 29(Suppl 1): 77–84.
85. Park K, Ahn K, Lee S et al. Decreased circulating levels of estrogen alter vaginal and clitoral blood flow and structure in the rabbit. Int J Impot Res 2001; 13(2): 116–24.
86. Onol FF, Ercan F, Tarcan T. The effect of ovariectomy on rat vaginal tissue contractility and histomorphology. J Sex Med 2006; 3(2): 233–41.
87. Bachmann GA. Androgen cotherapy in menopause: evolving benefits and challenges. Am J Obstet Gynecol 1999; 180(3 Pt 2): S308–11.
88. Kim HW, Kim SC, Seo KK, Lee MY. Effects of estrogen on the relaxation response of rabbit clitoral cavernous smooth muscles. Urol Res 2002; 30(1): 26–30.
89. Al Hijji J, Batra S. Downregulation by estrogen of nitric oxide synthase activity in the female rabbit lower urinary tract. Urology 1999; 53(3): 637–41.
90. Kim SC, Seo KK, Myung SC, Lee MY. Relaxation of rabbit cavernous smooth muscle to 17beta-estradiol: a non-genomic, NO-independent mechanism. Asian J Androl 2004; 6(2): 127–31.
91. Slob AK, Ernste M, van der Werff ten Bosch JJ. Menstrual cycle phase and sexual arousability in women. Arch Sex Behav 1991; 20(6): 567–77.
92. Dorfman RI, Shipley RA. Androgens: Biochemistry, Physiology and Clinical Significance. New York: Wiley; 1956.
93. Wagner G, Levin RJ. Effect of atropine and methylatropine on human vaginal blood flow, sexual arousal and climax. Acta Pharmacol Toxicol (Copenh) 1980; 46(5): 321–5.

94. Ottesen B, Gerstenberg T, Ulrichsen H et al. Vasoactive intestinal polypeptide (VIP) increases vaginal blood flow and inhibits uterine smooth muscle activity in women. Eur J Clin Invest 1983; 13(4): 321–4.
95. Ottesen B, Pedersen B, Nielsen J et al. Vasoactive intestinal polypeptide (VIP) provokes vaginal lubrication in normal women. Peptides 1987; 8(5): 797–800.
96. Angulo J, Cuevas P, Cuevas B, Bischoff E, Saenz dT, I. Vardenafil enhances clitoral and vaginal blood flow responses to pelvic nerve stimulation in female dogs. Int J Impot Res 2003; 15(2): 137–41.
97. Min K, Kim NN, McAuley I et al. Sildenafil augments pelvic nerve-mediated female genital sexual arousal in the anesthetized rabbit. Int J Impot Res 2000; 12(Suppl 3): S32–9.
98. Park JK, Kim JU, Lee SO et al. Nitric oxide–cyclic GMP signaling pathway in the regulation of rabbit clitoral cavernosum tone. Exp Biol Med (Maywood) 2002; 227(11): 1022–30.
99. Berman JR, Berman LA, Lin H et al. Effect of sildenafil on subjective and physiologic parameters of the female sexual response in women with sexual arousal disorder. J Sex Marital Ther 2001; 27(5): 411–20.
100. Kaplan SA, Reis RB, Kohn IJ et al. Safety and efficacy of sildenafil in postmenopausal women with sexual dysfunction. Urology 1999; 53(3): 481–6.
101. Laan E, van Lunsen RH, Everaerd W et al. The enhancement of vaginal vasocongestion by sildenafil in healthy premenopausal women. J Womens Health Gend Based Med 2002; 11(4): 357–65.
102. Becker JB, Rudick CN, Jenkins WJ. The role of dopamine in the nucleus accumbens and striatum during sexual behavior in the female rat. J Neurosci 2001; 21(9): 3236–41.
103. Matuszewich L, Lorrain DS, Hull EM. Dopamine release in the medial preoptic area of female rats in response to hormonal manipulation and sexual activity. Behav Neurosci 2000; 114(4): 772–82.
104. Pfaus JG, Damsma G, Wenkstern D, Fibiger HC. Sexual activity increases dopamine transmission in the nucleus accumbens and striatum of female rats. Brain Res 1995; 693(1–2): 21–30.
105. Paredes RG, Agmo A. Has dopamine a physiological role in the control of sexual behavior? A critical review of the evidence. Progr Neurobiol 2004; 73(3): 179–226.
106. Apostolakis EM, Garai J, Fox C et al. Dopaminergic regulation of progesterone receptors: brain D5 dopamine receptors mediate induction of lordosis by D1-like agonists in rats. J Neurosci 1996; 16(16): 4823–34.
107. Mani SK, Allen JM, Clark JH, Blaustein JD, O'Malley BW. Convergent pathways for steroid hormone- and neurotransmitter-induced rat sexual behavior. Science 1994; 265(5176): 1246–9.
108. Ben Zion IZ, Tessler R, Cohen L et al. Polymorphisms in the dopamine D4 receptor gene (DRD4) contribute to individual differences in human sexual behavior: desire, arousal and sexual function. Mol Psychiatry 2006; 11(8): 782–6.
109. Ashton A, Hamer R, Rosen RC. Serotonin reuptake inhibitor-induced sexual dysfunction and its treatment: a large retrospective study of 596 psychiatric outpatients. J Sex Marital Ther 1997; 23: 165–75.
110. Alcantara AG. A possible dopaminergic mechanism in the serotonergic antidepressant-induced sexual dysfunctions. J Sex Marital Ther 1999; 25(2): 125–9.
111. Kennedy SH, Eisfeld BS, Dickens SE, Bacchiochi JR, Bagby RM. Antidepressant-induced sexual dysfunction during treatment with moclobemide, paroxetine, sertraline, and venlafaxine. J Clin Psychiatry 2000; 61(4): 276–81.
112. Montejo-Gonzalez AL, Llorca G, Izquierdo JA et al. SSRI-induced sexual dysfunction: fluoxetine, paroxetine, sertraline, and fluvoxamine in a prospective, multicenter, and descriptive clinical study of 344 patients. J Sex Marital Ther 1997; 23(3): 176–94.
113. Marson L, McKenna KE. A role for 5-hydroxytryptamine in descending inhibition of spinal sexual reflexes. Exp Brain Res 1992; 88(2): 313–20.
114. Marson L, McKenna KE. Stimulation of the hypothamus initiates the urethrogenital reflex in male rats. Brain Res 1994; 638(1–2): 103–8.
115. Gorzalka BB, Mendelson SD, Watson NV. Serotonin receptor subtypes and sexual behavior. Ann NY Acad Sci 1990; 600: 435–44.
116. Mendelson SD, Gorzalka BB. 5-HT1A receptors: differential involvement in female and male sexual behavior in the rat. Physiol Behav 1986; 37(2): 345–51.
117. Ahlenius S, Fernandez-Guasti A, Hjorth S, Larsson K. Suppression of lordosis behavior by the putative 5-HT receptor agonist 8-OH-DPAT in the rat. Eur J Pharmacol 1986; 124(3): 361–3.
118. Wolf A, Jackson A, Price T et al. Attenuation of the lordosis-inhibiting effects of 8-OH-DPAT by TFMPP and quipazine. Brain Res 1998; 804(2): 206–11.
119. Wolf A, Caldarola-Pastuszka M, Uphouse L. Facilitation of female rat lordosis behavior by hypothalamic infusion of 5-HT(2A/2C) receptor agonists. Brain Res 1998; 779(1–2): 84–95.
120. Georgescu M, Pfaus JG. Role of glutamate receptors in the ventromedial hypothalamus in the regulation of female rat sexual behaviors I. Behavioral effects of glutamate and its selective receptor agonists AMPA, NMDA and kainate. Pharmacol Biochem Behav 2006; 83(2): 322–32.
121. McCarthy MM, Malik KF, Feder HH. Increased GABAergic transmission in medial hypothalamus facilitates lordosis but has the opposite effect in preoptic area. Brain Res 1990; 507(1): 40–4.
122. McCarthy MM, Masters DB, Rimvall K, Schwartz-Giblin S, Pfaff DW. Intracerebral administration of antisense oligodeoxynucleotides to GAD65 and GAD67 mRNAs modulates reproductive behavior in the female rat. Brain Res 1994; 636(2): 209–20.
123. Cragnolini A, Scimonelli T, Celis ME, Schioth HB. The role of melanocortin receptors in sexual behavior in female rats. Neuropeptides 2000; 34(3–4): 211–15.
124. Gonzalez MI, Celis ME, Hole DR, Wilson CA. Interaction of oestradiol, alpha-melanotrophin and noradrenaline within the ventromedial nucleus in the control of female sexual behaviour. Neuroendocrinology 1993; 58(2): 218–26.
125. Gonzalez MI, Vaziri S, Wilson CA. Behavioral effects of alpha-MSH and MCH after central administration in the female rat. Peptides 1996; 17(1): 171–7.
126. Nocetto C, Cragnolini AB, Schioth HB, Scimonelli TN. Evidence that the effect of melanocortins on female sexual behavior in preoptic area is mediated by the MC3 receptor; participation of nitric oxide. Behav Brain Res 2004; 153(2): 537–41.
127. Scimonelli T, Medina F, Wilson C, Celis ME. Interaction of alpha-melanotropin (alpha-MSH) and noradrenaline in the median eminence in the control of female sexual behavior. Peptides 2000; 21(2): 219–23.
128. Thody AJ, Wilson CA, Everard D. alpha-Melanocyte stimulating hormone stimulates sexual behaviour in the female rat. Psychopharmacology (Berl) 1981; 74(2): 153–6.
129. Pfaus JG, Shadiack A, Van Soest T, Tse M, Molinoff P. Selective facilitation of sexual solicitation in the female rat by a melanocortin receptor agonist. Proc Natl Acad Sci USA 2004; 101(27): 10201–4.
130. Rossler AS, Pfaus JG, Kia HK et al. The melanocortin agonist, melanotan II, enhances proceptive sexual behaviors in the female rat. Pharmacol Biochem Behav 2006; 85: 514–21.
131. Gelez H, Jacubovich M, Ismail N et al. Melanocortin agonists facilitate solicitation in female rats through a central mechanism of action. Proceedings Annual Meeting of the Society for Behavioral Neuroendocrinology, Pittsburgh 2006.
132. Diamond LE, Earle DC, Heiman JR et al. An effect on the subjective sexual response in premenopausal women with sexual arousal disorder by bremelanotide (PT-141), a melanocortin receptor agonist. J Sex Med 2006; 3(4): 628–38.
133. Caldwell JD, Prange AJ Jr, Pedersen CA. Oxytocin facilitates the sexual receptivity of estrogen-treated female rats. Neuropeptides 1986; 7(2): 175–89.

134. Caldwell JD, Jirikowski GF, Greer ER, Pedersen CA. Medial preoptic area oxytocin and female sexual receptivity. Behav Neurosci 1989; 103(3): 655–62.
135. Caldwell JD, Johns JM, Faggin BM, Senger MA, Pedersen CA. Infusion of an oxytocin antagonist into the medial preoptic area prior to progesterone inhibits sexual receptivity and increases rejection in female rats. Horm Behav 1994; 28(3): 288–302.
136. Witt DM, Insel TR. A selective oxytocin antagonist attenuates progesterone facilitation of female sexual behavior. Endocrinology 1991; 128(6): 3269–76.
137. Pedersen CA, Boccia ML. Vasopressin interactions with oxytocin in the control of female sexual behavior. Neuroscience 2006; 139(3): 843–51.
138. Sodersten P, Henning M, Melin P, Ludin S. Vasopressin alters female sexual behaviour by acting on the brain independently of alterations in blood pressure. Nature 1983; 301(5901): 608–10.
139. Caldwell JD, Barakat AS, Smith DD, Hruby VJ, Pedersen CA. A uterotonic antagonist blocks the oxytocin-induced facilitation of female sexual receptivity. Brain Res 1990; 512(2): 291–6.
140. Pfaus JG, Gorzalka BB. Opioids and sexual behavior. Neurosci Biobehav Rev 1987; 11(1): 1–34.
141. Pfaus JG, Gorzalka BB. Selective activation of opioid receptors differentially affects lordosis behavior in female rats. Peptides 1987; 8(2): 309–17.
142. Acosta-Martinez M, Etgen AM. The role of delta-opioid receptors in estrogen facilitation of lordosis behavior. Behav Brain Res 2002; 136(1): 93–102.
143. Pfaus JG, Pfaff DW. Mu-, delta-, and kappa-opioid receptor agonists selectively modulate sexual behaviors in the female rat: differential dependence on progesterone. Horm Behav 1992; 26(4): 457–73.
144. Sinchak K, Mills RH, Eckersell CB, Micevych PE. Medial preoptic area delta-opioid receptors inhibit lordosis. Behav Brain Res 2004; 155(2): 301–6.
145. Hull EM, Muschamp JW, Sato S. Dopamine and serotonin: influences on male sexual behavior. Physiol Behav 2004; 83(2): 291–307.
146. Segraves RT. Effects of psychotropic drugs on human erection and ejaculation. Arch Gen Psychiatry 1989; 46(3): 275–84.
147. Rosen RC, Lane RM, Menza M. Effects of SSRIs on sexual function: a critical review. J Clin Psychopharmacol 1999; 19(1): 67–85.
148. Giuliano F. 5-hydroxytryptamine in premature ejaculation: opportunities for therapeutic intervention. Trends Neurosci 2007; 30(2): 79–84.
149. Mooradian AD, Morley JE, Korenman SG. Biological actions of androgens. Endocr Rev 1987; 8(1): 1–28.
150. Halata Z, Munger BL. The neuroanatomical basis for the protopathic sensibility of the human glans penis. Brain Res 1986; 371(2): 205–30.
151. Christ GJ. K+ channels and gap junctions in the modulation of corporal smooth muscle tone. Drug News Perspect 2000; 13(1): 28–36.
152. Andersson KE. Pharmacology of penile erection. Pharmacol Rev 2001; 53(3): 417–50.
153. Hedlund P, Alm P, Ekstrom P et al. Pituitary adenylate cyclase-activating polypeptide, helospectin, and vasoactive intestinal polypeptide in human corpus cavernosum. Br J Pharmacol 1995; 116(4): 2258–66.
154. Burnett AL, Lowenstein CJ, Bredt DS, Chang TS, Snyder SH. Nitric oxide: a physiologic mediator of penile erection. Science 1992; 257(5068): 401–3.
155. Ignarro LJ, Bush PA, Buga GM et al. Nitric oxide and cyclic GMP formation upon electrical field stimulation cause relaxation of cor pus cavernosum smooth muscle. Biochem Biophys Res Commun 1990; 170(2): 843–50.
156. Steers WD. Viagra – after one year. Urology 1999; 54(1): 12–17.
157. Padma-Nathan H, Hellstrom WJ, Kaiser FE et al. Treatment of men with erectile dysfunction with transurethral alprostadil. Medicated Urethral System for Erection (MUSE) Study Group. N Engl J Med 1997; 336(1): 1–7.
158. Hancock MB, Peveto CA. A preganglionic autonomic nucleus in the dorsal gray commissure of the lumbar spinal cord of the rat. J Comp Neurol 1979; 183(1): 65–72.
159. Giuliano F, Bernabe J, Brown K et al. Erectile response to hypothalamic stimulation in rats: role of peripheral nerves. Am J Physiol 1997; 273(6 Pt 2): R1990–7.
160. Steers WD, Mallory B, de Groat WC. Electrophysiological study of neural activity in penile nerve of the rat. Am J Physiol 1988; 254(6 Pt 2): R989–1000.
161. McKenna KE, Nadelhaft I. The pudendo-pudendal reflex in male and female rats. J Auton Nerv Syst 1989; 27(1): 67–77.
162. Lavoisier P, Proulx J, Courtois F. Reflex contractions of the ischiocavernosus muscles following electrical and pressure stimulations. J Urol 1988; 139(2): 396–9.
163. Ertekin C, Reel F. Bulbocavernosus reflex in normal men and in patients with neurogenic bladder and/or impotence. J Neurol Sci 1976; 28(1): 1–15.
164. Hart BL. Hormones, spinal reflexes, and sexual behaviour. In: Hutchison JB, editor. Biological Determinants of Sexual Behaviour. Chichester, UK: Wiley and Sons; 1978, p. 319–47.
165. Beach FA. Cerebral and hormonal control of reflexive mechanisms involved in copulatory behavior. Physiol Rev 1967; 47(2): 289–316.
166. KUHN RA. Functional capacity of the isolated human spinal cord. Brain 1950; 73(1): 1–51.
167. Chapelle PA, Durand J, Lacert P. Penile erection following complete spinal cord injury in man. Br J Urol 1980; 52(3): 216–19.
168. Sachs BD. Contextual approaches to the physiology and classification of erectile function, erectile dysfunction, and sexual arousal. Neurosci Biobehav Rev 2000; 24(5): 541–60.
169. Marson L, Platt KB, McKenna KE. Central nervous system innervation of the penis as revealed by the transneuronal transport of pseudorabies virus. Neuroscience 1993; 55(1): 263–80.
170. Coolen LM, Peters HJ, Veening JG. Distribution of Fos immunoreactivity following mating versus anogenital investigation in the male rat brain. Neuroscience 1997; 77(4): 1151–61.
171. Hamson DK, Watson NV. Regional brainstem expression of Fos associated with sexual behavior in male rats. Brain Res 2004; 1006(2): 233–40.
172. Giuliano F, Rampin O, Brown K et al. Stimulation of the medial preoptic area of the hypothalamus in the rat elicits increases in intracavernous pressure. Neurosci Lett 1996; 209(1): 1–4.
173. Stefanick ML, Davidson JM. Genital responses in noncopulators and rats with lesions in the medial preoptic area or midthoracic spinal cord. Physiol Behav 1987; 41(5): 439–44.
174. Shimura T, Yamamoto T, Shimokochi M. The medial preoptic area is involved in both sexual arousal and performance in male rats: re-evaluation of neuron activity in freely moving animals. Brain Res 1994; 640(1–2): 215–22.
175. Liu YC, Salamone JD, Sachs BD. Lesions in medial preoptic area and bed nucleus of stria terminalis: differential effects on copulatory behavior and noncontact erection in male rats. J Neurosci 1997; 17(13): 5245–53.
176. Monaghan EP, Arjomand J, Breedlove SM. Brain lesions affect penile reflexes. Horm Behav 1993; 27(1): 122–31.
177. Liu YC, Salamone JD, Sachs BD. Impaired sexual response after lesions of the paraventricular nucleus of the hypothalamus in male rats. Behav Neurosci 1997; 111(6): 1361–7.
178. Chen KK, Chan SH, Chang LS, Chan JY. Participation of paraventricular nucleus of hypothalamus in central regulation of penile erection in the rat. J Urol 1997; 158(1): 238–44.
179. Liu YC, Sachs BD. Erectile function in male rats after lesions in the lateral paragigantocellular nucleus. Neurosci Lett 1999; 262(3): 203–6.
180. Marson L, List MS, McKenna KE. Lesions of the nucleus paragigantocellularis alter ex copula penile reflexes. Brain Res 1992; 592(1–2): 187–92.

181. Kondo Y, Sachs BD, Sakuma Y. Importance of the medial amygdala in rat penile erection evoked by remote stimuli from estrous females. Behav Brain Res 1997; 88(2): 153–60.
182. Steers WD. Neural pathways and central sites involved in penile erection: neuroanatomy and clinical implications. Neurosci Biobehav Rev 2000; 24(5): 507–16.
183. Argiolas A. Neuropeptides and sexual behaviour. Neurosci Biobehav Rev 1999; 23(8): 1127–42.
184. Pfaus JG. Neurobiology of sexual behavior. Curr Opin Neurobiol 1999; 9(6): 751–8.
185. Lee RL, Smith ER, Mas M, Davidson JM. Effects of intrathecal administration of 8-OH-DPAT on genital reflexes and mating behavior in male rats. Physiol Behav 1990; 47(4): 665–9.
186. Millan MJ, Peglion JL, Lavielle G, Perrin-Monneyron S. 5-HT2C receptors mediate penile erections in rats: actions of novel and selective agonists and antagonists. Eur J Pharmacol 1997; 325(1): 9–12.
187. Uitti RJ, Tanner CM, Rajput AH et al. Hypersexuality with antiparkinsonian therapy. Clin Neuropharmacol 1989; 12(5): 375–83.
188. Melis MR, Argiolas A, Gessa GL. Apomorphine-induced penile erection and yawning: site of action in brain. Brain Res 1987; 415(1): 98–104.
189. Giuliano F, Allard J, Rampin O et al. Spinal proerectile effect of apomorphine in the anesthetized rat. Int J Impot Res 2001; 13(2): 110–5.
190. Melis MR, Succu S, Mascia MS, Argiolas A. PD-168077, a selective dopamine D4 receptor agonist, induces penile erection when injected into the paraventricular nucleus of male rats. Neurosci Lett 2005; 379(1): 59–62.
191. Heaton JP, Morales A, Adams MA, Johnston B, el Rashidy R. Recovery of erectile function by the oral administration of apomorphine. Urology 1995; 45(2): 200–6.
192. Kaplan SA, Reis RB, Kohn IJ, Shabsigh R, Te AE. Combination therapy using oral alpha-blockers and intracavernosal injection in men with erectile dysfunction. Urology 1998; 52(5): 739–43.
193. Bitran D, Hull EM. Pharmacological analysis of male rat sexual behavior. Neurosci Biobehav Rev 1987; 11(4): 365–89.
194. Melis MR, Argiolas A, Gessa GL. Oxytocin-induced penile erection and yawning: site of action in the brain. Brain Res 1986; 398(2): 259–65.
195. Giuliano F, Bernabe J, McKenna K, Longueville F, Rampin O. Spinal proerectile effect of oxytocin in anesthetized rats. Am J Physiol Regul Integr Comp Physiol 2001; 280(6): R1870–7.
196. Melis MR, Succu S, Spano MS, Argiolas A. Morphine injected into the paraventricular nucleus of the hypothalamus prevents noncontact penile erections and impairs copulation: involvement of nitric oxide. Eur J Neurosci 1999; 11(6): 1857–64.
197. Melis MR, Argiolas A. Nitric oxide donors induce penile erection and yawning when injected in the central nervous system of male rats. Eur J Pharmacol 1995; 294(1): 1–9.
198. Melis MR, Argiolas A. Role of central nitric oxide in the control of penile erection and yawning. Progr Neuro-Psychopharmacol Biol Psychiatry 1997; 21(6): 899–922.
199. Argiolas A, Melis MR. The role of oxytocin and the paraventricular nucleus in the sexual behaviour of male mammals. Physiol Behav 2004; 83(2): 309–17.
200. Serra G, Fratta W, Collu M, Gessa GL. Hypophysectomy prevents ACTH-induced yawning and penile erection in rats. Pharmacol Biochem Behav 1987; 26(2): 277–9.
201. Vergoni AV, Bertolini A, Mutulis F, Wikberg JE, Schioth HB. Differential influence of a selective melanocortin MC4 receptor antagonist (HS014) on melanocortin-induced behavioral effects in rats. Eur J Pharmacol 1998; 362(2–3): 95–101.
202. Diamond LE, Earle DC, Rosen RC, Willett MS, Molinoff PB. Double-blind, placebo-controlled evaluation of the safety, pharmacokinetic properties and pharmacodynamic effects of intranasal PT-141, a melanocortin receptor agonist, in healthy males and patients with mild-to-moderate erectile dysfunction. Int J Impot Res 2004; 16(1): 51–9.
203. Doherty PC, Baum MJ, Todd RB. Effects of chronic hyperprolactinemia on sexual arousal and erectile function in male rats. Neuroendocrinology 1986; 42(5): 368–75.
204. Clark JT, Kalra PS. Effects on penile reflexes and plasma hormones of hyperprolactinemia induced by MtTW15 tumors. Horm Behav 1985; 19(3): 304–10.
205. Ra S, Aoki H, Fujioka T et al. In vitro contraction of the canine corpus cavernosum penis by direct perfusion with prolactin or growth hormone. J Urol 1996; 156(2 Pt 1): 522–5.
206. Keast JR. Pelvic ganglia. In: McLachlan EM, editor. Autonomic Ganglia. Luxembourg: Harwood Academic; 1995: 445–79.
207. Andersson KE, Wagner G. Physiology of penile erection. Physiol Rev 1995; 75(1): 191–236.
208. Hoyle CHV. Transmission: purines. In: Burnstock G, Hoyle CHV, eds. Autonomic Neuroeffector Mechanisms. Chur, Switzerland: Harwood Academic; 1992: 367–408.
209. Morris JL, Gibbins IL. Co-transmission and neuromodulation. In: Burnstock G, Hoyle CHV, editors. Autonomic Neuroeffector Mechanisms. Chur, Switzerland: Harwood Academic; 1992: 31–117.
210. Grundemar L, Hakanson R. Effects of various neuropeptide Y/peptide YY fragments on electrically-evoked contractions of the rat vas deferens. Br J Pharmacol 1990; 100(1): 190–2.
211. Zoubek J, Somogyi GT, De Groat WC. A comparison of inhibitory effects of neuropeptide Y on rat urinary bladder, urethra, and vas deferens. Am J Physiol 1993; 265(3 Pt 2): R537–43.
212. Dail WG, Moll MA, Weber K. Localization of vasoactive intestinal polypeptide in penile erectile tissue and in the major pelvic ganglion of the rat. Neuroscience 1983; 10(4): 1379–86.
213. Domoto T, Tsumori T. Co-localization of nitric oxide synthase and vasoactive intestinal peptide immunoreactivity in neurons of the major pelvic ganglion projecting to the rat rectum and penis. Cell Tissue Res 1994; 278(2): 273–8.
214. el Badawi A, Schenk EA. The distribution of cholinergic and adrenergic nerves in the mammalian epididymis: a comparative histochemical study. Am J Anat 1967; 121(1): 1–14.
215. Dun NJ, Dun SL, Huang RL et al. Distribution and origin of nitric oxide synthase-immunoreactive nerve fibers in the rat epididymis. Brain Res 1996; 738(2): 292–300.
216. Torres G, Bitran M, Huidobro-Toro JP. Co-release of neuropeptide Y (NPY) and noradrenaline from the sympathetic nerve terminals supplying the rat vas deferens; influence of calcium and the stimulation intensity. Neurosci Lett 1992; 148(1–2): 39–42.
217. Yamamoto M, Kondo H. Occurrence of a dense plexus of sensory nerve fibers immunoreactive to calcitonin-gene-related peptide in the cauda epididymidis of rats. Acta Anat 1988; 132(2): 169–76.
218. Carvalho TL, Hodson NP, Blank MA et al. Occurrence, distribution and origin of peptide-containing nerves of guinea-pig and rat male genitalia and the effects of denervation on sperm characteristics. J Anat 1986; 149: 121–41.
219. Dail WG. Autonomic innervation of male genitalia. In: Maggi CA, editor. Nervous Control of the Urogenital System. Chur, Switzerland: Harwood Academic; 1993: 69–102.
220. Sjostrand NO, Ehren I, Eldh J, Wiklund NP. NADPH-diaphorase in glandular cells and nerves and its relation to acetylcholinesterase-positive nerves in the male reproductive tract of man and guinea-pig. Urol Res 1998; 26(3): 181–8.
221. Stjernquist M, Owman C, Sjoberg NO, Sundler F. Coexistence and cooperation between neuropeptide Y and norepinephrine in nerve fibers of guinea pig vas deferens and seminal vesicle. Biol Reprod 1987; 36(1): 149–55.
222. Vaalasti A, Linnoila I, Hervonen A. Immunohistochemical demonstration of VIP, [Met5]- and [Leu5]-enkephalin immunoreactive nerve fibres in the human prostate and seminal vesicles. Histochemistry 1980; 66(1): 89–98.
223. Uckert S, Stanarius A, Stief CG et al. Immunocytochemical distribution of nitric oxide synthase in the human seminal vesicle: a

light and electron microscopical study. Urol Res 2003; 31(4): 262–6.
224. Vaalasti A, Hervonen A. Nerve endings in the human prostate. Am J Anat 1980; 157(1): 41–7.
225. Nadelhaft I. Cholinergic axons in the rat prostate and neurons in the pelvic ganglion. Brain Res 2003; 989(1): 52–7.
226. Chapple CR, Aubry ML, James S et al. Characterisation of human prostatic adrenoceptors using pharmacology receptor binding and localisation. Br J Urol 1989; 63(5): 487–96.
227. Dube D, Poyet P, Pelletier G, Labrie F. Radioautographic localization of beta-adrenergic receptors in the rat ventral prostate. J Androl 1986; 7(3): 169–74.
228. Adrian TE, Gu J, Allen JM et al. Neuropeptide Y in the human male genital tract. Life Sci 1984; 35(26): 2643–8.
229. Aumuller G, Jungblut T, Malek B, Konrad S, Weihe E. Regional distribution of opioidergic nerves in human and canine prostates. Prostate 1989; 14(3): 279–88.
230. Bloch W, Klotz T, Loch C et al. Distribution of nitric oxide synthase implies a regulation of circulation, smooth muscle tone, and secretory function in the human prostate by nitric oxide. Prostate 1997; 33(1): 1–8.
231. Dail WG, Hamill RW. Parasympathetic nerves in penile erectile tissue of the rat contain choline acetyltransferase. Brain Res 1989; 487(1): 165–70.
232. Morrison J, Steers WD, Brading A et al. Neurophysiology and neuropharmacology. In: Abrams P, Cardozo L, Khoury S, Wein A, eds. Incontinence. Plymouth, UK: Health Publication; 2002: 85–164.
233. Monneron MC, Gillberg PG, Ohman B, Alberts P. In vitro alpha-adrenoceptor autoradiography of the urethra and urinary bladder of the female pig, cat, guinea-pig and rat. Scand J Urol Nephrol 2000; 34(4): 233–8.
234. Alm P, Alumets J, Hakanson R et al. Origin and distribution of VIP (vasoactive intestinal polypeptide)-nerves in the genito-urinary tract. Cell Tissue Res 1980; 205(3): 337–47.
235. Crowe R, Milner P, Lincoln J, Burnstock G. Histochemical and biochemical investigation of adrenergic, cholinergic and peptidergic innervation of the rat ventral prostate 8 weeks after streptozotocin-induced diabetes. J Auton Nerv Syst 1987; 20(2): 103–12.
236. Grozdanovic Z, Baumgarten HG, Bruning G. Histochemistry of NADPH-diaphorase, a marker for neuronal nitric oxide synthase, in the peripheral autonomic nervous system of the mouse. Neuroscience 1992; 48(1): 225–35.
237. Crowe R, Burnstock G. A histochemical and immunohistochemical study of the autonomic innervation of the lower urinary tract of the female pig. Is the pig a good model for the human bladder and urethra? J Urol 1989; 141(2): 414–22.
238. Hokfelt T, Schultzberg M, Elde R et al. Peptide neurons in peripheral tissues including the urinary tract: immunohistochemical studies. Acta Pharmacol Toxicol (Copenh) 1978; 43(Suppl 2): 79–89.
239. Su HC, Wharton J, Polak JM et al. Calcitonin gene-related peptide immunoreactivity in afferent neurons supplying the urinary tract: combined retrograde tracing and immunohistochemistry. Neuroscience 1986; 18(3): 727–47.
240. Johnson RD, Halata Z. Topography and ultrastructure of sensory nerve endings in the glans penis of the rat. J Comp Neurol 1991; 312(2): 299–310.
241. Nunez R, Gross GH, Sachs BD. Origin and central projections of rat dorsal penile nerve: possible direct projection to autonomic and somatic neurons by primary afferents of nonmuscle origin. J Comp Neurol 1986; 247(4): 417–29.
242. Kaleczyc J, Scheuermann DW, Pidsudko Z et al. Distribution, immunohistochemical characteristics and nerve pathways of primary sensory neurons supplying the porcine vas deferens. Cell Tissue Res 2002; 310(1): 9–17.
243. Pennefather JN, Lau WA, Mitchelson F, Ventura S. The autonomic and sensory innervation of the smooth muscle of the prostate gland: a review of pharmacological and histological studies. J Auton Pharmacol 2000; 20(4): 193–206.
244. Baron R, Janig W. Afferent and sympathetic neurons projecting into lumbar visceral nerves of the male rat. J Comp Neurol 1991; 314(3): 429–36.
245. Morgan C, deGroat WC, Nadelhaft I. The spinal distribution of sympathetic preganglionic and visceral primary afferent neurons that send axons into the hypogastric nerves of the cat. J Comp Neurol 1986; 243(1): 23–40.
246. Nadelhaft I, McKenna KE. Sexual dimorphism in sympathetic preganglionic neurons of the rat hypogastric nerve. J Comp Neurol 1987; 256(2): 308–15.
247. Owman C, Stjernquist M. The peripheral nervous system. In: Bjorklund A, Hokfelt T, Owman C, editors. Handbook of Chemical Neuroanatomy. Amsterdam, The Netherlands: Elsevier Science; 1988: 445–544.
248. Schroder HD. Anatomical and pathoanatomical studies on the spinal efferent systems innervating pelvic structures. 1. Organization of spinal nuclei in animals. 2. The nucleus X-pelvic motor system in man. J Auton Nerv Syst 1985; 14(1): 23–48.
249. Johnson RD, Hubscher CH. Brainstem microstimulation differentially inhibits pudendal motoneuron reflex inputs. Neuroreport 1998; 9(2): 341–5.
250. Nordling J, Andersen JT, Walter S et al. Evoked response of the bulbocavernosus reflex. Eur Urol 1979; 5(1): 36–8.
251. Opsomer RJ, Caramia MD, Zarola F, Pesce F, Rossini PM. Neurophysiological evaluation of central-peripheral sensory and motor pudendal fibres. Electroencephalogr Clin Neurophysiol 1989; 74(4): 260–70.
252. Shafik A, El Sibai O. Mechanism of ejection during ejaculation: identification of a urethrocavernosus reflex. Arch Androl 2000; 44(1): 77–83.
253. Brackett NL, Ferrell SM, Aballa TC et al. An analysis of 653 trials of penile vibratory stimulation in men with spinal cord injury. J Urol 1998; 159(6): 1931–4.
254. Sonksen J, Biering Sorensen F, Kristensen JK. Ejaculation induced by penile vibratory stimulation in men with spinal cord injuries. The importance of the vibratory amplitude. Paraplegia 1994; 32(10): 651–60.
255. Kimura Y, Adachi K, Kisaki N, Ise K. On the transportation of spermatozoa in the vas deferens. Andrologia 1975; 7(1): 55–61.
256. Kolbeck SC, Steers WD. Neural regulation of the vas deferens in the rat: an electrophysiological analysis. Am J Physiol 1992; 263(2 Pt 2): R331–8.
257. Fedan JS, Besse JC, Carpenter FG, Teague RS. Motor innervation of the smooth muscle of the rat seminal vesicle. J Pharmacol Exp Ther 1977; 201(2): 285–97.
258. Terasaki T. Effects of autonomic drugs on intraluminal pressure and excretion of rat seminal vesicles in vivo. Tohoku J Exp Med 1989; 157(4): 373–9.
259. Kontani H, Shiraoya C. Method for simultaneous recording of the prostatic contractile and urethral pressure responses in anesthetized rats and the effects of tamsulosin. Jpn J Pharmacol 2002; 90(3): 281–90.
260. Watanabe H, Shima M, Kojima M, Ohe H. Dynamic study of nervous control on prostatic contraction and fluid excretion in the dog. J Urol 1988; 140(6): 1567–70.
261. Stjernquist M, Hakanson R, Leander S et al. Immunohistochemical localization of substance P, vasoactive intestinal polypeptide and gastrin-releasing peptide in vas deferens and seminal vesicle, and the effect of these and eight other neuropeptides on resting tension and neurally evoked contractile activity. Regul Pept 1983; 7(1): 67–86.
262. Kurokawa M, Tsunoo A. Parasympathetic depression of vas deferens contraction in the guinea-pig involves adenosine receptors. J Physiol 1988; 407: 135–53.

263. Creed KE, Tulloch AG. The effect of pelvic nerve stimulation and some drugs on the urethra and bladder of the dog. Br J Urol 1978; 50(6): 398–405.
264. Moss HE, Crowe R, Burnstock G. The seminal vesicle in eight and 16 week streptozotocin-induced diabetic rats: adrenergic, cholinergic and peptidergic innervation. J Urol 1987; 138(5): 1273–8.
265. Sjostrand NO, Hammarstrom M. Sympathetic regulation of fructose secretion in the seminal vesicle of the guinea-pig. Acta Physiol Scand 1995; 153(2): 189–202.
266. Lepor H, Kuhar MJ. Characterization of muscarinic cholinergic receptor binding in the vas deferens, bladder, prostate and penis of the rabbit. J Urol 1984; 132(2): 392–6.
267. Smith ER, Miller TB, Wilson MM, Appel MC. Effects of vasoactive intestinal peptide on canine prostatic contraction and secretion. Am J Physiol 1984; 247(4 Pt 2): R701–8.
268. Ventura S, Dewalagama RK, Lau LCL. Adenosine 5′-triphosphate (ATP) is an excitatory cotransmitter with noradrenaline to the smooth muscle of the rat prostate gland. Br J Pharmacol 2003; 138(7): 1277–84.
269. Meldrum LA, Burnstock G. Evidence that ATP is involved as a co-transmitter in the hypogastric nerve supplying the seminal vesicle of the guinea-pig. Eur J Pharmacol 1985; 110(3): 363–6.
270. Allcorn RJ, Cunnane TC, Kirkpatrick K. Actions of alpha, beta-methylene ATP and 6-hydroxydopamine on sympathetic neurotransmission in the vas deferens of the guinea-pig, rat and mouse: support for cotransmission. Br J Pharmacol 1986; 89(4): 647–59.
271. May AG, DeWeese JA, Rob CG. Changes in sexual function following operation on the abdominal aorta. Surgery 1969; 65(1): 41–7.
272. Weinstein MH, Machleder HI. Sexual function after aortoiliac surgery. Ann Surg 1975; 181(6): 787–90.
273. Pocard M, Zinzindohoue F, Haab F et al. A prospective study of sexual and urinary function before and after total mesorectal excision with autonomic nerve preservation for rectal cancer. Surgery 2002; 131(4): 368–72.
274. Sugihara K, Moriya Y, Akasu T, Fujita S. Pelvic autonomic nerve preservation for patients with rectal carcinoma. Oncologic and functional outcome. Cancer 1996; 78(9): 1871–80.
275. Brindley GS, Sauerwein D, Hendry WF. Hypogastric plexus stimulators for obtaining semen from paraplegic men. Br J Urol 1989; 64(1): 72–7.
276. Bohlen JG, Held JP, Sanderson MO. The male orgasm: pelvic contractions measured by anal probe. Arch Sex Behav 1980; 9(6): 503–21.
277. Gerstenberg TC, Levin RJ, Wagner G. Erection and ejaculation in man. Assessment of the electromyographic activity of the bulbocavernosus and ischiocavernosus muscles. Br J Urol 1990; 65(4): 395–402.
278. Grossiord A, Chapelle PA, Lacert P, Pannier S, Durand J. The affected medullary segment in paraplegics. Relation to sexual function in men. Rev Neurol (Paris) 1978; 134(12): 729–40.
279. Vinik AI, Maser RE, Mitchell BD, Freeman R. Diabetic autonomic neuropathy. Diabetes Care 2003; 26(5): 1553–79.
280. Xu C, Yaici ED, Conrath M et al. Galanin and neurokinin-1 receptor immunoreactivity spinal neurons controlling the prostate and the bulbospongiosus muscle identified by transsynaptic labeling in the rat. Neuroscience 2005; 134(4): 1325–41.
281. Coolen LM, Veening JG, Wells AB, Shipley MT. Afferent connections of the parvocellular subparafascicular thalamic nucleus in the rat: evidence for functional subdivisions. J Comp Neurol 2003; 463(2): 132–56.
282. Marberger H. The mechanisms of ejaculation. In: Coutinho EM, Fuchs F, eds. Physiology and Genetics of Reproduction. New York, USA: Plenum Press; 1974: 99–110.
283. Levin RJ. The mechanisms of human ejaculation – a critical analysis. Sex Relationship Ther 2005; 20(1): 123–31.
284. Holmes GM, Sachs BD. The ejaculatory reflex in copulating rats: normal bulbospongiosus activity without apparent urethral stimulation. Neurosci Lett 1991; 125(2): 195–7.
285. Hermabessiere J, Guy L, Boiteux JP. [Human ejaculation: physiology, surgical conservation of ejaculation]. Prog Urol 1999; 9(2): 305–9.
286. Gil-Vernet JM Jr, Alvarez-Vijande R, Gil-Vernet A, Gil-Vernet JM. Ejaculation in men: a dynamic endorectal ultrasonographical study. Br J Urol 1994; 73(4): 442–8.
287. Heeb MM, Yahr P. Anatomical and functional connections among cell groups in the gerbil brain that are activated with ejaculation. J Comp Neurol 2001; 439(2): 248–58.
288. Coolen LM, Olivier B, Peters HJ, Veening JG. Demonstration of ejaculation-induced neural activity in the male rat brain using 5-HT1A agonist 8-OH-DPAT. Physiol Behav 1997; 62(4): 881–91.
289. Meisel R, Sachs B. The physiology of male sexual behavior. In: Knobil E, Neill J, eds. The Physiology of Reproduction. New York, USA: Raven; 1994: 3–105.
290. Coolen LM, Peters HJ, Veening JG. Anatomical interrelationships of the medial preoptic area and other brain regions activated following male sexual behavior: a combined fos and tract-tracing study. J Comp Neurol 1998; 397(3): 421–35.
291. Arendash GW, Gorski RA. Effects of discrete lesions of the sexually dimorphic nucleus of the preoptic area or other medial preoptic regions on the sexual behavior of male rats. Brain Res Bull 1983; 10(1): 147–54.
292. Hull EM, Eaton RC, Markowski VP et al. Opposite influence of medial preoptic D1 and D2 receptors on genital reflexes: implications for copulation. Life Sci 1992; 51(22): 1705–13.
293. Pehek EA, Thompson JT, Hull EM. The effects of intracranial administration of the dopamine agonist apomorphine on penile reflexes and seminal emission in the rat. Brain Res 1989; 500(1–2): 325–32.
294. Larsson K, van Dis H. Seminal discharge following intracranial electrical stimulation. Brain Res 1970; 23(3): 381–6.
295. Simerly RB, Swanson LW. Projections of the medial preoptic nucleus: a *Phaseolus vulgaris* leucoagglutinin anterograde tract-tracing study in the rat. J Comp Neurol 1988; 270(2): 209–42.
296. Rizvi TA, Ennis M, Shipley MT. Reciprocal connections between the medial preoptic area and the midbrain periaqueductal gray in rat: a WGA-HRP and PHA-L study. J Comp Neurol 1992; 315(1): 1–15.
297. Murphy AZ, Rizvi TA, Ennis M, Shipley MT. The organization of preoptic-medullary circuits in the male rat: evidence for interconnectivity of neural structures involved in reproductive behavior, antinociception and cardiovascular regulation. Neuroscience 1999; 91(3): 1103–16.
298. Swanson LW, Sawchenko PE. Hypothalamic integration: organization of the paraventricular and supraoptic nuclei. Annu Rev Neurosci 1983; 6: 269–324.
299. Saper CB, Loewy AD, Swanson LW, Cowan WM. Direct hypothalamo-autonomic connections. Brain Res 1976; 117(2): 305–12.
300. Bancila M, Verge D, Rampin O et al. 5-Hydroxytryptamine2C receptors on spinal neurons controlling penile erection in the rat. Neuroscience 1999; 92(4): 1523–37.
301. Ackerman AE, Lange GM, Clemens LG. Effects of paraventricular lesions on sex behavior and seminal emission in male rats. Physiol Behav 1997; 63(1): 49–53.
302. Canteras NS, Simerly RB, Swanson LW. Organization of projections from the medial nucleus of the amygdala: a PHAL study in the rat. J Comp Neurol 1995; 360(2): 213–45.
303. Marson L, McKenna KE. CNS cell groups involved in the control of the ischiocavernosus and bulbospongiosus muscles: a transneuronal tracing study using pseudorabies virus. J Comp Neurol 1996; 374(2): 161–79.
304. Marson L, McKenna KE. The identification of a brainstem site controlling spinal sexual reflexes in male rats. Brain Res 1990; 515(1–2): 303–8.

305. Marson L. Lesions of the periaqueductal gray block the medial preoptic area-induced activation of the urethrogenital reflex in male rats. Neuroscience Lett 2004; 367(3): 278–82.
306. Murphy AZ, Hoffman GE. Distribution of gonadal steroid receptor-containing neurons in the preoptic–periaqueductal gray–brainstem pathway: a potential circuit for the initiation of male sexual behavior. J Comp Neurol 2001; 438(2): 191–212.
307. Holstege G, Georgiadis JR, Paans AMJ et al. Brain activation during human male ejaculation. J Neurosci 2003; 23(27): 9185–93.
308. Arnow BA, Desmond JE, Banner LL et al. Brain activation and sexual arousal in healthy, heterosexual males. Brain 2002; 125(Pt 5): 1014–23.
309. Perretti A, Catalano A, Mirone V et al. Neurophysiologic evaluation of central-peripheral sensory and motor pudendal pathways in primary premature ejaculation. Urology 2003; 61(3): 623–8.
310. Bazzett TJ, Eaton RC, Thompson JT et al. Dose dependent D2 effects on genital reflexes after MPOA injections of quinelorane and apomorphine. Life Sci 1991; 48(24): 2309–15.
311. Hull EM, Warner RK, Bazzett TJ et al. D2/D1 ratio in the medial preoptic area affects copulation of male rats. J Pharmacol Exp Ther 1989; 251(2): 422 7.
312. Clement P, Bernabe J, Denys P, Alexandre L, Giuliano F. Ejaculation induced by i.c.v. injection of the preferential dopamine D(3) receptor agonist 7-hydroxy-2-(di-N-propylamino)tetralin in anesthetized rats. Neuroscience 2007; 145(2): 605–10.
313. Hillegaart V, Ahlenius S. Facilitation and inhibition of male rat ejaculatory behaviour by the respective 5-HT1A and 5-HT1B receptor agonists 8-OH-DPAT and anpirtoline, as evidenced by use of the corresponding new and selective receptor antagonists NAD-299 and NAS-181. Br J Pharmacol 1998; 125(8): 1733–43.
314. Rowland DL, Houtsmuller EJ. 8-OH-DPAT interacts with sexual experience and testosterone to affect ejaculatory response in rats. Pharmacol Biochem Behav 1998; 60(1): 143–9.
315. Rehman J, Kaynan A, Christ G et al. Modification of sexual behavior of Long-Evans male rats by drugs acting on the 5-HT1A receptor. Brain Res 1999; 821(2): 414–25.
316. Foreman MM, Hall JL, Love RL. The role of the 5-HT2 receptor in the regulation of sexual performance of male rats. Life Sci 1989; 45(14): 1263–70.
317. Hull EM, Bitran D, Pehek EA et al. Brain localization of cholinergic influence on male sex behavior in rats: agonists. Pharmacol Biochem Behav 1988; 31(1): 169–74.
318. Arletti R, Bazzani C, Castelli M, Bertolini A. Oxytocin improves male copulatory performance in rats. Behav 1985; 19(1): 14–20.
319. Pfaus JG, Kippin TE, Centeno S. Conditioning and sexual behavior: a review. Horm Behav 2001; 40(2): 291–321.
320. Barnas JL, Pierpaoli S, Ladd P et al. The prevalence and nature of orgasmic dysfunction after radical prostatectomy. BJU Int 2004; 94(4): 603–5.
321. Koeman M, van Driel MF, Schultz WC, Mensink HJ. Orgasm after radical prostatectomy. Br J Urol 1996; 77(6): 861–4.
322. Newman HF, Reiss H, Northup JD. Physical basis of emission, ejaculation, and orgasm in the male. Urology 1982; 19(4): 341–50.
323. Pfaus JG, Frank A. Beach award. Homologies of animal and human sexual behaviors. Horm Behav 1996; 30(3): 187–200.
324. McKenna K. The brain is the master organ in sexual function: central nervous system control of male and female sexual function. Int J Impot Res 1999; 11(Suppl 1): 48–55.

Part II

Functional pathology of the lower urinary tract

9

Epidemiology of the neurogenic bladder

Patrick B Leu and Ananias C Diokno

Introduction

The neurogenic bladder is an entity with many different characteristics. It is not a disease in and of itself, but rather the manifestation of multiple different neurologic processes capable of exerting effects on the bladder by way of its innervation. The outward expression of these effects by the bladder is as varied as the conditions that cause them, ranging from essentially no bladder function at all to extreme overactivity. The long-term consequences cover a spectrum just as broad, ranging from little to no consequence to the patient to severe debility and even death.

This chapter aims to outline for the reader the many neurologic processes which can affect the bladder. While a brief description of some diseases will be given, the main focus is the prevalence and type of neurogenic bladder involvement in many of these conditions. Prevalence of neurogenic bladder is the frequency with which bladder dysfunction is observed among the population of neurologically impaired patients at a given time period. Organization of this chapter is based on location of neurologic injury: above the brainstem, the spinal cord, and the peripheral nervous system.

Cerebrovascular accident

Cerebrovascular accident (CVA) or 'stroke' is a major cause of morbidity and mortality, especially among the elderly. It is defined as the acute onset of a focal neurologic deficit. Causes include cerebral embolus, atherosclerotic thrombus, and hemorrhage. The prevalence is approximately 60/1000 patients older than 65 years and 95/1000 in those older than 75 years.[1] More than 500 000 cerebrovascular accidents occur annually in the United States. One-third are fatal, one-third necessitate long-term nursing care, and another third allow patients to return to home with normal or near-normal ability to function. Risk factors include hypertension, diabetes mellitus, smoking, high serum cholesterol, alcohol consumption, obesity, stress, and a sedentary lifestyle.[2]

Cerebrovascular accidents can have profound effects on the genitourinary system. Voiding dysfunction can range from urinary retention to total incontinence. Evaluation and management can be complicated due to associated comorbidities, which may also contribute to voiding dysfunction in this patient population.

Many studies have demonstrated urologic findings as predictors of prognosis in stroke patients. In an analysis of 532 stroke patients, Wade and Hewer noted that of those with urinary incontinence within the first week after the event, half died within 6 months.[3] They also noted an association between early incontinence and decreased chance of regaining mobility. Taub et al evaluated 639 CVA patients and found that initial incontinence was the best single indicator of future disability.[4]

Acute urinary retention, commonly known as cerebral shock, is often seen immediately after stroke. The neurophysiologic mechanism of this is unknown and it may not necessarily be the result of the stroke. It may be the consequence of inability to communicate the need to void, impaired consciousness, temporary overdistention, restricted mobility, associated comorbidities (i.e. diabetes, benign prostatic hyperplasia (BPH)) or medications. Urodynamic studies soon after unilateral CVA have demonstrated a 21% prevalence of overflow incontinence due to detrusor hyporeflexia; however, several of these patients were either diabetic or receiving anticholinergics.[5]

Urinary incontinence is common after stroke. It may be due to detrusor hyperreflexia secondary to loss of cortical inhibition, cognitive impairment with normal bladder function, or overflow incontinence secondary to detrusor hyporeflexia secondary to neuropathy or medication. Underlying dementia, BPH, or stress urinary incontinence may also contribute.[2]

Incontinence after stroke is frequently transitory. While the incidence of early post-stroke urinary incontinence is 57–83%, many of these patients have been found to recover continence with time, with as many as 80% being continent at 6 months post-CVA.[6]

Irritative voiding symptoms of frequency, urgency, and incontinence are most commonly seen after resolution of the cerebral shock. These are manifestations of detrusor hyperreflexia. In a review of recent literature, Marinkovic and Badlani found that 69% of patients had detrusor hyperreflexia, 10% had detrusor hypocontractility, 31% had uninhibited external sphincter relaxation, and 22% had detrusor-sphincter dyssynergia (DSD). Furthermore, they note that attempts at correlating either the site or mechanism (ischemic vs hemorrhagic) of injury with urodynamic findings have been inconclusive.[2]

Cerebellar ataxia

Ataxia refers to a heterogeneous spectrum of abnormal motor phenomena associated with cerebellar deficiency. Histologically, Purkinje's cells are abnormal and decreased in number. The location of nervous system involvement may extend from the cerebellum to the brainstem, spinal cord, and dorsal nerve roots. The disease is classified based on etiologies. Acute ataxia is secondary to various intoxicants, cerebellar tumors, viral infections, hyperpyrexia, demyelinating diseases, and vascular accidents. Subacute ataxia may be secondary to alcohol abuse, paraneoplastic syndromes, or cerebellar tumors. Chronic childhood ataxias may include Friedreich's ataxia, ataxia telangiectasia, and ataxias associated with inherited metabolic derangements. Adult forms include olivopontocerebellar atrophy and cortical cerebellar degeneration.

On examination, these patients manifest initially with poor leg coordination, with subsequent involvement of the upper extremities. Decreased deep tendon reflexes with decreased vibratory sensation and proprioception can be seen. Dysmetria of the arms, dysarthria, choreiform movements, and horizontal nystagmus may also be present.

Urodynamic evaluation by Leach et al of 15 ataxic patients, ranging in age from 8 to 58 years, found that 8 (53%) had hyperreflexia with bladder-sphincteric coordination, 1 (7%) had hyperreflexia without bladder-sphincteric coordination, 2 (13%) had normal bladder contraction without sphincteric coordination, and 4 (27%) had acontractile bladders.[7]

Tumors of the cerebrum

Incontinence of urine can occur in frontal tumors as part of a frontal lobe syndrome of indifference, disinhibition, and self-neglect. However, it can also present with urinary frequency, urgency, and incontinence without signs of cognitive or intellectual impairment. This was first described by Andrew and Nathan in 1964, who reported this with a variety of frontal lobe lesions and concluded what is known to be true today: there exists a micturition control center in the superomedial part of the frontal lobes.[8] Ten years later, 7 further cases were reported by Maurice-Williams in a series of 50 consecutive frontal lobe tumors (14%) over a 29-month time span. After evaluation of 100 consecutive intracranial tumors he observed that this constellation of symptoms was seen only with frontal tumors.[9]

Blaivas reported results of urodynamic studies on 550 patients. Twenty-seven (4.9%) of them had pathologic cystometric findings attributable solely to a focal suprapontine lesion. Thirteen of these patients had brain tumors and 14 of them had strokes. Incontinence was their only clinical manifestation, although not all of them were able to void.[10]

Lang et al reported on two cases of urinary retention and space-occupying lesions of the frontal cortex in 1996. The first case involved an 87-year-old woman who regained her ability to void with minimal post-void residual after evacuation of a subdural hematoma. The second patient was a 63-year-old woman who presented with increasing difficulty voiding over $2^1/_2$ years. She was found to have detrusor hypocontractility and mild bilateral hyperreflexia. She refused surgery for a large left frontal meningioma. During the 4-year follow-up she eventually required suprapubic catheterization before dying of increasing intracranial pressure from the expanding tumor.[11]

Normal pressure hydrocephalus

Normal pressure hydrocephalus (NPH) is a syndrome of progressing dementia and gait disturbance in patients with normal spinal fluid pressure yet distended cerebral ventricles. This was first described in 1965. While some patients can have an identifiable mechanical reason for dilation of cerebral ventricles (obstructing tumor, subarachnoid hemorrhage), the cause of this disease is not identifiable in many patients. Some have suggested failure of cerebrospinal fluid (CSF) to flow into the parasagittal subarachnoid space (where most fluid resorption occurs) as the most likely mechanism.

In 1975, Jonas and Brown evaluated 5 NPH patients with urinary incontinence by performing cystometry. These patients had urinary frequency, urgency, and urge incontinence. Four of the patients exhibited pressure spikes from involuntary bladder contractions. The other patient exhibited low-volume involuntary voiding at 200 ml of fluid. These findings are consistent with the so-called 'uninhibited neurogenic bladder,' as described by Lapides. This is secondary to loss of cortical inhibition of primitive bladder reflex contractions.[12]

Cerebral palsy

Cerebral palsy (CP) is a nonprogressive disorder of the brain, resulting in a variety of motor abnormalities often accompanied by intellectual impairment, convulsive disorders, or other cerebral dysfunction. Strict definitions exclude spinal cord involvement. Approximately one-third of children with CP have lower urinary tract symptoms.

McNeal et al published urodynamic results on 50 patients between the ages of 8 and 29 years. They found enuresis in 28%, stress incontinence in 26%, urgency in 18%, and dribbling in 6%. Overall, 36% had some form of voiding dysfunction and some had multiple symptoms.[13]

Decter et al evaluated 57 children with cerebral palsy and lower urinary tract symptoms. Incontinence occurred in 49/57 (86%) patients. Eleven of the children had wetting limited to day or night, while the remaining 38 experienced wetting during both the day and night. Of the 8 who were totally continent, 3 suffered from severe urgency and frequency, 2 presented with urinary tract infections, 2 complained of difficulty initiating urination, and 1 was in urinary retention.

Although general neurologic examination revealed only minor findings in some patients, urodynamic studies identified definite abnormalities in a majority of patients. On urodynamic evaluation, 70% of the incontinent patients had uninhibited contractions that could not be suppressed, 6% had overflow incontinence with incomplete emptying secondary to detrusor-sphincter dyssynergia (DSD), 4% had hypertonia causing intermittent leaking, and 2% had periodic relaxation of the external sphincter during filling. Overall, 49 of the 57 (86%) patients (continent and incontinent) were found to have purely upper motor neuron lesions.

Urinary tract infection was seen in 11% of the patients. Four of the 6 had bladder outlet obstruction secondary to DSD and 1 had elevated residual volumes owing to poor detrusor contraction. Radiologic abnormalities were seen in all 6 children.[14]

Mental retardation

Mental retardation may result from a heterogeneous group of disorders and is seldom the result of deficient intelligence alone.[15] Etiologies include infection, toxin exposure (maternal overdose), perinatal injury, metabolic disturbances (hypercalcemia, hypoglycemia, phenylketonuria), malformations (hydrocephaly, microcephaly, and others), genetic disorders (Down's syndrome), and cerebral palsy.[16]

In 1981 Mitchell and Woodthorpe published data on prevalence and disability of mentally handicapped people born between 1958 and 1963 in three London boroughs. They reported that nocturnal enuresis occurred in over a quarter of patients and 12% experienced both day and nighttime incontinence.[16] Another British study by Reid et al evaluated behavioral syndromes in a sample of 100 severely (49) and profoundly (51) retarded adults. Sixtyfive percent of patients in this study of hospitalized patients were incontinent.[17]

Hellstrom et al studied 21 mentally retarded patients (16 men, 5 women; average age 36 years) referred for longstanding urinary problems. The most common urinary symptoms were incontinence, nocturnal enuresis, and urinary retention/poor bladder emptying. The most common urodynamic findings were detrusor areflexia (7) and detrusor hyperreflexia (5). Four patients had normal urodynamic studies. High micturition pressure was found in 3 patients and large bladder capacity in 1 patient. Poor flow with high residual volume was seen in 2 patients. Some patients had more than one finding.[15]

Parkinson's disease

Parkinson's disease is a leading cause of neurologic disability among the elderly population. The estimated prevalence of the disease in the United States is 100 to 150 per 100,000 population and the incidence per annum is 20 per 100,000. Pathogenesis of the disease involves degeneration of the pigmented dopamine-rich substantia nigra of the brain. The resultant dopamine deficiency results in imbalance between dopamine and acetylcholine concentrations. This manifests clinically as tremor, rigidity and bradykinesia.[18] Urinary symptoms associated with onset of tremor in some Parkinsonian patients were described as early as 1936 and later studies in the 1960s and 1970s demonstrated a 37–71% incidence of bladder dysfunction with Parkinson's disease.[19–21] It is felt that the effect of the normal basal ganglia on micturition is inhibitory in nature.

Pavlakis et al in 1983 reported urodynamic findings on 30 patients (22 men and 8 women) with Parkinson's disease and voiding dysfunction. Fifty-seven percent complained of irritative symptoms, 23% obstructive symptoms and 20% had a combination of the two.

Ninety-three percent of the 30 CO_2 cystometrographs (CMGs) performed demonstrated detrusor hyperreflexia and 7% (women only) detrusor areflexia. No patient had a normal CMG. Of patients with detrusor hyperreflexia, 75% demonstrated appropriate sphincter relaxation, 7% showed pseudo-dyssynergia (voluntary contraction of the perineal floor at the time of detrusor contraction in an attempt to prevent leakage), 11% demonstrated sphincter bradykinesia (involuntary electromyographic (EMG) activity persisting through at least the initial part of the expulsive phase of the CMG), and 7% showed neuropathic sphincter potentials. In the two women with detrusor areflexia there was no evidence of detrusor denervation based on supersensitivity testing, nor was there any evidence of sphincter denervation based on EMG studies. These two patients were on anticholinergics, and this may have been the etiology of their areflexia.

Maximum flow rate was decreased in 10 of the 17 men who underwent uroflow analysis. All 10 had prostatic enlargement and 8 presented with obstructive symptoms. Eight of the 10 demonstrated detrusor hyperreflexia with normal sphincter relaxation and the other 2 had pseudo-dyssynergia.[18]

A more recent study from Araki et al reported urodynamic findings on 70 patients (30 men and 40 women) with Parkinson's disease. No male with evidence of prostatic enlargement based on transrectal ultrasound and retrograde urethrocystography was included.

Detrusor hyperreflexia was present in 67% of patients and hyporeflexia or areflexia was seen in 16%. Other findings were hyperreflexia with impaired contractile function in 9%, hyperreflexia with detrusor-sphincter dyssynergia in 3%, and normal detrusor function in 6%. Detrusorsphincter dyssynergia and detrusor hyperreflexia with impaired contractile function were observed only at advanced stages, whereas bladder function was normal only at mild or moderate stages. Abnormal urodynamic findings increased with disease severity.[22]

Shy–Drager syndrome

Shy–Drager syndrome is a rare syndrome which manifests as orthostatic hypotension, urinary incontinence and retention, and associated neurologic dysfunction. It was first described in 1960. The complete syndrome may also include rectal incontinence, anhydrosis, iris atrophy, external ocular palsies, rigidity, tremor, impotence, fasciculations, myasthenia, and anterior horn cell neuropathy. Although the disease mostly affects men, it can also affect women; it is a slowly progressive disease. Urinary symptoms occur early and orthostatic hypotension appears later.[23]

Salinas et al studied 9 patients (7 men and 2 women, mean age 71 years) referred for urologic evaluation. Thirtythree percent of patients had difficulty or inability to void, 44% had stress urinary incontinence, 33% had urinary frequency, and 33% had urge incontinence. Two-thirds of patients had lax anal tone and 45% had absent voluntary anal control. Electromyography of the periurethral striated muscle revealed normal response to cough/Valsalva in 56% and weak or absent activity in the remaining patients. Voluntary sphincter control, likewise, was present in 56% and weak or absent in 44%. Two of the three patients who were able to void had synchronous cessation of EMG activity and the other patient exhibited sporadic sphincteric activity. On CMG, 67% failed to demonstrate reflex or voluntary detrusor contractions. Poor bladder compliance was seen in 4 out of the 9 patients. Involuntary contractions were seen in one-third of patients.[24]

Multiple sclerosis

Multiple sclerosis (MS) is a disabling neurologic disease caused by a demyelinating process affecting the central nervous system. It is characterized by exacerbations and remissions, with associated changes in signs and symptoms. It is the most common neurologic disorder in the 20–45-year-old age group and affects women and men in a 2:1 ratio. It affects 1 of 1000 Americans.[25] Eighty to 90% of patients with MS will have urologic manifestations, and as many as 10% will present with urologic dysfunction. Patients may exhibit symptoms of urgency, urge incontinence, frequency and urinary retention. These are secondary to detrusor hyperreflexia, detrusor-sphincter dyssynergia, and hypocontractility.[26] Litwiller et al performed a review of the literature on multiple sclerosis and the involvement of the genitourinary system. In evaluating 22 studies involving 1882 patients, they found urodynamic evidence of detrusor hyperreflexia in 62% of patients, detrusor-sphincter dyssynergia in 25%, and detrusor hypocontractility in 20% of patients. Less than 1% of patients had renal deterioration.[27]

The manifestations of the disease can also change during its course. Ciancio et al published data on urodynamic pattern changes in multiple sclerosis. They evaluated 22 patients with MS who underwent at least 2 urodynamic evaluations with a mean follow-up interval of 42 45 months between the studies. Overall, 55% of the patients demonstrated a change in their urodynamic patterns and/or compliance. Sixty-four percent of patients had the same or worsening of the same symptoms and 36% had new urologic symptoms. Forty-three percent of patients with no new symptoms and 75% of patients with new symptoms had significant changes found with followup urodynamic testing.[28]

Myelodysplasia

Myelodysplasia, also known as spina bifida, is a condition of malformation of the caudal end of the neural tube and vertebral arches. It is the most common cause of neuropathic bladder in children. Spina bifida cystica refers to protrusion of a sac through the vertebral arch defect. This sac may contain parts of nervous tissue, meninges, spinal fluid, and fat. If this sac contains only meninges, the condition is referred to as a meningocele. If there is some element of spinal cord present with the meninges, it is referred to as a myelomeningocele. This is the case in 90% of patients with spina bifida cystica. A lipomyelomeningocele occurs if a fatty growth of tissue is protruding into the sac with spinal cord elements. Myeloschisis occurs when the spinal cord is completely open without any meningeal covering.

Myelodysplasia occurs in approximately 1 in 1000 births in the United States. It can involve all levels of the spinal column, including the lumbar 26%, lumbosacral 47%, sacral 20%, thoracic 5%, and cervical spine 2%. Eighty-five percent of children have an associated Arnold–Chiari malformation.

The neurologic lesion produced can be quite variable and depends on which neural elements have everted with the meningocele sac. The level of the bony defect gives little clue to the clinical manifestation of the patient. The height of the bony level and the highest extent of the neurologic lesion may vary from 1 to 3 vertebral levels in either direction. Furthermore, the differential growth rates between the veterbral bodies and the elongating spinal cord add a factor of dynamism in the developing child. Because of fibrosis surrounding the spinal cord at the site of meningocele closure, the cord can become tethered during growth, leading to changes in bowel, bladder, and lower extremity function. Urodynamic evaluation of these patients is therefore a critical component of their management.[29]

Urodynamic studies in the newborn period have shown that 57% of myelodysplastic infants have bladder contractions. In children with upper lumbar or thoracic lesions where the sacral cord is spared, 50% have bladder contractions.[30] EMG studies of the external sphincter demonstrate 48% of newborns with intact sacral reflex arcs and no lower motor neuron denervation, 23% with partial denervation, and 29% with complete loss of sacral cord function.[31]

In 1981, McGuire et al demonstrated the relation between intravesical pressure at the time of urethral leakage and presence/development of upper tract changes in myelodysplastic patients. No patient with an intravesical pressure less than 40 cmH_2O at the time of urethral leakage developed vesicoureteral reflux and only 10% demonstrated ureteral dilatation on excretory urography. Sixty-eight percent of patients with higher leak point pressures developed vesicoureteral reflux and 81% showed ureteral dilatation on excretory urography.[32]

A major problem and risk factor for developing upper urinary tract deterioration is the presence of dyssynergia between the external sphincter and the bladder. Urodynamic evaluation of 36 infants with myelodysplasia demonstrated 50% with dyssynergia, 25% with synergy, and 25% with no sphincter activity. Seventy-two percent of the group with dyssynergia were found to exhibit hydroureteronephrosis by 2 years of age. This was present in only 22% of those with synergy and 11% with absent activity. Of those patients with synergy who went on to develop upper tract deterioration, it occurred only after development of incoordination between the detrusor and external sphincter. The one patient with absent sphincter activity who developed upper tract changes had an elevated fixed urethral resistance at 1 year of age. This is felt to be secondary to fibrosis of the striated external urethral sphincter. Treatment by catheterization or cutaneous vesicostomy improved drainage of the urinary tract in each patient.[33]

The tethered cord syndrome, resulting from fibrosis around the cord and differential growth rates of vertebral bodies and the spinal cord, can be seen in children and adults after neurosurgical closure of the primary defect. Symptoms of bladder dysfunction may be seen in 56% of patients at presentation.[34] Adamson et al reported on 5 adults with tethered cord syndrome revealing a full spectrum of bladder dysfunction ranging from retention in 2 of the 5 and frequency and or urgency/incontinence in 3 of the 5 patients.[35] Flanigan et al reported urodynamic results of 24 children prior to operative cord release. Seventyone percent had areflexia and 29% had hyperreflexic bladders.[36] Pang and Wilberger reported preoperative urodynamic study results on 8 patients. Five demonstrated small capacity, spastic unstable bladders while 3 had hypotonic bladders.[34]

Sacral agenesis

Sacral agenesis is defined as the absence of all or part of two or more vertebral bodies at the lower end of the spinal column. Defective development of the second to fourth sacral nerves accompanying the bony abnormalities leads to variable patterns of neuropathic bladder. The incidence of sacral agenesis is about 0.09–0.43% of births. It is seen more frequently in children of diabetic mothers. It is also seen in 12% of children with high imperforate anus. Approximately 20% of children with sacral agenesis are not identified until they are 3–4 years old and present with difficulty in toilet training.[29]

The urodynamic pattern in children with sacral agenesis is varied. Guzman et al reported upper motor lesions at a rate of 35%, including detrusor hyperreflexia, detrusor-sphincter dyssynergia, exaggerated sacral reflexes, and no voluntary control over sphincter function. Forty percent demonstrated lower motor lesions, including detrusor areflexia and absent sacral reflexes. The remaining 25% were unaffected.[37]

Another study by Koff and Deridder evaluated 13 patients with sacral agenesis. Urodynamic studies revealed a 31% rate of lower motor lesions (flaccid bladder), 23% had an upper motor lesion, and 31% had a mixed pattern.[38]

Spinal cord injury

Spinal cord injury (SCI) affects over 200,000 persons in the United States, with an estimated 8000–10,000 new cases occurring annually.[39] Bladder dysfunction after SCI can be classified as either lower motor neuron (LMN) dysfunction or upper motor neuron (UMN) dysfunction.[40]

In patients with hyperreflexia following spinal cord injury, it is imperative to know whether the external sphincter is coordinated (synergic) with the detrusor contraction or if the sphincter is uncoordinated (dyssynergic) with the involuntary detrusor contraction. Diokno et al reported a 66% rate of dyssynergia among 47 patients with a reflex neurogenic bladder.[41]

Kaplan et al reported videourodynamic results obtained from 489 patients with spinal cord lesions secondary to a variety of causes: trauma (284), myelomeningocele (75), spinal stenosis (54), tumors (39), sacral agenesis (5), and other conditions (34). Their analysis found that while there was a general correlation between the neurologic level of injury and the expected vesicourethral function, it was neither absolute nor specific. For example, some patients with cervical cord lesions exhibited detrusor areflexia and some with sacral cord lesions exhibited detrusor hyperreflexia or DSD.[42]

In 2000, Weld and Dmochowski reported urodynamic findings of 243 SCI patients. All but 3 patients were male. Of 196 patients with suprasacral injuries, 95% demonstrated hyperreflexia and/or DSD. Forty-two percent had low bladder compliance and 40% had high detrusor leak point pressures. Of 14 patients with sacral injuries, 86% manifested areflexia, 79% had low compliance, and 86% had high leak point pressures. Of 33 patients with combined suprasacral and sacral injuries, 68% demonstrated hyperreflexia and/or DSD, 27% exhibited areflexia, 58% had low compliance, and 61% had high leak point pressures. Hyperreflexia was seen in 42%, 54%, 32%, 14%, and 33% of cervical, thoracic, lumbar, sacral, and multilevel cord injuries, respectively. Detrusor-sphincter dyssynergia was seen in 68%, 50%, 39% 14%, and 45% of these same lesions. Areflexia was seen in 0%, 0%, 21%, 86%, and 27%, respectively. Normal urodynamic findings were found in 1%, 4%, 4%, 0%, and 3% of injuries at the aforementioned levels. These findings further reinforce that while general correlations between level of injury and the clinical manifestation exist, they are not exact or exclusive.[43]

The central cord syndrome is caused by incomplete cervical spinal cord injury and is characterized by incomplete quadriplegia with disproportionately worse impairment of the upper than the lower extremities. Central cord syndrome may involve 9–16% of all spinal cord injuries and is more predominant in the elderly. Smith et al reported videourodynamic testing results from 22 men with central cord syndrome. Studies were done an average of 34.5 months after injury and after spinal shock had resolved. Results demonstrated normal evaluations in 14%, detrusor areflexia in 18%, detrusor hyperreflexia with synergy in 5%, DSD in 50%, and detrusor hypocontractility in 5%.[44]

Nath et al reported different findings based on urodynamic studies of 20 men with central cord syndrome and voiding difficulties. Carbon dioxide cystometrography with EMG revealed detrusor hyperreflexia without dyssynergia in 15 (75%) patients and DSD in 5 patients (25%). The differences in these studies may be based on methodology (videourodynamics vs CO_2) or timing of the study with respect to injury. Regardless, urodynamic evaluation is important in evaluating and forming appropriate treatment strategies for these patients.[45]

The status of innervation and function of the external sphincter or periurethral striated muscle is as important as the type of detrusor innervation and function following a spinal cord injury, or for that matter any neurologic condition affecting the lower urinary tract. A paralytic external sphincter due to total or partial injury to the anterior motor neuron will certainly cause reduction to the urethral resistance at the sphincteric level, predisposing the individual to stress incontinence. In patients with areflexic bladder, Diokno et al reported 60% of patients with complete denervation of the external sphincter and the rest had partial denervation.[41]

Diabetes

Diabetes is the most common metabolic disease and affects over 5 million people in the United States. Neuropathy is the most frequent of the many complications associated with the disease. The cause is thought to be due to a combination of ischemic nerve injury secondary to vasculopathy associated with the disease, as well as nerve injury secondary to deranged metabolic function. Neuropathy can occur in either insulin-dependent or non-insulin-dependent diabetes. Tests of autonomic function have shown impairment in roughly 20–40% of diabetic patients.[46]

Diabetic cystopathy is the constellation of clinical and urodynamic findings associated with long-term diabetes mellitus. Classically, it has been described as decreased bladder sensation, increased bladder capacity, and impaired detrusor contractility. It is frequently insidious in onset and progression and many patients may have minimal symptoms. Impaired bladder sensation is the most common initial presentation. Patients may void only once or twice a day. Eventually, they may have difficulty initiating and maintaining voiding. Urodynamic testing of unselected diabetics reveals diabetic cystopathy in 26–87% of patients. The finding of cystopathy correlates directly with the duration of symptoms, which generally occur about 10 years after the onset of diabetes. It frequently coexists with signs of peripheral neuropathy. Many diabetics have coexisting other urologic problems such as benign prostatic hyperplasia, stress incontinence, bladder or prostate cancer or infection, causing voiding symptoms which may be similar to or different from the classically described diabetic bladder.[47]

Kaplan et al reported urodynamic findings of 115 male and 67 female consecutive diabetic patients referred for evaluation of voiding symptoms. Mean duration of diabetes was 58 months, and mean duration of voiding symptoms was 27 months. The most common symptoms were nocturia greater than 2 times in 87%, urinary frequency in 78%, urinary hesitancy in 62%, decreased force of stream in 52%, and sensation of incomplete emptying in 45%. No differences between men or women in the above symptoms were noted.

First sensation of filling was 298 ml. Mean bladder capacity was 485 ml. Fifty-two percent had detrusor instability, 23% had impaired detrusor contractility, 11% had indeterminate findings, 10% had detrusor areflexia, 24% had poor compliance, and 1% was normal. Of the 47 patients with peripheral neuropathy, 70% had detrusor instability, 57% had bladder outlet obstruction, 13% had indeterminate findings, 30% had detrusor areflexia, and 66% had evidence of sacral cord signs.

Bladder outlet obstruction was present in 36% of men. It was an isolated finding in 36% of them and associated with another urodynamic finding in 67%. Nine percent of patients (13) had urinary retention, which in men was secondary to bladder outlet obstruction in 7 and detrusor areflexia in 5. All 4 women with retention had areflexia. Patients with sacral cord signs were more likely to exhibit intermittent detrusor contractions/impaired contractility and detrusor areflexia, while those without sacral cord signs were more likely to demonstrate detrusor instability.[48]

Kitami performed urodynamic studies on 173 diabetics. Patients in this study did have classic findings of increased volume at first desire and decreased maximum vesical pressure (67%), but they also demonstrated overactive bladder (14.5%), low-compliance bladder (11%), and detrusorexternal sphincter dyssynergia (32%).[49]

Frimodt-Moller, who coined the term 'diabetic cystopathy', reported on 124 patients with diabetes. Thirty-eight percent had what are now recognized as classic cystopathic findings and 26% had bladder outlet obstruction.[50]

Disc disease

Symptoms from lumbar disc protrusion are most often secondary to posterolateral protrusion, occurring frequently at the L4–L5 and L5–S1 levels. However, more central (posterior) protrusion may disturb nerves leading to the bladder, perineal floor, and cavernous tissue of the penis. The intrathecal sacral nerve roots have been affected in 1–15% of reported cases of lumbar disc prolapse verified at operation, and the most common associated disorder is urinary retention. Fanciullacci et al studied 22 patients with lumbar central disc protrusion and neuropathic bladder. All patients except 2 women with urinary incontinence had urinary retention at presentation. Urodynamic studies performed at the onset of disease revealed areflexia with normal compliance in all patients. Bladder sensation was absent in 16 (73%) and reduced in 6 (27%). EMG showed signs of severe denervation. Postoperative urodynamic evaluation in 17 patients revealed 65% had persistent areflexia, 29% had normoreflexia, 6% had areflexia, and all had normal compliance. Bladder sensation was absent in 35%, reduced in 47%, and normal in 18%. EMG studies of the periurethral muscles showed good recovery of voluntary contraction in 76% of patients.[51]

O'Flynn et al reviewed the records of 30 patients with lumbar disc prolapse and bladder dysfunction who underwent laminectomy and disc removal. Preoperatively, 87% of the patients developed urinary symptoms. Fifty-three percent required catheterization for urinary retention. Postoperative urodynamics revealed 37% of patients had areflexic bladders and voided by straining, 13% exhibited detrusor hyperreflexia with urinary incontinence, and 7% had low compliance with opening of the bladder neck during filling. Thirty-seven percent demonstrated genuine stress incontinence at bladder volumes greater than 300 ml. Only one patient regained normal detrusor activity postoperatively.[52]

Bartolin et al prospectively analyzed 114 patients with lumbar intervertebral disc protrusion requiring surgical treatment. Patients with acute central disc protrusion (cauda equina syndrome) were not included. Urodynamic studies revealed detrusor areflexia in 27.2% of patients. They did not find a significant difference in the rate of areflexia based on the level of disc herniation (L5 vs L4). All patients with detrusor areflexia reported difficult voiding with straining.[53]

The same author evaluated bladder function after surgery. Ninety-eight patients underwent urodynamic evaluation before and after surgery. Twenty-eight percent of patients exhibited detrusor areflexia preoperatively. Only 22% of these patients had a return to normal function after surgery. Of the 71 patients with normal urodynamic findings preoperatively, 4 (6%) developed detrusor hyperreflexia and 3 (4%) developed areflexia postoperatively.[54]

The cauda equina syndrome is a relatively rare constellation of symptoms for herniated lumbar discs. It is characterized by bilateral sciatica, lower extremity weakness, saddle-type hypesthesia, and bowel and bladder dysfunction. Cauda equina syndrome occurs in approximately 1–10% of cases of lumbar disc herniation. Early operative decompression is advocated, but may not always restore normal function. Chang et al evaluated the incidence and long-term outcome of patients with this condition. They identified 4 of 144 (2.8%) consecutive surgical cases of lumbar disc herniation with urinary retention. All patients regained voluntary voiding within 6 months, 1, 3, and 4 years of surgery.[55]

Infectious diseases

Acquired immune deficiency syndrome

Patients with acquired immune deficiency syndrome (AIDS) have not made up a large portion of most urologists' practices. However, due to the large number of people with this disease and increased survival with new medications, urologists can expect to see more patients with AIDS.

Neurologic involvement occurs in 30–40% of patients with AIDS, and involves the central and peripheral nervous systems.[56–58] Neurologic involvement may be the result of infection, immunologic injury to target organs, or neoplasia.

Khan et al performed urodynamic studies on 11 of 677 AIDS patients. Voiding dysfunction secondary to neurogenic bladder was found in 9 of 11 (82%) patients. Urinary retention in 6 of the 11 (55%) patients was the most common presenting symptom. Three patients (27%) presented with urinary incontinence, 1 (9%) with urinary frequency, 1 (9%) with poor urinary flow. Urodynamic study demonstrated areflexia in 4 (36%) patients, hyperreflexia in 3 (27%), hyporeflexia in 2 (18%), and urinary outflow obstruction without evidence of neurologic involvement in 2 (18%).

Electromyographic studies of the urinary sphincter were done in 8 of the patients. Only 2 of them had abnormalities: one with myelopathy exhibited poor recruitment of neuronal activity and the remaining patient with cauda equina syndrome had many fibrillatory potentials.[59]

Menendez et al reported urodynamic evaluations of 3 patients with AIDS and neurogenic bladder. Two of the patients had areflexic bladder secondary to ascending myelitis by herpes simplex virus type II in 1 patient, and cerebral abscess from toxoplasmosis in the other patient. A third patient with AIDS dementia complex exhibited a hyperreflexic detrusor. Voiding symptoms improved in all 3 patients with institution of antiviral, antibiotic, and anticholinergic medications, respectively.[60]

Guillain–Barré syndrome

Guillain–Barré syndrome is an idiopathic polyradiculopathy frequently related to viral illnesses or vaccination. Lesions of the motor neuron in the spinal nerve are seen on pathological examination. Clinically, it is characterized by motor paralysis initially in the lower extremities and progressing cephalad.

Kogan et al first reported urodynamic findings in 2 patients with Guillain–Barré syndrome in 1981. Both patients were found to have motor paralytic bladders on cystometrogram evaluation.[61]

Wheeler et al reported urodynamic findings on 7 patients with Guillain–Barré syndrome. Impaired voiding with large residuals was present in all 7 patients. Urodynamic studies revealed 4 patients with detrusor areflexia and nonrelaxation of the perineal muscles with a positive bethanechol supersensitivity test. Three of these 4 patients had abnormal perineal EMG studies that demonstrated a decreased interference pattern with polyphasic potentials, which is characteristic of motor denervation. Three of the 7 patients had detrusor hyperreflexia with appropriate sphincter relaxation. Intravesical sensation, although decreased, was present in 6 patients and completely absent in 1 patient.[62]

Another study by Sakakibara et al described urologic findings in 28 patients with Guillain–Barré syndrome. Micturitional symptoms were seen in 25% of patients and included voiding difficulty in 6, transient urinary retention in 3, nocturnal urinary frequency in 3, urinary urgency in 3, diurnal urinary frequency in 2, urge incontinence in 2, and stress incontinence in 1. Urodynamic evaluation in 4 patients revealed disturbed sensation in 1 patient, bladder areflexia in 1, and absence of bulbocavernosus reflex in another. Cystometry showed decreased bladder volume in 2 and bladder overactivity in 2, one of whom had urge urinary incontinence and the other urinary retention.[63]

Herpes

Herpes zoster infection is a viral syndrome characterized by a painful vesicular eruption involving one or more dermatomes and inflammation of the corresponding dorsal root ganglia. Both sensory and motor neurons can be affected.

Cohen et al reviewed the literature of herpes zoster associated with bladder and/or bowel dysfunction since 1970. Thirty-two cases had been reported. Urinary retention was present in 28 (88%), symptoms of cystitis (dysuria, frequency, hesitancy) in 13 (41%), symptoms of both retention and cystitis in 11 (34%), and constipation and/or fecal incontinence in 20 (63%) patients. Sacral dermatomes (S2–S4) were involved in 78% of cases; lumbar and thoracic dermatomes were affected in 16% and 2% of patients, respectively. Men were affected more commonly than women (66% vs 34%). Patients tended to present in the sixth to eighth decades of life, although some women in their twenties have been reported. Cystometrograms typically show absent detrusor spikes or flaccid neurogenic bladders.[64]

In 1993, Brosetta et al published urologic findings on 57 patients diagnosed with and treated for herpes zoster infection. Fifty-four percent of the patients were men and the mean age was 51 years. Thirty-seven percent of patients had some type of immunodeficiency (HIV, hepatic disease, lymphoproliferative disorder). Fifteen of the 57 (26%) had urologic manifestations. Two of the 15 (13%) exhibited urinary retention and were found to have detrusor areflexia on CMG. Three of the 15 (20%) exhibited incontinence and detrusor hyperreflexia on CMG.[65]

Human T-lymphotropic virus

HTLV-I-associated myelopathy (HAM) is a slowly progressive spastic paraparesis caused by infection with human

T-lymphotropic virus type I (HTLV-I) and less frequently with HTLV type II. Clinical manifestations result from demyelination and eventual atrophy of the thoracic spinal cord. The myelopathy has a peak incidence in HTLVinfected patients age 40–50 years and women are affected more than men. Co-infection with HIV results in an increased rate of myelopathy among those with HTLV infection. Murphy et al performed a cross-sectional analysis of HTLV-seropositive subjects who were detected from 5 blood donor centers in the United States. Myelopathy was confirmed in 4 of 166 (2.4%) HTLV-I-positive subjects and in 1 of 404 (0.25%) HTLV-II-positive subjects. All 5 patients diagnosed with HAM underwent urodynamic evaluation and all were found to have dyssynergic bladder contractions. In fact, urinary urgency and incontinence were the most common presenting symptoms and 2 of the patients had undergone urodynamic evaluation prior to enrollment in the study.[66]

Lyme disease

Lyme disease is caused by the spirochete *Borrelia burgdorferi.* It is the most common tick-borne disease in the United States and is associated with a variety of neurologic sequelae. Chancellor et al evaluated 7 patients with confirmed Lyme disease and associated lower urinary tract dysfunction. Most of the patients had paraparesis with partial sensory loss and 1 was temporarily in a coma. Two patients had urinary retention, 4 patients had one or more irritative symptoms (frequency, urge incontinence, nocturia), and 1 patient had enuresis. On urodynamic evaluation, 5 of the patients demonstrated detrusor hyperreflexia and 2 had detrusor areflexia. Detrusor-sphincter dyssynergia was not observed in any patient. Of the five patients with detrusor hyperreflexia, 2 were aware of the involuntary contractions but could not inhibit them and 3 were unaware of the involuntary contractions. With follow-up after intravenous antibiotics ranging from 6 months to 2 years, urologic symptoms resolved completely in 4 patients, while in 3 patients, symptoms improved but with residual urgency and frequency.[67]

Poliomyelitis

Acute poliomyelitis is often associated with urinary retention owing to detrusor areflexia, although bladder function is generally recovered. Uninhibited detrusor contractions with urge incontinence or an atonic bladder with weak, ineffective detrusor contractions may also be seen.[68] Howard et al reported an 11% prevalence of retention in 23 of 203 patients during the acute polio episode, whereas 69/203 (34%) had chronic urinary symptoms persisting after resolution of the acute episode.[69]

Progressive functional deterioration occurring years after an acute episode of poliomyelitis is termed postpolio syndrome (PPS). It manifests as new-onset or progressive motor or visceral dysfunction, or as joint or limb deterioration. It may be present in as many as 78% of patients with a history of polio. Symptoms can be classified into two categories: those associated with orthopedic and joint deterioration and those caused by neurologic deterioration. The symptoms are exacerbated by physical activity or fatigue. The mechanism is not known but may be secondary to premature or accelerated loss of anterior horn cells that innervate large numbers of muscle fibers, loss of neuronal cell terminals that had sprouted to innervate muscle fibers, reactivation of the virus, deterioration of the immune system, and intercurrent neurologic or nonneurologic diseases.[69]

Johnson et al evaluated 330 completed questionnaires mailed randomly to subjects in West Texas with a history of polio. Eighty-seven percent of women and 74% of males reported symptoms of PPS. The mean age of responders was 55 years. The mean age at acute attack was 10 years and the mean interval between the acute episode and the development of PPS was 33 years for females and 36 years for males. Three hundred and six (93%) patients reported urologic symptoms which included change in bladder function, change in sexual function, frequency 8 voids/day, nocturia 2 voids/night, hesitancy, urgency, intermittency, post-void dribbling, and decreased force of stream. Thirty-five patients (10.6%) reported detrusor instability Only a few had symptoms compatible with hypocontractile or areflexic bladders, requiring catheterization.

The prevalence of incontinence among females was similar among those with and without PPS (72% vs 77%, respectively); however, the severity of incontinence was worse in those with PPS. Incontinence in men was limited to post-void dribbling or urge incontinence. These symptoms were worse in men with PPS.[70]

Syphilis

Voiding dysfunction related to neurosyphilis had a high prevalence in the pre-penicillin era. Voiding dysfunction caused by decreased vesical sensation resulted in large residual urine and bladder decompensation. Fortunately, improvements in medical care have made neurosyphilis arare entity.

Neurosyphilis affects males more than females and presents in middle-aged years after a period of latency. Roughly 10% of patients infected with primary syphilis later develop neurosyphilis. Lumbosacral meningomyelitis with involvement of the dorsal cord and/or spinal roots (tabes dorsalis) results in bladder dysfunction. This manifests as decreased bladder sensation, large bladder capacity, and high post-void residuals. In some patients, typically those with general paresis of the insane, incontinence can occur which is usually functional or possibly the result of uninhibited detrusor activity as seen in upper motor neuron lesions.[71]

Brodie reported on 13 patients with neurosyphilis and bladder involvement. Twelve of the 13 had classic detrusor areflexia and decreased bladder sensation, leading to overdistention. One patient had detrusor hyperreflexia.[72]

Garber et al reported on 3 patients with tertiary syphilis. All 3 were found to have hypocompliant bladders with detrusor hyperreflexia, detrusor-sphincter dyssynergia, and elevated residual volumes on videocystometrography. This small group of patients demonstrates how tertiary syphilis can manifest with upper motor neuron bladder dysfunction.[73]

Tuberculosis

Tuberculosis can affect the spine. Spinal tuberculosis is more severe, dangerous, and disabling in children than in adults. Mushkin and Kovalenko studied 32 patients under the age of 16 years with thoracic and lumbar spinal tuberculosis who underwent antibiotic and surgical treatment. Paraplegia occurred in 8 patients and was always associated with bladder and bowel dysfunction. Three other patients without paraplegia also had bladder and bowel dysfunction (34%, overall). Eight of the 11 recovered bladder and bowel function postoperatively. Urodynamic evaluations were not included in this report.[74]

Radical pelvic surgery

Rectal carcinoma/resection

Urinary dysfunction as a consequence of damage to important neuroanatomic structures remains a common complication of radical pelvic surgery, particularly in abdominoperineal resection (APR) for rectal carcinoma. The extent of primary resection and lymphadenectomy are major determinants of degree of postoperative urologic morbidity. The incidence of *de-novo* urinary dysfunction following APR has been reported to be as high as 70%. Urinary retention caused by detrusor denervation is the most common type of voiding dysfunction after APR, and is the result of disruption of detrusor branches of the pelvic nerve. Less commonly, stress urinary incontinence secondary to denervation of the external sphincter or direct injury to the muscle itself can occur.[75]

Voiding dysfunction is more severe after APR than after rectal sphincter-preserving procedures, such as low anterior resection (LAR), and degree of dysfunction is related to the extent of dissection. In a study by Hojo et al, 22 of 25 patients (88%) who underwent preservation of the autonomic nerves were voiding spontaneously by postoperative day 10, whereas 28 of 36 patients (78%) with complete resection of the pelvic autonomic nerves still had urinary retention and were dependent on indwelling catheter drainage by postoperative day 60.[76]

Similar studies by Mitsui et al and Sugihara et al demonstrated that 100% of patients undergoing bilateral nerve sparing with radical resection for rectal carcinoma regained spontaneous voiding postoperativley.[77,78] When unilateral pelvic plexus preservation is performed, over 90% are able to void spontaneously. Thirty percent of patients undergoing complete resection of pelvic autonomic nerves in Sugihara's study required self-catheterization. In Mitsui's series, only 30% of patients in the nonpreserved group voided normally. Interestingly, they noted no significant difference in lower urinary tract function between patients receiving LAR vs APR.

Michelassi and Block reported on 27 patients who underwent either conventional (10) or wide (17) pelvic lymphadenectomy with radical resection for carcinoma of the rectum. They noted that 18% of patients undergoing wide pelvic lymphadenectomy required intermittent self-catheterization postoperatively. All patients in this group were able to stop catheterization within 8 months of thesurgery.[79]

Cosimelli et al reported minimal urologic morbidity in 57 male patients undergoing LAR and limited lumboaortic lymphadenectomy. Less than 3% had urinary incontinence and 4.2% experienced urinary retention.[80]

Radical hysterectomy

Voiding dysfunction after radical hysterectomy and pelvic lymphadenectomy for carcinoma of the cervix has typically manifested as bladder atonia. An early report by Ketcham et al revealed an 8% rate of atonia requiring Foley catheter drainage postoperatively.[81]

Seski and Diokno prospectively studied 10 patients before and after radical hysterectomy. Results suggest that a hypertonic phase immediately postoperatively is transient and secondary to myogenic tonicity. By 6–8 weeks postoperatively, bladder capacity and compliance returned to the preoperative level. Only 1/10 (10%) developed significant detrusor denervation, as demonstrated by a positive bethanechol supersensitivity test.[82]

A more recent report by Lin et al reported urodynamic results on patients who underwent either radical hysterectomy, pelvic radiation, or both, and compared them to a control group of patients with cervical cancer before treatment. Detrusor instability or low bladder compliance was found in 57%, 45%, 80%, and 24% of patients, respectively. Each group was found to have decreased bladder capacity. The frequency of abdominal strain voiding was 100% in all treatment groups, but was 0% in the pretreatment group. Abnormal residual urine was seen in 41%, 27%, 40%, and 24% of patients, respectively.[83]

Spinal stenosis

Lumbar spinal stenosis does not often cause chronic bladder dysfunction. However, when it does, it is considered to be an advanced form and is related to compression of the cauda equina. Kawaguchi et al evaluated 37 patients with lumbar spinal stenosis before and after decompressive laminectomy. Twenty-nine patients had subjective urinary complaints. Preoperative CMG studies revealed 23 patients (62%) with neuropathic bladders (18 underactive, 5 overactive). Thirty-eight percent had normal CMG studies. Postoperative CMG studies in 9 patients with neuropathic bladders demonstrated a normal pattern in 6 patients, with 3 exhibiting a persistent underactive bladder.[84]

Cervical spondylosis is a generalized disease process which can affect all levels of the cervical spine. When the pathology is located laterally, spondylosis causes only radicular symptoms, whereas a central or paracentral location can cause cord compression in addition to root lesions. Lower urinary tract sphincter disturbances and bladder dysfunction (frequency, urgency, urge incontinence) can be seen along with lower extremity signs such as gait disturbance, lower extremity spasticity, and hyperactive tendon reflexes. Tammela et al performed urodynamic studies on 30 consecutive patients with clinically and radiologically verified cervical spondylosis causing radiculopathy and/or myelopathy. Sixty-one percent of patients complained of irritative bladder symptoms, and detrusor hyperactivity was demonstrated urodynamically in 46%. Twenty-five percent had hyperreflexic detrusor contractions with ice water provocation. Sensitivity to cold was lacking in 39%. Eleven percent described difficulty emptying the bladder and all were found to have hypotonic detrusors.[85]

Spine surgery

The incidence of voiding dysfunction after spinal surgery has been shown to be as high as 60%.[86] Boulis et al reported an incidence of 38% of 503 patients undergoing routine cervical or lumbar laminectomy or discectomy. Neither the rate nor the duration of retention between men and women was significantly different. Patients undergoing cervical or lumbar laminectomy were found to have longer duration of retention than those undergoing cervical or lumbar discectomy. Preoperative use of beta-blockers was associated with increased risk of urinary retention postoperatively. Patients who developed urinary retention were older on average than those who did not develop retention (51.9 years vs 48.4 years). The rate of retention did not differ significantly between groups who did and did not have intraoperative Foley catheters placed.[87]

Brooks et al performed urodynamic evaluations on 74 patients who complained of new onset (69) voiding symptoms or exacerbation of underlying voiding symptoms (5) after undergoing lumbosacral laminectomy, discectomy, or both. Sixty percent were found to have pathologic urodynamic findings. Sixteen percent were found to have a hypoesthetic bladder and 24% demonstrated a hyperesthetic bladder. Fourteen percent had bladder capacities less than 200 ml while another 14% had capacities greater than 500 ml.[86]

Other causes of neurogenic bladder

Non-neurogenic neurogenic bladder

Non-neurogenic neurogenic bladder, also known as Hinman's syndrome is a functional bladder outlet obstruction caused by voluntary contractions of the external urethral sphincter during voiding. It is a learned voiding dysfunction developed early in life by children in response to uncontrolled bladder contractions. Typically, patients present with frequency, urgency, urinary incontinence, recurrent urinary tract infections, or occasionally encopresis. The voiding dysfunction is usually acquired after toilet training and tends to resolve after puberty.[88,89] The syndrome is rare in children. Reports on the prevalence of Hinman's syndrome in adults vary. Jorgensen et al reported a 0.5% prevalence rate among patients referred for urodynamic evaluation.[90]

In scanning a urodynamic database of 1015 consecutive adults referred for evaluation of voiding dysfunction, Groutz et al identified 21 (2%) patients (13 women, 8 men) who met criteria for Hinman's syndrome. Ninety-five percent of the patients exhibited obstructive symptoms and more than half had frequency, nocturia, and urgency. On non-invasive uroflow evaluation, all patients exhibited an intermittent flow pattern. On urodynamic study, firstsensation volume was significantly lower in women than in men (123 vs 272 ml). This trend was also seen in first urge, strong urge, and bladder capacity volumes. Fourteen percent (3) were also found to have detrusor instability. Detrusor pressure at maximum flow and maximum detrusor pressure during voiding were both found to be significantly higher in men than in women. The authors concluded that the prevalence of this condition among the adult population may actually be higher than 2%.[89]

Myasthenia gravis

Myasthenia gravis (MG) is an autoimmune disorder whereby antibodies against the nicotinic cholinergic receptors of neuromuscular transmission result in muscle weakness and easy fatigability. It typically affects striated muscle, although antibodies against smooth muscle muscarinic receptors have been identified as well. Voiding dysfunction in association with the disease is rare.[91]

There are reports in the literature which note an association between MG and incontinence in men with prostatic bladder outlet obstruction. It has been hypothesized that thorough resection led to injury to a sphincter already compromised by the underlying neurologic disorder and the authors recommended incomplete resection to prevent this complication.[92] Another small series of 8 men with MG and prostatic resection found that patients who underwent TURP (transurethral resection of the prostate) with blended current all became incontinent, but men who underwent TURP with either high-frequency unblended current, partial proximal resection, or open prostatectomy remained dry.[93] Khan and Bhola published a report of 1 patient who underwent open prostatectomy and remained dry. EMG studies revealed that although his sphincter functioned normally, it did demonstrate easy fatigability.[94]

There are 4 reports in the literature of voiding dysfunction in patients with no history of TURP. Howard et al reported a 31-year-old female with recurrent incontinence after undergoing bladder neck suspension for stress incontinence. She was found to have an open bladder neck, inability to sustain a pelvic floor contraction, and hyperreflexia which occurred concomitantly with deterioration of her myasthenia gravis.[95] Three other publications reported patients with myasthenia gravis and voiding dysfunction with either detrusor hyporeflexia or areflexia.[96–98]

References

1. Nitti VW, Adler H, Combs AJ. The role of urodynamics in the evaluation of voiding dysfunction in men after cerebrovascular accident. J Urol 1996; 155: 263–266.
2. Marinkovic SP, Badlani G. Voiding and sexual dysfunction after cerebrovascular accidents. J Urol 2001; 165: 359–370.
3. Wade DT, Hewer RL. Outlook after an acute stroke: urinary incontinence and loss of consciousness compared in 532 patients. Q J Med 1985; 56: 601–608.
4. Taub NA, Wolfe CD, Richardson E, Burney PG. Predicting the disability of first-time stroke sufferers at 1 year. 12-month follow-up of a population-based cohort in Southeast England. Stroke 1994; 25: 352–357.
5. Gelber DA, Good DC, Laven LJ, Verhulst SJ. Causes of urinary incontinence after acute hemispheric stroke. Stroke 1993; 24: 378–382.
6. Brocklehurst JC, Andrews K, Richards B, Laycock PJ. Incidence and correlates of incontinence in stroke patients. J Am Geriatr Soc 1985; 33: 540–542.
7. Leach GE, Farsaii A, Kark P, Raz S. Urodynamic manifestations of cerebellar ataxia. J Urol 1982; 128: 348–350.
8. Andrew J, Nathan PW. Lesions of the anterior frontal lobes and disturbances of micturition and defaecation. Brain 1964; 87: 233–262.
9. Maurice-Williams RS. Micturition symptoms in frontal tumors. J Neurol Neurosurg Psychiatr 1974; 37: 431–436.
10. Blaivas JG. The neurophysiology of micturition: a clinical study of 550 patients. J Urol 1982; 127: 958–963.
11. Lang EW, Chestnut RM, Hennerici M. Urinary retention and spaceoccupying lesions of the frontal cortex. Eur Neurol 1996; 36: 43–47.
12. Jonas S, Brown J. Neurogenic bladder in normal pressure hydrocephalus. Urology 1975; 5: 44–50.
13. McNeal DM, Hawtrey CE, Wolraich ML, Mapel JR. Symptomatic neurogenic bladder in a cerebral-palsied population. Dev Med Child Neurol 1983; 25: 612–616.
14. Decter RM, Bauer SB, Khoshbin S, et al. Urodynamic assessment of children with cerebral palsy. J Urol 1987; 138: 1110–1112.
15. Hellstrom PA, Jarvelin M, Kontturi MJ, Huttunen NP. Bladder function in the mentally retarded. Br J Urol 1990; 66: 475–478.
16. Mitchell SJF, Woodthorpe J. Young mentally handicapped adults in three London boroughs: prevalence and degree of disability. J Epidemiol Comm Health 1981; 35: 59–64.
17. Reid AH, Ballinger BR, Heather BB. Behavioural syndromes identified by cluster analysis in a sample of 100 severely and profoundly retarded adults. Psychol Med 1978; 8: 399–412.
18. Pavlakis AJ, Siroky MB, Goldstein I, Krane RJ. Neurourologic findings in Parkinson's disease. J Urol 1983; 129: 80–83.
19. Langworthy OR, Lewis LG, Dees JE, Hesser FH. Clinical study of control of bladder by central nervous system. Bull Johns Hopkins Hosp 1936; 58: 89.
20. Murnaghan GF. Neurogenic disorders of the bladder in parkinsonism. Br J Urol 1961; 33: 403–409.
21. Porter RW, Bors E. Neurogenic bladder in parkinsonism: effect of thalamotomy. J Neurosurg 1971; 34: 27–32.
22. Araki I, Kitahara M, Oida T, Kuno S. Voiding dysfunction and Parkinson's disease: urodynamic abnormalities and urinary symptoms. J Urol 2000; 164: 1640–1643.
23. Shy GM, Drager GA. A neurological syndrome associated with orthostatic hypotension: a clinico-pathologic study. Arch Neurol 1960; 2: 511–527.
24. Salinas JM, Berger Y, De La Rocha RE, Blaivas JG. Urological evaluation in the Shy Drager syndrome. J Urol 1986; 135: 741–743.
25. Fingerman JS, Finkelstein LH. The overactive bladder in multiple sclerosis. JAOA 2000; 100: S9–S12.
26. Rashid TM, Hollander JB. Multiple sclerosis and the neurogenic bladder. Phys Med Rehabil Clin N Am 1998; 9: 615–629.
27. Litwiller SE, Frohman EM, Zimmern PE. Multiple sclerosis and the urologist. J Urol 1999; 161: 743–757.
28. Ciancio SJ, Mutchnik SE, Rivera VM, Boone TB. Urodynamic pattern changes in multiple sclerosis. Urology 2001; 57: 239–245.
29. Selzman AA, Elder JS, Mapstone TB. Urologic consequences of myelodysplasia and other congenital abnormalities of the spinal cord. Urol Clin N Am 1993; 20: 485–504.
30. Pontari MA, Keating M, Kelly M, et al. Retained sacral function in children with high level myelodysplasia. J Urol 1995; 154: 775–777.
31. Spindel MR, Bauer SB, Dyro FM, et al. The changing neurourologic lesion in myelodysplasia. JAMA 1987; 258: 1630–1633.
32. McGuire EJ, Woodside JR, Borden TA, Weiss RM. Prognostic value of urodynamic testing in myelodysplastic patients. J Urol 1981; 126: 205–209.
33. Bauer SB, Hallett M, Khoshbin S, et al. Predictive value of urodynamic evaluation in newborns with myelodysplasia. JAMA 1984; 252: 650–652.
34. Pang D, Wilberger JE. Tethered cord syndrome in adults. J Neurosurg 1982; 57: 32–47.
35. Adamson AS, Gelister J, Hayward R, Snell ME. Tethered cord syndrome: an unusual cause of adult bladder dysfunction. Br J Urol 1993; 71: 417–421.

36. Flanigan RC, Russell DP, Walsh JW. Urological aspects of tethered cord. Urology 1989; 33: 80–82.
37. Guzman L, Bauer SB, Hallet M, et al. Evaluation and management of children with sacral agenesis. Urology 1983; 22: 506–510.
38. Koff SA, Deridder PA. Patterns of neurogenic dysfunction in sacral agenesis. J Urol 1977; 118: 87–89.
39. Waites KB, Canupp KC, DeVivo MJ, et al. Compliance with annual urologic evaluations and preservation of renal function in persons with spinal cord injury. J Spinal Cord Med 1995; 18: 251–254.
40. Burns AS, Rivas DA, Ditunno JF. The management of neurogenic bladder and sexual dysfunction after spinal cord injury. Spine 2001; 26: S129–S136.
41. Diokno AC, Koff SA, Anderson W. Combined cystometry and perineal electromyography in the diagnosis and treatment of neurogenic urinary incontinence. J Urol 1976; 115: 161–163.
42. Kaplan SA, Chancellor MB, Blaivas JG. Bladder and sphincter behavior in patients with spinal cord lesions. J Urol 1991; 146: 113–117.
43. Weld KJ, Dmochowski RR. Association of level of injury and bladder behavior in patients with post-traumatic spinal cord injury. Urology 2000; 55: 490–494.
44. Smith CP, Kraus SR, Nickell KG, Boone TM. Video urodynamic findings in men with the central cord syndrome. J Urol 2000; 164: 2014–2017.
45. Nath M, Wheeler JS, Walter JS. Urologic aspects of traumatic central cord syndrome. J Am Paraplegia Soc 1993; 16: 160–164.
46. Ross MA. Neuropathies associated with diabetes. Med Clin N Am 1993; 77: 111–124.
47. Kaplan SA, Blaivas JG. Diabetic cystopathy. J Diabet Complications 1988; 2: 133–139.
48. Kaplan SA, Te AE, Blaivas JG. Urodynamic findings in patients with diabetic cystopathy. J Urol 1995; 153: 342–344.
49. Kitami K. Vesicourethral dysfunction of diabetic patients. Nippon Hinyokika Gakkai Zasshi 1991; 82: 1074–1083.
50. Moller CF. Diabetic cystopathy. I: A clinical study of the frequency of bladder dysfunction in diabetics. Dan Med Bull 1976; 23: 267–278.
51. Fanciullacci F, Sandri S, Politi P, Zanollo A. Clinical, urodynamic and neurophysiological findings in patients with neuropathic bladder due to a lumbar intervertebral disc protrusion. Parapelgia 1989; 27: 354–358.
52. O'Flynn KJ, Murphy R, Thomas DG. Neurogenic bladder dysfunction in lumbar intervertebral disc prolapse. Br J Urol 1992; 69: 38–40.
53. Bartolin Z, Gilja I, Bedalov G, Savic I. Bladder function in patients with lumbar intervertebral disk protrusion. J Urol 1998; 159: 969–971.
54. Bartolin Z, Vilendecic M, Derezic D. Bladder function after surgery for lumbar intervertebral disk protrusion. J Urol 1999; 161: 1885–1887.
55. Chang HS, Nakagawa H, Mizuno J. Lumbar herniated disc presenting with cauda equina syndrome: long-term follow-up of four cases. Surg Neurol 2000; 53: 100–105.
56. Britton CB, Miller JR. Neurologic complications in acquired immunodeficiency syndrome (AIDS). Neurol Clin 1984; 2: 315–339.
57. Levy RM, Bredesen DE, Rosenblum ML. Neurological manifestations of acquired immunodeficiency syndrome: experiences at UCSF and review of the literature. J Neurosurg 1985; 62: 475–495.
58. Snider WD, Simpson DM, Nielsen S, et al. Neurological complications of acquired immune deficiency syndrome: analysis of 50 patients. Ann Neurol 1983; 14: 403–418.
59. Khan Z, Singh VK, Yang WC. Neurogenic bladder in acquired immune deficiency syndrome (AIDS). Urology 1992; 40: 289–291.
60. Menendez V, Valls J, Espuna M, et al. Neurogenic bladder in patients with acquired immunodeficiency syndrome. Neurourol Urodyn 1995; 14: 253–257.
61. Kogan BA, Solomon MH, Diokno AC. Urinary retention secondary to Landry–Guillain–Barré syndrome. J Urol 1981; 126: 643–644.
62. Wheeler JS, Siroky MB, Pavlakis A, Krane RJ. The urodynamic aspects of the Guillain–Barré syndrome. J Urol 1984; 131: 917–919.
63. Sakakibara R, Hattori T, Kuwabara S, et al. Micturitional disturbance in patients with Guillain–Barré syndrome. J Neurol Neurosurg Psychiatr 1997; 63: 649–653.
64. Cohen LM, Fowler JF, Owen LG, Callen JP. Urinary retention associated with herpes zoster infection. Int J Dermatol 1993; 32: 24–26.
65. Broseta E, Osca JM, Morera J, et al. Urological manifestations of herpes zoster. Eur Urol 1993; 24: 244–247.
66. Murphy EL, Fridey J, Smith JW, et al. HTLV-associated myelopathy in a cohort of HTLV-I and HTLV-II-infected blood donors. Neurology 1997; 48: 315–320.
67. Chancellor MB, McGinnis DE, Shenot PJ, et al. Urinary dysfunction in Lyme disease. J Urol 1993; 149: 26–30.
68. Timmermans L, Bonnet F, Maquinay C. Urological complications of poliomyelitis and their treatment. Acta Urol Belg 1965; 33: 409–426.
69. Howard RS, Wiles CM, Spencer GT. The late sequelae of poliomyelitis. Q J Med 1988; 66: 219–232.
70. Johnson VY, Hubbard D, Vordermark JS. Urologic manifestations of postpolio syndrome. JWOCN 1996; 23: 218–223.
71. Wheeler JS, Culkin DJ, O'Hara RJ, Canning JR. Bladder dysfunction and neurosyphilis. J Urol 1986; 136: 903–905.
72. Brodie EL, Helfert I, Phifer IA. Cystometric observations in asymptomatic neurosyphilis. J Urol 1940; 43: 496–510.
73. Garber SJ, Christmas TJ, Rickards D. Voiding dysfunction due to neurosyphilis. Br J Urol 1990; 66: 19–21.
74. Mushkin AY, Kovalenko KN. Neurological complications of spinal tuberculosis in children. Int Orthop 1999; 23: 210–212.
75. Hollabaugh RS, Steiner MS, Sellers KD, et al. Neuroanatomy of the pelvis: implications for colonic and rectal resection. Dis Colon Rectum 2000; 43: 1390–1397.
76. Hojo K, Vernava AM, Sugihara K, Katumata K. Preservation of urine voiding and sexual function after rectal cancer surgery. Dis Colon Rectum 1991; 34: 532–539.
77. Mitsui T, Kobayashi S, Matsuura S, et al. Vesicourethral dysfunction following radical surgery for rectal carcinoma: change in voiding pattern on sequential urodynamic studies and impact of nerve-sparing surgery. Int J Urol 1998; 5: 35–38.
78. Sugihara K, Moriya Y, Akasu T, Fujita S. Pelvic autonomic nerve preservation for patients with rectal carcinoma: oncologic and functional outcome. Cancer 1996; 78: 1871–1880.
79. Michelassi F, Block GE. Morbidity and mortality of wide pelvic lymphadenectomy for rectal adenocarcinoma. Dis Colon Rectum 1992; 35: 1143–1147.
80. Cosimelli M, Mannella E, Giannarelli D, et al. Nerve-sparing surgery in 302 resectable rectosigmoid cancer patients: genitourinary morbidity and 10-year survival. Dis Colon Rectum 1994; 37: S42–46.
81. Ketcham AS, Hoye RC, Taylor PT, et al. Radical hysterectomy and pelvic lymphadenectomy for carcinoma of the uterine cervix. Cancer 1971; 28: 1272–1277.
82. Seski JC, Diokno AC. Bladder dysfunction after radical abdominal hysterectomy. Am J Obstet Gynecol 1977; 128: 643–651.
83. Lin HH, Sheu BC, Lo MC, Huang SC. Abnormal urodynamic findings after radical hysterectomy or pelvic irradiation for cervical cancer. Int J Gynaecol Obstet 1998; 63: 169–174.
84. Kawaguchi Y, Kanamori M, Ishihara H, et al. Clinical symptoms and surgical outcome in lumbar spinal stenosis patients with neuropathic bladder. J Spinal Disord 2001; 14: 404–410.
85. Tammela TLJ, Heiskari MJ, Lukkarinen OA. Voiding dysfunction and urodynamic findings in patients with cervical spondylotic spinal stenosis compared with severity of the disease. Br J Urol 1992; 70: 144–148.
86. Brooks ME, Moreno M, Sidi A, Braf ZF. Urologic complications after surgery on lumbosacral spine. Urology 1985; 26: 202–204.
87. Boulis NM, Mian FS, Rodriguez D, et al. Urinary retention following routine neurosurgical procedures. Surg Neurol 2001; 55: 23–28.
88. Hinman F. Nonneurogenic neurogenic bladder (the Hinman syndrome): 15 years later. J Urol 1986; 136: 769–777.

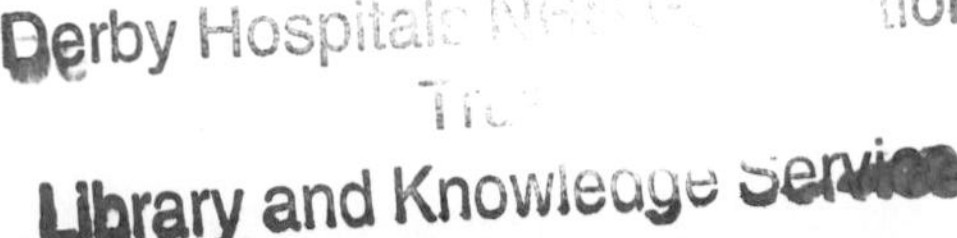

89. Groutz A, Blaivas JG, Pies C, Sassone AM. Learned voiding dysfunction (non-neurogenic, neurogenic bladder) among adults. Neurourol Urodynam 2001; 20: 259–268.
90. Jorgensen TM, Djurhuus JC, Schroder HD. Idiopathic detrusor sphincter dyssynergia in neurologically normal patients with voiding abnormalities. Eur Urol 1982; 8: 107–110.
91. Sandler PM, Avillo C, Kaplan SA. Detrusor areflexia in a patient with myasthenia gravis. Int J Urol 1998; 5: 188–190.
92. Greene LF, Ghosh MK, Howard FM. Transurethral prostatic resection in patients with myasthenia gravis. J Urol 1974; 12: 226–227.
93. Wise GJ, Gerstenfeld JN, Brunner N, Grob D. Urinary incontinence following prostatectomy in patients with myasthenia gravis. Br J Urol 1982; 54: 369–371.
94. Khan Z, Bhola A. Urinary incontinence after transurethral resection of prostate in myasthenia gravis patients. Urology 1989; 34: 168–169.
95. Howard JF, Donovan MK, Tucker MS. Urinary incontinence in myasthenia gravis: a single-fiber electromyographic study. Ann Neurol 1992; 32: 254(abstr).
96. Matsui M, Enoki M, Matsui Y et al. Seronegative myasthenia gravis associated with atonic urinary bladder and accommodative insufficiency. J Neurol Sci 1995; 133: 197–199.
97. Berger AR, Swerdlow M, Herskovitz S. Myasthenia gravis presenting as uncontrollable flatus and urinary/fecal incontinence. Muscle Nerve 1996; 19: 113–114.
98. Sandler PM, Avillo C, Kaplan SA. Detrusor areflexia in a patient with myasthenia gravis. Int J Urol 1998; 5: 188–190.

10

Ultrastructure of neurogenic bladders

Axel Haferkamp

Introduction

Functional pathology of the detrusor has evolved as a new paradigm for the clinical study of voiding dysfunction.[1,2] It defines altered microstructure of the detrusor and how it impacts on abnormalities of its function, as a corollary to the premise that normal detrusor microstructure and function are closely interrelated, if not interdependent.[3] This approach has led to a better understanding of various voiding dysfunctions, including incontinence, in the elderly, and promises to be equally valuable in similar disorders in younger patients.

Three distinctive ultrastructural patterns occurring separately or in combination have been described: the degeneration, dysjunction, and myohypertrophy patterns, respectively associated with impaired detrusor contractility (IDC), detrusor overactivity (DO), and detrusor with bladder outlet obstruction (BOO). A fourth so-called 'dense-band' pattern with depleted caveolae and elongated intervening dense bands of muscle cell membranes (sarcolemmas) appears to be characteristic of the aged detrusor, whether it is normal or dysfunctional.

To date, intrinsic structural defects in neurogenic bladder dysfunction (NBD) have been described in feline models, and proposed as the structural basis of the dysfunction associated with lower motoneuron injury or deficit.[4–6] Intrinsic structural defects of longstanding neurogenic bladder dysfunction due to an upper motoneuron lesion (spinal cord injury, brain disorder) or from a combined lower and upper motoneuron deficit (meningomyelocele) have been investigated in humans.[7–10]

Tissue preparation for ultrastructural evaluation

An endoscopic cold cup biopsy should be obtained extra-trigonally from the bladder wall. The open biopsy from the bladder wall should be excised by scalpel to obviate tissue destruction and artefacts of electrocautery. Each biopsy should be placed immediately in chilled fixative (2.5% glutaraldehyde in 0.1 M phosphate buffer containing 0.02% magnesium sulfate heptahydrate), and later processed for electron microscopy by a standardized procedure:[1,2,11] Specimen processing includes trimming of each specimen to yield 5–10 tissue blocks (~1 mm^3), postfixation in 1% osmium tetroxide, dehydration in ascending concentrations of ethanol, and embedment in Epon® or Araldite®. Semithin (1–2 μm) sections can be stained, for example with toluidine blue, and examined by light microscopy in order to select from each biopsy two blocks best suitable for electron microscopy (ample diagonally and longitudinally sectioned smooth muscle). Ultrathin (60 nm thick) sections of the selected blocks can be obtained by a diamond knife, mounted on uncoated 150-mesh copper grids, and stained by a standard uranyl acetate/lead citrate sequence. Between 8 and 12 sections on two grids from each tissue block should be examined and photographed by an electron microscope.

Following the MIN approach to structural study of the detrusor,[3] the ultrastructure of smooth muscle (M), interstitium (I), and intrinsic nerves (N) should be examined at various magnifications (×2500–100 000), both qualitatively and quantitatively.

Criteria for ultrastructural evaluation

Smooth muscle

The detrusor should be examined for grouping arrangement of the muscle cells as compact, intermediate, or loose fascicles[2] (Figure 10.1), and the various ultrastructural patterns of nonneuropathic vesical dysfunction.[1,2,12] Three distinctive ultrastructural patterns occurring separately or in combination have been described:

- Impaired detrusor contractility (IDC) is characterized structurally by a widespread marked degeneration of intrinsic muscle cells and axons (full degeneration pattern).[13,2]

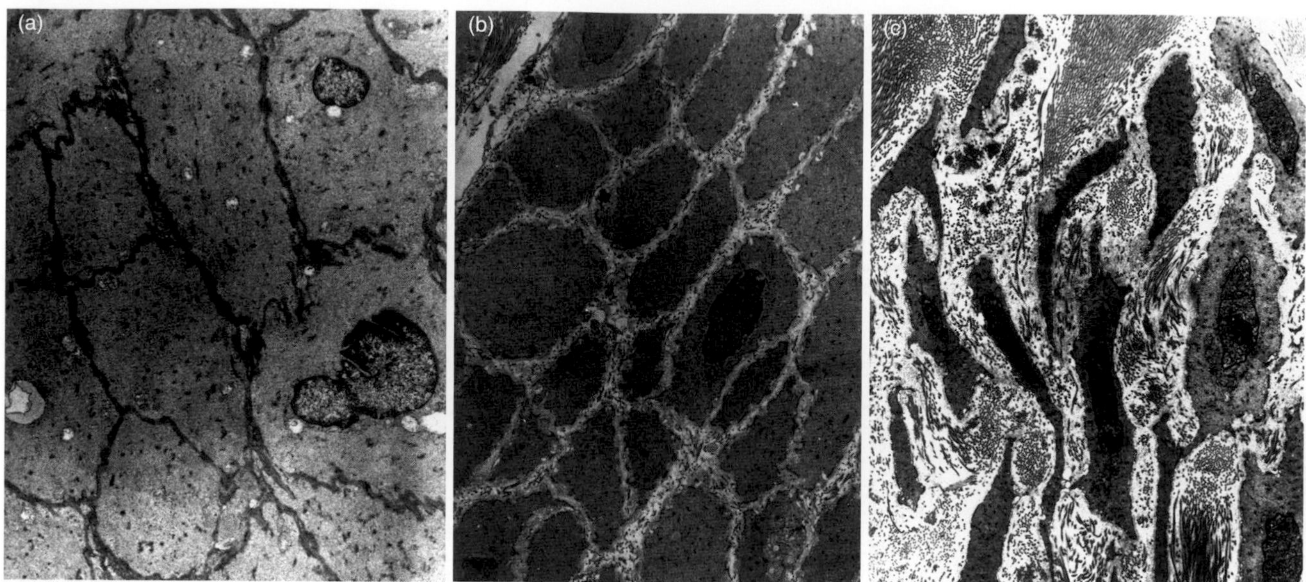

Figure 10.1
Fascicular arrangement of detrusor smooth muscle. (a) Compact (near-normal) fascicles with closely packed muscle cells: shortest intercellular distance 90 nm (Neg. # 45296; ×4109). (b) Intermediate fascicles with mild muscle cell separation: shortest intercellular distance 285 nm (Neg. # 46551; ×3897). (c) Loose fascicles; arrangement of widely separated muscle cells with lots of intercellular collagen fibrils: intercellular distance up to 1 μm or more (Neg. # 68816; ×4141).

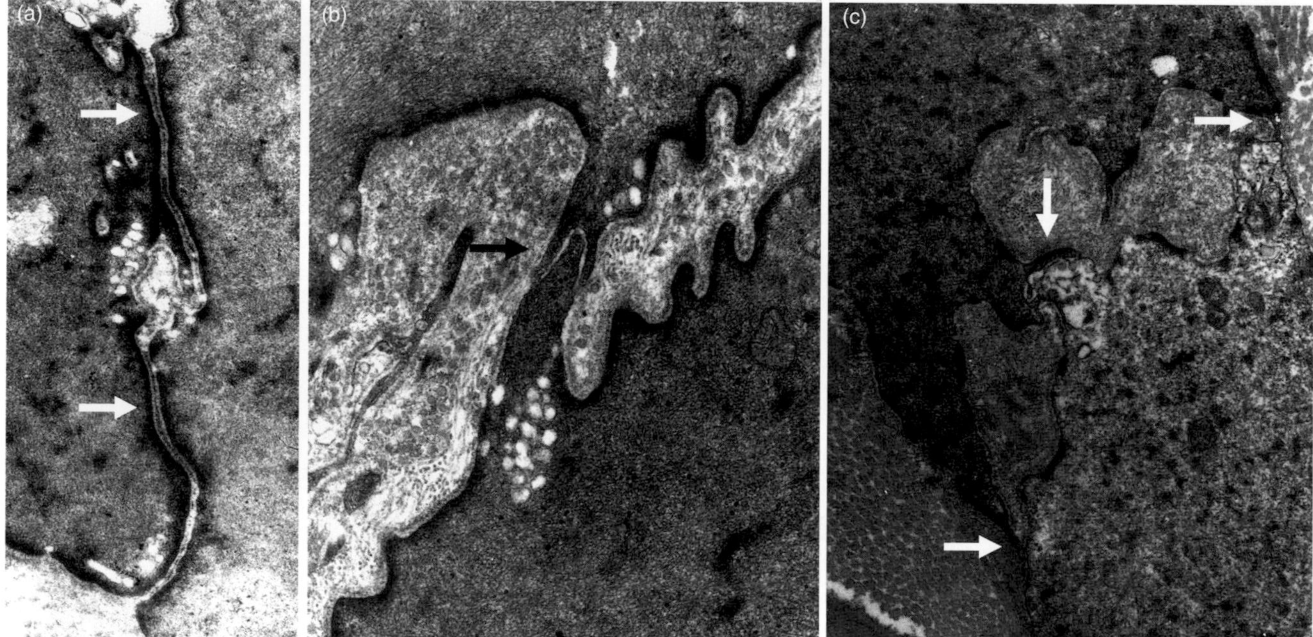

Figure 10.2
Muscle cell junctions. (a) Normal intermediate junctions (white arrows); note strictly parallel sarcolemmas with uniform 56 nm wide cell separation containing central linear density (Neg. # 45688; ×15 790). (b) Finger-like intimate cell apposition (ICA) (black arrow) (Neg. # 47271; ×27 900). (c) Finger-like intimate cell appositions (ICAs) (white arrows) (Neg. # 46718; ×17 860).

- BOO presents with muscle cell hypertrophy and increased collagen content of widened spaces between individual cells (myohypertrophy pattern).[14]
- Geriatric and obstructive DO has been associated with altered muscle cell junctions.

Intermediate junctions (IJs) of muscle cells predominate in normal detrusor, and mediate contraction coupling of muscle cells mechanically.[15] The IJ consists of strictly parallel sarcolemmas with paired symmetric dense plaques in the subsarcolemmal sarcoplasm, separated by a

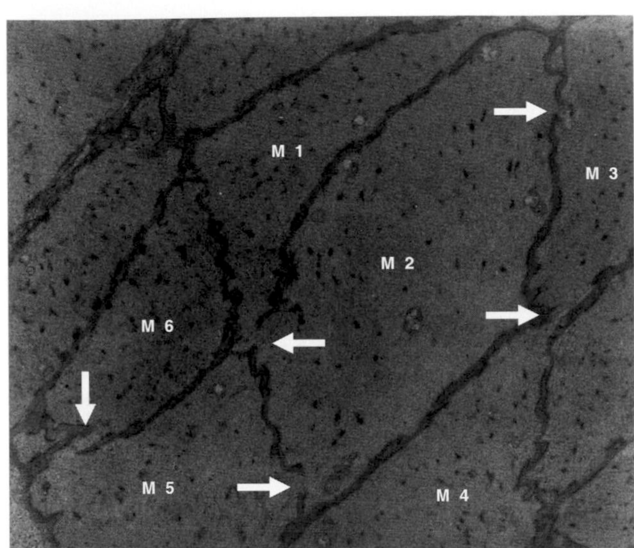

Figure 10.3
Muscle cell chain: six muscle cells (M1–6) chain-linked by finger-like protrusion junctions (white arrows) (Neg. # 45295; ×7425).

25–60 nm junctional gap containing a central linear density (Figure 10.2). The overactive detrusor has a distinctive ultrastructural pattern (complete dysjunction) of three essential components.[1,2,10,12,16] These are reduction or loss of IJs, abundance (or exclusive presence) of new cell junctions with very close separation gaps, introduced as protrusion junctions and ultraclose abutments and collectively designated as intimate cell appositions (ICAs) (Figure 10.2), and chain-like linkage of five or more muscle cells by these close junctions (Figure 10.3). With very close gaps (6–12 nm) between apposed sarcolemmas, these junctions were suggested as the myogenic basis of involuntary contractions during bladder filling (detrusor overactivity), mediating electrical coupling of muscle cells.[17]

A fourth (dense-band) pattern with depleted caveolae and elongation of intervening dense bands of musle cell membranes (sarcolemmas) was recognized as characteristic of the aged detrusor, be it normal or dysfunctional.[12]

Disruptive muscle cell degeneration is recognized by the disarray of sarcoplasmic myofilaments and dense bodies, sarcoplasmic vacuolation, sequestration or blebbing, and cell shrinkage or fragmentation (Figure 10.4).[1,2,12] The degeneration is considered rare when observed in one-quarter or less of the examined microscopic fields, focal when in one-quarter to one-half of the fields, widespread when in one-half to all the fields, and generalized when observed in every muscle cell – generally with condensation, intensified electron density, or disruption of its sarcoplasm. Muscle cells were also examined for features of regeneration, including nucleoli, expanded endoplasmic reticulum, and abundant mitochondria.

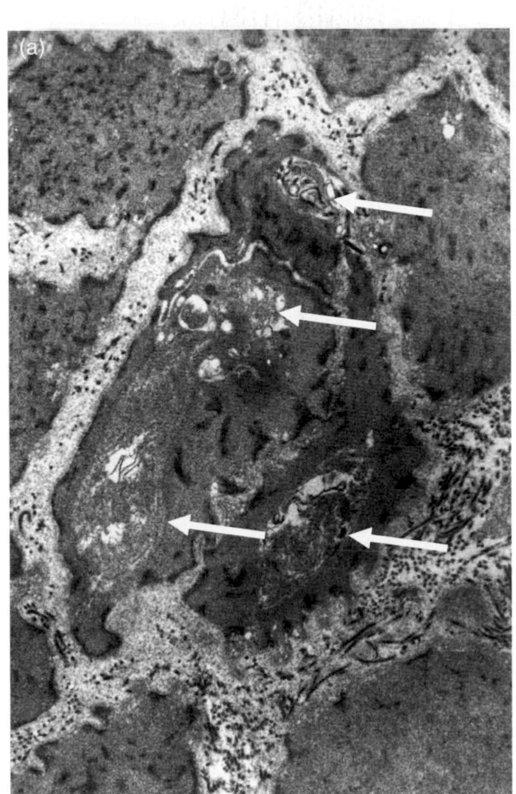

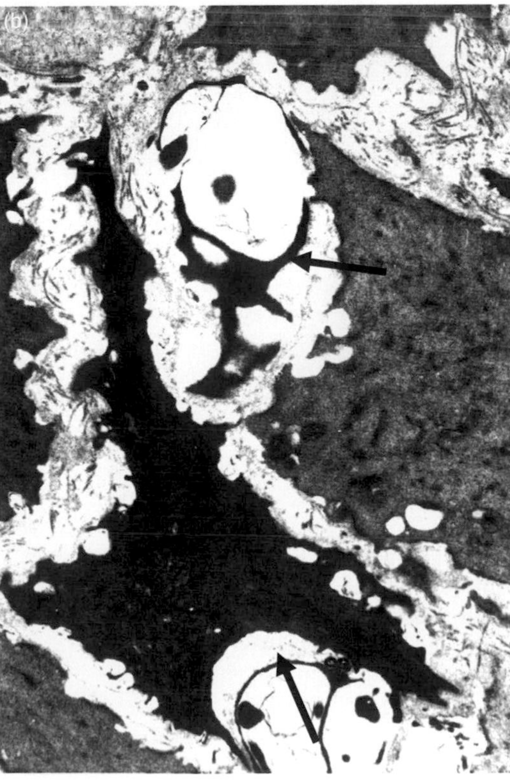

Figure 10.4
Disruptive muscle cell degeneration. (a) Vacuolated sarcoplasm: arrows (Neg. # 45803; ×7425). (b) Intensely electron-dense sarcoplasm of shrunken muscle cells: arrows (Neg. # 46694; ×7965).

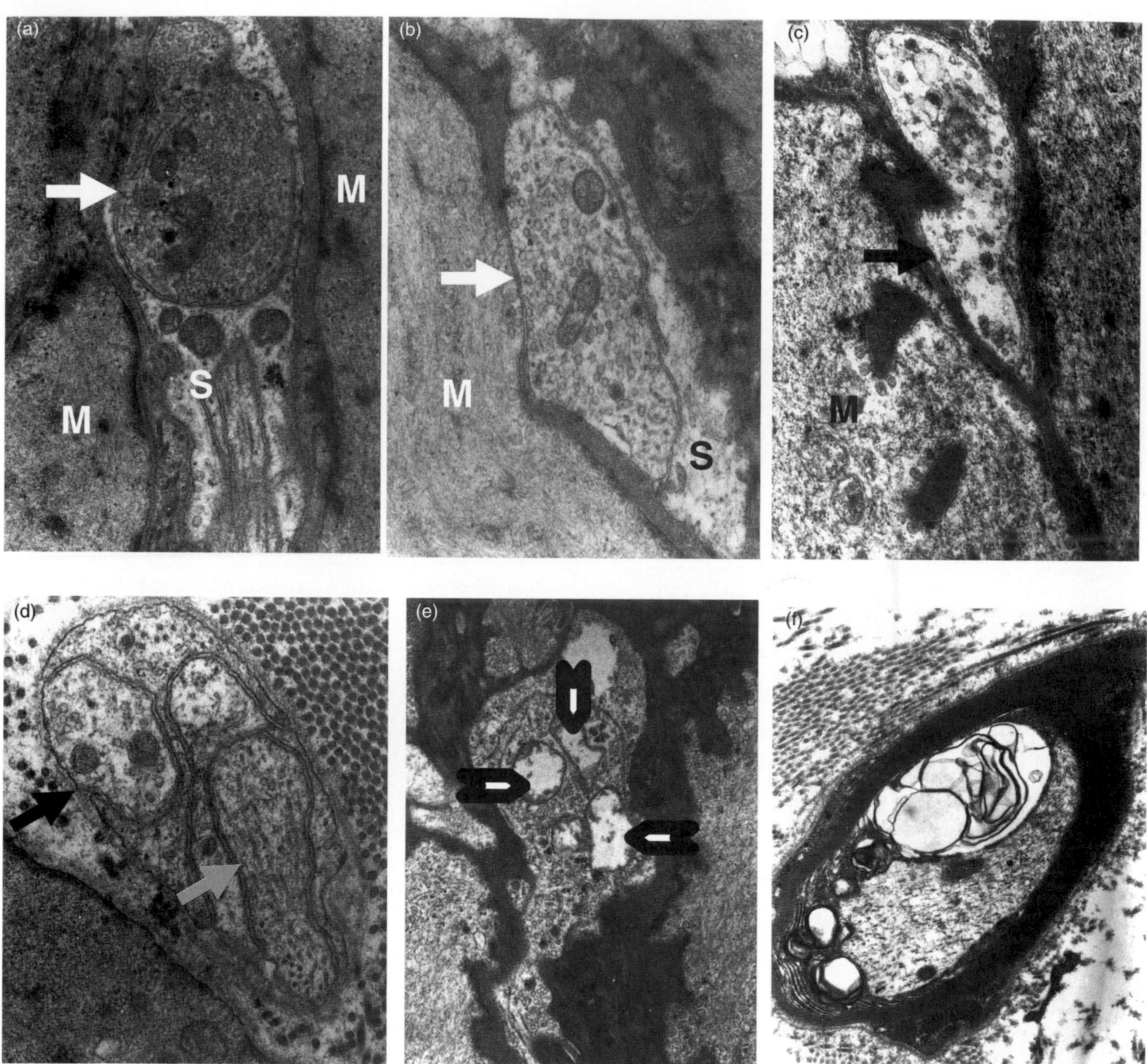

Figure 10.5 Intrinsic nerve profiles. (a) Normal axon terminal (cholinergic; white arrow), partially ensheated by a Schwann cell (S) at a neuroeffector junction with a muscle cell (M) (Neg. # 45304; ×21 649). (b) Axon terminal partially ensheathed by a Schwann cell (S) with a very small neuroeffector junctional gap (Neg. # 45368; ×25 200). (c) Degenerated axon terminal with reduced (black arrow) clear small vesicles at a neuroeffector junction (Neg. # 45646; ×26 069). (d) Schwann cell ensheathed (S) axon preterminals: degenerated with reduced (black arrow) or nearly depleted (white arrow) vesicles. (Neg. # 45269; ×29 077). (e) Degenerated axon terminal: bloated disrupted mitochondria (arrow) (Neg # 45562; ×16 614). (f) Nonvaricose segment of myelinated axon within nerve bundle, with features of degeneration: irregularly split myelin sheath, and collapsed axoplasm (Neg. # 46729; ×15 007).

Intrinsic neural elements

The ultrastructural morphology and content of axon terminals at neuroeffector junctions (axon–muscle cell contacts) and Schwann cells, together with their ensheathed unmyelinated and myelinated axons (axon preterminals and nonvaricose segments), should be evaluated. Profiles of unmyelinated axon terminals and preterminals can be defined as normal, degenerated, or regenerated.

Normal axon terminals within the detrusor (Figure 10.5) are unmyelinated and bare (without a Schwann cell sheath), are packed with small vesicles (SVs; approximately 60 nm diameter), contain 1–3 rodlet-shaped mitochondria with defined cristae, and contact muscle cells with 15–25, >25–40, or >40–80 nm gaps, respectively, at close, almost close, or *en passant* neuroeffector junctions.[9,18] Cholinergic axons contain clear (empty) and adrenergic axons dense-cored (granular) small vesicles. The latter vesicles are often

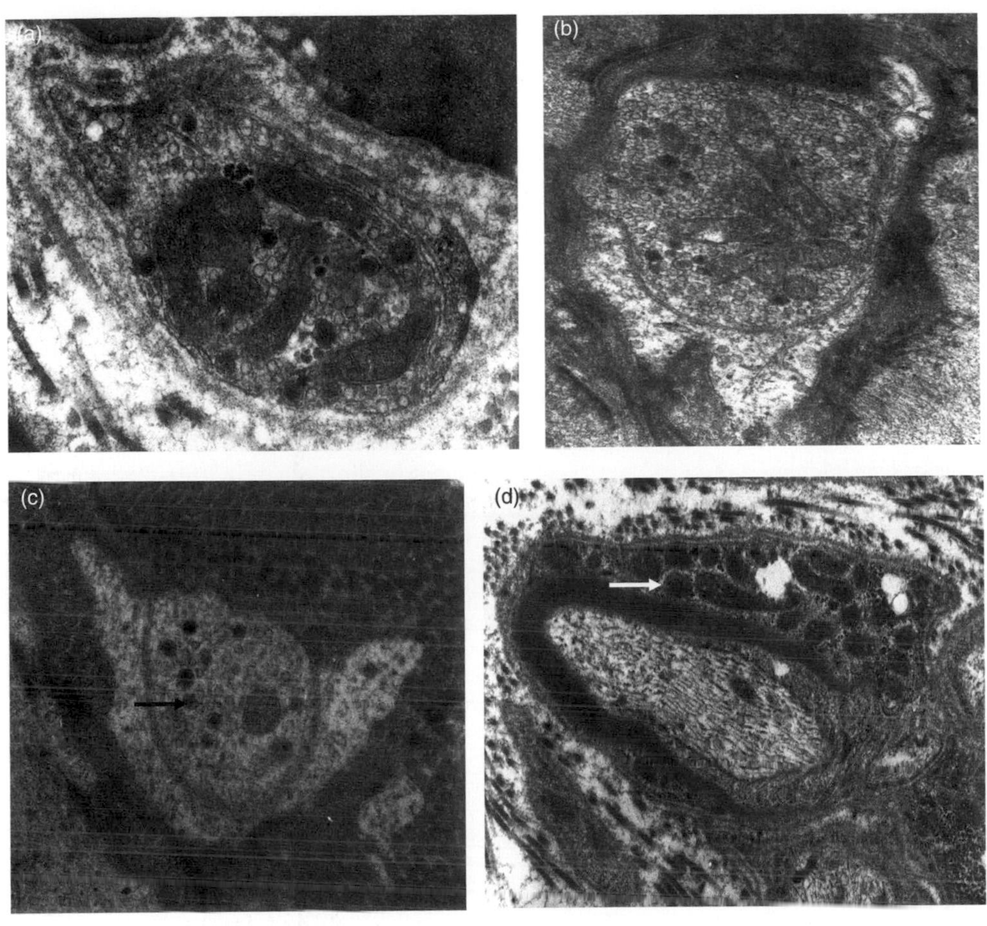

Figure 10.6 Regenerated nerve profiles. (a and b) Axon sprout replete with mitochondria and LDCV (Neg. # 45361,47197; ×41 850). (c) Copeptidergic axon profile with few mitochondria and abundant LDCVs (black arrow) (Neg. # 45184; ×36 260). (d) Activated Schwann cell ensheathing myelinated axon segment with abundant neurotubules; cytoplasm contains abundant mitochondria (arrow) (Neg. # 45711; ×26 460).

indiscernible in tissues fixed *in vitro* because of the rapid release of the neurotransmitter norepinephrine (responsible for the dense cores), so that the content of adrenergic axons in human biopsies processed routinely *in vitro* tends to be underestimated. Unfortunately, corrective procedures to intensify the dense cores ensuring their visualization (e.g. injection of 5-hydroxydopamine *in vivo* prior to biopsy[4–6]) are inapplicable to the human. Axon terminal profiles often contain one or two large dense-cored vesicles (LDCVs; approximately 120 nm diameter) that are believed to store purinergic and/or peptidergic neurotransmitters in the same terminals containing acetylcholine in cholinergic or norepinephrine in adrenergic small vesicles.[5,19] Preterminal axons resemble terminals but have Schwann cell sheaths and lack contact with muscle cells (Figure 10.5). More central normal unmyelinated and myelinated nonvaricose axon segments within nerve bundles are also ensheathed, but their axoplasms abound in neurotubules and neurofilaments, and contain few SVs but no LDCVs (Figure 10.5).

Degenerated axon terminal profiles have much fewer to depleted SVs (Figure 10.5), often with neuroeffector junctional gaps >80 nm – even exceeding 200 nm. Wide gaps alone, however, cannot be considered a sign of axonal degeneration. Globoid (empty) mitochondria with distorted cristae[20] were an ancillary feature of axonal degeneration when not attributable to artefacts of bladder/tissue manipulation at open surgery, causing similar involvement of other tissue elements. Degeneration of myelinated axons (within nerve bundles) can be identified by changes resembling Wallerian degeneration, including collapse of nonvaricose axon segments, and angulated, bean-shaped, or split myelin sheaths (Figure 10.5).[7,9,21]

The cardinal feature of growing and regenerating axons is a general increase in axoplasmic organelles. Sprouting axons have been characterized ultrastructurally by having abundant mitochondria and LDCVs, in addition to increased neurofilaments and neurotubules in the axoplasm. In the absence of available standards, abundant mitochondria have been defined in the studies presented by Elbadawi et al[7] and Haferkamp et al[9] as ≥4, and abundant LDCV as ≥3 per axon profile. Profiles with both features were considered as axon sprouts (Figure 10.6), and those with abundant LDCVs only (i.e. with ≤3 mitochondria) as copeptidergic axons (Figure 10.6). Sprouts were assumed to represent active, ongoing regeneration. Terminal profiles designated as copeptidergic were considered normal (representing stable regeneration) when also packed with SVs, or degenerating (presumably representing 'regressed' regeneration) when SVs were reduced or depleted. Abundant neurotubules/neurofilaments were discounted when observed as the only axoplasmic change in single cross-sectioned profiles of nonvaricose axon segment profiles since these are indistinguishable from cross-sectioned processes of activated Schwann cells containing abundant ultrastructurally similar microtubules and microfilaments.[24]

Schwann cells can be evaluated for changes similar to those following peripheral nerve transection[24,25] occurring in conjunction with axonal degeneration and regeneration. Normal cells contain few mitochondria, underdeveloped endoplasmic reticulum, and few ribosomes.[22] Activated Schwann cells (Figure 10.6) have abundant mitochondria, ribosomes, microfilaments, and microtubules, and dilated endoplasmic reticulum, cell processes mimicking axon profiles,[24] and outlying dense collagen deposits.[26]

Gap widths at neuroeffector junctions were based on the measurement of the shortest distances between axon terminals and adjacent muscle cells.

Short- and long-term ultrastructural changes in lower motoneuron neurogenic bladder dysfunction in a feline model

Elbadawi and coworkers[4,6] and Atta et al[5] evaluated the ultrastructural changes of the detrusor muscle and its cholinergic and adrenergic innervation in a feline animal model. All animals had undergone bladder decentralization by unilateral sacral ventral rhizotomy (deterioration of the preganglionic peripheral axon). In a short-term evaluation (2–4 weeks after surgery) in all samples a widespread transsynaptic degeneration of cholinergic axon terminals and varicosities occurred together with a loss of neuroeffector junctions, characterized by a widening of the axon terminal to a muscle cell cleft (up to ± 500 nm). The herein observed degenerative changes in (postganglionic) axons of the decentralized bladder represent the first example of transsynaptic degeneration in an autonomically innervated mammalian smooth muscle system. This was associated with a preservation of most adrenergic axons and especially starting in the 4-week samples with concurrent early regeneration or sprouting in many cholinergic and adrenergic axons. In the long-term evaluation (8–10 weeks after surgery) there was a widespread regeneration of cholinergic axons that displayed initial transsynaptic degeneration shortly after operation, with reformation of cholinergic neuroeffector junctions. This was associated with reactive sprouting of adrenergic axons leading to adrenergic hyperinnervation, as well as the emergence of a population of cholinergic and adrenergic axons containing strikingly abundant LDCV. These findings suggest that the degeneration of cholinergic axons occurring after rhizotomy is reversible, and is compensated by the development of adrenergic hyperinnervation and by an emergent probable 'peptidergic' axonal influence.

These neural changes were associated with both degenerative and regenerative ultrastructural changes in smooth muscle cells, indicating transjunctional changes in an effector tissue. Degenerative muscle cell profiles presented with myofilament disruption with reduced electron density, granular disintegration, flocculent degeneration, vacuolar degeneration, or generalized increase of sarcoplasmic electron density with aggregation of myofilaments, and were much more frequent in short- than in long-term samples. Although the muscle cell changes had no constant relationship with neural changes in their spatially close axon bundles, most degenerative profiles were observed next to degenerating cholinergic neuroeffector junctions.

In contrast, regenerative muscle cell profiles were much more frequent and widespread in the long-term samples. These profiles were recognized by their overall intact ultrastructure with 'active' nuclei and proliferation of some organelles.

Long-term ultrastructural changes in human upper motoneuron neurogenic bladder dysfunction

Haferkamp et al[8,9] undertook the ultrastructural evaluation of detrusor biopsies of 9 patients with meningomyelocele (MMC), 25 patients with spinal cord injury (SCI), and 12 patients with different brain disorders (BD). In these patients the neurogenic hyperreflexic bladder dysfunction had been present for between 3 months and 43 years.

The most frequent fascicle structure was compact; it tended to be more common in biopsies of the SCI group than those of either the MMC ($p = 0.011$) or the BD group ($p = 0.026$).

Biopsies from four patients with BOO (BD group) displayed the ultrastructural myohypertrophy pattern, with broadly undulated or crenelated cell contours. This observation confirms the previously described ultrastructural myohypertrophy patterns in outlet obstruction. In contrast, detrusor–sphincter–dyssynergia, which is tantamount to 'functional obstruction' of the outlet, was not associated with the myohypertrophy pattern in the present study.

The dense-band pattern of aged detrusor was identified in 14 biopsies obtained from 65- to 96-year-old patients (2 SCI, 12 BD group). None of the MMC group biopsies had this pattern, but a similar pattern was also observed in a patchy distribution in four more SCI group biopsies from 50–65-year-old patients.

The complete dysjunction pattern of detrusor overactivity with chain-like linkage of ≥5 muscle cells was observed in all biopsies. One BD group biopsy had dominant IJs with a 0.8 ICA:IJ ratio. This ratio was elevated (range: 2–45) in the other 45 biopsies. An ICA:IJ ratio ≥3 thus had 91% sensitivity as an ultrastructural marker of neurogenic detrusor overactivity. Our observations confirm abnormal junctions (protrusion and other forms of similarly close ICA) as a constant feature of detrusor overactivity, be it non-neuropathic idiopathic or obstructive or neuropathic.

Some degree of disruptive muscle cell degeneration was observed in all biopsies. The degree of degeneration in SCI group biopsies had no association with the anatomic level of spinal cord injury or its degree (complete versus incomplete). Nor had it any association with impaired detrusor contractility in collective analysis of all biopsies – unlike previously reported findings in non-neuropathic dysfunctional detrusor.

The observed neural changes comprised widespread axonal degeneration, far in excess of concomitant muscle cell degeneration, and restricted regeneration with activated related Schwann cells: Most evaluated axon profiles (64%) had features of axonal degeneration, 20% had features of axonal regeneration, and 16% normal ultrastructural morphology. Axonal degeneration and regeneration coexisted in 75% of biopsies, of which 57% also had admixed axon profiles of normal morphology. Regeneration was not identified or indeterminate in 24% of biopsies.

Reduction/depletion of SVs was the dominant feature of transsynaptic axonal degeneration in MMC (median 87% of axon terminals) and SCI (median 84%) group biopsies, but was less prominent in BD (median 60%) group biopsies. This may be attributed to the greater number of synaptic relays (at least three) in neural pathways in biopsies of the BD than in the other two groups. Another feature of axonal degeneration, i.e. widening of axon/muscle cell separation gaps at neuroeffector junctions, was very frequently observed (71% of junctions), with clefts often exceeding 200 nm, but does not indicate whether the degeneration was present at the time of biopsy or had happened some time before and persisted, since gaps between regenerating axons and related muscle cells were also widened.

Distorted axonal mitochondria were observed in 38 biopsies (90.5%). Seven mixed nerve bundles contained degenerated myelinated axons. Axonal collapse and irregularities of myelin sheaths were present in all, and split sheaths in five biopsies.

Axon sprouts and/or copeptidergic axons were restricted, but observed in 76% of the 45 biopsies with discernible neural elements. The prevalence of regeneration was rather similar in the three biopsy groups, and it had no association with the duration of NBD.

Axon sprout profiles were identified in 17 biopsies (38%), and copeptidergic axon profiles in the 34 biopsies. A characteristic component of the regeneration was the obvious increase in copeptidergic axons (median 18% of axons versus only <1% in normal detrusor[19]). There were no significant differences between the three biopsy groups in the prevalence of either sprout or copeptidergic profiles.

The observed regeneration was restricted. It was limited to small populations of axon profiles, was incomplete (represented by either copeptidergic axons or sprouts), even in cases with longstanding NBD, and coexisted with features of degeneration in many. Most copeptidergic axons (73%) had reduced SVs (similar to degenerated axons), despite an evident increase in LDCVs. These probably represent initial regeneration that subsequently 'regressed'. The remainder (27%) had abundant LDCVs and were filled with SVs (like morphologically normal axons), and thus probably represented 'stable' regenerated axons. The duration of NBD had no association with the presence or absence of sprouts or copeptidergic axons. Sprouts and normal or regressed copeptidergic axons in variable proportions were present in biopsies from bladders with 3–10 months' as well as in those with 1 to >10 years' duration of NBD. The lack of a relationship of axonal degeneration to duration of NBD despite its wide range, together with the associated restricted regeneration, suggests a persistent – or continuing – degenerative process.

Activated Schwann cells were observed within nerve bundles and around ensheathed preterminals in 11 of the 45 biopsies with discernible neural elements. Their presence had no association with the biopsy groups, duration of NBD, or axonal regeneration. Abundant mitochondria were present in 13 (29%), dilated endoplasmic reticulum in 6 (13%), and increased microfilaments and microtubules in all 44 biopsies (98%). Abundant outlying collagen was observed within the perineurium of the eight identified nerve bundles.

Summary

Characteristic ultrastructural findings have been described for lower and upper motoneuron bladder dysfunction in animal models or human specimens. These findings represent morphologic markers to indicate not only the presence of such dysfunction, but also the anatomic level of its causative neural deficit, i.e. spinal versus supraspinal (cephalic). The possible contribution of an occult neurologic factor to clinically non-neurogenic vesical dysfunction in both the young and the elderly has so far eluded clinical and urodynamic recognition. The usefulness of the suggested morphologic markers in the clinical management of vesical dysfunction, whether overtly neurogenic or non-neurogenic, remains to be investigated in future studies.

References

1. Elbadawi A. Functional pathology of urinary bladder muscularis: the new frontier in diagnostic uropathology. Semin Diagn Pathol 1993; 10: 314–54.
2. Hailemariam S, Elbadawi A, Yalla SV, Resnick NM. Structural basis of geriatric voiding dysfunction. V. Standardized protocols for routine ultrastructural study and diagnosis of endoscopic detrusor biopsies. J Urol 1997; 157: 1783–801.
3. Elbadawi A. Microstructural basis of detrusor contractility. The 'MIN' approach to its understanding and study. Neurourol Urodyn 1991; 10: 77–85.
4. Elbadawi A, Atta MA, Franck JI. Intrinsic neuromuscular defects in the neurogenic bladder. I. Short-term ultrastrucutral changes in muscular innervation of the decentralized feline bladder base following unilateral sacral ventral rhizotomy. Neurourol Urodyn 1984; 3: 93–113.
5. Atta MA, Franck JI, Elbadawi A. Intrinsic neuromuscular defects in the neurogenic bladder. II. Long-term innervation of the unilaterally decentralized feline bladder base by regenerated cholinergic, increased adrenergic and emergent probable 'peptidergic' nerves. Neurourol Urodyn 1984; 3: 185–200.
6. Elbadawi A, Atta MA. Intrinsic neuromuscular defects in the neurogenic bladder. III. Transjunctional, short- and long-term ultrastructural changes in muscle cells of the decentralized feline bladder base following unilateral sacral ventral rhizotomy. Neurourol Urodyn 1984; 3: 245–70.
7. Elbadawi A, Resnick NM, Dorsam J, Yalla SV, Haferkamp A. Structural basis of neurogenic bladder dysfunction. I. Methods of prospective ultrastructural study and overview of the findings. J Urol 2003; 169: 540–6.
8. Haferkamp A, Dorsam J, Resnick NM, Yalla SV, Elbadawi A. Structural basis of neurogenic bladder dysfunction. II. Myogenic basis of detrusor hyperreflexia. J Urol 2003; 169: 547–54.
9. Haferkamp A, Dorsam J, Resnick NM, Yalla SW, Elbadawi A. Structural basis of neurogenic bladder dysfunction. III. Intrinsic detrusor innervation. J Urol 2003; 169: 555–62.
10. Haferkamp A, Dorsam J, Elbadawi A. Ultrastructural diagnosis of neuropathic detrusor overactivity: Validation of a common myogenic mechanism. Adv Exp Med Biol 2003; 539: 281–91.
11. Elbadawi A, Yalla SV, Resnick NM. Structural basis of geriatric voiding dysfunction. I. Methods of a prospective ultrastructural/urodynamic study and an overview of the findings. J Urol 1993; 150: 1650–6.
12. Elbadawi A, Hailemariam S, Yalla SV, Resnick NM. Structural basis of geriatric voiding dysfunction. VI. Validation and update of diagnostic criteria in 71 detrusor biopsies. J Urol 1997; 157: 1802–13.
13. Elbadawi A, Yalla SV, Resnick NM. Structural basis of geriatric voiding dysfunction. II. Aging detrusor: normal versus impaired contractility. J Urol 1993; 150: 1657–67.
14. Elbadawi A, Yalla SV, Resnick NM. Structural basis of geriatric voiding dysfunction. IV. Bladder outlet obstruction. J Urol 1993; 150: 1681–95.
15. Elbadawi A. Functional anatomy of the organs of micturition. Urol Clin N Am 1996; 23: 177–210.
16. Elbadawi A, Yalla SV, Resnick NM. Structural basis of geriatric voiding dysfunction. III. Detrusor overactivity. J Urol 1993; 150: 1668–80.
17. Elbadawi A. The neostructural myogenic mechanism of detrusor overactivity. Urology 1997; 50(Suppl 6A): 71–2.
18. Elbadawi A. Autonomic muscular innervation of the vesical outlet and its role in micturition. In: Hinman F Jr (ed.). Benign Prostatic Hypertrophy. New York: Springer, 1983: 330–48.
19. Daniel EE, Cowan W, Daniel VP. Structural bases for neural and myogenic control of human detrusor muscle. Can J Physiol Pharmacol 1983; 61: 1247–73.
20. Mugnaini E, Friederich VL. Electron microscopy. Identification and study of normal and degenerating neural elements by electron microscopy. In: Heimer L, Robards MJ eds. Neuroanatomical Tract – Tracing Methods. New York: Plenum Press, 1981: 377–406.
21. Friede RL, Martinez AJ. Analysis of axon-sheath relations during early Wallerian degeneration. Brain Res 1970; 19: 199–212.
22. Blümcke S, Niedorf HR. Elektronenoptische Untersuchungen an Wachstumsendkolben regenerierenden peripherer Nervenfasern. Virchows Arch Pathol Anat 1965; 340: 93–104.
23. Lampert PW. A comparative electron microscopic study of reactive, degenerating, regenerating and dystrophic axons. J Neuropathol Exper Neurol 1967; 26: 345–68.
24. Payer AF. An ultrastructural study of Schwann cell response to axonal degeneration. J Comp Neurol 1979; 183: 365–84.
25. Knoche H, Terwort H. Elektronenmikroskopischer Beitrag zur Kenntnis von Degenerationsformen der vegetativen Endstrecke nach Durchschneidung postganglionärer Fasern. Z Zellforsch 1973; 141: 181–202.
26. Nathaniel EJH, Pease DC. Collagen and basement membrane formation by Schwann cells during nerve regeneration. J Ultrastruct Res 1963; 9: 550–60.

11

Pathophysiology of the overactive bladder

Alison F Brading

Introduction

In the proceedings of the Second International Consultation on Incontinence, the overactive bladder is described as one which fails to remain relaxed until an appropriate time for urination.[1] The resulting symptom syndrome includes the symptoms of urgency, with or without urge incontinence, usually with frequency and nocturia. International Continence Society (ICS) terminology in 2002[2] classifies the overactive bladder as one in which the symptoms are suggestive of urodynamically demonstrable detrusor overactivity (involuntary detrusor contraction) during the filling phase, which may be spontaneously provoked. Detrusor overactivity is thus a urodynamic observation, and the term replaces detrusor instability. It can be subdivided into neurogenic (when there is a relevant neurologic condition) or non-neurogenic (including idiopathic overactivity, and overactivity related to outflow obstruction and aging).

The very fact that the symptom syndrome is found in patients with all the different associations of detrusor overactivity suggests that there may well be common underlying pathologic changes in the bladder wall, and indeed examination of the physiologic properties and ultrastructure of bladder wall obtained from human overactive bladders or bladder from animal models of overactivity supports this assertion. In this chapter the common pathophysiologic features of the overactive bladder will be discussed and their significance examined. The possible causes of the changes will then be explored, and the chapter will end with a consideration of the origin of probably the most 'bothersome' of the symptoms, that is urgency.

The following changes in the detrusor are routinely seen:

- increased spontaneous myogenic activity
- fused tetanic contractions
- altered responsiveness to stimuli
- characteristic changes in smooth muscle ultrastructure.

Examination of the bladder wall, peripheral innervation, and the micturition reflex in animals and humans with overactive bladders also shows common changes:

- patchy denervation of the bladder wall
- increased numbers of interstitial cells
- enlarged sensory neurons
- enlarged parasympathetic ganglion cells
- increased effectiveness of a spinal micturition pathway.

All these common features make it very likely that whatever the etiology of the condition, the underlying causative mechanisms are the same or very similar. I will first discuss the normal bladder and then consider the changes seen in the overactive bladder in more detail.

The normal bladder

The normal bladder fills at low pressure, whilst keeping its surface area:volume ratio minimal, so that synchronous contraction of the detrusor through parasympathetic innervation can rapidly increase intravesical pressure when micturition is initiated. The maintenance of a minimum surface area:volume ratio with little pressure rise is achieved by spontaneous contractile activity of the smooth muscle bundles combined with relatively poor electrical coupling between the myocytes, allowing them to adjust to the changing volume of the bladder without the synchronous activity necessary to raise the intravesical pressure. This type of spontaneous activity has been examined in some detail in the isolated bladders of small mammals, in which individual areas of the bladder wall can be seen contracting independently, and has been called 'autonomous activity'.[3] Interstitial cells between the smooth muscle bundles may play a role in coordinating such activity.[4,5] The urothelium is an active tissue that can respond to changes in stretch and the composition of the urine, communicating with the suburothelium by secreting chemical mediators such as NO and ATP.[6,7] The suburothelium contains a network of capillaries, interstitial cells,[5] and tachykinin-containing sensory nerve terminals,[8] and is thought to be able to modulate the behavior of sensory nerves and the underlying detrusor to induce sensations of fullness and urgency and trigger micturition in an appropriate way.

Normal properties of the detrusor

Smooth muscle strips dissected from normal animal or human detrusor have characteristic properties. A proportion of them, presumably reflecting the degree of cellular coupling in that strip, will develop spontaneous contractile behavior, featuring small transient rises in pressure from a low or zero baseline tone, the size of which is considerably smaller than that of evoked contractions (Figure 11.1). These spontaneous contractions are not abolished either by tetrodotoxin, which blocks conducted action potentials in nerves, or by blocking activation of muscarinic or purinergic receptors that normally mediate the parasympathetic nerve activity,[9] although they can be modulated by drugs affecting the interstitial cells.[10] The strips can be activated by transmural stimulation of the intrinsic nerves with short electrical current pulses in a frequency-dependent manner, or directly activated by longer current pulses. Contraction mediated by intrinsic nerves can be totally abolished in normal human bladder by the muscarinic receptor antagonist atropine[11] (Figure 11.2), although in animal bladders there is usually an atropine-resistant component which predominates at low frequencies and is mediated by neuronal release of ATP (Figure 11.3; for references see Brading[9]).

This purinergic innervation may be used to produce small spurts of urine without bladder emptying for territorial marking. Strips from animal and human bladders will also respond by contracting in a dose-dependent manner to depolarization with high potassium solutions and application of muscarinic and P2x purinoceptor agonists, although activation of purinoceptors cannot initiate the full contractile response available to the strip.

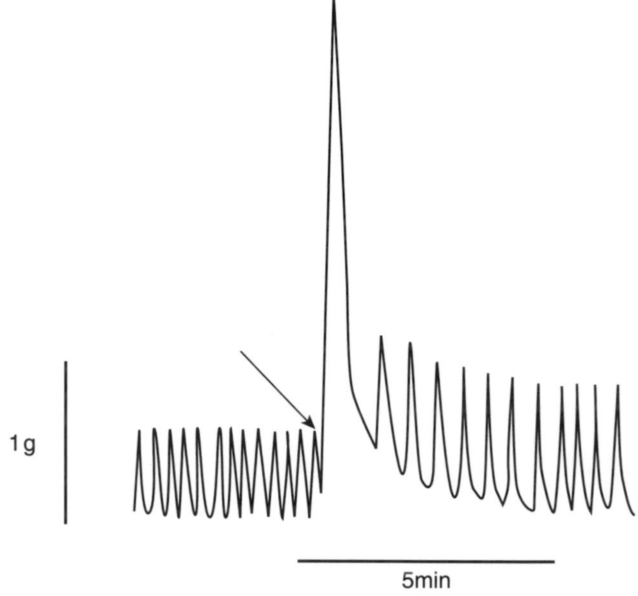

Figure 11.1
Spontaneous contractile activity in a strip of smooth muscle dissected from the detrusor of a pig bladder. At the arrow the intramural nerves were stimulated for 5 s at 50 Hz.

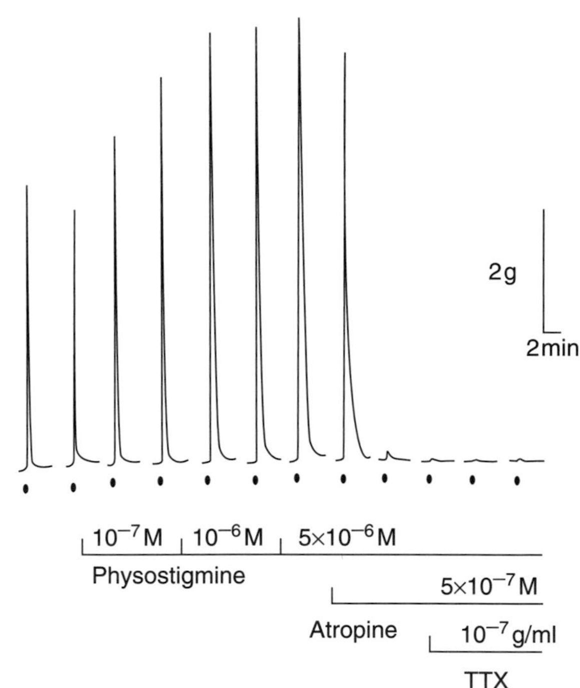

Figure 11.2
Contractile responses in a strip of human detrusor to transmural field stimulation (20 Hz, 5 s) of the intrinsic nerves. Note that the size of the response is enhanced by the cholinesterase inhibitor physostigmine, and almost completely blocked by the muscarinic antagonist atropine. (Reproduced from Sibley with permission.)[12]

The overactive bladder

The overactive bladder often develops spontaneous rises in pressure during filling which may lead to leakage of urine, normally triggers micturition at lower volumes, and, if the pathways are intact, initiates the sensation of urge and urgency more readily than the normal bladder.

Changes to the smooth muscle of the bladder wall

Spontaneous activity

Smooth muscle strips dissected from overactive bladders often show increases in spontaneous contractile activity. This has been seen in human bladder strips from obstructed overactive bladders[11] and from neuropathic

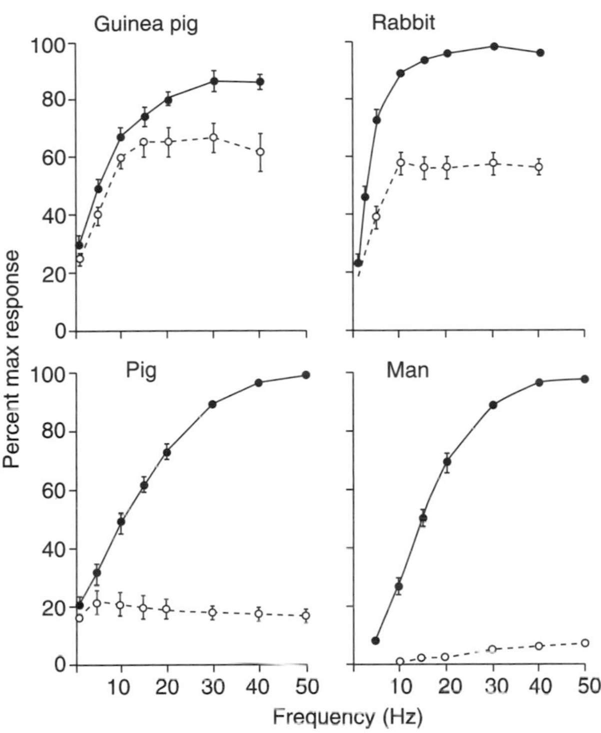

Figure 11.3
Frequency–response curves of detrusor strips from various animals under control conditions (filled symbols) and in the presence of atropine (open symbols). Note the species dependency of the size of the atropine-resistant responses. These curves were further suppressed in the presence of tetrodotoxin with the exception of the human bladder, where the atropine-resistant contractions were also TTX resistant, and presumably due to direct smooth muscle stimulation (not shown).

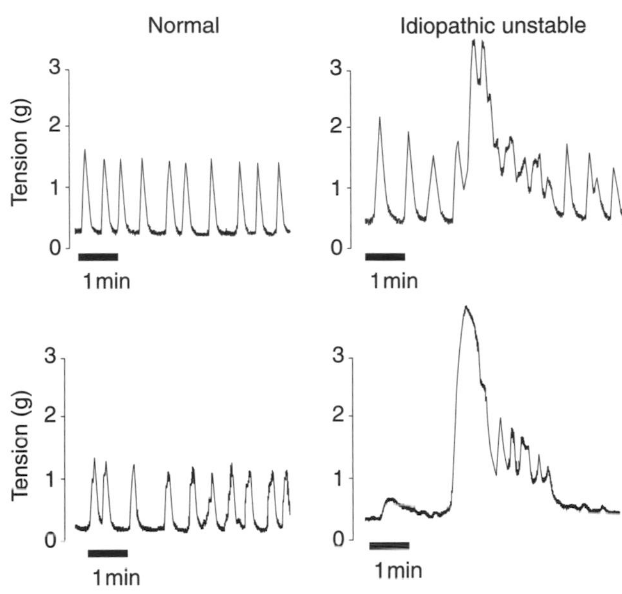

Figure 11.4
Spontaneous contractile activity in detrusor strips dissected from normal (left) and idiopathically overactive (right) human bladders. Note the typical small phasic contractions of the normal detrusor strips, and the larger fused contractions in strips from overactive bladders. (Reproduced from Mills with permission.)[19]

overactive bladders.[13] A change in the pattern of the spontaneous activity is also seen which is very characteristic of bladder overactivity. Strips from overactive bladders show fused tetanic contractions[14–17] (Figure 11.4), reminiscent of the activity typically shown by well-coupled smooth muscles such as in the gut. Similar fused tetanic contractions are seen in bladders from pigs with instability secondary to outflow obstruction; indeed, in those with well-developed instability, bizarre patterns are often observed[11] (Figure 11.5). More recently, recording from human bladders with multiple electrodes has also demonstrated increased spontaneous activity associated with sensory urgency.[18]

Altered responsiveness to stimuli

Alterations are also seen in the responses of overactive detrusor to stimulation with agonists and to transmural electrical stimulation (either direct or via activation of intrinsic nerves). In this case, there are differences in the patterns seen in tissues from overactive bladders of different etiology. In obstructed bladders there is a supersensitivity to muscarinic agonists and KCl with a reduced contraction to intrinsic nerve stimulation.[12,21–23] Similar changes are seen in animal models of bladder overactivity (pig[24,25] and rabbit[26]) (Figure 11.6). In neuropathic bladders from patients with spina bifida (Figures 11.7 and 11.8), supersensitivity is again seen to cholinergic agonists and KCl, but there is no change in the sensitivity of the contractile response to intrinsic nerve stimulation, although the size of the response is smaller.[13] In idiopathic overactivity, bladder strips show supersensitivity to KCl, but not to muscarinic agonists (Figure 11.9) and there is a reduced contractile response to intrinsic nerve stimulation.[16] We have also found evidence that overactive strips are more easily activated by direct electrical stimulation of the smooth muscle (contractions elicited by transmural nerve stimulation that are resistant to the nerve blocking action of tetrodotoxin (TTX) (Figure 11.10).[27]

Ultrastructural changes

At an ultrastructural level, a common feature seen in neurogenic detrusor overactivity is the presence of protrusion junctions and ultraclose abutments between the

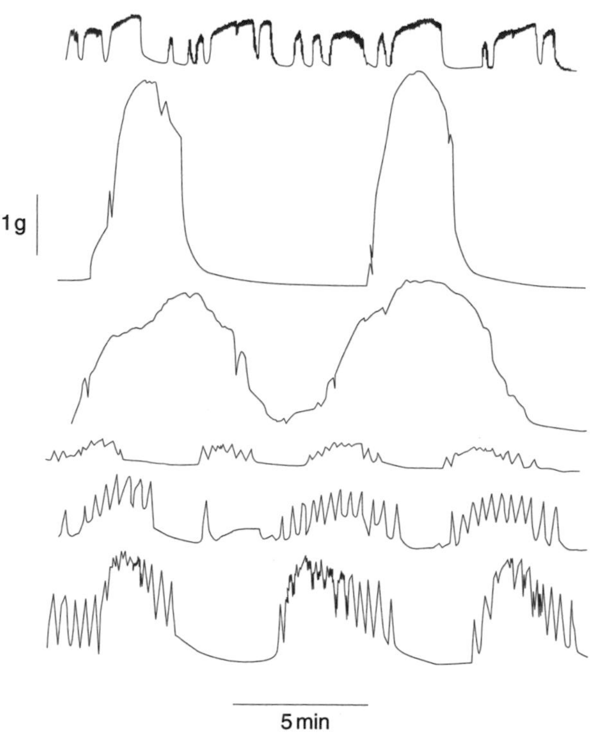

Figure 11.5
Bizarre spontaneous contractile activity in strips of smooth muscle dissected from the bladders of pigs with an overactive bladder due to partial bladder outlet obstruction. Note the spontaneous large fused tetanic contraction, which can reach an amplitude larger than the response to transmural stimulation (not shown). (Reproduced from Turner with permission.)[20]

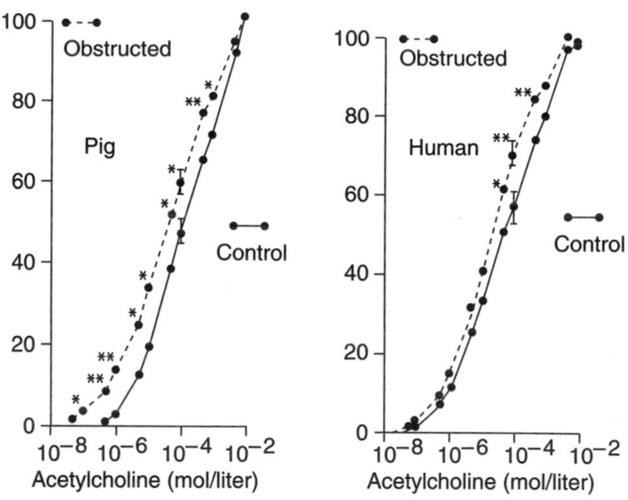

Figure 11.6
Concentration–contractile response curve to 10 s applications of carbachol to strips from normal human (right) and pig (left) bladders (continuous line curve) and bladders from patients and pigs with overactive bladders secondary to bladder outflow obstruction (dotted line curve). Note the increased sensitivity of the smooth muscle to the muscarinic agonist. (Stars indicate significant difference from control.) (Reproduced from Sibley.)[12]

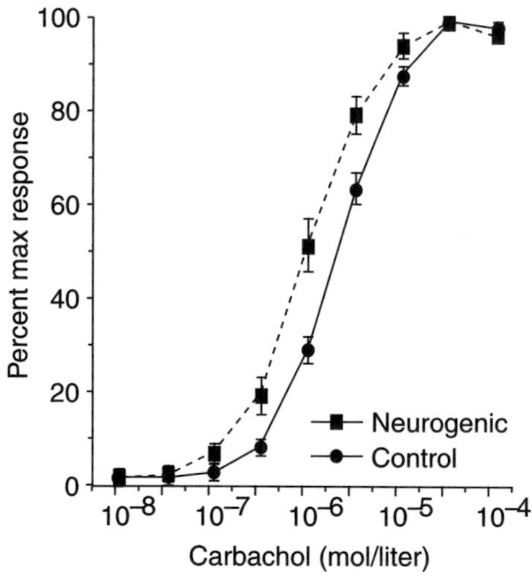

Figure 11.7
Concentration–contractile response curve to 10 s applications of carbachol to strips from normal human bladders (circles) and bladders from spina bifida patients with neurogenic overactive bladders (squares). Expressed as a percentage of the maximal response of each strip, strips from the overactive bladders are significantly more sensitive to muscarinic agonists. (Reproduced from German et al with permission.)[13]

smooth muscle cells, features occurring only rarely in normal tissue.[28–30] Again, development of these junctions has been seen in animal models.[31]

Significance of these changes

The properties of the normal detrusor support the suggestion that the smooth muscle bundles are not as well coupled electrically as are most visceral smooth muscles. This is supported by the fact that spontaneous myogenic contractions only produce a fraction of the tension available on synchronous activation of the whole strip and by the lack of clearly defined gap junctions between the smooth muscle cells (for example see Daniel et al[32]). Immunohistochemical studies do, however, demonstrate the presence of connexins (the gap-junction proteins) in the detrusor, and an increase in patients suffering from urge[33,34] and electrophysiologic measurements in the guinea pig[35–37] show that individual cells within a bundle are electrically coupled to their neighbors, but that spread of current between cells in the axial direction is poor, with current spread rarely occurring between pairs of cells separated by more than 40 μm in the axial direction. This poorly developed electrical coupling prevents synchronous

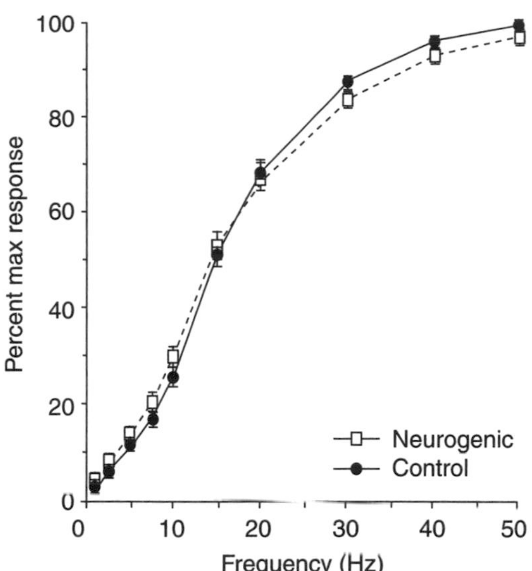

Figure 11.8
Frequency–response curve to transmural nerve stimulation of strips from normal human bladders (circles) and bladders from patients with overactive bladders secondary to spina bifida (squares). Expressed as a percentage of the maximal response of each strip, there is no significant difference between the two curves, indicating that the sensitivity to stimulation is unchanged, although the absolute size of the response is smaller in strips from the overactive bladders. (Reproduced from German et al with permission.)[13]

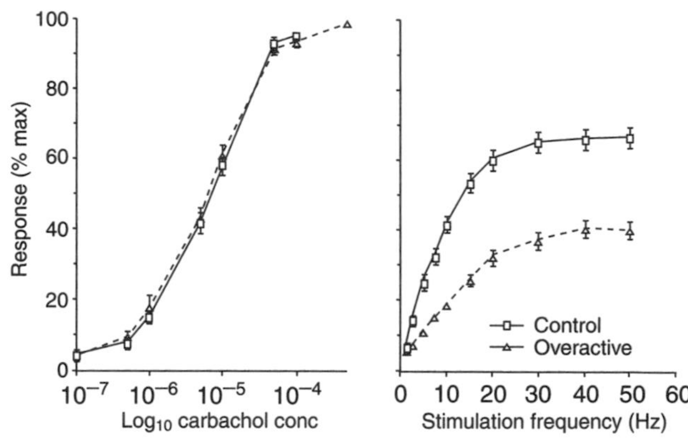

Figure 11.9
Log concentration–response curves (to 10 s carbachol) and frequency response curves of human bladder strips from normal (continuous line curve) bladders and bladders from patients with idiopathic detrusor overactivity (dotted line curve).

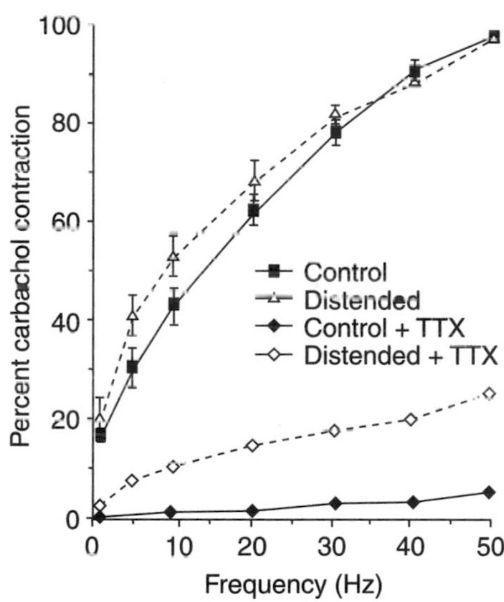

Figure 11.10
Frequency–response curves of strips from pig bladders to electrical field stimulation and the effects of tetrodotoxin (TTX) in normal pigs (squares) and those with overactive bladders secondary to previous overdistention (dots). Note the TTX-resistant contractions in the strips from overactive bladders. (Reproduced from Sethia with permission.)[27]

activation of all the smooth muscles in the strip from spontaneous action potentials, and is likely to account for the small size of the spontaneous contractions. In the whole bladder, the great compliance of the bladder wall means that intravesical pressure will only rise when there is synchronous contraction of the majority of smooth muscle cells in the wall. The lack of good coupling means that *in-vivo* electrical activity will be able to control the length of individual cells without the risk of generating a rise in intravesical pressure. Synchronous activation of the muscle and a rise in intravesical pressure during micturition requires coordinated activation of the smooth muscle, and is achieved through the dense parasympathetic innervation in which varicosities form close junctions with the great majority of the smooth muscle cells.[32,38]

The changes that occur in the smooth muscle of the overactive bladders strongly suggest that the cells are better coupled by some means, so that spontaneous activity will spread and initiate synchronous contractions in many more smooth muscle cells. This would account for the fused tetanic contractions seen in the overactive bladder strips; the close abutments and protrusion junctions seen ultrastructurally may be the morphologic correlates of this connectivity, although the increase in interstitial cells may play a role (see below). In the whole bladder, the increased excitability of the smooth muscle combined with the greater connectivity results in the situation where a focus of electrical activity can spread to activate the whole detrusor and produce an overactive contraction. Such a focus of activity could arise myogenically or could be evoked by activation of a few motor nerves, which in the normal bladder would not elevate intravesical pressure. A myogenic origin of the spontaneous pressure rises seen in pigs with grossly overactive bladders is certainly suggested since they persist after section of the sacral

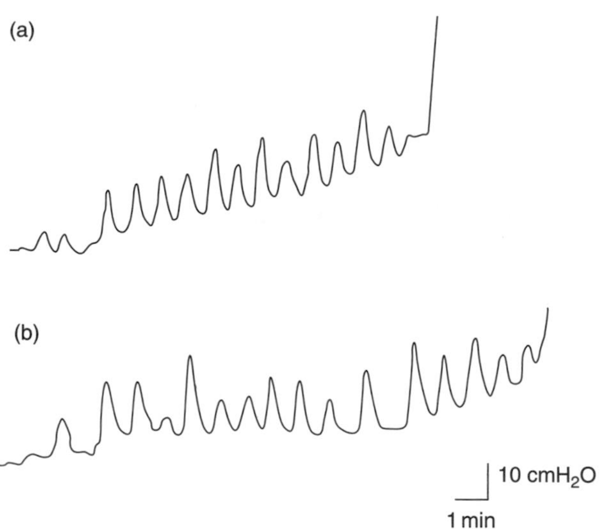

Figure 11.11
Overactive pressure rises in a pig during artificial filling. This animal had been made overactive by a partial bladder outflow obstruction several months earlier. (a) The situation when the spinal roots are intact and (b) after section of the dorsal and ventral spinal roots L7–S3. (Reproduced from Sethia with permission.)[27]

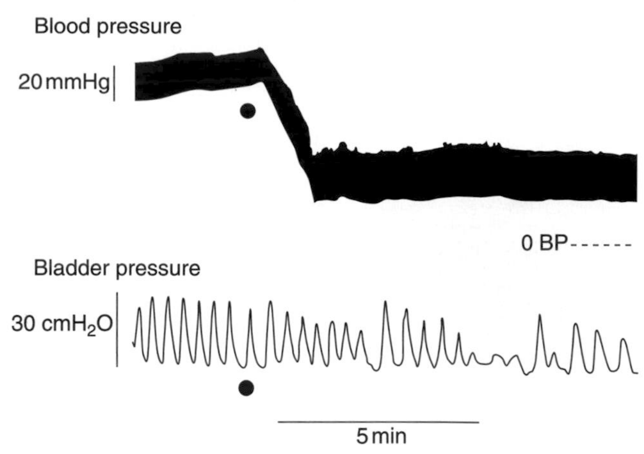

Figure 11.12
Urodynamic experiment in an anesthetized mini-pig. Upper trace, blood pressure; lower trace, intravesical pressure. The animal had an overactive bladder secondary to bladder outflow obstruction. At the dot, tetrodotoxin (TTX) was infused in an amount sufficient to prevent action potentials in the autonomic and somatic nerves. Note the rapid fall in blood pressure (removal of sympathetic tone), but persistence of bladder overactivity. Artificial ventilation was applied after TTX infusion, since respiration stopped. (Reproduced from Turner with permission.)[20]

roots[27] (Figure 11.11), and can still occur in the presence of TTX[20] (Figure 11.12).

Why should such changes occur in the smooth muscle of overactive bladders? Smooth muscle, along with most innervated tissues, is capable of altering its responses to changes in its pattern of activation. The types of change that are seen in the detrusor smooth muscle are reminiscent of the changes due to experimental denervation.[39] It seems very likely that the changes in detrusor properties are caused by altered patterns of activation. This will be explored below.

Changes in peripheral innervation and the micturition reflex

Changes in the bladder wall

Another common feature of overactive detrusor is a change in the macroscopic structure of the bladder wall. Regardless of the etiology of the condition, sections of the bladder wall from overactive human bladder frequently show patchy denervation of the muscle bundles. Some muscle bundles may be completely denervated, whereas neighboring ones appear normal (Figures 11.13 and 11.14) and in other areas sparser innervation is also seen.[13,16,31,40,41] A similar pattern is seen in animal models (pigs,[42] guinea pigs,[43] and rabbit[26]), although interestingly not in the rat,[38] where the postganglionic neurons are all in the pelvic ganglia and not in the bladder wall. The denervated and sparsely innervated areas of the bladder wall become infiltrated with connective tissue elements such as collagen and elastin (Figure 11.15),[13,31,40] and in the completely denervated areas in tissue from idiopathic and neuropathic overactive bladders, hypertrophy of the smooth muscle cells is seen.[40] Between the smooth muscle bundles and under the urothelium, an increase in the number of cells showing immunohistochemical staining for the kit receptor is also seen in sections of human bladder from all types of bladder overactivity (Figure 11.16). This marker is located on interstitial cells and demonstrates that there is a large increase in their number.

Changes in neuronal structure

Animal experiments (carried out mainly in the rat) have demonstrated that procedures such as spinal section or urethral obstruction, as well as leading to the development of bladder instability, also lead to an increase in size of both the afferent neurons in the dorsal root ganglia (L6–S1[44]) and the efferent neurons in the pelvic plexus (after obstruction[45,46] and after spinal section[47]). We have seen a similar increase in the size of the neurons in bladder wall ganglia in the obstructed guinea pig (unpublished work).

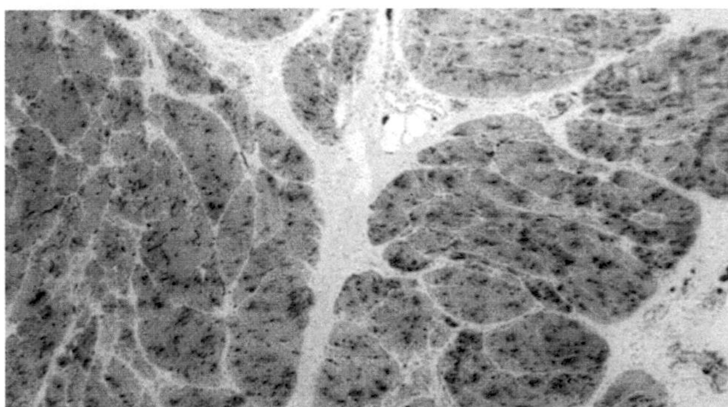
Control

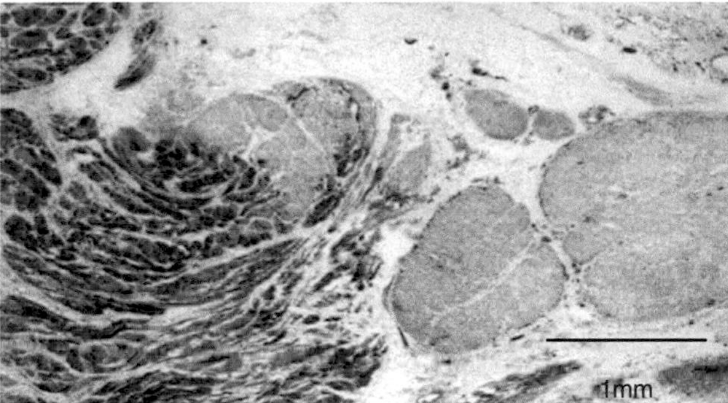

Overactive idiopathic

Figure 11.13
Sections of human detrusor stained to show the presence of acetylcholinesterase on the axons of intramural nerves. Upper trace from a normal bladder: note uniform dense staining of the smooth muscle bundles. Lower trace from a patient with idiopathic instability (note the patchy denervation of the smooth muscle bundles). (Reproduced from Mills et al with permission.)[16]

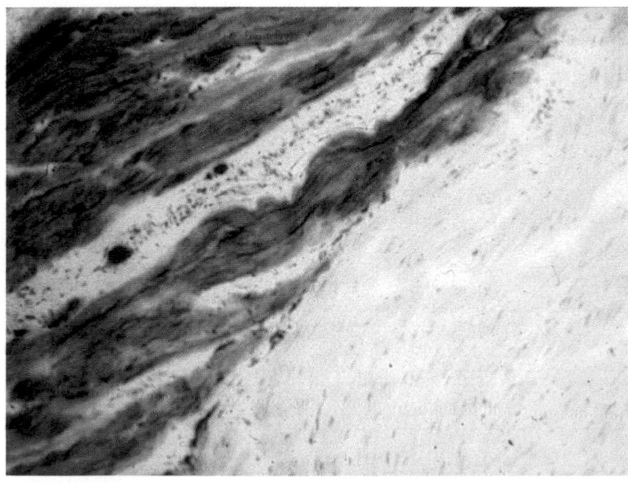

Figure 11.14
Section of a human detrusor from a patient with an unstable bladder secondary to spina bifida. Note the exceptionally dense brown innervation of one muscle bundle adjacent to another completely denervated bundle.

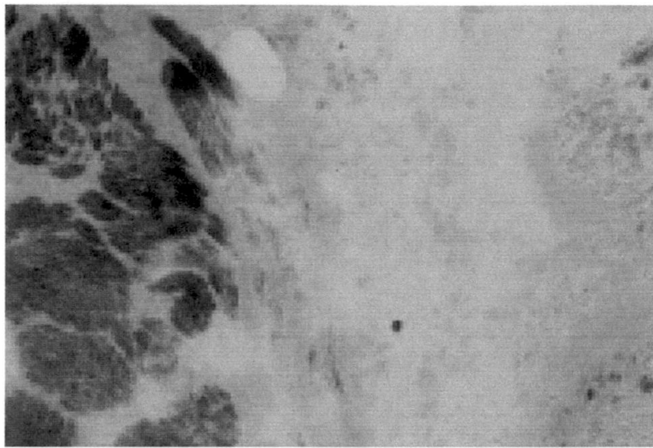
Smooth muscle (pink)

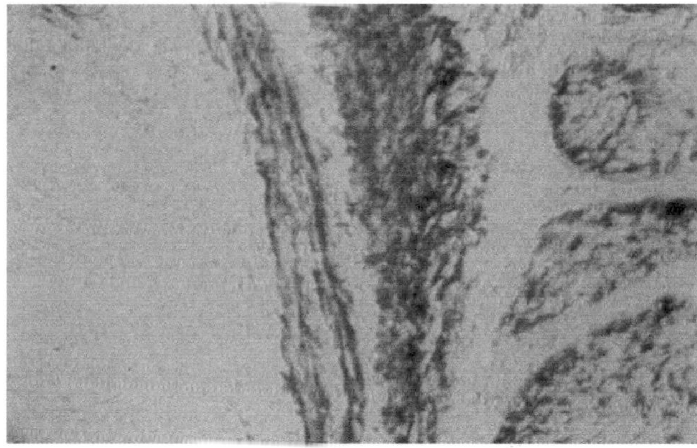
Elastin (pink)

Figure 11.15 Two adjacent sections of human detrusor from a spina bifida patient with an overactive bladder. Top panel stained with Masson's trichrome (smooth muscle seen in pink); bottom panel stained for the presence of elastin. In these sections normal muscle bundles are present on the left, and on the right damaged bundles with less smooth muscle, and also denervation (not shown). Note the increased elastin distribution in the damaged bundles.

Changes in the interstitial cells

It has recently been suggested that interstitial cells in the bladder wall may play a role in interconnection of the smooth muscle cells and propagation of action potentials in the bladder wall (for references see Brading and McCloskey[5]). In overactive bladders, there is a large increase in their number,[10] as illustrated in Figure 11.16. Functional studies on the effects of the kit inhibitor Glivec suggest that these cells may play some role in the activity of the tissues, since Glivec reduces spontaneous activity, and is effective at lower concentrations in the overactive bladder. However, overactive bladders frequently show an increase in the extracellular matrix surrounding the smooth muscle and it is possible the interstitial cells are responsible for secreting this.

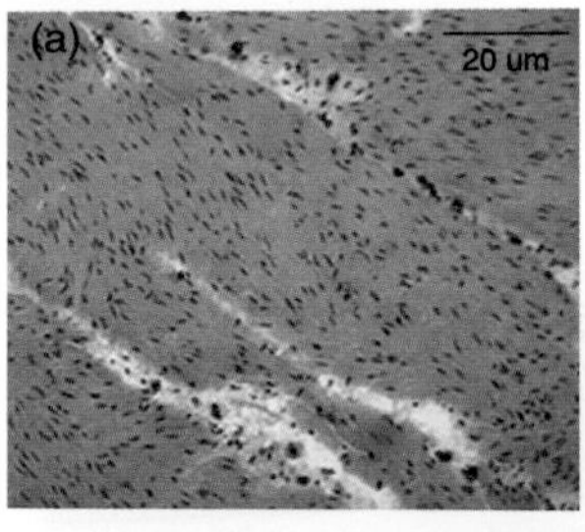

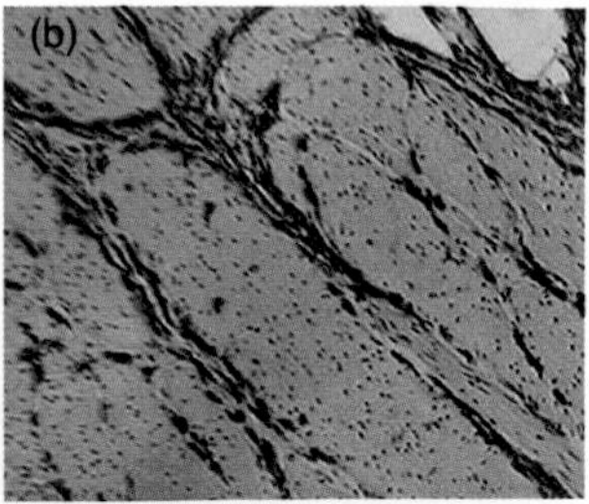

Figure 11.16
Sections from human bladder stained to show the presence of the kit receptor. Brownish red staining localizes the receptor and is presumably on interstitial cells. (a) Normal bladder. (b) Neurogenic unstable bladder. Note labeled cells are sparse around the bundles in normal tissue, but densely packed around the muscle bundles in the overactive tissue. Sections kindly provided by Philippa Cheetham.

Changes in the micturition reflex

Changes have also been seen in the micturition reflex in animals after recovery from spinal shock following spinal injury. Electrophysiologic measurements of the central delay in the micturition reflex show a shorter delay in animals with spinal injury (for references see de Groat[48]) than in intact animals, suggesting that there has been reorganization of the micturition pathway from a spinobulbospinal pathway to a purely spinal pathway. Also, activation of specific C-fiber afferents can trigger micturition in overactive bladders but not in normal bladders. This latter observation is thought to be true in humans, since in normal humans the ice water test (instillation of the bladder with cold water), which is thought to activate specific C fibers, does not trigger micturition, but does so in many patients with overactive bladders.[49,50] In fact, intravesical administration of selective C-fiber neurotoxins such as capsaicin and resiniferatoxin is an effective treatment in many patients with neuropathic instability.[51]

Possible causes of these changes

It seems inherently likely that the changes associated with the overactive bladder are the result of alterations in the activity in the neuronal pathways controling the detrusor. The sensory neurons are likely to encounter increased stimulation after outflow obstruction or inflammation of the urothelium, which could result in the hypertrophy of the dorsal root ganglion neurons and also of the autonomic ganglia, since presumably increased parasympathetic activation will result. The patchy denervation suggests that there has been death of some of the intrinsic neurons in the bladder wall. The most likely cause of this is bladder wall ischemia. The bladder has been shown to be susceptible to ischemia,[19,52,53] since anything that raises intravesical pressure to more than 30–40 cmH_2O seriously compromises blood flow in the wall. Enhanced intravesical pressure and bladder wall ischemia could result from prostatic obstruction or, in cases of spinal injury, from detrusor sphincter dyssynergia. In outflow obstruction where there is a significant hypertrophy of the wall, increased metabolic demands[54] and reduced blood flow[53] can lead to significant periods of anoxia, which might result eventually in neuronal death (Figure 11.17). We have shown that 1

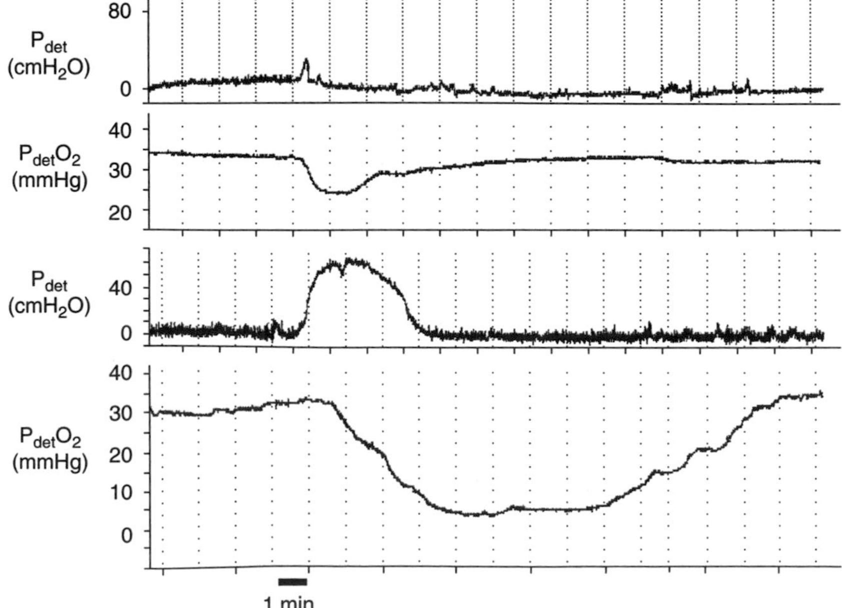

Figure 11.17
Urodynamic tracings from pigs. The top of each pair of tracings is the intravesical pressure, and the bottom trace is oxygen tension in the bladder wall, recorded with an oxygen electrode. The traces show bladder filling and a micturition. The top traces are from a normal pig, and show a small rise in intravesical pressure during voiding, and an associated more prolonged reduction in oxygen tension. The bottom traces are from a pig with a bladder outflow obstruction. Note the increased and prolonged pressure rise during the void, and the drastic extended fall in oxygen tension, which does not return to baseline for about 14 min. (Reproduced from Greenland and Brading with permission.)[56]

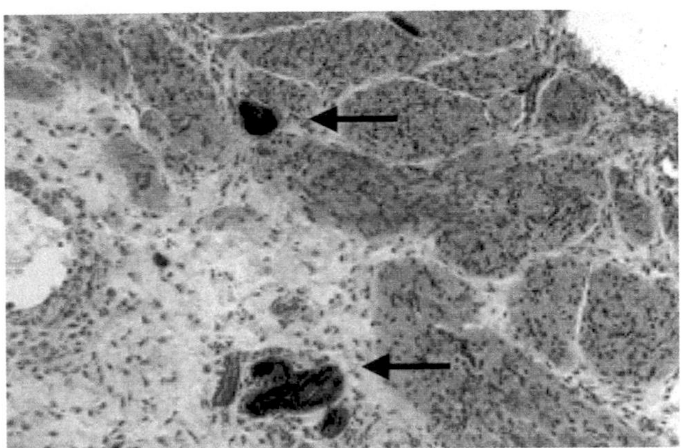
Acetylcholinesterase stain

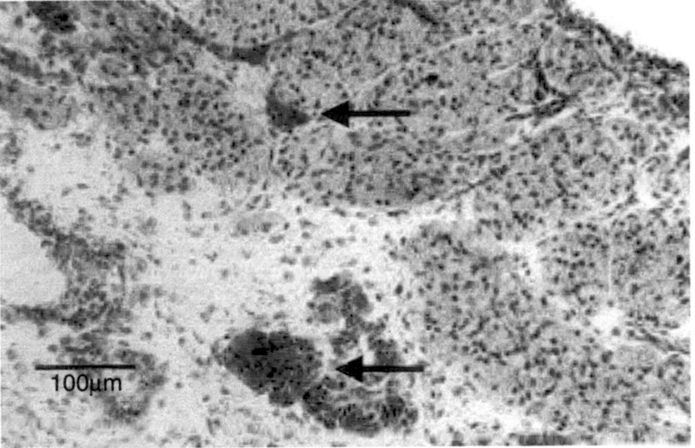

Caspase 3 immunoreactivity

Figure 11.18
Two adjacent sections from a guinea pig bladder that had been subjected to ischemic conditions. The top section localizes intramural ganglia which show acetylcholinesterase activity. In the bottom section the ganglia can be seen to react with antibodies to caspase 3, a pro-apoptotic marker. (Reproduced from Symes[55] with permission; sections prepared by Lucia Esposito.)

hour of bladder ischemia produced in anesthetized guinea pigs by occlusion of the terminal aorta, followed by 1 hour reperfusion, resulted in expression of apoptotic-associated markers in the ganglia in the bladder wall[55] (Figure 11.18).

The changes in the reflex pathway that occur after spinal injury probably result from the loss of descending pathways. This may trigger the production of growth factors and the resultant sprouting of axon terminals in surviving pathways to make new and abnormal connections; for instance, the C fibers may increase their connections to the interneurons or motor neurons in the segmental spinal parasympathetic pathways. The enhanced size of the efferent postganglionic neurons in obstructed bladders appears to be the result of the liberation of nerve growth factor (NGF) by the detrusor, since autoimmunization of rats against NGF reduces the neuronal hypertrophy.[57] Presumably, the stimulus for the production of NGF may be the increased work load of the obstructed bladder.[58]

The problem of urgency

Everyday experience would suggest that urgency is a separate sensation from that of bladder fullness. Animal experiments recording from afferent nerves during bladder filling and contraction[58–61] have shown increased activity in a unimodal population of small myelinated and unmyelinated (Aδ and C) fibers in response to intravesical pressure and detrusor contraction, suggesting that there are in-series stretch receptors in the bladder wall whose activity correlates with the sensations of bladder filling and fullness. However, it seems unlikely that fibers with such properties mediate the sensation of urgency. Again, from everyday experience, urgent desire to void disappears as soon as micturition starts at a time when intravesical pressure and detrusor activity will both be high. Unfortunately, the relationship between urgency and detrusor activity cannot be investigated in animals, since we cannot know what sensations they perceive. In humans, however, it is clear from both normal and ambulatory cystometry that overactive pressure rises may occur without eliciting any apparent sensations. A sensible theory about urgency has been proposed by Coolsaet et al.[62] They suggest that urgency is triggered by local distortions in the bladder wall, caused by activity in some muscle bundles but not others. Such a condition would arise in normal bladders if a small population of low-threshold postganglionic parasympathetic neurons were activated, e.g. towards the end of bladder filling. Because of relatively poor coupling between bundles, such diffuse activity would not cause a rise in intravesical pressure, but could activate a population of sensory nerve fibers that might specifically mediate the sensation of urgency and play a useful role in encouraging the initiation of normal micturition. In overactive bladders, however, such diffuse activation of some muscle bundles might spread because of the increased connectivity to give rise to the overactive pressure rises. An increase in the sensitivity of fibers mediating urgency may be responsible for the enhanced urgency seen in inflammatory conditions, interstitial cystitis, and other examples of sensory urgency. The role of the urothelium and its secretory products is of interest here, and the arrangement of the suburothelial nerve plexus and interstitial cells. The interactions between the various elements are currently the focus of intense research by several groups.

Conclusions

It is clear that we are still some way from really understanding what causes bladder overactivity. However, there are sufficient clues from the observations and experimental results described above to suggest that we are dealing with the consequences of altered patterns of activation of the nerves in the micturition pathways and the resultant effects of this on the smooth muscle in the detrusor. In cases of severe overactivity and urge incontinence, the process has probably been ongoing for years. Some factors such as detrusor-sphincter dyssynergia, outflow obstruction, or abnormal rises in intra-abdominal pressure have caused periodic bladder wall ischemia and this has reached a stage in which neurons in the bladder wall have actually died; the smooth muscle in the detrusor has then become able to generate synchronous contractions and these result in the overactive pressure rises seen. What precise mechanism triggers these overactive contractions is not yet clear, although it is likely that premature activation through some local or supraspinal pathway of the remaining parasympathetic ganglia is usually involved.

It may be that the most likely scenario for urge incontinence which is associated with overactive contractions is as follows: activity in some muscle bundles generated either by stretch or by diffuse activity in parasympathetic fibers causes local distortions of the bladder wall; this both activates the sensation of urgency and spreads to cause synchronous activation of the bladder wall, resulting in an overactive pressure rise. The sequence of events recorded should be urgency occurring first, followed almost immediately by an overactive contraction. What happens after this may vary. If the contraction is large enough to overcome the outflow resistance, leakage will occur. This could, in its turn, activate receptors in the urethra and trigger secondary changes (transient opening of the bladder neck, etc.), but often the pressure and sensation of urgency will subside. Synchronous detrusor contraction will itself reduce the sensation of urgency and the bladder pressure may return to normal. Activation of the detrusor smooth muscle, unless supported by continuous neural input, is self-limiting, since the muscles possess calcium-activated potassium channels which ensure that the membrane hyperpolarizes and spontaneous action potentials will be switched off transiently.[63] Normally, urge incontinence does not result in complete bladder emptying, but if there is a well-developed segmental spinal micturition reflex and loss of any descending control, activation of the pressure/stretch receptors may reinforce the activity and produce bladder emptying.

References

1. Koelbl H, Mostwin JL, Boiteux JP et al. Pathophysiology. In: Abrams P, Cardozo L, Khoury S, Wein A (eds): Incontinence. Plymouth UK: Health Publications 2002: 205–41.
2. Abrams P, Cardozo L, Fall M et al. The standardisation of terminology of lower urinary tract function: report from the Standardisation Sub-committee of the International Continence Society. Neurourol Urodyn 2002; 21: 167–78.
3. Drake MJ, Harvey IJ, Gillespie JI. Autonomous activity in the isolated guinea pig bladder. Exp Physiol 2003; 88: 19–30.
4. Hashitani H, Yanai Y, Suzuki H. Role of interstitial cells and gap junctions in the transmission of spontaneous Ca^{2+} signals in detrusor smooth muscles of the guinea-pig urinary bladder. J Physiol 2004; 559: 567–81.
5. Brading AF, McCloskey KD. Mechanisms of disease: specialized interstitial cells of the urinary tract – an assessment of current knowledge. Nat Clin Pract Urol 2005; 2: 546–55.
6. Ferguson DR. Urothelial function. BJU Int 1999; 84: 235–42.
7. Birder L. Role of the urothelium in bladder function. Scand J Urol Nephrol Suppl 2004: 48–53.
8. Wiseman OJ, Fowler CJ, Landon DN. The role of the human bladder lamina propria myofibroblast. BJU Int 2003; 91: 89–93.
9. Brading AF. Physiology of bladder smooth muscle. In: Torrens MJ, Morrison JFB (eds). The Physiology of the Lower Urinary Tract. New York: Springer Verlag, 1987: 161–91.
10. Biers SM, Reynard JM, Doore T, Brading AF. The functional effects of a c-kit tyrosine inhibitor on guinea-pig and human detrusor. BJU Int 2006; 97: 612–16.
11. Sibley GNA. A comparison of spontaneous and nerve-mediated activity in bladder muscle from man, pig and rabbit. J Physiol (Lond) 1984; 354: 431–43.
12. Sibley GNA. The response of the bladder to lower urinary tract obstruction [DM]. Oxford, 1984.
13. German K, Bedwani J, Davies J, Brading AF, Stephenson TP. Physiological and morphometric studies into the pathophysiology of detrusor hyperreflexia in neuropathic patients. J Urol 1995; 153: 1678–83.
14. Kinder RB, Mundy AR. Pathophysiology of idiopathic detrusor instability and detrusor hyper-reflexia. An in vitro study of human detrusor muscle. Br J Urol 1987; 60: 509–15.
15. Mills IW, Greenland JE, McMurray G, Noble JG, Brading AF. Spontaneous myogenic contractile activity of isolated human detrusor smooth muscle in idiopathic instability. BJU 1999; 83: 20.
16. Mills IW, Greenland JE, McMurray G et al. Studies of the pathophysiology of idiopathic detrusor instability: the physiological properties of the detrusor smooth muscle and its pattern of innervation. J Urol 2000; 163: 646–51.
17. Turner WH, Brading AF. Smooth muscle of the bladder in the normal and the diseased state: pathophysiology, diagnosis and treatment. Pharmacol Ther 1997; 75: 77–110.
18. Drake MJ, Harvey IJ, Gillespie JI, Van Duyl WA. Localized contractions in the normal human bladder and in urinary urgency. BJU Int 2005; 95: 1002–5.
19. Mills IW. The Pathophysiology of Detrusor Instability and the Role of Bladder Ischaemia in its Aetiology. MS Thesis, Pharmacology Department. Oxford, 1999.
20. Turner WH. An experimental urodynamic model of lower urinary tract function and dysfunction [DM]. Cambridge, 1997.
21. Brading AF. Alterations in the physiological properties of urinary bladder smooth muscle caused by bladder emptying against an obstruction. Scand J Urol Nephrol Suppl 1997; 184: 51–8.
22. Brading AF, Turner WH. The unstable bladder: towards a common mechanism. Br J Urol 1994; 73: 3–8.
23. Sibley GNA. Developments in our understanding of detrusor instability. BJU 1997; 80: 54–61.
24. Sibley GNA. An experimental model of detrusor instability in the obstructed pig. Br J Urol 1985; 57: 292–8.
25. Speakman MJ, Brading AF, Gilpin CJ et al. Bladder outflow obstruction – a cause of denervation supersensitivity. J Urol 1987; 138: 1461–6.
26. Harrison SC, Ferguson DR, Doyle PT. Effect of bladder outflow obstruction on the innervation of the rabbit urinary bladder. Br J Urol 1990; 66: 372–9.
27. Sethia KK. The pathophysiology of detrusor instability [DM]. Oxford, 1988.

28. Elbadawi A, Resnick NM, Dorsam J, Yalla SV, Haferkamp A. Structural basis of neurogenic bladder dysfunction. I. Methods of prospective ultrastructural study and overview of the findings. J Urol 2003; 169: 540–6.
29. Haferkamp A, Dorsam J, Resnick NM, Yalla SV, Elbadawi A. Structural basis of neurogenic bladder dysfunction. III. Intrinsic detrusor innervation. J Urol 2003; 169: 555–62.
30. Haferkamp A, Dorsam J, Resnick NM, Yalla SV, Elbadawi A. Structural basis of neurogenic bladder dysfunction. II. Myogenic basis of detrusor hyperreflexia. J Urol 2003; 169: 547–54.
31. Brading AF, Speakman MJ. Pathophysiology of bladder outflow obstruction. In: Whitfield H, Kirby R, Hendry WF, Duckett J (eds). Textbook of Genitourinary Surgery, 2nd edn. Oxford: Blackwell Science, 1998: 465–79.
32. Daniel EE, Cowan W, Daniel VP. Structural bases for neural and myogenic control of human detrusor muscle. Can J Physiol Pharmacol 1983; 61: 1247–73.
33. Neuhaus J, Weimann A, Stolzenburg JU et al. Smooth muscle cells from human urinary bladder express connexin 43 in vivo and in vitro. World J Urol 2002; 20: 250–4.
34. Neuhaus J, Pfeiffer F, Wolburg H, Horn LC, Dorschner W. Alterations in connexin expression in the bladder of patients with urge symptoms. BJU Int 2005; 96: 670–6.
35. Bramich NJ, Brading AF. Electrical properties of smooth muscle in the guinea-pig urinary bladder. J Physiol 1996; 492(Pt 1): 185–98.
36. Fry CH, Cooklin M, Birns J, Mundy AR. Measurement of intercellular electrical coupling in guinea-pig detrusor smooth muscle. J Urol 1999; 161: 660–4.
37. Hashitani H, Fukuta H, Takano H, Klemm MF, Suzuki H. Origin and propagation of spontaneous excitation in smooth muscle of the guinea-pig urinary bladder. J Physiol 2001; 530: 273–86.
38. Gabella G. The structural relations between nerve fibres and muscle cells in the urinary bladder of the rat. J Neurocytol 1995; 24: 159–87.
39. Westfall DP. Supersensitivity of smooth muscle. In: Bülbring E, Brading AF, Jones AW, Tomita T (eds). Smooth Muscle: An Assessment of Current Knowledge. London: Arnold, 1981: 285–309.
40. Charlton RG, Morley AR, Chambers P, Gillespie JI. Focal changes in nerve, muscle and connective tissue in normal and unstable human bladder. BJU Int 1999; 84: 953–60.
41. Drake MJ, Hedlund P, Mills IW et al. Structural and functional denervation of human detrusor after spinal cord injury. Lab Invest 2000; 80: 1491–9.
42. Speakman MJ. Studies on the physiology of the normal and obstructed bladder [MS]. London, 1988.
43. Williams JH, Turner WH, Sainsbury GM, Brading AF. Experimental model of bladder outflow tract obstruction in the guinea-pig. Br J Urol 1993; 71: 543–54.
44. Steers WD, Ciambotti J, Etzel B, Erdman S, de Groat WC. Alterations in afferent pathways from the urinary bladder of the rat in response to partial urethral obstruction. J Comp Neurol 1991; 310: 401–10.
45. Steers WD, Ciambotti J, Erdman S, de Groat WC. Morphological plasticity in efferent pathways to the urinary bladder of the rat following urethral obstruction. J Neurosci 1990; 10: 1943–51.
46. Gabella G, Berggren T, Uvelius B. Hypertrophy and reversal of hypertrophy in rat pelvic ganglion neurons. J Neurocytol 1992; 21: 649–62.
47. Kruse MN, Belton AL, de Groat WC. Changes in bladder and external sphincter function after spinal injury in the rat. AM J Physiol 1993; 264: 1157–63.
48. de Groat WC. A neurological basis for the overactive bladder. Urology 1997; 50: 36–52.
49. Geirrson G, Lindstrom S, Fall M. The bladder cooling reflex in man – characteristics and sensitivity to temperature. Br J Urol 1993; 71: 675–80.
50. Geirsson G, Fall M, Lindstrom S. The ice-water test – a simple and valuable supplement to routine cystometry. Br J Urol 1993; 71: 681–5.
51. de Ridder D, Baert L. Vanilloids and the overactive bladder. BJU Int 2000; 86: 172–80.
52. Greenland JE, Brading AF. Urinary bladder blood flow changes during the micturition cycle in a conscious pig model. J Urol 1996; 156: 1858–61.
53. Brading AF, Greenland JE, Mills IW, McMurray G, Symes S. Blood supply to the bladder during filling. Scand J Urol Nephrol Suppl 1999; 201: 25–31.
54. Levin RM, Haugaard N, Hypolite JA, Wein AJ, Buttyan R. Metabolic factors influencing lower urinary tract function. Exp Physiol 1999; 84: 171–94.
55. Symes SE. Effects of ishaemic-like conditions on guinea-pig urinary bladder [DPhil]. Oxford, 2002: 246.
56. Greenland JE, Brading AF. The effect of bladder outflow obstruction on detrusor blood flow changes during the voiding cycle in conscious pigs. J Urol 2001; 165: 245–8.
57. Steers WD, Creedon DJ, Tuttle JB. Immunity to nerve growth factor prevents plasticity following urinary bladder hypertrophy. J Urol 1996; 155: 379–85.
58. Iggo A. Tension receptors in the stomach and the urinary bladder. J Physiol 1955; 128: 593–607.
59. Jänig W, Morrison JFB. Functional properties of spinal visceral afferents supplying abdominal and pelvic organs, with special emphasis on visceral nociception. Progr Brain Res 1986; 67: 87–114.
60. Morrison JFB. Sensations arising from the lower urinary tract. In: Torrens M, Morrison JFB (eds). The Physiology of the Lower Urinary Tract. Berlin: Springer-Verlag, 1987: 89–131.
61. Namasivayam S, Eardley I, Morrison JF. A novel in vitro bladder pelvic nerve afferent model in the rat. Br J Urol 1998; 82: 902–5.
62. Coolsaet BL, Van Duyl WA, Van Os-Bossagh P, De Bakker HV. New concepts in relation to urge and detrusor activity. Neurourol Urodyn 1993; 12: 463–71.
63. Wellner MC, Isenberg G. Stretch effects on whole-cell currents of guinea-pig urinary bladder myocytes. J Physiol (Lond) 1994; 480: 439–48.

12

Pathophysiology of detrusor underactivity/acontractile detrusor

Dae Kyung Kim and Michael B Chancellor

Introduction

According to the standardization of terminology from the International Continence Society,[1] detrusor underactivity (DU) is urodynamically defined as a contraction of reduced strength and/or duration, resulting in prolonged bladder emptying and/or a failure to achieve complete bladder emptying within a normal time span. Acontractile detrusor (AD) is one that cannot be demonstrated to contract during urodynamic studies. DU or AD (DU/AD) can be developed from various kinds of conditions, when afferent and/or efferent pathways innervating the bladder are mainly damaged. Various myogenic factors in detrusor muscles also cause AD as well as DU.

The mechanism of micturition reflexes

Pelvic afferent pathways

Efferent outflow to the lower urinary tract can be activated reflexively by spinal afferent pathways as well as by input from the brain. Afferent input from the pelvic visceral organs and somatic afferent pathways from the perineal muscle and skin are very important.[2] Somatic afferent pathways in the pudendal nerves, which transmit noxious or non-noxious information from the genital organs, urethra, prostate, vagina, anal canal, and skin, can modulate voiding function.[3–5]

Bladder afferent nerves are critical for sending signals of bladder fullness and discomfort to the brain and for initiating the micturition reflex. The bladder afferent pathways are composed of two types of axons: large/medium diameter myelinated Aδ fibers and unmyelinated C fibers.[6] Aδ fibers transmit signals mainly from mechanoreceptors that detect bladder fullness or wall tension. C fibers, on the other hand, mainly detect noxious signals and initiate painful sensations. The bladder C fiber nociceptors perform a similar function and signal the central nervous system when we have an infection or irritative condition in the bladder.

C fiber bladder afferents also have reflex functions to facilitate or trigger voiding.[7–9] This can be viewed as a defense mechanism to eliminate irritants or bacteria from the body. C fiber bladder afferents have been implicated in the triggering of reflex bladder overactivity associated with neurologic disorders such as spinal cord injury and multiple sclerosis.

Micturition reflexes

Normal micturition is completely dependent on neural pathways in the central nervous system. These pathways perform three major functions: *amplification, coordination,* and *timing.*[3] The nervous control of the lower urinary tract must be able to *amplify* weak smooth muscle activity to provide sustained increases in intravesical pressure sufficient to empty the bladder. The bladder and urethral sphincter function must be *coordinated* to allow the sphincter to open during micturition but to be closed at all other times. *Timing* represents the voluntary control of voiding in the normal adult and the ability to initiate voiding over a wide range of bladder volumes (Figure 12.1).

In this regard, the bladder is a unique visceral organ, which exhibits predominantly voluntary rather than involuntary (autonomic) neural regulation. A number of important reflex mechanisms contribute to the storage or elimination of urine and modulate the voluntary control of micturition.[5]

Guarding reflexes (guarding against stress urinary incontinence)

There is an important bladder to urethral reflex that is mediated by sympathetic efferent pathways to the urethra. This is

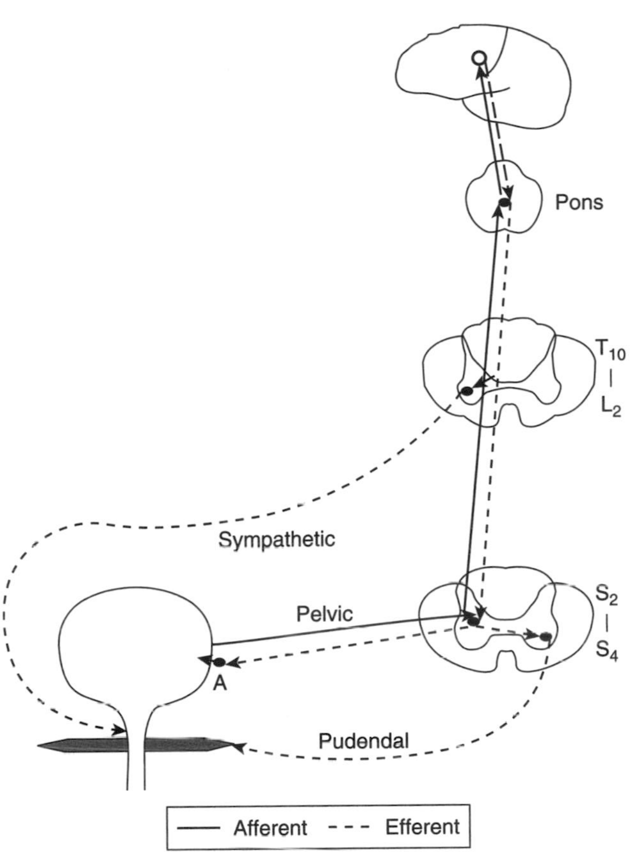

Figure 12.1
Micturition requires positive feedback to ensure complete bladder emptying. As the bladder fills, myelinated Aδ tension receptors are activated. This afferent signal must reach the pontine micturition center with subsequent activation of parasympathetic efferent outflow.

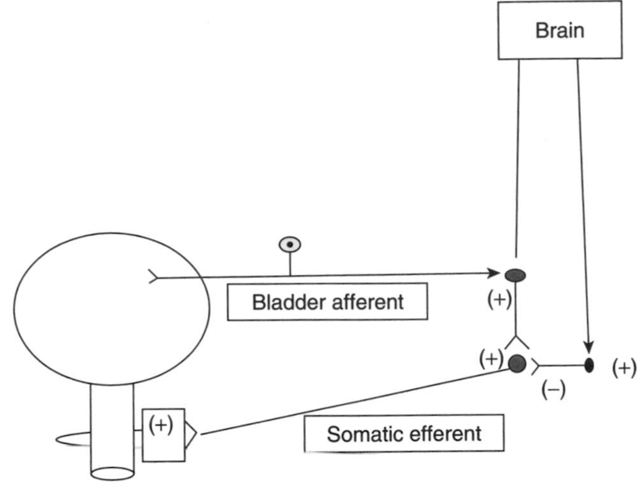

Figure 12.2
The guarding reflex prevents urinary incontinence. When there is a sudden increase in intravesical pressure, such as cough, the urinary sphincter contracts via the spinal guarding reflex to prevent urinary incontinence. The spinal guarding reflex can be turned off by the brain to urinate.

an excitatory reflex that contracts the urethral smooth muscle and thus is called a guarding reflex.[10,11] The positive reflex is not activated during micturition but when bladder pressure is increased such as during a cough or exercise. A second guarding reflex is triggered by the bladder afferents, which synapse with sacral interneurons that in turn activate urethral external sphincter efferent neurons that send axons into the pudendal nerves.[12] The activation of pudendal urethral efferent pathways contracts the external urinary sphincter, and prevents stress urinary incontinence (Figure 12.2). The brain inhibits the guarding reflexes during micturition.

Conditions or diseases developing DU/AD

DU/AD is usually observed when the following mechanisms are damaged:[13]

- bladder peripheral afferent pathways
- bladder peripheral efferent pathways
- lumbosacral spinal cord (micturition center)
- myogenic failure.

These four factors are often mixed in the condition of DU/AD. In this section, we discuss several kinds of diseases that develop DU/AD, including the pathogenesis, urodynamic findings, and treatments. Future treatment strategies are also presented.

Diabetes mellitus (diabetic cystopathy)

Bladder dysfunction associated with the complication of diabetes mellitus (DM), classically called diabetic cystopathy, has been described as impaired sensation of bladder fullness, increased bladder capacity, reduced bladder contractility, and increased residual urine.[14–16]

However, these classic symptoms are not always observed in diabetic patients and symptom presentations are quite variable. Moreover, common concomitant diseases such as urinary tract infection, benign prostatic hyperplasia, and stress urinary incontinence may obscure underlying diabetic cystopathy. Therefore, it is important to discern the major factor from the complex presentation of symptoms in an individual patient. It has also been reported that diabetic cystopathy can occur silently and early in the course of diabetes.[17] In such cases, it is not rare for bladder dysfunction induced by diabetes not to be found without careful questions and/or urodynamic testing.

The sex and age of patients are not the factors related to prevalence, whereas the duration of diabetes is bound up with the prevalence rate of diabetic cystopathy.[17]

Pathogenesis of diabetic cystopathy

Pathophysiology of diabetic cystopathy has multifocal aspects. Traditionally, diabetic cystopathy was thought to result from polyneuropathy that predominantly affects sensory and autonomic nerve fibers.[18,19] Some of the proposed pathogenesis includes altered metabolism of glucose, ischemia, superoxide-induced free radical formation, impaired axonal transport, and metabolic derangement of the Schwann cells.[20,21] In addition to neuronal changes, many recent studies suggest that diabetic cystopathy can result from an alteration in the physiology of the detrusor smooth muscle cell, or urothelial dysfunction.[21]

Detrusor smooth muscle function has shown altered physiology in streptozotocin (STZ)- or alloxan-induced DM animal models. Major physiologic alterations are changes in sensitivity and contractile forces. Although there is some controversy on the responsiveness to muscarinic agonists, most agree on the increased responsiveness of DM bladder strip to electrical field stimulation.[22,23] These changes are suggested to reflect increased calcium channel activity and enhanced calcium sensitivity.[23] Myocytes from DM rats have also shown increased depolarization to externally applied acetylcholine and decreased spontaneous activity, presumably related to altered purinergic transmission.[24] Changolkar et al[25] reported that diabetes induced a decrease in detrusor smooth muscle contractility and an increase in oxidative stress factors, an increase in lipid peroxidase/sorbitol, and concomitant overexpression of the aldose reductase/polyol pathway activation. The same group also reported increased expression of thin filament proteins, calponin, tropomyosin, and caldesmon, in DM rabbit bladder, which might alter the contractile and cytoskeletal structure.[26]

The changes in tissue neurotrophic factors such as nerve growth factor (NGF) have been focused on as a convincing pathogenesis of diabetic neuropathy.[27–32] In STZ-DM rats, the decrease in tissue NGF levels in the bladder and bladder afferent pathways is associated with diabetic cystopathy.[33] Changes in another neurotrophic factor, neurotrophin-3 (NT-3), have also been reported.[34–36] It is promising for future treatment strategies that the changes in tissue neurotrophic factor could play a critical role in inducing diabetic cystopathy.

Studies have shown that the urothelium is not a passive barrier but rather it can take an active role in bladder physiology.[21] The urothelium can release many mediators including ATP, NO, and prostanoid.[37,38] Pinna et al[39] reported that, in isolated urothelial layer preparations from STZ-DM rats, levels of endogenous prostaglandins E2 and F2α were higher than in preparations from normal rats. ATP and bradykinin significantly increased the endogenous release of prostaglandins E2 and F2α from the urothelium when compared with the basal release level. This time-dependent increase was higher in diabetic tissues than in controls. Prostaglandins may have a role in the sensitization of sensory nerves and may increase the sensitivity of DM bladder to contractile stimuli.

The formation of nitric oxide synthase (NOS) and reactive nitrogen species also change during DM-related bladder remodeling. Poladia and Bauer[40] reported that endothelial NOS is significantly upregulated in the lamina propria, neuronal NOS is upregulated in the urothelium, lamina propria, and smooth muscle, while inducible NOS is upregulated only in the urothelium. They suggested that impaired NO control is an early event leading to increased oxidative stress and proteasomal activation in the pathogenesis of diabetic cystopathy.

Urodynamic testing on diabetic cystopathy

In most typical cases with diabetic cystopathy, cystometry shows a long curve with lack of sensation, often until bladder capacity is reached, with a low detrusor pressure.[16,41,42] However, it has been reported that this classical type of underactive diabetic cystopathy is sometimes modified by concomitant lesions such as bladder outlet obstruction (BOO) or a history of cerebrovascular disease. For example, previous studies have reported a high incidence of detrusor overactivity (DO), of up to 50–60%, when bladder function was examined in a selected population of diabetic patients presenting with positive lower urinary tract symptoms or with a history of stroke.[43,44] BOO should also be considered as a differential diagnosis for DO in diabetic patients.[41] BOO is documented by measuring a high or normal pressure in the presence of an impaired urinary flow rate. Some patients with both diabetic cystopathy and BOO exhibit DO and elevated detrusor pressure during low-flow voiding.

However, despite reports of a relatively high incidence of DO in symptomatic diabetic patients,[43] one should be aware that autonomic and sensory neuropathy with diminished bladder sensation and bladder contractility is the predominant urologic manifestation of diabetic cystopathy when unselected diabetic patients are examined[14–16] (Figures 12.3 and 12.4).

Electromyography (EMG) is usually normal but sometimes exhibits sphincter denervation and uninhibited sphincter relaxation. Uroflowmetry shows low peak flow and prolonged duration of flow associated with increased

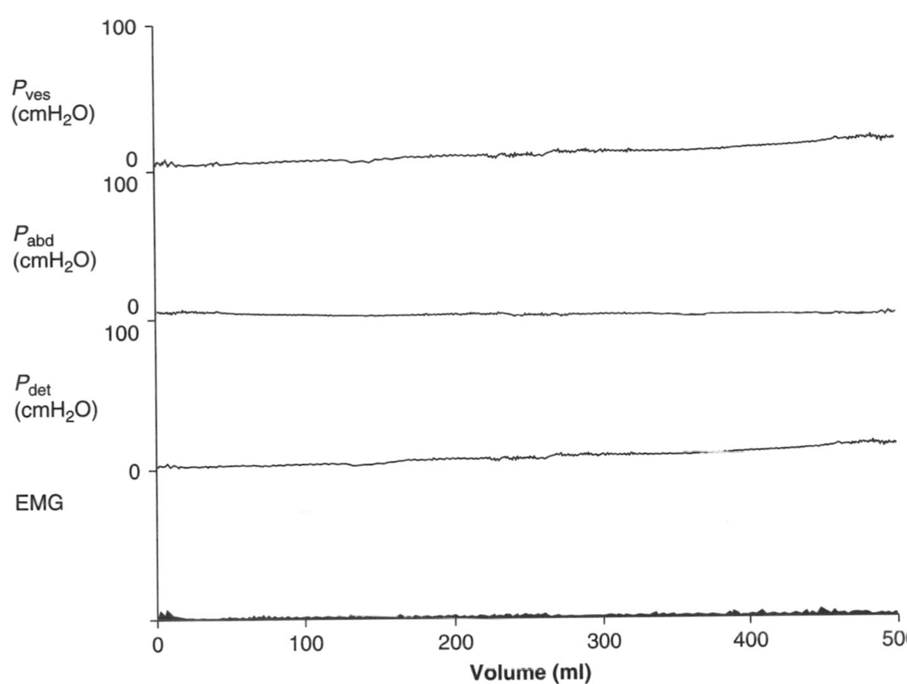

Figure 12.3
Acontractile detrusor in a 62-year-old insulin-dependent diabetic woman. The patient is on intermittent catheterization approximately 4 times per 24 hours. P_{ves}, intravesical pressure; P_{abd}, abdominal pressure; P_{det}, detrusor pressure.

residual urine. Urethral pressure profiles have not been well studied or validated in diabetic cystopathy.[16,45]

Treatment of diabetic cystopathy

The first and most important step in the management of diabetes is to control the blood glucose level. Hyperglycemia has been proved to be related to neuropathy and other complications of diabetes. However, the control of blood glucose level does not mean the prevention of diabetic cystopathy.[17] Other preventive general management techniques include hypertension and hyperlipidemia control and education on non-smoking.

The main goal in treatment for diabetic cystopathy is basically to avoid overdistention of the bladder and to decrease residual urine. Since diabetic cystopathy usually has an insidious onset, scheduled voiding should be recommended to all diabetic patients regardless of symptom presence. If needed, double or triple voiding may also be recommended.[46] Manual compression of the lower abdomen (Credé's maneuver) or abdominal straining (Valsalva maneuver) may be helpful to decrease residual urine in selected patients. However, these maneuvers are contraindicated in the presence of increased intravesical pressure, vagal reflux, and vesico-ureteral reflux. Alpha-blockers have some benefit in diabetic cystopathy concomitant with BOO. Cholinergic receptor agonists such as bethanechol chloride or urecholine have been used with inconsistent results in diabetic cystopathy.[47]

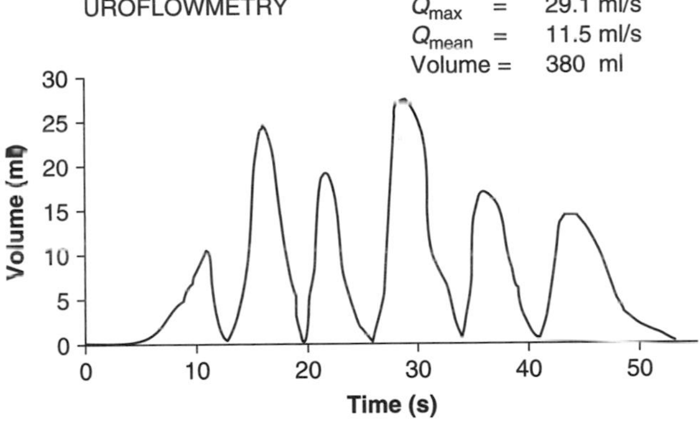

Figure 12.4
Straining uroflowmetry of the diabetic woman in Figure 12.3. The patient complained of a sensation of incomplete emptying postmicturition, occasional incontinence, and straining to urinate. Although her maximum flow rate (Q_{max}) is normal (29.1 ml/s), the voiding pattern is classic for Valsalva voiding without true detrusor contractility.

Loss of bladder sensation is irreversible in diabetes and long-term follow-up is necessary. In addition, many patients with diabetic cystopathy may delay seeking urologic evaluation because of the insidious development of diabetic cystopathy that induces diminished sensation and increased bladder capacity. Thus, careful surveillance for voiding symptoms and screening for elevated residual urine, including urodynamic studies, should be done regularly to prevent long-term complications secondary to diabetic cystopathy.

Future treatment strategies

Conservative treatments for diabetic cystopathy are limited and cannot restore bladder function, as mentioned previously. Recently, new treatment approaches for diabetic polyneuropathy, including diabetic cystopathy, have been reported in both the basic and clinical fields. Following the efficacy of nerve growth factor (NGF) treatment in basic studies,[48–50] the efficacy of NGF treatment in the clinical field has been reported.[51–53]

The feasibility of gene therapy using replication-deficient herpes simplex virus (HSV) encoding *rhNGF* genes has been reported. Four weeks after HSV–*rhNGF* injection into the STZ-DM rat bladder, a significant increase of NGF levels in the bladder and the L6 dorsal root ganglion (DRG) was detected. DM rats on HSV-NGF gene therapy also had a smaller bladder capacity and less residual urine than untreated DM rats.[54,55] Studies using neurotrophic factors other than NGF, such as glial cell line-derived neurotrophic factor (GDNF) or neurotrophin-3 (NT-3), have also demonstrated significant efficacy in restoring nerve function in diabetic animals.[56,57]

Thus, in the future, neurotrophic factors or other growth factors combined with targeted gene therapy techniques may be beneficial for the therapy of patients with diabetic cystopathy.

Conclusions

Diabetic cystopathy, which is characterized by loss of bladder sensation and DU/AD, is common and can develop insidiously. Tests, including urodynamic studies in the early stages of diabetes, are needed. Exciting new approaches to the treatment of diabetic cystopathy are being investigated.

Injury to the spinal cord, cauda equina, and pelvic plexus

Any injury to the spinal cord, such as blunt, degenerative, developmental, vascular, infectious, traumatic, and idiopathic injury, can cause voiding dysfunction. In this section we will discuss the urodynamic manifestations of some common spinal and cauda equina neurologic processes.

Injury to the cauda equina or peripheral sacral nerves can have a devastating effect on bladder and urethral sphincter function. The resulting urinary dysfunction can be a major cause of morbidity in these cases. Lumbosacral spinal cord injury and herniated intervertebral disc are the two most common etiologic factors.[58,59] Other etiologic causes include lumbar spinal stenosis, myelodysplasia, spinal arachnoiditis, arteriovenous malformation, and primary or metastatic tumors of the lumbar spine. It is also a rare complication of regional anesthesia.

Injury to the pelvic plexus is not common. It is usually iatrogenic, most often occurring after major abdominal and pelvic surgery such as abdominoperineal resection or radical hysterectomy. Sometimes the problem may result from a pelvic fracture, or the trauma may be intentional (e.g. transvesical phenol injection) to abolish neurogenic DO in patients who have failed standard treatment regimens.

Neuroanatomy and pathophysiology

Although it is well established that the pelvic plexus is derived from the ventral rami of S2–4 nerves,[58–60] there is contradictory information on sacral nerve connections and collateralization.[59–61] The precise branching and interconnections among the sacral plexus are important because of increasing interest in dorsal rhizotomy and functional electrical stimulation for bladder control.

The pelvic plexus lies deep in the pelvis, oriented in a parasagittal plane alongside the rectum. On most occasions, injury to this structure is iatrogenically induced following major pelvic ablative surgery. A malignant process involving the pelvis or invasive rectal neoplasms in the lateral and posterior or rectal wall may infiltrate the adjacent pararectal autonomic nerves, thus causing pelvic plexus injury.[62–64]

Marani et al[61] reported the surgical dissection of the cauda equina and pelvic plexus of 10 human cadavers (5 males and 5 females). In 9 (4 males and 5 females) a branch connecting the ventral rami of the second and third sacral spinal nerves was found. Electron microscopy demonstrated the presence of thick myelinated fibers in this branch. This may contribute to the interaction between detrusor and sphincter contractions. The branches contributing to the pelvic plexus have individual and intersexual differences. It is important to be aware of the wide range of branches when decisions have to be made concerning the strategy of neurostimulation or dorsal rhizotomy.

Voiding dysfunction after major pelvic surgery is usually caused by intraoperative injury to pelvic, hypogastric, and pudendal nerves.[64,65] The neuroanatomic basis for the denervation of the bladder has been described on the basis of detailed anatomic dissections.[66] Direct damage to the parasympathetic nerves and the posterior part of the pelvic plexus may occur during dissection on the anterolateral aspect of the lower rectum. In addition, traction injury may occur during mobilization of the lower rectum due to the relationship of the pelvic nerves with the fascial capsule investing the rectum.[67]

During hysterectomy, the main factor producing bladder denervation appears to be extensive dissection inferolateral to the cervix.[63] Damage to the sympathetics in the hypogastric plexus may occur at the pelvic brim medial to the ureters and also in the region lateral to the rectum. Extensive dissection in the vicinity of the cardinal ligaments at the time of radical hysterectomy may also produce sympathetic denervation.[64]

During the perineal portion of an abdominoperineal resection at the time of mobilization of the anus, injury to the pudendal nerve may occur. It is therefore apparent that varying degrees of damage to parasympathetic, sympathetic, and somatic nerves may occur, which can range from neural traction injury, to incomplete or complete nerve ablation.

Pelvic surgery

The incidence of vesico-ureteral dysfunction has been reported to be 20–68% of patients after abdominal perineal resection, 16–80% after radical hysterectomy, 10–20% after proctocolectomy, and 20–25% after anterior resection.[64,65,67–70] However, the true incidence of lower urinary tract dysfunction after pelvic plexus injury is still unknown, mainly because it is very difficult to make prospective studies with pre- and postoperative neurourologic evaluation of the patients. Three additional factors make the issue more complex. Firstly, most patients in the age group requiring treatment for abdominal or pelvic malignancy may have pre-existing BOO or another pathology responsible for the functional derangement of the lower urinary tract. Secondly, in a significant percentage of patients, recovery of bladder function may occur as time goes on. Up to 80% of the patients with bladder dysfunction resulting from major pelvic surgery will resume normal voiding within 6 months from the procedure. Lastly, in most early series the technical means for a comprehensive urodynamic evaluation were not available at that time.

Regarding the complexity of neural injuries in these cases, which can involve parasympathetic, sympathetic, as well as somatic nerve fibers, it is evident that only modern urodynamic techniques can provide the exact information on the nature and the extent of an individual case.[62,65]

Pelvic and sacral fractures

Pelvic trauma can result in cauda equina and pelvic plexus injury. The frequency of neurologic injury after pelvic fractures is estimated at between 0.75 and 11%.[71–73] Autopsy findings and clinical studies have shown that neurologic injury accompanying sacral fractures occurs either intradurally or extradurally within the sacral canal. Sacral fractures are associated with pelvic fractures in 90% of the cases.[71,72] Approximately 25% of sacral fractures will result in permanent neurologic deficit.[74,75] Transverse fractures are most closely correlated with neurologic injury. Approximately two-thirds of these patients will have neurogenic bladder.[76]

Because most of the injuries are incomplete, the majority of patients with neuro-urologic injury after pelvic and sacral fractures will notice improvement with time. However, delayed neurologic deficits may occur after sacral fracture as a late complication.[77,78] These delayed deficits result from various causes: scarring, hematoma formation at the fracture site, and untreated spinal instability.

Herniated disc

Some reports indicate that the incidence of voiding dysfunction as a result of disc prolapse may approach 20% of patients.[79,80] Since the data demonstrated that detrusor recovery was rare after treatment once patients showed bladder dysfunction following lumbar disc prolapse, cauda equina syndrome from lumbar disc herniation might be a diagnostic and surgical emergency.[81,82]

Lesions of the pudendal nerve

The pudendal nerve arises from anterior primary rami of S2–4, leaves the pelvis through the greater sciatic foramen below the piriformis muscle, and passes forward into the ischiorectal fossa. The nerve is occasionally injured in fractures of the pelvis. Damage produces sensory loss in the perineum and scrotum on the side of the lesion. Bilateral lesions produce bladder disturbances, with urinary retention and overflow incontinence.

Clinical findings

Patients with known or suspected neurologic injury due to pelvic or sacral injury should have a careful physical examination. The integrity of the sacral dermatomes is tested by assessing perianal sensation, anal sphincter tone, and the bulbocavernosus reflex.

The type of the resulting functional disturbance will depend on the nature and extent of nerve injury. Parasympathetic denervation causes AD, whereas sympathetic damage will produce loss of proximal urethral pressure as a result of the compromised alpha-mediated innervations to the smooth muscle fibers of the bladder neck and urethra.[83,84]

Many patients complain of straining to urinate, incontinence, and a sensation of incomplete emptying. The urinary stream may be diminished and interrupted, as many of these patients rely on abdominal straining to urinate. On occasions, symptoms of voiding dysfunction can be the only initial clinical manifestation of a cauda equina lesion.[85] The varied and mixed symptomatologies emphasize the need for a complete neuro-urologic evaluation.

The physical examination may reveal a distended bladder, but the most characteristic features are elicited on a careful neurologic examination. Sensory loss in the perineum or perianal area is associated with S2–4 dermatomes. The extent of perineal anesthesia can be a useful predictive clinical index in patients with lumbar disc prolapse. If 'saddle' anesthesia of the S2–4 dermatomes continues after surgical laminectomy and decompression, the urinary bladder rarely recovers.[86] On the contrary, a unilateral or mild sensory disturbance indicates a better prognosis. Deep tendon reflexes in the lower extremities, clonus, and plantar responses, as well as the bulbocavernosus reflex, should be routinely evaluated.

In a series of patients with cauda equina injury of various etiologies, the bulbocavernosus reflex was absent or significantly diminished in 84% of the cases, whereas the perineal sensation and muscle stretch reflexes were compromised in 77% of the patients.[76] In addition, it was noted that absence of the reflex correlated well with perineal floor denervation.[87]

It is of interest that parasympathetic denervation itself may actually increase adrenergic activity by unmasking already existing alpha-receptors or inducing alpha-receptors. It has been demonstrated by histochemical fluorescence studies that the adrenergic nerve terminals of denervated human detrusors were thicker and denser than those of neurologically normal detrusors. A complete injury of both pelvic plexuses disrupts the nerve supply to the bladder and the urethra, but most injuries are incomplete. Since most ganglia lie close to or within the bladder wall and large numbers of postganglionic neurons remain intact, any denervation is followed by reinnervation,[88] so that some residual lower tract activity remains. Sensation may be preserved, but, if it is lost, the resultant symptoms are usually urinary retention and overflow incontinence.

Peripheral sympathetic injury results in an open, nonfunctional bladder neck and proximal urethra. Although this could occur as an isolated injury, it typically occurs in association with partial detrusor denervation, but with preservation of sphincter function.[84] The combination of decreased compliance, open bladder neck, and fixed external sphincter resistance results in the paradoxic symptomatology of both leaking across the distal sphincter and the inability to empty the bladder. Under these circumstances, the optimal management is a combination of anticholinergics and intermittent catheterization.

Urodynamic findings

The typical cystometrogram (CMG) finding of cauda equina injury is loss of detrusor contraction.[62,76] On the uroflowmetry, an abdominal straining saw-tooth pattern is generally seen when the patients claim they can urinate. Urodynamic abnormalities may be the only aberration documented without other overt neurologic manifestations in some patients with cauda equina injury. On herniated disc, which is not induced by trauma or acute conditions, the protrusion is usually slow and progressive. In these cases, it may result in nerve irritation and consequently detrusor DO.[89]

Sphincter denervation – as documented on EMG by a decreased interference pattern, fibrillation, positive sharp waves, and polyphasic potentials – has also been reported.[76] This observation can be attributed to the different location of the detrusor and pudendal motor nuclei within the sacral cord,[90] as well as to the fact that the dominant segment of the pelvic nerve usually arises one segment higher than that of the pudendal nerve.[91]

The predominant CMG/EMG pattern is AD associated with sphincter neuropathy. Bladder sensation, however, is preserved in a significant number of patients because there are numerous exteroceptive sensory nerves in the bladder trigone and bladder neck entering the thoracolumbar spinal segments, thus bypassing the sacral cord.[92]

The integrity of the sacral reflex may be further studied with the evaluation of the latency time of the sacral evoked potentials by stimulating the penile skin and recording the response with a needle electrode in the bulbocavernosus muscle.[66,93] In patients with complete cauda equina lesions, the sacral evoked response is either absent or significantly prolonged,[94] and this represents a more sensitive indicator of neuropathy than the classic EMG changes.

Rockswold and Bradley[95] reported the use of evoked EMG responses in diagnosing lesions of the cauda equina in 110 patients and correlated the results with clinical myelographic and operative findings. Absent evoked EMG responses were consistently correlated with urinary retention. Delayed evoked EMG responses were less consistently associated with urinary retention and lesions along this reflex pathway. However, normal responses do not exclude significant pathology of the cauda equina. Four patients with normal preoperative evoked EMG responses had arachnoiditis, a congenital lipoma, or a myelomeningocele at the time of the operation. Therefore, the technique cannot be considered in isolation. The technique does provide information regarding lesions involving the sacral nerves distal to the dural sac that were not accessible to myelography. Routine magnetic resonance imaging (MRI) was not available at that study. In conclusion, the major urodynamic features in patients with cauda equina injury are an absent or diminished bulbocavernosus reflex, AD, neuropathic changes on perineal floor EMG, and absent evoked EMG responses.

Treatment

Individualization of treatment is necessary according to the underlying abnormality. Indwelling or intermittent catheterization should be instituted in the postoperative period. Urodynamic evaluation should be performed after a few weeks. It is better to perform a urodynamic study after the patients have had a chance to recover from the major pelvic injury. If the bladder is acontractile, clean intermittent self-catheterization is recommended. If bladder compliance diminishes or DO develops, anticholinergics should be started in order to prevent upper tract damage.[62,84]

If the DO or poor filling compliance is unresponsive to aggressive anticholinergic trials, bladder augmentation using a detubularized bowel segment may be used. Prostatectomy in a man who develops urinary retention immediately after a major pelvic operation must be avoided. Not only does resection of the prostate not help a man to urinate, it may also result in stress urinary incontinence when there is underlying denervation of the external sphincter.[53] Even when there is clearly documented benign prostatic hyperplasia (BPH) prior to cauda equina surgery or injury, resection of the internal sphincter, the bladder neck, in light of a denervated external sphincter, can render the unhappy patient who has a bladder that does not work worse, because now not only can he not void but he is also completely incontinent and wearing an adult diaper. It is medically unsound to perform a prostatectomy without careful urodynamic testing in this scenario.

The most commonly used pharmacologic agent in the treatment of AD is the cholinergic agent bethanechol chloride. Although the drug increases intravesical pressure, it has not been shown beneficial in promoting adequate bladder emptying.[96,97] In fact, there are no single prospective randomized studies that demonstrate any clinical efficacy of bethanechol chloride in AD. Bethanechol chloride is especially contraindicated in patients with AD and BOO such as BPH, urethral stricture, or sphincter dyssynergia. In this scenario, increasing intravesical pressure with the existing increased outlet resistance may hasten vesicoureteral reflux, urinary sepsis, and renal damage. Similarly, the performance of Credé's maneuver for AD may trigger a reflex contraction of the perineal floor, thus increasing bladder outlet resistance, a phenomenon that can also impede renal function. An adequate Credé's maneuver or abdominal straining voiding is only effective when both smooth and skeletal muscle resistance are significantly reduced. This is feasible in some women but rarely effective or safe in men. Finally, external stimulation with implantable electrodes has met with many problems, making its routine use impractical.

Stress urinary incontinence secondary to pelvic floor denervation may be difficult to manage. In men, the application of an external condom-type collecting device is the most common solution. In women, however, no external urinary collection device has ever proven effective. Many women choose an indwelling Foley catheter, but this is associated with bladder irritation, chronic bacterial colonization, destruction of the sphincter mechanism, and even squamous cell carcinoma of the bladder with prolonged indwelling bladder catheterization.

Treatment options for the destroyed urethral sphincter require major reconstructive urologic surgery such as the artificial urinary sphincter implantation, pubovaginal sling procedures, or supravesical urinary diversion such as the ileocystostomy, bladder chimney procedure. Finally, in patients with detrusor and perineal floor denervation but preservation of urethral smooth muscle function, the combination of bladder augmentation with a continent stoma and intermittent catheterization provides a reasonable therapeutic alternative.

Conclusions

Neuro-urologic dysfunction secondary to injury to the cauda equina and pelvic plexus can result in devastating urologic dysfunction, the loss of volitional micturition, and the risk of upper tract damage. Fortunately, most of the initial bladder and urethral dysfunction will recover within 6–12 months unless the injury is severe and bilateral. Conservative bladder management such as clean intermittent self-catheterization guided by urodynamic evaluation is the preferred management. Permanent solutions should be deferred until after the recovery or stabilization of the general neurologic status.

Infectious neurologic problems

Acquired immune deficiency syndrome

The acquired immune deficiency syndrome (AIDS) is caused by human immunodeficiency virus (HIV) and commonly associated with neurologic dysfunction. Neurologic involvement occurs in as many as 40% of patients with AIDS.[98] It involves both central and peripheral nervous systems, causing various neurologic manifestations: HIV dementia, encephalopathy, myelopathy, and peripheral neuropathy. Voiding symptoms are very common in AIDS patients, especially at the late stages of the disease or when associated with neurologic manifestations.

Urodynamic evaluation in a series of 18 AIDS patients with voiding symptoms revealed neurogenic bladder in 11 patients.[99] Urinary retention was the most common presenting symptom, and was seen in 6 of the 11 patients (55%). Urodynamic study revealed AD in 36%, DO in 27%, and BOO in 18%. The remaining 19% had normal urodynamic findings.

Neurosyphilis (tabes dorsalis)

Neurosyphilis has long been recognized as a cause of central and peripheral nerve abnormalities. Voiding dysfunction related to neurosyphilis was common in the era before penicillin use.

Hattori and associates[100] reported decreased bladder sensation in tabes dorsalis. Six of 8 patients had increased bladder capacity at first desire to void and 3 also had an increased maximum cystometric capacity. The most common urodynamic finding in neurosyphilis is AD. Sphincteric EMG activity is generally normal, as the corticospinal tracts are not involved in the disorder.[101]

Herpes zoster and herpes simplex

Herpes zoster is an acute, painful mononeuropathy associated with a vesicular eruption in the distribution of the affected nerve. The viral activity is predominantly located in the dorsal root ganglia or sensory ganglia of the cranial nerves. However, sacral nerve involvement may be associated with loss of bladder and anal sphincter control.[102]

When viral invasion of the lumbosacral dorsal roots occurs there may be visible skin vesicles along the corresponding dermatome, and cystoscopy may reveal a similar grouping of vesicles in the urethral and bladder mucosa. The early stages of lower urinary tract involvement with herpes are manifested as symptomatic detrusor instability with urinary frequency and urgency, but the latter stages include decreased sensation of filling and elevated residual urine or urinary retention.[103] On the positive side, the problem is only temporary and generally recovers spontaneously over several months.

Guillain–Barré syndrome

Guillain–Barré syndrome, also known as postinfectious polyneuritis, is an acute symmetric ascending polyneuropathy occurring 1–4 weeks after an acute infection. The syndrome is characterized by rapidly progressive signs of motor weakness and paresthesias progressing from the lower to upper extremities. Paralysis may progress for about 10 days and then remains relatively unchanged for about 2 weeks. The recovery is gradual and may take from 6 months to 2 years for completion. Autonomic disorders are not unusual.

The inflammatory process may involve the afferent sensory neurons as well and produce loss of position and vibration sense. This may explain the urodynamic findings of detrusor motor and sensory deficits with Guillain–Barré syndrome.[104] Retention of urine may occur in the early stages and require bladder catheterization.[105] Long-term urologic dysfunction is uncommon.

Lyme disease

Lyme disease, caused by the spirochete *Borrelia burgdorferi*, is associated with a variety of neurologic sequelae. The urologic manifestation of Lyme disease can be the primary or late manifestation of the disease affecting both sexes and all ages. Urinary urgency, nocturia, and urge incontinence are the most common urological symptoms.[106]

Urodynamic evaluation in a series of 7 patients revealed DO in 5 patients and AD in 2 patients.[107] Detrusor-external sphincter dyssynergia was not noted on EMG in any patient. The urinary tract may be involved in two different ways in the course of Lyme disease. There may be neurogenic voiding dysfunction as a part of neuroborreliosis and there may also be direct invasion of the urinary tract by the spirochete. This is analogous to voiding dysfunction secondary to other neurologic diseases such as multiple sclerosis. Only one patient had direct bladder invasion by the spirochete and he was an unusual case of Lyme disease with a fulminate presentation and multisystem involvement.

Other conditions causing DU/AD

Acute cerebrovascular accidents

Cerebrovascular accident (CVA) is a serious neurologic event and it can cause temporary or permanent voiding dysfunction to the victims. It is generally accepted that the most common urodynamic finding in CVA patients is DO. However, most reports in CVA patients have been done in a retrospective analysis and often months to years after the acute episode.[108–110]

After the initial stroke episode, patients are in a state of 'cerebral shock' and urinary retention commonly occurs. Burney et al[111] reported urodynamic evaluations in 60 CVA patients, performed within 72 hours from the accident. In their series, 47% of patients had urinary retention, mainly due to AD (75%). AD was found more commonly in patients with hemorrhagic infarcts (85%), compared to only in 10% with ischemic infarct. While most cortical and internal capsular lesions resulted in DO, all cerebellar infarcts resulted in AD.

Multiple sclerosis

Multiple sclerosis (MS) is a chronic disease with focal demyelinization of the central nervous system at various levels, causing a wide spectrum of neurologic manifestation. Urologic problems are reported in up to 90% of patients and represent the most troublesome and socially disabling feature of the disease course.[112] The storage symptoms such as frequency, urgency, and urge incontinence are more common, but voiding symptoms such as weak stream, straining, and large residual urine are also common manifestations in MS patients.

In MS patients, large residual urine generally means inefficient voiding from either detrusor contraction problems or sphincteric dyssynergia. It may be caused by concomitant BOO such as BPH. Therefore, thorough urodynamic evaluation is mandatory in MS patient management. Since cervical lesions predominate in MS, DO with/without dyssynergia is the most common urodynamic finding in 50–80% of cases. DU/AD has been reported up to 30% of cases when the plaques involve lumbosacral lesions.[113,114]

Parkinson's disease

Parkinson's disease is a degenerative disorder of the central nervous system (CNS) characterized by muscle rigidity, tremor, and a slow physical movement. These symptoms result from decreased stimulation of the motor cortex by the basal ganglia, usually caused by the insufficient formation and action of dopamine, which is produced in the dopaminergic neurons of the brain.

Most patients with Parkinson's disease complain of lower urinary tract symptoms, and the degree of symptoms reported correlates with the severity and duration of the disease.[115] The most common finding in a urodynamic study is DO, which reflects the involvement of the CNS in this condition. However, DU/AD has also been reported in up to 16% of patients.[116] These findings may result from a deterioration in bladder contractile function in the late stages of Parkinson's disease, or from possible adverse effects of anticholinergic agents, which are commonly used in these patients for CNS symptom control.

Systemic sclerosis

Systemic sclerosis is a connective tissue disease characterized by thickening and fibrosis of the skin. It also shows abnormalities of the small arteries involving the gastrointestinal tract, heart, lung, and kidney. Typical histopathologic findings are arteritis and periarteritis with leukocyte infiltrates and deposition of fibrous tissues.

Although bladder involvement in systemic sclerosis is an uncommon manifestation, there are some reports of DU/AD from systemic sclerosis patients with LUTS. In a series of 9 patients, urodynamic evaluation revealed normal findings in 5 patients and AD in 4 patients.[117] Bladder biopsies from acontractile patients demonstrated a derangement of the capillary bed of the muscle tissue, atrophy of the muscularis, and fibrotic replacement of the smooth muscle with attenuation of the lumen of the small arteries.

Sacral nerve stimulation

Sacral afferent input-modifying micturition reflexes

The guarding and voiding reflexes are activated at different times under completely different clinical scenarios. However, anatomically they are located in close proximity in the S2–4 levels of the human spinal cord.[118] Both sets of reflexes are modulated by a number of centers in the brain. Thus, these reflexes can be altered by a variety of neurologic diseases, some of which can unmask involuntary bladder activity mediated by C fibers.

It is possible to modulate these reflexes via sacral nerve stimulation (SNS) and restore voluntary micturition. Experimental data from animals indicate that somatic afferent input to the sacral spinal cord can modulate the guarding and bladder–bladder reflexes. Sacral preganglionic outflow to the urinary bladder receives inhibitory inputs from various somatic and visceral afferents, as well as a recurrent inhibitory pathway.[119] Electrical stimulation of somatic afferents in the pudendal nerve elicits inhibitory mechanisms.[120] This is supported by the finding that interneurons in the sacral autonomic nucleus exhibiting firing correlated with bladder activity and were inhibited by activation of somatic afferent pathways. This electrical stimulation of somatic efferent nerves in the sacral spinal roots could inhibit reflex of DO mediated by spinal or supraspinal pathways.

In neonatal kittens and rats, micturition as well as defecation are elicited when their mother licks the perineal region.[120] This reflex appears to be the primary stimulus for micturition, since urinary retention occurs when the young kittens and rat pups are separated from their mother.

To induce micturition the perineal afferents must activate the parasympathetic excitatory inputs to the bladder but also suppress the urethral sympathetic and sphincter somatic guarding reflexes. A suppression of guarding reflexes by SNS contributes to the enhancement of voiding in patients with urinary retention.

The perineal-to-bladder reflex is very prominent during the first 4 postnatal weeks and then becomes less effective and usually disappears in kittens by the age of 7–8 weeks, which is the approximate age of weaning. In adult animals and humans, perineal stimulation or mechanical stimulation of the sex organs (vagina or penis) inhibits the micturition reflex.[5,10,11]

Besides the strong animal research that identified somatic afferent modulation of bladder and urethral reflexes, there are also data from clinical physiologic studies supporting the view that stimulation of sacral afferents

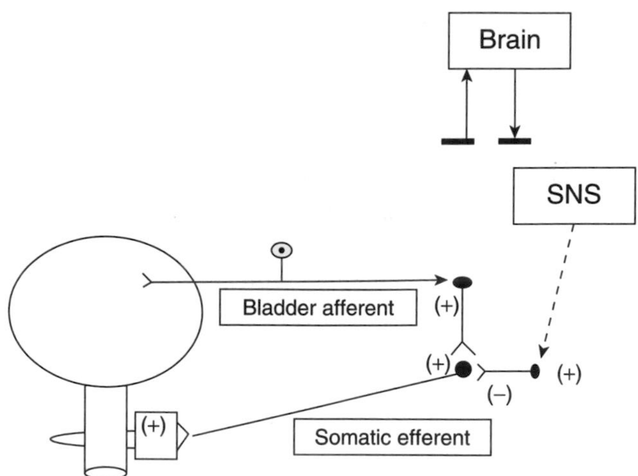

Figure 12.5
In cases of neurologic diseases, the brain cannot turn off the guarding reflex and retention can occur. Sacral nerve stimulation restores voluntary micturition in cases of voiding dysfunction and urinary retention but inhibits the guarding reflex.

can modify bladder and urethral sphincter reflexes. Functional electrical stimulation appears to be a favorable nonsurgical treatment for many patients with detrusor instability.

Hypotheses of sacral nerve stimulation mechanisms

How do sacral somatic afferents alter lower urinary tract reflexes to promote voiding? To understand this mechanism, it should be recognized that, in adults, brain pathways are necessary to turn off sphincter and urethral guarding reflexes to allow efficient bladder emptying.

Thus, spinal cord injury produces bladder sphincter dyssynergia and inefficient bladder emptying by eliminating the brain mechanisms (Figure 12.5). This may also occur after more subtle neurologic lesions in patients with idiopathic urinary retention, such as after a bout of prostatitis or urinary tract infection. Before the development of brain control of micturition, at least in animals, that stimulation of somatic afferent pathways passing through the pudendal nerve to the perineum can initiate efficient voiding by activating bladder efferent pathways and turning off the excitatory pathways to the urethral outlet.[3,4,8] Tactile stimulation of the perineum in the cat also inhibits the bladder–sympathetic reflex component of the guarding reflex mechanism.

With the hypothesis that SNS can elicit similar responses in patients with urinary retention and turn off excitatory outflow to the urethral outlet and promote bladder emptying, Tanagho and Schmidt[121] demonstrated the efficacy of sacral nerve stimulation for AD, not only in animal studies but also in clinical studies. Jonas et al[122] reported the efficacy of SNS for idiopathic urinary retention in a prospective, randomized multicenter trial, which is the largest one so far. At 6 months after implantation, 69% of the patients treated eliminated catheterization and an additional 14% had a 50% or greater reduction in catheter volume per catheterization. However, patients in this trial were a mixed population with DU, AD, or functional outlet obstruction due to urethral overactivity, and no subgroup analysis was reported.

The methods for nerve stimulation also vary, including intraspinal transplantation, nerve root implantation, and transcutaneous stimulation.[121,123,124] Because sphincter activity can generate afferent input to the spinal cord that can, in turn, inhibit reflex bladder activity, an indirect benefit of suppressing sphincter reflexes would be a facilitation of bladder activity. This may also be useful in this patient population.

Myogenic sections

Degeneration of or damage to bladder smooth muscle is also an important factor that induces DU/AD. Diabetes is the most common disease that shows these conditions. Chronic overdistention can result in detrusor myogenic failure even if the neurologic disease is treated or reversed. Bladder management to avoid overdistention, such as institution of intermittent catheterization after spinal cord injury, may protect the bladder from permanent myogenic damage.

At the present time, detrusor myogenic failure has been impossible to treat or reverse. This is why catheterization, either intermittent or indwelling, has been the most commonly used management. There is potential hope for the future, however, of transplanting muscle stem cells to repair the damaged bladder with or without *ex-vivo* gene therapy.

The aim of *ex-vivo* cell therapy is to replace, repair, or enhance the biologic function of damaged tissue or organs. An *ex-vivo* process involves harvesting cells from patients or donors, *in-vitro* manipulation to enhance the therapeutic potential of the harvested cells (*ex-vivo* gene therapy), and subsequent injection or implantation of the cells into the patient. One particular advantage of cellular based *ex-vivo* gene therapy is that the manufactured cells act like bioreactors. At any stage of the process, cells can be cryopreserved so that therapy can be scheduled according to the patient's requirements.[125] A safety feature of the *ex-vivo* approach is that all genetic manipulation involving viral vectors is performed *in vitro* in a controlled fashion. Therefore, the patients are not directly exposed to the viral vectors. In addition, the amount of gene product expression can be quantitated, leading to controlled protein production at specific sites with decreased system side-effects.[126]

Cell transplantation is not a new concept; however, the field of urologic tissue engineering has just recently grown to new and exciting levels. Because there is a general lack of regenerative ability in the bladder and urethral smooth muscle, research has centered on tissue repair by using pluripotent stem cells derived from other lineages. Our laboratory has focused on the isolation and characterization of a small population of these pluripotent stem cells that were derived from skeletal muscle. Using the preplate technique, we can purify and isolate cells that are highly capable of surviving post-transplantation and differentiating into other lineages.[127]

The rationale for using skeletal muscle for cellular-based gene therapy for the urinary tract is two-fold. In contrast to smooth muscle, skeletal muscle is constantly undergoing repair of its damaged tissue due to the presence of satellite cells.[128] These cells are fusion-competent skeletal muscle precursors and, when differentiated, fuse to form myofibers capable of muscle contraction. Secondly, some purified satellite cells behave like pluripotent stem cells that may differentiate into another lineage.

We and other investigators have previously demonstrated the ability to harvest muscle-derived cells (MDCs) which contain satellite cells and stem cells from a skeletal muscle biopsy.[127,129–131] MDCs have been used for the delivery of secretory nonmuscle protein products, such as human growth hormone and coagulation factor IX, to the circulation.[132,133] In addition, when MDCs differentiate, they form myofibers that become postmitotic and consequently exhibit long-term transgene persistence.[134]

We have also demonstrated that MDC transplantation increased muscle contractility in a cryo-injured detrusor model and nerve, or a sphincter-injured incontinence model.[135–139] Thus, transplantation of MDCs from skeletal muscle might be a promising treatment strategy for DU or AD.

Summary

DU/AD can be observed in many neurologic conditions. Careful neurologic and urodynamic examinations are necessary for the diagnosis. Proper management is focused on prevention of upper tract damage, avoidance of overdistention, and decrease of residual urine. Scheduled voiding, double voiding, α_1-blockers, and self-intermittent catheterization are the typical conservative treatment options. Sacral nerve stimulation may be an effective treatment option for DU/AD. New promising concepts such as stem cell therapy and neurotrophic gene therapy are being explored.

References

1. Abrams P, Cardozo L, Fall M et al. The standardisation of terminology in lower urinary tract function: report from the standardisation sub-committee of the International Continence Society. Urology 2003; 61: 37–49.
2. de Groat WC, Theobald RJ. Reflex activation of sympathetic pathways to vesical smooth muscle and parasympathetic ganglia by electrical stimulation of vesical afferents. J Physiol 1976; 259: 223–37.
3. de Groat WC. Central nervous system control of micturition. In: O'Donnell PD, ed. Urinary Incontinence. St Louis: Mosby, 1997: 33–47.
4. Yoshimura N, de Groat WC. Neural control of the lower urinary tract. Int J Urol 1997; 4: 111–25.
5. de Groat WC, Araki I, Vizzard MA et al. Developmental and injury induced plasticity in the micturition reflex pathway. Behav Brain Res 1998; 92: 127–40.
6. Yoshimura N, Chancellor MB. Current and future pharmacological therapy for overactive bladder. J Urol 2002; 168: 1897–913.
7. Cheng CL, Ma CP, de Groat WC. Effect of capsaicin on micturition and associated reflexes in rats. Am J Physiol 1993; 265: R132–138.
8. Kruse MN, de Groat WC. Spinal pathways mediate coordinated bladder/urethral sphincter activity during reflex micturition in normal and spinal cord injured neonatal rats. Neurosci Lett 1993; 152: 141–4.
9. Cheng CL, Ma CP, de Groat WC. Effect of capsaicin on micturition and associated reflexes in chronic spinal rats. Brain Res 1995; 678: 40–8.
10. de Groat WC, Nadelhaft I, Milne RJ et al. Organization of the sacral parasympathetic reflex pathways to the urinary bladder and large intestine. J Auton Nerv Syst 1981; 3: 135–60.
11. de Groat WC, Vizzard MA, Araki I, Roppolo JR. Spinal interneurons and preganglionic neurons in sacral autonomic reflex pathways. In: Holstege G, Bandler R, Saper C, eds. The Emotional Motor System. Progress in Brain Research. New York: Elsevier Science, 1996; 107: 97.
12. de Groat WC. Inhibitory mechanisms in the sacral reflex pathways to the urinary bladder. In: Ryall RW, Kelly JS, eds. Iontophoresis and Transmitter Mechanisms in the Mammalian Central Nervous System, Holland: Elsevier, 1978. 366–8.
13. Chancellor MB, Blaivas JG. Classification of neurogenic bladder disease. In: Chancellor MB, eds. Practical Neuro-urology. Boston: Butterworth-Heinemann, 1995: 25–32.
14. Frimodt-Moller C. Diabetic cystopathy: I. A clinical study of the frequency of bladder dysfunction in diabetics. Dan Med Bull 1976; 23: 267–78.
15. Ellenburg M. Development of urinary bladder dysfunction in diabetes mellitus. Ann Intern Med 1980; 92: 321–3.
16. Ueda T, Yoshimura N, Yoshida O. Diabetic cystopathy: relationship to autonomic neuropathy detected by sympathetic skin response. J Urol 1997; 157: 580–4.
17. Frimodt-Moller C. Diabetic cystopathy: epidemiology and related disorders. Ann Intern Med 1980; 92: 318–21.
18. Mastri AR. Neuropathology of diabetic neurogenic bladder. Ann Intern Med 1980; 92: 316–18.
19. Van Poppel H, Stessens R, Van Damme B et al. Diabetic cystopathy: neuropathological examination of urinary bladder biopsy. Eur Urol 1988; 15: 128–31.
20. Apfel SC. Neurotrophic factors and diabetic peripheral neuropathy. Eur Neurol 1999; 41(Suppl): 27–34.
21. Yoshimura Y, Chancellor MB, Andersson KE et al. Recent advances in understanding the biology of diabetes-associated bladder complications and novel therapy. BJU Int 2004; 95: 733–8.
22. Longhurst PA, Kauer J, Levin RM. The ability of insulin treatment to reverse or prevent the changes in urinary bladder function

caused by streptozotocin-induced diabetes mellitus. Gen Pharmacol 1991; 22: 305–11.
23. Waring JV, Wendt IR. Effect of streptozotocin-induced diabetes mellitus on intracellular calcium and contraction of longitudinal smooth muscle from rat urinary bladder. J Urol 2000; 163: 323–30.
24. Hashitani H, Suzuki H. Altered electrical properties of bladder smooth muscle in streptozotocin-induced diabetic rats. Br J Urol 1996; 77: 798–804.
25. Changolkar AK, Hypolite JA, Disanto M et al. Diabetes induced decrease in detrusor smooth muscle force is associated with oxidative stress and overactivity of aldose reductase. J Urol 2005; 173: 309–13.
26. Mannikarottu AS, Changolkar AK, Disanto ME et al. Overexpression of smooth muscle thin filament associated proteins in the bladder wall of diabetics. J Urol 2005; 174: 360–4.
27. Kasayama S, Oka T. Impaired production of nerve growth factor in the submandibular gland of diabetic mice. Am J Physiol 1989; 257: E400–4.
28. Hellweg R, Hartung HD. Endogenous levels of nerve growth factor (NGF) are altered in experimental diabetes mellitus: a possible role of NGF in the pathogenesis of diabetic neuropathy. J Neurosci Res 1990; 26: 258–67.
29. Fernyhough P, Diemel LT, Brewster WJ, Tomlinson DR. Deficits in sciatic nerve neuropeptide content coincide with a reduction in target tissue nerve growth factor messenger RNA in streptozotocin-diabetic rats: effects of insulin treatment. Neuroscience 1994; 62: 337–44.
30. Steinbacher BC, Nadelhaft I. Increased level of nerve growth factor in the urinary bladder and hypertrophy of dorsal root ganglion neurons in the diabetic rat. Brain Res 1998; 782: 255–60.
31. Diemel LT, Cai F, Anand P et al. Increased nerve growth factor mRNA in lateral calf skin biopsies from diabetic patients. Diabet Med 1999; 16: 113–18.
32. Schmid H, Forman LA, Cao X et al. Heterogenous cardiac sympathetic denervation and decreased myocardial nerve growth factor in streptozotocin-induced diabetic rats: implications for cardiac sympathetic dysinnervation complicating diabetes. Diabetes 1999; 48: 603–8.
33. Sasaki K, Chancellor MB, Phelan MW et al. Diabetic cystopathy correlates with long-term decrease in nerve growth factor (NGF) levels in the bladder and lumbosacral dorsal root ganglia. J Urol 2002; 168: 1259–64.
34. Ihara C, Shimatsu A, Mizuta H. Decreased neurotrophin-3 expression in skeletal muscles of streptozotocin-induced diabetic rats. Neuropeptides 1996; 30: 309–12.
35. Fernyhough P, Diemel LT, Tomlinson DR. Target tissue production and axonal transport of neurotrophin-3 are reduced in streptozotocin diabetic rats. Diabetologia 1998; 41: 300–6.
36. Cai F, Tomlinson DR, Fernyhough P. Elevated expression of neurotorophin-3 mRNA in sensory nerve of streptozotocin-diabetic rats. Neurosci Lett 1999; 263: 81–4.
37. Vlaskovska M, Kasakov L, Rong W et al. P2X3 knock-out mice reveal a major sensory role for urothelially released ATP. J Neurosci 2001; 21: 5670–7.
38. Birder LA, Nealen ML, Kiss S et al. Beta-adrenocepter agonists stimulate endothelial nitric oxide synthase in rat urinary bladder urothelial cells. J Neurosci 2002; 15: 8063–70.
39. Pinna C, Zanardo R, Puglisi L. Prostaglandin-release impairment in the bladder epithelium of streptozotocin-induced diabetic rats. Eur J Pharmacol 2000; 388: 267–73.
40. Poladia DP, Bauer JA. Early cell-specific changes in nitric oxide synthase, reactive nitrogen species formation, and ubiquitinylation during diabetes-related bladder remodeling. Diabetes Metab Res Rev 2003; 19: 313–19.
41. Frimodt-Moller C. Diabetic cystopathy: a review of the urodynamic and clinical features of neurogenic bladder dysfunction in diabetes mellitus. Dan Med Bull 1978; 25: 49–60.
42. Blaivas JG. Neurogenic dysfunction. In: Yalla SU, McGuire EJ, Elbadawi A, Blaivas JG, eds. Neurourology and Urodynamics: Principles and Practice. New York: Macmillan, 1988: 347–50.
43. Kaplan SA, Te AE, Blaivas JG. Urodynamic findings in patients with diabetic cystopathy. J Urol 1995; 153: 342–4.
44. Starer P, Libow L. Cystometric evaluation of bladder dysfunction in elderly diabetic patients. Arch Intern Med 1990; 150: 810–13.
45. Bradley WE. Diagnosis of urinary bladder dysfunction in diabetes mellitus. Ann Intern Med 1980; 92: 323–6.
46. Kaplan SA, Blaivas JG. Diabetic cystopathy. J Diabet Compl 1988; 2: 133–9.
47. Hunter KF, Moore KN. Diabetes-associated bladder dysfunction in the old adult. Geriatr Nurs 2003; 24: 138–47.
48. Apfel SC, Arezzo JC, Brownlee M et al. Nerve growth factor administration protects against experimental diabetic sensory neuropathy. Brain Res 1994; 634: 7–12.
49. Delcroix JD, Michael GJ, Priestley JV et al. Effect of nerve growth factor treatment on $p75^{NTR}$ gene expression in lumbar dorsal root ganglia of streptozotocin-induced diabetic rats. Diabetes 1998; 47: 1779–85.
50. Unger JW, Klitzsch T, Pera S, Reiter R. Nerve growth factor (NGF) and diabetic neuropathy in the rat: morphological investigation of the sural nerve, dorsal root ganglion, and spinal cord. Exp Neurol 1998; 153: 23–34.
51. Petty BG, Comblath DR, Adornato BT et al. The effect of systemically administered recombinant human nerve growth factor in healthy human projects. Ann Neurol 1994; 36: 244–6.
52. Apfel SC, Kessler JA, Adomato BT et al. The NGF study group: recombinant human nerve growth factor in the treatment of diabetic polyneuropathy. Neurology 1998; 51: 695–702.
53. Apfel SC, Schwartz S, Adomato BT et al. The rhNGF clinical investigator group: efficacy and safety of recombinant human nerve growth factor in patients with diabetic polyneuropathy. A randomized control trial. JAMA 2000; 284: 2215–21.
54. Goins WF, Yoshimura N, Phelan MW et al. Herpes simplex virus mediated nerve growth factor expression in bladder and afferent neurons: potential treatment for diabetic bladder dysfunction. J Urol 2001; 165: 1748–54.
55. Sasaki K, Chancellor MB, Goins WF et al. Gene therapy using replication defective herpes simplex virus (HSV) vectors expressing nerve growth factor (NGF) in a rat model of diabetic cystopathy. Diabetes 2004; 53: 2723–30.
56. Akkina SK, Patterson CL, Wright DE. GDNF rescues nonpeptidergic unmyelinated primary afferents in streptozotocin-treated diabetic mice. Exp Neurol 2001; 167: 173–82.
57. Pradat PF, Kennel P, Naimi-Sadaoui S et al. Continuous delivery of neurotrophin 3 by gene therapy has a neuroprotective effect in experimental models of diabetic and acrylamide neuropathies. Hum Gene Ther 2001; 12: 2237–49.
58. Bradley WE, Andersen JT. Neuromuscular dysfunction of the lower urinary tract in patients with lesions of the cauda equina and conus medullaris. J Urol 1976; 116: 620–1.
59. Hellstrom P, Kortelainen P, Kontturi M. Late urodynamic findings after surgery for cauda equina syndrome caused by a prolapsed lumbar intervertebral disk. J Urol 1986; 135: 308–12.
60. Gray H. In: Williams PL, Warwick R, eds. Gray's Anatomy, 36th edn. Edinburgh: Churchill Livingstone, 1984: 1110–23.
61. Marani E, Pijl ME, Kraan MC et al. Interconnections of the upper ventral rami of the human sacral plexus: a reappraisal for dorsal rhizotomy in neurostimulation operations. Neurourol Urodyn 1993; 12: 585–98.
62. Woodside JR, Crawford ED. Urodynamic features of pelvic plexus injury. J Urol 1980; 124: 657–8.
63. Forney JP. The effect of radical hysterectomy on bladder physiology. Am J Obstet Gynecol 1980; 138: 374–82.

64. Yalla SV, Andriole GL. Vesicourethral dysfunction following pelvic visceral ablative surgery. J Urol 1984; 132: 503–9.
65. Blaivas JG, Barbalias GA. Characteristics of neural injury after abdominoperineal resection of the rectum. J Urol 1983; 129: 84–7.
66. Siroky MB, Sax DS, Krane RJ. Sacral signal tracing: the electrophysiology of the bulbocavernosus reflex. J Urol 1979; 122: 661–4.
67. Smith PH, Ballantyne B. The neuroanatomical basis for denervation of the urinary bladder following major pelvic surgery. Br J Surg 1968; 55: 929–33.
68. McGuire EJ. Urodynamic evaluation after abdominal-perineal resection and lumbar intervertebral disc herniation. Urology 1975; 6: 63–70.
69. Seski JC, Diokno AC. Bladder dysfunction after radical abdominal hysterectomy. Am J Obstet Gynecol 1977; 128: 643–51.
70. Mundy AR. An anatomical explanation for bladder dysfunction following rectal and uterine surgery. Br J Urol 1982; 54: 501–4.
71. Patterson FP, Morton KS. Neurologic complications of fractures and dislocations of the pelvis. Surg Gynecol Obstet 1961; 112: 702.
72. Brynes DP, Russo GL, Dunker TB, Cowley RA. Sacrum fractures and neurological damage. J Neuorsurg 1977; 47: 459–62.
73. Heckman JD, Keats PK. Fracture of the sacrum in children. J Bone Joint Surg Am 1978; 60: 404–5.
74. Goodell CL. Neurological deficit associated to pelvic fractures. J Neurosurg 1966; 24: 837–42.
75. Fountain SS, Hamilton RD, Jameson RM. Transverse fractures of the sacrum: a report of six cases. J Bone Joint Surg Am 1977; 59: 486–9.
76. Pavlakis AJ. Cauda equina and pelvic plexus injury. In: Krane RJ, Siroky MB, eds. Clinical Neuro urology. Boston: Little Brown, 1991: 333–4.
77. Dewey P, Browne PSH. Fractures and dislocation of the lumbosacral spine with cauda equina lesion. J Bone Joint Surg Br 1968; 50: 635–8.
78. Fardon DF. Displaced fractures of the lumbosacral spine with delayed cauda equina deficit. Clin Orthop 1976; 120: 155–8.
79. Scott PJ. Bladder paralysis in cauda equina lesions from disc prolapse. J Bone Joint Surg 1965; 47: 244.
80. Bartolin Z, Vilendecic M, Derezic D. Bladder function after surgery for lumber intervertebral disk protrusion. J Urol 1999; 161: 1885–7.
81. O'Flynn KJ, Murphy R, Thomas DG. Neurogenic bladder dysfunction in lumbar intervertebral disc prolapse. Br J Urol 1992; 69: 38–40.
82. Shapiro S. Medical realities of cauda equina syndromes secondary to lumbar disc herniation. Spine 2000; 25: 348–52.
83. Albert NE, Sparks FC, McGuire EJ. Effect of pelvic and retroperitoneal surgery on the urethral pressure profile and perineal floor electromyogram in dogs. Invest Urol 1977; 15: 140–2.
84. McGuire EJ, Wagner FC. The effects of sacral denervation on bladder and urethral function. Surg Gynecol Obstet 1977; 144: 343–6.
85. Blaivas JG, Scott MR, Labib KB. Urodynamic evaluation as neurologic test for sacral cord function. Urology 1979; 8: 682–7.
86. Scott M. Surgery of the spinal column. Prog Neurol Psychiatry 1965; 20: 509–23.
87. Lapides J, Babbitt JM. Diagnostic value of bulbocavernosus reflex. JAMA 1956; 162: 971.
88. Neal DE, Bogue PRI, Williams RE. Histological appearances of the nerves of the bladder in patients with denervation of the bladder after excision of the rectum. Br J Urol 1982; 54: 658–66.
89. Jones DL, Moore T. The types of neuropathic bladder dysfunction associated with prolapsed lumbar intervertebral discs. Br J Urol 1973; 45: 39–43.
90. Kuru M. Nervous control of micturition. Physiol Rev 1965; 45: 425.
91. Bradley WE, Teague C. Spinal cord representation of the peripheral neural pathways of the micturition reflex. J Urol 1969; 101: 220–3.
92. Bradley WE, Timm GM, Scott FB. Cystometry: V. Bladder sensation. Urology 1975; 6: 654–8.
93. Blaivas JG, Zaved AAH, Labib KB. The bulbocavernosus reflex in urology: a prospective study of 299 patients. J Urol 1981; 126: 197–9.
94. Krane RJ, Siroky MB. Studies on sacral evoked potentials. J Urol 1980; 124: 872–6.
95. Rockswold GL, Bradley WE. The use of evoked electromyographic responses in diagnosing lesions of the cauda equina. J Urol 1977; 118: 629–31.
96. Blaivas JG, Labib KB, Michalik SJ, Zayed AA. Failure of bethanechol denervation supersensitivity as a diagnostic aid. J Urol 1980; 123: 199–201.
97. Wein A, Raezer D, Malloy T. Failure of the bethanechol supersensitivity test to predict improved voiding after subcutaneous bethanechol administration. J Urol 1980; 123: 302–3.
98. Levy R, Janssen R, Bush T et al. Neuroepidemiology of acquired immunodeficiency syndrome. In: Rosenblum ML, ed. AIDS and the Nervous System. New York: Raven Press, 1998: 13–40.
99. Kahn Z, Singh VK, Yang WE. Neurogenic bladder in acquired immune deficiency syndrome (AIDS). Urology 1992; 40: 289–91.
100. Hattori T, Yasuda K, Kita K, Hirayama K. Disorders of micturition in tabes dorsalis. Br J Urol 1990; 65: 497–9.
101. Wheeler JS Jr, Culkin DJ, O'Hara RJ, Canning JR. Bladder dysfunction and neurosyphilis. J Urol 1986; 136: 903–5.
102. Cohen LM, Fowler JF, Owen LG, Callen JP. Urinary retention associated with herpes zoster infection. Int J Dermatol 1993; 32: 24–6.
103. Yamanishi T, Yasuda K, Sakakibara R et al. Urinary retention due to herpes virus infections. Neurol Urodyn 1998; 17: 613–19.
104. Wheeler JS Jr, Siroky MB, Pavlakis A, Krane RJ. The urodynamic aspects of the Guillain–Barré syndrome. J Urol 1984; 137: 917–19.
105. Kogan BA, Solomon MH, Diokno AC. Urinary retention secondary to Landry Guillain–Barré syndrome. J Urol 1981; 126: 643–4.
106. Chancellor MB, McGinnis DE, Shenot PJ et al. Lyme cystitis and neurogenic bladder dysfunction. Lancet 1992; 339: 1237–8.
107. Chancellor MB, McGinnis DE, Shenot PJ et al. Urinary dysfunction in Lyme disease. J Urol 1993; 149: 26–30.
108. Tsuchida S, Noto H, Yamaguchi O, Itoh M. Urodynamic studies on hemiplegic patients after cerebrovascular accident. Urology 1983; 21: 315–18.
109. Gelber DA, Good DC, Laven LJ, Verhulst SJ. Causes of urinary incontinence after acute hemispheric stroke. Stroke 1993; 24: 378–82.
110. Khan Z, Starer P, Yang WC, Bhola A. Analysis of voiding disorders in patients with cerebrovascular accidents. Urology 1990; 35: 265–70.
111. Burney TL, Senapati M, Desai S et al. Acute cerebrovascular accident and lower urinary tract dysfunction: a prospective correlation of the site of brain injury with urodynamic findings. J Urol 1996; 156: 1748–50.
112. Haensch CA, Jorg J. Autonomic dysfunction in multiple sclerosis. J Neurol 2006; 253(Suppl 1): 1/3–1/9.
113. Wheeler JS Jr. Multiple sclerosis. In: Krane RJ, Siroky MB, eds. Clinical Neuro-urology. Boston: Little Brown, 1991: 353–63.
114. Barbalias GA, Nikiforidis G, Liatsikos EN. Vesicourethral dysfunction associated with multiple sclerosis: Clinical and urodynamic perspectives. J Urol 1998; 160: 106–11.
115. Araki I, Kuno S. Assessment of voiding dysfunction in Parkinson's disease by the international prostate symptom score. J Neurol Neurosurg Psychiatry 2000; 68: 429–33.
116. Araki I, Kitahara M, Oida T, Kuno S. Voiding dysfunction and Parkinson's disease: urodynamic abnormalities and urinary symptoms. J Urol 2000; 164: 1640–3.
117. Lazzeri M, Beneforti P, Benaim G et al. Vesical dysfunction in systemic sclerosis. J Urol 1995; 153: 1184–7.
118. Chancellor MB, Chartier-Kastler EJ. Principles of sacral nerve stimulation (SNS) for the treatment of bladder and urethral sphincter dysfunctions. J Neuromod 2000; 3: 15–26.

119. de Groat WC. Nervous control of the urinary bladder of the cat. Brain Res 1975; 87: 201–11.
120. de Groat WC. Changes in the organization of the micturition reflex pathway of the cat after transection of the spinal cord. In: Veraa RP, Grafstein B, eds. Cellular mechanisms for recovery from nervous systems injury: a conference report. Exp Neurol 1981; 71: 22.
121. Tanagho EA, Schmidt RA. Electrical stimulation in the clinical management of the neurogenic bladder. J Urol 1988; 140: 1331–9.
122. Jonas U, Fowler CJ, Chancellor MB et al. Efficacy of sacral nerve stimulation for urinary retention: results 18 months after implantation. J Urol 2001; 165: 15–19.
123. Heine JP, Schmidt RA, Tanagho EA. Intraspinal sacral root stimulation for controlled micturition. Invest Urol 1977; 15: 78–82.
124. Crocker M, Doleys DM, Dolce JJ. Transcutaneous electrical nerve stimulation in urinary retention. South Med J 1985; 78: 1515–16.
125. Huard J, Acsadi G, Jani A et al. Gene transfer into skeletal muscles by isogenic myoblasts. Hum Gene Ther 1994; 5: 949–58.
126. Schindhelm K, Nordon R. Ex Vivo Cell Therapy. San Diego: Academic Press, 1999: 1–4.
127. Lee JY, Qu-Petersen Z, Cao B et al. Clonal isolation of muscle-derived cells capable of enhancing muscle regeneration and bone healing. J Cell Biol 2000; 150(5): 1085–100.
128. Campion DR. The muscle satellite cell: a review. Int Rev Cytol 1984; 87: 225.
129. Rando TO, Blau HM. Primary mouse myoblast purification, characterization, and transplantation for cell-mediated gene therapy. J Cell Biol 1994; 125: 1275–87.
130. Qu Z, Balkir L, van Deutekom JC, Robbins PD et al. Development of approaches to improve cell survival in myoblast transfer therapy. J Cell Biol 1998; 142: 1257.
131. Yokoyama T, Huard J, Yoshimura N et al. Muscle derived cells transplantation and differentiation into the lower urinary tract smooth muscle. Urology 2001; 57: 826–31.
132. Dhawan J, Pan LC, Pavlath GK et al. Systemic delivery of human growth hormone by injection of genetically engineered myoblasts. Science 1991; 254: 1509.
133. Dai Y, Schwarz EM, Gu D et al. Cellular and humoral immune responses to adenoviral vectors containing factor IX gene: tolerization of factor IX and vector antigens allow for long-term expression. Proc Natl Acad Sci USA 1995; 92: 1401.
134. Jiao S, Guerich V, Wolffe JA. Long-term correction of rat model of Parkinson's disease by gene therapy. Nature 1993; 362: 450.
135. Chancellor MB, Yokoyama T, Tirney S et al. Preliminary results of myoblast injection into the urethra and bladder wall: a possible method for the treatment of stress urinary incontinence and impaired detrusor contractility. Neurourol Urodyn 2000; 19: 279–87.
136. Yokoyama T, Dhir R, Qu Z et al. Persistence and survival of autologous muscle derived cells versus bovine collagen as possible treatment of stress urinary incontinence. J Urol 2001; 165: 271–6.
137. Lee JY, Cannon TW, Pruchnic R et al. The effects of periurethral muscle-derived stem cell injection on leak point pressure in a rat model of stress urinary incontinence. Int Urogynecol J Pelvic Floor Dysfunct 2003; 14(1): 31–7.
138. Cannon TW, Lee JY, Somogyi G et al. Improved sphincter contractility after allogenic muscle-derived progenitor cell injection into the denervated rat urethra. Urology 2003; 62(5): 958–63.
139. Kwon D, Kim Y, Pruchnic R et al. Periurethral cellular injection: comparison of muscle-derived progenitor cells and fibroblasts with regard to efficacy and tissue contractility in an animal model of stress urinary incontinence. Urology 2006; 68(2): 449–54.

13

Pathophysiology of the low compliant bladder

Emmanuel Chartier-Kastler, Jean-Marc Soler, and Pierre Denys

Introduction and physiology

Bladder compliance is defined by the ratio of the increase in intravesical pressure over the increase in bladder volume ($\Delta V/\Delta P$). It reflects the capacity of the detrusor to allow bladder filling at low pressure in order to maintain the functional properties of the urinary system and to avoid deterioration of these properties (vesicorenal reflux, deterioration of the bladder wall, incontinence). It is dependent on both the physical reservoir qualities and the qualitative and quantitative innervation of the bladder (autonomic nervous system).

The urodynamic definition of bladder compliance was proposed by the International Continence Society (ICS) and its various clinical study reports. The individual definition of compliance has been shown to vary as a function of bladder volume at the time of measurement, the filling rate,[1,2] the technique used to measure compliance,[3] repetition of urodynamic investigations,[4] and filling conditions (physiological versus artificial).[5]

The detrusor is normally composed of 70% elastic tissue, consisting of smooth muscle cells, and 30% viscous tissues, consisting of collagen fibers. Smooth muscle fibers behave like elastic elements, i.e. they are able to return to their initial state as soon as the stretching force is removed. Smooth muscle fiber lengthening is proportional to the tension applied. By Hooke's law:

$$T \text{ (tension)} = f \text{ (elastic module)} \times L \text{ (lengthening)}$$

Collagen fibers present the property of being able to delay deformation in response to stretch. Linear viscosity is governed by Newton's law, which states that the deformity of a fiber is directly proportional to the rate of tension. For more than 25 years, there has been an ongoing debate concerning whether bladder tone is determined by the passive properties of the bladder wall or by the autonomic nervous system. In this chapter, we will see that arguments derived from clinical experience of neurogenic bladder and its natural history, as well as our knowledge of detrusor innervation, now explain the important role of the nervous system in disorders of compliance.

In 1994, in an editorial devoted to this subject, McGuire[6] summarized the history of these concepts. The interaction between reflex detrusor contraction and failure of sphincter opening mechanisms inevitably leads to the appearance of disorders of compliance. Introduction of self-catheterization into the management of neurogenic bladder, in which there is no longer any detrusor-sphincter synergy, has demonstrated the positive effect on improvement of bladder compliance. An increase in intravesical pressure, for whatever reason, is universally accepted to be a major factor in disorders of compliance. Various diseases can be responsible for increased intravesical pressure, including myelomeningocele, spinal cord injury, multiple sclerosis, obstructive uropathy, including benign prostatic hyperplasia, and radiotherapy-induced lesions. All of the treatments proposed below are designed to decrease intravesical pressures, as clinical experience has demonstrated the major role of raised intravesical pressure in deterioration of the upper tract and the appearance of voiding disorders with severe repercussions on quality of life.

Natural history of compliance in neurogenic bladder: prognostic factors related to the mode of drainage

Clinical experience provides pathophysiological information about disorders of compliance in neurogenic bladder. A review of large cohorts analyzed according to the level of the spinal cord lesion and the treatment used demonstrates a correlation between high intravesical pressure and disorders of compliance. In a series of 316 patients, Weld et al[7] showed that patients treated by self-catheterization had a significantly higher incidence of normal bladder compliance than those with indwelling catheter, regardless of the level of the lesion. With a follow-up ranging between 16 and 20 years, 75% of patients treated by self-catheterization had normal compliance (>12.5 ml/cm) vs 20% of patients with an indwelling catheter and 60% of patients with reflex voiding. The rate of clinical complications was also proportional to the state of compliance. The level of the lesion also influences the incidence of low compliant bladder, which are less frequent in the case of a suprasacral vs sacral lesion, or an incomplete vs complete lesion.

These data were confirmed by other cohort studies.[8–11] Particular attention must be paid to cauda equina lesions, which may be associated with low compliance in up to 55% of cases,[12] representing a major threat for the upper urinary tract, requiring strict surveillance and screening. More recently, Beric and Light[13] emphasized the need to clearly distinguish between cauda equina lesions and conus lesions, especially by neurological or electrophysiological examinations. Pure conus lesions without detrusor areflexia may present various abnormalities of compliance on urodynamic studies (5 patients), including decreased compliance with a high risk of functional impairment. This finding has also been reported even more recently by Shin et al.[14]

Myelomeningocele must also be considered separately. Although the extent of the neurological lesions can vary considerably, 40–48%[15] of patients develop upper urinary tract lesions over a period of 7 years. A correlation has been demonstrated between the level of the malformation, as 57% of patients present with upper urinary tract dilatation in the case of thoracolumbar lesion and 90% in the case of thoracic lesion. This is particularly true during early childhood, whereas puberty and the growth period constitute the second high-risk period for the appearance of a major compliance disorder, even despite well-conducted treatment, especially self-catheterization. Boys are more particularly concerned (65%) and the presence of a tethered spinal cord, destabilized by growth, must be detected and treated if necessary, but this does not always prevent the risk of deterioration of probably 'acquired' bladder compliance. This problem must be carefully assessed before treatment of sphincter incompetence, especially by artificial urinary sphincter. De Badiola et al[16] demonstrated the importance of precise preoperative assessment of compliance, which, when abnormal (<2 ml/cm), must be treated by bladder enlargement associated with artificial urinary sphincter in a population predominantly composed of patients with myelomeningocele (18/23). This demonstrates the major role of raised intravesical pressure on deterioration of bladder compliance in the case of artificial increase of sphincter resistance on a reservoir with limited properties. Kaufman et al,[17] in a cohort of 214 children with myelomeningocele, confirmed the often irreversible nature of the disorder of compliance in this population (only 42% improvement after treatment based on a radiologically documented urological indication). Upper tract deterioration, reflecting increased resistance to bladder emptying, should not be detected by radiological surveillance alone, but especially by urodynamic studies.

Clinical experience has confirmed the higher incidence of compliance disorders according to the level (topography) and complete or incomplete nature of the neurological lesion. The available treatments for hyperreflexia and low compliance were limited to bladder enlargement surgery in the case of failure of self-catheterization and parasympatholytics, which have been shown to improve intravesical pressure and compliance.[7,18]

New conservative treatments for hyperreflexia more clearly illustrate the role of neurological tone in the pathogenesis of disorders of compliance.

Data on disorders of compliance derived from conservative treatments of neurogenic bladder

Old data concerning improvement of compliance by urethral dilatation in children with myelomeningocele support the important role of high intravesical pressure as a factor predisposing to disorders of compliance. A short series of 18 children out of 350[19] treated by dilatation (12F to 38F dilators) showed improvement of compliance by 11.66–27.41 ml/cmH_2O. The urodynamic results of open or endoscopic sphincterotomy do not specifically concern compliance, but may nevertheless indicate similar changes.

Disafferentation induced by section of the posterior nerve roots performed in the context of implantation of a Brindley stimulator[20] induced a marked improvement of compliance. Brindley,[20] Koldewijn et al,[21] and Madersbacher have reported their experience with this technique. In a publication specifically devoted to this aspect of neurogenic bladder, Koldewijn et al[21] reported a dramatic improvement of compliance at 6 months in 27 patients, which remained less than 20 ml/cmH_2O in only 2 patients. This result was not constantly observed at the 5th postoperative day, while hyperreflexia was abolished in the great majority of patients and an increase of compliance was even observed in some cases during the very first postoperative days. Detrusor denervation interrupts the reflex arc and consequently reduces or even abolishes detrusor hyperreflexia and high pressures. Previous denervation techniques failed, probably due to incomplete rhizotomy.

Few papers have reported the use of α-blockers in neurogenic bladder, particularly concerning their effects on bladder compliance. Swierzweski et al[22] prospectively studied the effect of terazosin on compliance in 12 spinal cord injury patients after failure of self-catheterization and maximal pharmacological blockade. Terazosin, at a dosage of 5 mg/day (by month) for 4 weeks, significantly improved bladder compliance during treatment, suggesting an α-blocking effect on detrusor receptors. The bladder compliance of 22 patients was improved by an average of 73% with return to baseline after stopping treatment, reflecting an 'on-off' effect. The feedback effect induced on the urethra could not be analyzed, but cannot be excluded, as indicated by the authors. The authors also reported a significant reduction of episodes of incontinence and dysreflexia. More recently, Schulte-Baukhloh et al[23] reported a study concerning alfuzosin. Seventeen children, mostly with myelomeningocele, with a mean age of 6.3 years, obtained an increase in bladder compliance from 9.3 to 19.6 ml/cmH_2O (111%).

The use of adrenergic blocking agents appears to clinically confirm the neurogenic interference on disorders of compliance, which may be due to a cholinergic activity, myogenic activity, or fibrosis, but it can also be mediated by activation of α-adrenergic receptors.[22] The reduction of bladder outlet obstruction has been shown to improve compliance of neurogenic bladders, but these clinical data on alpha blockers tend to suggest a direct effect on detrusor α-adrenergic receptors. None of the patients in this study developed incontinence as a result of terazosin. A more precise pathophysiological explantation cannot be proposed in the absence of a study of bladder leak point. Sundin et al,[24] in 1977, demonstrated the presence of adrenergic nerve endings in the detrusor, specifically in the case of parasympathetic denervation.

The use of vanilloids (resiniferatoxin and capsaicin) is still under evaluation. The treatment strategy consists of inducing pharmacological bladder disafferentation of silent type C afferent fibers. Resiniferatoxin has been demonstrated to be effective on detrusor hyperreflexia,[25] and was able to improve the disorder of compliance of a patient with myelomeningocele not presenting hyperreflexia.[26] According to the authors, this result appears to suggest that type C fibers are partially responsible for signals participating in deterioration of bladder compliance in some patients with myelomeningocele. This result needs to be confirmed on larger cohorts, especially including spinal cord injury patients.

The use of intravesical botulinum toxin is much more interesting in terms of pathophysiology and treatment. Schurch et al reported the effects of intravesical botulinum toxin on continence in spinal cord injury patients,[27] as blockade of the release of acetylcholine into the neuromuscular junction (efferent) induces a variable duration of bladder paralysis, with an estimated mean duration of 6–8 months. The results obtained on bladder compliance in adults and, more recently, in children with myelomeningocele are particularly demonstrative. Bladder compliance was improved from 20.39 to 45.18 ml/cmH_2O, i.e. by 121%. Botulinum toxin induces a marked reduction of intravesical pressure by inhibiting reflex contractions, but by acting on the efferent pathway of the reflex arc, thereby transforming the disorder of compliance, provided there is no pre-existing disorder of the bladder wall.

The effect of continuous intrathecal baclofen on compliance has been studied in neurogenic bladder. Steers et al[28] in 1992 and Bushman et al[29] in 1993, respectively, demonstrated the marked effects on bladder compliance in a population of patients with spastic spinal cord injury or hereditary spastic paraplegia. The effect of baclofen may be related to relaxation of the striated sphincter, leading to decreased resistance and/or a central neurological effect.

Data derived from experimental studies

Morphometric studies on human bladder strips and animal models now provide a better understanding of the cellular and intercellular mechanisms of neurological disorders of compliance.

The study published by Backhaus et al[30] is particularly important. Although an increased intravesical pressure participates in the disorder of compliance, and although it is not always easy to distinguish the respective roles of bladder wall disorders and purely neurological disorders, these authors developed, for the first time, an experimental model designed to correlate pressure and the expression of proteolytic enzymes and their endogenous inhibitors (tissue metalloproteinase MMP-1 inhibitors). On human bladder cells, they demonstrated that pressures of 20 or 40 cmH_2O interfered with MMP-1 production. The molecular mechanisms responsible for the turnover of intercellular matrix have not been clearly elucidated, but this study showed the link between the pressure applied and the rate of release into the medium of these enzymes responsible for destruction of types I and III collagen. Earlier studies[31] demonstrating that the urothelium could be involved in the production of type I collagen suggest the role of these cells in the synthesis of extracellular matrix also needs to be studied.

The direct participation of type III collagen was demonstrated on human bladder chips by the elevated levels of mRNA observed in the case of non-compliant bladder.[32] Older morphometric studies[33] demonstrated a significant increase of connective tissue with no loss of muscle tissue on neurogenic non-compliant bladder, already suggesting participation of the bladder wall in the disorder of compliance with very probable functional alterations. The chronology of the disorders and their reversible or irreversible nature has not been studied *in vitro*.

Several studies have tried to elucidate the role of blood flow and possible slowing of blood flow on these disorders of the bladder wall. In general and independently of any neurogenic cause for detrusor dysfunction, Kershen et al[34] studied the effect of bladder filling on the blood supply of the wall in 17 conscious patients (Doppler transducer introduced by endoscopy). Blood flow tended to increase with increasing bladder volume and pressure and was mediated by local control mechanisms. In contrast, when the bladder reached its full capacity, blood flow decreased followed by a rebound increase after bladder emptying. The authors found a strong correlation between reduction of detrusor blood flow and bladder wall compliance, suggesting that ischemia participates in structural modifications of the bladder wall. This study provides different, but complementary data, concerning the role of ischemia due to high intravesical pressure in neurogenic bladder. Ohnishi et al[35] had already studied this hypothesis on neurogenic bladders presenting disorders of compliance vs a control group using laser Doppler measurement of blood flow, confirming that blood flow was highly significantly decreased in full non-compliant bladders.

The role of innervation has been studied on models of bilateral hypogastric nerve transection in spinal cord injury rats,[36] as these nerves provide the major sympathetic input to the bladder neck and urethra. Transection of these nerves reduces detrusor dysfunction in paraplegic patients, but did not alter the effects of dopaminergic receptor antagonists on the micturition reflex in spinal cord injury rats. Ten years earlier, the same mechanism was studied in anesthetized, non-spinal cord injury cats. Nerve section induced a reduction of bladder compliance at the end of filling, reflecting the inhibitory effect of sympathetic innervation during the second phase of filling, which probably helps to explain the mechanism of action of α-blockers[22,23] in this type of dysfunction.

Gloeckner et al[37] confirmed that bladder wall disorders induced a loss of viscoelastic properties of the bladder. They used biaxial mechanical testing to study the bladders of spinal cord injury rats vs a control group and demonstrated marked differences, with muscle hypertrophy, in rats with central neurogenic bladder. Human morphometric studies also provide similar findings, showing a significant increase of connective tissue with no loss of muscle tissue in neurogenic bladders. Landau et al[38] studied bladder biopsies in a population of 29 consecutive patients with neurogenic bladder requiring bladder enlargement and demonstrated an increase in the percentage of connective tissue and the connective tissue/muscle tissue ratio.

Hormonal factors also probably play a role. Experiments conducted on pregnant and virgin female rabbits demonstrated loss of compliance in response to hormonal impregnation. Electrical or pharmacological stimulation of bladder strips also considerably altered compliance.[39]

Conclusion

The pathophysiology of disorders of bladder compliance is still poorly understood. Although the presence of high intravesical pressure, facilitated by uncontrolled detrusor hyperreflexia or high sphincter resistance, is certainly still poorly elucidated (Table 13.1). All of the treatments used in routine clinical practice demonstrate that the main factor ensuring improvement of the disorder of compliance is an action on high intravesical pressure. Studies on bladder biopsies in patients with neuro-urological disease could provide greater insight, especially concerning collagen deposits. New treatments, particularly botulinum toxin, may be useful in the context of a test of reversibility of the disorder of compliance. In the future, molecular biology and the study of cellular interactions should provide a better understanding of the mechanism linking raised intravesical pressure and loss of compliance. A number of aspects remain to be elucidated,[40] especially cellular interactions in wall changes, the reversible or irreversible nature of the various changes observed, the role of local neurotrophic factors, and changes induced on bladder afferent pathways. Similar questions have yet to be resolved concerning bladder aging or abnormalities induced by non-neurological obstruction.

Table 13.1 *Clinical factors influencing low compliant neurogenic bladder*

Type of drainage of the bladder
Type of neurogenic lesion
Location
Completeness
Type of treatment of hyperreflexia (bladder pressure)

Further studies need to be conducted to develop a preventive treatment for disorders of compliance in neurogenic bladder, other than specific treatment of the underlying disease or bladder drainage, and to determine the adjuvant role of α-blocking drugs in this setting.

References

1. Coolsaet B. Bladder compliance and detrusor activity during the collection phase. Neurourol Urodyn 1985; 4: 263–73.
2. Coolsaet B, Elhilali M. Detrusor overactivity. Neurourol Urodyn 1988; 7: 541–61.
3. Nordling J, Walter S. Repeated, rapid fill CO_2-cystometry. Urol Res 1977; 5: 117–22.
4. Sorensen S, Nielsen J, Norgaard J et al. Changes in bladder volumes with repetition of water cystometry. Urol Res 1984; 12: 205–8.
5. Webb R, Griffiths C, Ramsden P, Neal D. Ambulatory monitoring of bladder pressure in low compliance neurogenic bladder dysfunction. J Urol 1992; 148(5)1477–81.
6. McGuire E. Editorial: bladder compliance. J Urol 1994; 151: 955–6.
7. Weld KJ, Graney MJ, Dmochowski RR. Differences in bladder compliance with time and associations of bladder management with compliance in spinal cord injured patients. J Urol 2000; 163(4): 1228–33.
8. Soler J-M, Amarenco G, Lemaitre D et al. Corrélations entre données cystométriques et sphinctérométriques et lésions médullaires. Ann Readap Med Phys 1988; 31: 465–71.

9. Hackler R, Hall M, Zampieri T. Bladder hypocompliance in the spinal cord injury population. J Urol 1989; 141: 1390–3.
10. Light J, Beric A. Detrusor function in suprasacral spinal cord injuries. J Urol 1992; 148: 355–8.
11. Cardenas D, Mayo M, Turner L. Lower urinary changes over time in suprasacral spinal cord injury. Paraplegia 1995; 33: 326–9.
12. Rhein F, Audic B, Bor Y, Perrigot M. Etude clinique de la récupération des syndromes de la queue de cheval par hernie discale. A propos de 65 cas. Ann Readapt Med Phys 1985; 28: 153–68.
13. Beric A, Light J. Detrusor function with lesions of the conus medullaris. J Urol 1992; 148(1): 104–6.
14. Shin J, Parc C, Kim H, Lee I. Significance of low compliance bladder in cauda equina injury. Spinal Cord 2002; 40(12): 650–5.
15. Anderson P, Travers A. Development of hydronephrosis in spina bifida patients: predictive factors and management. Br J Urol 1993; 72: 958–61.
16. de Badiola F, Castro-Diaz D, Hart-Austin C, Gonzalez R. Influence of preoperative bladder capacity and compliance on the outcome of artificial urinary sphincter implantation in patients with neurogenic sphincter incompetence. J Urol 1992; 148(5): 1493–5.
17. Kaufman A, Ritchey M, Roberts A et al. Decreased bladder compliance in patients with myelomeningocele treated with radiological observation. J Urol 1996; 156(6): 2031–3.
18. Weld KJ, Dmochowski RR. Effect of bladder management on urological complications in spinal cord injured patients. J Urol 2000; 163(3): 768–72.
19. Bloom D, Knechtel J, McGuire E. Urethral dilation improves bladder compliance in children with myelomeningocele and high leak point pressures. J Urol 1990; 144: 430–3.
20. Brindley G. The first 500 patients with sacral anterior root stimulator implants: general description. Paraplegia 1994; 32(12): 795–805.
21. Koldewijn E, van Kerrebroeck P, Rosier P et al. Bladder compliance after posterior sacral root rhizotomies and anterior sacral root stimulation. J Urol 1994; 151: 955–60.
22. Swierzewski S, Gormely E, Belville W et al. The effect of terazosin on bladder function in the spinal cord injured patient. J Urol 1994; 151(4): 951–4.
23. Schulte-Baukloh H, Michael T, Miller K, Knispel H. Alfuzosin in the treatment of high leak-point pressure in children with neurogenic bladder. BJU Int 2002; 90(7): 716–20.
24. Sundin T, Dahlstrom A, Norlin L, Svedmyr N. The sympathetic innervation and adrenoreceptor function of the human lower urinary tract in the normal state and after parasympathetic denervation. Invest Urol 1977; 14: 322–5.
25. Chancellor M, de Groat W. Intravesical capsaicin and resiniferatoxin therapy: spicing up the ways to treat the overactive bladder. J Urol 1999; 162: 3.
26. Seki N, Ikawa S, Takano N, Naito S. Intravesical instillation of resiniferatoxin for neurogenic dysfunction in a patient with myelodysplasia. J Urol 2001; 166: 2368–9.
27. Schurch B, Hauri D, Rodic B et al. Botulinum-A toxin as a treatment of detrusor-sphincter dyssynergia: a prospective study in 24 spinal cord injury patients. J Urol 1996; 155: 1023–9.
28. Steers W, Meythalter J, Haworth C et al. Effects of acute and chronic continuous intrathecal baclofen on genitourinary dysfunction due to spinal cord pathology. J Urol 1992; 148(6): 1849–55.
29. Bushman W, Steers W, Meythalter J. Voiding dysfunction in patients with spastic paraplegia: urodynamic evaluation and response to continuous intrathecal baclofen. Neurourol Urodyn 1993; 12(2): 163–70.
30. Backhaus B, Kaefer M, Haberstroh K et al. Alterations in the molecular determinants of bladder compliance at hydrostatic pressures less than 40 cm H_2O. J Urol 2002; 168: 2600–4.
31. Baskin L, Howard P, Macarak E. Effect of physical forces on bladder smooth muscle and urothelium. J Urol 1993; 150: 601–5.
32. Kaplan E, Richier J, Howard P et al. Type III collagen messenger RNA is modulated in non-compliant human bladder tissue. J Urol 1997; 157(6): 2366–9.
33. Ohnishi N, Kishima Y, Hashimoto K et al. Morphometric study of low compliant bladder [in Japanese]. Hinyokika Kiyo 1994; 40(8): 657–61.
34. Kershen R, Azadzoi K, Siroky M. Blood flow, pressure and compliance in the male human bladder. J Urol 2002; 168: 121–5.
35. Ohnishi N, Kishima Y, Hashimoto K et al. A new method of measurement of the urinary bladder blood flow in patients with low compliant bladder [in Japanese]. Hinyokika Kiyo 1994; 40(8): 663–7.
36. Yoshiyama M, de Groat W. Effect of bilateral hypogastric nerve transection on voiding dysfunction in rats with spinal cord injury. Exp Neurol 2002; 175(1): 191–7.
37. Gloeckner D, Sacks M, Fraser M et al. Passive biaxial mechanical properties of the rat bladder wall after spinal cord injury. J Urol 2002; 167(5): 2247–52.
38. Landau E, Jayanthi V, Churchill B et al. Loss of elasticity in dysfunctional bladders: urodynamic and histochemical correlation. J Urol 1994; 152: 702–5.
39. Lee J, Wein A, Levin R. Effects of pregnancy on urethral and bladder neck function. Urology 1993; 42(6): 747–52.
40. Koebl H, Mostwin J, Boiteux J-P et al. Pathophysiology. In: Abrams P, Cardozo L, Khoury S, Wein A, eds. Incontinence. Plymouth: Health Publications, 2002: 203–41.

14

Pathophysiology of the vesico-sphincteric dyssynergia

Helmut G Madersbacher

Detrusor external sphincter dyssynergia (DSD) is defined as the presence of an involuntary contraction of the external sphincter during an involuntary detrusor contraction, and is therefore neurogenic. More recently, DSD has been simply characterized as intermittent or continuous according to the consistency of the sphincter contraction during the detrusor contraction.[1]

Coordinated micturition – vesico-sphincteric synergia

Normal micturition is controlled by neural circuits in the spinal cord and in the brain that coordinate the activity of visceral smooth muscle in the urinary bladder and urethra with activity of striated muscle in the urethral sphincter.[2] Normal micturition is preceded by relaxation of the external urethral sphincter.[3] The main reflex components of these switching circuits are, that high level afferent activity (pelvic nerve) results in inhibition of external sphincter activity via a spino-bulbospinal reflex, inhibition of sympathetic outflow reflexes, activation of parasympathetic outflow to the bladder, and activation of parasympathetic outflow to the urethra via a spinal reflex. When the volume of urine in the bladder exceeds the micturition threshold increased afferent firing from tension receptors in the bladder reverses the pattern of efferent outflow, producing firing in the sacral parasympathetic pathways and inhibition of sympathetic and somatic pathways. Relaxation of the urethral smooth muscle is mediated in the animal model by activation of a parasympathetic pathway to the urethra that triggers the release of nitric oxide, an inhibitory transmitter, and by removal of adrenergic and somatic cholinergic excitatory inputs to the urethra. Secondary reflexes elicited by flow of urine through the urethra facilitate further bladder emptying. These reflexes need the integrative action of the neuronal population at various levels of the neuraxis.

Within the spinal cord, afferent neurons from the bladder and other segmentally innervated structures synapse on interneurons, that send the axons to the brain. These ascending neurons connect with structures in the brainstem, including the pons and the periaqueductal gray (PAG) of the midbrain. There is good evidence that ascending afferent input from the spinal cord may pass through relay neurons in the PAG before reaching the pontine micturition center (PMC).[4] The PMC has a modulating effect on reflexes such as those mediating excitatory outflow to the sphincter and sympathetic inhibitory outflow to the bladder, which are organized at the spinal level.

The dorsolateral pontine tegmentum is established as an essential control center for micturition in the normal subject. It was first described by Barrington[5] in the cat, and has subsequently been called 'Barrington's nucleus', the 'pontine micturition center', or the 'M region'.[6] In the animal (cat) pons a region, which is located laterally to the pontine micturition center – hence the term 'L region' – has an important input to the external urethral sphincter motoneurons in the Onuf's nucleus as well as a projection to the thoracolumbar parasympathetic preganglianic neurons. Experimental findings let us assume that the M region is necessary to voiding and the L region is part of a larger, less specific area that probably serves sphincter control in various circumstances, when increased activation is required, such as during respiration, coughing, sneezing, or sexual activity. The fact that there is an area in the pons that is active during bladder storage suggests that the 'switching mechanism' originally proposed by De Groat,[6] instead of switching the PMC on and off, switches between the L and M regions during storage and voiding, respectively.

Uncoordinated micturition – vesico-sphincteric dyssynergia/detrusor-sphincter dyssynergia

With acute spinal cord injury the normal connections between the sacral cord and the supraspinal circuits that

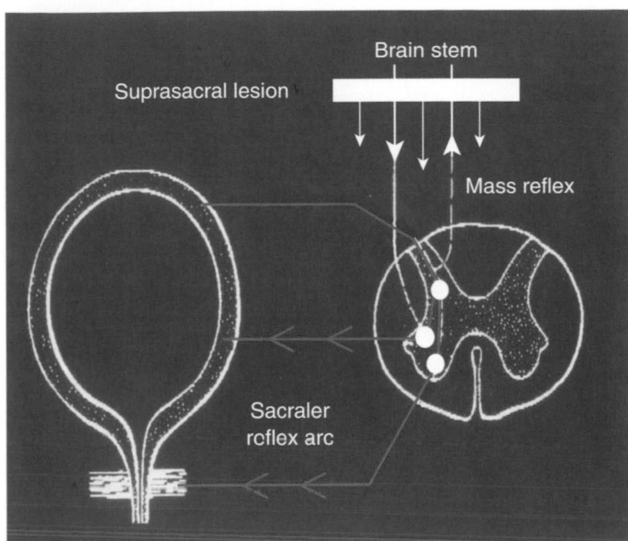

Figure 14.1
Schematic (simplified) drawing of sacral reflex voiding with DSD.

control urine storage and release are disrupted. After the so-called spinal shock phase, detrusor overactivity develops. This overactivity is mediated by a spinal micturition reflex that emerges in response to a reorganization of synaptic connections in the spinal cord.[15] Bladder afferents that are normally unresponsive to low intravesical pressures become more mechano-sensitive, leading to the development of detrusor overactivity. Normal micturition is associated with a spino-bulbo-spinal reflex mediated by myelinated Aδ afferents. These fibers represent about 20% of bladder afferents in some species. Compared to Aδ fibers, the more prevalent unmyelinated C fibers are relatively insensitive to gradual distention of the urinary bladder, they remain silent during normal filling, and it is only after spinal cord injury that a capsaicin-sensitive C fiber-mediated spinal reflex develops. The C fiber afferents obviously play a role in the development of bladder overactivity after spinal cord injury. Due to the increased mechanosensitivity of C fibers after spinal cord injury the cells in the dorsal root ganglion supplying the bladder are enlarged and show increased electrical excitability. Nitric oxide has been suggested as an important inhibitory transmitter in the lower urinary tract. Nerves with the capacity to synthesize nitric oxide supply the urethra and the urinary bladder. Nitric oxide seems to be important for the relaxation of the striated external sphincter.[14] It has been shown that oral nitric oxide donors decrease significantly the resting sphincter pressure within 10 to 15 minutes after intake. In addition, the contractile ability of the external urethral sphincter seems to be influenced by nitric oxide donors.

When the spinal cord injury is suprasacral and complete (neurologically defined as ASIA A) there is no modulation of pelvic floor reflexes such as the pudendo-anal (or urethral) reflex, whereas in incomplete injuries the reflex activity is variably facilitated. *Spinal neurogenic detrusor overactivity* is therefore often accompanied by *detrusor-sphincter dyssynergia,* defined as a neurogenically-determined failure of coordination of detrusor and urethra (Figure 14.1). Patients with brain lesions rostral to the pons with an intact detrusor–brainstem reflex do not show detrusor sphincter dyssynergia, their micturition remains coordinated. When the sacral cord and the PMC are separated, reflex voiding is initiated by an involuntary detrusor contraction rather than by relaxation of the external urethral sphincter. The failure of the urethral sphincter to relax, when the detrusor contracts, causes a functional urethral obstruction which may not only hinder bladder emptying, but may also permit the development of high detrusor pressures. If high pressures are present for prolonged periods in daily life, renal function is in danger (see below). From pediatric studies there is level 3 evidence that upper urinary tract deterioration is more probable when detrusor leak point pressure is elevated.[8]

How to diagnose detrusor-sphincter dyssynergia

Normally, voiding is characterized by cessation of EMG activity in the urethral sphincter prior to detrusor contraction. This coordination is impaired with lesions between the lower sacral segments and the upper pons. Consequently, sphincter EMG activity is not inhibited and is often increased before detrusor contraction, characteristic for detrusor-sphincter dyssynergia.

> Bladder outlet obstruction may be anatomic or functional in nature. An anatomic obstruction creates a urethral segment with a small and fixed diameter that does not dilate during voiding. As a result, the flow pattern is plateau shaped, with a low and constant maximum flow rate, despite high detrusor pressure and complete relaxation of the urethral sphincter. In a functional obstruction, however, it is the active contraction of the urethral sphincter during passage of urine that creates a narrow urethral segment, constantly or intermittently.

To differentiate anatomic from functional obstruction, information is needed about the activity of the urethral sphincter during voiding. This information can be obtained, and recorded together with pressure and flow, by monitoring the urethral pressure at the level of urethral sphincter, and by recording a continuous electromyogram (EMG) of the striated urethral sphincter. Also the use of videourodynamics can be very helpful in this respect, as contractions of the pelvic floor muscles and the external sphincter can actually be seen during the voiding phase.

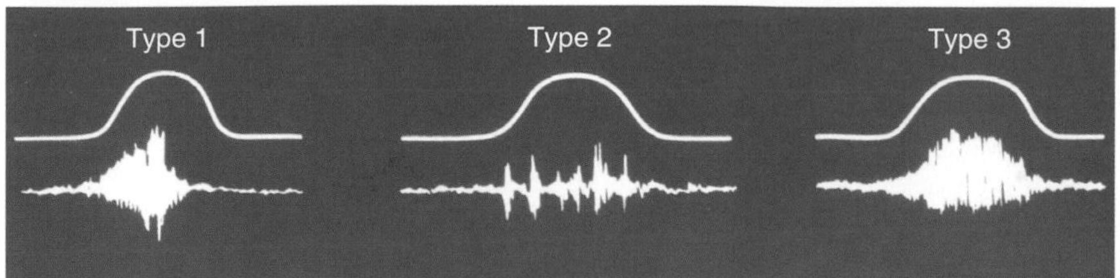

Figure 14.2
On the basis of the temporal relationship between urethral and detrusor contractions, these three types of dyssynergia have been described by Blaivas et al[11] (see text).

EMG of the striated sphincter/pelvic floor muscle

For clinical purposes surface (patch) electrodes are often used in order to achieve a quantitative 'random' EMG of the pelvic floor striated muscle. Where the urethral sphincter is not really accessible, the EMG of the striated anal sphincter is often used to monitor activity of the striated urethral sphincter. We use lac-isolated wire electrodes,[10] as originally described by Scott et al,[9] in patients with analgesia in the pelvic floor area to register striated anal sphincter and pelvic floor striated muscle EMG activity.

On the basis of the temporal relationship between urethral and detrusor contractions, Blaivas et al[11] described three types of dyssynergia (Figure 14.2). Type 1 had a crescendo increase in electromyographic activity that reached a maximum at the peak of the detrusor contraction, type 2 had clonic sphincter contractions interspersed throughout the detrusor contraction, and type 3 was characterized by a sustained sphincter contraction that coincided with a detrusor contraction. However, there is no correlation between the clinical neurologic level and the type of dyssynergia.[11] Also, Weld et al[1] found no significant differences between the DSD type and the level of injury (cervical, thoracic, or lumbar spinal cord). However, continuous DSD was strongly associated with complete spinal cord injuries. The more severe injuries probably result in more neural sprouting or other neural reorganization that fosters the development of continuous DSD. There are also no data on the effect of time on DSD type from published reports.

Videourodynamic findings in DSD

The characteristic radiologic sign consistently observed in men is an intermittent or constant narrowing of the urethra below the veromontanum, where it passes through the pelvic floor musculature. This narrowing of the urethra is clearly seen on the voiding cystourethrography; the most distal part of the posterior urethra is often as narrow as a thread, whereas widening of the proximal part of the posterior urethra is similar to a prestenotic dilatation. The weakly-muscled posterior wall is more distended than the anterior wall. The bladder neck seems narrowed and the posterior urethra shortened. Because of this, the urethra takes on a typical shape similar to an 'amphora' or 'spinning top'. This transformation prohibits the physiologic funneling of the bladder outlet, which normally occurs during micturition and which normally enables the wash-out of bacteria. The same is true for female patients with a functional obstruction located in the midurethra.

Differential diagnosis to detrusor-sphincter dyssynergia

A neurogenic uncoordinated sphincter behavior has to be differentiated from 'voluntary' contractions, e.g. due to anxiety, which may occur in the unnatural labaratory setting of urodynamics. 'Pseudodyssynergia' may be seen during abdominal straining, coughing, or attempted inhibition of an involuntary bladder contraction. Non-neurogenic sphincter contraction during micturition may also be a learned abnormal behavior, and may be encountered particularly in children with dysfunctional voiding. Such voluntary contractions may also be seen in patients with suprapontine detrusor overactivity in order to prevent incontinence, and may eventually become a reflex behavior. Sphincter contraction, or at least failure of relaxation during involuntary detrusor contractions, has also been reported in patients with Parkinson's disease. Striated sphincter behavior in this disease has also been named bradykinesia.

Prevalence of detrusor-sphincter dyssynergia

Of the 269 patients with suprasacral spinal cord injuries investigated by Weld et al,[1] 12.3% had no dyssynergia, 7.4% had intermittent, and 80.3% continuous DSD. Again, there was no significant association between the specific level of injury and the DSD type. Blaivas et al[11] found that 94.9% of patients with suprasacral injuries demonstrated detrusor overactivity and/or detrusor-sphincter dyssynergia, 41.8% had low bladder compliance, and 40% had high detrusor leak point pressures.

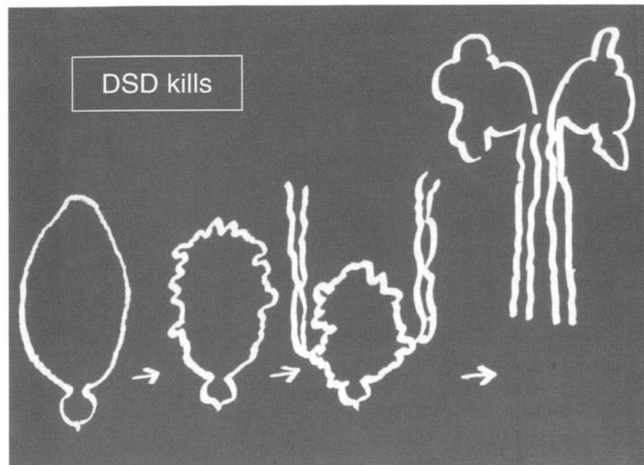

Figure 14.3
The impact of untreated DSD on the urinary tract (Drawing by M Stoehrer, 1985).

The clinical impact of detrusor-sphincter dyssynergia

Patients with DSD are at an increased risk of elevated intravesical pressure. Elevated residual urine, structural bladder damage, and vesico-ureteral reflux, when combined with recurrent infections, cause renal failure (Figure 14.3). This is more common with continuous than intermittent DSD. More than half of men with DSD develop urologic complications.[12]

A comparison of voiding cystourethrograms of patients with different illness duration showed clearly that the amphora shape of the posterior urethra was especially pronounced in patients who were paraplegic for a relatively short time (5 years).[13] With ongoing DSD this characteristic shape became less evident, whereas other striking findings become more evident: in 40% of our patients with

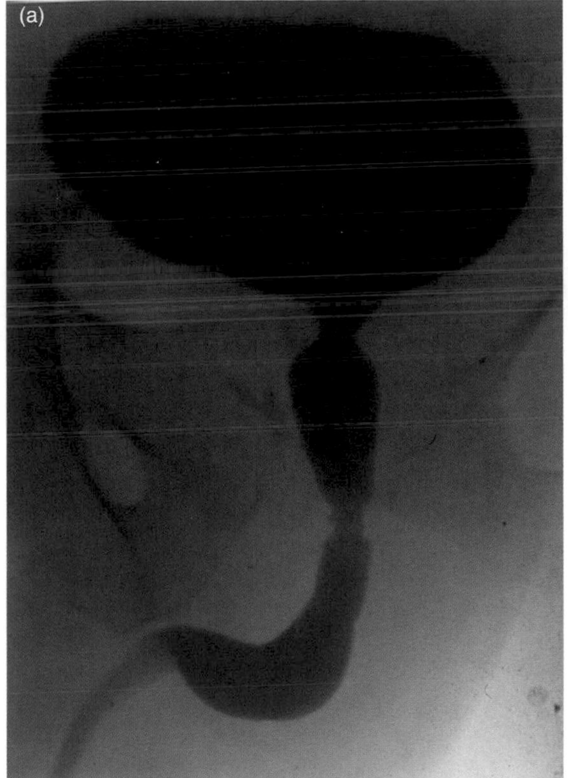

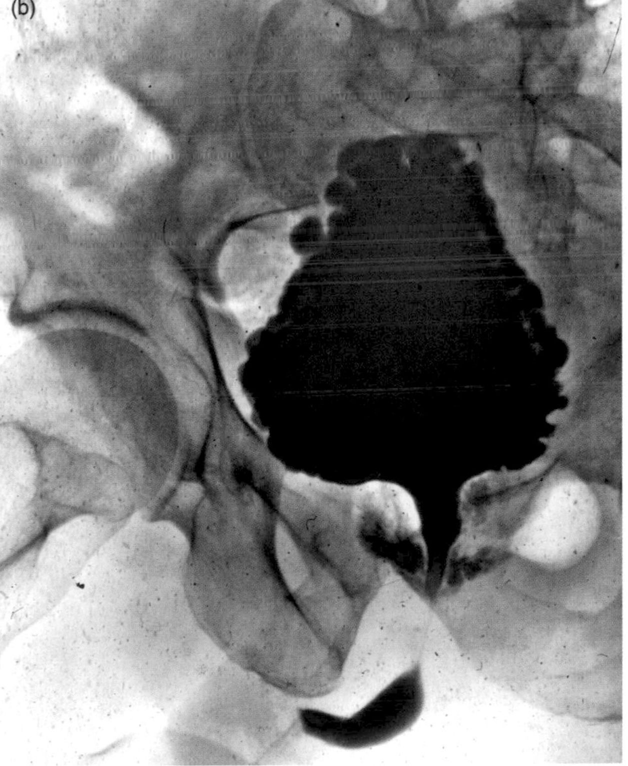

Figure 14.4
Voiding cystourethrograms (VCUGs) of the same patient (a) 6 months after spinal cord injury and (b) 5 years later without treatment of DSD. (a) Already on the VCUG 6 months postinjury there is a narrowing of the posterior urethra at the level of the external striated sphincter/pelvic floor musculature. There is slight influx of contrast medium into the prostate, indicating the presence of DSD; the bladder still has a normal shape. (b) 5 years later there is now massive influx into the prostate, the ballooning of the posterior urethra has decreased, the detrusor has become heavily trabeculated, and the bladder outline shows saculations as a result of untreated DSD.

spinal reflex voiding, extensive influx into the prostate and into the seminal vesicles, indeed even into the vas deferens and into the epididymis, occurred. Prostatic stones and caverns were also noted (Figure 14.4).

In men with early paraplegia (up to 1 year) we found such changes in 16% (4 of 25); in men who were paraplegic for up to 5 years in 28% (7 of 24), and for those with paraplegia of between 5 and 15 years' duration in 47% (8 of 17). In paraplegics of more than 15 years' duration 84% (11 of 13) showed the above-mentioned changes. These findings date back to 1977, when not much attention was yet paid to DSD. In children with non-neurogenic detrusor-sphincter dysfunction as well as in children with neurogenic DSD, the proximal urethra also showed the so-called 'spinning top' configuration during voiding, sometimes also already during filling. With detrusor and pelvic floor muscles contracting at the same time, the force of the detrusor contraction will dilate the proximal urethra down to the level of the closed striated external sphincter. The resulting 'spinning top' configuration is a sign of distal urethral stenosis, and may also be responsible for recurrent urinary tract infections in these children due to impaired wash-out of bacteria.

References

1. Weld KJ, Graney MJ, Dmochowski RR. Clinical significance of detrusor sphincter dyssynergia type in patients with post-traumatic spinal cord injury. Urology 2000; 56: 565–8.
2. Morrison JFB. Physiology of the striated muscles of the pelvic floor. In: Corcos J, Schick E, eds. The Urinary Sphincter. New York: Marcel Dekker, 2001.
3. Vereecken RL, Verduyn H. The electrical activity of the paraurethral and perineal muscle in normal and pathologic conditions. Br J Urol 1970; 42: 457–60.
4. Blok BFM. Central pathways controlling micturition and urinary continence. Urology 2002; 59: 13.
5. Barrington F. The relation of the hindbrain for micturition. Brain 1971; 44: 23–53.
6. De Groat WC. Nervous control of the urinary bladder of the cat. Brain Res 1975; 87: 201.
7. Araki I, de Groat WC. Developmental synaptic depression underlying reorganization of visceral reflex pathways in the spinal cord. J Neurosci 1997; 17: 8402.
8. McGuire EJ, Woodside JR, Borden TA et al. Prognostic value of urodynamic testing in myelodysplastic patients. J Urol 1981; 126: 205–9.
9. Scott FB, Quesada EM, Cardus D. Studies on the dynamics of micturition. Observations on healthy men. J Urol 1964; 90: 455.
10. Madersbacher H. The neuropathic urethra: urethrogram and pathophysiologic aspects. Eur Urol 1977; 3: 321–32.
11. Blaivas JG, Sinha IHB, Zeyed AAH et al. Detrusor-external sphincter dyssynergia: a detailed electromyographic study. J Urol 1981: 545–8.
12. Chancellor NB, Rivas DA. Current management of detrusor-sphincter dyssynergia. In: McGuire EJ, Bloom D, Catalone WE et al, eds. Advance in Urology. St Louis: Mos, 1995, 8: 291–324.
13. Madersbacher H. Combined pressure flow EMG and X-ray studies for the evaluation of neurogenic bladder disturbance. Urol Int 1977; 32: 176–83.
14. Ho KM, McMurray G, Brading AF et al. Nitric oxide synthase in the heterogeneous population of intramural striated muscle fibres of the human membranous urethral sphincter. J Urol 1998; 159(3): 1091–6.
15. Sekhon I, Fehling M. Epidemiology, demographics and pathophysiology of acute spinal cord injury. Spine 2001; 26: 2–12.

15

Pathophysiology of the autonomic dysreflexia

Inder Perkash

Historical overview

In 1860, Hilton[1] was the first to report a case consistent with autonomic dysreflexia (AD). He described recurrent chills and hot flushes in a C5 injured patient. In 1890, Bowlby[2] quoted hot flushes and sweating in C7 injured patients after catheter passage.

In 1917, Head and Riddoch[3] observed episodes of intense sweating associated with slowing pulse in association with bladder filling, blocked catheter, or administration of an enema in spinal cord injury (SCI) patients.

In 1938, Talaat[4] found distention of the bladder with increased blood pressure. Guttmann and Whitteridge reported the relationship between bladder distention and excessive rise in blood pressure in SCI patients in 1947.[5] They described, in a series of SCI patients, how distention of the viscera led to an autonomic response which induced profound effects on cardiovascular activity in parts of the body above the level of the spinal cord lesion. In 1951, Pollock and his group[6] reported defective regulatory mechanisms of autonomic nervous system function after SCI. Subsequently, many publications have described AD, its pathophysiology, and treatment, including reviews by Trop and Bennett,[7] Vaidyanathan et al,[8] and Karlsson.[9] The association between AD and detrusor-sphincter dyssynergia (DSD) has now been well recognized[10] and the therapeutic role of transurethral sphincterotomy (TURS) in relieving AD has been well documented.

Paroxysmal hypertension with pounding headache has been reported as the usual presenting symptom of AD. This is usually related to bladder distention and quite often accompanied by profuse sweating and bradycardia and sometimes tachycardia.[5,11] Other infrequent causes of AD are a loaded rectum, high bowel impaction, ureteric calculi, fractured long bones, and perforated abdominal viscera. Additionally, it has also been reported during extracorporeal shock wave lithotripsy (ESWL) for kidney stone patients[12] and during childbirth.[13] Appreciation of the pathophysiology of AD is important since it is preventable and failure to recognize it may result in hypertensive seizure and stroke.

Symptoms

SCI patients may present with one or more of the following signs or symptoms when experiencing an AD episode. However, the symptoms may be minimal or absent, despite the significantly increased blood pressure. Usually, the symptoms start after the spinal shock period. However, AD can be seen at an early stage and it should be considered in the differential diagnosis of patients immediately after SCI.[14]

AD symptoms are diverse and include:

- profuse sweating above the level of the injury, mainly the face, neck, and shoulders, but it could also occur below the level of injury
- pounding headaches
- hot flushes above the injury, especially the face and neck
- piloerection or goose bumps above or below the lesion
- blurred vision and the appearance of spots in the visual field
- nasal congestion and anxiety
- severe headaches, usually occipital, bitemporal, and bifrontal in location, in more than 50% of patients.[15]

Signs

Systolic and diastolic blood pressure increases can be severe and sudden, frequently associated with bradycardia. Usually, patients with SCI above T6 have normal systolic blood pressure in the range of 90–110 mmHg. Therefore, a blood pressure 20–40 mmHg above baseline may be a sign of AD.[9] However, systolic blood pressures above 300 mmHg and diastolic blood pressures above 220 mmHg have been reported.[16,17]

Other objective signs that might be associated with AD include:

- tachycardia
- atrial fibrillation, premature ventricular contraction, atrioventricular conduction abnormalities
- cutaneous vasodilatation or vasoconstriction
- penile erection
- changes in skin and rectal temperature and changes in the level of consciousness.

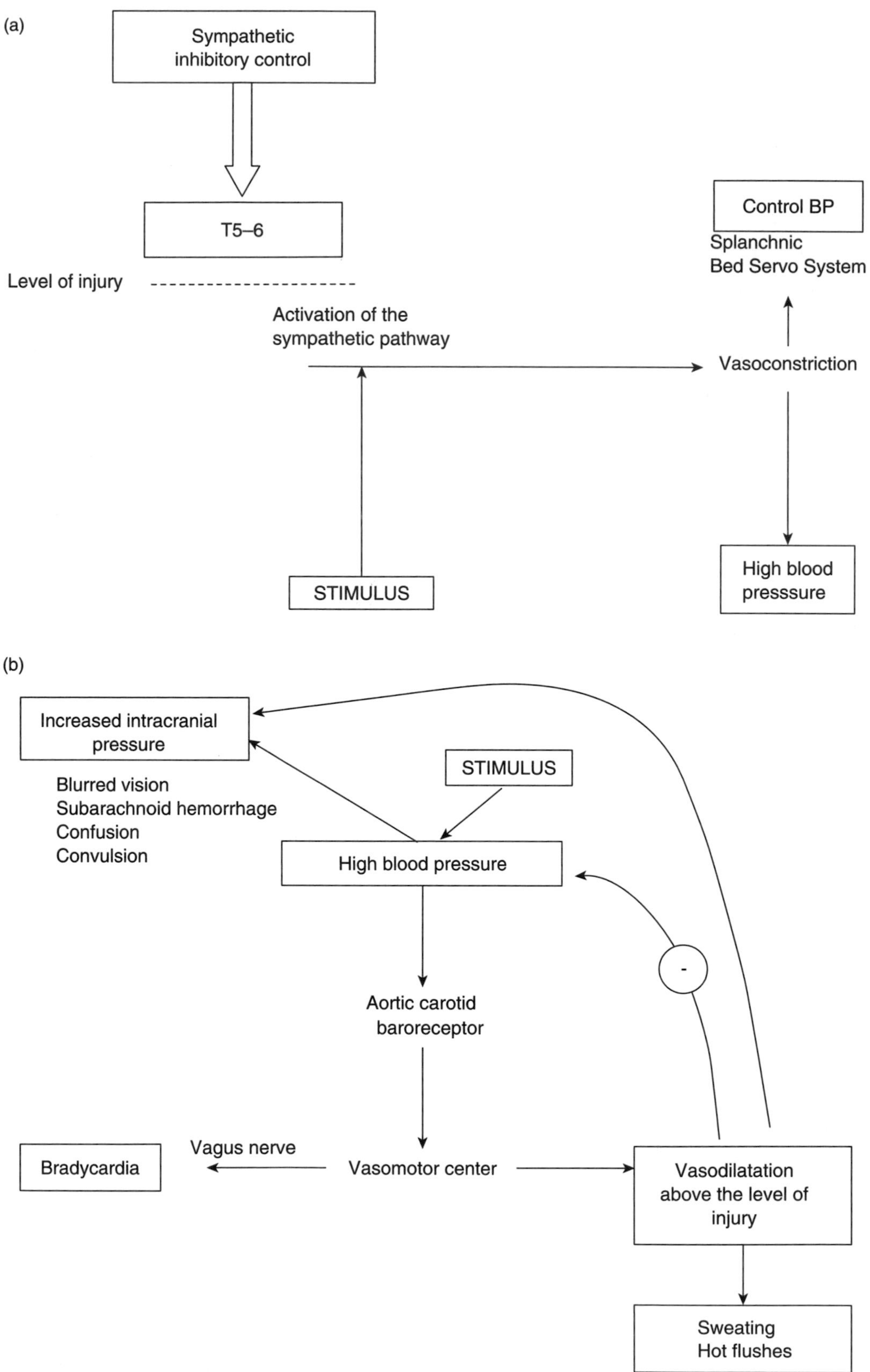

Figure 15.1
Sympathetic and parasympathetic activity leading to AD. (a) Illustrates the mechanism whereby blood pressure rises; (b) shows the manifestation of AD and the parasympathetic activity to control blood pressure.

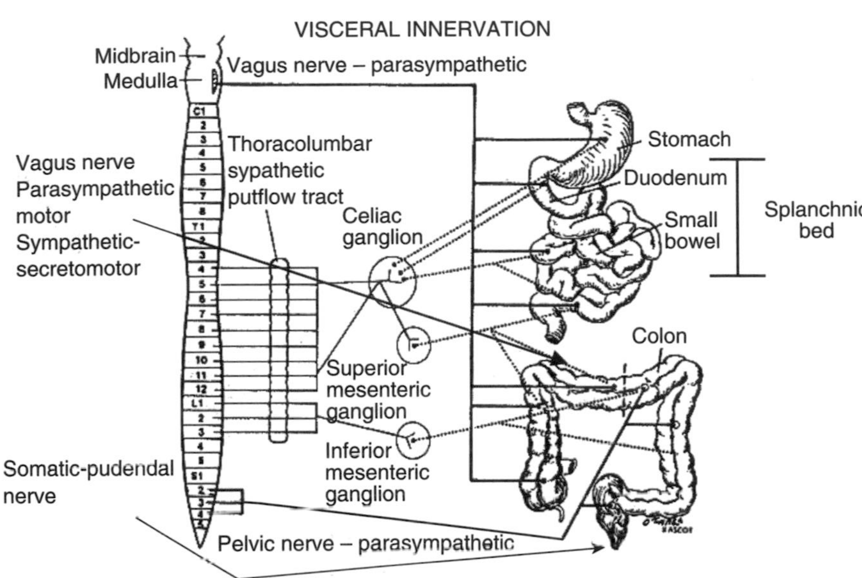

Figure 15.2
Sympathetic and parasympathetic visceral innervation (with permission from Gore RM; Mintzer RA. Gastrointestinal complications. In: Calenoff L, ed. Radiology of Spinal Injury. St Louis: CV Mosby, 1981).

Neurophysiologic basis of autonomic dysreflexia after spinal cord injury

AD usually occurs after the shock phase following SCI. About 90% of tetraplegics show positive cystometrographic (CMG) results for AD within 6 months of injury.[16] Sympathetic preganglionic vasoconstrictor fibers pass through the paravertebral ganglions to synapse with post-ganglionic neurons. Experimental studies in rats have shown that, soon after SCI, bulbospinal pathways are damaged and this disrupts the control of sympathetic preganglionic neurons.[17] This renders the neurons less receptive to any excitatory input, and explains why there is no AD during the shock phase. In about 30 days there is significant recovery in the rat in the preganglionic fibers, and reorganization of the synaptic input with the return of the excitatory sympathetic responses. The recovery of morphology and spinal circuitry change herald the occurrence of AD, which signals the development of abnormal synaptic connections within the spinal cord. The preganglionic neurons may express new receptors or probably upregulate normally expressed receptors in response to their initial deafferentation. Thus AD is time dependent[18] (for its intensity and magnitude) after injury in clinical patients. It has also been observed that there is hypersensitivity of vascular α-adrenorceptors in tetraplegics in the manifestation of AD.[19] The major splanchnic (sympathetic) outflow from the spinal cord is from T5 to T12. Patients with lesions above T5–6 have no control on the splanchnic bed. Full bladder, any other pelvic visceral distention, or other noxious stimuli below the level of SCI can reflexly stimulate peripheral vasoconstriction, resulting in increased venous return and a rise in blood pressure. It has been shown to be associated with an increase in plasma norepinephrine[18] and with no elevation in plasma renin during or after an episode of AD,[20] indicating that it is the increased sympathetic activity which leads to the rise in blood pressure and not the increased adrenal activity (see Figures 15.1 and 15.2).

Sympathetic skin responses seem to be sensitive in determining the degree of damage to the descending spinal sympathetic system. In their evaluation they did not find any SCI patient with hand and foot somatic skin responses (SSRs) intact who had an episode of AD. However, all patients with pathologic SSRs in the hands and feet exhibited AD. It seems to be a requisite for AD.[21] The authors also reported that 70% of AD patients had a pathologic circadian rhythm for blood pressure (there was no difference between day and night mean blood pressure). In a study in tetraplegics, the circadian rhythm for blood pressure was abolished but was preserved for heart rate.[22]

The blood pressure is autoregulated through sensory impulses passing through the carotid bodies and aortic arch to the hypothalamus, with negative feedback through the sympathetic pathways, and this leads to pooling of blood in the splanchnic bed, which could be as much as 1 or more liters – an enormous reduction in the circulating blood volume. This autoregulation is not possible with lesions above T5–6. However, the intact vagus nerve does lead to slowing of the heart rate, but the blood pressure is maintained due to the peripheral vasoconstriction and increased venous return. This manifests with signs and symptoms of AD. In one study, a large number of patients with injuries above the T6 spinal level only had a rise in blood pressure in the absence of symptoms of AD.[23] The

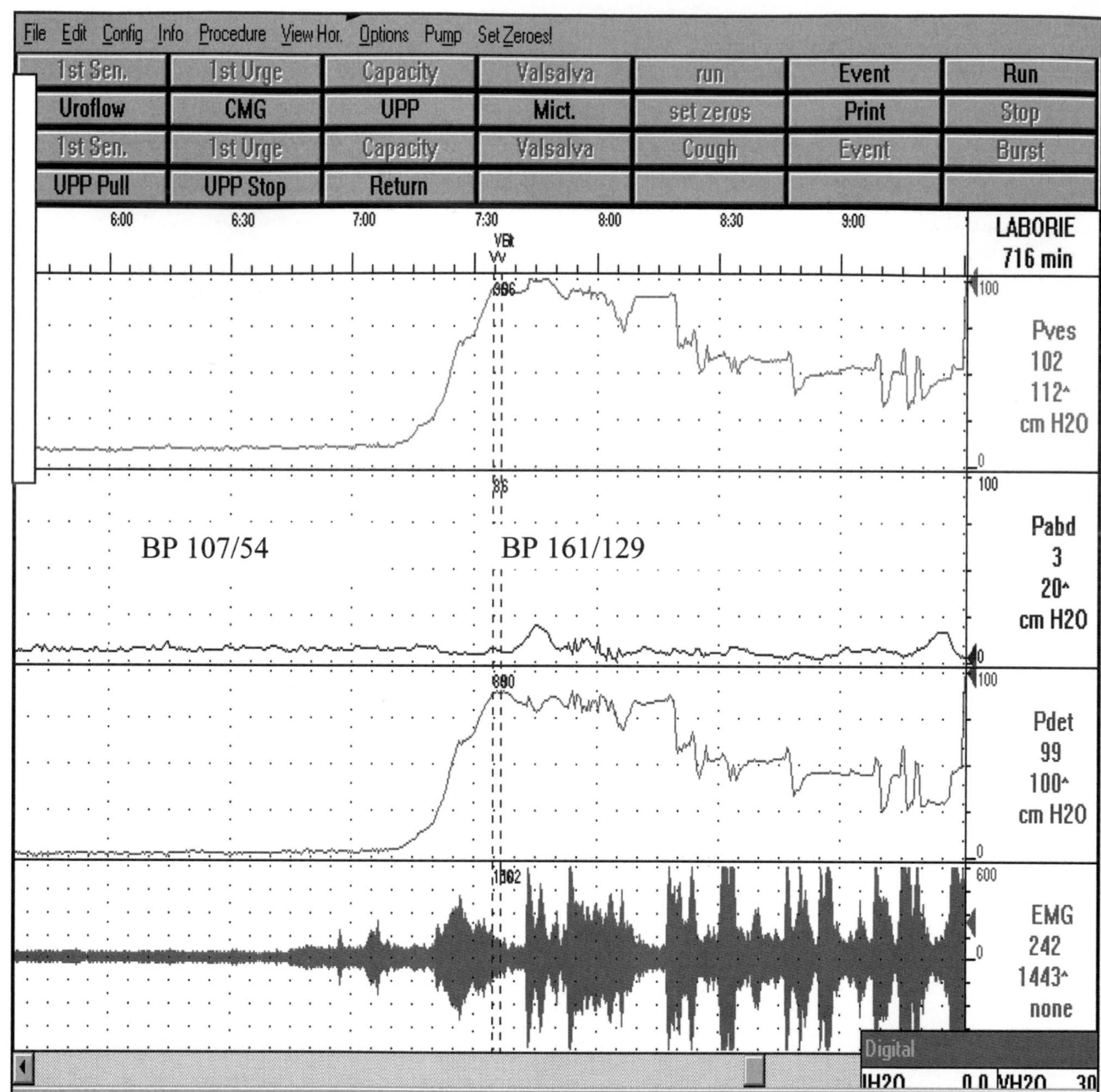

Figure 15.3
Rise in blood pressure with bladder contractions during CMG in a tetraplegic patient.

patients might, therefore, be wrongly diagnosed as suffering from essential hypertension unless urodynamic evaluation is done with BP monitoring to evaluate the effect of bladder distention on BP rise and occurrence of AD. In this study, urodynamics were critical to confirm the patients prone to AD (see Figure 15.3). During urodynamic evaluation of SCI patients, a significant rise in blood pressure was noticed in patients with DSD.[24,25] AD is thus associated with DSD in SCI patients.[19] Persistence of AD after TURS has not been adequately evaluated.

The failures of TURS have been reported as due to abnormal bladder contractions and bulbar urethral strictures. They could also be due to possible failed or inadequate TURS. Following an electrocautery incision there is a high incidence of urethral stricture, particularly when the incision is made into the bulbous urethra. Repeated urinary tract infections and urethral trauma can also lead to a urethral stricture. The availability of laser for TURS has reduced the incidence of urethral strictures and TURS failures.[26,27]

References

1. Hilton J. Pain and therapeutic influence of mechanical physiological rest in accident and surgical disease. Lancet 1860; 2: 401.
2. Bowlby AA. The reflexes in cases of injury to the spinal cord. Lancet 1890; 1: 1071.
3. Head H, Riddoch G. The autonomic bladder, excessive sweating, and some other reflex conditions in gross injuries of the spinal cord. Brain 1917; 40: 188.
4. Talaat M. Afferent impulses in nerves supplying the bladder. J Physiol 1938; 32: 121.
5. Guttmann L, Whitteridge D. Effects of bladder distension on autonomic mechanisms after spinal cord injuries. Brain 1947; 70: 361.
6. Pollock LJ, Boshes B, Chor H. Defects in the regulatory mechanism of autonomic function in injuries to the spinal cord. Neurophysiology 1951; 14: 85.
7. Trop CS, Bennett CJ. Autonomic dysreflexia and urological implications. A review. J Urol 1991; 146: 1461.
8. Vaidyanathan S, Soni BM, Sett P et al. Pathophysiology of autonomic dysreflexia: long term treatment with terazosin in adult and pediatric spinal cord injury patients manifesting recurrent dysreflexic episodes. Spinal Cord 1998; 36: 761.
9. Karlssan AK. Autonomic dysreflexia. Spinal Cord 1999; 37: 363.
10. Perkash I. Transurethral sphincterotomy provides significant relief in autonomic dysreflexia in spinal cord injured male patient: long-term follow up results. J Urol 2007; 177: 1026–9.
11. Silver JR. Vascular reflexes in spinal shock. Paraplegia 1971; 8: 231.
12. Kabalin JN, Lennon S, Gill HS, Wolfe V, Perkash I. Incidence and management of autonomic dysreflexia and other intraoperative problems encountered in spinal cord injury patients undergoing extracorporeal shock wave lithotripsy without anesthesia on a second generation lithotripter's. Urology 1993; 149: 1064.
13. Wanner MB, Rageth CJ, Zach GA. Pregnancy and autonomic hyperreflexia in patients with spinal cord lesions. Paraplegia 1987; 25: 482.
14. Silver JL. Early autonomic dysreflexia. Spinal Cord 2000; 38: 229.
15. Kewalramani LS. Autonomic dysreflexia in traumatic myelopathy. Am J Phys Med 1980; 59: 1.
16. Lindon R, Joiner E, Freehafer AA, Hazel C. Incidence and clinical features of autonomic dysreflexia in patients with spinal cord injury. Paraplegia 1980; 18: 285.
17. Krassioukov AV, Weaver LC. Morphological changes in sympathetic preganglionic neurons after spinal cord injury in rats. Neuroscience 1996; 70: 211–25.
18. Mathias CJ, Christensen NJ, Corbett JL et al. Plasma catecholamine during paroxysmal neurogenic hypertension in quadriplegic man. Circ Res 1976; 39: 204.
19. Arnold JMO, Feng Q-P, Delaney GA, Teasell RW. Autonomic dysreflexia in tetraplegic patients: evidence for alpha-adrenoceptor hyperresponsiveness. Clin Auton Res 1995; 5: 267–70.
20. Nanninga JB, Rosen JS, Krumlovsky F. Effect of autonomic hyperreflexia on plasma renin. Urology 1997; 7: 638.
21. Curt A, Nitsche B, Schurch B, Dietz V. Assessment of autonomic dysreflexia in patients with spinal cord injury. J Neurol Neurosurg Psychiatry 1997; 62(5): 473–7.
22. Nitsche B, Pershak H, Curt A, Dietz V. Loss of circadian blood pressure variability in complete tetraplegia. J Hum Hypertens 1996; 10(5): 311–7.
23. Linsenmeyer TA, Campagnolo DI, Chou IH. Silent autonomic dysreflexia during voiding in men with spinal cord injuries. J Urol 1996; 155(2): 519–22.
24. Perkash I. Pressor response during cystomanometry in spinal injury patients complicated with detrusor-sphincter dyssynergia. J Urol 1979; 121: 778.
25. Perkash I. Autonomic dysreflexia and detrusor-sphincter dyssynergia in spinal cord injury patients. J Spinal Cord Med 1997; 20: 365.
26. Perkash I. Abalation of urethral strictures using contact chisel crystal firing neodymium: YAG laser J Urol 1997; 157: 809.
27. Noll F, Sauerwein D, Stohrer M. Transurethral sphincterotomy in quadriplegic patients: long-term follow-up. Neurourol Urodyn 1995; 14: 351.

16

Pathophysiology of spinal shock

Magdy Hassouna, Nader Elmayergi, and Mazen Abdelhady

Introduction

The functions of the lower urinary tract are to store and periodically eliminate urine. This function implies a reciprocal relation between the reservoir (bladder) and outlet (urethra and sphincter) component of the lower urinary tract. The functions of the bladder and urethral sphincter are regulated by a complex neural control system located in the brain and spinal cord.[1,2] Spinal cord injury (SCI) initially induces an areflexic bladder and urinary retention due to loss of supraspinal excitatory stimulation.

Recognition of the problem of SCI and the associated lower urinary tract dysfunction dates back to at least 1700 BC, with the description in the *Edwin Smith Surgical Papyrus*: 'One having a dislocation in a vertebra of his neck while he is unconscious of his two legs and his two arms, and his urine dribbles. An ailment not to be treated.'[3]

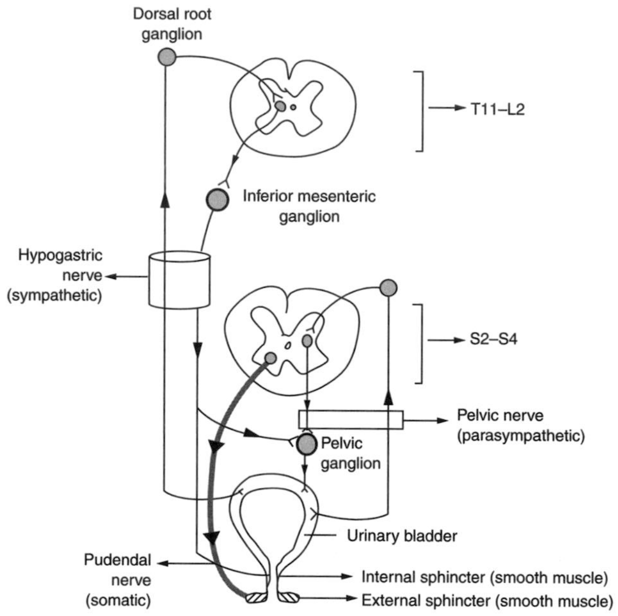

Figure 16.1
Innervation of bladder by parasympathetic, sympathetic and somatic nerves.

Innervation of the lower urinary tract

The bladder is innervated by three sets of peripheral nerves: parasympathetic (pelvic), sympathetic (hypogastric), and somatic (pudendal) nerves[4] (Figure 16.1). Afferent sensory fibers from the bladder can exit along either the sympathetic or parasympathetic pathway. Also, these nerves contain afferent axons innervating the lower urinary tract and the most important afferents for initiating micturition are those carried in the pelvic nerve[1,5] (Figure 16.1).

Parasympathetic preganglionic axons originate in the intermediolateral column of the S2–S4 spinal cord and terminate on postganglionic neurons in the bladder wall and in the pelvic plexus, which is a rectangular network located on the lateral surface of the rectum in humans (Figure 16.1). The portion of the pelvic plexus that specifically supplies the bladder is sometimes called the vesical plexus. The plexus receives input from the S2–S4 spinal cord segments by means of the presacral nerve. The primary supply to the detrusor is by parasympathetic nerves, which are uniformly and diffusely distributed throughout the detrusor.[6]

A rich plexus of sympathetic nerve terminals supplies the bladder neck smooth muscle in males. In contrast, in the female numerous parasympathetic nerves, which are identical to that innervating the detrusor, supply the bladder neck and urethral muscle. In the female the bladder muscle and the urethra receive a poor supply of sympathetic innervation.[7]

The sympathetic preganglionic nuclei are located in the first and second lumbar segments, and possibly the twelfth thoracic segment.

The superior hypogastric plexus is a fenestrated network of fibers anterior to the lower abdominal aorta. The hypogastric nerves exit bilaterally at the inferior poles of

Table 16.1 *Receptors in peripheral nervous pathways regulating lower urinary tract function. Facilitatory and inhibitory responses are indicated by plus and minus in parentheses, respectively*

		Efferent			
		Parasympathetic	Sympathetic	Somatic	Afferent
Ganglia	(+)	N, M, VIP	N, M, α_1[a], β[b]		
	(–)	ENK δ[a]	α_2[b]		
Bladder	(+)	M_2, M_3, P_{2X}, M_1[a]			NK_1, NK2, CGRP, H_1, B_2, vanilloid
	(–)	M_1[a], NPY[a]	β_1, β_2, NPY[a]		VIP
Bladder neck and urethra	(+)	M_2, M_3	α_1, α_2		
	(–)	NO			
Striated urethral sphincter	(+)			N	
	(–)				

[a]Presynaptic receptors.
[b]Heterosynaptic inputs onto parasympathetic ganglion cells.Abbreviations: ENK, enkephalin; VIP, vasoactive intestinal peptide; NO, nitric oxide; NPY, neuropeptide Y; N, nicotinic receptor; M_1, M_2, and M_3, muscarinic receptors; α_1, α_2, β_1 and β_2, adrenergic receptors; P_{2X}, purinergic receptor; CGRP, calcitonin gene-related peptide receptors; NK_1 and NK_2, tachykinin receptors; δ, opioid receptors; H_1, histamine receptor; B_2, bradykinin receptor.

the superior hypogastric plexus, which lie at the level of the sacral promontory. The network of nerve structures is located between the endopelvic fascia and the peritoneum. The hypogastric nerves unite the superior hypogastric plexus and the inferior hypogastric plexus or pelvic plexus bilaterally.[8] The superior hypogastric plexus and hypogastric nerves are mainly sympathetic, the pelvic splanchnic nerves are mainly parasympathetic, and the inferior hypogastric plexus has both types of nerves.

Bladder afferent fibers convey mechanoreceptive input essential for voiding. These visceral afferent fibers also transmit sensations of bladder fullness, urgency, and pain.

The pudendal nerve is a mixed nerve carrying motor and sensory fibers. It is a part of the pelvic plexus, and its fibers are derived from the somatic components of the 2nd, 3rd, and 4th sacral nerves. Nerve branches combine to form one major trunk of the pudendal nerve.[9]

The parasympathetic preganglionic axons release acetylcholine (ACh) which activates postsynaptic nicotinic receptors.[10,11] Nicotinic transmission at ganglionic synapses can be regulated by various modulatory synaptic mechanisms which involve muscarinic, adrenergic, and enkephalinergic receptors[1] (Table 16.1). Parasympathetic postganglionic neurons in turn provide an excitatory input to the bladder smooth muscle. Parasympathetic postganglionic nerve terminals release ACh, which can excite different types of muscarinic receptors (M_2 and M_3) which are present in the detrusor muscle[12–14] (Table 16.1). Muscarinic receptors are also involved in a presynaptic inhibition (M_2) and facilitation (M_1) of ACh release from postganglionic nerve terminals in the bladder[15,16] (Table 16.1). Adenosine triphosphate (ATP), which is a cotransmitter also released from parasympathetic postganglionic terminals, induces a rapid onset, transient contraction of the bladder[17] (Table 16.1). On the other hand, the parasympathetic input to the urethra elicits inhibitory effects mediated at least in part via the release of nitric oxide (NO), which directly relaxes the urethral smooth muscle.[9,17,18] In contrast to other transmitters which are stored and released from synaptic vesicles by exocytosis, NO is not stored but is synthesized immediately prior to release by the enzyme nitric oxide synthase (NOS). NOS-containing nerve terminals are found more densely in the bladder base and urethra than in the detrusor.[19] Thus, it seems reasonable to assume that the excitation of sacral parasympathetic efferent pathways induces a bladder contraction via ACh/ATP release and urethral relaxation via NO release (Table 16.1). Sympathetic preganglionic neurons located within the intermediolateral cell column of the T11–L2 spinal cord make synaptic connections with postganglionic neurons in the inferior mesenteric ganglion as well as with postganglionic neurons in the paravertebral ganglia and pelvic ganglia[1,8,20] (Figure 16.1). Ganglionic transmission in sympathetic pathways is also mediated by ACh acting on nicotinic receptors. Sympathetic postganglionic terminals, which release norepinephrine, elicit contractions of the bladder base and urethral smooth muscle and relaxation of the bladder body mediated though adrenoceptors[17,20] (Table 16.1). In addition, postganglionic sympathetic input to bladder parasympathetic ganglia can facilitate and inhibit parasympathetic ganglionic transmission.[20] Somatic efferent pathways which originate from the motoneurons in Onuf's nucleus of the anterior horn of the S2–S4 spinal cord innervate the external striated urethral

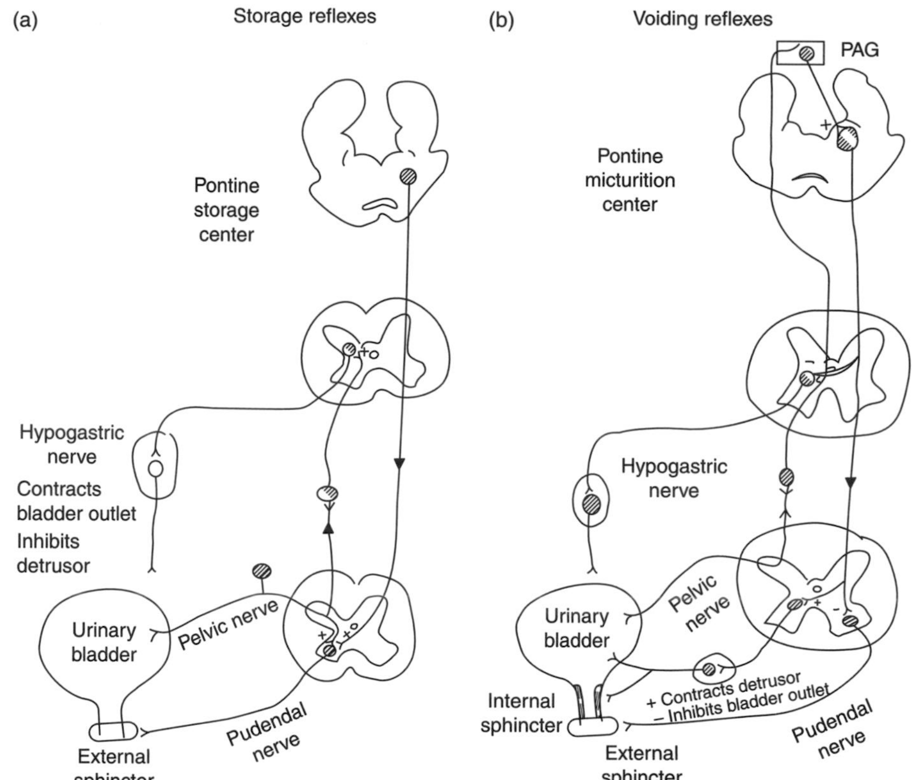

Figure 16.2
Storage and voiding reflexes of the bladder.

sphincter muscle and the pelvic floor musculature (Figure 16.1). Somatic nerve terminals release ACh that acts on nicotinic receptors to induce a muscle contraction (Table 16.1). Combined activation of sympathetic and somatic pathways elevates bladder outlet resistance and contributes to urinary continence. Several other nonadrenergic–noncholinergic transmitters such as leucine enkephalin (ENK), vasoactive intestinal polypeptide (VIP), and neuropeptide Y have been identified as modulators of efferent inputs to the lower urinary tract[20,21] (Table 16.1).

Physiology of urine storage and micturition

The bladder functions as a low-pressure reservoir during urine storage. The bladder pressures remain low and relatively constant when bladder volume is below the threshold for inducing voiding. This is mainly due to the combined effect of the viscoelastic properties of the bladder wall and quiescence of the parasympathetic pathway to the bladder.[1,2] During urine storage, the bladder outlet is closed and the bladder smooth muscle is quiescent, allowing intravesical pressure to remain low over a wide range of bladder volumes. Sensory information including the feeling of bladder fullness or bladder pain is conveyed to the spinal cord via afferent axons in the pelvic and hypogastric nerves.[5,24] Neuronal bodies of these afferent nerves are located in the dorsal root ganglia (DRG) at S2–S4 and T11–L2 spinal segmental levels (Figure 16.1). The afferent fibers carry impulses from tension receptors and nociceptors in the bladder wall to neurons in the dorsal horn of the spinal cord. Afferent fibers passing in the pelvic nerve to the sacral cord are responsible for initiating the micturition reflex. These bladder afferents have myelinated (Aδ fiber) or unmyelinated (C fiber) axons.[23,25]

In addition, during bladder filling, afferent activity derived from the bladder activates a sacral to thoracolumbar intersegmental spinal reflex pathway which triggers firing in sympathetic pathways to the bladder.[26] Activation of sympathetic efferents then mediates an inhibition of bladder activity and contraction of the bladder neck and proximal urethra.[27] Pudendal motoneurons are also activated by vesical afferent input as the bladder fills, thereby inducing a contraction of the striated sphincter muscle which contributes to urinary continence.[28,29] Thus urine storage is mainly controlled by reflexes integrated in the spinal cord (Figure 16.2). However, it is also reported that a supraspinal urine storage center is located in the dorsolateral pons. Descending inputs from this region activate the pudendal motoneurons to increase urethral resistance[30] (Figure 16.2).

When bladder volume reaches the micturition threshold, afferent activity originating in bladder mechanoceptors triggers micturition reflexes, which consist of firing in the sacral parasympathetic pathways and inhibition of sympathetic and somatic pathways. This leads to a contraction of the bladder and a concomitant relaxation of the urethra. The afferent fibers which trigger micturition in the rat and cat are myelinated Aδ fibers.[23,24] These bladder afferents in the pelvic nerve synapse on neurons in the sacral spinal cord, which then send their axons rostrally to a micturition center in the dorsolateral pons. This center contains neurons which are essential for inducing voiding reflexes.[30–33] It has been demonstrated that activity ascending from the spinal cord may pass through a relay center in the periaqueductal gray before reaching the pontine micturition center.[28,29] Thus voiding reflexes depend on a spino-bulbospinal pathway which passes through an integrative center in the brain (Figure 16.2). This center functions as an 'on-off' switch, activated by afferent activity derived from bladder mechanoceptors, and also receives inhibitory and excitatory inputs from the brain regions rostral to the pons. Reflex voiding is also facilitated by afferent inputs from the urethra. This urethrovesical reflex triggered by urine flow into the urethra enhances bladder contractions.[1] During voiding reflexes, activity in the pudendal efferent pathway to the striated urethral sphincter is suppressed to reduce outlet resistance.[1,33] This mechanism is mainly due to an inhibition of the pudendal motoneurons by the descending inputs from the dorsolateral pons.[24,34,35] An excitation of the sacral parasympathetic pathway also directly induces a relaxation of urethral smooth muscle mediated by the release of NO.

During voluntary voiding, relaxation of the pelvic floor and striated urethral sphincter muscles occurs, followed by a detrusor muscle contraction and opening of the bladder neck. Reflex inhibition of the smooth and striated urethral sphincter muscles also occurs during micturition.

In the human bladder smooth muscle, only two muscarinic receptor subtypes (M_2 and M_3) have been identified. Although the M_2 receptor subtype is the predominant subtype in the bladder (approximately 80%), the contractions of the bladder are mediated by M_3 receptors.[36] Muscarinic receptors (M_1 subtype) are also located prejunctionally on cholinergic nerve terminals in the bladder.[37] Voiding reflexes are mediated by myelinated (Aδ fiber) bladder afferents, which activate a supraspinal micturition reflex that passes through neural circuits in the rostral brainstem.[38] Also, unmyelinated (C fiber) bladder afferents are present and they are found to be silent in normal cats and do not respond to bladder distention.

Effects of spinal cord injury on micturition

The spinal cord is divided into 31 segments, each with a pair of anterior (motor) and dorsal (sensory) spinal nerve roots. On each side, the anterior and dorsal nerve roots combine to form the spinal nerve as it exits from the vertebral column through the neuroforamina. The spinal cord extends from the base of the skull and terminates near the lower margin of the L1 vertebral body. Thereafter, the spinal canal contains the lumbar, sacral, and coccygeal spinal nerves that comprise the cauda equina. Therefore, injuries below L1 are not considered SCIs because they involve the segmental spinal nerves and/or cauda equina. Spinal injuries proximal to L1, above the termination of the spinal cord, often involve a combination of spinal cord lesions and segmental root or spinal nerve injuries.

The primary watershed area of the spinal cord is the midthoracic region. Vascular injury may cause a cord lesion at a level several segments higher than the level of spinal injury. For example, a lower cervical spine fracture may result in disruption of the vertebral artery that ascends through the affected vertebra. The resulting vascular injury may cause an ischemic high cervical cord injury. At any given level of the spinal cord, the central part is a watershed area. Cervical hyperextension injuries may cause ischemic injury to the central part of the cord, causing a central cord syndrome.

The effect of SCI on the lower urinary tract depends on the level, duration, and completeness of the cord lesion. According to the level, it may give the picture of an upper motor neuron lesion, which corresponds with damage to the spinal cord rostral to the sacral cord, and lower motor neuron diseases in which damage occurs to the sacral cord and/or cauda equina that give rise to the parasympathetic and somatic pathway to the bladder and urethral sphincter.[39,40] Among patients with SCI, upper motoneuron disease such as cervical and thoracic vertebral injuries forms the major group.[39] Upper motoneuron type of SCI initially leads to a phase of spinal shock which is followed by a recovery phase during which neurologic changes emerge. During the period of spinal shock immediately after SCI, there is a flaccid paralysis and absence of reflex activity below the level of the lesion; thus the urinary bladder becomes areflexic. However, activity of the internal and external sphincter persists or rapidly recovers after suprasacral injuries. Therefore, because sphincter tone is present, urinary retention develops and patients have to be treated with intermittent or continuous catheterization to eliminate urine from the urinary bladder. Following the spinal shock phase, reflex detrusor activity reappears after 2–12 weeks in most cases.[39,40]

Pathophysiology of spinal cord injury

The pathophysiology of SCI is a two-step process involving primary and secondary mechanisms.[41,42]

Table 16.2 *Primary mechanisms of acute spinal cord injury*

- Acute compression
- Impact
- Missile
- Distraction
- Laceration
- Shear

Primary mechanism

The primary mechanism of SCI (see Table 16.2) is a combination of both the initial impact as well as the subsequent persisting compression. This is common in injuries like fracture dislocation, missile injuries, ruptured discs, and burst fractures. Clinical scenarios where impact alone occurs without ongoing compression may include severe ligamentous injuries in which the spinal column dislocates and then spontaneously reduces.[43] Similarly, spinal cord laceration from sharp bone fragments or missile injuries can produce a mixture of spinal cord laceration, contusion, and compression or concussion.[44]

Secondary mechanisms

The primary mechanical injury initiates a cascade of secondary injury mechanisms (Table 16.3), including the following:

1. vascular changes[42,45,47]
2. free radical production[47–49]
3. ionic derangements[50,51]
4. programmed cell death or apoptosis[52,53]
5. neurotransmitter accumulation (excitotoxic cell injury)[54,55]
6. inflammation
7. loss of ATP-dependent cellular processes[56]
8. edema[57]
9. endogenous opioids.[58,59]

Table 16.3 *Secondary mechanisms of spinal cord injury*

Systemic vascular effects:

- Heart rate: brief tachycardia then prolonged bradycardia
- Blood pressure: brief hypertension then prolonged hypotension
- Peripheral resistance: decreased
- Cardiac output: decreased
- Hypoxia
- Hyperthermia
- Injudicious movement of the unstable spine leading to worsening compression

Local vascular changes:

- Loss of autoregulation
- Systemic hypotension (neurogenic shock)
- Hemorrhage
- Loss of microcirculation
- Reduction in blood flow
  - Vasospasm
  - Thrombosis

Free radical production:

- Lipid peroxidation

Ionic derangements:

- Increased intracellular calcium
- Increased intracellular potassium
- Increased intracellular sodium and sodium permeability

Apoptosis

Neurotransmitter accumulation:

- Excitotoxic amino acids

Inflammation

Loss of energy metabolism:

- Decreased ATP production

Edema

Endogenous opioids:

- Endorphins

Vascular changes

One of the most critical elements in the evolution of biochemical and morphologic alterations following spinal cord trauma is the condition of vascular flow to the tissue. Blood flow, which is present or lacking in the spinal cord tissue after trauma, is a reflection of the damage provoked.[53]

Blood supply of the spinal cord

Blood is supplied to the vertebral column by way of segmental arteries that arise near it from the aorta, or from adjacent arteries in the areas beyond the extent of the aorta. These include the costocervical and intercostal arteries in the thorax, the lumbar and iliolumbar arteries in the lumbar region, and the lateral sacral arteries in the pelvis.

The anterior spinal artery (ASA) is supplied by a series of 5–10 unpaired radicular arteries (that originate from the vertebral arteries, and aorta and its branches). This single artery runs in the ventral midline from the foramen magnum to the filum terminale. The posterior spinal arteries are fed by smaller radicular arteries at nearly every spinal level.

Table 16.4 *Systemic and local vascular effects with acute SCI*

Systemic effects (neurogenic shock)	Local effects (cord microcirculation)
Heart rate (increased then decreased)	Mechanical disruption of spinal cord vessels
Blood pressure (brief increase then prolonged decrease)	Hemorrhage
Peripheral resistance (decreased)	Loss of microcirculation
Cardiac output (decreased)	Loss of autoregulation
Catecholamines (increased then decreased)	Reduction of spinal cord blood flow (SCBF)
	Vasospasm
	Thrombosis

The centripetal blood supply is derived from the posterior spinal and pial arteries. The pial arteries are lateral branches from the ASA and they communicate extensively with lateral branches originating from the posterior spinal arteries. The centrifugal supply is by the sulcal arteries. These arteries number approximately 4–5 per centimeter of spinal cord, and often bifurcate in the anterior median sulcus. The centrifugal sulcal arterial system supplies the anterior gray matter, the anterior half of the posterior gray matter, the inner half of the anterior and lateral white columns, and the anterior half of the posterior white columns.[46] The intervening watershed zones are supplied by both the centripetal and centrifugal systems.

After an acute SCI, both local and systemic changes occur to affect the spinal cord blood flow (SCBF) (see Table 16.4).

Systemic effects

Acute SCI can cause numerous cardiovascular and hemodynamic effects, the magnitude of which is related directly to the level and severity of the SCI, with the largest changes occurring in complete cervical injuries.[45] It is also one of the causes of neurogenic shock,[60] typically being related to the magnitude and severity of the cord injury. Neurogenic shock is characterized by severe autonomic dysfunction, resulting in hypotension, relative bradycardia, peripheral vasodilation, and hypothermia. It usually does not occur with SCI below the level of T6. Decreased sympathetic tone, unopposed cardiac vagal tone, and other cardiac changes are all contributory.[61] At its extreme, systemic effects including hypotension and bradycardia may be profound. These changes may persist for an extended period of time, sometimes months. In concert with these changes, total peripheral resistance and cardiac output may also remain depressed for a prolonged period of time.

The main cause for most of these effects is impairment of autoregulation following an acute SCI.[62–64] The systemic hypotension (preceded by a transient hypertension) that occurs as a result of this can cause further decreases in SCBF with induced hypertension (see Endogenous Opioids section) not necessarily reversing the ischemia, but rather causing marked hyperemia at adjacent sites.[42,65] The reason for this transient hypertension is unknown but may be mediated by both the thoracic sympathetic ganglions and the adrenal glands.[66] Experimentally, it has been shown in animal studies that autoregulation is intact during the initial 60 to 90 minutes after SCI but is then lost coincident with the onset of ischemia. It has been suggested that the ischemic response to SCI is mediated both by the loss of autoregulation and by relative constriction of the resistance vessels.[63]

Disturbances of venous drainage may play a role in the secondary damage that occurs after acute SCI, particularly in terms of exacerbating ischemia of the posterior columns.[67–69] This hypothesis gains weight by studies that show that venous occlusion in various pathologic conditions causes white matter lesions.[70–72] It may be that peculiarities of the venous drainage of the spinal cord make it more susceptible to damage.[68]

Local effects

Microcirculation There is a major reduction in the microcirculation of the traumatized spinal cord and lack of perfusion. Also, major areas lack filling of the arterioles, capillaries, and venules. This occurs both at the injury site, and for a considerable distance cephalad and caudad in the cord. The ischemic zones encompass a large portion of the gray matter and the surrounding white matter, and are especially severe in white matter adjacent to hemorrhages in the gray matter.[46] This may be due to obstruction of the anterior sulcal arteries that leads to the hemorrhagic necrosis and subsequent central myelomalacia seen at the site of injury.

There also seems to be a secondary injury to the microcirculation such as thrombosis or vasospasm of arterioles traversing the gray matter to supply the white matter. The large vessels of the cord such as the anterior spinal artery and the anterior sulcal arteries, however, almost always remain patent even after severe cord injury.

Axonal conduction The relationships among the severity of acute SCI, motor and somatosensory evoked potentials

(MEPs and SSEPs), and SCBF were studied. A linear relationship was found between the severity of acute SCI and the reduction in SCBF at the injury site. Also the reduction in amplitude of the MEP and SSEP was significantly correlated with the reduction of post-traumatic SCBF. Both the severity of cord injury and the degree of post-traumatic ischemia were significantly related to post-traumatic axonal dysfunction. Thus, these studies provide quantitative evidence linking post-traumatic ischemia to axonal dysfunction following acute SCI.[45]

Histology Histologically, there are many changes that occur after an SCI. Though there are petechial and more confluent hemorrhages in the gray matter, there is an initial absence of cellular and tissue necrosis. A progressive necrotizing process and an inflammatory cell infiltration that affects the gray matter and extends into the white matter follows this early period. Throughout these changes the main arteries remain patent, and this has led to the conclusion that much of the vascular damage occurs primarily in the intramedullary vascular system.

Also, the principle site of vascular damage is the endothelial cells, either by direct physical trauma or secondary to the resultant ischemia. These alterations in endothelial cell function cause an increase in vascular permeability and edema formation.[73–75] Endothelial damage occurs early, with the formation of craters, adherence of noncellular debris, over-riding of endothelial cell junctions, and microglobular formations occurring 1–2 hours after acute SCI.[76]

Free radical pathology and lipid peroxidation

Molecules are composed of atoms bonded together. This bonding process is accomplished by the sharing of electrons. When two atoms come together and their electrons pair up, a bond is created. Paired electrons are quite stable; nearly 100% of all electrons in the human body exist in a paired state, and a general principle of quantum chemistry is that only 2 electrons can exist in one bond.

If the bond between atoms is broken, the electrons either stay together (i.e. one atom gets both electrons and the other atom gets none) or they split up (each atom gets one electron). If the electrons split up, the atoms are called *free radicals* (molecules with an unpaired electron). This electron split is what makes free radicals both useful and dangerous.

It is important to mention that there are several essential biochemical pathways and cell biologic phenomena that depend on free radicals. Examples include (but are not limited to) mitochondrial electron transport, phagocytosis by macrophages and polymorphonuclear leukocytes, and hydroxylation reactions in the endoplasmic reticulum.

However, among biomolecules, the unsaturated acyl chains in cell membrane phospholipids and cholesterol in membranes are highly susceptible to pathologic free radical damage. This is due to:

1. Their inherent structure (polyunsaturated acyl chains are normally unconjugated and the α-methylenic carbons between carbons with double bonds have allylic hydrogen that can readily enter into free radical reactions).
2. The 700% greater solubility of molecular oxygen within nonpolar compared to aqueous environments (the most nonpolar regions of a cell are generally the hydrophobic portion of the membranes; the phospholipid acyl chains and the cholesterol comprise the hydrophobic portion of cell membranes, with the exception that organelle membranes are usually devoid of cholesterol, which is usually found in close association with phospholipids only in the plasma membrane and myelin).
3. Molecular oxygen has outer orbitals that have unpaired electrons, thereby conferring upon oxygen certain properties of free radicals such as magnetic susceptibility (due to the magnetic moment of an unpaired electron in orbit) and the ability to initiate free radical chain reactions among susceptible molecules that lack sufficient antioxidant neighboring molecules.[47]

The consumption of a major CNS antioxidant, ascorbic acid, in the ischemic or traumatized tissues occurs before the loss of the lipids, and is an important factor in establishing the free radical nature of some of the pathologic changes.

Free radicals most commonly form from molecular oxygen. Superoxide (O_2) is formed by incomplete electron transport in mitochondria. Superoxide is converted to H_2O_2 by superoxide dismutase and this in turn to H_2O and O_2 by catalase. In the presence of free iron, released from hemoglobin, transferrin, or ferritin by either lowered pH or oxygen radicals, H_2O_2 forms highly reactive hydroxyl radicals (HO). These, if unchecked, can cause geometrically progressive lipid peroxidation, spreading over the cellular surface and causing impairment of phospholipid-dependent enzymes, disruption of ionic gradients, and, if severe enough, membrane lysis. This process also forms more lipid peroxides and consequently more free radicals.[47]

After experimental SCI, there appears to be a persistent accumulation of cyclooxygenase-1 (COX-1)-expressing microglia/macrophages and upregulation of COX-1 expression by the endothelium.[77] This substance, produced by the conversion of arachidonic acid, contributes to reduced blood flow by causing platelet aggregation and vasoconstriction.[78] It can also contribute to an inflammatory response and lipid peroxidation.[79]

Cyclooxygenase-2 (COX-2) has been studied recently as a putative contributor to secondary injury. COX-2 mRNA and protein expression is also induced after experimental SCI.[80] It may represent a common substrate linking membrane damage and excitotoxicity in SCI. Indeed, selective inhibition of COX-2 improves outcome after spinal cord insult in preliminary animal investigations.[79,80]

Though still not completely established, in SCI the initiation of the free radical reactions following impact is probably mediated by the initial extravasation of blood in the central gray matter and perhaps by coenzyme Q autoxidation when spinal cord ischemia (hypoxia) occurs. The hemorrhages are minute and petechial, but they provide inorganic iron and copper from the plasma, as well as iron and copper from RBCs that extravasate and lyse. Iron compounds such as hematin can accelerate the autoxidation of unsaturated lipids by five orders of magnitude. Further, the concentration of highly polyunsaturated fatty acyl (PUFA) chains in membrane phospholipids is greatest in the central gray matter; PUFAs are very susceptible to free radical reactions, particularly in the presence of iron, or copper.[47]

Ionic derangements

Potassium and calcium Potassium ions (K^+) and calcium ions (Ca^{2+}) play important roles in the central nervous system (CNS). Intracellular K^+ activity ($[K^+]i$) is normally at least 20 times greater than extracellular K+ activity ($[K^+]e$). The resultant transmembrane K^+ gradient controls membrane potentials, action potential conduction, and active transport of sodium ions (Na^+). Increases in cell membrane permeability to K^+ produce rises in $[K^+]e$. Because normal $[K^+]e$ is 3–4 mmol/liter (mM), small changes in $[K^+]e$ profoundly alter neuronal activity. Cells typically maintain very low intracellular Ca^{2+} activity ($[Ca^{2+}]i$), <100 nmol/liter (nM) in contrast to extracellular Ca^{2+} activity ($[Ca^{2+}]e$) of >1.0 mM. Owing to this very large gradient, Ca^{2+} ions readily enter cells when membrane permeability increases. Ca^{2+} entry into cells links membrane activity with cellular functions. Large Ca^{2+} influxes into cells have been postulated to kill hepatocytes, myocytes, peripheral nerves, myelin, and spinal axons.[51]

Potassium changes Contusion that occurs causes a disruption of a large proportion of cells at the impact site. This disruption leads to a large increase in extracellular K, with a rise from 4 mM to 54 mM. One hour after impact, approximately 50% of K is lost from the impact site. By 3 hours, only 35% of pre-injury tissue K remains at the impact site.

Consequences of potassium depletion Cells do not repossess K^+ ions released into the extracellular space at the impact site. K is gone from the impact site, not merely equilibrated between the intra- and extracellular compartments. The cells not initially disrupted by the contusion also lose intracellular K^+, due to increased permeability of cell membranes depolarized by elevated $[K^+]e$.

The surviving cells tend to distribute in the outer rim of the spinal cord, the part least susceptible to ischemia. Note that the effects of $[K^+]i$ depletion are likely to outlast the $[K^+]e$ changes. K^+ ions released into extracellular space should be rapidly cleared by diffusion and glial transport.[81,85] $[K^+]i$ restoration depends on active ionic transport.

Ironically, rapid recovery of $[K^+]e$ to normal levels will force ionic restitution mechanisms to work against steeper transmembrane ionic gradients. One consequence of low $[K^+]i$ will be depolarization of cells in the presence of normal $[K^+]e$. This may explain the paradoxical loss of spontaneous activity or conduction block occasionally observed in ischemia and SCI even when $[K^+]e$ appears to be normalized.[51]

Potassium diffusion The K^+ spilt from the damaged cells is absorbed either into the spinal cord itself, into the CSF, or into the blood. The far majority (70%) of K^+ is absorbed into the cord surrounding the impact site. Three hours after the injury (the time it takes for the blood–brain barrier to break down) increased amounts of K^+ are lost into the CSF. However, diffusion into the CSF and blood is negligible during the periods of ischemia[86,87] and spreading depression.[82,84,89] Spreading depression is a transient, slowly propagating wave of tissue depolarization that can be evoked by mechanical stimulation, and has been associated with ischemia or traumatic brain injury. Each wave lasts for 1–2 minutes; waves of spreading depression have been observed to occur for several days after injury. In a model of ischemia, these waves have been shown by MRI to precede neural damage, with infarct volume increasing by up to 23% after each wave. Spreading depression is of non-neuronal origin, being mediated by astrocytes, and neurons are only secondarily affected. Two different, interacting mechanisms help to propagate spreading depression from cell to cell: a gap junction-mediated pathway and an ATP-purinergic pathway. While most of the work on spreading depression has been done in the brain, recent studies have shown that spinal cord astrocytes can mediate spreading depression via the ATP-purinergic pathway after edema.

Calcium changes Extracellular calcium $[Ca^{2+}]e$ recorded with ion-selective microelectrodes is typically greater than 1.2 mM in uninjured spinal cords and brain. $[Ca^{2+}]i$ in the spinal cord is not known with certainty, but some estimates suggest <100 nM[3], negligible compared to $[Ca^{2+}]e$. The amounts of Ca changes at the impact site appear small when compared with the K changes. On an ion-by-ion basis, the Ca shifts constitute a minor fraction of the ionic changes at the impact site. But the Ca changes must be considered in light of the lower pre-injury $[Ca^{2+}]e$ levels and the higher proportion of bound Ca versus free Ca^{2+} in the spinal cord. $[Ca^{2+}]e$ remains at <0.1 mM for hours after the injury at the impact site.

Calcium diffusion Uptake of Ca by intact cells plays only a small role in the persistent low $[Ca^{2+}]e$ levels found after injury at the impact site. Active uptake into the CSF is very difficult, due to the large concentration gradient and rapid drop of $[Ca^{2+}]e$. Inorganic phosphate plays a major role.

Phosphate binds strongly with Ca^{2+} to form phosphate complexes, most notably hydroxyapatite or $Ca_5(PO_4)_3(OH)$. The association constant of Ca^{2+} with the phosphate ion (H_2PO_4) is pK −7.2.[90,91] Tissue concentrations of inorganic phosphates often exceed 5 mM. Calcium phosphate is quite insoluble. Hydroxyapatite has a solubility product of pK 58.6 and is less sensitive to pH than other Ca complexes.[92] At pH <6.5, other Ca complexes transform to hydroxyapatite when phosphates are available.[93–95] Ca^{2+} ions diffusing to the impact site sequester inorganic phosphates and precipitate as hydroxyapatites or other complexes, i.e. 'amorphous calcium deposits'.

There are sufficient phosphates in the tissue to buffer large quantities of Ca^{2+}. ATP turnover, for example, can provide 1–2 mM of phosphate. Extreme depletion of cellular phosphates due to sequestration by Ca^{2+} explains the rapid losses of ATP and other metabolic derangements in injured spinal cords.[96,97]

Pathologic consequences of calcium influx The finding of early Ca accumulation at the impact site preceding onset of gross tissue necrosis argues for a causative role of Ca^{2+} in cell damage. The intracellular volume of axons at the impact site is likely to be a tiny fraction of the total axoplasm available to buffer Ca^{2+} ions entering the axon. Furthermore, the critical metabolic apparatus of cells giving rise to the axons is situated far from the lesion site and therefore is not as accessible to the entering Ca^{2+} ions. In contrast, cell bodies situated at the lesion site are more vulnerable to the damaging effects of Ca^{2+} influx.[51]

Apoptosis (programmed cell death)

Cell death that occurs after SCI occurs either through necrosis or apoptosis. Necrotic cell death occurs passively, resulting from the actual tissue mechanical damage and resultant release of destructive lysozymes, ion fluxes, and disturbed cell membranes producing an inflammatory response that has long been understood to be the sole component of neuronal tissue death and the ultimate clinical neurologic ramifications of acute SCI.

In contradistinction to necrotic cell injury, apoptosis is associated with physiologic or programmed cell death.[98,99] It is an actively regulated response and there are a variety of morphologic criteria that distinguish apoptotic from necrotic cell death.

Apoptotic cell death occurs a single cell at a time, while necrotic cells normally die in groups. Although cell membranes may undergo blebbing during apoptotic cell death, they do not lose their structural integrity as do cells undergoing necrotic cell death. Cells undergoing apoptotic death actually shrink, forming apoptotic cell bodies which contain cleaved DNA. In contrast, necrotic cells swell and lyse which incites a significant inflammatory response. Thus, although both apoptotic cell bodies and necrotic cells may be phagocytosed by tissue macrophages, apoptotic cell bodies do not incite any type of inflammatory response and thus undergo a 'silent' cell death.

At the molecular level, there are many distinct morphologic and biochemical changes occurring during apoptosis, including chromatin condensation, DNA fragmentation into oligonucleosome-sized fragments, and the compaction of chromatin into uniformly dense masses. The constant biochemical event which occurs in apoptosis is the activation of an endonuclease which cleaves DNA at internucleosomal linker sites.

The biochemical criteria for distinguishing apoptotic from necrotic cell death are also quite well established. Apoptotic cell death is induced by physiologic stimuli, either external or internal, while necrotic cell death arises from nonphysiologic disturbances. Apoptotic cell death is a tightly regulated process with a sequence of activation steps that requires energy and specific macromolecular synthesis as well as *de-novo* gene transcription.[100] This precedes the nonrandom oligonucleosomal length DNA fragmentation which is the common final pathway of eventual apoptotic cell death. In contrast, during necrotic cell death there are no energy requirements because there is no *de-novo* gene transcription, and thus no new protein or nucleic acid synthesis occurring.[101,103] The cellular DNA is randomly digested following cell lysis by macrophages that are solicited following the inflammatory response.

There are several features of SCI that suggest apoptosis plays a key role in the pathophysiology.

Increases in intracellular Ca^{2+} occur after SCI and are important in post-traumatic cell death. Ca^{2+}-dependent breakdown of DNA and protein also occurs in apoptosis. Hypoxia and free radical formation follow SCI, and are processes known to trigger p53-mediated DNA repair and apoptosis. Glutamate excitotoxicity has been established as a key event following neural trauma and has also been linked to apoptosis.[52] (see Excitotoxins section).

It is thought that oligodendrocytes are the major cell type in compressive SCI that undergoes apoptosis[102,103] seen in areas of wallerian degeneration and detectable between 24 hours and 3 weeks postinjury.[104] The mechanism behind this is unclear, but it may occur as a result of adverse changes in the cellular environment resulting in axonal demyelination or as a result of wallerian degeneration, or by a combination of both of these processes.[105,106] Apoptosis occurs around the lesion epicenter as well as within areas of wallerian degeneration in both ascending and descending white matter tracts.[107]

Another component playing a role in apoptosis is the calpains (calcium-activated neutral proteases). They degrade cytoskeletal proteins and mediate necrotic and apoptotic cell death.[108] Their activation is triggered by calcium influx and oxidative stress, resulting in neurodegeneration. Calpeptin (a calpain inhibitor) and methylprednisolone administered after SCI resulted in diminished protein breakdown.[108] Calpeptin was associated with a reduction in the internucleosomal DNA fragmentation indicative of apoptotic cell death. The inhibition of cytoskeletal protein degradation suggests that calpeptin may be neuroprotective by decreasing cellular death and inhibition of cytoskeletal breakdown.[109]

Some forms of experimental treatment of SCI are aimed at limiting the histologic injury, such as the oncogene Bcl-2, which regulates the antioxidant pathway, thus limiting free radical generation. Similarly, cycloheximide treatment can improve outcome after contusion trauma in the spinal cords of rats.[110]

Excitotoxins

Endogenously released excitatory amino acids may contribute to injury in the CNS in several different disorders, including epilepsy, neurodegenerative diseases, and cerebral ischemia.[113] The acidic amino acids glutamate and aspartate are widely distributed within the CNS and serve as excitatory neurotransmitters. It has long been recognized that these substances may be neurotoxic.[55]

N methyl D aspartate (NMDA), quisqualate, and kainite are receptors of excitatory amino acids. Selective NMDA receptor antagonists, injected directly into the brain, protect hippocampal neurons from cell death following cerebral ischemia[114] and hypoglycemia.[113] NMDA receptors also play a role in neurotransmission in the spinal cord.[114,115]

Most selective NMDA antagonists do not readily cross the blood–brain barrier, and hence their effects only appear after direct CNS administration. MK-801 [(+)-5-methyl-10,11-dihydro-5H-dibenzol [a,d]cyclo-hepten-5,10-imine maleate] is centrally active following systemic administration. It is a selective, noncompetitive antagonist that is use-dependent, requiring activation of receptors for its effect to be demonstrated.[116]

MK-801 significantly improves neurologic outcome after traumatic spinal cord injury. Moreover, NMDA, but not its levo isomer, significantly exacerbates the consequences of traumatic injury. From these data it is suggested that excitotoxins, released in response to injury and acting in part through the NMDA receptor, contribute to the secondary pathophysiologic effects after trauma that lead to irreversible tissue damage.[55] These findings extend the excitotoxin hypothesis of CNS injury to trauma, in addition to their proposed role in neurodegenerative diseases, epilepsy, and ischemia.[111]

The exact mechanism of how these excitatory amino acids produce their neurotoxic actions is still not clear. One hypothesis suggests that such a toxicity is a result of neuronal depolarization and sustained excitation, leading to accumulation of intracellular Na and Cl and loss of energy reserves, then to cellular edema and lysis.[117] A second hypothesis proposes that neurotoxicity of excitatory amino acids is mediated by an influx of extracellular calcium. A third hypothesis is a mixture of the previous two, with an early response, associated with neuronal swelling, which is dependent upon extracellular sodium and chlorine and can be demonstrated in the absence of extracellular calcium; a more delayed response, leading to cell death, is dependent upon the presence of extracellular calcium.[118]

Inflammation

The CNS is relatively 'immune privileged', meaning that under normal conditions there is minimal immune surveillance. This is partly due to the blood–brain barrier, a specialized structure made up of endothelia and astrocytic end-feet that separates the circulatory and the central nervous systems, and tightly regulates passage of molecules and cells between them. Thus, few immune cells are found in the healthy CNS. Upon injury, however, the blood–brain barrier is physically and functionally altered, blood vessels become leaky, and cells of the immune system invade the CNS, triggering an inflammatory response. The immediate, but transient, appearance of neutrophils characterizes the early immune response. The next phase of the immediate early inflammatory response that follows SCI is mediated mainly by two groups of leukocytes – T lymphocytes (or T cells) and macrophages. T cells are antigen-specific; each is activated by a specific stimulus (or antigen) that is frequently just a part of a molecule. They reside in the major immune organs, circulate through the body in the lymphatic system, and can home in to sites of injury where they migrate into the surrounding tissue. If activated by binding to their respective antigen, they increase their release of cytokines and are cytotoxic to target cells. Macrophages, on the other hand, are not antigen-specific. They circulate, but also reside in various tissues. Best known for their phagocytic properties, macrophages also have important functions in antigen presentation, cytokine secretion, and cytotoxicity. Quiescent macrophages residing within the CNS are known as microglia.

The molecular basis of spinal cord inflammation draws from a vast arsenal of known immunologic molecules, including cytokines and chemokines, as well as growth factors, trophic factors, and other agents. Cytokines, of which there are about 60, regulate cell–cell communication between immune cells. They are small proteins that produce local and transient effects. Chemokines are chemotactic molecules that attract immune cells, helping them to 'home' to sites of inflammation. Frequently, the cells producing these regulatory molecules also bear receptors for them, participating in a complex network of self-regulating and local interactions that orchestrate the proliferation of immune cells and then the subsequent decline of immune activity.

TNF-α (tumor necrosis factor-α) is perhaps the most extensively studied cytokine amongst the many involved in SCI. It can be produced by a number of different cell populations, including neutrophils, astrocytes, macrophages and microglia, and T cells,[119] and has been shown to accumulate rapidly at the site of spinal cord injury.[120]

There are studies that have revealed both the neurotoxic and neuroprotective properties of TNF-α.[121] For example, inhibiting TNF-α after CNS injury with antibodies or other cytokines has been shown to promote functional recovery, suggesting a cytotoxic role for TNF-α.[117,118] Conversely, some *in-vitro* studies have demonstrated TNF-α to be neuroprotective against excitotoxic death.[122,123] Along the same line, transgenic mice lacking TNF-α receptors (making them presumably insensitive to the effects of endogenous TNF-α) have actually demonstrated greater tissue loss and functional deficits than wild-type mice after spinal cord injury, suggesting that TNF-α would have mediated a neuroprotective effect.[119]

TNF-α clearly has beneficial and deleterious effects, probably dependent on the timing of its release after the injury, and on which cellular populations it is acting. Other cytokines, such as interleukin (IL)-10 (which is produced by many of the same cells as TNF-α), are considered to have potent anti-inflammatory properties.[124] The administration of (IL)-10 has been shown to be neuroprotective after experimental spinal cord injury, possibly by inducing anti-apoptotic genes.[118] Also, although phagocytic macrophages that rapidly invade the SCI site have traditionally been implicated in the further destruction of neural tissue, it has recently been suggested that the macrophage response to CNS injury is in fact an inadequate one, and that the poor regenerative response after SCI as compared with peripheral nerve injury is related in part to the more pronounced macrophage invasion in the latter.[118,125] This line of investigation has led to a phase I human clinical trial in which activated macrophages have been implanted into the spinal cords of acutely injured patients.

These examples provide some insights into the enormous complexity of the inflammatory and immune response to SCI. The conflicting actions of TNF-α and other factors described above reflect a growing awareness that the view of inflammation as a detrimental, neurotoxic process best inhibited by anti-inflammatory agents, such as corticosteroids, is a gross oversimplification.[118,126] If the inflammatory response is deleterious to recovery, one approach might be to eliminate the immune cells that mediate this response. This is still under research.

Loss of ATP-dependent cellular processes

The ATP-dependent cellular processes are affected in SCI in two successive stages, one in the first 4 hours and the second between 4 and 24 hours. Throughout the 24-hour period, the total adenylates and concentrations of ATP, P-creatine, and lactic acid are relatively constant. However, the difference between the two stages is in the sequence of changes in the lactate/pyruvate ratio, the energy change, and the tissue levels of pyruvate and glucose.

After the first 15 minutes, there is a decline in glucose concentration in the spinal cord. This is due to both the utilization of glucose stores and the impediment of proper glucose transport to the impact site. However, after the initial 15 minutes up till 4 hours there is a rise in glucose as replenishment occurs.

The tissue levels of both glucose and pyruvate become supranormal between 4 and 24 hours. Also, there is a slight rise in energy changes and the lactate/pyruvate ratio falls to normal levels.

The increase in tissue glucose and pyruvate levels suggested a stimulation or release of the glycolytic rate from its previously depressed state. Decline in the lactate/pyruvate ratio implies that oxidative pathways are operative. The mechanism(s) responsible for the increased metabolic rate are not known.[56] In those areas where edema was minimal or diminishing, some recovery of metabolic rate would be expected.[127] The rise in tissue glucose levels between 4 and 24 hours may be due to increased perfusion to microregions within the injured segment, perhaps coupled with an augmented glucose transport from blood.[128]

Two theories have previously been advanced to explain the prolonged depression of the adenylate pool and tissue ATP levels in the oligemic cerebrum. First, during ischemia, ATP is dephosphorylated to ADP and AMP, and the size of the adenine nucleotide pool is diminished secondary to the degradation of AMP to inosine monophosphate (IMP) and adenosine.[129] Since many of the AMP metabolites are diffusible and resynthesis of adenine nucleotides is slow, the size of the adenylate pool may be subnormal for extended periods.[130] Consequently, insufficient levels of ADP and AMP may prevent adequate resynthesis of ATP.[131] Second, it has been suggested that lack of ATP resynthesis and persistent depression of total adenylates reflect irreversible tissue damage.[127,131,132] Histologic studies after compression injury of the spinal cord showed hemorrhagic necrosis of gray and white matter and prominent ischemic nerve cell change.[133,134] Thus, the injured segment may present a spectrum of tissue injury ranging from normal to necrotic. Consequently, the sequence of metabolic changes may reflect an averaging of these necrotic, anaerobic, and aerobic areas. For the initial 4 hours, anaerobic metabolism likely predominates. However, between 4 and 24 hours there appears to be an increasing percentage of oxidative metabolism in the remaining metabolically viable tissue.[56]

Edema

Edema in the spinal cord is defined as a significant increase in the water content of the tissue. Impact trauma to the spinal cord causes vascular damage at the site of injury, which results in extravasation of serum proteins and an increase in tissue water. There is a direct relationship between the formation and spread of edema and the magnitude of trauma leading to the SCI.

The spread of edema longitudinally, rostrally, and caudally in the white matter after trauma is likely to be associated with the development of tissue pressure gradients between the area adjacent to the injury site and areas more rostral and caudal.

Endogenous opioids

Following SCI, significant vascular changes occur (see Vascular changes section). There is a reduction in SCBF, which begins in the central gray region shortly after trauma and progresses in a centripetal fashion to involve the long white matter tracts in the early hours after injury.[135–137] Since autoregulation of SCBF is often impaired following spinal injury,[138,139] blood flow depends more directly upon blood pressure; thus, the hypotension that often accompanies injuries to the cervical and upper thoracic spinal cord[142] may potentiate the progressive ischemia initiated by spinal trauma. Under these conditions, restoration of blood pressure should augment SCBF and reduce subsequent ischemia, thereby improving neurologic outcome. Unfortunately, pressor agents have not been helpful in improving blood pressure after spinal injury,[141,142] probably due to the rapid development of tachyphylaxis.[143]

It is suggested that endogenous opioid peptides (endorphins) contribute to the hypotension in spinal injury. Naloxone (an opiate antagonist) treatment improves blood pressure and SCBF and is associated with less prominent spinal cord changes and significantly improved neurologic recovery.

References

1. de Groat WC, Booth AM, Yoshimura N. Neurophysiology of micturition and its modification in animal models of human disease. In: Maggi CA, ed. The Autonomic Nervous System, Vol. 3, Nervous Control of the Urogenital System. London: Harwood Academic Publishers, 1993: 227–90.
2. Chai TC and Steers WC. Neurophysiology of micturition and continence. Urol Clin North Am 1996; 23: 221–36.
3. Breasted JH. The Edwin Smith Surgical Papyrus. Chicago, IL: University of Chicago Press, 1930.
4. Yoshimura N and de Groat WC. Neural control of the lower urinary tract. Int J Urol 1997; 4: 111–25.
5. Jänig W, Morrison JFB. Functional properties of spinal visceral afferents supplying abdominal and pelvic organs, with special emphasis on visceral nociception. Progr Brain Res 1986; 67: 87–114.
6. Gosling J. The structure of the bladder and urethra in relation to function. Urol Clin North Am 1979; 6: 31–8.
7. ACOG technical bulletin. Chronic pelvic pain, No 223. Int J Gynecol Obstet 1996; 54: 59–68.
8. Havenga K, DeRuiter MC, Enker WE, Welvaart K. Anatomical basis of autonomic nerve-preserving total mesorectal excision for rectal cancer. Br J Surg 1996; 83: 384–8.
9. Juenemann KP, Lue TF, Schmidt RA, Tanagho EA. Clinical significance of sacral and pudendal nerve anatomy. J Urol 1988; 139: 74–80.
10. Jänig W and McLachlan EM. Organization of lumber spinal outflow to distal colon and pelvic organs. Physiol Rev 1987; 67: 1332–440.
11. Lundberg JM. Pharmacology of cotransmission in the autonomic nervous system: integrative aspects on amines, neuropeptides, adenosine triphosphate, amine, acids and nitric oxide. Pharmacol Rev 1996; 48: 113–78.
12. Yamaguchi O, Shishido K, Tamura K et al. Evaluation of mRNAs encoding muscarinic receptor subtypes in human detrusor muscle. J Urol 1996; 156: 1208–13.
13. Kondo S, Morita T, Tashima Y. Muscarinic cholinergic receptor subtypes in human detrusor muscle studies by labelled and nonlabelled pirenzepine, AF-DX116 and 4DAMP. Urol Int 1995; 54: 150–3.
14. Wang P, Luthin GR, Ruggieri MR. Muscarinic acetylcholine receptor subtypes mediating urinary bladder contractility and coupling to GTP proteins. J Pharmacol Exp Ther 1995; 273: 959–66.
15. Somogyi GT, de Groat WC. Evidence for inhibitory nicotinic and facilitatory muscarinic receptors in cholinergic nerve terminals of the rat urinary bladder. J Auton Nerv Syst 1992; 37: 89–97.
16. Somogyi GT, Tanowitz M, de Groat WC. M 1 muscarinic receptor mediated facilitation of acetylcholine release in the rat urinary bladder but not in the heart. J Physiol 1994; 80: 81–9.
17. Hoyle CHV, Burnstock GP. Postganglionic efferent transmission in the bladder and urethra. In: Maggi CA, ed. The Autonomic Nervous System, Vol. 3, Nervous Control of the Urogenital System. London: Harwood Academic Publishers, 1993: 349–82.
18. Andersson KE. Pharmacology of lower urinary tract smooth muscles and penile erectile tissues. Pharmacol Rev 1993; 45: 253–308.
19. Bennett BC, Roppolo JR, Kruse MN, de Groat WC. Neural control of urethral smooth and striated muscle activity in vivo: role of nitric oxide. J Urol 1995; 153: 2004–9.
20. Persson K, Alm P, Johansson K, Larsson B, Andersson KE. Nitric oxide synthase in pig lower urinary tract: immunohistochemistry, NADPH diaphorase histochemistry, and functional effects. Br J Pharmacol 1993; 110: 521–30.
21. de Groat WC, Booth AM. Synaptic transmission in pelvic ganglia. In: Maggi CA, ed. The Autonomic Nervous System, Vol. 3, Nervous Control of the Urogenital System. London: Harwood Academic Publishers, 1993: 291–347.
22. Tran LV, Somogyi GT, de Groat WC. Inhibitory effects of neuropeptide Y on cholinergic and adrenergic transmission in the rat urinary bladder and urethra. Am J Physiol 1994; 266: R1411–17.
23. Häbler HJ, Jänig W, Koltzenburg M. Activation of unmyelinated afferent fibres by mechanical stimuli and inflammation of the urinary bladder in the cat. J Physiol 1990; 425: 545–62.
24. Mallory B, Steers WD, de Groat WC. Electrophysiological study of micturition reflexes in rats. Am J Physiol 1989; 257: R410–21.
25. de Groat WC, Nadelhaft I, Milne RJ et al. Organization of the sacral parasympathetic reflex pathways to the urinary bladder and large intestine. J Auton Nerv Syst 1981; 3: 135–60.

26. Vera PL, Nadelhaft I. Conduction velocity distribution of afferent fibers innervating the rat urinary bladder. Brain Res 1990; 520: 83–9.
27. de Groat WC, Lalley PM. Reflex firing in the lumbar sympathetic outflow to activation of vesical afferent fibers. J Physiol 1972; 226: 289–309.
28. de Groat WC, Theobald RJ. Reflex activation of sympathetic pathways to vesical smooth muscle and parasympathetic ganglia by electrical stimulation of vesical afferents. J Physiol 1976; 259: 223–37.
29. Shimoda N, Takakusaki K, Nishizawa O, Tsuchida S, Mori S. The changes in the activity of pudendal motoneurons in relation to reflex micturition evoked in decerebrated cats. Neurosci Lett 1992; 135: 175–8.
30. Fedirchuk B, Shefchyk SJ. Membrane potential changes in sphincter motoneurons during micturition in the decerebrate cat. J Neurosci 1993; 13: 3090–4.
31. Holstege G, Griffiths D, de Wall H, Dalm E. Anatomical and physiological observations on supraspinal control of bladder and urethral sphincter muscles in cat. J Comp Neurol. 1986; 250: 449–61.
32. Nishizawa O, Sugaya K, Noto H, Harada T, Tsuchida S. Pontine micturition center in the dog. J Urol 1988; 140: 872–4.
33. Noto H, Roppolo JR, Steers WD, de Groat WC. Electrophysiological analysis of ascending and descending components of the micturition reflex pathway in the rat. Brain Res 1991; 549: 95–105.
34. Kruse MN, Noto H, Roppolo JR, de Groat WC. Pontine control of the urinary bladder and external urethral sphincter in the rat. Brain Res 1990; 532: 182–90.
35. Shimoda N, Takakusaki K, Nishizawa O, Tsuchida S, Mori S. The changes in the activity of pudendal motoneurons in relation to reflex micturition evoked in decerebrated cats. Neurosci Lett 1992; 135: 175–8.
36. Fedirchuk B, Shefchyk SJ. Membrane potential changes in sphincter motoneurons during micturition in the decerebrate cat. J Neurosci 1993; 13: 3090–4.
37. Hedge SS, Eglen RM. Muscarinic receptor subtypes modulating smooth muscle contractility in the urinary bladder. Life Sci 1999; 64: 419–28.
38. Somogyi GT, de Groat WC. Function, signal transduction mechanisms and plasticity of presynaptic muscarinic receptors in the urinary bladder. Life Sci 1999; 64: 411–18.
39. Yoshimora N. Bladder afferent pathway and spinal cord injury: possible mechanisms including hyperreflexia of the urinary bladder. Progr Neurobiol 1999; 57: 583–606.
40. Fam BA, Sarkarati M, Yalla SV. Spinal cord injury. In: Yalla SV, McGuire EJ, Elbadawi A and Blaivas JG, eds. Neurourology and Urodynamics. New York: Macmillan Publishing Company, 1988: 291–302.
41. Chancellor MB, Blaivas JG. Spinal cord injury. In: Chancellor MB and Blaivas JG, eds. Practical Neuro-Urology: Genitourinary Complications of Neurologic Disease. Butterworth-Heinemann, Newton. 1996: 99–118.
42. Fried LC, Goodkin R. Microangiopathic observations of the experimentally traumatized spinal cord. J Neurosurg 1971; 35: 709–14.
43. Tator CH, Fehlings MG. Review of the secondary injury theory of acute spinal cord trauma with emphasis on vascular mechanisms. J Neurosurg 1991; 75: 15–26.
44. Sekhon L, Fehling M. Epidemiology, demographics, and pathophysiology of acute spinal cord injury. Spine 2001; 26: S2–12.
45. Tator CH. Update on the pathophysiology and pathology of acute spinal cord injury. Brain Pathol 1995; 5: 407–13.
46. Tator CH. Review of experimental spinal cord injury with emphasis on the local and systemic circulatory effects. Neurochirurgie 1991; 37: 291–302.
47. Tator CH, Koyanagi I. Vascular mechanisms in the pathophysiology of human spinal cord injury. J Neurosurg 1997; 86: 483–92.
48. Demopoulos HB, Flamm ES, Pietronigro DD et al. The free radical pathology and the microcirculation in the major central nervous system disorders. Acta Physiol Scand Suppl 1980; 492: 91–119.
49. Hall ED, Yonkers PA, Horan KL et al. Correlation between attenuation of posttraumatic spinal cord ischemia and preservation of tissue vitamin E by the 21-aminosteroid U74006F: evidence for an in vivo antioxidant mechanism. J Neurotrauma 1989; 6: 169–76.
50. Hung TK, Albin MS, Brown TD et al. Biomechanical responses to open experimental spinal cord injury. Surg Neurol 1975; 4: 271–6.
51. Agrawal SK, Fehlings MG. Mechanisms of secondary injury to spinal cord axons in vitro: role of Na+, Na(+)-K(+)-ATPase, the Na(+)-H+ exchanger, and the Na(+)-Ca2+ exchanger. J Neurosci 1996; 16: 545–52.
52. Young W, Kerch I. Potassium and calcium changes in injured spinal cords. Brain Res 1986; 365: 42–53.
53. Casha S, Yu WR, Fehlings MG. Oligodendroglial apoptosis occurs along degenerating axons and is associated with FAS and P75 expression following spinal cord injury. Neuroscience 2001; 103: 203–18.
54. De La Torre JC. Spinal cord injury: review of basic and applied research. Spine 1981; 6: 315–35.
55. Agrawal SK, Fehlings MG. The role of NMDA and non-NMDA inotropic glutamate receptors in traumatic spinal cord axonal injury. J Neurosci 1997; 17: 1055–63.
56. Faden AI, Simon RP. A potential role for excitotoxins in the pathophysiology of spinal cord injury. Ann Neurol 1988; 23: 623–6.
57. Anderson DK, Means ED, Waters TR et al. Spinal cord energy metabolism following compression trauma to the feline spinal cord. J Neurosurg 1980; 53: 375–80.
58. Wagner FC Jr, Stewart WB. Effect of trauma dose on spinal cord edema. J Neurosurg 1981; 54: 802–6.
59. Faden AI, Jacobs TP, Holaday JW. Comparison of early and late naloxone treatment in experimental spinal injury. Neurology 1982; 32: 677–81.
60. Faden AI, Jacobs TP, Smith MT. Evaluation of calcium channel antagonist nimodipine in experimental spinal cord ischemia. J Neurosurg 1984; 60: 796–9.
61. Atkinson PP, Atkinson JL. Spinal shock. Mayo Clin Proc 1996; 71: 384–9.
62. Guha A, Tator CH. Acute cardiovascular effects of experimental spinal cord injury. J Trauma 1988; 28: 481–90.
63. Kobrine Al, Doyle TF, Rizzoli HV. Altered spinal cord blood flow as affected by changes in systemic arterial blood pressure. J Neurosurg 1975; 42: 144–9.
64. Senter HJ, Venes JL. Loss of autoregulation and posttraumatic ischemia following experimental spinal cord trauma. J Neurosurg 1979; 50: 198–206.
65. Young W, Decrescito V, Tomasula JJ. Effect of sympathectomy on spinal blood flow autoregulation and posttraumatic ischemia. J Neurosurg 1982; 56: 706–10.
66. Guha A, Tator CH, Rochon J. Spinal cord blood flow and systemic blood pressure after experimental spinal cord injury in rats. Stroke 1989; 20: 372–7.
67. Young W, Decrescito V, Tomasula JJ et al. The role of the sympathetic nervous system in pressor responses induced by spinal injury. J Neurosurg 1980; 52: 473–81.
68. Koyanagi I, Tator CH, Lea PJ. Three-dimensional analysis of the vascular system in the rat spinal cord with scanning electron microscopy of vascular corrosion casts: 2. Acute spinal cord injury. Neurosurgery 1993; 33: 285–92.
69. Koyanagi I, Tator CH, Theriault E. Silicone rubber microangiography of acute spinal cord injury in the rat. Neurosurgery 1993; 32: 260–8.
70. Shingu H, Kimura I, Nasu Y et al. Microangiographic study of spinal cord injury and myelopathy. Paraplegia 1989; 27: 182–9.
71. Kim RC, Smith HR, Henbest ML et al. Nonhemorrhagic venous infarction of the spinal cord. Ann Neurol 1984; 15: 379–85.

72. Ohshio I, Hatayama A, Kaneda K et al. Correlation between histopathologic features and magnetic resonance images of spinal cord lesions. Spine 1993; 18: 1140–9.
73. Rao KR, Donnenfeld H, Chusid JG et al. Acute myelopathy secondary to spinal venous thrombosis. J Neurol 1982; 56: 107–13.
74. Griffiths IR, Miller R. Vascular permeability to protein and vasogenic edema in experimental concussive injuries to the canine spinal cord. J Neurol Sci 1974; 22: 291–304.
75. Hsu CY, Hogan EL, Gadsden RHS et al. Vascular permeability in experimental spinal cord injury. J Neurol Sci 1985; 70: 275–82.
76. Stewart WB, Wagner FC. Vascular permeability changes in the contused feline spinal cord. Brain Res 1979; 169: 163–7.
77. Demopoulos HB, Yoder M, Gutman EG et al. The fine structure of endothelial surfaces in the microcirculation of experimentally injured feline spinal cords. In: Becker RP, Johari O, eds. Scanning Electron Microscopy II. AMF O'Hare, IL: Scanning Electron Microscopy, O'Hare IL 1978: 677–82.
78. Schwab JM, Brechtel K, Nguyen TD et al. Persistent accumulation of cyclooxygenase 1 (COX-1) expressing microglia/macrophages and upregulation by endothelium following spinal cord injury. J Neuroimmunol 2000; 111: 122–30.
79. Boucher BA, Phelps SJ. Acute management of the head injury patient. In: DiPiro JT, Talbert RL, Yee GC et al., eds. Pharmacotherapy: A Pathophysiological Approach. Stamford: Appleton & Lange, 1997: 1229–42.
80. Dumont RJ, Okonkwo DO, Verma S et al. Acute spinal cord injury, part I: pathophysiologic mechanisms. Clin Neuropharmacol. 2001; 24(5): 254–64.
81. Resnick DK, Graham SH, Dixon CE et al. Role of cyclooxygenase 2 in acute spinal cord injury. J Neurotrauma 1998; 15: 1005–13.
82. Cordingley GE, Somjen GG. The clearing of excess potassium from extracellular space in spinal cord and cerebral cortex. Brain Res 1978; 151: 291–306.
83. Gardner-Medwin AR, Gibson JL, Willshaw DJ. The mechanism of potassium dispersal in brain tissue. J Physiol (Lond) 1979; 293: 37–8P.
84. Gardner-Medwin AR. Analysis of potassium dynamics in mammalian brain tissue. J Physiol (Lond), 1983; 335: 393–426.
85. Nicholson C. Dynamics of the brain cell microenvironment. Neurosci Res Bull 1980; 18: 177–322.
86. Nicholson C, Philips JM, Gardner-Medin A. Diffusion from an iontophoretic point source in the brain: a role of tortuosity and volume fraction. Brain Res 1979; 164: 580–4.
87. Hansen AJ, Gjedde A, Siemkowicz E. Extracellular potassium and blood flow in the post-ischemic rat brain. Pfluger's Arch 1980; 389: 1–7.
88. Hansen AJ, Lund-Andersen H, Crone C. K+ permeability of the blood brain barrier investigated by aid of a K+-sensitive microelectrode. Acta Physiol Scand 1977; 101: 438–45.
89. Hansen AJ. The potassium concentration in cerebrospinal fluid in young and adult rats following complete brain ischemia – effects of pre-treatment with hypoxia. Acta Physiol Scand 1976; 97: 519–22.
90. Nicholson C. Modulation of extracellular calcium and functional implications. Fed Proc Fed Am Soc EP Biol 1980; 39: 1519–23.
91. Betts F, Blumenthal NC, Posner AS, Becker GL, Lehninger AL. Atomic structure of intracellular amorphous calcium phosphate deposits. Proc Natl Acad Sci USA 1975; 72: 2088–90.
92. Brown WE. Solubility of phosphates and other sparingly soluble compounds. In: Griffin EJ, Beeton A, Spencer JM, Mitchell DT eds. Environmental Phosphorus Handbook. John Wiley NY, 1973: 203.
93. Balentine JD, Spector M. Calcifications of axons in experimental spinal cord trauma. Ann Neurol 1977; 2: 520–3.
94. Kretsinger RH. Calcium in neurobiology: a general theory of its function and evolution. In Schmitt FO and Worden FG eds. The Neurosciences – Fourth Study Program, MIT Press, Cambridge, 1979: 617–22.
95. Sillen SG. The physical chemistry of sea water. In: Sears M eds Oceanography, American Association for the Advancement of Science. Pub No 67, 1961; 549–81.
96. Astrup J. Energy-requiring cell functions in the ischemic brain: their critical supply and possible inhibition in protective therapy. J Neurosurg 1982; 56: 482–97.
97. Braughler JM, Hall ED. Lactate and pyruvate metabolism in the injured cat spinal cord before and after a single large intravenous dose of methylprednisolone. J Neurosurg 1983; 59: 256–61.
98. Abrams JM, White K, Fessler LI, Steller H. Programmed cell death during Drosophila embryogenesis. Development 1993; 117: 29–43.
99. Bargmann Cl. Death from natural and unnatural causes. Elegant studies of the nematode are providing answers to the question of how programmed cell death and neurodegeneration are regulated. Curr Biol 1991; 1: 388–90.
100. Kerr JFR, Wyllie AH, Currie AR. Apoptosis. A basic biological phenomenon with wide-ranging implications in tissue kinetics. Br J Cancer 1972; 26: 239–57.
101. Collins WF, Piepmeir J, Ogle E. The spinal cord injury problem. A review. Central Nery Syst Trauma 1986; 3: 317–31.
102. Collins WF. A review and update of experimental and clinical studies of spinal cord injury. Paraplegia 1983; 21: 204–19.
103. Li GL, Brodin G, Farooque M et al. Apoptosis and expression of Bcl-2 after compression trauma to rat spinal cord. J Neuropathol Exp Neurol 1996; 55: 280–9.
104. Crowe MJ, Bresnahan JC, Shuman SL et al. Apoptosis and delayed degeneration after spinal cord injury in rats and monkeys. Nat Med 1997; 3: 73–6.
105. Barres BA, Jacobson MD, Schmid R. Does oligodendrocytes survival depend on axons? Curr Biol 1993; 3: 489–97.
106. Dusart I, Schwab ME. Secondary cell death and the inflammatory reaction after dorsal hemisection of the rat spinal cord. Eur J Neurosci 1994; 6: 712–24.
107. Emery E, Aldana P, Bunge MB et al. Apoptosis after traumatic human spinal cord injury. J Neurosurg 1998; 89: 911–20.
108. Chan SL, Mattson MP. Caspase and calpain substrates: roles in synaptic plasticity and cell death. J Neurosci Res 1999; 58(1): 167–90.
109. Carlson GD, Gorden C. Current developments in spinal cord injury research. Spine J 2002; 2(2): 116–28.
110. Liu XZ, Xu XM, Hu R et al. Neuronal and glial apoptosis after traumatic spinal cord injury. J Neurosci 1997; 17: 5395–406.
111. Meldrum B. Possible therapeutic applications of antagonists of excitatory amino acid neurotransmitters. Clin Sci 1985; 68: 113–22.
112. Feden AI. Pharmacotherapy in spinal cord injury: a critical review of recent developments. Clin Neuropharmacol 1987; 10: 193–204.
113. Wieloch T. Hypoglycemia-induced neuronal damage prevented by N-methyl-D-aspartate antagonist. Science 1985; 230: 681–3.
114. Davies J, Watkins JC. Role of excitatory amino acid receptors in mono- and polysynaptic excitation in the cat spinal cord. Exp Brain Res 1983; 49: 280–90.
115. Ganoug AH, Lanthorn TH, Cotman CW. Kynurenic acid inhibits synaptic and acidic amino acid-induced responses in the rat. Brain Res 1983; 273: 170–4.
116. Wong EHF, Kemp JA, Priestley T. The novel anticonvulsant MK-801 is a potent N-methyl-aspartate antagonist. Proc Natl Acad Sci USA 1986; 83: 7104.
117. Olney JW, Ho OL, Rhee V. Cytotoxic effects of acidic and sulphur containing amino acids on the infant mouse central nervous system. Exp Brain Res 1971; 14: 61–76.
118. Rivlin AS, Tator CH. Objective clinical assessment of motor function after experimental spinal cord injury in the rat. J Neurosurg 1977; 47: 577–81.
119. Yan P, Li Q, Kim GM et al. Cellular localization of tumor necrosis factor-alpha following acute spinal cord injury in adult rats. J Neurotrauma 2001; 18(5): 563–8.

120. Bethea JR, Nagashima H, Acosta MC et al. Systemically administered interleukin 10 reduces tumor necrosis factor-alpha production and significantly improves functional recovery following traumatic spinal cord injury in rats. J Neurotrauma 1999; 16(10): 851–63.
121. Kwon BK, Tetzlaff W, Grauer JN et al. Pathophysiology and pharmacologic treatment of acute spinal cord injury. Spine J 2004; 4(4): 451–64.
122. Barger SW, Horster D, Furukawa K et al. Tumor necrosis factors alpha and beta protect neurons against amyloid beta-peptide toxicity: evidence for involvement of a kappa B-binding factor and attenuation of peroxide and Ca^{2+} accumulation. Proc Natl Acad Sci USA 92 20 1995; 9328–32.
123. Cheng B, Christakos S, Mattson MP. Tumor necrosis factors protect neurons against metabolic-excitotoxic insults and promote maintenance of calcium homeostasis. Neuron 1994; 12(1): 139–53.
124. Knoblach SM, Faden AI. Interleukin-10 improves outcome and alters proinflammatory cytokine expression after experimental traumatic brain injury. Exp Neurol 1998; 153(1): 143–51.
125. Schwartz M, Moalem G, Leibowitz-Amit R et al. Innate and adaptive immune responses can be beneficial for CNS repair. Trends Neurosci 1999; 22(7): 295–9.
126. Lazarov-Spiegler O, Rapalino O, Agranov G et al. Restricted inflammatory reaction in the CNS: a key impediment to axonal regeneration? Mol Med Today 1998; 4(8): 337–42.
127. Welsh FA, Ginsberg MD, Rieder W et al. Diffuse cerebral ischemia in the cat. II. Regional metabolites during severe ischemia and recirculation. Ann Neurol 1978; 3: 493–501.
128. Gatfield PD, Lowry OH, Schulz DW et al. Regional energy reserves in mouse brain and changes with ischemia and anaesthesia. J Neurochem 1966; 13: 185–95.
129. Smith AL, Wollman H. Cerebral blood flow and metabolism. Anesthesiology 1972; 36: 378–400.
130. Siesjo BK. Brain Energy Metabolism. London/New York: John Wiley and Sons, 1978.
131. Nordstrom CH, Rehncrona S, Seisjo BK. Effects of pentobarbital in cerebral ischemia. Part II: Restitution of cerebral energy state, as well as glycolytic metabolites, citric acid cycle intermediates and associated amino acids after pronounced incomplete ischemia. Stroke 1978; 9: 335–43.
132. Atkinson DE. Cellular Energy Metabolism and its Regulation. New York: Academic Press, 1977.
133. Means ED, Anderson DK. Histopathology of experimental spinal cord compression injury. Fifth Annual Meeting of the Society for Neuroscience. New York City, Nov 2–6 1975 New York (Hilton Hotel), Vol 1, 1975: 698.
134. Means ED, Anderson DK, Gutierrez C. Light and electron microscopy of gray matter following experimental spinal cord compression injury. J Neuropathol Exp Neurol 1976; 35: 348.
135. Dohrmann GJ. Wick KM, Bucy PC. Spinal cord blood flow patterns in experimental traumatic paraplegia. J Neurosurg 1973; 38: 52–8.
136. Ducker TB, Salcman M, Lucas JT et al. Experimental spinal cord trauma. II: Blood flow, tissue oxygen, evoked potentials in both paretic and plegic monkeys. Surg Neurol 1978; 10: 64–70.
137. Sandler AN, Tator CH. Effect of acute spinal cord compression injury on regional spinal cord blood flow in primates. J Neurosurg 1976; 45: 660–76.
138. Ducker TB, Perot PL. Spinal cord blood flow compartments. Trans Am Neurol Assoc 1971; 96: 229–31.
139. Osterholm JL. The pathophysiological response to spinal cord injury. J Neurosurg 1974; 40: 5–33.
140. Yashon D. Spinal Injury. New York: Appleton-Century-Crofts, 1978: 248–54.
141. Ducker TB, Salcapan M, Daniell HB. Experimental spinal cord trauma. III: Therapeutic effect of immobilization and pharmacologic agents. Surg Neurol 1978; 10: 71–6.
142. Faden AI, Jacobs TP, Woods M. Cardioacceleratory sites in the zona intermedia of the cat spinal cord. Exp Neurol 1978; 61: 301–10.
143. Faden AI, Jacobs TP, Mougey MS, Holaday JW. Endorphins in experimental spinal injury: therapeutic effect of naloxone. Ann Neurol 1981; 10: 326–32.

Part III

Neurologic pathologies responsible for the development of the neurogenic bladder

17

Systemic illnesses (diabetes mellitus, sarcoidosis, alcoholism, and porphyrias)

Ditlev Jensen and Bjørn Klevmark

This chapter on peripheral neuropathies comprises four systemic illnesses. Among these diseases, diabetes mellitus is the only one where a neurogenic bladder is a well-known complication. Hence, there is a separate summary after the diabetes mellitus section, and a short conclusion for the three other conditions at the end of the chapter.

Diabetes mellitus

The two major forms of diabetes mellitus (diabetes) are type 1 (A and B) and type 2. Type 1A is caused by an autoimmune destruction of the pancreatic Langerhans islet beta cells. Type 1B affects few patients and is without immunologic markers. Insulin deficiency is common for 1A and 1B. Type 2 is a heterogeneous disease characterized by insulin resistance, impaired insulin secretion, and increased glucose production.[1] Type 2 usually occurs at an older age. The two types affect men and women almost evenly, and seem to be equally susceptible to complications, which are similar for both.[2]

The prevalence of diabetes is difficult to ascertain. For all age groups, a world-wide estimate of 2.8% was given for 2000.[3] In 2005, also concerning all ages, 7% of the population in the USA had diabetes.[4] Among adults the world-wide estimated prevalence was 5.1.[5] The prevalence for both types is increasing, and a more rapid increase in type 2 is expected.[1,6,7] Among school-age children in the USA the prevalence of type 1 is 1.9 per 1000. It is increasing with age, from 1 in 1430 children at age 5 to 1 in 360 at age 16; both sexes are almost equally affected. In Western Europe the prevalence among children is markedly highest in Denmark and Finland.[8]

Complications

The main complications are the vascular and the neurogenic ones; the latter are probably the most common.[6]

Table 17.1 *Clinical syndromes of diabetic peripheral neuropathy*

Mononeuropathy of cranial, trunk, or limb nerves
Mononeuropathia multiplex
Painful lumbosacral radiculoplexus neuropathy
Atrophic lumbosacral radiculoplexus neuropathy (diabetic amyotrophy)
Symmetric lower limb proximal neuropathy
Symmetric upper and lower limb distal polyneuropathy (most common)
Autonomic neuropathy
Mixed forms

Diabetic neuropathy occurs throughout the world, and is equally distributed among men and women. Available information indicates a prevalence of about 50% for patients with diabetes of 25 years' duration. Neuropathy is present in less than 10% when diabetes is discovered.[9] In children the most common complication is peripheral neuropathy, which was found in 11% of diabetic patients from 8 to 15 years of age.[10]

Diabetic peripheral neuropathy can be separated into eight clinical syndromes (Table 17.1).[11–13] Autonomic neuropathy is the cause of the neurogenic bladder. It is often combined with one of the other syndromes, most often with the symmetric upper and lower limb distal polyneuropathy. In that case the clinical manifestations of autonomic neuropathy usually appear at a later stage than those of the other syndromes.

Peripheral innervation

The lower urinary tract has autonomic innervation of the bladder and urethra, and somatic innervation of the striated part of the urethral wall and of the striated periurethral sphincter (m. pubococcygeus). In peripheral neuropathies only lesions of the parasympathetic nerves to the bladder (nn. pelvici) will result in a neurogenic bladder. Both the afferent and efferent arms of the micturition reflex are located in the pelvic nerves. Lesions of somatic nerves (n. pudendalis) can influence voiding by changing the striated sphincter function. Lesions of the sympathetic nerves (nn. hypogastrici) can alter tension in the bladder neck and urethra. Sympathectomy in humans does not change the clinical pattern of voiding. Peripheral local reflexes and feedback mechanisms can be disturbed by peripheral neuropathies.

Pathologic anatomy and pathogenesis

In the diabetic autonomic neuropathy, neuron degeneration as well as neurons with vacuoles and granular deposits are found. There is a loss of myelinated nerve fibers in the vagus and splanchnic nerves, and a neuronal loss in the spinal cord intermediolateral columns.[12] Alterations such as beading, thickening, and fragmentation of postganglionic sympathetic axons adjacent to the bladder have been demonstrated.[14] Also shown is a reduced density of acetylcholinesterase-positive-staining parasympathetic nerves in the bladder wall.[15] If the impairment of mechano-responsive nociceptors found in diabetic small-fiber neuropathy[16] also applies to the bladder receptors, this may explain some afferent aspects of the diabetic bladder.

The pathogenesis of the neuropathologic changes may be related to the functional state of the vasa nervorum. If these are blocked by atherosclerosis, ischemia is the cause of the degenerative changes. If the vessels are open, another pathologic nerve metabolism will take place. However, divergent study conclusions confuse the role of microvascular transformation.[17–19] Four hypotheses have been put forward to explain how hyperglycemia may lead to chronic complications in diabetes.[1]

The first hypothesis suggests that increased intracellular glucose gives rise to an advanced glycosylation end product that crosslinks proteins, accelerates atherosclerosis, promotes glomerular dysfunction, and induces endothelial dysfunction. The second hypothesis assumes that in the state of increased intracellular glucose, some of the glucose is converted to sorbitol. This substance acts as a tissue toxin, and may be a factor in the pathogenesis of retinopathy, neuropathy, cataracts, nephropathy, and aortic disease.[2,14] The third hypothesis proposes that hyperglycemia increases the formation of diacylglycerol, leading to activation of isoforms of protein kinase C, which in turn alters, among others, extracellular matrix proteins around endothelial cells and neurons. The fourth hypothesis suggests that hyperglycemia may alter the function of the hexosamine pathway. This can change the gene expression of the transforming growth factor beta. The transforming growth factor beta, together with other growth factors, is suspected of playing an important role in the proliferative deviations demonstrated in different tissues.

Whether all pathophysiologic processes are responsible for all complications, or whether certain processes predominate in certain organs is so far not fully understood.[1] According to present knowledge, diabetic autonomic neuropathy may be of multifactorial origin.[20] Hyperglycemia is still considered to be a possible common cause by way of increasing the production of mitochondrial superoxide. The superoxide may activate all four pathways.[1] Concerning the detrusor muscle, after studying a rat model of diabetes, the authors suggested that changes in the length–tension ratio may be due to an adaptation to the increased diuresis following diabetes.[21] Another rat model has revealed an increase in a marker of sympathetic innervation as well as a decrease in a marker of parasympathetic innervation (tyrosine hydroxylase and vesicular acetylcholine transporter, respectively). These are early events during diabetes-related bladder dysfunction and remodeling.[22]

No exact data on the prevalence, incidence, and risk factors of the diabetic neurogenic bladder (diabetic cystopathy) are available.[23,24] In different studies, the figures vary between 20 and 80%,[25,26] and are even quoted by other authors as between 2 and 83%.[27] Most patients with a diabetic neurogenic bladder show prominent signs of other long-term diabetic complications. Their bladder dysfunction appears to be related to the severity of diabetes, not to its duration.[28]

Little information has been obtained on the diabetic neurogenic bladder among children. The few cases found are anecdotal.[29,30]

Examinations

To diagnose dysfunction of the lower urinary tract, some or most of the investigations shown in Table 17.2 may be necessary. The bladder symptoms have an insidious onset, characterized by a progressive failure of bladder emptying. Sensory nerve function is usually impaired at an early stage. Patients are not adequately warned to empty the bladder, and a situation occurs which may lead to increased voiding intervals, difficult initiation, and increasing volumes of residual urine. This can sometimes result in chronic total retention with overflow incontinence. Males may already have noticed an impairment of erection before the occurrence of bladder symptoms.[27,31–37]

In diabetes, isolated autonomic neuropathy is rare. Most common is the mixed form. At the clinical neurourologic investigation of this condition, a diminished superficial and deep sensation may be found in the lower limbs and in the perianal region. Knee and ankle jerks are depressed or

Table 17.2 *Neurogenic bladder: examinations*

History
Clinical examination
Frequency volume chart
Pad test (in cases of incontinence)
Residual urine
Uroflowmetry
Uroflowmetry with rectal pressure recording (eventually with electromyography (EMG))
Pressure flow study (eventually with EMG)
Cystometry
Cystometry with rectal pressure (eventually with EMG)
Ambulatory monitoring
Urethral pressure profile
EMG
Evoked responses
Urethrocystoscopy
Ultrasonography
Radiology (urography, micturition urethrocystography, CT, MRI)

wholly absent, and a similar lack of reaction is found in the anal skin reflex and the bulbocavernosus reflex. The digital exploration of the rectum may show a reduced external anal sphincter tonus, with no response to cough and voluntary contraction.

In cases of reduced sensory function the frequency volume chart will show either infrequent voiding of large volumes or frequent voiding of small volumes (chronic retention of urine). Residual urine is measured with ultrasonography. If uroflowmetry is not normal (Figure 17.1) a flowmetry with rectal pressure recording should be done. This can demonstrate the use of abdominal straining during voiding (Figure 17.2). To evaluate the strength of detrusor and a bladder outlet obstruction, a pressure flow study is necessary. Cystometry has been performed as conventional cystometry, usually with the nonphysiologic filling rate of 50 ml/min. However, conventional cystometry is considered traumatic to bladder afferents and impairs detrusor contractility.[38] The Standardisation Sub-Committee of the International Continence Society recommends now that filling rates are divided into physiologic and nonphysiologic rates.[39] All the three urodynamic studies can be combined with electromyography (EMG) from urethral or periurethral striated muscles (Table 17.2). The usual finding in a patient with a diabetic neurogenic bladder is a sensory hypoactive bladder with desire to void at a larger volume than normal, and often reduced detrusor contractility (Figure 17.3).

However, some elderly diabetic patients have suffered vascular complications affecting the brain or the spinal cord above the conus medullaris. In such cases the central nervous lesion may cause increased tendon reflexes and neurogenic overactive detrusor (Figure 17.4).[40]

The urethral pressure profile is usually normal. When the striated muscles of the external anal sphincter, the male bulbocavernosus muscle and the female urethral wall striated muscle are investigated with needle electrode EMG, denervation potentials can be demonstrated (Figure 17.5).

Pseudomyotonic activity may also be a sign of peripheral nerve affection of the pelvic floor muscles (Figure 17.6).[41] The latency of the first component of the evoked bulbocavernosus reflex is delayed only in patients with an advanced peripheral neuropathy. This reflex investigation only assesses conduction velocity in somatic nerves, not in

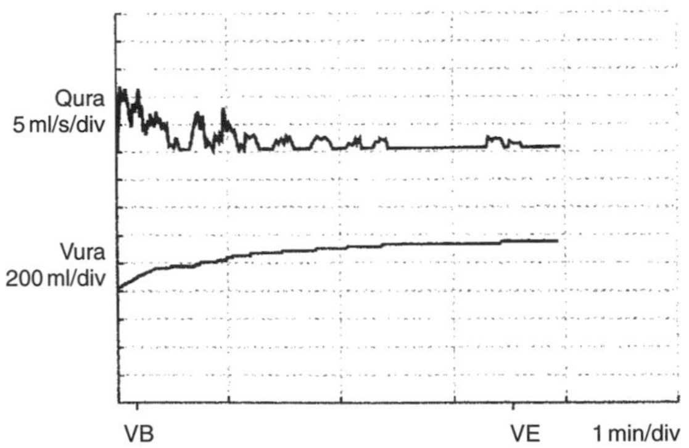

Figure 17.1
Uroflowmetry. Emptying with interrupted flow (Qura) causing a prolonged voiding time of 216 s. The voided volume (Vura) is 341 ml, maximum flow rate 12.5 ml/s, average flow rate 3.0 ml/s, and residual urine 118 ml. VB: void begins, VE: void ends. Prolonged interrupted voiding in a patient with sensory hypoactive neurogenic bladder. Same patient as in Figures 17.3 and 17.5.

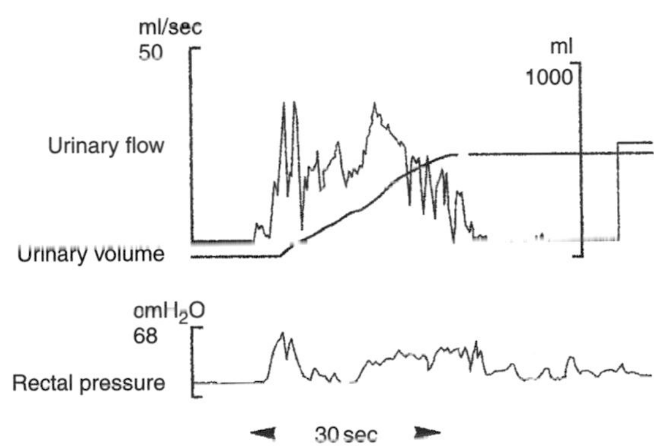

Figure 17.2
Uroflowmetry with rectal pressure measurement. Voiding starts with abdominal straining and continues with a combination of detrusor contraction and abdominal straining. Most probably motor hypoactive neurogenic bladder.

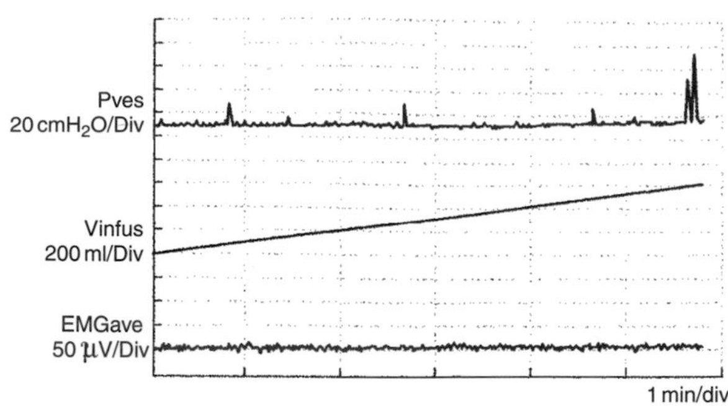

Figure 17.3
Cystometrogram with electromyography (EMG). Cystometry with filling rate 100 ml per minute. Moderate intravesical pressure rise (Pves) of 10 cmH_2O at 600 ml of filling (Vinfus). Filling stopped. No feeling of filling and no detrusor contraction. Small artifacts due to coughing. The electromyographic activity from the female urethral wall striated muscle is minimal and does not show the normal increase during filling (concentric needle recording, integrated signal, EMGave). Sensory hypoactive neurogenic bladder with peripheral neurogenic striated muscle affection.

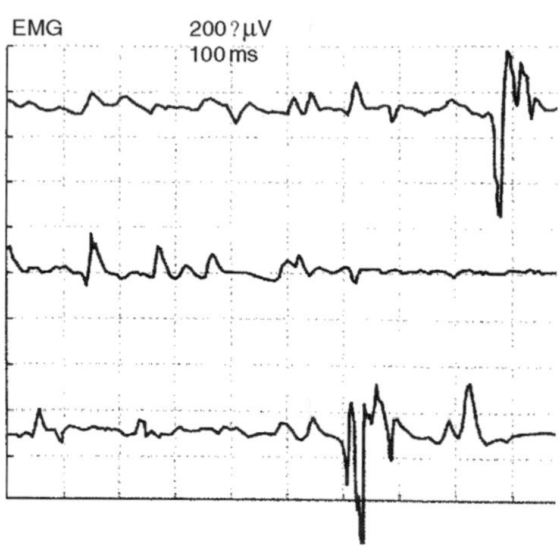

Figure 17.5
Electromyography from the female urethral wall striated muscle. Concentric needle electromyographic recording. Two bursts of polyphasic denervation potentials are consistent with peripheral neurogenic striated muscle affection.

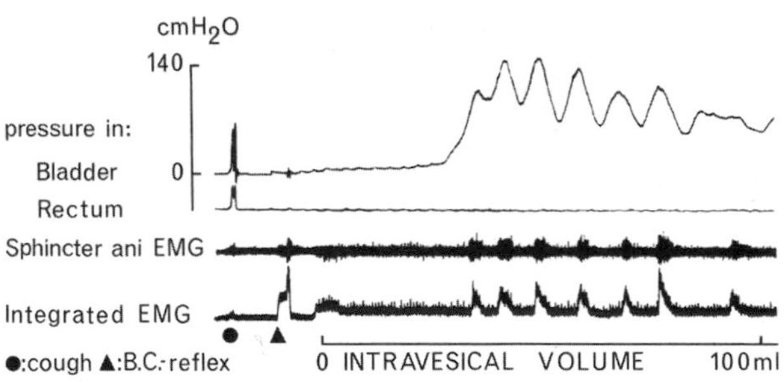

Figure 17.4
Cystometrogram with rectal pressure recording and electromyography (EMG). Recorded are bladder and intra-abdominal (rectum) pressures, concentric needle EMG from external anal sphincter (sphincter ani EMG) and the same sampling as an integrated EMG. After filling of nearly 50 ml an uninhibited bladder contraction is elicited. A repeated rise in bladder pressure as well as a synchronous increase in EMG activity occurs. There is no sign of voluntary contraction, the rectum pressure remains flat. Intravesical pressure increases during coughing; the EMG activity boosts by eliciting the bulbocavernosus reflex. Neurogenic overactive detrusor with detrusor-sphincter dyssynergia in patient with encephalopathy.

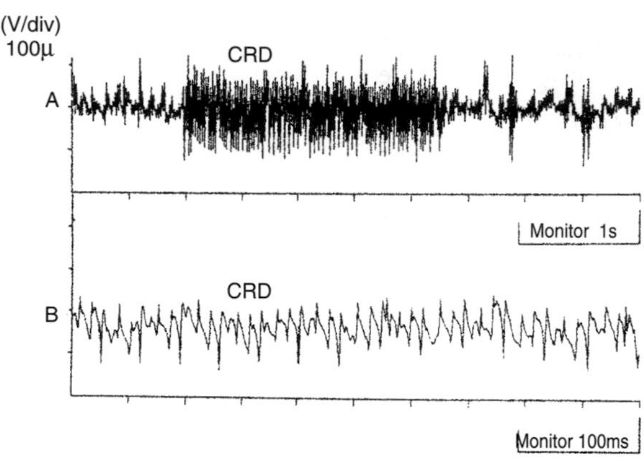

Figure 17.6
Electromyography from the female urethral wall striated muscle. Concentric needle electromyographic recording. A: The normal resting activity is interrupted by bursts of complex repetitive discharges (CRD) of almost regular amplitude and rate. B: The CRD potentials depicted at high speed monitoring. The finding, also called pseudomyotonic activity, is consistent with peripheral neurogenic striated muscle affection.

autonomic fibers.[42,43] In men, during urethrocystoscopy, at a level just below the pelvic floor, the voluntary and reflex contraction of the periurethral striated sphincter can be visually evaluated. The bladder wall is usually smooth without trabeculation. In females, the bladder neck may be open or closed. Ultrasonography gives information about the caliber of the upper urinary tract, and the size, form, and consistency (cysts) of the kidney. Urography may often be a necessary screening investigation of the kidneys and the upper urinary tract. Vesicoureteral reflux can, however, only be demonstrated by micturition urethrocystography (MUCG). If a urethral dysfunction is suspected, MUCG is the necessary radiologic investigation.[44] At all anatomic levels of the urinary tract, X-ray can be supplemented by CT and MRI.

Autonomic neuropathy in a patient with diabetes can have many other etiologies. The main groups of such conditions are metabolic, infectious, spinal, and degenerative. Examples are vitamin B12 deficiencies, herpes infections, lumbar disc prolapse, and multiple system atrophy.[45] Therefore, a detailed case history and thorough clinical examination is mandatory.

Diagnosis and treatment

The cardinal clinical symptoms of diabetes mellitus are polyuria, polydipsia, and weight loss. Further diagnostic criteria are a random blood glucose of 11.1 mmol/l or higher, or a fasting plasma glucose of 7.0 mmol/l or higher, or during the oral glucose tolerance test, a two-hour plasma glucose of at least 11.1 mmol/l. In asymptomatic individuals, a positive fasting plasma glucose will be sufficient. If necessary repeated tests have to be performed before a proper diagnosis can be made. For type 1 diabetes, insulin is vital for survival. Type 2 is usually treated with peroral antidiabetics. Insulin may, however, be added to control hyperglycemia.[1] Additional risk factors for neuropathy are hypertension, smoking, and alcohol consumption as well as high cholesterol and triglyceride levels.[20] In order to control the disease, it is important to modify these factors by securing a strict dietetical regimen. All patients will benefit from physical exercise. Recent studies have shown that islet cell transplantation can result in insulin independence with an excellent metabolic control.[46] This method has even effectively restored the liver to coordinated pulsatile insulin delivery.[47]

The diabetic neurogenic bladder with residual urine is treated with bladder training and eventually intermittent catheterization (CIC). In cases of motor hypoactive bladder, cholinergic agonists may be tried. If detrusor-sphincter dyssynergia is present, α_1-adrenergic blockers may be indicated. In cases of neurogenic overactive detrusor, anticholinergic drugs (antimuscarinics) are appropriate. For some patients, a urinary diversion may be the preferred treatment. Details are given elsewhere in this book.

Summary

Diabetic peripheral neuropathy has eight clinical syndromes. Autonomic neuropathy is the cause of the diabetic neurogenic bladder, and results from pathologic metabolic processes in the parasympathetic pelvic nerves and/or the central nervous system. The bladder is usually sensory hypoactive and, to a lesser degree, motor hypoactive. Neurogenic bladder is often combined with one of the other clinical syndromes. Clinical neurourologic and urodynamic investigations show characteristic findings. However, many etiologies other than diabetes are possible. Treatment is usually by means of a bladder-emptying regimen, supplemented by CIC if necessary.

Sarcoidosis

Prevalence

Sarcoidosis, known as Mb Boeck or Besnier–Boeck–Schaumann disease [Boeck, Caesar, 1845–1917, Professor of Dermatology, Christiania (Oslo)],[48] is a relatively common disease that affects individuals of both sexes, and most ages, races, and geographic locations. Females seem to be slightly more susceptible than males.[49] Among adults, the prevalence is from 10 to 40 per 100 000 in both the USA and Europe. A high prevalence is found in The Netherlands, Great Britain, and the Scandinavian countries.[50] The peak incidence in both sexes is around the age of 25–30 years. In Scandinavia and Japan there is a second peak of incidence in women who have passed 50 years of age.[51] The disease is infrequent below the age of 15, and especially below 9 years of age. It is estimated that about 6% of all affected by the disease are children.[52]

Pathologic anatomy

Sarcoidosis is a chronic, multisystem disorder of unknown etiology. The disease may be a result of an exaggerated acquired or inherited cellular immune response to a limited class of persistent antigens or self-antigens.[49] Invading antigen is recognized by helper T-lymphocytes and antigen presenting cells. Influenced by a complex cytokine cascade, monocyte macrophages fuse to form multinucleated giant cells and epithelioid cells. Conchoid, stellate, and residual inclusion bodies are often found in the giant cells.[53] Characteristics are an accumulation of lymphocytes and mononuclear phagocytes, noncaseating epithelioid granulomas, as well as derangements of the normal tissue architecture. Most organs are involved, the disease, however, only manifests itself in organs where it affects function, or is otherwise easily observed.[49] No disease has more multifarious manifestations.[53]

Neurosarcoidosis

Neurogenic damage can occur at any site along the whole neuraxis. In adults, the prevalence of neurogenic complication is 5%, for 48% of these it was the initial manifestation of sarcoidosis.[54] The proportion of peripheral nervous involvement is 25–67%.[50,55,56] The central nervous system is often assailed. Among 68 patients with neurosarcoidosis, 38% had a central nervous basal leptomeningeal MRI enhancement, and 43% had multiple cerebral or spinal white-matter lesions.[57] In some rare cases, multiple sarcoidosis lesions can clinically mimic multiple sclerosis or spinal cord abnormalities.[49] Neurosarcoidosis is unusual in children,[58] but the precise prevalence is not known.[59]

Pathologic anatomy

The pathologic findings in peripheral nerves are scattered perineural changes and sarcoid granuloma infiltration between nerve fibers,[50,56] giving rise to practically all types of nerve involvement. This includes focal and multifocal sensorimotor neuropathy, multifocal subacute or chronic sensorimotor neuropathy, chronic symmetric sensory polyneuropathy, subacute multifocal sensorimotor neuropathy with conduction block, and progressive lesion of the cauda equina. The type of neuropathy is most consistent with axonal degeneration with a multifocal pattern.[60] When granulomas infiltrate the epineurium, little or no nerve fiber damage occurs, except in cases where the granulomas induce necrotizing vasculitis giving rise to nerve ischemia. If the endoneurium and the surrounding blood vessels are infiltrated, serious damage to the nerve fibers and their function is the consequence.[56]

Neurogenic bladder

If the autonomic nerves innervating the lower urinary tract are affected, a neurogenic bladder, as described in the section on diabetes mellitus, can occur. Likewise, if the central nervous system is affected, detrusor overactivity can be found. Only a few cases of neurogenic bladder due to neurosarcoidosis have been urodynamically investigated and reported: one patient showed neurogenic detrusor overactivity due to a cerebral frontal lobe lesion, two patients suffered from neurogenic detrusor overactivity with detrusor-sphincter dyssynergia caused by thoracic intramedullary lesions, and one patient had neurogenic detrusor overactivity without dyssynergia due to a cervical lesion, and an autonomic dysreflexia as well.[61–64] Seeding of granulomas in the subarachnoidal space has caused polyradiculopathy, simulating the demyelinating polyradiculoneuropathy Guillain–Barré syndrome. Among 17 patients, 6 were noted with micturition difficulties.[65] According to the clinical information given, they probably had both the upper and lower types of the neurogenic bladder.

Diagnosis and treatment

The acute or subacute sarcoidosis manifests itself in 20–40% of the cases during some weeks with fever, fatigue, malaise, anorexia, or weight loss. These complaints are mostly mild, but in nearly 25% they are pronounced.[49] Respiratory problems and polyarthritis may accompany. Scandinavian and Irish females are frequently stricken by Löfgren's syndrome of sarcoidosis with erythema nodosum, bilateral X-ray hilar adenopathy, and joint symptoms. The Heerfordt–Waldenström syndrome of sarcoidosis includes fever, parotid gland enlargement, anterior uveitis, and peripheral facial nerve palsy, usually of a bilateral kind. The insidious progress develops over months in 40–70% of patients, a period most often associated with respiratory symptoms only. In 10% of patients, organs other than the lungs give rise to the initial inconvenience. Patients with an insidious presentation commonly evolve the chronic disease with permanent damage to the organs affected.

The erythrocyte sedimentation rate is raised in the active phase. Anemia, neutropenia, lymphopenia, hypergammaglobulinemia, and hypercalcemia may also be present. The angiotensin-converting enzyme (ACE) is raised in 60% of cases, but is also present in other conditions, like diabetes and alcoholic liver disease.[53] The most important single criterion for the diagnosis of sarcoidosis is the histologic finding of typical granulomas in more than one organ, and an exclusion of other granulomatous diseases.[66] Even if sarcoid granulomas are rarely found in nerve biopsy specimens, this procedure is of importance when combined with biopsy of the corresponding muscle. In patients with sarcoid neuropathy, this muscle is nearly always affected. Finding granulomas in muscle tissues will always exclude tuberculoid leprosy, since leprous granulomas never affect muscles.[56]

Sarcoidosis is often self-limiting, and the prognosis on the whole is good.[49] When indicated, the therapy includes the use of glucocorticoids, methotrexate, azathioprine, cyclophosphamide, or hydroxychloroquine, which is an antimalarial drug. For patients in a final stage of the disease, a bilateral lung transplantation is a possible therapy. A recurrence of sarcoid in the transplant is, however, to be expected in 30–80% of cases.

Handling the neurogenic urinary bladder caused by this illness is according to the recommendations given in the diabetes section.

Alcoholism

Definition and prevalence

The drinking of ethanol (alcohol) is a universal behavior, and is performed by 80% of all people. One definition of alcoholism (the primary type) is when there is physical evidence that alcohol has harmed a person's health, including signs of an alcoholic withdrawal syndrome. According to the fourth edition of the *American Diagnostic and Statistical*

Manual of Mental Disorders (*DSM-IV*), alcohol dependence is repeated alcohol-related difficulties in at least three of seven areas of functioning that cluster together over any 12-month period.[67,68] Alcoholism is seen in all races, ethnic, and socioeconomic groups. The exact prevalence of alcoholism is, however, difficult to determine. An estimate is that 10 million men and women in the USA, or approximately 10% of the nation's labor force, has a drinking problem.[69] In most Western countries the lifetime risk for alcohol dependence is 10–15% in men and 5–8% in women. In addition to the ethanol, the congeners found in alcoholic beverages which may contribute to body injuries with heavy drinking are methanol, butanol, aldehydes, esters, histamine, phenols, tannins, iron, lead, and cobalt.

Biochemistry

Ethanol is absorbed from the mucous membranes through the whole digestive tract. The molecule is weakly charged and moves easily through cell membranes, rapidly equilibrating between blood and tissues. A certain amount of ethanol is excreted directly through lungs, urine, and sweat. In the liver, the major portion is metabolized in the cell cytosol by alcohol dehydrogenase (ADH) to acetaldehyde. This, in turn, is rapidly destroyed by aldehyde dehydrogenase (ALDH) in the cytosol and mitochondria. In high blood alcohol concentrations, microsomes are responsible for some disintegration by oxidation. The cellular effects of chronic ethanol consumption may remain several weeks after the cessation of drinking. In the interim, neurons require ethanol to function optimally at this stage. The person has in that way developed physical dependence.[68]

Clinical neuropathology

Alcohol-related neurologic disorders affect the brain, brainstem, cerebellum, and the peripheral nerves. Polyneuropathy is the most common chronic disease,[70] affecting 5–15% of alcoholics.[68] The precise prevalence is unknown. In some reports men and women seem to be nearly equally affected, even though three-quarters of alcoholics are men, which suggests that women may be more susceptible to alcoholic polyneuropathy than men.[71] Alcohol can also interfere with the absorption of various vitamins, e.g. folate, pyridoxine (B6), thiamine (B1), nicotinic acid (B3), and vitamin A.[68] Polyneuropathy is a result of thiamine deficiency and/or a direct toxic effect of ethanol and acetaldehyde.[67] The body's storage of thiamine is low. The half-life of thiamine is only about 14 days. A continuous intake of food is therefore vital to prevent lack of this important vitamin.[72]

Alcoholic polyneuropathy usually presents as a gradual development of a distal, symmetric, sensoric, and motoric disease. Axonal degeneration, as well as segmental demyelination, are the main factors in this pathologic process.[6,70] The degenerative process is most intense in the distal direction; the nerve roots are spared, except in advanced cases. Unmyelinated fibers are also involved.[11] A loss of sympathetic and parasympathetic nerve fibers as well as ganglion neurons has also been observed.[73]

Autonomic dysfunction

Clinical manifestations of autonomic dysfunction are unusual in uncomplicated alcoholic peripheral neuropathy.[74] Previous references to affection of the lower urinary tract are sparse; a peripheral as well as a myelopathic neurogenic overactive bladder has been reported.[33,34,75] More recently, three more cases have been reported, all with a peripheral nervous lesion, two with huge urinary retention.[76,77] Interestingly, one woman also developed a severe distended bladder. The time of onset, however, suggested that this was induced by alcohol withdrawal.[78] This conclusion is according to the statement that neurons need alcohol in order to function optimally in the phase of abstinence.

Diagnosis and treatment

The identification of alcohol abuse is often problematic. Information from relatives and questionnaires can be helpful. Attention to alcohol-related problems as well as laboratory tests may expose the actual situation. Elevated levels of gamma-glutamyl transferase (GGT) and carbohydrate-deficient transferrin (CDT) are nearly 80% sensitive for the diagnosis. High normal values of erythrocyte mean corpuscular volume (MCV) and serum uric acid may also indicate an abnormal use of alcohol.[68] The clinical symptoms develop gradually over weeks or months, but may also arise acutely within days. Fatigue, irritability, and muscle cramps appear at an early stage of nutritional deficiency. Signs of neuropathy follow a more prolonged state. A mild sensory loss and dysesthesias associated with aching and cramping in the legs often precede distal sensory loss and weakness in both feet and hands.

In cases with neurogenic bladder, a clinical neurourologic and urodynamic investigation will show the same findings as for diabetic neurogenic bladder. The latency of the evoked bulbocavernosus reflex is shown to be least normal in patients with alcoholic polyneuropathy.[79]

The therapy of alcoholics is a very demanding task, and is here only intimated. Motivational interviews as well as courses for detoxification are crucial. Preventing a withdrawal syndrome is also essential. It is equally important to substitute vitamins, particularly thiamine. Tranquilizers and the ALDH inhibitor disuliram or acamprosate may be added. The exact mechanism of action of acamprosat is as yet unknown. It may, however, stimulate the GABA (gamma-aminobutyric acid) system, and inhibit the NMDA (*N*-methyl-D-aspartate) reseptor system.

The therapy of the neurogenic bladder is as described in the section on diabetes.

Porphyrias

Definition and biochemistry

Porphyrias comprise a group of eight hereditary disorders – five hepatic and three erythropoietic – with porphyrin accumulation in either the hepatic or erythropoietic tissues. The disease is due to inherent or acquired enzymatic disturbances in heme biosynthesis. Each of the eight types is characterized by a specific pattern of overproduction, accumulation, and excretion of metabolic products of heme. In the acute hepatic porphyrias, an overproduction of porphyrin precursors occurs, whereas the substance is porphyrin in the cutaneous types.[9,80–82] The synthesis of heme involves cooperation between the mitochondrial and cytosolic compartments, and is controlled by the hepatic free intracellular heme in a negative feedback loop. Initially, succinyl coenzyme A and glycine combine to form delta-aminolevulinic acid (ALA) catalyzed by ALA synthase. Then two molecules of ALA are condensed to the circular structure of porphobilinogen (PGB). The intermediates of porphyrinogens arise through six further stages, resulting in the iron-containing terminal product heme. As a major part of the hepatic heme is used to synthesize cytochrome P-450 enzymes, the hepatic ALA synthase and cytochrome P-450s are regulated in an integrated way.[82] P-450 is a protein complexed to cytochrome oxidase, located in hepatic microsomes. Functioning as a catalyst, it decomposes various endogenous and exogenous substances, including drugs.

Types and attacks

Neurologic symptoms are present in four of the hepatic porphyrias: delta-aminolevulinic acid dehydratase deficient porphyria (ADP), acute intermittent porphyria (AIP), variegate porphyria (VP), and hereditary coproporphyria (HCP). The two latter types also have cutaneous manifestations.[83] ADP is an autosomal recessive disorder described in only a few patients. The three other hepatic types in question are transmitted as autosomal dominant disorders. The acute attacks of symptoms are similar, often precipitated by intake of a vast number of different drugs, including barbiturates, estrogens, contraceptives, sulfonamides, griseofulvin, meprobamate, phenytoin, valproic acid, ergots, steroids, and succinamides. These attacks are caused by an imbalance in the ALA synthase and P-450 system released by the drugs, giving rise to increased ALA production. By the same mechanism, alcohol, starvation, infections, and fever may also provoke the attacks.[80,84,85]

Prevalence and distribution

AIP (Swedish porphyria) is the most common of the three relevant hepatic types with neurogenic affection, occurring world-wide with a prevalence estimated to be between 1 in 5000 and 1 in 50 000. This type of disorder becomes clinically manifest after puberty, with an onset usually between 20 and 50 years of age. It is far more frequent in females (65%) than in males (35%). The highest prevalence occurs in Scandinavia and the United Kingdom.[80,81,86] VP (South African genetic porphyria) has a higher prevalence of 3 in 1000 in South Africa than elsewhere. Affected individuals in South Africa have been identified as descendants of a Dutch female settler who immigrated in 1688. The disease is, however, distributed world-wide. It is probably less common than AIP, and has no racial or geographic predilection.[80,81] HCP seems to occur less frequently than AIP, but since the disease is more gentle and more likely to express itself only in a latent form, the true frequency is difficult to ascertain. Racial predilections are unknown.[81,84]

Neuropathology

In rapidly fatal cases the central and peripheral nervous systems may be without traceable pathologic lesions. Otherwise, patchy areas of demyelination with or without destruction of the axis cylinders can be observed throughout the nervous system. Chromolysis may appear in the neurons of the anterior horns, in the cranial nerve nuclei, the spinal ganglia, the celiac ganglion, and the cerebral cortex. The most dramatic changes will, however, be seen in the peripheral nerves and supporting cells. Here, a degeneration of the axons with secondary demyelination is found, whereas inflammatory or vascular lesions are lacking.[12,84,86] Autonomic function studies have demonstrated abnormalities of both sympathetic and parasympathetic nerves.[87]

The mental disturbances seen in porphyrias may be due to an elevated PBG that mimics serotonin, thereby acting as a false neurotransmitter. Another pathway may be that ALA blocks normal GABA neurotransmission. ALA is structurally related to GABA and is a partial agonist of GABA, which is the major inhibitory neurotransmitter in the central nervous system.[84] The mechanisms behind the second type of abnormality, the structural neuronal damage, are so far not understood. They may be related to a direct neurotoxicity of elevated levels of ALA.[88]

Two further modes of action also warrant discussion.[84] The first one suggests that, due to the enzyme deficiency, there will be a lack of heme-containing proteins for the transportation of oxygen and electrons, and for the cytochrome P-450 system. A widespread disturbance of the neuronal function due to a failure in the oxidative energy metabolism is consequently to be expected. But no morphologic changes resembling the effects of hypoxia or hypoglycemia have been found.

The second mechanism suggested also seems rather unlikely. A failure of the cytochrome P-450 system might lead to axonal damage due to an inability to detoxify drugs or their metabolites. The AIP-inducing drugs are, however, not neurotoxic, and many of them have effects contrary to those seen in AIP. The final action requires neurotoxicity of the accumulated ALA and PBG. In humans, no evidence has so far proved that these metabolites are directly neurotoxic in the amount found during porphyric attacks. This is also the case in mice porphyric models. The primary motor axon neuropathy histologically demonstrated in the animal developed chronically and progressively, and with normal or slightly increased plasma and urine levels of ALA. These data suggest that heme deficiency and a consequent dysfunction of heme proteins can cause porhyric neuropathy.[89]

Table 17.3 *Autonomic neuropathies which may cause neurogenic bladder*

Disorders without associated somatic peripheral neuropathy: primary disorders

- Acute and subacute autonomic neuropathy
  - Pure pandysautonomia
  - Pure cholinergic dysautonomia
- Chronic
  - Pure autonomic failure

Disorders associated with somatic peripheral neuropathy: secondary disorders

- Hereditary
  - Amyloid disease (also secondary amyloidosis)
  - Porphyrias
- Metabolic
  - Diabetes mellitus
  - Chronic renal failure
  - Chronic hepatic failure
  - Vitamin B12 deficiency
- Alcoholism and nutritional disorders
- Sarcoidosis
- Connective tissue disorders: immune-complex diseases?
  - Systemic lupus erythematosus
  - Rheumatoid arthritis
  - Mixed connective tissue disease
  - The vasculitis syndromes
- Malignancy: paraneoplastic remote effect of cancer
- Toxins
  - Antineoplastic agents, certain other drugs, heavy metals, organic solvents

Diagnosis and treatment

Clinical symptoms are similarly distributed in the three types of porphyrias in question. Recurrent attacks are reported lasting from days to months, varying in frequency and severity. The main features are initial abdominal pain, psychotic symptoms, peripheral acute or subacute proximal or distal polyneuropathy or mononeuritis multiplex, trunkal sensory loss, and the excretion of colorless porphyrinogens in urine, turning red or purple when exposed to light and air.[9,12,80,84] In the acute attack, progressive muscle weakness can give rise to a respiratory and bulbar paralysis, and can be fatal without a correct diagnosis and treatment. The most common manifestations, including abdominal pain, however, are a result of autonomic neuropathy. Other symptoms due to autonomic failure include tachycardia, postural hypotension, hypertension, fever, sweating, retinal artery spasm, and urinary retention.[86] In two female patients with porphyria and acute urinary retention cystoscopy was normal, whereas the cystometrogram shifted to the right.[90] The same diagnostic considerations as described for the diabetic neurogenic bladder apply for the porphyrias.

In serum, severe hyponatremia and hypomagnesemia may be present. In reference laboratories the porphyrin isomers in urine and feces can be separated and defined by high-performance liquid chromatography. Molecular genetic and enzyme analysis makes a precise identification of the genetic basis of each porphyria possible.[82–84] In the third step of the heme metabolic pathway, failure of porphobilinogen deaminase causes AIP. In urine the excretion of PBG exceeds that of ALA. Failure of coproporphyrinogen oxidase in the sixth step results in HCP with ALA, PBG, and coproporphyrin III in the urine. In the seventh step, failure of the protoporphyrinogen oxidase enzyme leads to VP. The urine amount of ALA is higher than that of PBG. Coproporphyrin III is also present.

It is important to avoid porphyrogenic drugs and prolonged starvation as well as excessive physical stress without consuming carbohydrates. During an acute attack, hyponatremia has to be regulated slowly to prevent central pontine myelinolysis. Carbohydrate nutrition is important, if necessary administered as a glucose infusion. The most direct and immediate therapy is intravenous heme. The mortality rate due to acute attacks is less than 10%.[82,84]

If a neurogenic bladder is present, the same therapy as proposed in the diabetes section is recommended.

Conclusion

Autonomic neuropathy with a neurogenic bladder has only rarely been shown in sarcoidosis, alcoholism, and porphyrias. Different classifications of autonomic neuropathy are accounted for in tabular versions.[12,34,74,91,92] A selection relevant for this chapter is given in Table 17.3.

A correct diagnosis of the four conditions of this chapter is often dependent on vital investigations not mentioned so far. In clinical practice, spinal fluid analysis, depiction of the central nervous system with computer tomography as well as magnetic resonance imaging, extremity nerve conduction measurement, and electromyography of skeletal muscle studies, among others, may be required.

References

1. Powers AC. Diabetes mellitus. In: Kasper DL, Fauci AS, Longo DL et al, eds. Harrison's Principles of Internal Medicine, 16th edn. New York: McGraw-Hill, 2005: 2152–80.
2. Windebank AJ, McEvoy KM. Diabetes and the nervous system. In: Aminoff MJ, ed. Neurology and General Medicine. New York: Churchill Livingstone, 1989: 273–304.
3. Wild S, Green A, Sicree R, King H. Global prevalence of diabetes. Estimates for the year 2000 and projections for 2030. Diabetes Care 2004; 27: 1047–53.
4. National Diabetes Statistics. National Diabetes Information Clearinghouse. NIH publication No 06–3892, November 2005.
5. Diabetes Atlas. International Diabetes Federation, Belgium, 2005. www.eatlas.idf.org/Prevalence/All_diabetes
6. Bosch EP, Mitsumoto H. Disorders of peripheral nerves, plexuses, and nerve roots. In: Bradley WG, Daroff RB, Fenichel GM, Marsden CD, eds. Neurology in Clinical Practice. Boston: Butterworth-Heinemann, 1991: 1719–818.
7. Herman WH, Sinnock P, Brenner E et al. An epidemiologic model for diabetes mellitus: incidence, prevalence, and mortality. Diabetes Care 1984; 7: 367–71.
8. Sperling MA. Diabetes mellitus. In: Behrman RE, Kliegman RM, Jenson HB, eds. Nelson Textbook of Paediatrics, 16th edn. Philadelphia: WB Saunders, 2000: 1767–91.
9. Schaumburg HH, Berger AR, Thomas PK, eds. Disorders of Peripheral Nerves, 2nd edn. Philadelphia: FA Davis, 1992.
10. Eeg-Olofsson O, Petersen I. Childhood diabetic neuropathy. Acta Ped Scand 1966; 53: 163–7.
11. Dyck PJ, Low PA, Stevens JC. Diseases of peripheral nerves. In: Joynt RJ, ed. Clinical Neurology. Philadelphia: JB Lippincott, 1990: 1–126.
12. Adams RD, Victor M, Ropper AH. Principles of Neurology, 6th edn. New York: McGraw-Hill, 1997.
13. Thomas PK, Tomlinson DR. Diabetic and hypoglycemic neuropathy. In: Dyck PJ, Thomas PK, Griffin JW et al, eds. Peripheral Neuropathy, 3rd edn. Philadelphia: WB Saunders, 1993: 1219–50.
14. Low PA, Dyck PJ. Pathologic studies and the nerve biopsy in autonomic neuropathies. In: Low PA, ed. Clinical Autonomic Disorders Boston: Little, Brown, 1993: 331–44.
15. Faerman I, Glocer L, Celener D et al. Autonomic nervous system and diabetes. Histological and histochemical study of the autonomic nerve fibers of the urinary bladder in diabetic patients. Diabetes 1973; 22: 225–37.
16. Ørstavik K, Namer B, Scmidt R et al. Abnormal function of C-fibers in patients with diabetic neuropathy. J Neurosci 2006; 26: 11287–94.
17. Powell HC, Rosoff J, Myers RR. Microangiopathy in human diabetic neuropathy. Acta Neuropathol 1985; 68: 295–305.
18. Walker D, Carrington A, Cannan SA et al. Structural abnormalities do not explain the early functional abnormalities in the peripheral nerves of the streptozotocin diabetic rat. J Anat 1999; 195: 419–27.
19. Malik RA, Newrick PG, Sharma AK et al. Microangiopathy in human diabetic neuropathy: relationship between capillary abnormalities and the severity of neuropathy. Diabetologia 1989; 32: 92–102.
20. Llewelyn JG, Tomlinson DR, Thomas PK. Diabetic neuropathies. In: Dyck PJ, Thomas PK, eds. Peripheral Neuropathy, 4th edn. Philadelphia: Elsevier Saunders, 2005: 1951–91.
21. Andersson PO, Malmgren A, Uvelius B. Cystometrical and in vitro evaluation of urinary bladder function in rats with streptozotocin-induced diabetes. J Urol 1988; 139: 1359–62.
22. Poladia DP, Schanbacher B, Wallace LJ, Bauer JA. Innervation and connexin isoform expression during diabetes-related bladder dysfunction: early structural vs. neuronal remodeling. Acta Diabetol 2005; 42: 147–52.
23. Frimodt-Møller C. Diabetic cystopathy I: A clinical study of the frequency of bladder dysfunction in diabetics. Dan Med Bul 1976; 23: 267–78.
24. Yoshimura N, Chancellor MB, Andersson K-E, Christ GJ. Recent advances in understanding the biology of diabetes-associated bladder complications and novel therapy. BJU Int 2005; 95: 733–8.
25. Hilsted J, Low PA. Diabetic autonomic neuropathy. In: Low PA, ed. Clinical Autonomic Disorders. Boston: Little, Brown, 1993: 423–43.
26. Kaplan SA, Blaivas JG. Urodynamic findings in patients with diabetic cystopathy. J Urol 1995; 153: 342–44.
27. Bors E, Comarr AE. Neurological Urology. Basel: S. Karger, 1971.
28. Buck AC, McRae CU, Chisholm GD. The diabetic bladder. Proc R Soc Med 1974; 67: 81–3.
29. Ouvrier RA. Peripheral neuropathy. In: Berg BO, ed. Principles of Child Neurology. New York: McGraw-Hill, 1996: 1607–55.
30. Garg BP. Disorders of micturition and defecation. In: Swaiman KF, ed. Pediatric Neurology, Principles and Practice, 2nd edn. St Louis: Mosby, 1994: 271–84.
31. Hopkins WF, Pierce JM. The neurogenic bladder in diabetes mellitus. In: Boyarsky S, ed. The Neurogenic Bladder. Baltimore: Williams and Wilkins, 1967: 155–7.
32. Kendall AR, Karafin L. Classification of neurogenic bladder disease. In: Lapides J, ed. Symposium on Neurogenic Bladder. The Urologic Clinics of North America. Philadelphia: WB Saunders, 1974: 37–44.
33. Bradley WE. Neurologic disorders affecting the urinary bladder. In: Krane RJ, Siroky MB, eds. Clinical Neurourology. Boston: Little, Brown, 1979: 245–55.
34. Hald T, Bradley WE. The Urinary Bladder, Neurology and Dynamics. Baltimore: Williams and Wilkins, 1982.
35. Dasgupta P, Thomas PK. Peripheral neuropathy. In: Fowler CJ, ed. Neurology of Bladder, Bowel, and Sexual Dysfunction. Boston: Butterworth-Heinemann, 1999: 339–52.
36. Szabo L, Barkai L, Lombay B. Urinary flow disturbance as an early sign of autonomic neuropathy in diabetic children and adolescents. Neurourol Urodyn 2007; 26: 218–21.
37. Yamaguchi C, Sakakibara R, Uchiyama T et al. Bladder sensation in peripheral nerve lesions. Neurourol Urodyn 2006; 25: 763–9.
38. Klevmark B. Volume threshold for micturition. Influence of filling rate on sensory and motor bladder function. Scand J Urol Nephrol 2002; 210(Suppl): 6–10.

39. Abrams P, Cardozo L, Fall M et al. The standardisation of terminology of lower urinary tract function: Report from the Standardisation Sub-Committee of the International Continence Society. Neurourol Urodyn 2002; 21: 167–78.
40. Starer P, Libow L. Cystometric evaluation of bladder dysfunction in elderly diabetic patients. Arch Intern Med 1990; 150: 810–13.
41. Jensen D, Stien R. The importance of complex repetitive discharges in the striated female urethral sphincter and the male bulbocavernosus muscle. Scand J Urol Nephrol 1996; 179(Suppl): 69–73.
42. Vodusek DB, Fowler CJ. Clinical neurophysiology. In: Fowler CJ, ed. Neurology of Bladder, Bowel, and Sexual Dysfunction. Boston: Butterworth-Heinemann, 1999: 109–43.
43. Beck RO. Investigation of male erectile dysfunction. In: Fowler CJ, ed. Neurology of Bladder, Bowel, and Sexual Dysfunction. Boston: Butterworth-Heinemann, 1999: 145–60.
44. Jensen D, Aasen S, Talseth T. Uroflowmetry with simultaneous electromyography versus voiding video cystourethrography. Scand J Urol Nephrol 2006; 40: 232–7.
45. Appel RA, Whiteside HV. Diabetes and other peripheral neuropathies affecting lower urinary tract function. In: Krane RJ, Siroky MB, eds. Clinical Neurourology, 2nd edn. Boston: Little, Brown, 1991: 365–73.
46. Shapiro J, Lakey JRT, Ryan EA et al. Islet transplantation in seven patients with type 1 diabetes mellitus using a glucocorticoid free immunosuppressive regimen. N Engl J Med 2000; 343: 230–8.
47. Meier JJ, Hong-McAtee I, Galasso R et al. Intrahepatic transplanted islets in humans secrete insulin in a coordinate pulsatile manner directly into the liver. Diabetes 2006; 55: 2324–32.
48. Boeck C. Multiple benign sarkoid of the skin. J Cutan Genitourin Dis 1899; 17: 543–50.
49. Crystal RG. Sarcoidosis. In: Kasper DL, Fauci AS, Longo DL, et al, eds. Harrison's Principles of Internal Medicine, 16th edn. New York: McGraw-Hill, 2005: 2017–23.
50. Silberberg DH. Sarcoidosis of the nervous system. In: Aminoff MJ, ed. Neurology and General Medicine. New York: Churchill Livingstone, 1989: 701–12.
51. Alsbirk PH. Epidemiologic studies on sarcoidosis in Denmark based on a nation-wide register. A preliminary report. Acta Med Scand Suppl 1964; 425: 106–9.
52 Dyken PR. Neurosarcoidosis. In: Berg BO, ed. Principles of Child Neurology. New York: McGraw-Hill, 1996: 889–99.
53. Gawkrodger DJ. Sarcoidosis. In Burns T, Breathnach S, Cox N, Griffiths C, eds. Rook's Textbook of Dermatology, 7th edn. Oxford: Blackwell, 2004: 58.1–58.24.
54. Stern BJ, Krumholz A, Johns C, Scott P, Nissim J. Sarcoidosis and its neurological manifestations. Arch Neurol 1985; 42: 909–17.
55. Delaney P. Neurologic manifestations in sarcoidosis: review of the literature, with a report of 23 cases. Ann Intern Med 1977; 87: 336–45.
56. Said G, Lacroix C. Sarcoid neuropathy. In: Dyck PJ, Thomas PK, eds. Peripheral Neuropathy, 4th edn. Philadelphia: Elsevier Saunders, 2005: 2415–25.
57. Zajicek JP, Scolding NJ, Foster O et al. Central nervous system sarcoidosis – diagnosis and management. Q J Med 1999; 92: 103–17.
58. Weil ML, Levin M. Infections of the nervous system. In: Menkes JH, ed. Textbook of Child Neurology, 5th edn. Baltimore: Williams and Wilkins, 1995: 379–509.
59. Ashwal S, Schneider S. Neurologic complications of vasculitic disorders of childhood. In: Swaiman KF, ed. Pediatric Neurology, Principles and Practice, 2nd edn. St Louis: Mosby, 1994: 841–63.
60. Scott TS, Brillman J, Gross JA. Sarcoidosis of the peripheral nervous system. Neurol Res 1993; 15: 389–90.
61. Sakakibara R, Hattori T, Uchiyama T, Yamanishi T. Micturitional disturbance in a patient with neurosarcoidosis. Neurourol Urodyn 2000; 19: 273–7.
62. Fitzpatrick KJ, Chancellor MB, Rivas DA et al. Urologic manifestation of spinal cord sarcoidosis. J Spinal Cord Med 1996; 19: 201–3.
63. Kim IY, Elliott DS, Husmann DA, Boone TB. An unusual presenting symptom of sarcoidosis: neurogenic bladder dysfunction. J Urol 2001; 165: 903–4.
64. Sakakibara R, Uchiyama T, Kuwabara S et al. Autonomic dysreflexia due to neurogenic bladder dysfunction; an unusual presentation of spinal cord sarcoidosis. J Neurol Neurosurg Psychiatry 2001; 71: 819–20.
65. Koffman B, Junck L, Elias SB, Feit HW, Levine SR. Polyradiculopathy in sarcoidosis. Muscle Nerve 1999; 22: 608–13.
66. Burns TM. Neurosarcoidosis. Arch Neurol 2003; 60: 1166–8.
67. Schuckit MA. Alcohol and alcoholism. In: Braunwald E, Isselbacher KJ, Petersdorf RG, Wilsone JD, Martin JB, Fauci AS, eds. Harrison's Principles of Internal Medicine, 11th edn. New York: McGraw-Hill, 1987: 2106–11.
68. Schuckit MA. Alcohol and alcoholism. In: Kasper DL, Fauci AS, Longo DL et al, eds. Harrison's Principles of Internal Medicine, 16th edn. New York: McGraw-Hill, 2005: 2562–6.
69. Victor M. Neurologic disorders due to alcoholism and malnutrition. In: Joynt RJ, ed. Clinical Neurology. Philadelphia: JB Lippincot, 1990: 1–94.
70. Messing RO, Greenberg DA. Alcohol and the nervous system. In: Aminoff MJ, ed. Neurology and General Medicine. New York: Churchill Livingstone, 1989: 533–47.
71. Layzer RB. Neuromuscular Manifestations of Systemic Disease. Philadelphia: FA Davis, 1985.
72. Saperstein DS, Barohn RJ. Polyneuropathy caused by nutritional and vitamin deficiency. In: Dyck PJ, Thomas PK, eds. Peripheral Neuropathy, 4th edn. Philadelphia: Elsevier Saunders, 2005: 2051–62.
73. Windebank AJ. Polyneuropathy due to nutritional deficiency and alcoholism. In: Dyck PJ, Thomas PK, Griffin JW, Low PA, Poduslo JF, eds. Peripheral Neuropathy, 3rd edn. Philadelphia: WB Saunders, 1993: 1310–21.
74. McLeod JG. Autonomic dysfunction in peripheral nerve disease. In: Bannister R (Sir Roger), Mathias CJ, eds. Autonomic Failure, 3rd edn. Oxford: Oxford University Press, 1993: 659–81.
75. Sheremata WA, Sherwin I. Alcoholic myelopathy. With spastic urinary bladder. Dis Nerv Syst 1972; 33: 136–9.
76. Tjandra BS, Janknegt RA. Neurogenic impotence and lower urinary tract symptoms due to vitamin B1 deficiency in chronic alcoholism. J Urol 1997; 157: 954–5.
77. Ruiyong Y, Caracciolo VJ, Kulaga M. Chronic abdominal distension secondary to urinary retention in a patient with alcoholism. JAMA 2002; 287: 318–19.
78. Iga J-I, Taniguchi T, Ohmori T. Acute abdominal distention secondary to urinary retention in a patient after alcohol withdrawal. Alcohol Alcoholism 2005; 40: 86–7.
79. Ertekin C, Reel F. Bulbocavernosus reflex in normal men and in patients with neurogenic bladder and/or impotence. J Neurol Sci 1976; 28: 1–15.
80. Meyer UA. Porphyrias. In: Braunwald E, Isselbacher KJ, Petersdorf RG et al, eds. Harrison's Principles of Internal Medicine, 11th edn. New York: McGraw-Hill, 1987: 1638–43.
81. Sassa S. The porphyrias. In: Behrman RE, Kliegman RM, Jenson HB, eds. Nelson Textbook of Pediatrics, 16th edn. Philadelphia: WB Saunders, 2000: 430–9.
82. Desnick RJ. The porphyrias. In: Kasper DL, Fauci AS, Longo DL et al, eds. Harrison's Principles of Internal Medicine, 16th edn. New York: McGraw-Hill, 2005: 2303–8.
83. Sarkany RPE. The cutaneuos porphyries. In: Burns T, Breathnach S, Cox N, Griffiths C, eds. Rook's Textbook of Dermatology, 7th edn. Oxford: Blackwell, 2004: 57.1–57.124.
84. Windebank AJ, Bonkovsky HL. Porphyric neuropathy. In: Dyck PJ, Thomas PK, eds. Peripheral Neuropathy, 4th edn. Philadelphia: Elsevier Saunders, 2005: 1883–92.
85. Evans OB, Bock H-GO, Parker C, Hanson RR. Inborn errors of metabolism of the nervous system. In: Bradley WG, Daroff RB,

Fenichel GM, Marsden CD, eds. Neurology in Clinical Practice. Boston: Butterworth-Heinemann, 1991: 1269–322.
86. Glaser GH, Pincus JH. Neurologic complications of internal disease. In: Joynt RJ, ed. Clinical Neurology. Philadelphia: JB Lippincott, 1990: 1–57.
87. Laiwah AC, Macphee GJ, Boye P, Moore MR, Goldberg A. Autonomic neuropathy in acute intermittent porhyria. J Neurol Neurosurg Psychiat 1985; 48: 1025–30.
88. Albers JW, Fink JK. Porphyric neuropathy. Muscle Nerve 2004; 30: 410–22.
89. Lindberg RLP, Martini R, Baumgartner M et al. Motor neuropathy in porphobilinogen deaminase-deficient mice imitates the peripheral neuropathy of human acute porphyria. J Clin Invest 1999; 103: 1127–34.
90. Redeker AG. Atonic neurogenic bladder in porphyria. J Urol 1956; 75: 465–9.
91. Low PA, McLeod JG. The autonomic neuropathies. In: Low PA, ed. Clinical Autonomic Disorders. Boston: Little, Brown, 1993: 395–421.
92. Mathias CJ. Autonomic neuropathy: aspects of diagnosis and management. In: Asbury AK, Thomas PK, eds. Peripheral Nerve Disorders 2. Oxford: Butterworth-Heinemann, 1998: 95–117.

18

Other peripheral neuropathies (lumbosacral zoster, genitourinary herpes, tabes dorsalis, Guillain–Barré syndrome)

Vincent WM Tse and Anthony R Stone

Introduction

Peripheral neuropathy is a rare but significant cause of storage and voiding dysfunction. An adequate working knowledge of the underlying pathophysiology, clinical presentation, diagnosis, and management of such a dysfunction is essential in any urologist's armamentarium. The neuropathy affecting the bladder often takes the form of an autonomic neuropathy, which may involve both the sympathetic and parasympathetic, as well as afferent and efferent, innervation of the bladder and urethra, leading to alteration of bladder sensation, the sacral reflex arc, detrusor-sphincter synergy, and detrusor contractility. The cause of the neuropathy can be metabolic, iatrogenic, traumatic, infective, or immunologic. The focus of this chapter is on the infective and immunologic disorders which may lead to peripheral neuropathy: namely, lumbosacral herpes zoster, genitourinary herpes simplex, tabes dorsalis, and Guillain–Barré syndrome.

Neuropathic bladder associated with infection by the herpes virus family

The herpes virus family consists of DNA viruses which are relatively large and made up of 162 cylindrical capsomeres. Four members of this family affect humans: namely, herpesvirus hominis (herpes simplex virus (HSV) types 1 and 2), herpes varicellae (varicella-zoster virus), cytomegalovirus, and infectious mononucleosis virus. The first two types are more commonly encountered clinically. However, with respect to neuropathic bladder dysfunction, varicella-zoster infection is a more common cause than anogenital herpes simplex (type 2), although the latter can present with acute urinary retention as a result of micturitional pain rather than a direct viral neurogenic inflammation.[1] Cytomegalovirus and infectious mononucleosis have not been reported to cause neuropathic bladder dysfunction.

Lumbosacral herpes zoster

Pathophysiology

Herpes zoster is a varicella-zoster virus infection manifested by circumscribed painful vesicular eruption of the skin and mucous membrane. Urinary retention afflicts 3.5% of patients with active herpes zoster infection, and is most commonly seen in infection of the sacral dorsal root ganglia (78%), followed by thoracolumbar (11%), and higher thoracic levels (11%).[2] The urinary retention typically presents concurrently with or within a few days following the onset of the rash,[3] and is thought to be due to a sensory neuropathy from inflammatory reaction in the dorsal nerve roots and ganglia, which spreads proximally and distally to the sacral segments of the cord, with interruption of the micturition reflex.[4] If the sacral micturition center is involved, a parasympathetic motor neuropathy may also contribute to the urinary retention.[5] In herpes zoster affecting the thoracic and lumbar segments, urinary retention has been explained by activation of the lumbar sympathetic outflow, resulting in increased tone of the bladder neck and internal urethral sphincter.[6] Virus particles and neurotropic factors have been identified in neurons and supporting satellite cells in the sensory ganglia and within peripheral sensory nerves of the corresponding dermatome, thus explaining the origin of the dermatomal distribution of the rash and associated pain.[7] The virus may also cause inflammation of the spinal cord,[8] which may manifest as a myelitic disorder of the long tracts.[9]

Clinical features

Herpes zoster infections can occur sporadically in healthy subjects with previous exposure to varicella (chickenpox), or in the immunocompromised, most notably the elderly, diabetics, transplant patients, and patients with the acquired immunodeficiency syndrome (AIDS). A distinctive feature is the localization of the rash, which may involve one or two, and sometimes more, adjacent dermatomes. Those with bladder involvement usually have a classic zoster skin eruption in a sacral dermatomal distribution, typically affecting one or more of adjacent S2, S3, or S4 areas. The lesions can be either unilateral or bilateral, though the former predominates. In unilateral skin or bladder mucosal involvement, bilateral depression of the reflex arc, resulting in urinary retention, may still occur. This is because the virus affects not only the ipsilateral dorsal root ganglion and nerve but may also involve the meninges and the contralateral nerve roots.[1] Both sexes are affected equally but bladder involvement is more common in males.[1] There is no age predilection for bladder dysfunction, which may even occur in the pediatric population as young as the neonate or infant.[10]

Focused neurologic examination may reveal reduced or absent sensation to light touch and pinprick in the perineal or perianal areas. The anal and bulbocavernosus reflexes are often depressed or absent. The patellar (L2, 3, 4) and Achilles tendon (S1) reflexes may also be impaired, depending on the level of the neuritic inflammation. The Babinski sign is usually negative. Motor function is rarely affected.[1] Digital rectal examination may reveal a loaded rectum consistent with neurogenic rectal involvement.[3,11] Cystoscopy may reveal mucosal eruptions ipsilateral to the side of skin involvement.[12]

Clinical and urodynamic diagnosis

The diagnosis should be suspected in any young, healthy, sexually active individual as well as in those who are immunocompromised and present with acute urinary retention. Attention should be directed at examination of the perineal and perianal skin areas for the typical skin eruptions, which, together with antibodies against the virus (in cerebrospinal fluid and serum), would be diagnostic. Midstream urine should be collected to exclude bacterial infection. Urodynamic study in the acute phase typically reveals detrusor areflexia or hyporeflexia with decreased sensation of bladder filling.[13] Electromyography (EMG) is often difficult to perform in the acute phase due to painful blistering perineal skin. It has been reported that external anal sphincter EMG and bulbocavernosus reflex latency were often normal.[14] All urodynamic changes are reversible and usually resolve within 4–8 weeks. A urinary tract ultrasound, or intravenous pyelography (IVP) if evidence of hematuria, should be performed to exclude upper tract or pelvic pathology such as hydronephrosis or pelvic mass. A cystoscopy is recommended if there is associated hematuria to exclude bladder involvement or the presence of other intravesical pathology.

Treatment and prognosis

Management of zoster-induced urinary retention consists of simple analgesics, antiviral medications, and clean intermittent catheterization (CIC) for a period of 4–8 weeks during which the detrusor slowly returns to normal. Patients should be reassured that the voiding dysfunction is transient and full return to normal detrusor behavior is expected. Repeat urodynamics should be performed on follow-up to confirm this. Dermatologic opinion should be sought at the outset so that appropriate topical management for the blistering rash can be instituted to prevent development of superimposed bacterial cellulitis. Postherpetic neuralgia is rare but may occur.

Genitourinary herpes simplex

Pathophysiology

Infections with the HSV are common in humans. Like varicella-zoster, the virus may afflict the young and healthy as well as the immunocompromised. There are two types: type 1 is associated with orofacial infections and rarely involves the genitals, whereas type 2 is anogenital and often occurs after the onset of sexual activity.[15] The rash of herpes simplex is very similar to varicella-zoster but the distribution of the former is different, being limited to the face for type 1 and to the genitalia for type 2. Both HSV and the varicella-zoster virus may become dormant in the dorsal root ganglia after the initial infection, a feature called neurotropism. Within the cutaneous nerves that are afferent to the infected ganglia, viral proteins as well as perineural and intraneural inflammation have been demonstrated,[16] giving evidence that neurotropic factors may be transported between cutaneous nerve endings and the corresponding dorsal root ganglia, thus explaining the dermatomal distribution of postherpetic neuralgia and the development of the characteristic eruption in varicella-zoster.

Clinical features

Urinary retention in patients with anogenital herpes is not uncommon. Most cases are due to severe dysuria caused by direct contact of urine with the blistering urethral mucosa.[17] It is often seen in sexually active young adults, with no sexual predilection; though in men, it is often in the homosexual population. True neurogenic urinary retention in anogenital HSV infection is rare and occurs in less than 1% of cases.[18] In these cases, the onset of bladder dysfunction occurs typically 1–2 weeks after the onset of a vesicular and painful rash in the anogenital region. The pathogenesis of the neurogenic retention with HSV is localized lumbosacral meningomyelitis, with involvement of mainly sacral nerve roots, or infectious neuritis that affects the pelvic nerves,[1] thus resembling varicella-zoster. Aseptic meningoencephalitis and myelitis may occur. Neurogenic bowel may supervene, leading to constipation.

The neurologic findings are similar to those of its varicella-zoster counterpart. There may be blunting of sensation to light touch and pinprick over the sacral dermatomes. The bulbocavernous and anal reflexes are often intact, but may be reduced or absent, which suggests sacral involvement. Motor function is not affected.

Clinical and urodynamic diagnosis

The diagnosis can be clinched from the history, characteristic rash, and raised level of anti-HSV immunoglobulin M (IgM) titers. Depending on the patient's sexual habits, a full oropharyngeal, rectal, genital, and vaginal speculum examination should be performed to assess disease extent and to exclude other sexually transmitted diseases. Midstream urine should be collected to exclude bacterial infection, and appropriate investigations should be performed if other sexually transmitted diseases are suspected. Counseling is advised for contact tracing and treatment.

Urodynamically, there is often detrusor areflexia with impaired or absent sensation of bladder fullness. The detrusor is also acontractile. These changes are fully reversible, often within 4–8 weeks, but recovery taking up to months has been reported.[17,19]

Treatment and prognosis

Treatment is directed towards effective bladder drainage during the areflexic and acontractile phase by CIC for about 4–8 weeks. Any superimposed urine infection should be treated, but prophylactic antibiotics are not necessary. Follow-up should include repeat urodynamics to document full recovery of both storage and voiding phases of the micturition cycle. The patient should be reassured that the bladder dysfunction is temporary and reversible. Systemic antiviral therapy may be indicated in some patients to shorten the course of skin lesions. Postherpetic neuralgia is a rare but significant complication.

Caveat

Although the pathology and management of HSV and HZV are similar, it is important to point out that bladder dysfunction is an uncommon complication of herpes virus infection. Any patients, especially in the younger age group, who present with unexplained bladder dysfunction without the typical skin lesions should be investigated for neurologic pathology, some of which includes multiple sclerosis, lumbosacral disc prolapse, lumbar canal stenosis, spinal cord or brain tumors, other forms of viral sacral radiculomyelitis, spina bifida occulta, primary bladder neck obstruction, or Fowler's syndrome.

Neuropathic bladder dysfunction from tabes dorsalis

Pathophysiology

Syphilis is a sexually transmitted disease caused by the spirochete *Treponema pallidum*. Voiding dysfunction secondary to neurosyphilis is nowadays a very rare finding in the developed world, but may still be endemic in some underdeveloped countries. Approximately 10% of patients with primary syphilis will develop neurosyphilis. More males are affected than females. There are different types of neurosyphilis: asymptomatic, meningovascular, and parenchymatous.[20] The asymptomatic form only has positive cerebrospinal fluid. The meningovascular form involves the vasculature and meninges. If it affects the lumbosacral spinal cord, bladder dysfunction may result. As the posterior spinal cord mediates sensation, lumbosacral meningomyelitis may cause decreased bladder sensation and increased bladder capacity. Parenchymatous neurosyphilis includes syndromes known as tabes dorsalis and general paresis of the insane. Tabes dorsalis is a demyelinating atrophy of the dorsal spinal cord that affects the posterior column, resulting in impaired bladder sensation, detrusor areflexia, and hence overdistention and eventual detrusor decompensation if left untreated. Out of the three forms of neurosyphilis, parenchymatous neurosyphilis presents the latest, occasionally up to 20 years after the primary infection.

Clinical and urodynamic diagnosis

Definitive diagnosis of syphilis is done by darkfield examination or direct immunofluorescent antibody tests of lesion exudates. Serologic diagnosis is complementary. The rapid plasma reagin (RPR) and Venereal Disease Research Laboratory (VDRL) tests are not antibody-based and can be used to gauge disease activity as results are reported quantitatively, whereas the fluorescent treponemal antibody absorption test (FTA-ABS) is antibody-based and its level correlates poorly with disease activity.[21] False-negatives may occur with the FTA-ABS during the window period of initial infection and in immunocompromised patients. Hence a combination of both antibody and nonantibody-based tests is often necessary in patient management.

Urodynamics often demonstrate detrusor areflexia with reduced or absent bladder sensation and increased bladder capacity. Suprasacral as well as sacral cord involvement may occur, leading to reduced bladder compliance, detrusor hyperreflexia with detrusor-sphincter dyssynergia, or detrusor hypocontractility with large postvoid residual urine.[22,23]

Treatment and prognosis

Detrusor areflexia, bladder sensation, and bladder capacity often improve with time after treatment with penicillin, but may not return entirely to normal.[20] Timed voiding can be used to promote bladder drainage in those where contractility is not affected. Intermittent catheterization is necessary if hypocontractility with large postvoid residuals is present. A case of hyperreflexia requiring urinary diversion was reported.[23] Appropriate bladder management will facilitate bladder drainage, prevent urinary tract infection, and avoid renal damage.

Neuropathic bladder due to Guillain–Barré syndrome

Pathophysiology

Guillain–Barré syndrome (GBS) is an immune-mediated neurologic disorder affecting both small and large myelinated axons, causing acute progressive weakness, usually an ascending paralysis, with 30% of the affected having respiratory paralysis necessitating mechanical ventilation.[24,25] Complete or substantial recovery is the rule. It may manifest either as a demyelinating form or an axonal form. The pathophysiologic mechanism is an autoimmune destruction of myelin by antiganglioside antibodies. Activated T cells, macrophages, and increased matrix metalloproteinases may also play a role.[26] Autonomic neuropathy may be present in up to 50% of patients.[27] The lumbosacral spinal roots and thoracolumbar sympathetic chain may be involved, leading to lower urinary tract dysfunction.[28] It is likely that the condition of acute distal autonomic neuropathy is a form of GBS and may affect the pelvic plexus and its associated nerves (sympathetic and parasympathetic), which may result in lower urinary tract dysfunction.[29]

Clinical and urodynamic features

GBS is not directly genetically inherited, but presumed to be an individual's idiosyncratic response to a preceding infection, which may have a genetic basis. It affects both the pediatric and adult populations.[30] Typical presenting signs and symptoms include paresthesia of hands and feet, acute symmetric ascending weakness of limbs with areflexia, and reduced proprioception. Gait disorder is common in all age groups. Autonomic neuropathy may manifest as labile blood pressure, cardiac arrhythmias, paralytic ileus, or bladder dysfunction. Approximately 25% of patients with GBS show micturition symptoms.[31] These may include hesitancy, poor and prolonged flow, urinary retention, urgency, nocturnal frequency, and urge incontinence, reflecting that both storage and emptying function can be affected. These symptoms are more common in patients with severe weakness (especially those requiring ventilatory assistance) than in those with a mild form of neuropathy, typically present after onset of muscular weakness, and improve gradually with the neurologic signs over time.[32] Constipation as well as erectile dysfunction may also occur.

The diagnosis is made with nerve conduction studies, which are the most sensitive test. Lumbar puncture may show elevated protein, with normal white cell count.[33]

Urodynamics commonly reveal detrusor areflexia and impaired bladder sensation with large postvoid residuals.[34] Detrusor hyperreflexia, both with and without sphincter dyssynergia, has been reported.[35,36] Decreased bladder capacity may occur with hyperreflexia without radiologic evidence of spinal cord involvement, indicating that the overactivity may occur at the peripheral nerve level with probable pelvic nerve irritation.[31]

Treatment and prognosis

From a neurologic aspect, the principle of management is hospitalization with monitoring of respiratory function and elective endotracheal intubation for impending respiratory failure. Intravenous immunoglobulin with plasmapheresis is indicated for patients with severe weakness and rapid progression.[37] With respect to autonomic neuropathy, cardiac monitoring is required for arrhythmias, strict bowel regime for constipation and ileus, and CIC or indwelling urethral catheter for detrusor areflexia or detrusor hyperreflexia with sphincter dyssynergia. Urodynamic parameters improve during the course of the disease approximately 6–8 weeks after the onset of weakness. All patients should be educated that full or significant recovery is expected.

References

1. Yamanishi T, Yasuda K, Sakakibara R, et al. Urinary retention due to herpes virus infections. Neurourol Urodyn 1998; 17: 613–19.
2. Broseta E, Osca JM, Martinez-Agullo J, Jimenez-Cruz JF. Urological manifestations of herpes zoster. Eur Urol 1993; 24: 244–7.
3. Cohen LM, Fowler JF, Owen LG, Callen JP. Urinary retention associated with herpes zoster infection. Int J Dermatol 1993; 32(1): 24–6.
4. Gibbon N. A case of herpes zoster with involvement of urinary bladder. Br J Urol 1956; 28: 417–21.
5. Kendall AR, Karafin L. Classification of neurogenic bladder disease. Urol Clin N Am 1974; 1: 45.

6. Rankin JT, Sutton RA. Herpes zoster causing retention of urine. Br J Urol 1969; 41: 238–41.
7. Bastian FO, Rabson AS, Yee CL, Tralka TS. Herpesvirus varicellae: isolated from human dorsal root ganglia. Arch Pathol 1974; 97: 331–3.
8. Jellinek EH, Tulloch WS. Herpes zoster with dysfunction of bladder and anus. Lancet 1976; 2: 1219–22.
9. Richmond W. The genitourinary manifestations of herpes zoster. Three case reports and a review of the literature. Br J Urol 1974; 46: 193–200.
10. Gold I, Azizi E, Eshel G. Neurogenic bladder due to herpes zoster infection in an infant. Eur J Pediatr 1989; 148(5): 468–9.
11. Ginsberg PC, Harkaway RC, Elisco AJ III, Rosenthal BD. Rare presentation of acute urinary retention secondary to herpes zoster. J Am Osteopath Assoc 1998; 98(9): 508–9.
12. Ray B, Wise G. Urinary retention associated with herpes zoster. J Urol 1970; 104: 422–5.
13. Tsai HN, Wu WJ, Huang SP, et al. Herpes zoster induced neuropathic bladder – a case report. Kaohsiung J Med Sci 2002; 18(1): 39–44.
14. Herbaut AG, Nogueira MC, Wespes E. Urinary retention due to sacral myeloradiculitis: a clinical and neurophysiological study. J Urol 1990; 144: 1206–8.
15. Oates JK, Greenhouse PR. Retention of urine in anogenital herpetic infection. Lancet 1978; 1: 691–2.
16 Worrell JT, Cockerell CJ. Histopathology of peripheral nerves in cutaneous herpes virus infection. Am J Dermatopathol 1997; 19: 133–7.
17. Clason AE, McGeorge A, Garland C, Abel BJ. Urinary retention and granulomatous prostatitis following sacral herpes zoster infection. Br JUrol 1982; 54: 166–9.
18. Greenstein A, Matzkin H, Kaver I, Braf Z. Acute urinary retention in herpes genitalis infection. Urology 1988; 31(5): 453–6.
19. Riehle RA Jr, Williams JJ. Transient neuropathic bladder following herpes simplex genitalis. J Urol 1979; 122(2): 263–4.
20. Wheeler JS Jr, Culkin DJ, O'Hara RJ, Canning JR. Bladder dysfunction and neurosyphilis. J Urol 1986; 136: 903–5.
21. Krieger JN. Sexually transmitted diseases. In: Tanagho E, McAninch J, eds. Smith's General Urology, 15th edn. Columbus: McGraw-Hill, 2000: 287–99.
22. Garber SJ, Christmas TJ, Rickards D. Voiding dysfunction due to neurosyphilis. Br J Urol 1990; 66(1): 19–21.
23. Hattori T, Yasuda K, Kita K, Hirayama K. Disorders of micturition in tabes dorsalis. Br J Urol 1990; 65(5): 497–9.
24. Fowler CJ. Neurological disorders of micturition and their treatment. Brain 1999; 122(7): 1213–31.
25. Arnason BGW, Soliven B. Acute inflammatory demyelinating polyradiculoneuropathy. In: Dyck PJ, Thomas PK, eds. Peripheral Neuropathy, 3rd edn. Philadelphia: WB Saunders, 1993: 1437–97.
26. Pascuzzi R, Fleck J. Acute peripheral neuropathy in adults. Neurol Clin 1997; 15(3): 529–48.
27. Tuck RR, McLeod JG. Autonomic dysfunction in Guillain–Barré syndrome. J Neurol Neurosurg Psychiatry 1981; 52: 857–64.
28. Honavar M, Tharakan JKJ, Hughes RAC, et al. A clinicopathological study of the Guillain–Barré syndrome; nine cases and literature review. Brain 1991; 114: 1245–69.
29. Kirby RS, Fowler CJ, Gosling JA, Bannister R. Bladder dysfunction in distal autonomic neuropathy of acute onset. J Neurol Neurosurg Psychiatry 1985; 48: 762–7.
30. Evans O, Vedanarayanan V. Guillain–Barré syndrome. Pediatr Rev 1997; 18(1): 10–17.
31. Zochodne D. Autonomic involvement in Guillain–Barré syndrome: a review. Muscle Nerve 1994; 17: 1145–55.
32. Sakakibara R, Hattori T, Kuwabara S, et al. Micturitional disturbance in patients with Guillain–Barré syndrome. J Neurol Neurosurg Psychiatry 1997; 63: 649–53.
33. Wexler I. Serial sensory and motor conduction measurement in Guillain–Barré syndrome. Clin Neurophysiol 1980; 20(2): 87–103.
34. Wheeler JS Jr, Siroky MB, Pavlakis A, Krane RJ. The urodynamic aspects of Guillain–Barré syndrome. J Urol 1984; 131(5): 917–19.
35. Grbavac Z, Gilja I, Gubarev N, Bozicevic D. Neurologic and urodynamic characteristics of patients with Guillain–Barré syndrome. Lijec Vjesn 1989; 111(1–2): 17–20.
36. Kogan BA, Soloman MH, Diokno AC. Urinary retention secondary to Landry–Guillain–Barré syndrome. J Urol 1981; 126: 643–4.
37. Bella I, Chad D. Neuromuscular disorders and acute respiratory failure. Neurol Clin 1998; 6(2): 391–417.

19

Peripheral neuropathies of the lower urinary tract following pelvic surgery and radiation therapy

Richard T Kershen and Timothy B Boone

Introduction

Though control and coordination of micturition is relegated to higher centers in the brain and spinal cord, the lower urinary tract is ultimately innervated by the 'hard wiring' of peripheral nerves, conveying essential neurotransmission of the autonomic and somatic nervous systems. Iatrogenic damage to peripheral nerves of the bladder, urethra, and pelvic floor during the course of surgical endeavors or radiotherapy may result in significant patient morbidity in terms of resultant vesicourethral dysfunction. Voiding dysfunction resulting from extirparative or ablative therapies aimed at the treatment of cancer may be physically and socially devastating for a patient. It is important for the pelvic surgeon and radiotherapist alike to be familiar with the complex innervation of the bladder and urethra in order to reduce the likelihood of injury to peripheral nerves during the course of therapy. In addition, the urologist must be familiar with the signs, symptoms, and typical urodynamic manifestations of peripheral nerve injury in order to facilitate precise physiologic diagnosis and optimize treatment strategies. It is appropriate to begin our discussion with a review of the anatomy of the peripheral nervous system as it pertains to innervation and neural control of the lower urinary tract.

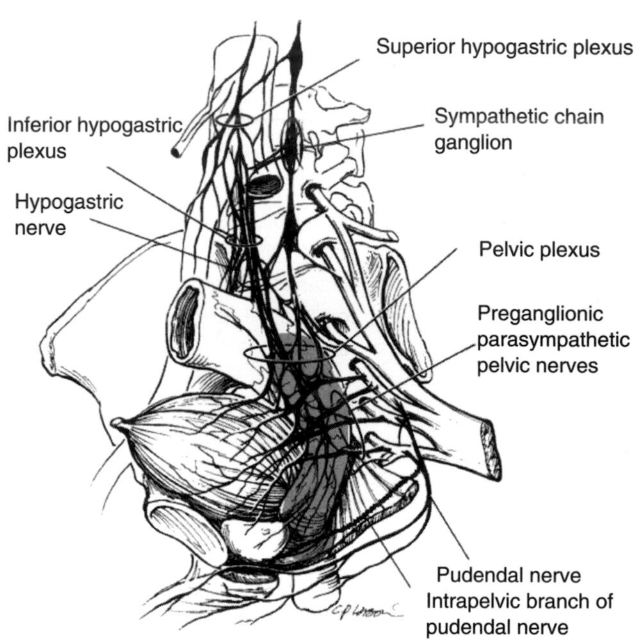

Figure 19.1
Peripheral innervation of the lower urinary tract.

Anatomic considerations in lower urinary tract innervation

Both the autonomic and somatic nervous systems are integrally responsible for innervation of the lower urinary tract. In essence, the lower urinary tract is innervated by three sets of peripheral nerves, representing the parasympathetic, sympathetic, and somatic nervous systems (Figure 19.1).[1] Each nerve conveys both sensory and motor fibers to and from the central nervous system. The parasympathetic input originates from the sacral spinal cord (S2–4) in the sacral parasympathetic nucleus located in the intermediolateral cell column.[2] Long, preganglionic parasympathetic nerve fibers travel within the pelvic nerve to synapse with their short, postganglionic counterparts in the pelvic plexus or detrusor muscle itself. Stimulation of the parasympathetic system results in detrusor contraction and urethral relaxation. Consequently, damage to the parasympathetic input will result in detrusor hyporeflexia or areflexia.[3] The sympathetic input arises in the intermediolateral cell columns of the thoracolumbar spinal cord (T11–12, L1–3). Preganglionic sympathetic nerve fibers arise from lumbosacral sympathetic chain ganglia traveling in lumbar spanchnic nerves composing the superior hypogastric plexus, which then bifurcates below the great vessels, forming paired hypogastric nerves which ultimately synapse with postganglionic sympathetic neurons in the pelvic plexus. Short postganglionic sympathetic nerves then go on to innervate the bladder body, neck, and proximal urethra.[4]

Of note, this arrangement is somewhat atypical for sympathetic nerves, which usually have short preganglionic nerves that synapse far from their target organs. In addition, multiple regions of crossover exist between opposing sides via branches coursing through the inferior mesenteric ganglion. Stimulation of the sympathetic system results in inhibition of bladder contractility as well as an increase in bladder outlet resistance. Damage to the sympathetic input will result in impaired compliance, bladder outlet incompetence, and retrograde ejaculation. Somatic input arises from motor neurons in Onuf's nucleus at the lateral border of the ventral horn of the sacral spinal cord (S2–4). Sacral nerve roots coalesce, forming the pudendal nerve, which travels through the pelvis and perineum, innervating the striated muscle of the external urethral sphincter.

Afferent information from the lower urinary tract is transmitted via pelvic, hypogastric, and pudendal nerves to the lumbosacral spinal cord. Bladder receptors sensing bladder volume and contractility travel in the pelvic nerve to the spinal cord via myelinated Aδ fibers and unmyelinated C fibers. C fibers are also recruited after neurologic insult (spinal cord injury), during times of obstruction or bladder inflammation to convey nociceptive responses.[1]

In the last several years, great strides have been made in our understanding of gross pelvic neuroanatomy due to the work of surgeons who understand the potential for iatrogenic injury during radical pelvic surgery. Hollabaugh and colleagues performed meticulous intrapelvic and perineal dissections under magnification on male and female cadavers hemisected at the level of the sacral promontory.[5] They traced the course of what they called the 'pelvic nerve' which, by description, appears to be the confluence of nerves arising from the pelvic plexus, going on to innervate the pelvic viscera. This nerve, originating over the hypogastric artery, represents a confluence of postganglionic sympathetic and parasympathetic fibers running together from the pelvic plexus. This dense intermingling of sympathetic and parasympathetic nerve fibers arising from the pelvic plexus has been described by other authors.[6] As the nerve enters the pelvis, it gives off multiple web-like branches which travel within the endopelvic fascial sleeve, innervating the detrusor muscle, and other pelvic viscera (colon, rectum, prostate, vagina, and uterus).

The main branch of the nerve was found to travel inferiolateral to the rectum, deep to the levator ani fascia, coursing through the pelvis towards the external sphincter, where it gives off its terminal innervating branches, anterior to the rectum. The pudendal nerve was also traced from its point of origin in the pelvis through its path in Alcock's canal.

It was noted that the pudendal nerve gives off an intrapelvic branch which courses beneath the levator ani fascia and joins the distal aspect of the pelvic nerve at the level of the prostatic apex to innervate the external urinary sphincter. The main trunk of the pudendal nerve then enters Alcock's canal and gives off numerous variable branches within the canal and in the perineum, ultimately terminating in the perineal nerve, providing somatic innervation to the urinary rhabdosphincter. Thus, the external urinary sphincter appears to have a dual innervation, both autonomic from the pelvic nerve and somatic from the intrapelvic and perineal branches of the pudendal nerve.

Strasser and colleagues sought to clarify the neuromuscular function and physiology of the urethra and external urinary sphincter.[7] Performing human cadaveric dissections as well as functional studies in sheep they found, similarly to Hollabaugh's group, that the autonomic fibers that supply the pelvic viscera course as a confluence of nerves lateral to the rectum within the envelope of the levator fascia. In the male, the smooth muscle within the membranous urethra was found to be innervated by autonomic fibers arising from this 'pelvic nerve' via branches derived from a prostatic plexus as well as the periprostatic cavernous nerves, which pass through the urogenital hiatus. In the female, the autonomic nerves to the proximal urethral smooth muscle arose from the pelvic nerve and traveled along the lateral aspects of the uterus and vagina to their point of insertion dorsolaterally.

Functionally, Strasser and colleagues found that stimulation of the pelvic plexus generated strong responses in the proximal urethra, but little in the distal urethra or external rhabdosphincter. Pudendal nerve stimulation, however, resulted in distal urethral smooth muscular contraction as well as the expected rhabdosphincter response. These findings suggest autonomic control over proximal urethral function with the somatic nervous system controling distal urethral function. It is obvious that the peripheral nerves serving the lower urinary tract are diverse, representing multiple targets for injury.

Peripheral neuropathies of the lower urinary tract as a consequence of pelvic surgery

Although peripheral neuropathies affecting bladder and urethral function may result from a variety of causes, including metabolic or infectious disease, degenerative disorders, systemic illnesses, or disc disease, for the purposes of this discussion we will focus on those that arise subsequent to surgical endeavors in the pelvis or ablative radiotherapy.

We will discuss specific mechanisms for injury as well as reported clinical and urodynamic findings correlating with the site of injury. In addition, we will elaborate on methods to prevent and reduce potential injury. Peripheral neuropathy will commonly distort normal motor, sensory, and/or autonomic functions. As the lower urinary tract is limited in its ability to express functional pathology, the presence of neurologic injury will manifest in a finite number of ways, including voiding dysfunction, incontinence, and/or pain. Predicting urodynamic findings for individual cases on the basis of symptomatology and neurologic examination alone is often impossible, and therefore therapy should be directed on the basis of clinical history and thorough urodynamic testing.

Extirpative pelvic surgery has long been associated with lower urinary tract dysfunction. The incidence of vesicourethral dysfunction has been reported to be 8–70% postabdominoperineal resection (APR),[5,8–13] 16–80% posthysterectomy,[14–16] and 20–25% after low anterior resection.[17] The manifestations of, and mechanisms for dysfunction are broad and may vary with the specific type of surgery performed and the initial indication for surgery (as pelvic malignancies themselves have been implicated in vesicourethral dysfunction).[18]

In general, notwithstanding iatrogenic injury resulting in gross anatomic derangements of the bladder, urethra, or sphincter themselves, neurologic injury is usually implicated as the causative factor. The exact nature of the neurological lesion may be difficult to predict by history alone however, due to the potential for partial or complete autonomic and/or somatic denervation. Transient neuropraxic injuries may occur due to neural traction during surgery. Urodynamic evaluation has proven invaluable for proper assessment of these patients, aiding in precise characterization of the neurologic lesion. As detailed earlier, our expanding knowledge of pelvic neuroanatomy and the neurophysiology of normal voiding has, in recent years, allowed modifications of extirpative surgical procedures which may reduce or eliminate negative iatrogenic sequelae on the lower urinary tract.

For the purposes of this chapter we will discuss specific surgical procedures, elucidating the mechanisms for injury and the clinical spectra of the subsequent neuropathies that develop. Neurologically-induced voiding dysfunction from peripheral neuropathy may either resolve during the early postoperative period (weeks to months) or stabilize and persist for years postoperatively. The most typical clinical manifestations of enduring peripheral nerve injury affecting the lower urinary tract after pelvic extirpative surgery will include large urinary residuals, incomplete emptying, and Valsalva voiding.[19] The classic functional pathology will include a noncontractile bladder (areflexic or underactive detrusor) with or without a relaxed urinary sphincter (denervated or underactive).[20] Generally, a parasympathetic injury will result in detrusor hypoactivity with varying degrees of bladder paralysis. Sympathetic injury may manifest as alpha- or beta-adrenergic denervation. Beta-adrenergic denervation may result in poor bladder compliance and occasionally detrusor hyperactivity.[19] Alpha-adrenergic denervation typically manifests as bladder neck incompetence. Of note, male patients with autonomic injury related to pelvic neuropathy often complain of coexistent erectile dysfunction.

Neurourologic examination

Iatrogenic peripheral nerve injury resulting in lower urinary tract dysfunction may have a variable presentation including sensory and/or motor neuropathy of the bladder with or without urethral sphincteric dysfunction. A focused neurourologic exam may provide clues to the underlying nature of the pathology, but may not necessarily be diagnostic. Unlike patients with spinal cord injuries, patients with peripheral nerve injury, with intact central nervous systems, will not exhibit abnormalities in lower extremity tone or reflex response. Competency of the sacral reflex arc may be assessed, however, via elicitation of the bulbocavernosus reflex. The glans penis or clitoris is manually stimulated and the anal sphincteric response is assessed. Absence or prolongation of this reflex suggests peripheral nerve injury in this subset of patients. Decreased or absent anal sphincteric tone may suggest pudendal motor nerve injury. Sensory examination of the perineum to assess vibratory and tactile sense should be performed to determine the likelihood of pudendal sensory neuropathy.

Urodynamic evaluation

The utility of preoperative urodynamics in any patient undergoing extirpative pelvic surgery cannot be adequately emphasized. Such studies may prove invaluable when faced with a patient complaining about postoperative voiding dysfunction. Preoperative voiding dysfunction due to pre-existing bladder outlet obstruction or, potentially, a preoperative peripheral nerve lesion from the primary pelvic pathologic process may be present, and complicate the interpretation of postoperative symptoms if previously undiagnosed. In addition, a pre-existing neuropathy related to tumor infiltration may indicate the potential risk for intraoperative injury during resection.

We typically perform initial postoperative urodynamic evaluations by the 3rd or 4th week after surgery. It is apparent that a variety of sympathetic, parasympathetic, and/or somatic injuries may occur and will require complete urodynamic evaluation to correctly identify the nature of the pathology. Videourodynamics with abdominal and vesical pressure monitoring as well as electromyography (EMG) of the pelvic floor/striated sphincter complex allows precise diagnosis. Abdominal pressure monitoring is essential for the determination of the true detrusor pressure, as many patients will suffer from areflexia.[21]

The absence of a detrusor contraction during urodynamics does not prove areflexia and the presence of abdominal straining will assist in the diagnosis. Pressure–flow evaluation will allow a precise diagnosis of obstruction if present. Indeed, Blaivas and Barbalias found significant obstruction from BPH in 4 of 5 males with urinary retention after APR.[13] Pelvic floor needle EMG will assist in determining the presence or absence of denervation potentials within the external sphincter. Sacral evoked potentials may also be performed to more accurately assess integrity of the sacral reflex arc.[22]

Abdominoperineal resection

It has long been recognized that radical rectal excision via abdominoperineal resection (APR) has been closely associated with postoperative voiding dysfunction.[23] McGuire performed the first urodynamic characterization of voiding dysfunction in these patients in 1975.[24] He described detrusor areflexia in all patients with variable degrees of internal and external sphincteric weakness. Blaivas and Barbalias subsequently performed videourodynamics on 13 men who had undergone APR.[13] Patients presented with a variety of symptoms including isolated storage problems (incontinence), isolated emptying problems (retention), or combined difficulties with storage and emptying. Interestingly, all patients demonstrated incompetence of the bladder neck (proximal sphincter) on videourodynamic testing, suggesting universal sympathetic denervation. Whether or not a patient was incontinent, however, was dependent upon the degree of concomitant parasympathetic and pudendal denervation. In fact, patients afflicted with the most troublesome sequelae of combined difficulties with storage and emptying (4/13 patients) had evidence of extensive neurologic injury, manifesting detrusor areflexia and an open bladder neck at rest, along with EMG and clinical evidence of a lower motor neuron lesion to the external sphincter (combined parasympathetic, sympathetic, and somatic/pudendal denervation). Overall, clinical and urodynamic evidence of parasympathetic denervation (impaired emptying/areflexia) was present in 38%, and somatic/pudendal denervation was present in 54%.

Yalla and Andriole were interested in the natural history of neurogenically-induced vesicourethral dysfunction in patients who had undergone radical pelvic surgery.[19] They performed both early (2 weeks to 4 months) and delayed (18 months to 3 years) postoperative urodynamic evaluations in patients with voiding dysfunction after APR. Early evaluation revealed the presence of an incompetent bladder neck, detrusor hypertonia (impaired compliance), diminished proprioception, and detrusor hypoactivity or inactivity, suggesting combined parasympathethic and sympathetic denervation. Additionally, patients who demonstrated total incontinence manifested diminished urethral closure pressures with absent reflex activity of the external striated sphincter. Interestingly, a recovery phase was noted with 75% of incontinent patients regaining passive continence within 4 months. This corresponded with the finding of restored urethral closure pressure in the membranous urethra with return of peirurethral striated muscle reflex activity. The bladder neck and prostatic urethra remained incompetent, suggesting recovery of somatic innervation without return of sympathetic urethral innervation. Delayed evaluations revealed persistence of parasympathetic denervation, manifested in a large cystometric capacity with detrusor hypoactivity or inactivity. The presence of bladder neck incompetence, indicative of persistent sympathetic innervation, was variable. Ultimately, 21 of 22 patients had persistent vesicourethral dysfunction with large residuals, and Valsalva voiding after pelvic extirparative surgery.

In summary, the most common urodynamic findings after APR include detrusor hyporeflexia with impaired sensation, increased capacity, and compliance with concomitant incompetence of the bladder neck, suggesting a combined injury to both parasympathetic and sympathetic innervation. Most patients will be continent and have difficulties related to impaired emptying. Incontinent patients after APR will have commonly suffered additional injury to the pudendal nerve, resulting in external sphincteric dysfunction. The more severely incontinent patients may have a higher degree of sympathetic denervation, with a resultant loss of bladder compliance occurring concurrently with decreased or absent proximal and distal sphincteric function. Fortunately, most patients with somatic nerve injury will have recovery of function over time with the return of active and/or passive continence. This may be heralded by the reappearance of the bulbocavernosus reflex. Because slow recovery is the rule, at least a year should lapse after APR before consideration of surgical intervention.

Mechanism for, and means for prevention of neurologic injury during abdominoperineal resection

It is clear that the extent of pelvic dissection during APR relates directly to the degree of subsequent vesicourethral dysfunction.[25] Urologic morbidity may be avoided by a detailed understanding of pelvic neuroanatomy. Indeed,

Hojo and colleagues[25] demonstrated that complete preservation of autonomic innervation allowed 88% of patients undergoing APR to void spontaneously within 10 days of surgery. Conversely, 78% of patients who underwent complete resection of the pelvic autonomic nerves remained in urinary retention by 2 months postoperatively. Damage along the course of the pelvic nerve may result in isolated bladder dysfunction, proximal urethral dysfunction, and/or external sphincteric dysfunction. It appears that avoidance of dissection beneath the presacral fascia will protect the proximal portions of continence-preserving nerves during rectal resection and mesorectal lymphadenectomy. This may avoid damage to the sympathetic fibers of the hypogastric plexus at the level of the pelvic brim, where they course medial to the ureters. The pelvic nerve is susceptible to injury as it courses inferolateral to the rectum towards the prostatic apex. It may be injured during the course of circumferential rectal dissection and during levator ani muscular division, resulting in proximal urethral denervation. Levator ani muscle division will also result in damage to the intrapelvic branch of the pudendal nerve, abolishing its ability to provide innervation to the smooth muscular component of the distal urethral sphincter. Injury to these continence-preserving nerves may be averted by respecting the integrity of Denonviller's fascia near the prostatic apex, and carefully dividing the levator ani away from the intrapelvic branch of the pudendal nerve traveling close to the ischium.[5] In females, preservation of the vagina will also protect these nerves as they travel to the urethra. During perineal dissection, care should be taken to dissect cautiously near the ischial tuberosity, where the terminal branches of the pudendal nerve may be injured as they exit Alcock's canal.

Hysterectomy

Similar to previously outlined experience with APR, the performance of radical hysterectomy has long been associated with the development of postoperative bladder dysfunction.[16,26,27] This relationship owes much to the close anatomic associations between the pelvic plexus and uterosacral and cardinal ligaments.[28] The uterosacral and cardinal ligaments, historically resected in radical hysterectomy, carry autonomic nerve fibers which go on to innervate the bladder and urethra. The uterosacral ligaments themselves contain important pelvic parasympathetic and hypogastric nerve rami. The cardinal ligaments, located at the base of the broad ligaments, surround the cervix and extend laterally to the pelvic sidewalls. Each ligament lays in close proximity to the cervix, at whose inferomedial margin, fibers from the pelvic plexus – predominantly sympathetic in nature – advance in a palpable nerve bundle to eventually innervate the bladder and urethra. As with any radical pelvic operation, damage to the pelvic plexus itself can also occur with aggressive posterior dissection.

Yalla and Andriole noted that nearly all patients with vesicourethral dysfunction after radical hysterectomy suffered parasympathetic denervation.[19] Up to 50% of patients may also have additional sympathetic denervation with the resultant manifestation of vesical hypertonia and incompetency of the bladder neck.[14,15,6,29] Indeed, Iio and colleagues noted urodynamically evident decreases in detrusor compliance and maximal urethral closure pressures in 24 patients who underwent radical hysterectomy.[30] The frequency of sympathetic denervation may correspond to the extent of dissection of the cardinal ligaments and the amount these ligaments are resected.[15] To avoid this injury and spare the sympathetic innervation of the bladder and its base, maintaining proximal urethral function and continence, more conservative surgical approaches (if allowable by the stage of the cervical cancer involved), that preserve the inferior portions of the cardinal ligaments are warranted.

Todo et al recently reported prospective urodynamic data on 27 consecutive patients who underwent radical hysterectomy for cervical cancer using a 'nerve-sparing' technique.[31] Their technique consisted of lateralizing the hypogastric nerves and proximal pelvic plexus during dissection of the uterosacral and rectovaginal ligaments. These nerves were then preserved by selective resection of the remaining exposed portions of the ligaments. In addition, dissection of the pelvic splanchnic nerves was avoided during resection of the cardinal ligaments. The authors were able to implement this technique unilaterally or bilaterally in 22 of 27 patients. In the remaining 5 patients nerves could not be preserved due to bleeding or anatomic difficulties during dissection. Patients underwent pre- and postoperative urodynamics and were followed for one year. Patients who underwent a successful nerve-sparing hysterectomy did not demonstrate any significant changes in bladder compliance, maximal flow rates, or postvoid residual. Patients who failed to have nerves spared demonstrated reductions in bladder compliance and maximal flow rates, and had higher postvoid residuals. Though both groups demonstrated reduced voiding pressures at maximal flow compared to preoperatively, the non-nerve-sparing patients appeared to void predominantly via the Valsalva maneuver. This study, though preliminary and nonrandomized, implies that nerve-sparing hysterectomy may help to preserve vesicourethral function.

Kuwabara and colleagues were the first to propose using intraoperative electrical stimulation of the cardinal ligaments to identify the location of the vesical branches of the pelvic nerve to assist in nerve preservation.[32] Katahira et al implemented Kuwabara's technique in 17 patients undergoing nerve-sparing radical hysterectomy.[33] The technique involved electrical stimulation of the roots of the pelvic splanchnic nerves and the posterior and dorsal regions of the vesico-uterine ligaments. Simultaneous bladder cystometry was performed during nerve stimulation. An increase in intravesical pressure was observed in 13 of 17 patients with stimulation of these nerves after uterine resection. Of these 13 patients, both pre- and postoperative urodynamic data were available in 8 patients. In all of these patients detrusor contractility was preserved and there were no subjective complaints of voiding difficulties. In the remaining 4 patients, where nerves were apparently damaged (no increase in intravesical pressure was seen with nerve stimulation after uterine removal), all patients developed postoperative detrusor areflexia and voided either by Valsalva or intermittent catheterization. These results, though not conclusive, suggest that intraoperative electrical nerve stimulation may be a useful adjunct to nerve-sparing procedures.

It has been suggested that simple, supracervical hysterectomy may be a less destructive surgical approach, and may reduce the risk of posthysterectomy bladder dysfunction.[34] This, however, is not absolute, as evident in the manuscript by Parys and colleagues who analyzed the clinical spectra of bladder dysfunction after simple hysterectomy.[16] They performed urodynamic studies and sacral reflex latency studies on 126 women with lower urinary tract symptoms after hysterectomy. They found that 86% of patients had a demonstrable urodynamic abnormality, with 47% of patients having detrusor overactivity, 37% having evidence of urethral obstruction, and 25% having evidence of stress incontinence. Sacral reflex latencies were prolonged or absent in 80% of 25 patients studied, suggesting autonomic peripheral neuropathy due to pelvic plexus injury.

Radical prostatectomy

It is clear that incontinence after radical prostatectomy is related to intrinsic sphincter deficiency in the majority of patients. Urodynamic studies in postprostatectomy patients have revealed, however, a high prevalence of concomitant detrusor dysfunction, namely instability and impaired compliance.[35,36] Hubert and colleagues, performed pre- and postoperative bladder biopsies comparing nerve fiber density in the superficial trigone in men undergoing radical prostatectomy.[37] They found that nerve fiber density decreased postoperatively and regenerated over time. Patients with persistent incontinence had less than half the amount of nerve fiber regeneration than continent patients at 6 months postoperatively. Urinary incontinence was associated with trigonal denervation, a high sensory threshold, and a low maximal urethral closure pressure. The authors hypothesized that wide dissection around the prostate, bladder base, and seminal vesicles leads to disruption of bladder and proximal urethral innervation. They suggested that preservation of trigonal innervation may be important for maintenance of continence. When this technique was applied to nerve and seminal vesicle sparing cystectomy, high degrees of urinary continence were achieved, supporting that preservation of the pelvic plexus and trigonal innervation improves urinary continence.[38] Although the etiology may be multifactorial, detrusor dysfunction after radical prostatectomy may indeed be related to peripheral nervous denervation.

Recently, robotic-assisted laparoscopic radical prostatectomy has enabled enhanced, magnified three-dimensional vision and more precise identification and preservation of pelvic nerves.[39] This has led to modifications in surgical technique which may eventually be shown to result in improved outcomes in terms of preserving potency and perhaps vesicourethral function. To date, there are no prospective studies that have proven superiority of this technique in this arena in comparison to standard nerve-sparing radical retropubic prostatectomy. Kaul et al, however, reported on 154 consecutive patients who underwent nerve-sparing robotic-assisted laparoscopic radical prostatectomy using a 'veil of Aphrodite' technique.[40] This technique involves preservation of the lateral prostatic fascia and has been reported to provide 'enhanced nerve sparing' by preventing resection of small nerves relevant to cavernosal innervation, which run in this fascia.[41] The technique also limits the use of cautery around the seminal vesicle to prevent injury to the pelvic plexus. In Kaul's series patients completed self-administered urinary function questionnaires (IPSS) before and one year after surgery. Of the 154 patients, 127 completed the questionnaires. Average IPSS scores decreased from 6 to 3.4 postoperatively, indicating a general improvement in urinary symptoms. The authors reported that 97% of patients had complete urinary control at one year after surgery. Most impressively, 29% of patients were reported continent at the time of catheter removal (usually 7 days postoperatively). On average, most regained complete continence by one month postoperatively. These results suggest that enhanced attention to nerve preservation at the time of radical prostatectomy may result in improved outcomes in terms of lower urinary tract function. More detailed anatomic and prospective randomized studies are needed to elucidate this mechanism in the future.

Ureteral reimplantation

Voiding dysfunction and urinary retention rarely complicate antireflux surgery. This is most commonly encountered after bilateral extravesical ureteral reimplantation.[42–44] Although urinary retention is usually self-limited, it has been reported to occur in up to 26% of these patients.[45] Several investigators have pursued the etiology of this phenomenon from an anatomic standpoint. Barrieras and colleagues found that, by modifying their technique to minimize dissection below the ureteral hiatus, they were able to reduce the incidence of urinary retention.[44] They hypothesized that this technique limited injury to the autonomic nerve fibers coursing into the bladder in the region of the trigone. Leissner and colleagues went on to confirm this via cadaver dissections that revealed the location of the pelvic plexus to be 1.5 cm dorsomedial to the distal ureter.[42]

Terminal branches from the plexus were identified coursing towards the bladder trigone in a delicate network surrounding the distal ureter. These branches could easily be damaged by dissection outside the plane of the mesoureter or by dissection dorsal and medial to the ureterovesical hiatus. These data support the theory that bladder dysfunction postbilateral extravesical reimplantation may have a similar etiology to that following hysterectomy or APR, namely efferent nerve denervation. The same group of investigators created an animal model of neurologic injury resulting from ureteral dissection at the ureteral hiatus, confirming their previous anatomic findings.[46] Unilateral or bilateral efferent nerve blockade was accomplished via xylocaine (lidocaine (lignocaine)) injection at the ureterovesical junction, which resulted in complete abolishment of motor response to sacral anterior nerve root stimulation.

David et al reported a retrospective review of 50 patients who underwent bilateral nerve-sparing extravesical ureteral reimplantation by a single surgeon.[47] The surgical technique adhered to the principles of limited ureteral dissection, with division of lateral but not dorsomedial ureterovesical attachments, limited cautery use, and preservation of the ureterovesical hiatus. All patients were able to void spontaneously on postoperative day 1 except for one, who voided within 48 hours. The authors concluded that implementation of this technique should eliminate the risk of long-term urinary retention in patients who undergo bilateral extravesical ureteral reimplantation.

Radiation therapy

Radiation therapy (RT) kills neoplastic cells. Unfortunately, its curative potential is limited by its potential to damage normal tissues which lie within its path. For many years it was believed that peripheral nerves were relatively radioresistant and did not serve as 'dose-limiting' structures when planning a course of radiotherapy.[48] In the last decade, however, observation of postirradiation brachial and lumbosacral plexopathies has made it clear that peripheral nerve damage may occur after sufficient dose.[49,50] These plexopathies will result in parasthesias and/or paralysis.[51] In cancer patients, radiation-induced cellular alterations may render peripheral nerves more sensitive to the ill effects of chemotherapy. Alternatively, chemotherapeutic agents may sensitize neural tissues to the effects of radiation.[52] Of note, there is often a lag period between treatment/exposure and the development of symptoms of neurologic injury. This is largely due to the major mechanism by which ionizing radiation causes cellular damage, i.e. destruction of DNA. If sublethal damage incurred by a cell is not repaired, death will occur when the damaged cell attempts to reproduce. When RT has been directed at the peripheral nervous system, cell death may occur months to years later due to slow reproductive cycles of glial and Schwann cells.[53] Peripheral nerve injury may also be incurred by radiation-induced damage to vascular endothelium, obliterating critical neural blood supply. Radiation-induced perineural fibrosis may also result in compression and ischemia of peripheral nerves. Though studies reporting direct radiation-induced injury to the pelvic peripheral nervous system are scarce, there are numerous studies documenting the indirect damage inflicted, inferred by reports of erectile and bladder dysfunction postradiotherapy.[54–56] For the purposes of this discussion we shall focus on radiation-induced peripheral neuropathies leading to bladder dysfunction.

The pelvis is a relatively confined space that contains closely approximated visceral organs including the bladder, prostate, uterus, and rectosigmoid portions of the large intestine. As previously discussed, these organs are in close proximity to the autonomic and somatic nerves which innervate them. External beam RT designated for any one particular organ will therefore inevitably result in simultaneous radiation exposure to other vital structures, including blood vessels and peripheral nerves.

There have been successful attempts to limit radiation exposure to bystander tissues, including three-dimensional treatment plans, conformal radiation, stereotactic radiosurgery, and brachytherapy. Due to the anatomically close relationship between the pelvic viscera and their innervating nerves, however, it is likely that peripheral nerve exposure and subsequent injury will occur with any treatment modality implemented in the pelvis. In fact, Tait and colleagues did not find a significant difference in the prevalence of urinary symptoms in patients receiving conformal versus conventional pelvic RT for the treatment of pelvic malignancies.[57] Even low-dose radiotherapy can inflict significant damage. Indeed, animal studies have revealed the threshold dose for peripheral neuropathy following RT is merely 15–20 Gy, well below the normal dose utilized for most pelvic malignancies.[58,59] Unfortunately, the same anatomic relationships that render peripheral nerves susceptible to injury during RT lead to difficulties distinguishing whether peripheral nerve injury alone is responsible for dysfunctional changes within the lower urinary tract. The bladder and urethra themselves will often be incidentally exposed to RT (intentionally at times), resulting in direct radiation damage to microvascular, epithelial, and muscular components, and anatomically-mediated dysfunction.

Functional changes in the lower urinary tract have been reported after pelvic RT for the treatment of prostate, bladder, rectal, cervical, and uterine cancers.[57,60–63] Behr and colleagues performed urodynamic testing on 104 patients who received pelvic irradiation for cervical carcinoma with maximal follow-up of 10 years.[64] Sixty percent of patients developed *de-novo* urge incontinence related to detrusor instability concomitant with poor vesical compliance and diminished cystometric capacity. While maximal urethral closure pressures were initially unchanged by irradiation, the risk for stress urinary incontinence (SUI) increased over time and was significant by 6 years post-therapy. This suggests the possibility for neurogenically-mediated vesical and urethral dysfunction.

The delay in the development of SUI may be related to the gradual dying off of the sympathetic and pudendal nerve supply to the urethral sphincteric mechanism. In agreement with this theory are the observations of Litwin and colleagues, who showed that the time course for decline in urinary function in patients who received RT differed from that of patients who underwent radical prostatectomy for prostate cancer. Patients who received RT experienced a gradual decline in urinary function and an increase in urinary bother from irritative symptoms with time up to one year post-therapy where symptoms approached the severity of patients who underwent radical prostatectomy.[61]

Severe urgency/frequency syndrome and urge incontinence in post-RT patients were also identified by Parkin and colleagues.[60] Hanfmann and colleagues noted a decrease in micturitional volumes to 70% of that observed before RT for prostate cancer by 6 weeks after therapy.[63] At surgical exploration, Sindelar and colleagues identified perineural fibrosis in pelvic nerve trunks in patients who received RT for treatment of pelvic sarcomas.[65] This finding suggests RT-mediated peripheral nerve injury as a viable source for lower urinary tract dysfunction. Michailov and colleagues perfomed muscle bath contractile studies on rat detrusor strips exposed to external beam radiation. An increase in basal tone was noted occurring simultaneously with a decreased sensitivity to acetylcholine-mediated contraction. These data infer a possible mechanism for end-organ neurogenic injury to result in the observed clinical effects of hypertonia, decreased functional capacity, and diminished micturitional pressure.[66] It is evident that more studies need to be performed to evaluate the effects and functional consequences of RT on pelvic peripheral nerves. From indirect evidence, however, it is apparent that radiation-mediated peripheral nerve injury has a role in post-RT bladder dysfunction.

Managing the patient with vesicourethral dysfunction related to peripheral nerve injury

As a general rule, treatment of vesicourethral dysfunction after peripheral nerve injury should be directed by the urodynamic findings. As the time course and completeness of recovery after surgery or radiotherapy are not predictable, conservative treatment should be implemented initially prior to any irreversible surgical endeavors. For the patient in urinary retention, clean intermittent catheterization (CIC) is preferable to a chronic indwelling Foley catheter. The presence or absence of bladder outlet obstruction as well as sphincteric integrity should be established to determine the potential beneficial or harmful effects of transurethral resection. In the case of the hypocontractile detrusor, CIC may be continued indefinitely until the return of bladder contractility. A period of at least 6 months should pass before considering any definitive surgical intervention in the patient with sphincteric incontinence or poor compliance, as the natural history of peripheral nerve injury suggests that function may return over time.

Summary

Iatrogenic injury to peripheral nerves innervating the lower urinary tract during the course of pelvic surgery or radiotherapy may result in significant vesicourethral dysfunction. Detailed knowledge of the neuroanatomy and physiology of the bladder and urethra will help avoid these injuries in patients requiring these interventions. Should injury occur, urodynamic evaluation is key for the detection of concomitant pathology and planning management to restore vesicourethral function.

References

1. Chancellor MB, Yoshimura N. Physiology and pharmacology of the bladder and urethra. In Walsh PC, Retik AL, Vaughan ED et al, eds. Campbell's Urology, 8th edn. Philadelphia: WB Saunders, 2002: 846–8.
2. de Groat WC, Vizzard MA, Araki I, Roppolo JR. Spinal interneurons and preganglionic neurons in sacral autonomic reflex pathways. In Holstege G, Bandler R, Saper C (eds): The Emotional Motor System. Progr Brain Res 1996; 107: 97.
3. de Groat WC, Booth AM. Physiology of the urinary bladder and urethra. Ann Intern Med 1980; 92: 312.
4. Kihara K, de Groat WC. Sympathetic efferent pathways projecting to the bladder neck and proximal urethra in the rat. J Auton Nerv Syst 1997; 62: 134.
5. Hollabaugh, RS, Steiner MS, Sellers KD et al. Neuroanatomy of the pelvis: implications for colonic and rectal resection. Dis Colon Rectum 2000; 43(10): 1390–7.
6. Mundy AR. An anatomical explanation for bladder dysfunction following rectal and uterine surgery. BJU 1982; 54: 501–4.
7. Strasser H, Ninkovic M, Hess M et al. Anatomic and functional studies of the male and female urethral sphincter. World J Urol 2000; 8: 324–9.
8. Burgos FJ, Romero J, Fernandez E, Perales L, Tallada M. Risk factors for developing voiding dysfunction after abdominoperineal resection for adenocarcinoma of the rectum. Dis Colon Rectum 1988; 31: 682–5.

9. Kinn AC, Ohman U. Bladder and sexual function after surgery for rectal cancer. Dis Colon Rectum 1986; 29: 43–8.
10. Aagaard J, Gerstenberg TC, Knudsen JJ. Urodynamic investigation predicts bladder dysfunction at an early state after abdominoperineal resection of the rectum for cancer. Surgery 1986; 99: 564–8.
11. Gerstenberg TC, Neilsen ML, Clausen S et al. Bladder function after abdominoperineal resection of the rectum for anorectal cancer: urodynamic investigation before and after operation in a consecutive series. Ann Surg 1980; 191: 81.
12. Hojo K, Sawada T, Moriya Y. An analysis of survival and voiding, sexual function after wide iliopelvic lymphadenectomy in patients with carcinoma of the rectum, compared with conventional lymphadenectomy. Dis Colon Rectum 1989; 32: 128–33.
13. Blaivas JG, Barbalias GA. Characteristics of neural injury after abdominoperineal resection. J Urol 1983; 129: 84.
14. Seski JC, Diokno AC. Bladder dysfunction after radical abdominal hysterectomy. Am J Obstet Gynecol 1977; 128: 643.
15. Forney JP. The effect of radical hysterectomy on bladder physiology. Am J Obstet Gynecol 1980; 138: 374.
16. Parys BT, Woolfenden KA, Parsons KF. Bladder dysfunction after simple hysterectomy: urodynamic and neurological evaluation. Eur Urol 1990: 17: 129–33.
17. Kirkegaard P, Hjortrup A, Sanders S. Bladder dysfunction after low anterior resection for mid-rectal cancer. Am J Surg 1981; 141: 266.
18. Fowler JW, Bremner DN, Moffat LEF. The incidence and consequences of damage to the parasympathetic nerve supply to the bladder after abdominoperineal resection of the rectum for carcinoma. Br J Urol 1978; 50: 95.
19. Yalla SV, Andriole GL. Vesicourethral dysfunction following pelvic visceral surgery. J Urol 1981; 32: 503–9.
20. Norris JP, Staskin DR. History, physical examination, and classification of neurogenic voiding dysfunction. Urol Clin N Am 1996; 23(3): 337–43.
21. Nickell K, Boone TB. Peripheral neuropathy and peripheral nerve injury. Urol Clin N Am 1996; 23(3): 337–43.
22. Siroky MB, Sax DS, Krane RJ. Sacral signal tracing: the electrophysiology of the bulbocavernosus reflex. J Urol 1979; 122: 661–4.
23. Simmons HT. Retention of urine after excision of the rectum. Br Med J 1938; 1: 171.
24. Mcguire EJ. Urodynamic evaluation after abdominoperineal resection and lumbar intervertebral disk herniation. Urol 1975; 6: 63.
25. Hojo K, Vernava AM 3rd, Sugihara K et al. Preservation of urine voiding and sexual function after rectal cancer surgery. Dis Colon Rectum 1991; 34: 532–9.
26. Fishman IJ, Shabsigh R, Kaplan AL. Lower urinary tract dysfunction after radical hysterectomy for carcinoma of the cervix. Urol 1986; 28: 462–8.
27. Fraser AC. The late effects of Wertheims's hysterectomy on the urinary tract. J Obstet Gynaecol Br Commonw 1966; 73: 1002–7.
28. Tong XK, Huo RJ. The anatomical basis and prevention of neurogenic voiding dysfunction following radical hysterectomy. Surg Radiol Anat 1991; 13: 145–8.
29. Smith PH, Ballantyne B. The neuroanatomical basis for denervation of the urinary bladder following major pelvic surgery. Br J Surg 1968; 55: 929.
30. Iio S, Yoshioka S, Nishio S et al. Urodynamic evaluation for bladder dysfunction after radical hysterectomy. Jpn J Urol 1993; 84(3): 535–40.
31. Todo Y, Kuwabara H, Watari H et al. Urodynamic study on postsurgical bladder function in cervical cancer treated with systematic nerve-sparing radical hysterectomy. Int J Gynecol Cancer 2006; 16: 369–75.
32. Kuwabara Y, Suzuki M, Hashimoto M et al. New method to prevent bladder dysfunction after radical hysterectomy for uterine cervical cancer. J Obstet Gynecol Res 2000; 26(1): 1–8.
33. Katahira A, Nikura H, Kaiho Y et al. Intraoperative electrical stimulation of the pelvic splanchnic nerves during nerve-sparing radical hysterectomy. Gynecologic Oncology 2005; 98: 462–6.
34. Kilkku P, Hirvonen T, Gronoos M. Supra-vaginal uterine amputation vs. abdominal hysterectomy: the effects on urinary symptoms with special reference to pollakisuria, nocturia and dysuria. Maturitas 1981; 3: 197–204.
35. Ficazzola MA, Nitti VW. The etiology of post-radical prostatectomy incontinence and correlation of symptoms with urodynamic findings. J Urol 1998; 160(4): 1317–20.
36. Winters JC, Appell RA, Rackley RR. Urodynamic findings in post-prostatectomy incontinence. Neurourol Urodyn 1998; 17: 493–8.
37. Hubert J, Hauri D, Leuener M et al. Evidence of trigonal denervation and reinnervation after radical retropubic prostatectomy. J Urol 2001; 165: 111–13.
38. Columbo R, Bertini R, Salonia A et al. Nerve and seminal sparing radical cystectomy with orthotopic urinary diversion for select patients with superficial bladder cancer: an innovative surgical approach. J Urol 2001; 165: 51–5.
39. Takenaka A, Leung R, Fujisawa M et al. Anatomy of autonomic nerve component in the male pelvis: the new concept from a perspective for robotic nerve sparing radical prostatectomy. World J Urol 2006; 24: 136–43.
40. Kaul S, Savera A, Badani K et al. Functional outcomes and oncological efficacy of Vattikuti Institute prostatectomy with Veil of Aphrodite nerve-sparing: an analysis of 154 consecutive patients. BJU Int 2005; 97: 467–72.
41. Savera AT, Kaul S, Badani K et al. Robotic radical prostatectomy with the 'Veil of Aphrodite' technique: histologic evidence of enhanced nerve sparing. Eur Urol 2006; 49: 1065–74.
42. Leissner J, Allhoff EP, Wolff W et al. The pelvic plexus and antireflux surgery: topographical findings and clinical consequences. J Urol 2001; 165(5): 1652–5.
43. Fung LCT, McLorie GA, Jain U et al. Voiding efficiency after ureteral reimplantation: a comparison of extravesical and intravesical techniques. J Urol 1995; 153: 1972.
44. Barrieras D, Lapointe S, Reddy PP et al. Urinary retention after bilateral extravesical ureteral reimplantation: does dissection distal to the ureteral orifice have a role? J Urol 1999; 162: 1197.
45. Zaontz MR, Maizels M, Sugar EC et al. Detrusorraphy: extravesical ureteral advancement to correct vesicoureteral reflux in children. J Urol 1987; 138: 947.
46. Seif C, Braun PM, Martinez Portillo FJ et al. The risk of bladder denervation during antireflux surgery: a reliable neurophysiological model. J Urol 2002; 167(Suppl 4): 426.
47. David S, Kelly C, Poppas DP. Nerve sparing extravesical repair of bilateral vesicoureteral reflux: description of technique and evaluation of urinary retention. J Urol 2004; 172: 1617–20.
48. Rubin P, Cassarett GW eds. Central nervous system. In: Clinical Radiation Pathology. (Philadelphia: WB Saunders); 1968: 609–61.
49. Johnstone PAS, Wassermann EM, O'Connell PG et al. Lumbosacral plexopathy secondary to hyperfractionated radiotherapy: a case presentation and literature review. Radiat Oncol Invest Clin Basic Res 1993; 1: 126–30.
50. Olsen NK, Pfeiffer P, Johannsen L et al. Radiation-induced brachial plexopathy; neurological follow-up in 161 recurrence-free breast cancer patients. Int J Radiat Oncol Biol Phys 1993; 26: 43–9.
51. Esteban A, Traba A. Fasciculation-myokymic activity and prolonged nerve conduction block. A physiopathological relationship in radiation-induced brachial plexopathy. EEG Clin Neurophys 1993; 89(6): 382–91.
52. Keime-Guibert F, Napolitano M, Delattre JY. Neurological complications of radiotherapy and chemotherapy. J Neurol 1998; 245: 695–708.
53. Posner JB. Side effects of radiation therapy. In Posner JB: Neurologic Complications of Cancer. Philadelphia: FA Davis Company, 1995: 312.

54. Crook J, Esche B, Futter N. Effect of pelvic radiotherapy for prostate cancer on bowel, bladder and sexual function: the patient's perspective. Urol 1996; 47(3): 387–94.
55. Incrocci L, Koos Slob A. Incidence, etiology, and therapy for erectile dysfunction after external beam radiotherapy for prostate cancer. Urol 2002; 60: 107.
56. Nguyen LN, Pollack A, Zagars GK. Late effects after radiotherapy for prostate cancer in a randomized dose–response study: results of a self-assessment questionnaire. Urology 1998; 51(6): 991–7.
57. Tait DM, Nahum AE, Meyer LC et al. Acute toxicity in pelvic radiotherapy; a randomized trial of conformal versus conventional treatment. Radiother Oncol 1997; 42: 121–36.
58. Kinsella TJ, DeLuca AM, Barnes M et al. Threshold dose for peripheral neuropathy following intraoperative radiotherapy (IORT) in a large animal model. Int J Radiat Oncol Biol Phys 1991; 20: 697–701.
59. Johnstone PAS, DeLuca AM, Bacher JD et al. Clinical toxicity of peripheral nerve to intraoperative radiotherapy in a canine model. Int J Radiat Oncol Biol Phys 1995; 32(4): 1031–4.
60. Parkin DE, Davis JA, Symonds RP. Long-term bladder symptomatology following radiotherapy for cervical carcinoma. Radiother Oncol 1987; 9(3): 195–9.
61. Litwin MS, Pasta DJ, Yu J et al. Urinary function and bother after radical prostatectomy or radiation for prostate cancer: a longitudinal, multivariate quality of life analysis from the cancer of the prostate strategic urologic research endeavor. J Urol 2000; 164(6): 1973–7.
62. Maier U, Ehrenbock PM, Hofbauer J. Late urological complications and malignancies after curative radiotherapy for gynecological carcinomas: a retrospective analysis of 10,709 patients. J Urol 1997; 158(3): 814–17.
63. Hanfmann B, Engels M, Dorr W. Radiation-induced impairment of urinary bladder function. Assessment of micturition volumes. Strahlenther Onkol 1998; 174(Suppl 3): 96–8.
64. Behr J, Winkler M, Willgeroth F. Functional changes in the lower urinary tract after irradiation of cervix carcinoma. Strahlenther Onkol 1990; 166(2): 135–9.
65. Sindelar WF, Hoekstra H, Restrepo C et al. Pathological tissue changes following intraoperative radiotherapy. Am J Clin Oncol 1986; 9(6): 504–9.
66. Michailov MC, Neu E, Tempel K. Influence of x–irradiation on the motor activity of rat urinary bladder in vitro and in vivo. Strahlenther Onkol 1991; 167(5): 311–18.

20

Dementia and lower urinary tract dysfunction

Ryuji Sakakibara and Takamichi Hattori

Introduction

Urinary incontinence, dementia, and osteoporosis are major concerns in geriatric populations, which have grown rapidly in recent decades. Of the three, urinary incontinence is most often associated with dementia, since both conditions originate from the same underlying disorder and urinary incontinence occurs secondarily from dementia. Urinary incontinence can result in medical morbidity, impaired self-esteem, early institutionalization, stress on caregivers, and considerable financial cost. However, incontinence in persons with dementia has received limited study. In some nursing home settings, incontinence may be accepted as the norm and approached with therapeutic nihilism even though it is a potentially treatable condition. This chapter reviews the current concepts in lower urinary tract dysfunction associated with dementia, with particular reference to its prevalence, etiology, mechanism, and management.

Prevalence

Prevalence rate of urinary incontinence

Of the lower urinary tract dysfunctions in patients with dementia, urinary incontinence and its prevalence have been the focus of most investigators.[1–14] Many studies have relied on both patient and family/caregiver reports, since patients with dementia may underreport the problem owing to underrecognition, forgetfulness, or embarrassment. Possibly owing to differences in patient selection among these studies, incontinence prevalence rates have varied considerably, from 11% to 90% of individuals with dementia (Table 20.1). As expected, institutional samples had the highest prevalence (90%), with progressively lower rates reported for mixed institutional-community dwelling samples (around 40%) and individuals attending outpatient clinics and living at home (lowest prevalence, 11%).

The International Continence Society defines urinary incontinence as 'the involuntary loss of urine which is a social or hygienic problem and is objectively demonstrable'.[15,16] This definition implies a certain severity of incontinence, although many studies have looked at the presence or absence of urinary incontinence.

Ouslander et al[7] found that 65% of incontinent subjects had fewer than three episodes per week, 11% had three to six episodes per week, and 24% had incontinence once a day or more. McLaren et al[14] found that 90% of incontinent subjects had at least one episode during the 3-week assessment period, 78% had one episode a week, and 40% had incontinence once a day. Thus, according to these studies, more than two-thirds of incontinent patients with dementia have at least one episode a week. This figure contrasts with general population surveys of elderly individuals, of whom about 5% have urine loss at least once a week.[17] According to Campbell et al,[10] urinary incontinence was found in 53% of patients with dementia and in 13% of nondemented older individuals.

In post-stroke patients who were admitted to a rehabilitation program, Noto[12] found that urinary incontinence was present in 83% of patients with dementia and in 45% of nondemented patients. Institutional residents with dementia who were continent on admission were more likely to develop incontinence during a 12-month follow-up period, and incontinence was less likely to resolve in those individuals.[18,19] In addition, dementia is more prevalent in incontinent individuals than in those without. Palmer et al[18] and Ouslander et al[19] reported that 83% of incontinent nursing home residents had dementia, compared with only 58% of continent residents. Thus, these community-based and institutional studies confirm the frequent association between urinary incontinence and cognitive impairment.

However, it should be emphasized that association does not imply causation. Many studies were performed irrespective of underlying disease, even though it can considerably affect the prevalence rates of incontinence. As expected, compared with multi-infarct dementia, Berrios[6] found that incontinence was more prevalent in Alzheimer's

Table 20.1 *Prevalence of urinary incontinence in persons with dementia*

Study	Year	Setting	*n*	Mean age (years)	Dementia type	Rate of incontinence (%)	Reference
Teri	1989	Dementia clinic	56	71	AD	11	1
Teri	1988	Dementia clinic	127	77	AD	15	2
Teri	1990	Dementia clinic	106	77	AD	15	3
Swearer	1988	Dementia clinic	95	69	AD/MID/mixed	17	4
Udaka	1994	Neurology inpatients/outpatients	38	69	AD	21	5
Berrios	1986	Psychiatry outpatients	100	80	AD/MID/mixed	35	6
Ouslander	1990	Community	184	76	AD/MID/mixed	36	7
Rabins	1982	Psychiatry inpatients/outpatients	55	–	AD/MID/other	40	8
Burns	1990	Psychiatry inpatients/outpatients	178	80	AD	48	9
Campbell	1985	Random survey: home/institution	83	>64	–	53	10
Borrie	1992	Chronic care hospital	139	–	–	78	11
Noto	1994	Rehabilitation hospital	36	68	MID	83	12
Toba	1996	Chronic care hospital	867	>64	–	89	13
Mclaren	1981	Psychogeriatric inpatients	121	81	AD/MID	90	14

disease, which is the major etiology of severe cognitive decline. However, in dementia outpatient clinics, Teri et al[1–3] found urinary incontinence in only 11–15% of patients with Alzheimer's disease. On the other hand, Kotsoris et al[20] found urinary incontinence in up to 50% of 84 outpatients with multi-infarct dementia. Thus, urinary incontinence in multiple cerebral infarction tends to appear earlier than in Alzheimer's disease. Of particular importance is that urinary incontinence in those patients was not always accompanied by dementia and was often preceded by urinary frequency and urgency.[21] This implies that urinary incontinence in multiple cerebral infarction may have a different mechanism than in Alzheimer's disease, as will be discussed later.

Sex distribution

Among adults older than 60 years of age, urinary incontinence is twice as common in women as in men, reflecting anatomic differences in the urethra and the pelvic floor muscles that lead to stress urinary incontinence.[17] Alzheimer's disease also occurs more commonly in women. However, previous studies did not find a significant difference in the prevalence of incontinence between men and women with dementia.[6,7,9] On the contrary, Ouslander et al[19] reported that urinary incontinence was twice as prevalent in males as in females, and Palmer et al[18] found that male gender increased the probability of urinary incontinence by 68% 1 year after admission to a nursing home. These results are in line with the findings that men deteriorate mentally and physically more severely than women after admission to nursing homes.[18] The presence of prostatic hypertrophy predisposing to urinary overflow, combined with the male predominance of multi-infarct dementia, may explain these findings.[18,19]

Etiology

We now briefly discuss the underlying etiologies of both dementia and lower urinary tract dysfunction. It should be noted that in a clinical context, comorbidity of degenerative and vascular pathologies seems likely.

Alzheimer's disease

Alzheimer's disease is the most common cause of dementia in the elderly, and accounts for more than 50% of dementia patients.[22] The pathologic hallmarks of this disease include senile plaques and neurofibrillary tangles, together with neuronal degeneration, which appears initially in the temporal and parietal cortices.[23] Neurofibrillary tangles are tau-positive, whereas senile plaques are amyloid-beta1–42 positive, both of which can increase in the cerebrospinal fluid of patients with dementia. Recent positron emission tomography (PET) scans using Congo-red/thioflavin-T derivatives showed increased amyloid deposits in the parieto-temporal lobe of Alzheimer's disease patients *in vivo*.[24] Coronal and axial slices of magnetic resonance imaging (MRI) scans, or axial computed tomography (CT) scans, can reveal atrophy of the cerebral cortex and hippocampus (Figure 20.1); the latter accounts for memory impairment.

Dementia in Alzheimer's disease is characterized by loss of memory, intellectual dysfunction, disturbances in speech such as anomia (difficulty in word finding), and various types of apraxia and agnosia. In practice, dementia can be indicated by test scores, such as 23 or lower of 30 points on the mini-mental status examination (MMSE). Emotional disturbances include depression in about 25% of patients, with agitation and restlessness also common. Motor signs are particularly rare early in the course of the illness. Typical Alzheimer's disease patients have MMSE scores of less than 5, even though they can walk into the clinic without assistance. However, as the disease progresses, increased deep tendon reflexes and parkinsonian syndrome may develop. Myoclonus is occasionally reported. Decreased motivation and initiative are also significant features. In most advanced cases, abulia (loss of psychomotor activity) or apallic syndrome (akinetic mutism, vegetative state) occurs, making the patient totally dependent. As discussed earlier, prominent urinary disturbances do occur in Alzheimer's disease but are very uncommon at an early stage.

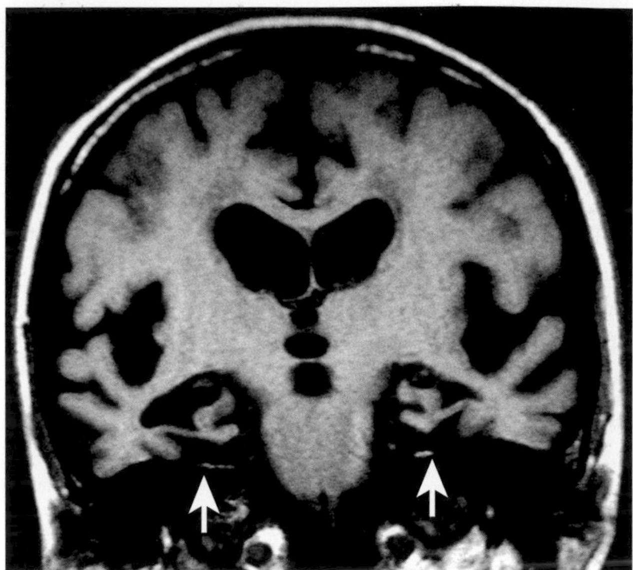

Figure 20.1
Magnetic resonance imaging of Alzheimer's disease. Atrophy in the hippocampus is the characteristic feature, and is typically observed in coronal planes (arrows) (image courtesy of Dr Shoichi Ito).

Dementia with Lewy bodies

Dementia with Lewy bodies (DLB) is a newly recognized entity that is considered to be the second most common degenerative cause of dementia.[25,26] In particular, DLB has attracted growing attention because the cognitive impairment that occurs with this disorder responds well to central cholinergic agents.[27] The name DLB is pathologically derived: Lewy bodies are cytoplasmic inclusion bodies, and they appear to be widespread in the cerebral cortex and basal ganglia in patients with this disorder.[28] Lewy bodies are alpha-synuclein-positive, presumably reflecting cytoskeletal alteration.[29] Lewy bodies are known as a pathologic hallmark of Parkinson's disease, but in Parkinson's they appear almost exclusively in the substantia nigra of the basal midbrain. Thus, the clinical features of DLB are a combination of dementia and parkinsonian syndrome, and visual hallucinations and fluctuation of the symptoms are common. In DLB, fluorodopa PET imaging reveals decreased dopaminergic neurons,[30] as is seen in Parkinson's disease. Brain MRI findings are not disease-specific for the diagnosis of DLB or Parkinson's disease. However, in DLB, brain perfusion imaging by single-photon emission computed tomography (SPECT) shows a diffuse decrease in perfusion, including the occipital lobe (Figure 20.2). This is in contrast to Alzheimer's disease, in which the occipital lobe is usually spared. This occipital lobe hypoperfusion may be relevant to the visual hallucinations in this disorder. Del-Ser et al[31] found that the onset of urinary incontinence was significantly earlier in patients with DLB (3.2 years after dementia onset) than in patients with Alzheimer's disease (6.5 years after dementia onset). In Alzheimer's disease, urinary incontinence is often associated with a severe cognitive decline, whereas in DLB it usually precedes severe mental failure. A significant though less common feature of DLB is widespread autonomic failure. In such cases, clinical presentations may mimic those of multiple system atrophy. When neuronal loss and Lewy bodies appear selectively in the peripheral nervous system, it is called 'pure autonomic failure (PAF)', which forms a spectrum of Lewy body diseases (Figure 20.3).

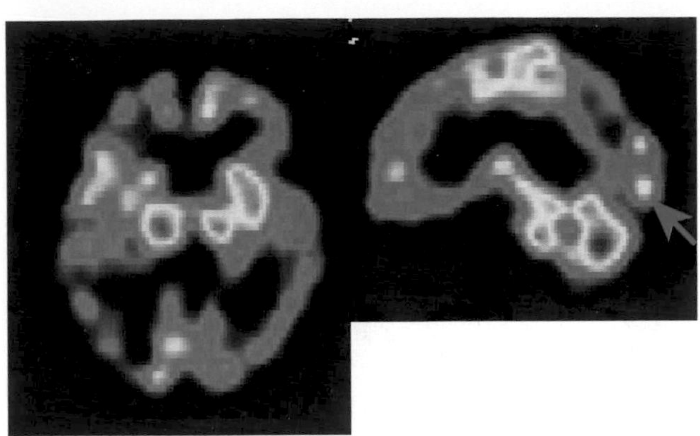

Figure 20.2
Brain perfusion single-photon emission computed tomography of dementia with Lewy bodies (DLB). Decreased brain perfusion including the occipital lobe is the characteristic imaging feature and is observed in axial and coronal planes (arrow). Decreased brain perfusion reflects the impairment of cortical activities resulting from this disorder.

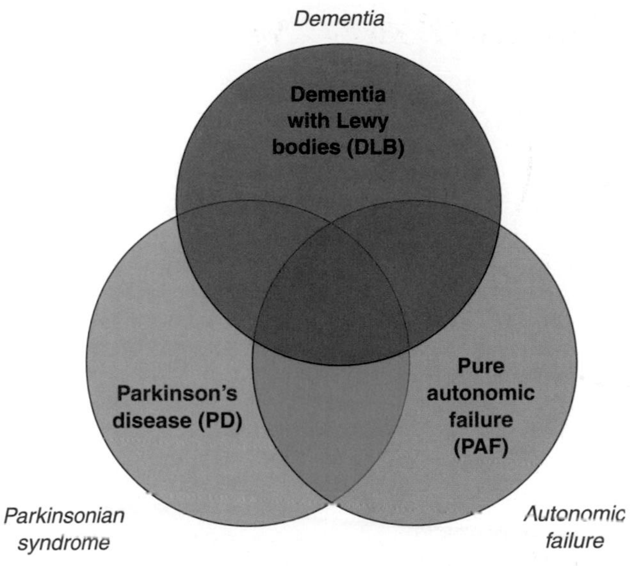

Figure 20.3
Spectrum of Lewy body diseases. When dementia is present, dementia with Lewy bodies is diagnosed (when motor disorder precedes dementia, it is also called Parkinson's disease with dementia). When motor disorder predominates, Parkinson's disease is diagnosed. When autonomic failure is the only manifestation, pure autonomic failure is diagnosed.

Multiple cerebral infarction

Multiple cerebral infarction is regarded as the third most common cause of dementia in the elderly, and, if dementia is the main problem, it is called a multi-infarct (vascular) dementia.[32] The cardinal features of multi-infarct dementia include history of stroke, stepwise deterioration, fluctuating course, focal neurologic symptoms, parkinsonian syndrome with wide-based gait, emotional incontinence, and the presence of arteriosclerotic risk factors such as hypertension. Of these features, Kotsoris et al[20] found that urinary disturbance, noted in 50% of patients, frequently preceded the development of dementia by 5 years or more. Similarly, gait disturbance, noted in 24%, preceded the development of dementia by 2 years or more. Even though two-thirds of men with urinary disturbance had been diagnosed with benign prostatic hypertrophy, urinary symptoms often persisted after prostatectomy. Fluid-attenuated inversion recovery (FLAIR) imaging of MRI scans is the most sensitive method for detecting and grading multiple cerebral infarction, particularly white-matter changes. Sakakibara et al[21] graded MRI-defined white-matter multi-infarction on a scale of 1 to 4, and found that urinary disturbance was more common than cognitive or gait disorders, particularly in patients with mild (grade 1) lesions. In addition, nocturnal urinary frequency was a more common and earlier feature than urinary incontinence (Figure 20.4).[33] Therefore, it is likely that urinary disturbance is the initial manifestation in a number of multi-infarction patients.

Other cerebral causes

Less common but potentially treatable causes of urinary incontinence/dementia should be addressed. Normal pressure (communicating) hydrocephalus is such a disorder in the elderly.[34] The clinical features of this disorder are often indistinguishable from those of multi-infarct dementia – parkinsonian syndrome, urinary incontinence, and dementia – the first two of which very often precede dementia.[35] However, in established cases the level of consciousness tends to decline, which is rarely seen in multi-infarct dementia. MRI scans reveal the presence of disproportionately dilated cerebral ventricles with cortical pressure signs. CT-ventriculography reveals a delayed disappearance (reflux) of contrast medium from lateral ventricles. A positive spinal tap test may predict successful outcome of shunt surgery. Chronic subdural hematoma is a cause of transient dementia and urinary incontinence. These signs usually appear several weeks after an episode of a fall, though they are not always apparent in elderly individuals. One-side-dominant pyramidal signs are common features, since this disease usually has laterality even though it occurs bilaterally. CT scans reveal crescent-like hematoma, particularly in the frontoparietal region.

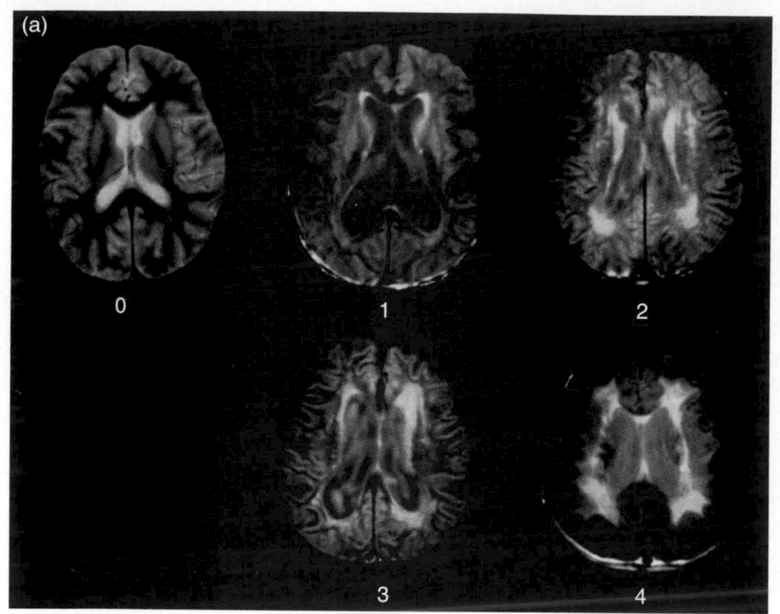

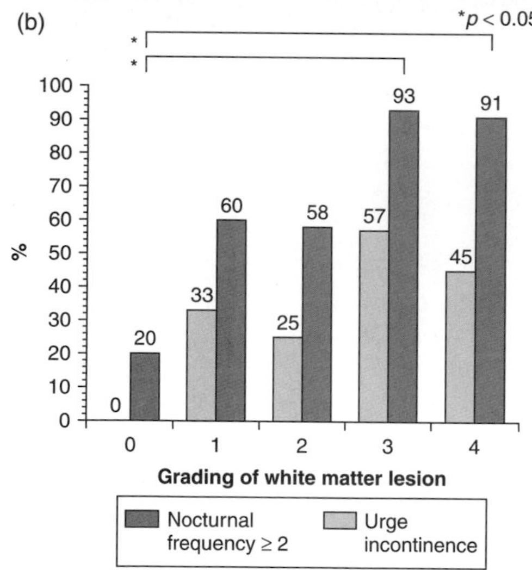

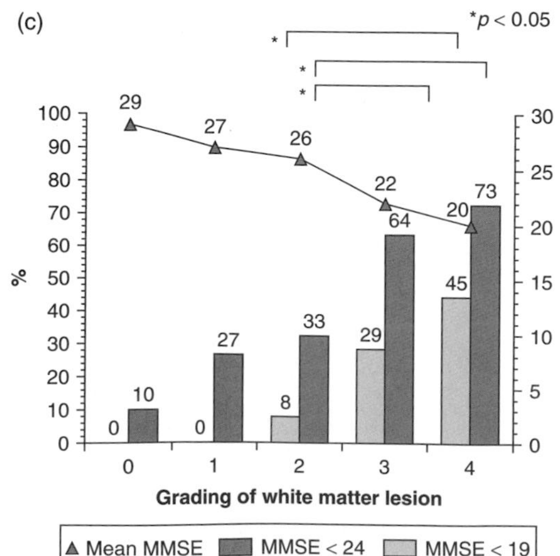

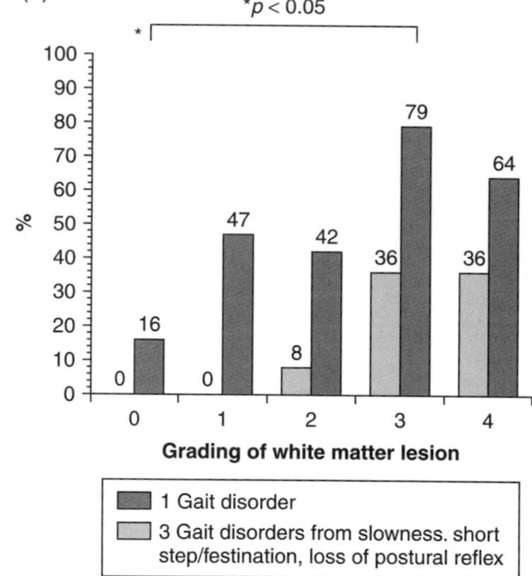

Figure 20.4

Cerebral white-matter lesions and urinary dysfunction. (a) Schematic presentation of the grading of white-matter lesions on magnetic resonance imaging (MRI) (according to Brand-Zawadzki et al[33]). Grade 1: punctate foci with high signal intensity in the white matter immediately at the top of the frontal horns of the lateral ventricles. Grade 2: white-matter lesions were seen elsewhere but remained confined to the immediate subependymal region of the ventricles. Grade 3: periventricular as well as separate, discrete, deep white-matter foci of signal abnormality. Grade 4: discrete white-matter foci had become large and coalescent. (b) Urinary dysfunction and white-matter lesions on MRI. (c) Cognitive disorder and white-matter lesion on MRI. MMSE: mini-mental state examination. (d) Gait disorder and white-matter lesion on MRI.

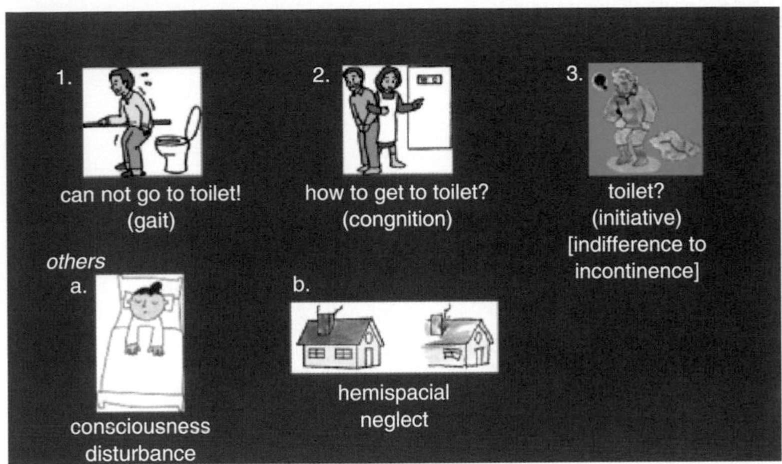

Figure 20.5
Functional incontinence: incontinence with normal LUT and innervation.

Mechanism

There are several prerequisites for maintaining continence in the elderly:

1. the presence of a normal lower urinary tract with intact innervation for both urinary filling and voiding
2. willingness to hold urine after having the first sensation and proper motivation to urinate in the toilet
3. a cognitive ability to know how to get to a toilet and how to adjust clothing
4. the physical ability to reach the toilet with hand dexterity sufficient to disrobe
5. an absence of medications that adversely affect the lower urinary tract innervation or alertness
6. a proper environment, including access to toilets and a lack of restraints.

It is very likely that incontinence in elderly demented patients is multifactorial, and often one factor relates to another.

Functional incontinence

Functional incontinence is the major cause of urinary incontinence in dementia. It refers to incontinence that is not derived from an abnormality in the lower urinary tract or its innervation, but from immobility, cognitive disability, and decreased motivation (Figure 20.5). Whereas patients with reduced mobility have a hard time going to the toilet, which seems farther away than it used to, patients with cognitive decline face a different problem: they do not know how to get to the toilet. In both cases, the patient worries over these difficulties. On the other hand, patients with less initiative – i.e., those with functional incontinence – may no longer worry about getting to the toilet or even about incontinence itself. In the most advanced cases, patients are indifferent to makeup, clothing, hygiene, and incontinence. They are akinetic, mute, and totally dependent. Disturbed consciousness may well lead to incontinence in patients with acute brain lesions. Similarly, left hemispacial neglect leads to incontinence in patients with brain lesions in the right hemisphere.

Among these factors, many studies have shown that the severity of immobility and that of dementia are positively correlated with functional incontinence.[36] The parkinsonian gait in these diseases is characterized as slow and short-stepped, with festination and postural instability. A wide-based ataxic gait often overlaps the short-stepped gait, particularly in cases of multiple cerebral infarction. The sites responsible for the gait disorder seem to be in the basal ganglia and medial frontal lobe, particularly the supplementary motor area or its pathways,[37] which partially overlaps the frontal micturition center. In addition, lesions in the basal ganglia cause both motor and micturition disorders, as seen in Parkinson's disease. In contrast, cognitive and motivation disorders are thought to reflect broad cortical dysfunction, as seen in Alzheimer's disease. Gait disorder and detrusor overactivity (DO) may be early and prominent features of multiple cerebral infarction and DLB, and may lead to functional incontinence and frequent falls, whereas they are very uncommon in the early stage of Alzheimer's disease. Taken together, these findings show that neurogenic urinary dysfunction (particularly DO) and gait disorder often appear together, as both reflect rather focal brain dysfunction (the basal ganglia and the medial frontal cortex). In contrast, functional incontinence appears secondarily from gait disorder and/or cognitive/motivation disorders, the latter reflecting more widespread brain dysfunction (Figure 20.6).

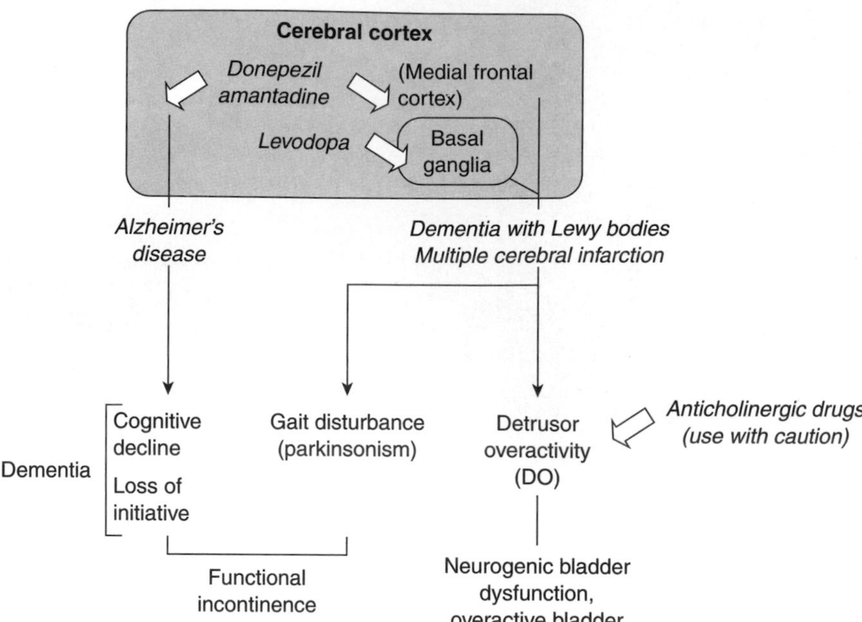

Figure 20.6
Relationship between functional incontinence and overactive bladder.

In addition, incontinence may develop because of confusion secondary to a superimposed delirium. Major depression occurs in up to 20% of patients with Alzheimer's disease, and apathy, psychomotor retardation, and lack of initiative may also precipitate immobility. Regression analysis by Resnick et al[38] revealed that cognitive impairment only doubled the risk of incontinence. Similarly, Jirovec and Wells[39] found that, in nursing home residents with dementia, immobility emerged as the best predictor of urinary incontinence. McGrother et al[40] found that 96% of subjects with dementia and incontinence were also dependent in getting to the toilet or dressing, and the combination of dementia and locomotor problems was 13 times more common among incontinent than continent individuals. Interestingly, post-stroke patients were incontinent and less active in daily living when they had left hemispacial neglect.[41] This finding suggests the importance of the right brain for general attention. In rehabilitation settings, urinary incontinence on admission predicted prolonged hospitalization and low scores in the Functional Independence Measure at discharge.[42] In post-stroke patients, those with cognitive impairment, pressure ulcer, urinary incontinence, or hearing impairment were more likely to significantly decline in physical functioning.[43] Falls during rehabilitation were strongly associated with bilateral motor deficit, male gender, and incontinence.[44] Cognitive decline after stroke was associated with high age and incontinence. These associations can be explained as follows. Patients with functional incontinence may well have larger, multiple brain lesions, and tend to have more severe cognitive and gait disorders. In other words, the important implication of these findings is that, in those patients, improvement in initiative and mobility for toileting may well lead to a reduction of incontinence. In particular, treatment will be successful insofar as persons with dementia alert their caregivers to urinary sensation and incontinence. Conversely, nocturia, a primary symptom of OAB, may result in sleep deprivation, which can have detrimental effects on psychologic performance (e.g., cognitive slowing, memory impairment).[45] Older people with cognitive impairment are at increased risk of falls, and elderly patients with urinary urge incontinence are also at increased risk of falls and fractures.[46]

Social and environmental factors also need to be considered. In some nursing home settings, diapers are automatically used for any patient, continent or not; if incontinence is found, balloon catheters are indwelled. Consequently, continence seems to be neither expected nor a high priority of care. In addition, toilet facilities may not be visible or easily accessible, thereby increasing the risk of incontinence. It should be mentioned that physical restraints can be iatrogenic causes of immobility. Behaviorally disturbed nursing home residents are more often restrained and unable to get to the toilet.

Overactive bladder

Besides functional incontinence, overactive bladder (OAB) is a major cause of urinary incontinence in dementia. When OAB is accompanied by incontinence, it is called OAB-wet; when not, it is called OAB-dry. OAB is a generic

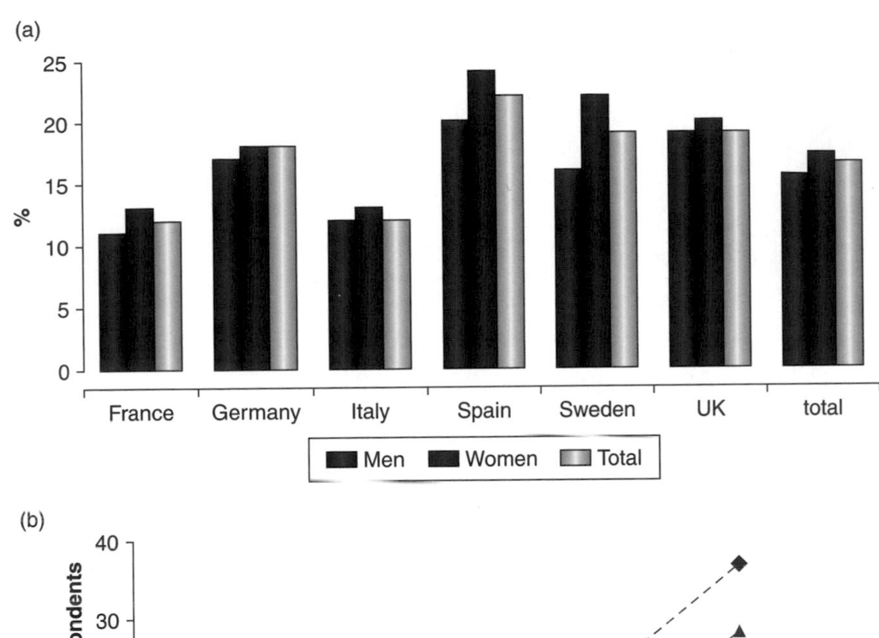

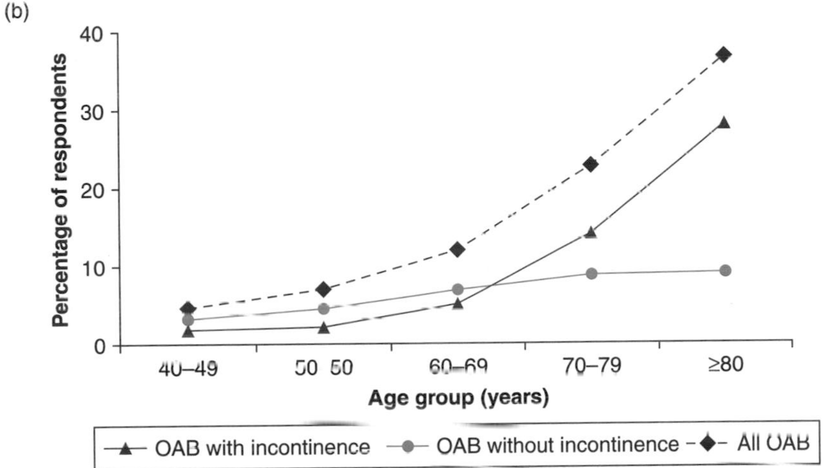

Figure 20.7
Frequency of overactive bladder (OAB) syndrome and its relation with age. (a) Frequency of OAB is around 12–22% in many countries.[49] (b) Frequency of OAB, particularly OAB-wet, increases with age.[50]

term that is now widely used to describe urgency (complaint of a sudden compeling desire to pass urine that is difficult to defer), with or without incontinence, usually with urinary frequency and nocturia.[16] OAB is common in the general population, with its prevalence in individuals aged 18 years and older being estimated as 16.5%, and this prevalence significantly increases with age (20–40%) (Figure 20.7).[47,48] Among the elderly, cognitive impairment might contribute to OAB-wet considerably.

Although urodynamic study is a gold standard for examining lower urinary tract (LUT) function, not many detailed studies have been made in cognitively impaired older subjects, because of methodologic (reliability) and ethical (feasibility and benefit) issues. To insure the accuracy of urodynamic results, the tests are better performed by physicians (with or without well-trained assistants) and by encouraging and communicating with the patient, particularly for assessing bladder capacity. In severely demented patients, we occasionally need to construe their urinary sensation based on their facial expression and body language. Rectal pressure monitoring is a necessity to subtract pressure changes that come from unwanted body movements and strains. Sphincter electromyography (EMG) recording is a matter of controversy since it is considered a bit harmful, although it may provide us with important information when there are large postvoid residuals. Considering these difficulties, there is an opinion that urodynamic testing should only be undertaken if empirical therapy has failed and other therapy approaches need to be tried, and if surgery is being considered. In addition, urodynamic testing has not been considered a prerequisite for a pharmacologic trial in patients with symptoms of OAB.

DO is urodynamically defined as an involuntary phasic increase in detrusor pressure > 10 cmH_2O during fillings; it is commonly associated with decreased bladder volumes at first sensation and maximum desire to void. DO is observed in a significant proportion of cognitively intact older subjects. In those subjects, two major etiologies for DO have been proposed: central and peripheral. Peripheral etiology includes detrusor muscle change, which may increase with age, as detected by electron microscopy.[51] Muscle cells from patients with DO *in vitro* have greater spontaneous contractile activity than those from normal detrusor, and greater sensitivity to electrical field stimulation and acetylcholine.[52] Attention has also been paid to men with outlet obstruction, in which increased α-adrenergic receptors and morphologic–biochemical changes of the detrusor muscles may lead to increased contractile activity and possible DO.[53] In such cases, surgical treatment of the obstruction may lessen DO.

Central etiology is thought to be more significant for DO. It is well known that cerebral diseases can lead to a loss of the brain's inhibitory influence on the spino-bulbo-spinal micturition reflex. The information that arises from the lower urinary tract reaches the pontine micturition center (PMC), which then activates the descending pathway to the sacral preganglionic neurons innervating the bladder.[54] The anteromedial frontal cortex is thought to be the higher center for micturition, since lesions in this area lead to DO and urinary retention (Figure 20.8); the latter occurs particularly in the initial phase. Recent PET studies have shown that during bladder filling the frontal micturition center is tonically active, together with activation in the basal ganglia and the pontine storage center adjacent to the PMC.[55,56] Griffiths et al[57] studied 128 geriatric incontinent patients, half of whom had dementia, and found that half of the 128 patients had DO by video-urodynamic study. In addition, SPECT imaging showed that patients with DO had significant underperfusion in the right frontal lobe. Similarly, cognitively intact, community dwelling older individuals commonly show 'silent' multiple cerebral infarction by MRI scans.[20,58] Detailed examination in that study revealed the presence of gait disorder, which is suggestive of the disease. Most of the individuals were continent, but often had nocturnal urinary frequency and urgency due in part to DO. In urodynamic studies of 133 incontinent female nursing home residents, 88% of whom had dementia, Yu et al[36] found normal bladder function in 41%, DO in 38%, stress incontinence in 16%, and overflow incontinence from outlet obstruction in 5%. Resnick et al[59] reported that 64% of nursing home residents with dementia had DO, compared with 47% of those who were cognitively intact. In women, a positive correlation was found between the presence of DO and dementia. These findings suggest a correlation between these two conditions, and that demented patients often have DO as a significant cause of incontinence.

Although not many studies have specified the types of dementia, Mori et al[62] examined 46 institutionalized dementia patients, 31 of whom had Alzheimer's, 11 of whom had multi-infarct dementia, and 4 of whom had both; they found DO in 58%, 91%, and 50%, respectively. Sugiyama et al[63] found DO in 40% of 20 patients with Alzheimer's disease. In particular, DO was noted in 8 of 13 incontinent patients and in 0 of 7 continent patients. We examined LUT function in 11 DLB patients.[64] All patients had LUT symptoms: urinary incontinence, 10 (urgency type, 7; functional type due to dementia and immobility, 2; both urgency and stress type, 1) and OAB symptoms in 9. Postvoid residual was noted in 7, and residual urine volume >100 ml was noted in 3. Decreased urinary flow was noted in all of the 5 patients who underwent flowmetry. DO was revealed in 5 of the 7 patients undergoing EMG-cystometry: a low compliance detrusor in 2 (storage phase); an underactive detrusor in 4, an acontractile detrusor in 1, and detrusor-sphincter dyssynergia in 1 (voiding phase). Bethanechol supersensitivity of the bladder was noted in the 2 patients with low compliance detrusor. Neurogenic changes were revealed in 2 of the 3 patients undergoing motor unit potential analysis. These peripheral features may need differential diagnosis from multiple system atrophy.

Sphincter EMG also revealed uninhibited sphincter relaxation (USR) in the patients. When USR occurs together with DO, incontinence becomes more prominent, which is thought to be a feature of cerebral diseases. The pathology of Alzheimer's disease involves the medial frontal lobe, which receives various inputs from another brain area. Of particular importance is the cholinergic pathway that originates from the nucleus basalis Meynert (Ch4 cell group). In experimental studies, lesions in this small nucleus give rise to DO, suggesting cortical cholinergic neurons have an inhibitory role in the micturition reflex.[65] Sakakibara et al[66] examined 19 patients with multi-infarct dementia. All of them had nocturnal frequency and urgency, and 70% had urinary incontinence of the urgency and stress types. Urodynamic studies revealed DO in 70% and a low compliance curve in 10%. Sakakibara et al[21] urodynamically studied 22 elderly subjects with white-matter multi-infarction and 11 subjects without. DO was significantly more prevalent in those with white-matter lesions (82%) than in those with normal MRI (9%). Although the difference was not statistically significant, USR was more common in subjects with white-matter lesions. Thus, according to these reports, DO contributes to urinary frequency and urgency incontinence more in multi-infarct dementia than in Alzheimer's disease.

Bladder underactivity

Resnick and Yalla[67] reported that a subgroup of incontinent elderly individuals with DO, most of whom were women, had bladder underactivity that led to post-micturition residuals (PMRs) with an average volume of 95 ml; they called this detrusor hyperactivity with impaired contractile function (DHIC). Although Eastwood and Lord[68] were not able to replicate these findings, Elbadawi et al[69] found that patients with DHIC could be differentiated from those with DO and normal contractility on the basis of the detrusor ultrastructure. Another important finding by Resnick and Yalla[67] was that sphincter EMG of patients with DHIC did not show detrusor-sphincter dyssynergia. We previously performed pressure–flow analysis in 8 patients with Alzheimer's disease who had neither PMR nor detrusor-sphincter dyssynergia. However, the mean voiding pressure

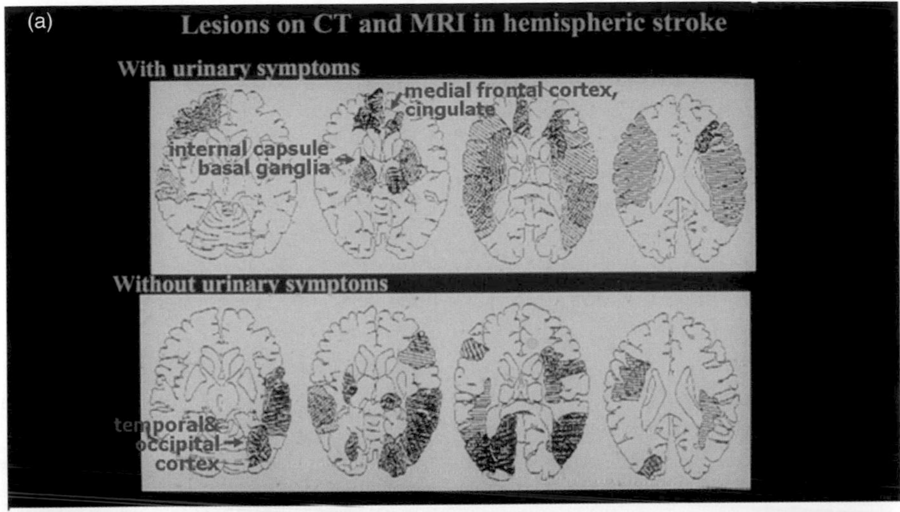

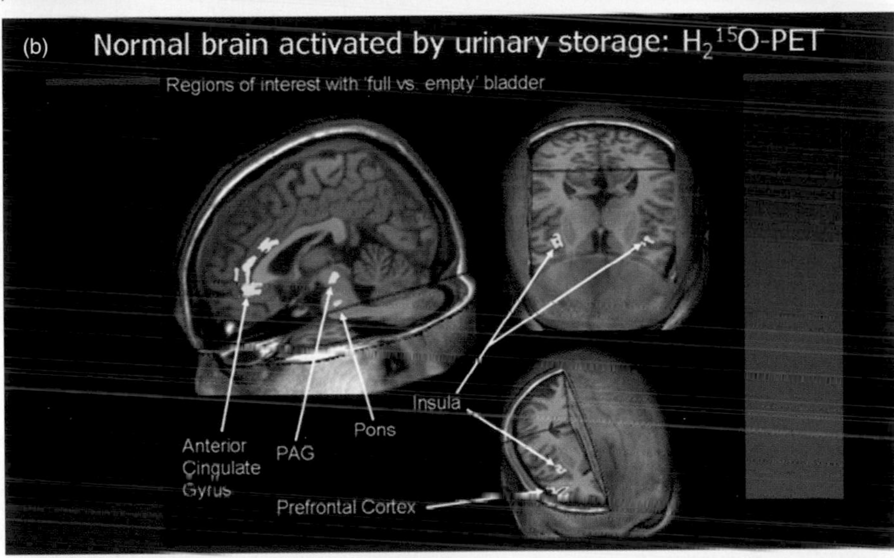

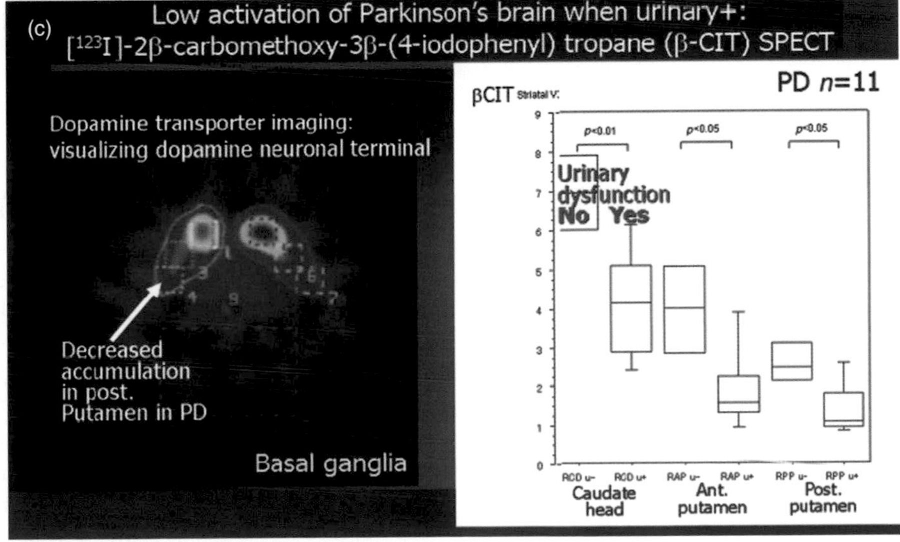

Figure 20.8
Neural mechanism of overactive bladder syndrome. (a) Location of brain lesions that caused or did not cause urinary dysfunction (with permission from reference 60) (b) Brain areas activated by urinary storage in normal volunteers (with permission from reference 56) (c) Marked depletion of basal ganglia activity in Parkinsonian brain when urinary dysfunction was present (with permission from reference 61)

of the patients was 54 cmH_2O (range 20–101 cmH_2O), and 5 of the 8 had weak detrusor.

Sakakibara et al[21] also found that persons with multi-infarction were more likely to have PMR with an average volume of 93 ml than those without (50% vs 9%, respectively). Correctly diagnosing the impaired contractility group with urodynamic testing is of therapeutic importance, because such patients may be at risk of acute urinary retention if given anticholinergic medication.[67] Kuwabara et al[70] studied PMR volumes by portable echography (BV5000) in 82 institutionalized dementia patients; 45 had Alzheimer's disease, 19 had multi-infarct dementia, 5 had normal pressure hydrocephalus, 2 had Pick's disease, and 11 had other causes. Eighty-three percent of the patients had urinary urgency or incontinence. They found PMR >100 ml in 6 patients (8%), consisting of Alzheimer's disease in 5 and multi-infarct dementia in 1. However, the cause of the high PMR in those patients was assumed to be drug-induced in 1, prostate hypertrophy in 1, frontal lobectomy for pre-existing schizophrenia in 1, and unknown in 2.

DHIC is recognized in various brain diseases (parkinsonian syndrome, Alzheimer's disease, etc.) and spinal cord diseases (cervical spondylotic myelopathy, etc.).[71] However, the exact pathophysiology of DHIC is still uncertain. In brain diseases, one explanation is that two separate brain areas (the facilitatory and inhibitory brain sites for micturition) might be involved that lead to DHIC. In contrast, in spinal cord lesions, a single partial lesion in the spinal autonomic pathways could cause DHIC, since it disrupts the spino-bulbo-spinal micturition reflex arc, and could cause the emergence of a C-fiber-mediated novel sacral micturition reflex arc below the lesion.[54] In the clinical context, the prevalence of a combination of multiple diseases, such as multiple cerebral infarction and diabetic neuropathy, or cervical and lumbar spondylotic radiculopathy, seems to be high. These combinations can lead to DHIC by lesions in the central (mostly inhibitory) and peripheral (facilitatory) nervous systems. Among comorbid conditions, lumbar spondylosis and diabetic polyneuropathy are common in the elderly. Examination of the lower extremities for sensation and deep tendon reflexes may provide cues to suspect these disorders. These issues are particularly problematic in patients who have undergone prostate hypertrophy for large PMR or retention, since impaired detrusor contractility during voiding is a significant factor that may lead to an unsuccessful surgical outcome.[67]

Stress urinary incontinence

It is important to evaluate patients for comorbid stress incontinence, since it is a very common condition due to pelvic floor weakness in older women and is potentially treatable. In an older incontinent population, Payne[72] found that half of the patients suffered from pure stress incontinence, 10–20% had pure urge incontinence, and the remaining patients had both. Resnick et al[59] noted that a significant proportion of women with dementia also had stress urinary incontinence. Although the reliability of stress incontinence diagnoses decreased as the severity of dementia increased, 80% of those with MMSE scores of 10–23 and 66% of those with scores of 9 or lower were still able to perform a stress maneuver.

Nocturnal polyuria

Nocturnal polyuria is a common reason for nocturia in the elderly, and is potentially treatable. Nocturnal polyuria in older individuals seems to be multifactorial. It may result from congestive heart failure or liver cirrhosis, but may also have a cerebral etiology. Cerebrovascular disease may cause nocturnal polyuria, particularly when it involves the hypothalamic region that contains arginine vasopressin (AVP) neurons. We had such patients; they lost the circadian rhythm of plasma AVP, which normally rises at night. Diabetes is also a common cause of polyuria.

Drug-induced incontinence and retention

Drugs that may affect either the central nervous system or the lower urinary tract are potential causes of transient incontinence. In a study of 84 elderly, incontinent, female nursing home residents, Keister and Creason[73] found that 70% of subjects were taking a drug that could potentially cause incontinence. Antipsychotic medications, antidepressants, benzodiazepines, and sedatives are frequently used to treat agitation, insomnia, and depression, and may cause incontinence through increased confusion, sedation, parkinsonism, and immobility. Urinary retention and overflow may result from the anticholinergic side-effects of tricyclic antidepressants and antipsychotic medications.

Management

In general, management for lower urinary tract dysfunction in dementia patients needs to be individualized, and the risk/benefit ratio of these procedures, particularly invasive or irreversible treatments, needs to be carefully considered.

Treatment of transient causes

The first step in management is to identify and treat transient acute causes of incontinence. Acute causes may be recalled from the mnemonic 'DIAPERS' (Delirium, Infection, Atrophic vaginitis, Pharmaceuticals, psychologic factors, Endocrine conditions, Restricted mobility, Stool impaction).[74] Some factors are derived from the dementing illness, but others are from comorbid medical conditions, inappropriate environment, and medication. There are also interrelationships among these factors. An elderly patient's delirium may be secondary to, for example, a pharmacologic or infectious outcome.

Toileting/behavioral therapy

Toileting regimens (behavioral therapy) have been used to manage functional incontinence in elderly individuals. Patients with decreased motivation, cognitive disability, and gait disorder are highly likely to be incontinent. With prompted voiding, patients who have decreased motivation are asked on a regular schedule if they need toileting assistance, but are given such assistance only if they request it. Prompted voiding is usually combined with positive reinforcement, in the form of praise, for making appropriate toileting requests and for keeping themselves dry. On most occasions, patients require physical assistance with toileting because of comorbid gait disorder and cognitive disability. According to Skelly and Flint,[75] who carefully reviewed seven studies, patients were dry 64% of the time at baseline on average when they were checked every 1–2 hours during waking hours. After treatment, this figure rose to 76%. This translated into a 32% mean relative reduction in wet episodes. A better response to the treatment was obtained in less demented patients, i.e., those who could recognize the need to void, and had fewer than four episodes of incontinence per 12-hour period. As expected, normal bladder function also predicted better response. With scheduled toileting, patients who had little or no motivation were toileted on a regular schedule (fixed schedule), usually every 2 hours, or on a schedule that matched the patient's own voiding pattern (individualized schedule). Ouslander et al[76] examined the effects of a fixed, 2-hourly toileting schedule on 15 cognitively impaired patients with DO, of whom 53% needed physical assistance. Toileting significantly reduced the incidence of incontinence, from 43% to 32%. Flint and Skelly[77] reported that 55% of ambulatory dementia patients became dry or had a significant improvement in incontinence with a toileting schedule. However, Jirovec[78] reported that 6 weeks of scheduled toileting did not improve incontinence in a group of demented and dependent nursing home residents, although poor staff compliance with the toileting program contributed to the negative outcome. The results suggest that more severely demented and less mobile individuals with bladder abnormalities are the least likely to benefit from toileting programs. Cost/benefit studies have indicated that the labor costs of toileting programs may be higher than the savings in laundry costs to the nursing home.[79] However, carefully selecting patients who can most benefit from toileting regimens is one possible way of reducing conflict between the cost and dryness.

Environmental settings are also important for managing functional incontinence. Chanfreau-Rona et al[80] assessed whether enhanced visual cues, such as painting the toilet doors bright orange and displaying large pictures of a lady sitting on a toilet, would have an impact on incontinence in severely demented women in a psychogeriatric ward. However, when environmental changes were the only treatment intervention, incontinence did not improve. Nevertheless, recommended toilet settings may include mobility aids such as hallway handrails, canes, walkers, and wheelchairs; easy toilet access and visibility; improvements to toilet facilities such as better lighting, grab bars, and toilet seat height; automatic washing devices for the buttocks and lift-up commodes; and, finally, well-designed clothes to make disrobing easier. Also, to maximize continence, alternatives to physical restraints need to be sought.

Medication

Cognitive impairment and decreased motivation

Although the etiology of Alzheimer's disease remains uncertain, the cognitive deficits in Alzheimer's disease patients are thought to be due, at least in part, to a decrease in cholinergic innervation of the cerebral cortex and basal forebrain. The loss of cholinergic nerve terminals in Alzheimer's disease is detected *in vivo* by PET using acetylcholinesterase (AChE) activities. Central cholinergic agents are widely used in the treatment of cognitive decline in Alzheimer's disease. There are several central cholinomimetic agents, including donepezil hydrochloride and rivastigmine, both of which are central AChE inhibitors that decrease degradation of acetylcholine, thus increasing the concentration of acetylcholine in the synaptic cleft. These agents inhibit AChE selectively in the brain,[81] and this action reverses cognitive decline in mild to moderate Alzheimer's disease patients for at least 6–12 months.[82] Clinicians must be aware that these agents may cause adverse gastrointestinal effects as peripheral nervous system (PNS) effects. As mentioned above, a subgroup of Alzheimer's disease patients have urge incontinence and DO even at an early stage. Hashimoto et al[83] reported that 7% of patients taking 5 mg/day of donepezil showed urinary incontinence as a potential initial adverse effect. However, we recently showed that donepezil could ameliorate cognitive function without serious adverse effects on the LUT function in patients with Alzheimer's disease.[84] As regards the changes in urodynamic parameters, DO appeared to be augmented after donepezil treatment,

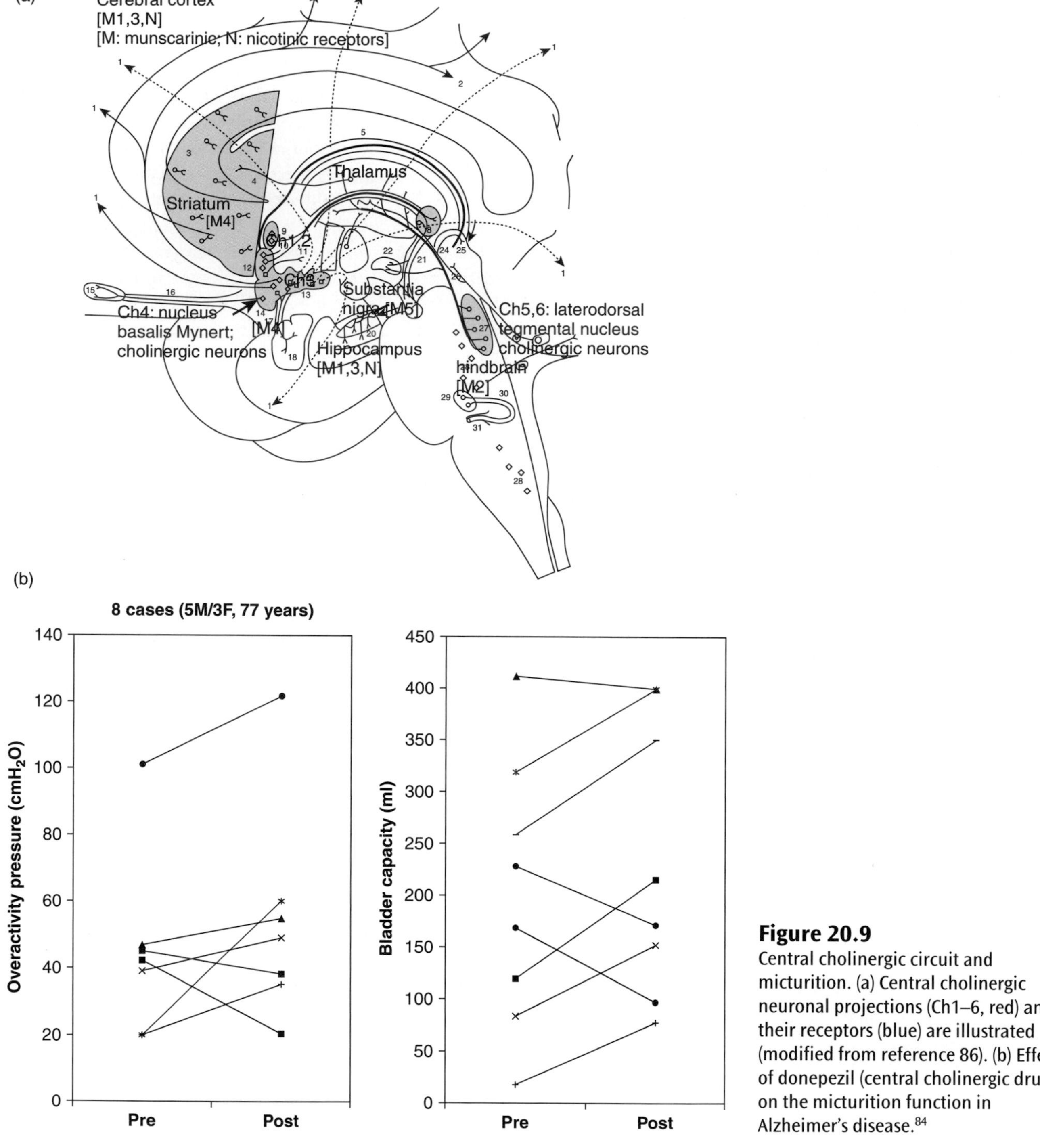

Figure 20.9
Central cholinergic circuit and micturition. (a) Central cholinergic neuronal projections (Ch1–6, red) and their receptors (blue) are illustrated (modified from reference 86). (b) Effect of donepezil (central cholinergic drug) on the micturition function in Alzheimer's disease.[84]

which is reasonably attributed to the PNS effects as seen with other cholinergic drugs. However, our patients with Alzheimer's disease showed a slight increase in bladder capacity, which cannot be explained by PNS effects alone. Although it is unknown to what extent the central cholinergic circuit may participate in the regulation of micturition, experimental studies showed that lesions in the nucleus basalis Meynert in the basal forebrain (central cholinergic nucleus projecting fibers to the frontoparietal cortex) lead to decreased bladder capacity.[85] In addition, improved cognitive status and alertness may well give the patient sufficient initiative to hold urine. Therefore central AchE inhibitors, including donepezil hydrochloride, may have complex effects on LUT function (Figure 20.9).

Cognitive impairment in patients with DLB also responded well to central cholinergic agents.[26] In patients with mild to moderate dementia, decreased motivation can be treated with 200–300 mg/day of amantadine hydrochloride. However, it has not been determined whether these drugs could improve patients' disability scale scores in toileting and functional incontinence. Aniracetam is a pyrrolidinone derivative and is thought to facilitate cholinergic neurotransmission. In an open study of 52 senile post-stroke patients, some of whom had dementia, Kumon et al[87] found that 600 mg/day of aniracetam improved urinary and fecal incontinence in 46% of the patients.

Gait disorder

Gait disorder is a symptom of parkinsonian syndrome in multi-infarct dementia and DLB, but it also occurs mildly in Alzheimer's disease. Although levodopa seems less effective in Alzheimer's than in Parkinson's disease, 200–300 mg/day (usually coupled with peripheral dopa-decarboxylase inhibitor) ameliorates gait disorder in dementia patients, and may be of benefit in treating functional incontinence. Levodopa is better prescribed in conjunction with rehabilitation programs, since Jirovec[88] found that, in cognitively impaired nursing home residents, a daily exercise program designed to improve walking significantly reduced daytime incontinence. Physicians should also be aware of the potential adverse effects of levodopa, such as postural hypotension and hallucinations. Although levodopa seems to ameliorate urinary urgency in early, untreated Parkinson's disease patients,[89,90] it may augment DO in a 1-hour time window in early[91] or advanced Parkinson's disease patients.[92]

Overactive bladder

Medications used to treat overactive bladder (OAB) or DO include anticholinergic agents such as propantheline, oxybutynin, and propiverine, and smooth muscle relaxants such as flavoxate. Mori et al[62] performed urodynamic studies in 46 dementia patients, and found DO in 58% of Alzheimer's patients and 91% of multi-infarct dementia patients. They conducted an open trial with 20 mg/day of propiverine hydrochloride for 2 weeks, irrespective of the presence of DO, and found increased bladder capacity or lessened frequency of incontinence in 40% of patients. Both types of dementia groups responded almost equally, and patients with DO showed the more satisfactory response.

Tobin and Brocklehurst[93] used a combination of propantheline bromide (15 mg/day) and flavoxate hydrochloride (200 mg/day) to treat urinary incontinence in a cognitively impaired nursing home population, of whom 95% were clinically diagnosed with overactive bladder. There was a significant reduction in nocturnal but not daytime incontinence compared with controls. Burgio et al[94] found that, in 197 cognitively intact elderly women with predominantly urge incontinence, either 7.5–15 mg/day of oxybutynin hydrochloride (68.5%) or behavioral treatment (80.7%) was more effective than placebo (39.4%) in randomized controlled trials. However, in dementia patients with DO, Zorzitto et al[95] found that 15 mg/day of propantheline was no more effective than placebo. When the dose of propantheline was increased to 30 mg, there was a statistically significant improvement, but the clinical benefit was outweighed by the presence of adverse effects in 50% of subjects. Although DO seems to be the cause of OAB-wet in those patients, the study's negative findings contrast with the reported efficacy of anticholinergic medications in approximately 50% of cognitively intact, independently mobile older outpatients with incontinence.[96] Therefore, treatment for OAB/DO may be of benefit only in mild to moderate dementia without marked immobility.

The use of medications with anticholinergic side-effects in older persons is a concern, particularly when there is a risk of exacerbating cognitive impairment. After they are ingested and absorbed from the intestine, anticholinergic drugs are systemically circulated. If they cross the blood–brain barrier (BBB), they reach the CNS and block cholinergic receptors, particularly M_1 muscarinic receptors in the cerebral cortex, or M_4 receptors in the basal ganglia. Previous data suggested that a centrally acting anticholinergic, trihexyphenidyl (for ameliorating Parkinson's disease), exacerbated cognitive function in experimental animals and humans. The same was reported for atropine (before endoscopy/surgery) and scopolamine (hyoscine) (for colicky pain or motion sickness). Although oxybutynin has been developed as a peripherally acting drug, recent research suggests that it has some adverse effects on cognitive function.[97] To a much lesser extent, tolterodine[98] and propiverine[99] also affect cognitive function. Factors underlying the cognitive effects of these medications include: (1) central muscarinic receptor affinity, e.g., high M_1 receptor selectivity, and (2) easy penetration of the BBB, e.g., high lipid solubility (water versus oil partition coefficient [log P] <3; number of hydrogen bonds <8); a neutral charge or low degree of ionization (polar surface area <90 A); and a less bulky (number of rotatable bonds <5) and smaller molecular size (<450 Da).[100] Regarding central muscarinic receptor affinity, most anticholinergics are nonselective muscarinic blockers. The exception is darifenacin, which is an M_3-selective antagonist (under manufacture). Regarding BBB penetration, most anticholinergics have a molecular size between 300 and 400 Da. However, among these, oxybutynin can readily penetrate the CNS, since it has high lipophilicity and neutrality. Other anticholinergics have less marked lipophilicity or neutrality. Trospium, a quaternary amine, has a particularly high polarity. Other common anticholinergic side-effects are dryness of the mouth (M_3) and constipation ($M_{2,3}$). Extended-release formulations may lessen these adverse effects.[101]

Stress incontinence

Tricyclic antidepressants are commonly used to treat both DO and stress incontinence, since they have both anticholinergic and α-adrenergic properties, the latter of which is expected to increase urethral tone. However, a randomized controlled study to examine the effect of a tricyclic on incontinence in an exclusively older group of patients did not find a statistically significant difference between imipramine hydrochloride (mean dose 54 mg) and placebo.[102] One has to exercise caution in using imipramine in older persons because of its sedative, hypotensive, and cardiac effects and because it increases the risk of falls. Alpha-adrenergic agonists, such as midodrine hydrochloride, have been shown to benefit some older women with stress incontinence.[96] The estrogen quinestradol was reported to be effective in reducing the frequency of incontinence in older women. However, prolonged estrogen therapy may increase the risk of endometrial carcinoma.

Outlet obstruction

Prazosin hydrochloride, a nonselective α_1-adrenergic antagonist, is effective in the symptomatic management of benign prostatic hypertrophy. However, adverse effects of α-adrenergic blockers may limit their use in frail elderly patients such as those with orthostatic hypotension. The proximal urethra has an abundance of α_{1A-D}-adrenergic receptors. In contrast, the vascular wall has an abundance of α_{1B} receptors, particularly in the elderly.[103] Prazosin may block both α_{1B} receptors in the vascular wall and α_{1A-D} receptors in the proximal urethra. Recently launched selective α_{1A-D}-adrenergic blockers, such as tamsulosin hydrochloride and naftopidil, are the drugs of choice because they have fewer side-effects.

Nocturnal polyuria

Desmopressin, a potent analog of AVP, has been used to treat patients with nocturnal polyuria due probably to impaired circadian rhythm of the plasma AVP.[104] We prescribed 5 μg of intranasal desmopressin once a night in post-stroke patients who had impaired circadian AVP rhythm, and noted improvement in nocturnal polyuria.[105] This small dose of desmopressin is unlikely to cause adverse effects, although hyponatremia and signs of cardiac failure should be checked regularly. A recently launched tablet form is feasible and may be of particular benefit.

Pelvic muscle exercises and biofeedback

Pelvic muscle exercises, sometimes combined with biofeedback, have been used successfully to treat stress incontinence in older women.[106] For the procedure to be effective, the patient must actively contract and relax the pubococcygeal muscles up to 80 times a day for several months. However, Tobin and Brocklehurst[93] note that, because most of their patients had severe cognitive and physical deterioration, they were unable to cooperate with treatment for stress incontinence.

Electrical stimulation

In an uncontrolled trial, Lamhut et al[107] studied the effectiveness of electrical stimulation in 9 incontinent female nursing home patients with DO. These patients had severe cognitive impairment, were bed-bound, and were completely dependent in activities of daily living. They were treated with stimulation for 15 min twice a week for 8 weeks using a rectal probe. In this group of subjects the treatment was not effective and was associated with a 20% increase in the average number of incontinent episodes. Two patients were withdrawn from the study because of agitation associated with the procedure.

Surgery

Surgery has been used to treat benign outlet obstruction and stress incontinence in older patients, when conservative methods and medications have failed or were not appropriate.[108] In some frail older persons, these problems can be corrected, or at least improved, by newer, less strenuous, brief surgical techniques such as transurethral incision of the prostate (TUIP) and tension-free vaginal tapes (TVT). However, whether or not the repair of these outlet lesions reliably restores continence in frail, demented individuals remains to be established.

Devices, pads, and catheters

Indwelling catheters are often used excessively and inappropriately in frail demented patients, even for the relief of incontinence, and are associated with a high rate of morbidity. Clean intermittent catheterization (CIC) is used to treat an underactive detrusor and other causes of urinary retention. The rates of symptomatic urinary tract infection and bladder stone formation are lower than those with indwelling catheters. However, it is often difficult to perform CIC in demented patients because of uncooperativeness, aggression, and agitation, and also because it increases demands on staff time. Indwelling catheterization should be restricted to persons who have urinary retention that cannot otherwise be treated, or to persons who are most severely demented with akinetic mutism, or as a short-term measure to allow for the healing of pressure sores. As one way of avoiding the use of catheters, absorbent pads and special undergarments are recommended for those patients whose incontinence has failed to respond to other treatment modalities.

Summary

Urinary incontinence is common in patients with dementia, and is more prevalent in demented than in nondemented older individuals. Since the etiology of incontinence is multifactorial, factors within and outside the lower urinary tract must be assessed in order to maximize continence in these patients. Patients with decreased motivation, cognitive disability, gait disorder, and detrusor overactivity (DO) are highly likely to be incontinent. However, a careful clinical evaluation with measurement of postvoid residuals seems to be sufficient to guide treatment in most cases. Most research on the management of urinary incontinence in dementia patients has focused on toileting programs for functional incontinence and on drug treatments for DO. To date, the use of anticholinergic medications for DO is still under consideration, although many studies have employed severely demented cases. It is possible that anticholinergic medication is of greater benefit to less-impaired individuals who are aware of, and able to tell the caregiver about, their urinary sensation or incontinence. Prompted and scheduled toileting for patients with decreased motivation and immobility appears to be an effective approach to managing incontinence. In the future, centrally acting drugs that can improve gait and cognitive function may become an option for the treatment of urinary incontinence in dementia patients.

References

1. Teri L, Borson S, Kiyak A, Yamagishi M. Behavioral disturbance, cognitive dysfunction, and functional skill; prevalence and relationship in Alzheimer's disease. J Am Geriatr Soc 1989; 37: 109–16.
2. Teri L, Larson EB, Reifler BV. Behavioral disturbance in dementia of the Alzheimer's type. J Am Geriatr Soc 1988; 36: 1–6.
3. Teri L, Hughes JP, Larson EB. Cognitive deterioration in Alzheimer's disease: behavioural and health factors. J Gerontol 1990; 45: P58–63.
4. Swearer JM, Drachman DA, O'Donnell BF, Mitchell AL. Troublesome and disruptive behaviors in dementia. J Am Geriatr Soc 1988; 36: 784–90.
5. Udaka F, Nishinaka K, Kameyama M et al. Urinary dysfunction in dementia; 1. dementia of Alzheimer type. Void Disord Dig 1994; 2: 271–5.
6. Berrios GE. Urinary incontinence and the psychopathology of the elderly with cognitive failure. Gerontology 1986; 32: 119–24.
7. Ouslander JG, Zarit SH, Orr NK, Muira SA. Incontinence among elderly community-dwelling dementia patients. J Am Geriatr Soc 1990; 38: 440–5.
8. Rabins PV, Mace NL, Lucas MJ. The impact of dementia on the family. JAMA 1982; 248: 333–5.
9. Burns A, Jacoby R, Levy R. Psychiatric phenomena in Alzheimer's disease. IV: Disorders of behaviour. Br J Psychiatry 1990; 157: S6–94.
10. Campbell AJ, Reinken J, McCosh L. Incontinence in the elderly: prevalence and prognosis. Age Ageing 1985; 14: 65–70.
11. Borrie MJ, Davidson HA. Incontinence in institutions: costs and contributing factors. Can Med Assoc J 1992; 147(3): 322–8.
12. Noto H. Urinary dysfunction in dementia; 2. multi-infarct dementia. Void Disord Dig 1994; 2: 277–84.
13. Toba K, Ouchi Y, Orimo H et al. Urinary incontinence in elderly inpatients in Japan; a comparison between general and geriatric hospitals. Aging Clin Exp Res 1996; 8: 47–54.
14. McLaren SM, McPherson FM, Sinclair F, Ballinger BR. Prevalence and severity of incontinence among hospitalised, female psychogeriatric patients. Health Bull 1981; 39: 157–61.
15. International Continence Society. Standardization of terminology of lower urinary tract function. Scand J Urol Nephrol 1988; 1 (Suppl 14): 5–19.
16. Abrams P, Cardozo L, Fall M et al. The standardization of terminology of lower urinary tract function: report from the standardization sub-committee of the International Continence Society. Neurourol Urodyn 2002; 21: 167–78.
17. Herzog AR, Fultz NH. Prevalence and incidence of urinary incontinence in community-dwelling populations. J Am Geriatr Soc 1990; 38: 273–81.
18. Palmer MH, German PS, Ouslander JG. Risk factors for urinary incontinence one year after nursing home admission. Res Nurs Health 1991; 14: 405–12.
19. Ouslander JG, Palmer MH, Rovner BW, German PS. Urinary incontinence in nursing homes: incidence, remission and associated factors. J Am Geriatr Soc 1993; 41: 1083–9.
20. Kotsoris H, Barclay LL, Kheyfets S et al. Urinary and gait disturbances as markers for early multi-infarct dementia. Stroke 1987; 18: 138–41.
21. Sakakibara R, Hattori T, Uchiyama T, Yamanishi T. Urinary function in elderly people with and without leukoaraiosis: relation to cognitive and gait function. J Neurol Neurosurg Psychiatry 1999; 67(5): 658–60.
22. American Psychiatric Association. Diagnostic and Statistical Manual of Mental Disorders, 4th edn. Washington, DC: American Psychiatric Association Press, 1994.
23. Braak H, Braak E. Diagnostic criteria for neuropathologic assessment of Alzheimer's disease. Neurobiol Aging 1997; 18(Suppl 1): S85–8
24. Kepe V, Huang SC, Small GW et al. Visualizing pathology deposits in the living brain of patients with Alzheimer's disease. Meth Enzymol 2006; 412: 144–1460.
25. McKieth IG, Galasko D, Kosaka K et al. Consensus guidelines for the clinical and pathologic diagnosis of dementia with Lewy bodies (DLB); report of the consortium on DLB International Workshop. Neurology 1996; 47: 1113–24.
26. McKeith IG, Dickson DW, Lowe J et al. Diagnosis and management of dementia with Lewy bodies: third report of the DLB Consortium. Neurology 2005; 65(12): 1863–72.
27. McKieth IG, Del-Ser T, Spano P et al. Efficacy of rivastigmine in dementia with Lewy bodies; a randomized, double-blind, placebo-controlled international study. Lancet 2000; 356(9247): 2024–5.
28. Braak H, Del Tredici K, Rüb U et al. Staging of brain pathology related to sporadic Parkinson's disease. Neurobiol Aging 2003; 24: 197–211.
29. Giorgi FS, di Poggio AB, Battaglia G et al. A short overview on the role of alpha-synuclein and proteasome in experimental models of Parkinson's disease. J Neural Transm Suppl 2006; 70: 105–9.
30. Hu XS, Okamura N, Arai H et al. 18F-Fluorodopa PET study of striatal dopamine uptake in the diagnosis of dementia with Lewy bodies. Neurology 2000; 55: 1575–7.
31. Del-Ser T, Munoz DG, Hachinski V. Temporal pattern of cognitive decline and incontinence is different in Alzheimer's disease and diffuse Lewy body disease. Neurology 1996; 46: 682–6.
32. Roman GC, Tatemichi TK, Erkinjuntti T et al. Vascular dementia, diagnostic criteria for research studies; report of the NINDS-AIREN International Workshop. Neurology 1993; 43: 250–60.

33. Brant-Zawadzki M, Fein G, Van Dyke C et al. MR imaging of the aging brain; patchy white-matter lesions and dementia. Am J Neuroradiol 1985; 6(5): 675–82.
34. Ahlberg J, Noren L, Blomstrand C, Wikkelso C. Outcome of shunt operation on urinary incontinence in normal pressure hydrocephalus predicted by lumbar puncture. J Neurol Neurosurg Psychiatry 1988; 51: 105–8.
35. Marmarou A, Black P, Bergsneider M et al. Guidelines for management of idiopathic normal pressure hydrocephalus: progress to date. Acta Neurochir Suppl 2005; 95: 237–40.
36. Yu LC, Rohner TJ, Kaltreider DL et al. Profile of urinary incontinent elderly in long-term care institutions. J Am Geriatr Soc 1990; 38: 433–9.
37. Della Sala S, Francescani A, Spinnler H. Gait apraxia after bilateral supplementary motor area lesion. J Neurol Neurosurg Psychiatry 2002; 72: 77–85.
38. Resnick NM, Baumann M, Scott M et al. Risk factors for incontinence in the nursing home: a multivariate study. Neurourol Urodyn 1988; 7: 274–6.
39. Jirovec MM, Wells TJ. Urinary incontinence in nursing home residents with dementia: the mobility-cognition paradigm. Appl Nurs Res 1990; 3: 112–17.
40. McGrother CW, Jagger C, Clarke M, Castleden CM. Handicaps associated with incontinence: implications for management. J Epidemiol Commun Health 1990; 44: 246–8.
41. Luk JK, Cheung RT, Ho SL, Li L. Does age predict outcome in stroke rehabilitation? A study of 878 Chinese subjects. Cerebrovasc Dis 2006; 21: 229–34.
42. Singh R, Hunter J, Philip A, Todd I. Predicting those who will walk after rehabilitation in a specialist stroke unit. Clin Rehabil 2006; 20: 149–52.
43. Landi F, Onder G, Cesari M et al. Functional decline in frail community-dwelling stroke patients. Eur J Neurol 2006; 13: 17.
44. Paolucci S, Antonucci G, Grasso MG, Pizzamiglio L. The role of unilateral special neglect in rehabilitation of right brain-damaged ischemic stroke patients; a matched comparison. Arch Phys Med Rehab 2001; 82: 743–9.
45. Himashree G, Banerjee PK, Selvamurthy W. Sleep and performance – recent trends. Ind J Physiol Pharmacol 2002; 46: 6–24.
46. Shaw FE. Falls in cognitive impairment and dementia. Clin Geriatr Med 2002; 18: 159–73.
47. Ouslander JG. Geriatric considerations in the diagnosis and management of overactive bladder. Urology 2002; 60(Suppl 1): 50–5.
48. Wein AJ, Rackley RR. Overactive bladder: a better understanding of pathophysiology, diagnosis, and management. J Urol 2006; 175: S5–10.
49. Milsom I, Abrams P, Cardozo L et al. How widespread are the symptoms of an overactive bladder and how are they managed? A population-based prevalence study. BJU Int 2001; 87: 760–6.
50. Homma Y, Yamaguchi O, Hayashi K et al. An epidemiological survey of overactive bladder symptoms in Japan. BJU Int 2005; 96: 1314.
51. Elbadawi A, Yalla SV, Resnick NM. Structural basis of geriatric voiding dysfunction. 3. Detrusor overactivity. J Urol 1993; 150: 1668–80.
52. Kinder RB, Mundy AR. Pathophysiology of idiopathic detrusor instability and detrusor hyper-reflexia; an in vitro study of human detrusor muscle. Br J Urol 1987; 60(6): 509–15.
53. Elbadawi A, Yalla SV, Resnick NM. Structural basis of geriatric voiding dysfunction. 4. Bladder outlet obstruction. J Urol 1993; 150: 1681–95.
54. de Groat WC, Booth AM, Yoshimura N. Neurophysiology of micturition and its modification in animal models of human disease. In: Maggi CA, ed. The Autonomic Nervous System: Nervous Control of the Urogenital System, Vol 3. London: Horwood Academic Publishers, 1993: 227–90; Griffiths D. Basics of pressure-flow studies. World J Urol 1995; 13: 30–3.
55. Aswal BS, Berkley KJ, Hussain I et al. Brain responses to changes in bladder volume and urge to void in healthy men. Brain 2001; 124; 369–77.
56. Kavia RBC, Dasgupta R, Fowler CJ. Functional imaging and the central control of the bladder. J Comp Neurol 2005; 493: 27–32.
57. Griffiths DJ, McCracken PN, Harrison GM et al. Cerebral etiology of urinary urge incontinence in elderly people. Age Ageing 1994; 23: 246–50.
58. Kitada S, Ikei Y, Hasui Y et al. Bladder function in elderly men with subclinical brain magnetic resonance imaging studies. J Urol 1992; 147: 1507–9.
59. Resnick NM, Yalla SV, Laurino E. The pathophysiology of urinary incontinence among institutionalized elderly persons. N Engl J Med 1989; 320: 1–7.
60. Sakakibara R, Hattori T, Yasuda K, Yamanishi T. Micturitional disturbance after acute hemispheric stroke; analysis of the lesion site by CT and MRI. J Neurol Sci 1996; 137: 47–56.
61. Sakakibara R, Shinotoh H, Uchiyama T et al. SPECT imaging of the dopamine transporter with [^{123}I]-β-CIT reveals marked decline of nigrostriatal dopaminergic function in Parkinson's disease with urinary dysfunction. J Neurol Sci 2001; 187: 55–9.
62. Mori S, Kojima M, Sakai Y, Nakajima K. Bladder dysfunction in dementia patients showing urinary incontinence; evaluation with cystometry and treatment with propiverine hydrochloride. Jpn J Geriatr 1999; 36: 489–94.
63. Sugiyama T, Hashimoto K, Kiwamoto H et al. Urinary incontinence in senile dementia of the Alzheimer type (SDAT). Int J Urol 1994; 1: 337–40.
64. Sakakibara R, Ito T, Uchiyama T et al. Lower urinary tract function in dementia of Lewy body type (DLB). J Neurol Neurosurg Psychiatry 2005; 76: 729–32.
65. Komatsu K, Yokoyama O, Otsuka N et al. Central muscarinic mechanism of bladder overactivity associated with Alzheimer type senile dementia. Neurourol Urodyn 2000; 4: 539–40.
66. Sakakibara R, Hattori T, Tojo M et al. Micturitional disturbance in patients with cerebrovascular dementia. Autonom Nerv Syst 1993; 30: 390–6.
67. Resnick NM, Yalla SV. Detrusor hyperactivity with impaired contractile function. JAMA 1987; 257: 3076–81.
68. Eastwood H, Lord A. Are there two types of detrusor hyperreflexia? Neurourol Urodyn 1990; 9: 415–16.
69. Elbadawi A, Yalla SV, Resnick NM. Structural basis of geriatric voiding dysfunction. 2. Ageing detrusor; normal versus impaired contractility. J Urol 1993; 150: 1657–67.
70. Kuwabara S, Naramoto C, Suzuki N et al. Silent post-micturition residuals in elderly subjects with dementia; a study with ultrasound echography. Senile Dementia 1997; 11: 417–21.
71. Yamamoto T, Sakakibara R, Uchiyama T et al. Neurological diseases that cause detrusor hyperactivity with impaired contractile function. Neurourol Urodyn 2006 [Epub ahead of print] PMID: 16532465.
72. Payne C. Epidemiology, pathophysiology and evaluation of urinary incontinence and overactive bladder. Urology 1998; 51(Suppl 2a): 3–10.
73. Keister KJ, Creason NS. Medications of elderly institutionalized incontinent females. J Adv Nurs 1989; 14: 980–5.
74. Resnick NM, Yalla SV. Current concepts; management of urinary incontinence in the elderly. N Engl J Med 1985; 313: 800–15.
75. Skelly J, Flint AJ. Urinary incontinence associated with dementia. J Austr Geriatr Soc 1995; 43: 286–94.
76. Ouslander JG, Blaustein J, Connor A, Pitt A. Habit training and oxybutynin for incontinence in nursing home patients: a placebo controlled study. J Am Geriatr Soc 1988; 36: 40–6.
77. Flint AJ, Skelly JM. The management of urinary incontinence in dementia. Int J Geriatr Psychiatry 1994; 9: 245–6.

78. Jirovec MM. Effect of individualized prompted toileting on incontinence in nursing home residents. Appl Nurs Res 1991; 4: 188–91.
79. Schnelle JF, Sowell VA, Hu TW, Traughber B. Reduction of urinary incontinence in nursing homes: does it reduce or increase costs? J Am Geriatr Soc 1988; 36: 34–9.
80. Chanfreau-Rona D, Bellwood S, Wylie B. Assessment of a behavioural programme to treat incontinent patients in psychogeriatric wards. Br J Clin Psychol 1984; 23: 273–9.
81. Shinotoh H, Aotsuka A, Fukushi K et al. Effect of donepezil on brain acetylcholinesterase activity in patients with AD measured by PET. Neurology 2001; 56: 408–10.
82. Burns A, Rossor M, Hecker J et al. The effects of donepezil in Alzheimer's disease; results from a multinational trial. Dementia Geriatr Cogn Disord 1999; 10: 237–44.
83. Hashimoto M, Imamura T, Tanimukai S et al. Urinary incontinence; an unrecognised adverse effect with donepezil. Lancet 2000; 356: 568.
84. Sakakibara R, Uchiyama T, Yoshiyama M et al. Preliminary communication: urodynamic assessment of donepezil hydrochloride in patients with Alzheimer's disease. Neurourol Urodyn 2005; 24: 273–5.
85. Komatsu K, Yokoyama O, Otsuka N et al. Central muscarinic mechanism of bladder overactivity associated with Alzheimer type senile dementia. Neurourol Urodyn 2000; 4: 539–40.
86. Nieuwenhuys R. Chemoarchitecture of the Brain. Springer-Verlag, Berlin, 1985.
87. Kumon Y, Sakaki S, Takeda S et al. Effect of aneracetam on psychiatric symptoms after stroke. J N Remedies Clin 1997; 46: 231–43.
88. Jirovec MM. The impact of daily exercise on the mobility, balance and urine control of cognitively impaired nursing home residents. Int J Nurs Stud 1991; 28: 145–51.
89. Aranda B, Cramer P. Effects of apomorphine and L-dopa on the parkinsonian bladder. Neurourol Urodyn 1993; 12: 203–9.
90. Sakakibara R, Uchiyama T, Hattori T, Yamanishi T. Urodynamic evaluation in Parkinson's disease before and after levodopa treatment. 9th International Catechecholamine Symposium, Kyoto, Japan, 2001.
91. Brusa L, Petta F, Pisani A et al. Central acute D2 stimulation worsens bladder function in patients with mild Parkinson's disease. J Urol 2006; 175: 202–6.
92. Uchiyama T, Sakakibara R, Hattori T et al. Short-term effect of a single levodopa dose on micturition disturbance in Parkinson's disease patients with the wearing-off phenomenon. Mov Disord 2003; 18: 573–8.
93. Tobin GW, Brocklehurst JC. The management of urinary incontinence in local authority residential homes for the elderly. Age Ageing 1986; 15: 292–8.
94. Burgio KL, Locher JL, Goode PS et al. Behavioural vs drug treatment for urge urinary incontinence in older women; a randomized controlled trial. JAMA 1998; 280: 1995–2000.
95. Zorzitto ML, Jewett MS, Fernie GR. Effectiveness of propantheline bromide in the treatment of geriatric patients with detrusor instability. Neurourol Urodyn 1986; 5: 133–40.
96. Ouslander JG, Sier HC. Drug therapy for geriatric urinary incontinence. Clin Geriatr Med 1986; 2: 789–807.
97. Donnellan CA, Fook L, McDonald P, Playfer JR. Oxybutynin and cognitive dysfunction. BMJ 1997; 315: 1363–4.
98. Womack KB, Heilman KM. Tolterodine and memory: dry but forgetful. Arch Neurol 2003; 60: 771–3.
99. Oka T, Nakano K, Kirimoto T, Matsuura N. Effects of antimuscarinic drugs on both urinary frequency and cognitive impairment in conscious, nonrestrained rats. Jpn J Pharmacol 2001; 87: 27–33.
100. Scheife R, Takeda M. Central nervous system safety of anticholinergic drugs for the treatment of overactive bladder in the elderly. Clin Ther 2005; 27: 144–53.
101. Chu FM, Dmochowski RR, Lama DJ, Anderson RU, Sand PK. Extended-release formulations of oxybutynin and tolterodine exhibit similar central nervous system tolerability profiles: a subanalysis of data from the OPERA trial. Am J Obstet Gynecol 2005; 192: 1849–55.
102. Castleden CM, Duffin HM, Gulati RS. Double-blind study of imipramine and placebo for incontinence due to bladder instability. Age Ageing 1986; 15: 299–303.
103. Schwinn DA. Novel role for α_1-adrenergic receptor subtypes in lower urinary tract symptoms. BJU Int 2000; 86(Suppl 2): 11–22.
104. Cannon A, Carter PG, McConnell PG, Abrams P. Desmopressin in the treatment of nocturnal polyuria in the male. BJU Int 1999; 84: 20–4.
105. Sakakibara R, Uchiyama T, Liu Z et al. Nocturnal polyuria with abnormal circadian rhythm of plasma arginin vasopressin in post-stroke patients. Intern Med 2005; 44: 281–4.
106. Wells TJ, Brink CA, Diokno AC et al. Pelvic muscle exercise for stress urinary incontinence in elderly women. J Am Geriatr Soc 1991; 39: 785–91.
107. Lamhut P, Jackson TW, Wall LL. The treatment of urinary incontinence with electrical stimulation in nursing home patients: a pilot study. J Am Geriatr Soc 1992; 40: 48–52.
108. Gillon G, Stanton SL. Long-term follow-up of surgery for urinary incontinence in elderly women. Br J Urol 1984; 56: 478–81.

21

Pathologies of the basal ganglia, such as Parkinson's and Huntington's disease

Satoshi Seki, Naoki Yoshimura, and Osamu Nishizawa

Introduction

It is well known that disorders of basal ganglia such as Parkinson's disease (PD) can affect lower urinary tract function. The basal ganglia are a group of anatomically closely related subcortical nuclei and have been implicated in a wide range of behavioral functions including motor, cognitive, and emotional functions. The prominent involvement of the basal ganglia in motor control has been recognized in clinical and experimental investigations.[1,2] Damage to these nuclei does not causes weakness, but usually causes dramatic motor abnormalities, as well as lower urinary tract dysfunction.[3,4] But the mechanisms that cause the clinical symptoms have not been completely clarified.

In this chapter an overview of the current concept of the contribution of the basal ganglia system to lower urinary tract function, as well as to general motor function, is given. Then, a review of the literature that describes lower urinary tract dysfunction in patients with disorders of the basal ganglia, such as PD and Huntington's disease (HD), is provided.

Functional anatomy of the basal ganglia

The basal ganglia consist of several subcortical nuclei including the striatum, the globus pallidus, the subthalamic nucleus, and the substantia nigra.

Striatum

Striatum, which consist of the caudate, the putamen, and the nucleus accumbens, is the main input structure of the basal ganglia. The caudate and putamen receive most of the afferents from the entire cerebral cortex, most probably using excitatory amino acids as transmitters; in this sense they are the doorway into the basal ganglia. The output neurons of the striatum use gamma-aminobutyric acid (GABA) as the principal transmitter,[5] co-localized with the neuropeptides enkephalin or substance P/dynorphin.[6–9]

Substantia nigra

The substantia nigra is divided into two parts: the substantia nigra pars compacta (SNpc) and the substantia nigra pars reticulata (SNpr). The SNpc receives input from the caudate and putamen and sends information right back. The SNpr also receives input from the caudate and putamen but sends information outside the basal ganglia. SNpc neurons produce dopamine as a transmitter, which is important for the micturition reflex as well as for normal movement.

Globus pallidus

The globus pallidus is also divided into two parts: the globus pallidus externa (GPe) and the globus pallidus interna (GPi). Both receive input from the caudate and putamen, and both communicate with the subthalamic nucleus (STN).

Physiology and pathophysiology of motor dysfunction in Parkinson's disease

The study of the circuitry of the basal ganglia has mainly been focused on the control of motor function.[10] The

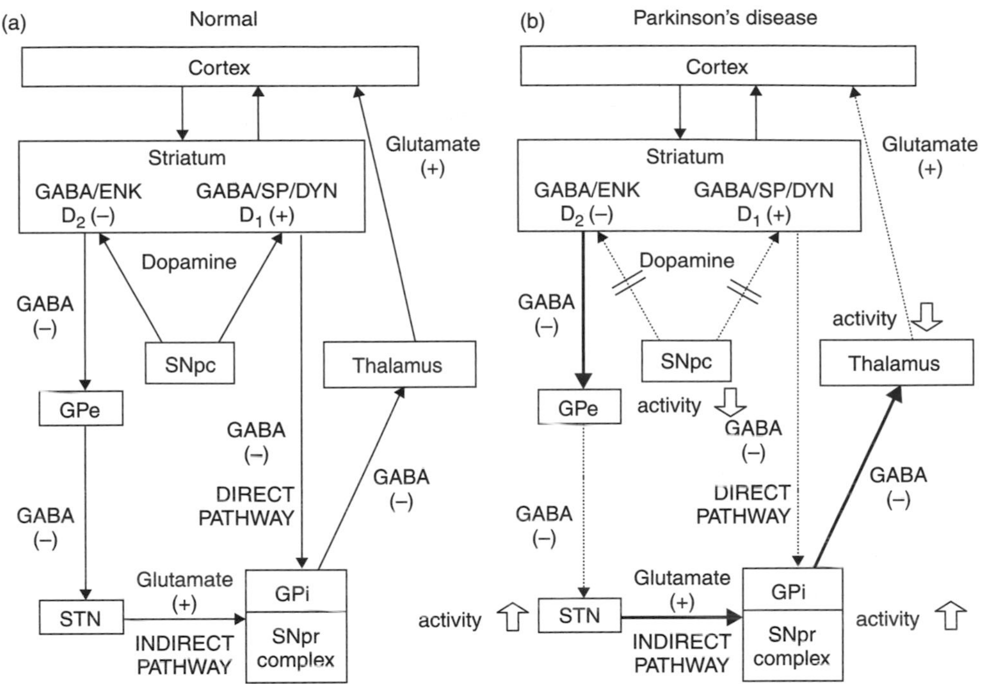

Figure 21.1
Simplified scheme of neural organization in the basal ganglia under (a) the normal conditions and (b) in Parkinson's disease. (a) The striatum receives multiple afferent inputs from the cerebral cortex. The GPi–SNpr complex exerts a tonic GABAergic inhibitory output upon excitatory premotor neurons located in the thalamus. The direct pathway arises from striatal neurons that contain GABA plus peptides substance P (SP) or dynorphin (DYN) and project monosynaptically to the GPi–SNpr complex. The indirect pathway originates from striatal neurons that contain GABA and enkephalin (ENK). Its output is conveyed polysynaptically to the GPi–SNpr complex via GPe and STN. Dopamine increases neuronal activity in the direct pathway via D_1 receptors and inhibits neurons in the indirect pathway via D_2 receptors. Bradykinesia or akinesia observed in Parkinson's disease is thought to result from increased GABAergic inhibition of thalamic premotor neurons. (Thick and broken arrows indicate increased and decreased activity, respectively). SNpr, substantia nigra pars reticulata; SNpc, substantia nigra pars compacta; GPe, globus pallidus externa; GPi, globus pallidus interna; STN, subthalamic nucleus; GABA, gamma-aminobutyric acid.

current model of the organization of the basal ganglia was proposed in the 1980s.

Physiology of the basal ganglia

Cortical information that reaches the striatum is conveyed to the basal ganglia output structure (GPi–SNpr complex) via two pathways (Figure 21.1a). One is an inhibitory direct pathway from the striatum to the GPi–SNpr complex, which mainly uses the inhibitory neurotransmitter GABA. Another is an indirect pathway, which includes (1) an inhibitory projection from the striatum to the GPe, (2) an inhibitory projection from the GPe to the subthalamic nucleus (STN), and (3) an excitatory projection from the STN to the GPi–SNpr complex. These two inhibitory pathways (striato–GPe and GPe–STN) use GABA as a transmitter and the excitatory pathway (STN to GPi–SNpr complex) is activated by glutamate (Figure 21.1a).[11]

The information is then transmitted back to the cerebral cortex via the thalamus. The activity of spiny striatal neurons, which are origin of the direct and indirect pathways, is modulated by dopamine released from nerve terminals of dopaminergic neurons in the SNpc. Dopamine D_2 receptors are expressed in striatopallidal neurons in the indirect pathway, while D_1 receptors are located on neurons in the direct pathway (striatonigral/striatoendopeduncular neurons)[12] (Figure 21.1a). Increased activity of the direct pathway is associated with facilitation of movement and activation of the indirect pathway is associated with inhibition of movement. Dopamine is thought to inhibit neuronal activity through dopamine D_2 receptors in the indirect pathway and to excite neurons via dopamine D_1 receptors in the direct pathway (Figure 21.1a). In conclusion, activation of D_1/D_2 receptors in the striatum provides excessive facilitation of motor systems by exerting the dual effect on the direct and indirect pathways.

Pathophysiology of motor dysfunction in Parkinson's disease

PD is a chronic progressive neurologic disease that is characterized by a decrease in spontaneous movements, gait difficulty, postural instability, rigidity, and tremor. Depigmentation, neuronal loss, and gliosis of the substantia nigra, particularly in the SNpc and locus ceruleus, are typical abnormalities found in the brain of patients with PD.

In PD, the normal inhibitory dopaminergic input to the indirect pathway is decreased, resulting in increased inhibition of GPe (Figure 21.1b). Because the GPe–STN pathway uses GABA as a transmitter, the STN becomes hyperactive. Hyperactivity of the STN results in increased activation of GPi–SNpr complex, leading to decreased activity of the thalamus and its cortical projection areas. This increased output from the indirect pathway is enhanced further by a reduction in the GABA mediated by the direct pathway.

Physiology and pathophysiology of lower urinary tract dysfunction in Parkinson's disease

Dopaminergic systems and micturition reflex

Among the brain structures that regulate micturition, the globus pallidus has been reported to suppress spontaneous detrusor contractions in early studies,[13,14] and the subthalamus and substantia nigra can reportedly inhibit reflex bladder contractions. Electrical stimulation of the basal ganglia, including the SNpc[15,16] and STN,[17] inhibits the micturition reflex in the cat. In addition, this inhibition of the micturition reflex by stimulation of the substantia nigra was blocked by an injection of the D_1-selective antagonist SCH 23390 into the lateral ventricle, and was also mimicked by an intracerebroventricular application of the D_1-selective agonist SKF 38393.[15] Thus, it is thought that dopaminergic neurons originating in the SNpc inhibit the micturition reflex via central dopamine D_1 receptors. Furthermore, a previous study revealed that a D_1 dopaminergic antagonist (SCH 23390) facilitated the micturition reflex, while a D_1 agonist (SKF 38393) had no effect on the reflex bladder contractions in awake rats, suggesting that dopaminergic neurons originating in the substantia nigra tonically inhibit the micturition reflex through dopamine D_1 receptors under normal conditions (Figure 21.2a).[18]

Disruption of this tonic dopaminergic inhibition, by destroying the nigrostriatal pathway with the neurotoxin 1-methyl-4-phenyl-1,2,3,6-tetrahydropyridine (MPTP), produces Parkinson-like motor symptoms in monkeys accompanied by hyperreflexic bladders,[19–21] as reported in patients with PD. The detrusor overactivity was suppressed by stimulation of D_1 receptors with SKF 38393 or pergolide (Figure 21.2b).[20,21] In addition, it has been reported that the striatal dopamine level is significantly increased in the storage phase as compared with that in the elimination phase in normal cats,[22] and that stimulation of D_1 receptors by intraventricular injection of SKF 38393 suppressed detrusor overactivity in a 6-hydroxydopamine (6-OHDA)-induced Parkinson rat model.[23] Thus, it is assumed that detrusor overactivity in patients with PD is due to activation failure of inhibitory mechanisms via dopamine D_1 receptors (Figure 21.2b).

While D_1 receptors mediate inhibition of the micturition reflex, stimulation of dopamine D_2 receptors facilitates the micturition reflex.[15,18,20,21,23,24] In awake rats, systemic application of a D_2 agonist (quinpirole) induced detrusor overactivity, which was blocked by a D_2 antagonist (remoxipride).[18] Similarly, systemic application of quinpirole induced detrusor overactivity in monkeys,[20,21] and treatment with bromocriptine, a D_2 receptor agonist, exacerbated urinary frequency in humans with PD.[25] However, since D_2 receptor-mediated facilitation of the micturition reflex was similarly found in normal and MPTP-induced parkinsonian monkeys,[20,21] and microinjection of dopamine to the pontine micturition center reduced bladder capacity and facilitated the micturition reflex in normal cats,[26,27] it is possible that D_2 receptor-mediated effects on bladder function might be mediated by dopaminergic mechanisms in systems other than the nigrostriatal dopaminergic pathways. A study by Yoshimura et al supports this assumption by demonstrating that detrusor overactivity induced by quinpirole was more pronounced after intrathecal application as compared with intracerebroventricular injection[23] (Figure 21.2a).

In addition, stimulation of D_3 receptors seems to have no influence on the micturition reflex.[23] On the other hand, nonselective dopamine agonists, such as apomorphine and levodopa, facilitate the micturition reflex in experimental animals, possibly via dopamine D_2 receptors.[20,28,29]

In humans, positron emission tomography (PET) has revealed that brain activation sites in response to bladder filling were altered in patients with PD.[30] Another imaging study, using single-photon emission computed tomography (SPECT), has also suggested that a reduction in nigrostriatal dopaminergic neurons is related to urinary disturbance in patients with PD.[31,32]

The ventral tegmentum area (VTA), that lies close to the substantia nigra and is abundant with dopaminergic and serotonergic neurons, seems to be functionally heterogeneous. Both inhibitory and facilitatory responses have been reported.[16,33] We do not know the exact mechanism by which

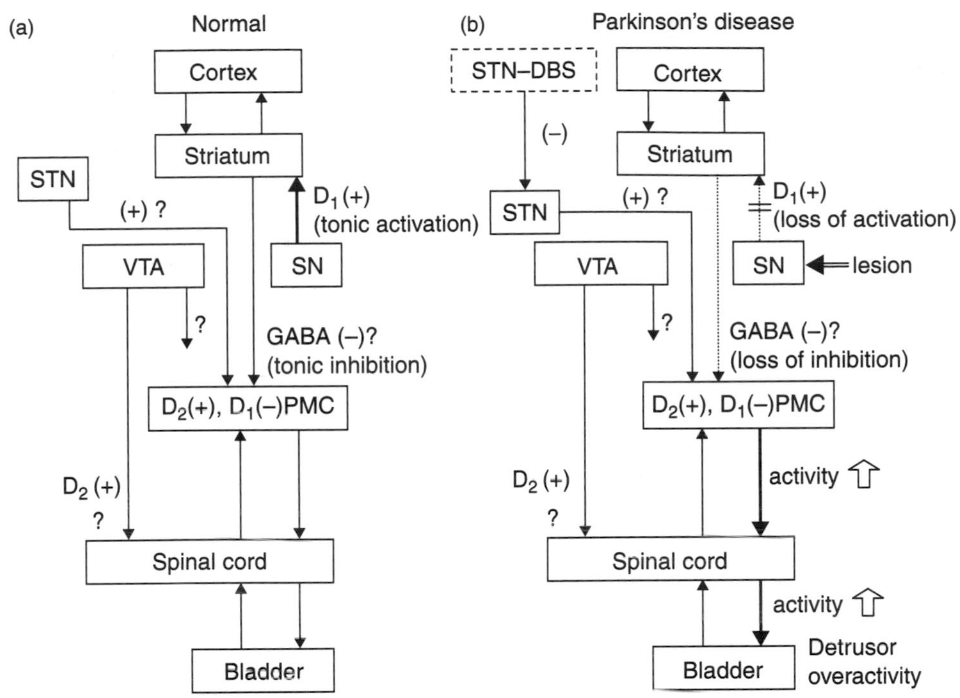

Figure 21.2
Hypothetic view of the relationship between the micturition reflex and dopaminergic systems (a) under normal conditions and (b) in Parkinson's disease. (a) Dopaminergic neurons originating in the substantia nigra pars compacta tonically activate dopamine D_1 receptors, leading to tonic inhibition of the pontine micturition center (PMC), probably through an activation of GABAergic inhibitory receptors. On the other hand, dopamine neurons arising from other brain areas such as the ventral tegmental area (VTA) might stimulate and suppress the micturition reflex via dopamine D_2 and D_1 receptors, respectively, in the PMC. They may also stimulate the micturition reflex via dopamine D_2 receptors in the spinal cord. The STN may directly or indirectly stimulate the PMC to facilitate the micturition reflex. (b) In patients with Parkinson's disease, neuronal cell loss in the substantia nigra pars compacta produces a deficit of dopamine and causes a failure of an activation of inhibitory mechanisms via dopamine D_1 receptors. This failure may be followed by a loss of GABAergic inhibition upon PMC, resulting in detrusor overactivity. (Thick and broken arrows indicate increased and decreased activity, respectively). GABA, gamma-aminobutyric acid; PMC, pontine micturition center; VTA, ventral tegmentum area, STN-DBS, deep brain stimulation of the subthalamic nucleus. Several studies have demonstrated that STN-DBS improved voiding dysfunction in PD patients. Although it is still uncertain whether suppression of neuronal activities in the subthalamic nucleus by STN-DBS directly or indirectly suppresses the pontine micturition center, the similar inhibitory effects were also observed in animal studies.

VTA neurons exert their effects. However, the inhibitory and facilitatory effects might be mediated via dopamine D_1 and D_2 receptors, respectively[33] (Figure 21.2a).

Clinical features of lower urinary tract dysfunction in patients with Parkinson's disease

Symptoms

Voiding dysfunction occurs in 35 to 70% of patients with PD,[34] and most of these patients are diagnosed as PD for several years before the onset of urinary symptoms.[35] Bonnet et al have reported that the age at onset of urinary tract symptoms was 58.7 years and the symptoms began approximately 6 years after onset of parkinsonian motor symptoms.[36] In a study using a symptom score questionnaire, Winge et al also showed that the time from onset of PD to the onset of lower urinary tract symptoms (LUTS) is 5 years.[37]

Storage symptoms, such as increased daytime frequency, nocturia, urgency, and urge urinary incontinence, are most commonly found in PD.[35,36,38–41] Patients also have voiding symptoms alone or in combination, although voiding symptoms that are secondary to PD are thought to be infrequent and moderate.[36] It should be noted that voiding function may be influenced by various types of treatments for the primary disease, PD, and that lower urinary tract dysfunction such as bladder outlet obstruction, which is common in the elderly, may coexist.

Several studies have also shown that the severity of urinary symptoms is related to the neurologic disability or disease severity.[31,36,37,42–44] Araki and Kuno reported that the International Prostate Symptom Score (I-PSS) correlated well with disease severity in patients with PD.[42] On the other hand, it has also been reported that bothersome bladder symptoms in PD correlated with disability due to PD, but there was no correlation between LUTS and stage of disease.[37,45] In any case, we should pay sufficient attention to various aspects of lower urinary tract function, since results of self-report measurements such as questionnaires are unlikely to reflect the real problems.

Bladder function

It is widely accepted that neurogenic detrusor overactivity during the filling phase[46] is most commonly found in urodynamic observations in patients with PD, ranging from 36 to 93%,[36,38,39,41,42,47–52] while bladder sensation is preserved. In the voiding phase, acontractile or underactive detrusor is also found (0 to 48%).[31,36,38,39,42,49,51] However, previous studies have shown that the diagnosis of multiple system atrophy (MSA) rather than PD is more likely made when residual urine greater than 100 ml is present[48,53] (see Chapter 22). Thus, the older studies may have included MSA patients, thereby affecting their results.

Because the incidence of detrusor overactivity with impaired contractile function increases with disease severity, it is possible that long-term detrusor overactivity may eventually lead to deteriorated bladder contractile function at late stages of PD.[42]

Urethral function

Previous studies have shown some disagreement on urethral dysfunction induced by PD. Detrusor-sphincter dyssynergia in patients with PD has been reported in some studies,[42,49] but not in others.[38,39,48,50] However, it seems likely that impaired relaxation or delay in striated sphincter relaxation might exist in patients with PD.[38,51] Pavlakis et al introduced the term 'sphincter bradykinesia', which is characterized by a normal guarding reflex during the filling phase of the CMG and by failure of the striated sphincter to relax rapidly before detrusor contraction,[38] suggesting that bradykinesia is a characteristic of PD and represents a manifestation of skeletal muscle hypertonicity involving pelvic floor muscles. In terms of the difference in detrusor-sphincter dyssynergia, Sakakibara et al demonstrated that it was not seen in patients with PD, but was present in 47% of those with MSA.[48] Therefore this discrepancy may be caused by misinterpretation of EMG or inclusion of patients with other neurologic disorders, such as MSA. In addition, Ogawa et al have demonstrated that activation of dopamine D_2 receptors at a supraspinal site can suppress activity of the striated muscle urethral sphincter in rats.[54] Thus, the presence of levodopa at the time of the studies, which is most commonly used as a therapeutic agent for PD, may also have affected the results in previous reports.

Several studies have also indicated that abnormal urethral and anal sphincter EMG in patients with parkinsonism is highly suggestive of MSA, and that it provides a useful method of distinguishing between idiopathic PD and MSA[48,55,56] (see Chapter 22).

Smooth muscle urethral sphincter dysfunction has not been reported in patients with PD.

Treatment

Various therapeutic options are available for voiding dysfunction in patients with PD, but it should be noted that these patients might have another cause leading to voiding dysfunction such as benign prostatic hyperplasia (BPH), which is common in the elderly. For example, questionnaire-based assessment of voiding dysfunction in patients with PD revealed that men with mild to moderate PD exhibited similar lower urinary tract symptoms to symptomatic patients with BPH.[40]

A high incidence of post-prostatectomy urinary incontinence has been reported by Staskin and coworkers. They reported that 28% of patients with PD who underwent transurethral prostatectomy (TUR-P) exhibited urinary incontinence, and they concluded that poor or absent voluntary sphincter control was the major risk factor of incontinence following TUR-P in the parkinsonian patients.[57] However, Chandiramani and associates pointed out that a poor outcome following prostatic surgery may be due to the inadvertent inclusion of some men with MSA,[35,58] which is a condition most frequently misdiagnosed, even by specialists, as PD.[59] The term 'multiple system atrophy' is synonymous with striatonigral degeneration (SND) when Parkinsonism predominates, olivopontocerebellar atrophy (OPCA) when cerebellar signs predominate, and Shy–Drager syndrome when autonomic failure is dominant. Voiding disturbance in MSA is characterized by a higher incidence of urinary incontinence, significant postvoid residual, and worsening urinary control after urologic surgery[58,60] (see Chapter 22). Although multiple factors may contribute to post-prostatectomy incontinence, it is essential to consider detrusor overactivity. It is unlikely that prostatic surgery for voiding dysfunction due to PD is a contraindication, since detrusor overactivity can be controlled by antimuscarinics.

Clinical studies, in which the effect of levodopa or apomorphine on bladder storage function in patients with PD was examined, have shown conflicting results. It is reasonable to assume that nonselective dopamine receptor agonists such as levodopa and apomorphine facilitates the micturition reflex via dopamine D_2 receptors, resulting in worsening of detrusor overactivity. However, some authors have demonstrated an improvement in detrusor overactivity with levodopa or apomorphine in some patients with PD,[39,47,61,62] and aggravation in others,[39,47,61–64] while Stocchi et al found no improvement in detrusor overactivity with apomorphine.[51] Brusa et al demonstrated that treatment using levodopa alone and levodopa with domperidone (a peripheral D_2 antagonist) worsened detrusor overactivity in patients with PD, while treatment using levodopa with sulpiride (a central and peripheral D_2 antagonist) counteracted the effect of levodopa in a dose dependent manner.[64] According to these results, they concluded that a central acute D_2 stimulation seems to be responsible for the worsening of detrusor overactivity. However, Benson et al reported that moderate doses of levodopa alleviated detrusor overactivity in patients with PD, but high doses of levodopa aggravated it.[62] Thus it is assumed that the dosage of these drugs also changes the response of storage function to the treatment.

In addition, metabolites of these agents, such as noradrenaline, or diversity of disease severity might have affected these results.

Previous studies have shown that administration of levodopa or apomorphine in patients with PD provided significant improvement in voiding dysfunction.[47,51,63] Christmas et al demonstrated that subcutaneous injection of apomorphine (a nonselective dopamine receptor agonist) improved flow rate and reduced postvoid residual in patients with PD, suggesting that bladder outlet obstruction secondary to BPH may be distinguished from voiding dysfunction secondary to PD.[47]

These effects on voiding function might be mediated by activation of dopamine D_2 receptors, which can enhance detrusor contractility to increase voiding efficiency. Furthermore, animal experiments have demonstrated that activation of D_2 receptors at a supraspinal site suppressed activity of the striated muscle urethral sphincter in the voiding phase.[54] Thus, the effects of levodopa or apomorphine on voiding function in patients with PD appear to be consequences of increased bladder contractility and decreased urethral resistance during voiding due to D_2 receptor stimulation.

Recently, deep brain stimulation of the subthalamic nucleus (STN-DBS) has been established as a surgical treatment of motor symptoms in PD patients. In addition, several studies have demonstrated that STN-DBS improved voiding dysfunction in PD patients. In these studies the main effect of STN-DBS seems to be a normalization of urodynamic parameters in the storage phase.[65–67] Although it is still uncertain whether suppression of neuronal activities in the subthalamic nucleus by STN-DBS directly or indirectly suppresses the pontine micturition center, the similar inhibitory effects were also observed in animal studies.[17,68]

Various antimuscarinic agents are currently available for the treatment of detrusor overactivity. The clinical and urodynamic data suggest that they can provide significant improvements in patients with PD.[4,69] However, it should be noted that these patients might have bowel dysfunction such as constipation secondary to PD.[70] If medical treatment fails and patients have large residual volumes, introduction of clean intermittent catheterization is an option.

Alpha-blockers are also preferred as the first-line treatment, especially for male patients with voiding and even storage symptoms, although patients may have orthostatic hypotension due to PD and/or its medication.

Huntington's disease

HD is a degenerative disease with autosomal dominant inheritance characterized by progressive neuronal loss in the basal ganglia, especially in the caudate nucleus and cerebral cortex.[71,72] The exact mechanisms underlying neuronal death in HD are still unknown. Although the disease may begin any time from childhood to old age (average age of onset is approximately 40 years), adult-onset HD is characterized by a triad of progressive motor, cognitive, and emotional symptoms.

There has been little investigation regarding urinary tract dysfunction in patients with HD. Wheeler et al reviewed the neurourologic findings in 6 patients with HD, who complained of lower urinary tract symptoms, and found that 4 out of 6 patients had detrusor overactivity with a normal sphincter, while the remaining 2 patients exhibited no abnormal findings. Symptoms include urinary frequency, urgency, nocturia, and incontinence, and the onset of these symptoms was 6.1 years after the onset of HD.[73] A survey of 1283 symptomatic individuals with HD found that lower urinary tract symptoms occurred in the late stage of HD, typically more than 10 years after onset.[74]

Anticholinergic agents could be useful to alleviate urologic symptoms. However, in patients with severe neurologic disability, a permanent indwelling catheter or urosheath drainage may be required.

References

1. Flowers KA. Visual 'closed-loop' and 'open-loop' characteristics of voluntary movement in patients with Parkinsonism and intention tremor. Brain 1976; 99(2): 269–310.
2. Evarts EV, Teravainen H, Calne DB. Reaction time in Parkinson's disease. Brain 1981; 104(Pt 1): 167–86.
3. Fowler CJ. Update on the neurology of Parkinson's disease. Neurourol Urodyn 2007; 26(1): 103–9.

4. Winge K, Fowler CJ. Bladder dysfunction in Parkinsonism: mechanisms, prevalence, symptoms, and management. Mov Disord 2006; 21(6): 737–45.
5. Kita H, Kitai ST. Glutamate decarboxylase immunoreactive neurons in rat neostriatum: their morphological types and populations. Brain Res 1988; 447(2): 346–52.
6. Vincent SR, Hokfelt T, Christensson I, Terenius L. Dynorphin-immunoreactive neurons in the central nervous system of the rat. Neurosci Lett 1982; 33(2): 185–90.
7. Vincent S, Hokfelt T, Christensson I, Terenius L. Immunohistochemical evidence for a dynorphin immunoreactive striato-nigral pathway. Eur J Pharmacol 1982; 85(2): 251–2.
8. Beckstead RM. Complementary mosaic distributions of thalamic and nigral axons in the caudate nucleus of the cat: double anterograde labeling combining autoradiography and wheat germ-HRP histochemistry. Brain Res 1985; 335(1): 153–9.
9. Kanazawa I, Emson PC, Cuello AC. Evidence for the existence of substance P-containing fibres in striato-nigral and pallido-nigral pathways in rat brain. Brain Res 1977; 119(2): 447–53.
10. Obeso JA, Rodriguez-Oroz MC, Rodriguez M et al. Pathophysiology of the basal ganglia in Parkinson's disease. Trends Neurosci 2000; 23(Suppl): S8–19.
11. Levy R, Hazrati LN, Herrero MT et al. Re-evaluation of the functional anatomy of the basal ganglia in normal and Parkinsonian states. Neuroscience 1997; 76(2): 335–43.
12. Le Moine C, Bloch B. D1 and D2 dopamine receptor gene expression in the rat striatum: sensitive cRNA probes demonstrate prominent segregation of D1 and D2 mRNAs in distinct neuronal populations of the dorsal and ventral striatum. J Comp Neurol 1995; 355(3): 418–26.
13. Lewin RJ, Dillard GV, Porter RW. Extrapyramidal inhibition of the urinary bladder. Brain Res 1967; 4: 301–7.
14. Raz S. Parkinsonism and neurogenic bladder. Experimental and clinical observations. Urol Res 1976; 4(3): 133–8.
15. Yoshimura N, Sasa M, Yoshida O, Takaori S. Dopamine D1 receptor-mediated inhibition of micturition reflex by central dopamine from the substantia nigra. Neurourol Urodyn 1992; 11: 535–45.
16. Sakakibara R, Nakazawa K, Uchiyama T et al. Micturition-related electrophysiological properties in the substantia nigra pars compacta and the ventral tegmental area in cats. Auton Neurosci 2002; 102(1–2): 30–8.
17. Sakakibara R, Nakazawa K, Uchiyama T et al. Effects of subthalamic nucleus stimulation on the micturition reflex in cats. Neuroscience 2003; 120(3): 871–5.
18. Seki S, Igawa Y, Kaidoh K et al. Role of dopamine D1 and D2 receptors in the micturition reflex in conscious rats. Neurourol Urodyn 2001; 20(1): 105–13.
19. Albanese A, Jenner P, Marsden CD, Stephenson JD. Bladder hyperreflexia induced in marmosets by 1-methyl-4-phenyl-1,2,3,6-tetrahydropyridine. Neurosci Lett 1988; 87(1–2): 46–50.
20. Yoshimura N, Mizuta E, Kuno S, Sasa M, Yoshida O. The dopamine D1 receptor agonist SKF 38393 suppresses detrusor hyperreflexia in the monkey with parkinsonism induced by 1-methyl-4-phenyl-1,2,3,6-tetrahydropyridine (MPTP). Neuropharmacology 1993; 32: 315–21.
21. Yoshimura N, Mizuta E, Yoshida O, Kuno S. Therapeutic effects of dopamine D1/D2 receptor agonists on detrusor hyperreflexia in 1-methyl-4-phenyl-1,2,3,6-tetrahydropyridine-lesioned parkinsonian cynomolgus monkeys. J Pharmacol Exp Ther 1998; 286(1): 228–33.
22. Yamamoto T, Sakakibara R, Hashimoto K et al. Striatal dopamine level increases in the urinary storage phase in cats: an in vivo microdialysis study. Neuroscience 2005; 135(1): 299–303.
23. Yoshimura N, Kuno S, Chancellor MB, de Groat WC, Seki S. Dopaminergic mechanisms underlying bladder hyperactivity in rats with a unilateral 6-hydroxydopamine (6-OHDA) lesion of the nigrostriatal pathway. Br J Pharmacol 2003; 139(8): 1425–32.
24. Kontani H, Inoue T, Sakai T. Dopamine receptor subtypes that induce hyperactive urinary bladder response in anesthetized rats. Jpn J Pharmacol 1990; 54: 482–6.
25. Kuno S, Mizuta E, Yoshimura N. Different effects of D1 and D2 agonists on neurogenic bladder in Parkinson's disease and MPTP-induced parkinsonian monkeys. Mov Disord 1997; 12(S1).
26. de Groat WC, Booth AM, Yoshimura N. Neurophysiology of micturition and its modification in animal models of human disease. In: Maggi CA, ed. The Autonomic Nervous System, Vol. 3, Nervous Control of the Urogenital System. London: Harwood Academic Publishers, 1993; 227–90.
27. Roppolo JR, Noto H, Mallory BS, de Groat WC. Dopaminergic and cholinergic modulation of bladder reflexes at the level of the pontine micturition center in the cat. Soc Neurosci Abstr 1987; 13: 733.
28. Ishizuka O, Pandita RK, Mattiasson A, Steers WD, Andersson KE. Stimulation of bladder activity by volume, L-dopa and capsaicin in normal conscious rats – effects of spinal alpha 1-adrenoceptor blockade. Naunyn Schmiedebergs Arch Pharmacol 1997; 355(6): 787–93.
29. Sillen U, Rubenson A, Hjalmas K. Central cholinergic mechanisms in L-DOPA induced hyperactive urinary bladder of the rat. Urol Res 1982; 10(5): 239–43.
30. Kitta T, Kakizaki H, Furuno T et al. Brain activation during detrusor overactivity in patients with Parkinson's disease: a positron emission tomography study. J Urol 2006; 175(3 Pt 1): 994–8.
31. Sakakibara R, Shinotoh H, Uchiyama T et al. SPECT imaging of the dopamine transporter with [(123)I]-beta-CIT reveals marked decline of nigrostriatal dopaminergic function in Parkinson's disease with urinary dysfunction. J Neurol Sci 2001; 187(1–2): 55–9.
32. Winge K, Friberg L, Werdelin L, Nielsen KK, Stimpel H. Relationship between nigrostriatal dopaminergic degeneration, urinary symptoms, and bladder control in Parkinson's disease. Eur J Neurol 2005; 12(11): 842–50.
33. Hashimoto K, Oyama T, Sugiyama T, Park YC, Kurita T. Neuronal excitation in the ventral tegmental area modulates the micturition reflex mediated via the dopamine D1 and D2 receptors in rats. J Pharmacol Sci 2003; 92(2): 143–8.
34. Wein A. Neuromuscular dysfunction of the lower urinary tract and its management. In: Walsh PC, Retik AB, Vaughan C, Wein A, eds. Campbell's Urology, 8th edn. Philadelphia: Saunders, 2002: 931–1026.
35. Chandiramani VA, Palace J, Fowler CJ. How to recognize patients with parkinsonism who should not have urological surgery. Br J Urol 1997; 80(1): 100–4.
36. Bonnet AM, Pichon J, Vidailhet M et al. Urinary disturbances in striatonigral degeneration and Parkinson's disease: clinical and urodynamic aspects. Mov Disord 1997; 12(4): 509–13.
37. Winge K, Skau AM, Stimpel H, Nielsen KK, Werdelin L. Prevalence of bladder dysfunction in Parkinsons disease. Neurourol Urodyn 2006; 25(2): 116–22.
38. Pavlakis AJ, Siroky MB, Goldstein I, Krane RJ. Neurologic findings in Parkinson's disease. J Urol 1983; 129: 80–3.
39. Fitzmaurice H, Fowler CJ, Rickards D et al. Micturition disturbance in Parkinson's disease. Br J Urol 1985; 57(6): 652–6.
40. Lemack GE, Dewey RB Jr, Roehrborn CG, O'Suilleabhain PE, Zimmern PE. Questionnaire-based assessment of bladder dysfunction in patients with mild to moderate Parkinson's disease. Urology 2000; 56(2): 250–4.
41. Defreitas GA, Lemack GE, Zimmern PE et al. Distinguishing neurogenic from non-neurogenic detrusor overactivity: a urodynamic assessment of lower urinary tract symptoms in patients with and without Parkinson's disease. Urology 2003; 62(4): 651–5.
42. Araki I, Kuno S. Assessment of voiding dysfunction in Parkinson's disease by the international prostate symptom score. J Neurol Neurosurg Psychiatry, 2000; 68(4): 429–33.

43. Hattori T, Yasuda K, Kita K, Hirayama K. Voiding dysfunction in Parkinson's disease. Jpn J Psychiatry Neurol 1992; 46(1): 181–6.
44. Winge K, Werdelin LM, Nielsen KK, Stimpel H. Effects of dopaminergic treatment on bladder function in Parkinson's disease. Neurourol Urodyn 2004; 23(7): 689–96.
45. Hobson P, Islam W, Roberts S, Adhiyman V, Meara J. The risk of bladder and autonomic dysfunction in a community cohort of Parkinson's disease patients and normal controls. Parkinsonism Relat Disord 2003; 10(2): 67–71.
46. Abrams P, Cardozo L, Fall M et al. The standardisation of terminology of lower urinary tract function: report from the Standardisation Sub-committee of the International Continence Society. Neurourol Urodyn 2002; 21(2): 167–78.
47. Christmas TJ, Kempster PA, Chapple CR et al. Role of subcutaneous apomorphine in parkinsonian voiding dysfunction. Lancet 1988; 2(8626–8627): 1451–3.
48. Sakakibara R, Hattori T, Uchiyama T, Yamanishi T. Videourodynamic and sphincter motor unit potential analyses in Parkinson's disease and multiple system atrophy. J Neurol Neurosurg Psychiatry 2001; 71(5): 600–6.
49. Khan Z, Starer P, Bhola A. Urinary incontinence in female Parkinson disease patients. Pitfalls of diagnosis. Urology 1989; 33(6): 486–9.
50. Gray R, Stern G, Malone-Lee J. Lower urinary tract dysfunction in Parkinson's disease: changes relate to age and not disease. Age Ageing 1995; 24(6): 499–504.
51. Stocchi F, Carbone A, Inghilleri M et al. Urodynamic and neurophysiological evaluation in Parkinson's disease and multiple system atrophy. J Neurol Neurosurg Psychiatry 1997; 62(5): 507–11.
52. Myers DL, Arya LA, Friedman JH. Is urinary incontinence different in women with Parkinson's disease? Int Urogynecol J Pelvic Floor Dysfunct 1999; 10(3): 188–91.
53. Hahn K, Ebersbach G. Sonographic assessment of urinary retention in multiple system atrophy and idiopathic Parkinson's disease. Mov Disord 2005; 20(11): 1499–502.
54. Ogawa T, Seki S, Masuda H et al. Dopaminergic mechanisms controlling urethral function in rats. Neurourol Urodyn 2006; 25(5): 480–9.
55. Eardley I, Quinn NP, Fowler CJ et al. The value of urethral sphincter electromyography in the differential diagnosis of parkinsonism. Br J Urol 1989; 64(4): 360–2.
56. Vodusek DB. How to diagnose MSA early: the role of sphincter EMG. J Neural Transm 2005; 112(12): 1657–68.
57. Staskin DS, Vardi Y, Siroky MB. Post-prostatectomy continence in the parkinsonian patient: the significance of poor voluntary sphincter control. J Urol 1988; 140(1): 117–18.
58. Fowler CJ. Urinary disorders in Parkinson's disease and multiple system atrophy. Funct Neurol 2001; 16(3): 277–82.
59. Quinn N. Parkinsonism – recognition and differential diagnosis. BMJ 1995; 310(6977): 447–52.
60. Beck RO, Betts CD, Fowler CJ. Genitourinary dysfunction in multiple system atrophy: clinical features and treatment in 62 cases. J Urol 1994; 151(5): 1336–41.
61. Aranda B, Cramer P. Effects of apomorphine and L-dopa on the parkinsonian bladder. Neurourol Urodyn 1993; 12(3): 203–9.
62. Benson GS, Raezer DM, Anderson JR, Saunders CD, Corriere JN Jr. Effect of levodopa on urinary bladder. Urology 1976; 7(1): 24–8.
63. Uchiyama T, Sakakibara R, Hattori T, Yamanishi T. Short-term effect of a single levodopa dose on micturition disturbance in Parkinson's disease patients with the wearing-off phenomenon. Mov Disord 2003; 18(5): 573–8.
64. Brusa L, Petta F, Pisani A et al. Central acute D2 stimulation worsens bladder function in patients with mild Parkinson's disease. J Urol 2006; 175(1): 202–6; discussion 206–7.
65. Finazzi-Agro E, Peppe A, D'Amico A et al. Effects of subthalamic nucleus stimulation on urodynamic findings in patients with Parkinson's disease. J Urol 2003; 169(4): 1388–91.
66. Seif C, Herzog J, van der Horst C et al. Effect of subthalamic deep brain stimulation on the function of the urinary bladder. Ann Neurol 2004; 55(1): 118–20.
67. Herzog J, Weiss PH, Assmus A et al. Subthalamic stimulation modulates cortical control of urinary bladder in Parkinson's disease. Brain 2006; 129(Pt 12): 3366–75.
68. Dalmose AL, Bjarkam CR, Sorensen JC, Djurhuus JC, Jorgensen TM. Effects of high frequency deep brain stimulation on urine storage and voiding function in conscious minipigs. Neurourol Urodyn 2004; 23(3): 265–72.
69. Palleschi G, Pastore AL, Stocchi F et al. Correlation between the Overactive Bladder questionnaire (OAB-q) and urodynamic data of Parkinson disease patients affected by neurogenic detrusor overactivity during antimuscarinic treatment. Clin Neuropharmacol 2006; 29(4): 220–9.
70. Sakakibara R, Shinotoh H, Uchiyama T et al. Questionnaire-based assessment of pelvic organ dysfunction in Parkinson's disease. Auton Neurosci 2001; 92(1–2): 76–85.
71. Feigin A, Zgaljardic D. Recent advances in Huntington's disease: implications for experimental therapeutics. Curr Opin Neurol 2002; 15(4): 483–9.
72. Walker FO. Huntington's disease. Lancet 2007; 369(9557): 218–28.
73. Wheeler JS, Sax DS, Krane RJ, Siroky MB. Vesico-urethral function in Huntington's chorea. Br J Urol 1985; 57(1): 63–6.
74. Kirkwood SC, Su JL, Conneally P, Foroud T. Progression of symptoms in the early and middle stages of Huntington disease. Arch Neurol 2001; 58(2): 273–8.

22

Urinary dysfunction in multiple system atrophy

Ryuji Sakakibara, Clare J Fowler, and Takamichi Hattori

Introduction

Multiple system atrophy (MSA) is an uncommon but well-recognized disease entity that both neurologists and urologists may encounter. The term MSA was introduced by Graham and Oppenheimer in 1969 to describe a disorder of unknown cause affecting extrapyramidal, cerebellar, and autonomic pathways.[1] MSA includes the disorders previously called striatonigral degeneration (SND),[2] sporadic olivopontocerebellar atrophy (OPCA),[3] and Shy–Drager syndrome.[4] The discovery in 1989 of glial cytoplasmic inclusions in the brains of patients with MSA[5] provided a pathologic marker for the disorder (akin to Lewy bodies in idiopathic Parkinson's disease (IPD)), and confirmed that SND, OPCA, and Shy–Drager syndrome are the same disease with differing clinical presentations. Immunocytochemistry showed that the glial cytoplasmic inclusions of MSA are ubiquitin-, tau-, and alpha-synuclein- positive, possibly representing a cytoskeletal alteration in glial cells that results in neuronal degeneration.[6] Familial occurrence is estimated to account for 1.6% of all cases, and data on such cases are being accumulated to identify a possible causative gene for this disorder.[7]

Autonomic failure (postural hypotension and urinary dysfunction) is fundamental to the diagnosis of MSA: it is diagnosed when the criteria of either postural hypotension (systolic blood pressure fall > 30 mmHg or diastolic > 15 mmHg) or urinary dysfunction (persistent, involuntary urinary incontinence/incomplete bladder emptying) or both are fulfilled, along with poorly levodopa-responsive parkinsonism or cerebellar dysfunction.[8] Based on the major motor deficits, MSA can be classified as MSA-P (parkinsonism-predominant) or MSA-C (cerebellar-predominant).[1] Clinical differential diagnosis between MSA-P, the most common clinical form, and IPD is difficult even for specialists. However, the lack of one-side dominance and resting tremor, poor response to levodopa, and rapid progression are all red flags indicating MSA.[9] MSA-C can mostly be distinguished from hereditary spinocerebellar ataxias, although some individuals with such disorders do not have apparent heredity. Autonomic failure (AF) is almost invariably present[10] and can be an initial manifestation (AF-MSA).[11] Autonomic failure occurs in other neurodegenerative diseases, for example in a subset of patients with IPD (AF-PD) as well as in pure autonomic failure (PAF), both of which are considered Lewy body diseases. This chapter reviews the current concepts of urinary dysfunction in MSA, with particular reference to urinary symptoms, (video-)urodynamic assessment and sphincter electromyography (EMG), and patient management.

Urinary symptoms

Urinary dysfunction and postural hypotension

Of various symptoms due to AF (erectile dysfunction, urinary dysfunction, postural hypotension, respiratory stridor) in patients with MSA, urinary dysfunction has been attracting less attention than postural hypotension, although urinary dysfunction may result in recurrent urinary tract infection and may be a cause of morbidity.[12] In addition, urinary incontinence results in impaired self-esteem, stress on the caregiver, and considerable financial cost. Postural hypotension was pointed out first in AF-MSA, which turned out to be a marker of autonomic involvement in this disorder. Both of the original 2 patients discussed by Shy and Drager had urinary frequency, incontinence, and urinary retention.[4] Other variants (MSA-P and MSA-C) rarely develop postural hypotension in their early stage. However, in the original reports, 3 of 4 patients with MSA-P showed voiding difficulty, retention, and urinary incontinence,[2] and both patients with MSA-C had voiding difficulty and urinary incontinence.[3] Thus, what are the most common and earliest autonomic features of MSA?

In our previous study of 121 patients with MSA,[13] urinary symptoms (96%) were more common than orthostatic symptoms (43%) ($p < 0.01$) (Figure 22.1). The most frequent urinary symptom was difficulty voiding in 79% of the patients, followed by nocturnal urinary frequency in 74%. Other symptoms included sensation of urgency

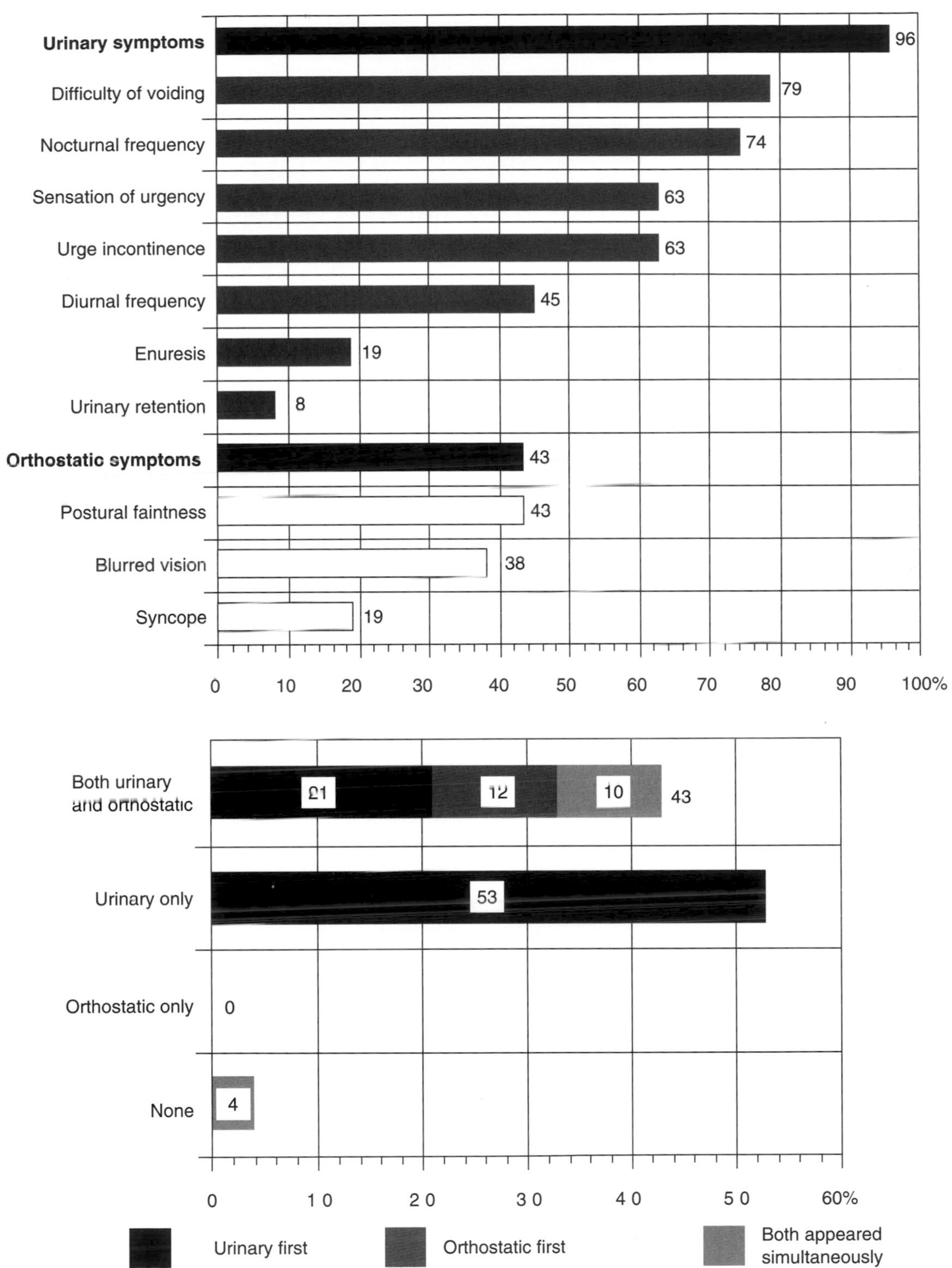

Figure 22.1
Urinary dysfunction and postural hypotension in MSA.

in 63%, urgency incontinence in 63%, diurnal urinary frequency in 45%, nocturnal enuresis in 19%, and urinary retention in 8%. The most frequent orthostatic symptom was postural faintness in 43%, followed by blurred vision in 38% and syncope in 19%. These figures are similar to those of Wenning et al,[14] who noted urinary incontinence in 71%, urinary retention in 27%, postural faintness in 53%, and syncope in 15% of 100 patients with MSA; these figures were recently confirmed by a larger study.[15] In our previous study mentioned above,

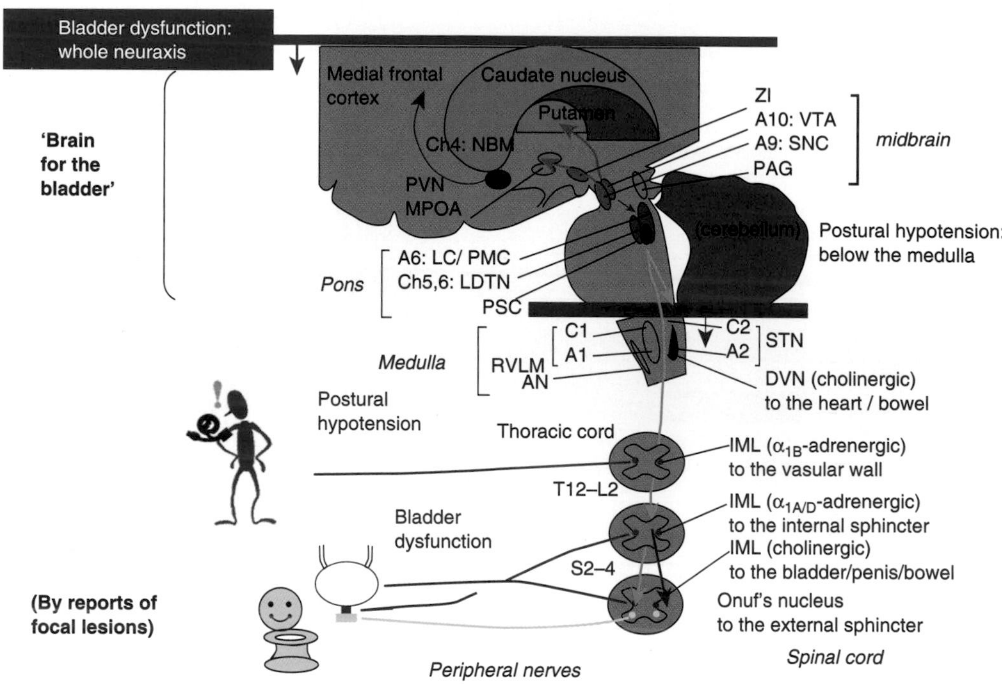

Figure 22.2
Why does bladder dysfunction occur more commonly and earlier than postural hypotension in MSA?

among 53 patients with both urinary and orthostatic symptoms, those who had urinary symptoms first (48%) were more common than those who had orthostatic symptoms first (29%), and some patients developed both symptoms simultaneously (23%).[13]

These findings indicate that urinary dysfunction is a more common and often earlier manifestation than postural hypotension in MSA. Many factors might be involved in this phenomenon. Reports of focal lesions have shown that postural hypotension occurs in lesions below the medulla, whereas urinary dysfunction occurs in lesions at any site in the neuraxis. MSA lesions involve the pons, the hypothalamus, and the basal ganglia, all of which might affect the lower urinary tract function as described below (Figure 22.2).

Urinary dysfunction and motor disorders

Looking at both urinary and motor disorders, approximately 60% of patients with MSA develop urinary symptoms either prior to or at the time of presentation with the motor disorder[12,13] (Figure 22.3). This indicates that many of these patients seek urologic advice early in the course of their disease. Since the severity of urinary symptoms is severe enough for surgical intervention, male patients with MSA may undergo urologic surgery for prostatic outflow obstruction before the correct diagnosis has been made. The results of such surgery are often transient or unfavorable because of the progressive nature of this disease. Male erectile dysfunction is often the first presentation,[12,13,16] possibly preceding the occurrence of urinary dysfunction in MSA. The urologist confronted with a patient showing these features should be cautious about embarking on an operative approach. The neurologist encountering a patient with marked urinary symptoms might consider future investigation by brain magnetic resonance imaging (MRI) and sphincter EMG.

Since motor disorders in MSA mostly mimic those in IPD, the urogenital distinction between these two diseases is worth considering, although a number of earlier studies on 'Parkinson's disease and the bladder' might inadvertently include patients with MSA. The prevalence rate of urinary dysfunction in MSA is higher than the 58–71% rate reported in IPD,[13,17–19]; similarly, that of urgency incontinence in MSA is higher than the 33% rate reported in IPD. In addition, urinary dysfunction is never the initial presentation in IPD.

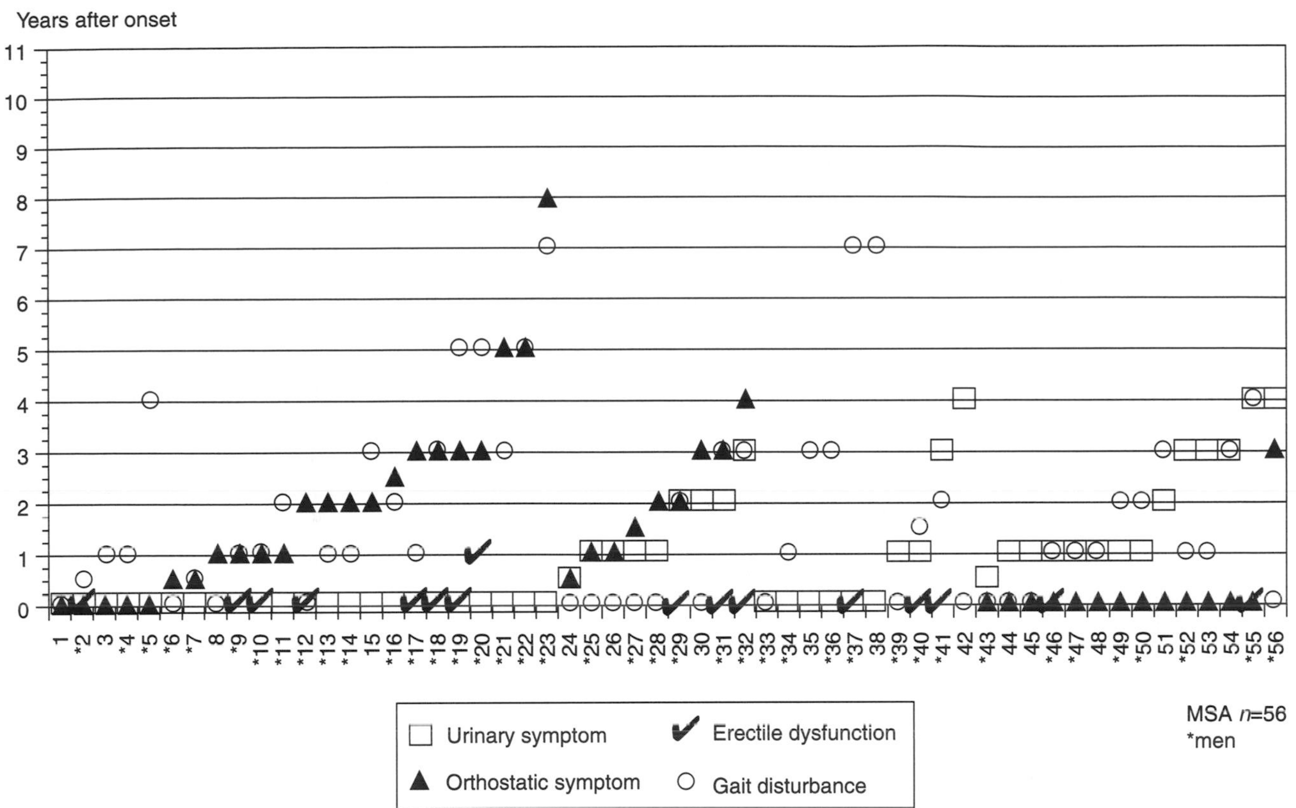

Figure 22.3
Autonomic and motor disorders in MSA.

Videourodynamic and sphincter electromyography assessments

Since MSA is a neurodegenerative disease that affects multiple brain regions, patients with the disease may have a wide range of urodynamic abnormalities that change with progression of the illness. Videourodynamics and sphincter EMG also enable us to assess the lumbosacral cord functions, which help to distinguish MSA from other parkinsonian disorders.

Bladder overactivity

Filling phase abnormalities included bladder overactivity in 33–100% and uninhibited external sphincter relaxation in 33% of MSA cases,[12,19–21] figures similar to those reported in IPD[10,12–16] (Figure 22.4). Bladder overactivity is urodynamically defined as an involuntary phasic increase in detrusor pressure (naïve bladder pressure – abdominal pressure) >10 cmH_2O during bladder filling, which is commonly associated with decreased bladder volumes at first sensation and bladder capacity. It is bladder overactivity that seems to be the major cause of urgency incontinence in patients with MSA. But when coupled with uninhibited sphincter relaxation, incontinence may worsen.[22]

It is well known that cerebral diseases can lead to a loss of the brain's inhibitory influence on the spino-bulbo-spinal micturition reflex. The information that arises from the lower urinary tract reaches the periaqueductal gray matter (PAG), then goes down to the pontine micturition center (PMC), an area identical or just adjacent to the locus ceruleus, which then activates the descending pathway to the sacral preganglionic neurons innervating the bladder.[23] The basal ganglia are thought to be one of the higher centers for micturition, since lesions of this area lead to bladder overactivity.[24–27] Recent positron emission tomography (PET) studies have shown that the hypothalamus, PAG, midline pons, and cingulate cortex are activated during urinary filling.[28,29] The central pathology of MSA includes neuronal loss of neuromelanin-containing cells in the locus ceruleus[30,31] as well as in the nigrostriatal dopaminergic system ('putaminal slit sign')[6,27] and cerebellum, and to a lesser extent in the ponto-medullary raphe ('pontine cross sign')[6,32] and the frontal cortex.[33,34] Recent experimental studies have suggested that the raphe modulates micturition function.[35] Experimental studies have also suggested that the cerebellum controls micturition function.[36]

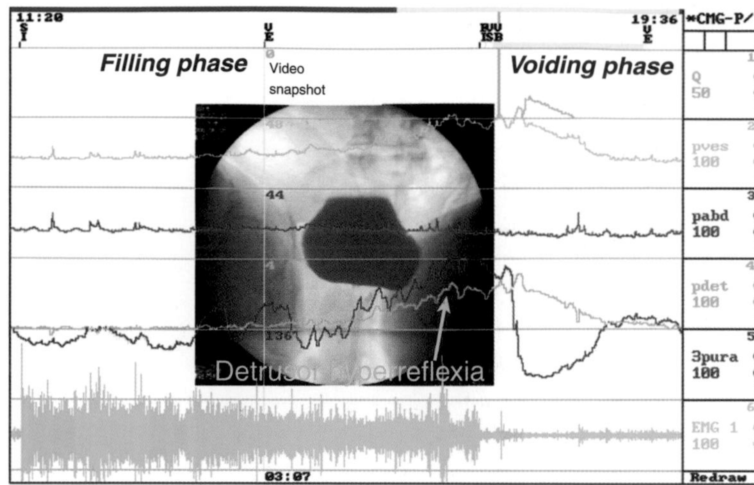

Figure 22.4
Bladder overactivity.

A single photon emission computed tomography (SPECT) study has shown that in the urinary storage and micturition phases, but not in the resting phase, activation of the cerebellar vermis was significantly lower in MSA patients than in control subjects (Figure 22.5).[37] These areas seem to be responsible for the occurrence of bladder overactivity and uninhibited sphincter relaxation in MSA patients.

Bladder underactivity and detrusor-sphincter dyssynergia

Incomplete bladder emptying is a significant feature in MSA. In fact, 47% of patients with MSA had a postvoid residual (PVR) >100 ml, whereas no patients with IPD had such levels (p <0.01).[19] The mean PVR volume was 71 ml in the first year, 129 ml in the second year (which exceeded the threshold volume for the start of clean intermittent catheterization (CIC)), and 170 ml in the fifth year from the onset of illness (Figure 22.6).[38]

Factors relevant to the voiding disorder in MSA include the bladder and the urethral outlet. Pressure–flow analysis refers to the simultaneous monitoring of detrusor pressure and urinary flow, and to drawing the relation curve between them (Figure 22.7). Although it was originally developed for diagnosing outlet obstruction due to prostatic hypertrophy,[39,40] pressure–flow analysis is useful for evaluating neurogenic voiding difficulty.[41]

Pressure–flow analysis showed that bladder underactivity (a weak detrusor contraction) during voiding is more common in MSA (71% in women and 63% in men) than in IPD (66% in women and 40% in men).[19] The AG number represents a grade of urethral obstruction, and an AG number >40 means outflow obstruction in men.[39] The mean AG numbers were smaller in patients with MSA (12 in women and 28 in men) than in those with IPD (40 in women and 43 in men).[19] However, a subset of patients with MSA may have an obstructive pattern, the reason for which is unknown. Detrusor-external sphincter dyssynergia is a factor contributing to neurogenic urethral relaxation failure,[41] which is noted in 47% of MSA patients.[19,42] Therefore, it is likely that bladder underactivity accounts mostly for voiding difficulty and elevated PVR in MSA. A subset of patients with MSA has bladder overactivity during storage and underactivity during voiding (detrusor hyperactivity with impaired contractile function, DHIC).[43] The exact mechanism of this phenomenon has yet to be ascertained. However, it has been recognized that the central mechanisms underlying bladder filling and voiding are distinct from each other; i.e., the area promoting micturition is located in the PMC and the frontal cortex, whereas that promoting urinary storage is in the pontine storage center, basal ganglia, raphe, and frontal cortex.[23] Lesions in these areas may cause various combinations of urinary filling and voiding disorders, such as DHIC.

Open bladder neck

The bladder neck, also known as the internal (smooth) urethral sphincter, is a component in the maintenance of continence that is innervated by the sympathetic hypogastric nerve. Videourodynamic study is an established method for evaluating bladder neck function. It is a combination of visualizing the lower urinary tract simultaneously with EMG cystometry; urethral pressure at the external urethral sphincter can be obtained with visual guidance using a radiopaque marker. In normal subjects,

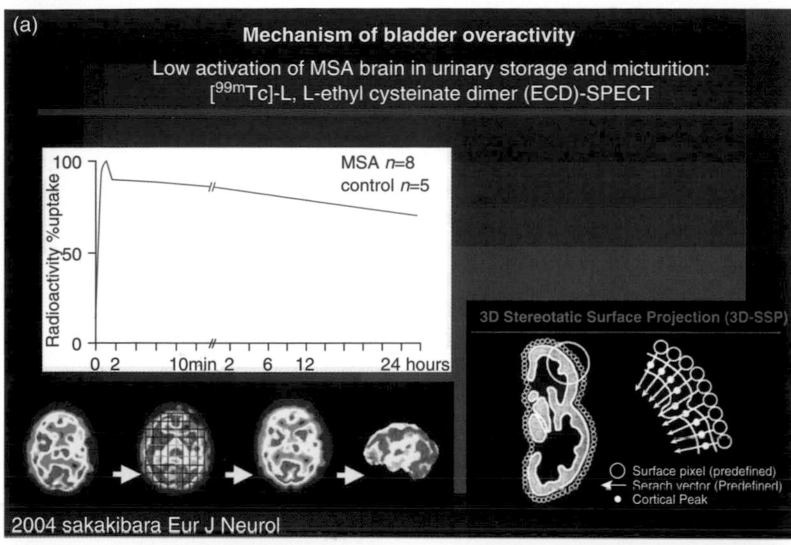

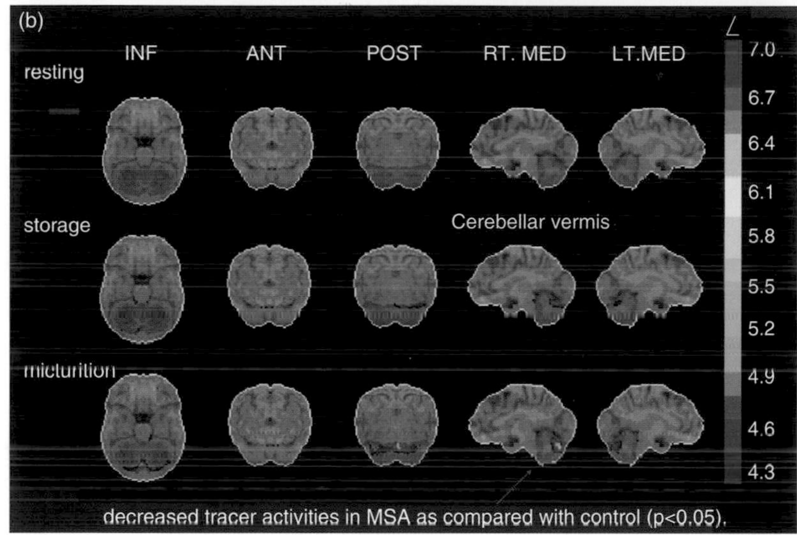

Figure 22.5
Reduced cerebellar vermis activation in urinary storage and micturition phases in MSA.

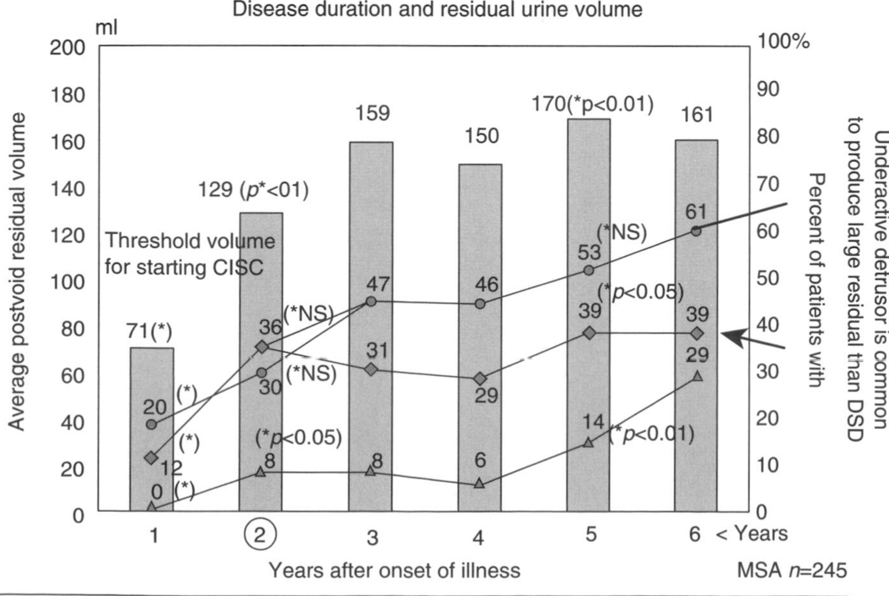

Figure 22.6
Incomplete bladder emptying in MSA.

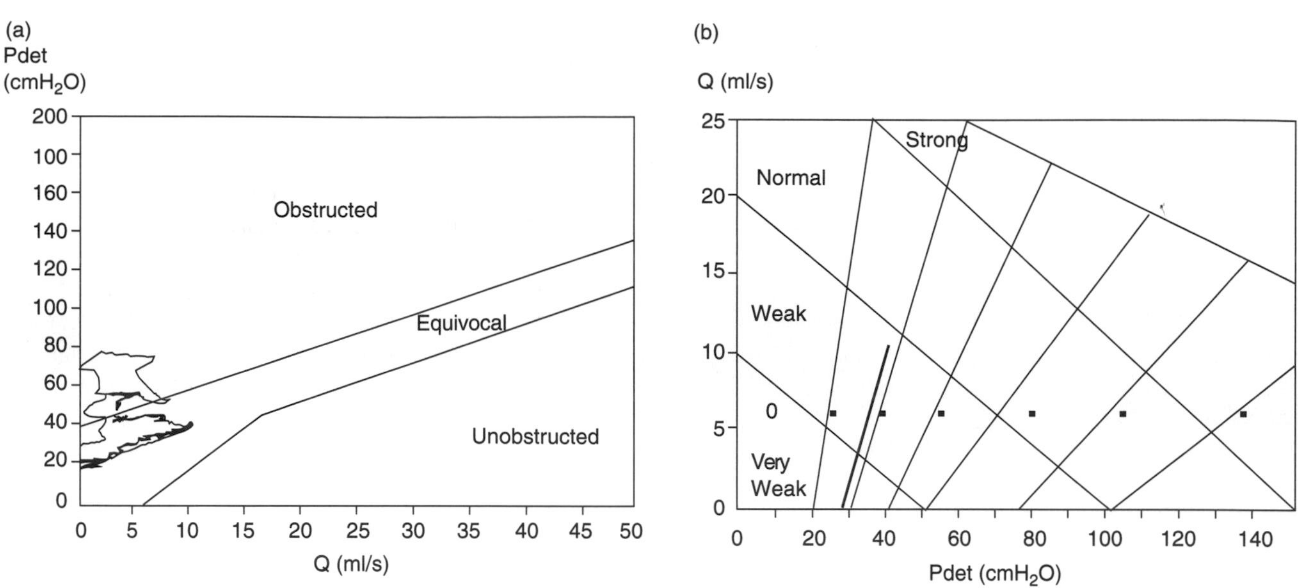

Figure 22.7
Two pressure–flow nomograms: (a) Abrams–Griffiths nomogram; (b) Schafer nomogram. Pdet, detrusor pressure; Q, urinary flow rate.

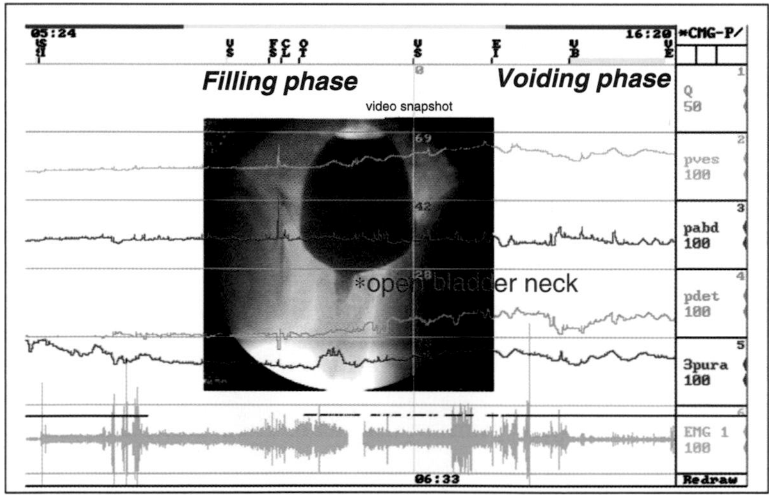

Figure 22.8
Open bladder neck.

the bladder neck is closed throughout filling so as to avoid leaking. However, an open bladder neck is found in 46–100% of MSA patients and in 23–31% of PD patients, and an open bladder neck at the start of bladder filling, even without the accompaniment of bladder overactivity, was noted in no PD patients but in 53% of MSA patients ($p < 0.01$) (Figure 22.8).[19] Because open bladder neck is common in patients with myelodysplasia or a lower thoracic cord lesion at T12–L2 (where sympathetic thoracolumbar intermediolateral [IML] nuclei are located) and is reproduced by systemic or intraurethral application of α_1-adrenergic blockers,[44] it is likely that an open bladder neck reflects the loss of sympathetic innervation. An open bladder neck is usually considered asymptomatic, but may cause incontinence and reduce bladder capacity.

Neurogenic changes in sphincter EMG

Of particular importance is the group of anterior horn cells in the sacral spinal cord, which project fibers to the external sphincters. They were first described by

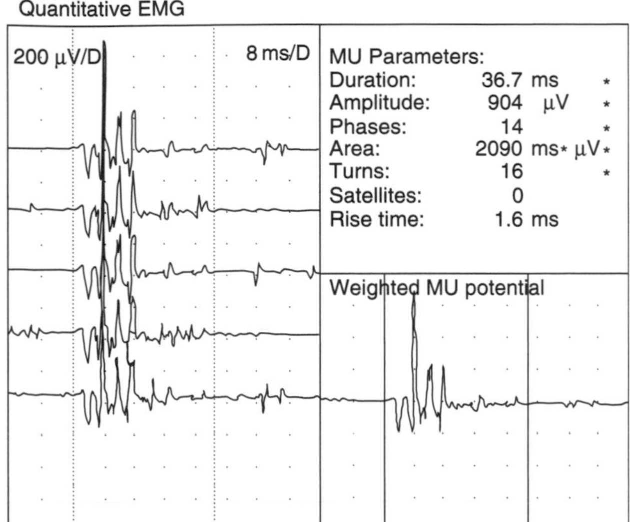

Figure 22.9
External sphincter EMG. A motor unit recorded from the anal sphincter of a patient with multiple system atrophy shows an abnormally prolonged duration (upper range of normal is <10 ms) and stable low-amplitude late components. D, division; EMG, electromyography; MU, motor unit.

Onufrowicz in 1900 and hence became known as 'Onuf's nuclei'. Postmortem studies in patients dying with MSA demonstrated a selective loss of anterior horn cells in Onuf's nuclei; such cells are spared in amyotrophic lateral sclerosis.[45,46] Since in IPD the anterior horn cells of Onuf's nuclei are also spared, sphincter EMG can be a means of distinguishing between MSA-P and IPD. The external (striated) urethral sphincter is another component in the maintenance of continence, and is innervated by the somatic pudendal nerve. The changes in chronic reinnervation that occur in the motor units of the external sphincter have been demonstrated by EMG.[47,48] Similar neurogenic changes have been demonstrated in the anal and urethral sphincters in MSA. As the anal sphincter is more superficial, needle EMG causes less discomfort and is therefore the preferred test. By varying the position of the needle electrode, 10 different motor units can be identified and the overall mean duration calculated. In the measurement of duration, it is important to include highly stable but low-amplitude late (satellite) components that may be separated from the initial part of the complex by an isoelectric period of several milliseconds (Figure 22.9). The control range of values for the duration of motor units is wide,[48] but a mean duration of motor unit potentials >10 ms or more than 20% of motor unit potentials with a duration >10 ms is most sensitive for diagnosing chronic reinnervation.[49] Previous reports showed neurogenic motor unit potentials in 75–100% of patients with MSA[11,19–21,49–51] and in 0–17% of those with IPD.[19–21] In MSA, neurogenic motor unit potentials occurred in 52% in the first year, which increased to 83% in the fifth year from the onset of illness.[52] Although denervation can be found in the other skeletal muscles in MSA, it occurs much earlier in the external sphincter muscles,[53] in contrast to the case in amyotrophic lateral sclerosis.

Up to 40% of patients with MSA may have low resting urethral pressure,[12] which most probably reflects sphincter weakness. The resulting denervation of the urethral sphincter, together with detrusor overactivity, is a reason why urgency incontinence is such a pronounced and early feature of MSA.[11] Sphincter weakness in MSA may also result in stress urinary incontinence, which occurs particularly in female patients.[54]

Changing bladder patterns

The sites responsible for cardiovascular autonomic failure in MSA are mostly central, in contrast to the peripheral lesions in PAF.[10] However, 31–45% of patients with MSA also had low-compliance detrusor, defined as a maximum bladder capacity/tonic detrusor pressure increase <20 ml/cmH_2O.[13] Low-compliance detrusor is known to occur in patients with spina bifida or in animals with experimental cauda equina lesions, most probably reflecting neuronal loss of bladder preganglionic neurons in the sacral IML nucleus and their fibers (pelvic nerve).[55,56] The bethanechol test is the established method to detect lesions in the most peripheral site.[57] A minimum amount (2.5 mg) of bethanechol, a cholinergic agent, is injected subcutaneously; this amount is not sufficient to evoke bladder contraction in normal subjects. However, when the bladder is denervated, cholinergic receptor densities in the postsynaptic membrane increase, increasing abnormal detrusor pressure upon bethanechol injection. Nineteen percent of MSA patients showed denervation supersensitivity of the detrusor.[13]

Repeated urodynamic studies in MSA patients showed that the cystometrogram changed from bladder overactivity to low-compliance or atonic detrusor, and from negative to positive bethanechol supersensitivity.[13] In fact, as the disease progresses, symptoms may change from urinary urgency and frequency to those due to incomplete bladder emptying.[12] These findings suggest that the responsible sites of the bladder cholinergic disorder may change from the 'center' (supranuclear) to the 'periphery' (nuclear sacral IML and/or infra-nuclear) during the course of the illness. Since MSA primarily affects the preganglionic neurons in the autonomic nervous system,[10] bladder findings that suggest postganglionic lesions might reflect trans-synaptic degeneration of the cholinergic fibers.

Nocturnal polyuria

Other than bladder disorders, patients with MSA may have nocturnal polyuria, which results in nocturnal urinary frequency and morning hypotension. In normal children over 7 years and adults, the circadian release of arginine vasopressin (AVP) from the posterior pituitary gland into plasma peaks at night. This leads to a nocturnal decrease in urine formation. The ratio of nighttime to daytime urine production is usually <1:2, which can be estimated by a frequency volume chart. This circadian rhythm can be impaired in cases of congestive heart failure, nephrosis, or cirrhosis with ascites. However, a postmortem study of the brains of patients with MSA revealed the degeneration of AVP neurons in the suprachiasmatic nucleus,[58] leading to impairment of the circadian rhythm of the plasma AVP concentration in MSA.[59,60] In addition, daytime postural hypotension may also cause nocturnal polyuria in patients with MSA.[61] This is probably due to a combination of factors that include compensatory supine hypertension at night, leading to increased glomerular filtration.

Management of urinary dysfunction

Incomplete bladder emptying

More than half of patients with MSA have urinary dysfunction either prior to or at the time of presentation with motor disorder. Since many of these patients develop incomplete bladder emptying, they may be misdiagnosed as having prostatic hypertrophy. In fact, the results of urologic surgery are not always favorable, since bladder underactivity contributes more to voiding difficulty than does outflow obstruction. Therefore, it is important to avoid inappropriate urologic surgery in patients with MSA.[62] In men with MSA, effects of transurethral resection of the prostate lasted for less than 2 years.[38] A conservative approach with medical measures to manage urinary problems can be effective.

Estimation of the PVR volume is a simple and useful test in patients with MSA; even though their urinary complaints are solely urinary urgency/frequency, they may be unaware that their bladders do not empty completely. PVR can be measured by ultrasound echography, either with specific machines (bladder manager BVI3000, for example) or abdominal echography (multiplied 3-direction diameters*0.5). Transurethral catheterization is also available in the clinic but causes slight discomfort. If the patient has a significant PVR and is symptomatic, this aspect of the problem should be managed using CIC performed by either the patient or the caregiver. However, in patients with advanced disease and severe neurologic disability, a permanent indwelling catheter, either transurethral or suprapubic, or urosheath drainage may be required.

Bladder overactivity

The bladder is innervated by the parasympathetic pelvic nerve and has an abundance of $M_{2/3}$ muscarinic receptors. Bladder overactivity may reflect an increased micturition reflex via either the brainstem or the sacral cord, which can be treated with anticholinergic medication such as tolterodine, oxybutynin, propiverine, or propantheline. These drugs diminish the parasympathetic tone on bladder smooth muscle, and are usually tried in patients with urinary urgency and frequency. However, anticholinergic side-effects, particularly dry mouth (probably mediated by M_3 receptors) and constipation ($M_{2/3}$ receptors), may limit their use in a proportion of the patients. A subset of patients with MSA may develop mild cognitive decline at an advanced stage of the disease. Since the use of anticholinergic drugs carries a risk of cognitive impairment (M_1 receptors),[63] though this is much less common than the drugs' peripheral effects, we have to be careful to manage urinary dysfunction in such patients. Anticholinergic drugs do ameliorate urgency and frequency, but may also reduce bladder contractility during voiding.[11] Therefore, it should be better to measure PVR regularly. If PVR exceeds 100 ml, the medication should be withdrawn or CIC should be added. If nighttime urinary urgency/frequency is the problem, a night balloon is a good alternative to drugs for patients who are performing CIC.[38]

Interactions between drugs to treat bladder, postural hypotension, and motor disorder

α-Adrenergic receptors

Since incomplete bladder emptying in patients with MSA is due mostly to bladder underactivity, drugs acting on outflow obstruction are unlikely to benefit all patients. However, in some patients, α-adrenergic blockers may be effective in lessening PVR volumes, due probably to detrusor-sphincter dyssynergia.[64] Uroselective blockers such as tamsulosin and naftopidil may be of choice because they have fewer side-effects such as postural hypotension. The effects of α-adrenergic blockers were reported to last for less than 2 years.[38]

In contrast, the drugs most commonly used to treat postural hypotension in MSA are adrenergic agonists.

However, administration of amezinium, an adrenergic drug, may increase the risk of retention and PVR volume compared to that before treatment.[65] Amezinium most probably stimulates the α receptors, both in the vascular wall (α_{1B} receptors, particularly in the elderly[66]) and the proximal urethra ($\alpha_{1A/D}$-adrenergic receptors).

Cholinergic receptors

Both postural hypotension and bladder dysfunction are common clinical features in MSA. Pyridostigmine, an acetylcholinesterase inhibitor, can be effective in lessening PVR volume, since it stimulates muscarinic acetylcholine receptors on the bladder ($M_{2/3}$ muscarinic receptors) that are innervated by parasympathetic cholinergic neurons.[67] Pyridostigmine also lessens postural hypotension, presumably by enhancing nicotinic acetylcholine receptor transmission in the sympathetic ganglia.[68,69]

Dopaminergic receptors

Whether centrally acting drugs, such as pergolide (a dopaminergic $D_{1/2}$ receptor agonist) for parkinsonism, might ameliorate urinary dysfunction in MSA has not been fully studied.[70,71] Early untreated IPD patients with mild urgency and frequency tend to benefit from levodopa ($D_{1/2}$) treatment. However, in a one-hour time window, levodopa may augment bladder overactivity in early[72] or advanced[73] IPD patients. Since D_1-selective stimulation inhibits the micturition reflex that D_2-selective stimulation facilitates, the balance of these stimulations may explain the various effects of the drugs. Levodopa ($D_{1/2}$) and its metabolites, such as norepinephrine (noradrenaline), may also contract the bladder neck by stimulating α_1-adrenergic receptors.[65]

Nocturnal polyuria (vasopressin receptors)

Desmopressin is a potent analog of AVP (hypertensive and antidiuretic effects: 100 vs 100 in AVP; 0.39 vs 1200 in desmopressin, respectively), and it is used in the treatment of diabetes insipidus due to a loss of posterior pituitary AVP secretion. Mathias et al[60] used 2–4 µg of intramuscular desmopressin in patients with autonomic failure including MSA. We also prescribed 5 µg of intranasal desmopressin once a night in MSA patients with impaired circadian rhythm of AVP and nocturnal polyuria, with benefit.[74] This small dose of desmopressin is unlikely to cause adverse effects. However, hyponatremia and signs of cardiac failure should be checked for regularly. A tablet form is available and may be more convenient for patient use. Desmopressin could also ameliorate morning hypotension resulting from the abnormal loss of body fluid at night.[60]

Micturition syncope

Well-known triggers for syncope in MSA include (1) standing (postural syncope), (2) eating (post-prandial syncope), and (3) exercise (postexertional syncope).[10] We found that syncope in patients with MSA is also triggered by (4) voiding (micturition syncope). In our patients, the systolic blood pressure increase was less pronounced during storage, whereas the systolic blood pressure decrease was significant during and after voiding as compared with controls.[75] The detailed link between the bladder and the cardiovascular system is still uncertain in this condition. However, particularly in patients who experience abdominal strain upon voiding, CIC could lessen micturition syncope.

Summary

Urinary dysfunction is a prominent autonomic feature in patients with MSA, and it is more common (above 90%) and occurs earlier than postural hypotension in this disorder. Since the clinical features of MSA may mimic those of IPD, a distinctive pattern of urinary dysfunction in both disorders is worth looking at. In contrast to IPD, MSA patients have more marked urinary dysfunction, which consists of both urgency incontinence and PVR >100 ml. Videourodynamic and sphincter EMG analyses are important tools for understanding the extent of these dysfunctions and for determining both the diagnosis and management of the disorders. The common finding in both disorders is bladder overactivity, which accounts for urinary urgency and frequency. However, detrusor-sphincter dyssynergia, open bladder neck at the start of bladder filling (internal sphincter denervation), and neurogenic sphincter EMG (external sphincter denervation) are all characteristics of MSA. These features may reflect pathologic lesions in the basal ganglia, pontine tegmentum, raphe, intermediolateral cell column, and sacral Onuf's nuclei. During the course of the disease, the pathophysiologic balance shifts from central to peripheral, with bladder emptying disorder predominating.

Since MSA is a progressive disorder and impaired detrusor contractility is common, it is important to avoid inappropriate urologic surgery in patients with MSA. A conservative approach with medical measures includes anticholinergics for urinary urgency and frequency, desmopressin for nocturnal polyuria, uroselective α-blockers and cholinergic stimulants for voiding difficulty, and CIC for large PVR.

References

1. Graham JG, Oppenheimer DR. Orthostatic hypotension and nicotinic sensitivity in a case of multiple system atrophy. J Neurol Neurosurg Psychiatry 1969; 32: 28–34.
2. Adams RD, van Bogaert L, Eecken HV. Striato-nigral degeneration. J Neuropathol Exp Neurol 1964; 23: 584–608.
3. Dejerine J, Thomas A. L'atrophie olivo-ponto-cérébelleuse. Nouvelle Iconographie de la Salpêtriére 1900; 13: 30–70.
4. Shy GM, Drager GA. A neurological syndrome associated with orthostatic hypotension; a clinical-pathologic study. Arch Neurol 1960; 2: 511–27.
5. Papp MI, Kahn JE, Lantos PL. Glial cytoplasmic inclusions in the CNS of patients with multiple system atrophy (striatonigral degeneration, olivopontocerebellar atrophy and Shy–Drager syndrome). J Neurol Sci 1989; 94: 79–100.
6. Wenning GK, Colosimo C, Geser F et al. Multiple system atrophy. Lancet Neurol 2004; 3: 93–103.
7. Soma H, Yabe I, Takei A, Fujiki N et al. Heredity in multiple system atrophy. J Neurol Sci 2006; 240: 107–10.
8. Gilman S, Low PA, Quinn N et al. Consensus statement on the diagnosis of multiple system atrophy. Clin Auton Res 1998; 8: 359–62.
9. Quinn N. Parkinsonism – recognition and differential diagnosis. BMJ 1995; 310: 447–52.
10. Bannister R, Mathias CJ. Clinical features and investigation of the primary autonomic failure syndromes. In: Bannister R, Mathias CJ, eds. Autonomic Failure, 3rd edn. Oxford: Oxford Medical Publications, 1992: 531–47.
11. The Consensus Committee of the American Autonomic Society and the American Academy of Neurology. Consensus statement on the definition of orthostatic hypotension, pure autonomic failure, and multiple system atrophy. Neurology 1996; 46: 1470.
12. Beck RO, Betts CD, Fowler CJ. Genito-urinary dysfunction in Multiple System Atrophy: clinical features and treatment in 62 cases. J Urol 1994; 151: 1336–41.
13. Sakakibara R, Hattori T, Uchiyama T et al. Urinary dysfunction and orthostatic hypotension in multiple system atrophy; which is the more common and earlier manifestation? J Neurol Neurosurg Psychiatry 2000; 68: 65–9.
14. Wenning GK, Ben Shlomo Y, Magalhaes M et al. Clinical features and natural history of multiple system atrophy: an analysis of 100 cases. Brain 1994; 117: 835–45.
15. Gilman S, May SJ, Shults CW et al. The North American Multiple System Atrophy Study Group. J Neural Transm 2005; 112: 1687–94.
16. Kirchhof K, Apostolidis AN, Mathias CJ et al. Erectile and urinary dysfunction may be the presenting features in patients with multiple system atrophy: a retrospective study. Int J Impot Res 2003; 15: 293–8.
17. Christmas TJ, Chapple CR, Lees AJ et al. Role of subcutaneous apomorphine in parkinsonian voiding dysfunction. Lancet 1998; Dec 24/31: 1451–3.
18. Fitzmaurice H, Fowler CJ, Richards D et al. Micturition disturbance in Parkinson's disease. Br J Urol 1985; 57: 652–6.
19. Sakakibara R, Hattori T, Uchiyama T et al. Videourodynamic and sphincter motor unit potential analyses in Parkinson's disease and multiple system atrophy. J Neurol Neurosurg Psychiatry 2001; 71: 600–6.
20. Berger Y, Salinas JM, Blaivas JG. Urodynamic differentiation of Parkinson disease and the Shy–Drager syndrome. Neurourol Urodyn 1990; 9: 117–21.
21. Stocchi F, Carbone A, Inghilleri M et al. Urodynamic and neurophysiological evaluation in Parkinson's disease and multiple system atrophy. J Neurol Neurosurg Psychiatry 1997; 62: 507–11.
22. Sand PK, Bowen LW, Ostergard DR. Uninhibited urethral relaxation; an unusual cause of incontinence. Obstet Gynecol 1986; 68: 645–8.
23. de Groat WC, Booth AM, Yoshimura N. Neurophysiology of micturition and its modification in animal models of human disease. In: Maggi CA, ed. The Autonomic Nervous System: Nervous Control of the Urogenital System, Vol 3. London: Harwood Academic Publishers, 1993: 227–90.
24. Yoshimura N, Mizuta E, Kuno S et al. The dopamine D1 receptor agonist SKF 38393 suppresses detrusor hyperreflexia in the monkey with parkinsonism induced by MPTP. Neuropharm 1993; 32: 315–21.
25. Sakakibara R, Fowler CJ. Cerebral control of bladder, bowel, and sexual function and effects of brain disease. In: Fowler CJ, ed. Neurology of Bladder, Bowel, and Sexual function. Boston: Butterworth-Heinemann, 1999: 229–43.
26. Sakakibara R, Nakazawa K, Uchiyama T et al. Micturition-related electrophysiological properties in the substantia nigra pars compacta and the ventral tegmental area in cats. Auton Neurosci Basic Clin 2002; 102: 30–8.
27. Yamamoto T, Sakakibara R, Hashimoto K et al. Striatal dopamine level increases in the urinary storage phase in cats: an *in vivo* microdialysis study. Neuroscience 2005; 135: 299–303.
28. Aswal BS, Berkley KJ, Hussain I et al. Brain responses to changes in bladder volume and urge to void in healthy men. Brain 2001; 124: 369–77.
29. Kavia RBC, Dasgupta R, Fowler CJ. Functional imaging and the central control of the bladder. J Comp Neurol 2005; 493: 27–32.
30. Daniel SE. The neuropathology and neurochemistry of multiple system atrophy. In: Bannister R, Mathias CJ, eds. Autonomic Failure, 3rd edn. Oxford: Oxford Medical Publications, 1992: 564–85.
31. Benarroch EE, Schmeichel AM. Depletion of corticotrophin-releasing factor neurons in the pontine micturition area in multiple system atrophy. Ann Neurol 2001; 50: 640–5.
32. Benarroch EE, Schmeichel AM, Low PA et al. Involvement of medullary serotonergic groups in multiple system atrophy. Ann Neurol 2004; 55: 418–22.
33. Fujita T, Doi M, Ogata T et al. Cerebral cortical pathology of sporadic olivopontocerebellar atrophy. J Neurol Sci 1993; 116: 41–6.
34. Andrew J, Nathan PW. Lesions of the anterior frontal lobes and disturbances of micturition and defaecation. Brain 1964; 87: 233–62.
35. Ito T, Sakakibara R, Nakazawa K et al. Effects of electrical stimulation of the raphe area on the micturition reflex in cats. Neuroscience 2006 [Epub ahead of print] PMID: 16996219.
36. Nishizawa O, Ebina K, Sugaya K et al. Effect of cerebellectomy on reflex micturition in the decerebrate dog as determined by urodynamic evaluation. Urol Int 1989; 44: 152–6.
37. Sakakibara R, Uchida Y, Uchiyama T et al. Reduced cerebellar vermis activation in response to micturition in multiple system atrophy; 99mTc-labeled ECD SPECT study. Eur J Neurol 2004; 11: 705–8.
38. Ito T, Sakakibara R, Yasuda K et al. Incomplete emptying and urinary retention in multiple system atrophy: when does it occur and how do we manage it? Mov Disord 2006 [Epub ahead of print] PMID: 1651–1861.
39. Abrams P. Objective evaluation of bladder outlet obstruction. Br J Urol 1995; 76(Suppl 1): 11–15.
40. Shäfer W. Principles and clinical application of advanced urodynamic analysis of voiding dysfunction. Urol Clin North Am 1990; 17: 553–66.
41. Sakakibara R, Fowler CJ, Hattori T et al. Pressure–flow study as an evaluating method of neurogenic urethral relaxation failure. J Auton Nerv Syst 2000; 80: 85–8.
42. Blaivas JG, Sinha HP, Zayed AAH et al. Detrusor-sphincter dyssynergia; a detailed electromyographic study. J Urol 1981; 125: 545–8.
43. Resnick NM, Yalla SV. Detrusor hyperactivity with impaired contractile function. JAMA 1987; 257: 3076–81.
44. Yamanishi T, Yasuda K, Sakakibara R et al. The effectiveness of terazosin, an α1-blocker, on bladder neck obstruction as assessed by urodynamic hydraulic energy. BJU Int 2000; 85: 249–53.

45. Mannen T, Iwata M, Toyokura Y et al. Preservation of a certain motor neurone group in amyotrophic lateral sclerosis: its clinical significance. J Neurol Neurosurg Psychiatry 1977; 4: 464–9.
46. Sakuta M, Nakanishi T, Toyokura Y. Anal muscle electromyograms differ in amyotrophic lateral sclerosis and Shy–Drager syndrome. Neurology 1978; 28: 1289–93.
47. Fowler CJ, Kirby RS, Harrison MJG[ ]et al. Individual motor unit analysis in the diagnosis of disorders of urethral sphincter innervation. J Neurol Neurosurg Psychiat 1984; 47: 637–41.
48. Fowler CJ. Pelvic floor neurophysiology. In: Binnie C, ed. Clinical Neurophysiology, Vol. 1. Oxford: Butterworth-Heinemann, 1995: 233–50.
49. Palace J, Chandiramani VA, Fowler CJ. Value of sphincter electromyography in the diagnosis of multiple system atrophy. Muscle Nerve 1997; 20: 1396–1403.
50. Vodusek DB. Sphincter EMG and differential diagnosis of multiple system atrophy. Mov Disord 2001; 16: 600–7.
51. Paviour DC, Williams D, Fowler CJ et al. Is sphincter electromyography a helpful investigation in the diagnosis of multiple system atrophy? A retrospective study with pathological diagnosis. Mov Disord 2005; 20: 1425–30.
52. Yamamoto T, Sakakibara R, Uchiyama T et al. When is Onuf's nucleus involved in multiple system atrophy? A sphincter electromyography study. J Neurol Neurosurg Psychiatry 2005; 76: 1645–8.
53. Pramstaller PP, Wenning GK, Smith SJM et al. Nerve conduction studies, skeletal muscle EMG, and sphincter EMG in multiple system atrophy. J Neurol Neurosurg Psychiatry 1995; 580: 618–21.
54. Sakakibara R, Hattori T, Kita K et al. Stress-induced urinary incontinence in patients with spinocerebellar degeneration. J Neurol Neurosurg Psychiatry 1998; 64: 389–91.
55. Morgan C, Nadelhaft I, de Groat WC. Location of bladder preganglionic neurones within the sacral parasympathetic nucleus of the cat. NeurosciLett 1979; 14: 189–94.
56. Sleehan AM, Downie JW, Awad SA. The pathophysiology of contractile activity in the chronic decentralized feline bladder. J Urol 1993; 149: 1156–64.
57. Lapides J, Friend CR, Ajemian EP et al. Denervation supersensibility as a test for neurogenic bladder. Surg Gyn Obst 1962; 114: 241–4.
58. Ozawa T, Oyanagi K, Tanaka H et al. Suprachiasmal nucleus in a patient with multiple system atrophy with abnormal circadian rhythm of arginine vasopressin secretion into plasma. J Neurol Sci 1998; 154: 116–21.
59. Ozawa T, Tanaka H, Nakano R et al. Nocturnal decrease in vasopressin secretion into plasma in patients with multiple system atrophy. J Neurol Neurosurg Psychiatry 1999; 67: 542–5.
60. Mathias CJ, Fosbraey P, DaCosta DF et al. The effect of desmopressin on nocturnal polyuria, overnight weight loss, and morning postural hypotension in patients with autonomic failure. BMJ 1986; 293: 353–6.
61. Wilcox CS, Aminoff MJ, Penn W. Basis of nocturnal polyuria in patients with autonomic failure. J Neurol Neurosurg Psychiatry 1974; 37: 677.
62. Chandiramani VA, Palace J, Fowler CJ. How to recognize patients with parkinsonism who should not have urological surgery. Br J Urol 1997; 80: 100–4.
63. Donnellan CA, Fook L, McDonald P et al. Oxybutynin and cognitive dysfunction. BMJ 1997; 315: 1363–4.
64. Sakakibara R, Hattori T, Uchiyama T et al. Are alpha-blockers involved in lower urinary tract dysfunction in multiple system atrophy? A comparison of prazosin and moxisylyte. J Auton Nerv Syst 2000; 79: 191–5.
65. Sakakibara R, Uchiyama T, Asahina M et al. Amezinium metilsulfate, a sympathomimetic agent, may increase the risk of urinary retention in multiple system atrophy. Clin Auton Res 2003; 13(1): 51–3.
66. Schwinn DA. Novel role for alpha 1-adrenergic receptor subtypes in lower urinary tract symptoms. BJU Int 2000; 86(Suppl 2): 11–22.
67. Yamanishi T, Yasuda K, Kamai T et al. Combination of a cholinergic drug and an alpha-blocker is more effective than monotherapy for the treatment of voiding difficulty in patients with underactive detrusor. Int J Urol 2004; 11: 88–96.
68. Sandroni P, Opfer-Gehrking TL, Singer W et al. Pyridostigmine for treatment of neurogenic orthostatic hypertension. A follow-up survey study. Clin Auton Res 2005; 15: 51–3.
69. Yamamoto T, Sakakibara R, Yamanaka Y et al. Pyridostigmine in autonomic failure: can we treat postural hypotension and bladder dysfunction with one drug? Clin Auton Res 2006; 16: 296–8.
70. Yamamoto M. Pergolide improves neurogenic bladder in patients with Parkinson's disease. Movem Dis 1997; 12(Suppl): 328.
71. Kuno S, Mizutaa E, Yamasakia S et al. Effects of pergolide on nocturia in Parkinson's disease: three female cases selected from over 400 patients. Parkinsonism Relat Disord 2004; 10: 181–7.
72. Uchiyama T, Sakakibara R, Yamanishi T et al. Short-term effect of l-dopa on the micturitional function in patients with Parkinson's disease. Mov Disord 2003; 18: 573–8.
73. Brusa L, Petta F, Pisani A et al. Central acute D2 stimulation worsens bladder function in patients with mild Parkinson's disease. J Urol 2006; 175: 202–6.
74. Sakakibara R, Matsuda S, Uchiyama T et al. The effect of intranasal desmopressin on nocturnal waking in urination in multiple system atrophy patients with nocturnal polyuria. Clin Auton Res 2003; 13: 106–8.
75. Uchiyama T, Sakakibara R, Asahina M et al. Post-micturitional hypotension in patients with multiple system atrophy. J Neurol Neurosurg Psychiatry 2005; 76: 186–90.

23

Multiple sclerosis

Line Leboeuf, Brian Cohen, and Angelo E Gousse

Introduction

Multiple sclerosis (MS) is a complex, autoimmune relapsing–remitting disorder of the central nervous system (CNS) that results in disabling neurologic deficits. The etiology and pathogenesis of the disease are still unknown, but there is increasing evidence that the primary disease mechanism of MS is related to an autoimmune attack on the CNS myelin, although genetic, environmental, and viral factors have all been implicated. The clinical course of the disease is extremely variable and unpredictable from one individual to the other, but voiding dysfunction is present in the majority of these patients at some point in time during the evolution of the illness. Not only does voiding dysfunction represent a considerable psychosocial burden to affected individuals but it also poses great challenges to the treatment team. In that regard, knowledge of the pathophysiology and clinical evolution of MS, as well as proper evaluation and individualized treatments, is essential to the urologist to prevent complications and increase the quality of life of these patients.

History and epidemiology of multiple sclerosis

We owe to Jean-Martin Charcot in 1868 the correlation between the clinical presentation of MS and its pathologic description.[1] However, the first identification of the lesions in MS was presented by Cruveilhier (1835) and Carswell (1838) 30 years earlier.[2]

The disease has an incidence of about 7 in 100 000 every year, with a prevalence of 120 per 100 000, and a lifetime risk of 1 in 400.[3] A clear gender difference exists, females being more commonly affected than men by a ratio of 2:1. Populations vary in their susceptibility to MS; the prevalence is approximately 1 per 1000 in Americans, and 2 per 1000 in northern Europeans. In contrast with Caucasians, MS is less common in Orientals.[4,5] Prevalence rates are also reported to be greatest at the extremes of latitudes in both the northern and southern hemispheres.[6] This uneven geographic distribution of the disease has been attributed to environmental factors, but recent studies have demonstrated that genetic susceptibility may play a more important role in determining the prevalence of the disease in a particular location than was previously believed.[7] The risk of MS in monozygotic twins seems to be in favor of this argument; hence, the concordance rate for monozygotic twins is approximately 30% compared to 3–5% in dizygotic twins and 0.1–0.4% in nontwin siblings and the general population.[8] Multiple sclerosis is diagnosed most often between the ages of 20 and 50 years old, with pediatric and geriatric populations being rarely affected by the disease.[9,10]

Pathogenesis of multiple sclerosis

The pathologic hallmarks of multiple sclerosis are, as described by Charcot, the zones of acute focal inflammatory demyelination or plaques in the white matter of the brain and spinal cord. At the present time, the precise etiology of MS remains unknown, although numerous studies have implicated, alone or in combination, genetic, environmental, viral, and autoimmune factors. Growing experimental evidence points, however, toward an autoimmune mechanism for the chronic multifocal plaques from which the disease gets its name.

Immunopathology

The autoimmune attack on CNS myelin in MS leads to a loss of saltatory conduction and velocity in axonal pathways. The oligodendrocyte, which is primarily responsible for synthesis and maintenance of the myelin sheath around nerve axons in the CNS, is phagocytosed, and subsequently this event leads to demyelination. The resultant edema worsens the neurologic impairment. Chronic attacks will eventually lead to scarring of nerves, with associated severe and often permanent neurologic dysfunction.[3,9–11] The phenomenon of acute demyelination is believed to be the first event leading to neurologic dysfunction in MS. However, with successive offences, repetitive cell reactivity will isolate the nerve lesions, further reducing remyelination potential and the capacity of damaged nerves to accommodate cumulative deficits. This second phase seems to mark the transition from temporary to persistent neurologic deficit.[3]

Cell-mediated autoimmunity

The contribution of autoreactive T lymphocytes to the demyelinating process appears crucial.[12] In the peripheral circulation, T lymphocytes, activated by unknown mechanisms, will migrate through the blood–brain barrier, where they will be stimulated by binding of the T-cell receptor with class II major histocompatibility complex to the antigen on the surface of an antigen-presenting cell. Release of proinflammatory cytokines by the activated T lymphocytes will then enhance macrophage activity that may injure the myelin processes or oligodendroglial cells.[10]

Humoral and antibody-mediated autoimmunity

The association of T cells and antigen in the CNS activates B-lymphocyte cells, which subsequently differentiate into antibody-secreting plasma cells. The potential for damage from those antibodies resides in the opsonization of the autoimmune target and the activation of the complement membrane attack complex; all of these phenomena subsequently cause damage to myelin and the myelin oligodendrocyte glycoprotein (MOG).[13] Antibodies to MOG have been demonstrated within human MS lesions.[14]

Genetics

The question of genetic predisposition to MS has been raised by reports from twin and sibling studies. As previously mentioned, concordance rates between monozygotic twins are approximately 30%, compared with 5% for dizygotic twins and nontwin siblings.[8] It has also been found that the risk of MS for genetically unrelated family members living with an index case is the same as the risk in the general population.[15] Several chromosomal linkages have also been associated with multiple sclerosis, notably at the 1p, 6p, 10p, 17q, and 19q sites.[16] The disease seems to conform to the inheritance pattern of a polygenic disease.[17]

Although genetic predisposition seems to play a prominent role in the physiopathology of MS, at this time genetic factors are not yet clearly determined and explain only part of the susceptibility to MS. Lack of identification of a major susceptibility gene and the discordance rate of 70% between monozygotic twins despite identical genetic background remain to be explored.

Infectious agents

Multiple infectious agents have been proposed to be linked to the physiopathology of MS. Agents currently under investigation include Epstein–Barr virus (EBV), human herpesvirus 6 (HHV-6), and *Chlamydia pneumoniae*.[18] It has been proposed that a genetically susceptible individual could be exposed to an infectious agent at a critical time, leading subsequently to development of MS, with acute attacks possibly related to reactivation of the latent infection.[10] Also, autoimmune offence against self-antigens could be triggered by infectious agents that are antigenically similar to normal tissue.[19] Wandinger et al[20] have reported 100% EBV seropositivity for immunoglobulin G (IgG) antibodies in MS patients, compared with 90% IgG and 4% IgM in normal controls. Also, the same authors found that acute relapses of MS were associated with the presence of reactivation of EBV DNA within blood. Moreover, other investigators have found HHV-6 in actively demyelinating plaques.[21] The bacteria *Chlamydia pneumoniae* were cultured from the cerebrospinal fluid of 64% of MS patients and from 11% of controls.[22]

As these results have not been invariably confirmed by other laboratories at this time, most authors agree that more studies are necessary to delineate the mechanisms of action of those infectious agents, and even more work is required to link these agents to the pathogenesis of MS.

Clinical presentation and course of multiple sclerosis

The neurologic symptoms and signs of MS reflect the location of the affected site within the CNS and are the consequences of demyelination on axon conduction (Figure 23.1). Involvement of the cerebrum can lead to cognitive, sensory, and motor impairment, with or without epilepsy and focal cortical deficits.[3] When assessed with magnetic resonance imaging (MRI), the cerebrum is almost always involved, but usually most abnormalities cannot be linked to specific clinical symptoms.[23] Lesions of the optic nerve typically lead to painful loss of vision, whereas those of the cerebellum and brainstem may present with tremor, ataxia, vertigo, diplopia, and impaired speech and swallowing. The spinal cord is frequently affected with subsequent alterations of motor, sensory, and autonomic function, with or without bowel, bladder, and erectile dysfunction.[3,10] Other symptoms such as debilitating fatigue,

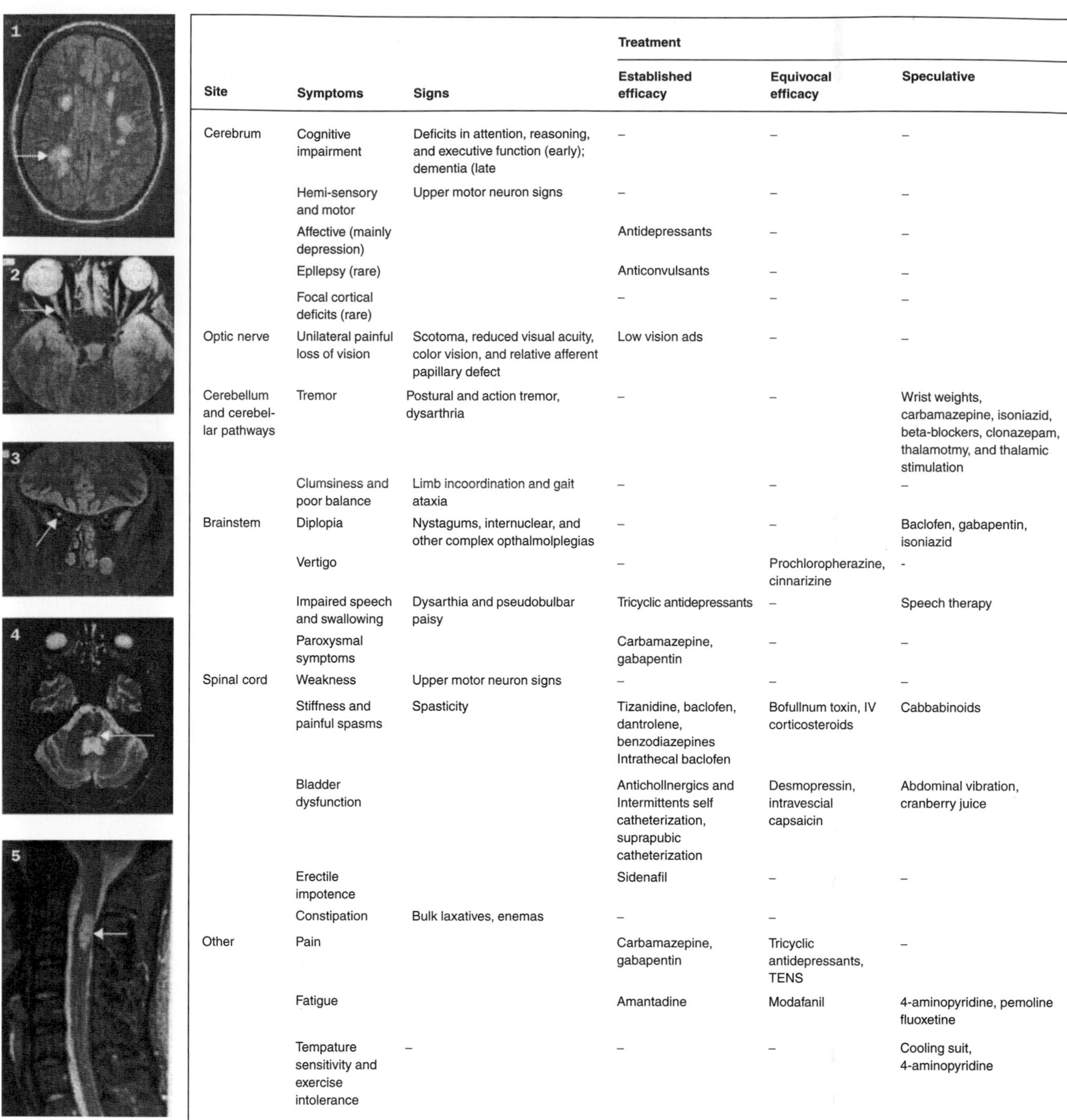

Site	Symptoms	Signs	Treatment: Established efficacy	Treatment: Equivocal efficacy	Treatment: Speculative
Cerebrum	Cognitive impairment	Deficits in attention, reasoning, and executive function (early); dementia (late	–	–	–
	Hemi-sensory and motor	Upper motor neuron signs	–	–	–
	Affective (mainly depression)		Antidepressants	–	–
	Epllepsy (rare)		Anticonvulsants	–	–
	Focal cortical deficits (rare)		–	–	–
Optic nerve	Unilateral painful loss of vision	Scotoma, reduced visual acuity, color vision, and relative afferent papillary defect	Low vision ads	–	–
Cerebellum and cerebel-lar pathways	Tremor	Postural and action tremor, dysarthria	–	–	Wrist weights, carbamazepine, isoniazid, beta-blockers, clonazepam, thalamotmy, and thalamic stimulation
	Clumsiness and poor balance	Limb incoordination and gait ataxia	–	–	–
Brainstem	Diplopia	Nystagums, internuclear, and other complex opthalmolplegias	–	–	Baclofen, gabapentin, isoniazid
	Vertigo		–	Prochloropherazine, cinnarizine	-
	Impaired speech and swallowing	Dysarthia and pseudobulbar paisy	Tricyclic antidepressants	–	Speech therapy
	Paroxysmal symptoms		Carbamazepine, gabapentin	–	–
Spinal cord	Weakness	Upper motor neuron signs	–	–	–
	Stiffness and painful spasms	Spasticity	Tizanidine, baclofen, dantrolene, benzodiazepines Intrathecal baclofen	Bofullnum toxin, IV corticosteroids	Cabbabinoids
	Bladder dysfunction		Antichollnergics and Intermittents self catheterization, suprapubic catheterization	Desmopressin, intravescial capsaicin	Abdominal vibration, cranberry juice
	Erectile impotence		Sidenafil	–	–
	Constipation	Bulk laxatives, enemas	–	–	
Other	Pain		Carbamazepine, gabapentin	Tricyclic antidepressants, TENS	–
	Fatigue		Amantadine	Modafanil	4-aminopyridine, pemoline fluoxetine
	Tempature sensitivity and exercise intolerance	–	–	–	Cooling suit, 4-aminopyridine

Figure 23.1
Lesion sites, syndromes, and symptomatic treatments in multiple sclerosis. T2-weighted magnetic resonance imaging (MRI) abnormalities (arrows) in the cerebrum (1), right optic nerve, longitudinal section, (2), transverse section (3), brainstem and cerebellar peduncle (4), and cervical spinal cord (5). TENS, transcutaneous electric nerve stimulation. Reproduced from Compston[8] with permission from *Journal of Neurology*.

paresthesias on neck flexion (Lhermitte's symptoms) and heat-exacerbated symptomatic worsening (Uhthoff's symptom) may be present.[10] As many lesions can be clinically silent, other causes for the symptom complex must be sought before considering the diagnosis of MS, all of which are beyond the scope of this chapter and are covered comprehensively elsewhere.[24]

Current accepted clinical diagnostic categories for MS present as follows: relapsing–remitting (RRMS), secondary progressive (SPMS), primary progressive (PPMS), and progressive-relapsing (PRMS).[25] Approximately 80% of patients present with RRMS, typically described as discrete clinical attacks followed by full recovery. RRMS is mostly encountered in the younger population. Years after

Table 23.1 *Factors of good and poor prognosis in multiple sclerosis (adapted from Keegan and Noseworthy)*[10]

Good prognosis	Poor prognosis
Female gender	Male gender
Younger age of onset Optic neuritis	Predominant cerebellar and motor involvement
Sensory attacks	
Complete recovery from attacks	Incomplete resolution of attacks
Few attacks	Progressive course from onset Frequent early attacks
Long interattacks interval	Short interattacks interval

Reproduced from Compston[8] with permission from *Journal of Neurology.*

onset, approximately 30–40% of RRMS patients will develop a more progressive chronic course characterized by progressive persistent deficits with or without acute clinical attacks; hence, it is termed secondary progressive MS. In 20% of patients, the disease is primary progressive from onset, without clinically evident relapses.[26] Alternatively, these patients can later experience superimposed exacerbation of neurologic dysfunction, a condition referred to as PRMS.

Overall life expectancy from disease onset is estimated to be approximately 25 years, death being almost invariably caused by unrelated events. Due to the wide variety of clinical features and presentations, prognosis varies widely. Isolated sensory and visual symptoms have been associated with good prognosis and with complete recovery.[3] On the other hand, motor involvement with coordination and balance deficits has been linked with poorer prognosis. Clinical indicators of good and poor prognosis has been described by some authors[27] and are presented in Table 23.1.

Diagnosis of multiple sclerosis

Diagnosis of MS is based on clinical evidence of symptoms and is facilitated by paraclinical data: i.e. MRI, cerebrospinal fluid (CSF) analysis with oligoclonal bands, and visually evoked potentials (Figure 23.2).[23] A purely clinical diagnosis of MS is made upon the occurrence of two or more distinct attacks, affecting more than one anatomic site within the myelinated regions of the CNS (cerebral white matter, brainstem, cerebellar tracts, optic nerves, spinal cord). Also, a single clinical attack with additional lesions discovered by paraclinical evidence can suggest the diagnosis.

MRI of the brain and spinal cord is the most sensitive investigational technique in the diagnosis of MS. More than 95% of patients with MS have T2-weighted white matter abnormalities, although these are not always diagnostic.[3] MRI can also help predict the risk of progression to clinically definite MS in a patient with a single episode; monosymptomatic patients with one or no brain MRI lesions are at low risk of developing a second clinical attack in the subsequent decade (15–20%), in contrast to patients with two or more cerebral MRI lesions, who are at high risk (85%) for a second .attack over the same period.[28] However, imaging is most useful in the investigation of individuals with clinically isolated lesions or insidious progressive disease at a single site.

CSF protein electrophoresis shows oligoclonal IgG bands in more than 90% of cases of MS.[3] Its role in the pathogenesis of MS is unresolved but confirms the inflammatory nature of the underlying pathology, therefore excluding alternative explanations. Evoked potentials measure conduction along afferent CNS pathways following stimulation of a sensory receptor.[3] Abnormal conduction may identify a clinically occult demyelinated lesion and provide evidence in diagnostically difficult situations. Finally, before attributing the diagnosis of MS, the clinician must exclude other causes of focal or multifocal CNS disease.[24]

Neurologic effect of multiple sclerosis on the urinary tract

Neuroanatomy and neurophysiology of normal lower urinary tract

Bladder and sphincter function is considered a single physiologic unit whose purpose is the efficient, low-pressure storage and expulsion of urine. These rather discrete and simple functions are achieved through the complex coordination of the autonomic, somatic, and central nervous systems (Figure 23.3). The parasympathetic and sympathetic divisions of the autonomic nervous system produce, via their action through neurotransmitters and receptors in the bladder and urethral sphincter, bladder emptying and storage (Table 23.2). The somatic innervation of the lower urinary tract is provided by neurons in spinal segments S2 to S4. Through the pudendal nerve these fibers activate contraction of the external urethral sphincter, producing retention of urine and continence.

Bladder function is also controlled by centers in the brainstem, as reported from mammalian animal experiments,[29] and later confirmed in human studies.[30] The so-called pontine micturition center provides coordination between the autonomic and somatic nervous systems involved in voiding, providing a ‘switch’ phenomenon between the storage and emptying phases of micturition.

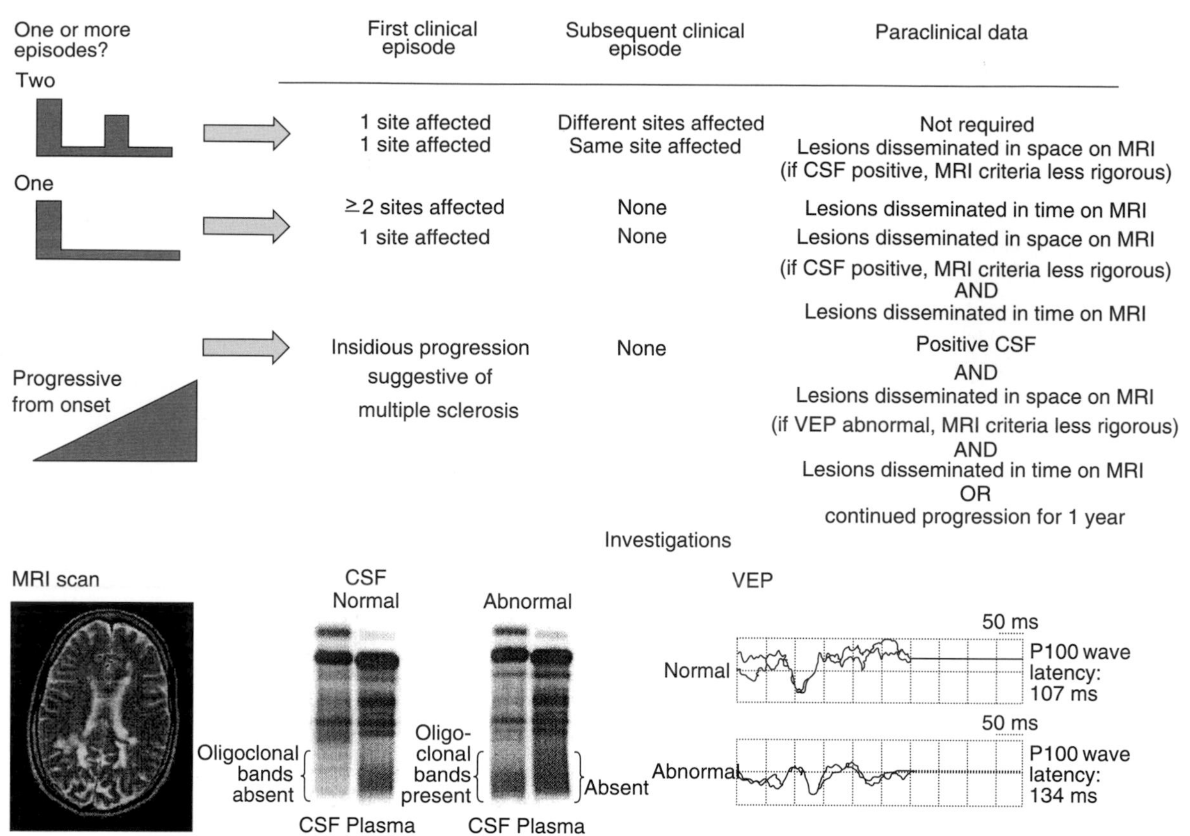

Figure 23.2
Criteria for diagnosis of multiple sclerosis. The principle is to establish that two or more episodes affecting separate sites within the central nervous system have occurred at different times, using clinical analysis or laboratory investigations. Dissemination in space based on MRI requires: any three features from (1) one gadolinium (Gd)-positive or nine T2 MRI lesions; (2) ≥1 infratentorial lesion; (3) ≥1 juxtacortical lesion; or (4) ≥3 periventricular lesions. If VEPs or CSF are positive, ≥2 MRI lesions consistent with multiple sclerosis are sufficient. Dissemination in time of MRI lesions requires: one Gd-positive lesion at >3 months after the onset of the clinical event; or a Gd-positive or new T2 lesion on a second scan repeated 3 months after the first. Patients having an appropriate clinical presentation, but who do not meet all of the diagnostic criteria, can be classified as having possible multiple sclerosis. MRI, magnetic resonance imaging; CSF, cerebrospinal fluid; VEP, visually evoked potential test. (Reproduced with permission from Compston and Coles.[3])

Higher control of micturition is located in the medial frontal cortex and the diencephalon; these regions are responsible for voluntary control of the initiation and cessation of micturition. Detailed description of voiding and storage pathways are beyond the scope of this chapter and are comprehensively covered elsewhere in this book.

Suprasacral, sacral, and intracranial plaques' effects

Oppenheimer, in an autopsy study of patients with multiple lesions, demonstrated that almost all exhibited cervical spinal cord demyelination with marked involvement of lateral corticospinal and reticulospinal tracts. Moreover, the lumbar and sacral cord were involved in 40% and 18% of patients, respectively.[31] Because innervation of the detrusor and external urethral sphincter is mediated via these lateral spinal tracts, and knowing the predilection of demyelinating plaques for the cervical spinal cord, most MS patients have lower urinary tract dysfunction. Litwiller et al have divided the effects of MS on the urinary tract into suprasacral, sacral, and intracranial.[11]

Suprasacral plaques

Interruption of the reticulospinal pathways between the pontine and sacral micturition centers may cause loss of

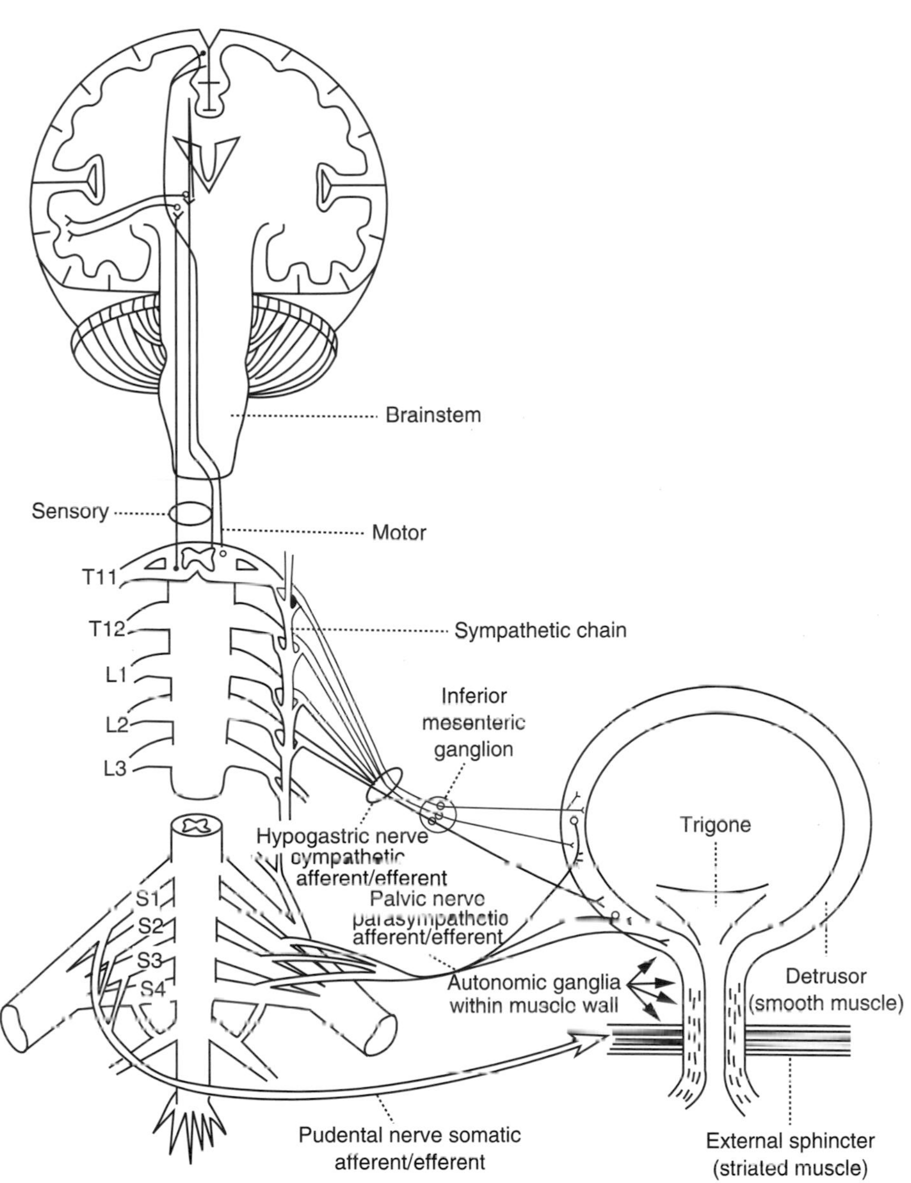

Figure 23.3
Normal bladder neuroanatomy. (Reproduced from Fernandez with permission.)[35]

Table 23.2 *Innervation of the bladder (modified from Fernandez)*[35]

Division	Spinal cord	Nerve	Neurotransmitter	Receptor	Mechanism	Effect
Parasympathetic	S2 to S4	Pelvic	Acetylcholine	Muscarinic	Contraction of detrusor Relaxation of outlet (urethra)	Bladder emptying Bladder emptying
Sympathetic	T10 to L2	Hypogastric	Norepinephrine	Beta Alpha	Relaxation of detrusor Contraction of outlet (urethra)	Retention of urine Retention of urine
Somatic	Efferent S2 to S4 Afferent S2 to S4	Pudendal	Acetylcholine	Nicotinic	Contraction of external sphincter	Retention of urine

Table 23.3 *Percentage of patients affected by symptoms of bladder dysfunction in multiple sclerosis (modified from Fernandez and Quarto.[35,40])*

Study		No. of patients	Urgency	Frequency	Urge incontinence	Hesitancy	Retention
Sachs	1921	57	31	–	37	49	–
Langworthy	1938	97	54	33	34	40	–
Carter	1950	36	24	17	50	–	17
Miller	1965	321	60	50	36	33	2
Bradley	1973	90	86	60	–	28	20
Philp	1981	52	61	59	47	25	8
Goldstein	1983	86	32	32	49	–	–
Awad	1984	47	85	65	72	36	–
Gonor	1985	64	70	48	56	30	–
Betts	1992	170	85	82	63	49	–
Hennessey	1999	191	71	76	19	48	–
Borello-France	2004	133	61	71	83	–	–
Ukkonen	2004	24	83	54	75	58	–
Quarto	2007	107	61	83	32	–	–

synergistic activity between the urethral sphincter and the detrusor, possibly resulting in detrusor-external sphincter dyssynergia (DESD).[32] On the other hand, the lack of supraspinal suppression of autonomous bladder contraction may result from lesions in the corticospinal tract.

Sacral plaques

Studies have demonstrated a 20% incidence of involvement of the sacral cord in autopsy patients.[33] Moreover, Mayo and Chetner reported that almost two-thirds of patients with sacral plaques had detrusor hypocontractility and 5% had areflexia.[34] Hence, it has been postulated that plaques located in the spinal afferents and efferents of the sacral reflex arc may inhibit bladder contraction and therefore result in impaired emptying or urinary retention.

Intracranial plaques

Intracranial plaques can be found in approximately 60–80% of patients;[11] their location involves any area of the white matter, but particularly the periventricular zone. In those patients affected with this type of lesion, the micturition reflex as well as the synergistic integration of bladder and urethral sphincter function remain intact. Micturition is thus physiologically unimpaired. However, perception of fullness and ability to inhibit bladder contraction are dependent on an alert and normally functioning sensorium. Intracranial plaques may result in loss of voluntary control of initiation or prevention of voiding. Disease in the supraspinal CNS may account for detrusor hyperreflexia.

Urologic symptoms associated with multiple sclerosis

Urologic symptoms in patients with MS are shown to vary greatly from study to study, their incidence ranging from 52% to 97%. The best-known series addressing urinary symptoms in MS are summarized in Table 23.3.[11,35,36] Frequency and urgency are the most frequent, manifested in 31–86% of patients, whereas incontinence and obstructive symptoms with or without urinary retention are reported in 34–72% and 2–49%, respectively.[11,35,36] Although lower urinary tract symptoms are frequent in the MS population, voiding problems are rarely the sole initial presentation of the disease:[32,37] only about 10% of patients present solely with voiding symptoms at the time of initial clinical manifestation of MS.[32,37,38] Additionally, MRI findings correlate poorly with the presence of frequency, nocturia, and stress or urge incontinence.[39]

Moreover, correlation between urologic symptoms and urodynamic evaluation has been reported unreliable as an indicator of the extent of vesical dysfunction.[41–43] Koldewijn et al have demonstrated urodynamic evidence of urinary dysfunction in 100% of symptomatic patients and in 50% of asymptomatic ones.[41] Also, in another study, nearly half of the patients with elevated postvoid residual (PVR) felt sensation of incomplete emptying as compared with nearly all patients who expressed complaints of incomplete emptying and were found to have elevated PVR.[43] Some authors have postulated that the poor correlation between objective clinical findings and subjective symptoms may be explained by the chronicity of the disease and subsequent adaptation to the symptom complex. Failure or denial to recognize symptoms is another explanation.[44] Of upmost importance is the study of Bemelmens et al showing that MS patients without urologic symptoms can have urologic pathology. Hence, 52% of asymptomatic patients had anomalies on urodynamic evaluation, suggesting that the corticospinal and reticulospinal tracts are commonly involved at a subclinical level and that this involvement can be found quite early in the demyelinating process. Patients who deny urologic problems can still have significant urodynamically verifiable pathology.

Finally, studies have reported that patients older than 50 years of age seem to be more bothered by bladder symptoms.[43] An explanation for this is the possible cumulative effect of other diseases causing bladder dysfunction such as benign prostatic hyperplasia (BPH), pelvic relaxation associated with stress incontinence, and longer duration of disease in older patients. No significant relationship between overall incidence of symptoms and gender exists, but men with MS have a higher incidence of obstructive symptoms and complications, possibly related to age-related changes in the prostate or severity of DESD in men.[41]

Studies have demonstrated that lower urinary symptoms were strongly related to disability status, as measured by the expanded disability status scale[11,13] with weaker relation to disease duration and age, as it was previously reported. The extent of pyramidal dysfunction also seems to be a strong predictor of urologic pathology.[45] Finally, the disease presentation may influence bladder function, as SPMS shows increased risk of bladder function deterioration.[45]

Urologic complications such as urinary tract infection (UTI), stones, renal impairment, incontinence, and deaths associated with lower urinary tract dysfunction in MS are decreasing as knowledge of the course of the disease, sophisticated evaluation, follow-up, and intermittent catheterization are becoming widespread. Although the incidence of MS is higher in women than in men, urologic complications occur more frequently in the latter, and about half of the affected men have DESD. It is believed that the high prevalence of incontinence in women may protect them by decreasing the risk of developing dangerously elevated intravesical pressures, hence impeding severe bladder or renal function.[46] Also, one has to be careful in attributing urologic symptoms in MS patients to their underlying neurologic disease, as common urologic disorders may coexist, mimic, or aggravate the neurologic dysfunction. Although only 7% of patients with MS will develop serious bladder or renal problems in the course of the disease, it is important to recognize the impact of morbidity from urologic symptoms, especially UTI and incontinence. These factors pose a great burden on the patients and every effort should be made to address them.

Evaluation of urinary tract dysfunction in patients with multiple sclerosis

History

Initial assessment of MS patients should include a comprehensive history and physical examination. The history aims to ascertain whether urologic symptoms exist and should begin by emphasis on description of irritative or obstructive symptoms and urinary incontinence. Temporal and spatial characterization of symptoms, use of a protective device, assessment of fluid intake, and quality of life should also be addressed.[11] One should also determine the presence or absence of urologic complications: upper or lower urinary tract infection, hematuria, and stones. Past medical and surgical history is mandatory, since urologic pathologies like BPH or stress incontinence are common in the older population and may confuse the neurourologic profile. Medication should be noted, as many drugs may affect bladder function. Of particular importance is the young patient with unexplained urologic symptoms. In those patients, every effort should be made to elicit neurologic symptoms suggestive of MS, and prompt referral is mandatory.[11]

Physical examination

The genitourinary evaluation begins with an abdominal examination to ensure that there is no overt evidence of bladder distention. Careful inspection of external genitalia may reveal hypospadias or urethral erosion in patients with an indwelling catheter. Prostate and testicular palpation may aid in cancer screening and BPH detection. The pelvic examination should be performed to evaluate sensory and motor function of the pelvic floor and sacral dermatomes. Determination of the anal sphincter tone and reflex and perineal sensation may help to evaluate the presence of neurologic disease of the bladder, since absent anal reflexes, lax anal tone, or absent perineal sensation may be associated with neurologic disease of the bladder. Also, pelvic evaluation is important to determine the presence of concomitant urethral hypermobility or vaginal prolapse, the latter itself being able to cause irritative or obstructive voiding symptoms.

A directed neurologic examination can not only help understand the extent of the disease but can also help to predict urologic dysfunction. For instance, investigators have noted an association between hyperactive deep tendon reflexes and DESD.[38] Betts et al have reported a high correlation between cerebellar signs such as ataxia and dysdiadochokinesis and detrusor areflexia.[44] Finally, as mentioned earlier, the degree of lower extremity motor dysfunction may be the best predictor of urologic and bladder dysfunction.[45]

After the preliminary history and physical examination, routine laboratory tests include urine analysis and culture and serum creatinine. Urinary tract infection is common in MS patients and has been reported in as many of 60% of patients.[46] Also, an elevated serum creatinine may herald renal insufficiency in an asymptomatic patient. A voiding diary may also be useful to objectively assess the voiding complaints and evaluate the extent of the incontinence problem.

Although the definite diagnosis of MS is based on clinical judgment, MRI is used routinely and is diagnostic in 70–95% of patients with clinically confirmed MS.[47] The most common MRI abnormality associated with MS, although nonspecific for the disease, is a focus of increased signal intensity on T2-weighted scans corresponding to a plaque demyelination.[48] However, many patients are found to have lesions on MRI without clinical evidence of the disease as reported in imaging studies of normal subjects.[49] Conversely, the absence of lesions on MRI does not exclude the diagnosis of MS, as illustrated in the criteria used for the diagnosis of the disease. Finally, there does not seem to exist any correlation between MRI findings and specific urodynamic parameters.[50]

Cerebrospinal fluid analysis and evoked responses provide additional evidence for the diagnosis of MS. However, although abnormal findings are common, no characteristic of these tests is specific, neither to the disease itself nor to the urologic dysfunctions associated with it.

Koldewijn et al have reported an incidence of upper tract abnormalities of 7% in a study of 2076 patients with MS,[41] showing that upper tract deterioration is the exception rather than the rule. DESD, the presence of an indwelling catheter, and poor bladder compliance are risk factors that have been strongly linked to upper tract deterioration.[32,42] Although baseline radiographic assessment remains an integral part of initial evaluation, the low incidence of upper tract deterioration has led many urologists to abandon routine yearly upper tract imaging unless baseline studies are abnormal or there is a change in clinical status.[43]

Lower tract imaging seldom helps with the management of patients with MS. However, it may be beneficial to discriminate between neurogenic voiding and other lower urinary tract lesions in the genesis of voiding dysfunction.

Urodynamic evaluation

A thorough urodynamic evaluation is mandatory for effectively diagnosing urinary tract dysfunction and planning urinary tract management. The purposes of urodynamic testing are to determine and classify the type of voiding dysfunction and to identify risks factors such as DESD, decreased bladder compliance, and high detrusor filling pressures. All these factors are known to predispose to upper tract problems, including vesicourethral reflux, bladder and kidney stones, hydronephrosis, pyelonephritis, and renal insufficiency. However, a recent retrospective analysis of 66 MS patients revealed no predictive urodynamic parameters for upper tract deterioration as identified by ultrasound.[51]

The incidence of abnormal urodynamic findings in patients with voiding symptoms and MS approaches 100%. The incidence of normal urodynamic findings in symptomatic patients, on the other hand, is approximately 10%, as revealed by a meta-analysis of 1900 patients[11,39,51] (Table 23.4). Bemelmans et al have addressed the particular situation of MS patients without urinary complaints; in their study, they demonstrated a 52% incidence of clinically silent urodynamic abnormalities.[52] This study stresses that even MS patients who deny urologic symptoms can have significant urodynamic pathology.

The relationship between urodynamic and MRI findings has also been investigated. Ukkonen et al evaluated 24 patients with primary progressive MS and found that patients with urodynamically proven DSD had a higher volume of T2-weighted plaques on brain MRI compared to MS patients with normal urodynamic studies. Additionally, these investigators found that patients with hypotonic detrusors had smaller brain volumes than those with normal bladder function.[39]

Three major patterns of urodynamic dysfunction have been described in MS patients and are reported in Table 23.4:

1. detrusor hyperreflexia without bladder outlet obstruction
2. detrusor hyperreflexia with outlet obstruction (DESD)
3. detrusor hypocontractility or areflexia.

Detrusor hyperreflexia without bladder outlet obstruction

The most common urodynamic abnormality in MS is detrusor hyperreflexia, which is manifested symptomatically by urinary urgency, frequency, nocturia, and incontinence (Figure 23.4). These findings correlate well with the high incidence of intracranial and cervical spinal plaques.[31] In a meta-analysis of 22 published series, Litwiller et al reported that 62% of patients had detrusor hyperreflexia on urodynamic findings.[11]

Detrusor hyperreflexia with bladder outlet obstruction

Detrusor hyperreflexia with DESD is the second most common urodynamic finding in patients with neurogenic

Table 23.4 *Published series of urodynamic patterns in multiple sclerosis (modified from Litwiller et al)*[11]

Study		No. of patients	Hyperreflexia		DSD		Hyporeflexia		Normal	
			No.	%	No.	%	No.	%	No.	%
Anderson and Bradley	1973	52	33	(63)	16	(31)	21	(40)	2	(4)
Awad et al	1984	57	38	(66)	30	(52)	12	(21)	7	(12)
Beck et al	1981	46	40	(87)	–	(–)	6	(13)	–	(–)
Betts et al	1993	70	63	(91)	–	(–)	–	(–)	7	(10)
Blaivas et al	1979	41	23	(56)	12	(30)	16	(40)	2	(4)
Bradley et al	1973	99	58	(60)	20	(20)	40	(40)	1	(1)
Bradley	1978	302	127	(62)	–	(–)	103	(34)	10	(24)
Ciancio et al	2001	22	10	(45)	5	(23)	4	(18)	3	13
Eardley et al	1991	24	15	(63)	6	(27)	3	(13)	6	(25)
Goldstein et al	1982	86	65	(76)	57	(66)	16	(19)	5	(6)
Gonor et al	1985	64	40	(78)	8	(12)	13	(20)	1	(2)
Hinson and Boone	1996	70	44	(63)	15	(21)	20	(28)	6	(9)
Koldewijn et al	1995	212	72	(34)	27	(13)	32	(8)	76	(36)
Mayo and Chetner	1992	89	69	(78)	5	(6)	5	(6)	11	(12)
McGuire and Savastano	1984	46	33	(72)	21	(46)	13	(28)	0	(0)
Petersen and Pederson	1984	88	73	(83)	36	(41)	14	(16)	1	(1)
Philip et al	1981	52	51	(99)	16	(37)	0	(0)	1	(2)
Piazza and Diokno	1997	31	23	(74)	9	(47)	2	(6)	3	(9)
Schoenburg et al	1979	39	27	(69)	20	(5)	2	(6)	6	(15)
Sirls et al	1994	113	79	(70)	15	(28)	17	(15)	7	(6)
Summers	1978	50	26	(52)	6	(12)	6	(12)	9	(18)
Van Poppel and Baert	1987	160	105	(66)	38	(24)	38	(24)	16	(10)
Weinstein et al	1988	91	64	(70)	16	(18)	15	(16)	11	(12)
Ukkonen et al	2004	24	14	(58)	17	(71)	4	(17)	3	(13)
Lemack et al	2005	66	49	(74)	22	(33)	5	(8)	–	(–)
Total/Total No. (%)		1994	1267	(63.54)	417/1559	(26.74)	407	(20.0)	191	(10)

DSD, detrusor-sphincter dyssynergia; No, number.

bladder associated with MS (Figure 23.5) and is reported in 25% of patients.[11] The hyperreflexic contraction occurs without proper relaxation of the external urethral sphincter. DESD usually presents with obstructive symptoms and incomplete emptying, the latter being possibly related to sphincteric dysfunction or incomplete bladder contraction. As opposed to DESD in spinal cord patients, DESD in MS patients is rarely associated with upper tract dysfunction, suggesting that the hyperreflexia and extent of external sphincter spasms may be less severe than in spinal cord injury (SCI) patients.[41,53]

Detrusor hyporeflexia

Finally, detrusor hyporeflexia (Figure 23.6) is reported in approximately 20% of patients[11] and symptoms include straining or incapacity to void and/or overflow incontinence. Mayo and Chetner have reported that almost two-thirds of patients with sacral plaques had detrusor hyporeflexia and 5% had detrusor areflexia.[34]

As neurologic patterns in MS are known to change over time, since the disease is dynamic and is characterized by exacerbations and remissions, changes in urodynamic patterns have also been reported. Changes in lower urinary tract function with time and in response to treatment can occur. No generalizations concerning patterns of changes can be drawn, but a significant proportion of patients (15–55%) will develop changes on urodynamic testing, undermining the need for repeat urodynamic studies, even in patients with persistent stable symptomatology.[54,55]

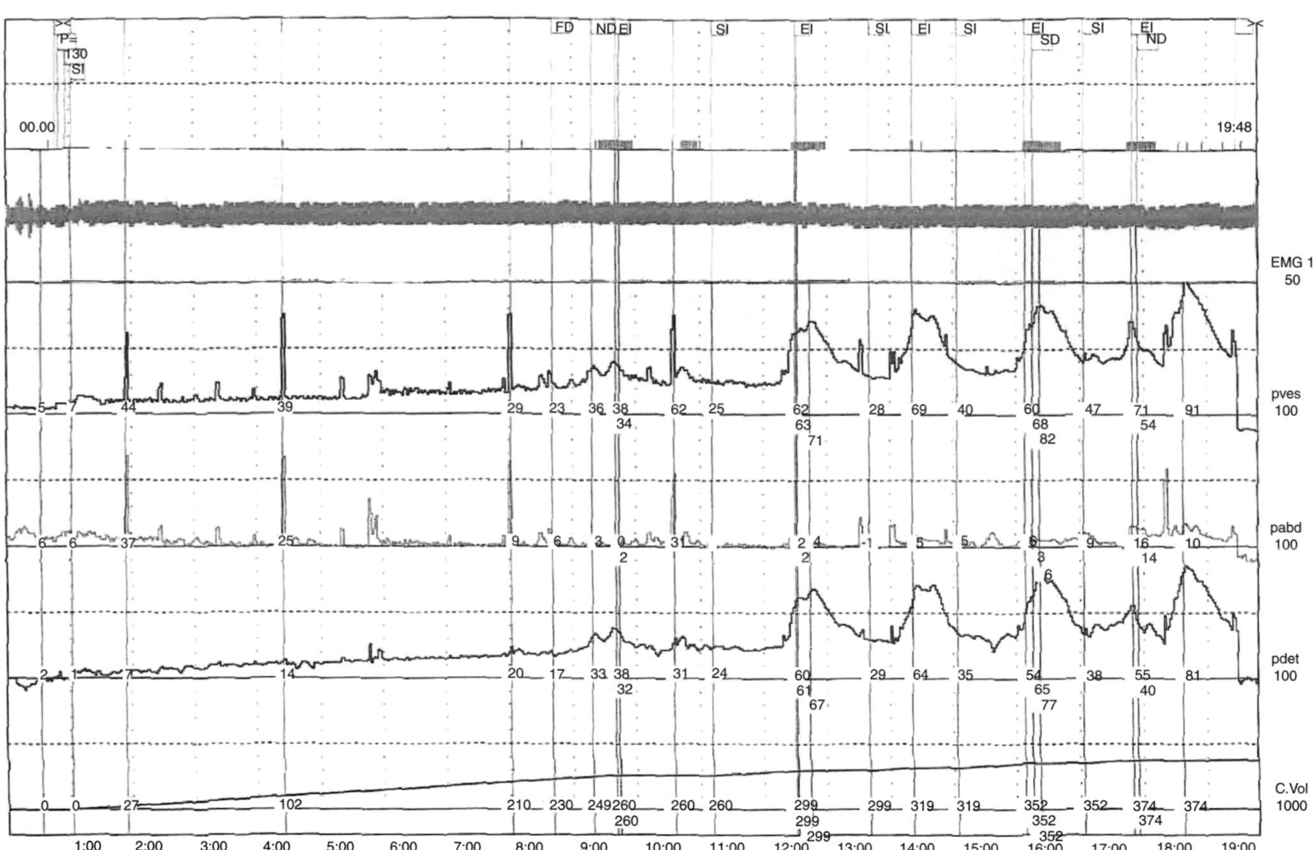

Figure 23.4
Detrusor hyperreflexia without bladder outlet obstruction.

Management of urinary manifestations of multiple sclerosis

The aim of treatment of the neurogenic patient is management of lower urinary tract symptoms, prevention of urinary tract infections, preservation of the upper urinary tract, and improvement of the quality of life. The choice of treatment should be based on a clear understanding of the pathology and on objective parameters, as well as on the patient's disability, autonomy, manual dexterity, and motivation. Since symptoms of MS can change over time due to its remission–exacerbation pattern, treatment modalities should preferably be reversible and permanent surgical procedures should be avoided as much as possible. Table 23.5 is a summary of the different options presented below.

Detrusor hyperreflexia without bladder outlet obstruction

Behavioral modifications and pelvic floor rehabilitation

Voiding symptoms can often be improved by simple behavioral manipulations, but the success of voiding mostly relies on the patient's motivation. Regular voiding may reduce hyperreflexic contraction by emptying the bladder before a critical state of filling is reached. Limitation of fluids may help prevent irritative symptoms, as well as avoidance of beverages such as coffee, tea, cola, and alcohol that may cause diuresis or irritation of the bladder.[56] Although behavioral modification is a conservative treatment modality, objective evaluation should not be

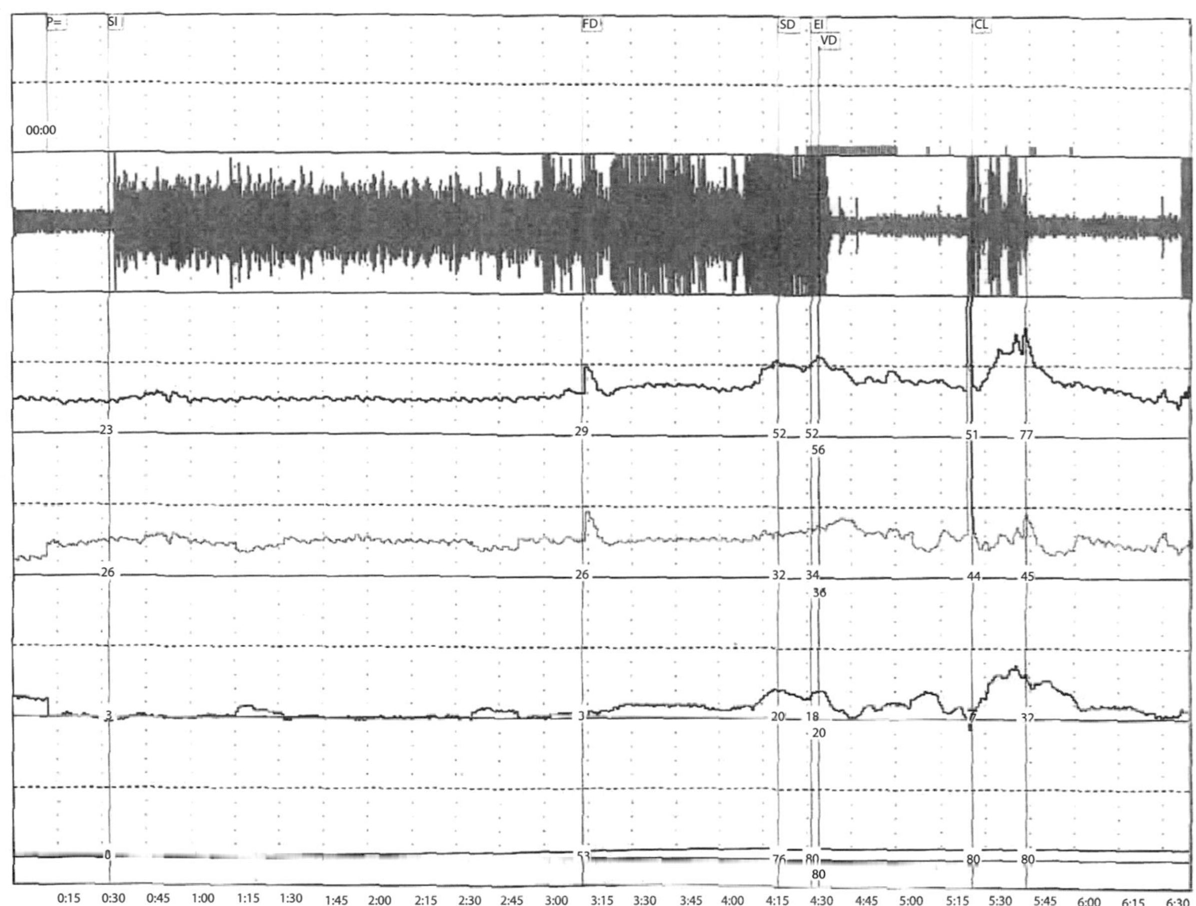

Figure 23.5
Detrusor hyperreflexia with bladder outlet obstruction.

overlooked. Empirical treatment trials without proper evaluation should be avoided, as it may lead to improper care and complications.[11]

Suppression of an involuntary detrusor contraction by stimulation of the perineal musculature is the physiologic principle underlying pelvic floor rehabilitation. This modality has already been part of the treatment of many problems, such as stress incontinence, urgency, sexual dysfunction, and fecal incontinence. Pelvic floor rehabilitation has been reported to be of some value in the treatment of detrusor instability and urgency, by influencing the sacral micturition reflex arc and thus inhibiting detrusor hyperreflexia. De Ridder et al have noted a subjective improvement in 76.7% of patients, with significant improvement in functional bladder capacity, frequency, and incontinence, as evaluated by urodynamic study.[57]

Clean intermittent catheterization and catheter drainage

Clean intermittent catheterization (CIC) is a simple and very effective treatment modality for neurogenic voiding dysfunction, either in patients with primary emptying difficulties or after pharmacologic therapy in patients with detrusor hyperreflexia.[42,45] Urodynamic evaluation is required to define bladder storage capabilities and to select the optimum catheterization interval. Chronic catheter drainage after pharmacologic therapy in patients with detrusor hyperreflexia should be considered only after all the treatment options have been evaluated since indwelling catheters have been associated with multiple problems such as urethral erosion in males, bladder neck and urethral damage in females, and urinary tract infections.[58]

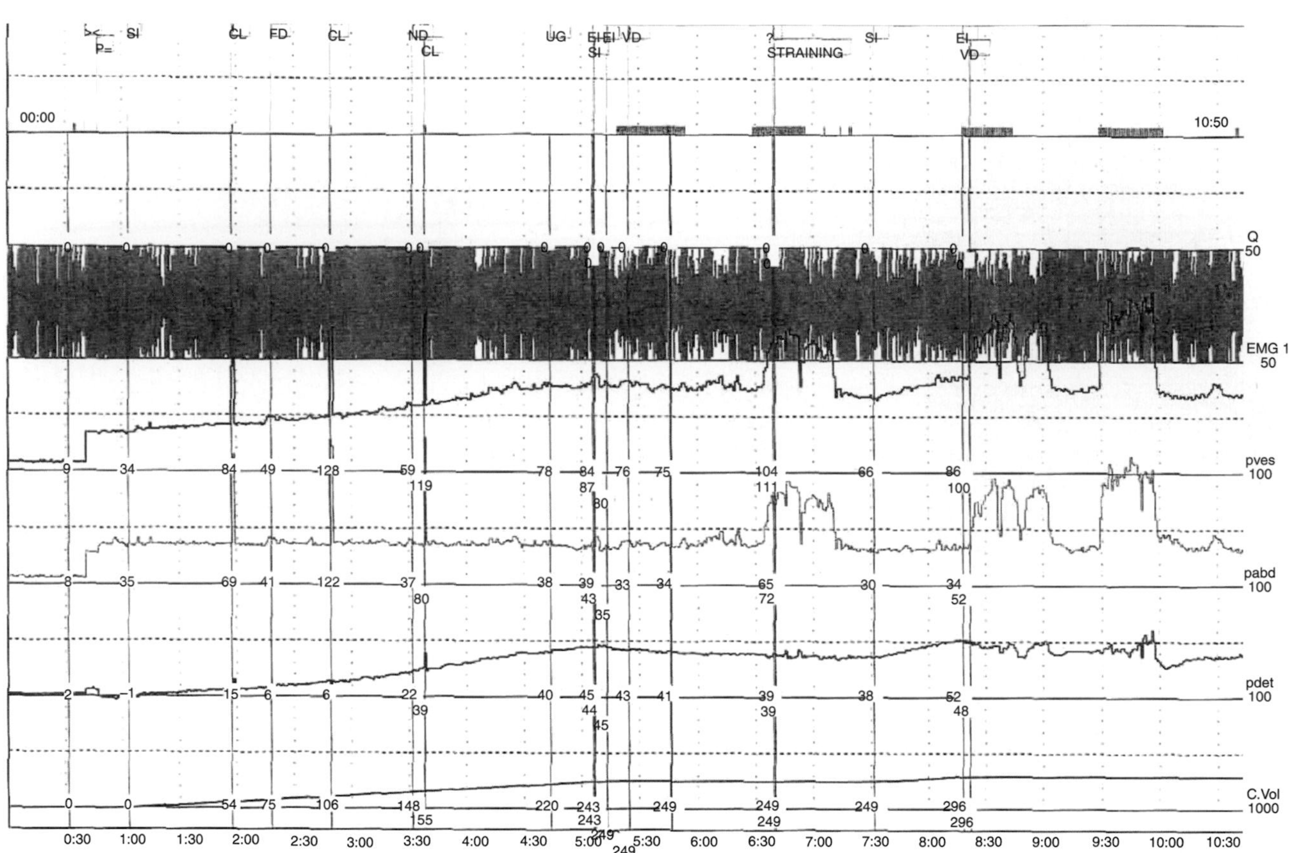

Figure 23.6
Detrusor hyperreflexia.

Pharmacologic therapy

Since almost two-thirds of patients with MS have detrusor hyperreflexia, treatment often involves pharmacologic therapy to suppress uninhibited bladder contractions. Traditionally, oxybutynin chloride has been among the most widely used drugs. It binds competitively to the muscarinic receptor, thus suppressing bladder contractions. Response rates in MS patients have been reported in the range of 65–80%.[1] However, because of the anticholinergic profile of its side-effects – namely, decreased salivation, constipation, and blurred vision – discontinuation of treatment was reported in as many as 50% of patients.[57] Tolterodine, a potent antimuscarinic agent, was specifically developed for the treatment of the overactive bladder. It is a selective muscarinic receptor blocker with efficacy proven equivalent to oxybutynin but with a more favorable tolerability profile.[59,60] In patients who tolerate these medicines, recent research indicates that additional benefit can be achieved (decreased incontinence episodes, increased cystometric capacity) by doubling the recommended dosages.[61] Newer antimuscarinic agents (darifenacin and solifenacin) have not been studied specifically in the MS population, but remain potential treatment options. In certain patients with combined storage and emptying failure, CIC may be used in concert with anticholinergic therapy. In these patients, urinary retention is promoted by anticholinergics and the 'paralyzed' bladder is hence drained by CIC.

Experimental treatment with sublingually-delivered cannabis extracts has also been demonstrated to alleviate urinary symptoms in MS patients.[62] Urinary urgency, number and volume of incontinence episodes, frequency, and nocturia episodes all decreased in the cannabis extract group, and patients also reported decreased pain and spasticity with improved quality of sleep on the drug.[62] This remains an area of future study.

Intravesical instillation of oxybutynin is another treatment option for detrusor hyperreflexia, and is reported to alleviate side-effects of oral medication.[63,64] Capsaicin and resiniferatoxin, the newer intravesical agents, are thought to exert a selective neurotoxic action on axons of C sensory fibers. These fibers appear to play an important role in bladder reflex pathways following spinal cord insult. Intravesical capsaicin and resiniferatoxin are known to reduce the amplitude of hyperreflexic contractions and

Table 23.5 *Management options of MS patients based on urologic dysfunction*

Detrusor hyperreflexia without bladder outlet obstruction:

- Behavioral modification and pelvic floor rehabilitation
- Clean intermittent catheterization/catheter drainage
- Pharmacologic therapy
- Surgical management
  - Denervation procedures
  - Augmentation cystoplasty
- Neuromodulation
- Botulinum toxin

Detrusor hyperreflexia with bladder outlet obstruction:

- Clean intermittent catheterization/catheter drainage
- External sphincterotomy
- Augmentation cystoplasty
- Ileal conduit
- Cutaneous ileovesicostomy
- Neuromodulation
- Botulinum toxin

Detrusor hyporeflexia:

- Clean intermittent catheterization/catheter drainage
- Credé's maneuver (women)
- Urinary diversion

have been used in selective research centers for the treatment of intractable detrusor hyperreflexia.[65,66]

Nocturia and enuresis are common problems in MS and the effect of sleep disturbance may be detrimental to the patient's functional level. Desmopressin, a synthetic analog of vasopressin, has been proven efficacious and safe in the management of these problems in that population.[67,68]

Surgical management

The role of surgical intervention in the management of patients with neurogenic dysfunction secondary to MS has been reduced dramatically with the advent of CIC. As a general rule, nonoperative treatment should be used as long as possible. As the course of the disease is dynamic and progressive, permanent procedures should be performed only after stabilization of the neurologic status and after all other conservative options have been exhausted. Evaluation of manual dexterity, disability, life expectancy, and social support should be undertaken as well as a thorough urodynamic characterization of the neurogenic voiding dysfunction.

Denervation procedures of the bladder have been reported for treatment of detrusor hyperreflexia and include selective dorsal rhizotomy, subtrigonal injection of phenol or alcohol, and bladder myotomy and transection. These techniques, although displaying good short-term results, have not proven to produce satisfactory long-term effects.[69]

Augmentation cystoplasty with or without a catheterizable limb (using the ileocecal valve or intussuscepted portion of the small bowel) is usually reserved for the patient with refractory detrusor hyperreflexia in whom all other nonoperative options have failed. Bladder augmentation will allow attainment of large volumes of urine in the bladder with low filling pressures. Excellent results can be expected in at least 80% of patients, but most will require CIC; thus, the ability to perform CIC is mandatory if one is to consider this type of procedure.[70,71] Careful evaluation of sphincteric competence may also obviate the need for a concomitant outlet procedure such as pubovaginal sling or sphincter prosthesis.

Neuromodulation

Sacral nerve stimulation (SNS) modulates dysfunctional voiding behavior in patients by a mechanism not fully understood, but comprising detrusor inhibition via afferent and/or efferent stimulation of sacral nerves.[72] Although the Food and Drug Administration (FDA)-approved indications for SNS are urge incontinence, urgency-frequency syndrome, and non-neurogenic urinary retention, sacral nerve stimulation has been evaluated as a reversible treatment option for neurogenic refractory urge incontinence related to detrusor hyperreflexia. Chartier-Kastler et al have reported a 43.6-month long-term efficacy of this technique in 7 out of 9 patients with urodynamically demonstrable detrusor hyperreflexia, with or without DESD.[73] Although sacral neuromodulation seems to be a promising therapy for neurogenic disease, further studies and long-term results with an extended cohort of SCI and MS patients are yet to be obtained.

Additional means of neuromodulation to control voiding symptoms are being evaluated. Transcutaneous electrical nerve stimulation (TENS) has been evaluated in MS patients with improvement in irritative voiding symptoms, diminished 24-hour micturition frequency, and incontinence episodes.[74] Placement of TENS units on either the sacral dermatomes or doral nerve of the penis or clitoris has been successful.[74,75] However, placement of the TENS unit on the dorsal nerve of the penis or clitoris may have the added benefit of inhibiting detrusor contractions.[76] Additional study is required to place this method into everyday clinical practice.[76]

Botulinum-A toxin

Botulinum-A toxin inhibits calcium-mediated release of acetylcholine vesicles at the neuromuscular junction, which results in reduced muscle contractility and atrophy at the injection site.[77] Injections into the detrusor muscle seem to be a safe conservative treatment for detrusor hyperreflexia in SCI patients. In a study of 21 patients, Schurch et al found that 19 of them achieved complete continence at 6 weeks and 11 out of 22 at 36 weeks.[78] Schulte-Baukloh et al[79] evaluated 16 MS patients with frequency, urgency, and urge incontinence who were refractory to anticholinergics. Botulinum-A toxin was injected into 40 sites of the detrusor muscle for a total dose of 300 units. Patients had an increase in postvoid residual urine, with one woman needing to perform CIC for an extended period of time. Both daytime and night-time micturition frequency decreased to a statically significant lower amount. Incontinence was improved, and patients also required fewer pads per day at the 3-month visit. Urodynamic parameters were also measured and demonstrated increased reflex volume, mean cystometric capacity, and decrease in mean detrusor pressure. Patient satisfaction was evaluated with validated questionnaires. Patients indicated improvement in quality of life and overall satisfaction, and all patients indicated a willingness to undergo repeated procedures.[79] Other studies evaluating botulinum-A toxin in neurogenic patients typically include patients with MS and show good results, but do not stratify the results as to the cause of the dysfunction.[80,81] Based on the limited results that currently exist, botulinum-A toxin seems to be a promising treatment that requires further multi-institutional studies.

Detrusor hyperreflexia with bladder outlet obstruction

Behavioral modifications and pelvic floor rehabilitation

Pelvic floor spasticity and DESD are both predictors of poor prognosis, and behavioral modifications and pelvic floor rehabilitation should be reserved for mildly symptomatic patients. Some women may be guided in voiding by Credés maneuver, but this may put the upper urinary tract at risk.[42] Although the maneuver appears easier and less invasive, in women, with time, a significant number of patients develop daytime and night-time frequency and stress incontinence. Consequently, CIC should be the method of choice.

Clean intermittent catheterization and catheter drainage

Patients with detrusor hyperreflexia have higher treatment failures and more upper tract damage.[32] The most reasonable treatment is CIC. The alternative, in the male, if he cannot perform CIC is external sphincterotomy, which is discussed below. The other alternative for both sexes is indwelling catheter, but these patients, as mentioned earlier, have a higher incidence of upper tract changes.[32]

Pharmacologic therapy

Symptoms of neurogenic voiding dysfunction complicated by bladder outlet obstruction may be treated by alpha antagonists (terazosin, doxazosin, tamsulosin) or muscle relaxants (diazepam, baclofen, dantrolene). Alpha antagonists aim at blockage of the sympathetic receptors of the smooth muscle component of the proximal urethra and bladder neck, thereby decreasing the sphincter tone and relieving bladder outlet obstruction. These treatments have had mixed results in MS patients.[82] Commonly encountered side-effects include orthostatic hypotension, dizziness, and lassitude.

Surgical management

Patients with DESD are at higher risk of upper tract damage.[32] In those males who cannot be treated with conservative measures, outlet-reducing procedures such as transurethral external sphincterotomy, self-expandable urethral stents, or balloon dilatation may be necessary. The conventional and most-used technique is external sphincterotomy, which typically involves transurethral incision of the external sphincter. These procedures allow for total urinary incontinence, which can afterward be managed by condom catheter drainage. They are best reserved for the patient with limited hand function for whom CIC is not an option or for patients who do not have caretakers that can provide this service.[83,84] The performance of supravesical diversion (ileal conduit) has decreased with the widespread acceptance of augmentation cystoplasty. The latter, constructed with or without a continent stoma, is the preferred method. These procedures should be reserved for patients with failure of conservative therapy who lack the fine motor skills to do CIC.[71] Cutaneous ileovesicostomy has been used successfully for storage or emptying abnormalities. In this procedure, a segment of ileum is used to construct a 'chimney' from the bladder to allow cutaneous drainage to an external collection device.[85] Such procedure should be reserved for individuals who cannot have CIC performed, either by themselves or by others, and who wish to avoid chronic indwelling catheter drainage.

Botulinum-A toxin

Phelan et al evaluated prospectively 22 SCI patients with DESD who were voiding by indwelling catheters or by CIC. After botulinum-A toxin injection in the external sphincter, all patients except 2 were able to void without catheterization.[77] For treatment of DESD, the duration of botulinum effect has been reported to be approximately 3 months for a single injection,[77,86] but monthly intervals for 3 months resulted in clinical effects up to 9 months.[77] Hence, botulinum-A toxin may be an alternative to external sphincterotomy for men with neuropathic DESD. It produces a reversible chemical sphincterotomy, which avoids the risks associated with the surgical procedure. However, the main disavantage is the need for repeated injections to maintain results. This treatment has to be considered in cases of failure of more traditional conservative modalities and before definitive surgery.

A recent multi-institutional placebo-controlled trial of 86 patients recruited from six centers in Europe randomized patients with MS and urodynamically proven DESD to injection of the striated sphincter with placebo or botulinum-A toxin.[87] The authors found no difference in postvoid residual volumes between the treatment and placebo groups ($p = 0.45$) However, the botulinum-A toxin group had significantly increased voided volumes (197 ml vs 128 ml) and decreased maximal detrusor pressures (52 vs 66 cm water pressure). No serious side adverse events were attributable to the botulinum-A toxin.[87] Further study is warranted in this patient population.

Neuromodulation

Chartier-Kastler et al have evaluated the use of SNS for patients with detrusor hyperreflexia. They implanted a sacral neurostimulator into 9 patients, of whom 5 had detrusor hyperreflexia with DESD. Four of these patients had improvement in frequency, volume voided, and urinary incontinence.[73] Long-term results have to be carefully evaluated, particularly in the light of an evolving disease such as MS. However, it could become a minimally invasive therapy used in the armamentarium of modalities for the disease.

Detrusor hyporeflexia

Behavioral modifications and pelvic floor rehabilitation

In certain patients with high postvoid residuals, behavioral modifications such as bladder emptying maneuvers (Credé), double-voiding, and Valsalva can all assist with bladder emptying. Also, timed voiding may also be helpful by avoidance of overdistention of the bladder. Pelvic floor stimulation in the hyporeflexic bladder has been proven to play a very limited role.[88]

Clean intermittent catheterization and catheter drainage

For some patients with more advanced disease and/or poor hand dexterity, catheterization may be a problem. These patients may require an indwelling catheter or suprapubic cystostomy. The latter is an attractive option as it has several advantages over a conventional indwelling catheter: urethral erosion and traumatic hypospadias may be avoided and personal hygiene and catheter care are simplified because of the accessibility of the catheter and its position remote from perineal or vaginal soilage. Also, the external genitalia can be free of foreign bodies and may render sexual activity possible.[69,88]

Chronic catheter drainage should be considered only after all the treatment options have been exhausted. The risks of bladder calculi, infection, and squamous cell carcinoma[88–90] should be weighed against the advantages for the patient.

Pharmacologic therapy

There is no proven pharmacologic therapy for detrusor hyporeflexia or areflexia. Bethanechol chloride, a cholinergic agonist, was used in the past, but no prospective placebo-controlled trial has ever demonstrated its efficacy in MS.[91]

Surgical management

When MS patients present symptoms, have urologic complications, or cannot perform CIC, urinary diversion is to be considered. However, the risks and benefits of this major surgical procedure must be carefully evaluated, especially in those patients with advanced disease.

Neuromodulation

Detrusor areflexia or hyporeflexia, i.e. impaired detrusor function of neurogenic origin, as a cause of voiding dysfunction, is a contraindication for sacral neuromodulation therapy. Destruction of the peripheral innervation will not allow neuromodulation therapy to be effective.[72]

Conclusion

Urinary tract dysfunction is the fate of the majority of patients suffering from MS with the advancing course of their disease. Due to the poor correlation between subjective symptoms and objective parameters, a thorough evaluation of the urinary tract is mandatory in patients with and without urinary symptoms. Although many options exist for treatment of the neurogenic bladder, a stepwise approach with conservative and initially reversible therapy is important considering the waxing and waning course of the disease. Long-term follow-up aims at preserving renal function while minimizing symptoms and enhancing quality of life.

References

1. Charcot M. Histologie de la sclerose en plaques. Gaz Hop Paris 1868; 141: 554.
2. McDonald WI. The dynamics of multiple sclerosis. The Charcot Lecture. J Neurol 1993; 240: 28.
3. Compston A, Coles A. Multiple sclerosis. Lancet 2002; 359: 1221–31.
4. Shibasaki H, McDonald WI, Kurojwa Y. Racial modifications of clinical picture of multiple sclerosis: comparison between British and Japanese patients. J Neurol Sci 1981; 49: 253–71.
5. Kira J, Kanai T, Nishimura Y et al. Western versus Asian types of multiple sclerosis: immunogenetically and clinically distinct disorders. Ann Neurol 1996; 40: 569–74.
6. Compston A. Risks factors for multiple sclerosis: race or place? J Neurol Neurosurg Psychiatry 1990; 53: 821–3.
7. Poser CM. The epidemiology of multiple sclerosis: a general overview. Ann Neurol 1994; 36(S2): S180–93.
8. Sadovnick A, Eberg G, Dyment D, Rish N, and Canadian Collaborative Study Group. Evidence for genetic basis of multiple sclerosis. Lancet 1996; 347: 1728–30.
9. Hinson JL, Boone TB. Urodynamics and multiple sclerosis. Urol Clin N Am 1996; 23(3): 475–81.
10. Keegan BM, Noseworthy JH. Multiple sclerosis. Annu Rev Med 2002; 53: 285–302.
11. Litwiller SE, Frohman EM, Zimmern PE. Multiple sclerosis and the urologist. J Urol 1999; 161: 743–57.
12. Zhang J, Markovic-Plese S, Lacet B et al. Increased frequency of interleukin 2-responsive T cells specific for myelin basic protein and proteolipid protein in peripheral blood and cerebrospinal fluid of patients with multiple sclerosis. J Exp Med 1994; 179: 973–84.
13. Archelos JJ, Storch MK, Hartung HP. The role of B cells and autoantibodies in multiple sclerosis. Ann Neurol 2000; 47: 694–706.
14. Genain CP, Cannella B, Hauser SL, Raine CS. Identification of autoantibodies associated with myelin damage in multiple sclerosis. Nat Med 1999; 5: 170–5.
15. Ebers G, Sadovnick A, Rish N. Canadian Collaborative Study Group. A genetic basis for familial aggregation in multiple sclerosis. Nature 1995; 377: 150–1.
16. Sawcer S, Meranian M, Setakis E et al. A whole genome screen for linkage disequilibrium in multiple sclerosis confirms disease associations with regions previously linked to susceptibility. Brain 2002; 125: 1337–47.
17. Compston A. The genetic epidemiology of multiple sclerosis. Phil Trans R Soc Lond, B Biol Sci 1999; 354: 1623–34.
18. Hunter SF, Hafler DA. Ubiquitous pathogens – links between infection and autoimmunity in MS? Neurology 2000; 55: 164–5.
19. Albert LJ, Inman RD. Molecular mimicry and autoimmunity. N Engl J Med 1999; 341: 2068–74.
20. Wandinger KB, Jabs W, Siekhaus A et al. Association between clinical disease activity and Epstein–Barr virus reactivation in MS. Neurology 2000; 55: 178–84.
21. Challoner P, Smith K, Parker J et al. Plaque-associated expression of human herpesvirus 6 in multiple sclerosis. Proc Natl Acad Sci USA 1995; 92: 7440–4.
22. Sriram S, Stratton C, Yao S et al. *Chlamydia pneumoniae* infection of the central nervous system in multiple sclerosis. Ann Neurol 1999; 46: 6–14.
23. McDonald WI, Compston A, Edan G et al. Recommended diagnostic criteria for multiple sclerosis: guidelines from the International Panel on the diagnosis of multiple sclerosis. Ann Neurol 2001; 50: 121–7.
24. Weinshenker B, Lucchinetti C. Acute leukoencephalopathies: differential diagnosis and investigation. Neurologist 1998; 4: 148–66.
25. Lublin FD, Reingold SC. Defining the clinical course of mutiple sclerosis: results of an international survey. Neurology 1996; 46: 907–11.
26. Werring DJ, Bullmore ET, Toosy AT et al. Recovery from optic neuritis is associated with a change in the distribution of cerebral response to visual stimulation: a functional magnetic resonance imaging study. J Neurol Neurosurg Psychiatry 2000; 68: 441–9.
27. Weinshenker BG, Rice GPA, Noseworthy JH et al. The natural history of multiple sclerosis: a geographically based study. III. Multivariate analysis of predictive factors and models of outcome. Brain 1991; 114: 1045–56.
28. O'Riordan JI, Thompson AJ, Kingsley DP et al. The prognostic value of brain MRI in clinically isolated syndromes of the CNS. A 10-year follow-up. Brain 1998; 121: 495–503.
29. Griffiths D, Holstege G, de Wall H, Dalm E. Control and coordination of bladder and urethral function in the brain stem of the cat. Neurourol Urodyn 1990; 9: 63–82.
30. Blok B, Willemsen T, Holstege G. A PET study of brain control of micturition in humans. Brain 1997; 129: 111–21.
31. Oppenheimer DR. The cervical cord in multiple sclerosis. Neuropathol Appl Neurobiol 1978; 4: 151–62.
32. Blaivas JG, Barbalias GA. Detrusor external sphincter dyssynergia in men with multiple sclerosis: an ominous urologic condition. J Urol 1984; 131: 91–4.
33. Philip T, Read DJ, Higson RH. The urodynamic characteristics of multiple sclerosis. Br J Urol 1981; 53: 672–5.
34. Mayo ME, Chetner MP. Lower urinary tract dysfunction in multiple sclerosis. Urology 1992; 39: 67–70.
35. Fernandez O. Mechanisms and current treatments of urogenital dysfunction in multiple sclerosis. J Neurol 2002; 249: 1–8.
36. Hennessey A, Robertson NP, Swingker R et al. Urinary, faecal and sexual dysfunction in patients with multiple sclerosis. J Neurol 1999; 246: 1027–32.
37. Beck RP, Warren KG, Whitman P. Urodynamic studies in female patients with multiple sclerosis. Am J Obstet Gynecol 1981; 139: 273–6.
38. Goldstein I, Siroky MB, Sax DS, Krane RJ. Neurourologic abnormalities in multiple sclerosis. J Urol 1982; 128: 541–5.
39. Ukkonen M, Elovaara I, Dastidar P, Tammela TLJ. Urodynamic findings in primary progressive multiple sclerosis are associated with increased volumes of plaques and atrophy in the central nervous system. Acta Neurol Scand 2004; 109: 100–5.
40. Quarto G, Autorino R, Gallo A et al. Quality of life in women with multiple sclerosis and overactive bladder syndrome. Int Urogynecol J 2007;18: 189–94.
41. Koldewijn EL, Hommes OR, Lemmens AJG et al. Relationship between lower urinary tract abnormalities and disease-related parameters in multiple sclerosis. J Urol 1995; 154: 169–73.
42. McGuire EJ, Savastano JA. Urodynamic findings and long-term outcome management of patients with multiple sclerosis induced lower urinary tract dysfunction. J Urol 1984; 132: 713–15.
43. Sirls LT, Zimmern PE, Leach GE. Role of limited evaluation and aggressive medical management in multiple sclerosis: a review of 113 patients. J Urol 1994; 151: 946–50.
44. Betts CD, D'Mellow MT, Fowler CJ. Urinary symptoms and the neurological features of bladder dysfunction in multiple sclerosis. J Neurol Neurosurg Psychiatry 1993; 56: 245–50.
45. Awad SA, Gajewski JB, Sogbein SK et al. Relationship between neurological and urological status in patients with multiple sclerosis. J Urol 1984; 132: 499–502.
46. Chancellor MB, Blaivas JG. Urological and sexual problems in multiple sclerosis. Clin Neurosci 1994; 2: 189–95.
47. Lee KH, Hashimoto SA, Hooge JP et al. Magnetic resonance imaging of the head in the diagnosis of multiple sclerosis: a prospective 2-year follow-up with comparison of clinical evaluation, evoked potentials, oligoclonal banding, and CT. Neurology 1991; 41: 657–60.
48. Goodkin DE, Rudick RA, Ross JS. The use of brain magnetic resonance imaging in multiple sclerosis. Arch Neurol 1994; 51: 505–16.
49. Prineas JW, Barnard RO, Kwon EE et al. Multiple sclerosis: remyelination of nascent lesions. Ann Neurol 1993; 33: 137–51.

50. Kim YH, Goodman C, Omessi E et al. The correlation of urodynamic findings with cranial magnetic resonance imaging findings in multiple sclerosis. J Urol 1998; 159: 972–6.
51. Lemack GE, Hawker K, Frohman E. Incidence of upper tract abnormalities in patients with neurovesical dysfunction secondary to multiple sclerosis: analysis of risk factors at initial urologic evaluation. Urology 2005; 65(5): 854–7.
52. Bemelmans BL, Hommes OR, Van Kerrebroek PEV et al. Evidence for early lower urinary tract dysfunction in clinically silent multiple sclerosis. J Urol 1991; 145: 1219–24.
53. Gonor SE, Carroll DJ, Metcalfe JB. Vesical dysfunction in multiple sclerosis. Urology 1985; 25: 429–31.
54. Wheeler JS Jr, Siroky MB, Pavlakis AJ et al. The changing neurourologic pattern of multiple sclerosis. J Urol 1983; 130: 1123–6.
55. Ciancio SJ, Mutchnik SE, Rivera VM, Boone TB. Urodynamic pattern changes in multiple sclerosis. Urology 2001; 57: 239–45.
56. McClurg D, Ashe RG, Marshall K, Lowe-Strong AS. Comparison of pelvic floor muscle training, electromyography biofeedback, and neuromuscular electrical stimulation for bladder dysfunction in people with multiple sclerosis: a randomized pilot study. Neurourol Urodyn 2006; 25: 337–48.
57. De Ridder D, Vermeulen C, Ketelaer P et al. Pelvic floor rehabilitation in multiple sclerosis. Acta Neurol Belg 1999; 99: 61–4.
58. De Ridder D, Ost D, Van der Aa F et al. Conservative bladder management in advanced multiple sclerosis. Mult Scler 2005; 11: 694–9.
59. Thuroff JW, Bunke B, Ebner A et al. Randomized, double-blind, multicenter trial on treatment of frequency, urgency and incontinence related to detrusor hyperactivity: oxybutynin versus propantheline versus placebo. J Urol 1991; 145: 813–17.
60. Abrams P, Freeman R, Anderstrom C, Mattiasson A. Tolterodine, a new antimuscarinic agent: as effective but better tolerated than oxybutynin in patients with an overactive bladder. Br J Urol 1998; 81(6): 801–10.
61. Horstmann M, Schaefer T, Aguilar Y, Stenzl A, Sievert KD. Neurogenic bladder treatment by doubling the recommended antimuscarinic dosage. Neurourol Urodyn 2006; 25: 441–5.
62. Brady CM, DasGupta R, Dalton C et al. An open-label pilot study of cannabis-based extracts for bladder dysfunction in advanced multiple sclerosis. Mult Scler 2004; 10: 425–33.
63. Madersbacher H, Jilg G. Control of detrusor hyperreflexia by the intravesical instillation of oxybutynin hydrochloride. Paraplegia 1991; 29: 84–90.
64. Weese DL, Roskamp DA, Leach GE, Zimmern PE. Intravesical oxybutynin chloride: experience with 42 patients. Urology 1993; 41(6): 527–30.
65. de Ridder D, Chandiramani V, Dasgupta P et al. Intravesical capsaicin as a treatment for refractory detrusor hyperreflexia: a dual center study with long-term follow up. J Urol 1997; 158: 2087–92.
66. Lazzeri M, Beneforti P, Spinelli M et al. Intravesical resiniferatoxin for the treatment of hypersensitive disorder: a randomized placebo controlled study. J Urol 2000; 164: 676–9.
67. Valiquette G, Herbert J, Meade-D'Alisera P. Desmopressin in the management of nocturia in patients with multiple sclerosis. Arch Neurol 1996; 53: 1270–5.
68. Eckford SD, Swami KS, Jackson SR, Abrams PH. Desmopressin in the treatment of nocturia and enuresis in patients with multiple sclerosis. Br J Urol 1994; 74(6): 733–5.
69. Chancellor MB, Blaivas JG. Multiple sclerosis. Probl Urol 1993; 7(1): 15–33.
70. Goldwasser B, Webster GD. Augmentation and substitution enterocystoplasty. J Urol 1986; 135: 215–24.
71. Luangkhot R, Peng BCH, Blaivas JG. Ileocecocystoplasty for the management of refractory neurogenic bladder: surgical technique and urodynamic findings. J Urol 1991; 146: 1340–4.
72. Scheepens WA, van Kerrebroeck PEV. Indications and predictive factors. In: Udo J, Grunewald V, eds. New Perspectives in Sacral Nerve Stimulation. London: Martin Dunitz, 2002: 89–98.
73. Chartier-Kastler E, Ruud Bosch JLH, Perrigot M et al. Long-term results of sacral nerve stimulation (S3) for the treatment of neurogenic refractory urge incontinence related to detrusor hyperreflexia. J Urol 2000; 164: 1476–80.
74. Skeil D, Thorpe AC. Transcutaneous electrical nerve stimulation in the treatment of neurological patients with urinary symptoms. BJU Int 2001; 88: 899–908.
75. Fjorback MV, Van Rey FS, Riijkhoff NJM, Nohr M, Petersen T, Heesakkers JP. Electrical stimulation of sacral dermatomes in multiple sclerosis patients with neurogenic detrusor overactivity. Neurourol Urodyn 2007; 26: 525–30.
76. Fjorback MV, Riijkhoff N, Petersen T, Nohr M, Sinkjaer T. Event driven electrical stimulation of the dorsal penile/clitoral nerve for management of neurogenic detrusor overactivity in multiple sclerosis. Neurourol Urodyn 2006; 25: 349–55.
77. Phelan MW, Franks M, Somogyi GT et al. Botulinum toxin urethral sphincter injection to restore bladder emptying in men and women with voiding dysfunction. J Urol 2001; 165: 1107–10.
78. Schurch B, Stohrer M, Kramer G et al. Botulinum-A toxin for treating detrusor hyperreflexia in spinal cord injured patients: a new alternative to anticholinergic drugs? Preliminary results. J Urol 2000; 164: 692–7.
79. Schulte-Baukloh H, Schobert J, Stolze T, Sturzebecher B, Weiss C, Knispel HH. Efficacy of botulinum-A toxin bladder injections for the treatment of neurogenic detrusor overactivity in multiple sclerosis patients: an objective and subjective analysis. Neurourol Urodyn 2006; 25: 110–15.
80. Schurch B, de Seze M, Deys P et al. Botulium toxin type A is a safe and effective treatment for neurogenic urinary incontinence: results of a single treatment, randomized, placebo controlled 6-month study. J Urol 2005; 174: 196–200.
81. Smith CP, Nishiguchi J, O' Leary M. Yoshimura N. Chancellor MB. Single-institution experience in 110 patients with botulinum toxin A injection into bladder or urethra. Urology 2005; 65(1): 37–41
82. O'Riordan JI, Doherty C, Javed M et al. Do alpha-blockers have a role in lower urinary tract dysfunction in multiple sclerosis? J Urol 1995; 153: 1114–16.
83. Lockhart JL, Vorstman B, Weinstein D, Politano VA. Sphincterotomy failure in neurogenic bladder disease. J Urol 1986; 135: 86–9.
84. Sauerwein D, Gross AJ, Kutzenberger J, Ringert RH. Wallstents in patients with detrusor-sphincter dyssynergia. J Urol 1995; 154: 495–7.
85. Schwartz SL, Kennely MJ, McGuire EJ, Farber GJ. Incontinent ileovesicostomy urinary diversion in the treatment of lower urinary tract dysfunction. J Urol 1994; 152: 99.
86. Schurch B, Hauri D, Rodic B et al. Botulinum-A toxin as a treatment of detrusor-sphincter dyssynergia: a prospective study in 24 cord injury patients. J Urol 1996; 155: 1023–9.
87. Gallien P, Reymann J-M, Amarenco G et al. Placebo controlled, randomized, double blind study of the effects of botulinum A toxin on detrusor sphincter dyssynergia in multiple sclerosis patients. J Neurol Neurosurg Pschiaty 2005; 76: 1670–6.
88. Rashid TM, Hollander JB. Multiple sclerosis and the neurogenic bladder. Phys Med Rehab Clin N Am 1998; 9(3): 615–29.
89. Broecker BH, Klein FA, Hackler RH. Cancer of the bladder in spinal cord injury patients. J Urol 1981; 125: 196–7.
90. Bejany DE, Lockhart JL, Rhamy RK. Malignant vesical tumors following spinal cord injury. J Urol 1987; 138: 1390–2.
91. Finkbeiner AE. Is bethanechol chloride clinically effective in promoting bladder emptying? A literature review. J Urol 1985; 134: 443–9.

24

Other diseases (transverse myelitis, tropical spastic paraparesis, progressive multifocal leukoencephalopathy, Lyme´s disease)

Tomáš Hanuš

Transverse myelitis

Incidence

Acute transverse myelitis (ATM) has an incidence of one to four new cases per million people per year, affecting individuals of all ages, with bimodal peaks between the ages of 10 and 19 years and 30 and 39 years. There is no sex or familial predisposition to ATM. The characteristics and natural history, particularly in relation to neurologic outcome, have already been described in a pediatric population in recent years, as well; however, it is a relatively rare condition in children.

Etiology and pathogenesis

Transverse myelitis (TM) is a clinical syndrome, whereby an immune-mediated process causes a neural injury to the spinal cord, resulting in varying degrees of weakness, sensory alterations, and autonomic dysfunction. TM may exist as part of a multifocal disease of the central nervous system (CNS) (e.g. multiple sclerosis (MS)), as a multisystemic disease (e.g. systemic lupus erythematosus), or as an isolated, idiopathic entity.

Acute TM is commonly parainfectious. Recurrent ATM occurs in connective tissue disease (CTD), infective myelitis, and idiopathic inflammatory demyelinating disorders (IIDD), including MS and neuromyelitis optica (NMO). With improved understanding of the underlying neurophysiology, only true spinal inflammatory processes are designated *myelitis.* Myelitis is classified either according to the speed of symptom progression (acute, subacute, or chronic) or according to the etiology (viral, bacterial, parasitic, tuberculosis, and idiopathic). These disorders may selectively affect different parts of the nervous system, spinal cord and meninges (meningomyelitis), or meninges and roots (meningoradiculitis). The inflammatory distribution is termed poliomyelitis when it is confined to the gray matter and leukomyelitis if it affects the white matter. When the entire thickness of the spinal cord is involved it is called transverse myelitis.

Diagnosis

ATM is characterized clinically by an acute or subacute onset of symptoms and signs of neurologic dysfunction in motor, sensory, and autonomic nerves and nerve tracts of the spinal cord. There is often a clearly defined upper border of sensory dysfunction, and spinal magnetic resonance imaging (MRI) and lumbar puncture often show signs of acute inflammation. When the maximal level of deficit is reached, approximately 50% of patients lose all movements of their legs, virtually all patients have bladder dysfunction, and 80 to 94% of patients have numbness, paresthesias, or band-like dysesthesias. Autonomic symptoms consist variably of increased urinary urgency, bowel or bladder incontinence, difficulty or inability to void, incomplete evacuation, or constipation.

The Transverse Myelitis Consortium Working Group suggested a set of uniform diagnostic criteria and nosology for ATM, which is a focal inflammatory disorder of the spinal cord, resulting in motor, sensory, and autonomic dysfunction.[1] This set was proposed to avoid the confusion that inevitably results when investigators use differing criteria. This set will ensure a common language of classification, reduce diagnostic confusion, and will lay the groundwork necessary for multicenter clinical trials. In addition, a framework is suggested for evaluation of individuals presenting with signs and symptoms of ATM. The best treatment often depends on a timely and accurate diagnosis.

Table 24.1 *Criteria for idiopathic ATM*
A Inclusion criteria
Development of sensory, motor, or autonomic dysfunction attributable to the spinal cord
Bilateral signs and/or symptoms (though not necessarily symmetric)
Clearly defined sensory level
Exclusion of extra-axial compressive etiology by neuroimaging (MRI or myelography; CT of spine not adequate)
Inflammation within the spinal cord demonstrated by CSF pleocytosis or elevated IgG index or gadolinium enhancement. If none of the inflammatory criteria is met at symptom onset, repeat MRI and lumbar puncture evaluation between 2 and 7 days following symptom onset
Progression to nadir between 4 hours and 21 days following the onset of symptoms
B Exclusion criteria
History of previous radiation to the spine within the last 10 years
Clear arterial distribution clinical deficit consistent with thrombosis of the anterior spinal artery
Abnormal flow voids on the surface of the spinal cord c/w AVM
Serologic or clinical evidence of connective tissue disease (sarcoidosis, Behçet's disease, Sjögren's syndrome, SLE, mixed connective tissue disorder, etc.)
CNS manifestations of syphilis, Lyme disease, HIV, HTLV-1, Mycoplasma, other viral infection (e.g. HSV-1, HSV-2, VZV, EBV, CMV, HHV-6, enteroviruses)
Brain MRI abnormalities suggestive of MS
History of clinically apparent optic neuritis

Because acute transverse myelopathies are relatively rare, delayed and incomplete work-up often occurs. Rapid and accurate diagnosis will ensure not only that compressive lesions are detected and treated but also that an idiopathic ATM is distinguished from ATM secondary to known underlying disease. Identification of etiologies may suggest medical treatment, whereas no clearly established medical treatment currently exists for idiopathic ATM. Establishment of a diagnostic algorithm will likely lead to improved care, although it is recognized that the entire evaluation may not be performed for every patient.

The diagnostic criteria for idiopathic ATM are listed in Table 24.1. Diagnosis of idiopathic ATM should require that all of the inclusion criteria and none of the exclusion criteria are fulfilled. Diagnosis of disease-associated ATM should require that all the inclusion criteria are met and that the patient is identified as having an underlying condition listed in the disease-specific exclusions.

Voiding dysfunctions

Transverse myelitis has various neurologic manifestations. Bladder dysfunction is common and may be the only sequel. The neurologic events during normal micturition that culminate in a detrusor contraction and urethral relaxation are integrated in the rostral brainstem in the area designated as the pontine micturition center. Any lesion within the spinal cord, such as trauma, multiple sclerosis, myelodysplasia and myelitis, which causes a disruption of this pathway, may result in detrusor-external sphincter dyssynergia (DSD). If the disease involves the sacral (S2 to S4) cord or roots a lower motor neuron lesion may occur as well, with pudendal or parasympathetic dysfunction. If the thoracolumbar cord is affected sympathetic dysfunction may occur. Urodynamic study is helpful in evaluating the bladder dysfunction and also in its management.

Ganesan and Borzyskowski described the characteristics and course of urinary tract dysfunction after acute transverse myelitis in 10 children, with ages ranging from 8 months to 16 years.[2] Patients were studied with videourodynamics and followed at a pediatric neurourology clinic. Nine of 10 children had obstructive urinary tract symptoms at presentation and all developed irritative urinary tract symptoms (frequency and urgency) about 1 month after the initial presentation. Videourodynamics showed a combination of irritative (detrusor overactivity) and obstructive (DSD) abnormalities in most patients and enabled management to be specifically directed towards these. The patients' progress was followed for a median duration of 36 months. All had residual bladder dysfunction, only 4 were asymptomatic on treatment. The degree of recovery of bladder function was not related to the degree of motor recovery.

In the study of Cheng et al, the long-term urologic outcome of children with ATM was assessed.[3] Medical records of children with ATM over last 15 years were reviewed. The median age of the 5 children with ATM at the time of onset was 6 years (range 2 to 12 years). The median length of follow-up was 5 years (range 2 to 10 years). Four children recovered completely from paraparesis; 2 had no urinary symptoms with normal voiding. However, videourodynamic studies 3 years after the acute onset revealed that 4 out of the 5 children, including one without any urinary symptom, suffered from residual bladder dysfunction – two from contractile neurogenic bladder and two from intermediate type neurogenic bladder.

Leroy-Malherbe et al studied retrospectively the records of 21 children admitted at the mean age of 8 years 5 months (range 2 to 14 years 8 months) for acute transverse myelopathy.[4] Bladder sphincter dysfunction occurred on the first days of the disease in 85% of these patients. Abnormal perception of micturition was one of the most constant and specific symptoms. Anorectal function was also impaired. A complete regressive course was noted in 38% of patients, minor sequelae in 39%, and major sequelae after 6 months in 23%. No upper tract deterioration was noted after 3 years. Factors of favorable prognosis were early motor function recovery (especially recommencement of walking before 20 days) and early management of bladder dysfunction (inability to void had better prognosis than urinary incontinence). Early systematic bladder drainage in case of inability to void might be essential for improved prognosis. Voiding dysfunction secondary to schistosomal myelopathy was also described by Gomes et al. *Schistosomiasis mansoni* is an endemic fluke infection in South America, the Caribbean, and Africa. In the United States and Europe, people may become infected mainly after traveling to endemic areas and after immigration of infected individuals. Clinical involvement of the spinal cord is a well-recognized complication of the disease. The typical presentations are those of an acute TM with sudden onset of lower extremity neuropathy associated with bladder and bowel dysfunction. The authors reviewed records and urodynamic studies of 14 consecutive patients (10 men and 4 women, aged 23 to 49 years) with schistosomal myelopathy confirmed by cerebrospinal fluid (CSF) serology for *S. mansoni*, who were referred for evaluation of voiding dysfunction during a 2-year period. At the time of the urologic evaluation, 9 patients had chronic neurologic and urinary symptoms and 5 had recent onset of acute symptoms. History of voiding function, urologic complications, and outcomes after therapy for schistosomiasis were also reviewed. Of the patients with acute disease (5 patients), the urologic symptoms included urinary retention (3 patients) and incontinence (2 patients). Three of them had concurrent lower back pain and lower extremity neurologic deficits. Urodynamic studies were performed in 3 patients and revealed bladder acontractility in 2 patients and detrusor overactivity with external sphincter dyssynergia in 1 patient.

The patients were started on clean intermittent catheterization (CIC) and received praziquantel and corticosteroids. Three patients had complete resolution of their symptoms, one recovered normal voiding function but the neurologic deficits persisted, and one had no clinical improvement. All patients with chronic schistosomal myelopathy presented with lower limb neurologic deficits of varying degrees and urinary symptoms, including difficulty in bladder emptying (7 patients), urinary incontinence (6 patients), and urgency and frequency (2 patients). Laboratory and radiographic investigations of patients with chronic disease revealed urinary tract infection in 5 patients, hydronephrosis in 2 patients, and bladder calculi in 2 patients. Urologic management consisted of antibiotics, CIC, anticholinergic medication, and stone removal, as appropriate. In 1 patient, conservative treatment failed and the patient required ileocystoplasty. Schistosomal myelopathy is a potential cause of severe voiding dysfunction secondary to spinal cord disease. A high index of suspicion is of paramount importance because early medical intervention can abort the progression of neurologic deterioration.

Kalita et al evaluated voiding abnormalities in ATM and correlated these with evoked potentials, MRI, and urodynamic findings.[5] Of 18 patients with ATM aged 4 to 50 years, 15 had a paraparesis and three quadruparesis. Patients with ATM had a neurologic examination and tibial somatosensory and motor evoked potential studies in the lower limbs. Spinal MRI was carried out using a 1.5 T scanner. Urodynamic studies were done using a Dantec UD 5500 machine. Neurologic outcome was classified on the basis of the Barthel index score at 6 months as poor, partial, or complete. In some patients, urodynamic studies were repeated at 6 and 12 months. Spinal MRI in 14 of 18 patients revealed T2 hyperintense signal changes, extending over at least three spinal segments in 13 patients. One patient had normal MRI. In the acute phase, 17 patients had a history of urinary retention and one had urge incontinence. At 6 months' follow-up 2 patients had regained normal voiding, retention persisted in 6, and storage symptoms had developed in 10, of whom 5 also had emptying difficulties. Urodynamic studies showed an acontractile or hypocontractile bladder in 10, detrusor overactivity with poor compliance in 2, and DSD in 3 patients. Early abnormal urodynamic findings commonly persisted at the 6- and 12-month examinations. Persistent abnormalities included detrusor overactivity, dyssynergia, and acontractile bladder. The urodynamic abnormalities correlated with muscle tone and reflex changes, but not with sensory or motor evoked potentials, muscle power, MRI signal changes, sensory level, or 6-month outcome.

Sakakibara et al reported on 10 patients with ATM.[6] Seven patients had urinary retention and 3 patients had voiding difficulties within 1 month after the onset of the disease. Five patients with retention became able to void. After the mean follow-up of 40 months, 9 still had urinary symptoms, including difficult voiding in 5 and urinary frequency, urgency, and incontinence in 4 patients. Four patients had urinary disturbance as a sole sequel of ATM. Urodynamic studies performed on 9 patients revealed that all of the 3 patients with the urgent incontinence had detrusor overactivity, all of the 4 patients with retention had an acontractile cystometrogram as well as sphincter overactivity, and 3 of 5 patients with voiding difficulty had DSD. The acontractile cystometrogram tended to change to a low compliance bladder, followed by detrusor overactivity or a normal cystometrogram. Analysis of the motor unit potentials of the external sphincter revealed that 2 of the 3 patients had high-amplitude or polyphasic neurogenic changes. Supranuclear as well as nuclear types of parasympathetic and somatic nerve dysfunctions seemed to be responsible for voiding disturbances in the patients with ATM.

Chan et al reported the case of a 63-year-old Chinese man who presented with quadruparesis and urinary incontinence.[7] The initial diagnosis was a cord compression from cervical spondylosis. The patient relapsed 3 months after cervical laminectomy. The TM picture, left optic atrophy, and suggestive brainstem evoked potentials led to treatment of a presumptive demyelinating process. The presence of vitiligo, however, led to the detection of high titers of antinuclear antibodies (ANAs) and the presence of anti-nonhistone antibodies. The patient was then diagnosed to have a lupus (SLE)-like disease, which has not fully developed. He was prescribed pulsed cyclophosphamide and prednisolone, with significant gains both neurologically and functionally up to 1 year of follow-up. It can occur in men in the seventh decade of life, heightening the need for awareness in our approach to the myelopathic patient.

The following year, Chan et al published clinical features of 9 lupus patients who presented with TM and documented functional outcomes of early treatment with high-dose corticosteroids and/or cyclophosphamide.[8] These 9 patients who developed a total of 14 episodes of TM were retrospectively reviewed. All patients were females aged 21 to 59 years. Nine episodes of paraparesis, 3 of quadruparesis, 1 of numbness, and 1 of neurogenic bladder were reported early in the diagnosis of SLE (median of 2 years). Neurogenic bowel and bladder and the presence of antibodies ANA and anti-ds-DNA were invariable.

Berger et al found abnormal detrusor function in all 6 patients with TM.[9] CT scans and myelograms were inconclusive and CSF studies were normal. ESR and complement levels were insensitive as markers of disease activity. The treatment regimens included pulses of methylprednisolone and/or cyclophosphamide followed by prednisolone and high-dose prednisolone from the onset. The functional outcomes were uniformly good, with independent ambulation in all except 3 (who needed assistive devices) and improvement of motor scores. Acute hospital stay was short (range 3 to 45 days) and only two were referred for inpatient rehabilitation. Bladder abnormalities persisted despite motor recovery. Six men and 2 women with a history of TM and persistent lower urinary tract symptoms underwent neurourologic evaluation. Of the patients, 4 were neurologically intact, while the remainder had residual neurologic deficits. Urodynamic studies revealed detrusor-external sphincter dyssynergia in 6 patients. Two patients had detrusor overactivity, of whom 1 also had an incompetent sphincter. Erectile or ejaculatory dysfunction was reported by 3 men. They concluded that prolonged bladder and sexual dysfunction, caused by spinal cord inflammatory insult, may persist despite a systemic neurologic recovery. Therefore, bladder management guided by initial and follow-up urodynamics is recommended.

Chartier-Kastler et al in 2000 assessed clinical and urodynamic results of sacral nerve stimulation for patients with neurogenic (spinal cord disease) urge incontinence and detrusor overactivity resistant to parasympatholytic medications.[10] Nine women with a mean age of 42.6 years (range 26 to 53 years) had been treated since 1992 for refractory neurogenic urge incontinence with sacral nerve stimulation. Neurologic spinal diseases included viral and vascular myelitis in 1 patient each, MS in 5, and traumatic spinal cord injury in 2. The mean time since neurologic diagnosis was 12 years. All patients had incontinence with chronic pad use related to neurogenic detrusor overactivity. Intermittent self-catheterization for external detrusor-sphincter dyssynergia was used by 5 patients. Social life was impaired and these patients were candidates for bladder augmentation. A sacral (S3) lead was surgically implanted and connected to a subcutaneous neurostimulator after a positive stimulation trial. Mean follow-up was 43.6 months (range 7 to 72 months). All patients had clinically significant improvement of incontinence and 5 were completely dry. The average number of voids per day decreased from 16.1 to 8.2. Urodynamic parameters at 6 months after implant improved significantly from baseline, including maximum bladder capacity from 244 to 377 ml, and volume at first uninhibited contraction from 214 to 340 ml. Maximum detrusor pressure at first uninhibited contraction increased in 3, stabilized in 2, and decreased in 4 patients. Urodynamic results returned to baseline when stimulation was inactivated. All patients subjectively reported improved visual analog scale results by at least 75% at the last follow-up. It was concluded that sacral nerve stimulation can be used as a reversible treatment option for refractory urge incontinence related to detrusor overactivity in selected patients with spinal lesions.

Das and Jaykumar reported a case of TM with urinary retention in Nepal following typhoid vaccination.[11] The prognosis is unsatisfactory and there tends to be a prolonged period with residual paralysis.

Tsiodras et al reviewed all available literature on cases of *Mycoplasma* spp. associated ATM with dominant spinal cord pathology and classified those cases according to the strength of evidence implicating *M. pneumoniae* as the cause.[12] A wide range of data on diagnosis, epidemiology, immuno-pathogenesis, clinical picture, laboratory diagnosis, neuroimaging, and treatment of this rare entity has been presented. The use of highly sensitive and specific molecular diagnostic techniques may assist to clearly elucidate the role of *M. pneumoniae* in ATM/ADEM syndromes in the near future. Myelitis is one of the most severe central nervous system complications seen in association with *Mycoplasma pneumoniae* infections, and ATM has been observed. Immunomodulating therapies may have a role in the treatment of such cases. A case of TM with urinary retention in a 16-year-old man caused by *Mycoplasma pneumoniae* was also reported. He was discharged from hospital after 2 months. However, since urinary frequency, urge incontinence, and a weak urinary stream persisted, he was referred to a pressure–flow study examination that showed overactive detrusor and DSD. He improved after 8 months of oral propiverin hydrochloride and imipramine hydrochloride treatment, but still had nighttime incontinence. Another case described a 9-year-old girl with urinary retention 16 days after measles and rubella vaccination. Her illness was diagnosed as TM. She was treated with steroids and discharged with only mild lower limb weakness.

Krishnan et al described the clinical manifestations of TM as a consequence of a dysfunction of motor, sensory, and autonomic pathways.[13] At peak deficit, 50% of patients with TM were completely paraplegic (with no volitional leg movement), virtually all had some degree of bladder dysfunction, and 80 to 94% had numbness, paresthesias, or band-like dysesthesias. Recent studies have shown that the cytokine interleukin-6 may be a useful biomarker, as the levels of interleukin-6 in the cerebrospinal fluid of acute TM patients correlate strongly with and are highly predictive of disability. Clinical trials testing the efficacy of promising axonoprotective agents in combination with intravenous steroids in the treatment of TM are currently underway.

Prognosis

A longitudinal case series of ATM revealed that approximately one-third of patients recovered with little to no sequelae, one-third were left with a moderate degree of permanent disability, and one-third had severe disabilities. Rapid progression of symptoms, back pain, and spinal shock predict poor recovery. Paraclinical findings such as absent central conduction on evoked potential testing and the presence of 14-3-3 protein, a marker of neuronal injury, in the CSF during the acute phase predict a poor outcome. Some authors have reported that the recovery rate is generally complete. Long-term follow-up of urologic function in all patients with TM is recommended.

Tropical spastic paraparesis

HAM: human T-cell lymphotropic virus type 1-associated myelopathy.

Etiopathogenesis and epidemiology

Tropical spastic paraparesis (TSP) is a condition associated with and probably caused by the retrovirus human T-cell lymphotropic virus type 1 (HTLV-1).[14,15] HTLV-1 is a retrovirus with affinity for CD-4 cells.

It is a common cause of paraparesis in the West Indies,[16] where it was formerly known as Jamaican neuropathy or myelopathy, and in the southern islands of Japan, where it is called HTLV-1-associated myelopathy or HAM,[17] but it is also found widely in the tropics and subtropics and in immigrants to northern Europe from endemic areas.[15,18]

The first description of HTLV-1 was made in 1980, followed closely by the discovery of HTLV-2, in 1982. Since then, the main characteristics of these viruses, commonly referred to as HTLV-1/2, have been thoroughly studied. Central and South America and the Caribbean are areas of high prevalence of HTLV-1 and HTVL-2 and have clusters of infected people. The major modes of transmission have been through sexual contact, blood, and mother to child via breast-feeding. HTLV-1 is associated with adult T-cell leukemia/lymphoma (ATL), HTLV-associated myelopathy/tropical spastic paraparesis (HAM/TSP), and HTLV-associated uveitis, as well as infectious dermatitis of children. More clarification is needed in the possible role of HTLV in rheumatologic, psychiatric, and infectious diseases. Since cures for ATL and HAM/TSP are lacking and no vaccine is available to prevent HTLV-1 and HTLV-2 transmission, these illnesses impose enormous social and financial costs on infected individuals, their families, and health-care systems. For this reason, public health interventions aimed at counseling and educating high-risk individuals and populations are of vital importance. In the Americas this is especially important in the areas of high prevalence.[19]

Pathology

Meningomyelitis with demyelination and axonal loss, particularly affecting the corticospinal tracts, is usually present. These findings are most prominent in the lower thoracic and upper lumbar regions.[15,16,20]

Symptoms

This infection may give rise to a broad spectrum of disorders including T-cell leukemia/lymphoma, the myelopathy/tropical spastic paraparesis complex (M/TSP), and, to a lesser extent, uveitis, arthritis, polymyositis, and peripheral neuropathy. M/TSP is a progressive, chronic myelopathy characterized by spasticity, hyperreflexia, muscle weakness, and sphincter disorders. Much less frequently it may precede, or give rise to, a cerebellar syndrome with ataxia and intention tremor. The widespread nature of the pathologic changes within the nervous system results in a complex variety of urodynamic and neurophysiologic features. Gait disturbance is a main symptom of HAM, however bladder dysfunction is one of the major symptoms characteristic to HAM and these patients frequently complain of voiding disturbances.

Fujiki et al 1999 reported the case of a 75-year-old woman with HAM presenting with cerebellar signs.[21] She was admitted because of walking unsteadiness, which initially appeared 3 years previously with gradual worsening. Neurologic examination revealed limb and truncal ataxia, cerebellar type dysfunction of eye movements, pyramidal signs, diminished vibration sense, and neurogenic bladder. Serum and CSF titers of anti-HTLV-1 antibody were markedly elevated. MRI revealed abnormal signals in cerebral white matter, mild cerebellar atrophy, and thoracic cord atrophy. Cerebellar signs and symptoms were initial and main neurologic manifestations in this patient, which were improved by steroid therapy. They considered this case was unique among HAM, because the cerebellum was considered to be the main site of her lesions.

The presence of a cerebellar syndrome or neuropathy of uncertain origin, in endemic areas, should lead to the inclusion of HTLV-1 infection in the differential diagnosis, even in the absence of pyramidal symptoms or defined M/TSP. Maternal seropositivity supports the hypothesis of mother–daughter transmission during breast-feeding. Anti-HTLV-1 antibodies and ATL-like cells can be present in the peripheral blood of patients with HAM.

A clinical case with a cerebellar syndrome and peripheral neuropathy as manifestations of infection by HTLV-1 was described by Carod-Artal et al.[22] This was the case of a 13-year-old adolescent girl who presented with a neurologic syndrome which had started with head and limb tremor, ataxia, dysmetria, frequent falls, and sphincter disorders. During the two and a half years that she had had this illness she developed spastic paraparesis of the legs and had repeated urinary infections. Blood and CSF serology was positive for HTLV-1 using the ELISA technique and confirmed by Western blot. Electromyography (EMG) showed predominantly axonal sensomotor neuropathy. Neurogenic bladder was detected on urodynamic studies. MRI revealed moderate atrophy of the thoracic spinal cord and slight alterations of the subcortical white matter.

Urodynamic findings

The condition is characterized by a progressive paraparesis associated with back pain and voiding disturbances. While there have been many reports concerning the clinical and immunologic features of this condition, little attention has been paid to the bladder dysfunction which commonly accompanies it. Most patients had urodynamic evidence of overactivity and DSD. The supranuclear type of voiding dysfunction seems to be in accordance with the known pathologic lesions of this disease.

Sakiyama et al evaluated symptoms and urodynamic examinations in 21 untreated patients with HAM.[23] Although 2 cases (11%) had no urinary symptoms, 19 cases (89%) suffered from dysuria, frequency, incontinence, or urgency. The combination of irritative and obstructive urinary disturbance was a characteristic symptom in the HAM patients. In 3 cases the urinary symptoms preceded the gait disturbance which is the main symptom of HAM. Urodynamics revealed bladder overactivity in 14 cases (66%), although 3 cases (15%) showed underactive or acontractile bladder with a decrease in urinary sensation. The urethral pressure profile (UPP) was normal, but DSD was found frequently at EMG. This typical dysfunction of the HAM patients was thought to be caused by destruction of the lateral column of the spinal cord.

Eardley et al reported the clinical features, urodynamic results and neurophysiologic findings in 6 patients with urinary symptoms related to TSP.[24] Voiding dysfunction was also evaluated in 26 patients (9 males and 17 females) with HAM by Yamashita and Kumazawa.[25] Of 26 patients, 22 (85%) had voiding difficulties, 15 (58%) had urinary frequency, and 9 (35%) had urge incontinence. Cystograms showed trabeculated bladder in 5 patients, vesicoureteral reflux in 3, and bladder neck obstruction in 5. In 25 patients (96%), urodynamic studies showed detrusor overactivity with normal urethral function during storage. Of these patients, 17 had detrusor underactivity with DSD during micturition. One patient had normal detrusor function during storage and detrusor acontractility during voiding. In 1991, Imamura et al performed clinical surveys and urodynamic examinations in 25 untreated patients with HAM.[26] Although 4 cases (16%) were entirely aware of urinary symptoms, the onset of urinary symptoms preceded other pyramidal symptoms in 6 cases (24%). All cases suffered from dysuria. The cause of dysuria was thought mainly to be detrusor-external sphincter dyssynergia, but in some cases underactive detrusor and poor opening of the bladder neck at voiding were also the causes.

Again, in 1994, Imamura (1994) evaluated 50 patients with untreated HAM by urodynamic studies to clarify the nature of the urinary disturbance and to determine suitable urologic treatment.[27] Both irritative and obstructive symptoms coexisted in the HAM patients. Thirty-eight percent of patients experienced urinary symptoms only throughout the affected period. The main cause of frequency was neurogenic detrusor overactivity during the filling phase, which was found in 58% of patients. However, decreased effective bladder capacity due to a large amount of residual urine was possibly another cause of frequency. DSD was the main cause of voiding symptoms, but in some cases underactive detrusor at voiding phase was also present. Hydronephrosis was observed in only 5 kidneys, although as many as 30 out of 46 cases (65.2%) showed bladder deformities. Seventeen patients (34%) had urinary tract infection at the first visit. As the activities of daily living deteriorated, the mean postvoid residual volume, incidence of detrusor hyperreflexia, and DSD were all increased. Medical treatment was effective to relieve subjective symptoms, but urodynamic examination did not necessarily confirm improvement. Intermittent catheterization was needed, and was successful in 64% of all cases.

Walton and Kaplan presented urodynamic findings in 4 females and 1 male with TSP.[28] Of the 5 patients, 4 presented with detrusor-external sphincter dyssynergia and 1 had detrusor overactivity with coordinated sphincter contraction.

Hattori et al reported the findings of voiding histories and urodynamic studies in 5 patients with HAM.[29] Histories showed that all patients had obstructive as well as irritative voiding symptoms, and symptoms were present from the onset of the disease in 4 patients. Urodynamic studies showed that 4 patients had residual urine (average 170 ml), all had detrusor overactivity, and two had DSD. No patient had neurogenic changes in external urethral sphincter electromyography. The findings of supranuclear type of voiding dysfunction seemed to be in accordance with the known pathologic lesions of this disease.

Matsumoto et al performed clinical and electrophysiologic studies in 9 cases of HAM (7 females and 2 males).[30] Spastic paraparesis and neurogenic bladder were present in 8 patients and sensory disturbances were detected in only 4. The conduction velocities of the posterior tibial and sural nerves were reduced in 2 cases. Median nerve somatosensory nerve potentials (SSEP) revealed a delay of N11, N13, N14, and N20 peak latencies, and an increase of N9–N20, N13–N14, and N13–N20 interpeak latencies. The electrophysiologic studies are the most accurate indicators of the diffuse involvement not only of central motor and sensory pathways but also of the peripheral nervous system.

Complications

Lower urinary symptoms associated with HAM/TSP are common, but have been regarded as 'neurogenic' due to spinal involvements. However, in some cases, these symptoms are persistent, progressive, and do not correlate directly with the severity of other neurologic symptoms of the lower spinal cord. These findings prompted Nomata et al to locate organic lesions in the lower urinary tract and to correlate them with HTLV-1 infection.[31] Among 35 HAM patients with lower urinary symptoms, they found 4 cases with persistent and progressive symptoms, 3 with contracted bladder, and another with persistent prostatitis. Histologic or cytologic investigations indicated local lymphocyte infiltrations in the lower urinary tract in all cases, with bladder infiltration in 3 cases and high lymphocyte concentration in expressed prostatic secretions in others. Of 3 cases whose urine samples were available, urinary concentration of anti-HTLV-1 IgA antibodies were significantly increased in 2 cases. The urinary IgA antibodies were not elevated in the third case, but the sample had been obtained after resection of the affected bladder. None of the control cases showed significant levels of anti-HTLV-1 IgA antibodies in urine except for a case of gross hematuria due to chemotherapy for adult T-cell leukemia. The authors suggested inclusion of these processes into the spectrum of complications for HAM/TSP. The elevated level of anti-HTLV-1 IgA antibodies in the urine may be an indicator of these complications. There is a tendency for urinary dysfunction to become worse as the primary disease progresses.

Treatment

Idiopathic or HTLV-1 associated progressive spastic paraparesis does not have a clear treatment. Cartier et al assessed the effects of a medication containing cytidine monophosphate, uridine triphosphate, and vitamin B12 in the treatment of progressive spasticity.[32] Patients with the disease were randomly assigned to receive Nucleus CMP forte (containing dysodium cytidine monophosphate 5 mg, trisodium uridine triphosphate 3 mg, and hydroxycobalamin 2 mg) three times a day or placebo for 6 months. Gait, spasticity, degree of neurogenic bladder, and somatosensitive evoked potentials were assessed during treatment. Forty-six patients aged 25 to 79 years old were studied: 24 were female and 29 were HTLV-1 positive. Twenty-two patients were treated with the drug and in the rest with placebo. Gait and spasticity improved in 7 of 22 patients receiving the drug and in 1 of 24 receiving placebo (p <0. 05). Neurogenic bladder improved in 10 of 22 receiving the drug and in 4 of 24 receiving placebo (NS). Somatosensitive evoked potentials improved in 4 of 7 patients treated with the drug and in 2 of 7 treated with placebo. The medication resulted in a modest improvement in patients with progressive spastic paraparesis and was free of side-effects.

Harrington et al used danazol for the treatment of urinary incontinence in tropical spastic paraparesis.[33]

Saito et al reported 4 patients (3 females and 1 male) diagnosed by neurologists to have HAM with spastic gait disturbance and increased titer of anti-HTLV-1 antibodies.[34] They complained of urge incontinence, bed wetting, voiding difficulties, and/or frequency. Urodynamically, severe uninhibited detrusor contractions were observed in 3 of them. On the other hand, in one case detrusor contractility during voiding was completely lost. Bladder sensation was well preserved in all patients. Corticosteroids and interferon could not improve their urologic symptoms. CIC in 3 patients with a significant amount of postvoid residual urine volume relieved their urinary incontinence. The authors believed that HAM in patients suffering from severe voiding disturbances is a good indication for CIC.

Namima et al presented 2 case reports with HAM. Patient 1 (a 24-year-old female) had complained of slowly progressive urinary incontinence (since age 14) and gait disturbance (since age 18).[35] Marked pyramidal disorder was observed, and anti-HTLV-1 antibodies (1:640) were present in her peripheral blood. She was diagnosed as having HAM. Repeated urodynamic studies revealed exacerbation of overactive bladder and DSD with progression of the disease. Patient 2 (a 48-year-old male) had complained of gait disturbance (since age 32) and progressive urinary hesitancy (since age 46). Physical examination revealed a significant pyramidal disorder. Anti-HTLV-1 antibodies (1:200) and ATL-like cells were present in his peripheral blood. He was diagnosed as having HAM. Voiding cystourethrography demonstrated an abnormal change of the bladder wall. Urodynamic studies revealed overactive bladder and marked DSD. Medications based on adrenocortical steroids and urologic care have improved urinary symptoms, in both cases.

Conclusions

In summary, TSP is a spinal cord disorder caused by the retrovirus HTLV-1. Patients commonly have urinary symptoms that usually begin simultaneously with complaints of limb weakness. This process must be distinguished from MS. Up to 80% of patients suffering from symptoms due to TSP are affected by detrusor-external sphincter dyssynergia (DESD). Thus, it seems justifiable that patients with TSP who have urinary symptoms are evaluated aggressively. These patients are at high risk for detrusor-external sphincter dyssynergia and they should undergo urodynamic evaluation before appropriate therapy is instituted. This is particularly true in men with TSP to prevent the potentially deleterious effects of untreated and unrecognized detrusor-external sphincter dyssynergia on the upper tract. Patients with HAM must be carefully followed by urologists in order to prevent deterioration of the urinary tract.

Progressive multifocal leukoencephalopathy

PML is an infectious demyelinating brain disease, caused by the JCV which is associated with significant morbidity and mortality in the immunocompromised host.

The polyomaviruses BK virus (BKV), JC virus (JCV), and simian virus 40 (SV40) have been known to be associated with diseases in humans for over 30 years. BKV-associated nephropathy and JCV-induced progressive multifocal leukoencephalopathy (PML) were rare diseases for many years, occurring only in patients with underlying severe impaired immunity. Over the past decade, the use of more potent immunosuppression in transplantations and acquired immune deficiency syndrome (AIDS) have coincided with a significant increase in the prevalence of these viral complications.

PML is an infectious demyelinating brain disease caused by JCV that is associated with significant morbidity and mortality in the immunocompromised host. It is a destructive demyelinating infection which vitiates oligodendrocytes. The dramatic increase in the incidence of PML that occurred as a consequence of the AIDS pandemic and the recent association of PML with the administration of natalizumab, a monoclonal antibody against α4 integrin that blocks entry of inflammatory cells into the brain, has stimulated a great deal of interest in this previously obscure viral demyelinating disease. The etiology of this disorder is JCV observed in 80% of the population world-wide. Seroepidemiologic studies indicate that infection with this virus typically occurs before the age of 20 years. No primary illness owing to JCV infection has been recognized and the means of spread from person to person remains obscure. Following infection, the virus becomes latent in bone marrow, spleen, tonsils, and other tissues. Periodically the virus reactivates, during which time it can be demonstrated in circulating peripheral lymphocytes. The latter is significantly more commonly observed in immunosuppressed populations compared to normal subjects. Despite the large pool of people infected with JCV, PML remains a relatively rare disease. It is seldom observed in the absence of an underlying predisposing illness, typically one that results in impaired cellular immunity. A variety of factors are likely responsible for the unique increase in the frequency of PML in HIV infection relative to other underlying immunosuppressive disorders. Preliminary data suggest that natalizumab appears to distinctively predispose recipients to PML relative to other infectious complications. Studies in these populations will be invaluable in understanding the mechanisms of disease pathogenesis.[36]

Bartt et al, over a period of 6 years at the Gay Men's Health Clinic in Sweden, used the polymerase chain reaction (PCR) to investigate approximately 400 cerebrospinal fluid samples from immunosuppressed individuals with neurologic symptoms for the presence of polyomaviruses.[37] BKV and JCV establish latency in the urinary tract and can be reactivated in AIDS. JCV might cause PML, but although up to 60% of AIDS patients excrete BKV in the urine, there have been few reports of BKV-related renal and/or neurologic diseases. BKV could be demonstrated in the brain, cerebrospinal fluid, eye tissue, kidneys, and peripheral blood mononuclear cells. BKV DNA has, so far, only been found in one case. They also analyzed brain, eye tissue, cerebrospinal fluid, urine, and peripheral blood mononuclear cells by nested PCR for polyomavirus DNA. Macroscopic and microscopic examinations were performed on renal and brain tissue obtained postmortem. Immunohistochemical staining for the two BKV proteins, the VP1 and the agnoprotein, was performed on autopsy material and virus-infected tissue culture cells. Although reports of BKV infections in the nervous system are rare, there is now evidence for its occurrence in immunocompromised patients and the diagnosis should be considered in such patients with neurologic symptoms and signs of renal disease. It is easy to verify and also important to establish this diagnosis

Robinson et al reported a case of successful treatment with highly active antiretroviral therapy and cidofovir in an adolescent patient perinatally infected with HIV that caused PML.[38] Aksamit described PML in patients treated with natalizumab.[39] MRI imaging of the brain gives clues to the diagnosis, but is nonspecific in distinguishing MS from PML. Spinal fluid detection of JCV is specific, but has insufficient sensitivity. Associated immunosuppression is typically of the cell-mediated type but can be poorly defined on clinical grounds. It is apparent that natalizumab is a predisposing factor for the development of PML from the 3 cases of natalizumab-treated patients. There is no reliable presymptomatic way to detect PML or JCV infection of the brain by virologic or imaging surveillance techniques. One patient with MS and natalizumab treatment has survived, indicating that withdrawal of antibody, possibly in combination with antiviral therapy, may permit survival. However, immune reconstitution disease is a risk after immune restoration and withdrawal of natalizumab. PML deficits would be expected to be permanent. The estimated incidence of PML in natalizumab-treated patients is 1 per 1000. The duration of natalizumab treatment may be an independent risk factor for the development of PML. PML, a usually fatal neurologic infection, should be considered as a risk factor when using natalizumab. The treatment of MS patients with natalizumab is a matter of informed risk, individualized for each patient. Prophylactic and therapeutic interventions for human polyomavirus diseases are limited by our current understanding of polyomaviral pathogenesis. Clinical trials are limited by the small numbers of patients affected with clinically significant diseases, the lack of defined risk factors and disease definitions, the lack of proven effective treatment, and the overall significant morbidity and mortality associated with these diseases.[40]

Lyme disease

Etiology and epidemiology

Lyme disease (LD) is an infection caused by *Borrelia burgdorferi*, the type of bacterium called a spirochete that is carried by deer ticks. Infected ticks can transmit the spirochete to humans and animals by its bites. Untreated, the bacterium travels through the bloodstream, gets into various body tissues, and can cause a number of symptoms, some of which are severe. Lyme borreliosis is a multiorgan infection caused by spirochetes of the *Borrelia burgdorferi sensu lato* group with its species *B. burgdorferi sensu stricto*, *B. garinii*, and *B. afzelii*, which are transmitted by ticks of the species *Ixodes*. This multisystemic infection may cause skin, neurologic (including neurogenic bladder), cardiac, or rheumatologic disorders.

Manifestations of what we now call LD were first reported in the medical literature in Europe in 1883. Over the years, various clinical signs of this illness have been noted as separate medical conditions: acrodermatitis chronica atrophicans, lymphadenosis benigna cutis, erythema migrans, and lymphocytic meningoradiculitis (Bannwarth's syndrome). However, these diverse manifestations were not recognized as indicators of a single infectious illness until 1975, when LD was described following an outbreak of apparent juvenile arthritis, preceded by a rash, among residents of Lyme, Connecticut.

Lyme borreliosis caused by the spirochete *B. burgdorferi* is now the most common vector-borne disease in North America, Europe, and Asia. It is a potentially serious infection, common in many countries of the world, but few data about its incidence, distribution, and clinical manifestations are available. Since very little is known about the clinical expression of Lyme borrleiosis in Western Europe, a 3-year prospective study was conducted by Attali et al, who studied the expression of this disease in northeastern France.[41] This study included all patients seen for suspected Lyme borreliosis at the Strasbourg University Hospital in northeastern France. The diagnosis was made on the basis of the presence of erythema migrans (EM) or on the basis of another suggestive clinical manifestation and laboratory confirmation. A total of 132 patients, 70 women and 62 men, mean age 54 years, had Lyme borreliosis according to these criteria. Within this study group, 77% of the patients were regularly exposed to tick bites and 64% could remember one. EM, the most frequent clinical manifestation, occurred in 60% of the patients and was the only sign of Lyme borreliosis in 40%. Lymphocytoma and acrodermatitis chronica atrophicans were rare (1 and 3 patients, respectively). Nervous system involvement (mainly radiculoneuropathy), the second most common clinical manifestation, was found in 40% of the patients and was the only sign of Lyme borreliosis in 22%. Musculoskeletal involvement was present in 26% of the patients and was an isolated finding in 14%. During the study period, no patient was diagnosed with Lyme carditis. There was serologic evidence of Lyme borreliosis in 75% of the cases and direct evidence of borrelial infection in 10 patients (7.5%). The results show that the clinical expression of Lyme borreliosis in northeastern France is similar to that in other European countries, but different from that in North America.

Data on disease expression and epidemiologic characteristics of Lyme borreliosis in southeastern Europe are scarce. To reveal features of Lyme borreliosis in Bulgaria, clinical data and epidemiologic characteristics of 1257 patients reported between 1999 and 2002 were analyzed by Christova and Komitova.[42] The most affected age group was 5–9 years, followed by 45–49 years, 50–54 years, and 10–14 years. Most of the patients (68%) lived in a rural area or were attacked by ticks during activities in a rural area. Lyme borreliosis cases occurred throughout the year with two peaks – one in June and a second smaller one in September. The most common clinical manifestation was EM diagnosed in 868 (69.1%) of the patients. Rashes had a median diameter of 11 cm and were predominantly located on the lower extremities. Forty-four percent of the rashes consisted of homogenous erythema and 56% had central clearing. Multiple EM was detected in 4.3% of the EM cases. Neuroborreliosis including voiding disorders was the second most common presentation of Lyme borreliosis, and was diagnosed in 19% of the patients. Lyme arthritis was found in 8% of the patients. Cardiac and ocular manifestations were recorded in 1.1% and 0.9% of the patients, respectively. Borrelial lymphocytoma and acrodermatitis chronica atrophicans were very rare (0.3%). Twenty-seven patients (2.1%) had multiple organ involvement. The results of the study show that epidemiology and clinical manifestations of Lyme borreliosis in Bulgaria are similar to those in the majority of European countries, but possess some distinguishing characteristics.

In order to improve the notification in Germany, 6 of Germany's 16 states – Berlin, Brandenburg, Mecklenburg-Vorpommern, Sachsen, Sachsen-Anhalt, and Thuringen – have enhanced notification systems, which include Lyme borreliosis. The efforts made in these states to monitor confirmed cases through notification are therefore an important contribution to the understanding of the epidemiology of Lyme borreliosis in Germany. The report of Mehnert and Krause summarizes the analysis of Lyme borreliosis cases sent to the Robert Koch Institute during 2002–03.[43] The average incidence of Lyme borreliosis in the six East German states was 17.8 cases per 100 000 people in 2002, which increased by 31% to 23.3 cases in 2003. Patient ages were bimodally distributed, with a peak incidence among children aged 5 to 9 years and elderly patients, aged 60 to 64, in 2002, and 65 to 69 in 2003. For both years, 55% of the patients were female. Around 86% of notified cases occurred from May to October. EM affected 2697 patients (89.3%) in 2002 and 3442 (86.7%) in 2003. For a vector-borne disease such as Lyme borreliosis, the risk of infection depends on the degree and duration of contact between humans and ticks harboring *B. burgdorferi.* As infected ticks probably occur throughout Germany, it is likely that the situation in the remaining 10 German states is similar to that of the states in this study.

Nygarg et al confirmed in their study that Lyme borreliosis is also the most common tick-borne infection in Norway.[44] All clinical manifestations of Lyme borreliosis other than EM are notifiable to Folkehelseinstituttet, the Norwegian Institute of Public Health. During the period 1995–2004 a total of 1506 cases of disseminated and chronic Lyme borreliosis were reported. Serologic tests were the basis for laboratory diagnosis in almost all cases. Annual statistics showed no clear trend over the period, but varied each year between 120 and 253 cases, with the highest number of cases reported in 2004. Seventy-five percent of cases with information on time of onset were in patients who fell ill during the months of June to October. There was marked geographic variation in reported incidence rates, with the highest rates reported from coastal counties in southern and central Norway. Fifty-six percent of the cases were in males and 44% in females. The highest incidence rate was found in children aged between 5 and 9 years. Neuroborreliosis was the most common clinical manifestation (71%), followed by arthritis/arthralgia (22%) and acrodermatitis chronica atrophicans (5%). Forty-six percent of patients were admitted to hospital. Prevention of borreliosis in Norway relies on measures to prevent tick bites, such as the use of protective clothing and insect repellents, and the early detection and removal of ticks. Antibiotics are generally not recommended for prophylaxis after tick bites in Norway.

Symptoms

LD presents as a multisystemic inflammatory disease that affects skin in its early, localized stage, and spreads to the joints, nervous system, and, to a lesser extent, other organ systems in its later, disseminated stages. Early symptoms of LD can be mild and easily overlooked. People who are aware of the risk of LD in their communities and who do not ignore the sometimes subtle early symptoms are most likely to seek medical attention and treatment early enough to be assured of a full recovery. The first symptom is usually an expanding rash (EM) which is thought to occur in 80 to 90% of all LD cases.

As the LD spirochete continues disseminating through the body, a number of other symptoms including severe fatigue, a stiff aching neck, and peripheral nervous system involvement such as tingling or numbness in the extremities or facial palsy (paralysis) can occur.

The more severe, potentially debilitating symptoms of later stage LD may occur weeks, months, or in a few cases years after a tick bite. These can include severe headaches, painful arthritis and swelling of joints, cardiac abnormalities, and central nervous system involvement leading to cognitive (mental) disorders.

The following is a checklist of common symptoms seen in various stages of LD:

- *Localized early (acute) stage:* solid red or bull's-eye rash, usually at the site of the bite, swelling of lymph glands near the tick bite, generalized aches, and headache.
- *Early disseminated stage:* two or more rashes not at the site of the bite, migrating pains in joints/tendons, headache, stiff aching neck, facial palsy (facial paralysis similar to Bell's palsy), tingling or numbness in extremities, multiple enlarged lymph glands, abnormal pulse, sore throat, changes in vision, fever of 100–102°F, severe fatigue.
- *Late stage*: arthritis (pain/swelling) of one or two large joints, disabling neurologic disorders (disorientation, confusion, dizziness, short-term memory loss, inability to concentrate, finish sentences, or follow conversations; mental 'fog'), numbness in arms/hands or legs/feet.

It was observed that the urinary tract may be involved in two respects in the course of LD: (1) voiding dysfunction may be part of neuroborreliosis and (2) the spirochete may directly invade the urinary tract. Several neurologic manifestations of LD, both central and peripheral, have been described. Associated neurologic symptoms fall broadly into three syndromes: (1) encephalopathy, (2) polyneuropathy, and (3) leukoencephalitis.

Common skin manifestations of Lyme borreliosis include EM, lymphocytoma, and acrodermatitis chronica atrophicans. The last two conditions are usually caused by *B. garinii* and *B. afzelii*, respectively, which are seen more frequently in Europe than in America. Late extracutaneous manifestations of Lyme borreliosis are characterized by carditis, neuroborreliosis, and arthritis.[45]

Diagnostic methods

Laboratory testing of Lyme borreliosis includes culture, antibody detection using ELISA with whole extracts or recombinant chimeric borrelia proteins, immunoblot, and PCR with different levels of sensitivity and specificity for each test.

The EM rash, which may occur in up to 90% of reported cases, is a specific feature of LD, and treatment should begin immediately. Even in the absence of an EM rash, diagnosis of early LD should be made solely on the basis of symptoms and evidence of a tick bite, not blood tests, which can often give false results if performed in the first month after initial infection (later on, the tests are considered more reliable). If early symptoms are undetected or ignored it is recommended to use the ELISA and Western blot blood tests. These tests are considered more reliable and accurate when performed at least a month after initial infection, although no test is 100% accurate.

If neurologic symptoms or swollen joints are present, in addition a PCR test via a spinal tap or withdrawal of synovial fluid from an affected joint can be performed. This test amplifies the DNA of the spirochete and will usually indicate its presence.

The aims of the thesis presented by Lebech[46] were: (1) to develop a PCR assay for direct detection of *B. burgdorferi* DNA and to evaluate the diagnostic utility of PCR in clinical specimens from patients with Lyme borreliosis, and (2) to study the taxonomic classification of *B. burgdorferi* isolates and its implications for epidemiology and clinical presentation. Laboratory diagnosis of Lyme borreliosis by direct demonstration of *B. burgdorferi* in clinical specimens compared to current serology would allow (1) optimal specificity, (2) increased sensitivity during the first weeks of infection, when the antibody response is not yet detectable, and (3) discrimination between ongoing and past infection.[46] Due to the extreme paucity of spirochetes in clinical specimens, neither *in-vitro* culture nor antigen detection had yielded a sufficient diagnostic sensitivity. The recently introduced highly sensitive PCR methodology was thus employed. Assays for PCR amplification and subsequent identification of *B. burgdorferi*-specific sequences were established and used. For all assays the analytic sensitivity was a few genome copies using purified DNA as template.

The efficacy of PCR was initially evaluated using tissue samples from experimentally infected gerbils in order to start with biological samples *a priori* known to contain *B. burgdorferi. B. burgdorferi* DNA was detectable in 88% of the specimens. Thus the diagnostic sensitivity of PCR was comparable to and even higher than *in-vitro* culture. PCR was significantly more sensitive than in the histologic *B. burgdorferi*-specific immunophosphatase staining method. PCR was then used to identify *B. burgdorferi* DNA in skin biopsies from 31 patients with EM. The sensitivity of PCR was 71%, which was superior to culture and serology. Based on our own and other published results there is clear evidence for PCR being the most sensitive and specific test for detection of *B. burgdorferi* in skin biopsies from patients with both early and late dermatoborreliosis. However, since the clinical diagnosis of dermatoborreliosis is, in most instances, straightforward, an invasive procedure such as skin biopsy will only be justified in patients with an atypical clinical presentation.

The most frequent and serious manifestation of disseminated Lyme borreliosis is neuroborreliosis. PCR was used in 190 patients with untreated and confirmed neuroborreliosis and *B. burgdorferi* DNA was detectable in 17–21% of CSF samples. In patients with very early neuroborreliosis (<2 weeks), still negative for specific intrathecal antibody synthesis, a positive PCR was more frequent than in patients with a longer disease duration. PCR can be used as a diagnostic aid in these patients. However, in general the measurement of specific intrathecal antibody production in patients with neuroborreliosis was superior to PCR.

In urine samples from patients with Lyme borreliosis the diagnostic sensitivity varied, generally showing a low reproducibility. Urine is thus not regarded as a suitable sample source for *B. burgdorferi* PCR. The reason may be the variable presence of Taq polymerase inhibitors. Based on a semiquantitative detection system for amplicons, reflecting the input amount of specific DNA and thus the density of spirochetes in the clinical samples, high levels of DNA were found in skin biopsies, whereas in urine the DNA levels were low.

When Lebech's present study[46] was initiated there was no accepted classification of *B. burgdorferi*. Heterogeneity among *B. burgdorferi* strains might have important implications for understanding the epidemiology and different clinical presentations (dermatoborreliosis versus neuroborreliosis) and courses (self-limiting versus chronic disease). Furthermore, strain differences are of importance in the selection of suitable antigens for diagnostic assays and for vaccine development. Since then, *B. burgdorferi* isolates have been studied by phenotypic and genotypic traits and have been shown to be highly heterogeneous. The first approach of Lebech[46] was to genotype a panel of human *B. burgdorferi* isolates by restriction fragment length polymorphism (RFLP) of three genes. Thereafter, sequencing and dideoxy fingerprinting of ospA was applied. By RFLP the strains could be differentiated into two to five groups. The RFLP classification was compared with four different phenotypic and genotypic methods, including the rRNA typing. Results obtained with the different methods correlated highly and confirmed the taxonomic classification by Baranton et al.[47] According to this, the term *B. burgdorferi sensu lato* comprises three different human pathogenic genospecies – *B. burgdorferi sensu stricto*, *B. garinii*, and *B. afzelii*. All three genospecies have been isolated among Danish patients with Lyme borreliosis and are thus prevalent in Denmark. Since the isolation of *B. burgdorferi* from patients with Lyme borreliosis is laborious and often unsuccessful, molecular typing methods based on PCR are recommended to obviate the need for isolation by prior culture. It was of particular interest to study the possible association of neuroborreliosis with certain *B. burgdorferi* genospecies, indicating species-dependent organotropism. By RFLP all six CSF isolates tested belonged to *B. garinii*, and 6 out of 7 isolates from patients with acrodermatitis chronica atrophicans belonged to *B. afzelii*. Due to the low culture yield of *B. burgdorferi* from CSF, the association of *B. garinii* and neuroborreliosis was further studied by sequence analysis and dideoxy fingerprinting analysis of ospA PCR amplicons obtained from CSF samples from patients with neuroborreliosis. Phylogenetic analysis showed that, in 11 out of 13 patients *B. garinii* DNA was found in CSF. These data strongly support the hypothesis that *B. garinii* is the principal agent of Lyme neuroborreliosis in Europe. Similarly it was shown that *B. afzelii* is associated with acrodermatitis chronica atrophicans and thus dermatoborreliosis. Due to a strain dependent selection pressure in culture, only PCR-based methods can be used to determine whether mixed infections occur in patients. Our data indicate that mixed infections in humans are likely to be rare.

Schwan et al experimentally infected white-footed mice, *Peromyscus leucopus*, in the laboratory with *B. burgdorferi*.[48] The mice were infected by intraperitoneal or subcutaneous inoculation, or by tick bite, attempts were then made to culture spirochetes from the urinary bladder, spleen, kidney, blood, and urine. Spirochetes were most frequently isolated from the bladder (94%), followed by the kidney (75%), spleen (61%), and blood (13%). No spirochetes were isolated from the urine. Tissue sectioning and immunofluorescence staining of the urinary bladder demonstrated spirochetes within the bladder wall. The results demonstrate that cultivation of the urinary bladder is a very effective means to isolate *B. burgdorferi* from experimentally infected white-footed mice and that culture of this organ may be productive when surveying wild rodents for infection with this spirochete.

Druschky et al reported the case of a 57-year-old patient suffering from the typical symptoms of normal pressure hydrocephalus (NPH), including gait disturbance, urinary incontinence, and mental deterioration.[49] CSF analysis established the diagnosis of chronic active Lyme neuroborreliosis with lymphocytic pleocytosis and intrathecal *B. burgdorferi* antibody production. After several weeks of iv antibiotic treatment the CSF parameters normalized and there was a clear improvement in clinical symptoms so that surgical shunting was no longer indicated. Interference with the subarachnoid CSF flow may be a possible cause of the observed symptomatic NPH in a patient with chronic Lyme neuroborreliosis.

Pavia et al showed the efficacy of an evernimicin (SCH27899) *in vitro* and in an animal model of Lyme disease.[50] The minimal inhibition concentrations (MICs) of evernimicin at which 90% of *B. burgdorferi* patient isolates were inhibited ranged from 0.1 to 0.5 μg/ml. Evernimicin was as effective as ceftriaxone against *B. burgdorferi* in a murine model of experimental Lyme disease. As assessed by culturing the urinary bladders of infected C3H mice, no live *Borrelia* isolates were recoverable following antibiotic treatment. These authors also collected 34 small mammals in the vicinity of Ljubljana and tested them for the presence of *B. burgdorferi sensu lato* by PCR of urinary bladder tissues, using universal flagellin primers and species-specific rRNA primers. Seventeen small mammals (50%) were found to be positive and 7 small mammals were infected with two species of *B. burgdorferi sensu lato* simultaneously. The most commonly found species was *B. afzelii* ($n = 14$), followed by *B. burgdorferi sensu stricto* ($n = 7$) and *B. garinii* ($n = 3$), as determined by species-specific primers. They concluded that PCR is a rapid and reliable method to detect infection with *B. burgdorferi sensu lato* in small mammals.[49]

Since the possibility of asymptomatic infection with *B. burgdorferi* has been suggested by positive serology found in healthy subjects, others have hypothesized that these subjects might excrete borrelial DNA sequences in urine, as happens in patients with Lyme borreliosis. Borrelial sequences have been found by nested PCR in the urine samples from 3 of 13 healthy *B. burgdorferi* antibody positive adults, but not in urine samples from 79 antibody-negative healthy controls. Following doxycycline therapy, urine samples were repeatedly negative for *B. burgdorferi* DNA. It seems that urinary excretion of borrelial DNA sequences may occur in seropositive healthy subjects during asymptomatic infection. Demonstration of such sequences in urine must be interpreted cautiously and may not necessarily prove a borrelial cause of disease.

The studies of Czub et al have demonstrated that the urinary bladder is a consistent source for isolates of *B. burgdorferi*, from both experimentally infected and naturally exposed rodents.[51] They examined histopathologic changes in the urinary bladder of different types of rodents experimentally infected with Lyme spirochetes, including BALB/c mice (*Mus musculus*), nude mice (*M. musculus*), white-footed mice (*Peromyscus leucopus*), and grasshopper mice (*Onychomys leucogaster*). Animals were inoculated intraperitoneally, subcutaneously, or intranasally with low-passaged spirochetes, high-passaged spirochetes, or phosphate-buffered saline. At various times after inoculation, animals were killed and approximately one-half of each urinary bladder and kidney were cultured separately in BSK-II medium, while the other half of each organ was prepared for histologic examination. Spirochetes were cultured from the urinary bladder of all 35 mice inoculated with low-passaged spirochetes while we were unable to isolate spirochetes from any kidneys of the same mice. The pathologic changes observed most frequently in the urinary bladder of the infected mice were the presence of lymphoid aggregates, vascular changes, including an increase in the number of vessels and thickening of the vessel walls, and perivascular infiltrates. Our results demonstrate that nearly all individuals (93%) of the four types of mice examined had a cystitis associated with spirochetal infection. The heart can also be severely affected in humans with Lyme disease, causing conduction defects and, rarely, heart failure. Although immunodeficient and young mice may develop cardiac lesions, cultivation of *B. burgdorferi* from cardiac tissues of experimentally infected animals has not been previously reported.

Goodman et al infected Syrian hamsters with *B. burgdorferi* 297 and found marked tropism of the spirochete for myocardial and urinary tract tissues.[52,53] Fifty-six of 57 hearts (98%) and 52 of 58 bladders (90%) were culture positive. The cardiac infection was persistent and could be documented in 21 of 22 hearts (96%) cultured from days 28 to 84 postinfection. The urinary tract was also a site of persistent infection in most animals, with 18 of 23 bladders (78%) being culture positive from days 28 to 84. The persistence of spirochetes was specific for the heart and bladder, as indicated by negative cultures of specimens from the liver and spleen, in which only 1 of 23 cultures was positive from days 28 to 84. Because of the high isolation rates, tropism, and persistence that we found for *B. burgdorferi* in the hamster heart and bladder, these sites will be useful and important for the cultivation of spirochetes in experimental studies that evaluate the efficacies of both candidate vaccines in preventing infection and of antibiotics in eradicating organisms from privileged sites. In addition, the clear demonstration of persistent cardiac infection with *B. burgdorferi* may provide a useful model for studying the pathogenesis of cardiac Lyme disease.

Chancellor et al described patients with neuroborreliosis who also had lower urinary tract dysfunction.[54,55] Urodynamic evaluation revealed neurogenic detrusor overactivity or detrusor acontractility. Neurologic and urologic symptoms in all patients were slow to resolve and convalescence was protracted.

Aberer et al reported the case of a 38-year-old male patient with coexisting acrodermatitis chronica atrophicans, lichen sclerosus et atrophicus, and recurrent diabetic metabolic disorders since 9 years of age.[56] Serologically, IgG antibodies against *B. burgdorferi* could be detected. Structures, morphologically resembling borreliae, could be demonstrated in the urine sediment by dark field microscopy. Additionally a tubulointerstitial nephritis was diagnosed by the presence of dysmorphic hematuria, pathologic polyacrylamide gel electrophoresis, and raised α_1- and β_2-microglobulin in the urine. The authors suggested that the excreted spirochete-like structures were borreliae, which may be the putative infectious agent for the development of lichen sclerosus et atrophicans in the genital area.

Treatment

Early treatment of LD (within the first few weeks after initial infection) is straightforward and almost always results in a full cure. Treatment begun after the first 3 weeks will also likely provide cure, but the cure rate decreases the longer treatment is delayed.

Doxycycline, amoxicillin, and ceftin are the three oral antibiotics most highly recommended for treatment of all but a few symptoms of LD. A 4-week course of oral doxycycline is just as effective in treating late LD, and much less expensive, than a similar course of intravenous ceftriaxone (Rocephin) unless neurologic or severe cardiac abnormalities are present. If these symptoms are present, the study recommends immediate intravenous treatment. Conservative bladder management including CIC guided by urodynamic evaluation is recommended. Chancellor et al published the first report of urinary retention as the initial clinical presentation of Lyme disease. Paralysis and urinary retention resolved with intravenous ceftriaxone treatment.[57]

Olivares et al reported a case of ATM related to Lyme neuroborreliosis that presented with isolated acute urinary retention and no lower extremity impairment.[58] This case, documented by urodynamic and electrophysiologic investigations, partially resolved after 6 weeks of intravenous ceftriaxone, affording removal of the indwelling catheter. Alpha-blocker therapy was needed for 3 months, until complete normalization of urodynamic and electrophysiologic findings. This case study indicates that whenever urinary retention is encountered, either associated with ATM or alone, the patient should be investigated for LD. Relapses of active LD and residual neurologic deficits are common. Urologists practicing in areas endemic for LD need to be aware of *B. burgdorferi* infection in the differential diagnosis of neurogenic bladder dysfunction.

Taylor et al emphasized that Lyme borreliosis is the most common tick-borne bacterial infection and that incidence is increasing in parts of Europe and the USA.[59] They suggested a prompt antimicrobial therapy using oral agents such as doxycycline or amoxicillin, which is successful in more than 90% of patients. Inadequate penetration of oral agents into the CNS may result in the development of overt neuroborreliosis. The parenteral agent ceftriaxone is the drug of choice for severe acute and chronic infections, due to its good penetration into the CSF, convenient single daily dosage regimen, and proven high efficacy in clinical trials involving a wide variety of disseminated infections. Regardless of the therapeutic agent, there appears to be a small minority of patients (<10%) who do not respond. Such cases may be due to long-term persistence of borrelial cysts and to misdiagnoses based solely on seropositivity. Several adjunct therapies are available, including hyperbaric oxygen therapy and immune system supplements, but clinical trials have yet to be conducted. If diagnosed and treated early with antibiotics, LD is almost always readily cured. Generally, LD in its later stages can also be treated effectively; however, because the rate of disease progression and individual response to treatment vary from one patient to another, some patients may have symptoms that linger for months or even years following treatment. In rare instances, LD causes permanent damage.

References

1. Transverse Myelitis Consortium Working Group. Proposed diagnostic criteria and nosology of acute transverse myelitis. Neurology 2002; 59: 499–505.
2. Ganesan V, Borzyskowski M. Characteristics and course of urinary tract dysfunction after acute transverse myelitis in childhood. Dev Med Child Neurol 2001; 43(7): 473–5.
3. Cheng W, Chiu R, Tam P. Residual bladder dysfunction 2 to 10 years after acute transverse myelitis. J Paediatr Child Health 1999; 35(5): 476–8.
4. Leroy-Malherbe V, Sebire G, Hollenberg H, Tardieu M, Landrieu P. Neurogenic bladder in children with acute transverse myelopathy. Arch Pediatr 1998; 5(5): 497–502.
5. Kalita J, Shah S, Kapoor R, Misra UK. Bladder dysfunction in acute transverse myelitis: magnetic resonance imaging and neurophysiological and urodynamic correlations. J Neurol Neurosurg Psychiatry 2002; 73(2): 154–9.
6. Sakakibara R, Hattori T, Yasuda K, Yamanishi T. Micturition disturbance in acute transverse myelitis. Spinal Cord 1996; 34(8): 481–5.
7. Chan KF, Kong KH, Boey ML. Great mimicry in a patient with tetraparesis: a case report Arch Phys Med Rehabil 1995; 76(4): 391–3.
8. Chan KF, Boey ML. Transverse myelopathy in SLE: clinical features and functional outcomes. Lupus. 1996; 5(4): 294–9.
9. Berger Y, Blaivas JG, Oliver L. Urinary dysfunction in transverse myelitis. J Urol 1990; 144(1): 103–5.
10. Chartier-Kastler EJ, Bosch JLHR, Perrigot M, Chancellor MB, Richard F, Denys P. Long-term results of sacral nerve stimulation (S3) for the treatment of neurogenic refractory urge incontinence related to detrusor hyperreflexia. J Urol 2000; 164(5): 1476–80.
11. Das RN, Jaykumar J. Acute transverse myelitis following typhoid vaccination. Ulster Med J 2007; 76(1): 39–40.
12. Tsiodras S, Kelesidis T, Kelesidis I,Voumbourakis K, Giamarellou H. *Mycoplasma pneumoniae*-associated myelitis: a comprehensive review. Eur J Neurol 2006; 13(2): 112 –24.
13. Krishnan C, Kaplin AI, Pardo CA, Kerr DA, Keswani SC. Demyelinating disorders: update on transverse myelitis. Curr Neurol Neurosci Rep 2006; 6(3): 236–43.
14. Gessaia A, Barin F, Vemant JC et al. Antibodies to human T-lymphotropic virus type-1 in patients with tropical spastic paraparesis. Lancet B, 1985; 5: 407–9.
15. Cruickshank JK, Rudge P, Dalgkish AG et al. Tropical spastic paraparesis and human T cell lymphotropic virus type 1 in the United Kingdom. Brain 1989; 112: 1057–90.
16. Montgomery RD, Cruickshank EK, Robertson WB et al. Clinical and pathological observations on Jamaican neuropathy. A report of 206 cases. Brain 1964; 87: 425–60.
17. Roman GC, Roman LN. Tropical spastic paraparesis. A clinical study of 50 patients from Tumaco (Columbia) and review of the worldwide literature features of the syndrome. J Neurol Sci 1988; 87: 121.
18. Gout O, Gessaia A, Bolgert F et al. Chronic myelopathies associated with human T-cell lymphotropic virus type-1. A clinical serological and immunovirological study of ten patients in France. Arch Neur 1989; 46: 255–60.
19. Carneiro-Proietti AB, Catalan-Soares BC, Castro-Costa CM et al. HTLV in the Americas: challenges and perspectives. Rev Panam Salud Pub 2006; 19(1): 44–53.
20. Iwasaki Y. Pathology of chronic myelopathy associated with HTLV1 infection (HAM/TSP). Neurol Sci 1990; 6: 103–23.
21. Fujiki N, Oikawa O, Matsumoto A, Tashiro KA case of HTLV-I associated myelopathy presenting with cerebellar signs as initial and principal manifestations. Rinsho-Shinkeigaku. 1999; 39(8): 852–5.
22. Carod-Artal FJ, Del-Negro MC, Vargas AP, Rizzo I. Cerebellar syndrome and peripheral neuropathy as manifestations of infection by HTLV-I human T-cell lymphotropic virus. Rev Neurol 1999; 29(9): 932–5.
23. Sakiyama H, Nishi K, Kikukawa H, Ueda S. Urinary disturbance due to HTLV-1 associated myelopathy. Nippon Hinyokika Gakkai Zasshi 1992; 83(12): 2058.
24. Eardley I, Fowler CJ, Nagendran K, Kirby RS, Rudge P. The neurourology of tropical spastic paraparesis. Br J Urol 1991; 68(6): 598–603.
25. Yamashita H, Kumazawa J. Voiding dysfunction: patients with human T-lymphotropic-virus-type-1 associated myelopathy. Urol Int 1991; 47(Suppl 1): 69–71.
26. Imamura A, Kitagawa T, Ohi Y, Osame M. Clinical manifestation of human T-cell lymphotropic virus type-I-associated myelopathy and vesicopathy. Urol Int 1991; 46(2): 149–53.
27. Imamura A. Studies on neurogenic bladder due to human T-lymphotropic virus type-I associated myelopathy (HAM). Nippon Hinyokika Gakkai Zasshi 1994; 85(7): 1106–15.

28. Walton GW, Kaplan SA. Urinary dysfunction in tropical spastic paraparesis: preliminary urodynamic survey. J Urol 1993; 150(3): 930–2.
29. Hattori T, Sakakibara R, Yamanishi T, Yasuda K, Hirayama K. Micturitional disturbance in human T-lymphotropic virus type-1-associated myelopathy. J Spinal Disord 1994; 7(3): 255–8
30. Matsumoto SC, Nakasato O, Kataoka A, Inayoshi S, Okajima T. Myelopathy associated with HTLV-1: clinical electrophysiologic study. Neurologia 1993; 8(9): 291–4.
31. Nomata K, Nakamura T, Suzu H et al. Novel complications with HTLV-1-associated myelopathy/tropical spastic paraparesis: interstitial cystitis and persistent prostatitis. Jpn J Cancer Res 1992; 83(6): 601–8.
32. Cartier L, Castillo JL, Verdugo R. Effect of the Nucleus CMP forte in 46 patients with progressive spastic paraparesis. Randomized and blind study. Rev Med Chile 1996; 124(5): 583–7.
33. Harrington WJ Jr, Sheramata W, Cabral L. Danazol for urinary incontinence in tropical spastic paraparesis. Lancet 1992; 339(8789): 368.
34. Saito M, Kato K, Kondo A, Miyake K. Neurogenic bladder in HAM (HTLV-I associated myelopathy). Hinyokika Kiyo 1991; 37(9): 1005–8.
35. Namima T, Sohma F, Imabayashi K, Nishimura Y, Orikasa S. Two cases of neurogenic bladder due to HTLV-1 associated myelopathy (HAM). Nippon Hinyokika Gakkai Zasshi 1990; 81(3): 475–8.
36. Berger JR, Houff S. Progressive multifocal leukoencephalopathy: lessons from AIDS and natalizumab. Neurol Res 2006; 28(3): 299–305.
37. Bratt G, Hammarin A.L, Grandien M et al. BK virus as the cause of meningoencephalitis, retinitis and nephritis in a patient with AIDS. AIDS 1999; 13(9): 1071–5.
38. Robinson, LG, Chiriboga CA, Champion SE et al. Progressive multifocal leukoencephalopathy successfully treated with highly active antiretroviral therapy and cidofovir in an adolescent infected with perinatal human immunodeficiency virus (HIV). J Child Neurol 2004; 19(1): 35–8.
39. Aksamit AJ. Review of PML and natalizumab. Neurologist 2006; 12(6): 293–8.
40. Roskopf J, Trofe J, Stratta RJ, Ahsan N. Pharmacotherapeutic options for the management of human polyomaviruses.Adv Exp Med Biol 2006; 577: 228–54.
41. Attali P, Frey M, Kubina M et al. Gebly Study Group for Lyme borreliosis. Disease expression of Lyme borreliosis in northeastern France. Eur J Clin Microbiol Infect Dis 2001; 20(4): 225–30.
42. Christova I, Komitova R. Clinical and epidemiological features of Lyme borreliosis in Bulgaria. Wien Klin Wochenschr 2004; 31,116 (1–2): 42–6.
43. Mehnert WH, Krause G. Surveillance of Lyme borreliosis in Germany, 2002–2003. Euro Surveill 2005; 10(4): 83–5.
44. Nygarg K, Bransaeter AB, Mehl A. Disseminated and chronic Lyme borreliosis in Norway, 1995–2004. Euro Surveill 2005; 10(10): 83–5.
45. Hengge UR, Tannapfel A, Tyring SK et al. Lyme borreliosis. Lancet Infect Dis 2003; 3(8): 489–500.
46. Lebech AM. Polymerace chain reaction in diagnosis of *Borrelia burgdorferi* infections and studies on taxonomic classification. APMIS Suppl 2002; 105: 1–40.
47. Schwan TG, Burgdorfer W, Schrumpf ME, Karstens RH. The urinary bladder, a consistent source of *Borrelia burgdorferi* in experimentally infected white-footed mice (*Peromyscus leucopus*). J Clin Microbiol 1988; 26(5): 893–5.
48. Druschky K, Stefan H, Grehl H, Neundorfer B. Secondary normal pressure hydrocephalus. A complication of chronic neuroborreliosis. Nervenarzt 1999; 70(6): 556–9.
49. Pavia CS, Wormser GP, Nowakowski J, Cacciapuoti A. Efficacy of an evernimicin (SCH27899) in vitro and in an animal model of Lyme disease. Antimicrob Agents Chemother 2001; 45(3): 936–7.
50. Czub S, Duray PH, Thomas RE, Schwan TG. Cystitis induced by infection with the Lyme disease spirochete, *Borrelia burgdorferi*, in mice. Am J Pathol 1992; 141(5): 1173–9.
51. Goodman JL, Jurkovich P, Kramber JM, Johnson RC. Molecular detection of persistent *Borrelia burgdorferi* in the urine of patients with active Lyme disease. Infect Immun 1991; 59(1): 269–78.
52. Goodman JL, Jurkovich P, Kodner C, Johnson RC. Persistent cardiac and urinary tract infections with *Borrelia burgdorferi* in experimentally infected Syrian hamsters. J Clin Microbiol 1991; 29(5): 894–6.
53. Chancellor MB, McGinnis DE, Shenot PJ, Kiilholma P, Hirsch IH. Urinary dysfunction in Lyme disease. J Urol 1993; 149(1): 26–30.
54. Chancellor MB, McGinnis DE, Shenot PJ, Hirsch IH, Kiilholma PJ. Lyme cystitis and neurogenic bladder dysfunction. Lancet 1992; 339(8803): 1237–8.
55. Aberer E, Neumann R, Lubec G. Acrodermatitis chronica atrophicans in association with lichen sclerosus et atrophicans: tubulo-interstitial nephritis and urinary excretion of spirochete-like organisms. Acta Derm Venereol 1987; 67(1): 62–5.
56. Chancellor MB, Dato VM, Yang JY. Lyme disease presenting as urinary retention. J Urol 1990; 143(6): 1223–4.
57. Olivares JP, Pallas F, Ceccaldi M et al. Lyme disease presenting as isolated acute urinary retention caused by transverse myelitis: an electrophysiological and urodynamical study. Arch Phys Med Rehabil 1995; 76(12): 1171–2.
58. Taylor RS, Simpson IN. Review of treatment options for Lyme borreliosis. J Chemother 2005; 17(Suppl 2): 3–16.

25

Cerebrovascular accidents, intracranial tumors, and urologic consequences

Christopher E Wolter, Harriette Scarpero, and Roger Dmochowski

Introduction

Intact cerebral cortical function is crucial for normal voiding function and urinary continence. Cerebrovascular accidents (CVAs) and intracranial tumors are the most common processes that will alter normal higher cortical function and normal micturition. These disease entities and their subsequent effects on urinary tract function therefore are clinically important to urologists.

For practical purposes, these two disease processes will be dealt with together as they commonly manifest in similar ways. Clinical evidence suggests that CVAs, or strokes, and their effects on micturition, are commonly associated with voiding dysfunction, while data relating to intracranial masses are more sparse. Herein, this chapter will focus on the lesion location and its consequences, regardless of the underlying etiology.

The most pressing urologic consequence of cortical disease is voiding dysfunction, usually inclusive of urinary incontinence, urinary frequency, and often (although not universally) urinary urgency. While incontinence is the most common and disruptive concern, patients with acute intracranial lesions can also be found to be in urinary retention, especially in the acute phase of an event. In addition, there can be an element of sexual dysfunction present from cortical lesions. Genitourinary dysfunction arising from acute intracranial lesions is commonly complicated by the patient's premorbid level of functioning. The pre- and postmorbid voiding dysfunction poses a serious diagnostic and therapeutic challenge to those who treat and manage this patient population.

Incidence

Approximately 700 000 CVAs occur in the United States each year. Of these, about 500 000 are initial episodes, and the balance are recurrent strokes. This equates to one stroke occurring every 45 seconds.[1] Of those who suffer a CVA, about one-third will die from the acute event, another third will require long-term rehabilitation, and the rest will return to their homes, some at their previous level of function eventually. More specifically, of the survivors, 10% will have no residual effects, 40% will have mild disability, 40% will have significant disability, and 10% will require nursing home care. Additionally, CVA is the number one cause of disability in adults.[2] CVA is the third leading cause of death in the United States, following heart disease and cancer.[3]

With the population as a whole increasing in age, the cumulative number of post–CVA patients is expected to increase in the future. It has been estimated that there are roughly 3 800 000 stroke survivors currently alive in North America. In addition to the disease burden that CVA poses, there are serious healthcare cost implications. Estimates range up to $40 billion annually in the United States.[4] Despite declining mortality rates, the accumulation of survivors leaves a large number of individuals needing post-stroke care.[5]

There are several risk factors associated with CVAs. The most common etiologies include: age, hypertension, diabetes, hypercholesterolemia, tobacco abuse, obesity, alcohol consumption, and stress, with age being the highest independent risk factor.[2] Two primary mechanisms account for stroke-related phenomena: occlusive lesions, either embolic or thrombotic, and hemorrhagic lesions, produced from trauma or vascular malformation.

The resulting ischemia and/or mass effect from these insults produce the signs and symptoms that comprise a stroke. The pathophysiology of micturition disturbance after CVA involves two separate mechanisms. First, there is decreased sensation or awareness of bladder filling, which would normally lead to a desire to micturate. Second, damage to higher cortical centers, especially in the frontal lobe, leads to inability to suppress a bladder contraction, sometimes leading to incontinence. Therefore, either bladder overflow due to incomplete emptying or detrusor overactivity produce voiding dysfunction after cortical events.[2]

A diagnostic dilemma can often present itself in the poststroke patient with urinary incontinence. Prostatic disorders, overactive bladder, and stress incontinence are all commonly seen in this patient population and may obfuscate the clinical presentation. Daily urinary incontinence in the general population under the age of 65 can be as high as 1 in 20, and this increases to 1 in 12 over the age of 75.[6] Overall, the prevalence of incontinence in the general population is estimated to be 6%; in older people it can range from 11% to 29%. This compares to rates ranging from 12% to 79% in the stroke population, depending on the time after onset of stroke.[7] Also, the incidence of uninhibited detrusor contractions in the elderly is 10% in women and 25% to 35% in men,[3] further complicating the presentation.

Presentation

Urinary retention may be the first event to occur after a CVA. The exact mechanism is not clear but has been termed 'cerebral shock'. Retention may not necessarily be a direct result of the neurologic lesion itself, but rather from the impaired consciousness, immobility, and inability to communicate the need to void, with resultant overdistention of the bladder and failure to void.[8] This lack of appreciation of bladder events appears to be more commonly associated with certain cortical insults. Burney et al also showed a high incidence of retention and areflexia (85%) in patients with hemorrhagic CVAs. The authors were unable to explain these findings, however these more serious events and large infarcts could contribute to stroke sequelae leading to retention.[9] Premorbid detrusor dysfunction or concomitant medications may also cause and/or contribute to retention in the acute setting.[10]

In a prospective study, the rate of urinary retention was 29% at 13 days after CVA.[11] In these patients, there was a higher rate of diabetes, cognitive impairment, aphasia, and decreased functional status. The retention resolved in 96% of the patients within 2 months after discharge. These results should be contrasted to other studies where the rate of retention seen at 72 hours was 47%, and 21% at 3 weeks.[9,10] Thus, there appears to be a decrease in the rate of urinary retention after the onset of acute CVA over time.

Incontinence can also be seen in the acute phase. Additionally, mixed detrusor overactivity and incomplete emptying have also been reported after acute cortical events. These findings are partially dependent on the premorbid urinary function of the patient and the overall size of the stroke and affected area of the brain.

Incontinence and stroke

Over time, after the retention resolves, not all patients return to normal voiding. There appears to be an evolution from retention to a more fixed dysfunction, usually manifested by urinary urgency, frequency, and urinary incontinence. These findings have been attributed to detrusor overactivity in clinical series. As mentioned previously, the prevalence of incontinence in stroke patients can vary widely. For example, frequency and urgency with urge incontinence was seen in 67% of patients at an average of 19 months after CVA.[12]

Other studies have evaluated the occurrence of incontinence at various times after stroke. Overall the trend falls from the upward rate of 79% in elderly patients (over 75) in the more acute setting,[13] to a rate of 25% to 28% at discharge,[6] to a low of 12% several months postCVA.[14] Although the incidence of incontinence may decrease with time, there are still a significant number of patients with abnormal and chronic storage and voiding parameters.

Incontinence is a major predictive factor in the overall health quality outcome of CVA patients. It is a prognostic indicator for both mortality and for quality of life. The mortality rate for continent patients in the first few days after a CVA is much lower than in those with incontinence. Patients with incontinence had a 52% mortality rate at 6 months, whereas those who remained continent experienced a 7% mortality rate.[15] In another series, at 1 year poststroke, the relative risk of death was 3.9 (95% confidence interval, 1.4–10.6) in subjects with incontinence, and was significantly higher than for patients without incontinence.[16]

Patel et al evaluated stroke patients with incontinence within 7 days of CVA onset. Of the 511 subjects, the rate of incontinence was 39% in this period. The mortality rate of these patients at 3 months was 32%. The functional status and institutionalization rate of those who survived were compared between the continent and incontinent groups. The group that regained continence (127/207 patients) had overall better functional status and a lower institutionalization rate than those who remained incontinent.[17] The presence of incontinence is an indicator of a more severe CVA, and thus patients with this can be expected to have worse overall outcomes.

Pettersen et al assessed the types of urinary incontinence and how these related to outcomes in CVA patients. An assessment of 315 patients with acute stroke, including mental status and functional testing, and frequent checks of urinary symptoms, was performed in this study. These evaluations were repeated at 3 months. Those with impaired awareness were found to have the poorest outcomes, and the least improvement in urinary function at 3 months.[18] The authors attributed this impairment in awareness to anosognosia, which is an unawareness or denial of a neurologic deficit. Other studies have attributed anosognosia to more severe overall disability, and this finding is an independent predictor in these patients.[19]

That decreased awareness of self and basic needs (for example, hygiene) leads to worse outcome seems intuitive, yet this finding is consistent in postCVA patients. This is not an all-or-none phenomenon in CVA patients, but rather a continuum of decreased awareness from mild to complete neglect.[18] Patients with any degree of self-neglect have worse attention deficits and are more functionally impaired than those without neglect.[20] When patients with a CVA develop neglect as a consequence, their inability to recognize basic needs, such as the need to void and perform hygiene, adds to their overall disability, and leads to a worse outcome than those in whom these executive functions are intact. Executive functions are those that are involved in planning and initiating complex activities, such as voiding. These functions are strongly related to basic and essential activities of daily living.[21] So, when a patient does not sense that his bladder is full until the sudden onset of voiding, the event can be characterized as urge, but may more so reflect the lack of recognition by the patient. Further, this finding probably indicates a more severe CVA.[18]

Indeed, urinary symptoms also play a major role in the quality of life and overall wellbeing of patients after stroke. In a population based study by Brittain et al, 10 000 community members underwent evaluation for the incidence of stroke and urinary symptoms.[7] When specifically evaluating incontinence, the authors found that 64% of the stroke survivors had lower urinary tract symptoms. Of these, 49% had nocturia, 33% had incontinence, 19% had urgency, 15% had frequency, 3.5% had straining, and 2.5% had pain. There was significant overlap of symptoms among the patients. Overall, the more severe the patients self-rated their symptoms, the greater degree of disability and negative effect on quality of life was identified. These subjects also had greater difficulty with activities of daily living.[7]

In addition to worse outcomes, the presence of incontinence after a CVA can also predict impaired recovery in these patients. In a study by Turhan et al, the presence of poststroke incontinence was evaluated and found to be an important negative predictive factor in recovery from stroke from a functional standpoint, though it did not affect length of stay in a rehabilitation unit.[22] This finding of impaired functional recovery with incontinence after CVA has been supported in several other studies as well.[17,23–26]

Incontinence can cause a loss of up to 11 hours per week of therapy in patients in an inpatient rehabilitation setting.[27] In a study by Eldar et al, patients with incontinence in an inpatient rehabilitation setting were assessed.[27] In the study population, at an average of 38 days postCVA, the incontinence rate was 24% on admission. Of these patients, a significantly longer rehabilitative stay (114 days) was found as compared to those who were continent (91 days). Also, 20% of the incontinent patients regained continence at 6 weeks, and 25% at discharge.

Looking at the functional independence measure (FIM),[28] those who regained continence had a higher FIM physical score at admission, though their FIM cognitive scores were similar to those who remained incontinent. This seems to indicate that in a rehabilitation setting, physical function is important for regaining continence. At 6 months' follow-up, the continence rate rose to 55%.[27] This continued improvement in continence over time has been seen previously, with 42% of patients being incontinent at 4 weeks, and the rate dropping to 20% at 6 months.[15]

There are also morale and social issues regarding incontinence in postCVA patients. Depression is a common finding in the poststroke population and appears to be related to the level of disability seen. It is also a factor affecting functional and social outcomes[29] in stroke patients. Since patients who remain continent or regain continence after stroke have better outcomes than those who do not, it has been suggested that recovery of continence improves morale and self-esteem among these patients and may even expedite recovery.[30] From a social standpoint, the rate of institutionalization after stroke is much higher if incontinence is present. In one large study, the rate of patients returning home from rehab after a CVA was 79% if they were continent, and dropped to 45% if they were not.[31] Incontinent patients had lower emotional wellbeing, more stroke-related symptoms, and less satisfaction with their reintegration into home and society.[32] Incontinence can also affect the home family members and caregivers of stroke patients. In a study where predominantly female caregivers were given questionnaires to identify their wellbeing, the subjects scored below acceptable levels for both emotional distress and anger.[33] The presence of incontinence may also lead to caretakers seeking nursing home placement for these patients.[34]

In summary, incontinence is a common and very important problem in patients who suffer a CVA. Incontinence portends a higher mortality rate and more severe physical and mental dysfunction. While recovery of continence can be seen, there are still a significant number of patients with residual micturition disturbances afterwards, and this disability can hamper their recovery. Finally, incontinence after a CVA can affect the morale, social placement, and caregivers of the patient.

Neuroanatomy and imaging

When a CVA occurs, it can disrupt the complex interactions in the central nervous system that regulate voiding. The bladder's main functions are to store and empty urine. This is under control at several levels: the cerebral cortex (suprapontine), the pons, and at the spinal level. The pontine micturition center is where regulation and coordination of voiding occurs.[35] During normal storage, there is a net inhibitory effect of the central nervous system on the detrusor, and the external sphincter is closed. When the need to void is sensed, the central nervous system 'allows' the urethral sphincter to relax, the detrusor to contract reflexively, and voiding is initiated.[3] This is an overly simplified view of this, but disturbances at the level of the CNS (CVA, tumor) cause a significant breakdown in this normal control.

With the loss of the main inhibitory input, especially the frontal lobes, the net result is usually a hyperreflexic detrusor, which results in clinical overactivity and urge incontinence.[36] There are several complex interactions in the central nervous system that all contribute to normal voiding function, and it is important to gain an understanding of this in order to see how lesions in the CNS such as CVAs and tumors can affect voiding. In a review by Kavia et al, the various regions of the brain and their activity during the micturition cycle are thoroughly described.[37]

As mentioned before, central regulation and control of voiding occurs in the pons. More specifically, this occurs in the pontine micturition center. This was the first structure to be shown to control micturition and was first described by Barrington in 1921.[37] This area is also known as the 'M-region' from animal studies, as it is medially located, and is essential in the regulation of voiding.[38] A homologous region exists in humans in the dorsal pontine tegmentum and was found by Blok et al to be activated in functional studies.[39] De Groat reported that stimulation of this area in the feline caused relaxation of the urinary sphincter and led to a coordinated detrusor contraction, thus initiating voiding.[40] Ablation of this area disabled sphincter relaxation and detrusor contraction, causing retention.[37]

Another region in the pons that is less understood is the 'L-region', or lateral in animal studies. Stimulation of this area in cats demonstrates activation of the urethral sphincter, and is thought to serve its purpose more for continence and not necessarily for micturition.[41] This region has been found to be activated when patients are unable to void during positron emission tomography (PET) studies, and because of this it is suspected that this region acts as a continence center.[37,39] Another study demonstrated the L-region to be more activated when the bladder was full compared to when it was empty.[42]

The pons receives afferent information from the periaqueductal gray (PAG), a region that is activated during both the filling and micturition phases. That the PAG is active during both phases suggests that it serves as an interface between the afferent and efferent information involved in micturition.[37] The PAG indeed has robust interconnections with higher brain centers and the sacral spinal cord, as well as with the pons in humans.[37] The net sum of this is that the PAG receives sensory input from the viscera, and relays this information to higher centers and the pons, and is important in the control of micturition.

The thalamus serves as an important relay center for sensory afferent information. This part of the brain has been shown by PET and functional MRI studies to be activated during bladder filling.[43,44] It has also been shown to have interconnections with the prefrontal cortex, and with the PAG.[37] Although this is not its only role, this gives the thalamus a key role in conveying information from the bladder.[45]

After information is relayed to the thalamus, it is carried to the insula, where information from organ sensation is sensed, otherwise termed interoception.[46] The anterior insula becomes activated when unpleasant sensations occur, such as the strong desire to void.[44] Griffiths et al and Blok et al showed that, on functional MRI and PET studies, respectively, the insula is activated when the bladder is full.[39,44] Integration of autonomic response and the limbic system involves the insula. Sympathetic activation in the bladder inhibits the detrusor, causing relaxation, thus distending the bladder, which is why the insula becomes activated when the bladder is full.[37]

In the limbic system, the anterior cingulate gyrus is involved in emotions, pleasure, and memory formation, as well as control of the autonomic nervous system. It also appears to be involved in cognitive functions, such as conflict.[37,47] The conflict during the micturition cycle is the desire to void versus social appropriateness. In the anterior cingulate gyrus, the anterior portion is more affective, while the posterior portion is cognitive. Thus, during the desire to void, a cognitive function, the posterior portion is activated, whereas during voiding itself, the anterior portion is activated.[37,42,43]

The frontal cortex is where cognitive control of voiding is located. The functions of this region determine when it is and is not appropriate to void, and any decision to initiate voiding is carried out through the frontal lobe.[48] The main effect on voiding from the frontal cortex is inhibition of the detrusor to facilitate storage of urine and elimination at an appropriate time. If this function is not present, the patient may not be able to suppress the urge to void when it occurs.[39]

When a CVA occurs, or when there is a brain mass causing micturition disturbance, the location of the lesion can give some indication of what types of voiding disturbances can occur. Single photon emission computed tomography (SPECT) studies in elderly patients revealed information about underperfused areas in relation to incontinence. When compared to normal subjects, those with incontinence showed significantly decreased perfusion to their frontal lobes, namely the right superior frontal and left cortical areas, especially in cases of reduced awareness.[49] Therefore, when the underlying underperfusion is a result of a CVA, it is believed that the CVA caused the incontinence.

One of the earliest studies done was by Tsuchida et al looking at CT findings after hemiplegic stroke and comparing them with urodynamic studies on these patients.[12] All patients in this study had some form of micturition disturbance, and

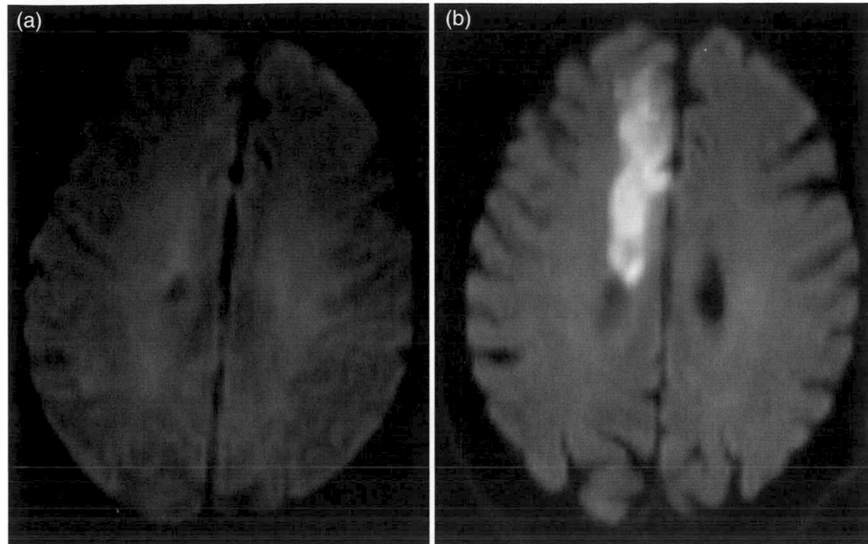

Figure 25.1
MRI of normal brain (a) and brain with acute ischemic frontal lobe stroke (b).

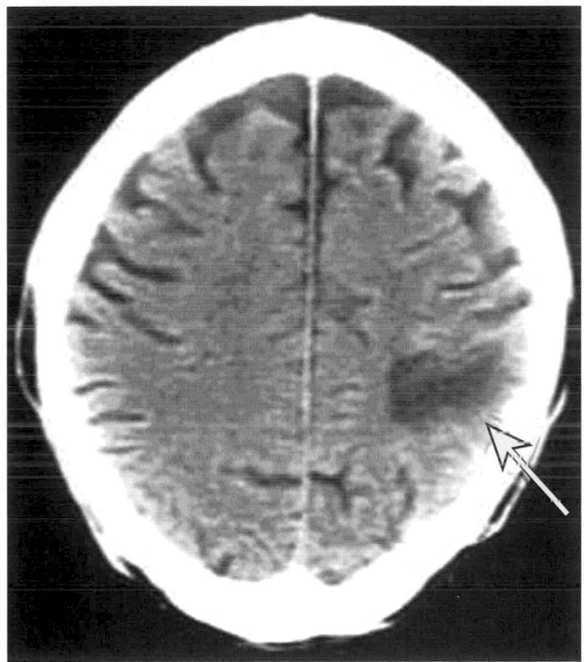

Figure 25.2
Fronto-parietal-temporal lobe ischemic stroke.

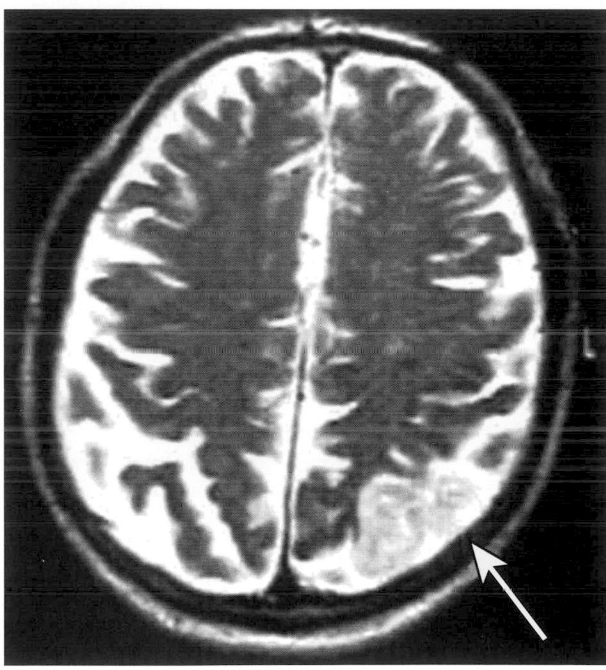

Figure 25.3
Occipital lobe ischemic stroke.

their CVAs occurred an average of 19 months prior to being studied. The most common symptoms seen were frequency with urge incontinence in 26/39 patients, and the rest complained of dysuria or retention. While the results of the CT findings were not consistent in 16 of their patients, there were some subgroups where there was consistency of findings.[12] Patients with frontal lobe and internal capsule lesions showed detrusor hyperactivity and an increased rate of uninhibited sphincter relaxation. Detrusor external sphincter dyssynergia (DESD) was a rare occurrence in their study population.

Another study looked at CT and MRI findings in CVA patients within 3 months after their insult. The findings in this study were similar as well. Their study population had a urinary symptom rate of 53%, and patients with symptoms had significantly more lesions located in the frontal lobe (Figure 25.1), large lesions in the fronto-parietal-temporal (Figure 25.2) and fronto-parietal-occipital area than in the temporal, parietal, and occipital areas alone[50] (Figure 25.3). The consistency of involvement with the frontal lobe above all other areas shows the

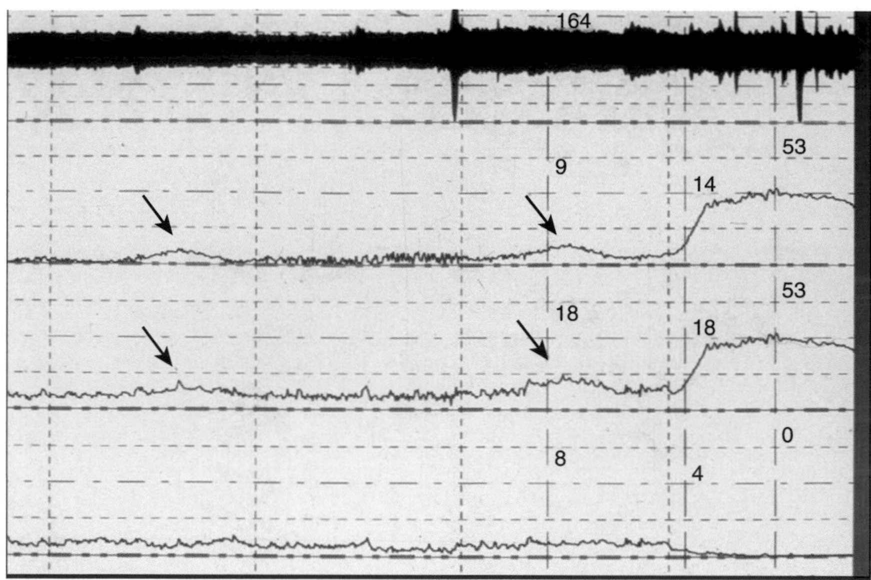

Figure 25.4
Cystometrogram tracing demonstrating phasic detrusor contractions. Note that contractions are initially suppressed, a good prognostic indicator.

importance of this region in normal voiding and how disturbances of this can cause symptoms in these patients. This patient population also commonly demonstrated uninhibited sphincter relaxation in frontal lobe lesions, and additionally showed DESD frequently in patients with basal ganglia lesions.

Pathways from the frontal cortex affected by CVA can also manifest as detrusor hyperreflexia with absence of sphincter control. Suprapontine lesions often lead to this loss of sphincter control, especially when this sensorimotor cortex and the corticospinal tracts are affected.[9] This was indeed the case in a study by Burney et al, where they looked at patients in the acute phase of stroke and performed urodynamics in this time period and correlated them to brain imaging. Patients with sphincter abnormality had uninhibited relaxation in 83% and the lesions in these patients were heavily concentrated in the frontal cortex and internal capsule.[9]

The cerebellum also has a role in normal bladder storage and emptying. The function of this part of the brain on voiding lies in coordination between the cortical centers and detrusor nuclei in the brainstem, and its main effect is to prevent reflexic contractions from occurring.[36] In a previously mentioned study, all of the patients with cerebellar infarctions, however, had detrusor areflexia with normal sphincters, which seems counterintuitive given the normally inhibitory function of the cerebellum on the bladder.[9] In another study, functional MRI (fMRI) was used to study activation of brain regions and the cerebellum was found to be involved in inhibition of the micturition reflex as well.[51] So, while the cerebellum's normal function is inhibitory on the detrusor, its role after a CVA to this part of the brain is not well understood.

There has been some question as to whether the sidedness of the brain lesion matters. One study reported that urgency, frequency, and incontinence were more common in right-sided lesions.[52] This would appear to agree with the SPECT findings by Griffiths mentioned earlier, where incontinence was seen frequently when the right frontal lobe was underperfused.[49] Other authors assessed this concept and found that the side of the lesion did not matter where incontinence was concerned. Burney et al evaluated hemispheric dominance in CVA patients and found no difference among patients with regard to continence and the side of the lesion.[2] Gelber et al analyzed lesion sidedness and found no correlation between the side of the lesion and incontinence.[10]

Urodynamics

When incontinence occurs after a CVA, the main urodynamic finding is attributed to detrusor overactivity. Cystometrogram tracings representative of detrusor dysfunction typically found can be seen in Figures 25.4 and 25.5. In Figure 25.4, it can be seen from this tracing that there are multiple phasic episodes of detrusor activity that eventually culminate in a large sustained contraction. While this finding is related to incontinence in this patient, there is some evidence of suppression of the contractions in this patient, which may be a good prognostic indicator for future social continence. In Figure 25.5, the hyperreflexia is more pronounced, causing a much higher amplitude contraction at a certain threshold volume that the patient sensed and had difficulty suppressing. This is the pattern of loss of inhibitory control normally performed by the frontal cortex. Detrusor areflexia can also be seen, though it may be

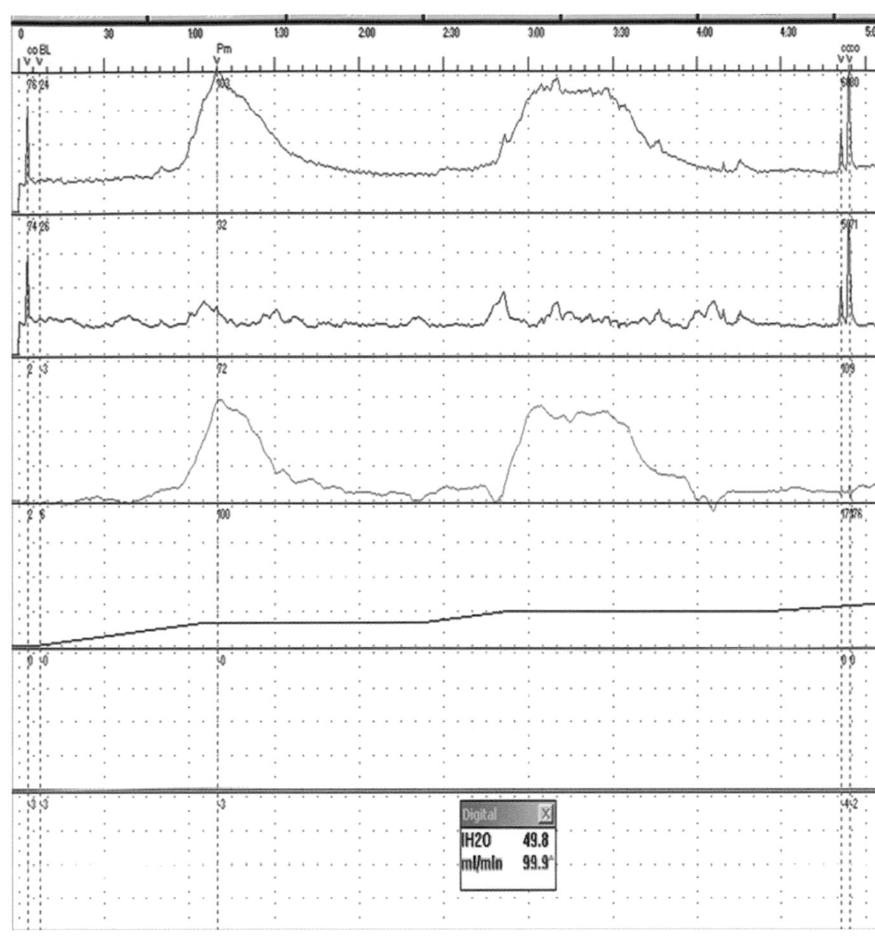

Figure 25.5
Cystometrogram demonstrating large amplitude detrusor contractions. Note how the contraction is not suppressed, indicating loss of frontal lobe input.

limited to the acute phase related to cerebral shock, and can resolve over time to normal voiding or hyperreflexia.

Another common urodynamic finding is uninhibited sphincter relaxation. In many studies, this finding is consistently present with detrusor hyperreflexia, and seen in the frontal lobe lesions.[9,12,50] This finding is rare in basal ganglia lesions.[50] This indicates that control of the external sphincter is under higher cortical functioning, and when uninhibited relaxation happens, it is often associated with more profound urine loss and reduced awareness.[49,50]

The other sphincter finding that is of concern is that of DESD. Fortunately, DESD is a rare finding after CVA and is usually confused with pseudodyssynergia.[53] True DESD usually implies a contemporaneous cord lesion occurring with the cortical lesion. This is the presence of increased EMG activity during filling in response to an involuntary detrusor contraction where the patient is voluntarily contracting the sphincter to avoid urinary loss. In previously reported studies, the presence of sphincteric dysfunction ranged from 8.3% to 17%.[9,12,50,54] When present, sphincteric dysfunction is frequently seen when there is involvement of the basal ganglia, in contrast to the situation of uninhibited sphincter relaxation.

Treatment

There is a relative paucity of information on treatment of incontinence in patients who have suffered from a CVA or tumor. The presence of hypocontractility and restricted mobility is detrimental to regaining normal voiding function.[55] In the acute phase, when there may be retention and loss of consciousness, indwelling or intermittent catheterization is an acceptable strategy. Indwelling catheterization should be discontinued as early as reasonably possible. Access to toileting should be optimized. Behavioral therapies such as timed voids (especially in aphasic patients) and fluid restriction can be of assistance.[2] Pelvic floor muscle training in women has been shown to be effective in reducing incontinence episodes in the poststroke time frame.[56]

Medical management of symptoms can be difficult in this patient population, and surgical management can be fraught with complications.[3] Alpha-blockers can have the unfortunate side-effect of dizziness and hypotension, which is especially detrimental to functioning and rehabilitation in these patients. Additionally, anticholinergic medications can have effects on cognitive functioning, especially when there is baseline impairment.[57] Imipramine is another drug

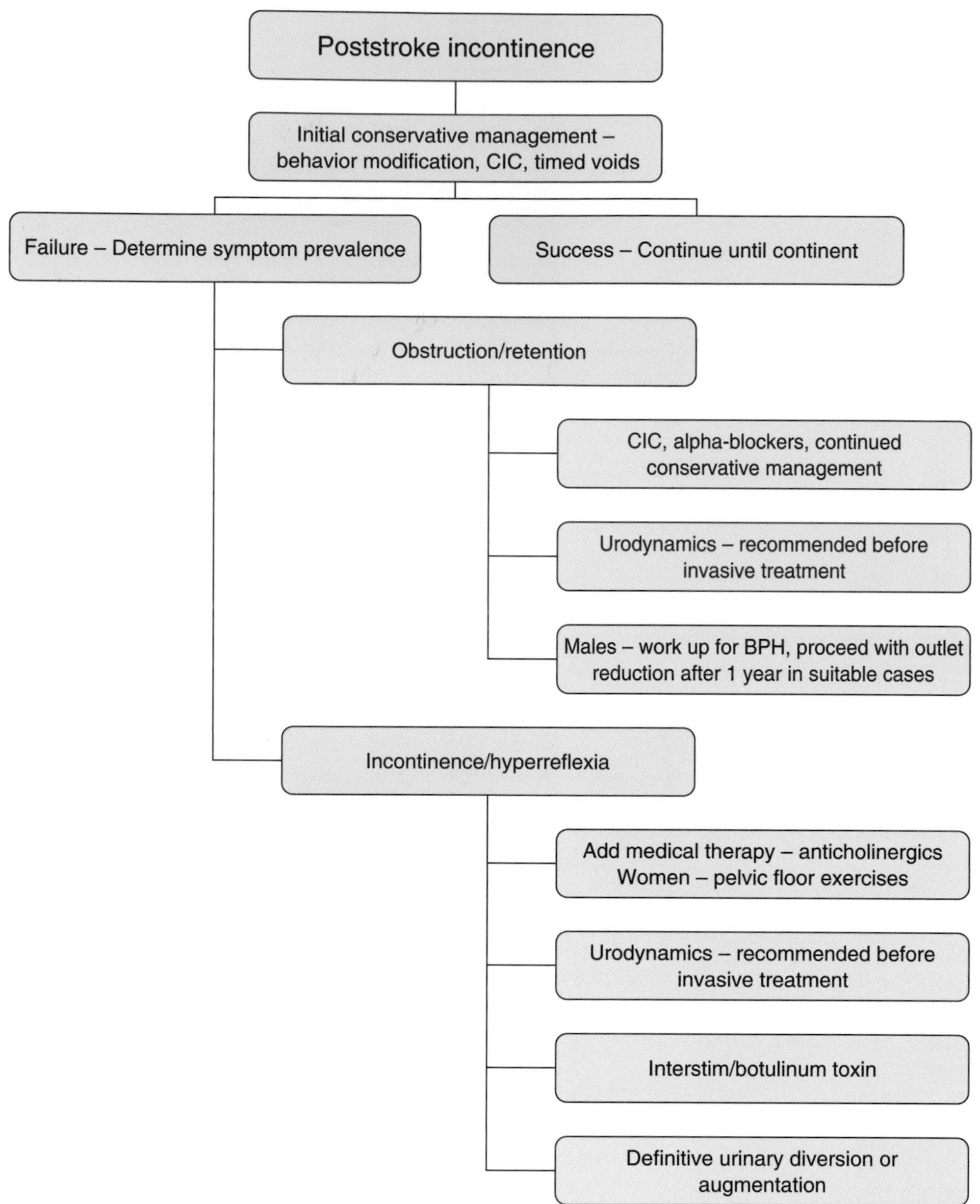

Figure 25.6
Proposed treatment algorithm for post-CVA incontinence.

that can be used for patients with urge and/or mixed incontinence. It has anticholinergic properties, and it also prevents reuptake of norepinephrine, which will increase bladder outlet resistance.[58] Duloxetine is another drug agent which may have benefit for women with mixed symptoms, but remains unavailable for this indication in the United States.

Surgical management is complicated by underlying comorbidities. The treatment of the CVA itself often involves antiplatelet and anticoagulant drugs, and these need to be addressed before therapy. Outlet therapy should be delayed in men with prostatic obstruction for at least 6 months after their CVA.[3] In a study by Natsume et al, the experience of TURP in postCVA patients in the chronic phase of their disease was reviewed and they found that 92% achieved successful micturition.[59] A contrasting study by Lum and Marshall, however, found satisfactory results in only 50% of patients, and surgery less than 1 year from the time of CVA was associated with a worse outcome, namely, continued incontinence and increased complication rates.[60] There are several minimally invasive therapies available now, including laser and microwave prostatectomy, and these may be considered in patients not medically fit for a TURP under anesthesia.[3]

For patients in whom incontinence is the problem, there are many surgical therapies available as well. Intravesical botulinum type A toxin (Botox) injections have been used for the treatment of detrusor hyperreflexia and urge incontinence. In a prospective study comparing the effects of botox on patients with true neurogenic incontinence in two groups (spinal cord injury patients and CVA patients), it was found to be 91.6% effective in increasing bladder volume and decreasing incontinence episodes in the spinal cord injury group, but only 50% effective in the CVA group.[61] Sacral neuromodulation is another possible form of treatment. It is approved for the treatment of neurogenic and idiopathic detrusor overactivity; however, in patients with neurologic disease it may not be as effective when dealing with refractory patients.[62] If the patient has an otherwise good life expectancy, is medically stable, and has refractory incontinence with poor urodynamic findings, augmentation cystoplasty or urinary diversion should be considered as well. (A treatment algorithm can be found in Figure 25.6.)

Conclusion

Patients with intracranial pathologies such as CVAs and brain tumors often develop a disturbance in their voiding habits. Any form of incontinence can occur in early periods after an acute event. Subsequently, the typical presentation is an overactive detrusor, often resulting in urgency and urge incontinence. Incontinence after a CVA is a very important prognostic factor for the mortality, severity of the stroke, and recovery of the patient. Though management can be challenging in these patients, social continence should be the ultimate goal, as this can affect their overall sense of wellbeing and outcome. Through a thorough understanding of the anatomy and behavior of brain lesions, the urologist should be able to understand and anticipate the needs of these often disabled patients.

References

1. Thom T, Haase N, Rosamond W et al. Heart disease and stroke statistics – 2006 update: a report from the American Heart Association Statistics Committee and Stroke Statistics Subcommittee. Circulation 2006; 113(6): e85–151.
2. Burney TL, Senapati M, Desai S, Choudhary ST, Badlani GH. Effects of cerebrovascular accident on micturition. Urol Clin North Am 1996; 23(3): 483–90.
3. Marinkovic S, Badlani G. Voiding and sexual dysfunction after cerebrovascular accidents. J Urol 2001; 165(2): 359–70.
4. Sacco RL. Risk factors, outcomes, and stroke subtypes for ischemic stroke. Neurology 1997; 49(5 Suppl 4): S39–44.
5. May DS, Kittner SJ. Use of Medicare claims data to estimate national trends in stroke incidence, 1985–1991. Stroke 1994; 25(12): 2343–7.
6. Brittain KR, Peet SM, Castleden CM. Stroke and incontinence. Stroke 1998; 29(2): 524–8.
7. Brittain KR, Perry SI, Peet SM et al. Prevalence and impact of urinary symptoms among community-dwelling stroke survivors. Stroke 2000; 31(4): 886–91.
8. Borrie MJ, Campbell AJ, Caradoc-Davies TH, Spears GF. Urinary incontinence after stroke: a prospective study. Age Ageing 1986; 15(3): 177–81.
9. Burney TL, Senapati M, Desai S, Choudhary ST, Badlani GH. Acute cerebrovascular accident and lower urinary tract dysfunction: a prospective correlation of the site of brain injury with urodynamic findings. J Urol 1996; 156(5): 1748–50.
10. Gelber DA, Good DC, Laven LJ, Verhulst SJ. Causes of urinary incontinence after acute hemispheric stroke. Stroke 1993; 24(3): 378–82.
11. Kong KH, Young S. Incidence and outcome of poststroke urinary retention: a prospective study. Arch Phys Med Rehabil 2000; 81(11): 1464–7.
12. Tsuchida S, Noto H, Yamaguchi O, Itoh M. Urodynamic studies on hemiplegic patients after cerebrovascular accident. Urology 1983; 21(3): 315–18.
13. Kalra L, Smith DH, Crome P. Stroke in patients aged over 75 years: outcome and predictors. Postgrad Med J 1993; 69(807): 33–6.
14. Brocklehurst JC, Andrews K, Richards B, Laycock PJ. Incidence and correlates of incontinence in stroke patients. J Am Geriatr Soc 1985; 33(8): 540–2.
15. Nakayama H, Jorgensen HS, Pedersen PM, Raaschou HO, Olsen TS. Prevalence and risk factors of incontinence after stroke. The Copenhagen Stroke Study. Stroke 1997; 28(1): 58–62.
16. Anderson CS, Jamrozik KD, Broadhurst RJ, Stewart-Wynne EG. Predicting survival for 1 year among different subtypes of stroke. Results from the Perth Community Stroke Study. Stroke 1994; 25(10): 1935–44.
17. Patel M, Coshall C, Lawrence E, Rudd AG, Wolfe CD. Recovery from poststroke urinary incontinence: associated factors and impact on outcome. J Am Geriatr Soc 2001; 49(9): 1229–33.
18. Pettersen R, Wyller TB. Prognostic significance of micturition disturbances after acute stroke. J Am Geriatr Soc 2006; 54(12): 1878–84.
19. Hartman-Maeir A, Soroker N, Oman SD, Katz N. Awareness of disabilities in stroke rehabilitation – a clinical trial. Disabil Rehabil 2003; 25(1): 35–44.
20. Buxbaum LJ, Ferraro MK, Veramonti T et al. Hemispatial neglect: subtypes, neuroanatomy, and disability. Neurology 2004; 62(5): 749–56.
21. Pohjasvaara T, Leskela M, Vataja R et al. Post-stroke depression, executive dysfunction and functional outcome. Eur J Neurol 2002; 9(3): 269–75.
22. Turhan N, Atalay A, Atabek HK. Impact of stroke etiology, lesion location and aging on post-stroke urinary incontinence as a predictor of functional recovery. Int J Rehabil Res 2006; 29(4): 335–8.
23. Thommessen B, Bautz-Holter E, Laake K. Predictors of outcome of rehabilitation of elderly stroke patients in a geriatric ward. Clin Rehabil 1999; 13(2): 123–8.
24. Tilling K, Sterne JA, Rudd AG et al. A new method for predicting recovery after stroke. Stroke 2001; 32(12): 2867–73.
25. van Kuijk AA, van der Linde H, van Limbeek J. Urinary incontinence in stroke patients after admission to a postacute inpatient rehabilitation program. Arch Phys Med Rehabil 2001; 82(10): 1407–11.
26. Samanci N, Dora B, Kizilay F et al. Factors affecting one year mortality and functional outcome after first ever ischemic stroke in the region of Antalya, Turkey (a hospital-based study). Acta Neurol Belg 2004; 104(4): 154–60.
27. Eldar R, Ring H, Tshuwa M, Dynia A, Ronen R. Quality of care for urinary incontinence in a rehabilitation setting for patients with stroke. Simultaneous monitoring of process and outcome. Int J Qual Health Care 2001; 13(1): 57–61.
28. Granger CV, Ottenbacher KJ, Fiedler RC. The Uniform Data System for Medical Rehabilitation. Report of first admissions for 1993. Am J Phys Med Rehabil 1995; 74(1): 62–6.
29. Haacke C, Althaus A, Spottke A et al. Long-term outcome after stroke: evaluating health-related quality of life using utility measurements. Stroke 2006; 37(1): 193–8.
30. Barer DH. Continence after stroke: useful predictor or goal of therapy? Age Ageing 1989; 18(3): 183–91.

31. Ween JE, Alexander MP, D'Esposito M, Roberts M. Incontinence after stroke in a rehabilitation setting: outcome associations and predictive factors. Neurology 1996; 47(3): 659–63.
32. Edwards DF, Hahn M, Dromerick A. Post stroke urinary loss, incontinence and life satisfaction: when does post-stroke urinary loss become incontinence? Neurourol Urodyn 2006; 25(1): 39–45.
33. Williams AM. Caregivers of persons with stroke: their physical and emotional wellbeing. Qual Life Res 1993; 2(3): 213–20.
34. Noelker LS. Incontinence in elderly cared for by family. Gerontologist 1987; 27(2): 194–200.
35. Carlsson CA. The supraspinal control of the urinary bladder. Acta Pharmacol Toxicol (Copenh) 1978; 43(Suppl 2): 8–12.
36. Bradley WE, Sundin T. The physiology and pharmacology of urinary tract dysfunction. Clin Neuropharmacol 1982; 5(2): 131–58.
37. Kavia RB, Dasgupta R, Fowler CJ. Functional imaging and the central control of the bladder. J Comp Neurol 2005; 493(1): 27–32.
38. Blok BF, Holstege G. Direct projections from the periaqueductal gray to the pontine micturition center (M-region). An anterograde and retrograde tracing study in the cat. Neurosci Lett 1994; 166(1): 93–6.
39. Blok BF, Willemsen AT, Holstege G. A PET study on brain control of micturition in humans. Brain 1997; 120(Pt 1): 111–21.
40. De Groat WC. Nervous control of the urinary bladder of the cat. Brain Res 1975; 87(2–3): 201–11.
41. Griffiths DJ. The pontine micturition centres. Scand J Urol Nephrol Suppl 2002; (210): 21–6.
42. Athwal BS, Berkley KJ, Hussain I et al. Brain responses to changes in bladder volume and urge to void in healthy men. Brain 2001; 124 (Pt 2): 369–77.
43. Matsuura S, Kakizaki H, Mitsui T et al. Human brain region response to distention or cold stimulation of the bladder: a positron emission tomography study. J Urol 2002; 168(5): 2035–9.
44. Griffiths D, Derbyshire S, Stenger A, Resnick N. Brain control of normal and overactive bladder. J Urol 2005; 174(5): 1862–7.
45. Chandler MJ, Hobbs SF, Fu QG et al. Responses of neurons in ventroposterolateral nucleus of primate thalamus to urinary bladder distension. Brain Res 1992; 571(1): 26–34.
46. Craig AD. Interoception: the sense of the physiological condition of the body. Curr Opin Neurobiol 2003; 13(4): 500–5.
47. Kerns JG, Cohen JD, MacDonald AW 3rd et al. Anterior cingulate conflict monitoring and adjustments in control. Science 2004; 303(5660): 1023–6.
48. Fukuyama H, Matsuzaki S, Ouchi Y et al. Neural control of micturition in man examined with single photon emission computed tomography using 99mTc-HMPAO. Neuroreport 1996; 7(18): 3009–12.
49. Griffiths D. Clinical studies of cerebral and urinary tract function in elderly people with urinary incontinence. Behav Brain Res 1998; 92(2): 151–5.
50. Sakakibara R, Hattori T, Yasuda K, Yamanishi T. Micturitional disturbance after acute hemispheric stroke: analysis of the lesion site by CT and MRI. J Neurol Sci 1996; 137(1): 47–56.
51. Zhang H, Reitz A, Kollias S et al. An fMRI study of the role of suprapontine brain structures in the voluntary voiding control induced by pelvic floor contraction. Neuroimage 2005; 24(1): 174–80.
52. Kuroiwa Y, Tohgi H, Ono S, Itoh M. Frequency and urgency of micturition in hemiplegic patients: relationship to hemisphere laterality of lesions. J Neurol 1987; 234(2): 100–2.
53. Wein A, Barrett DM. Etiologic possibilities for increased pelvic floor electromyography activity during cystometry. J Urol 1982; 127(5): 949–52.
54. Khan Z, Hertanu J, Yang WC, Melman A, Leiter E. Predictive correlation of urodynamic dysfunction and brain injury after cerebrovascular accident. J Urol 1981; 126(1): 86–8.
55. Natsume O, Yoshii M, Takahashi S et al. [Urological management for stroke patients; relation between brain lesions and establishment of micturitional modality]. Hinyokika Kiyo 1991; 37(12): 1651–5.
56. Tibaek S, Gard G, Jensen R. Pelvic floor muscle training is effective in women with urinary incontinence after stroke: a randomised, controlled and blinded study. Neurourol Urodyn 2005; 24(4): 348–57.
57. Bottiggi KA, Salazar JC, Yu L et al. Long-term cognitive impact of anticholinergic medications in older adults. Am J Geriatr Psychiatry 2006; 14(11): 980–4.
58. Hunsballe JM, Djurhuus JC. Clinical options for imipramine in the management of urinary incontinence. Urol Res 2001; 29(2): 118–25.
59. Natsume O, Yasukawa M, Yoshii M et al. [Transurethral resection of the prostate in the urological management for patients with stroke]. Hinyokika Kiyo 1992; 38(10): 1123–7.
60. Lum SK, Marshall VR. Results of prostatectomy in patients following a cerebrovascular accident. Br J Urol 1982; 54(2): 186–9.
61. Kuo HC. Therapeutic effects of suburothelial injection of botulinum a toxin for neurogenic detrusor overactivity due to chronic cerebrovascular accident and spinal cord lesions. Urology 2006; 67(2): 232–6.
62. Amundsen CL, Romero AA, Jamison MG, Webster GD. Sacral neuromodulation for intractable urge incontinence: are there factors associated with cure? Urology 2005; 66(4): 746–50.

26

Intervertebral disc prolapse

Erik Schick and Pierre E Bertrand

Introduction

Intervertebral disc prolapse causes direct neurologic damage by mechanical compression of the spinal cord or the nerve roots emerging from it. This damage is proportional to the severity and length of compression on these structures. Table 26.1 summarizes the consequences of these events. The chances for recovery are inversely proportional to the duration and degree of neural compression.[1]

The most frequent site of disc herniations is lumbar, followed by cervical and thoracic spine; some are asymptomatic. By age 60, nearly one-third of asymptomatic patients have one or more herniated lumbar discs.[2] About 90% of symptomatic herniated discs occur at the L4–L5 or L5–S1 level,[3] and 90% inside the spinal canal.[4] A strong correlation was observed between the level of herniation and age: lumbar disc herniation is more cranially localized in older patients.[5] In the cervical spine C6–C7 is the site of 60–70% of herniated discs, and C5–C6 accounts for 20–30%.[6] About 15% of asymptomatic adults have thoracic disc herniation in magnetic resonance imaging (MRI) studies.[7] On the other hand, symptomatic thoracic disc herniations represent only 0.25–0.57% of all symptomatic disc herniations.[7,8]

Cervical spine

Dong et al[9] reported recently on 12 patients with cervical disc herniation. Ten of them had detrusor hyperreflexia (8 with and 2 without associated detrusor-external sphincter dyssynergia) and 2 had areflexic bladder. Upper urinary tract pathology was detected in 71.43% of patients in this group.

Thoracic spine

Stillerman et al[10] analyzed their own series of 82 symptomatic herniated thoracic discs in 71 patients, and made an extensive review of the recent literature (from 1986 to 1997). Among the 71 patients they operated on, they noted bladder dysfunction in 24% (17 out of 71), with urgency being the most common complaint. The incidence of

Table 26.1 *Nerve lesions according to the severity and length of compression*

Compression	Consequences	Recovery	Pathology
Short and mild	Nerve impulse blocked	Almost immediate	Local ischemia
Moderate	Nerve impulse blocked	Several weeks; depends on remyelinization	Local demyelinization axon preserved
Local, progressive, chronic	Progressive decrease in motor impulse transmission	Depends on degree of remyelinization	Segmental demyelinization, between Ranvier's node, at the site of compression and its vicinity
Severe, but temporary	Section of nerve fibers	Depends on axonal regeneration in Schwann's cell sheath	Wallerian degeneration distally
Severe and chronic	Section of nerve fibers	None; Schwann's cell sheath remains blocked by compression; retrograde axonal degenerescence	Wallerian degeneration

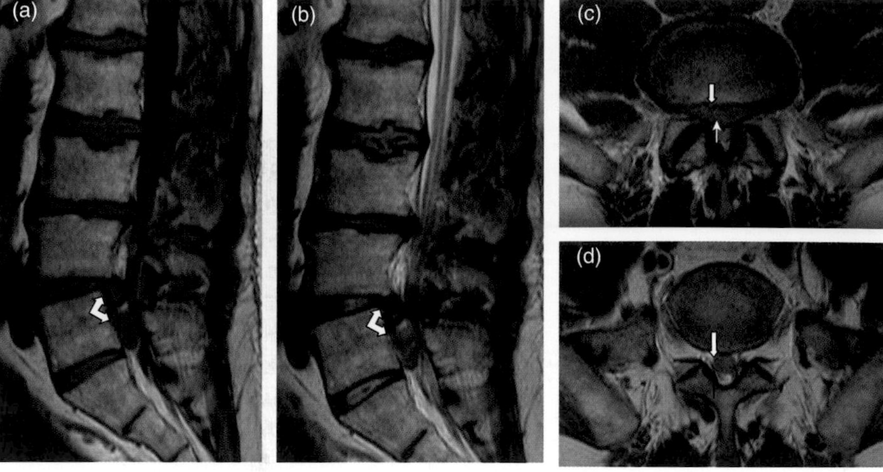

Figure 26.1
(a and b) L4–L5 sequestered disc herniation (linked white arrows); (c) protruded disc (thick white arrow) and displaced dural sac (thin white arrow); (d) sequestered disc fragment (thick white arrow). (Courtesy of Dr Marie-Josée Berthiaume).

bladder/bowel dysfunction in the reviewed literature was somewhat higher, 35% (72 out of 208). The review did not mention the type of bladder dysfunction encountered.

Lumbar spine

As 95% of disc prolapses are in the lumbar and lumbosacral region, we focus our discussion mainly on this region. Scutellari et al[11] studied more than 2000 patients with low back pain, using computed tomography, and in 15% of them found a significant pathologic condition, including mechanical compression, inflammatory and neuropathic factors. Presentation of lumbar disc prolapses can be divided into two categories: those with major symptoms other than urologic (sciatic neuralgia, cauda equina syndrome, etc.) and those showing only urologic manifestations (vesicourethral dysfunction).

The level of termination of the spinal cord, the conus medularis, is between T12 and L1–L2, most frequently at the mid-portion of L1.[12] The descending nerve bundles run posterior to the lumbar vertebral bodies until they exit the spinal canal, and are called cauda equina. Central protrusion of the disc occurs in 1–15% of cases and fibers of the cauda equina can thus be compressed[13] (Figure 26.1). Cauda equina syndrome is discussed in more detail in Chapter 27. Most disc prolapses occur at the L4–L5 or L5–S1 level (Figure 26.2) and, when central, they can affect nerve roots exiting at S2–S4 sacral levels, interfering with normal vesicourethral function (Figures 26.3 and 26.4).

Jennet[14] estimates that in the majority of lumbar disc prolapses the cauda equina is involved. This opinion is challenged by others. In a series of 121 patients operated on by Tay and Chacha,[15] only 8 patients presented with compression of the cauda equina. In a large series of 1972 patients who underwent lumbar discoidectomy, as reported by Nielsen et al,[16] only 26 (1.32%) presented with cauda equina syndrome. It is, however, difficult to distinguish in the literature patients with lumbar disc prolapse who have, or have not an associated cauda equina lesion.

Recent imaging studies suggest that no differences in cross-sectional area of the dural sac on CT scan exist between patients with or without neurogenic bladder dysfunction. However, in patients with bladder dysfunction the anteroposterior diameter of the dural sac was significantly shorter, 8 mm or less.[17]

Nerve bundles of the cauda equina contain parasympathetic and somatic fibers. The clinical presentation is often dominated by the effects of compression of the somatic fibers. This may explain why vesicourethral and rectal dysfunctions have been studied less frequently. Classically, vesicourethral dysfunction in this syndrome is estimated to have a frequency rate of 1–16%.[14,18–27] Rosomoff et al[28] were the first to include cystometry in the routine preoperative evaluation of patients with disc prolapse. They found a 96% incidence of hypotonic bladder. Andersen and Bradley[29] studied urethral and bladder innervation in 8 patients with protruded lumbar disc documented by myelography and found detrusor areflexia in all of them. Among the 30 patients with lumbar disc disease reported by Mosdal et al,[30] 18 patients had lower urinary tract symptoms, six patients had areflexic bladder, and 13 patients had hyposensitive and/or hypotonic detrusor. These data suggest that a significant proportion of patients with symptomatic lumbar disc prolapse will also have bladder dysfunction, even if lower urinary tract disturbances are not the predominant symptoms.

A relatively small number of patients with disc prolapse will not have symptoms related to somatic nerve compression, and will become clinically manifest exclusively by urinary symptoms. These cases are of particular interest for the urologist, aware of the neurologic bases for lower urinary tract symptoms.

Jennet[14] was first to suggest that urinary retention might be the only symptom of a prolapsed disc, followed by Gangai[31] 10 years later. Emmett and Love[32,33] analyzed in detail the urologic manifestations of disc prolapse.

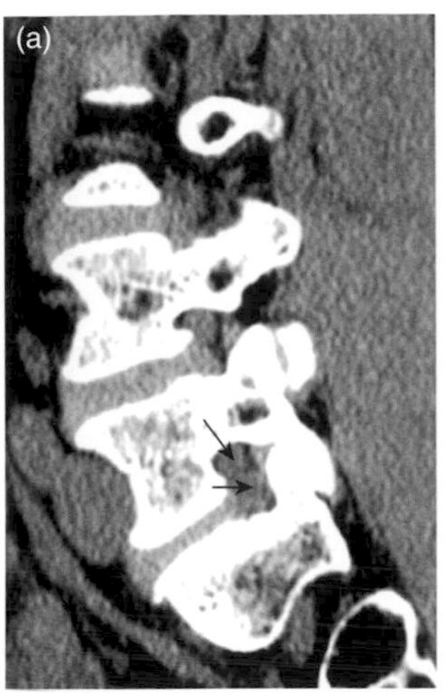

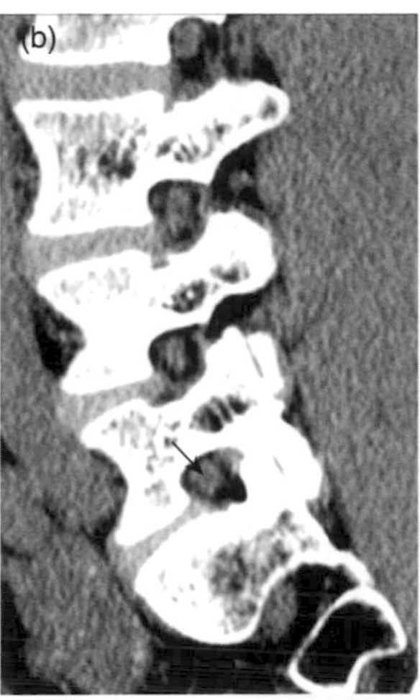

Figure 26.2
L4–L5 left foraminal disc herniation (oblique straight black arrow) obliterating the L4 exiting nerve root (straight black arrow). (Courtesy of Dr Marie-Josée Berthiaumeé).

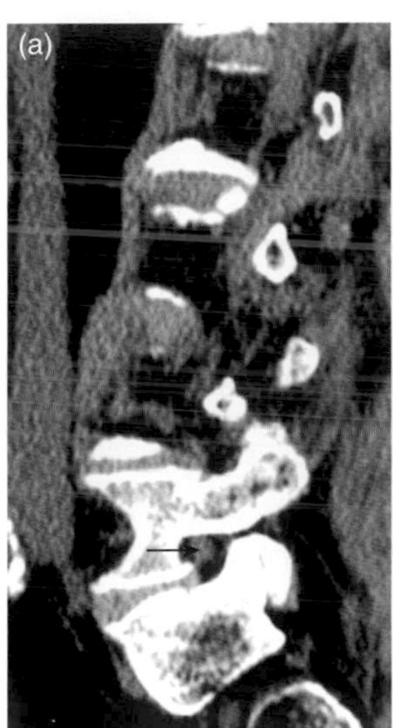

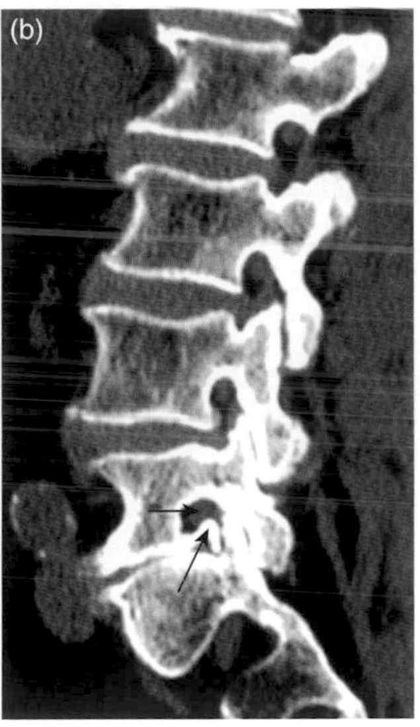

Figure 26.3
(a) Right L5–S1 foraminal stenosis from foraminal disc herniation (horizontal black arrow) just below the right L5 exiting nerve root; (b) normal left L5–S1 foramina with left L5 exiting nerve root (oblique black arrow). (Courtesy of Dr Marie-Josée Berthiaume.)

Subsequently, several other case reports or small series have been published.[34–43] It is worthwhile to note that in these reports females often outnumbered males.[36,40]

Urinary symptoms

Only a small number of patients will report urinary symptoms spontaneously. A more probing questionnaire, however, will reveal lower urinary tract disturbances in many patients.[38,44] No pathognomonic urinary symptom exists for lumbar disc prolapse. The most frequent symptom is acute or chronic urinary retention.[15,32,34,35,39,42–47]

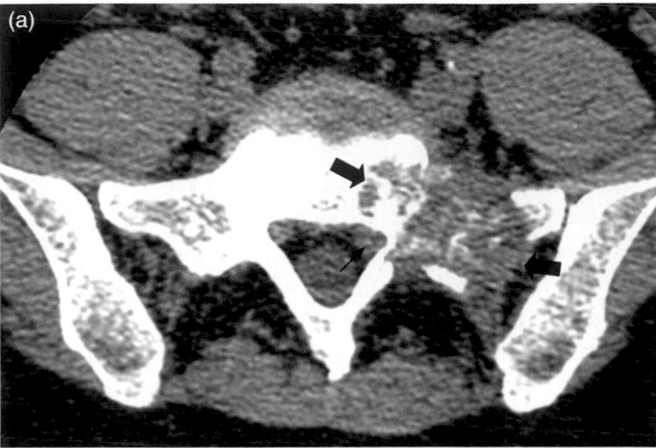

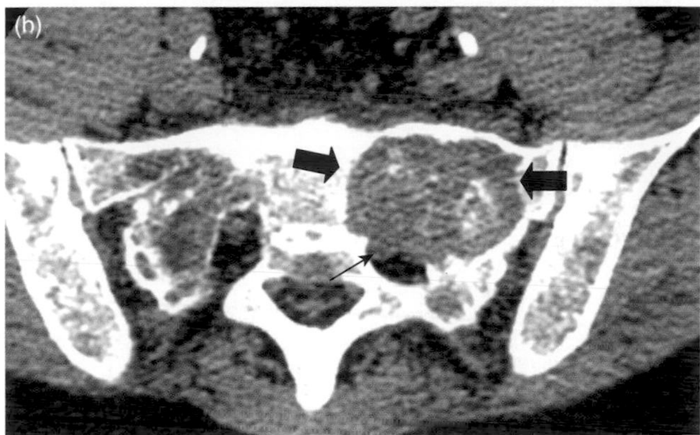

Figure 26.4
(a) L5–S1 posterior parasagittal disc herniation (dark thick arrow); (b) displaced left L5 root (thin oblique dark arrow). (Courtesy of Dr Marie-Josée Berthiaume.)

Irritative symptoms sometimes precede urinary retention.[32,45] Dysuria,[30,36,38–40] disappearance of normal desire to void,[38–40,45] decreased flow,[38,41] and urinary incontinence related to stress,[38,46] or by overflow[40] have also been described.

An important neurourologic study was published more than 30 years ago by Gunterberg et al.[48] This study is important because, to the best of our knowledge, up to now this is the only urologic investigation in patients who underwent uni- or bilateral division of sacral nerves during sacral resection for tumor. Five patients had bilateral, and 4 unilateral, precisely defined nerve lesions. This offered a unique opportunity to the authors to study the clinical (symptomatic) and cystometric (functional) consequences of uni- and bilateral sacral nerve injuries. Some important pathophysiologic conclusions may be drawn from this study. Bilateral division of the sacral nerves below the S2 level abolished detrusor contraction, suggesting that bilaterally preserved S2 nerves alone cannot insure bladder contractility. In contrast, unilateral division of S1 to S5, or

S2 to S5 resulted in a normal micturition reflex. The appearance of the detrusor contraction on the cystometrograms during micturition in these patients was indistinguishable from that of normal persons.

All patients with unilateral sacral nerve resection considered their bladder function to be essentially normal and had no complaints concerning their bowel or sexual function. Also, cystoscopic findings in this group of patients were essentially normal.

These observations are particulary important from the medicolegal point of view. If history, clinical evaluation, imaging studies, and operative reports clearly indicate that the patient has purely unilateral nerve lesion(s) as a sequel of the treatment of his/her initial pathology, urinary, bowel, and/or sexual symptoms are probably not a consequence of this nerve injury.

Urologic investigations

Cystoscopy

A number of observations can be made in a patient with lumbar disc prolapse:

1. a decrease or absence of sensation during the passage of the instrument through the urethra and less discomfort with movement of the instrument or touching of the trigone
2. a sensation of hypogastric fullness rather then real desire to void during bladder filling
3. the absence of bladder wall trabeculation, even in the presence of a large residual urine.

This triade should evoke the possibility of a lumbar disc prolapse as the cause of urinary symptoms,[32,33,37] even with a negative neurologic examination. Susset et al[41] reported a case of partial bladder denervation secondary to a disc prolapse in which mild bladder wall trabeculation was present and desire to void preserved.

Urodynamics

This is probably the best diagnostic tool to evaluate visceral innervation originating from the lumbosacral spine. Rosomoff[49] suggested that cystometry was the best test to diagnose cauda equina lesions. This opinion has been challenged by few. Emmett and Love[32] reported that cystoscopy can give the same, and sometimes more, diagnostic information than does cystometry. According to Cheek et al,[39] urodynamics are more useful in the postoperative period to document treatment outcome, mainly because before treatment it cannot distinguish between an areflexic neurogenic bladder and a decompensated, noncontractile bladder resulting from chronic overdistention.

Experimental animal studies suggest that the cystometrogram is only sensitive to severe compression of the cauda equina. Detrusor areflexia appears to occur with blockage of axoplasmic flow and early sensory changes occur with neurovenous congestion.[50]

Detrusor areflexia develops in approximately 25% of patients with lumbar intervertebral disc protrusion. Capacity is significantly increased;[27,36,38,49,51,52] during the filling phase the curve is flat, hypotonic,[36,48,50] and the first desire to void is delayed or abolished.[30,36,38,46,49,51] During voiding the detrusor is hypocontractile.[29,36,38,46,49] It should be noted, however, that in a few, well-documented lumbar disc prolapses, bladder capacity and filling phase were normal.[30,36] In a prospective study of 122 patients, Bartolin et al[53] found only 32 patients (26%) with areflexic bladder, the remaining 90 (74%) had normal detrusor function on urodynamic evaluation. Studying 31 patients with intervertebral disc prolapse, Murayama et al[54] found that those with perineal hyposensitivity should be suspected of having voiding dysfunction.

Jones and Moore[45] were first to describe the coexistence of lumbar disc prolapse and bladder hyperreflexia. In a series of 81 patients with neurogenic bladder secondary to disc prolapse or spinal degeneration, 22 patients had hyperreflexic bladders.[55] Mosdal et al[30] described an identical case and Hellström et al[56] added 3 other cases. In these cases there was usually no postvoid residual urine, and bladder sensitivity was normal. Hyperreflexia was not secondary to outflow obstruction but presumably due to 'irritation of the nerve root'.[55] This opinion is shared by Yamanishi et al,[57] who analyzed the urodynamic studies of 80 patients with spinal lesions below the L3 level, including 31 with intervertebral disc prolapse and 49 with spinal canal stenosis. Thirty-one percent of them had detrusor overactivity. Only 10 of the 80 patients were followed up after surgery, but in 5 of them overactivity disappeared. This suggests that, at least in some of these patients, the protruded disc was responsible for the overactivity because, with its removal, detrusor function returned to normal.

Shin et al[58] studied 50 patients with complete cauda equina injury. Bladder compliance was decreased in 28% (14/50) and normal in 72% (36/50). Detrusor hyperreflexia was observed in 6 out of the 14 patients with low-compliant bladder, but none in the normal-compliant group. Hyperreflexia disappeared with the normalization of compliance and capacity. These authors concluded that low compliance appeared to be the main cause of hyperreflexia.

Norlèn et al[59] reported α-adrenergic activity in the bladder of cats who underwent parasympathetic denervation. The same phenomenon was observed in humans as well. This α-adrenergic activity can be responsible for detrusor contractions during the filling phase which can be misinterpreted as being true hyperreflexia due to parasympathetic activity.

It is interesting to observe that bladder compliance is normal in areflexic bladders secondary to disc prolapse.[46] This is in contrast with the areflexic bladder resulting from trauma or myelodysplasia, where compliance is often decreased.

Murnaghan et al[60] transsected the cauda equina in monkeys and obtained low-compliant bladders. The compliance

Table 26.2 *Usual urologic manifestations of cauda equina syndrome*

	Compression of the sensory fibers of the sacral roots	Consequences of the motoricity of the detrusor
Endoscopy	Hyposensitivity of the urethra and the trigone Bladder proprioception delayed or abolished Cystoscopic capacity increased	Bladder wall without trabeculations Increased postvoid residual urine
Cystometry	Proprioception (B_1) delayed or abolished Cystometric capacity increased	Bladder wall compliance normal. Hypo- or acontractile detrusor
Free flowmetry		Maximum flow rate and mean flow rate decreased
Urethral pressure profilometry		Maximum urethral closure pressure normal or decreased (depends on pudendal nerve injury)
Electrophysiology	Sensory threshold of penis (or clitoris) altered	Bulbocavernosus (or clitorido-anal) reflex latency increased or abolished Denervation (to various extent) of pelvic floor muscles

of these bladders could be improved by administration of phentolamine and emepromium bromide.[59] This suggests that the decreased compliance was of neurogenic origin, due to both α-adrenergic and cholinergic activities.

The areflexic bladder, as observed in disc protrusion, has a normal compliance. This areflexia is thus not motor in origin – as in the experiences of Murnaghan et al,[60] or reported by Sandri et al[61] – but secondary to lesions of the sensory fibers of the bladder, or to incomplete lesions of the parasympathetic preganglionic fibers.[46] The bethanechol supersensitivity test is positive in 100% of areflexic and low-compliant bladders from other causes, but it is significantly less positive in those when areflexia is secondary to lumbar disc prolapse. This suggests that in the latter situation motor impairment is not primary, but a consequence of sensory impairment.[62] The injury to the muscle fibers of these large decompensated bladders probably results from chronic overdistention and not from a direct neurologic lesion.[47]

Bladder dysfunction, primarily sensitive and secondarily motor in nature, explains the urinary symptoms encountered and the observations made during urodynamic testing (Table 26.2).

Flowmetry

Few authors have studied free flowmetry in lumbar disc prolapse. As expected, in the majority of cases the maximum and mean flows are decreased.[29,30,38,39,41] Kontturi[38] established a relation between the degree of nerve compression and the decrease in mean flow. This, however, does not seem to be the rule, because Andersen and Bradley[29] and Mosdal et al[30] reported that 50% of their patients had normal flowmetry. Sometimes the flow curve undulates, suggesting Valsalva maneuvers during micturition.[30,39]

Urethral pressure profilometry

Kontturi[38] found a normal sphincteric tone in every patient. He was unable to establish any relation between urethral pressure profile (UPP) parameters and the severity of neural injury as demonstrated clinically or radiologically on myelography. He noted, however, that in the group of patients with the most severe neurologic impairment, sphincter tonus was abnormally high in patients with urinary retention and the sphincter was hypotonic in those patients with urinary incontinence.

McGuire[63] analyzed UPP in 6 patients with disc prolapse. Proximal urethral pressure was normal, an expected finding since herniated lumbar discs do not interfere with hypogastric plexus activity. McGuire also noted a decrease in tone at the membraneous urethra in 2 patients in whom electromyographic activity was poor in the striated sphincter. Chuang et al[52] reported on 14 patients who had lesions below the conus medullaris and had anal sphincter abnormalities. All the patients showed a significant decrease in maximum urethral closure pressure, which suggested injury to the pudendal nerve by the protruded disc.

Electromyography

Recently many authors have expressed an increasing interest regarding anal sphincter electromyography as an indicator of pudendal nerve activity, mainly as a result of the group from Ljubljana, in Slovenia.[64–67] Andersen and Bradley[29] could not register any electrical activity in 1 of 18 patients. Fanciullacci et al[46] analyzed 22 patients and found no electrical activity in 16 patients and an abnormal EMG in 6 patients.

Electromyelography

Susset et al[41] found an increased bulbocavernosus latency time in their patients. Urethroanal reflex was perturbed in two-thirds of the patients studied by Andersen and Bradley,[29] as well as by Fanciullacci et al.[46] These observations suggest an alteration in the somatic segmental innervation of the vesicourethral unit. The sensory threshold of the penis (or clitoris) was often altered.[46] Amarenco and Kerdraon[68] suggested that a difference of >3 ms in the latency time of the bulbocavernosus reflex between the left and right side can be indicative of a significant alteration in the conduction over the sacral reflex arc. (The mean interlatency difference between the two sides in 10 normal males was 1.8±0.4 ms.) These data might be important from the medico-legal standpoint when determination of isolated nerve root function is a key element in the evaluation of the patient.

Table 26.2 summarizes the urologic manifestations of cauda equina syndrome.

Postoperative results

When conservative measures fail, the treatment of herniated discs is surgical, with excision of the disc(s).

The evaluation of immediate and long-term results is difficult because subjective improvement does not necessarily match functional recuperation, as demonstrated by urodynamics and electrophysiologic studies.[39] Several authors reported significant improvement, even complete recovery, of preoperative lower urinary tract symptoms.[15,28,30,32,34,36,37,41,47,69] Scott,[26] however, found no noticeable improvement, especially when perianal anesthesia persisted.

Urodynamic evaluation can return to normal.[35,38,41,63] However, normal detrusor function preoperatively can become abnormal in up to 10% of cases following surgery.[70] Recovery of vesical function is poor or even nonexistent when neurologic signs, particularly perianal anesthesia, remain.[26–38] Perianal anesthesia is considered the most important prognostic indicator.[51] However, Hellström et al[56] reported 3 patients with persistant bilateral perianal anesthesia and a contractile detrusor. Gleave and Macfarlane[47] found no relation between bladder recovery and persisting saddle anesthesia. It should be noted, however, that about 10% of patients with clinical, electrodiagnostic, and radiologic findings compatible with cauda equina or conusmedullaris lesions will exhibit normal saddle sensation.[71] Seventy-nine percent of their patients had no urinary symptoms, but 78% remained with perianal sensory deficit. (These patients, however, did not have a urodynamic evaluation.) For several authors, detrusor areflexia has a tendency to remain permanent.[29,46,70,72] In a small series of 8 patients (follow-up 1 month to 6 years) Yamanishi et al[73] demonstrated that urethral function showed a better recovery after surgery than did bladder function in patients with acute urinary retention due to central lumbar disc protrusion. Fanciullacci et al[46] demonstrated that the afferent branch of the pudendal reflex arc is more vulnerable than its efferent branch. This might explain why perianal anesthesia rarely recovers. Detrusor recovery is not proportional to the dimension of the disc prolapse.[74]

Opinions are divided as to what extent this pathology should be considered as a surgical emergency. Some researchers[17,53,75–77] advocate rapid decompression because it improves the chances of detrusor recovery. Other researchers[14,47,51,78,79] found no relation between the delay to surgery and normalization of bladder function. One possible exception could be decompression in an acute episode within the first 6 hours, the limit of time for axone ischemia to become irreversible.[47] In all reported series, such rapid intervention is exceptional.

Short-term recovery of bladder function is often poor after lumbar disc surgery; indeed, the recovery of bladder function may be very slow, taking months to years.[79,80] From the urologic point of view, these patients need careful long-term follow-up.

Conclusions

Lateral intervertebral disc prolapse compressing unilateral nerve root(s) does not give rise to urinary, bowel, and/or sexual dysfunction. Detrusor contractions on urodynamic studies are indistinguishable from those of normal persons.

Intervertebral disc prolapse of the lumbar spine compressing bilateral nerve roots or the cauda equina can lead to urethrovesical dysfunction. In the great majority of cases it results in an areflexic detrusor. This areflexia is secondary to an impairment of the afferent, sensitive, branch of the sacral reflex arc which, in turn, influences its efferent, motor branch. The distal urethral sphincteric mechanism is usually intact.

There exists a particular form of lumbar disc protrusion that is well documented in the literature, with about 100 cases published, the majority in females in which the only clinical symptom is urinary retention. The desire to void is modified, with the patient describing hypogastric fullness. Physicians should suspect this condition when the bladder has a huge capacity, a significant postvoid residual urine, no bladder wall trabeculation, and a hyposensitive urethra and trigone during cystoscopy. Urodynamics will demonstrate a flat curve during the filling phase and an increased bladder wall compliance. The first desire to void is delayed, or even abolished. Electrophysiologic studies show an increased bulbocavernosus (or clitoridoanal) latency time. Radiologic exploration, CT scan and/or MRI, should confirm the clinical diagnosis (Figures 26.5 and 26.6).

Treatment is the surgical removal of the protruded disc. There is no consensus in the literature on the degree of urgency of this condition. Common sense dictates rapid intervention, when possible. Complete recovery of urethrovesical function may take months, or even years. An extended follow-up is indicated.

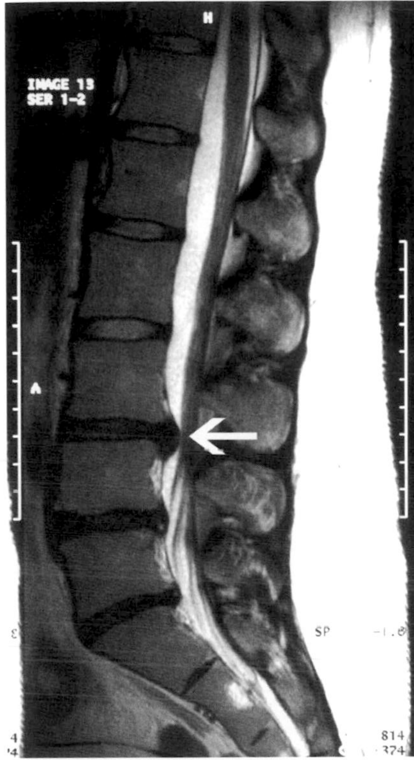

Figure 26.5

Magnetic resonance image (sagittal plane) of a sequestered discal fragment (arrow). Note the difference on MRI of the degenerated disc at the L3–L4 level, compared with normal intervertebral discs at more proximal levels. (Courtesy of Dr Marie-Christine Roy.)

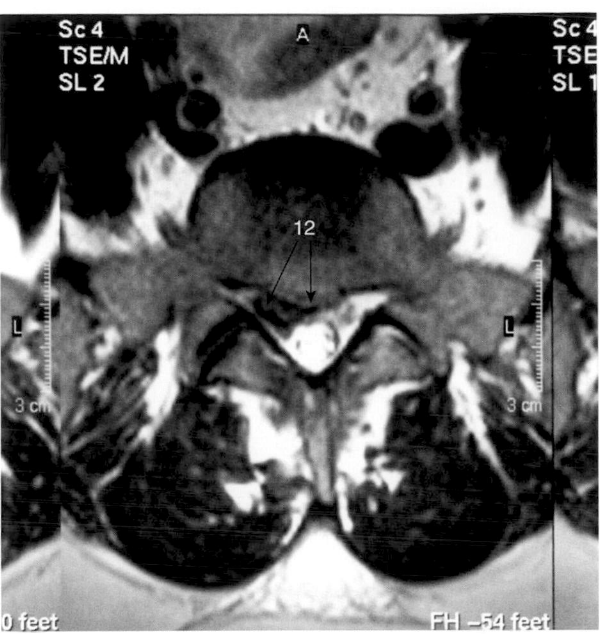

Figure 26.6

Magnetic resonance image (transverse plane). Right lateral protrusion of the herniated intervertebral disc: (1) disc fragment on the right side; (2) mid-line exophytic growth. (Courtesy of Dr Mario Séguin.)

References

1. Spinner M, Spencer PS. Nerve compression lesions of the upper extremity. A clinical and experimental review. Clin Orthop 1974; 104: 46–67.
2. Boden SD, Davis DO, Dina TS et al. Abnormal magnetic-resonance scans of the lumbar spine in asymptomatic subjects. A prospective investigation. J Bone Joint Surg Am 1990; 72: 403–8.
3. Williams AL, Haughton VM. Disc herniation and degenerative disc disease. In: Newton TH, Potts DG, eds. Modern Neuroradiology, Vol. 1, Computed Tomography of the Spine and Spinal Cord. 1983: 213–49.
4. Siebner HR, Faulhauer K. Frequency and specific surgical management of far lateral lumbar disc herniations. Acta Neurochir (Wien) 1990; 105: 124–31.
5. Dammers R, Koehler PJ. Lumbar disc herniation: level increases with age. Surg Neurol 2002; 58: 209–12.
6. Russell EG. Cervical disc disease. Radiol 1990; 177: 313–25.
7. Williams MP, Cherryman GR, Husband JE. Significance of thoracic disc herniation demonstrated by MR imaging. J Comput Assist Tomogr 1989; 13: 211–14.
8. Awwad EE, Martin DS, Smith KR Jr, Baker BK. Asymptomatic versus symptomatic herniated thoracic discs: their frequency and characteristics as detected by computed tomography after myelography. Neurosurgery 1991; 28: 180–6.
9. Dong D, Xu Z, Shi B et al. Urodynamic study in the neurogenic bladder dysfunction caused by intervertebral disk hernia. Neurourol Urodyn 2006; 25: 446–50.
10. Stillerman CB, Chen TC, Couldwell WT, Zhang W, Weiss MH. Experience in the surgical management of 82 symptomatic herniated thoracic discs and review of the literature. J Neurosurg 1998; 88: 623–33.
11. Scutellari PN, Rizzati R, Antinolfi G, Malfaccini F, Leprotti S, Campanati P. The value of computed tomography in the diagnosis of low back pain. A review of 2012 cases. Minerva Med 2005; 96: 41–59
12. Toribatake Y, Baba H, Kawahara N et al. The epiconus syndrome presenting with radicular-type neurological features. Spinal Cord 1997; 35: 163–70.
13. Goldman HB, Appell RA. Lumbar disc disease. In: Appell RA, ed. Voiding Dysfunction. Totowa, NJ. Humana, 2000: 149–62.
14. Jennet WB. A study of 25 cases of compression of the cauda equina by prolapsed intervertebral disc. J Neurol Neurosurg Psychiatry 1956; 19: 109–16.
15. Tay EC, Chacha PB. Midline prolapse of a lumbar intervertebral disc with compression of the cauda equina. J Bone Joint Surg Br 1979; 61–B: 43–6.
16. Nielsen B, de Nully M, Schmidt K, Iversen-Hansen RI. A urodynamic study of cauda equina syndrome due to lumbar disc herniation. Urol Int 1980; 35: 167–70.
17. Inui Y, Doita M, Ouchi K et al. Clinical and radiological features of lumbar spinal stenosis and disc herniation with neuropathic bladder. Spine 2004; 29: 869–73.
18. Mixter WJ, Barr JS. Rupture of the intervertebral disc with involvement of the spinal canal. N Engl J Med 1934; 211: 210–15.
19. Dandy WB. Serious complications of ruptured intervertebral disc. JAMA 1942; 119: 474–7.
20. Ver Brugghen A. Massive extrusions of the lumbar intervertebral disc. Surg Gyn Obstet 1945; 81: 269–77.
21. Waris W Lumbar disc herniation. Acta Chir Scand 1948 (Suppl 140): 1–134.
22. O'Connell JE. Protrusion of the lumbar intervertebral discs. A clinical review based on 500 cases treated by excision of the protrusion. J Bone Joint Surg Br 1951; 33–B: 8–30.
23. Eyre-Brook AL. A study of late results from disc operations. Br J Surg 1952; 39: 289.
24. Shephard RH. Diagnosis and prognosis of cauda equina syndrome produced by protrusion of lumbar disc. Br Med J 1959; 2: 1434–9.

25. Wilson PJ. Cauda equina compression due to intrathecal herniation of an intervertebral disk: a case report. Br J Surg 1962; 49: 423–6.
26. Scott PJ. Bladder paralysis in cauda equina lesions from disc prolapse. J Bone Joint Surg 1965; 47–B: 224–35.
27. Aho AJ, Auranen A, Pesonen K. Analysis of cauda equina symptoms in patients with lumbar disc prolapse. Preoperative and follow-up clinical and cystometric studies. Acta Chir Scand 1969; 135: 413–20.
28. Rosomoff HL, Johnson JD, Gallo AE et al. Cystometry in the evaluation of nerve root compression in the lumbar spine. Surg Gyn Obstet 1963; 117: 263–70.
29. Andersen JT, Bradley WE. Neurogenic bladder dysfunction in protruded lumbar disc and after laminectomy. Urology 1976; 8: 94–6.
30. Mosdal C, Iversen P, Iversen-Hansen R. Bladder neuropathy in lumbar disc disease. Acta Neurochir (Wien) 1979; 46: 281–6.
31. Gangai M. Acute urinary obstruction secondary to neurologic diseases. J Urol 1966; 95: 805–8.
32. Emmett JL, Love JG. Urinary retention in women caused by asymptomatic protruded lumbar disc: report of 5 cases. J Urol 1968; 99: 597–606.
33. Emmett JL, Love JG. Vesical dysfunction caused by protruded lumbar disc. J Urol 1971; 105: 86–91.
34. Malloch JD. Acute retention due to intervertebral disc prolapse. Br J Urol 1965; 37: 578.
35. Yarxley RP. Note on urinary retention due to intervertebral disc prolapse. Br J Urol 1966; 38: 324–5.
36. Ivanovici F. Urine retention: an isolated sign in some spinal cord disorders. J Urol 1970; 104: 284–6.
37. Ross JC, Jameson RM. Vesical dysfunction due to prolapsed disc. Br Med J 1971; 3: 752–4.
38. Kontturi M. Investigations into bladder dysfunction in prolapse lumbar intervertebral disc. Ann Chir Gynaecol Fenn Suppl 1968; 162: 1–53.
39. Cheek WR, Anchondo H, Raso E, Scott B. Neurogenic bladder and lumbar spine. Urology 1973; 2: 30–3.
40. Dan N, Golovsky D, Sharpe D. Urinary retention and intervertebral disc protrusion. Med J Aust 1980; 2: 258–60.
41. Susset JG, Peters ND, Cohen SI, Ghonhem GM. Early detection of neurogenic bladder dysfunction caused by protruded lumbar disc. Urology 1982; 20: 461–3.
42. Hsu CH. Herniated disk: an obscure cause of neurogenic bladder in males. Kans Med 1996; 97: 16–17.
43. Sylvester PA, McLoughlin J, Sibley GN et al. Neuropathic urinary retention in the absence of neurological signs. Postgrad Med J 1995; 71: 747–8.
44. Kontturi M, Harviainen S, Larmi TK. Atonic bladder in lumbar disc herniation. Acta Chir Scand Suppl 1966; 357: 232–5.
45. Jones DL, Moore T. The types of neuropathic bladder dysfunction associated with prolapsed lumbar intervertebral discs. Br J Urol 1973; 45: 39–43.
46. Fanciullacci F, Sandri S, Politi P, Zanollo A. Clinical, urodynamic and neurophysiological findings in patients with neuropathic bladder due to a lumbar intervertebral disc protrusion. Paraplegia 1989; 27: 354–8.
47. Gleave JR, Macfarlane R. Prognosis for recovery of bladder function following lumbar central disc prolapse. Br J Neurosurg 1990; 4: 205–9.
48. Gunterberg B, Norlén L, Stener B, Sundin T. Neurourologic evaluation after resection of the sacrum. Invest Urol 1975; 13: 183–8.
49. Rosomoff HL. The neurogenic bladder of lumbar disc syndromes. Trans Am Neurol Assoc 1964; 89: 249–51.
50. Delamarter RB, Bohlman HH, Bodner D, Biro C. Urologic function after experimental cauda equina compression. Cystometrograms versus cortical-evoked potentials. Spine 1990; 15: 864–70.
51. Kostuik JP, Harrington I, Alexander D et al. Cauda equina syndrome and lumbar disc herniation. J Bone Joint Surg Am 1986; 68: 386–91.
52. Chuang TY, Cheng H, Chan RC et al. Neurourologic findings in patients with traumatic thoracolumbar vertebra junction lesions. Arch Phys Med Rehabil 2001; 82: 375–9.
53. Bartolin Z, Savic I, Persec Z. Relationship between clinical data and urodynamic findings in patients with lumbar intervertebral disc protrusion. Urol Res 2002; 30: 219–22.
54. Murayama N, Yamanishi T, Yashuda K et al. Urodynamic studies in patients with intervertebral prolapse. Nippon Hinyokika Gakkai Zasshi 1991; 82: 607–12.
55. Jameson RM. Urological management in non-traumatic paraplegia: disc protrusions, multiple sclerosis and spinal metastasis. Paraplegia 1976; 13: 228–34.
56. Hellström P, Kortelainen P, Kontturi M. Late urodynamic findings after surgery for cauda equina syndrome caused by a prolapsed lumbar intervertebral disc. J Urol 1986; 135: 308–12.
57. Yamanishi T, Yasuda K, Sakakibara R et al. Detrusor overactivity and penile erection in patients with lower spine lesions. Eur Urol 1998; 34: 360–4.
58. Shin JC, Park CI, Kim HJ, Lee IY. Significance of low compliance bladder in cauda equina injury. Spinal Cord 2002; 40: 650–5.
59. Norlèn L, Dahlstrom A, Sundin T, Svedmyr N. The adrenergic innervation and adrenergic receptor activity of the feline urinary bladder and urethra in the normal state and after hypogastric and/or parasympathetic denervation. Scand J Urol Nephrol 1976; 10: 177–84.
60. Murnaghan GF, Gowland SP, Rose M et al. Experimental neurogenic disorders of the bladder after section of the cauda equina. Br J Urol 1979; 51: 518–23.
61. Sandri SD, Fanciullacci F, Zanollo A. Pharmacologic tests in low compliance areflexic bladders. Proc 15th Annual Meeting ICS, London, 1987: 162.
62. Sandri SD, Fanciullacci F, Politi P, Zanollo A. Urinary disorders in intervertebral disc prolapse. Neurourol Urodyn 1987; 6: 11–19.
63. McGuire EJ. Urodynamic evaluation after abdomino-perineal resection and lumbar intervertebral disc herniation. Urology 1975; 6: 63–70.
64. Vodušek DB, Fowler CJ, Deletis V, Podnar S. Clinical neurophysiology of pelvic floor disorders. Suppl Clin Neurophysiol 2000; 53: 220–7.
65. Podnar S. Clinical reappraisal of referrals to electromyography and nerve conduction studies. Eur J Neurol 2005; 12: 150–5.
66. Podnar S, Tršinar B, Vodušek D. Bladder dysfunction in patients with cauda equina lesions. Neurourol Urodyn 2006; 25: 23–31.
67. Podnar S. Nomenclature of electrophysiologically tested sacral reflexes. Neurourol Urodyn 2006; 25: 95–7.
68. Amarenco G, Kerdraon J. Clinical value of ipsi- and contralateral sacral reflex latency measurement: a normative data study in man. Neurourol Urodyn 2000; 19: 565–76.
69. Rosomoff HL, Johnston JD, Gallo HE et al. Cystometry as an adjunct in the evaluation of lumbar disc syndromes. J Neurosurg 1970; 33: 67–74.
70. Bartolin Z, Vilendecic M, Derezic D. Bladder function after surgery for lumbar intervertebral disc protrusion. J Urol 1999; 161: 1885–7.
71. Podnar S. Saddle sensation is preserved in a few patients with cauda equina or conus medullaris lesions. Eur J Neurol 2007; 14: 48–53.
72. Guest J, Eleraky MA, Apostolides PJ, Dickman CA, Sonntag VK. Traumatic central cord syndrome: results of surgical management. J Neurosurg 2002; 97(1 Suppl): 25–32.
73. Yamanishi T, Yasuda K, Yuki T et al. Urodynamic evaluation of surgical outcome in patients with urinary retention due to central lumbar disc prolapse. Neurourol Urodyn 2003; 22: 670–5.
74. Robinson RG. Massive protrusions of lumbar discs. Br J Surg 1965; 52: 858–65.
75. Dinning TA, Schaeffer HR. Discogenic compression of the cauda equina: a surgical emergency. Aust NZ J Surg 1993; 63: 927–34.
76. Kennedy JG, Soffe KE, McGrath A et al. Predictors of outcome in cauda equina syndrome. Eur Spine J 1999; 8: 317–22.
77. Shapiro S. Medical realities of cauda equina syndrome secondary to lumbar disc herniation. Spine 2000; 25: 348–51.
78. Gleave JR, Macfarlane R. Cauda equina syndrome: what is the relationship between timing of surgery and outcome? Br J Neurosurg 2002; 16: 325–8.
79. Leroi AM, Berkelmans I, Rabehenoina C et al. Results of therapeutic management of vesico-urethral and anorectal disorders in 20 patients with cauda equina syndrome. Neurochirurgie (Paris) 1994; 40: 301–6.
80. Chang HS, Nakagawa H, Mizuno J. Lumbar herniated disc presenting with cauda equina syndrome. Long-term follow-up of four cases. Surg Neurol 2000; 53: 100–4.

27

The cauda equina syndrome

Tala AL Afraa, Abdulrahman J. Sabbagh, and Line Leboeuf

Cauda equina refers to that part of the nervous system which is situated below the level of the conus medullaris, within the spinal canal. It consists of both sensory and motor nerve bundles.[1] The length of the spinal cord is shorter than the vertebral canal. As a consequence of the relative inequality in the rates of growth of the spinal cord and the vertebral column, the nerve roots, which in the early embryo passed transversally outward to reach their respective intervertebral foramina, become more and more oblique in direction from above downward during normal development, so that the lumbar and sacral nerves descend almost vertically to reach their point of exit from the vertebral canal. From the appearance of these nerves at their attachment to the spinal cord, and from their great length, they are collectively named the cauda equina.[2] Injury to the nerves of the cauda equina can result in the so-called cauda equina syndrome (CES), which refers to the simultaneous compression of multiple lumbosacral nerve roots below the level of the conus medullaris. This is typically characterized by low back pain, sciatalgia, saddle and perineal hypoesthesia or anesthesia, decreased anal tone, absent ankle, knee, or bulbocavernosus reflexes, variable lower extremity motor and sensory loss, as well as bowel and bladder dysfunction.[2] Mixter and Barr are thought to be the first to report this clinical syndrome, in 1934.[3–5] Diagnosis of a cauda equina lesion may be complicated and require neuroradiologic imaging together with bladder, bowel, sexual, and somatic function tests. Management may be difficult and require prolonged intensive and long-term rehabilitation.[2,6]

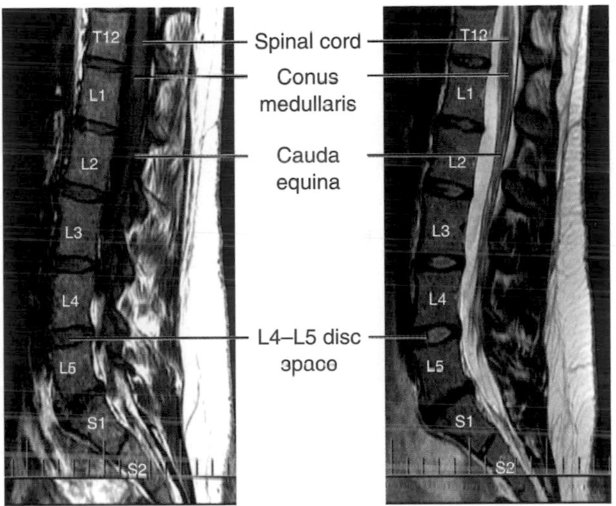

Figure 27.1
Normal MRI of the lumbosacral region.

Neuroanatomy

The relationship between the terminal part of the spinal cord, the conus terminalis, and the vertebral column changes during intrauterine development, in the neonate, in infancy, and in the adult. This is because the vertebral column grows more rapidly in the longitudinal direction than does the spinal cord.[7,8] In the third month of intrauterine life, the spinal cord fills the whole length of the vertebral canal. In neonates, the spinal cord terminates at the lumbosacral junction.[7] During infancy and early childhood, the spinal cord terminates between the first and third lumbar vertebrae,[7,8] whereas in adults, it may terminate at a level anywhere from the T12 vertebral body to the L2 and L3 intervertebral space.[1,2,7–9] Arai et al studied 602 patients aged between 8 months and 84 years and found the location of the conus medullaris at the middle one-third of L1[10] (Figure 27.1).

The S2–S5 sacral roots are located in the dorsal aspect of the thecal sac. The lumbar and the first sacral roots have an oblique, layered pattern as they ascend. Within each root the motor bundle is situated anteromedially to its respective sensory bundle. Invaginations of arachnoid keeps the nerve roots in a fixed relationship to one another.

The lower part of the cord is tapered to form the conus medullaris from which a prolongation of the pia mater forms the filum terminale, which extends downwards to be

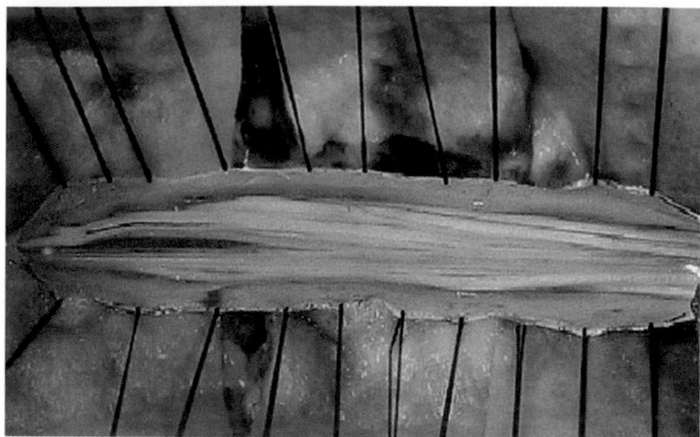

Figure 27.2
Intraoperative picture shows the cauda equina nerve fibers.

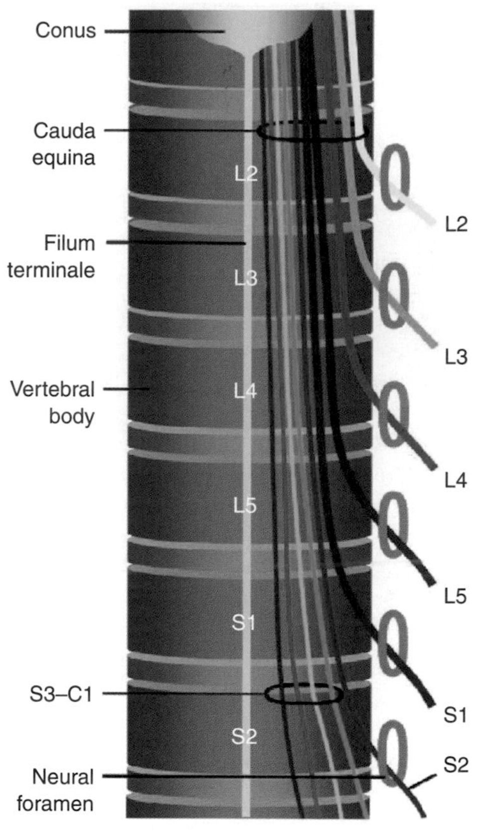

Figure 27.3
The cauda equina nerves. L, lumbar; S, sacral; C, coccygeal.

attached to the coccyx.[1,2] The conus medullaris contains the myelomeres of the five sacral nerve roots S1–S5.[1,2,7] The cauda equina is the site of transition from the central to the peripheral nervous system[1,2,7] (Figures 27.2 and 27.3).

The cauda equina nerve roots give the sensory and motor innervation to the lower urinary tract, lower bowel, urethral and anal sphincter, sexual organs, lower extremities, and the pelvic floor[1] (Table 27.1).

The sacral parasympathetic plexus arise from S2, S3, and S4 sacral nerve roots and join the sympathetic fibers to form the pelvic plexuses branches to give innervations to the bladder, urethra, male and female genital organs, rectum, and blood vessels.[11–18] The somatic nerve which originates from Onuf's nucleus (S2–4) via the pudendal nerve supplies the rhabdosphincter of the urethral sphincter and anal sphincter, and the levator ani and transversus perinei muscle.[19–22]

Pathophysiology

CES is a result of compression of the cauda equina nerve roots within the spinal canal, below the level of L1.[25] Any space-occupying lesion that causes narrowing of the anteroposterior diameter of the dural sac can directly exert a mechanical effect on the nerve root.[4,7,26,27] This compression will be responsible for Wallerian degeneration, decreased blood flow, intraneuronal edema, and axonal transport block, resulting in neural dysfunction.[28]

Kobayashi et al, in a study using 12 dogs, applied mechanical compression on lumbar nerves at the level of L7. They concluded that Wallerian degeneration, macrophage aggregation, inflammatory reaction, breaking of the blood–nerve barrier, and increased vascular permeability led to intraradicular edema. This may be responsible for radiculitis and pain.[29,30]

In a study on 21 rats, Igarashi et al demonstrated that acute compression on nerve roots caused an increase in endoneurial flow pressure, a decrease in blood flow within the nerve fiber, and endoneurial edema, thus possibly causing nerve dysfunction and pain.[31]

Delamarter et al[32] and Bodner et al,[33] in a study using 20 pure bred female beagles, constricted the cauda equina at the 7th lumbar level by 25%, 50%, and 75%. The three groups were evaluated by cystometrogram (CMG) and cortical-evoked potential. The first two groups had normal CMGs but significant changes in the cortical-evoked potential. They also found mild motor weakness, but no urinary incontinence. However, in the 75% constricted group there was urinary and fecal incontinence, as well as paraparesis of the lower limbs. The CMG and cortical-evoked potential curves appeared flat. They concluded that cystometry was not sensitive enough until the nerve roots were severely compressed. The cortical-evoked potential was the most sensitive indicator of neural compression.

McGuire studied the effect of sacral denervation on the bladder and urethra. They found that complete sacral denervation caused loss of anal sphincter tone, as well as loss

Table 27.1 *Lumbosacral nerves and their distribution*[23,24]

	Origin	Motor	Sensory
Iliohypogastric nerve	L1	Internal and external oblique muscle	Lower anterior abdominal wall and pubis
Ilioinguinal nerve	L1		Sensation to the mons pubis and anterior scrotum or libia majora
Genitofemoral nerve	L1, L2	Genital branch to the cremaster and dartos muscles	Femoral part transmits sensation from the anterior thigh below the inguinal ligament and from the anterior scrotum
Femoral nerve	L2, L3, L4	Psoas muscle and iliacus muscle Extensor of the knee	Sensation from the anteromedial portion of the lower extremity
Obterator nerve	L2, L3, L4	Adductor muscle of the thigh	
Lumbosacral trunk	L4, L5	Posterior thigh and lower leg	Posterior thigh and lower leg
Posterior femoral cutaneous	S2, S3		Anterior part of the perineum and posterior part of the scrotum
Pudendal nerve	S2, S3, S4	Erectile tissue External anal sphincter Ischiocavernosus Bulbospongiosus Transverses perinei muscles Levator ani and striated urethral sphincter	Sensation from the penis, perianal skin and posterior part of the scrotum
The nervi erigentes	S2, S3, S4 (pelvic plexus)	Rectum Bladder Seminal vesicle Prostate	
Pelvic somatic efferent nerve	S2, S3, S4	Levator ani and striated urethral sphincter	

of detrusor and external urethral sphincter activity. The internal urethral sphincter was not affected.[34]

Two types have been described: cauda equina syndrome incomplete (CESI), characterized by altered urinary sensation, loss of desire to void, weak urinary stream, and straining during micturition; and cauda equina syndrome retention (CESR), characterized by painless urinary retention, dribbling, and overflow incontinence.[35]

Incidence and prevalence of CES

The incidence and prevalence of CES in the general population are not known. Podnar reported an incidence rate of 3.4 cases per million and a prevalence of 8.9 per 100 000.[36] The prevalence is much higher among patients with lower back pain, about 40 in 100 000.[37,38] The incidence of CES in spinal pathology ranges from 1 to 5%, depending on the origin of the disease.[3,39–41] Males in the fourth and fifth decades of life are most prone to CES secondary to intervertebral disc herniation.[3,25,40,42–46]

Etiology of CES

Any lesion causing narrowing of the spinal canal and compression of the cauda equina nerves below the level of the conus medullaris can lead to CES. Table 27.2 summarizes the different etiologies of CES.

Congenital causes

Meningomyelocele, spina bifida, dystematomyelia, congenital dermoid sinus, or congenital midline tumor (dermoid, epidermoid, teratoma, lipoma).[1,2]

Table 27.2 *Causes of CES*

Congenital	Spina bifida, meningomyelocele, congenital midline tumors
Degenerative disease	Central lumbar disc herniation, spondylosis, spondylolisthesis, Paget's disease
Traumatic	MVA, GSW, fall from height
Neoplasia	Primary or metastatic
Iatrogenic	Spinal anesthesia, orthopedic and neurosurgical procedures
Vascular	Arteriovenous malformation
Infection	TB of spine, Herpes simplex infection, etc.
Miscellaneous	Leukemia, lymphoma, rheumatoid arthritis, neurosarcoidosis, etc.

MVA, motor vehicle accident; GSW, gun shot wound; TB, tuberculosis.

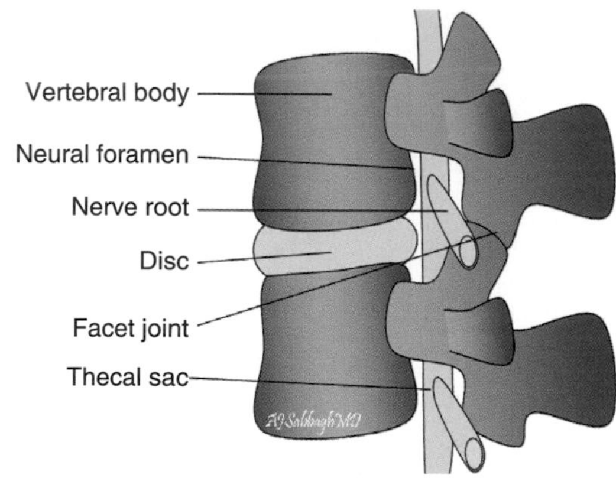

Figure 27.4
L4 and L5 vertebrae, the intervertebral disc, and the relation to the thecal sac (cauda equina nerves are within the sac and not shown here).

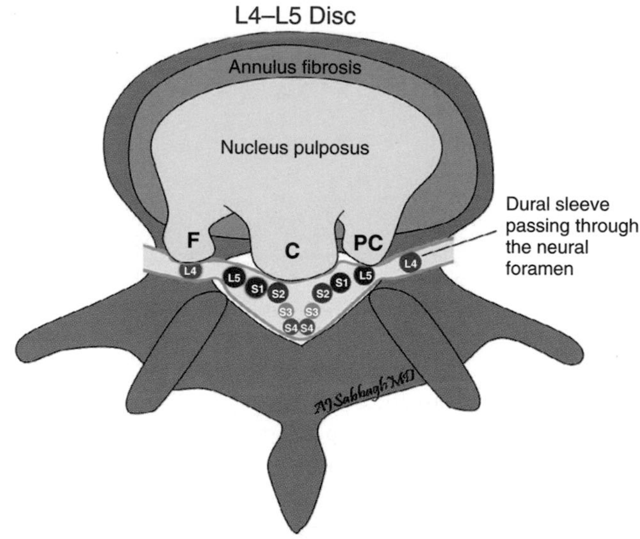

Figure 27.5
Types of disc herniation. Foraminal disc herniation (F) compresses the L4 root as it exits the spinal canal. Paracentral herniation (PC) compresses the L5 root. Central disc herniation (C) compresses the remaining sacral roots. Foraminal and paracentral herniation will not compress nerve roots bilaterally, so cannot result in CES. On the contrary, central herniation compresses nerve roots bilaterally, so being responsible for CES. L lumbar; S sacral.

Lumbar disc herniation

It is well known that lumbar disc herniation can cause compression of the cauda equina.[3,27,40,46–48] About 60–85% of lumbar disc herniations occur centrally.[48] Central disc protrusion is the most common cause of CES[39] (Figure 27.4). The most frequent intervertebral space involved is L4–L5, followed by L5–S1 and L3–L4[4,39,40,46,48–50] (see Figure 26.8, Chapter 26). CES is a serious complication of lumbar disc herniation.[42] About 1 to 2% of lumbar disc herniation cases will present with CES.[46] About 2–6% of lumbar discoidectomies are performed because of CES.[45]

Median disc herniation causes significant urinary symptoms compared with paramedian and lateral herniation.[51] This may be due to the direct effect the median compression exerts on the parasympathetic fibers bilaterally which are located at the postero-median side in the dural sac[26,27] (Figure 27.5).

Traumatic injury

Trauma of the lower lumbar spine is the second most common cause of CES.[41,42,52,53] Thongtrangan et al reported 17 patients who developed CES from postspinal trauma occurring as a result of motor vehicle accidents, falls from height, and gun shot wounds. The severity of the initial injury has a role in recovery, with gun shot wounds tending to be the more severe, and often leading to a less complete recovery.[41] Sacral fractures have also been reported as causes of CES.[54,55]

Iatrogenic injury

During spinal anesthesia nerve damage can be due to needle trauma, neurotoxicity, hematoma, or abscess formation.[56] Loo et al presented 6 patients with CES after spinal anesthesia where hyperbaric 5% lignocaine was used. Direct neurotoxicity was most likely the cause of the syndrome.[57] Rigler et al also reported 4 cases due to continuous spinal anesthesia.[58] Subdural hematoma may be secondary to spinal anesthesia,[59] and epidural catheter placement or removal.[60] CES may follow orthopedic and/or neurosurgical procedures. It is a rare complication of disc hernia surgery, ranging between 0.2 and 1%.[61,62] McLaren and Bailey reported on 6 patients with CES after lumbar discoidectomy. Four factors could be responsible for CES including postoperative edema, haematoma, retained disc fragments, and Gelfoam.[63] It should be noted that large amounts of Gelfoam by itself can lead to CES.[64] Schoenecker et al reported on12 patients who developed CES after vertebral arthrodesis for spondylolisthesis.[65] Another possible cause may be free fat grafts following discoidectomy.[66]

Neoplasia

Tumors of the lower spine can cause compression of the nerve roots leading to CES. Patients with CES caused by neoplasm usually have a nonspecific disease, long history of back pain, or paresthesia.[67] Tumors of the spine can be primary (myxopapillary ependymomas, schwannomas, paragangliomas, astrocytomas, chordomas, giant cell tumors,[67] meningeal carcinomatosis,[68] spinal epidural lipomatosis,[69] etc. The metastatic tumors which can be responsible for the development of CES include lung cancer, breast cancer, lymphoma, colorectal cancer, prostate cancer, thyroid cancer,[67] renal cell carcinoma,[70] etc. Leukemia and lymphoma are rare causes of CES but they had been reported (for example: leukemia,[71] epidural lymphoma,[72,73] non-Hodgkin lymphoma involving the cauda equina,[74] Hodgkin's disease[75]). A few benign lesions have been reported to cause CES, such as intrathecal sacral cyst[76] and lumbosacral arachnoid cyst.[77]

Spinal stenosis

There are two types of spinal stenosis, congenital and acquired, both of which can cause CES. The congenital type includes dysplastic spondylolisthiasis[65] and congenital spinal stenosis.[78] Acquired spinal stenosis, the more common form, can also contribute to CES and includes spondylosis, ankylopoetic spondylolisthesis, Paget's disease,[48] longstanding ankylosing spondylitis,[79] and spondylolytic spondylolisthesis.[80]

Miscellaneous causes

Vascular causes: Only a few cases of CES caused by vascular disease have been reported, such as arteriovenous malformation,[2] inferior vena cava thrombosis,[81] lumbar vertebral hemangioma,[82–85] and hemorrhage from spinal ependymoma.[85]

Infectious causes: Infection can lead to the formation of abscesses that can cause compression of the nerve roots. Some reported cases include gnathostomiasis,[86] epidural abscess,[87] tuberculosis of the spine,[88] pneumococcal meningitis,[89] and herpes viral infection (viral sacral myeloradiculitis).[90]

Inflammatory causes: More rarely, inflammation may cause CES. This may include: primary angiitis of the central nervous system,[91] lumbar spinal rheumatoid discitis, neurosarcoidosis,[92,93] etc.

Clinical manifestations

CES includes several symptoms and signs, characteristic of this entity.[38,10,42,46,49,86,94] Commonly, patients present with a triad of symptoms: saddle anesthesia , lower extremity weakness, and bladder and/or bowel dysfunction,[38] but may also exhibit sexual dysfunction as well.[26,27,35]

The symptoms and signs develop within a few hours in more than 85% of patients.[39,46] Tandon and Sankaran described three different presentations, which are: sudden onset of symptoms; a long history of lower back pain (LBP) followed by a sudden onset of bladder disturbance; and chronic lower back pain with sciatalgia which gradually progress to CES.[95] The type of presentation defines the prognosis and outcome.[39,49] Most patients present with a combination of sacral dysfunctions (LUT, bowel, and sexual dysfunction).[53]

The incidence of the most frequent clinical presentations is summarized in Table 27.3.

Low back pain and sciatalgia

More than 83% of CES patients present with LBP and uni- or bilateral sciatalgia.[38,39,43,45,46,53] About 70% of the patients have a past history of LBP, while 30% of them have sudden onset of pain within a period of 1 or 2 days.[42,46,49,53,79] A history of chronic LBP increases the risk of permanent urinary dysfunction by 11 times and rectal dysfunction by 25 times.[79] Radiculopathy appeared in 90% of patients.[49] Such radiculopathy, projecting pain to the corresponding dermatomal area, is due to compression of

Table 27.3 *Summary of common clinical presentations*	
Low back pain	83%
Bilateral or unilateral sciatalgia	90%
Saddle anesthesia	96%
Lower limb weakness	84%
Urinary retention	90%
Incontinence	74%
Fecal incontinence	85%
Constipation	70%
Sexual dysfunction	85%

the dorsal root associated with an inflammatory reaction (radiculitis).[48] Pain may also be due to ischemia resulting from compression of the sacral nerve roots.[94] Kennedy et al reported sciatalgia in all their patients except one. They found that bilateral sciatalgia is a common presenting symptom. It is considered to be a poor prognostic factor.[39]

Motor deficit

Motor deficit can present as a progressive lower extremity weakness and may progress to paraparesis.[39,41–43,45,49,62,63,96,97] Shapiro reported on 44 patients with CES; 84% of them were unable to stand or walk because of pain and foot weakness.[46] The deep tendon reflex may also be weak or even absent.[39,41,43,45,49,63,98]

Sensory deficit

Cauda equina patients usually present with numbness, anesthesia in the corresponding dermatome of the lower limbs, and saddle hypoesthesia.[50] Saddle sensory loss is a useful clinical sign for CES diagnosis, identifying patients who need immediate lumbosacral imaging.[99] Saddle hypoesthesia is present in almost all these patients.[39,41,45,46] Decreased sensation starts at the perineal and sacral regions, and then progresses to the feet.[63] Podnar and colleagues reported perianal sensory loss in 96% of patients and this significantly correlated with lower urinary tract dysfunction.[53,99] Kennedy et al concluded that the presence of complete perineal sensation loss is significantly correlated with a poor outcome following decompression.[39] However, when only saddle hypoesthesia and not complete anesthesia was present, this was not an indicator for poor outcome.[39] Buchner and Schittenwolf found that the absence of complete perianal and saddle anesthesia correlated with a better outcome after decompression.[43]

Vesicourethral dysfunction

There are a variety of lower urinary tract symptoms commonly found in patients with CES.[42] These symptoms may be found in as many as 89% of patients.[98] CES patients may experience a disturbance in bladder emptying, including acute urinary retention, a feeling of retention, loss of desire to void, micturition with straining, poor stream, and altered urethral sensation.[3,25,27,39,41,46,63,98]

The presence of both LBP and urinary retention is an extremely strong indicator of CES in most cases (sensitivity: 90%, specificity 95%).[38,46] Urinary incontinence, specifically overflow incontinence, is another symptom which may be present in patients with CES.[38,41,43,45,46,53] Podnar et al noted that stress urinary incontinence was the second most common complaint in these patients, more pronounced in women than in men (74% in women and 54% in men). Furthermore, lower urinary tract symptoms affect quality of life in 88% and interfere with sexual activity in 71% of patients.[53]

In a study of 56 patients with CES, McCarthy found 55% had urinary incontinence and 60% had urinary retention.[34] It should be noted that bladder dysfunction is significantly related to the degree of cauda equina compression.[27,32]

Bowel dysfunction

Cauda equina patients may present with fecal incontinence or constipation, incontinence being more frequent and occurring in as many as 85% of cases.[42,43,98,100] Patients may present with intermittent fecal incontinence, liquid stool incontinence, or flatus incontinence; the latter is the most common type.[49,100]

Podnar studied bowel dysfunction in 67 patients with CES. He found that fecal incontinence and constipation were more frequent than in the general population. Fecal incontinence was significantly associated with decreased perianal sensation. Constipation was found mostly in women. Furthermore, 39% of patients reported loss of sensation during defecation. In these cases, constipation may be due to damage to the sacral parasympathetic nerves and slow colon transit.[100]

Anal sphincter tone is diminished or absent in up to 80% of patients. [38,41,49] There is a significant correlation between anal sphincter weakness and poor prognosis.[39]

Sexual dysfunction

Sexual dysfunction is also a common symptom of CES:[25,53,62,94,98] It could be due to damage to the parasympathetic nerves S2–S4.[53,98] About 85% of patients have some degree of sexual dysfunction, including erectile dysfunction and impairment of ejaculation.[53,98] Women experience vaginal anesthesia and numbness; whereas in men the problem manifests as a failure to begin or maintain erection.[46] Prolonged cauda equina compression may be responsible for increased male sexual dysfunction.[46] However, age is strongly associated with the severity of sexual dysfunction in these patients.[53,98]

Investigation

Clinical diagnosis

Clinical history: Early recognition and diagnosis is very important because CES can lead to significant physical and mental disability.[49] Late or missed diagnoses may have significant medicolegal consequences as well.[49,101] A detailed voiding history should be obtained.[3,25,53] Podnar et al used the International Continence Society's Lower Urinary Tract Symptom Questionnaire to evaluate the urinary symptoms of their patients,[53] but other similar questionnaires may also be useful.

Physical examination: A neurologic examination should be performed to evaluate the motor and sensory deficit including deep tendon reflex (knee and ankle), perianal sensation, and anal sphincter tone.[46,49,53,98,100]

Laboratory work-up: A full blood count, chemistry, electrolyte, fasting blood sugar, and sedimentation rate should be considered. In cases where infectious causes are suspected, the following tests are recommended: syphilis, lyme serology,[2,48] cerebrospinal fluid analysis, bacteriology, viral studies, and venereal serology.[90]

Radiologic evaluation

Plain film: This may indicate areas that need further investigation.[38]

Magnetic resonance imaging: MRI of the spine proved to be effective in viewing the cauda equina region,[102] and is considered to be the gold standard today for confirmation and localization of the lesion, especially in patients with disc herniation and where soft tissue visualization may be important.[7,38] MRI does not expose patients to radiation, but it does have several disadvantages. It is not available in every medical center, it requires more time to deliver complete images, it is not suitable for patients with ferromagnetic implants, and finally it is not suitable for claustrophobic patients.[7]

Computed tomography: CT scan is the best way to assess bone anatomy, especially in cases of spinal trauma;[7,41] however, it has limitations when used to examine disc herniation and epidural or subdural hematoma.

Computed tomography combined with myelography: CT-MG has been used as a diagnostic tool by several authors.[7,27,38,40,48,61] Narrowing of the anteroposterior diameter of the dural sac to less than 8 mm is significantly correlated with neuropathic bladder dysfunction.[27]

Urologic evaluation

Cystoscopy: When performing cystoscopy in patients with CES, characteristic signs include decreased or absent urethral sensation during instrumentation, suprapubic fullness, rather than real desire to void at capacity, and absence of bladder wall trabeculation.[103]

Flowmetry: Only a few authors have studied free flowmetry in patients with CES. In the majority of cases, the maximum and average flow rates were reduced.[3,25,27,47,94] However, Mosdal et al reported normal flowmetry in 50% of their patients.[47] The shape of the flowmetry curve can indicate abdominal straining during micturition, in case of which a pressure–flow study should demonstrate hypo- or acontractile detrusor.[3,25,47,94]

Postvoid residual urine: This can be measured with a catheter or by ultrasound. Although if Mosdal et al[47] and Nielsen et al[3] reported that all their patients were able to empty the bladder completely, Podnar et al found that about 40% of males with CES had a postvoid residual urine of more than 100 ml Repeated postvoid residual measurements are therefore recommended.[53]

Urodynamic studies: These are the best diagnostic tool to evaluate lower urinary tract function. Rosomoff studied 100 patients with lumbar disc herniation. Abnormal urodynamic studies were found in 83% of them. The authors suggested that cystometry was the best test to diagnose bladder abnormality in patients with CES.[104] Inui et al studied 34 patients with CES secondary to lumbar disc herniation and/or lumbar spinal stenosis. They found that 60% of patients had subjective urinary symptoms which were confirmed by urodynamic studies, whereas the other 40% had no urologic symptoms but urodynamic studies revealed neuropathic bladder.[27] Kennedy et al recommended performing urodynamic studies at initial presentation when CES is suspected.[39]

Videourodynamics: During the filling phase, bladder sensitivity, manifested by a delay in the sensation of first desire to void,[3,47] increased bladder capacity, and increased bladder wall compliance will be noted. The detrusor is usually stable,[3,25,47] however detrusor overactivity, low compliance, and reduced bladder capacity may also be found in cauda equina patients. This may be due to decentralization of parasympathetic ganglia or irritation of the lower sacral roots, occurring in about 20% of patients.[25,53,105] Hellstrom et al, in a study of 20 patient with CES, did not find patients with low bladder compliance and detrusor-sphincter dyssynergia.[25] Light et al studied 13 patients with traumatic CES via videourodynamics and found that all 13 patients had bladder neck incompetence. In these patients, neurophysiologic tests revealed evidence of lower motor neuron lesions.[106] Similar findings have been previously reported by Nordling et al.[107] Most authors report either detrusor underactivity or acontractile detrusor during pressure–flow studies.[3,25,47,53,90,94,104,106,108,109] Pavlakis et al studied 56 patients with conus medullaris or cauda equina injury by cystometry and electromyography (EMG). They found that 93% of them had noncontractile detrusor, together with abnormal perineal EMG changes.[9] There is a strong correlation between the presence of saddle anesthesia and detrusor areflexia. The presence of both these symptoms is associated with poor outcome.[94]

Urethral pressure profile: Hellstrom et al, in a study of 20 patients, reported normal UPP in all patients except one, who had low maximum urethral closure pressure.[25] Kontturi reported normal UPP in all his patients.[109] McGuire reported that complete sacral denervation does not cause a loss of urethral profile unless it is close to the area of the pelvic muscle innervation.[34]

Ice water test: The IWT has been reported to differentiate upper from lower motor neuron lesions. It is performed by rapidly filling the bladder with 100 ml of 4°C sterile saline solution. The test is positive in more than 90% of patients with upper motor neuron lesions, whereas it is almost always negative in lower motor neuron lesions.[110–113] Bradley and Andersen studied 21 patients with cauda equina and conus medullaris lesions by means of urodynamics, EMG, and the IWT. They found that the IWT was less indicative of lower motor lesions than were the other tests.[114]

Neurophysiologic evaluation

The neurophysiologic tests can be used to evaluate patients with sacral dysfunction, i.e. lower urinary tract, anorectal, and sexual dysfunction. In this respect, useful tests include EMG, concentric needle EMG (CNEMG), motor unit potential (MUPs), interference pattern (IP), motor evoked potential (MEP), and evoked pressure curve (EPC).[115] These tests are highly specialized and should be done in conjunction with a clinical neurophysiologist.[115]

EMG allows evaluation of the bulbocavernosus reflex. It is sensitive in revealing the integrity of the S2–S4 reflex arc.[115]

CNEMG is commonly used to evaluate the striated urethral and anal sphincters. It was reported to be helpful in diagnosing dysfunctional voiding in females.[115] Podnar and colleagues used CNEMG to evaluate bladder, bowel, and sexual (dys)function. They found that CNEMG was abnormal in more than 80% of patients with CES.[53,98–100] CNEMG is the most informative test to detect both denervation and reinnervation in cauda equina lesions.[116]

MUP and IP are sophisticated tests used to evaluate the external anal sphincter. MUPs are prolonged and polyphasic in the case of CES.[115]

MEP and EPC: Schmid et al studied 33 patients (14 with cauda equina lesions) with MEP responses from the urethral compressive muscle by inserting a bipolar ring electrode mounted on a catheter and positioned at the level of the external urethral sphincter during a urodynamic study. They found the EPC latencies were significantly delayed in patients with cauda equina lesions. This procedure has several advantages, including painless stimulation, atraumatic recording, only one catheterization, and simultaneous measurement of intra-sphincter pressure and EMG.[117] MEP is a useful test in CES because it can reveal abnormalities of nerve root conduction shortly after the onset of symptoms and may identify the site of the lesion. EMG requires 2–3 weeks to exhibit a positive result.[118]

Evaluation of bowel dysfunction

Podnar studied bowel dysfunction in 88 patients by means of a questionnaire which included 18 questions to assess consistency of feces, sensation during defecation, pain, constipation, and other bowel-related medical problems; an EMG; and the assessment of perianal sensation. The study showed that constipation is more common in females and significantly associated with low or absent perianal sensation.[100]

Evaluation of sexual dysfunction

The evaluation of sexual dysfunction is mainly undertaken through a detailed history. Podnar and colleagues studied the sexual function of 46 patients with documented CES. They used the International Index of Erectile Function (IIEF), which consists of 15 questions (6 questions to assess erectile function, 3 questions regarding intercourse satisfaction, 2 questions for orgasmic function, 2 questions concerning sexual desire, and 2 questions about overall satisfaction). Evaluation of the deep tendon reflex and the sensation of the perianal region, and EMG of the external anal sphincter completed the investigation. The authors concluded that sexual dysfunction is strongly correlated with age of the patient, but not with sensory loss or EMG findings.[98,100]

Table 27.4 *Recovery of bladder function following decompression (modified from Buchner and Schiltenwolf[43])*

Authors	No of patients	Decompression within 48 hours	Decompresion after 48 hours	Mean follow up (years)	Percent recovery
Kostuik et al 1986[97]	31	10 patients	21 patients	8	77
Hellstrom et al 1986[25]	17	14 patients	3 patients	2.8	59
Shapiro 1993[40]	14	7 patients	7 patients	3.3	72
Kennedy et al 1999[39]	19	14 patients	5 patients	2	70
Shapiro 2000[46]	44	20 patients	24 patients	5.3	95 in early surgery 63 in delayed surgery
Buchner and Schiltenwolf 2002[43]	22	18 patients	4 patients	3.9	77
Thongtrangan et al 2004[41]	17	All patients		1	100
McCarthy et al 2007[49]	42	26 patients	16 patients	5	88

Management

Management of CES should be directed toward the underlying causes. Detailed treatment options are beyond the scope of this chapter. Some general principles and controversial aspects in the timing of surgical intervention will be discussed.

Nonsurgical management

Some cases of CES can be treated medically, for instance infectious causes, which can be treated with antibiotics or antiviral medications.[90] Upon diagnosis of CES, and while the patient waits for a more definitive therapy, he/she will receive a high dose of intravenous steroid, analgesia, and catheterization if retention or high residual urine is present.[38]

Surgical management

The timing of early or delayed surgical decompression is still controversial. Several authors support early decompression, while others report favorable outcome with delayed decompression.[7,41,42,49]

Early decompression within 48 hours: CES is considered to be a surgical emergency.[3,7,41,43,46] Dinning and Schaeffer reported that decompression performed within 24 hours of diagnosis improved urological outcome.[119] Kennedy et al reported good sexual recovery after early decompression.[39] They studied 19 patients, and they recommend decompression within 24 hours of presentation, especially when saddle anesthesia and/or bladder dysfunction are present.[39] According to these authors, resolution of sensory and motor deficit, as well as bladder and bowel dysfunction, is significantly related to early decompression, within 48 hours. Patients who wait more than 48 hours have a higher risk of permanent impairment.[42]

Delayed decompression after 48 hours: Kostuik et al reported clinical improvement when decompression was done several days after the onset of symptoms. They believed that the timing of surgery is less important than the severity of the initial symptoms.[97] Stephenson et al studied 45 patients with CES, divided into two groups in which surgery was done within or after 24 hours. They found that there was no difference in the outcome between the two groups.[120] Radulovic et al examined 47 patients who underwent surgery for CES; in 27 of the cases this was secondary to a herniated disc (57%). Decompression was done after the 7th day of the onset of symptoms. The authors concluded that there was no statistically significant difference in outcome between the onset of symptoms and the time of surgical decompression. Proper diagnosis and adequate treatment gave satisfactory outcome regardless of the timing of surgery.[4] Gleave and Macfarlane advocate that a delay worsens the outcome for patients with CESI, but once CES evolves to urinary retention (CESR), the timing of surgery does not influence the final outcome. Thus, they recommended urgent surgery for patients who are still in the CESI stage.[35]

Outcome

Bladder function and sexual function take time to recover. This process may even take several years.[25,49,121] Sensory recovery is less complete than motor recovery.[42] Saddle sensation is least likely to improve.[49] The recovery from urologic symptoms in most cases is greater than 70% (Table 27.4).

Poor outcome factors include longer time delay since the onset of symptoms,[3,122] saddle anesthesia, noncontractile detrusor,[94] bilateral sciatalgia or chronic LBP, old age,[39,42] and sudden onset of symptoms.[39] Following surgery, the persistence of saddle anesthesia[43] and severe motor weakness,[61] and the presence of urinary retention are bad prognostic factors as far as complete rehabilitation is concerned. Favorable outcome factors include prompt recognition of the correct diagnosis, absence of sensory deficit, and early treatment.[25,46]

Summary

CES is a relatively rare condition caused by any space-occupying lesion that leads to compression of the nerve fibers which constitute the cauda equina. The lesion must compromise the nerve fibers within the cauda equina bilaterally to be responsible for CES. This condition is characterized by LBP, saddle hypoesthesia or anesthesia, and sacral (i.e. lower urinary tract, bowel, and sexual) dysfunction. Early diagnosis and treatment can improve the outcome of these patients. Timing of surgery, however, is still subject to controversy.

References

1. Richard LM. Macroscopic anatomy of the spinal cord and spinal nerves. In: Standing S, ed. Gray's Anatomy, 39th edn. London: Churchill Livingstone, 2005: 775–87.
2. Hussain I. Cauda equina damage and its management. In: Fowler CJ, ed. Neurology of Bladder, Bowel and Sexual Dysfunction. London: Butterworth-Heinemann, 1999.
3. Nielsen B de NM, Schmidt K, Hansen RI. A urodynamic study of cauda equina syndrome due to lumbar disc herniation. Urol Int 1980; 35(3): 167–70.
4. Radulovic D, Tasic G, Jokovic M, Nikolic I. The role of surgical decompression of cauda equina in lumbar disc herniation and recovery of bladder function. Med Pregl 2004; 57(7–8): 327–30.
5. Mixter WJ, Barr J. Rupture of the intervertebral disc with involvement of the spinal canal. N Engl J Med 1934; 211: 210–5.
6. Hussain I. Cauda equina lesion. In: Fowler CJ, ed. Neurology of Bladder, Bowel, and Sexual Dysfunction, 23rd edn. Butterworth-Heinemann; 1999: 325–37.
7. Harrop JS, Hunt GE Jr, Vaccaro AR. Conus medullaris and cauda equina syndrome as a result of traumatic injuries: management principles. Neurosurg Focus 2004; 16(6): e4.
8. Malas MA, Salbacak A, Buyukmumcu M et al. An investigation of the conus medullaris termination level during the period of fetal development to adulthood. Kaibogaku Zasshi 2001; 76(5): 453–9.
9. Pavlakis AJ, Siroky MB, Goldstein I, Krane RJ. Neurourologic findings in conus medullaris and cauda equina injury. Arch Neurol 1983; 40(9): 570–3.
10. Arai Y, Shitoto K, Takahashi M, Kurosawa H. Magnetic resonance imaging observation of the conus medullaris. Bull Hosp Jt Dis 2001; 60(1): 10–12.
11. Creed KE. Innervation of the smooth muscle of the lower urinary tract. J Smooth Muscle Res 1995; 31(1): 1–4.
12. de Groat WC, Nadelhaft I, Milne RJ et al. Organization of the sacral parasympathetic reflex pathways to the urinary bladder and large intestine. J Auton Nerv Syst 1981; 3(2–4): 135–60.
13. deGroat WC, Booth AM. Physiology of male sexual function. Ann Intern Med 1980; 92(2): 329–31.
14. deGroat WC, Booth AM. Physiology of the urinary bladder and urethra. Ann Intern Med 1980; 92(2): 312–15.
15. Giuliano F, Rampin O, Allard J. Neurophysiology and pharmacology of female genital sexual response. J Sex Marital Ther 2002; 28(Suppl 1): 101–21.
16. Giuliano F, Rampin O. Neural control of erection. Physiol Behav 2004; 83(2): 189–201.
17. Hollabaugh RS Jr, Steiner MS, Sellers KD, Samm BJ, Dmochowski RR. Neuroanatomy of the pelvis: implications for colonic and rectal resection. Dis Colon Rectum 2000; 43(10): 1390–7.
18. Lue TF, Zeineh SJ, Schmidt RA, Tanagho EA. Neuroanatomy of penile erection: its relevance to iatrogenic impotence. J Urol 1984; 131(2): 273–80.
19. Hollabaugh RS Jr, Dmochowski RR, Steiner MS. Neuroanatomy of the male rhabdosphincter. Urology 1997; 49(3): 426–34.
20. Juenemann KP, Lue TF, Schmidt RA, Tanagho EA. Clinical significance of sacral and pudendal nerve anatomy. J Urol 1988; 139(1): 74–80.
21. Zvara P, Carrier S, Kour NW, Tanagho EA. The detailed neuroanatomy of the human striated urethral sphincter. Br J Urol 1994; 74(2): 182–7.
22. Zachoval R, Zalesky M, Lukes M et al. Lower urinary tract function and its disorders. Cesk Fysiol 2000; 49(3): 134–44.
23. Brooks J. Anatomy of the lower urinary tract and male genitalia. In: Walsh P, Retik A, Vaughan E, Wein A, eds. Campbell's Urology, 8th ed. Philadelphia: Elsevier Science, 2002: 41–80.
24. Kabalin J. Surgical anatomy of the retroperitoneum, kidney, and ureters. In: Walsh P, Retik A, Vaughan E, Wein A, editors. Campbell's Urology, 8th ed. Philadelphia: Elsevier Science, 2002: 3–40.
25. Hellstrom P, Kortelainen P, Kontturi M. Late urodynamic findings after surgery for cauda equina syndrome caused by a prolapsed lumbar intervertebral disk. J Urol 1986; 135(2): 308–12.
26. Cohen M. The anatomy of cauda equina on CT scan and MRI. J Bone Joint Surg Am 1991; 73(B): 381–4.
27. Inui Y, Doita M, Ouchi K et al. Clinical and radiologic features of lumbar spinal stenosis and disc herniation with neuropathic bladder. Spine 2004; 29(8): 869–73.
28. Rydevik B, Brown MD, Lundborg G. Pathoanatomy and pathophysiology of nerve root compression. Spine 1984; 9(1): 7–15.
29. Kobayashi S, Yoshizawa H, Yamada S. Pathology of lumbar nerve root compression. Part 2: morphological and immunohistochemical changes of dorsal root ganglion. J Orthop Res 2004; 22(1): 180–8.
30. Kobayashi S, Yoshizawa H, Yamada S. Pathology of lumbar nerve root compression. Part 1: Intraradicular inflammatory changes induced by mechanical compression. J Orthop Res 2004; 22(1): 170–9.
31. Igarashi T, Yabuki S, Kikuchi S, Myers RR. Effect of acute nerve root compression on endoneurial fluid pressure and blood flow in rat dorsal root ganglia. J Orthop Res 2005; 23(2): 420–4.
32. Delamarter RB, Sherman JE, Carr JB. Volvo Award in experimental studies. Cauda equina syndrome: neurologic recovery following immediate, early, or late decompression. Spine 1991; 16(9): 1022–9.
33. Bodner DR, Delamarter RB, Bohlman HH et al. Urologic changes after cauda equina compression in dogs. J Urol 1990; 143(1): 186–90.
34. McGuire EJ. The effects of sacral denervation on bladder and urethral function. Surg Gynecol Obstet 1977; 144(3): 343–6.
35. Gleave JR, Macfarlane R. Cauda equina syndrome: what is the relationship between timing of surgery and outcome? Br J Neurosurg 2002; 16(4): 325–8.

36. Podnar S. Epidemiology of cauda equina and conus medullaris lesions. Muscle Nerve 2007; 35: 529–31.
37. Deyo RA, Rainville J, Kent DL. What can the history and physical examination tell us about low back pain? JAMA 1992; 268(6): 760–5.
38. Small SA, Perron AD, Brady WJ. Orthopedic pitfalls: cauda equina syndrome. Am J Emerg Med 2005; 23(2): 159–63.
39. Kennedy JG, Soffe KE, McGrath A et al. Predictors of outcome in cauda equina syndrome. Eur Spine J 1999; 8(4): 317–22.
40. Shapiro S. Cauda equina syndrome secondary to lumbar disc herniation. Neurosurgery 1993; 32(5): 743–6.
41. Thongtrangan I, Le H, Park J, Kim DH. Cauda equina syndrome in patients with low lumbar fractures. Neurosurg Focus 2004; 16(6): e6.
42. Ahn UM, Ahn NU, Buchowski JM et al. Cauda equina syndrome secondary to lumbar disc herniation: a meta-analysis of surgical outcomes. Spine 2000; 25(12): 1515–22.
43. Buchner M, Schiltenwolf M. Cauda equina syndrome caused by intervertebral lumbar disk prolapse: mid term results of 22 patients and literature review. Orthopedics 2002; 25(7): 727–31.
44. Henriques T, Olerud C, Petren-Mallmin M, Ahl T. Cauda equina syndrome as a postoperative complication in five patients operated for lumbar disc herniation. Spine 2001; 26(3): 293–7.
45. Hussain SA, Gullan RW, Chitnavis BP. Cauda equina syndrome: outcome and implications for management. Br J Neurosurg 2003; 17(2): 164–7.
46. Shapiro S. Medical realities of cauda equina syndrome secondary to lumbar disc herniation. Spine 2000; 25(3): 348–51.
47. Mosdal C, Iversen P, Iversen-Hansen R. Bladder neuropathy in lumbar disc disease. Acta Neurochir (Wien) 1979; 46(3–4): 281–6.
48. Orendacova J, Cizkova D, Kafka J et al. Cauda equina syndrome. Prog Neurobiol 2001; 64(6): 613–37.
49. McCarthy MJ, Aylott CE, Grevitt MP, Hegarty J. Cauda equina syndrome: factors affecting long-term functional and sphincteric outcome. Spine 2007; 32(2): 207–16.
50. Mangialardi R, Mastorillo G, Minola L et al. Lumbar disc herniation and cauda equina syndrome. Considerations on a pathology with different clinical manifestations. Chir Organi Mov 2002; 87(1): 35–42.
51. Perner A, Andersen JT, Juhler M. Lower urinary tract symptoms in lumbar root compression syndromes: a prospective survey. Spine 1997; 22(22): 2693–7.
52. Ahn UM, Ahn NU, Buchowski JM et al. Cauda equina syndrome secondary to lumbar disc herniation: a meta-analysis of surgical outcomes. Spine 2000; 25(12): 1515–22.
53. Podnar S, Trsinar B, Vodusek DB. Bladder dysfunction in patients with cauda equina lesions. Neurourol Urodyn 2006; 25(1): 23–31.
54. Muthukumar T, Butt SH, Cassar-Pullicino VN, McCall IW. Cauda equina syndrome presentation of sacral insufficiency fractures. Skeletal Radiol 2007; 36(4): 309–13.
55. Martineau PA, Ouellet J, Reindl R, Arlet V. Surgical images: musculoskeletal. Delayed cauda equina syndrome due to a sacral insufficiency fracture missed after a minor trauma. Can J Surg 2004; 47(2): 117–18.
56. Wills JH, Wiesel S, Abram SE, Rupp FW. Synovial cysts and the lithotomy position causing cauda equina syndrome. Reg Anesth Pain Med 2004; 29(3): 234–6.
57. Loo CC, Irestedt L. Cauda equina syndrome after spinal anaesthesia with hyperbaric 5% lignocaine: a review of six cases of cauda equina syndrome reported to the Swedish Pharmaceutical Insurance 1993–1997. Acta Anaesthesiol Scand 1999; 43(4): 371–9.
58. Rigler ML, Drasner K, Krejcie TC et al. Cauda equina syndrome after continuous spinal anesthesia. Anesth Analg 1991; 72(3): 275–81.
59. Ozgen S, Baykan N, Dogan IV, Konya D, Pamir MN. Cauda equina syndrome after induction of spinal anesthesia. Neurosurg Focus 2004; 16(6): e5.
60. Standring S. Central nervous system. In: Standing S, ed. 39th edn. Churchill Livingstone, 2005.
61. Henriques T, Olerud C, Petren-Mallmin M, Ahl T. Cauda equina syndrome as a postoperative complication in five patients operated for lumbar disc herniation. Spine 2001; 26(3): 293–7.
62. Jensen RL. Cauda equina syndrome as a postoperative complication of lumbar spine surgery. Neurosurg Focus 2004; 16(6): e7.
63. McLaren AC, Bailey SI. Cauda equina syndrome: a complication of lumbar discectomy. Clin Orthop Relat Res 1986, 2004: 143–9.
64. Friedman J, Whitecloud TS, III. Lumbar cauda equina syndrome associated with the use of gelfoam: case report. Spine 2001; 26(20): E485–7.
65. Schoenecker PL, Cole HO, Herring JA, Capelli AM, Bradford DS. Cauda equina syndrome after in situ arthrodesis for severe spondylolisthesis at the lumbosacral junction. J Bone Joint Surg Am 1990; 72(3): 369–77.
66. Imran Y, Halim Y. Acute cauda equina syndrome secondary to free fat graft following spinal decompression. Singapore Med J 2005; 46(1): 25–7.
67. Bagley CA, Gokaslan ZL. Cauda equina syndrome caused by primary and metastatic neoplasms. Neurosurg Focus 2004; 16(6): e3.
68. Lakkis S, Afeiche N, Ashkar K. Meningeal carcinomatosis: a rare cause of cauda equina syndrome. Ann Saudi Med 2003; 23(6): 391–3.
69. Lisai P, Doria C, Crissantu L et al. Cauda equina syndrome secondary to idiopathic spinal epidural lipomatosis. Spine 2001; 26(3): 307–9.
70. Gaetani P, Di IA, Colombo P et al. Intradural spinal metastasis of renal clear cell carcinoma causing cauda equina syndrome. Acta Neurochir (Wien) 2004; 146(8): 857–61.
71. Onal IK, Shorbagi A, Goker H et al. Cauda equina syndrome as a rare manifestation of leukemia relapse during postallograft period. J Natl Med Assoc 2006; 98(5): 808–10.
72. Bachmeyer C, Kazerouni F, Langman B, Daumas L, Hessler P. A rare cause of cauda equina syndrome: primary epidural lymphoma. Presse Med 2005; 34(15): 1082–3.
73. Ooi GC, Peh WC, Fung CF. Case report: magnetic resonance imaging of primary lymphoma of the cauda equina. Br J Radiol 1996; 69(827): 1057–60.
74. Zagami AS, Granot R. Non-Hodgkin's lymphoma involving the cauda equina and ocular cranial nerves: case reports and literature review. J Clin Neurosci 2003; 10(6): 696–9.
75. Riffaud L, Adn M, Brassier G, Morandi X. Acute cauda equina compression revealing Hodgkin's disease: a case report. Spine 2003; 28(14): E270–2.
76. Hamlat A, Saikali S, Lakehal M, Pommereuil M, Morandi X. Cauda equina syndrome due to an intra-dural sacral cyst in type-1 Gaucher disease. Eur Spine J 2004; 13(3): 249–52.
77. Ziv T, Watemberg N, Constantini S, Lerman-Sagie T. Cauda equina syndrome due to lumbosacral arachnoid cysts in children. Eur J Paediatr Neurol 1999; 3(6): 281–4.
78. Johnsson KE, Sass M. Cauda equina syndrome in lumbar spinal stenosis: case report and incidence in Jutland, Denmark. J Spinal Disord Tech 2004; 17(4): 334–5.
79. Ahn NU, Ahn UM, Nallamshetty L et al. Cauda equina syndrome in ankylosing spondylitis (the CES-AS syndrome): meta-analysis of outcomes after medical and surgical treatments. J Spinal Disord 2001; 14(5): 427–33.
80. Miyamoto M, Genbum Y, Ito H. Diagnosis and treatment of lumbar spinal canal stenosis. J Nippon Med Sch 2002; 69(6): 583–7.
81. Mohit AA, Fisher DJ, Matthews DC, Hoffer E, Avellino AM. Inferior vena cava thrombosis causing acute cauda equina syndrome. Case report. J Neurosurg 2006; 104(1 Suppl): 46–9.
82. Ahn H, Jhaveri S, Yee A, Finkelstein J. Lumbar vertebral hemangioma causing cauda equina syndrome: a case report. Spine 2005; 30(21): E662–4.

83. Ghazi NG, Jane JA, Lopes MB, Newman SA. Capillary hemangioma of the cauda equina presenting with radiculopathy and papilledema. J Neuroophthalmol 2006; 26(2): 98–102.
84. Roncaroli F, Scheithauer BW, Deen HG Jr. Multiple hemangiomas (hemangiomatosis) of the cauda equina and spinal cord. Case report. J Neurosurg 2000; 92(2 Suppl): 229–32.
85. Tait MJ, Chelvarajah R, Garvan N, Bavetta S. Spontaneous hemorrhage of a spinal ependymoma: a rare cause of acute cauda equina syndrome: a case report. Spine 2004; 29(21): E502–5.
86. Sawanyawisuth K, Tiamkao S, Nitinavakarn B, Dekumyoy P, Jitpimolmard S. MR imaging findings in cauda equina gnathostomiasis. Am J Neuroradiol 2005; 26(1): 39–42.
87. Lenehan B, Sullivan P, Street J, Dudeney S. Epidural abscess causing cauda equina syndrome. Ir J Med Sci 2005; 174(3): 88–91.
88. Kapoor SK, Garg V, Dhaon BK, Jindal M. Tuberculosis of the posterior vertebral elements: a rare cause of compression of the cauda equina. A case report. J Bone Joint Surg Am 2005; 87(2): 391–4.
89. Kikuchi M, Nagao K, Muraosa Y, Ohnuma S, Hoshino H. Cauda equina syndrome complicating pneumococcal meningitis. Pediatr Neurol 1999; 20(2): 152–4.
90. Herbaut AG, Nogueira MC, Wespes E. Urinary retention due to sacral myeloradiculitis: a clinical and neurophysiological study. J Urol 1990; 144(5): 1206–8.
91. Paisansinsup T, Manno EM, Moder KG. Cauda equina syndrome as a clinical presentation of primary angiitis of the central nervous system (PACNS). J Clin Rheumatol 2004; 10(5): 265–8.
92. Verma KK, Forman AD, Fuller GN, Dimachkie MM, Vriesendorp FJ. Cauda equina syndrome as the isolated presentation of sarcoidosis. J Neurol 2000; 247(7): 573–4.
93. Kaiboriboon K, Olsen TJ, Hayat GR. Cauda equina and conus medullaris syndrome in sarcoidosis. Neurologist 2005; 11(3): 179–83.
94. Smith AY, Woodside JR. Urodynamic evaluation of patients with spinal stenosis. Urology 1988; 32(5): 474–7.
95. Tandon P, Sankaran B. Cauda equina syndrome due to disc prolapse. Ind J Orthop 1967; 1: 112–19.
96. Choudhury AR, Taylor JC. Cauda equina syndrome in lumbar disc disease. Acta Orthop Scand 1980; 51(3): 493–9.
97. Kostuik JP, Harrington I, Alexander D, Rand W, Evans D. Cauda equina syndrome and lumbar disc herniation. J Bone Joint Surg Am 1986; 68(3): 386–91.
98. Podnar S, Oblak C, Vodusek DB. Sexual function in men with cauda equina lesions: a clinical and electromyographic study. J Neurol Neurosurg Psychiatry 2002; 73(6): 715–20.
99. Podnar S. Saddle sensation is preserved in a few patients with cauda equina or conus medullaris lesions. Eur J Neurol 2007; 14(1): 48–53.
100. Podnar S. Bowel dysfunction in patients with cauda equina lesions. Eur J Neurol 2006; 13(10): 1112–17.
101. Kostuik JP. Medicolegal consequences of cauda equina syndrome: an overview. Neurosurg Focus 2004; 16(6): e8.
102. Monajati A, Wayne WS, Rauschning W, Ekholm SE. MR of the cauda equina. Am J Neuroradiol 1987; 8(5): 893–900.
103. Schick E, Bertrand PE. Intervertebral disc prolapse. In: Cocos J, Schick E, eds. Textbook of The Neurogenic Bladder Adults and Children. London: Martin Dunitz, 2004: 315–23.
104. Rosomoff H. The neurogenic bladder of lumber disc syndrome. Trans Am Neurol Assoc 1964; 89: –249.
105. Shin JC, Park CI, Kim HJ, Lee IY. Significance of low compliance bladder in cauda equina injury. Spinal Cord 2002; 40(12): 650–5.
106. Light JK, Beric A, Petronic I. Detrusor function with lesions of the cauda equina, with special emphasis on the bladder neck. J Urol 1993; 149(3): 539–42.
107. Nordling J, Meyhoff HH, Olesen KP. Cysto-urethrographic appearance of the bladder and posterior urethra in neuromuscular disorders of the lower urinary tract. Scand J Urol Nephrol 1982; 16(2): 115–24.
108. Kontturi M, Harviainen S, Larmi TK. Atonic bladder in lumbar disk herniation. Acta Chir Scand Suppl 1966; 357: 232–5.
109. Kontturi M. Investigations into bladder dysfunction in prolapse of lumbar intervertebral disc. Ann Chir Gynaecol Fenn Suppl 1968; 162: 1–53.
110. Wang TG, Hsu TC, Wang YH, Lai JS, Lien IN. [Clinical application of the ice water test in evaluation of neurogenic bladder dysfunction.] J Formos Med Assoc 1994; 93(Suppl 2): S115–19.
111. Geirsson G, Fall M, Lindstrom S. The ice-water test – a simple and valuable supplement to routine cystometry. Br J Urol 1993; 71(6): 681–5.
112. Balmaseda MT Jr, Reynolds HT, Gordon C. The value of the ice water test in the management of the neurogenic bladder. Am J Phys Med Rehabil 1988; 67(5): 225–7.
113. Ronzoni G, Menchinelli P, Manca A, De GL. The ice-water test in the diagnosis and treatment of the neurogenic bladder. Br J Urol 1997; 79(5): 698–701.
114. Bradley WE, Andersen JT. Neuromuscular dysfunction of the lower urinary tract in patients with lesions of the cauda equina and conus medullaris. J Urol 1976; 116(5): 620–1.
115. Vodusek DB, Fowler CJ, Deletis V, Podnar S. Clinical neurophysiology of pelvic floor disorders. Suppl Clin Neurophysiol 2000; 53: 220–7.
116. Podnar S, Vodusek DB. Protocol for clinical neurophysiologic examination of the pelvic floor. Neurourol Urodyn 2001; 20(6): 669–82.
117. Schmid DM, Curt A, Hauri D, Schurch B. Motor evoked potentials (MEP) and evoked pressure curves (EPC) from the urethral compressive musculature (UCM) by functional magnetic stimulation in healthy volunteers and patients with neurogenic incontinence. Neurourol Urodyn 2005; 24(2): 117–27.
118. Di L V, Pilato F, Oliviero A et al. Role of motor evoked potentials in diagnosis of cauda equina and lumbosacral cord lesions. Neurology 2004; 63(12): 2266–71.
119. Dinning TA, Schaeffer HR. Discogenic compression of the cauda equina: a surgical emergency. Aust NZ J Surg 1993; 63(12): 927–34.
120. Stephenson G, Gibson R, Sonntag V. Who is to blame for the morbidity of acute cauda equina compression? J Neural Neurosurg Psychiatry 1994; 57: 388.
121. Chang HS, Nakagawa H, Mizuno J. Lumbar herniated disc presenting with cauda equina syndrome. Long-term follow-up of four cases. Surg Neurol 2000; 53(2): 100–4.
122. Haldeman S, Rubinstein SM. Cauda equina syndrome in patients undergoing manipulation of the lumbar spine. Spine 1992; 17(12): 1469–73.

28

Tumors of the spinal cord

Homero Bruschini, J Pindaro P Plese, and Miguel Srougi

Tumors compromising the neural transmission at the spinal cord can originate in the bone structures or tissue extensions involving the spinal cord and in the neural structures existing inside the bone framework.

Spinal cord tumors constitute 15% of the central nervous system neoplasias. They are divided according to their relation to the duramater into extradural, intradural but extramedullary, and intramedullary[1] (Figure 28.1). Intradural spinal cord tumors are less common.[2] In a few cases an intramedullary and an extramedullary component may coexist, with communication through the entrance of the nerve root or at the conus medullaris–filum terminale transition. Some intradural tumors extend through the nerve root sheaths to the extradural space. Intradural extramedullary tumors comprise about 45% of intradural tumors in children.[3]

An accurate diagnosis is crucial to determine the prognosis and direct therapy. Magnetic resonance imaging has revolutionized the diagnosis of intraspinal tumors, allowing for early detection and improved anatomic localization.[4] It has also become fundamental for staging primary and metastatic neoplasms.

Bladder and sphincter dysfunctions are rarely the first symptoms in these patients, but they may coexist with other complaints, usually as a late presentation. Scientific communications specifically on this topic are scarce in the literature.

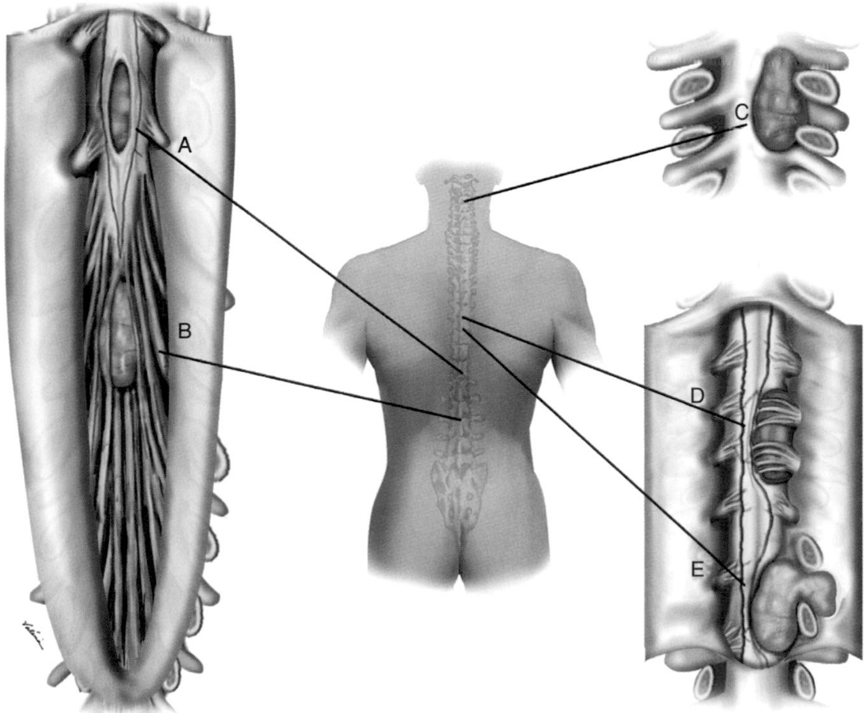

Figure 28.1
Anatomic relationship of spinal tumors with other spine structures: (A) intramedullary tumor; (B) filum terminale ependymoma; (C) extradural neurofibroma; (D) intradural extramedullary meningioma; (E) schwannoma growing through the vertebral foramina.

Table 28.1 *Incidence of tumors in adults (after Schwartz and McCormick[1])*

Extramedullary (two-thirds of cases)	%	Intramedullary (one-third of cases)	%
Nerve sheath tumors	40	Ependymoma	45
Meningioma	40	Astrocytoma	40
Filum ependymoma	15	Hemangioblastoma	5
Miscellaneous	5	Miscellaneous	10

Intradural extramedullary tumors

About two-thirds of the so-called adult spinal cord tumors are extramedullary (Table 28.1). Schwannomas, meningiomas, and ependymomas comprise 95% of the extraspinal tumors. The other 5% are intradural metastases, inclusion cysts, paragangliomas, and melanocystic neoplasias. With few exceptions, intradural extramedullary tumors are benign and surgically excisable.

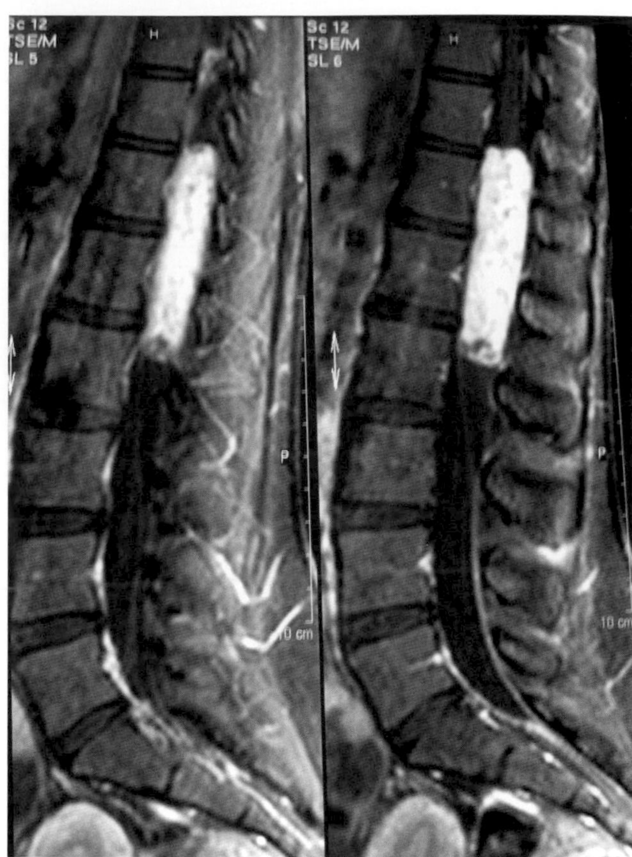

Figure 28.2
MRI of a large neurinoma.

Types of tumor

Tumors derived from the neural sheath

These consist of neurinomas or schwannomas. They constitute about 25% of all the intradural adult tumors and the annual incidence is 0.3 to 0.4 per 100 000 of the population. The most frequent presentation is as a single lesion in the vertebral channel, in the 4th to 6th decades of life, with no gender differentiation (Figure 28.2). The most affected regions are the dorsal roots, with 30% growing through the vertebral foramina in an hourglass shape. About 10% can be exclusively extradural. Only 1% originate from the perivascular neural sheaths of the penetrating medullary circulation vessels. Malignant tumors comprise only 2.5%, mostly associated with neurofibromatosis, and they have a poor prognosis, with an average survival of one year.

Meningiomas

These originate from the arachnoid cells close to the nerve exit, which explains its lateral localization. They occur in a frequency similar to the neural sheath tumors. They can affect people of any age; however, most arise in the 5th to 7th decade, with 80% in the thoracic segment (Figure 28.3). They sometimes occur in the high cervical area, and at the craniovertebral junction, such as the magnum foramina. About 90% of spinal meningiomas are intradural. They are more suitable for surgical excision than the intracranial meningiomas, since they do not invade the pia mater. This is due to the presence of a leptomeningeal cellular layer between the pia mater and the arachnoid in the spinal area, different from the cranial region.

Ependymomas

The filum terminale ependymomas correspond to 40% of spinal ependymomas (Figure 28.4). Other rare presentations of filum terminale tumors are astrocytomas, paragangliomas, and oligodendrogliomas. The usual histologic pattern is a benign myxopapillary ependymoma, which is more aggressive in young patients.

Other tumors

Less common tumors are those derived from embryologic disorders, such as dermoid cysts, lipomas, teratomas, and

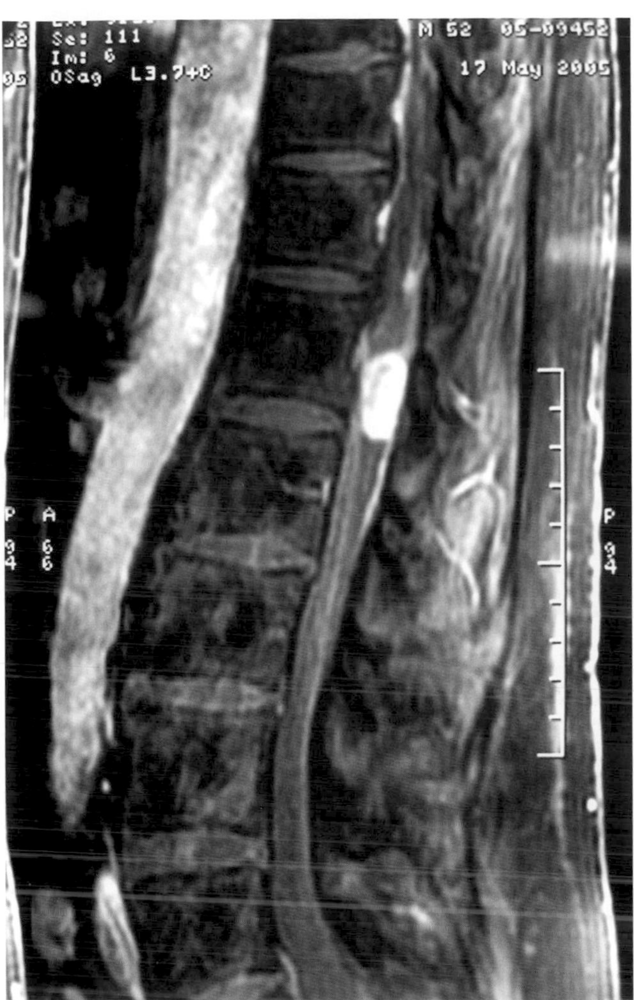

Figure 28.3
MRI of an extramedullary intradural thoracic meningioma.

neuroenteric cysts. They occur mainly in the lumbar and thoraco-lumbar areas. Other causes are malformations such as spina bifida and occult racheschises. Some non-neoplastic lesions can simulate tumors, such as arachnoid cysts[5] and dural inflammations such as sarcoidosis and tuberculosis.

Clinical findings and treatment

These tumors grow slowly. The clinical findings are mainly a consequence of compression and depend on its localization. The usual complaint is pain and some enervation impairment of the corresponding area. Tumors of the craniovertebral junction and magnum foramina are mostly ventral, causing suboccipital pain and weakness of the arm, with atrophy of the intrinsic muscular components of the hands. The physiopathology may be related to local venous insufficiency. Tumors in a high cervical position may cause hydrocephaly due to higher levels of protein and decreased liquor absorption. Segmental motor deficiency together with signs and symptoms of the involvement of the spinothalamic and corticospinal tracts suggests lesions of the medium and low cervical segments. They generally cause premature and asymmetric symptoms. Thoracic tumors particularly compromise the corticospinal tract. This is usually signaled by complaints of rigidity and spasticity together with distal weakness of the arms, as a consequence of the initial participation of the peripheral fibers. Tumors of the dorsal median line initially cause gait ataxia due to compression and loss of sensitivity of the posterior column. Bladder and sphincter dysfunction is unusual and may present only as a late symptom. Filum terminale ependymomas usually present as lumbar pain, with irradiation to the legs. In these cases, worsening of symptoms when taking the horizontal dorsal position is indicative of large extramedullary tumors, especially at the cauda equina. Intraoperative monitoring of bladder function during spinal cord surgery in a few cases including ependymoma of the cauda equina and cervical intramedullary tumors has been reported.[6] This method proved unsuitable for intramedullary tumors, but is an effective tool for identifying bladder efferent nerves at the cauda equina. The practical use of this approach has yet to be tested.

Intramedullary tumors

Around 80% of spinal cord intramedullary tumors are glials (originating from the central nervous system) and histologically benign. They include astrocytomas, ependymomas, and, less frequently, gangliogliomas, oligodendrogliomas, and subependymomas. Hemangioblastomas comprise 3 to 8% of intramedullary tumors. Less than 5% of these tumors are metastatic lesions, usually from primary tumors of the lung and breasts. The other 10 to 15% of these tumors are inclusion cysts, tumors from the neural sheath, neurocytomas, and melanocytomas. Some lesions, such as tuberculosis, bacterial abscesses, sarcoidosis, and multiple sclerosis, can simulate neoplasia. Differential diagnosis is suggested by the rapid course of symptoms in the real tumors. A recent series of 48 patients with intramedullary tumors presented ependymoma in 67% of cases, followed by lipomas, gangliomas, astrocytomas, and hemangioblastomas.[7]

Three percent of all astrocytomas are located at the spinal cord. They can be found at any age, being more frequent in the first three decades of life. Ninety percent of the pediatric intramedullary tumors in the first 10 years of life are astrocytomas. They are associated with syringomyelia in 20% of cases. Around 60% of them occur at the cervical or

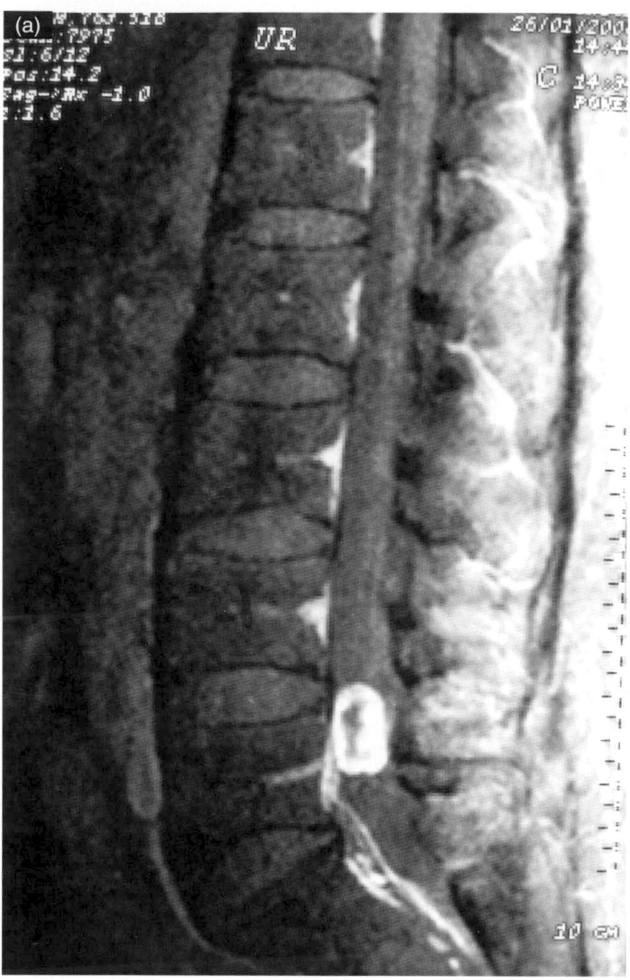

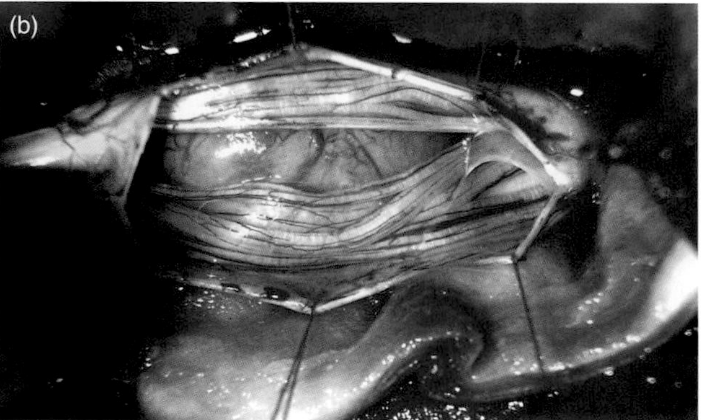

Figure 28.4
(a) MRI of an ependymona of cauda equina. (b) Surgical aspect of the tumor.

cervico-thoracic transition. It is known that intramedullary astrocytomas tend to be associated with neurofibromatosis type 1.

Malignancy varies from low-grade pyelocystic astrocytomas to anaplastic astrocytoma or glioblastomas. Malignant tumors are more frequent in the pediatric population. In adults, 25% of tumors are malignant, whilst ependymomas are the most frequent tumor, with equal gender commitment. They occur in association with syringomyelia in 65% of patients, especially in those tumors located at the cervical area. Mutations of gene NF 2 are associated with ependymomas. Most of the wide variety of histologic presentations are benign. The most frequent is the fibrillar ependymoma. Besides the absence of a true capsule, they are well limited and without infiltrating adjacent structures.

Hemangioblastomas are intramedullary in 3 to 8% of cases. They are present in 15 to 25% of cases of von Hippel–Lindau syndrome, occurring in all ages except in childhood. Implantation in the pia mater is the rule, mainly in the dorsal and dorsolateral areas. They also do not have a true capsule, being localized and benign lesions.

Intramedullary metastatic lesions are unusual, occurring in less than 5% of cases.

Clinical findings and treatment

Clinical manifestations of these tumors are quite variable. Initial complaints are nonspecific and start 3 to 4 years before the diagnosis. There have been cases diagnosed at a chiropractic clinic after intermittent backache for some years, without any other symptom or with mild and irrelevant bowel and bladder dysfunction.[8] In adults, pain and weakness are the most frequent initial symptoms. Malignant neoplasias have a shorter evolutionary course. A sudden neurologic impairment suggests intratumoral bleeding, being more frequent in ependymomas (Figure 28.5). The pain is usually in accordance with the level of the lesion. Upper extremity symptoms predominate in cervical lesions. Thoracic tumors cause spasticity and sensorial problems due to involvement of the posterior portion of the medulla and thalamo-spinal tracts. Lumbar tumors promote pain in the posterior areas of the thighs and feet, simulating radicular pain. Bladder and sphincter symptom participation is unusual, occurring most in advanced stages of medullary and cauda equina compression. A review of 48 patients showed pain as the first symptom in 50%, sensory alterations such as paresthesias and dysesthesias in 35%, and gait problems in 15%, with no urinary or bowel complaints as first manifestation.[7]

Magnetic resonance imaging is the method of choice to detect these tumors. Early detection favors a curative therapeutic approach. Subtotal aggressive surgical excision seems feasible in two-thirds of cases, and should be the target when possible, with an improved or stable situation resulting in over 65% of patients.[7]

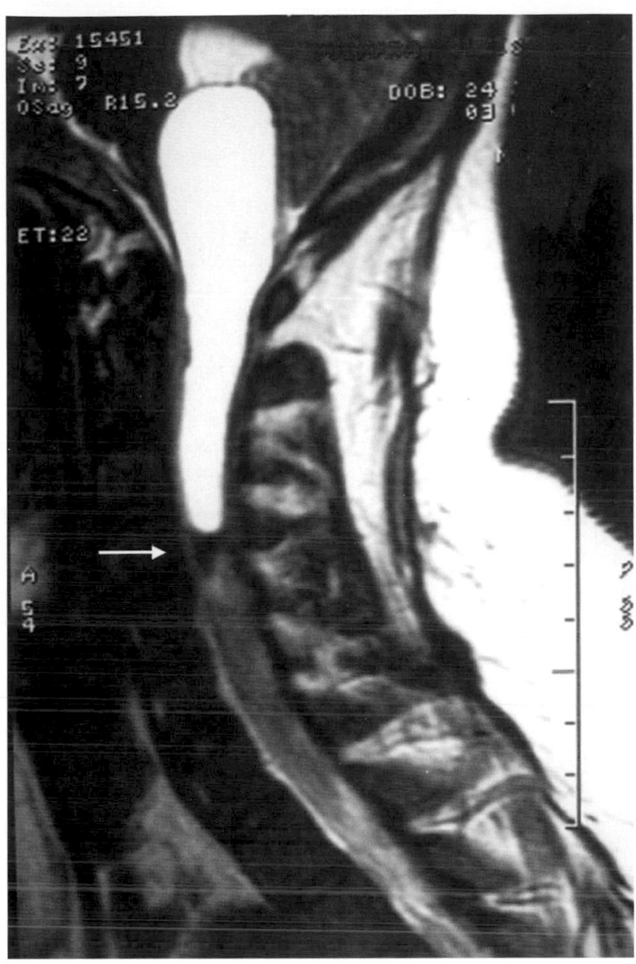

Figure 28.5
MRI of an intramedullary cervical ependymoma. Bleeding of the tumor, as seen in the upper portion of the figure, caused a sudden worsening of symptoms.

Metastatic spinal lesions

The spinal muscular and bone structures are the third most common place for metastasis, after the lungs and liver. Vertebral bone metastasis occurs in 10% of malignancies, being the most common spinal tumors. Extradural compression represents 97% of spinal cord metastatic lesions.[9] Metastasis usually arises in the posterior aspect of the vertebral body, with later invasion of the epidural space (Figure 28.6). Pathophysiologically, vascular insufficiency is more important than direct spinal cord compression.[10]

Neoplastic cells reach the spine through the arterial or venous hematogenic pathway, or through direct extension. The vertebral venous plexus of Batson is the main route for dissemination of breast, intrathoracic, intra-abdominal, and pelvic tumors to this area. The absence of valves in these blood vessels allows neoplastic cells to disseminate to the bone, without passing through lung and liver filters. The most frequent primary tumors to give metastasis to this area are breast,[11] lung,[12–14] uterus,[15] kidney, and prostate.[16] In around 10% of metastases, a primary tumor is not immediately found. Recently, with the evolution of neoplasia, 50% of undetectable primary tumors show a lung origin. Anecdotal cases of primary nervous system tumors such as multiform glioblastomas causing vertebral metastasis have been reported.[17]

Clinical findings and treatment

Insidious and progressive pain is the first complaint in vertebral metastasis in 90% of patients, followed by weakness, sensory complaints, and lost of voluntary control of sphincters. In a study of symptoms carried out in 153 patients with metastatic compression of the spinal cord or cauda equina,[18] radicular pain was predominant in cases with metastases located in the lumbar area, while the severity of motor symptoms was positively correlated with thoracic metastases. The most frequent initial symptom was radicular pain, followed with decreasing frequency by motor weakness, sensory complaints, and bladder dysfunction.

The nocturnal worsening of symptoms is very characteristic. A sudden aggravation of pain suggests pathologic fractures and additional compressions. Increased pain with movement means vertebral instability. Around 87% of the patients receive an initial diagnosis of fibromuscular pain. Recent dorsal pain in oncologic patients should be investigated as potential metastasis. Early diagnosis is related to better treatment evolution. Concomitant activation of Herpes zoster, the Brown–Sequard syndrome, or ataxia at the level of medullary compression is unusual.

Surgery for treatment of intramedullary spinal cord metastasis is controversial. Sporadic cases have been reported, with pain relief and improvement in bladder dysfunction.[19] This procedure was recommended by Faillot et al in selected cases, which might benefit from an improvement in the quality and comfort of life, although it does not seem to affect the duration of survival.

A retrospective analysis of clinical data concerning 140 patients with spinal cord compression compared those submitted to surgical decompressive laminectomy followed by radiation therapy (127 cases) to those treated by primary radiation alone (26 cases).[20] Combined therapy offered sphincter function improvement in 68% of cases, compared to an improvement in 33% with radiation alone. It seems that the treatment of choice for each patient must take into account his general condition, life expectancy, and the origin of the primary tumor.[21]

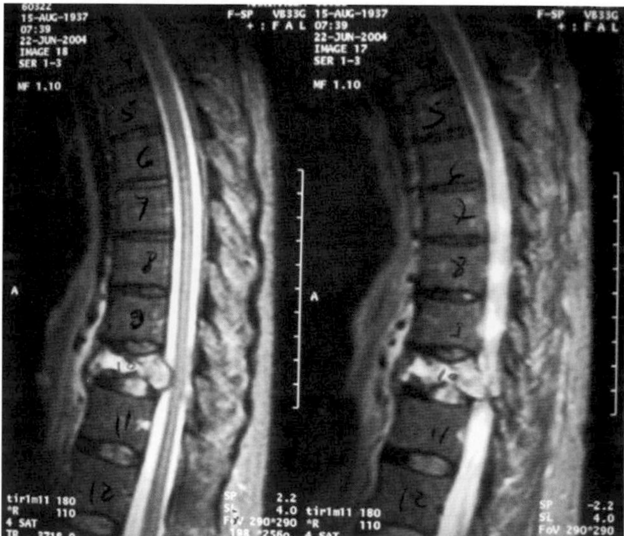

Figure 28. 6
Breast neoplasia causing bone metastasis to T10 and invading the medullary space.

Conclusions

Bladder and sphincter complaints are seldom the first and sole symptom of spinal tumors.[22] Usually other signs of neural impairment, such as pain, or sensory or motor weakness, precede it. The urinary dysfunction is initially overlooked in these patients and total attention is in general directed to the tumor itself and its treatment. The urologists rarely see these patients before the neurosurgical approach.

When urinary dysfunction results, it is related to the localized area involved rather than to the tumor type. Urodynamic examination should be employed to identify the level of the lesion and the urotherapeutic approach. Underlying disease and life expectancy should establish the type of bladder management in patients with neoplastic spinal cord involvement.[23] Those with stabilized sequel lesions and potentially curative disease should be submitted to a full bladder rehabilitation program, as described in other chapters of this book. Those with spinal tumors not eligible for bladder rehabilitation and needing only temporary urinary care may be managed with a transurethral, or preferably a suprapubic, catheter.

References

1. Schwartz H, McCormick PC. Spinal cord tumors in adults. In: Winn HR, ed. Neurological Surgery, 5th edn, Vol 4. Philadelphia, WB Saunders Co, 2004: 4817–34.
2. Traul DE, Shaffrey ME, Schiff D. Part I: Spinal-cord neoplasms – intradural neoplasms. Lancet Oncol 2007; 8(1): 35–45.
3. Jallo GI, Kothbauer KF, Epstein FJ. Intraspinal tumors in infants and children . In: Neurological Surgery, 5th edn, Vol 3. Philadelphia, WB Saunders Co, 2004: 3707–15.
4. Bloomer CW, Ackerman A, Bhatia RG. Imaging for spine tumors and new applications. Top Magn Reson Imaging 2006; 17(2): 69–87.
5. Dulou R, Blondet E, Dutertre G et al. Spinal cord compression by arachnoid cysts. Neurochirurgie 2006; 52(4): 381–6.
6. Schaan M, Boszczyk B, Jaksche H et al. Intraoperative urodynamics in spinal cord surgery: a study of feasibility. Eur Spine J 2004; 13(1): 39–43.
7. Taricco MA. Post-operative follow-up of the intramedullary tumors evolution. PhD thesis, University of Sao Paulo School of Medicine, 2006.
8. Lensgraf AG, Young KJ. Ependymoma of the spinal cord presenting in a chiropractic practice: 2 case studies. J Manipul Physiol Ther 2006; 29(8): 676–81.
9. Spinazze S, Careceni A, Schrijvers D. Epidural spinal cord compression. Crit Rev Oncol Hematol 2005; 56(3): 397–406.
10. Mut M, Schiff D, Shaffrey ME. Metastasis to nervous system: spinal epidural and intramedullary metastases. J Neurooncol 2005; 75(1): 43–56.
11. Luvin R, Cornu P, Philippon J et al. Isolated cervical intramedullary metastasis from breast cancer. Value of magnetic resonance imaging. Rev Neurol (Paris) 1988; 144(1): 40–2.
12. Wada H, Ieki R, Ota T et al. Intramedullary spinal cord metastasis of lung adenocarcinoma causing Brown–Sequard syndrome. Nihon Kokyuki Gakkai Zasshi 2001; 39(8): 590–4.
13. Takahima M, Ono N, Noguchi T et al. Two cases of intramedullary spinal cord metastasis of lung cancer detected with MRI. Nihon Kokyuki Gakkai Zasshi 2003; 41(4): 320–3.
14. Kato A, Katayama H, Nagao T et al. A case of small cell lung cancer with intramedullary spinal cord metastasis. Nippon Ronen Igakkai Zasshi 2005; 42(5): 567–70.
15. Sakuma S, Iwasaki Y, Isu T et al. A case of intramedullary spinal cord metastasis from adenocarcinoma of corpus uteri. No Shinkei Geka 1990; 18(7): 653–7.
16. Maranzano E, Latini P, Beneventi S et al. Comparison of two different radiotherapy schedules for spinal cord compression in prostate cancer. Tumori 1998; 84(4): 472–7.
17. Slowik F, Balogh I. Extracranial spreading of glioblastoma multiforme. Zentralbl Neurochir 1980; 41(1): 57–68.
18. Helweg-Larsen S, Sorensen PS. Symptoms and signs in metastatic spinal cord compression: a study of progression from first symptom until diagnosis in 153 patients. Eur J Cancer 1994; 30(3): 396–8.
19. Faillot T, Roujeau T, Dulou R, Blanc JL, Chedru F. Intramedullary spinal cord metastasis: is there a place for surgery? Case report and review of literature. Neurochirurgie 2002; 48(6): 533–6.
20. Landmann C, Hunig R, Gratzi O. The role of laminectomy in the combined treatment of metastatic spinal cord compression. Int J Radiat Oncol Biol Phys 1992; 24(4): 627–31.
21. Byrne TN, Borges LF, Loeffler JS. Metastatic epidural spinal cord compression: update on management. Semin Oncol 2006; 33(3): 307–11.
22. Perea J, Romero Maroto J, Ruiz C, Fernandez A, Perales Cabanas L. Urologic symptoms as first clinical manifestation of tumors of the nervous system. Apropos of 2 cases. Actas Urol Esp 1989; 13(1): 71–4.
23. Reitz A, Haferkamp Am, Wagener N, Gerner HJ, Hohenfellner M. Neurogenic bladder dysfunction in patients with neoplastic spinal cord compression: adaptation of the bladder management strategy to the underlying disease. NeuroRehabilitation 2006; 21(1): 65–9.

29

Tethered cord syndrome

Shokei Yamada, Brian S Yamada, and Daniel J Won

Introduction

Tethered cord syndrome (TCS) is a stretch-induced functional disorder of the spinal cord caused by the anchoring of its caudal end by an inelastic structure. The neurologic dysfunction with TCS can be attributed to lumbosacral cord lesions, and is reversible if cord-untethering surgery is done at an appropriate time. Clinical and basic research has indicated that oxidative metabolism is impaired in the tethered spinal cord and that there is a link between recovery from the neurologic dysfunction and oxidative metabolism when the stretched cord is released.[1]

This chapter seeks to increase urologists' understanding of TCS and the importance of early diagnosis and treatment in patients with associated urinary incontinence. The discussion includes pathophysiology, symptomatology, treatment, and prognosis of TCS patients. Since TCS is associated with anatomic abnormalities, many clinicians still believe erroneously that the congenital dysraphic anomalies are synonymous with TCS. This misunderstanding of TCS is accentuated by the terms derived from visual impressions of anatomic abnormalities, such as 'cord tethering' and 'tethered cord.' To clarify these expressions, the authors formulate three categories and define those patients in category 1 as clearly representing TCS.[2]

History of TCS

In the early twentieth century, several surgeons and radiologists suggested the concept of a tethering-induced spinal cord lesion.[3–8] In 1940, Lichtenstein[9] attributed paraplegia and Chiari malformation to the downward spinal cord traction by the caudally located spinal dysraphism (e.g. myelomeningocele). This hypothesis was not accepted by Barry et al,[10] Barson,[11] or Gardner et al.[12] Two major questions were unanswered: first, if tethering-induced symptoms exist, what part of the nervous system is affected? Second, what is the pathophysiologic basis for any reversible lesion?

In 1976 Hoffman et al[13] localized reversible lesions in the lumbosacral cord anchored by an inelastic thickened filum, and adopted the term 'tethered spinal cord'. In 1981, Yamada et al[1] demonstrated that oxidative metabolism was impaired in the lumbosacral cord of TCS patients and that neurologic improvement from untethering was accompanied by parallel metabolic improvement. Since then, articles referring to 'TCS' and 'tethered spinal cord' have increasingly appeared in the neurosurgical literature.[14,15]

Categorization of TCS and similar disorders

Yamada and Won[2] divided the conditions visually described by 'cord tethering' or 'tethered cord' into three pathophysiologic categories.

- Category 1: The mechanical tethering site is located at the caudal end of the spinal cord. Lumbosacral cord dysfunction can be reversible. Patients with an inelastic filum, sacral myelomeningocele (MMC), and caudal lipomyelomeningocele (LMMC) belong to this category.
- Category 2: The anomalies are attached or continuous to the dorsal aspect of the lumbosacral cord. Many MMCs and some of the dorsal or large transitional LMMCs belong to this category. The symptomatology may be partly the manifestation of TCS, and partly due to local compressive or ischemic effects, or it may result only from the latter. Impaired cerebrospinal fluid circulation may accentuate local cord dysfunction. Accordingly, signs and symptoms are only partially reversible, or unchanged after repair surgery. Some cases often require repeated surgery, sometimes resulting in progressive neurologic worsening, but not as a sign of TCS.
- Category 3: This category includes patients with no signs and symptoms of TCS, although the spinal cords in these patients appear to be tethered in MRI studies and at surgery. One subgroup of category 3 patients includes paraplegic and totally incontinent patients

associated with higher lumbar or thoracic MMCs or occasionally by LMMCs. No functional neurons exist in the lumbosacral cord. Another sub-group includes asymptomatic patients with an elongated cord and a thick filum because the syndrome is meant to be a special neurologic complex.

Embryology

The anomalies related to TCS originate in two developmental stages.[14–21] The first stage is complicated by incomplete neurulation during the 3rd to 4th week of gestation. Failure to connect two neural crests for the formation of the neural tube results in spinal dysraphism.[15,21] The 9th to 11th week of the gestation period corresponds to the second stage. At the 9th week, the permanent spinal cord forms, with its caudal end located in the coccygeal canal. Further caudally, the coccygeal medullary vestige is formed and then separated from the conus–filum complex.[16] If the vestige, which is surrounded by mesenchymal tissue, is not isolated, fibrous tissue may continue to grow into the filum, resulting in an inelastic filum.

Epidemiology

The epidemiology of the TCS is not clear, although the incidence of the midline dorsal anomalies has been reported. Demographic studies in the Unites States have shown that myelomeningoceles and other midline dorsal anomalies occur in 1 out of 1000 births.[14,22] A child with a sibling who was born with spinal dysraphism has a higher probability of this anomaly.

There are no generally accepted statistics available for the incidence of TCS. From our experiences, less than 10% of category–1 patients are found in the spina bifida clinic among newborns. It is not possible to determine whether neurologic deficits of newborns with category–2 patients are related to TCS at the MMC repair. Patients with LMMC are found less frequently than MMC, and the incidence of TCS is higher than that of MMC. Fifty percent of adult and late teenage patients with TCS associated with an inelastic filum (with or without filum thickening) were referred to our clinic as the diagnosis of failed back surgery syndrome (Yamada S, unpublished work). We believe that institutional studies are needed to collect systematically arranged data, based on populations of three categories.

Pathophysiology of TCS

The link between neurologic function and metabolic activity is not surprising since the central nervous system (CNS) relies absolutely on oxidative metabolism to produce ATP, which is the energy-donating molecule necessary for neuronal function and cell survival.[23] Experimental tethered spinal cords have shown that impairment of oxidative metabolism parallels that of glucose metabolism, and diminished interneuron activities in the spinal cord,[24] and blood flow decreases.[25–28] Of relevance to the impaired oxidative metabolism in human TCS,[29] mild to moderate spinal cord stretching had effects similar to mild hypoxemia,[30] while severe stretching had the effects expected from prolonged ischemia.[31]

Experimental cord traction studies have also indicated that, with increasing traction weight, there was greater cord elongation that paralleled greater metabolic changes. Such metabolic changes were more prominent in the caudal segments than in the cephalic segments (Figure 29.1a,b), and were not found above the lowest pair of the dentate ligaments (attachments to the T12–L1 cord segments).[32] Accordingly, the human conus medullaris is most vulnerable to traction at the caudal end.[1,33,34]

Symptomatology

Various authors have described signs and symptoms in children[1,13,35] and adults.[36,37,38] In infants, the signs and symptoms of TCS include dribbling of urine (constant wetting of diapers), foot deformity, skin stigmata, and a dysraphic dorsal midline spine or spinal cord. Skin abnormalities include a tuft of hair, fatty swelling, dimple, hemangioma, and dermal sinus in the lumbosacral areas. Young children with TCS show progression of the following signs and symptoms: (1) stumbling after walking normally for months or years; (2) dribbling urine after successful toilet training, (3) foot drop, (4) painless sore, (5) scoliosis and exaggerated lumbosacral lordosis. Early teenagers with TCS present with only a few mild symptoms, such as scoliosis, difficulty in bending over, or difficulty in running, often associated with thinning of lower limb muscles. A complaint of back and leg pain is more frequently found in this group than in the younger children, usually aggravated by exercises that include flexion–extension of the spine.

For diagnostic and prognostic purposes, Yamada et al divided adults and late teenage patients with TCS into two groups.[38,39] Group 1 patients have a prior history of spinal dysraphism associated with stabilized neurologic signs and symptoms from childhood. They usually present with subtle progression of the signs and symptoms in adulthood. Group 2 patients present with new subtle neurologic symptoms in adulthood without associated spinal dysraphism. Group 2 patients are easily overlooked because they present with subtle, specific symptomatology and radiologic findings. In particular, MRI studies show neither cord elongation nor filum thickening in 50% of the

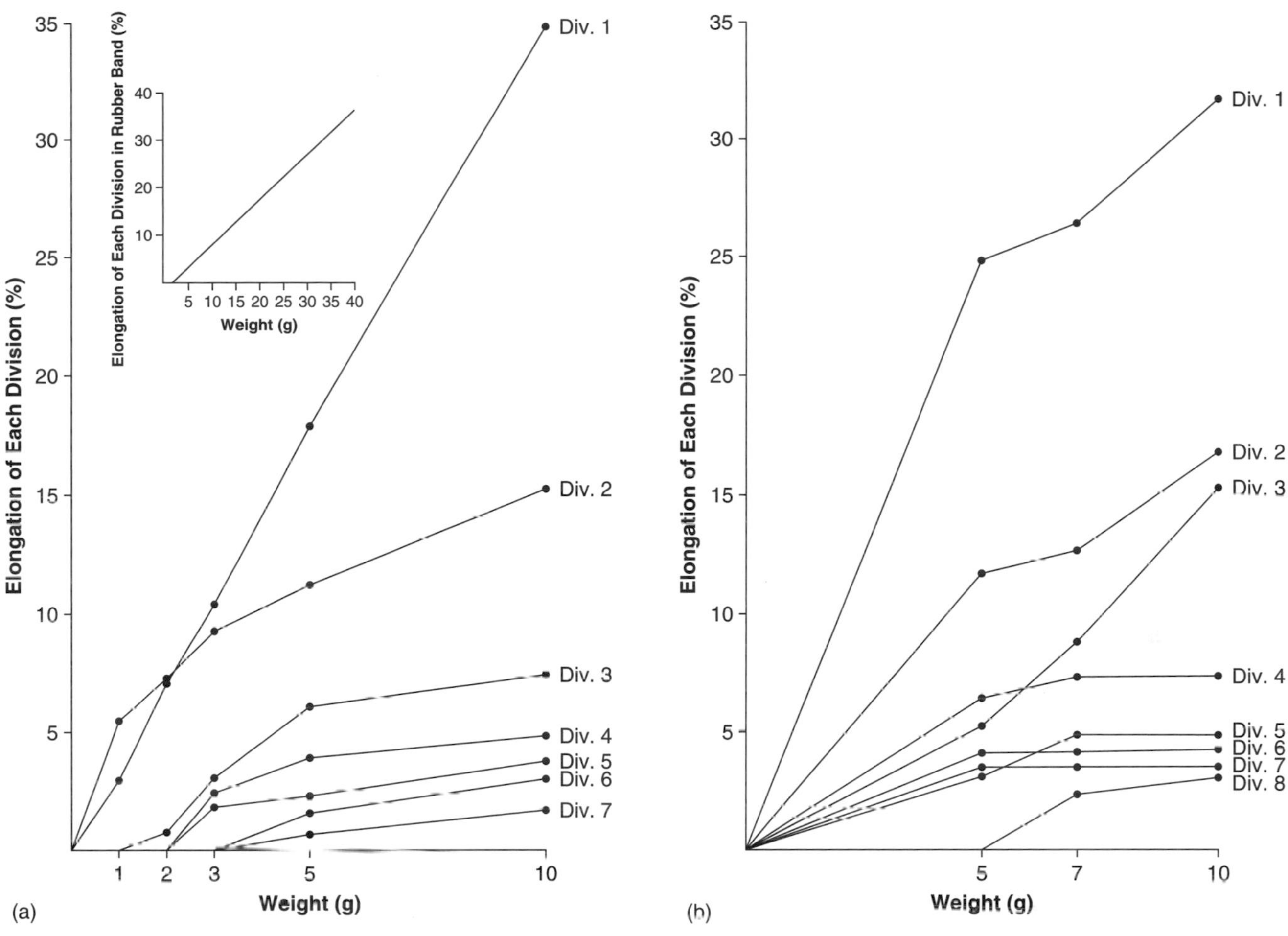

Figure 29.1
(a) By caudad traction of the filum, elongation of the filum and cord segments was measured in experimental cats. The graph shows the elongation rate of the filum (with a steep rise) and slow rise of the spinal cord segment (division 2 being the lowest and division 6 being the highest lumbar cord segment). Viscoelasticity of the filum is much greater than that of the spinal cord. This experimental model simulates the normal lumbosacral cord that is protected from overstretching when an intense vertical traction force is exerted. (b) By caudad traction of the spinal cord tip, the lowest cord segment elongates much more than when the filum was tractioned, but less than the filum in (a). The other cord segments also elongate more than in the case of filum traction. This model simulates the human tethered spinal cord, in which the conus is most vulnerable to stretching force exerted in the causal direction. (Reproduced with permission from the American Association of Neurological Surgeons, Rolling Meadows, IL, USA)

patients. In order to properly diagnose group 2 TCS patients, signs and symptoms common to the patients of this group were tabulated. More than 90% of signs and symptoms were positive in all the adult TCS patients.[40] Commom symptoms are:

1. back and leg pain, particularly aggravated by postural changes, and by other activities such as:
   - sitting with legs crossed in a Buddha pose
   - bending over the sink
   - holding a baby at waist level
   - lying supine
   - sitting in a slouching position.
2. increasing difficulty in urination and bowel control
3. physical stress-related complaints, such as decreased tolerance to running or walking, and driving a car, especially on bumpy roads.

Common signs of TCS in adults are:

1. weakness of distal muscles, e.g. extensor hallucis longus, or extensive muscle weakness in the lower limbs in scattered myotomes, and hypotrophic leg muscles
2. hyporeflexia in the lower limbs
3. sensory deficits in the distal lower limbs and perianal area, or extensive hypalgesia in lower limbs with patchy distribution

Table 29.1 *Combination of spinal cord tip location and filum thickness*
1. Normal range of caudal end (above L2–L3 interspace) and filum thickness < 2 mm: 30 cases (28.8%)
2. Normal range of caudal end and abnormally thick filum: 7 cases (6.7%)
3. Low-lying caudal end and normal range filum thickness: 30 cases (28.8%)
4. Low-lying caudal end and abnormally thick filum: 37cases (35.6%)

4. increases in postvoid residual urine
5. diminished sphincter tone: reflex (digital insertion, voluntary contraction, and wink reflex)
6. musculoskeletal deformities such as:
   - spinal: exaggerated lumbosacral lordosis and thoracolumbar scoliosis
   - leg or foot: high-arched feet, hammertoes.

Negative signs and symptoms such as no pain aggravation in lower limbs on coughing and straight leg raising are important for differential diagnosis from herniated lumbar disc.

Reflex changes are important signs for the diagnosis of TCS. Somatic reflex activities have been clearly explained by the facilitation and inhibition of reflex arcs.[41,42] Patients with TCS usually show hypoactive tendon reflexes in the lower limbs, since the lesions are located in the gray matter and the reflex arcs are inactivated. If hyperactive tendon reflexes are noted, another lesion must be suspected above the L2 cord segment, including diastomatomyelia, congenital spinal diplegia, and cerebral anomalies (e.g. Chiari malformation). Bladder control relies on complex reflex mechanisms through the parasympathetic, sympathetic, and somatic systems.

Imaging diagnosis

MRI is the most effective, noninvasive diagnostic technology for TCS, although radiography, CT scan, and ultrasound studies provide useful background information on the anomalies that may be related to TCS.[8,43–46] CT myelography is useful for patients with claustrophobia, or a cardiac pacemaker, and ultrasonography is useful for detecting an inelastic filum in newborns. It is important, however, to clinically assess imaging studies for correlation with the signs and symptoms of TCS.

Common MRI findings are:

1. an elongated cord[8] or thickened filum (> 2 mm) is frequently noted[35,43]
2. a consistent finding in TCS patients is the posterior displacement of the conus and filum, indicative of its inelastic nature.[38] The filum touches the posterior arachnoid membrane usually at the L5 or S1 lamina. Detailed axial T1 and T2 weighted views are mandatory
3. spinal dysraphism, such as MMC, LMMC, lipomas
4. a fat signal in the filum helps to confirm its posterior displacement.

The following imaging features can be indicative or suggestive of TCS:

- MMC, lipoma, and LMMC continuous to the caudal spinal cord (category 1, true TCS)
- MMC, lipoma, and LMMC attached to the dorsal aspect of the lumbosacral cord (category 2), a dermal sinus tract continuous to the caudal spinal cord
- epidermoid or dermoid tumor located in the sacral canal
- a bony septum or split cord.

An increasing number of patients with TCS who failed to show cord elongation (with the caudal end above the L1–2 or L2–3 interspace)[37,47] and filum thickening (<2 mm) have been reported. The location of the caudal end of the spinal cord and the diameter of the filum in 104 cases are shown in Table 29.1.[29,48] Of these cases, 16 (15%) had a caudal end located at the L3 vertebral level, which was not clearly identified by MRI studies, for the reason that the attachment of the 100–150 μm coccygeal nerve root was beyond the MRI resolution.

Diastemetomyelia and split cord

Pang extensively studied the split spinal cord and associated TCS.[49] Here spinal cord is divided into two halves, side by side. The partition can be a bony septum, dura, or arachnoid membrane. The tethering site can be the upper edge of the bony septum,[50] the lower edge of the bony septum,[51] or the junction of the conus and filum (or one of the double fila continuous to split hemicords).[50]

Surgical indications

Surgical treatment is indicated when there are consistent or progressive signs and symptoms of TCS such as those described above. Subtle neurologic changes, especially incontinence, and musculoskeletal deformity progression, must be watched carefully. In particular, TCS with incontinence should not be overlooked, because of its tendency to become quickly irreversible.[15,35,37,52]

The usefulness of prophylactic sectioning of the thick filum to prevent future development of TCS is debatable.[34,53,54] Based on their experience, however, Hoffman et al recommended surgical repair of LMMC for cord untethering at 4 years of age, even for asymptomatic patients.[55]

Surgical techniques

The basic techniques of untethering procedures of the spinal cord for treatment of TCS have been briefly described[14,15,39,49,52,56] in this section.

1. *Tethered cord syndrome with an inelastic filum, including a thickened filum continuous to the elongated cord.* The patients in this group belong to category 1. A 1-cm long segment of an inelastic filum is resected with its cephalic end 0.5 cm below the junction, and the specimen is histologically examined to prove that the filum is inelastic due to replacement of glial tissue by fibrous or fibroadipose tissue. The lowest coccygeal nerve root exit is a landmark for the junction of the conus and filum.[39]
2. *Lipoma or lipomyelomeningocele (LMMCs)* (Figure 29.1.) General surgical techniques consist of adequate resection of a fibroadipose mass for cord untethering. Total resection of the caudal lipoma and caudal LMMC can be accomplished without causing neural damage. The dorsal and transitional LMMC are usually resected flush to the spinal cord surface. Tight closure of meninges is mandatory after repair of LMMC for protection of neural structures.[15,56,57]
3. *Myelomeningoceles (MMCs).* Patients with the MMC located at the caudal end of the spinal cord (category 1) are expected to have the same excellent benefit from surgical repair as those with an inelastic filum. Those of category 2 or 3 require careful dissection of the neural placode to prevent further cord damage and postoperative adhesion.[14]

Incontinence

Pathophysiology of incontinence in TCS

Storage and emptying are the two fundamental functions in the human lower urinary tract. These are voluntarily controlled by the cerebral centers and by reflex coordination of the spinal cord centers through the parasympathetic and sympathetic systems which regulate bladder and sphincter contraction. The bladder's natural distensibility allows it to hold low intravesical pressure (<10 cmH_2O) without high sphincteric resistance until the urine volume reaches a certain amount.[58–61]

Studies indicate that the conus is highly vulnerable to cord traction.[1,33,47] Accordingly, control of bladder function is often lost earlier than motor and sensory function in the lower limbs. Since the main lesion of TCS is located in the gray matter,[1] and not in the long tract,[62] impaired synaptic transmission in the conus is likely responsible for loss of normal micturition.

Parasympathetic fibers are distributed to the bladder and urethral sphincter. Afferent fibers from the bladder travel in the pelvic nerve and enter the conus through the posterior sensory ganglia. These sensory fibers then reach the intermediolateral column, and synapse with the efferent fibers, forming the reflex arcs. The afferent fibers from the sphincter travel in the pudendal nerve, and enter the conus through the posterior sensory ganglia, and then to the intermediolateral column for synaptic connection to the efferent fibers. The efferent fibers reach the bladder and sphincter through the same pathways as in the reverse direction.

The sympathetic system, with its spinal cord center in the intermediolateral column of T10–L2 cord segments, is distributed to the bladder and sphincter through the hypogastric nerve. The efferent fibers join the parasympathetic fibers in the pelvic and pudendal nerves, and the afferent sympathetic fibers take similar pathways to those of the efferent fibers. Because of their much higher location than the conus, the sympathetic reflex arcs in the spinal cord are not involved in the TCS lesion.

Other reflex arcs are organized by the parasympathetic afferent system and central somatic efferent system. Impulses from the bladder and sphincter are carried through the parasympathetic afferent fibers, ascend in the spinal cord, and reach the cerebral and pontine micturition centers. The efferent fibers from these centers descend in the corticospinal tract and control bladder and sphincter balance.[58,60,63,64]

Although similar cerebral control mechanisms were found for excitation and inhibition of bladder activities between the somatic and autonomic systems, lesions in the spinal cord are manifested differently.[58] Considering the loss of motor innervation to the bladder caused by injuries of peripheral parasympathetic fibers,[59,65,66] Blaivas suggested from his own urodynamic studies that TCS results in one of two abnormalities; (1) areflexic, hypotonic bladder or (2) areflexic hypertonic bladder.[59] Although areflexic hypertonic bladder explains frequent micturition of a small amount of urine in patients with spinal cord injuries, how a conus lesion could result in this condition was not clarified. Ruch's analysis of hypertonic bladder (increased tonus) due either to the postgangionic parasympathetic excitation or to bladder muscle contracture may be responsible.[58]

Presentation of urinary control dysfunction

According to Hadley and Holevas,[60] bladder dysfunction is an associated complaint in 40% of patients with TCS, and the exclusive complaint in 4%. Yamada and Lonser reported that 78% of adults with TCS experienced difficulties with bladder control.[37]

A careful history and physical examination is required, especially related to the function of storing and emptying urine, including:

1. diurnal and nocturnal voiding patterns
2. urgency
3. dysuria
4. hesitation
5. sensation of fullness, and voiding
6. ability to interrupt or inhibit micturition
7. straining to void
8. incontinence
9. erection, emission, and ejaculation
10. bowel habits and continence
11. testing the bulbocavernosus muscle and anal wink reflex.[60]

From our experience, incontinence becomes evident when parents check diapers every 15 minutes for one hour, 3–4 times a day. After a few days, such parents typically report that the diapers are constantly wet. When children reach one year or older, the parents notice slow adjustment or fluctuation in the child's toilet training, or that the child has developed incontinence after successful toilet training.

As TCS patients grow older, they often exhibit a lack of normal urinary stream (as compared with other boys), difficulties with voiding (initiating or completing urination and dribbling postvoiding), or increasing frequency. Adult and late teenage patients and may complain of urinary hesitancy, slow urinary stream, or stress urinary incontinence.

Urodynamic studies

In separate reviews of urodynamic studies in TCS patients with urologic complaints, Hellstrom et al[67] found detrusor areflexia in 50%, hyperreflexia in 26%, mixed lesions (decreased compliance and involuntary contractions) in 12%, sensory urgency with decreased capacity in 12%, and normal studies in 12%.

Imaging studies

For urologic evaluation, Khoury et al recommend a lumbosacral X-ray and voiding cystourethrogram (VCUG).[61] Lumbosacral X-ray is helpful in identifying bone spinal abnormalities.[68] This test may also help establish the possibility of neurogenic bowel by identifying a significant amount of fecal material in the colon. VCUG helps to evaluate for vesicoureteral reflux, neurogenic or atonic bladder, and bladder outlet obstruction.

Treatment

Several studies have documented improved voiding function following surgical release of tethered cords. Khoury et al reported resolution of daytime incontinence and detrusor hyperreflexia in 72% and 59% of patients, respectively, as well as improved compliance in 66%.[69] Reviewing 15 adults with TCS, Kondo et al found 60% of patients improved following untethering surgery, and identified three factors among the remaining 40% that imparted a poor prognosis: (1) symptoms for longer than 3 years; (2) loss of bladder sensation; and (3) severe tethering with the conus fixed to the bottom of the dural sac.[70]

The baseline bladder function of patients who develop TCS is often abnormal, and a significant number of patients who do not respond to untethering surgery will have residual neurogenic bladder dysfunction. Addressing their urologic problems in terms of the storage and emptying functions of the bladder facilitates management of these patients. In emptying failure due to detrusor areflexia (the most common pattern seen in these patients), an intermittent catheterization program is often most effective. Some patients utilize abdominal straining augmented by the Crede's maneuver (manual abdominal compression) to attempt complete voiding. This technique rarely empties the bladder effectively and generates high intravesical pressures, which may ultimately be detrimental to the urinary system. Cholinergics (e.g. bethanechol) have been used in an effort to improve detrusor muscle contractility; however, they have not been shown to enhance bladder emptying.

Case reports

Two cases with TCS are presented, one representing category 1, and the other category 2 (Figure 29.2).

Case 1

A 4-year-old-girl began to have urinary dribbling after successful toilet training, starting 4 months before admission. Episodes of dribbling continued to increase. No other neurologic signs and symptom were noted. Spina bifida was demonstrated at S5 and the sacral spine on plain X-ray films (Figure 29.4). A large soft swelling of the left gluteal

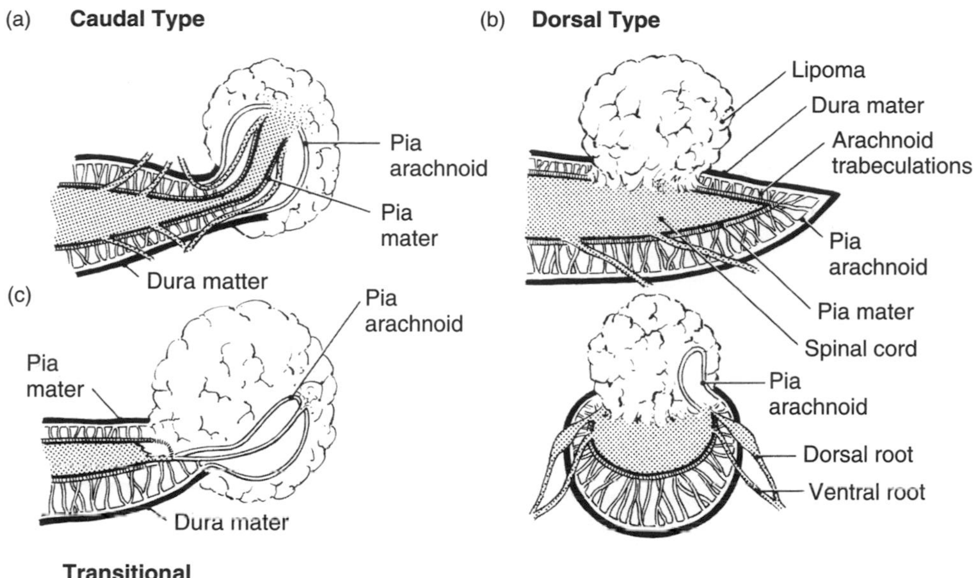

Figure 29.2
Schematic drawings of the three types of lipomyelomeningoceles (LMMCs) include, counterclockwise: (a) upper left: the caudal (terminal) type. The interface of the spinal cord and the lipoma is located at the caudal extremity of the lower sacral or coccygeal cord. The fusion of the meninges (dura and arachnoid) with the spinal cord is located slightly caudal to the interface. (b) Upper and lower right: the dorsal type. The interface of the spinal cord with the lipoma is found at its dorsal aspect. A usually small subarachnoid space extends into or surrounds the fatty mass. (c) Lower left: the transitional type. The interface of the cord and lipoma is located in the posterior part of the caudal extremity and extends to the dorsal aspect of the cord. The anterior part of the caudal extremity extends to the filum terminale that continues caudad and is surrounded by cerebrospnial fluid, the arachnoid, and dura, and ends at the fatty sac wall.

area (Figure 29.3) corresponded to the cerebrospinal fluid accumulation underneath the skin on myelography. Surgical repair of a caudal lipomyelomeningocele was performed and the caudal end of the spinal cord was disconnected from fat tissue in the wall of the anomaly. The patient regained continence in 2 weeks. Intraoperative redox studies before and after surgical untethering showed remarkable oxidative metabolic improvement from the reduced state to the normally oxidized state.

Case 2

A 14-year-old girl was known as an infrequent voider in early infancy. At 3 years of age, toilet training was successful except for occasional enuresis. A the age of 7, enuresis became frequent and progressed to total incontinence, associated with lack of urgency or sensation of a full bladder. Urinary loss was related to overflow and to stress or Valsalva manuevers, requiring continuous pad protection. On examination, minimal suprapubic pressure would express urine. Two small dimples in the sacral area and pes cavus were noted. Neurologic findings included weakness of extensor hallucis longus, bilaterally hypoactive Achilles tendon reflex, and analgesia in the perianal area. Postvoid urinary residual was >200 ml. The urine was sterile. Plain films revealed spina bifida at S1 through S5. VCUG showed bilaterally promptly functioning kidneys, a cellule and diverticula formation in the bladder, right vesicoureteral reflux, and a large postvoid residual. A myelogram showed LMMC in the sacral level with a cord tip at the S2 level. Surgical repair of a large transitional LMMC consisted of removal of the entire fibroadipose mass, with dissection from the caudal end of the spinal cord. Within one week after the operation, the patient began to regain bladder control without evidence of stress incontinence. VCUG clarified resolution of the reflux and a normal residual urine. This patient underwent 18 urologic procedures from the age of 7 to 14 to manage her neurogenic bladder and vesicoureteral reflux. Redox studies showed postuntethering metabolic improvement.

Discussion for isolated incontinence with TCS

Recently, three groups of authors discussed incontinence in patients with 'occult tethered cord syndrome'. These patients showed neither filum thickening nor cord elongation.[71–74] It is reasonable to assume that TCS may be

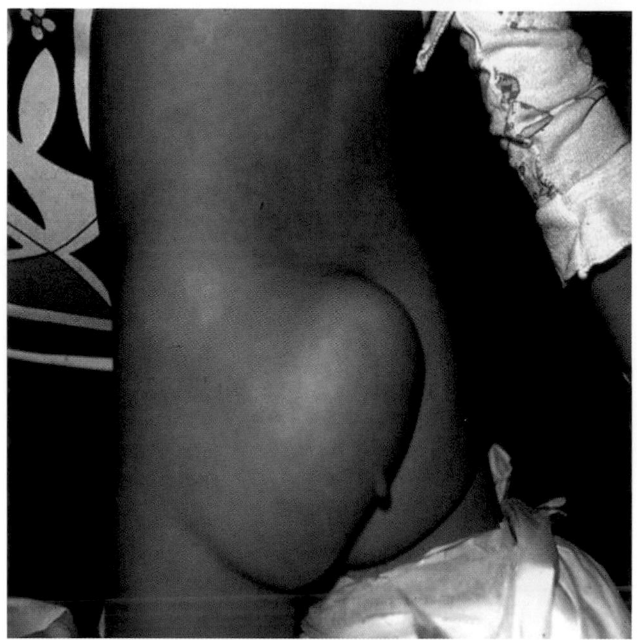

Figure 29.3
Photograph of a caudal-type LMMC. The left gluteal swelling fluctuated. (Reproduced with permission from the American Association of Neurological Surgeons, Rolling Meadows, IL, USA).

manifested by incontinence alone, because our experimental work has indicated that the conus medullaris is most vulnerable to traction-induced dysfunction. When the reliability of MRI findings was discussed by the questionnaire,[73] all neurosurgeons agreed to surgical intervention in the presence of positive findings such as elongated cord, thick filum, fat signal in the filum on the patients who showed incontinence, along with motor and sensory dysfunction. Without such MRI signs, the neurosurgeons' opinions were divided. To enhance the diagnosis of TCS in these patients, Yamada et al directed that special attention be given to MRI studies to detect posterior displacement of the conus and filum. Additionally in surgery, subarachnoid endoscopy confirmed this finding, and further stretch test proved a lack of filum elasticity.[34,74]

Subsequently the three groups of authors advocate that extensive lower urinary tract testing be done before decision-making.[74] In our experience, however, most adult and late teenage patients showed negative renal and bladder tests. The most frequent positive finding was an elevated postvoid urinary residual. There were 50 group-2 patients of whom 36 complained of urinary incontinence; 92% of incontinent patients had a postvoid residual of greater than 50 ml. After untethering surgery, more than 94% of them reported resolution of incontinence within 2 days to 1 week, and had an associated decrease in residual to 0–20 ml (Yamada S, Yamada BS, unpublished work).

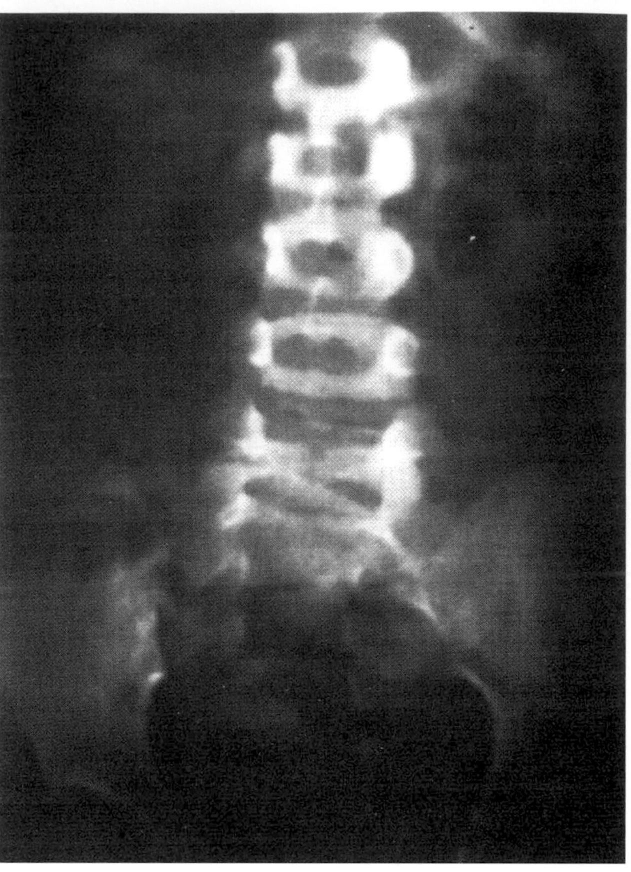

Figure 29.4
A plain film shows spina bifida of the sacral spine. (Reproduced with permission from the American Association of Neurological Surgeons, Rolling Meadows, IL, USA).

Voiding symptoms and incontinence after surgical untethering

The majority of patients regained control of bladder function after untethering procedures, as described earlier by Khoury,[69] and by Fukui and Kakizaki[75] who showed resolution of incontinence associated with detrusor-external urethral sphincter dyssynergy. However, the baseline bladder function in patients who develop TCS is often abnormal, whilst 30–40% of patients do not respond to cord release.[61] A significant number of patients will have residual neurogenic bladder dysfunction. The surgical outcome of Kondo et al[70] supports this data. From our experience, those cases probably belonged to category 2, for example with a large transitional LMMC.[2] Another logical explanation is drawn from our experimental studies,[24,76] suggesting that neuronal degeneration develops in the conus after sudden cord stretching caused by extreme spinal flexion and extension in TCS patients.

Addressing their urologic problems in terms of the storage and emptying functions of the bladder facilitates management of these patients. In emptying failure due to detrusor areflexia, the most common pattern seen in these patients, an intermittent catheterization program is often most effective.

Conclusion

TCS is defined as a stretch-induced functional disorder of the spinal cord with its caudal part anchored by inelastic structures. Clinical findings such as motor and sensory deficits in the lower limbs, incontinence, and musculoskeletal deformities allow for the localization of the lesions in the lumbosacral cord. These clinical impressions are compatible with findings of spinal cord traction in experimental animals. In TCS patients and in experimental animals, impaired oxidative metabolism and electrophysiologic activities within the lumbosacral cord were linked to neurologic dysfunction. These changes occurred without observable histologic damage to neurons. Many patients with TCS have associated voiding dysfunction and incontinence. In some patients, urinary incontinence is the sole complaint. The urologist must have a high index of suspicion for a neurologic etiology for the urinary incontinence. Prompt recognition of the neurologic disorder is of paramount importance. With early intervention, neurosurgic untethering of the spinal cord in category 1 patients can result in complete resolution of neurologic deficit, including urinary symptoms. The surgical results for category 2 patients are not as good as in the former patients. Nevertheless, the diagnosis and treatment must not be delayed or irreversible urinary tract dysfunction may occur.

Acknowledgment

The authors acknowledge Dr Myron Rosenthal, Professor of Physiology and Neurology at the University of Miami School of Medicine, for his continued support and advice for our research in tethered cord syndrome.

References

1. Yamada S, Zinke DE, Sanders D. Pathophysiology of 'tethered cord syndrome'. J Neurosurg 1981; 54: 494–503.
2. Yamada S, Won DJ. What is the true tethered cord syndrome? Childs' Nerv Syst 2007; 23: 371–5.
3. Fuchs A. Über Beziehungen der Enuresis nocturna zu Rudimentarformen der Spina bifida occulta (myelodysplasie). Wien Med Wochenschr 1910; 80: 1569–73.
4. Garceau GJ. The filum terminale syndrome (The cord-traction syndrome). Bone Joint Surg (Am) 1953; 35: 711–16.
5. Hoffmann GT, Hooks CA, Jackson IJ, Thompson IM. Urinary incontinence in myelomeningoceles due to a tethered spinal cord and its surgical treatment. Surg Gynecol Obstet 1956; 103: 618–24.
6. Jones PH, Love JG. Tight filum terminale. Arch Surg 1956; 73: 556–66.
7. James CCM, Lassman LP. Spinal dysraphism. The diagnosis and treatment of progressive lesions in spina bifida occulta. J Bone Joint Surg (Br) 1962; 44: 828–40.
8. Fitz C, Harwood-Nash DC. Tethered conus, AJR 1975; 125: 515–23.
9. Lichtenstein BW. Distant neuroanatomic complications of spina bifida (spinal dysraphism), hydrocephalus, Arnold–Chiari deformity, stenosis of the aqueduct of Sylvius, etc; pathogenesis and pathology. Arch Neurol Psychiatry 1940; 47: 195–214.
10. Barry A, Pattern BM, Stewart BH. Possible factors in the development of the Arnold–Chiari malformation. J Neurosurg 1957; 14: 285–301.
11. Barson AJ. The vertebral level of termination of the spinal cord during normal and abnormal chemical development. J Anat 1970; 106: 489–97.
12. Gardner WJ, Smith JL, Padget DH. The relationship of Arnold–Chiari and Dandy–Walker malformations. J Neurosurg 1972; 36: 481–9.
13. Hoffman HJ, Hendrick EB, Humpreys RJ. The tethered spinal cord: its protean manifestations, diagnosis and surgical correction. Childs Brain 1976; 2: 145–55.
14. Reigel DH. Spinal bifida. In: McLaurin RL, Schut L, Venes JL, Epstein F, eds, Pediatric Neurosurgery, 2nd edn. Philadelphia: WB Saunders, 1989: 35–52.
15. McLone DG, Naidich TP, The tethered spinal cord. In: McLaurin RL, Schut I, Venes JL, Epstein F, eds. Pediatric Neurosurgery, 2nd edn. Philadelphia: WB Saunders 1989: 76–96.
16. Kunitomo K. The development and reduction of the tail and of the caudal end of the spinal cord. Contrib Embryol Carnegie Inst 1978; 8: 161–98.
17. Streeter GI. Factors involved in the formation of the filum terminale. Am J Anat 1919; 25: 1–12.
18. Lemire RI, Shepard TH, Ellsworth CA Jr. Caudal myeloschisis (lumbo-sacral spina bifida cystica) in five millimeter (Horizen XIV) human embryo. Anat Rec 1965; 192: 9–16.
19. French BN. The embryology of spinal dysraphism. Clin Neurosurg 1983; 3: 295–340.
20. Marin Padilla M. The tethered cord syndrome: developmental consideration. In: Holtzman RNN, Stein BM, eds. The Tethered Spinal Cord. New York: Thieme-Stratton, 1985: 1–13.
21. Newgreen DF, McKeown ASJ. The neural crest: a model developmental EMT. In: Savagner P, ed. Rise and Fall of Epithelial Phenotype: Concepts of Epithelial Mesenchymal Transition. New York: Kluwer Academic/Academic/Plenum, 2005: 29–39.
22. Shurtleff DB, Lemire RL. Epidemiology, etiologic factors, and prenatal diagnosis of open spinal dysraphism. Neurosurg Clin North Am 1995; 6: 183–93.
23. Rosenthal M, LaManna J, Yamada S, Somjen G. Oxidative metabolism, extracellular potassium and sustained potential shifts in cat spinal cord in situ. Brain Res 1979; 162: 113–27.
24. Yamada S, Iacono R, Yamada BS. Pathophysiology of tethered cord syndrome. In: Yamada S, ed. Tethered Cord Syndrome Park Ridge, IL: American Association of Neurological Surgeons, 1996: 29–48.
25. Turnbull IM, Breig A, Hassler O. Blood supply of cervical spinal cord in man. A microangiographic cadaver study. J Neurosurg 1966; 24: 951–65.
26. Yamada S, Knierim D, Yonekura M, Schultz R, Maeda G. Tethered cord syndrome. J Am Paraplegia Soc 1983; 6: 58–61.
27. Kang JK, Kim MC, King DS, Song JU. Effects of tethering on regional spinal cord blood flow and sensory-evoked potentials in growing cats. Childs Nerv Syst 1987; 3: 35–9.
28. Schneider SJ, Rosenthal AD, Greenberg VM, Danto J. A preliminary report on the use of laser-Doppler flowmetry during tethered spinal cord release. Neurosurgery 1983; 32: 214–17.

29. Yamada S, Won DJ, Yamada SM. Pathophysiology of tethered cord syndrome and clinical correlation. Neurosurg Forum 2004; 16: 1–5.
30. Yamada S, Sanders DC, Haugen GE. Functional and metabolic responses of the spinal cord to anoxia and asphyxia. In: Austin GM, ed. Contemporary Aspects of Cerebrovascular Disease. Dallas, TX: Professional Information Library, 1976: 239–46.
31. Yamada S, Sanders DC, Maeda G. Oxidative metabolism during and following ischemia of cat spinal cord. Neurol Res 1981; 3: 1–16.
32. Yamada S, Perot PL, Ducker TB, Lockard I. Myelotomy for control of mass spasms in paraplegia. J Neurosurg 1976; 45: 681–3.
33. Tani S, Yamada S, Knighton R. Extensibility of the lumbar and sacral spinal cord – pathophysiology of tethered spinal cord. J Neurosurg 1987; 66: 116–23.
34. Yamada S, Won DJ, Pezeshkpour G et al. Pathophysiology of tethered cord syndrome and similar disorders. Neurosug Focus 2007; 23(2): E6: 1–10.
35. Pang D, Tethered cord syndrome. In: Hoffman HJ, ed. Advances in Neurosurgery, Vol 1, No 1. Philadelphia: Hanley & Belfus, 1986: 45–79.
36. Pang D, Wilberger JE Jr. Tethered cord syndrome in adults. J Neurosurg 1982; 57: 32–47.
37. Yamada S, Lonser RR. Adult tethered cord syndrome. J Spinal Disord 2000; 13: 319–23.
38. Yamada S, Won DJ, Kido DK. Adult tethered cord syndrome: new classification correlated with symptomatology, imaging and pathophysiology. Neurosurg Q 2001; 11: 260–75.
39. Yamada S, Iacono R, Douglas C, Lonser RR, Shook J. Tethered cord syndrome in adults. In: Yamada S, ed. Tethered Cord Syndrome. Park Ridge, IL: American Association of Neurological Surgeons, 1996: 149–65.
40. Yamada S, Siddiqi J, Won DJ et al. Symptomatic protocols for adult tethered cord syndrome. Neurol Res 2004; 26: 741–4.
41. Grew TJ, Spinal cord II: Reflex action. In: Kandel EP, Schwartz JH, eds. Principles of Neural Science. New York: Elsevier/North Holland, 1981: 293–304.
42. Haines DE, Mihailoff GA, Yerzierski RP. The spinal cord. In: Haines DE, ed. Fundamental Neuroscience, 2nd edn. New York: Churchill Livingston, 2002: 294–357.
43. Harwood-Nash D, Neuroradioogy A: Computed tomography. In: Holtzman RNN, Stein BM, eds. The Tethered Spinal Cord. New York: Thieme-Stratton, 1985: 41–6.
44. Naidich P, McLone DG. Neuroradiology B: Ultrasonography. In: Holtzman RNN, Stein B, eds. The Tethered Spinal Cord. New York: Thieme-Stratton, 1985: 47–58.
45. Hinshaw DB Jr, Engelhart JA, Kaminsky CK. Imaging of the tethered spinal cord. In: Yamada S, ed. Tethered Cord Syndrome. Park Ridge, IL: American Association of Neurological Surgeons, 1996: 55–70.
46. Nelson MD. Ultrasonic evaluation of the tethered cord syndrome. In: Yamada S, ed. Tethered Cord Syndrome. Park Ridge, IL: American Association of Neurological Surgeons, 1996: 71–8.
47. Tubbs RS. Oakes WJ: Can the conus medullaris in normal position be tethered? Neurol Res 2004; 26: 727–31.
48. Wehby MC, O'Hollaren PS, Abtin K, Hune JL, Richards BJ. Occult tight filum terminale syndrome: results of surgical untethering, Pediatr Neurosurg 2004; 40: 51–7.
49. Pang D. Split cord malformation. In: Pang D ed. Disorders of the Pediatric Spine. New York: Raven Press, 1995: 203–52.
50. Yamada S, Yamada SM, Mandybur GM, Yamada BS. Conservative versus surgical treatment and tethered cord syndrome prognosis. In: Yamada S, ed. Tethered Cord Syndrome. Park Ridge, IL: American Association of Neurological Surgeons, 1996: 183–202.
51. Guthkelch AN, Hoffmann GT. Tethered spinal cord in association with diastematomyelia, Surg Neurol 1981; 15: 352–4.
52. Hoffman HJ. Indication and treatment of the tethered spinal cord. In: Yamada S, ed. Tethered Cord Syndrome. Park Ridge, IL: American Association of Neurological Surgeons, 1996: 29–48.
53. Till K. Spinal dysraphism. A study of congenital malformations of the lower back. J Bone Joint Surg (Br) 1969; 51: 415–22.
54. Till K. Occult spinal dysraphism, The value of prophylactic surgical treatment. In: Sano K, Ishii S, Le Vay D, eds. Recent Progress in Neurological Surgery. New York: Elsevier, 1973: 61–6.
55. Hoffman HJ, Taecholarn C, Hendrick EB, Humphreys RP. Management of lipomyelomeningoceles. Experience at the Hospital for Sick Children. Toronto J Neurosurg 1985; 62: 1–8.
56. Yamada S, Lonser RR, Yamada SM, Iacono RP. Tethered cord syndrome associated with myelomeningoceles and lipomyelomeningoceles. In: Yamada S, ed Tethered Cord Syndrome. Park Ridge, IL: American Association of Neurological Surgeons, 1996: 103–23.
57. Sakamoto H, Hakuba A, Fujitani K, Nishimura S. Surgical treatment of the tethered spinal cord after repair of lipomyelomeningocele. J Neurosurg 1991; 74: 709–14.
58. Ruch TC. The urinary bladder. In: Ruch TC, Fulton JF, eds, Medical Physiology and Biophysics. Philadelphia: W.B Saunders, 1960: 955–62.
59. Blaivas JG. Urological abnormalities in the tethered spinal cord. In: Holtzman RNN, Stein BM, eds. The Tethered Spinal Cord. New York: Thieme-Stratton, 1985: 41–6.
60. Hadley R, Holevas RE. Lower urinary tract dysfunction in tethered cord syndrome. In: Yamada S, ed. Tethered Cord Syndrome. Park Ridge, IL: American Association of Neurological Surgeons, 1996: 79–88.
61. Khoury AE, Balcom A, LcLorie GA, Churchill BM. Clinical experience in urological involvement with tethered cord syndrome. In: Yamada S, ed. Tethered Cord Syndrome. Park Ridge, IL: American Association of Neurological Surgeons, 1996: 89–98.
62. Fuse T, Patrickson J, Yamada S. Axonal transport of horseradish peroxidase in the experimental tethered spinal cord. Pediatr Neurosci 1989; 15: 296–301.
63. Murphy JJ, Wein AJ. Urologic aspects of surgery. In: Austin GM, ed. The Spinal Cord, 3rd edn. New York: Igaku-Shoin, 1983: 664–76.
64. Hardy SGP, Naftel JP. Viscerosensory pathway. In: Haines DE, ed. Fundamental Neuroscience. New York: Churchill Livingstone, 2002: 293–322.
65. Kuru M. Nervous control of micturition. Physiol Rev 1965; 45: 425–94.
66. McGuire EJ, Woodside JR, Borden TA, Weiss RM. Prognostic value of urodynamic testing in myelodysplastic patients. J Urol 1981; 126: 205–9.
67. Helstrom WJG, Edwards MSB, Kogan BA. Urological aspects of the tethered cord syndrome. J Urol 1986; 135: 317–20.
68. Pippi Salle JL, Capolicchi Edwards MSB, Kogan BA. Urological aspects of the tethered cord syndrome. J Urol 1986; 135: 317–20.
69. Khoury AE, Hendrick EB, McLorie GA, Kulkami A, Churchill BM. Occcult spinal dysraphism: clinical and urodynamic outcome after division of the filum terminale. J Urol 1990; 144: 426–9.
70. Kondo A, Kato K, Kanai, Sakakibara T. Bladder dysfunction secondary to tethered cord syndrome in adults: is it curable? J Urol 1986; 135: 313–16.
71. Drake JM. Occult tethered cord syndrome: not an indication for surgery, J Neurosurg 2006; 104(5 Suppl Pediatrics): 305–8.
72. Selden NR. Occult tethered cord syndrome: the case for surgery, J Neurosurg 2006; 104(5 Suppl Pediatrics): 302–4.
73. Steinbok P, Garton HJL, Gupta N. Occulta tethered cord syndrome: a survey of practice pattern, J Neurosurg 2006; 104(5 Suppl Pediatrtics): 309–13.
74. Yamada S, Won DJ. Neurosurgical forum, Letters to the editor. Occult tethered cord syndrome. J Neurosurg 2007; 106: 411–14.
75. Fukui J, Kakizaki TL. Urodynamic evaluation of tethered cord syndrome including tight filum terminale. Urology 1980; 16: 539–52.
76. Yamada S, Schultz RL, Mandybur GT et al. Axonal degeneration after sudden forceful traction of the spinal cord: is it the cause of permanent neurological deficit? J Neurosurg 2003; 98: 681.

30

Spinal cord injury and cerebral trauma

Jerzy B Gajewski and John W Downie

Introduction

Disturbances of micturition are very common with head and spinal cord injuries. The range of bladder symptoms caused by neurologic lesions is wide and determined by whether the lesion primarily affects supraspinal control, the pontine–sacral neural circuit, or the sacral nerves and whether these lesions are predominantly motor or sensory, or both. The role of this innervation in bladder physiology is the key to understanding bladder dysfunction in head trauma and spinal cord injury.

Neuroanatomy

The function of the lower urinary tract is storage of urine and emptying when socially accepted. This is controlled and coordinated by the neurologic system. Micturition is a coordinated contraction of the detrusor muscle of the bladder and relaxation of the proximal (smooth muscle of the bladder neck and urethra) and distal (striated muscle) external urethral sphincters following release of cortical inhibition. Control of micturition is localized in the cortical, pontine, and sacral centers connected by a neural circuit that extends from the cortex through the pons to the sacral cord.[1,2] The cortical areas influencing bladder control include the limbic lobes and paracentral lobules from which fibers pass to the pons and downward in the corticospinal tracts to the anterior and lateral horn cells at S2–4. In rat, the locus ceruleus may be involved in arousal, which is mediated by bladder distention.[3]

Human positron emission tomography (PET) scans have shown two distinct cortical areas involved in micturition and contraction of the pelvic floor (Figure 30.1).[4] The right prefrontal cortex showed increased activity during micturition and during attempts to voluntarily inhibit voiding. Activity in the anterior cingulate gyrus is decreased during inhibition of voiding. Voluntary contraction of the female pelvic floor causes increased activity in the superomedial precentral gyrus (part of the primary motor cortex).[5] Others have shown in functional magnetic Resonance imaging (fMRI) studies that pelvic floor contractions result in an increased desire to void and activation of the 'continence areas', which include the medial premotor cortex, basal ganglia, and cerebellum.[6]

The basal ganglia, hypothalamus, and cerebellum all modulate function of the lower urinary tract through the pontine micturition center (PMC). Early brain transection experiments indicated that the basic micturition reflex was subject to modulation by higher levels of the neuraxis.[7] The identities of some of the specific modulatory areas have been postulated based on experiments in animals and on imaging in humans. However, the roles of these areas are not always clear, and in most cases the pathways by which they affect micturition are not yet established. For example, the cerebellum seems to be important in facilitating voiding in dogs,[8] but is active during both urine storage[9,10] and voiding in humans.[11] Due to extensive connections between the cerebellum and the rest of the neuraxis, the pathway through which it modulates micturition is unclear at present.[12] The hypothalamus, particularly the preoptic area, has been considered an important regulator of bladder function because of its extensive projection to the micturition center in the pons of the cat and rat.[13,14] Some imaging studies in humans have demonstrated hypothalamic activation during micturition,[15] but in the other clinical studies, the response is less clear.[14,15] The hypothalamus appears not to be activated during urine storage.[4,5,9,10] The role of functional imaging in identifying brain areas important for micturition has been reviewed.[16,17]

Coordination of the detrusor contraction and sphincter relaxation is mainly done by the PMC located in the brainstem.[18] Normally, the external sphincter activity increases during bladder distention by a spinal reflex mechanism, then ceases through descending inhibition when a bladder contraction occurs.[19] In the cat, there appears to be a spinal neural organization that can mediate coordinated activity in the bladder preganglionic neurons and pudendal interneuron pools independently from the PMC.[18,19]

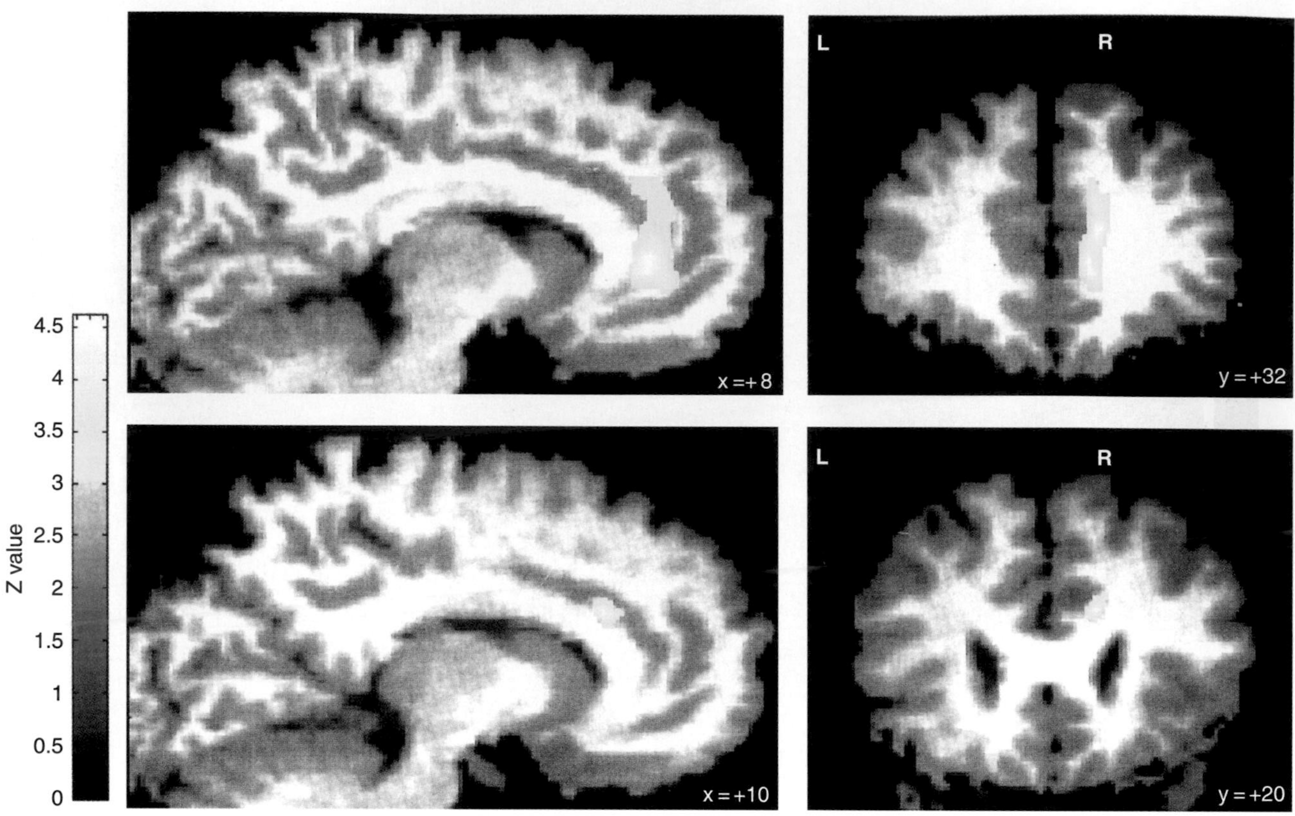

Figure 30.1
Top: Significant differences in rCBF in the anterior cingulated gyrus, comparing successful micturition with voluntary withholding of urine (scan 2 – scan 1; average of 10 subjects). *Bottom:* Significant differences in rCBF in the anterior cingulated gyrus, comparing unsuccessful micturition with voluntary withholding of urine (scan 2 – scan 1; average of 7 subjects). Uncorrected threshold of $p < 0.001$. (Reproduced with permission from Blok et al.[4])

There seem to be two centers in the pontine region; first, the PMC, which is responsible for emptying, is located in Barrington's nucleus or the M region, and, secondly, the pontine urine storage facilitator center (PUSFC), which is located in the nucleus locus subceruleus (Lsc) L region.[20,21] PET study in healthy men and women confirmed the presence of the L region and the M region (Figure 30.2).[3,4] Experimental study on cats showed that an ascending projection from the lumbosacral region reaches the periaqueductal gray (PAG), and a group of PAG neurons, in turn, project to the M region of the PMC (Figure 30.3).[22] Although transmission of bladder-related afferent information by this pathway has yet to be confirmed in the cat,[23] a crucial role for the ventrolateral periaqueductal gray matter (PAGvl) in micturition has been demonstrated in rats.[24,25] Facilitatory and inhibitory influences from the cortical and subcortical centers are exerted on this neural circuit, with the overall effect being inhibitory. Normal micturition is believed to involve a spino-bulbo-spinal reflex activation of parasympathetic preganglionic neurons (to the bladder) and inhibition of pudendal motoneurons – Onuf's nucleus (to the striated urethral sphincter).[26,27] PMC projection to the Onuf's nucleus is not direct and may involve interneurons in sacral intermediomedial (IMM) cell columns.[28] Afferent (sensory) and efferent (motor) nerve fibers connect the bladder and urethra to the sacral and thoracolumbar segments. Interneurons involved in bladder reflexes are located in the region of the sacral parasympathetic nucleus (SPN), the dorsal commissure (DCM), and superficial laminae of the dorsal horn.[29,30] In cats, Aδ fibers comprise the peripheral afferent pathway involved in the reflex.[31–33]

Sensory fibers subserving proprioception and muscle stretch sensation from the lower urinary tract travel in the pelvic, hypogastric, and pudendal nerves to the sacral (S2, 3, and 4) and thoracolumbar (T11–L2) cord. Sensory impulses of touch, pain, and fullness from bladder mucosa travel via pelvic nerves. Most of these fibers are thin Aδ-myelinated axons and some are unmyelinated C-fiber axons. Most Aδ-myelinated axons connect to mechanoreceptors in the detrusor (cats) and are involved in the normal micturitional reflex[34] (Figure 30.4). C fibers in the pelvic nerve normally do not transmit impulses from

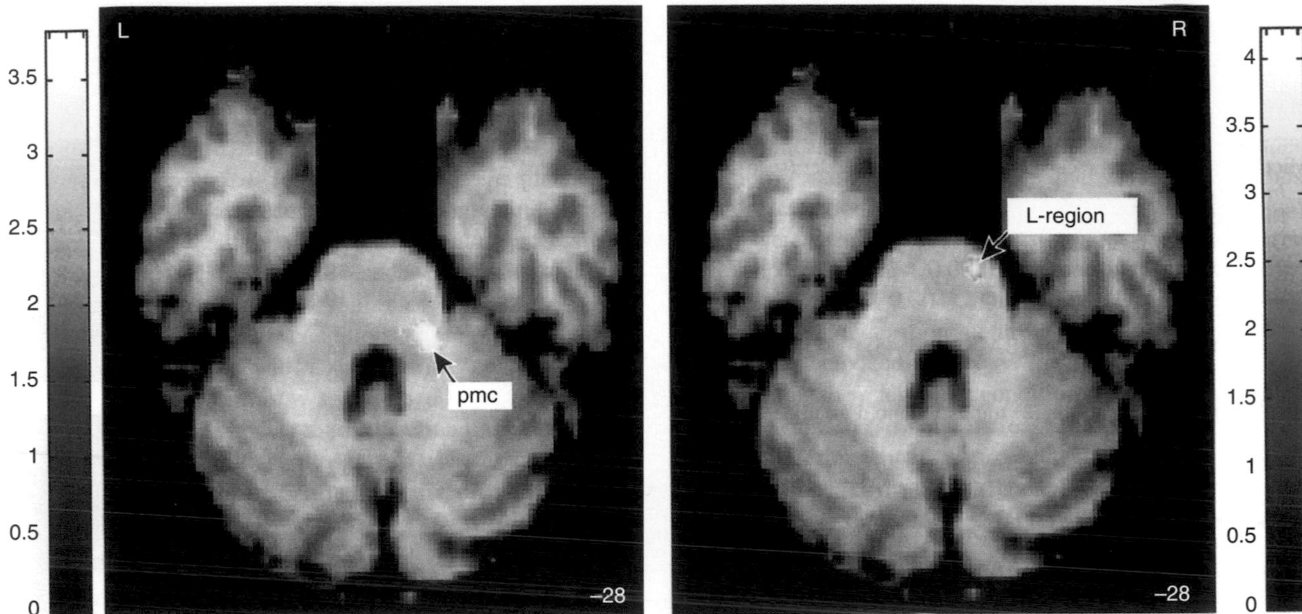

Figure 30.2
Left: Significant differences in rCBF in the right dorsal pontine tegmentum (indicated by pmc = pontine micturition center) after the comparison between conditions 'successful micturition' (scan 2) and 'empty bladder' (scan 3). *Right:* Significant differences in rCBF in the right ventral pontine tegmentum (indicated by L-region) after the comparison between conditions 'successful micturition' (scan 2) and 'empty bladder' (scan 3). The threshold used for display is uncorrected (p <0.005). The number –28 refers to the distance in millimeters relative to the horizontal plane through the anterior and posterior commissures (z direction). The numbers on the color scale refer to the corresponding Z scores. Areas with significant activity are superimposed on the average MRI scan (from 6 normal subjects) and have been transformed stereotactically to fit a standard atlas. L, left side of the brain; R, right side. (Reproduced with permission from Blok.[5])

the bladder distention or contraction and are 'silent';[35] they have been found to be sensitized by intravesical chemical irritation or after spinal cord injury. Some other reports indicated that both C fibers and Aδ-myelinated neurons can be silent.[36] Sensory impulses of temperatures and distention, particularly from the trigone, pass centrally in sympathetic nerves (hypogastric nerves and/or sacral sympathetic chain) and are relayed to the cortex for conscious awareness through the dorsal columns and spinothalamic tracts. This conscious awareness produces the feeling of bladder fullness, the desire to void, or pain.

Motor fibers pass distally along the same paths. The parasympathetic system via pelvic nerves exerts a contractile effect on detrusor muscle (muscarinic receptors). Parasympathetic preganglionic motoneurons are located in the S2–S4 segments in humans[37] and S1–S3 in cats[38] and reside in the sacral intermediolateral (IML) cell group. Parasympathetic neurons (releasing nitric oxide) also mediate relaxation of the urethral smooth muscles during voiding.[39] The sympathetic system, via hypogastric nerves and sympathetic chain, innervates smooth muscles of the bladder (β_1 receptors), bladder neck, and urethra (α_1 receptors). Human sympathetic preganglionic motoneurons are located in the lumbar intermediolateral area at the level of the L1–L4 cord.[37] The somatic system, via pudendal nerves (nicotinic receptors), controls the external striated urethral sphincter (rhabdosphincter). Although the pontine–sacral neural circuit for micturition can function autonomously, it is controlled after infancy by higher inhibitory influences from the brain, which are under conscious, or at least preconscious, control.[40]

Normally, the bladder will fill with urine slowly, stretching the detrusor muscle to accommodate a larger volume with low pressure. This bladder property is called compliance and depends on both neural and non-neural factors. During storage, parasympathetic activity is low, allowing the detrusor muscle to relax. Simultaneously, sympathetic activity is high, causing the smooth muscle of the bladder neck and urethra to contract. Sympathetic activity also inhibits parasympathetic ganglia (α_2 receptors) and relaxes detrusor directly (β receptors). Somatic activity increases with increased bladder volume, allowing the rhabdosphincter to remain contracted. When the bladder contains 400–500 ml of urine, there is cortical awareness of a desire to void. Micturition is initiated by voluntary inhibition of the rhabdosphincter activity followed by deinhibition of the

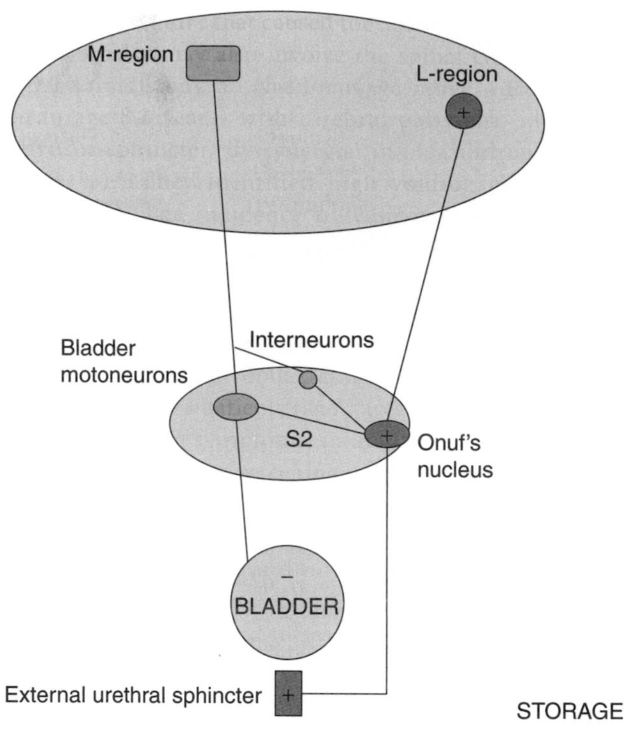

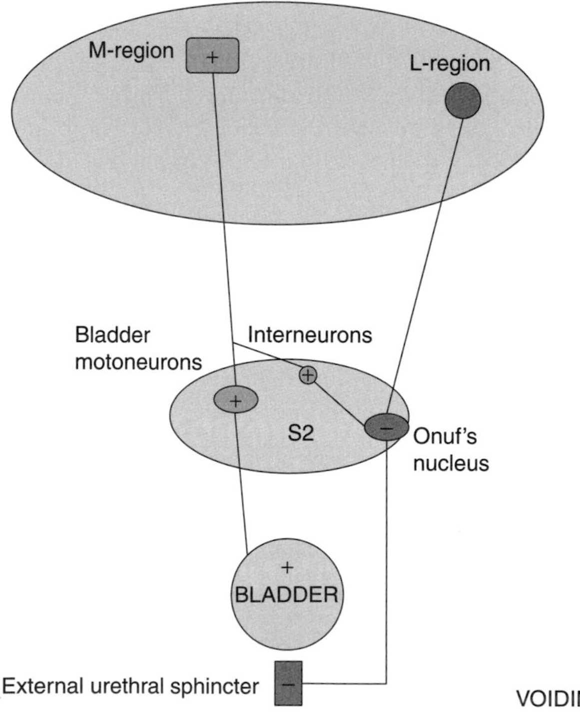

Figure 30.3
Arrangement of the ponto-sacral axis during storage and voiding.

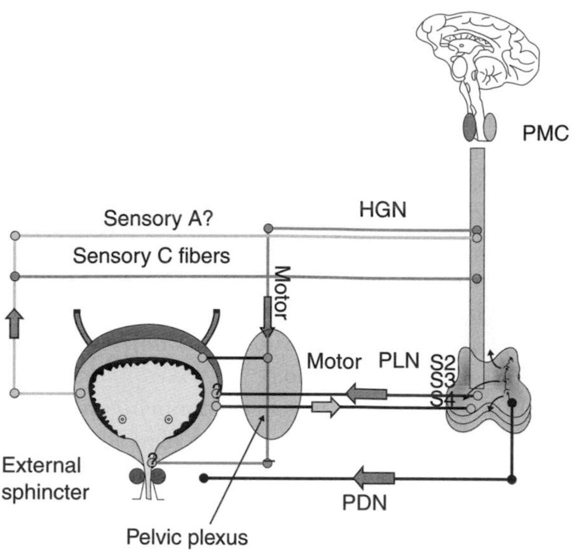

Figure 30.4
Innervation of the lower urinary tract. PMC, pontine micturition center; PDN, pudendal nerve (somatic); HGN, hypogastric nerve (sympathetic); PLN, pelvic nerve (parasympathetic).

bladder reflexes. Parasympathetic activity increases and sympathetic and somatic activity decreases, allowing the detrusor to contract against little resistance and the bladder empties completely.

Central nervous system neuropharmacology

Catecholamines

Pelvic preganglionic and pudendal motoneuron areas in the sacral spinal cord receive catecholamine projections from pontine centers.[41,42] Thus, it would be expected that bladder and sphincter reflexes would be affected by adrenergic influences. Dorsal horn interneurons are subject to descending modulation from the raphe magnus and locus ceruleus, implying mediation by a primary amine.[43] α_2-Agonists selectively suppress noxious inputs to dorsal horn projection neurons.[44] Whether the selective effect is also expressed on visceral inputs to such cells, or onto other cells in visceral spinal pathways, is unknown. The influence of norepinephrine (noradrenaline) on motor function may be due to a widespread action on interneurons in the ventral horn.[47] Central α adrenoceptors do influence somatic and viscerosomatic reflexes related to the external sphincter in animals[46–48] and probably in man.[51] It has been suggested that dorsal horn neurons can exhibit different or additional afferent inputs after spinal transection.[50] Anatomic plasticity of spinal synaptic contacts may underlie this phenomenon. α_2-Agonists also have a beneficial effect on bladder-sphincter dyssynergia[47] and on spasticity associated with spinal injury.[51]

Serotonin

The raphe magnus, raphe obscurus, and raphe pallidus provide the serotonergic innervation of the spinal cord[52] through a descending path in the dorsolateral funiculus.[53] Serotonin (5-hydroxytryptamine or 5-HT) is released in the dorsal horn by stimulation within the nucleus raphe magnus,[54] and stimulation of this area suppresses bladder reflex activity.[55] Multiple 5-HT receptor subtypes have been located in the spinal cord.[56–58] Serotonin inhibits ascending bladder afferent activity[59] at the spinal level, but facilitates pudendal nerve reflexes.[60] Both a serotonergic agonist and a precursor inhibit bladder contractions in rats.[61] A 5-HT antagonist (methysergide) decreases the volume threshold of the micturition reflex in cats.[62] At the supraspinal level, however, in normal conscious rats, 5-HT receptors can enhance the micturition reflex induced by bladder filling.[63] The roles that various 5-HT receptor subtypes may play in micturition have been reviewed.[64]

Gamma aminobutyric acid

Gamma aminobutyric acid (GABA), or a GABA agonist, suppresses reflex bladder activity and increases voiding threshold when injected into the brainstem, and the GABA antagonists have an opposite action.[65] Thus there appears to be a tonic GABAergic supraspinal inhibition of the micturition reflex. GABA also acts at a spinal level to suppress bladder preganglionic neurons[66] and it suppresses reflex micturition.[67] This was confirmed in clinical studies.[68] Glycine may also contribute to inhibition of pudendal motoneurons.[69]

Dopamine

Parkinson's disease and experimentally-induced parkinsonism in primates are both associated with bladder overactivity.[70,71] However, the symptoms may also be related to cortical dysfunctions.[72] The administration of a D1 dopamine agonist suppresses bladder activity,[73] whereas D2 agonists facilitate it.[74]

Opioid peptides

Opioid peptides and related drugs are well-known modulators of nociception. They also influence somatic reflex mechanisms by a spinal action.[75] The pharmacology of opioids is complicated by the existence of several receptor types and subtypes,[76] and the three major opioid receptor types, μ, δ, and κ, are present in the spinal cord.[77,78] Although there is evidence that there are at least two subtypes of κ receptor,[79] appropriately selective blocking drugs are available only for the κ_1 subtype.

Immunohistochemistry in the sacral spinal cord has demonstrated that both the parasympathetic nucleus (preganglionic neurons of the pelvic nerve) and Onuf's nucleus (motoneuron pool of the pudendal nerve to the external sphincter) are richly innervated by opioid-containing nerve terminals.[80] However, the details of the opioid pharmacology in these two areas differ.

The susceptibility of bladder function to depression by opioid peptides or morphine is well known in both animals and man.[81–87] The depression may be reversed by opioid antagonists or by increasing bladder pressure (i.e. bladder contraction can be obtained), but the volume threshold is increased.[85,87,88] Pharmacologic analysis in animals has indicated that, at the spinal cord level, the inhibition of micturition is attributable to activation of δ-opioid receptors.[89] However, in man the involvement of μ-opioid receptors cannot be discounted due to the activity of epidural morphine.[82] It should be noted that epidural pentazocine, a κ-opioid agonist, does not produce urinary retention.[90] Also, it has been shown that while μ or δ opioids suppress micturition, they do not inhibit reflex-evoked pudendal nerve activity.[91,92] On the other hand, pudendal nerve activity is suppressed by ethylketocyclazocine, a fairly selective κ-opioid agonist.[92] The presence of opioid receptor subtypes selectively associated with different components of the sacral spinal mechanisms for bladder and sphincter control may make it possible to differentially affect the components.

Head injury

Coma

Head injury can cause temporary dysfunction (coma) or permanent lesion. Unconsciousness after cerebral injury relates to compression, hemorrhage, or ischemia. The brainstem can be displaced downwards or the temporal lobe herniates through the tentorial opening. Classification of the different stages of coma is best described by the Glasgow Scale.[93] In most cases of coma, spontaneous micturition is possible and there seems to be some perception of bladder fullness in lighter stages.[94] Because only the suprapontine area is affected, coordination between the detrusor and sphincter remains. Voiding is synergistic, with no residual. Most patients, however, show decreased detrusor compliance. An indwelling Foley catheter, which patients usually have, may cause detrusor irritation and may explain increased stiffness of the bladder. Lack of sympathetic inhibition of bladder activity by the cerebrum, as in progressive autonomic and multiple system failure,[95,96] can be another explanation. In some comatose patients, however, there is temporary bladder retention. It is not clear whether this is related to bladder overstretching immediately after the accident or to active cerebral bladder

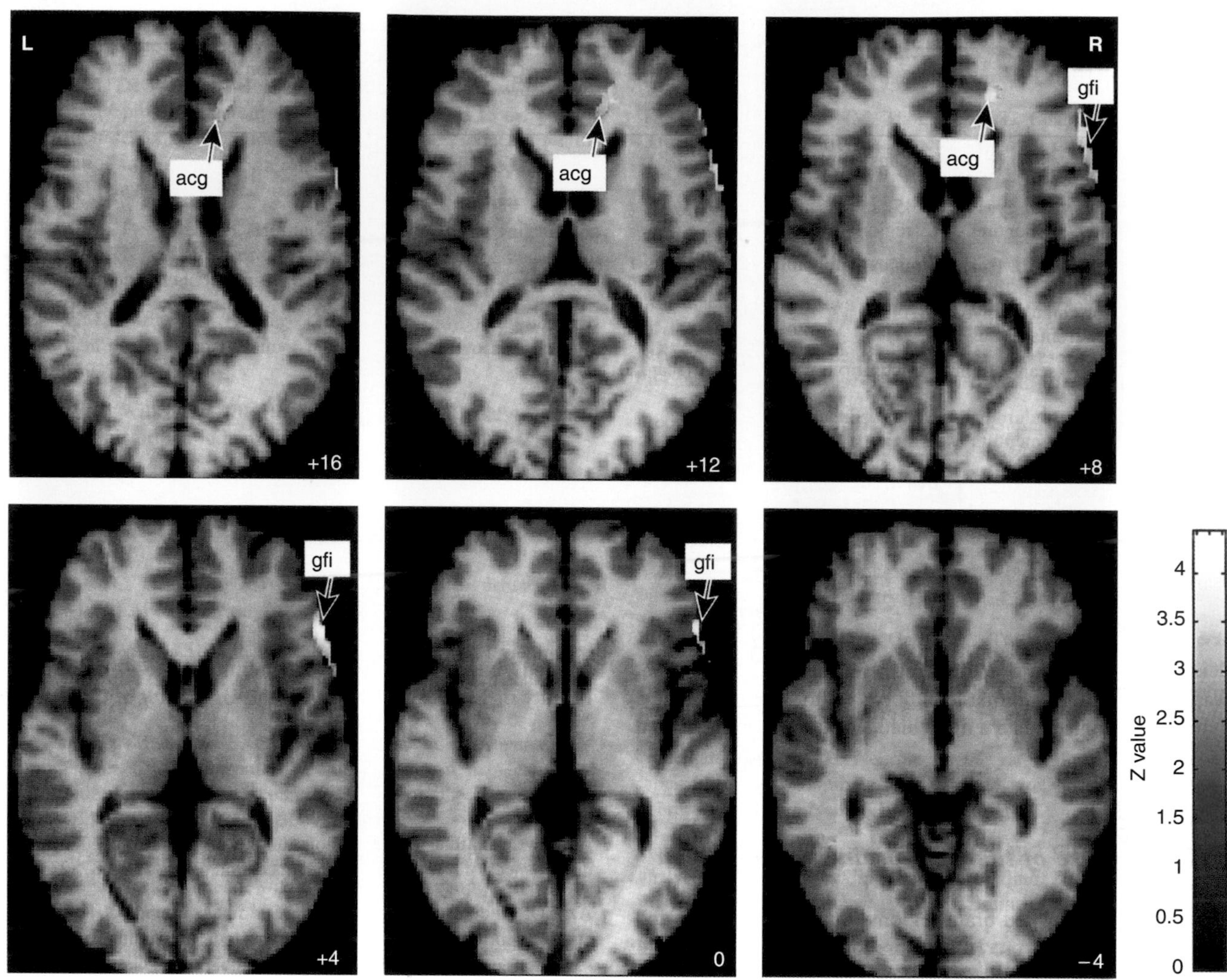

Figure 30.5
Significant differences in rCBF in the cortical areas after the comparison between the conditions 'successful micturition' (scan 2) and 'urine withholding' (scan 1). Note the activation of the right anterior cingulated gyrus (acg) in z planes +8 to +16, and the right inferior frontal gyrus (gfi) in *z* planes 0 to +12. (Reproduced with permission from Blok.[5])

inhibition. The possibility of temporary pontine shock similar to spinal shock cannot be excluded.

Suprapontine neurogenic detrusor overactivity

If the amount of cortical inhibition running in descending pathways is reduced by a suprapontine injury, there will be diminished ability to inhibit the micturition reflex. This results in an uninhibited detrusor contraction, with synergistic relaxation of the proximal and distal sphincter. Animal studies showed that injury above the inferior colliculus eliminated the inhibitory effect on the micturition center, whereas a lesion below this point abolished the normal micturition reflex.[97] Human PET study showed that the control areas of micturition are mostly located on the right side of the brain (Figure 30.5).[4,5] Some clinical reports indicate that urge incontinence is more commonly associated with right-sided damage.[98] Other clinical observations suggest that unilateral right cortical lesions (prefrontal damage) produce transient dysfunction, whereas bilateral lesions produce permanent dysfunction.[99]

Experimental results indicate that supraspinal nitric oxide has an important role in bladder overactivity after cerebral infarction, but it does not affect normal micturition in rats. This finding suggests a central mechanism sensitive to nitric oxide for bladder overactivity after cerebral infarction.[100]

During the filling phase, when the bladder contains a comparatively small volume of urine, inhibition of the suprapontine reflex arc will fail and the detrusor muscle will contract. There is no resistance from the urethra because of adequate relaxation of the sphincters due to the preserved sacro-pontine reflex arc. Patients with suprapontine

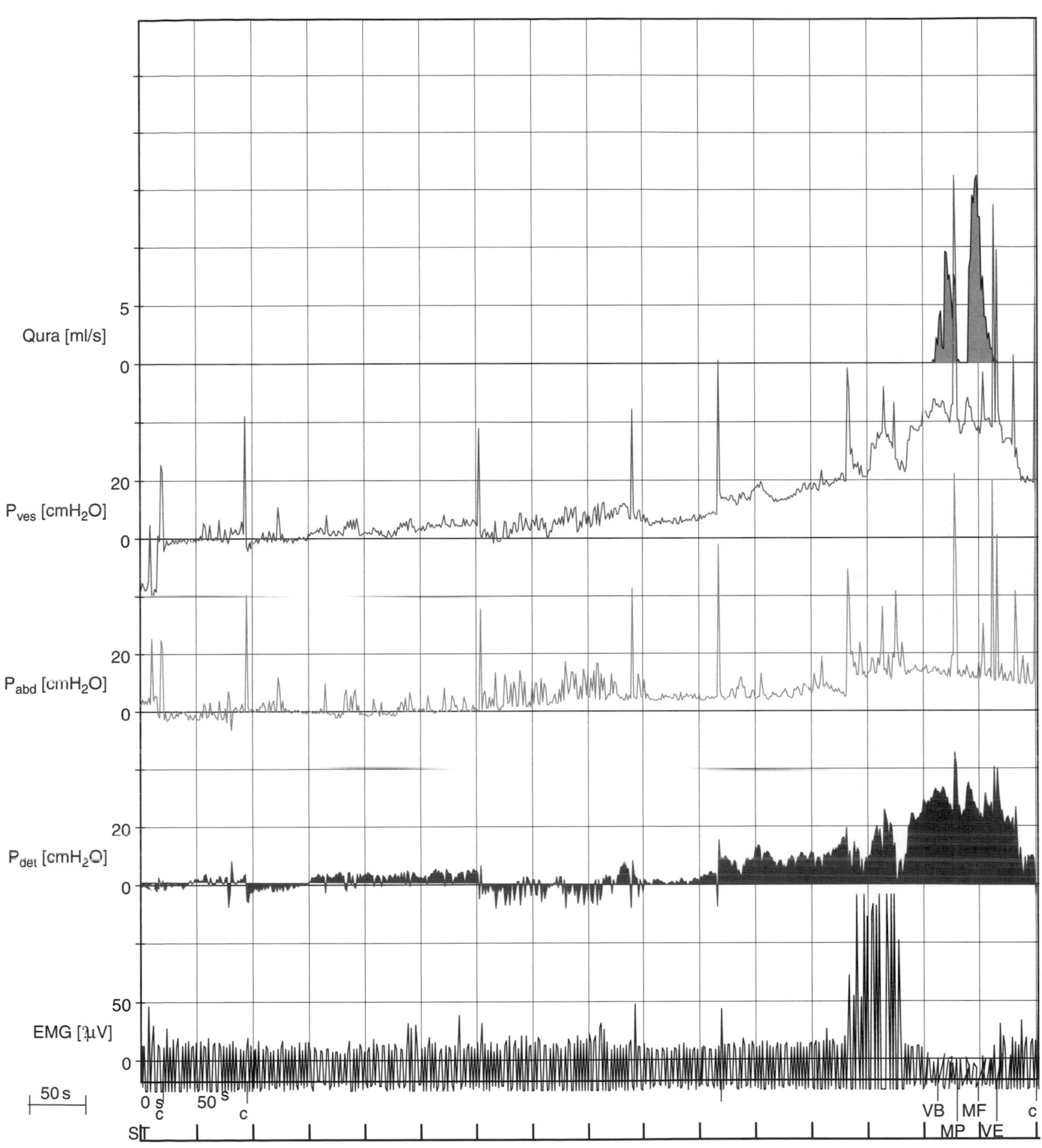

Figure 30.6

Pressure–flow study in a patient with a suprapontine lesion. The patient has no sensation; however, voiding is coordinated between the detrusor (P_{det}) and external sphincter EMG. EMG activity decreases during detrusor contraction. Qura, flow rate; P_{ves}, bladder pressure; P_{abd}, abdominal pressure.

detrusor overactivity will complain of frequency, urgency, and incontinence and, in severe cases, lack of sensory or motor control of the micturition reflex. They have no residual urine and thus are not prone to bladder infections.

Urodynamic studies may show early (small-volume) detrusor contractions, no detrusor-sphincter dyssynergia (the sphincter relaxes during detrusor contraction), and voiding without residual (Figure 30.6).

ASIA IMPAIRMENT SCALE

- ☐ A = Complete: No motor or sensory function is preserved in the sacral segments S4–S5.
- ☐ B = Incomplete: Sensory but not motor function is preserved below the neurological level and includes the sacral segments S4–S5.
- ☐ C = Incomplete: Motor function is preserved below the neurological level, and more than half of key muscles below the neurological level have a muscle grade less than 3.
- ☐ D = Incomplete: Motor function is preserved below the neurological level, and at least half of key muscles below the neurological level have a muscle grade of 3 of more.
- ☐ E = Normal: Motor and sensory function are normal.

CLINICAL SYNDROMES

- ☐ Central cord
- ☐ Brown-Sequard
- ☐ Anterior cord
- ☐ Conus medullaris
- ☐ Cauda equina

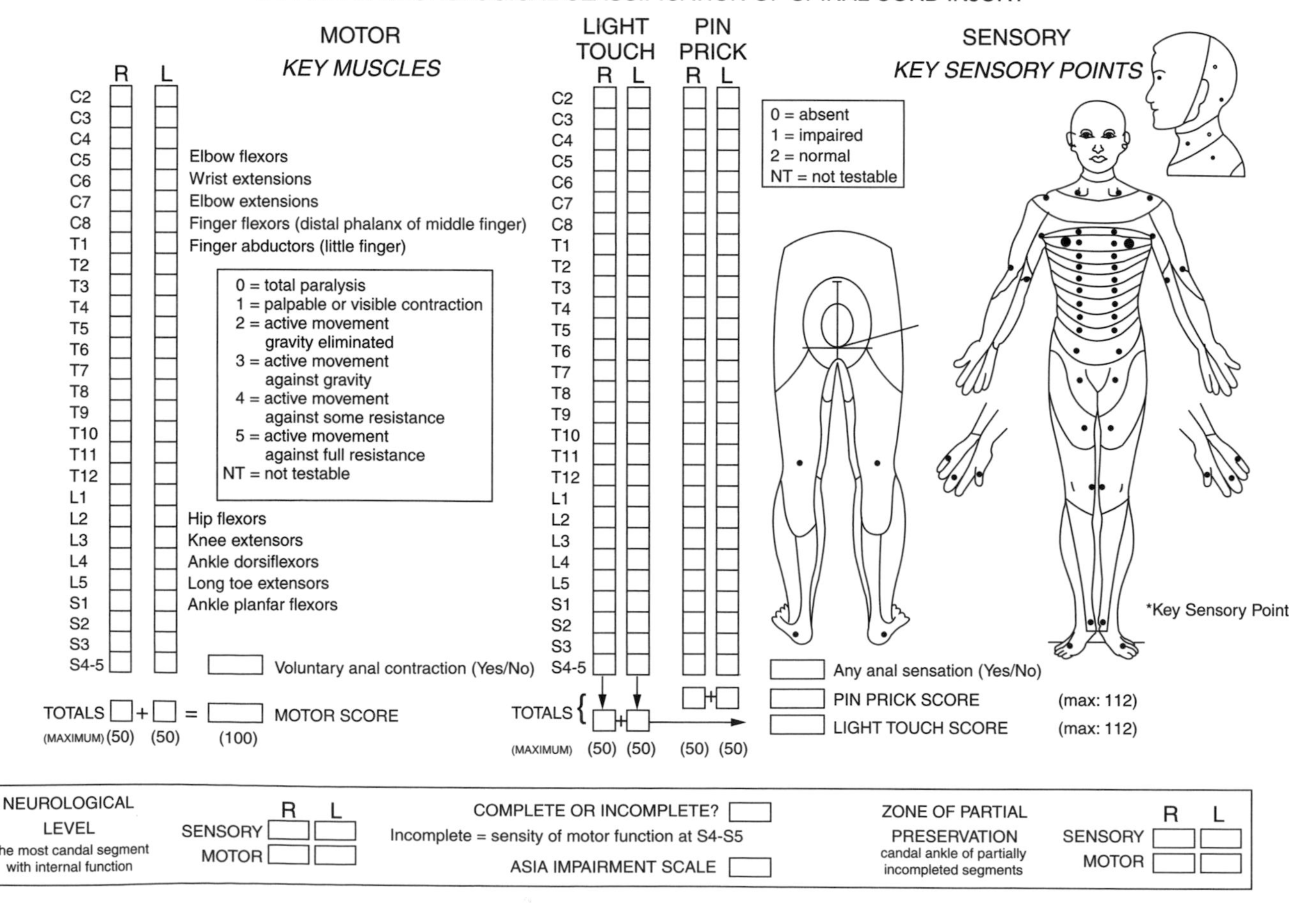

ASIA

STANDARD NEUROLOGICAL CLASSIFICATION OF SPINAL CORD INJURY

MOTOR — *KEY MUSCLES* (R L)

C2, C3, C4
C5 Elbow flexors
C6 Wrist extensions
C7 Elbow extensions
C8 Finger flexors (distal phalanx of middle finger)
T1 Finger abductors (little finger)
T2, T3, T4, T5, T6, T7, T8, T9, T10, T11, T12, L1
L2 Hip flexors
L3 Knee extensors
L4 Ankle dorsiflexors
L5 Long toe extensors
S1 Ankle planfar flexors
S2, S3, S4-5

0 = total paralysis
1 = palpable or visible contraction
2 = active movement gravity eliminated
3 = active movement against gravity
4 = active movement against some resistance
5 = active movement against full resistance
NT = not testable

☐ Voluntary anal contraction (Yes/No)

TOTALS ☐ + ☐ = ☐ MOTOR SCORE
(MAXIMUM) (50) (50) (100)

LIGHT TOUCH (R L) — PIN PRICK (R L)

C2, C3, C4, C5, C6, C7, C8, T1, T2, T3, T4, T5, T6, T7, T8, T9, T10, T11, T12, L1, L2, L3, L4, L5, S1, S2, S3, S4-5

TOTALS { ☐ + ☐ ☐ + ☐
(MAXIMUM) (50) (50) (50) (50)

SENSORY — *KEY SENSORY POINTS*

0 = absent
1 = impaired
2 = normal
NT = not testable

☐ Any anal sensation (Yes/No)
☐ PIN PRICK SCORE (max: 112)
☐ LIGHT TOUCH SCORE (max: 112)

*Key Sensory Points

NEUROLOGICAL LEVEL — The most candal segment with internal function: SENSORY R ☐ L ☐; MOTOR R ☐ L ☐

COMPLETE OR INCOMPLETE? ☐
Incomplete = sensity of motor function at S4-S5
ASIA IMPAIRMENT SCALE ☐

ZONE OF PARTIAL PRESERVATION — candal ankle of partially incompleted segments: SENSORY R ☐ L ☐; MOTOR R ☐ L ☐

Figure 30.7
Classification developed by the American Spinal Injury Association (ASIA).

Spinal cord injury

Classification

The most comprehensive classification is that developed by the American Spinal Injury Association (ASIA) (Figure 30.7). It utilizes the examination of dermatomes and myotomes to determine the level and completeness of the sensory and motor functions and distinguishes four classes of spinal cord injury based on the Frankel system and five clinical syndromes:

- *Central cord syndrome* is a result of hemorrhagic necrosis of the central gray matter and some of the medial white matter and is most commonly due to hyperextension injury. More caudal fibers of the corticospinal and spinothalamic tract are localized in the spine more lateral (from the centre), and hence are better protected from the central necrosis; consequently, arms are more affected than legs. Bladder dysfunction is also less common.
- *Brown–Séquard syndrome* is a rare unilateral cord condition which can result from penetrating injury or asymmetric disc herniation. It presents as ipsilateral motor weakness and sense impairment of fine touch and position and contralateral sensory impairment of pain and temperature. Bladder dysfunction in the pure condition is uncommon.
- *Anterior cord syndrome* is characterized by injury to the anterior aspects of the cord, with preservation of the posterior columns and dorsal horns. There is a motor deficit and loss of pain and temperature sensation below the level of the injury.
- *Conus medullaris and cauda equina syndrome* result from damage to the conus and spinal nerve roots, leading to flaccid paraplegia and sensory loss. Sacral reflexes can be partially or totally lost.

The bladder in 'spinal shock'

Following an acute spinal cord injury (the first 2 weeks to 3 months) at a level above the sacral segments, the central synapses between the afferent and efferent arms of the micturition reflex will be rendered inactive. The mechanism of the spinal shock is unclear and may relate to lack of supraspinal facilitation or to total depression of the interneuronal activity due to release of inhibitory transmitters. The detrusor will be paralyzed (acontractile detrusor), and there will be no conscious awareness of bladder fullness. However, the bladder neck and proximal urethra remain closed and the bladder will continue to distend because the reflex arc does not function. The resulting retention of urine is followed by dribbling incontinence as a consequence of an overflow. This retention cannot be avoided or managed by muscarinic stimulation with bethanechol.[101,102] Infection resulting from the large amount of residual urine may become a serious recurrent problem. The only reflex activity which is preserved or returns almost immediately is anal and bulbocavernosus reflex. Bladder reflex activity recovers usually within 2–3 months. It has been shown that sacral root stimulation during spinal shock facilitates recovery of the reflex activity of the detrusor.[103] We have also found that perineal and urethral stimulation is necessary for recovery of bladder reflex activity in spinally transected cats.[104]

Upper motor neuron lesion

Suprasacral neurogenic detrusor overactivity

This follows the stage of spinal shock resulting from a *cord injury above the S1 level.* Reflex bladder function eventually occurs in experimental animals and in man after suprasacral cord injury. This function is different from normal in that:

- it involves different afferent fibers (C fibers in the cat)[109]
- bladder contractions are poorly sustained[105]
- the urethra and bladder become discoordinated[106]
- previously 'irrelevant' stimuli influence the bladder[26] and/or external sphincter activity.[107]

Consciousness of bladder sensation may not be totally absent but voluntary inhibition of the micturition reflex arc is lost. The initial retention of urine with accompanying overflow incontinence during the stage of spinal shock gives way to the effects of an augmented reflex arc and results in a small, spastic, and overactive bladder. The bladder empties incompletely because of the dyssynergic contraction of the external sphincter, reflex inhibition from the dyssynergic sphincter, and primary detrusor failure (discoordinated contraction).[108] Overall, this alteration in central organization results in a high voiding pressure, residual urine, and incontinence. These subsequently lead to recurrent infection, hydronephrosis, and finally to renal failure. In some instances of an incomplete suprasacral lesion, synergistic relaxation of the external sphincter is preserved. In these patients, given time, reflex bladder contraction in response to skin stimulation may be learned, thus allowing the patient some voluntary control.

Afferent fibers

Normal micturition reflex involves Aδ-fiber afferents. Only in inflammatory states are C-fiber afferents involved

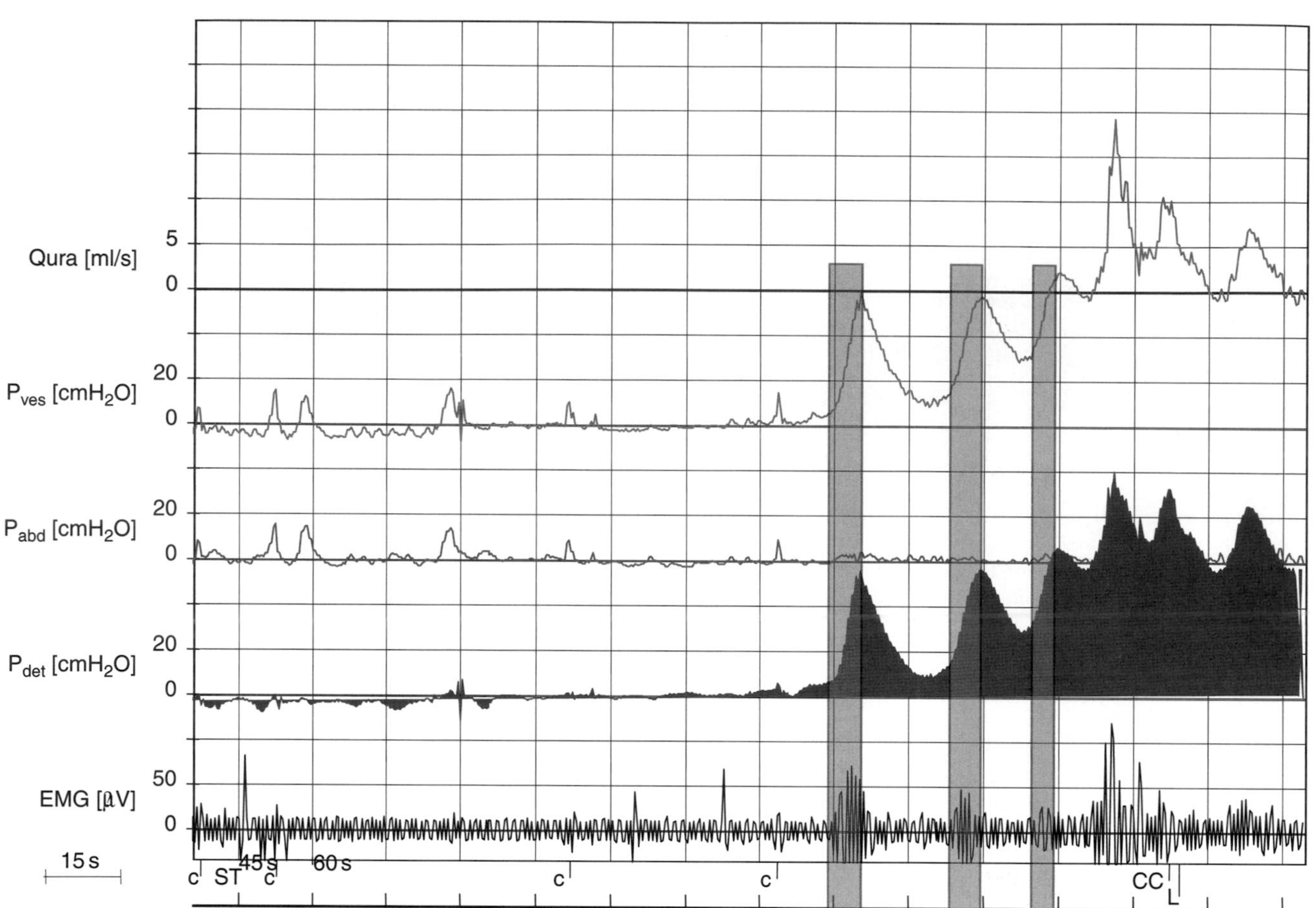

Figure 30.8
Pressure–flow study in a patient with a suprasacral complete lesion. The patient has detrusor-sphincter dyssynergia (DSD). Increase in external sphincter EMG activity is during the ascending phase of detrusor contraction (P_{det}) – shaded area. There is no urine flow because of severe bladder outlet obstruction due to DSD. Qura, flow rate; P_{ves}, bladder pressure; P_{abd}, abdominal pressure.

(chemosensitivity). After spinal cord injury C-fiber afferents mediate (mechanosensitivity) the abnormal sacral segmental bladder reflex.[31,109] The mechanism of this change from chemosensitivity to mechanosensitivity of C fibers is unclear. In rats, the timing of recovery of bladder contractile activity after spinal cord injury coincides with sacral primary afferent terminal sprouting.[110]

Detrusor underactivity

The normal micturition reflex is controlled by spinal (sacral) and supraspinal centers.[111] After suprasacral spinal cord injury some reflex bladder function persists. However, the bladder contractions are ineffective and poorly sustained[105] and the urethra and bladder become uncoordinated.[106] It has been assumed that poor detrusor function is primarily due to reflex inhibition from the dyssynergic sphincter.[112] There are suggestions that primary detrusor failure might also be of significance.[113] In some instances of cervical and high thoracic spinal cord injury (10–20%) detrusor acontractility and external sphincter denervation are present, indicating a distinct and separate lesion in the sacral area.[114–116]

Detrusor-sphincter dyssynergia (internal and external)

The pons coordinates the micturition reflex. Any lesion between the sacral and pontine level may produce discoordinated voiding, which results in increased external sphincter activity during detrusor contraction. Detrusor-sphincter dyssynergia (DSD) correlates with completeness but not the level of the upper motor neuron lesion.[117] DSD is responsible for the bladder outlet obstruction and, in combination with neurogenic detrusor overactivity, for high, sustained intravesical pressure, which is the most common cause of upper tract complications in spinal cord injury.[118,119] Diagnosis of DSD is based on electromyography (EMG)

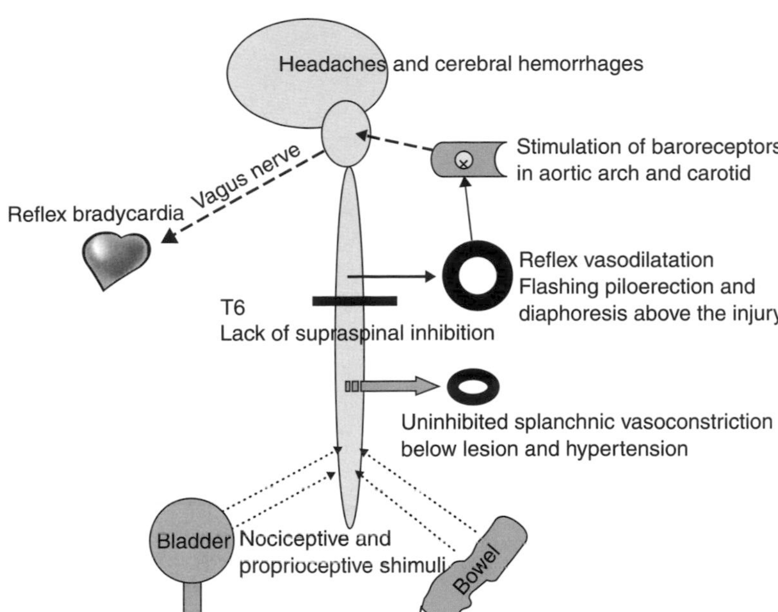

Figure 30.9
Autonomic dysreflexia.

recording during cystometography (CMG) and voiding. There is an increased EMG activity during bladder contraction. In true DSD, increased EMG activity correlates with an ascending portion of the detrusor contraction curve, as opposed to dysfunction voiding, in which the EMG increase is more random (Figure 30.8).[120]

A normal constant increase in the activity of the smooth and striated urethral sphincter accompanies bladder filling in response to the activation of bladder afferents.[117,121] This reflex is mainly driven by afferents conveyed through the pelvic nerves; it is lost in patients with complete upper motor neuron lesions and correlates well with DSD.[121]

The sympathetic system controls the bladder neck and proximal urethra from the T10 to L2 spinal cord segments.[122] A spinal cord lesion above T10 removes supraspinal inhibitory control of the sympathetic vesicourethral neurons, resulting in bladder neck functional obstruction (smooth muscle dyssynergia).[123] Urologic manifestations of smooth muscle dyssynergia are the same as with detrusor-external sphincter dyssynergia. Outflow obstruction is at the level of the bladder neck and proximal urethra and adds to the obstruction at the level of the external sphincter.[124]

Abnormal reflex activity after spinal injury

Bladder activity can be influenced not only by its own sensory inputs but also by those from the colon and anal sphincter,[125,126] and from somatic structures (e.g. perineum).[127] Visceral afferents can also have effects on somatic reflexes, particularly polysynaptic ones.[127] Sacral spinal interneurons appear to be one site for these interactions.[128,129] After acute suprasacral spinal transection, the external urethral sphincter quickly recovers its response to bladder distention. However, the absence of the normal suppression of this reflex during bladder contraction creates inefficient voiding. In chronic suprasacral spinal injury, previously 'irrelevant' stimuli to the penis, perineal skin, etc., can cause bladder contraction[26,127] and/or external sphincter activity[107] in both man and animals.

The 'skin–CNS–bladder reflex', in animal experiments, is effective in initiating bladder contractions after acute transection of the lumbar spinal cord. It is suggested that somatic motor axons can innervate bladder parasympathetic ganglion cells and thereby transfer somatic reflex activity to the bladder smooth muscle.[130]

Autonomic dysreflexia

In the patient with a neurologic midthoracic or higher spinal lesion, autonomic dysreflexia may occur.[131,132] These syndromes are secondary to loss of supraspinal inhibitory control of a thoracolumbar sympathetic outflow and result from massive discharge of the sympathetic system. Systemic manifestation of the autonomic dysreflexia (usually with a lesion above T6) includes sweating below and cutaneous flushing above the level of the neurologic lesion, pounding headache, nasal congestion, and piloerection.[133,134] Splanchnic vasoconstriction occurs rapidly, causing hypertension which may be life threatening due to intracranial hemorrhage. There is a bradycardia, mediated through vagus nerves (Figure 30.9). Autonomic dysreflexia can be triggered by a noxious stimulus below the level of the spinal cord injury, and includes bladder distention, urologic manipulations, constipation, and skin irritation.[135] The severity of the dysreflexia depends on the sprouting of myelinated and unmyelinated primary afferents below the injury. Although there is no evidence that sprouting reaches directly autonomic or motor neurons, an increased pool of interneurons contributes to exaggerated autonomic reflexes (dysreflexia).[136] An animal study showed that blocking intraspinal sprouting minimized dysreflexia.[137] In the case of so-called malignant autonomic dysreflexia, supraspinal autonomic control is also lost.[138]

Lower motor neuron lesion

Spinal cord injury to the *sacral paths at S1–4* results in parasympathetic decentralization of the bladder detrusor and somatic denervation of the external urethral sphincter, and loss of some afferent pathways. In a complete lesion, conscious awareness of bladder fullness will be lost and the micturition reflex is absent. Some pain sensation can be preserved because the hypogastric (sympathetic) nerve is intact.

Bladder

Parasympathetic decentralization results in degeneration and regeneration changes in the muscle cells of the bladder detrusor as well as in their innervating axons,[139] and that can account for the abnormal physiologic and pharmacologic behaviour observed. In the chronic decentralized human and feline bladder, an increase in adrenergic innervation to the detrusor has been reported.[140–142] This results in the outgrowth of sympathetic fibers in the detrusor and the conversion of their functional role from β-adrenoreceptor-mediated relaxation to α-adrenoreceptor-mediated contraction.[140,141,143] This change in sympathetic function appeared only after complete lesions.[145] On the other hand, deGroat and Kawatani[144] postulated that unilateral parasympathetic preganglionic denervation of the detrusor leads to a reinnervation of the denervated cholinergic ganglions by sympathetic preganglionic pathways. This new pathway provides a means for eliciting excitatory bladder muscle responses.

It has been suggested that an altered sympathetic pathway could explain the decrease in detrusor compliance associated with lower motor neuron (LMN) lesions in monkeys[145] and dogs.[146] McGuire and Morrissey[145] demonstrated in monkeys that complete intradural sacral rhizotomy produced hypertonic areflexic bladder, whereas selective dorsal root damage produced hypotonic areflexic detrusor. Further studies showed that α-adrenergic blockade partially reversed the effect of chronic denervation on detrusor compliance in these animals[147] and in dogs.[146] Gunasekera et al[148] reported decreased bladder compliance in more than half of patients with acquired LMN lesions. More than 70% of patients with myelodysplasia have bladders with low compliance.[149] In our study[150] of patients with LMN lesions, all of whom were on intermittent catheterization, we could not demonstrate any changes in detrusor compliance, regardless of whether the lesion was complete or incomplete. This is in agreement with a laboratory study[151] in which compliance was not decreased 3 months after sacral root injury in cats. These findings imply that ongoing activity from the sacral cord or pelvic afferent nerve traffic is not required for the maintenance of normal detrusor compliance in this situation. The role of the sympathetic system, however, in the parasympathetically decentralized bladder detrusor is still unclear.

The chronic complete parasympathetically decentralized bladder develops supersensitivity to muscarinic stimulants[152] which can be demonstrated as a marked increase in the intravesical pressure, in response to subcutaneous bethanechol. In partial LMN lesions, supersensitivity was not detected in rats[153] or dogs.[154] Using an alternative way of performing the bethanechol test (reduction in threshold dose of bethanechol rather than an increase in bladder pressure used as an indicator), El-Salmy et al[155] demonstrated supersensitivity of the detrusor in cats with partial sacral rhizotomies. In our study,[150] patients with complete or incomplete lesions responded to bethanechol injection with bladder pressure increase, although the more dramatic response was seen in patients with complete lesions. These findings dispute the validity of the bethanechol test in differentiating between complete and incomplete lesions.

Urethra and external urinary sphincter

The urethra is mainly innervated by the sympathetic system and only sparsely by the parasympathetic system. Maximum urethral pressure (MUP) values were low, however, in our patients[150] when compared with our normal values or other[156] standards. There was no significant difference between complete and incomplete lesions. Mattiasson et al[157] also reported that MUP was significantly lower in patients with parasympathetic decentralization than in volunteers. Loss of somatic innervation to the external sphincter may account for this finding. Phentolamine had little effect on MUP in our study, in contrast to the finding in volunteers with normal lower urinary tracts.[156] There is a possibility that sympathetic influence over urethral closure pressure has been lost in this situation. Other researchers have reported variable urethral pressure profile responses to α-adrenergic blockers in LMN lesions.[158] In a complete LMN lesion due to somatic denervation of the external sphincter, striated muscle activity is abnormal. EMG is characterized by individual action potentials which are of increased amplitude and duration, and are polyphasic with some abnormal spontaneous activity in the form of positive waves and fibrillation potentials.[159] Conscious control is lost; however, some muscle tone is preserved. Narrowing in the region of the external urethral sphincter is not an uncommon finding. Proposed mechanisms include:

- fibrosis of the urethral sphincter[160]
- sympathetic dyssynergia[161]
- denervation supersensitivity[162] or autonomic reinnervation of the rhabdosphincter.[163,164]

Bladder neck and proximal urethra

The bladder neck and proximal urethra receive a dual cholinergic and adrenergic innervation from the pelvic and hypogastric nerve, respectively.[143,165–167] Laboratory studies have demonstrated a predominance of α-adrenergic receptors in that area.[168–170] Normally, the bladder neck should remain closed except during voiding.[171] Neurogenic and non-neurogenic factors influence competence of the bladder neck. The hydromechanical effect of Credé's maneuver has been shown to reduce proximal urethral closure pressure in cats with a sacral injury.[172] It is not clear whether an open bladder neck in an LMN lesion is a primary neurologic defect or is secondary to associated detrusor dysfunction (increased stiffness or autonomous waves) or treatment. There are conflicting reports regarding which neurologic lesion causes an open bladder neck.[149,173,174] McGuire and Wagner[174] found that a complete, isolated sacral decentralization of the parasympathetic and pudendal nerves did not result in an open bladder neck, which conflicts with our results.[150] We have shown that bladder neck incompetence is related to completeness of the LMN lesion and that sympathetic blockade (phentolamine) had an effect on the bladder neck closing mechanism only in incomplete lesions. The data imply that, in addition to sympathetic function, some sacral root activity takes part in the maintenance of bladder neck closure, either through efferent parasympathetic activity or by providing an afferent link to a sympathetic reflex. Kirby et al[175] found the bladder neck open in all patients with pelvic nerve injury or cauda equina lesion. Open bladder neck was also found in almost 90% of children with myelodysplasia.[149] Extensive autonomic system damage (after A-P resection) was found to be associated with open bladder neck, probably due to sympathetic denervation.[176] However, a contribution from the increased intravesical pressure cannot be ruled out.

Neurogenic bladder dysfunction is more common than was previously diagnosed. A report by Ahlberg et al[177] showed that up to 82% of patients with 'idiopathic bladder' dysfunction have pathologic neurologic findings, which indicates that patients with voiding dysfunction should be considered to have a neurologic underlying condition unless proven otherwise.

References

1. Barrington FJF. The effect of lesions of the hind and mid-brain on micturition in the cat. Quart J Exp Physiol 1925; 15: 81–102.
2. Bradley WE, Teague CT. Spinal cord representation of the peripheral neural pathways of the micturition reflex. J Urol 1969; 101: 220–3.
3. Imada N, Koyama Y, Kawauchi A et al. State dependent response of the locus caeruleus neurons to bladder distension. J Urol 2000; 164(5): 1740–4.
4. Blok BFM, Willemsen ATM, Holstege G. A PET study on the brain control of micturition in humans. Brain 1997; 120: 111–21.
5. Blok BFM, Sturms LM, Holstege G. Brain activation during micturition in women. Brain 1998; 121: 2033–42.
6. Zhang H, Reitz A, Kollias S et al. An fMRI study of the role of suprapontine brain structures in the voluntary voiding control induced by pelvic floor contraction. Neuroimage 2005; 24: 174–80.
7. Ruch TC, Tang PC. Localization of brain stem and diencephalic areas controlling the micturition reflex. J Comp Neurol. 1956; 106(1): 213–45.
8. Nishizawa O, Ebina K, Sugaya K et al. Effect of cerebellectomy on reflex micturition in the decerebrate dog as determined by urodynamic evaluation. Urol Int 1989; 44(3): 152–6.
9. Athwal BS, Berkley KJ, Hussain I et al. Brain responses to changes in bladder volume and urge to void in healthy men. Brain 2001; 124: 369–77.
10. Matsuura S, Kakizaki H, Mitsui T et al. Human brain region response to distention or cold stimulation of the bladder: a positron emission tomography study. J Urol 2002; 168: 2035–9.
11. Nour S, Svarer C, Kristensen JK, Paulson OB, Law I. Cerebral activation during micturition in normal men. Brain 2000; 123(Pt 4): 781–9.
12. Dietrichs E, Haines DE. Possible pathways for cerebellar modulation of autonomic responses: micturition. Scand J Urol Nephrol Suppl 2002; 210: 16–20.
13. Holstege G. Some anatomical observations on the projections from the hypothalamus to brainstem and spinal cord: an HRP and autoradiographic tracing study in the cat. J Comp Neurol 1987; 260: 98–126.
14. Rizvi TA, Ennis M, Aston-Jones G et al. Preoptic projections to Barrington's nucleus and the pericoerulear region: architecture and terminal organization. J Comp Neurol 1994; 347: 1–24.
15. Blok BFM, Willemsen ATM, Holstege G. A PET study on brain control of micturition in humans. Brain 1997; 120, 111–21.
16. Kavia RB, Dasgupta R, Fowler CJ. Functional imaging and the central control of the bladder. J Comp Neurol 2005; 493: 27–32.
17. Morrison JF, Birder LA, Craggs M et al. Neural control. In: Abrams P et al, eds. Incontinence. Paris: Health Publications Ltd, 2005: 363–422.
18. Shefchyk SJ. The effect of lumbosacral deafferentation on pontine micturition centre-evoked voiding in the decerebrate cat. Neurosci Lett 1989; 99: 175–80.
19. Fedirchuk B, Shefchyk SJ. Effects of electrical stimulation of the thoracic spinal cord on bladder and external urethral sphincter activity in the decerebrate cat. Exp Brain Res 1991; 84: 635–42.
20. Griffiths D, Holstege G, Dalm E, de Wall H. Control and coordination of the bladder and urethral function in the brainstem of the cat. Neurourol Urodyn 1990; 9: 63–82.
21. Nishizawa O, Sugaya K. Cat and dog: higher centre of micturition. Neurourol Urodyn 1994; 13: 169–79.

22. Blok BFM, de Weerd H, Holstege G. Ultrastructural evidence for a paucity of projections from the lumbosacral cord to the pontine micturition centre or M-region in the cat: a new concept for organization of micturition reflex with the periaqueductal gray as central relay. J Comp Neurol 1995; 359: 300–9.
23. Duong M, Downie JW, Du HJ. Transmission of afferent information from urinary bladder, urethra and perineum to periaqueductal gray of cat. Brain Res 1999; 819: 108–19.
24. Matsuura S, Allen GV, Downie JW. Volume-evoked micturition reflex is mediated by the ventrolateral periaqueductal gray in anesthetized rats. Am J Physiol 1998; 275: R2049–55.
25. Matsuura S, Downie JW, Allen GV. Micturition evoked by glutamate microinjection in the ventrolateral periaqueductal gray is mediated through Barrington's nucleus in the rat. Neuroscience 2000; 101: 1053–61.
26. De Groat WC, Ryall RW. Reflexes to sacral parasympathetic neurones concerned with micturition in the cat. J Physiol (Lond) 1969; 200: 87–108.
27. Blaivas JG. The neurophysiology of micturition: a clinical study of 550 patients. J Urol 1982; 127: 958–63.
28. Holstege G, Griffiths D, De Wall H, Dalm E. Anatomical and physiological observation on supraspinal control of bladder and urethral sphincter muscles in the cat. J Comp Neurol 1986; 250: 449–61.
29. De Groat WC, Araki I, Vizzard MA et al. Developmental and injury induced plasticity in micturition reflex pathway. Behav Brain Res 1998; 92: 127–40.
30. Nadelhaft I, Vera PL. Neurons in the rat brain and spinal cord labeled after pseudorabies virus injected into the external urethral sphincter. J Comp Neurol 1996; 375: 502–17.
31. De Groat WC, Nadelhaft I, Milne RJ et al. Organization of the sacral parasympathetic reflex pathways to the urinary bladder and large intestine. J Auton Nerv Syst 1981; 3: 135–60.
32. De Groat WC. Neuropeptides in pelvic afferent pathways. Experientia 1987; 43: 801–13.
33. De Groat WC. Spinal cord projections and neuropeptides in visceral afferent neurons. Progr Brain Res 1986; 67: 165–87.
34. Habler HJ, Janig W, Koltzenburg M. Myelinated primary afferents of the sacral spinal cord responding to slow filling and distension of the cat urinary bladder. J Physiol 1993; 463: 449–60.
35. Habler HJ, Janig W, Koltzenburg M. Activation of unmyelinated afferent fibers by mechanical stimuli and inflammation of the urinary bladder in the cat. J Physiol 1990; 425: 545–62.
36. Morrison JFB. The activation of bladder wall afferent nerves. Exp Physiol 1998; 84: 131–6.
37. Pick J. The Autonomic Nervous System: Morphological, Comparative, Clinical and Surgical Aspects. Philadelphia: Lippincott, 1970.
38. Morgan C, Nadelhaft I, De Groat WC. Location of bladder preganglionic neurons within the sacral parasympathetic nucleus of the cat. Neurosci Lett 1979; 14: 189–94.
39. Bennett BC, Kruse MN, Roppolo JR et al. Neural control of urethral outlet activity in vivo. Role of nitric oxide. J Urol 1995; 153: 2004–9.
40. De Groat WC. Anatomy and physiology of the lower urinary tract. Urol Clin N Am 1993; 20: 383–401.
41. Westlund KN, Coulter JD. Descending projections of the locus coeruleus and subcoeruleus/medial parabrachial nuclei in monkey: axonal transport studies and dopamine-β-hydroxylase immunocytochemistry. Brain Res Rev 1980; 2: 235–64.
42. Kojima M, Matsuura T, Kimura H et al. Fluorescence histochemical study on the noradrenergic control to the anterior column of the spinal lumbosacral segments of rats and dog, with special reference to motoneurons innervating the perineal striated muscles (Onuf' s nucleus). Histochem 1984; 81: 237–41.
43. Willis WD. Descending control of spinal cord nociceptive neurons. Prog Sens Physiol 1982; 3: 77.
44. Fleetwood-Walker SM, Mitchell R, Hope PJ, Molony V, Iggo A. An α_2 receptor mediates the selective inhibition by noradrenalin of nociceptive responses of identified dorsal horn neurones. Brain Res 1985; 334(2): 243–54.
45. Jordan LM, McCrea DA, Steeves JD, Menzies JE. Noradrenergic synapses and effects of noradrenalin on interneurons in ventral horn of the cat spinal cord. Can J Physiol Pharmacol 1977; 55(3): 399–412.
46. Gajewski JB, Downie JW, Awad SA. Experimental evidence for a central nervous system site of action in the effect of alpha-adrenergic blockers on the external urinary sphincter. J Urol 1984; 133: 403–9.
47. Galeano C, Jubelin B, Carmel M, Ghazal G. Urodynamic action of clonidine in the chronic spinal cat. Neurourol Urodyn 1986; 5: 475–92.
48. Downie JW, Bialik GJ. Evidence for a spinal site of action of clonidine on somatic and viscerosomatic reflex activity evoked on the pudendal nerve in cats. J Pharmacol Exp Ther 1988; 246: 352–8.
49. Nordling J, Meyhoff HH, Hald T. Sympatholytic effect on striated urethral sphincter. Scand J Urol Nephrol 1981; 15: 173–80.
50. Brenowitz GL, Pubols LM. Increased receptive field size of dorsal horn neurons following chronic spinal cord hemisections in cats. Brain Res 1981; 216: 45–59.
51. Tuckman J, Chu DS, Petrillo CR, Naftchi NE. Clinical trial of an alpha-adrenergic receptor stimulant drug (clonidine) for treatment of spasticity in spinal cord injured patients. In: Naftchi NE, ed. Spinal Cord Injury. New York: SP Medical and Scientific Books, 1982: 133–7.
52. Jones SL, Light AR. Serotoninergic medullary raphespinal projection to the lumbar spinal cord in the rat: a retrograde immunohistochemical study. J Comp Neurol 1992; 322: 599–610.
53. Westlund KN, Lu Y, Coggeshall RE, Willis WD. Serotonin is found in myelinated axons of the dorsolateral funiculus in monkeys. Neurosci Lett 1992; 141: 35–8.
54. Abhold RH, Bowker RM. Descending modulation of dorsal horn biogenic amines as determined by in vivo dialysis. Neurosci Lett 1990; 108: 231–6.
55. McMahon SB, Morrison JFB. Two groups of spinal interneurones that respond to stimulation of the abdominal viscera of the cat. J Physiol 1982; 322: 21–34.
56. Laporte AM, Koscielniak T, Ponchant M et al. Quantitative autoradiographic mapping of 5-HT3 receptors in the rat CNS using [125I]Iodo zacopride and [3H]Zacopride as radioligands. Synapse 1992; 10: 271–81.
57. Seybold VS. Distribution of histaminergic, muscarinic and serotonergic binding sites in cat spinal cord with emphasis on the region surrounding the central canal. Brain Res 1985; 342: 291–6.
58. Pubols LM, Bernau NA, Kane LA et al. Distribution of 5-HT1 binding sites in cat spinal cord. Neurosci Lett 1992; 142: 111–14.
59. Espey MJ, Du HJ, Downie JW. Serotonergic modulation of spinal ascending activity and sacral reflex activity evoked by pelvic nerve stimulation in cats. Brain Res 1998; 798: 101–8.
60. Danuser H, Thor KB. Spinal 5-HT2 receptor-mediated facilitation of pudendal nerve reflexes in the anaesthetized cat. Br J Pharmacol 1996; 118: 150–4.
61. Steers WD, de Groat WC. Effects of m-chlorophenylpiperazine on penile and bladder function in rats. Am J Physiol 1989; 257: R1441–1449.
62. Espey MJ, Downie JW, Fine A. Effect of 5-HT receptor and adrenoceptor antagonists on micturition in conscious cats. Eur J Pharm 1991; 195: 301–4.
63. Ishizuka O, Gu B, Igawa Y et al. Role of supraspinal serotonin receptors for micturition in normal conscious rats. Neurourol Urodyn 2002; 21: 225–30.
64. Ramage AG. The role of central 5-hydroxytryptamine (5-HT, serotonin) receptors in the control of micturition. Br J Pharmacol 2006; 147(Suppl 2): S120–131.

65. Mallory BS, Roppolo JR, de Groat WC. Pharmacological modulation of the pontine micturition center. Brain Res 1991; 546: 310–20.
66. Araki I. Inhibitory postsynaptic currents and the effects of GABA on visually identified sacral parasympathetic preganglionic neurons in neonatal rats. J Neurophysiol 1994; 72: 2903–10.
67. Igawa Y, Mattiasson A, Andersson KE. Effects of GABA-receptor stimulation and blockade on micturition in normal rats and rats with bladder outflow obstruction. J Urol 1993; 150: 537–42.
68. Nanninga JB, Frost F, Penn R. Effect of intrathecal baclofen on bladder and sphincter function. J Urol 1989; 142: 101–5.
69. Shefchyk SJ, Espey MJ, Carr P et al. Evidence for a strychnine-sensitive mechanism and glycine receptors involved in the control of urethral sphincter activity during micturition in the cat. Exp Brain Res 1998; 119: 297–306.
70. Andersen JT, Bradley WE. Cystometric, sphincter and electromyographic abnormalities in Parkinson's disease. J Urol 1976; 116: 75–8.
71. Albanease A, Jenner P, Marsden CD, Stephenson JD. Bladder hyperreflexia induced in marmosets by 1-methyl-4-phenyl-1,2,3,6-tetrahydropyridine. Neurosci Lett 1988; 87: 46–50.
72. Fowler CJ. Update on the neurology of Parkinson's disease. Neurourol Urodyn 2007; 26: 103–9.
73. Yoshimura N, Mizuta E, Kuno S, Sasa M, Yoshida O. The dopamine D1 receptor agonist SKF 38393 suppresses detrusor hyperreflexia in the monkey with parkinsonism induced by 1-methyl-4-phenyl-1,2,3,6-tetrahydropyridine (MPTP). Neuropharmacology 1993; 32: 315–21.
74. Kontani H, Inoue T, Sakai T. Dopamine receptor subtypes that induce hyperactive urinary bladder response in anesthetized rats. Jpn J Pharmacol 1990; 54: 482–6.
75. Zeigelgansberger W. Opioid actions on mammalian spinal neurons. Int Rev Neurobiol 1984; 25: 243.
76. Wood PL. Multiple opiate receptors: support for unique mu, delta and kappa sites. Neuropharmacology 1982; 21: 487–97.
77. Morris BJ, Herz A. Distinct distribution of opioid receptor types in rat lumbar spinal cord. Naunyn-Schmiedeberg's Arch Pharmacol 1987; 336: 240–3.
78. Traynor JR, Wood MS. Distribution of opioid binding sites in spinal cord. Neuropeptides 1987; 10: 313–20.
79. Wollemann M, Benyhe S, Simon J. The kappa-opioid receptor: evidence for different subtypes. Life Sci 1993; 52: 599–611.
80. Glazer E, Basbaum A. Leucine enkephalin: localization in and axoplasmic transport by sacral parasympathetic preganglionic neurons. Science 1980; 208: 1479–81.
81. Gustafsson LL, Schildt B, Jacobsen K. Adverse effects of extradural and intrathecal opiates: report of a nationwide survey in Sweden. Br J Anaesth 1982; 54: 479–86.
82. Rahwal N, Mollefors K, Axelsson K et al. An experimental study of urodynamic effects of epidural morphine and of naloxane reversal. Anesth Analg 1983; 62: 641–7.
83. De Groat WC, Kawatani M, Hisamitsu T et al. The role of neuropeptides in the sacral autonomic reflex pathways of the cat. J Autonom Nerv Syst 1983; 7: 339–50.
84. Jubelin B, Galeano C, Ladouceur D et al. Effect of enkephalin on the micturition cycle of the cat. Life Sci 1984; 34: 2015–27.
85. Dray A, Metsch R. Inhibition of urinary bladder contractions by spinal action of morphine and other opioids. J Pharmacol Exp Ther 1984; 231: 254–60.
86. Hisamitsu T, De Groat WC. The inhibitory effect of opioid peptides and morphine applied intrathecally and intracerebroventricularly on the micturition reflex in the cat. Brain Res 1984; 298: 51–65.
87. Bolam JM, Robinson CJ, Hofstra TC, Wurster RD. Changes in micturition volume thresholds in conscious dogs following spinal opiate administration. J Autonom Nerv Syst 1986; 16: 261–77.
88. Herman RH, Wainberg MC, delGiudice PF, Willscher MK. The effect of a low dose of intrathecal morphine on impaired micturition reflexes in human subjects with spinal cord lesion. Anesthesiology 1988; 69: 313–18.
89. De Groat WC, Kawatani M. Neural control of the urinary bladder: possible relationship between peptidergic inhibitory mechanisms and detrusor instability. Neurourol Urodyn 1985; 4: 285–300.
90. Kalia PK, Madan R, Saksena R et al. Epidural pentazocine for post-operative pain relief. Anesth Analg 1983; 62: 949–50.
91. Dray A, Metsch R. Spinal opioid receptors and inhibition of urinary bladder motility in vivo. Neurosci Lett 1984; 47: 81–4.
92. Thor KB, Hisamitsu T, Roppolo JR et al. Selective inhibitory effects of ethylketocyclazocine on reflex pathways to the external urethral sphincter of the cat. J Pharmacol Exp Ther 1989; 248: 1018–25.
93. Born JD. The Glasgow–Liege Scale. Prognostic value and evolution of motor response and brain stem reflexes after severe head injury., Acta Neurochir (Wien) 1988; 91(1–2): 1–11.
94. Wyndaele JJ. Urodynamics in comatose patients. Neurourol Urodyn 1990; 9: 43–52.
95. Kirby RS. Autonomic failure and the role of the sympathetic nervous system in the control of the lower urinary tract function. Clin Sci 1986; 70(Suppl 14): 45s–50s.
96. Shy GM, Drager GA. A neurological syndrome associated with orthostatic hypotension a clinical-pathologic study. Arch Neurol (Chicago) 1960; 2: 511–27.
97. Tang PC. Levels of brain stem and diencephalon controlling micturition reflex. J Neurophysiol 1955; 18: 583–95.
98. Kuroiwa Y, Tohgi H, Ono S, Itoh M. Frequency and urgency of micturition in hemiplegic patients: relationship to hemisphere laterality of lesions. J Neurol 1987; 234: 100–2.
99. Mochizuki H, Saito H. Mesial frontal lobe syndrome: correlations between neurological deficits and radiological localizations. Tohoku J Exp Med 1990; 161(Suppl): 231–9.
100. Kodama K, Yokoyama O, Komatsu K et al. Contribution of cerebral nitric oxide to bladder overactivity after cerebral infarction in rats. J Urol 2002; 167: 391–6.
101. Twiddy DA, Downie JW, Awad SA. Response of the bladder to bethanechol after acute spinal cord transection in cats. J Pharmacol Exp Ther 1980; 215: 500–6.
102. Downie JW. Bethanechol chloride in urology – a discussion of issues. Neurourol Urodyn 1984; 3: 211–22.
103. Hassuna M, Li JS, Sawan M et al. Effect of early bladder stimulation on spinal shock: experimental approach. Urology 1992; 40: 563–73.
104. Downie JW, Espey MJ, Gajewski JB. Contribution of perineal stimulation to the emergence of distension-evoked bladder contractions in spinal cats. Soc Neurosci Abstracts 1995; 21: 1201.
105. Blaivas JG. The neurophysiology of micturition: a clinical study of 550 patients. J Urol 1982; 127: 958–63.
106. Galeano C, Jubelin B, Germain L, Guenette L. Micturitional reflexes in chronic spinalized cats: the underactive detrusor and detrusor-sphincter dyssynergia. Neurourol Urodyn 1986; 5: 45–63.
107. Downie JW, Awad SA. The state of urethral musculature during the detrusor areflexia after spinal cord transection. Invest Urol 1979; 17: 55–9.
108. Nagatomi J, Toosi KK, Grashow JS, Chancellor MB, Sacks MS. Quantification of the bladder smooth muscle orientation in normal and spinal cord injured rats. Ann Biomed Eng 2005; 33: 1078–89.
109. De Groat WC, Kawatani M, Hisamitsu T et al. Mechanisms underlying the recovery of urinary bladder function following spinal cord injury. J Auton Nerv System 1990; 30: S71–7.
110. Zinck NDT, Rafuse VF, Downie JW. Sprouting of CGRP primary afferents in lumbosacral spinal cord precedes emergence of bladder activity after spinal injury. Exp Neuroll 2007; 204: 777–90.
111. Barrington FJF. The nervous mechanism of micturition. Q J Exp Physiol 1915; 8: 33–71.
112. Yalla SV, Blunt KJ, Fam BA et al. Detrusor-urethral sphincter dyssynergia, J Urol 1977; 118: 1026–9.
113. Griffiths DJ. Residual urine, underactive detrusor function and the nature of detrusor/sphincter dyssynergia. Neurourol Urodyn 1983; 2: 289–94.

114. Dimitrijevic MR, Larsson LE, Lehmkuhl D, Sherwood AM. Evoked spinal cord and nerve root potentials in human using a non-invasive recording technique. Electroencephalogr Clin Neurophysiol 1978; 45: 331–40.
115. Beric A, Dimitrijevic MR, Light JK. A clinical syndrome of rostal and caudal spinal injury: neurological, neurophysiological and urodynamic evidence for occult sacral lesion. J Neurol Neurosurg Psychiatry 1987; 50(5): 600–6.
116. Beric A, Light JK. Correlation of bladder dysfunction and lumbosacral somatosensory evoked potential S wave abnormality in spinal cord injured patients. Neurourol Urodyn 1988; 7: 131–40.
117. Siroky MB, Krane RJ. Neurologic aspects of detrusor sphincter dyssynergia, with reference to the guarding reflex. J Urol 1982; 127: 953–7.
118. McGuire EJ, Savastano JA. Long term follow-up of spinal cord injury patients managed by intermittent catheterization. J Urol 1983; 129: 775–6.
119. Wang SC, McGuire EJ, Bloom DA. A bladder pressure management system for myelodysplasia – clinical outcome. J Urol 1988; 140: 1499–502.
120. Rudy DC, Woodside JR. Non-neurogenic neurogenic bladder. The relationship between intravesical pressure and external sphincter electromyogram. Neurourol Urodyn 1991; 10: 169–76.
121. Rudy DC, Awad SA, Downie JW. External sphincter dyssynergia: an abnormal continence reflex. J Urol 1988; 140: 105–10.
122. De Groat WC, Lalley PM. Reflex firing in the lumbar sympathetic outflow to activation of vesical afferent fibres. J Physiol 1972; 226: 289–309.
123. Schurch B, Yasuda K, Rossier AB. Detrusor bladder neck dyssynergia revisited. J Urol 1994; 152: 2066–70.
124. Awad SA, Downie JW, Kiruluta HG. Alpha-adrenergic agents in urinary disorders of proximal urethra. Part II. Urethral obstruction due to 'sympathetic dyssynergia'. Br J Urol 1978; 50: 336–9.
125. Pedersen E. Regulation of bladder and colon–rectum in patients with spinal lesions. J Auton Nerv Syst 1983; 7(3–4): 329–38.
126. Floyd K, Hick VE, Morrison JF. The influence of visceral mechanoreceptors on sympathetic efferent discharge in the cat. J Physiol Lond 1982; 323: 65–75.
127. Sato A, Sato Y, Sugimoto H, Terui N. Reflex changes in the urinary bladder after mechanical and thermal stimulation of the skin at various segmental levels in cats. Neuroscience 1977; 2: 111–17.
128. McMahon SB, Morrison JFB. Two groups of spinal interneurones that respond to stimulation of the abdominal viscera of the cat. J Physiol 1982; 322: 21–34.
129. Coonan EM, Downie JW, Du H-J. Sacral spinal cord neurons responsive to bladder pelvic and perineal inputs in cats. Neurosci Lett 1999; 260: 137–40.
130. Xiao CG, De Groat WC, Godec CJ et al. 'Skin–CNS–bladder' reflex pathway for micturition after spinal cord injury and its underlying mechanisms. J Urol 1999; 162: 936–42.
131. Head H, Riddoch G. The autonomic bladder, excessive sweating and some other reflex conditions, in gross injuries of the spinal cord. Brain 1917; 40: 188.
132. Guttmann L, Whitteridge D. Effects of bladder distention on autonomic mechanisms after spinal cord injuries. Brain 1947; 70: 361.
133. Rossier A, Bors E. Urological and neurological observations following anesthetic procedures for bladder rehabilitation of patients with spinal cord injuries. I. Topical anesthesias. J Urol 1962; 87: 876–82.
134. Perkash I. An attempt to understand and to treat voiding dysfunction during rehabilitation of the bladder in spinal cord injury patients. J Urol 1976; 115: 36–40.
135. Yalla SV. Spinal cord injury. In: Krane RJ, Siroky MB, eds. Clinical Neuro-urology. Boston: Little, Brown and Company, 1979: 229–43.
136. Krenz NR, Weaver LC. Sprouting of primary afferent fibers after spinal cord transection in the rat. Neuroscience 1998; 85: 443–58.
137. Krenz NR, Meakin SO, Krassioukov AV, Weaver LC. Neutralizing intraspinal nerve growth factor blocks autonomic dysreflexia caused by spinal cord injury. J Neurosci 1999; 19: 7405–14.
138. Elliott S, Krassioukov A. Malignant autonomic dysreflexia in spinal cord injured men. Spinal Cord 2006; 44: 386–92.
139. Elbadawi A, Atta MA, Franck JI. Intrinsic neuromuscular defects in the neurogenic bladder. I. Short-term ultrastructural changes in muscular innervation of the decentralized feline border base following unilateral sacral ventral rhizotomy. Neurourol Urodyn 1984; 3: 93–113.
140. Sundin T, Dahlstrom A, Norlen LJ, Svedmyr N. The sympathetic innervation and adrenoreceptor function of the human lower urinary tract in the normal state and after parasympathetic denervation. Invest Urol 1977; 14: 322–8.
141. Norlen LJ, Dahlstrom A, Sundin T, Svedmyr N. The adrenergic innervation and adrenergic receptor activity of the feline urinary bladder and urethra in the normal state and after hypogastric and/or parasympathetic denervation. Scan J Urol Nephrol 1976; 10: 177–84.
142. Atta MA, Franck JI, Elbadawi A. Intrinsic neuromuscular defects in the neurogenic bladder. II. Long-term innervation of the unilaterally decentralized feline bladder base by regenerated cholinergic, increased adrenergic and emergent probable 'peptidergic' nerves. Neurourol Urodyn 1984; 3: 185–200.
143. Sundin T, Dahlstrom A. The sympathetic innervation of the urinary bladder and urethra in the normal state and after parasympathetic denervation at the spinal root level. An experimental study in cats. Scand J Urol Nephrol 1973; 7: 131–49.
144. deGroat WV, Kawatani M. Reorganization of sympathetic preganglionic connections in cat bladder ganglia following parasympathetic denervation. J Physiol 1989; 409: 431–49.
145. McGuire EJ, Morrissey SG. The development of neurogenic vesical dysfunction after experimental spinal cord injury or sacral rhizotomy in non-human primates. J Urol 1982; 128: 1390–3.
146. Ghoniem GM, Regnier HC, Biancani P et al. Effect of bilateral sacral decentralization on detrusor contractility and passive properties in dog. Neurourol Urodyn 1984; 3: 23–33.
147. McGuire EJ, Savastano JA. Effect of alpha-adrenergic blockade and anticholinergic agents on the decentralized primate bladder. Neurourol Urodyn 1985; 4: 139–42.
148. Gunasekera WSL, Richardson AE, Seneviratne KN, Eversden ID. Significance of detrusor compliance in patients with localized partial lesions of the spinal cord and cauda equina. Surg Neurol 1983; 20: 59–62.
149. McGuire EJ, Woodside JR, Borden TA, Weiss RM. Prognostic value of urodynamic testing in myelodysplastic patients. J Urol 1981; 126: 205–9.
150. Gajewski JB, Awad SA, Heffernan LPH et al. Neurogenic bladder in lower motor neuron lesion: long-term assessment. Neurourol Urodyn 1992; 11: 509–18.
151. Skehan AM, Downie JW, Awad SA. Control of bladder stiffness in normal and chronic decentralized feline bladder. J Urol 1993; 149: 1165–73.
152. Lapides J, French CR, Ajemian EP, Reus WF. A new method for diagnosis of the neurogenic bladder. Univ Mich Med Bull 1962; 28: 166–80.
153. Carpenter FG, Rubin RM. The motor innervation of the rat urinary bladder. J Physiol 1967; 192: 609–17.
154. Diokno AC, Davis R, Lapides J. Urecholine test for denervated bladders. Invest Urol 1975; 13: 233–5.
155. El-Salmy S, Downie JW, Awad SA. Bladder and urethral function and supersensitivity to subcutaneously administered bethanechol in cats with chronic cauda equina lesions. J Urol 1985; 134: 1011–18.
156. Donker PJ, Ivanovici F, Noach EL. Analysis of the urethral pressure profile by means of electromyography and the administration of drugs. Br J Urol 1972; 44: 180–93.
157. Mattiasson A, Andersson K-E, Sjogren C. Urethral sensitivity to alpha-adrenoceptor stimulation and blockade in patients with parasympathetically decentralised lower urinary tract and in healthy volunteers. Neurourol Urodyn 1984; 3: 223–33.
158. Clarke SJ, Thomas DG. Characteristics of the urethral pressure profile in flaccid male paraplegics. Br J Urol 1981; 53: 157–61.

159. Blaivas JG. A critical appraisal of specific diagnostic techniques. In: Krane RJ, Siroky MB, eds. Clinical Neuro-urology. Little, Brown and Company, 1979: 69–109.
160. Bauer SB, Labib KB, Dieppa RA, Retik AB. Urodynamic evaluation of the boy with myelodysplasia. Urology 1977; 10: 354–62.
161. Awad SA, Downie JW. Sympathetic dyssynergia in the region of the external sphincter: a possible source of lower urinary tract obstruction. J Urol 1977; 118: 636–40.
162. Parsons KF, Turton MB. Urethral supersensitivity and occult urethral neuropathy. Br J Urol 1980; 52: 131–37.
163. Elbadawi A, Atta MA. Intrinsic neuromuscular defect in the neurogenic bladder. V. Autonomic re-innervation of the male feline rhabdosphincter following somatic denervation by bilateral sacral ventral rhizotomy. Neurourol Urodyn 1986; 5: 65–85.
164. Flood HD, Downie JW, Awad SA. Urethral function after chronic cauda equina lesion in cats. II. The role of autonomically-innervated smooth and striated muscle in distal sphincter dysfunction. J Urol 1990; 144: 1029–35.
165. Kluck P. The autonomic innervation of the human urinary bladder, bladder neck and urethra. A histochemical study. Anat Rec 1980; 198: 439–47.
166. Elbadawi A. Neuromorphological basis of vesicourethral function I. Histochemistry, ultrastructure and function of intrinsic nerves of the bladder and urethra. Neurourol Urodyn 1982; 1: 3–50.
167. Awad SA, Downie JW, Kiruluta HG. Alpha adrenergic agents in urinary disorders of the proximal urethra. Part I. Sphincteric incontinence. Br J Urol 1978; 50: 332–5.
168. Awad SA, Downie JW. The adrenergic component in the proximal urethra. Urol Int 1977; 32: 192–7.
169. Nergardh A. The functional role of adrenergic receptors in the outlet region of the bladder. An in vitro and in vivo study in the cat. Scand J Urol Nephrol 1974; 8: 100–7.
170. Caine M, Raz S, Zeigler M. Adrenergic and cholinergic receptors in prostate, prostatic capsule and bladder neck. Br J Urol 1975; 47: 193–202.
171. Stephenson TP, Wein AJ. The interpretation of urodynamics. In: Mundy AR, Stephenson TP, Wein AJ, eds. Urodynamics: Principles, Practice and Application. London: Churchill-Livingstone, 1984: 93–115.
172. Flood HD, Downie JW, Awad SA. Urethral function after chronic cauda equina lesions in cats. I. The contribution of the mechanical factors and sympathetic innervation to proximal sphincter dysfunction. J Urol 1990; 144: 1022–8.
173. Barbalias GA, Blaivas JG. Neurologic implication of the pathologically open bladder neck. J Urol 1983; 129: 780–2.
174. McGuire EJ, Wagner FC. The effects of sacral denervation on bladder and urethral functions. Surg Gynecol Obstet 1977; 144: 343–6.
175. Kirby RS, Flower C, Gilpin S et al. Non-obstructive detrusor failure. A urodynamic, electromyographic, neurohistochemical and autonomic study. Br J Urol 1983; 55: 652–9.
176. Blaivas JG, Barbalias GA. Characteristics of neural injury after abdominoperineal resection of the rectum. J Urol 1983; 129: 84–7.
177. Ahlberg J, Edlund C, Wikkelsö C et al. Neurological signs are common in patients with urodynamically verified 'Idiopathic' bladder overactivity. Neurourol Urodyn 2002; 21: 65–70.

31

Cerebral palsy, cerebellar ataxia, AIDS, phacomatosis, neuromuscular disorders, and epilepsy

Mark W Kellett and Ling K Lee

Introduction

In previous chapters, authors have described neurologic disorders that are frequently associated with, or produce characteristic neurogenic bladder disturbances. In this chapter the authors review a number of miscellaneous conditions in which neurogenic disorders of the bladder may infrequently occur, either as a manifestation of the primary disease, or sometimes as a complication of disease treatment. Although urinary disturbance is well recognized in many of the conditions discussed, in others such as neuromuscular disorders cases are rare and reports are largely anecdotal.

Table 31.1 *The percentage of children aged 6 years old with cerebral palsy (CP) of different severity who were continent compared to normally developing children*[1]

At age 6 years old	Percent continent
Normally developing	92
Spastic hemiplegia	80
Spastic diplegia	84
Spastic tetraplegia	54
CP with IQ > 65	80
CP with IQ < 65	38
Spastic tetraplegia with IQ < 65	33

Cerebral palsy

Cerebral palsy is becoming increasingly common as more premature low birthweight infants are surviving in neonatal intensive care units and are prone to insults to their central nervous system. Adverse events such as infection, cerebral vascular accident, or anoxia, in the prenatal and perinatal period, can permanently damage areas in the brain which lead to the nonprogressive disorders of motor function seen in cerebral palsy. The most common manifestation is muscle spasticity (70–80%), with athetoid, hypotonic and ataxic motor disorders making up the rest. Intellectual capacity is directly related to the severity of physical impairment. The combination of mental, neurologic, and physical handicap means urinary symptoms and incontinence are commoner in patients with cerebral palsy.

Roijen et al[1] sent a continence questionnaire to the parents of 601 children (aged between 4 and 18 years) with cerebral palsy and received a response from 459 (76%). The prevalence for primary urinary incontinence in this study was 23.5%. Daytime continence usually preceded nocturnal continence and 85% of children gained nocturnal continence within the year of achieving daytime continence. In this study, 96% of all cerebral palsy children with normal intelligence (IQ >65) were continent, demonstrating the importance of comprehension and communication skills for continence training. The ability to achieve continence was related to the extent of both physical and mental handicap (Table 31.1) and, not surprisingly, children with spastic tetraplegia and low intelligence (IQ <65) were the least likely to become continent. The majority of children with cerebral palsy (89%) who were continent became so before 12 years old, and a small minority would continue to gain control spontaneously into their late teens.

Although urinary incontinence is the commonest reason for a urologic referral (Table 31.2), a significant number of patients with cerebral palsy have other lower urinary tract symptoms.[2–6] Over a 7-month period, McNeal et al[5] interviewed 50 patients (between 8 and 29 years old) with cerebral palsy who attended outpatient clinics and actively sought out symptoms of urinary dysfunction. More than a third (36%) had two or more urinary symptoms prompting referral for further urologic assessment. In reality, the overall incidence of lower urinary tract symptoms could be higher, as McNeal's study excluded patients with IQs <40.

Table 31.2 *The distribution of the common lower urinary tract symptoms in patients with cerebral palsy undergoing urological assessment. Some patients had multiple symptoms*

	McNeal et al[5]	Decter et al[4]	Mayo[3]	Reid and Borzyskowski[2]
Number of patients	50	57	33	27
Symptoms				
Incontinence[a]	54%	86%	48%	74%
Urgency	18%			37%
Frequency		51%		56%
Dribbling	6%			
Hesitancy/voiding difficulties		3.5%	46%	11%
Retention		2%	6%	7%

[a]Incontinence includes urge/stress/day and/or enuresis.

Table 31.3 *Urodynamic findings on patients with cerebral palsy*

	Reid and Borzyskowski[2]	Mayo[3]	Decter et al[4]	McNeal et al[5]	Drigo et al[7]	Karaman et al[6]
Number of patients	27	33	57	13	9	36
Hyperreflexic	21 (78%)	22 (67%)	35 (61%)	4 (31%)	9 (100%)	17 (47%)
End-fill instability				2 (15%)		
Detrusor sphincter dyssynergia	5 (19%)	1 (3%)	7 (17%)		2 (22%)	4 (11%)
Acontractile bladder	2		1			

Mayo[3] found an unusually high incidence of voiding difficulty in 17 of the 33 patients who underwent videocystometrogram. The patients predominantly had difficulty initiating a urinary stream and two adult patients were using catheters for urinary retention. His group of patients was older (10 patients >20 years old, 3 patients >55 years old) and Mayo postulated that obstructive symptoms might become more prevalent as patients with cerebral palsy progress into adult life. This, he felt, was due to lack of voluntary control over a 'spastic' pelvic floor.

A hyperreflexic bladder (involuntary contractions during bladder filling in the presence of a known neurologic disorder) consistent with an upper motor neuron injury was the commonest urodynamic finding in symptomatic patients with cerebral palsy[2–5,7] (Table 31.3). Symptoms of urgency and frequency appear to correlate well with an overactive detrusor. Mayo demonstrated hyperreflexia in 14 of the 16 patients with urge ± incontinence compared to only 8 out of the 17 with voiding difficulties. Reduced bladder capacity was also a common finding, and occasionally a noncompliant bladder with end-fill instability was found to be responsible for the patient's symptoms. A voiding study was more difficult to obtain, bearing in mind that a proportion of patients were wheelchair bound and had learning disabilities. Therefore, it is difficult to estimate the incidence of detrusor underactivity or bladder outlet obstruction in patients with cerebral palsy. Excluding 2 patients who were in retention and 1 with detrusor-sphincter dyssynergia, Mayo found the remaining 14 of 17 patients with voiding difficulties had low postvoid residual volumes, and none had significant trabeculation to suggest obstruction. During urodynamic evaluation on 57 children with cerebral palsy, Decter et al also carried out electromyography on the external sphincter using needle electrodes.[4] They identified 11 patients with incomplete lower motor neuron injury to the sphincter. This was defined as a partially denervated sphincter which, when stimulated, has a reduced number of motor units recruited to contract, but whose amplitude and duration of action potential may be increased during voiding simulating dyssynergia.[4] However, Decter et al did not comment as to whether these patients had outflow obstruction. Although uncommon, the finding of detrusor-sphincter dyssynergia and lower motor neuron lesions (acontractile bladder) implies that the perinatal injury that caused the abnormal neurology in cerebral palsy may also involve the spinal cord. Another urodynamic study on children (age range 4 to18 years, mean age 8.2 years) with cerebral palsy also identified detrusor-sphincter dyssynergia in 4 children out of 36 (11%).[6] They identified high voiding pressures of 90 cmH_2O. The incidence of vesicoureteric reflux on videourodynamics varied from 1.8 to 35%,[2–4,6,7] but none of the authors commented on renal impairment or the presence of reflux nephropathy.

Given the risk of upper tract damage in neurogenic voiding dysfunction, Brodak et al[8] prospectively screened on sonography 90 patients (age 1 to 25 years old), with or without urologic symptoms, in an attempt to determine whether urinary tract screening was necessary for patients with cerebral palsy. On first ultrasound, 7 of the 90 patients had renal abnormalities, which were hydronephrosis in 3, renal asymmetry in 2 and non-visualization in 2. On a follow-up ultrasound, only 2 of the 3 had persistent hydronephrosis and had ultrasound evidence of a neurogenic bladder, i.e. marked bladder wall trabeculation and/or resolution of hydronephrosis following catheterization. The authors concluded that routine urinary tract screening was not justified because urinary tract abnormalities were only detected in 2% of the patients studied.

Patients with cerebral palsy are more prone to UTIs[9] and should be investigated with ultrasound imaging of kidneys, bladder, and postmicturition residual volume. A plain kidney, ureter, and bladder (KUB) X-ray is useful, although renal tract stones are uncommon.[10] In the presence of abnormalities, further evaluation with videourodynamics, micturating cystourethrography, renogram, etc., should be performed. Decter et al[4] found that all 6 children with UTIs (single episode or recurrent) in their study had radiologic and urodynamic abnormalities, 4 had detrusor-sphincter dyssynergia, and one had chronic retention due to detrusor failure (one other not specified). In contrast, the study by Reid and Borzyskowski[2] involved 13 patients with a history of UTIs, but vesicoureteric reflux was demonstrated in only 1 patient who had hyperreflexia and detrusor-sphincter dyssynergia.

Treatment is primarily with anticholinergic drugs for hyperreflexic bladders and patients with symptoms of urge and frequency. Postmicturition bladder residuals should then be closely monitored, as clean intermittent catheterization may be necessary with increasing residuals. Prophylactic antibiotics are used for urinary tract infections and reflux nephropathy. Adrenergic drugs may be effective for a weak bladder neck causing stress incontinence.[2] Mayo advocated muscle relaxants (e.g. diazepam, baclofen) for his patients with voiding difficulties due to spasticity of their pelvic floor muscles.[3] Using a combination of medication and behavioral modification (e.g. frequent voiding schedule), Decter et al[4] were able to improve the incontinence in 21 of the 27 cerebral palsy patients (78%) who had adequate follow-up data. Cerebral palsy patients with detrusor-sphincter dyssynergia are most at risk of developing hydronephrosis and renal deterioration, and should have long-term upper tract monitoring. Karaman et al[6] advocated early intermittent catheterization with or without anticholinergics for increased residual urine and voiding biofeedback in the 4 children with detrusor-sphincter dyssynergy on urodynamic studies. In these patients with worsening renal function, and in whom intermittent catheterization is not a realistic alternative, a vesicostomy or urinary diversion (ileal conduit or continent diversion) should be performed.[2–4,11] Long-term catheterization for neuropathic bladders is generally not recommended because of the high complication rates of stone formation, urinary bypassing, and upper tract dilation.[12,13]

Selective sacral dorsal rhizotomy for controling lower limb spasticity in cerebral palsy patients may result in a lower motor neuron lesion of the bladder. Abbott noted urinary retention in 7% of the 200 patients who underwent this procedure, although it was transient in all but one of the 13 patients.[14] Houle et al demonstrated an increase in bladder capacity (p <0.005) by carrying out pre- and post-sacral rhizotomy urodynamic studies in 13 patients.[15] The resultant improved bladder storage and better mobility enabled some patients to become continent, and Sweetser et al found that the patients with milder forms of spasticity were most helped by this procedure.[15,16]

Cerebellar and spinocerebellar disorders

In cerebellar ataxia, the cerebellum and/or the pathways connecting the cerebellum with other parts of the nervous system undergo progressive, premature neuronal death and atrophy. The result is a heterogeneous spectrum of motor abnormalities, which is manifested in an abnormal broad-based gait, incoordination, tremor, dysarthria, and motor and autonomic dysfunction. The etiology in many cases is an underlying genetic abnormality, of which Friedreich's ataxia is the commonest and accounts for at least 50% of hereditary ataxias. The nonhereditary ataxias can present acutely, subacutely, or can also have a chronic course. The nature and extent of urinary disturbances depend on the site of involvement in the central nervous system. In isolated cerebellar disorders urinary disturbance is generally absent.[17] More frequently, the degenerative neuropathologic process affects multisystems including the brainstem, cerebrum, and spinal cord, in which case urinary symptoms are more likely.

In patients with spinocerebellar ataxia, urinary symptoms most commonly manifest as incontinence and urgency. Among 195 patients (aged between 8 and 54 years)

Table 31.4 *Urodynamic findings in patients with cerebellospinal ataxia*

	Leach et al[17]	Vezina et al[19]	Chami et al[18]
Number of patients	15	17	55
Hyperreflexia	8 (53%)	7 (41%)	14 (25%)
Detrusor-sphincter dyssnergia	3 (6%)	6 (37%)	
Detrusor acontractility	4 (27%)		9 (16%)

with hereditary spinocerebellar ataxia, Chami et al found 23% had urgency and 6% had urinary incontinence.[18] Reports on urodynamic findings on patients with ataxia are limited (Table 31.4), and in some the authors have found it difficult to classify the bladder disturbance.[17–19] Detrusor hyperreflexia appears to be the most common finding, which is not surprising as the cerebellum and basal ganglia are important in influencing the cerebral–brainstem loop that facilitates the coordinated voluntary control of the voiding reflex. Detrusor-sphincter dyssynergia and acontractility are less common and correlate with the extent of neuronal damage in the spinal cord. In Chami's paper, 36 of the 55 patients who had urodynamic studies had no urinary problems, and although 23 (64%) had normal urodynamic studies, detrusor hyperreflexia and detrusor acontractility were found in 6 and 2 patients, respectively.[18]

Treatment for urgency and urge incontinence in patients with ataxia ideally should be specific to the urodynamic findings. However, the likelihood is an underlying hyperreflexic bladder and these patients could be treated empirically with anticholinergics if they do not carry large residual volumes. Patients with under active detrusor can be treated with intermittent catheterization. Leach et al successfully treated their 3 patients with sphincter dyssynergia with a combination of α-sympathetic blockade (phenoxybenzamine), diazepam, and baclofen.[17]

Nonhereditary ataxias with a multitude of etiologies, e.g. alcohol intoxication, neurosarcoidosis, superficial siderosis, can present acutely or subacutely, with urinary incontinence as a common copresenting symptom.[20–24] Urodynamic studies are not commonly performed in the investigation of such patients, but when they have been done a hyperreflexic bladder has typically been identified.[20,21,24] Treatment will depend on the etiology and prognosis of the underlying condition. In some cases improvements in urinary control will occur as the underlying disease responds to specific treatment.[20,21,24]

Human immunodeficiency virus (HIV) infection and acquired immunodeficiency syndrome (AIDS)

LUTS in the well HIV-positive patient is uncommon and if present is usually due to UTI.[25] However, at the time of seroconversion to HIV, the patient may experience a variety of neurologic syndromes including acute urinary retention and sacral sensory loss.[28] Impaired micturition becomes more common with disease progression and can occur as part of a global neurologic dysfunction or due to infection.[25–28] Hermieu et al[27] undertook urodynamic and neurologic evaluation in 39 HIV-positive patients presenting with LUTS. A urodynamic abnormality, either an overactive or underactive detrusor or detrusor-sphincter dyssynergia, was identified in 87% of patients. Of these, 61% had AIDS-related neurologic problems such as cerebral toxoplasmosis, HIV demyelination disorders, motor dysfunction, and AIDS-related dementia. This heralded a poor prognosis as 43% in this group died after 2–24 months (mean 8 months).

Urinary sphincter abnormalities leading to either urinary incontinence or retention can occur as a result of spinal cord compression (e.g metastatic lymphoma, tuberculoma), or infection of the spinal cord (myelitis) or nerve roots (radiculitis) by opportunistic infections such as cytomegalovirus (CMV), toxoplasmosis, and herpes. Diagnosis of the underlying cause for the neurologic complication requires MRI of the spine, biopsies of abnormal spinal lesions, cerebrospinal fluid analysis, and also the identification of concurrent opportunistic infections.[29] CMV polyradiculopathy is very rare but eminently treatable and reversible if caught early. The patient presents with back and sciatica pain with bladder or bowel dysfunction. A lumbar puncture is performed and the diagnosis is made by finding a polymorphonuclear cell-predominant pleocytosis and by confirming the presence of CMV using PCR in the cerebrospinal fluid. Detrusor failure due to a lower motor lesion is uncommon and is usually caused by malignancy or infection such as herpes. These patients should be taught clean intermittent self-catheterization. Long-term indwelling catheters are best avoided in HIV-infected patients because of their vulnerability to *Staphylococcus aureus* bacteremia.

Neurocutaneous syndromes (phacomatosis)

Neurocutaneous syndromes encompass a number of congenital or hereditary conditions featuring involvement of nervous system, eyeball, retina, and skin. They present in childhood and slowly progress through adolescence, with many conditions demonstrating a propensity to malignant transformation. Most cases are genetically determined, although sporadic cases can occur.[30,31]Minor features are often present from birth, but with age neoplasia can often develop. Bladder disorders are unusual in many of these conditions, but the reported cases are discussed below. In some phacomatoses, such as tuberose sclerosis, bladder disorders have not been reported. Neurogenic bladder abnormalities have most commonly been reported in neurofibromatosis.

Neurofibromatosis types 1 (von Recklinhausens disease) and 2 (central type)

There are numerous reports of various neurofibromatosis type 1 associated tumors affecting the urinary system and particularly the bladder. They are usually derived from nerves of the pelvic, vesical, and prostatic plexuses,[32] and include benign and, less commonly, malignant neurofibromas,[32–52] paragangliomas,[53] and other occasional malignant tumors.[54] They should be suspected when patients with neurofibromatosis develop any urinary symptoms, as they may present in a multitude of ways. Lower urinary tract symptoms, enuresis, flank pain, incontinence, or symptoms related to urinary tract obstruction may occur, but in addition localized pain, low back pain, and lower limb dysesthesia can occur.[55] These symptoms may result from the tumor size[56] and/or neurogenic involvement.[57–59]

A conservative management approach to tumors causing urinary symptoms has been suggested due to likely damage to adjacent organs on attempted extirpation. However, careful follow-up is necessary to detect signs of upper tract obstruction, which may be a sign of tumor progression or malignant transformation.[56]

Neurofibromatosis type 2, and related conditions such as spinal schwannomatosis,[60] may also lead to upper motor neuron syndromes when tumors such as schwannomas, neurofibromas, meningiomas, or hamartomas[61] damage the spinal cord.[62–66] Neurofibromas or schwannomas,[66,67] or other tumors,[68] may involve the conus or cauda equina. In such cases, a mixture of upper and/or lower motor neuron bladder symptoms could occur. The typical presentation of conus and cauda equina lesions and the effects on the bladder have been described in earlier chapters.

Cobb syndrome

Cobb syndrome is a rare neurocutaneous syndrome manifest by cutaneous nevi and spinal angiomas within the same metaphere.[69] Wakabayarshi et al[70] reported an 8-year-old boy presenting with difficulty initiating micturition, constipation, low back pain, and a mild spastic paraparesis. Multiple angiokeratomas were present over dermatomes of the cervical region and lower sacral region on the right and over the lumbar and sacral areas on the left. Multiple angiomas were present in the cervicothoracic spinal cord and conus medullaris, with evidence of bleeding from an upper thoracic angioma that had probably produced his presenting symptoms. His symptoms gradually improved without surgical intervention. This phenotype most closely resembles Cobb syndrome, but unusually he also had cerebral angiomas that are rare in this condition.

Klippel–Trenaunay–Weber syndrome

In Klippel–Trenaunay–Weber syndrome intracranial and intraspinal angiomas may occur in association with hypertrophy of skeletal muscles and visceral involvement.[71–73] Urinary symptoms would be expected if symptomatic spinal cord pathology occurred due to pressure or bleeding from large spinal angiomas. Kojima et al[74] reported one such case with a nevus flammeus, varices, hypertrophy, and elongation of the left leg. The patient presented with a progressive paraparesis and urinary retention due to an extensive spinal arteriovenous malformation extending from T11 to L2. The arteriovenous malformation was treated surgically with an initial deterioration in bladder function, however, 6 months later her motor function improved to the preoperative state and the bladder dysfunction disappeared.

Various other non-neurogenic genitourinary manifestations may occur in Klippel–Trenaunay syndrome. They tend to occur in the more severe cases and usually involve cutaneous vascular malformations of the trunk, pelvis, and genitalia, sometimes with intra-abdominal and intrapelvic extension of the vascular malformations.[75]

Proteus syndrome

Proteus syndrome has numerous manifestations. It is characterized by massive tissue overgrowth and asymmetry. Frequent features include partial gigantism of hands and feet, nevi, and hemihypertrophy, as well as other multisystem involvement.[30] Neurogenic bladder symptoms are not a reported feature of this condition,[30] but urinary tract involvement may occur. In one case presenting with renal tract stones, left-sided ureterovesical reflux was found on the same side as hemihypertrophy. The authors postulated that the unilateral involvement was a feature related to hemihypertrophy,[76] however, similar cases have not been reported to further corroborate this. In another case, leiomyoma of the urinary bladder occurred.[77]

Neurocutaneous melanosis

Neurocutaneous melanosis is a form of phakomatosis in which there is a proliferation of melanocytes in skin and meninges. The most common skin lesion is a giant pigmented hairy nevus, but diffuse pigmentation can also occur. Infiltration of the pia and arachnoid by melanocytes can usually be seen macroscopically. There is an approximate 2 to 13% risk of malignant change in skin and a 50% risk of malignant change in the meninges. Typical neurologic abnormalities include hydrocephalus (probably due to vascular obstruction of the fourth ventricle), epilepsy, intracranial hemorrhage, cranial nerve palsies, and psychiatric disturbance. Neurogenic bladder has not been a feature except in one case reported by Sawamura et al.[78] The 13-year-old subject of their report presented with signs attributable to a large right frontal malignant leptomeningeal melanoma. Amongst his other clinical features was a neurogenic bladder, although, as there was no direct spinal involvement from the neurocutaneous melanosis, it was more likely to be attributable to his coexisting spina bifida. In 28 additional cases reviewed from the literature, neurogenic bladder disturbance was not reported, suggesting that it is unlikely to be a disease feature.[78]

Neuromuscular disorders

Neuromuscular junction disorders

Myasthenia gravis

Myasthenia gravis is an autoimmune disorder due to the presence of antiacetylcholine receptor antibodies that bind to the nicotinic cholinergic receptors at the motor endplate of the neuromuscular junction. It typically affects striated muscle, causing weakness with fatiguability. In 15% of patients its effects are confined to the ocular and facial muscles, causing ptosis and diplopia; however, more generalized weakness occurs in the majority of remaining patients. Although the antibodies act on nicotinic cholinergic receptors, antibodies have also been demonstrated against muscarinic cholinergic receptors.

Bladder disturbance attributable to myasthenia gravis is unusual, but a number of individual case reports have been published.[79–84] The clinical, urodynamic, and neurophysiologic findings in these cases are summarized in Table 31.5. The bladder dysfunction in all cases resembled a lower motor neuron pattern with variable degrees of detrusor areflexia/atonia. In the patient reported by Sandler et al,[83] the voiding dysfunction was complete and prolonged, and the patient required long-term intermittent catheterization. Unfortunately the authors do not report on the response of the original myasthenia gravis symptoms. In other patients, urinary symptoms have responded to medical therapy directed at the myasthenia gravis.[80,82] In some rare cases, voiding dysfunction may be the initial presenting symptom,[79,81] and in others may be associated with an exacerbation of generalized myasthenia gravis.[81,83] The detrusor muscle is predominantly under control of the parasympathetic nervous system with muscarinic innovation. Detrusor failure suggests involvement of acetylcholine receptor antibodies at muscarinic receptors on the detrusor muscle itself or in the pelvic ganglia. The fluctuation in severity related to drug treatment of myasthenia gravis suggests a causal relationship in some cases.

Urinary symptoms in myasthenia gravis have also been reported in male patients who have undergone prostatic surgery. Greene et al reported six men with bladder outflow obstruction who underwent a transurethral resection of the prostate (TURP) and subsequently developed urinary incontinence. They hypothesized that the resection led to some form of injury to the external sphincter that had already been compromised by the underlying myasthenia gravis. They therefore recommended an incomplete resection in order to leave distal tissue that they felt would prevent trauma to be sphincter. They later reported a seventh man with myasthenia gravis who underwent an incomplete resection who initially remained dry, but 3 months later developed urge incontinence. Subsequently, Wise et al found that incontinence after TURP was associated with the use of blended current, and that patients treated with either high frequency unblended current, partial proximal resection, or open prostatectomy remained dry.[85] Unfortunately urodynamic or EMG studies were not made in these cases and therefore the pathophysiologic mechanism is unclear. However, Khan and Bhola[86] reported another patient who remained continent after an open prostatectomy. Preoperative EMG of the external urinary sphincter revealed fatiguability and abnormal motor units, suggesting an underlying neurogenic weakness of the continence mechanism. The authors postulated that electrical current could further damage this mechanism, possibly by damaging residual acetylcholine receptors.[86]

Lambert–Eaton myasthenic syndrome

Lambert–Eaton myasthenic syndrome (LEMS) is characterized by muscle weakness as well as autonomic dysfunction; it is associated with small cell lung cancer in approximately 60% of cases and is often associated with the presence of anti-P/Q-type voltage-gated calcium

Table 31.5 *The clinical, urodynamic and neurophysiological findings of myasthenia gravis patients with bladder disturbance*

Reference	Age Sex	Myasthenia characteristics	Urinary symptoms	Urodynamic and EMG findings
80	59 Female	Generalized MG	Difficulty voiding Incomplete bladder emptying Frequency Severity related to treatment with pyridostigmine	Normal bladder capacity (430 ml). Normal filling sensation Atonic detrusor (pressure < 8 cmH_2O) during attempted void Voiding by abdominal pressure with poor flow and interrupted flow pattern
81	31 Female	Generalized MG	Stress incontinence Bladder neck suspension 8 months before MG diagnosed Associated with deterioration in MG condition	Open bladder neck Inability to sustain pelvic floor contraction Bladder hyperreflexia
82	20 Female	Seronegative Generalized MG	'Urinary disturbance' Symptoms responded to treatment with steroids and thymectomy	Atonic bladder
79	Elderly Male	Generalized MG	Urgency and urge incontinence Uncontrollable flatus and fecal incontinence on sneezing and coughing	Detrusor hyporeflexia
83	39 Female	Seropositive Generalized MG	Incontinence followed by retention with constipation at time of myasthenic crisis	Bladder capacity 662 ml Areflexic detrusor Unable to generate detrusor contraction and unable to void EMG – low intensity unchanged during bladder filling
84	61 Female	Generalized MG	Frequency Difficulty voiding Incomplete bladder voiding Recurrent urinary tract infections	Residual volume 100 ml Detruser underactivity Poor flow rates and voided by abdominal straining

channel antibodies.[87–89] Dysautonomia is frequent in LEMS and involves cholinergic and adrenergic systems,[90–94] but neurogenic bladder involvement is rare.

In one series of 50 patients, autonomic symptoms occurred in 80% of patients, with dry mouth and impotence being the most frequently experienced symptoms, followed by constipation, blurred vision, and sweating abnormalities; there were no reports of bladder dysfunction.[91] Another study involving 30 patients had similar findings.[92] Bladder dysfunction has been reported in five cases,[90,95,96] although detailed features, including urodynamic findings, have only been reported in one case.[96] In this report, Satoh et al described a 71-year-old Japanese woman with neurophysiologically and serologically confirmed LEMS. She was initially treated with anticholinesterase drugs, corticosteroids, and plasma exchange. Four years after presentation her condition deteriorated and she was unable to stand or walk. She complained of a dry mouth and urinary frequency greater than 15 times per day. Urodynamic studies consisting of uroflowmetry, cystometry, and urethral pressure recordings were made before and after treatment with 3,4-diaminopyridine. Maximum urinary flow rate was decreased at 12.8 ml/s, suggestive of an underactive detrusor. Bladder emptying was reasonable, with postvoid residual volumes of 37 ml, 170 ml, and 70 ml on three separate measurements. After treatment with 10 mg of 3,4-diaminopyridine muscle weakness and dry mouth dramatically improved and this was associated with reduced urinary frequency. Post-treatment anal sphincter EMG and detrusor and abdominal pressures also increased markedly during voiding, and the maximum urine flow rate normalized from 12.8 ml/s to

17.9 ml/s. The presentation with frequency is a little unusual in disorders manifest by detrusor underactivity; however, this patient's urinary symptoms undoubtedly improved with better detrusor contractility.

Detrusor muscle pressure and abdominal muscle pressure were reduced in voiding, suggesting that the neurogenic bladder was caused by defective neurotransmission in both autonomic detrusor muscle and skeletal abdominal muscle. Furthermore, the response to 3,4-diaminopyridine suggests that the neurogenic bladder was directly attributable to the dysautonomia of LEMS. The authors speculated that this was due to the action of anti-P/Q-type voltage-gated calcium channel antibodies on the bladder. In support of this theory they cited a number of animal studies suggesting an important role for these antibodies in mediating neurotransmitter release in the urinary bladder of mice, rats, and guinea pigs.[94,97,98]

Muscular dystrophies

Myotonic dystrophy

Myotonic dystrophy is a disorder characterized by myotonia (sustained contraction of muscle in response to electrical or percussive stimuli) and dystrophy (progressive loss of skeletal muscle with fibrosis and fatty infiltration). However, it is a multisystem disorder with the most prominent manifestations in skeletal muscle, the cardiac conduction system, brain, smooth muscle, and lens. It is inherited as an autosomal dominant trait with variable penetrance and phenotypic expression, and it demonstrates the phenomenon of anticipation with worsening of the disease in subsequent generations. The genetic mutation primarily responsible for the autosomal dominant inheritance of myotonic dystrophy is a variable triplet repeat (CTG) that is located on chromosome 19 in the 3′ untranslated region of a gene with protein kinase domains named myotonin protein kinase.[99]

Smooth muscle abnormalities are well recognized in myotonic dystrophy but predominantly affect the gastrointestinal tract. Urinary tract dysfunction is much less commonly encountered.[100] Urinary retention without evidence of other pathologic conditions was noted in a number of early reports.[101–103] Bundschu et al[104] described two brothers with myotonic dystrophy who developed dilatation of the renal pelvis, ureter, and bladder due to presumed smooth muscle involvement. However, in a more systematic study using cystomerograms involving 9 patients, Orndahl et al[105] found normal bladder function in all cases. More recently, in two systematic studies symptomatic bladder dysfunction was found in 6 of 16 patients.[106,107] Symptoms often occurred at a young age and included urinary urgency, frequency, and stress incontinence. Urodynamic investigation revealed reduced urethral pressures and abnormal motor units in the external sphincter. There was a suggestion that, in women in particular, pelvic floor muscle involvement may have been contributory.

Histopathologic findings in reported cases have been variable. The bladder was reported to be normal in one autopsied case,[108] however in another case, Harvey et al[101] found slight vacuolization of the bladder smooth muscle syncytium and an increased number of nuclei. Furthermore, Pruzanski and Huvos,[109] in another autopsy study, demonstrated muscle degeneration in the bowel and bladder. Histology of the bladder showed separation of myofibrils by edematous fibrous tissue, variation in muscle fiber size and shape, and longitudinal myofibers showed break-up with hypereosinophilia. Fibrous tissue replacement as seen in the bladder of the latter case is frequently seen in skeletal muscles of patients with myotonic dystrophy. However, it should be noted that this patient also had evidence of prostatic hyperplasia with some trabeculation of the bladder wall and thus the significance of these pathologic changes is uncertain.[109]

Limb-girdle muscular dystrophy

Limb-girdle muscular dystrophies (LGMD) are a group of genetically heterogenous disorders that share similar presenting features.[110] Their classification is based on mode of inheritance and chromosomal localization, with the gene product known in increasing numbers of subtypes in many, and currently 11 limb-girdle dystrophies can be defined by gene product, but identification of others is likely soon.[110–112] Limb girdle dystrophies occur in both sexes, with onset between the second and sixth decade, usually in late childhood or early adulthood, although onset can occur at almost any age. Weakness in many cases begins in the pelvic girdle musculature then spreads to the pectoral muscles, although the reverse is not unusual.

The various phenotypes have been widely characterized and urinary symptoms are unusual. However, Dixon et al[113] reported a 48-year-old woman with clinical, laboratory, and neurophysiologic evidence of LGMD with urinary symptoms that appeared to be related to the presence of LGMD. The patient was nulliparous and had originally developed stress incontinence at the age of 12 years when jumping. This progressed over subsequent years until it was present on coughing and walking. Videocystometogram showed marked bladder descent and stress incontinence with no detrusor instability and normal urethral sphincter EMG. Histology of pelvic floor muscles revealed changes consistent with LGMD: large variability of fiber size with hypertrophied and atrophic fibers and type 1 fiber predominance, frequent internal nuclei, and disruption of the myofibrillar pattern. Unfortunately, at the time this report was made it was impossible to identify the specific phenotype although it may represent a subtype with early and predominant involvement of pelvic muscles. Although not directly

Table 31.6 *Clinical features and neurophysiologic findings in seven patients with DMD (adapted from Caress et al[117])*

Patient	Age	History of spinal fusion	Symptoms	Urodynamic/ urethral EMG	Detrusor-sphincter dyssynergy	Uninhibited contractions	Motor unit appearance
1	17	Yes	Retention	Normal	No	No	Normal
2	14	Yes	Urgency, incontinence	UMN	No	Yes	Normal
3	11	Yes	Voiding difficulty	LMN	No	No	Long duration
4	17	Yes	Incontinence, frequent UTIs	UMN	Yes	Yes	Normal
5	8	No	Incontinence	UMN	No	Yes	Normal
6	16	?	Urgency, UTI. incontinence	UMN	Yes	Yes	Normal
7	16	Yes	Incontinence	UMN	Yes	Yes	Normal

neurogenic in etiology, the weak pelvic floor muscles led to abnormal positioning of the vesicourethral junction, which was the most likely cause of the incontinence in this case.

Duchenne muscular dystrophy

Duchenne muscular dystrophy (DMD) is an X-linked disorder that is the most common muscular dystrophy in children. It is characterized by progressive weakness of skeletal muscle with onset in early childhood. The disorder is caused by loss-of-function mutations of an extremely large gene located on the X-chromosome (Xp21). The protein product of the gene, dystrophin, is absent or markedly deficient. Dystrophin is a cytosolic protein associated with the external membrane of skeletal, cardiac, and smooth muscle cells and of some neurons. Lack of dystrophin ultimately leads to a chronic necrotizing myopathy with marked muscle wasting. The disease progresses over 20 years and is always associated with an inability to walk.[114]

Despite the fact that most patients with DMD have normal sphincter function, some patients will experience urinary incontinence. It is not uncommon for a short period of urinary and bowel incontinence to occur around the age of 12 years, as the child becomes wheelchair-dependent. This appears unrelated to structural pathology such as increasingly severe scoliosis, and is thought to be a manifestation of depression. It usually resolves within a few months.[115]

Neurogenic bladder disorders do also occur, albeit unusually. In one retrospective study from the Mayo Clinic in Rochester, 33 patients with DMD, born between 1953 and 1983 and followed during their second decade of life, were studied. Urinary disturbance was described in only two of the 33 cases (6%); it occurred relatively late in the disease course and in both cases was manifest by urinary retention. In one 12-year-old boy, acute urinary retention occurred several weeks following surgery for correction of scoliosis. In the other case, acute urinary retention appeared while the patient was undergoing an excretory cystourethrogram for nephrolithiasis. Although this settled, acute retention recurred several months later. Detailed urodynamic studies were not reported and the authors were unclear about the significance of these findings in view of the associated events.[116]

In another study, Caress et al[117] identified 7 boys with DMD who had undergone urodynamic tests at the Children's Hospital of Boston during the years 1978–94. The clinical, urodynamic, and neurophysiologic findings are summarized in Table 31.6. Five of the boys complained of urinary incontinence and 2 had difficulty initiating voiding consistent with urinary retention. Five of the boys had undergone a spinal fusion procedure, and in 2 of these there was a temporal relationship between their spinal fusion surgery and the onset of urinary dysfunction, similar to the case reported by Boland et al.[116] In one of these cases acute urinary retention and left lateral thigh and testicular numbness occurred immediately following his T4–L5 spinal fusion. In another case, bladder and bowel incontinence was associated with paraplegia and a T10 sensory level following a spinal fusion procedure. None of the other 6 patients had upper motor neurone signs, although the severe muscle wasting and weakness could have obscured subtle signs.

Sacral reflexes were preserved in all of the patients and bladder contractions were of normal or high pressures in all but one child. Urodynamic studies and EMG were abnormal in 6 cases, with 5 out of 6 exhibiting upper motor neuron dysfunction. There was no clear pattern of bladder size or postvoid residual volume in this group, but uninhibited contractions were a frequent finding (4/5), as was detrusor-sphincter dyssynergia (3/5). One patient had normal reflexes but enlarged motor units suggestive of reinnervation and was classified as having lower motor neuron dysfunction. This 11-year-old had a normal capacity bladder and an initial postvoid residual urine volume of 250 ml.[117] Despite the advanced disease course in most of the cases, unlike the previous case with LGMD[113] there was no evidence of myopathic motor units or abnormal spontaneous activity in the pelvic floor muscles. Furthermore, bladder pressures generated during voiding or during uninhibited contractions were normal or elevated, suggesting that no significant detrusor myopathy was present.[117]

The upper motor neuron lesions in these cases, and in the case of Boland and colleagues,[116] are most likely to be due to progressive scoliosis or complications of surgical treatment, or both. The temporal nature of urinary disturbance to a surgical procedure in at least 3 of 9 reported cases suggests a direct causal relationship. In the other cases that had undergone surgery, the lack of a clear temporal relationship does not exclude a similar mechanism. Caress and colleagues also postulated that upper motor neuron dysfunction could result from the action of DMD on the central nervous system.[117] Dystrophin is present in the normal brain and its presumed absence in DMD patients may be related to the cognitive deficiencies seen in many affected individuals. Thus they suggested that an absence of dystrophin in the brain or spinal cord could account for the upper motor neuron findings. However, they concluded that it is an unlikely explanation as there are no other upper motor neuron signs, and it would be unlikely to cause isolated bladder/sphincter dyssynergy.[117]

The treatment of bladder disturbance in these cases followed standard therapy and all patients were subsequently treated with anticholinergic medicines or clean intermittent catheterization, or both.

Epilepsy

Seizure classification

Seizures are symptoms of cerebral dysfunction, resulting from paroxysmal hyperexcitable and/or hypersynchronous discharges of neurones involving the cerebral cortex. Epilepsy is defined as a disorder characterized by recurrent epileptic seizures. The International Classification of Epileptic Seizures divides the clinical manifestations into partial seizures, which begin in a part of one hemisphere, and generalized seizures, which begin in both hemispheres simultaneously. The clinical manifestations of simple partial seizures are determined by the function of the cortical area involved and are divided by the International Classification into motor, sensory, autonomic, and psychic phenomena.[118] Accordingly, semiology in partial seizures can lateralize and sometimes localize seizure onset, which can be of relevance in patients undergoing presurgical evaluation.

Cortical bladder control and seizure localization

A number of regions within the brain are implicated in cortical control of urinary function. Functional studies using PET and SPECT suggest lateralization to the right hemisphere for cortical bladder control and more specifically involvement of the right medial temporal gyrus, right anterior cingulate gyrus, right inferior frontal gyrus, right frontal operculum, dorsomedial pontine tegmentum, periaqueductal gray, and rostral hypothalamus.[119–121] Furthermore, in patients with structural pathology, urinary incontinence usually correlates with right hemisphere involvement,[122,123] and in elderly patients, urge incontinence with reduced bladder filling sensation is associated with right frontal abnormalities on SPECT scanning.[124] Thus, given that semiology of partial seizures is dependent on the cortical function involved, it is not surprising that disorders of micturition are seen during seizures arising from the above regions of the brain.

Urinary symptoms in epilepsy

Urinary incontinence is a common and well-recognized feature of epileptic seizures. Indeed, enquiry into loss of continence during seizures or blackouts is a routine aspect of history taking. Incontinence during episodes of loss of consciousness is, however, not diagnostic of seizures, and must always be considered along with other ictal phenomena as incontinence can also occur in simple faints, and micturition can induce syncope in some patients.

Incontinence in seizures

During typical absence seizures, pressure recordings with catheterization reveal increased intravesicular pressure secondary to detrusor muscle contraction.[125] Enuresis following generalized tonic-clonic seizures is due to relaxation of the external sphincter.[126] During absence status, urinary incontinence occurs as a result of either micturitional automatism or neglect. Isolated ictal enuresis is rare. The exact frequency of incontinence in different seizure types is not known.

Micturition in localization related epilepsy (partial seizures)

The urinary system is primarily under the control of the autonomic nervous system and, therefore, seizures involving the autonomic nervous system are often associated with urinary symptoms. Autonomic seizures often arise from mesiobasal limbic, frontal, orbital, or opercular regions, with likely rapid spread of seizure activity into hypothalamic areas further contributing to autonomic symptoms. Autonomic seizures are more common in the presence of impairment of consciousness, but may also occur with apparently fully preserved awareness and responsiveness.[127–129] Symptoms in autonomic seizures include vomiting, pallor, flushing, sweating, piloerection, pupil dilatation, borborygmi, and incontinence. These may occur as simple partial seizures or sometimes as an aura prior to complex partial or secondary generalized seizures, but must be distinguished from secondary effects of other seizure types that invariably cause autonomic signs as a later feature.[127] Collectively, autonomic phenomena comprise an important and substantial portion of partial seizure symptoms, representing approximately one-third of all simple partial seizures.[128–130]

Early onset benign childhood seizures with occipital spikes (Panayiotopoulos syndrome)

Autonomic symptoms are particularly prominent in the so-called Panayiotopoulos syndrome.[131,132] Cardinal features of this condition include infrequent partial seizures that consist of a combination of autonomic and behavioral disturbances, vomiting, deviation of the eyes, often with impairment of consciousness, that can frequently progress to convulsions. Autonomic disturbances of pallor and sweating, alone or together with behavioral disturbances (mainly irritability), may predominate, particularly in the early stages of the ictus.[133–136] Incontinence of urine occurs in 10% of cases, usually when consciousness is impaired even without convulsions; less commonly, fecal incontinence can occur with other autonomic or behavioral features even in nocturnal seizures. Seizures are typically long, often lasting for 5 or more minutes and, in 40% for hours, consistent with partial status epilepticus. The condition is considered benign with an excellent prognosis. About half of all patients only have a single attack, and in the majority of the remainder spontaneous remission occurs within a few years. For this reason, antiepileptic drug treatment is rarely used.

Ictal urinary urge in partial seizures (auras)

An ictal desire to void is an infrequent but well-recognized feature of temporal lobe seizures, with a reported frequency of between 0.4 and 8%.[128,137–141] Baumgartner et al[139] reviewed video-EEG records of 277 patients with refractory temporal lobe epilepsy and found 6 (2.2%) reported an intense urge to urinate, which they termed 'ictal urinary urge'. The urge is usually accompanied by other auras, which in some can include genital automatisms.[138] EEG localization and imaging using high resolution MRI, supplemented by interictal SPECT studies in 4 patients and ictal SPECT studies in 2 patients, suggested onset in the right or left temporal lobes, with intracarotid amytal testing confirming that this was the nondominant temporal lobe in all cases.[139] Ictal and interictal EEG studies in a subsequent report of 6 patients with stereotyped ictal urinary urge also found onset in the nondominant, right, temporal lobe.[141] In the latter study, temporal lobe resection led to seizure freedom in two cases, confirming the localization to the temporal lobe.[141] The authors postulated an area in the nondominant temporal lobe involved in the initiation of micturition.[139,141] The recognition of this 'ictal urge' in seizure semiology may be of relevance when patients are being considered for epilepsy surgery.

Micturition-induced reflex epilepsy

Recently Glass et al[142] reported a 12-year-old girl with complex partial seizures beginning, at age 2. From age 10 years she had reflex seizures with every micturition and also with prayer. Seizures occurred 4 to 6 times per day and were refractory to treatment with multiple antiepileptic drugs and the ketogenic diet. Seizure semiology observed during video-EEG monitoring revealed pupil dilatation and staring, followed by loss of body tone and at times deviation of the head and eyes to the left, with occasional rhythmic clonic activity of both arms. Previously, micturition-induced seizures have been reported in a number of other children. Some have had learning difficulties[143,144] or structural pathology, such as a calcified granuloma in the right frontal lobe.[145] Most recently, Okumura et al[146] reported an 8-year-old girl with micturition-induced seizures and cited two previous cases from the Japanese literature.[147,148]

EEG recordings have suggested onset of seizures in the central anterior or right frontal lobe in some cases,[143,144] or in the deep midline structures with rapid spread to frontal regions in others.[142,146] Reports in other children with micturition-induced seizures have failed to demonstrate EEG localization, but semiology has suggested onset in the supplementary sensorimotor region.[147–149] Furthermore, in another patient who had reflex seizures induced by micturition and stepping into hot water, onset during video-EEG of immersion-induced attacks suggested the seizures arose in the central midline region.[143]

In the case reported by Glass and colleagues, ictal SPECT studies revealed activity in the anterior cingulate gyrus and anterolateral right frontal lobe.[142] The regulation of autonomic and endocrine function is one of a number of

Table 31.7 *Urinary disturbances associated with gabapentin treatment*[154]

Age/ Sex	Seizure type	Neurological status	Urinary disturbance	Gabapentin dose	Other anti-epileptic drugs	Outcome
43 Male	Secondary GTCS Atypical absence tonic	'Mental retardation' secondary to perinatal hypoxic ischemic brain injury	Daily bladder and rectal incontinence unrelated to seizures	600 mg tid	Carbamazepine 600 mg/day Phenytoin 300 mg/day	Incontinence resolved on reducing dose to 300 mg bid
34 Female	Secondary GTCS Complex partial	Congenital hemiplegia	Weekly bladder and rectal incontinence unrelated to seizures	1800 mg/day	Phenytoin 250 mg/day Phenobarbitone 180 mg/day	Resolved when dose reduced to 300 mg/day prior to discontinuation
12 Male	Complex partial	Hyperactivity and tics Convulsive status epilepticus age 4 years	Daily urinary incontinence unrelated to seizures	200 mg tid	Valproate 500 mg bid.	Resolved 2 days after gabapentin stopped

functions localized to the anterior cingulate gyrus,[150] and the cortical control of micturition itself is coordinated from the superomedial portion of the frontal lobe (mainly the right) and the anterior aspect of the cingulate gyrus.[151] Thus Glass et al postulated a region of hyperexcitability in the 'affect' component of the anterior cingulate gyrus, with seizures triggered by micturition and emotion in their patient.[142] In the case reported by Okumura et al,[146] subtraction ictal SPECT studies showed increased perfusion in the mesial frontal region, suggesting onset in the supplementary sensorimotor area of the right frontal lobe.

Urinary symptoms related to antiepileptic drugs

Urinary frequency and incontinence has also been reported as an adverse reaction to antiepileptic medication. Incontinence is an unusual side-effect of carbamazepine and valproic acid,[152] and was reported in a single case during a clinical trial of gabapentin,[153] however, details of the urinary disturbance and outcome are not available. Gil-Nagel et al[154] reported urinary incontinence in three of their 394 cases treated with gabapentin at their tertiary referral centre. The clinical details of the three cases are summarized in Table 31.7. Gabapentin-related incontinence included isolated urinary incontinence in one case with temporal lobe epilepsy and severe double incontinence in two cases with secondary generalized epilepsy. The problem persisted as long as patients were taking the drug and disappeared soon after it was discontinued or the dose was reduced. The three patients had medically refractory seizures and two adults had signs of generalized or multifocal neurologic dysfunction, including mental retardation and hemiplegia. Incontinence did not appear to be related to seizure activity in any patient and video-EEG recordings in one patient corroborated this. Unfortunately, urodynamic assessment was not undertaken in any of the cases and, therefore, the physiologic mechanism for the incontinence is unclear. However, the authors postulated that, because gabapentin is distributed in most organs and tissues, it could act at one or more sites involving not only the brain and spinal cord but also the gastrointestinal and urinary tracts. Gabapentin enhances the action of glutamate dehydrogenase and is a weak inhibitor of GABA transaminase and may therefore modulate glutamate and GABA. Both these neurotransmitters are involved in the regulation of micturition in the central nervous system. Thus, incontinence could be related to the effect of gabapentin in the cortex, interfering with the inhibition that the frontal lobe exerts on the pontine micturition center. It is possible that pre-existing damage to the cerebral cortex acts as a substrate for the development of gabapentin-induced incontinence.

Treatment of bladder symptoms in epilepsy

Treatment of incontinence related to epilepsy primarily involves optimization of antiepileptic drug treatment, or other therapies, to minimize the frequency and severity of seizures. However, Harari and Malone-Lee[155] reported beneficial effects of oxybutynin in one patient with epilepsy. The 30-year-old was invariably incontinent during seizures and also at night on occasions. On the assumption that incontinence was due to hyperreflexic detrusor contractions during seizures, the authors prescribed oxybutynin at a dose of 5 mg twice daily. On this dose he remained continent despite further seizures. From the earlier discussion it can be seen that incontinence in seizures has many potential mechanisms. In this case detrusor hyperreflexia may have been prominent, however oxybutynin may not be as effective if other mechanisms are operating, particularly if incontinence is a feature of autonomic seizures themselves.

References

1. Roijen LE, Postema K, Limbeek VJ, Kuppevelt VH. Development of bladder control in children and adolescents with cerebral palsy. Dev Med Child Neurol 2001; 43: 103–7.
2. Reid CJ, Borzyskowski M. Lower urinary tract dysfunction in cerebral palsy. Arch Dis Child 1993; 68: 739–42.
3. Mayo ME. Lower urinary tract dysfunction in cerebral palsy. J Urol 1992; 147: 419–20.
4. Decter RM, Bauer SB, Khoshbin S et al. Urodynamic assessment of children with cerebral palsy. J Urol 1987; 138: 1110–12.
5. McNeal DM, Hawtrey CE, Wolraich ML, Mapel JR. Symptomatic neurogenic bladder in a cerebral-palsied population. Dev Med Child Neurol 1983; 25: 612–16.
6. Karaman MI, Kaya C, Caskurlu T, Guney S, Ergenekon E. Urodynamic findings in children with cerebral palsy. Int J Urol 2005; 12: 717–20.
7. Drigo P, Seren F, Artibani W et al. Neurogenic vesico-urethral dysfunction in children with cerebral palsy. Ital J Neurol Sci 1988; 9: 151–4.
8. Brodak PP, Scherz HC, Packer MG, Kaplan GW. Is urinary tract screening necessary for patients with cerebral palsy? J Urol 1994; 152: 1586–7.
9. Moulin F, Quintart A, Sauvestre C et al. [Nosocomial urinary tract infections: retrospective study in a pediatric hospital.] Arch Pediatr 1998; 5 (Suppl 3): 274S–8S.
10. Kroll P, Martynski M, Jankowski A. [Staghorn calculi of the kidney and ureter as a urologic complication in a child with cerebral palsy.] Wiadomosci Lekarskie 1998; 51: 98–101.
11. Connolly B, Fitzgerald RJ, Guiney EJ. Has vesicostomy a role in the neuropathic bladder? Z Kinderchir 1988; 43 (Suppl 2): 17–18.
12. Honda N, Yamada Y, Nanaura H et al. Mesonephric adenocarcinoma of the urinary bladder: a case report. Hinyokika Kiyo 2000; 46: 27–31.
13. Tan PK, Edmond P. Longterm indwelling urethral catheterization for neuropathic bladders – an audit. J R Coll Surg Edin 1994; 39: 307–9.
14. Abbott R, Johann-Murphy M, Shiminski-Maher T et al. Selective dorsal rhizotomy: outcome and complications in treating spastic cerebral palsy. Neurosurg 1993; 33: 851–7.
15. Houle AM, Vernet O, Jednak R, Pippi Salle JL, Farmer JP. Bladder function before and after selective dorsal rhizotomy in children with cerebral palsy. J Urol 1998; 160: 1088–91.
16. Sweetser PM, Badell A, Schneider S, Badlani GH. Effects of sacral dorsal rhizotomy on bladder function in patients with spastic cerebral palsy. Neurourol Urodynam 1995; 14: 57–64.
17. Leach GE, Farsaii A, Kark P, Raz S. Urodynamic manifestations of cerebellar ataxia. J Urol 1982; 128: 348–50.
18. Chami I, Miladi N, Ben Hamida M, Zmerli S. Continence disorders in hereditary spinocerebellar degeneration. Comparison of clinical and urodynamic findings in 55 cases. Acta Neur Belg 1984; 84: 194–203.
19. Vezina JG, Bouchard JP, Bouchard R. Urodynamic evaluation of patients with hereditary ataxias. Can J Neurol Sci 1982; 9: 127–9.
20. Sakakibara R, Hattori T, Uchiyama T, Yamanishi T. Micturitional disturbance in a patient with neurosarcoidosis. Neurourol Urodyn 2000; 19: 273–7.
21. Carod-Artal FJ, del Negro MC, Vargas AP, Rizzo I. [Cerebellar syndrome and peripheral neuropathy as manifestations of infection by HTLV-1 human T-cell lymphotropic virus.] Revista Neurol 1999; 29: 932–5.
22. Nakane S, Motomura M, Shirabe S, Nakamura T, Yoshimura T. [A case of superficial siderosis of the central nervous system – findings of the neuro-otological tests and evoked potentials.] No to Shinkei – Brain & Nerve 1999; 51: 155–9.
23. Fujiki N, Oikawa O, Matsumoto A, Tashiro K. [A case of HTLV-I associated myelopathy presenting with cerebellar signs as initial and principal manifestations.] Rinsho Shinkeigaku – Clinical Neurology 1999; 39: 852–5.
24. Sakakibara R, Hattori T, Yasuda K et al. Micturitional disturbance in Wernicke's encephalopathy. Neurourol Urodyn 1997; 16: 111–15.
25. Gyrtrup HJ, Kristiansen VB, Zachariae CO et al. Voiding problems in patients with HIV infection and AIDS. Scand J Urol Nephrol 1995; 29: 295–8.
26. Zeman A, Donaghy M. Acute infection with human immunodeficiency virus presenting with neurogenic urinary retention. Genitourin Med 1991; 67: 345–7.
27. Hermieu JF, Delmas V, Boccon-Gibod L. Micturition disturbances and human immunodeficiency virus infection. J Urol 1996; 156: 157–9.
28. Menendez V, Valls J, Espuna M et al. Neurogenic bladder in patients with acquired immunodeficiency syndrome. Neurourol Urodyn 1995; 14: 253–7.
29. Thurnher MM, Post MJ, Jinkins JR. MRI of infections and neoplasms of the spine and spinal cord in 55 patients with AIDS. Neuroradiol 2000; 42: 551–63.
30. Baraister M. Neurocutaneous disorders. In: Baraister M, ed. The Genetics of Neurological Disorders, 3rd edn. Oxford: Oxford University Press, 1997: 85–101.
31. Dahan D, Fenichel GM, El-Said R. Neurocutaneous syndromes. Adolesc Med 2002; 13: 495–509.
32. Hintsa A, Lindell O, Heikkila P. Neurofibromatosis of the bladder. Scand J Urol Nephrol 1996; 30: 497–9.
33. Hulse CA. Neurofibromatosis: bladder involvement with malignant degeneration. J Urol 1990; 144: 742–3.
34. Nyholm HC. [Neurofibromatosis with bladder localization.] Ugeskr Laeger 1980; 142: 2426–7.
35. Kramer SA, Barrett DM, Utz DC. Neurofibromatosis of the bladder in children. J Urol 1981; 126: 693–4.
36. Aygun C, Tekin MI, Tarhan C et al. Neurofibroma of the bladder wall in von Recklinghausen's disease. Int J Urol 2001; 8: 249–53.
37. Miller WB Jr, Boal DK, Teele R. Neurofibromatosis of the bladder: sonographic findings. J Clin Ultrasound 1983; 11: 460–2.
38. Kargi HA, Aktug T, Ozen E, Kilicalp A. A diffuse form of neurofibroma of bladder in a child with von Recklinghausen disease. Turk J Pediatr 1998; 40: 267–71.
39. Jensen A, Nissen HM. Neurofibromatosis of the bladder. Scand J Urol Nephrol 1976; 10: 157–9.
40. Torres H, Bennett MJ. Neurofibromatosis of the bladder: case report and review of the literature. J Urol 1966; 96: 910–12.
41. Winfield HN, Catalona WJ. An isolated plexiform neurofibroma of the bladder. J Urol 1985; 134: 542–3.
42. Merksz M, Toth J, Kiraly L. Neurofibromatosis of the bladder. Int Urol Nephrol 1985; 17: 53–9.

43. Gold BM. Neurofibromatosis of the bladder and vagina. Am J Obstet Gynecol 1972; 113: 1055–6.
44. Dahm P, Manseck A, Flossel C, Saeger HD, Wirth M. Malignant neurofibroma of the urinary bladder. Eur Urol 1995; 27: 261–3.
45. Rober PE, Smith JB, Sakr W, Pierce JM Jr. Malignant peripheral nerve sheath tumor (malignant schwannoma) of urinary bladder in von Recklinghausen neurofibromatosis. Urology 1991; 38: 473–6.
46. Borden TA, Shrader DA. Neurofibromatosis of bladder in a child: unusual cause of enuresis. Urology 1980; 15: 155–8.
47. Pycha A, Klingler CH, Reiter WJ et al. Von Recklinghausen neurofibromatosis with urinary bladder involvement. Urology 2001; 58: 106.
48. Carlson DH, Wilkinson RH. Neurofibromatosis of the bladder in children. Radiol 1972; 105: 401–4.
49. Maneschg C, Rogatsch H, Bartsch G, Stenzl A. Treatment of giant ancient pelvic schwannoma. TechUrol 2001; 7: 296–8.
50. Mimata H, Kasagi Y, Ohno H, Nomura Y, Iechika S. Malignant neurofibroma of the urinary bladder. Urologia Internationalis 2000; 65: 167–8.
51. Sharma NS, Lynch MJ. Intrapelvic neurilemmoma presenting with bladder outlet obstruction. Br J Urol 1998; 82: 917.
52. Salvant JB Jr, Young HF. Giant intrasacral schwannoma: an unusual cause of lumbrosacral radiculopathy. Surg Neurol 1994; 41: 411–13.
53. Burton EM, Schellhammer PF, Weaver DL, Woolfitt RA. Paraganglioma of urinary bladder in patient with neurofibromatosis. Urology 1986; 27: 550–2.
54. Reich S, Overberg-Schmidt US, Leenen A, Henze G. Neurofibromatosis 1 associated with embryonal rhabdomyosarcoma of the urinary bladder. Pediatr Hematol Oncol 1999; 16: 263–6.
55. Dominguez J, Lobato RD, Ramos A et al. Giant intrasacral schwannomas: report of six cases. Acta Neurochirurgica 1997; 139: 954–9.
56. Chakravarti A, Jones MA, Simon J. Neurofibromatosis involving the urinary bladder. Int J Urol 2001; 8: 645–7.
57. Clark SS, Marlett MM, Prudencio RF, Dasgupta TK. Neurofibromatosis of the bladder in children: case report and literature review. J Urol 1977; 118: 654–6.
58. Daneman A, Grattan-Smith P. Neurofibromatosis involving the lower urinary tract in children. A report of three cases and a review of the literature. Ped Radiol 1976; 4: 161–6.
59. Cheng L, Scheithauer BW, Leibovich BC et al. Neurofibroma of the urinary bladder. Cancer 1999; 86: 505–13.
60. Evans DG, Mason S, Huson SM et al. Spinal and cutaneous schwannomatosis is a variant form of type 2 neurofibromatosis: a clinical and molecular study. J Neurol Neurosurg Psychiatry 1997; 62: 361–6.
61. Brownlee RD, Clark AW, Sevick RJ, Myles ST. Symptomatic hamartoma of the spinal cord associated with neurofibromatosis type 1. Case report. J Neurosurg 1998; 88: 1099–103.
62. Chaparro MJ, Young RF, Smith M, Shen V, Choi BH. Multiple spinal meningiomas: a case of 47 distinct lesions in the absence of neurofibromatosis or identified chromosomal abnormality. Neurosurgery 1993; 32: 298–301; discussion 301–292.
63. Babjakova L, Jurkovic I, Krajcar R, Kocan P. [Multiple intracranial and intraspinal meningiomas in the neurocristopathy (phacomatosis) type of neurofibromatosis.] Ceskoslovenska Patologie 2000; 36: 150–5.
64. Kawsar M, Goh BT. Spinal schwannoma as a cause of erectile dysfunction with urinary incontinence and groin and testicular pain. Int J STD AIDS 2002; 13: 584–5.
65. Honda E, Hayashi T, Goto S et al. [Two different spinal tumors (meningioma and schwannoma) with von Recklinghausen's disease in a case.] No Shinkei Geka – Neurological Surgery 1990; 18: 463–8.
66. Mizuo T, Ando M, Azima J, Ohshima H, Yamauchi A. [Manifestation of mictional disturbance in four cases of von Recklinghausen's disease.] Hinyokika Kiyo – Acta Urol Jap 1987; 33: 125–32.
67. Caputo LA, Cusimano MD. Schwannoma of the cauda equina. J Manipul Physiol Therapeutics 1997; 20: 124–9.
68. Acharya R, Bhalla S, Sehgal AD. Malignant peripheral nerve sheath tumor of the cauda equina. Neurol Sci 2001; 22: 267–70.
69. Kissel P, Dureurx JB. Cobb syndrome. Cutaneomeningospinal angiomatosis. In: Bruyn Gw, Vinken PJ, eds. Handbook of Clinical Neurology. New York: North Holland, 1972: 429–45.
70. Wakabayashi Y, Isono M, Shimomura T et al. Neurocutaneous vascular hamartomas mimicking Cobb syndrome. Case report. J Neurosurg 2000; 93: 133–6.
71. Klippel M, Trenaunay P. Du naevus variquex osteo-hypertropique. Arch Genet Med 1900; 3: 641–72.
72. Weber FP. Angioma formation in connection with hypertrophy of limbs and hemihypertrophy. Br J Dermatol 1907; 19: 231–5.
73. Weber FP. Hemangioectatic hypertrophy of limbs. Congenital phlebarteriectasia and so-called congenital varicose veins. Br J Child Dis 1918; 15: 13–17.
74. Kojima Y, Kuwana N, Sato M, Ikeda Y. Klippel–Trenaunay–Weber syndrome with spinal arteriovenous malformation – case report. Neurologia Medico-Chirurgica 1989; 29: 235–40.
75. Furness PD, 3rd Barqawi AZ, Bisignani G, Decter RM. Klippel–Trenaunay syndrome: 2 case reports and a review of genitourinary manifestations. J Urol 2001; 166: 1418–20.
76. Ben Becher S, Bouaziz A, Harbi MM, Hammou A, Boudhina T. [Protee syndrome associated with renal lithiasis and vesico-ureteral reflux.] Arch Franc Pediat 1993; 50: 599–601.
77. Horie Y, Fujita H, Mano S, Kuwajima M, Ogawa K. Regional Proteus syndrome: report of an autopsy case. Pathology Int 1995; 45: 530–5.
78. Sawamura Y, Abe H, Murai H, Tashiro K, Doi S. [An autopsy case of neurocutaneous melanosis associated with intracerebral malignant melanoma.] No to Shinkei – Brain & Nerve 1987; 39: 789–95.
79. Berger AR, Swerdlow M, Herskovitz S. Myasthenia gravis presenting as uncontrollable flatus and urinary/fecal incontinence. Muscle Nerve 1996; 19: 113–14.
80. Christmas TJ, Dixon PJ, Milroy EJ. Detrusor failure in myasthenia gravis. Br J Urol 1990; 65: 422.
81. Howard JFJ, Donovan MK, Tucker MS. Urinary incontinence in myasthenia gravis: a single fibre electromyographic study. Ann Neurol 1992; 32: 254.
82. Matsui M, Enoki M, Matsui Y et al. Seronegative myasthenia gravis associated with atonic urinary bladder and accommodative insufficiency. J Neurol Sci 1995; 133: 197–9.
83. Sandler PM, Avillo C, Kaplan SA. Detrusor areflexia in a patient with myasthenia gravis. Int J Urol 1998; 5: 188–90.
84. Kaya C, Karaman MI. Case report: a case of bladder dysfunction due to myasthenia gravis. Int Urol Nephrol 2005; 37: 253–5.
85. Wise GJ, Gerstenfeld JN, Brunner N, Grob D. Urinary incontinence following prostatectomy in patients with myasthenia gravis. Br J Urol 1982; 54: 369–71.
86. Khan Z, Bhola A. Urinary incontinence after transurethral resection of prostate in myasthenia gravis patients. Urology 1989; 34: 168–9.
87. Newsom-Davis J. Lambert–Eaton myasthenic syndrome. Curr Treat Options Neurol 2001; 3: 127–31.
88. Sanders DB. The Lambert–Eaton myasthenic syndrome. Adv Neurol 2002; 88: 189–201.
89. Vincent A, Lang B, Newsom-Davis J. Autoimmunity to the voltage-gated calcium channel underlies the Lambert–Eaton myasthenic syndrome, a paraneoplastic disorder. Trends Neurosci 1989; 12: 496–502.
90. Khurana RK, Koski CL, Mayer RF. Autonomic dysfunction in Lambert–Eaton myasthenic syndrome. J Neurol Sci 1988; 85: 77–86.
91. O'Neill JH, Murray NM, Newsom-Davis J. The Lambert–Eaton myasthenic syndrome. A review of 50 cases. Brain 1988; 111: 577–96.
92. O'Suilleabhain P, Low PA, Lennon VA. Autonomic dysfunction in the Lambert–Eaton myasthenic syndrome: serologic and clinical correlates. Neurology 1998; 50: 88–93.
93. Waterman SA. Autonomic dysfunction in Lambert–Eaton myasthenic syndrome. Clin Auton Res 2001; 11: 145–54.

94. Waterman SA, Lang B, Newsom-Davis J. Effect of Lambert–Eaton myasthenic syndrome antibodies on autonomic neurons in the mouse. Ann Neurol 1997; 42: 147–56.
95. Henriksson KG, Nilsson O, Rosen I, Schiller HH. Clinical, neurophysiological and morphological findings in Eaton Lambert syndrome. Acta Neurol Scand 1977; 56: 117–40.
96. Satoh K, Motomura M, Suzu H et al. Neurogenic bladder in Lambert–Eaton myasthenic syndrome and its response to 3,4-diaminopyridine. J Neurol Sci 2001; 183: 1–4.
97. Frew R, Lundy PM. A role for Q type Ca^{2+} channels in neurotransmission in the rat urinary bladder. Br J Pharmacol 1995; 116: 1595–8.
98. Houzen H, Hattori Y, Kanno M et al. Functional evaluation of inhibition of autonomic transmitter release by autoantibody from Lambert–Eaton myasthenic syndrome. Ann Neurol 1998; 43: 677–80.
99. Roses AD, Chang L. Myotonic dystrophy. In: Gilman S, ed. MedLink Neurology. San Diego: MedLink Corporation, 2002: Available at www.medlink.com.
100. Harper PS. Smooth muscle in myotonic dystrophy. In: Major Problems in Neurology, 37: Myotonic Dystrophy. 3rd ed. London: WB Saunders, 2001: 91–108.
101. Harvey JC, Sherbourne DH, Siegel CI. Smooth muscle involvement in myotonic dystrophy. Am J Med 1965; 39: 81–90.
102. Kohn NN, Faires JS, Chiu VSW. Unusual manifestations due to involvement of involuntary muscles in dystrophia myotonica. N Engl J Med 1964; 271: 1179.
103. Pruzanski W. Myotonic dystrophy – a multisystem disease: report of 67 cases and a review of the literature. Psychiatr Neurol 1965; 149: 302.
104. Bundschu HD, Hauger W, Lang HD. [Myotonic dystrophy (urological features and histochemical findings in muscle).] Deutsche Medizinische Wochenschrift 1975; 100: 1337–41.
105. Orndahl G, Kock NG, Sundin T. Smooth muscle activity in myotonic dystrophy. Brain 1973; 96: 857–60.
106. Bernstein IT, Andersen BB, Andersen JT et al. Bladder function in patients with myotonic dystrophy. Neurol Urodynam 1992; 11: 219–23.
107. Sakakibara R, Hattori T, Tojo M et al. Micturitional disturbance in myotonic dystrophy. J Aut Nerv Sys 1995; 52: 17–21.
108. Black WC, Ravin A. Studies in dystrophia myotonica. Arch Pathol 1947; 44: 176.
109. Pruzanski W, Huvos AG. Smooth muscle involvement in primary muscle disease. I. Myotonic dystrophy. Arch Path Lab Med 1967; 83: 229–33.
110. Bushby KM. Making sense of the limb-girdle muscular dystrophies. Brain 1999; 122: 1403–20.
111. Bushby K. The limb-girdle muscular dystrophies. Eur J Paediatr Neurol 2001; 5: 213–14.
112. Bushby K, Norwood F, Straub V. The limb-girdle muscular dystrophies – diagnostic strategies. Biochim Biophys Acta 2007; 1772: 238–42.
113. Dixon PJ, Christmas TJ, Chapple CR. Stress incontinence due to pelvic floor muscle involvement in limb-girdle muscular dystrophy. Br J Urol 1990; 65: 653–4.
114. Acsadi G. Duchenne muscular dystrophy. In: Gilman S, ed. MedLink Neurology. San Diego: MedLink Corporation, 2002: Available at www.medlink.com.
115. Brooke MH. Muscular dystrophies: Duchenne muscular dystrophy. In: Brooke MH, ed. A Clinicians View of Neuromuscular Diseases. 2nd ed. Baltimore: Williams and Wilkins, 1986: 117–54.
116. Boland BJ, Silbert PL, Groover RV, Wollan PC, Silverstein MD. Skeletal, cardiac, and smooth muscle failure in Duchenne muscular dystrophy. Ped Neurol 1996; 14: 7–12.
117. Caress JB, Kothari MJ, Bauer SB, Shefner JM. Urinary dysfunction in Duchenne muscular dystrophy. Muscle Nerve 1996; 19: 819–22.
118. Epilepsy CoCaTotILA. Proposal for revised clinical and electroencephalographic classification of epileptic seizures. Epilepsia 1981; 22: 489–501.
119. Blok BF, Sturms LM, Holstege G. Brain activation during micturition in women. Brain 1998; 121: 2033–42.
120. Blok BF, Willemsen AT, Holstege G. A PET study on brain control of micturition in humans. Brain 1997; 120 : 111–21.
121. Blok BF, Holstege G. The central control of micturition and continence: implications for urology. BJU Int 1999; 83(Suppl 2): 1–6.
122. Andrew J, Nathan PW. Lesions on the anterior frontal lobes and disturbances of micturition and defaecation. Brain 1964; 87: 233–62.
123. Maurice-Williams RS. Micturition symptoms in frontal tumours. J Neurol Neurosurg Psychiatry 1974; 37: 431–6.
124. Griffiths D. Clinical studies of cerebral and urinary tract function in elderly people with urinary incontinence. Behav Brain Res 1998; 92: 151–5.
125. Gastaut H, Batini C, Broughton R, Lob H, Roger J. Polygraphic study of enuresis during petit mal absences. Electroencephalogr Clin Neurophysiol 1964: 616–26.
126. Gastaut H, Broughton R, Roger J, Tassinari C. Generalized nonconvulsive seizures without local onset. In: Vinken P, Bruyn G, eds. Handbook of Clinical Neurology. New York, 1974: 130–44.
127. Liporace JD, Sperling MR. Simple autonomic seizures. In: Engel JJ, Pedley TA, eds. Epilepsy: The Comprehensive CD-ROM: Lippincott Williams and Wilkins, 1999.
128. Gupta AK, Jeavons PM, Hughes RC, Covanis A. Aura in temporal lobe epilepsy: clinical and electroencephalographic correlation. J Neurol Neurosurg Psychiatry 1983; 46: 1079–83.
129. Palmini A, Gloor P. The localizing value of auras in partial seizures: a prospective and retrospective study. Neurology 1992; 42: 801–8.
130. Devinsky O, Kelley K, Porter RJ, Theodore WH. Clinical and electroencephalographic features of simple partial seizures. Neurology 1988; 38: 1347–52.
131. Panayiotopoulos CP. Autonomic seizures and autonomic status epilepticus specific to childhood. Arch Pediatr Adolesc Med 2002; 156: 945.
132. Weig S. Panayiotopoulos syndrome: a common and benign childhood epileptic syndrome. J Neurol Sci 2002; 202: 99.
133. Panayiotopoulos CP. Early-onset benign childhood occipital seizure susceptibility syndrome: a syndrome to recognize. Epilepsia 1999; 40: 621–30.
134. Panayiotopoulos CP. Extraoccipital benign childhood partial seizures with ictal vomiting and excellent prognosis. J Neurol Neurosurg Psychiatry 1999; 66: 82–5.
135. Panayiotopoulos CP. Benign childhood epileptic syndromes with occipital spikes: new classification proposed by the International League Against Epilepsy. J Child Neurol 2000; 15: 548–52.
136. Panayiotopoulos CP. Panayiotopoulos syndrome. Lancet 2001; 358: 68–9.
137. Feindel W, Penfield W. Localization of discharge in temporal lobe automatism. Arch Neurol Psychiatry 1954; 72: 605–730.
138. Inthaler S, Donati F, Pavlincova E, Vassella F, Staldemann C. Partial complex epileptic seizures with ictal urogenital manifestation in a child. Eur Neurol 1991; 31: 212–15.
139. Baumgartner C, Groppel G, Leutmezer F et al. Ictal urinary urge indicates seizure onset in the nondominant temporal lobe. Neurology 2000; 55: 432–4.
140. O'Donovan C, Burgess R, Luders H. Aura in Temporal Lobe Epilepsy. New York: Churchill Livingstone; 2000.
141. Loddenkemper T, Foldvary N, Raja S, Neme S, Luders HO. Ictal urinary urge: further evidence for lateralization to the nondominant hemisphere. Epilepsia 2003; 44: 124–6.
142. Glass HC, Prieur B, Molnar C, Hamiwka L, Wirrell E. Micturition and emotion-induced reflex epilepsy: case report and review of the literature. Epilepsia 2006; 47: 2180–2.
143. Bourgeois BF. A retarded boy with seizures precipitated by stepping into the bath water. Semin Pediatr Neurol 1999; 6: 151–6; discussion 156–7.

144. Spinnler H, Valli G. Micturition 'reflex' epilepsy. Presentation of a clinical case. Riv Patol Nerv Ment 1969; 90: 212–20.
145. Pradhan S, Kalita J. Micturition induced reflex epilepsy. Neurol Ind 1993; 41: 221–3.
146. Okumura A, Kondo Y, Tsuji T et al. Micturition induced seizures: ictal EEG and subtraction ictal SPECT findings. Epilepsy Res 2007; 73: 119–21.
147. Ikeno T, Morikawa A, Kimura I. A case of epileptic seizure evoked by micturition. Rinsho Nouha 1998; 40: 205–8.
148. Yamatani M, Murakami M, Konda M et al. An 8-year-old girl with micturition-induced epilepsy. No To Hattatsu 1987; 19: 58–62.
149. Zivin I, Rowley W. Psychomotor epilepsy with micturition. Arch Intern Med 1964; 113: 8–13.
150. Devinsky O, Morrell MJ, Vogt BA. Contributions of anterior cingulate cortex to behaviour. Brain 1995; 118: 279–306.
151. Blok BF. Central pathways controlling micturition and urinary continence. Urology 2002; 59: 13–17.
152. Physicians' Desk Reference, 5th edn. Montvale: Medical Economics Company, 1996.
153. Handforth A, Treiman DM. Efficacy and tolerance of long-term, high-dose gabapentin: additional observations. Epilepsia 1994; 35: 1032–7.
154. Gil-Nagel A, Gapany S, Blesi K, Villanueva N, Bergen D. Incontinence during treatment with gabapentin. Neurology 1997; 48: 1467–8.
155. Harari D, Malone-Lee JG. Oxybutynin and incontinence during grand mal seizures. Br J Urol 1991; 68: 658.

32

Syringomyelia and lower urinary tract dysfunction

Marc Le Fort and Jean-Jacques Labat

Introduction

Syringomyelia manifests as a liquid cavity in the spinal cord. It may be accompanied by neurologic signs. This type of spinal cord cavity has been known for a long time through autopsies and dissections. The name 'syringomyelia' was coined by Olivier d'Angers in 1824 (*syrinx* = flute used by the Greek god Pan), described in 1867 by Bastian and only accepted as a real entity since the years 1950–1960 after Freeman's studies (1953) and the first report by Barnett and Jousse in 1966. Its evolution is classically slow and can become functionally disabling if untreated. Most syringomyelias occur in a congenital malformative context (primary syringomyelia), with a late clinical expression. A secondary syringomyelia can occur after spinal cord injury (SCI). The diagnosis is made by magnetic resonance imaging (MRI), but the mechanisms of syringomyelia occurrence are not perfectly understood.

Primary syringomyelia

Etiopathogeny

Dysraphic theory[1]

According to this ancient theory, syringomyelia would be due to a closing defect of the neural tube, which normally occurs between the 21st and 28th days of embryonal life. This embryopathy would arise from abnormal constitution of the posterior raphe. Bony anomalies associated with cervico-occipital transition and Chiari malformation would have no physiopathologic link.

Hydrodynamic theories

Gardner's theory.[2] In the 1950s, Gardner revolutionized the physiopathologic concepts of syringomyelia, introducing the notion of a pathogenic role of cerebrospinal fluid (CSF) dynamics. This primitive embryologic disorder comprises a lack or late opening of the roof orifices of the 4th ventricle that links the great cistern with the perimedullary and pericerebral subarachnoid spaces. Thus, a CSF hyperpressure is responsible for downward dilation of the spinal central canal. At birth, this hydromyelia bursts into a zone of lower resistance, the gray posterior commissure. It generates the syringomyelic cavity, which will have a permanent tendency to extend. Prolapse of the cerebellar tonsils, which by itself can hamper CSF circulation, and the cervico-occipital bony abnormalities would be consequences of the hydroencephalomyelia (Arnold–Chiari malformation).

Aboulker's theory.[3] This theory insists on the transition effect. Any effort generating veinous hyperpressure creates growth of CSF pressure in the perimedullary spaces. This hyperpressure is normally transmitted upwards to the cranious spaces. In the case of cervico-occipital bony abnormalities, CSF passage to the great cistern is held up, and the consequent hyperpressure furthers CSF entry into the medullary spaces, about the level of the posterior rootlets. Coalescence of the liquidian lakes forms the syringomyelic cavity.

Clinical signs

Physical examination may provide the diagnosis of medullary cavity and specify its extension that could even involve the high spinal cord (syringobulbomyelia). Its classic description is:

- An upper syndrome combining a lower motoneuron deficiency with dissociative sensory loss: abolished reflexes, amyotrophy, peripheral motor weakness, thermic and pain anesthesia but with relative sparing of light touch and perception.
- A lower syndrome under the lesion level: upper motoneuron weakness and vibratory sensory deficiency.

The clinical signs are not often as typical as the classical description. One symptom can raise suspicions of a spinal cord pathology and should lead to magnetic resonance imaging (MRI). However, CSF accumulation within the spinal cord does not necessarily result in clinical neurologic deterioration, and the time period between the first sign and the diagnosis is still 6–8 years.[1] Xenos et al[4] mention, in cases of spinal lipomas, a possible role for syringomyelia in accelerating clinical deterioration. The most frequent early functional signs are subjective sensitivity of an upper limb (paresthesiae, pain), walking incapacity, cervical or cephalic pain, vertigo, motor deficiency of a limb, trophic signs (painless burn), and rapidly progressing thoracic scoliosis of adolescence. Electrophysiologic exploration may contribute to the early diagnosis, not so much to affirm a syringomyelia as to suspect a pathology of the spinal cord.[5]

Radiologic signs

Standard radiography

There could be indirect signs of an expansive intraspinal process: interpedicle enlargement, pedicle thinning, and spinal scalloping. A cervico-occipital abnormality, an associated bony dysraphism (spina bifida occulta), or kyphoscoliosis should be investigated.

Neuroradiology

MRI supplants myelography. Myeloscans can be useful to study lower dysraphisms.

MRI[6,7] has close to 100% sensitivity and specificity. The signal of a syringomyelic cavity is the same as a CSF signal, and is better seen with T2 exploration. A syrinx is tube-shaped and extends beyond the SCI site to at least two vertebral levels. The signal is homogeneous and clearly delimits the upper and lower limits of the syringomyelia. The extension is always much more significant than the clinics suppose. The syringomyelic cavity may be multi-loculated, and neuroradiology also gives information on tension inside the syrinx. MRI can show the associated abnormalities, neuromeningeal or cerebellar.

There seems to be a significant correlation between the location of a segmental cavity in the spinal cord and the type of presenting symptomatology; however, in the case of a holocord cavity, the different types of signs may be evenly distributed.[8]

Urinary signs

Neuro-urologic disorders rarely reveal the development of a syringomyelia but are, on the contrary, regarded as a late symptomatology.[9] Nevertheless, they may be present at the time of the diagnosis and should be explored systematically, clinically, or through urodynamic studies. These urinary symptoms appeared after 5.3 years (ranging from 2 months to 13 years) from the occurrence of neurologic symptoms in a Japanese study.[9] Neuro-urologic signs readily coexist with bowel function and lower extremity abnormalities. Lower urinary tract dysfunction and spinal cord lesions may be suspected in patients with anorectal abnormalities: among 30 patients presenting with anorectal abnormalities, Taskinen et al[10] found 4 syringomyelias on systematic MRIs, with 2 normal on urodynamic evaluation and 2 overactive bladders.

The urinary signs are not specific most of the time, as they constitute a part of the lower syndrome syringomyelia, with an upper motor neuron bladder due to a suprasacral lesion. Their presentation is close to that of incomplete spinal cord lesions: urgency and eventually urge incontinence, pollakiuria, hesitancy, polyphasic micturition, occasional temporary urination impossibility, and even acute urine retention. Dysuria should provoke the search for other apparent causes such as prostate hypertrophy. Urodynamic studies argue in favor of such a spinal cord lesion, showing a poorly inhibited and/or dyssynergic bladder: lasting and wave-like high contractions are evocative.

Extension of the cavity into the sacral gray matter can give rise to signs of lower motor neuron bladder. Blunted micturition need, impaired perception of urine flow, or a progressively growing functional capacity of the bladder with a lower micturitional frequency can correspond to decreased bladder sensitivity or reflexivity on urodynamic assessment. Acute urinary retention has been described as the first manifestation of syringomyelia and can possibly be triggered by a well-defined factor – the Valsalva maneuver – which would acutely create increased pressure within the intraspinal space and the syrinx,[11] or a pharmacologic side-effect of cyproheptadine.[12]

These neurourologic disorders will progress in the same way as the disease. Serious disease forms will then combine with other functional incapacities and loss of autonomy. Sakakibara et al,[9] studying 11 primary and 3 secondary syringomyelias, tried to find a relationship between micturitional disturbance and neurologic signs. Besides detrusor hyperreflexia, common in patients with Babinski's sign (suprasacral lesion with pyramidal tract involvement), urinary disturbances (detrusor hyperreflexia or voiding difficulty) seem to be linked with other neurologic deficiencies, especially disturbed sleep sensation.

Patients are determined to be candidates for treatment on the basis of their clinical status and MRI findings. Surgery of a primary syringomyelia may be complex because of associated malformations. It is difficult to separate symptoms attributed to the syrinx alone, and, when associated with syringomyelia, lipoma excision, resection of an arachnoid cyst,[13] and cord untethering can, for instance, lead to a reduction in syrinx size: it is controversial whether syrinx cavities should be allowed to drain by themselves.[4] Intraoperative ultrasonography may be helpful in determining the optimal length of the dural opening.[13] In patients with Arnold–Chiari malformation and syringomyelia, suboccipital craniotomy seems to give the best chance for syrinx reduction, particulary in children younger than 10 years. Scoliosis correction without prior syrinx decompression carries a high neurologic risk.[14] The main goal of surgery is, however, to at least stabilize progression of the symptoms.[8] According to Oakes (editorial comment to La Marca et al[8]) the smaller a symptomatic syrinx is at the time of initial treatment, the more likely a successful therapeutic intervention will be.

Secondary syringomyelia

Syringomyelia can occur without any malformations due to spinal cord pathologies: arachnoiditis, tumors, or overall post-traumatic condition (Figure 32.1). The neurourologic status of SCI patients may change and raise suspicions of cavity occurrence.

Post-traumatic syringomyelia is defined as an intramedullary cavity that occurs secondarily to SCI. This etiology represents one-quarter of all syringomyelia cases. The incidence of post-traumatic syringomyelias is estimated to be 1.3–5%. Any spinal level can be affected by complete or incomplete lesions. The first clinical signs can occur between 2 months and 36 years.[15]

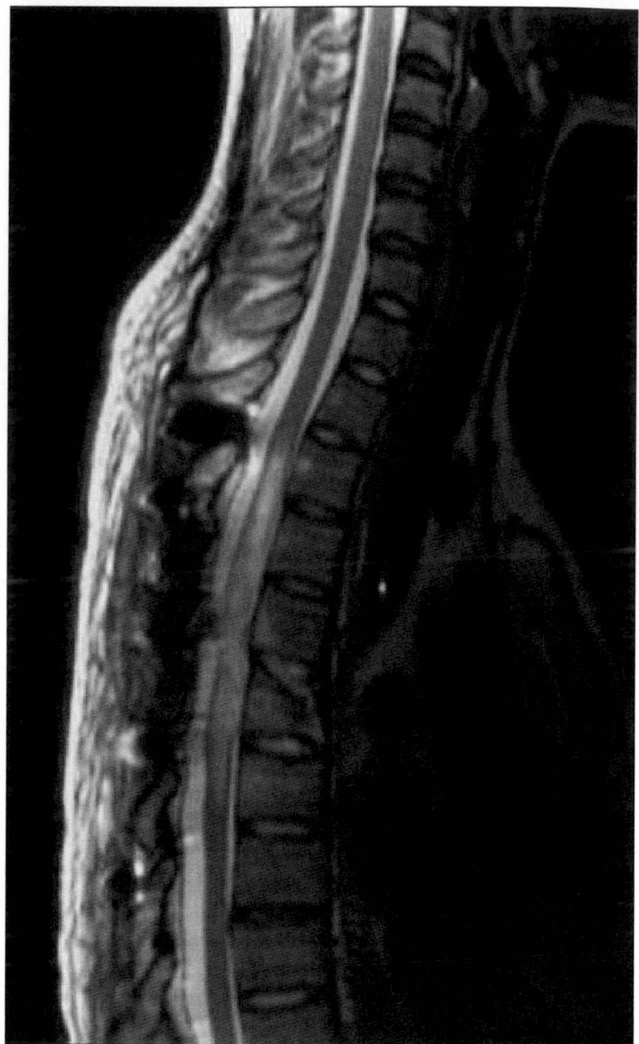

Figure 32.1
Post-traumatic syringomyelia.

Etiopathogeny

Pathogenesis theories are still being discussed, but two phases (initial formation and cavity extension) have to be taken into account.

Initial formation of the cavity

The mechanisms that lead to syrinx occurrence are not unequivocal. One is a vascular mechanism, especially secondary necrosis of a myelomalacic zone and a direct action of lysosomal enzymes on the injured parenchyma. The other mechanism is arachnoiditis, which is responsible not only for ischemia but also for permanent stretching of the injured zone during spinal movements.

Cavity extension

This mechanism is a more mechanical one. Williams et al[16] proposed the most compelling theory with a main role for variations in venous pressures. Any rise in pressure of the abdominal or thoracic cavity is transmitted to the epidural veins, squeezing the spinal cord and pushing the eventual intracystic fluid upwards. It is called the 'slosh' effect, an energetic and upward pulsatile movement of fluid, with energy so significant that blockage occurs at the lesion site. These phenomena dissect the spinal cord at the extremities of the cavity where the spinal cord parenchyma is more fragile. The downward extension can be explained by another mechanism – slush – a negative pressure gradient in relation to the upward movement, making liquid enter the cavity.[17,18] The extensions are favored by arachnoiditis, a tethered spinal cord, or persistent compression (Figure 32.2).

Treatment of post-traumatic syringomyelia is essential in cases of intractable pain and progression of a motor deficit, but it may also include the management of canal stenosis and arachnoiditis.[19]

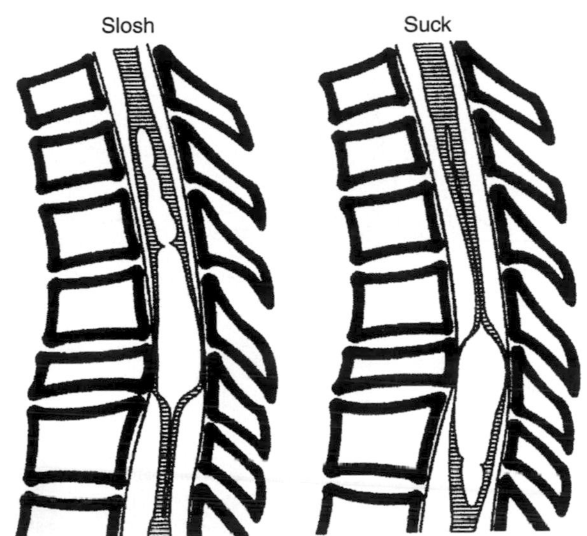

Figure 32.2
According to Williams' theory, secondary extension from the initial necrosis zone is a consequence of increased epidural venous pressure at the origin of intrachordal fluid movements. 'Slush' leads to rostral extension and breaks down the zones of structural weakness; 'slush' is the consequence of a pressure gradient at the origin of the caudal extension and filling of the cavity. These two phenomena are increased in the case of blockage in the subarachnoid space.[16] (Reproduced with permission from Macmillan Publishers Ltd.)

Clinical signs

Pain, the main sign, is often associated with paresthesiae and numbness; it is noted in more than one-half of patients: Rossier et al[20] reported pain in 17 out of 30 cases, dysesthesia in 8, and motor deficiency in 7. This pain may be impulsive. The other signs are rarely inaugural and isolated. Most of the time, sensitive signs consist of thermoalgesic dissociation with preservation of tactile sensitivity and proprioception. Preservation of normal sensitivity between the injury level and the upper sensory signs is often found.[21] Rossier et al[20] described an ascending sensory level in 28/30 patients; this ascending sensory level is generally unilateral. Increased motor weakness above the level of the lesion and loss of reflexes are early signs that can also be found.[19]

Radiologic signs

The diagnosis is also made by MRI, which can disclose the upper and lower levels, a multiloculated cavity, and intracystic turbulences. The signal criteria of syringomyelia are the same. Cross-sections transversely localize the cavity in the spinal cord. Perrouin-Verbe et al[22] reported a mean extension of 3.5 segments in asymptomatic patients and 10 segments in symptomatic cases. The persistent bony compression has also been assessed in the genesis of post-traumatic syringomyelia.[19,23]

Urinary signs

The urinary signs are not specific for post-traumatic syringomyelia, but their occurrence in an SCI patient must make them suspect. Dysuria may worsen, due to increased detrusor-sphincter dyssynergia or decreased bladder reflectivity; reflex voiding may disappear. Fading of reflex erections, difficult ejaculation, or deterioration of autonomic dysreflexia can also constitute an alert. These signs of lower motoneuron bladder lead to MRI, in a way investigating the downward extension of the syringomyelic cavity.

Possible lesion evolution imposes neuro-urologic follow-up in SCI patients. Clinical analysis must include determination of the level and flaccid or spastic character of the lesion, particularly in the sacral area. The mode of voiding and its eventual changes have to be assessed. Follow-up must be regular during the first 2 years; then, it should become annual, with clinical, urodynamic, and morphologic studies. Less frequent follow-up can be discussed in case there is no significant risk factor. The quality of the initial treament of a spinal cord injury is the first step in the prevention of a syrinx whose treatment, besides techniques of drainage, must also take into account the spinal realignment.[19]

Conclusion

Primary or secondary syringomyelia consists of an evolutive spinal cord syndrome that can lead to lower urinary tract dysfunction. MRI can easily confirm the diagnosis if it has previously been suspected by systematic clinical examination, or directed by functional symptoms. Most of the urinary signs are not specific. Primary syringomyelias correspond to an upper motor neuron bladder (suprasacral lesion), and in the secondary forms, modification of the voiding mode may be due to extension of the cavity into the sacral level. Treatment indications have not yet been perfectly determined, but surgery is decided on the basis of the patient's clinical status and MRI findings.

References

1. Sichez JP, Capelle L. Syringomyélie. Editions techniques, EMC Neurologie, 17077A10, 4–1990.
2. Gardner WJ, Angel J. The mechanism of syringomyelia and its surgical correction. Clin Neurosurg 1959; 6: 131–40.

3. Aboulker J. La syringomyélie et les liquides intra-rachidiens. Neurochirurgie (Paris) 1979; 25(S1): 9–22.
4. Xenos C, Sgouros S, Walsh R, Hockley A. Spinal lipomas in children. Pediatr Neurosurg 2000; 32: 295–307.
5. Anderson NE, Frith RW, Synek VM. Somatosensory evoked potentials in syringomyelia. J Neurol Neurosurg Psychiatry 1986; 49: 1407–10.
6. Wilberger JE, Maroon JC, Prostko ER et al. Magnetic resonance imaging and intraoperative neurosonography in syringomyelia. Neurosurg 1987; 20: 599–606.
7. Aubin ML, Baleriaux D, Cosnard G et al. IRM dans les syringomyélies d'origine congénitale, infectieuse, traumatique ou idiopathique. A propos de 142 cas. J Neuroradiol (Paris) 1987; 14: 313–36.
8. La Marca F, Herman M, Grant JA, MacLone DG. Presentation and management of hydromyelia in children with Chiari type II malformation. Pediatr Neurosurg 1997; 26: 57–67.
9. Sakakibara R, Hattori T, Yasuda K, Yamanishi T. Micturitional disturbance in syringomyelia. J Neurol Sci 1996; 143: 100–6.
10. Taskinen S, Valanne L, Rintala R. The effect of spinal cord abnormalities on the function of the lower urinary tract in patients with anorectal abnormalities. J Urol 2002; 168: 1147–9.
11. Amoiridis G, Meves S, Schöls L, Przuntek H. Reversible urinary retention as the main symptom in the first manifestation of a syringomyelia. J Neurol Neurosurg Psychiatry 1996; 61: 407–8.
12. Houang M, Leroy B, Forin V, et al. Rétention aiguë d'urines: un mode de révélation rare d'une syringomyélie cervicodorsale à l'occasion de la prise de cyproheptadine. Arch Pédiatrie (Paris) 1994; 1: 260–3.
13. Holly LT, Batzdorf U. Syringomyelia associated with intradural arachnoid cysts. J. Neurosurg. Spine 2006; 5: 111–16.
14. Ozerdemoglu RA, Transfeldt EE, Denis F. Value of treating primary causes of syrinx in scoliosis associated with syringomyelia. Spine 2003; 28(8): 806–14.
15. Umbach I, Heilporn A. Post spinal-cord injury syringomyelia. Review. Paraplegia 1991; 29: 219–21.
16. Williams B, Terry AF, Jones HWF, McSweeney T. Syringomyelia as a sequel to traumatic paraplegia. Paraplegia 1981; 19: 67–80.
17. MacLean DR, Miller JDR, Allen PBR, Ezzedin SA. Post traumatic syringomyelia. J Neurosurg 1973; 39: 485–92.
18. Ball MJ, Dayan AD. Pathogenesis of syringomyelia. Lancet 1972; 2: 799–800.
19. Perrouin-Verbe B, Lenne-Aurier K, Robert R, et al. Post-traumatic syringomyelia and post-traumatic spinal canal stenosis: a direct relationship: review of 75 patients with a spinal cord injury. Spinal Cord 1998; 36: 137–43.
20. Rossier AB, Foo D, Shillito J, Dyro FM. Post traumatic cervical syringomyelia: incidence, clinical presentation, electrological studies, syrinx protein and results of conservative and operative treatment. Brain 1985; 108: 439–61.
21. Vernon JD, Silver JR, Ohry A. Post traumatic syringomyelia. Paraplegia 1982; 20: 339–64.
22. Perrouin-Verbe B, Robert R, Le Fort M et al. Syringomyélie post-traumatique. Neurochirurgie (Paris) 1999; 45(S1): 58–66.
23. Schurch B, Wichmann W, Rossier AB. Post-traumatic syringomyelia (cystic myelopathy): a prospective study of 449 patients with spinal cord injury. J Neurol Neurosurg Psychiatry 1996; 60: 61–7.

Part IV

Evaluation of neurogenic bladder dysfunction

33

Clinical evaluation: history and physical examination

Gary E Lemack

Introduction

A thorough history and physical examination are the cornerstones of the initial evaluation of patients with neurologic diseases suffering from lower urinary tract symptoms. While more exact and specific means are often necessary to pinpoint the nature of bladder dysfunction in such patients, a directed, though thorough history and physical examination are essential to defining which patients require more costly and invasive testing, and which can be followed with alternative strategies. Advanced videourodynamic has allowed for a more precise characterization of bladder dysfunction in patients with neurologic disorders, but failing to know what questions to ask, and what signs to observe, can lead to erroneous diagnoses, and inappropriate testing. The focus of this chapter will be on obtaining as much information as possible on the initial visit by directed questioning and a focused examination, so as to be able to discern what testing, if any, is necessary on future visits.

History

Nature of neurologic disease

Most, though not all patients, will present to the urologist with a known neurologic condition. In patients with progressive conditions, it is useful to establish the onset of symptoms (often very different to the timing of diagnosis) as well as recent changes in symptom severity, as this information may clearly influence treatment recommendations. Even patients with a presumably fixed neurologic condition (i.e. spinal cord injury, myelomeningocele) may have symptomatic deterioration (e.g. due to development of a syrinx), and therefore any recent changes in sensory or motor function should be directly questioned. Often, patients or their caregivers will have tremendous insight into the medical condition and will, for example, know the Hoehn and Yahr stage of their Parkinson's disease (PD), which can be useful in predicting the severity of bladder dysfunction and prospects for further deterioration.[1] Patients with multiple sclerosis (MS) may give a history of recurrent flares in conjunction with worsening urinary symptoms, which should signal an investigation for recurrent urinary infections as a possible source. However, it is clear that the Expanded Disability Symptom Score (EDSS) status does not correlate with urodynamic (UD) findings, so that even in patients with fairly stable MS, bladder dysfunction may be present.[2] At the very least, initial screening for elevated postvoid residuals may also be appropriate, even among MS patients with few urinary symptoms.

In patients with more recent acute events, such as cerebrovascular accident, information about the stroke location and the recovery since the event can be useful, since stroke location can impact on prognosis.[3] It is also quite clear from several prospective population-based studies that post-stroke persistent incontinence is an ominous sign. Along with intermittent claudication, previous transient ischemic attacks, and prestroke disability, the finding of urinary incontinence after stroke is predictive of death within 5 years.[4]

Patients should also be specifically questioned regarding symptoms of intervertebral disc prolapse. Those with a history of sciatic-type pain or cauda equina syndrome (i.e. low back pain, perineal paresthesia, lower extremity weakness, diminution of sexual function) should be imaged to document possible lumbar disc prolapse, which can result in lower urinary tract dysfunction in up to 16% of patients. Patients with cervical disc herniation appear to be at even greater risk for both upper and lower urinary tract disorders and should certainly be monitored at periodic intervals with UD studies and upper tract imaging.[5]

Other medical conditions can have a tremendous impact on lower urinary tract symptoms (LUTS). Patients should be specifically questioned for the presence or history of diabetes mellitus, tabes dorsalis, herpes zoster, or extensive alcohol use. All of these conditions can result in peripheral neuropathies which may cause significant detrusor dysfunction. Anogenital herpes (simplex) can also result in LUT dysfunction or frank retention, typically due to severe urethral pain associated with vesicular eruptions.

Surgical history should also be elicited. Patients with a history of extensive pelvic surgery (i.e. radical hysterectomy, abdominoperineal resection, radical prostatectomy) as well as pelvic radiation may suffer from LUT dysfunction secondary to peripheral nerve damage. In addition, direct sphincteric damage may occur during surgery, resulting in urinary incontinence. While in certain instances these processes may cause progressive vesicosphincteric disorders, there is also evidence to suggest that nerve function may recover for a period of time following these insults (especially up to 6 months).[6]

Current medical treatments should also be documented. Medications with properties that can affect the bladder outlet (typically with either α-agonist or antagonist properties) or detrusor contractility (typically those with anticholinergic properties) should be recorded, along with narcotic and skeletal muscle relaxant use. Many commonly prescribed medications have anticholinergic properties (Table 33.1), even though their clinical utility may not be based on this attribute, and therefore careful documentation of all medications used may help to avoid adverse events related to the addition of a new agent.

Table 33.1 *Commonly prescribed medications with anticholinergic properties*

Anticholinergics
Atropine (Atropisol ophthalmic)
Scopolamine (Scopace)
Glycopyrrolate (Robinul)
Benztropine (Cogentin)
Trihexyphenidyl (Artane)
Anithistamines
Chlorpheniramine (Chlortrimeton and others)
Hydroxyzine (Atarax, Vistaril)
Diphenhydramine (Nytol, Sominex, and others)
Meclizine (Anitvert, Bonine, Dramamine)
Promethazine (Phernergan)
Antipsychotics
Chlorpromazine (Thorazine)
Clozapine (Clozaril)
Thioridazine (Mellaril)
Antispasmodic
Dicyclomine (Bentyl)
Hyoscyamine (Anaspaz, Cystospaz, Levsin)
Oxybutynin (Ditropan)
Propantheline (Pro-Banthine)
Cyclic antidepressants
Amitryptyline (Elavil)
Clomipramine (Anafranil)
Desipramine (Norpramine)
Imipramine (Tofranil)
Nortriptyline (Pamelor)
Mydriatics
Cyclopentolate (Ocu-Pentolate ophthalmic)
Tropicamide (Ocu-Tropic ophthalmic)

Nature of lower urinary tract symptoms

Duration of symptoms

Determining whether LUTS predate the neurologic disorder is often difficult, although it will help to clarify the etiology in many situations. In slowly progressive diseases, such as MS, a clear date of onset is often impossible to establish, although a general assessment of the time course over which the symptoms worsened is essential. Patients with PD also typically have pre-existing LUTS and therefore sorting out which symptoms are neurologically-based and which may be due to bladder outlet obstruction, for example, is difficult, even with the addition of UD studies. In some patients, the date of onset will be quite clear, though often, as is the case in patients with cerebrovascular accidents, the presence of pre-existing symptoms may be difficult to discern.

Previous urologic history

Patients will often come referred with a diagnosis of recurrent urinary tract infections, but precisely documenting the offending organism and its sensitivities is essential to discovering its source. Failure to clear an ongoing infection (persistence) and repeated bouts of new infections imply different etiologies. Clearly the method of bladder management will affect the susceptibility to infection, and the use of indwelling or intermittent catheterization should be documented. Additionally, the duration of each catheter use before change, and the cleaning technique used (intermittent catheterization), should be recorded, as well as a careful reassessment of catheterization technique. Patient education as to the correct techniques of intermittent catheterization is critical in minimizing infection risk, and it is clear that a sterile technique is not routinely warranted.[7] A history of previous bladder, prostate, or upper tract surgery must be carefully detailed, and operative notes of complex reconstructions reviewed.

Current urinary symptoms

While LUTS should be carefully assessed at the time of initial presentation, there is no doubt that the interpretation of urinary symptoms may be quite different (and masked) in patients with neurologic disease. Therefore, the reliability of LUT symptom questionnaires in most neurologic disorders has not been effectively established. Still, sensate patients should be questioned for the presence or progression of urinary urgency, frequency, and nocturia, in addition to other symptoms typically associated with disorders of bladder filling. Often, a 2- or 3-day voiding diary (see Chapter 34) can be of tremendous help in establishing micturition frequency and voided volumes.[8,9] In general, greater than 8 voids per day is considered abnormal, though clearly this finding is nonspecific. Urinary frequency may represent detrusor overactivity, impaired bladder capacity, excessive urine production (polyuria), impaired bladder emptying, urinary infection, stone disease, inflammatory bladder conditions, as well as many other possible etiologies.

LUTS typically associated with voiding, such as urinary hesitancy, straining, loss of stream, and interrupted urine flow, are also important to establish. A staccato type of voiding pattern (choppy, interrupted pattern) can be a warning sign indicating detrusor-sphincter dyssynergia, and should prompt a more through evaluation including UD testing. Excessive straining, too, is nonspecific and could represent detrusor failure or bladder outlet obstruction, and therefore should also prompt urodynamic testing in patients with known neurologic disease. However, as noted previously, patients with neurogenic bladder conditions may have elevated postvoid residuals and yet very little in the way of LUTS, so a high index of suspicion is required in their evaluation.

Incontinence, when present, should be characterized fully. Stress incontinence, occurring with increases in intra-abdominal pressure, and most frequently associated with physical activity, coughing, straining, and sneezing, should be assessed for severity, approximate time of onset, and degree of progression. During history taking, incontinence may be assessed by pad usage (nonspecific) and questionnaire response, although questionnaire response may not be a reliable indicator of severity of stress-related leakage.[10,11] Several validated questionnaires are available in men[12] and women,[13] though few were specifically designed for use in patients with neurogenic bladder conditions.[14] SCI patients with lower thoracic or lumbar lesions appear to be at greatest risk for stress incontinence due to intrinsic sphincteric insufficiency, and may note leakage upon transfer.

Urge incontinence, which is thought to be due to detrusor overactivity, loss of compliance, or heightened bladder sensation rather than pelvic floor hypermobility or intrinsic sphincteric weakness alone, as is the case with stress leakage, may be best assessed by a voiding diary and pad usage. In sensate patients, typical symptoms include the sudden, uncontrollable urge to urinate, night-time leakage episodes, and, sometimes, leakage during intercourse. This is the most common pattern among patients with MS, cerebrovascular accident, and PD, among whom the urodynamic finding of neurogenic detrusor overactivity is often noted.

Patients with overflow incontinence, may present with constant low-grade dribbling, recurrent urinary infections, or, at times, renal insufficiency due to the presence of significantly elevated postvoid residuals. In most instances, overflow incontinence is due to detrusor failure or severe bladder outlet obstruction. Patients in the spinal shock phase of spinal cord injury will typically present with this pattern (due to detrusor areflexia), which will often persist in those with lower lumbar and sacral cord injuries. Patients with continuous incontinence, which may be due to ureteral ectopy, fistula formation, bladder neck erosion (from long-term Foley catheter use), or occasionally a scarred, fixed urethra, will report constant urinary drainage, often with very infrequent voids due to the lack of urine accumulation in the bladder.

The development of new onset urinary symptoms in a neurogenic patient who has been followed for some time may reflect a new process and repeat evaluation should be considered. For example, a patient with spinal cord injury and stable LUT function who suddenly develops worsening incontinence may need to have repeated spinal cord imaging in addition to UD studies, while a patient with slowly improving urinary urgency following a stroke often can be safely followed with noninvasive monitoring. Similarly, neurogenic patients who develop verified recurrent urinary tract infections after a period of stability should be re-imaged and consideration given for repeat UD testing, in addition to cystoscopy to evaluate for intravesical sources of infection.

Nongenitourinary review of systems

An assessment of bowel function is imperative, as often bowel and bladder dysfunction parallel one another in patients with neurologic conditions. In patients with SCI, the nature of the bowel program should be established (i.e. digital stimulation, suppository use, etc.). The presence of fecal incontinence, tenesmus, chronic constipation, or obstipation should also be recorded.

A sexual history is also quite important, as sexual dysfunction is also extremely common among men and women with neurologic conditions.[15,16] Women may report lack of desire (loss of libido) or inability to have intercourse secondary to vaginal pain or dryness, or due to enhanced vaginal sensitivity (hyperasthesia), particularly in the case of MS. In women with SCI, disorders of arousal and orgasm appear to be the most prevalent conditions.[17] Men may report erectile dysfunction often secondary to altered penile sensation. Ejaculatory disturbances due to these changes in sensation (leading to either premature or delayed ejaculation), or bladder neck dysfunction (retrograde ejaculation) are also not uncommon. Patients with sympathetic outflow interruption, such as those with complete spinal cord lesions, will often experience anejaculation. In such instances, vibratory simulation to the penis or electrical stimulation applied transrectally can often result in successful ejaculation.

Physical examination

Neurologic assessment

A brief neurologic examination is essential when first evaluating patients with presumed neurovesical dysfunction. Mental status should be assessed, as significant cognitive dysfunction and memory disturbances have been independently associated with LUTS and incontinence. An appreciation of past and present intellectual capacity may also provide insight into the progression of lower urinary tract disorders, as well as guide the degree of complexity of treatment strategies. Both motor strength and sensory level should be determined, as the distribution of motor and sensory disturbances can often predict lower urinary tract dysfunction.[18]

There should also be a thorough evaluation of both cutaneous and motor reflexes at the time of the initial encounter. The bulbocavernosus reflex, which is elicited by gently squeezing the glans penis in men or gentle compression of the clitoris against the pubis in women and simultaneously feeling for an anal sphincter contraction (by placing a finger in the rectum), assesses the integrity of the S2–S4 reflex arc. The anal reflex, which assesses integrity of S2–S5, can be checked by applying a pinprick to the mucocutaneous junction of the anus and evaluating for anal sphincter contraction. The cremasteric reflex may be somewhat less reliable, but assesses sensory dermatomes supplied by L1–L2.

Muscle motor reflexes should also be routinely evaluated. The most common of these are the biceps reflex (assesses C5–C6), patellar reflex (L2–L4), and Achilles (ankle) reflex (L5–S2). Evidence of an upper motor neurologic injury would include spasticity of the involved skeletal muscle, heightened response to reflex testing, and an upgoing toe on gentle stroking of the plantar surface of the foot (positive Babinski).

General issues

Mode of ambulation and recent progression of ambulatory disturbances should be assessed at the initial visit. Clearly, the degree of physical independence of the patient, particularly as it relates to the ability to transfer oneself to the toilet, often affects the degree of urge-related leakage episodes. Additionally, certain patients who are nonambulatory may have great difficulty with self-urethral catheterization. Should that be the case, an abdominal catheterizable stoma may be a more reasonable option in the appropriately selected patient.

Hand function in patients with cervical SCI, and particularly the ability to grasp firmly between the thumb and index or middle finger, must be carefully judged in patients who may require intermittent catheterization following treatment. However, it is no longer mandatory that patients have use of both hands prior to such an intervention, as single unit catheter/collection systems have become commercially available.

An evaluation of the skin, particularly in the gluteal region, should be carried out, as localized skin and subcutaneous infections as well as more severe skin breakdown are not uncommon among patients with restricted mobility. Such issues will need to be addressed before major reconstructive procedures are considered. Some patients may also have intrathecal pumps in place and their location, as well as that of their tubing, should be assessed prior to surgical endeavors.

Pelvic examination

Pelvic examination should be carried out to assess for vaginal estrogenization (noting a loss of lubrication, rugation, and blanching of the mucosal surface), and pelvic prolapse. One should also observe for urine loss (either spontaneous or induced by Valsalva's maneuver or cough). An assessment of the urethra is essential in both men and women, particularly those with chronic indwelling catheters, as traumatic hypospadias in men and bladder neck erosion in women may require surgical repair or even closure for severe cases of erosion. A careful examination of sensation of the genitalia may provide insight into the nature of sexual dysfunction, as both hypo- and hyperasthesia have been described among patients with neurologic conditions. A rectal examination should assess for sphincter tone and for stool impaction, as chronic constipation often aggravates voiding dysfunction. In men, the prostate should be examined for areas of tenderness or fluctuance, since prostatitis and prostatic abscesses are not uncommon among men with severe neurovesical dysfunction, particularly those with chronic indwelling catheters.

Conclusion

As we try to provide a thorough, yet cost-effective evaluation of patients with neurovesical dysfunction, it has become apparent that our approach to the initial encounter is crucial in determining what further studies may be warranted. Not all patients with neurologic conditions and coexisting bladder dysfunction merit the same initial diagnostic evaluation, nor the same frequency of follow-up studies. The information obtained during history-taking and physical examination remains the framework for this type of ongoing decision-making.

References

1. Lemack GE, Dewey RB, Roehrborn CG, O'Suilleabhain PE, Zimmern PE. Questionnaire-based assessment of bladder dysfunction in patients with mild to moderate Parkinson's disease. Urology 2000; 56: 250–4.
2. Jolijn KJ, Hoogervorst ELJ, Uitdehaag BMJ, Polman CH. Relation between objective and subjective measures of bladder dysfunction in multiple sclerosis. Neurology 2004; 63: 1716–18.
3. Khan Z, Starer P, Yang YC, Bhola A. Analysis of voiding disorders in patients with cerebrovascular accidents, Urology, 1990; 32: 265–70.
4. Kolminsky-Rabas PL, Hilz MJ, Neunderfer B, Heuschmann PU. Impact of urinary incontinence after stroke: results from a prospective population-based stroke register. Neururol Urodyn 2003; 22: 322–6.
5. Dong D, Xu Z, Shi B et al. Urodynamic study in the neurogenic bladder dysfunction caused by intervertebral disk herniation. Neurourol Urodyn 2006; 25: 446–50.
6. Hubert J, Hauri K, Leuener M et al. Evidence of trigonal denervation and reinnervation after radical retropubic prostatectomy. J Urol 2001; 165: 111–13.
7. Moore KN, Burt J, Voaklander DC. Intermittent catheterization in the rehabilitation setting: a comparison of clean and sterile technique. Clin Rehab 2006; 20: 461–8.
8. Wyman JF, Choi SC, Harkins SW, Wilson MS, Fantl JA. The urinary diary in evaluation of incontinent women: a test-retest analysis. Obstet. Gynecol. 1988; 71: 812–17.
9. Groutz A, Blaivas JG, Chaikin DC et al. Noninvasive outcome measures of urinary incontinence and lower urinary tract symptoms: a multicenter study of micturition diary and pad tests. J. Urol. 2000, 164: 698–701.
10. Lemack GE, Zimmern PE. Predictability of urodynamic findings based on the Urogenital Distress Inventory questionnaire. Urology 1999; 54: 461–6.
11. Harvey MA, Kristjansson B, Griffith D, Versi E. The Incontinence Impact Questionnaire and the Urogenital Distress Inventory: a revisit of their validity in women without a urodynamic diagnosis. Am J Obstet Gynecol 2001; 185: 25–31.
12. Barry MJ, Fowler FJ Jr, O'Leary MP et al. and the Measurement committee of the American Urological Association: The American Urological Association symptom index for benign prostatic hyperplasia. J. Urol. 1992; 148: 1549–57.
13. Uebersax JS, Wyman FF, Shumaker SA, McClish DK, Fantl JA. Short forms to assess life quality and symptom distress for urinary incontinence in women: the incontinence impact questionnaire and urogenital distress inventory. Neurourol Urodyn 1995; 14: 131–9.
14. Sakakibara R, Shinotoh H, Uchiyama T et al. Questionnaire-based assessment of pelvic organ dysfunction in Parkinson's disease. Auton Neurosci Basic Clin 2001; 92: 76–85.
15. Lundberg PO, Hutler B. Female sexual dysfunction in multiple sclerosis: a review. Sex Dis 1996; 14: 65–72.
16. Aisen ML, Sanders AS. Sexual dysfunction in neurologic disease: mechanisms of disease and counseling approaches. Am Urol Assoc Update Ser 1998; 17: 274–9.
17. Forstythe E and Horsewell JE. Sexual rehabilitation of women with a spinal cord injury. Spinal Cord. 2006; 44: 234–1.
18. Betts CD, D'Mellow MT, Fowler CJ. Urinary symptoms and the neurological features of bladder dysfunction in multiple sclerosis. J Neurol Neurosurg Psychiatry. 1993; 56(3): 245–50.

34

The voiding diary

Martine Jolivet-Tremblay, Pierre E Bertrand, and Erik Schick

Introduction

Since the advent of urodynamic studies in clinical practice, urologists have tried to analyze voiding habits to better define lower urinary tract symptoms (LUTS). The bladder being an 'unreliable witness', diagnosis based solely on clinical symptoms was revealed to be inadequate.

The voiding diary is a well-known diagnostic tool for this purpose. However, in spite of the fact that the utilization of the voiding diary is recommended by multiple national and international associations in many treatment algorithms, it is still frequently overlooked by some, even if it is one of the simplest noninvasive tests to evaluate the function of the lower urinary tract (LUT). The patients complete it at home and/or at work, and it offers the advantage of assessing the severity of LUTS in their customary environment. By filling out the voiding diary, patients become active participants in the diagnostic process and their degree of motivation can be assessed. In our technologic era, patients often submit very complete voiding diaries done with home software on their personal computer. On this particular subject, Quinn et al,[1] in a small study of 35 patients, tried to assess the effectiveness of a portable electronic diary as a data collection device for overactive bladder symptoms, and also to evaluate its level of patient acceptability compared with a conventional written voiding diary. They confirmed that the electronic diary is a novel method of collecting clinically relevant symptom data from patients with an overactive bladder. In addition, the ease-of-use ratings support the electronic diary as a superior alternative to paper diaries, providing real-time data, which can be rapidly analyzed, and thus allowing a speedy review of data during ongoing clinical studies. This probably represents the future for voiding diaries.

The first studies published on voiding diaries were limited to urinary incontinence. However, since the late 1980s the voiding diary has become a widely accepted tool in the investigation of voiding dysfunctions in women, men, and children, including obstructive uropathy, urinary tract infection, vesicoureteral reflux, and neurogenic bladder.

The voiding diary is now a crucial part of most research protocols and has become an important criterion for the indication of treatments, such as injection of Botox (botulinum toxin A–hemagglutinin complex) or implantation of neurostimulation/neuromodulation devices.

Articles appearing in the literature since the first publication of this textbook are numerous and quite varied. In reviewing the present chapter we gave precedence to articles dealing with the validation of the voiding diary over those concerning its many applications.

Definition and terminology

The Abrams–Klevmark classification

In 1996, Abrams and Klevmark[2] were the first to describe four different voiding diaries in a laudable effort to standardize the terminology. This classification is based on the type and amount of information contained in each of them (Table 34.1). The charts give objective information on the number of voidings, the distribution of voiding between daytime and night-time, and each voided volume. The charts can also be used to record episodes of urgency and leakage and the number of incontinence pads used. The frequency–volume chart is not only useful in the assessment of voiding disorders but also in treatment follow-up.

The frequency chart

In this very simple chart only the number of micturitions and the number of incontinence episodes are registered per 24 hours. This limited information does not include urinary volume or the degree of incontinence.

The frequency–severity chart

In this chart, the number of micturitions and episodes of incontinence are noted plus the number of pads used or cloths changed. This diary is a better evaluation of the severity of incontinence. However, it does not provide

Table 34.1 *Voiding diaries: the Abrams–Klevmark classification*

Frequency chart	Frequency–severity chart	Frequency–volume chart	Urinary diary
Number of voidings + Number of incontinence episodes	Number of voidings + Number of incontinence episodes + Number of pads used Number of pads used	Time of each voiding + Volume of each voiding + Time of each incontinent episode	Time of each voiding + Volume of each voiding + Time of each incontinent episode + Types of drinks, foods, activities related to LUTS

Reproduced with modifications from Jolivet-Tremblay M, Schick E. The voiding diary. In: Corcos J, Schick E, eds. The Urinary Sphincter. New York:

Marcel Dekker, 2001: 262.

LUTS, lower urinary tract symptoms.

Table 34.2 *Voiding diaries: the ICS classification*

Micturition time chart	Frequency–volume chart	Bladder diary
Time of micturitions (minimum 24 hours)	Time of micturitions (minimum 24 hours) + Volume voided at each micturition	Time of micturitions + Volume voided at each micturition + Incontinence episodes + Pad usage, fluid intake, degree of urgency, degree of incontinence

information on urinary volume or quantity of urine lost. This voiding diary can be useful in a follow-up of patients after a more complete chart is filled originally.

The frequency–volume chart

This voiding diary is still the most widely used by urologists. It provides the maximum of information. Although it demands some effort on the part of the patient, it is an investment in his welfare. The time and the volume of urine voided at each micturition plus the number and the timing of each incontinent episode are registered on a chart. From this, the 24-hour diuresis, the frequency of micturition, the functional capacity of the bladder, and daytime diuresis, compared with nocturnal diuresis, etc., can be calculated. This type of voiding diary, however, does not provide information on fluid intake or its distribution through a 24-hour period.

The urinary diary

This is the most elaborate and complicated form of voiding diary. Besides its role as a frequency–volume chart, it also provides information on the types and number of beverages and foods taken every day. The patient also notes any activities related to LUTS. This type of chart is very onerous to the patient and is often difficult to analyze for the physician. Under normal circumstances, knowledge of fluid intake is not absolutely necessary since it generally parallels total diuresis.

The International Continence Society classification

In their report[3] a subcommittee of the International Continence Society in 2002 suggested three types of diaries (Table 34.2):

1. *micturition time chart*, which records only the times of micturition, day and night, for at least 24 hours
2. *frequency–volume chart*, which records the volumes voided as well as the times of micturition, day and night, for at least 24 hours
3. *bladder diary*, which records the times of micturition, voided volumes, incontinence episodes, pad usage, and other information such as fluid intake, the degree of urgency, and the degree of incontinence.

Rationale for the voiding diary

Routine use of the voiding diary in the investigation and follow-up of patients with LUTS will fulfill four objectives:

1. The voiding diary leads to an objective measurement of the patient's subjective complaints in a familiar environment. Patient perception of voiding habits may be misleading. For example, McCormack et al[4] studied 88 consecutive patients in whom urinary frequency was evaluated by a questionnaire at the first visit. This was compared with the frequency obtained by analyzing the frequency–volume chart filled out by the patient for 7 consecutive days. A very wide discrepancy was noted between subjectively estimated frequency and chart-determined frequency.
2. It can help the physician to identify the etiology of the patient's LUTS. The clinical examples are numerous. Urologists often encounter patients with a complaint of pollakiuria who complete a voiding diary revealing frank polyuria.
3. As previously mentioned, when taking an active role in the elaboration of his voiding calendar, the patient becomes a participant to the diagnosis and treatment of the urologic problem. This may serve as a measure of his motivation to get well.
4. The voiding diary is also an important tool in the follow-up of a medical treatment or a specific surgery. Siltberg et al[5] estimated that the voiding diary provided the best tool for follow-up in the treatment of the urge syndrome. It is now of common use in many clinical research protocols.

Data extracted from the voiding diary

Important parameters can be obtained about the frequency of micturition and the number of episodes of incontinence by careful examination of the data in the voiding diary. It also provides an accurate estimate of total diuresis during a 24-hour period. Nowadays, in the majority of urodynamic laboratories, all the parameters can be entered into a computer and, using a simple software program, a more precise and detailed analysis may be done. This kind of computer program, like the one developed in our laboratory, calculates the following parameters: the mean voided volume per micturitions (ml), the frequency (units), the diuresis (ml/min), the mean interval between micturition (min), and the voided volume during a specific period of the day (ml). All these parameters are calculated separately for daytime and night-time. On rising, the initial micturition is the first daytime voiding registered in the software. This first voided volume is considered part of nocturnal diuresis and is treated as such by the computer program. It is assumed that daytime lasts 16 hours (960 min) and night-time 8 hours (480 min). Therefore, the amount of urine voided during the day is divided by 960 and during the night by 480, to give the day and night diuresis in milliliters per minute. Further analysis produces two more parameters: output per 24 hours (ml), which is the total voided volume during a 24-hour period, and the ratio between night-time and daytime diuresis. In addition, the computer prints out the number of days analyzed, the number of incontinence episodes occurring during this period, and the number of micturitions for which volume was not measured by the patient. The computer program is designed to automatically correct daytime and night-time diuresis as well as the total volume voided (output per day, output per night, output per 24 hours) for micturition when volume was not measured. The mean voided volume is calculated from all recorded volumes. This mean volume is then substituted for each missing micturition volume to give the corrected output. The diuresis ratio (night/day) is derived from this corrected diuresis.[6]

To facilitate interpretation of the patient's data, the computer will print out the normal value for each parameter, along with the standard deviation (SD) and the standard normal deviation (Z-value), which is the number of SDs an observation lies away from the mean. A Z-value of 2.00 or more suggests a significant deviation from the mean[7] (Table 34.3).

Furthermore, this software is able to print a graph of the mean voided volumes over a 24-hour period as a function of time. Figures 34.1 to 34.6 represent mean hourly voided volumes.

We have used this computer program in our urodynamic laboratory for almost 25 years, analyzing more than 2500 frequency–volume charts.

Normal values

To obtain valuable information from a voiding diary, it is essential to know normal values. However, surprisingly, very few data are available concerning normal values. Fitzgerald and Brubaker[8] analyzed the variability of the

Table 34.3 *Basic data provided by software*

Parameter	Normal	1 SD
Day:		
Mean voided volume (ml)	2.37	67
Frequency	5.63	1.26
Diuresis (ml/min)	1.11	0.35
Corrected diuresis (ml/min)	1.11	0.35
Interval between micturitions (min)	222	60
Output (ml)	1005	497
Corrected output (ml)	1005	497
Night:		
Mean voided volume (ml)	379	132
Frequency	0.08	0.16
Diuresis (ml/min)	0.84	0.27
Corrected diuresis (ml/min)	0.84	0.27
Interval between micturitions (min)	454	50
Output (ml)	409	130
Corrected output (ml)	409	130
Output in 24 hours (ml)	1473	386
Corrected output in 24 hours (ml)	1473	386
Diuresis ratio (night/day)	0.81	0.30

Reproduced with modifications from Jolivet-Tremblay M, Schick E. The voiding diary. In: Corcos J, Schick E, eds. The Urinary Sphincter. New York: Marcel Dekker, 2001: 264.

24-hour voiding diary among asymptomatic women and introduced a new parameter, namely the number of voidings per liter of intake. Their study demonstrated that this parameter, together with mean and maximum voided volume, total intake, as well as daytime and night-time diuresis rates, remained stable under normal circumstances. Urinary frequency and urine volumes may vary significantly. The authors concluded that when urinary frequency is of interest, the number of voidings per liter of intake may represent the most reliable measure.

Normal values still remain an important issue, however, because baseline values are needed to compare them with data from patients with various LUTS.

Children

Bloom et al[9] analyzed the voiding habits of 1192 children without a history of urinary tract infection. They obtained a mean frequency of about 4–5 micturitions per day. Data were obtained by questionnaire, but no frequency–volume chart was filled out.

Mattsson[10] studied 206 children, aged 7–15 years, considered asymptomatic. All of them completed a 24-hour frequency–volume chart. They voided 2–10 times a day, but 95% of them had a voiding frequency of 3–8. About 10% voided once during the night. Voided volume varied greatly, the morning voiding being the largest, and the last voiding before bedtime, the smallest. Single voided volume varied between 20 and 800 ml, with total volumes over 24 hours between 325 and 2100 ml. Wan et al[11] estimated that voiding frequency for normal children was approximately 6 times daily. They used a frequency chart on which urine volume could be measured, but this was not mandatory. They found the diary particularly useful in infrequent voiding. Hellström et al,[12] studying the micturition habits of 3556 7-year-old children, found that the frequency of micturitions was 3–7 per day among those without symptoms of bladder disturbance and without previous urinary tract infection.

Esperanca and Gerrard[13] determined urinary frequency in 297 normal children aged 4–14 years. The average frequency for 4-year-olds was 5.3 micturitions, whereas for 12-year-olds it was 4.8.

Table 34.4 *Data obtained from frequency–volume charts of normal females*

	Boedker et al[18] (*n* = 123)	Larsson and Victor[16] (*n* = 151)	Siltberg et al[5] (*n* = 151)	Saito et al[17] (*n* = 20)[a]	Kassis and Schick[6] (*n* = 33)
Mean voided volume (day) in ml				179	237 (±67)
Mean voided volume (night) in ml		} 250 (±79)	} 240	230	379 (± 132)
Mean frequency (day)				6.8	5.63 (± 1.26)
Mean frequency (night)	} 5.7	} 5.8 (± 1.41)	} 5.5	0.5	0.08 (±0.16)
Diuresis in ml/min (day)					1.11 (±0.35)
Diuresis in ml/min (night)					0.84 (±0.27)
Excreta in ml (day)				1149	1.005 (± 497)
Excreta in ml (night)				234	409 (± 130)
Diuresis per 24 hours in ml	1350	1430 (±487)	1350	1272	1473 (± 386)
Night diuresis					
Day diuresis					0.81 (±0.30)
Functional capacity in ml		460 (± 174)	450		

[a] Also includes normal males.

Reproduced with permission from Jolivet-Tremblay M, Schick E. The voiding diary. In: Corcos J, Schick E, eds. The Urinary Sphincter. New York: Marcel Dekker, 2001: 266.

Bower et al[14] constructed nomograms for mean maximum voided volume, mean voided volume, and mean minimum voided volume for specific age groups using data obtained from 322 incontinent children, aged 6–11 years, who completed a 2-day frequency–volume chart. They noted a wide variation of voided volumes, very much as Mattsson and Lindström did in normal children.[15] Based on all these findings, frequency–volume charts by themselves seem to be an unsuitable screening tool for children.

Females

Most of the data on voiding diaries concern women. Several authors[5,6,16–18] have established normal values for healthy women. Comparison of these data is given in Table 34.4.

It was in studies done on women that authors began to analyze diurnal and nocturnal data separately. The first results were obtained by Saito et al[16] and Kassis and Schick.[6] This distinction is important because night-time diuresis may exceed daytime diuresis and be responsible for nocturia, especially in the elderly.

On this particular subject, according to Saito et al[17] an increase in urine volume during the night can be induced by three physiologic events related to aging. First, the circadian rhythm of antidiuretic hormone or atrial natriuretic hormone secretion may be abnormal.[19] Second, the glomerular filtration rate or renal plasma flow may be altered because of a reduction in the concentrating ability of the distal tubules. Finally, an impaired cardiovascular system may not be able to supply sufficient amounts of blood to the kidneys during waking hours, creating edema in the lower extremities, which becomes mobilized in the supine position.

The calculated ratio of night over day diuresis can draw attention to one of these phenomena, which is important to recognize, because its logical consequence, nocturia, has nothing to do with a vesicourethral pathology (such as outflow obstruction, unstable bladder function, etc.).

Amundsen et al[20] recently studied the effects of age and 24-hour voided volume on measurements of voiding frequency and also on functional bladder capacity in a cohort of asymptomatic females. They utilized computer-processed 3-day voiding diaries from 161 females, aged 19.6–81.8 years. Their findings demonstrated an increase with age in the 24-hour volume and functional bladder capacity, suggesting an adaptive mechanism because the frequency of micturition did not increase. They also suggested reference values for age and 24-hour voided volume by calculating 'normal limits'. However, there was a large overlap between normal and abnormal, which suggests that it may be more useful to report voiding diary measurements as reference population percentiles rather than to designate them normal or abnormal.

Males

An extensive revision of the recent literature did not reveal any precise data concerning reference values for frequency–volume charts in men. Published data for males mostly concern diseases like benign prostatic hypertrophy (BPH), nocturnal polyuria, and overactive bladder (OAB) in men. Latini et al[21] studied urinary habits of American men without LUTS by using a 24-hour voiding diary. Two hundred and eighty-four asymptomatic males, 18 to 66 years old, returned interpretable diaries. Subjects voided a median of 7 times in 24 hours. Median 24-hour urine volume was 1650 ml (range 290 to 6840 ml). Median fluid intake was 2747 ml (range 500 to 10 520). Of these men, 29% reported at least one nocturic episode. The authors concluded a threshold of 8 micturitions to define abnormal urinary frequency may not be correct, since more than a third of asymptomatic men voided more than 8 times daily. It is probably inadvisable to apply a single set of values to all American men because of significant variability in regional climates and populations.

The study by Saito et al[17] already quoted included males and females, but did not separate them into two subgroups. One reason for this lack of data may be the difficulty in defining the clinical characteristics of a normal male without LUTS. This 'normality' probably changes with age.

Recent data from the literature suggest that in men with LUTS suggestive of BPH, the urodynamically proven obstruction is the most important factor influencing voided volumes, cystometric capacity, and residual urine volume. By contrast, voiding frequency is not significantly influenced, because patients with small voided volumes minimize their fluid intake.[22] Using a 3-day frequency–volume chart, Blanker et al[23] showed that functional bladder capacity, i.e. the largest single voided volume, decreased with age. They also demonstrated that nocturnal urine production has only a modest influence on nocturnal voiding frequency. Therefore, nocturnal urine production seems to have little diagnostic value for increased nocturnal voiding frequency.[24] It should also be noted that in a large population-based study of 1688 men, circadian urine production could only be demonstrated in men younger than 65.[25]

Duration of the chart

After all these years of abundantly using voiding diaries there still is neither consensus nor clear guidelines in the literature on the minimum number of days necessary to produce a reliable diary. A wide range of 1–14 days exists. The gold standard for now is probably 7 days. Abrams[26] recommended a 7-day chart, Barnick and Cardozo[27] a 5-day chart, Sommer et al[28] a 3-day chart, and Larsson and Victor[15] a 48-hour chart.

Barnick and Cardozo[27] compared a 5-day chart with a 1-day chart in a group of 150 women attending a urodynamic clinic. They found a significant correlation between the two sets of results, with $p < 0.0001$.

Wyman et al[29] studied a 2-week diary in 55 incontinent women, and compared the first week with the second week. They concluded that a 1-week diary is sufficient to assess the frequency of micturition and incontinence episodes. The 7-day diary can consequently be considered as the gold standard for voiding diaries. Homma et al[30] reached the same conclusion.

Gisolf et al[31] studied the reliability of data obtained from the 24-hour frequency–volume charts of 160 men with LUTS secondary to BPH. Their study suggested that the 24-hour chart compared favorably to 3 days or more charts, and concluded that the 1-day chart provided sufficient insight into voiding habits of this group of patients. According to Matthiessen et al,[32] nocturia secondary to nocturnal polyuria can be detected by a 3-day frequency– volume chart in men with LUTS suggestive of BPH. van Melick et al[33] analyzed 2- or 3-day charts of 98 females with urodynamically proven motor urge incontinence and concluded that a single 24-hour chart is sufficient to gain insight into these patients' voiding habits. Locher et al[34] focused on the number of incontinence episodes in a group of 214 community-dwelling women, aged 40–90 years. Based on the number of days necessary to obtain an internal consistency of 0.90 for Cronbach's alpha, they estimated that a 7-day frequency–volume chart is needed to provide a stable and reliable measurement of the frequency of incontinence episodes. Nygaard and Holcomb[35] compared two 7-day diaries completed at 4-week intervals by 138 stress urinary incontinent women. They observed a good correlation for the number of incontinence episodes between the two diaries (0.831), and the results of the first 3-day diaries correlated well with those of the last 4-day diaries. They concluded that a 3-day diary is an appropriate measure in clinical trials evaluating treatments for stress incontinence, but a 7-day diary is preferable when the number of incontinence episodes is considered. Fitzgerald and Brubaker[7] introduced a new variable in the analysis of voiding diaries: the number of micturitions per liter of intake. They estimated that this represents the most reliable measure in comparing two 24-hour charts.

Schick et al[36] compared the standard 7-day chart to various lengths of frequency–volume charts analyzing 14 parameters. Overall results showed that a 4-day diary is almost identical to a 7-day diary. However, when the number of incontinence episodes was considered of primary importance, a 5-day diary was preferable. This reduction in duration made compliance to the voiding diary easier for patients. Ku et al,[37] who compared 2-day, 3-day, and 7-day voiding diaries, have confirmed this. Their results suggest that keeping a diary for 7 days may increase patient burden. They recommend that the 7-day diary should be reduced to fewer days.

Finally, Yap et al[38] made a good review of the literature up to 2006. They still were not able to recommend a definite number of days for the duration of the voiding diary, but 3 days seemed to be the norm.

Our voiding diary

Patients are invited to fill out a 4-day frequency–volume chart in which diurnal and nocturnal voiding is clearly identified. The patient is specifically asked to register the time and volume of each voiding as well as the time of each incontinence episode. When, for some reason, the patient is unable to measure a voided volume, he notes the time, and marks an 'X' instead of the volume. Volume can be expressed in milliliters (ml) or in fluid ounces (fl oz), but should remain uniform throughout the chart. The back of the chart offers simple instructions for completion, with examples for the patient.

It is clinically proven that patients easily understand the elaboration of the frequency–volume chart. More than 95% of our patients fill out the chart correctly. At the beginning we offered lengthy explanations to every patient. But, with time, written instructions proved to be clear enough to forego verbal explanations. The chart can be sent out by mail, fax, or even e-mailed, so that the patient arrives for a visit with complete frequency–volume information.

Reliability of the voiding diary

To be reliable, frequency–volume charts must be filled out correctly. In an effort to verify their accuracy, Palnaes Hansen and Klarskov[39] studied 18 subjects who noted their fluid intake and voided volumes and collected 24-hour urine samples for 3 consecutive days. They concluded that self-reported frequency–volume chart data are valid and useful for patients with voiding symptoms.

Barnick and Cardozo[27] studied 106 consecutive patients who received a 5-day frequency–volume chart by mail, to be filled out before their physical examination. Only 40% of them completed the chart correctly for the full 5 days.

Robinson et al[40] compared two 7-day diaries in 278 incontinent women. The first was completed with minimal instructions, the second after receiving extensive instructions. They concluded that a 7-day diary remained a reliable tool to assess urinary symptoms, even if patients received minimal instructions on filling out the chart.

Groutz et al[41] assessed the reliability of a micturition diary and pad test in patients referred for the evaluation of urinary incontinence and LUTS. They prospectively enrolled 109 patients in their study. The 24-hour micturition diary was a reliable instrument for assessing the number of incontinent episodes. Increasing the test duration to 48 and 72 hours increased reliability but resulted in decreased patient compliance.

According to our own experience, more than 1000 patients correctly completed the frequency–volume chart without extensive verbal instructions. The fact that we allow our patients to use milliliters or fluid ounces for volume measurements is probably helpful, because older people are less familiar with the metric system. Bailey et al[42] presented results similar to our own, with most patients completing the chart correctly before their first visit.

The frequency–volume chart as a diagnostic tool

The possibility of using the frequency–volume chart as a diagnostic tool is very tempting because of its simplicity and noninvasiveness. Several authors have explored this possibility. Larsson and Victor[43] compared the frequency–volume charts of 81 stress-incontinent patients with those of 151 asymptomatic women. Interestingly, all three parameters (total voided volume, frequency, and largest single voided volume) differed statistically between the two groups; however, because of marked overlapping, the frequency–volume chart was judged an unreliable diagnostic tool for stress incontinence.

Larsson et al[44] analyzed the frequency–volume chart in bladder overactivity, compared it with a group of women without LUTS, and related it to cystometric findings, to evaluate the quantitative aspects of urgency incontinence. A 2-day period on a 7-day chart was evaluated. None of the parameters of the frequency–volume chart (frequency of micturition, mean voided volume, largest single voided volume, and variability in voided volumes) were useful in differentiating between motor urgency and normal voiding habits. Moreover, no correlation was found between any of the data from the frequency–volume chart and the filling phase of urodynamic studies (first desire to void, bladder volume at first unstable contraction, bladder capacity, and bladder volume at first leakage). The authors concluded that frequency–volume charts did not help in differential diagnosis, but that mean voided volume represented a good measure of the severity of detrusor instability symptoms.

In another study, Fink et al[45] compared the 24-hour frequency–volume chart in stress-incontinent and urge-incontinent women. When applying logistic regression to these two groups, the frequency of micturition during night-time was the parameter that best discriminated between these medical conditions. Mean voided volume (over the 24-hour period) showed the highest differentiating power with $p < 0.0001$, but the large overlap between groups limited the value of the frequency–volume chart for differential diagnosis.

Siltberg et al[5] proposed a nomogram on which the frequency of micturition was plotted against the range of voided volumes. According to these authors, this plot could be used to determine the degree of certainty (with 10%

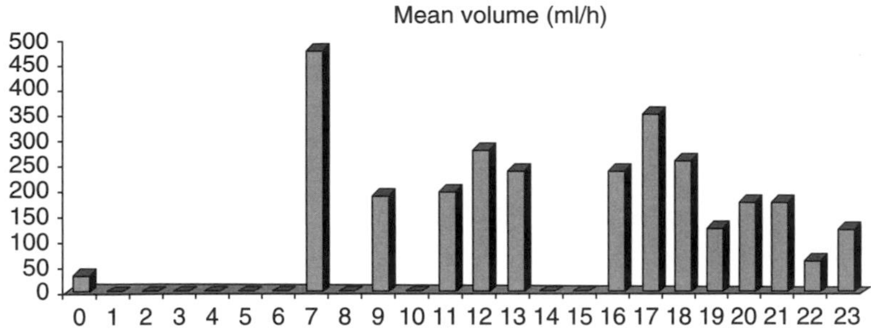

Figure 34.1
Graphic representation of a normal frequency–volume chart over a 3-day period.

intervals for probability) of having motor urgency incontinence vs stress incontinence. Tincello and Richmond[46] also tried to assess the reliability of the Larsson chart nomogram to predict the presence of detrusor overactivity or genuine stress incontinence without recourse to cystometry. Frequency–volume chart data were obtained from the records of 216 patients who had undergone multichannel urodynamics. In their study the Larsson chart did not provide diagnostic information and did not eliminate the need for formal cystometric evaluation of patients with urinary incontinence.

These observations are not surprising. Attempting to characterize such complex physiopathologic entities as continence and voiding with a single parameter is oversimplification. Although the voiding diary is found to have poor specificity and sensitivity in detecting overactive bladder vs stress incontinence, this simple tool remains a useful diagnostic aid in the current evaluation of urinary incontinence, imparting information regarding functional bladder capacity, urinary frequency, nocturia, and daily fluid intake. This diagnostic tool remains an important element in our understanding of patient symptomatology and is still one of the first tests to choose because of its simplicity and its usefulness in follow-ups. The gathered information can reveal the presence of specific entities such as diabetes insipidus, contracted bladder, and interstitial cystitis, and allow the physician to make simple adjustments in fluid intake to minimize incontinence, nocturia, and daytime diuresis. In accordance with other authors,[47] we continue to stress the importance of the voiding diary in clinical studies.

Interpretation of frequency–volume charts

In our department, the computer software we described above analyzes every frequency–volume chart filled out by a patient. The most important parameters in the clinical setting are the frequency of micturition (day and night), 24-hour urinary output, the ratio of night-time diuresis to daytime diuresis, and the mean voided volume (day and night). The hour-by-hour distribution is also very helpful.

Normal frequency–volume chart

Table 34.5 represents the results of a 3-day frequency–volume chart filled out by a 42-year-old lady who was referred because of incontinence. Three voided volumes were not recorded, representing 14.29% of the total number of micturitions during this 3-day period. The 24-hour corrected urinary output was within normal limits (1462 ml; Z-value: –0.03), as well as the night/day diuresis ratio (0.73; Z-value: –0.28). Daytime frequency (7.00; Z-value: 1.09) and night-time frequency (0.00; Z-value: –0.50) were almost within normal limits. Figure 34.1 illustrates the graphic representation of voidings and the mean voided volumes during a 24-hour period. The greatest single voided volume (480 ml), which represents in this example the daytime functional bladder capacity, was registered at 07:00 hours. No micturition occurred between midnight and 07:00 hours, and between 13:00 and 16:00 hours.

Increased 24-hour output (polyuria)

This type of pathology is relatively common and can be seen in patients with unbalanced diabetes or simple potomania of different magnitude.

This 45-year-old female consulted with symptoms suggestive of mixed urinary incontinence. She reported voiding about 20 times a day and 4–6 times at night. She complained of a sensation of incomplete emptying. Endoscopy revealed a bladder capacity of 300 ml and postvoid residual urine of 120 ml. The bladder wall was trabeculated, grade II. Gynecologic examination showed a grade II anterior vaginal wall prolapse, resulting from a lateral defect. The Q-tip test demonstrated a 25° urethral

Table 34.5 *Normal frequency–volume chart (for details see text)*

Parameter	Patient's data (±1 SD)	Normal (±1 SD)	Z-value
Day:			
Mean voided volume (ml)	187 (72)	273 (±67)	(0.75)
Voiding frequency	7.00 (0. 00)	5.63 (±1.26)	1.09
Diuresis (ml/min)	0.97	1.11 (±0.35)	(0.39)
Corrected diuresis (ml/min)	1.17	1.11 (±0.35)	0.17
Interval between micturitions (min)	192 (601)	222 (±60)	(0.50)
Output (ml)	935 (92)	1005 (±497)	(0.14)
Corrected output (ml)	1122(92)	1005 (±497)	0.24
Maximal voided volume (ml)	480		
Night:	340 (18)	379 (±132)	(0.30)
Mean voided volume (ml)	0.00	0.08 (±0.16)	(0.50)
Voiding frequency	0.71	0.84 (±27)	(0.49)
Diuresis (ml/min)	0.71	0.84 (±50)	(0.49)
Corrected diuresis (ml/min)	480 (0)	454 (±130)	(0.53)
Interval between micturitions (ml)	340 (102)	409 (±130)	(0.53)
Output (ml)	0.00	409 (±130)	(0.53)
Corrected output (ml)			
Maximal voided volume (ml)	0.00		
Output in 24 hours (ml)	1275	1473 (±386)	(0.51)
Corrected output in 24 hours (ml)	1462	1473 (±386)	(0.03)
Diuresis ratio (night/day)	0.73	0.81 (±0.3)	(0.28)

mobility (normal <30°). No urinary incontinence could be observed during cough in the supine position. On multichannel urodynamics, bladder capacity was 750 ml and the first desire to void occurred at 262 ml. Bladder wall compliance was normal. Maximum urethral closure pressure was 65 cmH_2O and the cough leak-point pressure was negative. No uninhibited detrusor contractions could be detected during the filling phase, but a strong postvoid contraction was registered which, in view of the clinical symptoms, was considered as a manifestation of unstable bladder.

The frequency–volume chart (Table 34.6) showed a tremendous increase in the corrected 24-hour urinary output (12 591 ml!) with a normal night/day diuresis ratio (0.91; Z-value: 0.33). Daytime voiding frequency was 18.71, not because of a decrease in mean voided volumes (494 ml; Z-value: 3.83), but due to an important daytime diuresis (8746 ml; Z-value: 15.58). Night-time diuresis was even more pronounced (3845 ml; Z-value: 26.43). In spite of this, voiding frequency was increased to a lesser degree (3.00; Z-value: 18.25), mainly because the mean nocturnal voided volume also increased (961 ml; Z-value: 4.41). The mean hourly voided volume (Figure 34.2) reflects the difference in mean voided volumes for night-time and daytime.

Nocturnal polyuria

A 69-year-old female consulted because of urgency and increased frequency. She claimed hourly micturitions during the day and 5–6 voidings each night. She was enuretic until the age of 9. Endoscopy revealed grade II bladder trabeculation associated with a cystoscopic capacity of 400 ml. Urodynamic study demonstrated an unstable bladder, with the first uninhibited contraction occurring at 60 ml. Cystometric capacity was 175 ml and the first desire to void occurred at 62 ml.

Her 7-day frequency–volume chart (Table 34.7) showed a slight increase in the 24-hour corrected output (1961 ml; Z-value: 1.15), but a significantly increased night/day ratio (4.66; Z-value: 12.84). Her daytime frequency was somewhat increased (7.43; Z-value: 1.43), but clearly less than the claimed frequency reported during the initial interview. Note that the decreased mean daytime voided volume (99 ml; Z-value: 2.06) is not very different from the bladder volume at the first desire to void (62 ml) and the appearance of the first uninhibited detrusor contraction (60 ml). The chart confirms the significantly increased night-time frequency (5.14; Z-value: 31.64), accompanied by a decreased mean voided volume (208 ml; Z-value: 1.29).

Table 34.6 *Increased 24-hour output (polyuria) (for details see text)*

Parameter	Patient's data (±1 SD)	Normal (±1 SD)	Z-value
Day:			
Mean voided volume (ml)	494 (205)	237 (±67)	3.83
Voiding frequency	18.71 (1075)	5.63 (±1.26)	10.38
Diuresis (ml/min)	8.82	1.11 (±0.35)	22.02
Corrected diuresis (ml/min)	9.11	1.11 (±0.35)	22.86
Interval between micturitions (min)	56 (222)	222 (±60)	(2.77)
Output (ml)	8464 (864)	1005 (±497)	15.01
Corrected output (ml)	8746 (1086)	1005 (±497)	15.58
Maximal voided volume (ml)	1350		
Night:			
Mean voided volume (ml)	961 (212)	379 (±132)	4.41
Voiding frequency	3.00 (0.00)	0.08 (±0.16)	18.25
Diuresis (ml/min)	8.01	0.84 (±0.27)	26.56
Corrected diuresis (ml/min)	8.01	0.84 (±0.27)	26.56
Interval between micturitions (ml)	120 (185)	454 (±50)	(6.68)
Output (ml)	3845 (617)	409 (±130)	26.43
Corrected output (ml)	3845 (617)	409 (±130)	26.43
Maximal voided volume (ml)	1380		
Output in 24 hours (ml)	12,309	1473 (±386)	28.07
Corrected output in 24 hours (ml)	12,591	1473 (±386)	28.80
Diuresis ratio (night/day)	0.91	0.81 (±0.3)	0.33

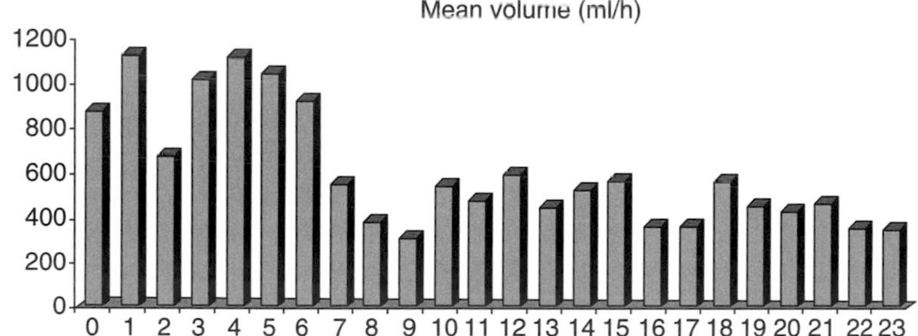

Figure 34.2
Graphic representation of the frequency–volume chart of a patient with an increased 24-hour output (polyuria).

On the graphical representation (Figure 34.3) one can easily see the predominantly nocturnal diuresis with the maximal functional capacity (325.31 ml) occurring during the second part of the night (04:00 hours).

Sensory urgency

A 73-year-old female patient complained of stress urinary incontinence but also experienced incontinence episodes, which were not associated with stress or urgency. Cystometric capacity was 800 ml with no postvoid residual urine. Her bladder was stable on multichannel urodynamics. Abdominal leak-point pressure was estimated between 100 and 150 cmH_2O, a grade III urethral incompetence,[47] explaining the clinical symptom of stress urinary incontinence.

Her 7-day frequency–volume chart (Table 34.8) demonstrated a 24-hour corrected urine output (1784 ml; Z-value 0.81) within normal limits. There was some degree of nocturnal polyuria (693 ml; Z-value: 2.18). Mean urinary frequency was 14.14 during daytime and 1.86 during night-time, with

Table 34.7 *Nocturnal polyuria (for details see text)*

Parameter	Patient's data (±1 SD)	Normal (±1 SD)	Z-value
Day:			
Mean voided volume (ml)	99 (48)	237 (±67)	(2.06)
Voiding frequency	7.43 (1.18)	5.63 (±1.26)	1.43
Diuresis (ml/min)	0.56	1.11 (±0.35)	(1.57)
Corrected diuresis (ml/min)	0.66	1.11 (±0.35)	(1.28)
Interval between micturitions (min)	177 (436)	222 (±60)	(0.75)
Output (ml)	537 (190)	1005 (±497)	(0.94)
Corrected output (ml)	635 (145)	1005 (±497)	(0.74)
Maximal voided volume (ml)	295.74		
Night:			
Mean voided volume (ml)	208 (64)	379 (±132)	(1.29)
Voiding frequency	5.14 (0.83)	0.08 (±0.16)	31.64
Diuresis (ml/min)	2.61	0.84 (±0.27)	6.54
Corrected diuresis (ml/min)	2.67	0.84 (±0.27)	6.77
Interval between micturition (ml)	80 (209)	454 (±50)	(7.48)
Output (ml)	1251 (103)	409 (±130)	6.47
Corrected output (ml)	1280 (156)	409 (±130)	6.70
Maximal voided volume (ml)	325.31		
Output in 24 hours (ml)	1787	1473 (±386)	0.81
Corrected output in 24 hours (ml)	1916	1473 (±386)	1.15
Diuresis ratio (night/day)	4.66	0.81 (±0.3)	12.84

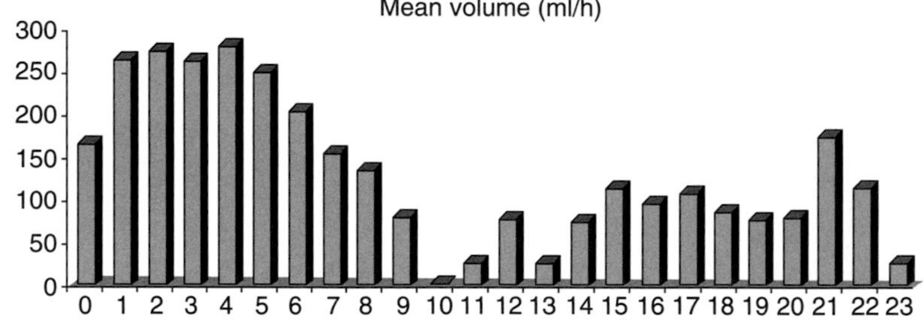

Figure 34.3
Graphic representation of the frequency–volume chart of a patient with significant nocturnal polyuria.

mean voided volumes of 83 and 243 ml, respectively (Figure 34.4). The functional bladder capacity was 395.74 ml in daytime and 709.77 ml during the night. This significant difference between mean voided volumes in the absence of an unstable bladder suggested sensory urgency.

Effect of neuromodulation

A 29-year-old female was investigated because of a significant increase in day and night urinary frequency, associated with urgency, but she did not complain of incontinence. She claimed daytime voidings every 20 min and about 15 micturitions per night. Endoscopy was unremarkable, the cystoscopic capacity being 250 ml. Multichannel urodynamics failed to reveal uninhibited detrusor contractions during the filling phase. Cystometric capacity was 220 ml and the first desire to void occurred at a 42 ml volume in the bladder. The urethra was hypertonic (maximal urethral closing pressure: 104 cmH_2O).

The 7-day frequency–volume chart (Table 34.9) showed a normal 24-hour corrected urine output (1267 ml; Z-value: 0.53) and a normal night/day diuresis ratio (0.50;

Table 34.8 *Sensory urgency (for details see text)*

Parameter	Patient's data (±1 SD)	Normal (±1 SD)	Z-value
Day:			
Mean voided volume (ml)	83 (63)	237 (±67)	(2.30)
Voiding frequency	14.14 (1.55)	5.63 (±1.26)	6.76
Diuresis (ml/min)	0.90	1.11 (±0.35)	(0.59)
Corrected diuresis (ml/min)	1.14	1.11 (±0.35)	0.08
Interval between micturitions (min)	92 (413)	222 (±60)	(2.17)
Output (ml)	866 (256)	1005 (±497)	(0.28)
Corrected output (ml)	1092 (237)	1005 (±497)	0.17
Maximal voided volume (ml)	295.74		
Night:			
Mean voided volume (ml)	243 (197)	379 (±132)	(1.03)
Voiding frequency	1.86 (0.35)	0.08 (±0.16)	11.11
Diuresis (ml/min)	1.44	0.84 (±0.27)	2.24
Corrected diuresis (ml/min)	1.44	0.84 (±0.27)	2.24
Interval between micturitions (ml)	168 (203)	454 (±50)	(5.72)
Output (ml)	693 (243)	409 (±130)	2.18
Corrected output (ml)	693 (243)	409 (±130)	2.18
Maximal voided volume (ml)	709.77		
Output in 24 hours (ml)	1559	1473 (±386)	0.22
Corrected output in 24 hours (ml)	1784	1473 (±386)	0.81
Diuresis ratio (night/day)	1.60	0.81 (±0.3)	2.63

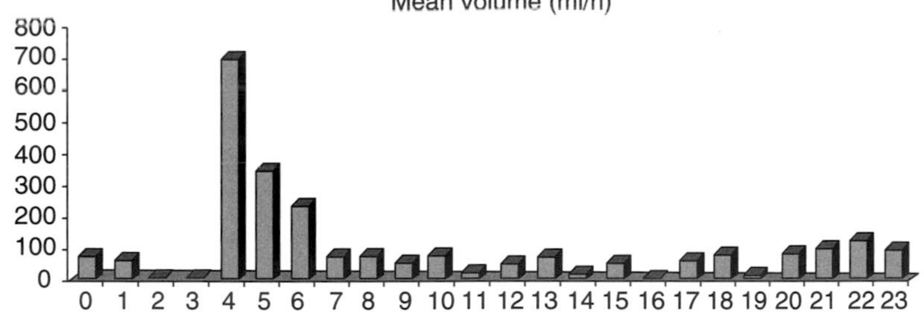

Figure 34.4
Graphic representation of the frequency–volume chart of a patient with sensory urgency. For differentiating between urge incontinence and SUI, the frequency of night-time micturition has been shown to be the most discriminating element.[48]

Z-value: 1.04). There was a very important decrease in the mean daytime (40 ml; Z-value: 2.94) and night-time (50 ml; Z-value: 2.49) voided volumes. The voiding frequency was 25.57 during the day, and 4.71 during the night. The functional bladder capacity was 110.00 ml and 80.00 ml, respectively. Graphic representation exhibits almost constant mean voided volumes throughout the 24-hour period (Figure 34.5).

Dramatic changes were observed in the different parameters of the frequency–volume chart during percutaneous nerve stimulation (Table 34.10). Despite an increase in the corrected 24-hour urinary output (1623 ml; Z-value: 0.39), the night/day ratio did not change (0.43; Z-value: 0.39). The mean daytime voided volume increased significantly (184 ml; Z-value: 0.79), as did the mean night-time voided volume (219 ml; Z-value: 1.21). Nocturia almost completely disappeared (0.29; Z-value: 1.29), as can also be seen in Figure 34.6. (Note the difference in the y-axis scale between Figures 34.5 and 34.6.) Daytime frequency was reduced by 60% (8.29; Z-value: 2.11). Functional bladder capacity also increased significantly.

Table 34.9 *Pre-neuromodulation (for details see text)*

Parameter	Patient's data (±1 SD)	Normal (±1 SD)	Z-value
Day:			
Mean voided volume (ml)	40	237 (±67)	(2.94)
Voiding frequency	25.57	5.63 (±1.26)	15.83
Diuresis (ml/min)	0.98	1.11 (±0.35)	(0.37)
Corrected diuresis (ml/min)	1.02	1.11 (±0.35)	(0.25)
Interval between micturitions (min)	41	222 (±60)	(3.02)
Output (ml)	943	1005 (±497)	(0.13)
Corrected output (ml)	983	1005 (±497)	(0.04)
Maximal voided volume (ml)	110		
Night:			
Mean voided volume (ml)	50	379 (±132)	(2.49)
Voiding frequency	4.71	0.08 (±0.16)	28.96
Diuresis (ml/min)	0.49	0.84 (±0.27)	(1.30)
Corrected diuresis (ml/min)	0.59	0.84 (±0.27)	(0.92)
Interval between micturitions (ml)	102	454 (±50)	(7.04)
Output (ml)	234	409 (±130)	(1.34)
Corrected output (ml)	284	409 (±130)	(0.96)
Maximal voided volume (ml)	80.00		
Output in 24 hours (ml)	1177	1473 (±386)	(0.77)
Corrected output in 24 hours (ml)	1267	1473 (±386)	(0.53)
Diuresis ratio (night/day)	0.50	0.81 (±0.3)	(1.04)

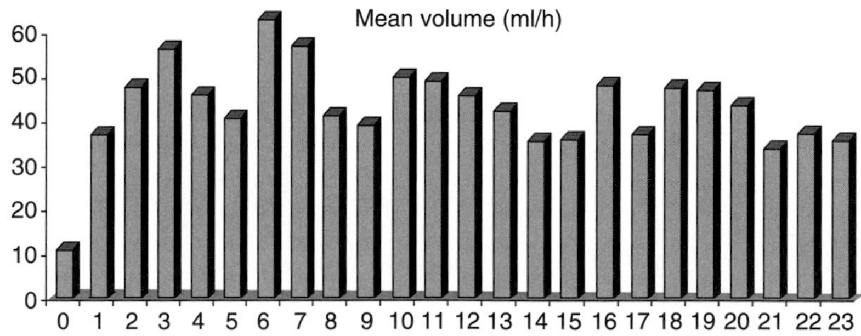

Figure 34.5
Graphic representation of the frequency–volume chart of a patient before testing for neuromodulation.

Conclusion

This overview of the literature on voiding diaries as well as our own experience leads us to the following conclusions. Frequency–volume charts are an invaluable and indispensable tool in the investigation of LUTS patients and in understanding their symptoms. Interpretation of the results is greatly simplified by simple computer software. The commercial unavailability of such software may explain why these charts are not more popular. Presently, in many research protocols, small user-friendly computers are used to ease the completion of frequency–volume charts.

Normal values for women are well known. However, more research should be done to study voiding diaries in children. Reference values for men are desperately needed.

Although the 7-day diary is currently considered the gold standard, comparative studies have begun to determine whether the minimum number of days for a frequency–volume chart completion could be less than 7 and still maintain reliability.

The voiding diary is a precious diagnostic tool, but it cannot guarantee a precise diagnosis. Because of the complex nature of LUT dysfunction, it has become evident that

Table 34.10 *Per-neuromodulation (for details see text)*

Parameter	Patient's data (±1 SD)	Normal (±1 SD)	Z-value
Day:			
Mean voided volume (ml)	184 (73)	237 (±67)	(0.79)
Voiding frequency	8.29 (1.67)	5.63 (±1.26)	2.11
Diuresis (ml/min)	1.21	1.11 (±0.35)	0.27
Corrected diuresis (ml/min)	1.40	1.11 (±0.35)	0.82
Interval between micturitions (min)	153 (506)	222 (±60)	(1.15)
Output (ml)	1158 (371)	1005 (±497)	0.31
Corrected output (ml)	1342 (371)	1005 (±497)	0.68
Maximal voided volume (ml)	400.00		
Night:			
Mean voided volume (ml)	219 (15)	379 (±132)	(1.21)
Voiding frequency	0.29 (1.70)	0.08 (±0.16)	1.29
Diuresis (ml/min)	0.52	0.84 (±0.27)	(1.18)
Corrected diuresis (ml/min)	0.59	0.84 (±0.27)	(0.94)
Interval between micturitions (ml)	420 (660)	454 (±50)	(0.68)
Output (ml)	250 (134)	409 (±130)	(1.22)
Corrected output (ml)	281 (199)	409 (±130)	(0.98)
Maximal voided volume (ml)	200.00		
Output in 24 hours (ml)	1408	1473 (±386)	(0.17)
Corrected output in 24 hours (ml)	1623	1473 (±386)	0.39
Diuresis ratio (night/day)	0.43	0.81 (±0.3)	(1.26)

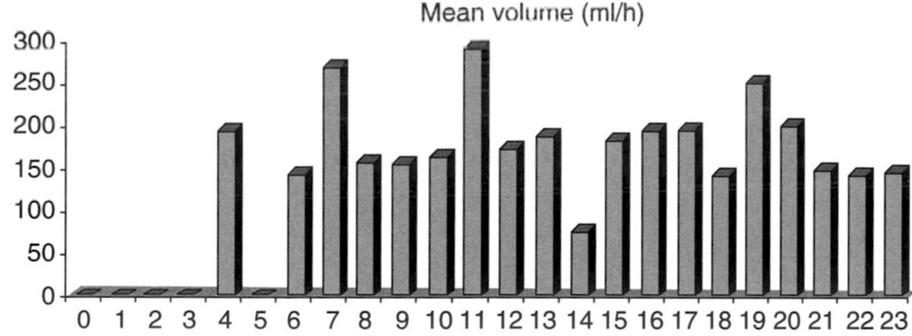

Figure 34.6
Graphic representation of the frequency–volume chart of the same patient as in Figure 34.5, but during neuromodulation.

frequency–volume charts by themselves will never replace urodynamic studies.

In addition to their value as a diagnostic tool, frequency–volume charts play an important role in evaluating the success of a surgical intervention (i.e. neuromodulation) or during follow-up of medical therapy.

In summary, the frequency–volume chart, although frequently overlooked, is a simple, objective, and noninvasive test for evaluating the function of the lower urinary tract. Although not perfect, it has proven its utility in the clinic and in research. It is presently part of most countries' guidelines for incontinence studies.[49]

References

1. Quinn P, Goka J, Richardson H. Assessment of an electronic daily diary in patients with overactive bladder. BJU Int 2003; 91: 647–52.
2. Abrams P, Klevmark B. Frequency–volume charts: an indispensable part of lower urinary tract assessment. Scand J Urol Nephrol Suppl 1996; 179: 47–53.
3. Abrams P, Cardozo L, Fall M et al. The standardization of terminology of lower urinary tract function: report from the standardization sub-committee of the International Continence Society. Neurourol Urodyn 2002; 21: 167–78.
4. McCormack M, Infante-Rivard C, Schick E. Agreement between clinical methods of measurement of frequency and functional bladder capacity. Br J Urol 1992; 69: 17–21.

5. Siltberg H, Larsson G, Victor A. Frequency/volume chart: the basic tool for investigating urinary symptoms. Acta Obstet Gynecol Scand 1997; 76(Suppl 166): 24–7.
6. Kassis A, Schick E. Frequency–volume chart pattern in a healthy female population. Br J Urol 1993; 72: 708–10.
7. Duncan RC, Knapp RG, Miller MC III. Introductory Biostatistics for the Health Sciences. New York: John Wiley & Sons, 1977.
8. Fitzgerald MP, Brubaker L. Variability of 24-hour voiding diary variables among asymptomatic women. J Urol 2003; 169: 207–9.
9. Bloom DA, Seeley WW, Ritchey ML et al. Toilet habits and continence in children: an opportunity sampling in search of normal parameters. J Urol 1993; 149: 1087–90.
10. Mattsson SH. Voiding frequency, volumes and intervals in healthy schoolchildren. Scand J Urol Nephrol 1994; 28: 1–11.
11. Wan J, Kaplinsky R, Greenfield S. Toilet habits of children evaluated for urinary tract infection. J Urol 1995; 154: 797–9.
12. Hellström AL, Hanson E, Hansson S et al. Micturition habits and incontinence in 7-year-old Swedish school entrant. Eur J Pediatr 1990; 149: 434–7.
13. Esperanca M, Gerrard JW. Nocturnal enuresis: studies in bladder function in normal children and enuretics. Can Med Assoc J 1969; 101: 324–7.
14. Bower WF, Moore KH, Adams RD et al. Frequency–volume chart data from incontinent children. Br J Urol 1997; 80: 658–62.
15. Mattsson S, Lindström S. Diuresis and voiding pattern in healthy schoolchildren. Br J Urol 1995; 76: 783–9.
16. Larsson G, Victor A. Micturition patterns in a healthy female population, studied with a frequency/volume chart. Scand J Urol Nephrol 1988; 114(Suppl 114): 53–7.
17. Saito M, Kondo A, Kato T et al. Frequency–volume charts comparison of frequency between elderly and adult patients. Br J Urol 1993; 72: 38–41.
18. Boedker A, Lendorf A, H-Nielsen A et al. Micturition pattern assessed by the frequency/volume chart in a healthy population of men and women. Neurourol Urodyn 1989; 8: 421–2.
19. Matthiesen TB, Rittig S, Norgaard JP et al. Nocturnal polyuria and natriuresis in male patients with nocturia and lower urinary tract symptoms. J Urol 1996; 156: 1292–9.
20. Amundsen CL, Parsons M, Tissot B et al. Bladder diary measurements in asymptomatic females: functional bladder capacity, frequency, and 24-hour volume. Neurourol Urodyn 2007; 26: 341–9.
21. Latini JM, Mueller E, Lux MM et al. Voiding frequency in a sample of asymptomatic American men. J Urol 2004; 172: 980–4.
22. Van Venrooij GE, Eckhardt MD, Boon TA. Data from frequency–volume charts versus maximum free flow rate, residual volume, and voiding cystometric estimated urethral obstruction grade and detrusor contractility in men with lower urinary tract symptoms suggestive of benign prostatic hyperplasia. Neurourol Urodyn 2002; 21: 450–6.
23. Blanker MH, Groeneveld FP, Bohnen AM et al. Voided volumes: normal values and relation to lower urinary tract symptoms in elderly men: a community-based study. Urology 2001; 57: 1093–8.
24. Blanker MH, Bernsen RM, Bosch JL et al. Relation between nocturnal voiding frequency and nocturnal urine production in older men: a population-based study. Urology 2002; 60: 612–16.
25. Blanker MH, Bernsen RM, Ruud Bosch JL et al. Normal values and determinants of circadian urine production in older men: a population-based study. J Urol 2002; 168: 1453–7.
26. Abrams P. Urodynamics, 2nd edn. London: Springer-Verlag, 1997.
27. Barnick C, Cardozo L. Unpublished data quoted by Barnick C. In: Cardozo L, ed. Urogynecology. London: Churchill Livingstone, 1997: 101–7.
28. Sommer P, Bauer T, Nielsen KK et al. Voiding patterns and prevalence of incontinence in women. A questionnaire survey. Br J Urol 1990; 66: 12–15.
29. Wyman JF, Choi SC, Harkins SW et al. The urinary diary in evaluation of incontinent women. A test-retest analysis. Obstet Gynecol 1988; 71: 812–17.
30. Homma Y, Ando T, Yoshida M et al. Voiding and incontinence frequencies: variability of diary data and required diary length. Neurourol Urodyn 2002; 21: 204–9.
31. Gisolf KW, van Venrooij GE, Eckhardt MD et al. Analysis and reliability of data from 24-hour frequency–volume charts in men with lower urinary tract symptoms due to benign prostatic hyperplasia. Eur Urol 2000; 38: 45–52.
32. Matthiessen TB, Rittig S, Mortensen JT et al. Nocturia and polyuria in men referred with lower urinary tract symptoms, assessed using a 7-day frequency–volume chart. BJU Int 1999; 83: 1017–22.
33. van Melick HH, Gisolf KW, Ecjhardt MD et al. One 24-hour frequency–volume chart in a woman with objective urinary motor urge incontinence is sufficient. Urology 2001; 58: 188–92.
34. Locher JL, Goode PS, Roth DL et al. Reliability assessment of the bladder diary for urinary incontinence in older women. J Gerontol A Biol Sci Med Sci 2001; 56: M32–5.
35. Nygaard I, Holcomb R. Reproducibility of the seven-day voiding diary in women with stress urinary incontinence. Int Urogynecol J Pelvic Floor Dysfunc 2000; 11: 15–17.
36. Schick E, Jolivet-Tremblay M, Dupont C et al. Frequency–volume chart: the minimum number of days required to obtain reliable results. Neurourol Urodyn 2003; 22: 92–6.
37. Ku JH, Jeong IG, Lim DJ et al. Voiding diary for the evaluation of urinary incontinence and lower urinary tract symptoms: prospective assessment of patient compliance and burden. Neurourol Urodyn 2004; 23: 331–5.
38. Yap T, Cromwell D, Emberton M. A systematic review of the reliability of frequency–volume charts in urological research and its implication for the optimum chart duration. BJU Int 2007; 99: 9–16.
39. Palnaes Hansen C, Klarskov P. The accuracy of the frequency–volume chart: comparison of self-reported and measured volumes. Br J Urol 1998; 81: 709–11.
40. Robinson D, McGlish DK, Wyman JF et al. Comparison between urinary diaries completed with and without intensive patient instructions. Neurourol Urodyn 1996; 15: 143–8.
41. Groutz A, Blaivas JG, Chaikin DC et al. Non-invasive outcome measures of urinary incontinence and lower urinary tract symptoms: a multicenter study of micturition diary and pad tests. J Urol 2000; 164: 698–701.
42. Bailey R, Shepherd A, Trike B. How much information can be obtained from frequency–volume charts? Neurourol Urodyn 1990; 9: 382–5.
43. Larsson G, Victor A. The frequency–volume chart in genuine stress incontinent women. Neurourol Urodyn 1992; 11: 23–31.
44. Larsson G, Abrams P, Victor A. The frequency–volume chart in detrusor instability. Neurourol Urodyn 1991; 10: 533–43.
45. Fink D, Perucchini D, Schaer GN et al. The role of the frequency–volume chart in the differential diagnosis of female urinary incontinence. Acta Obstet Gynecol Scand 1999; 78: 254–7.
46. Tincello DG, Richmond DH. The Larsson frequency/volume chart is not a substitute for cystometry in the investigation of women with urinary incontinence. Int Urogynecol J Pelvic Floor Dysfunct 1998; 9: 391–6.
47. Schick E. The objective assessment of the resistance of the female urethra to stress: a scale to establish the degree of urethral incompetence. Urology 1985; 26: 518–26.
48. Chapple CR, Wein AJ, Artibani W et al. A critical review of diagnostic criteria for evaluation of patients with symptomatic stress urinary incontinence. BJU Int 2005; 95: 327–34.
49. Corcos J, Gajewski J, Heritz D et al. Canadian Urological Association guidelines on urinary incontinence. Can J Urol 2006; 13: 3127–38.

35

The pad-weighing test

Martine Jolivet-Tremblay and Erik Schick

Introduction

Incontinence is not easy to quantify from patient interview or clinical examination.[1] Urinary incontinence, as defined by the International Continence Society (ICS) in 1988, is involuntary urine loss that is a social or hygienic problem.[2] This definition has been more recently modified[3] to state simply that 'urinary incontinence is the complaint of any involuntary leakage of urine'. This modification became necessary because the previous definition related to a complaint on quality of life issues. Quality of life instruments have been and are being developed in order to assess the impact of both incontinence and other lower urinary tract symptoms on patients.[4] The importance of this condition, as perceived by the patient, differs widely from one individual to another. Some patients cannot accept the loss of a few drops of urine happening only during some specific, often limited, circumstance, whereas others wear diapers for years before seeking medical advice.

The role of the pad-weighing test is to quantify urine loss. However, it does not evaluate the impact a given degree of incontinence has on the patient's quality of life. The Urodynamic Society recommended the use of the pad-weighing test in the pretreatment evaluation of incontinent patients as well as their post-treatment evaluation at each follow-up visit.[5] However, the Urodynamic Society did not specify the type of pad test to be used. On the other hand, the Agency for Health Care Policy and Research of the US Department of Health and Human Services did not mention the pad test for the identification and evaluation of urinary incontinence.[6] It is a tool that can be used for specific issues during the diagnostic process.

The aim of a diagnostic tool is its utility in clinic to make therapeutic decisions. Paick et al[7] tried to determine whether the severity of incontinence, measured objectively by the pad test, correlated with urethral parameters and, also, if it influenced the patient's clinical outcome. Two hundred and seventy-four female patients who had undergone a tension-free vaginal tape procedure between March 1999 and May 2003 were retrospectively reviewed. The 1-hour pad test was carried out as recommended by the International Continence Society, with some modification. On linear regression analysis, the Valsalva leak-point pressure (VLPP) was the only explanatory variable influencing the objective incontinence severity. The group of patients who failed had a more severe preoperative objective severity than the cured group. The findings suggest that the amount of urine leakage as measured during the pad test may be associated with the clinical outcome, after anti-incontinence surgery.

Abdel-Fattah et al[8] questioned the utility of this test in clinical practice. In a prospective cohort study they enrolled 90 female patients awaiting surgery for urodynamic stress urinary incontinence. The patients classified themselves on a 4-point scale (0: totally continent to urine, 1: mild/occasional urinary incontinence (UI), 2: moderate UI, 3: severe UI). They completed the King's Health Questionnaire (KHQ) and carried out the standard International Continence Society 1-hour pad test. A pad gain >1 g was considered a positive result. The women's self-assessment of UI (continent vs incontinent) had a good correlation with the pad test result (negative vs positive), and correlated well with the KHQ scores. This study suggests that simply asking a woman if she is continent for urine or not is as good as doing the pad test, and correlated better with the patient's quality of life.

Karantanis et al[9] also examined this assumption. They compared the International Consultation on Incontinence Questionnaire–Short Form (ICIQ-SF) and the 24-hour pad test with other measures that assess the severity of urine loss in women with urodynamic stress urinary incontinence. They found a strong correlation between the ICIQ-SF and the 24-hour pad test, and both also correlated with the mean frequency of urinary loss on a 3-day frequency–volume chart.

The result of a pad test can influence the treatment decision. In a study by Thomson and Tincello,[10] members of the International Continence Society in the United Kingdom were randomized to receive a scenario comprising clinical and urodynamic data of a woman with urodynamic stress incontinence, including a 1-hour pad loss of either 42 g (large loss) or 7 g (small loss). Members were

Table 35.1 *Discrimination between continence and incontinence*

Length of test	Authors	Suggested value for continence	Comments
No time	Hahn and Fall[11]	0 g	–
40 min	Martin et al[62]	<2 g	(With 75% of cystometric capacity)
1 hour	Kroman-Andersen et al[50]	≤1g	–
	Sutherst et al[1]	1 g	–
	Versi and Cardozo[63]	<0.94 g	–
	Ali et al[55]	<0.5g	–
2 hours	Walsh and Mills[65]	1.2 g (< 1.35 g)/2 hours	
2 4 hours	Mouritzen et al[60]	<5 g/24 hours	
	Lose et al[57]	4 g/24 hours	(max: 8 g)
	Versi et al[55]	7.13 g (<4.32 g)/24 hours	(95% upper confidence level < 15)
	Griffiths et al[12]	≤ 10 g/24 hours	

Reproduced with permission from Schick E, Jolivet-Tremblay M. Detection and quantification of urine loss: the pad-weighing test. In: Corcos J, Schick E, eds. The Urinary Sphincter. New York: Marcel Dekker, 2001: 276.

asked to indicate their initial management choice from a list of four options. Among the 72% who responded, significantly more opted for a surgical treatment in patients with a large pad loss, despite the poor reproducibility and reliability of the 1-hour pad test.

These observations suggest the need for further studies to determine the place of the pad-weighing test in the evaluation of the incontinent patient. For the time being, there is no better test described in the literature to quantify urine loss than this test. It should be mentioned, however, that the same amount of urine loss can affect the quality of life of two different people to different degrees.

Discrimination between continence and incontinence

Because perineal pads absorb perspiration, vaginal discharge, etc., results should be interpreted with caution. It is important to determine an upper limit of weight gain by a pad in continent subjects before interpreting pad test results.

Many authors have investigated this issue (Table 35.1). Usually, the extra-urinary weight increase will be directly proportional to the length of the test. In the protocol described by Hahn and Fall,[11] the length of the exercise program is very brief. Each and every gram of increase in the pad weight is considered a urine loss. Continent patients show no pad weight increase at the end of the test. Conversely, Griffiths et al, [12] investigating elderly patients for 10 days, considered a diagnosis of urinary incontinence only if pad weight exceeded 10 g per 24 hours.

The majority of authors estimate that during a 1-hour test the upper limit of pad weight gain in continent subjects is close to 1 g, whereas during a 24-hour test it is between 4 and 10 g, with an upper limit of 15 g in 24 hours. According to these authors, a weight gain of more than 1 g in a single pad or 8 g in 24 hours may be considered significant. It should be remembered, nonetheless, that weight gains less than the above-mentioned limits do not exclude incontinence, and supplementary investigations may be necessary to confirm the diagnosis.[13]

Nygaard and Zmolek[14] carefully assessed the reproducibility of three comparable exercise protocols, their relationship with voided volume, and Pyridium® (phenazopyridine) staining in 14 continent volunteers. The average pad weight gain during these three sessions was 3.19 g (± 3.16 g), with a range of 0.1–12.4 g. Because of the huge difference between subjects, they were unable to find a distinct cut-off value differentiating continence from incontinence. Similar experiences have been reported by others.[15] Adding Pyridium® did not improve the specificity of the test.

Karantanis et al[16] studied 140 continent women to obtain control values for the 24-hour pad test. They found that women lose only 0.3 g of vaginal secretions in 24 hours. This is much lower than previously reported. This might arise from the use of a highly accurate beam balance and the recruitment of a large sample of women with widely varying ages.

Types of pad tests

Pad tests can primarily be divided into two groups: qualitative tests and quantitative tests.

Qualitative tests

The qualitative test uses a substance to color urine orange: e.g. phenazopyridine (Pyridium), 200 mg three times a day. The patient is invited to wear hygienic pads and replace them periodically during normal daily activities. The degree of coloration on the pads is an assessment of incontinence.[17] This test is especially beneficial to document an insignificant urine loss which, however, may be quite bothersome for the patient, or when vaginal secretions cannot be differentiated easily from urinary incontinence.

A different approach was suggested by Mayne and Hilton,[18] who compared the distal urethral electrical conductance test (DUEC) with weighed perineal pads and discovered that the DUEC was extremely sensitive at detecting leakage (sensitivity 97%). Janez et al[19] reported similar observations.

Quantitative tests

One of the initial efforts to quantify urine loss, interestingly, involved an electric device, the so-called Urilos system, designed by James et al.[20] It incorporates a pad containing dry electrodes. The urinary electrolytes alter the capacitance of the aluminum strip electrodes in the pad proportionally to the quantity of urine. Stanton and coworkers[21,22] investigated this device in greater detail. They noticed problems with reproducibility in different groups. In a group of 26 women exhibiting symptoms of urinary incontinence with a negative stress test 9 proved leakage. In a further group of 30 patients with symptoms of stress incontinence, one-third had a negative clinical stress test, but presented leakage with the Urilos system. Eadie et al[23] concluded that the system was beneficial to confirm patient histories, in spite of the fact that it was laborious to achieve a quantitative measure of urine loss, particularly for volumes greater than 50 ml when the error range reached 35%. Presumably because of a lack of reliability, this device never gained wide acceptance.

A simpler and more efficient approach to the quantification of urine loss is to weigh perineal pads after different lengths of time during which patients are requested to execute standardized activities. This approach has resulted in a relatively large number of publications in which authors have experimented with various test durations, with or without different exercise protocols, in an attempt to define the optimal combination of reproducibility, reliability, and practicality.[24]

Patient populations

Children

Rare reports can be found in the literature on the use of pad tests in the pediatric population.

Hellström et al[25] compared a 2-hour pad test on the ward (with standardized activities and provoked diuresis) with a 12-hour pad test completed in the home environment. Both tests were similar in the detection of urine loss (68 and 70%, respectively), but the detection rate increased in about 10% of the 105 patients when fluid provocation was included in the home pad test.

Imada et al[26] studied 23 incontinent children with a 1-hour pad test, as recommended by the ICS,[2] and compared the results with an interval test during which the pad was utilized between three successive voidings and then weighed. They concluded that the interval test validates the clinical symptoms more appropriately than the 1-hour test. They advocated the former for the objective evaluation of urinary incontinence in children.

Bael et al[27]analyzed the relationship between self-reported and objective data on incontinence, voided volume, and voiding frequency, as part of the European Bladder Dysfunction Study. They concluded that the 12-hour pad test is not sensitive enough to complement self-reported symptoms of urinary incontinence in children with urge syndrome or dysfunctional voiding.

Adults

Many reports on the pad-weighing test for adults have been published in the literature: they vary mainly in the length of time the pad was employed. The short tests last 1 or 2 hours,[28–37] and are generally associated with a standardized exercise or activity program, but there can also be no time limit imposed with only an exercise protocol to follow.[11,38,39] The longer tests go from 12 hours up to 10 days.[12,40–44] Various authors compared tests of different lengths[35–37] or tests done in different environments.[45]

Exercise protocol without a fixed time schedule

The provocative pad test designed by Hahn and Fall[11] involves a sequence of exercises with the bladder filled to half of its cystometric capacity. The test–retest correlation is good ($r = 0.940$). The test takes about 20 minutes to complete. In control groups of clinically continent females, urine loss at the end of the exercise schedule was 0 g. The authors advocated the use of this test in incontinent females. However, because urge symptoms emerge at

Table 35.2 *Short-term pad test*

Authors	Sensitivity (%)	False-negative rate (%)	PPV (%)	NPV(%)	Comments
Anand et al[66]	70	30	92	53	Patients with LUTS
	81	19	91	72	Patients with SUI
Janez et al[67]	–	39.4	–	–	No fixed bladder
Cardozo and Versi[68]	68	32	91	48	No fixed bladder
Schüssler et al[69]	–	56.8	–	–	Fixed bladder
Jorgensen et al[34]	68	32	–	–	–
Lose et al[56]	58	42	–	–	Fixed bladder

PPV, positive predictive value; NPV, negative predictive value; LUTS, lower urinary tract symptoms; SUI, stress urinary incontinence. Reproduced with permission from Schick E, Jolivet-Tremblay M. Detection and quantification of urine loss: the pad-weighing test. In: Corcos J, Schick E, eds. The Urinary Sphincter. New York: Marcel Dekker, 2001:279.

irregular intervals and sometimes in particular situations in patients with bladder overactivity, a test of longer duration, for example 24 hours, seems to be more reliable.

Mayne and Hilton,[38] after filling the bladder with 250 ml of normal saline solution, compared a short pad test program with a 1-hour test in the same population. They could not find a notable difference between the two protocols.

Persson et al[46] proposed a rapid perineal pad test with a standardized bladder volume (300 ml) and a standardized physical activity of only 1 minute. They found the test reproducibility and feasibility acceptable, making it suitable for follow-up studies.

Miller et al[39] suggested the paper towel test to quantify urine loss associated with stress. After three deep coughs, the authors estimated the amount of urine loss by the wet area on a tri-folded paper towel placed on the perineal region. They found the test to be simple, with good test–retest reliability. They recommended its use for losses less than 10 ml because the paper towel becomes saturated with volumes exceeding 15 ml.

Neumann et al[47] investigated the repeatability of a short stress test, the so-called 'expanded paper towel test' (PTT). They measured the size of the wet area in 31 women who performed a provocative test on consecutive days. With the exclusion of one anomalous result, the repeatability proved to lie within 1 ml. They found that the 'expanded PTT' was a simple tool for quantification of urine loss (0.005–8 ml) in women with stress incontinence. The reliability of the test is dependent upon the use of a standard protocol and paper towel with a known volume–area ratio.

The 1-hour test

The 1-hour test is the one most extensively studied, since it was recommended by the Standardization Committee of the ICS.[2] Several authors have examined the reproducibility and reliability of this test. Klarskov and Hald[31] found the test to be reproducible and reliable when compared with subjective daytime incontinence. Jorgensen et al[34] advocated its reproducibility, particularly when bladder volume at the beginning of the test and diuresis during the test were taken into consideration ($r = 0.93$; $p < 0.0001$). When the test was achieved with a standardized bladder volume, the test–retest results were even superior ($r = 0.97$; $p < 0.001$), although personal variations of up to ±24 g were noted.[36]

Mayne and Hilton[38] accomplished the test with 250 ml of fluid in the bladder. Lose et al[32] filled the bladder up to 50% of its cystometric capacity, whereas Kinn and Larsson[48] favored 75%.

The sensitivity of the test (i.e. the proportion of patients with incontinence who have a positive result) varies between 58 and 81%. Its positive predictive values (i.e. the probability of a patient with a positive test being incontinent), which are more relevant to clinical practice, are over 90%. The false negative rate (i.e. incontinent patients with a negative pad test), nonetheless, is quite high (19–56.8%) (Table 35.2).

Simons et al[49] compared two 1-hour tests performed with natural diuresis, 1 week apart. They concluded that, with similar bladder volumes, the test–retest reliability was clinically inadequate, as the first and second pad test could differ by −44 to +66 g.

It appears that the 1-hour test proposed by the ICS is not optimal, and its reliability is weak.[49] This can be improved when bladder volume at the beginning and during the test is known and standardized.

Wu et al[50] tested a shorter pad test. They compared the sensitivity of the 20-minute pad test with a classic 1-hour pad test in women with stress urinary incontinence. One hundred women who underwent a urodynamic study were enrolled and each patient also underwent a 1-hour pad test before the urodynamic study. The infusion of 250 ml water into the bladder in the 20-minute pad test was performed after the urodynamic study. The results showed that the 20-minute pad test had a better sensitivity than the 1-hour one (46% versus 34%, p <0.001) in women with stress urinary incontinence. When the bladder was infused with sufficient quantity of water to elicit a strong desire to void, the latter had a better sensitivity measured by the 20-minute pad test in stress incontinent women (p =0.0004).[51]

The 2-hour test

Some authors proposed extending the test to 2 hours because they felt that its exactitude might be improved. The patient is asked to drink a given amount of water as quickly as feasible at the beginning of the first hour to induce a constant level of diuresis. The pad test itself starts at the second hour and involves a fixed exercise protocol. Richmond et al[37] studied two groups of incontinent patients who were submitted to the same protocol, except that the exercise sequence varied. They found that the sequence in which exercises were accomplished did not affect the overall identification of incontinent patients. They estimated that the ideal length of the test was 2 hours. Haylen et al[52] reached the same conclusions. Eadie et al,[53] comparing the 2-hour pad test with the Urilos system, demonstrated that the 2-hour test did not produce reproducible results, and confirmed that it was difficult to obtain quantitative measures of urine loss with the Urilos system.

The 12-hour test

When medium- or long-term pad tests are examined, it is important to ensure that no significant evaporation takes place between the end of the test and the time the pads are weighed. In an evaporation test, the mean weight loss of the pads, placed in a hermetically closed plastic container, is 0.2 g (0.1–0.3 g) after 24 hours, irrespective of the water volume in the pad. Mean weight loss after 48 hours and 6 days is 0.4 g (0.2–0.7 g) and 0.8 g (0.5–1.2 g), respectively.[54] Versi et al[55] noted no difference in weight after 1 week, and less than a 5% change in weight after 8 weeks (with the upper 95% confidence limit of less than a 10% loss).

The 12-hour test has not been investigated on its own, but has been compared with the 1-hour test by Ali et al,[56] who estimated that the 1-hour pad test on the ward was characteristic of the importance of urinary loss that patients encountered in their home environment. Thus, a 12-hour prolongation was not considered to add clinically relevant information to that obtained during the 1-hour test.

The 24-hour test

This test was examined in detail by Rasmussen et al[54] and found to be reproducible when there are only modest changes in physical activity and diuresis. With extreme reduction of fluid intake or excessive activity, differences in urine loss may be noted. Lose et al[57] compared this test with the 1-hour test. Among 31 stress or mixed incontinent women, 58% were categorized as incontinent with the 1-hour test and 90% with the 24-hour home test. The authors stated that the 24-hour test is effective as a discriminating tool for incontinence, but that its reproducibility is too low to be useful in scientific studies.

Matharu et al[58] compared the 1-hour and 24-hour pad tests in terms of the relationship with reported symptoms and urodynamic diagnosis. There was a significant difference between the proportion of women dry on a 1-hour pad test and those dry on a 24-hour pad test (26.0% versus 38.4%, difference 12.4%; CI 5.5; 19.4). The authors concluded that both pad tests bore little relationship to the underlying urodynamic diagnosis but there was a positive relationship with symptom severity, and they suggested that the 24-hour pad test appears to be clinically a more useful tool than the 1-hour test.

Versi et al[55] examined the 24- and 48-hour tests. Test–retest analysis demonstrated a strong correlation, with coefficients of 0.90 and 0.94, respectively. The reproducibility of the two time schedules was good, suggesting no additional benefit of a prolonged 48-hour test compared with a 24-hour schedule.

Assessing the test–retest reliability of 24-, 48-, and 72-hour pad tests, Groutz et al[59] found that the 24-hour pad test was a reliable instrument for defining the degree of urinary loss. Longer test duration increased reliability, but was associated with decreased patient compliance.

Mouritzen et al,[60] who compared the 1-, 24-, and 48-hour tests, drew similar conclusions. They found that the 1-hour test underestimated the degree of incontinence and related less with clinical parameters than did the 24-hour test. On the other hand, the 24-hour test was as informative as the 48-hour test, making the latter obsolete.

Considering these studies, the 24-hour pad test is considered by many as the gold standard for the quantification of urine loss.

The 48-hour test

The reproducibility of the 48-hour test appeared to be satisfactory (r = 0.90) and equivalent with the 1-hour test. Nevertheless, there was no relationship between these two tests (r = 0.10) according to Victor and Åsbrink.[61] Ekelund et al[43] showed this test can be successfully carried out in the patient's home, even with elderly women.

The elderly

Elderly patients represent a particular challenge to clinicians trying to quantify urine loss. There is a high incidence of urge incontinence among these patients. Also, some of them have notable mental impairment, making the completion of the test difficult. Finally, a number of these patients are unable to perform any formally designed exercise program.

Griffiths et al[12,40,41] studied the pad test thoroughly in the geriatric community. They established that physical examination often failed to show leakage in incontinent patients. The patient's voiding diary and the 1-hour pad-weighing test were often discordant and impractical. In their hands, the 24-hour pad test proved to be the best method to demonstrate and quantify incontinence. Combining this non-invasive test with invasive urodynamics, these authors identified the type of urinary incontinence in 100 elderly patients. They found that the 24-hour test had sufficient reproducibility and good sensitivity (88%) for detecting urine loss, which was mainly nocturnal urge incontinence. Its quantity depended, however, on the preceding evening's fluid intake and on nocturia. They concluded that nocturnal toileting and evening liquid limitation could diminish nocturnal incontinence by a tiny, but profitable, proportion of older patients with extreme urge incontinence.

O'Donnell et al[44] described a procedure which helps nursing personnel to recognize, grade, and register incontinence severity while supervising several patients. This procedure, however, has not been verified for its reproducibility.

Conclusion

From a clinician's perspective, the pad-weighing test is beneficial when the quantity of urine loss is a significant element of management decisions. It is useful in distinguishing urinary incontinence from excessive perspiration or vaginal secretions. In this respect, a 1-hour test, or even a briefer one (20 minutes) may be satisfactory. Under these circumstances, the test must be accomplished with a known bladder volume in order to provide reliable and objective information about the patient's condition.

For scientific and research purposes, the 24-hour pad test should be adopted, since it has good reproducibility, is simple to perform, and is done in the patient's own environment. It is better suited to detect and quantify urine loss secondary to urge incontinence than the 1-hour test. The 24-hour test should be used, along with other parameters, to assess success rates following various treatment modalities.

References

1. Sutherst JR, Brown MC, Richmond D. Analysis of the pattern of urine loss in women with incontinence as measured by weighing perineal pads. Br J Urol 1986; 58: 272–8.
2. Abrams P, Blaivas JG, Stanton SL, Andersen JT. The standardisation of terminology of lower urinary tract function. Scand J Urol Nephrol (Suppl 114): 1988: 5–19.
3. Abrams P, Cardozo L, Fall M et al. The standardisation of terminology of lower urinary tract function: Report from the Standardisation sub-committee of the International Continence Society. Neurourol Urodyn 2002; 21: 167–78.
4. Corcos J, Beaulieu S, Donovan J et al, and members of the Symptom and Quality of Life Assessment Committee of the First International Consultation on Incontinence. Quality of life assessment in men and women with urinary incontinence. J Urol 2002; 168: 896–905.
5. Blaivas JG, Appell RA, Fantl JA et al. Standards of efficacy for evaluation of treatment outcomes in urinary incontinence: recommendations of the Urodynamic Society. Neurourol Urodyn 1997; 16: 145–7.
6. Fantl JA, Newman DK, Colling J et al. Urinary incontinence in adults: acute and chronic management. Clinical Practice Guideline No 2, 1996 Update. Rockville, MD: Department of Health and Human Services. Public Health Service, Agency for Health Care Policy and Research. AHCPR Publication 96–0682, March 1996.
7. Paick JS, Ku JH, Shin JW et al. Significance of pad test loss for the evaluation of women with urinary incontinence. Neurourol Urodyn 2005; 24(1): 39–43.
8. Abdel-Fattah M, Barrington JW, Youssef M. The standard 1-hour pad test: does it have any value in clinical practice? Eur Urol 2004; 46(3): 377–80.
9. Karantanis E, Fynes M, Moore KH, Stanton SL. Comparison of the ICIQ-SF and 24-hour pad test with other measures for evaluating the severity of urodynamic stress incontinence. Int Urogynecol J Pelvic Floor Dysfunct. 2004; 15(2): 111–16.
10. Thomson AJ, Tincello DG. The influence of pad test loss on management of women with urodynamic stress incontinence. Br J Obstet Gynecol 2003; 110(8): 771–3.
11. Hahn I, Fall M. Objective quantification of stress urinary incontinence: a short, reproducible, provocative pad-test. Neurourol Urodyn 1981; 10: 475–81.
12. Griffiths DJ, McCracken PN, Harrison GM, Gormley EA. Relationship of fluid intake on voluntary micturition and urinary incontinence in geriatric patients. Neurourol Urodyn 1993; 12: 1–7.
13. Siltberg H, Victor A, Larsson G. Pad weighing test, the best way to quantify urine loss in patients with incontinence. Acta Obstet Gynecol Scand (Suppl) 1997; 166: 28–32.
14. Nygaard I, Zmolek G. Exercise pad testing test in continent exercisers: reproducibility and correlation with voided volume, pyridium staining and type of exercise. Neurourol Urodyn 1995; 14: 125–9.
15. Ryhammer AM, Djurhuus JC, Laurberg S. Pad testing in incontinent women: a review. Int Urogynecol J Pelvic Floor Dysfunc 1999; 10: 111–15.
16. Karantanis E, O'Sullivan R, Moore KH. The 24-hour pad test in continent women and men: normal values and cyclical alterations. Br J Obstet Gynecol 2003; 110(6): 567–71.
17. Iselin CE, Webster GD. Office management of female urinary incontinence. Urol Clin N Am 1998; 25: 625–45.
18. Mayne CJ, Hilton P. The distal urethral electric conductance test: standardization of method and clinical reliability. Neurourol Urodyn 1988; 7: 55–60.
19. Janez J, Rudi Z, Mihelic M et al. Ambulatory distal urethral electric conductance testing coupled to a modified pad test. Neurourol Urodyn 1993; 12: 324–6.
20. James ED, Flack FC, Caldwell KP, Martin MR. Continuous measurement of urine loss and frequency in incontinent patient. Preliminary report. Br J Urol 1971; 43: 233–7.

21. Stanton SL. Urilos: the practical detection of urine loss. Am J Obstet Gynecol 1977; 128: 461–3.
22. Robinson H, Stanton SL. Detection of urinary incontinence. Br J Obstet Gynecol 1981; 88: 59–61.
23. Eadie AS, Glen ES, Rowan D. The Urilos recording nappy system. Br J Urol 1983; 55: 301–3.
24. Soroka D, Drutz HP, Glazener CM et al. Perineal pad test in evaluating outcome of treatments for female incontinence: a systematic review. Int Urogynecol J Pelvic Floor Dysfunct 2002; 13: 165–75.
25. Hellström AL, Andersen K, Hjälmås K, Jodal U. Pad test in children with incontinence. Scand J Urol 1986; 20: 47–50.
26. Imada N, Kawauchi A, Tanaka Y, Watanabe H. The objective assessment of urinary incontinence in children. Br J Urol 1998; 81(Suppl 3): 107–8.
27. Bael AM, Lax H, Hirche H et al; the European Bladder Dysfunction Study (EC BMH1-CT94-1006). Self-reported urinary incontinence, voiding frequency, voided volume and pad-test results: variables in a prospective study in children. BJU Int 2007; 100: 651–6.
28. Sutherst J, Brown M, Shawer M. Assessing the severity of urinary incontinence in women by weighing perineal pads. Lancet 1981; 1: 1128–9.
29. Murray A, Price R, Sutherst J, Brown M. Measurement of the quantity of urine lost in women by weighing perineal pads. Proc Int Cont Soc Leiden 1982: 243–4.
30. Wood P, Murray A, Brown M, Sutherst J. Reproducibility of a one hour urine loss test (pad test). Proc Int Cont Soc Aachen 1983; II: 515–17.
31. Klarskov P, Hald T. Reproducibility and reliability of urinary incontinence assessment with a 60 min test. Scand J Urol Nephrol 1984; 18: 293–8.
32. Lose G, Gammelgaard J, Jorgensen TJ. The one-hour pad-weighing test: reproducibility and the correlation between the test result, the start volume in the bladder and the diuresis. Neurourol Urodyn 1986; 5: 17–21.
33. Christensen SJ, Colstrup H, Hertz JB et al. Inter and intradepartmental variations of the perineal weighing test. Neurourol Urodyn 1986; 5: 23–8.
34. Jorgensen L, Lose G, Andersen JT. One-hour pad weighing test for objective assessment of female urinary incontinence. Obstet Gynecol 1987; 69: 39–42.
35. Lose G, Rosenkilde P, Gammelgaard J, Schroeder T. Pad-weighing test performed with standardised bladder volume. Urology 1988; 32: 78–80.
36. Donnellan SM, Duncan HJ, MacGregor RJ, Russel JM. Prospective assessment of incontinence after radical retropubic prostatectomy: objective and subjective analysis. Urology 1997; 49: 225–30.
37. Richmond DH, Sutherst RJ, Brown MC. Quantification of urine loss by weighing perineal pads. Observations on the exercise regimen. Br J Urol 1987; 59: 224–7.
38. Mayne CJ, Hilton P. Short pad test: method and comparison with 1-hour test. Neurourol Urodyn 1988; 7: 443–5.
39. Miller J, Ashton-Miller JA, Delancey JOL. The quantitative paper towel test for measuring stress related urine loss. Proc Int Cont Soc Yokohama 1997: 43–4.
40. Griffiths DJ, McCracken PN, Harrison GM. Incontinence in the elderly: objective demonstration and quantitative assessment. Br J Urol 1991; 67: 467–71.
41. Griffiths DJ, McCracken PN, Harrison GM, Gormley EA. Characteristics of urinary incontinence in elderly patients studied by 24-hour monitoring and urodynamic testing. Age Aging 1992; 21: 195–201.
42. Ryhammer AM, Laurberg S, Djurhuus JC, Hermann AP. No relationship between subjective assessment of urinary incontinence and pad test weight gain in a random population sample of menopausal women. J Urol 1998; 159(3): 800–3.
43. Ekelund P, Bergstrom H, Milson I et al. Quantification of urinary incontinence in elderly women with the 48-hour pad test. Arch Gerontol Geriatr 1988; 7: 281–7.
44. O'Donnell PD, Finkbeiner AE, Beck C. Urinary incontinence volume measurement in elderly male inpatients. Urology 1990; 35: 499–503.
45. Wilson PD, Mason MV, Herbison GP, Sutherst JR. Evaluation of the home pad test for quantitative incontinence. Br J Urol 1989; 64: 155–7.
46. Persson J, Bergqvist CE, Wolner-Hanssen P. An ultra-short perineal pad-test for evaluation of female stress urinary incontinence treatment. Neurourol Urodyn 2001; 20: 277–85.
47. Neumann P, Blizzard L, Grimmer K, Grant R. Expanded paper towel test: an objective test of urine loss for stress incontinence. Neurourol Urodyn 2004; 23(7): 649–55.
48. Kinn A, Larsson B. Pad test with fixed bladder volume in urinary stress incontinence. Acta Obstet Gynecol Scand 1987; 66: 369–72.
49. Simons AM, Yoong WC, Buckland S, Moore KH. Inadequate repeatability of the one-hour pad test: the need for a new incontinence outcome measure. Br J Obstet Gynecol 2001; 108: 315–19.
50. Wu WY, Sheu BC, Lin HH. Comparison of 20-minute pad test versus 1-hour pad test in women with stress urinary incontinence. Urology 2006; 68(4): 764–8.
51. Kroman-Andersen B, Jakobsen H, Andersen J. Pad-weighing tests: a literature survey on test accuracy and reproducibility. Neurourol Urodyn 1989; 8: 237–42.
52. Haylen BT, Fraser MI, Sutherst JR. Diuretic response to fluid load in women with urinary incontinence; optimum duration of pad test. Br J Urol 1988; 62: 331–3.
53. Eadie AS, Glen ES, Rowan D. Assessment of urinary loss over a two hour test period: a comparison between Urilos recording nappy system and the weighed perineal pad method. Proc Int Cont Soc Innsbruck 1984: 94–5.
54. Rasmussen A, Mouritzen L, Dalgaard A, Frimond-Moller C. Twenty four hour pad weighing test: reproducibility and dependency activity level and fluid intake. Neurourol Urodyn 1994; 13: 261–5.
55. Versi E, Orrego G, Hardy E et al. Evaluation of the home pad test in the investigation of female urinary incontinence. Br J Obstet Gynaecol 1996; 103: 162–7.
56. Ali K, Murray A, Sutherst J, Brown M. Perineal pad weighing test: comparison of one hour ward pad test with twelve-hour home pad test. Proc Int Cont Soc Aachen 1983; I: 380–2.
57. Lose G, Jorgensen L, Thunedborg P. 24-hour home pad weighing test versus 1-hour ward test in the assessment of mild stress incontinence. Acta Obstet Gynecol Scand 1989; 68: 211–15.
58. Matharu GS, Assassa RP, Williams KS et al. Objective assessment of urinary incontinence in women: comparison of the one-hour and 24-hour pad tests. Eur Urol 2004; 45(2): 208–12.
59. Groutz A, Blaivas JG, Chaikin DC et al. Noninvasive outcome measures of urinary incontinence and lower urinary tract symptoms: a multicenter study of micturition diary and pad tests. J Urol 2000; 164: 698–701.
60. Mouritzen L, Berild G, Hertz J. Comparison of different methods for quantification of urinary leakage in incontinent women. Neurourol Urodyn 1989; 8: 579–87.
61. Victor A, Åsbrink AS. A simple 48-hour test for quantification of urinary leakage in incontinent women. Proc Int Cont Soc London 1985: 507–8.
62. Martin A, Halaska M, Voigt R. Our experience with modified pad weighing test. Proc Int Cont Soc Halifax 1992: 233–4.
63. Versi E, Cardozo L. One hour single pad test as a simple screening procedure. Proc Int Cont Soc Innsbruck 1984: 92–3.
64. Walsh JB, Mills GL. Measurement of urinary loss in elderly incontinent patients. A simple and accurate method. Lancet 1981; 1: 1130–1.
65. Anand D, Versi E, Cardozo L. The predictive value of the pad test. Proc Int Cont Soc London 1985: 290–1.
66. Janez J, Plevnik S, Vrtacnik P. Short pad test versus ICS pad test. Proc Int Cont Soc London 1985: 386–7.
67. Cardozo L, Versi E. The use of a pad test to improve diagnostic accuracy. Proc Int Cont Soc Boston 1986: 367–9.
68. Schüssler B, Hesse U, Horn J, Lentsch P. Comparison of two clinical methods for quantification of stress urinary incontinence. Proc Int Cont Soc Boston 1986: 563–5.

36

Endoscopic evaluation of neurogenic bladder

Saad Aldousari, Jacques Corcos, and Erik Schick

Introduction

Urethrocystoscopy is not useful in the initial evaluation of neurogenic bladder, but becomes very instrumental in the assessment of lower urinary tract complications. Urethrocystoscopy cannot, by any means, give information on lower urinary tract function. For example, external sphincter contractions and relaxation observed during voluntary movement do not reflect the real functional value of this complex unit. Another classic example is the examination of endoscopic aspects of the bladder neck, which cannot replace functional studies for the evaluation of its opening and closing.

Urethrocystoscopy helps in the appraisal of urethral and bladder anatomic anomalies, most of the time secondary to complications such as urethral strictures, trabeculations, bladder stones, and diverticula. The aim of this chapter is to review these different aspects with some illustrations.

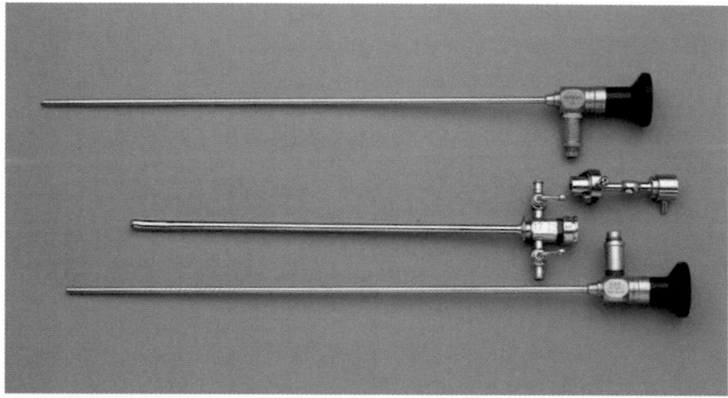

Figure 36.1
Rigid cystoscope.

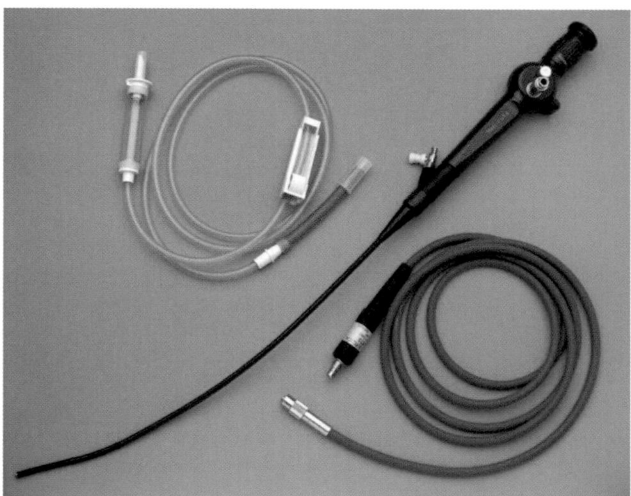

Figure 36.2
Flexible cystoscope.

Equipment

Different companies offer different types and sizes of extremely well-designed, rigid urethrocystoscopes (Figure 36.1), some with fixed lens (12–70°), others with exchangeable lens (0°, 30°, 70°, 120°). The choice of lens depends on the segment of urinary tract that we want to study: 0 or 30° for the urethra and 70 or 120° for the bladder in general.

Since sensitivity is often not a problem in neurogenic bladder patients, rigid urethrocystoscopes are often preferred. They give a much better optical field than flexible cystoscopes (Figure 36.2) and allow various manipulations through a bigger working channel (irrigation, washing, small stone extraction, etc.). Flexible cystoscopes are extremely useful in men with preserved sensitivity, and the test is usually painless. In our experience we do not use any local anesthetic, but only lubricating jelly. Others prefer to inject 2% Xylocaine (lidocaine) jelly transurethrally 2–4 minutes before the procedure. One of the biggest advantages of these cystoscopes is the possibility of introducing them in a supine as well as in a sitting position. Because of their deflection abilities, they allow a retrograde view of the bladder neck as well as the complete exploration of diverticulae, whatever the position.

Technique

Most of the time, the patient is installed in the lithotomy position, but, as mentioned earlier, a supine or a sitting position can be used with a flexible cystocope.

After the usual disinfection of the genitalia with a non-alcoholic solution, draping creates a sterile field around the genitalia.

Once the patient is informed of the beginning of the examination, the cystoscope, lubricated with sterile jelly, is very gently introduced into the meatus. A global view of the urethra permits the confirmation of penile urethra integrity in men. The cystoscope is then pushed forward into the membranous urethra, making the external sphincter visible. This concentric muscle closes the urethra, and can usually be passed by gentle pressure on the cystoscope. The prostatic urethra is then observed, and the anatomy of the prostate is then noted, mainly the size of the lateral lobes and the presence or absence of a median lobe.

Once into the bladder, the technique is slightly different, depending on the type of cystoscope. With a rigid cystoscope, we normally use a 70 or 120° lens. The instrument will have only in–out and rotating motions, allowing a complete view of the bladder without bending the unit, which may cause unnecessary pain and discomfort. With a flexible cystoscope, the same in–out motion is applied, but the rotation motion is replaced by deflections of the instrument's tip, which gives a complete view of the bladder wall. Observation of the ureteral orifices, urine efflux from these orifices, and exploration of bladder diverticulae may be necessary.

Washings, biopsies, etc., are performed at that time if indicated. Once the test is completed, the instrument is gently withdrawn after emptying of the bladder (when using a rigid instrument).

Drinking up to 6–8 glasses of water per day for 3 days is usually recommended and the patient is discharged. No antibiotics are required unless the patient has an artificial heart valve or it is considered necessary by the physician.

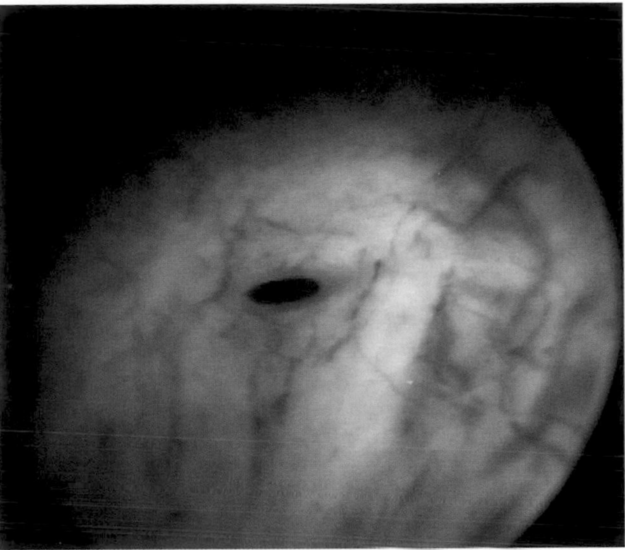

Figure 36.3
Urethral stricture.

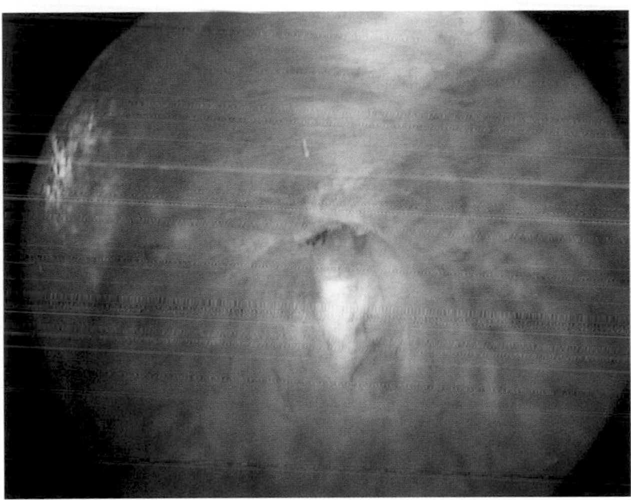

Figure 36.4
Urethral stricture.

Urethrocystoscopic findings

Urethral abnormalities

Urethral strictures

Indwelling catheters, multiple endoscopic manipulations, intermittent catheterizations, and neurogenic trophicity changes lead to frequent urethral strictures and false passages (Figures 36.3 and 36.4). For instance, in Goteborg, Sweden, a study was carried out to identify complications of clean intermittent catheterization in males and young boys with neurogenic bladder dysfunction. Major urethral lesions were seen on cystoscopy, and included urethral stricture, false passages, and meatal stenosis.[1]

Strictures can be short and sometimes easy to break just with the cystoscope, or solid, long and tight enough to not allow the cystoscope to pass through. Neglected, they can generate urethral diverticulae and urethroscrotal and urethrocutaneous fistulae.

Bladder neck cystoscopic evaluation

The degree of opening of the neurogenic bladder neck cannot be adequately evaluated by cystoscopy. False results can be induced by irrigation flow. These changes are dynamic and not anatomic. They should be evaluated by videourodynamic or simple voiding cystogram. In fact, a voiding cystourethrography (VCUG) might provide a tremendous amount of information useful in identifying multiple complications such as trabeculations, sacculations, diverticulae, vesicoureteric reflux, and postvoid residual, as well as the bladder's ability to empty.[2]

However, after bladder neck incision or resection to decrease bladder neck resistance, bladder neck strictures can be easily seen by cystoscopy, but, here again, their real impact on bladder function can be assessed only by voiding cystogram.

Endoscopic evaluation of urethral stents

Some specialized centers no longer perform incisional sphincterotomies, preferring endoluminal stents instead (i.e. Urolume – AMS). The techniques and results with these stents are detailed in Chapter 57.

It is usually easy to introduce a flexible cystoscope through these stents, which 'disappear' completely after a few months since the device is epithelialized through and in-between its pores: 90–100% of epithelialization of the stent has been demonstrated in 47.1% of cases 3 months after insertion, and in 87.7% of cases 12 months after insertion.

Mild epithelial hyperplasia can occur (34–44.4%) after stent insertion and may look like an obstructed urethra. Much less frequently, these strictures are severe (3.1%), requiring urethrotomy and sometimes insertion of a second stent at the same level as the first.[3]

Occasionally, however, and even several years later, part of the stent may remain visible, but usually does not cause any problems. Calcifications of the stents are rare. No stone formation has been reported.[3]

A study was carried out by Denys and colleagues,[4] in order to evaluate another type of urethral stent, the Ultraflex, for detrusor-sphincter dyssynergia. In that study, endoscopic evaluation proved to be very valuable. The mean follow-up of 39 patients was 1.73 ± 1.11 years. No stone encrustation or stenosis of stent extremities was observed. Nonobstructive granulation tissue was identified in 6.8%. The mean percentage of epithelialization of the stent was 90.8% ± 19.7%. No migration of the stent into the bladder was seen in that study, however minimal displacement of the stent compared to the initial position was observed in 21.7% of cases.

Structural bladder anomalies

The well-balanced bladder of a compliant patient looks normal (Figure 36.5) most of the time. However, it may show significant changes because of patient noncompliance with intermittent catheterization, medication, etc., or these treatments may have no effect.

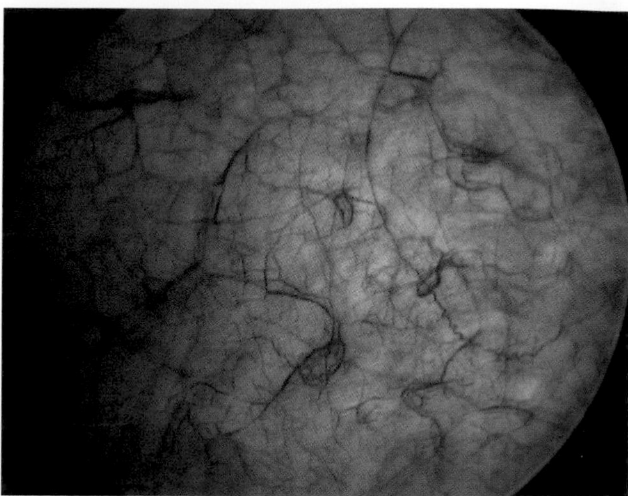

Figure 36.5
Normal bladder mucosa.

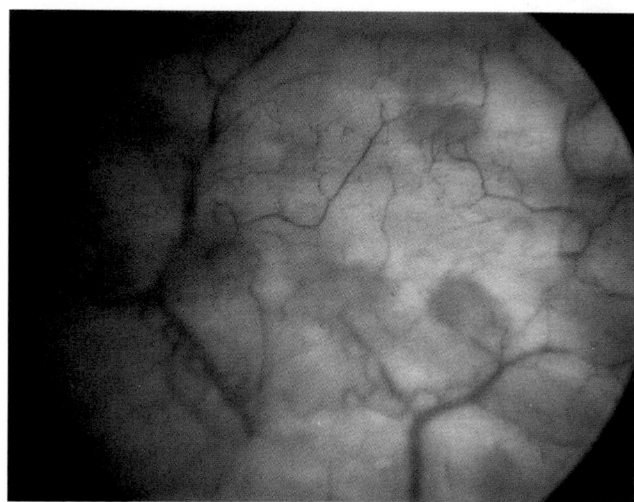

Figure 36.6
Cystitis glandularis.

Bladder wall abnormalities

Often associated with chronic infections but also often not related to any obvious disease, cystitis glandularis (Figure 36.6) and cystitis follicularis (Figure 36.7) can be found during systematic cystoscopic evaluation.

Bladder wall trabeculations

There is no consensus in the literature regarding the significance of bladder wall trabeculations (Figures 36.8 to 36.11). O'Donnell[5] suggested that they could be related to high bladder pressure.[3] To Brocklehurst,[6] McGuire,[7] Shah,[8] and O'Reilly[9] they are secondary to an infravesical obstruction. More authors believe that trabeculations reflect

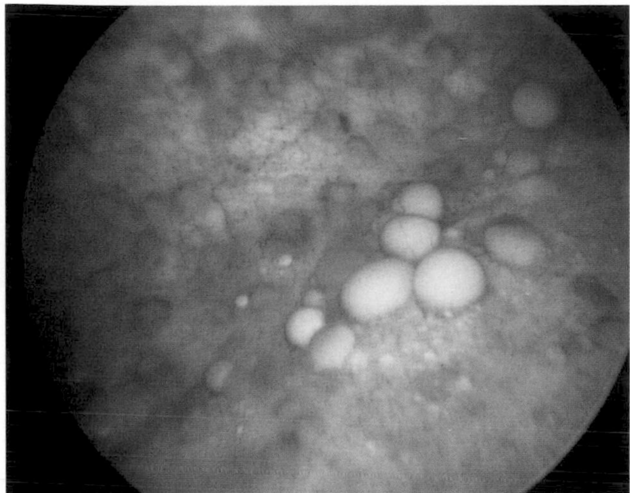

Figure 36.7
Cystitis follicularis.

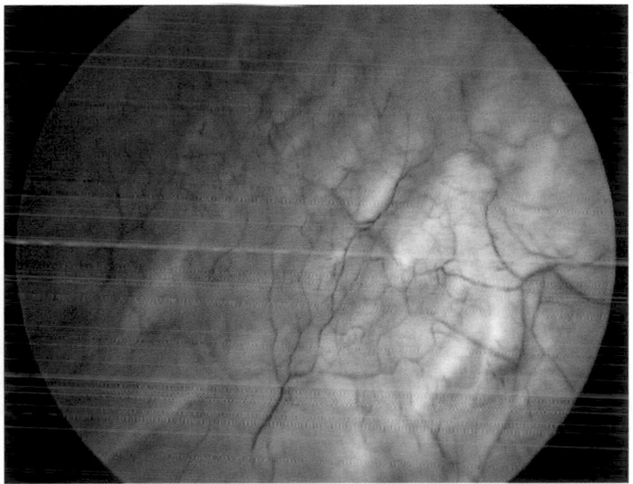

Figure 36.8
Trabeculation grade 1.

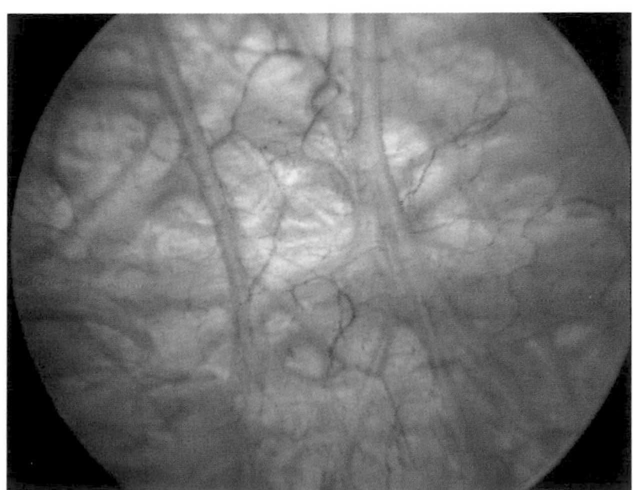

Figure 36.9
Trabeculation grade 2.

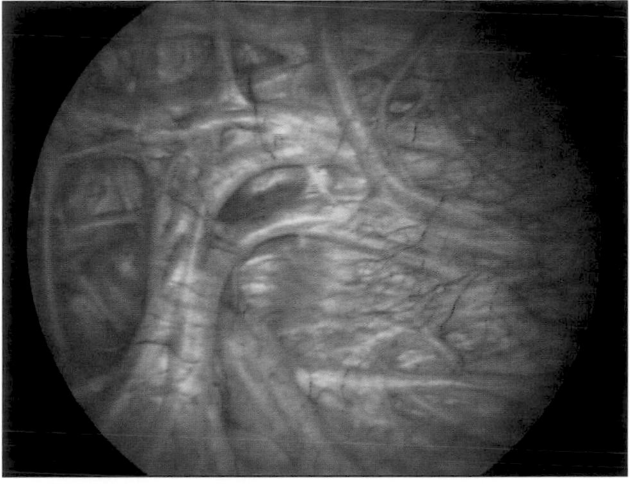

Figure 36.10
Trabeculation grade 3.

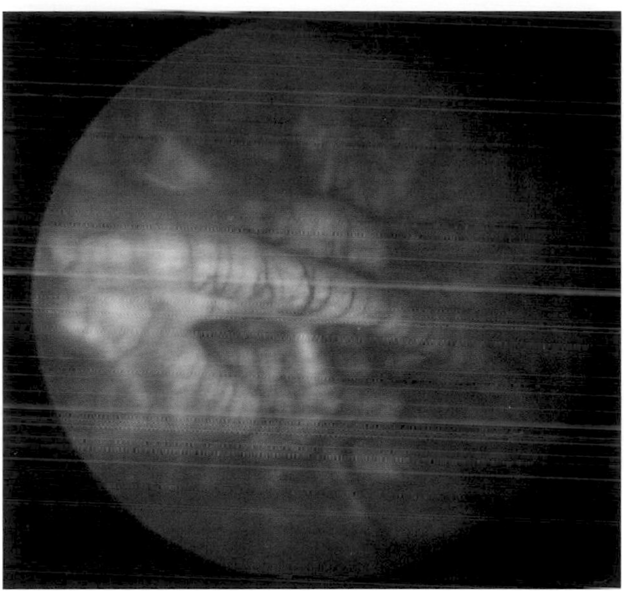

Figure 35.11
Trabeculation grade 4.

bladder overactivity and uninhibited contractions. Schick and Tessier[10] studied the correlation between the endoscopic aspects of bladder walls and urodynamic parameters in 220 women. They concluded that there is a close correlation between trabeculation grade and the percentage of unstable bladders (Figure 36.12).

Ureteral orifices

High bladder pressure, recurrent infections, and changes in bladder wall thickness may provoke alterations in the shape of the ureteral orifices. In some cases, they can look wide open. Their appearance cannot preclude the efficacy of the intramural ureteral valve mechanism and the presence of

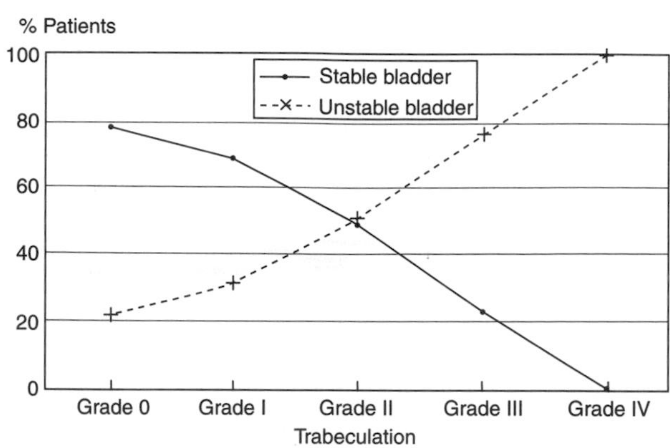

Figure 36.12
Correlation between the trabeculation grade and percentage of unstable bladders.

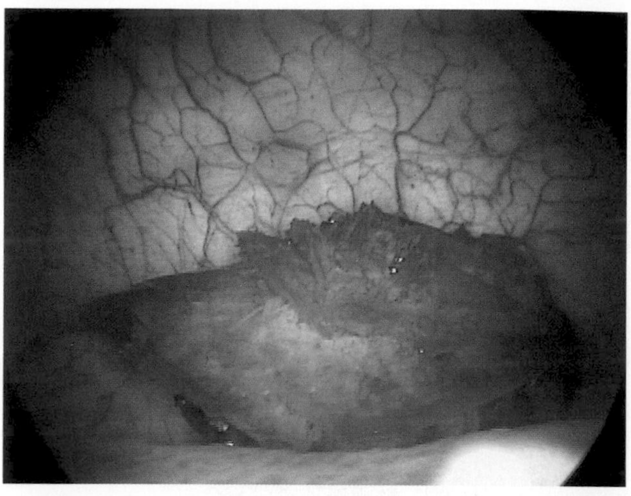

Figure 36.14
Bladder stone.

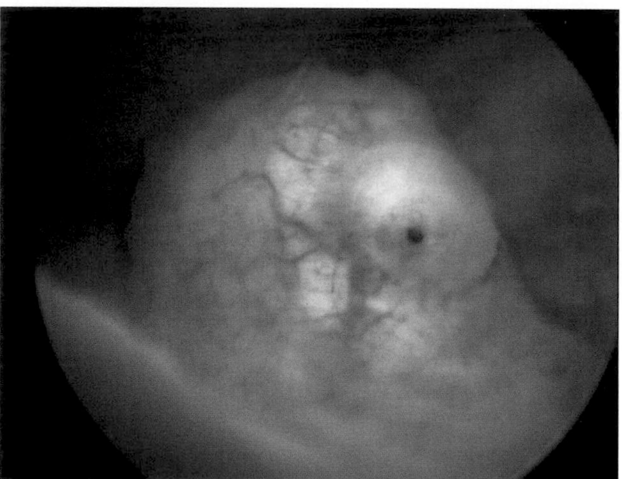

Figure 36.13
Ureterocele.

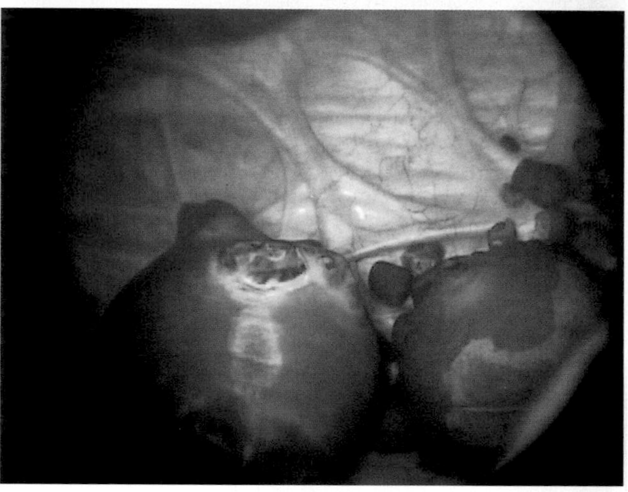

Figure 36.15
Bladder stone.

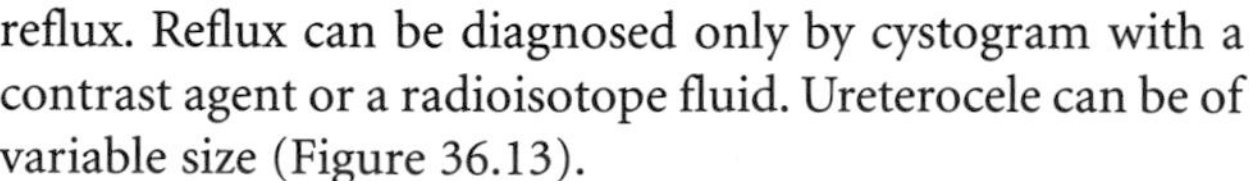

reflux. Reflux can be diagnosed only by cystogram with a contrast agent or a radioisotope fluid. Ureterocele can be of variable size (Figure 36.13).

Tumors, stones, and foreign bodies

Bladder stones

Usually secondary to infections, bladder stones are very frequent findings in neurogenic patients. They must be suspected in cases of recurrent *Proteus mirabilis* infections, increased spasticity or incontinence, elimination of small calcified fragments, etc. They are easy to diagnose by cystoscopy, and sometimes can be crushed for removal in the same set-up. Their aspects are extremely variable, from small, round, single, or multiple stones to huge 'egg-like' stones (Figures 36.14 and 36.15).

Bladder tumors

Patients with chronic indwelling catheters must undergo annual cystoscopic evaluation, which is the only way (with cytology) to detect suspicious lesions such as bladder carcinoma. Usually, these lesions start at the level of the trigone, where the catheter and the balloon lie down. In these patients, there is almost always a small reddish area

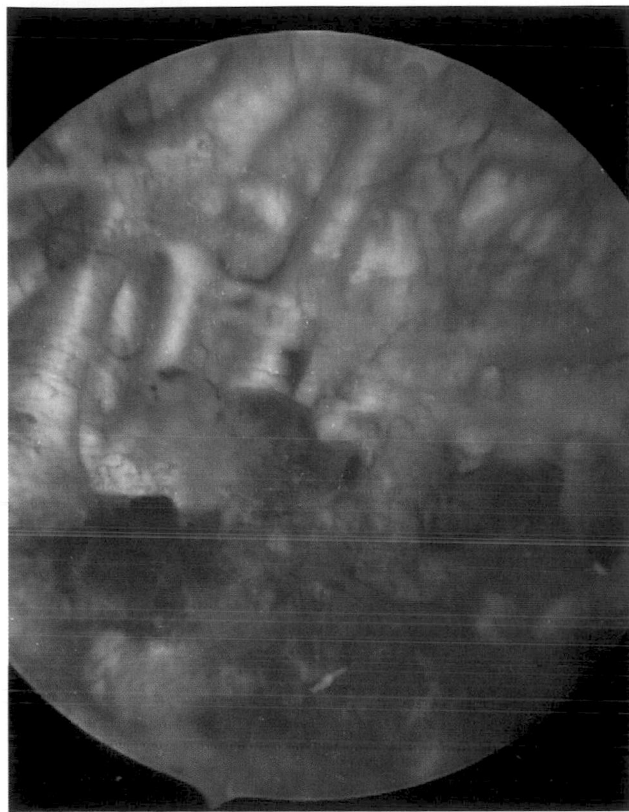

Figure 36.16
Mucosal catheter reaction.

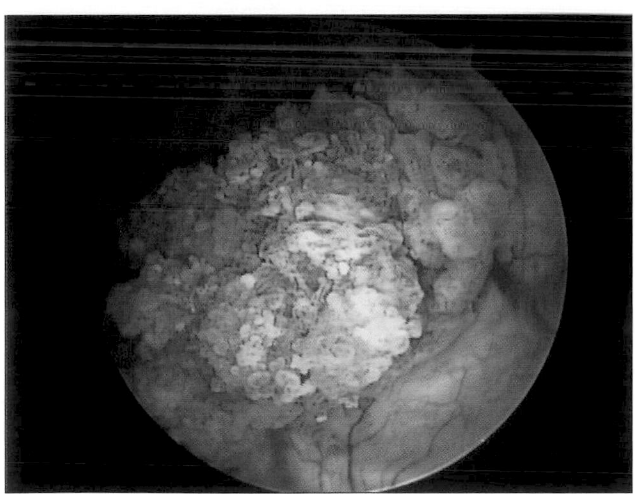

Figure 36.17
Bladder papillary tumor (partially calcified).

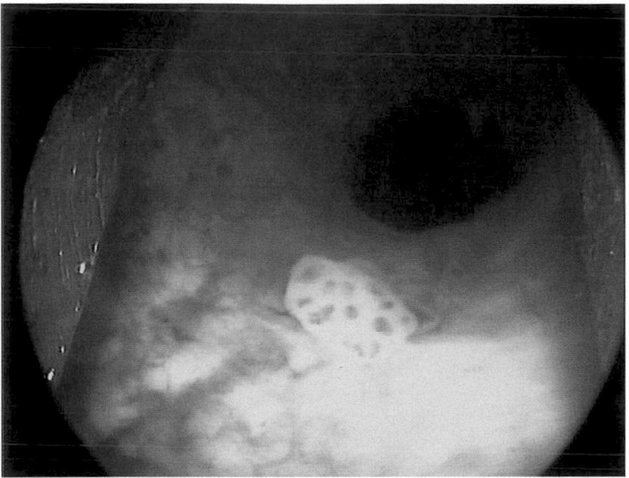

Figure 36.18
Urethral papillary tumor.

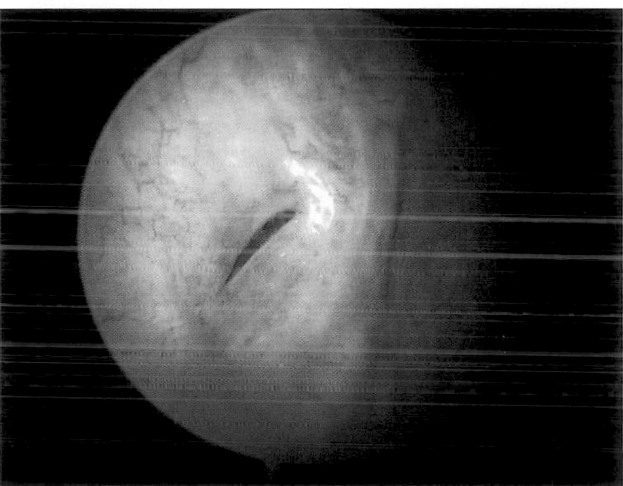

Figure 36.19
Stitch eroding the bladder wall.

which is difficult to differentiate from an early carcinoma (Figure 36.16). Biopsy of these lesions is a simple way of reassuring the physician and patient. Bladder tumors can be located anywhere in the bladder and have different aspects, but most frequently papillary (Figure 36.17). Much less frequent are urethral tumors (Figure 36.18).

Foreign bodies

Foreign bodies are rare. Not infrequently, hairs can be found in patients with intermittent catheterization. Sometimes, they start to be calcified, and always have to be removed. Even less frequently are iatrogenic foreign bodies. Pieces of Foley catheter balloons or sutures from urologic or nonurologic procedures are eroded into the bladder (Figures 36.19 and 36.20).

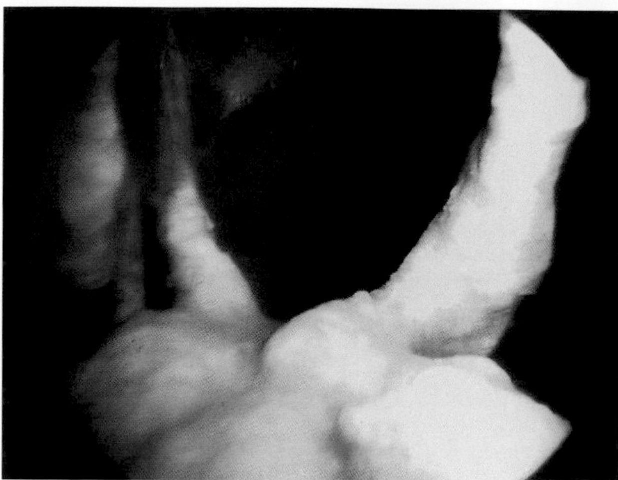

Figure 36.20
Calcified stitch into the bladder.

Conclusion

Urethrocystoscopy must be part of the regular evaluation of neurogenic bladders. It often allows us to understand the patient's worsening lower urinary tract function. Until now, and for most of the changes and abnormalities found by cystoscopy, no other test can replace it with the same accuracy and reliability.

References

1. Lindehall B, Abrahamsson K, Hjalmas K et al. Complications of clean intermittent catheterization in boys and young males with neurogenic bladder dysfunction. J Urol 2004; 172: 1686–8.
2. Palmer LS. Pediatric urologic imaging. Urol Clin N Am 2006; 33: 409–23.
3. Rivas DA, Chancelor MB. Sphincterotomy and sphincter stent prosthesis. In: Corcus J, Schick E, eds. The Urinary Sphincter. New York: Marcel Dekker, 2001: 565–82.
4. Denys P, Thiry-Escudie I, Ayoub N et al. Urethral stent for the treatment of detrusor-sphincter dyssynergia: evaluation of the clinical, urodynamic, endoscopic, and radiological efficacy after more than 1 year. J Urol 2004; 172: 605–7.
5. O'Donnell P. Water endoscopy. In: Rax S, ed. Female Urology. Philadelphia: WB Saunders, 1983: 51–60.
6. Brocklehurst JC. The genitourinary system. In: Brocklehurst JC, ed. Textbook of Geriatric Medicine and Gerontology. New York: Churchill Livingstone, 1978: 306–25.
7. McGuire EJ. Normal function of lower urinary tract and its relation to neurophysiology. In: Libertino IA, ed. Clinical Evaluation and Treatments of Neurogenic Vesical Dysfunction. International Perspectives in Urology. Baltimore: Williams & Wilkins, 1984: 1–15.
8. Shah PJR. Clinical presentation and differential diagnosis. In: Fitzpatrick JM, Krane RJ, eds. The Prostate. Edinburgh: Churchill Livingstone, 1989: 91–102.
9. O'Reilly PH. The effect of prostatic obstruction on the upper urinary tract. In: Fitzpatrick JM, Krane RJ, eds. The Prostate. Edinburgh: Churchill Livingstone, 1989: 111–18.
10. Schick E, Tessier J. Trabeculation de la paroi vesicale chez la femme: que signifie-t-elle? Presented at the 18th Annual Congress of the Association des Urologues du Quebec, Montreal, November 1993.

37

Imaging techniques in the evaluation of neurogenic bladder dysfunction

Walter Artibani and Maria A Cerruto

In the evaluation of neurogenic bladder dysfunction, imaging techniques have the following goals and roles:

- they can suggest a neurogenic etiology in voiding disorders
- they can assess the central nervous system (CNS) in order to confirm and identify the neurogenic lesion, and to relate level and type of neurogenic lesion to bladder dysfunction
- they can evaluate the morphologic status of the lower and upper urinary tract.

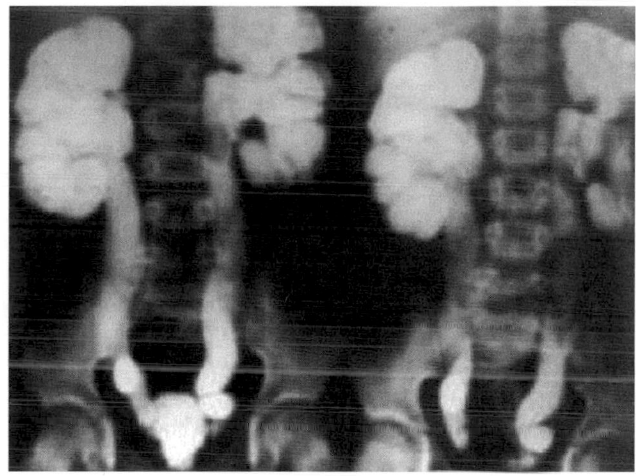

Figure 37.1
Sacral agenesis. Cystography: small retracted bladder and bilateral grade V vesicoureteric reflux.

Imaging techniques suggesting a neurogenic etiology

Lumbosacral spine X-rays

Lower urinary tract (LUT) dysfunction in children, and more rarely in young adults, can be the expression of an underlying spinal dysraphism. In the majority of cases, abnormalities of the gluteosacral region and/or legs and foot are visible (e.g. small dimples, tufts of hair, subcutaneous lipoma, dermal vascular malformations, one leg shortness, high arched foot or feet). However, in some cases these abnormalities may be minimal or absent. A careful evaluation of the anteroposterior and lateral film of the lumbosacral spine can identify vertebral anomalies commonly associated with nervous system anomalies.[1–5]

Sacral agenesis involves the congenital absence of part or all of two or more sacral vertebrae. The absence of two or more sacral vertebrae always implies the presence of a neurogenic bladder dysfunction (Figures 37.1 and 37.2).[6,7]

The significance of spina bifida occulta can vary. Simple failure to fuse the laminae of the 4th and 5th lumbar vertebrae is unlikely to be important, but when the spinal canal is noticeably widened, there may be cord involvement (diastematomyelia, tethered cord syndrome).[8]

Open bladder neck and proximal urethra at rest

Open bladder neck and proximal urethra at rest, during the storage phase, can be observed during cystography, videourodynamics, or bladder ultrasonography, both in patients with and without neurologic diseases.

Distal spinal cord injury has been associated with an open smooth sphincter area, but whether this is due to sympathetic or parasympathetic decentralization or defunctionalization is still unclear.[9]

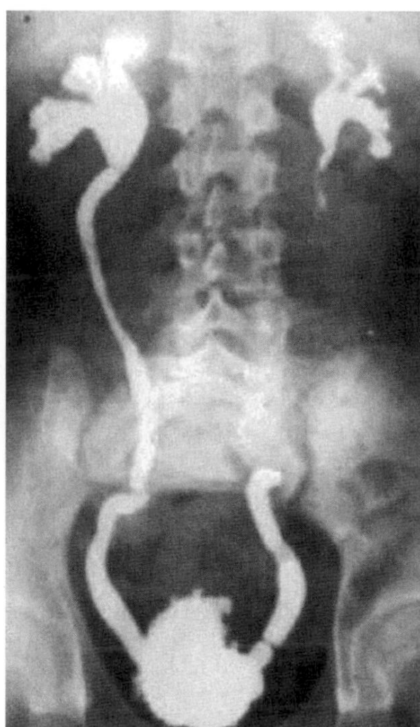

Figure 37.2
Sacral agenesis. Cystography: small sacculated bladder and bilateral grade III vesicoureteric reflux.

A relative incompetence of the smooth sphincter area may also result from interruption of the peripheral reflex arc, which is very similar to the dysfunction observed in the distal spinal cord injury. Twenty-one out of 54 patients with spinal stenosis were found to have an open bladder neck at rest.[10,11]

In a review of 550 patients,[12] 29 out of 33 patients with an open bladder neck had neurologic diseases. Although the association was more commonly seen in patients with thoracic, lumbar, and sacral lesions, when compared to cervical and supraspinal lesions the difference was not significant. Damage of sympathetic innervation to the bladder was also frequently observed in patients undergoing major pelvic surgery, such as abdominal perineal resection of the rectum.

Patients with myelodysplasia showed an inordinately high incidence of open bladder neck (10 out of 18 patients, vs 19 out of 290 with different neurologic disorders).

Patients with sacral agenesis are included in the larger category of myelodysplastic patients and suffer from open bladder neck with areflexic bladder.

Shy–Drager syndrome is a Parkinson-like status with peripheral autonomic dysfunction. A detrusor hyperreflexia (currently named neurogenic detruso overactivity – NDO) is usually found in association with an open bladder neck at rest and a denervated external sphincter.[13]

Peripheral sympathetic injury results in an open bladder neck and proximal urethra from damaged α-adrenergic innervation to the smooth muscle fibers of the bladder neck and proximal urethra.[14] Although it can occur as an isolated injury, this is usually associated with partial detrusor denervation and preservation of sphincter electromyographic (EMG) activity.

The loss of bladder neck closure suggests an autonomic neural deficit. The site and nature of the requisite deficit is unclear. Most authors agree on the importance of the sympathetic system in maintaining the integrity of the bladder neck,[15–19] although some authors have suggested the possible role of parasympathetic innervation.[20,21]

Open bladder neck at rest in children or in women with no neurologic diseases can represent a different disorder, either related to a congenital anomaly or secondary to an anatomic pelvic floor defect. Stanton and Williams[22] described an abnormality in girls with both diurnal incontinence and bed-wetting, based primarily on micturating cystourethrography, in which the bladder neck was wide open at rest. Murray et al[23] reported the 'wide bladder neck anomaly' in 24.5% of the girls (35) and 9.3% of the boys (10) amongst 251 children (143 girls and 108 boys) undergoing videourodynamics for the assessment of non-neuropathic bladder dysfunction (mainly daytime incontinence). The authors considered this anomaly as congenital and made the hypothesis that wide bladder neck anomaly in girls may provide a basis for the development of genuine stress incontinence in later life.

Chapple et al[24] reported that 21% of 25 totally asymptomatic women they investigated by transvaginal ultrasound had an open bladder neck at rest. Versi[25] found a 21% prevalence of open bladder neck at rest in 147 women visiting a urodynamic clinic and suggested that the finding is of little consequence.

Open bladder neck is a key point in defining type III stress incontinence according to the classification of Blaivas and Olsson.[26] This classification is based on history, imaging, and urodynamics, and distinguishes five diagnostic categories of stress incontinence. Incontinence type III is diagnosed by the presence of open bladder neck and proximal urethra at rest in the absence of any detrusor contraction, suggesting an intrinsic sphincter deficiency. The proximal urethra no longer functions as a sphincter. There is obvious urinary leakage, which may be gravitational in nature or associated with minimal increase in intravesical pressure.

In pelvic fracture with membranous urethral distraction defects, when cystography (and/or cystoscopy) reveals an open bladder neck before urethroplasty, the probability of postoperative urinary incontinence may be significant, although the necessity of a simultaneous (or sequential) bladder neck reconstruction is controversial.[27–29]

In summary, when observing an open bladder neck and proximal urethra at rest, during the storage phase, whatever imaging technique is used, it may be worthwhile to evaluate the possibility of an underlying autonomic neural deficit (occult spinal dysraphism, sacral agenesia, post-surgery peripheral neural damage, Shy–Drager syndrome). Previous pelvic trauma or female gender can lead to a different perspective.

In the case of a manifest diagnosed neurogenic disease, open bladder neck and proximal urethra stand for various pathophysiologic situations and require a thorough urodynamic investigation in order to be correctly interpreted (e.g. sympathetic damage, associated detrusor-sphincter dyssynergia, previous endoscopic manipulation).

Imaging techniques assessing the central nervous system

Imaging of the central nervous system, otherwise known as neuroimaging, is a valuable aid in the diagnosis of a variety of CNS diseases which may cause LUT dysfunctions. Computed tomography (CT), magnetic resonance imaging (MRI), single-photon emission computed tomography (SPECT), and positron emission tomography (PET) have been used and reported.

When LUT symptoms are just part of the many symptoms caused by a CNS disease, the diagnosis is made on clinical grounds and neuroimaging is carried out only to confirm it. In rare cases, LUT symptoms are the only presenting symptoms of an underlying neurologic disorder and neuroimaging is instrumental in the diagnosis.

The literature shows an endless list of rare neurologic conditions presenting with different symptoms, including LUT symptoms, in which CT scan, MRI, SPECT, and PET imaging were carried out to identify the underlying CNS disease.

After a cerebrovascular accident, the urodynamic behavior of the lower urinary tract has been correlated to CT pictures of the brain.[30,31]

The presence of significant cerebral lesions has been clearly demonstrated by CT, MRI, or SPECT in the absence of clinical neurologic symptoms and signs in patients complaining of urge incontinence.[32] This can be particularly significant in elderly patients. Griffiths et al,[33] studying 48 patients with a median age of 80 years, reported that the presence of urge incontinence was strongly associated with depressed perfusion of the cerebral cortex and midbrain as determined from the SPECT scan.

Kitaba et al,[34] using MRI, reported subclinical lesions in the brain in 40 out of 43 men more than 60 years old who complained of urinary storage symptoms; of these 40 patients, 23 (57.5%) had detrusor hyperreflexia (NDO).

In spinal cord injured patients, CNS MRI can detect unsuspected cerebral or spinal lesions (ischemic and hemorrhagic areas, syringomyelia, spinal compression, spinal stenoses) which provide explanations for the possible discrepancy between the clinically assessed level of neurologic lesion and the urodynamically observed LUT dysfunction.

Spinal MRI is instrumental in diagnosing a tethered cord syndrome, as a primary disorder due to dural adhesions or as the outcome of previous surgical manipulation of the distal spinal cord.

PET studies provide information on specific brain structures involved in micturition in humans. In men and women who are able to micturate during scanning, an increase in regional blood flow was shown in the dorsomedial part of the pons close to the 4th ventricle, the pontine micturition center (PMC). PET studies carried out in both men and women also showed an activation of the mesencephalic periacqueductal gray (PAG) area during micturition. Based on experiments on cats, this area is known to project specifically to the PMC and its stimulation elicits complete micturition. Experimental interruption of fibers from the PAG to the PMC results in a low-capacity bladder. PET studies during micturition in humans also showed an increased regional blood flow in the hypothalamus, including the preoptical area, which in cats can elicit bladder contractions.[35–37]

MRI is commonly used for diagnosis of multiple sclerosis (MS) and for measuring disease severity. Paradoxically, MRI-determined total lesion load in the brain correlates weakly with disability. The relatively low signal-to-noise ratios of MRI would require averaging data from many individuals, needing two methodologic developments: the registration of different brains into a standard stereotaxic space, and the application of statistical tests to the resultant data to generate so-called statistical parametric maps. Developing an automatic imaging algorithm for lesion detection in MS, Charil et al applied this automatic procedure to the MRI scans of 452 patients with relapsing-remitting MS,[38] demonstrating for the first time a relationship between the site of lesions and any type of disability in a large scale MRI data set in MS. In more detail, the authors found that bowel and bladder disability scores correlated with lesions in the medial frontal lobes, cerebellum, insula, dorsal midbrain, and pons, all areas known to be involved in the control of micturition.

The present functional neuroimaging technology shows great potential to improve our knowledge of nervous functional anatomy in relation to vesicourethral function and dysfunction.

Imaging techniques of the lower and upper urinary tract in neurogenic bladder

Imaging of the lower urinary tract

Imaging of the lower urinary tract in neurogenic bladder dysfunctions aims at visualizing the morphology of the bladder and urethra, locating infravesical obstruction, vesicoureteric reflux, diverticula, fistula, and stones, providing a reasonable assessment of residual urine, and demonstrating leakage.

Bors and Comarr[39] described in detail the use of (video)-cystourethrography, with natural or retrograde filling, with or without ice-cooled contrast medium: the use of ice-cooled contrast medium – iced cystourethrography – can be useful in some suprasacral neurogenic patients in order to elicit detrusor reflex and voiding. Changes are detectable in the urethra (diverticula and fistulae at the level of the penoscrotal junction, or a patulous urethra) and in the bladder (smooth overdistended bladder, trabeculation, wide open bladder neck, bladder asymmetry, 'Christmas Tree' bladder, thickened bladder wall, vesicoureteric reflux, paraureteric diverticula, bladder diverticula) (Figure 37.3). It is worthwhile to reread their description.

In expert hands ultrasonography can provide similar information. Color flow Doppler in combination with conventional B-mode sonography has been shown to be effective for detection and follow-up of vesicoureteric reflux in the neurogenic bladder, as an alternative to cystourethrography.[40]

LUT imaging by ultrasonography or cystourethrography can be performed as a separate test, but it is better performed at the time of urodynamic study (videourodynamics)[41] (Figure 37.4).

Videourodynamics is generally regarded as the 'gold standard' in the evaluation of LUT tract dysfunction. However, whether urodynamic and imaging testing should be performed simultaneously or on separate occasions is still controversial. An interesting tool in the evaluation of LUT function and dysfunction is the association between MRI and urodynamics. The concept of MRI videourodynamics would seem to be feasible and attractive. The combination of function and morphology allows us an innovative view of the pelvic floor, adding to our understanding of the various structure interactions. The development of MRI urodynamic examination gives the possibility to gather the objective functional test of bladder and urethra function provided by urodynamics and the best anatomical images of the pelvic floor offered by MRI together. This functional imaging techniques should currently be used only for research purposes.[42]

Urodynamic examinations must be repeated several times to obtain reproducibility. The more parameters are studied, the more complicated the examination becomes, with a correspondingly higher risk of bias. Nevertheless, simultaneous videomonitoring, along with tracings of detrusor pressure and possibly of EMG sphincter activity, is an important means to make sure that the imaging is performed at the appropriate times so that the morphologic features can be related to the various functional states.

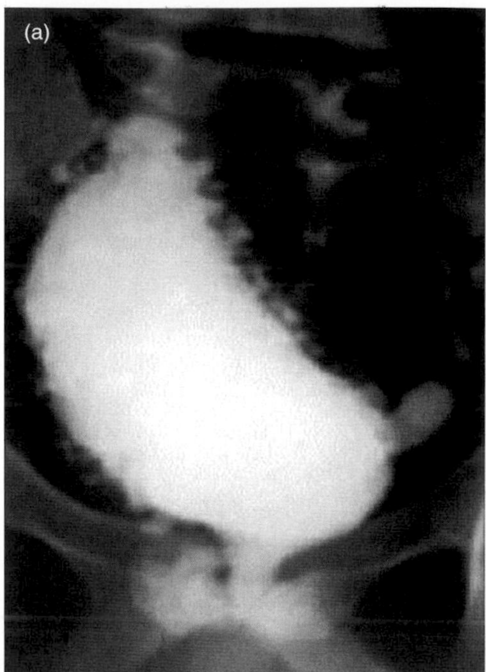

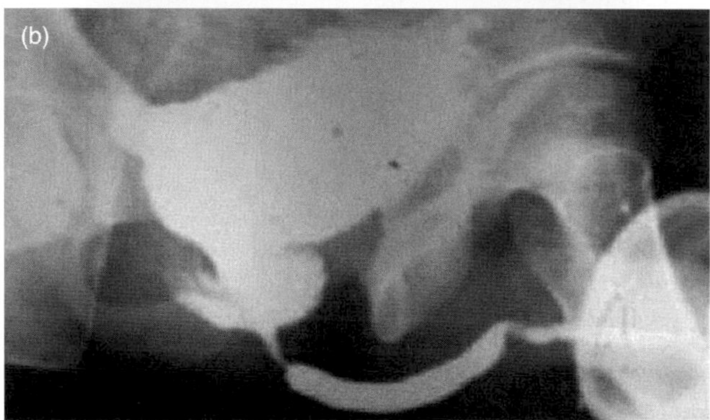

Figure 37.3
Myelomeningocele. Cystourethrography: (a) anteroposterior projection – 'Christmas tree' bladder, paraureteral diverticulum and grade I left vesicoureteric reflux, wide open bladder neck and proximal urethra, intraprostatic ducts visualization; (b) oblique projection during micturition – narrowed membranous urethra.

Severe bladder trabeculation with diverticula and pseudodiverticula, vesicoureteric reflux, wide bladder neck, and proximal urethra, and narrowing at the level of the membranous urethra can suggest, mainly in children, the presence of neurogenic LUT dysfunction (occult spinal dysraphism, non-neurogenic neurogenic bladder) even in the absence of neurogenic symptoms and signs.[43–45] In these cases imaging abnormalities indicate the need for urodynamic evaluation, electrophysiologic tests, and CNS imaging.

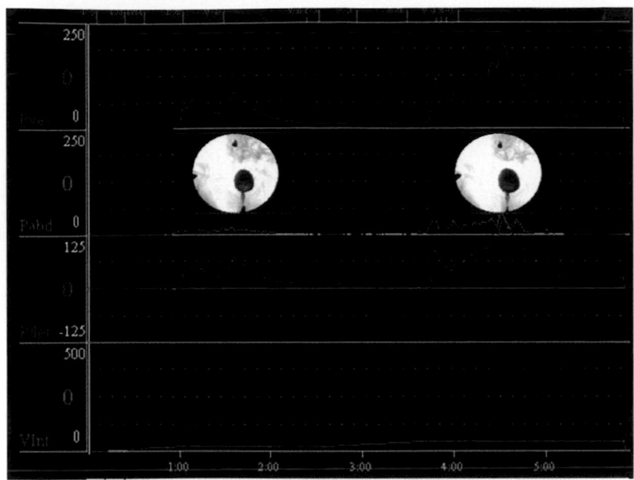

Figure 37.4
Spastic paraparesis secondary to herpetic encephalitis. Videourodynamics showed phasic neurogenic detrusor overactivity resulting in incontinence; during involuntary detrusor contractions a good bladder neck opening may be observed without any radiologic sign of detrusor-sphincter dyssynergia.

Residual urine evaluation can be worthwhile in neurogenic LUT dysfunctions. Residual urine is defined by the International Continence Society (ICS) as the volume of fluid remaining in the bladder immediately following completion of micturition.[46] Residual urine is usually referred to as an absolute value, but it can be measured also as a percentage of bladder capacity.

The measurement of postvoid residual urine (PVR) can be performed by invasive or noninvasive means: invasive means are in-and-out catheterization and endoscopy; noninvasive means are transabdominal ultrasonography and radioisotope studies.

In-and-out catheterization is indicated as the gold standard for the measurement of PVR. Its invasiveness is not an issue in patients who are or will be in a regimen of intermittent catheterization. This method is subject to inaccuracies if the person performing the catheterization is not fully instructed as to the procedures and techniques to assure complete emptying (moving the catheter in and out slowly, twisting it, suctioning with syringe, suprapubic pressure), especially in cases of bladder diverticula and vesicoureteric reflux.[47] Stoller and Millard[48] showed inaccuracies in 30% of 515 male patients evaluated by full-time urologic nurses, with a mean difference between the initial and the actual residual volume of 76 ml in 30% of inaccurate assessments. After further training by the nurses, inaccurate assessments were reduced to 14%, with a mean difference of 85 ml.

Before the era of ultrasonography, PVR was measured noninvasively by the phenolsulfonphthalein excretion test[49] or with isotopes.[50] These tools have now been practically abandoned.

Ultrasonography is the least-invasive method of determining the PVR. There are several methods for this measurement, which are based on transverse and longitudinal ultrasound bladder imaging. Using any of three parameters (length, height, width) or the surface area in the transverse image and the length obtained in the longitudinal image, various volume formulae for a spherical or an ellipsoid body are utilized to estimate the bladder volume. Currently, no single formula can be indicated as the best to calculate bladder volume.

Several studies report sufficient accuracy in the ultrasound estimation of PVR.[51–57] The intra-individual variability of PVR is high from day to day and even within a 24-hour period. This was reported in men with benign prostatic hypertrophy (BPH) by Birch et al[58] and by Bruskevitz et al.[59] Griffiths et al[60] examined the variability of PVR among 14 geriatric patients (mean age 77 years), measured by ultrasound at three different times of the day during each of two visits at 2–4-week intervals. Within-patient variability was large (SD 128 ml) because of a large systematic variation with time of the day, with greatest volumes in the early morning. The inherent random variability of the measurement was much smaller (SD 44 ml).

There are no data with regard to PVR variability in neurogenic bladders. The factors influencing the variability of PVR measurement are voiding in unfamiliar surroundings, voiding on command with a partially filled or overfilled bladder, the interval between voiding and the estimation of residual (it should be as short as possible), and the presence of vesicoureteric reflux or bladder diverticula.

Portable scanners have been introduced, with automatic measurement of bladder volume. In a prospective comparison,[61] where 100 measurements of PVR by portable ultrasound were compared with measurements by catheterization, the mean absolute error of the scanner was 52 ml. For volumes below 200 and 100 ml, the error was 36 and 24 ml, respectively. The portable scanner appears to be a valid alternative to in-and-out catheterization.

Imaging of the upper urinary tract

Imaging of the upper urinary tract is indicated in cases of neurogenic urinary incontinence with high risk of renal damage (due to high detrusor pressure, e.g. myelodysplasia, spinal cord injury, and low compliance bladder (Level of Evidence 3). Grade of Recommendations C according to the International Consultation on Urological Diseases (ICUD) system).[62]

Neurogenic bladder dysfunction, primarily in the case of low bladder compliance or detrusor-sphincter dyssynergia, or chronic retention with incontinence, can undermine urine transport through the ureterovesical junction from the kidneys to the bladder, resulting in hydronephrosis and renal damage. The relationship between high bladder storage pressure and renal deterioration has been well established by McGuire et al in a cohort of myelodysplastic children, showing that a detrusor leak point pressure >40 cmH_2O is detrimental to the upper urinary tract function.[63] Renal impairment is usually detectable at various stages by imaging of the kidneys and/or renal function tests.

Upper tract imaging is advisable at baseline and during follow-up in all cases of neurogenic bladder dysfunction, and most of all in urodynamic situations with high risk of renal damage (high bladder pressure and inefficient voiding, with or without vesicoureteric reflux and infection).

The upper tract imaging modalities most commonly used include ultrasonography, intravenous urography (IVU), isotope scanning, CT scanning, and MRI.

Ultrasonography is an excellent tool for imaging of the upper urinary tract. It is noninvasive, and successful imaging of the kidneys is independent of renal function. Ultrasound can be used to assess many features of renal anatomy, including renal size and growth, hydronephrosis, segmental anomalies, stones, and tumors. In the evaluation of the patient with neurogenic LUT dysfunction, the detection of hydronephrosis is extremely important and may be a marker for a badly managed LUT. Because ultrasonography cannot predict function or degree of obstruction or reflux, other imaging modalities are often used after hydronephrosis is initially diagnosed by ultrasound. Ultrasound is an excellent tool to follow the degree of hydronephrosis or the response to treatment over time.

IVU is the original radiographic examination of the upper (and lower) urinary tract. Successful examination is dependent upon adequate renal function. Renal dysfunction, obstruction, congenital anomalies, fistula, stones, and tumors may be detected.

In some neurogenic patients, both kidney ultrasonography and IVU can be difficult to perform and interpret due to chronic constipation, excessive bowel gas, severe kyphoscoliosis or other spinal deformities, and the presence of internal fixation devices.

Isotopes are used primarily to examine functional characteristics of the upper urinary tract. Isotope scanning can be used to evaluate renal morphology and location. Renography is used to examine the differential function of the two kidneys as well as how they drain. There are many physiologic factors and technical pitfalls that can influence the outcome, including the choice of radionuclide, timing of diuretic injection, state of hydration and diuresis, fullness or back pressure from the bladder, varying renal function, and compliance of the collecting system. Diuresis renography with bladder drainage is recommended when obstructive upper tract uropathy is suspected.[64–66]

CT scanning provides useful information about the anatomy of the upper urinary tract. Information can be independent of renal function; however, the addition of intravenous contrast can highlight specific anatomic characteristics (dependent upon renal function). CT scanning can be used as an alternative to ultrasonography or IVU, and in many cases provides additional information, although at a higher cost.

MRI offers some of the same benefits as CT in the evaluation of the upper urinary tract. Magnetic resonance urography is gaining popularity as an alternative to IVU, allowing multiplanar imaging and avoiding the intravenous injection of contrast media and the use of ionizing radiation. Its use in patients with neurogenic bladder due to spinal dysraphism with gross spinal deformity has been shown to be valuable and effective, even in the presence of gross spinal deformity.[67]

Conclusions

Upper urinary tract imaging, by means of ultrasonography or MRI urography, is recommended at baseline and during follow-up, as needed, in neurogenic LUT dysfunctions. Their implementation is mandatory when low bladder compliance and chronic retention with/without incontinence indicate a high risk of renal impairment.

In the evaluation of the LUT, the simultaneous performance of imaging and urodynamics (videourodynamics) is the gold standard.

Some morphologic findings at cystourethrography or ultrasonography – such as open bladder neck and proximal urethra at rest, heavily thickened sacculated and trabeculated asymmetric bladder, and membranous urethral narrowing – can have clinical and diagnostic relevance in raising the suspicion of a neurogenic disease, even in the absence of clear neurologic symptoms and signs.

Lumbosacral spine X-rays, followed when needed by MRI, have specific indications in children and young adults with suspected neurogenic LUT dysfunction, with or without gluteosacral stigmata.

CNS imaging should be considered when a neurologic disorder is suspected on the basis of clinical, imaging, and neurophysiologic findings.

Functional neuroimaging by PET is going to provide new insight into the functional anatomy of CNS related to vesicourethral function and dysfunction. Neuroimaging can cover the gap between clinical neurologic level assessment and the type of vesicourethral dysfunction.

Knowledge of functional and dysfunctional mechanisms will certainly increase, and together with developments in imaging techniques will enhance clinical understanding.

References

1. Anderson FM. Occult spinal dysraphism: a series of 73 cases. Pediatrics 1975; 55: 826.
2. Flanigan RF, Russel DP, Walsh JW. Urologic aspects of tethered cord. Urology 1989; 33: 80.
3. Kaplan WE, McLone DG, Richards I. The urologic manifestations of the tethered spinal cord. J Urol 1988; 140: 1285.
4. Kondo A, Kato K, Kanai S, Sakakibara T. Bladder dysfunction secondary to tethered cord syndrome in adults: is it curable? J Urol 1986; 135: 313.
5. Scheible W, James HE, Leopold GR, Hilton SW. Occult spinal dysraphism in infants: screening with high-resolution real-time ultrasound. Radiology 1983; 146: 743.
6. Jacobson H, Holm-Bentzen M, Hage T. Neurogenic bladder dysfunction in sacral agenesis and dysgenesis. Neurol Urodyn 1985; 4: 99.
7. Boemers TM, VanGool JD, DeJorg TPVM, Bax KMA. Urodynamic evaluation of children with caudal regression syndrome (caudal dysplasia sequence). J Urol 1994; 151: 1038–40.
8. Tarcey PT, Hanigan WC. Spinal dysraphism. Use of magnetic resonance imaging in evaluation. Clin Pediatr 1990; 29: 228–33.
9. Artibani W, Andersen JT, Gaiewsky JB et al. Imaging and other investigations. In: Abrams P, Cardozo L, Khoury S, Wein A, eds. Incontinence. 2nd International Consultation on Incontinence, 2001. Plymbridge Distributors, 2001: 427–34.
10. Wein AJ. Pathophysiology and categorization of voiding dysfunction. In: Campbell's Urology, 8th edn. Philadelphia: WB Saunders, 2002: 887–99.
11. Webster GD, Guralnick ML. The neurourologic evaluation. In: Campbell's Urology, 8th edn. Philadelphia: WB Saunders, 2002: 900–30.
12. Barbalias GA, Blaivas JG. Neurologic implications of the pathologically open bladder neck. J Urol 1983; 129(4): 780.
13. Salinas JM, Berger Y, De La Roche RE, Blaivas JG. Urological evaluation in the Shy–Drager syndrome. J Urol 1986; 135(4): 741.
14. Blaivas JG, Barbalias GA. Characteristics of neural injury after abdominoperineal resection. J Urol 1983; 129(1): 84.
15. de Groat WC, Steers WD. Autonomic regulation of the urinary bladder and sexual organs. In: Loewry AD, Spyers KM, eds. Central Regulation of the Autonomic Functions. Oxford: Oxford University Press, 1990: 313.
16. Nordling J. Influence of the sympathetic nervous system on lower urinary tract in man. Neurourol Urodyn 1983; 2: 3.
17. Woodside JR, McGuire EJ. Urethral hypotonicity after suprasacral spinal cord injury. J Urol 1979; 121(6): 783.
18. McGuire EJ. Combined radiographic and manometric assessment of urethral sphincter function. J Urol 1977; 118(4): 632.
19. McGuire EJ. The effects of sacral denervation on bladder and urethral function. Surg Gynecol Obstet 1977; 144(3): 343.
20. Nordling J, Meyhoff HH, Olesen KP. Cysto-urethrographic appearance of the bladder and posterior urethra in neuromuscular disorders of the lower urinary tract. Scand J Urol Nephrol 1982; 16(2): 115.
21. Gosling JA, Dixon JS, Lendon RG. The autonomic innervation of the human male and female bladder neck and proximal urethra. J Urol 1977; 118(2): 302.
22. Stanton SL, Williams D. The wide bladder neck in children. Br J Urol 1973; 45: 60.
23. Murray K, Nurse D, Borzykowski M, Mundy AR. The congenital wide bladder neck anomaly: a common cause of incontinence in children. Br J Urol 1987; 59(6): 533.
24. Chapple CR, Helm CW, Blease S et al. Asymptomatic bladder neck incompetence in nulliparous females. Br J Urol 1989; 64(4): 357.
25. Versi E. The significance of an open bladder neck in women. Br J Urol 1991; 68(1): 42.
26. Blaivas JG, Olsson CA. Stress incontinence: classification and surgical approach. J Urol 1988; 139: 737.
27. MacDiamis S, Rosario D, Chapple CR. The importance of accurate assessment and conservative management of the open bladder neck in patients with post-pelvic fracture membranous urethral distraction defects. Br J Urol 1995; 75: 65.
28. Isekin CE, Webster GD. The significance of the open bladder neck associated with pelvic fracture urethral distraction defects. J Urol 1999; 162: 347.
29. Shivde SR. The significance of the open bladder neck associated with pelvic fracture urethral distraction defects. J Urol 2000; 163: 552.
30. Tsuchida S, Noto H, Yamaguchi O, Itoh M. Urodynamic studies in hemiplegic patients after cerebrovascular accidents. Urology 1983; 21: 315.
31. Khan Z, Starer P, Yang WC, Bhola A. Analysis of voiding disorders in patients with cerebrovascular accidents. Urology 1990; 32: 256.
32. Andrew J, Nathan PW. Lesions of the frontal lobes and disturbances of micturition and defecation. Brain 1964; 87: 233–62.
33. Griffiths DJ, McCracken PN, Harrison GM, McEwan A. Geriatric urge incontinence: basic dysfunction and contributory factors. Neurourol Urodyn 1990; 9: 406–7.
34. Kitada S, Ikel Y, Hasui Y et al. Bladder function in elderly men with subclinical brain magnetic resonance imaging lesions. J Urol 1992; 147: 1507–9.
35. Blok BFM, Willemsen ATM, Holstege G. A PET study on brain control of micturition in human. Brain 1997; 120: 111.
36. Blok BFM, Holdstege G. The central control of micturition and continence: implications for urology. Br J Urol Int 1999; 83(Suppl 2): 1.
37. Nour S, Svarer C, Kristensen JKL et al. Cerebral activation during micturition in normal men. Brain 2000; 123: 781–9.
38. Charil A, Zijdenbos AP, Taylor J et al. Statistical mapping analysis of lesion location and neurological disability in multiple sclerosis: application to 452 patient data set. NeuroImage 2003; 19: 532–44.
39. Bors E, Comarr AE. Neurological urology, physiology of micturition, its neurological disorders and sequelae. Karger 1971: 157.
40. Papadaki PJ, Vlychou MK, Zavras GM et al. Investigation of vesicoureteral reflux with colour Doppler sonography in adult patients with spinal cord injury. Eur Radiol 2002; 12: 366–70.
41. Webster DG, Kreder KJ. The neurourologic evaluation. In: Campbell's Urology, 7th edn. Philadelphia: WB Saunders, 1998; 927–52.
42. Borghesi G, Simonetti R, Goldman SM et al. Magnetic resonance imaging urodynamics. Technique development and preliminary results. Int Braz J Urol 2006; 32: 336–41.
43. Hinman F. Urinary tract damage in children who wet. Pediatrics 1974; 54: 142.
44. Allen TD. The non-neurogenic bladder. J Urol 1977; 117: 232.
45. Williams DI, Hirst G, Doyle D. The occult neuropathic bladder. J Pediatr Surg 1975; 9: 35.
46. ICS Standardization of terminology of lower urinary tract function. Neurourol Urodyn 1998; 7: 403.
47. Purkiss SF. Assessment of residual urine in men following catheterisation. Br J Urol 1990; 66(3): 279.
48. Stoller ML, Millard RJ. The accuracy of a catheterized residual urine. J Urol 1989; 1741: 15.
49. Ruikka I. Residual urine in aged women and its influence on the phenolsulfonphthaleine excretion test. Gerontol Clin 1963; 5: 65–71.
50. Mulrow PJ, Huvos A, Buchanan DL. Measurement of residual urine with I-131-labeled Diodrast. J Lab Clin Med 1961; 57:
51. Piters K, Lapin S, Bessman AN. Ultrasonography in the detection of residual urine. Diabetes 1979; 28: 320–3.
52. Pedersen JF, Batrum RJ, Grytter C. Residual urine detection by ultrasonic scanning. Am J Roentgenol Rad Ther Nucl Med 1975; 125: 474–8.
53. Griffiths CJ, Muray A, Ramsden PD. Accuracy and repeatibility of bladder volume measurement using ultrasonic imaging. J Urol 1986; 136: 808.

54. Beacock CJM, Roberts EE, Rees RWM, Buck AC. Ultrasound assessment of residual urine. A quantitative method. Br J Urol 1985; 57: 410–13.
55. West KA. Sonocystography. A method for measuring residual urine. Scand J Urol Nephrol 1967; 1: 68.
56. McLean GK, Edell SL. Determination of bladder volumes by gray scale ultrasonography. Radiology 1978; 128: 181–2.
57. Widder B, Kornhuber HH, Renner A. Restharnmessung in der ambulanten Versorgung mit einem Klein-Ultrashallgerat. Dtsch Med Wochen-schr 1983; 108: 1552.
58. Birch NC, Hurst G, Doyle PT. Serial residual volumes in men with prostatic hypertrophy. Br J Urol 1998; 62: 571.
59. Bruskewitz RC, Iversen P, Madsen PO. Value of post-void residual urine determination in evaluation of prostatism. Urology 1982; 20: 602.
60. Griffiths DJ, Harrison G, Moore K, McCracken P. Variability of postvoid residual urine volume in the elderly. Urol Res 1996; 24(1): 23–6.
61. Ding YY, Sahadevan S, Pang WS, Choo PW. Clinical utility of a portable ultrasound scanner in the measurement of residual urine volume. Singapore Med J 1996; 37(4): 365–8.
62. Tubaro A, Artibani W, Bartram C et al. Imaging and other investigations. In: Abrams P, Cardozo L, Khoury S, Wein A, eds. Incontinence. 3nd International Consultation on Incontinence, 2005. Plymbridge Distributors, 2005: 710–14.
63. McGuire EM, Woodside JR, Borden TA. Prognostic value of urodynamic testing in myelodysplastic patients. J Urol 1981; 126: 205–9.
64. Conway JJ. 'Well-tempered' diuresis renography: its historical development, physiological and technical pitfalls, and standardized technique protocol. Semin Nuclear Med 1992; 22: 74–84.
65. Hvistendahl JJ, Pedersen TS, Schmidt F et al. The vesico-renal reflex mechanism modulates urine output during elevated bladder pressure. Scand J Urol Nephrol 1997; 186(31 Suppl): 24.
66. O'Reilly PH. Diuresis renography. Recent advances and recommended protocols. Br J Urol 1992; 69: 113–20.
67. Shipstone DP, Thomas DG, Darwent G, Morcos SK. Magnetic resonance urography in patients with neurogenic bladder dysfunction and spinal dysraphism. BJU Int 2002; 89: 658–64.

38

Evaluation of neurogenic bladder dysfunction: basic urodynamics

Christopher E Kelly and Victor W Nitti

Classification of neurogenic voiding dysfunction

The main objective in assessing patients with suspected neurogenic lower urinary tract (LUT) dysfunction is to determine what effect the neurologic disease has on the entire urinary tract so that treatment can be implemented to relieve symptoms and prevent upper and lower urinary tract damage. The functional classification system described by Wein (Figure 38.1) is a useful framework with which to conceptualize neurogenic voiding dysfunction and provides a basis for the discussion of various diagnostic and treatment modalities.[1] This simple and practical system can be easily applied to our diagnostic criteria (e.g. urodynamics). Of equal importance is the fact that treatment options can be chosen based on this system. The functional classification system is based on the simple concept that the LUT has two basic functions: storage of adequate volumes of urine at low pressures, and voluntary and complete evacuation of urine from the bladder. For normal storage and emptying to occur there must be proper and coordinated functioning of the bladder and bladder outlet (bladder neck, urethra, external sphincter). Hence, neurogenic LUT dysfunction can be classified under the following rubrics: 'failure to store', 'failure to empty', or a combination thereof. Abnormalities in LUT function may be the result of bladder dysfunction, bladder outlet dysfunction, or a combined dysfunction. Figure 38.2 summarizes how neurologic disease can adversely affect the bladder and/or the bladder outlet, causing storage and emptying dysfunction.

Prior to our discussion, it is important to emphasize that symptoms do not always indicate the magnitude to which the disease is affecting the urinary tract, especially in neurologic disorders. Serious urinary tract damage can result in the absence of symptoms. It is also vital to realize that patients with neurologic disease are at risk for developing

Functional classification:

1. Emptying abnormality (failure to empty)
2. Storage abnormality (failure to store)
3. Emptying and storage abnormality

Anatomic abnormality:

1. Bladder dysfunction
2. Bladder outlet dysfunction
3. Bladder and bladder outlet dysfunction

Figure 38.1
Functional classification of voiding disorders.

Failure to store

A. Bladder dysfunction:
   - Neurogenic detrusor overactivity
   - Impaired compliance

B. Bladder outlet dysfunction:
   - Neurogenic intrinsic sphincter deficiency

Failure to empty

A. Bladder dysfunction:
   - Detrusor underactivity
   - Acontractile detrusor

B. Bladder outlet dysfunction:
   - Detrusor-external sphincter dyssynergia
   - Bladder neck dyssynergia

Figure 38.2
Effects of neurologic disease on storage and emptying function.

the same urologic and gynecologic problems as persons of the same age without neurologic disease.[2] For example, just because a woman has had a cerebrovascular accident does not exclude her from having stress urinary incontinence. And, lastly, the clinician should remember that neurologic lesions may be 'complete' or 'incomplete'. Hence, urologic manifestations of neurologic disease may not always be predictable. A complete neuro-urologic evaluation of patients with neurogenic voiding dysfunction is therefore important.

In this chapter we will discuss the evaluation of patients with neurogenic LUT dysfunction with urodynamics. Prior to this discussion, a working knowledge of the neurophysiology of micturition is essential. This topic is covered in Chapter 7. Additionally, the effect of particular neurologic diseases on LUT function is covered elsewhere in the book.

Assessment of patients with neurogenic lower urinary tract dysfunction

History and physical examination

Any patient with obvious or suspected neurogenic voiding LUT dysfunction deserves a neurologic work-up. Controversy exists as to how often patients should be reassessed urologically. We recommend that patients be reviewed at least annually, and the complete work-up be repeated if significant changes occur in the neurologic status or LUT signs or symptoms.

Prior to urodynamic testing a complete history and physical examination are imperative. A thorough understanding of the patient's condition and symptoms is essential so that urodynamic investigations can be 'customized' to answer questions relevant to that particular patient. Initial evaluation of patients with suspected neurogenic LUT dysfunction should include a thorough history of the patient's general health and neurologic disease. It is important to understand how the neurologic disease affects daily activities, whether it affects other systems, and whether its course is stable or changing. In patients who do not have a history of neurologic disease (i.e. occult neurologic disease), it is important to carefully and directly question them even about their more subtle neurologic complaints.[2]

A standard and complete urologic examination should be performed on all patients with suspected neurogenic LUT dysfunction. A good general neurologic examination to assess sensation, strength, dexterity, and mobility is essential, as all of these can affect treatment of neurogenic LUT dysfunction. A specific and comprehensive evaluation of the sacral nerve (S2–S4) reflex arc is critical. A digital rectal examination will establish rectal tone and control. The bulbocavernosus reflex and perianal sensation should also be assessed. Finally, lower extremity spasticity along with patellar and ankle reflexes should be evaluated.

Laboratory studies

Basic serum and urine tests, including renal function tests and serum electrolytes, should be performed. Urinalysis and urine culture are essential, particularly in patients with an increased risk for developing urinary tract infections: those with chronic indwelling catheters, on intermittent self-catheterization, or those carrying high postvoid residual volumes.

Noninvasive urodynamic assessment

Noninvasive studies such as uroflowmetry and measurement of postvoid residual urine can be readily performed to give an initial assessment of the patient's ability to empty the bladder. While nonspecific for underlying dysfunction, uroflowmetry is often used as a screening test for voiding dysfunction and as a means for selecting patients for more sophisticated urodynamic studies. It also provides an objective way to monitor the emptying in patients who have specific diagnoses and are followed with observation or specific therapy.

Since the upper urinary tract in neurogenic voiding dysfunction can be adversely affected by secondary reflux, ascending infection, hydronephrosis, chronically elevated bladder storage pressure, or stones, we recommend some baseline imaging studies. The choice of study depends on the clinical question being answered. A renal ultrasound or intravenous pyelogram can be used to assess for anatomic abnormalities, hydronephrosis, or stones. Bladder ultrasound provides a noninvasive method of measuring residual bladder urine and may assist in ruling out bladder calculi, which are associated with chronic indwelling catheterization.[3] A voiding cystourethrogram, whether alone or as part of videourodynamics, can help diagnose vesicoureteral reflux.[4] Radionucleotide renography may be helpful when more detailed information on renal function is required, such as obstruction or cortical scarring.

Although it is an invasive technique, a few words on cystourethroscopy are important. It is indicated in those with indwelling catheters on a yearly basis. Besides evaluating for bladder calculi, epithelial changes can be detected.

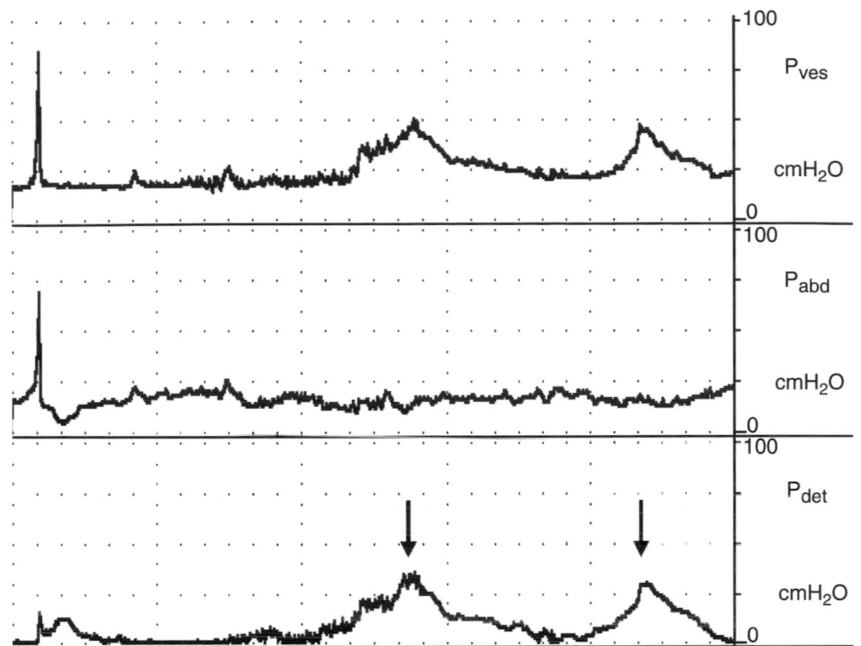

Figure 38.3
Filling phase of a urodynamic study in a 68-year-old woman with urge incontinence after cerebrovascular accident. Note the involuntary detrusor contractions (arrows). There is a rise in total bladder pressure (P_{ves}) and detrusor pressure (P_{det}), but no change in abdominal pressure (P_{abd}).

These patients carry a 5% lifetime risk of developing squamous cell carcinoma of the bladder.[5–7]

Urodyamics

Multichannel urodynamic evaluation is the mainstay of evaluation in patients with neurogenic LUT dysfunction. The goals of urodynamic testing in patients with neurologic disease are:

1. to provide documentation of the effect of neurologic disease on the LUT
2. to correlate the patient's symptoms with urodynamic events
3. to assess for the presence of urologic risk factors associated with urologic complications: detrusor striated sphincter dyssynergia (DESD), impaired bladder compliance, sustained high-pressure detrusor contractions, and vesicoureteral reflux.

The urodynamic evaluation consists of several components, including the uroflowmetry, cystometrogram (CMG), abdominal pressure monitoring, electromyography (EMG), and voiding pressure–flow studies. Simultaneous fluoroscopic imaging of the entire urinary tract during urodynamics (i.e. videourodynamics) can be helpful in cases of known or suspected neurogenic voiding dysfunction. It is not unusual to repeat a study several times in order to fulfill the above goals.

Cystometrogram

The filling CMG is used to mimic the bladder's filling and storage of urine while the pressure–volume relationship within the bladder is recorded. It is best to fill the bladder at a rate of 30 ml/min or less. In our experience, faster filling rates can exaggerate urodynamic observations. Important bladder parameters with respect to neurologic disease are bladder sensation, the presence of involuntary detrusor contractions (IDCs), compliance (storage pressures), and cystometric capacity. IDCs associated with neurologic disease are referred to as neurogenic detrusor overactivity according to the International Continence Society (Figure 38.3).[8] The magnitude, or pressure, of IDCs is often determined by the amount of resistance provided by the bladder outlet. For example, in cases of high outlet resistance such as DESD or anatomic obstruction, detrusor pressure with IDC can be quite high, whereas in cases of low outlet resistance, the IDC pressure is often low with subsequent incontinence. Neurogenic detrusor overactivity is caused by lesions above the sacral micturition center, including the spinal cord and brain. Simply stated, the inhibition of the spinal micturition reflex from suprapontine centers is blocked.

There are several very important points regarding involuntary contractions:

1. The clinician must be absolutely sure that the contraction is indeed involuntary. Sometimes a patient may become confused during the study and actually void as soon as he feels the desire.

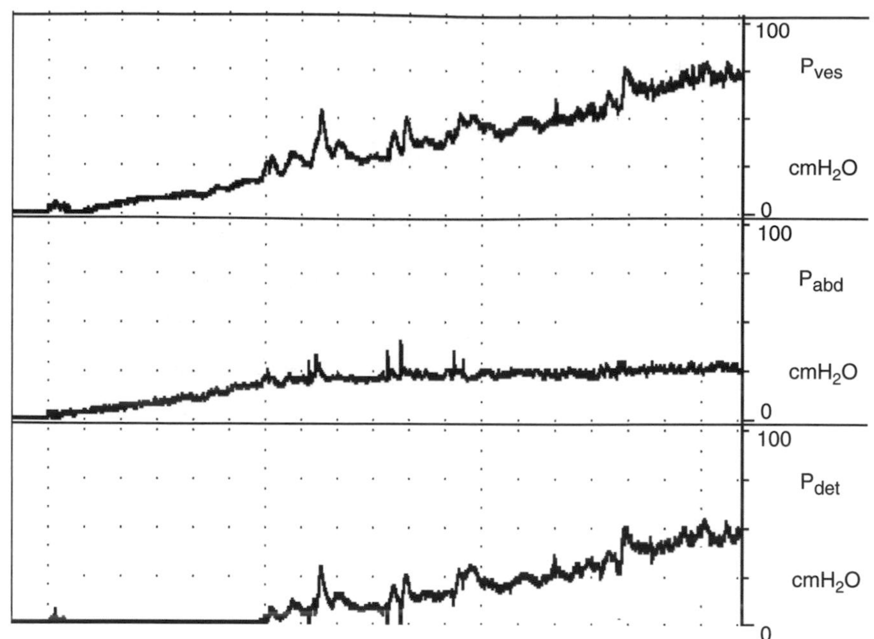

Figure 38.4
Impaired compliance in a 35-year-old male with a T8 spinal cord injury. Note that there is an initial rise in both total vesical pressure (P_{ves}) and abdominal pressure (P_{abd}), but the P_{ves} and, thus, the detrusor pressure (P_{det}) continue to rise to pressures exceeding 40 cmH_2O.

2. It is extremely important to determine whether or not a patient's symptoms are reproduced during the involuntary contraction. However, in cases of neurologic disease, IDCs can occur with symptoms and should not be discounted.
3. The volume at which contractions occur and the pressure of the contractions should be recorded.
4. It is often worthwhile to repeat the CMG at a slower filling rate if the patient experiences uncharacteristic symptoms (e.g. incontinence or spasms) or detrusor activity.
5. If the patient experiences incontinence during an involuntary contraction (urge incontinence), this should be noted. Sometimes the involuntary contraction will bring on involuntary voiding to completion (precipitant micturition).[9]

Compliance is defined as the change of volume for a change in detrusor pressure and is calculated by dividing the volume change (ΔV) by the change in detrusor pressure (ΔP_{det}) during that change in bladder volume. It is expressed in milliliters per centimeter H_2O (ml/cmH_2O). The spherical shape of the bladder as well as the viscoelastic properties of its components contribute to its excellent compliance, allowing storage of progressive volumes of urine at low pressure. When the pressure begins to rise with increasing volumes, compliance is decreased or 'impaired'. Impaired compliance is not uncommon in neurogenic voiding dysfunction and is potentially hazardous. The degree of impaired compliance in neurogenic voiding dysfunction is often dependent on outlet resistance. However, poor compliance can also occur with chronically catheterized bladders. Impaired compliance leads to high bladder storage pressures. The calculated value of compliance is probably less important than the actual bladder pressure during filling. This is because the compliance value can change, depending on the volume over which it is calculated. This is probably why compliance, despite being a well-known and accepted parameter, is rarely reported in terms of a discrete or well-defined value in the urologic literature.

Normal compliance has been difficult to establish. Toppercer and Tetreault evaluated a group of normal asymptomatic women and women with stress incontinence and found mean compliance to be 55.71 ± 27.37.[10] If two standard deviations are used, normal would be between 1 and 110 ml/cmH_2O. When compliance is calculated as a single point on the pressure–volume curve it becomes a 'static' property. Gilmour et al point out that this oversimplifies the concept of compliance and may lead to potentially erroneous conclusions.[11] For example, an abrupt and potentially dangerous rise in pressure may occur as compliance rapidly decreases. However, the value for compliance will be very different, depending on whether it is calculated over the entire filling volume or over the volume in which the change in pressure actually occurred.

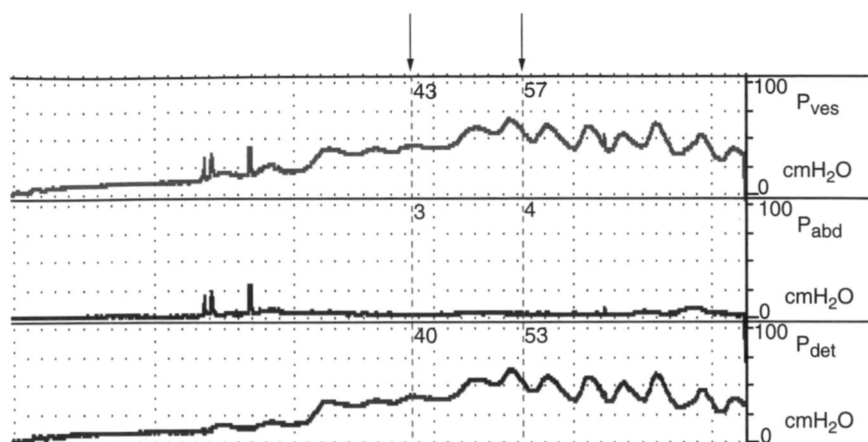

Figure 38.5
Involuntary detrusor contractions occurring in the face of impaired compliance in a teenage girl with myelomeningocele. The left arrow indicates where detrusor pressure equals and then exceeds 40 cmH_2O. The right arrow indicates where leakage occurs – at a bladder leak point pressure of 53 cmH_2O. P_{ves}, total vesical pressure; P_{det}, detrusor pressure; P_{abd}, abdominal pressure.

McGuire and associates have shown that sustained pressures of 40 cmH_2O or greater during storage can lead to upper tract damage.[12] Storage pressures in this range are dangerous, regardless of the volume in the bladder or calculated compliance value (Figure 38.4). In poorly compliant bladders in children, Gilmour et al have suggested determining compliance between initial filling and the point at which detrusor pressure exceeds 35 cmH_2O.[11] More recently, these investigators have applied the concept of dynamic compliance and argue that the amount of time spent with bladder compliance less than 10 ml/cmH_2O (an empirically derived value) will strongly influence upper tract deterioration.[13]

We would certainly agree that prolonged high-pressure storage is an ominous urodynamic finding, independent of any discrete value of compliance. One must remember that compliance may be dependent on filling rate during a urodynamic study; overly rapid filling rates may produce erroneously lower compliance values. Lastly, neurogenic detrusor overactivity can mimic impaired compliance. Two methods of differentiating these two entities are (1) stopping the infusion rate and, if necessary, (2) having the patient perform a sustained Kegel maneuver to suppress possible involuntary contractions. Involuntary detrusor contractions can also occur in the face of impaired compliance (Figure 38.5).

Storage parameters – leak-point pressures

During the filling portion of the CMG, urinary storage can also be assessed. Assessment of storage is important because patients with neurogenic bladders often have issues pertaining to urinary incontinence and/or storage pressures. Urinary leakage can be secondary to a bladder dysfunction (neurogenic detrusor overactivity or impaired compliance) and/or a sphincteric dysfunction (e.g. intrinsic sphincter deficiency). The bladder, or detrusor, leak-point pressure (DLPP) test measures the detrusor pressure required to cause urinary incontinence in the absence of increased abdominal pressure.[8] The DLPP is a direct reflection of the amount of resistance provided by the external sphincter. The higher the bladder outlet resistance (e.g. as in detrusor-sphincter dyssynergia), the higher the DLPP. High storage pressures and high DLPP are potentially dangerous to upper urinary tracts (Figure 38.5). Knowledge of the DLPP is useful because it allows the clinician to determine the volume at which detrusor pressure reaches dangerous levels.

Urinary leakage secondary to sphincteric dysfunction can be measured by the Valsalva or abdominal leak-point pressure (ALPP).[8,14] The ALPP is an indirect measure of the ability of the urethra to resist changes in abdominal pressure as an expulsive force.[15] Clinically, it is used to determine the presence of stress urinary incontinence and the degree of sphincter incompetence (Figure 38.6). Normally, there is no physiologic abdominal pressure that should cause incontinence, and therefore there is no 'normal ALPP'. Unlike the DLPP, an elevated ALPP does not indicate potential danger to the kidneys.

Voiding phase

As important as filling and storage is the voiding or emptying phase, known as micturition. Prior to urodynamic assessment, one must determine how the patient voids. If voiding is voluntary, the strength and duration of the detrusor contraction is assessed. Detrusor contractility may be impaired in particular types of neurologic disease,

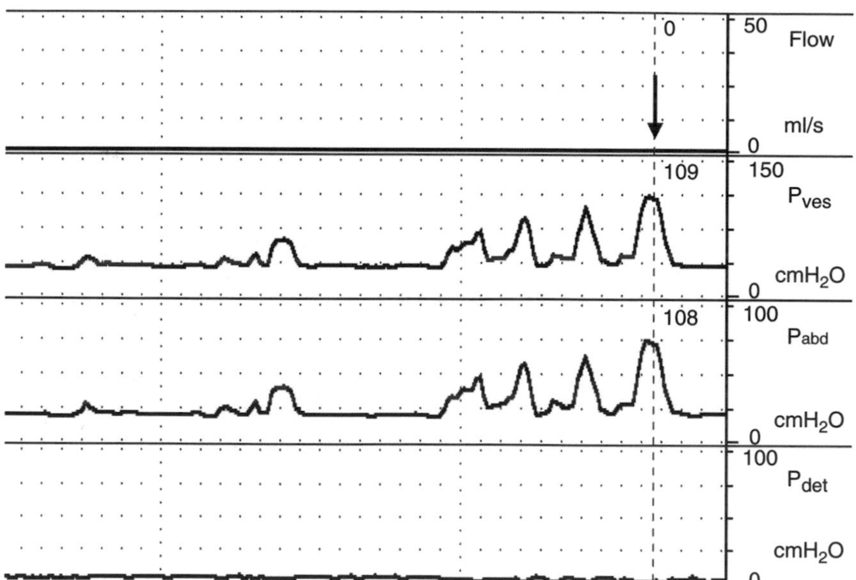

Figure 38.6
Urodynamic tracing of a female patient with stress incontinence. Tracing shows progressive Valsalva maneuvers until leakage occurs (arrow) at an abdominal pressure of 109 cmH_2O, which is the abdominal leak point pressure (ALPP). Note that there is no rise in detrusor pressure. P_{ves}, total vesical pressure; P_{det}, detrusor pressure; P_{abd}, abdominal pressure.

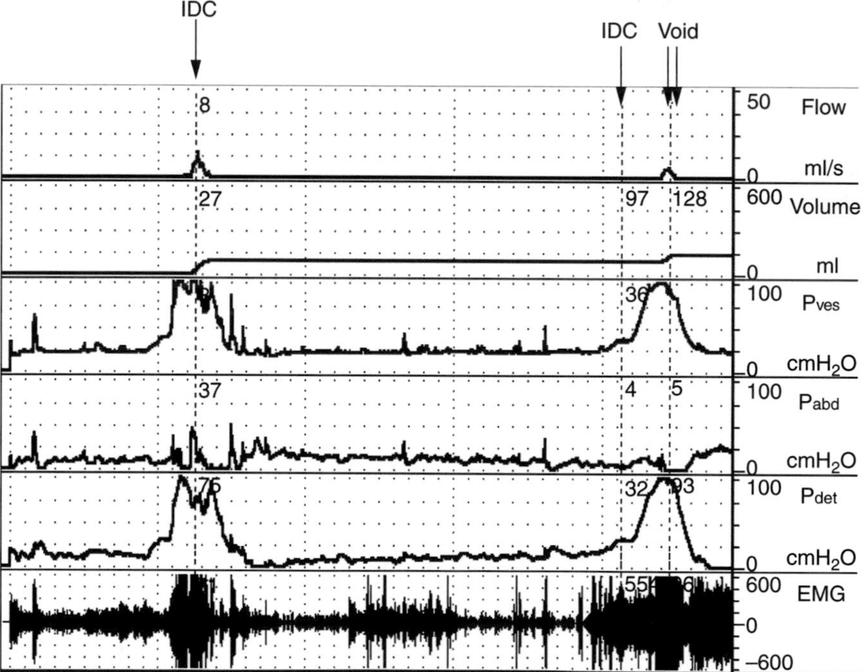

Figure 38.7
Urodynamic tracing of an 18-year-old woman with frequency, urgency, and urge incontinence who was diagnosed with a tethered cord. Note the involuntary detrusor contraction (IDC, arrow) associated with high-volume urine loss as registered in the flow meter. There is increased sphincter activity, as demonstrated by increased electromyograph (EMG) activity consistent with detrusor-external sphincter dyssynergia (DESD). On the second fill there is again an IDC, but this time the patient is instructed to void (double void). Note that there is increased EMG activity throughout the IC and 'voluntary void'. Detrusor pressures with IDCs are quite high because of the resistance of the contracting striated sphincter. P_{ves}, total vesical pressure; P_{det}, detrusor pressure; P_{abd}, abdominal pressure.

particularly with lower motor neuron or denervating lesions. This can cause impaired contractility or areflexia.

Aside from detrusor contraction, outlet resistance can be measured while voiding. Although the most common cause of outlet resistance in neurogenic voiding dysfunction is DESD, bladder outlet obstruction can occur anywhere distal to the bladder. Several nomograms and formulas exist to categorize pressure–flow relationships in terms of nonobstructed, obstructed, or equivocal.[16–20] It is important to note that interpretation of bladder outlet obstruction during urodynamics should be performed at the point at which the patient was actually given permission to void. If the patient has an involuntary bladder contraction and empties the bladder prematurely, this pressure–flow relationship should not be misinterpreted as being equivalent to normal physiologic voiding.

Electromyography during urodynamics permits the urologist to evaluate the striated sphincter function during

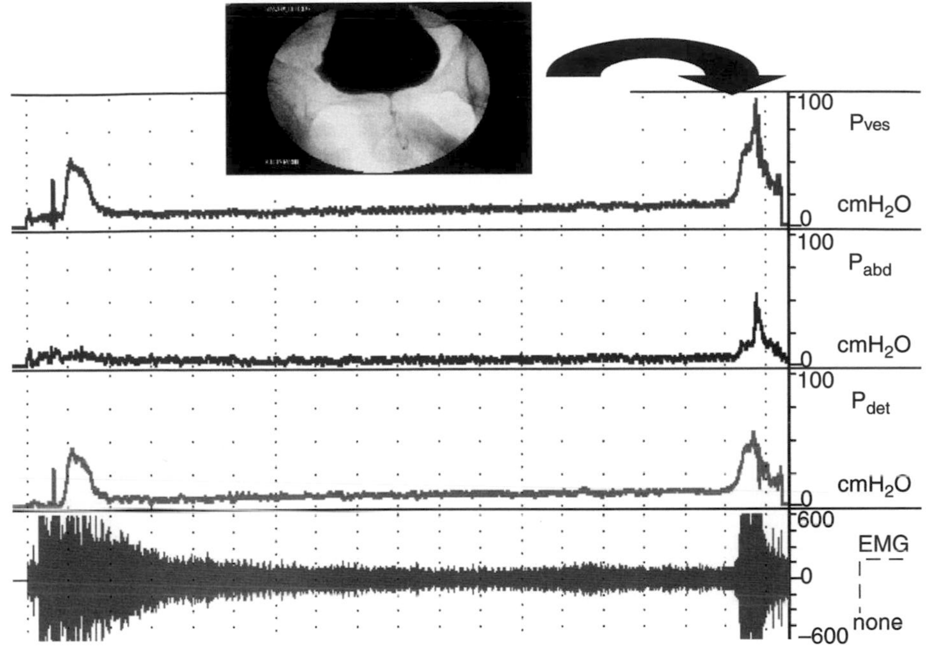

Figure 38.8
Detrusor-external sphincter dyssynergia (DESD) and detrusor-internal sphincter dyssynergia in a 35-year-old male with a high cervical spinal cord injury. There are two IDCs with associated increased electromyograph (EMG) activity consistent with DESD. However, the fluoroscopic picture taken at the time of the second IDC shows an incompletely opened bladder neck consistent with detrusor-internal sphincter dyssynergia. This patient underwent a striated sphincterotomy as well as a bladder neck incision to facilitate emptying and lower pressures. P_{ves}, total vesical pressure; P_{det}, detrusor pressure; P_{abd}, abdominal pressure.

micturition. Often, surface patch electrodes are used, but needle electrodes permit more accurate placement and more accurate recording. Normally, voluntary voiding is preceded by a complete relaxation of the striated sphincter. DESD refers to obstruction to the outflow of urine during bladder contraction caused by involuntary contraction of the striated sphincter during an IDC.[21,22] It is secondary to a neurologic lesion and is not associated with a learned voiding dysfunction such as dysfunctional voiding. DESD results in a functional obstruction that usually affects emptying, and ultimately leads to high storage pressures secondary to impaired compliance and incomplete emptying. True DESD is seen in patients with suprasacral spinal lesions (Figure 38.7). Depending on the level of the lesion, patients also may develop detrusor-internal sphincter dyssynergia. In such cases the bladder fails to open appropriately with a bladder contraction due to autonomic dysfunction. It typically occurs in lesions above T10. Detrusor-internal sphincter dyssynergia is best diagnosed by videourodynamics (Figure 38.8).

Videourodynamics

Videourodynamics, or simultaneous fluoroscopic monitoring of the urinary tract during urodynamics, is the most comprehensive and accurate way of assessing neurogenic lower urinary tract dysfunction (Figures 38.8 and 38.9).[23] During the evaluation of filling and storage, videourodynamics allows for the determination of vesicoureteral reflux and the pressure at which this occurs. Moreover, assessment of the DLPP or ALPP is facilitated as fluoroscopy is often more sensitive than direct observation in determining urinary leakage. Videourodynamics also permits the radiographic evaluation of the bladder neck during filling and anatomic abnormalities such as bladder and urethral diverticula and fistula. During the voiding phase, fluoroscopy permits an accurate determination of the site of obstruction when high-pressure/low-flow states exist. Videourodynamics also provides an excellent way of evaluating sphincter behavior during voiding, especially in cases where EMG tracing is imperfect or equivocal. Videourodynamics is the definitive test to determine the presence of detrusor-internal sphincter dyssynergia by the lack of opening of the bladder neck on fluoroscopy during a detrusor contraction. Using fluoroscopy with EMG can help make the diagnosis of detrusor-internal and detrusor-external sphincter dyssynergia.[24]

Conclusion

In patients with known neurologic disease, careful urodynamic evaluation may be necessary to gauge any deleterious effect on the urinary tract, to determine the etiology of LUT symptoms, and to screen for any urologic risk factors. Often times, urodynamics is necessary for the asymptomatic patient because the effects of the disease on the

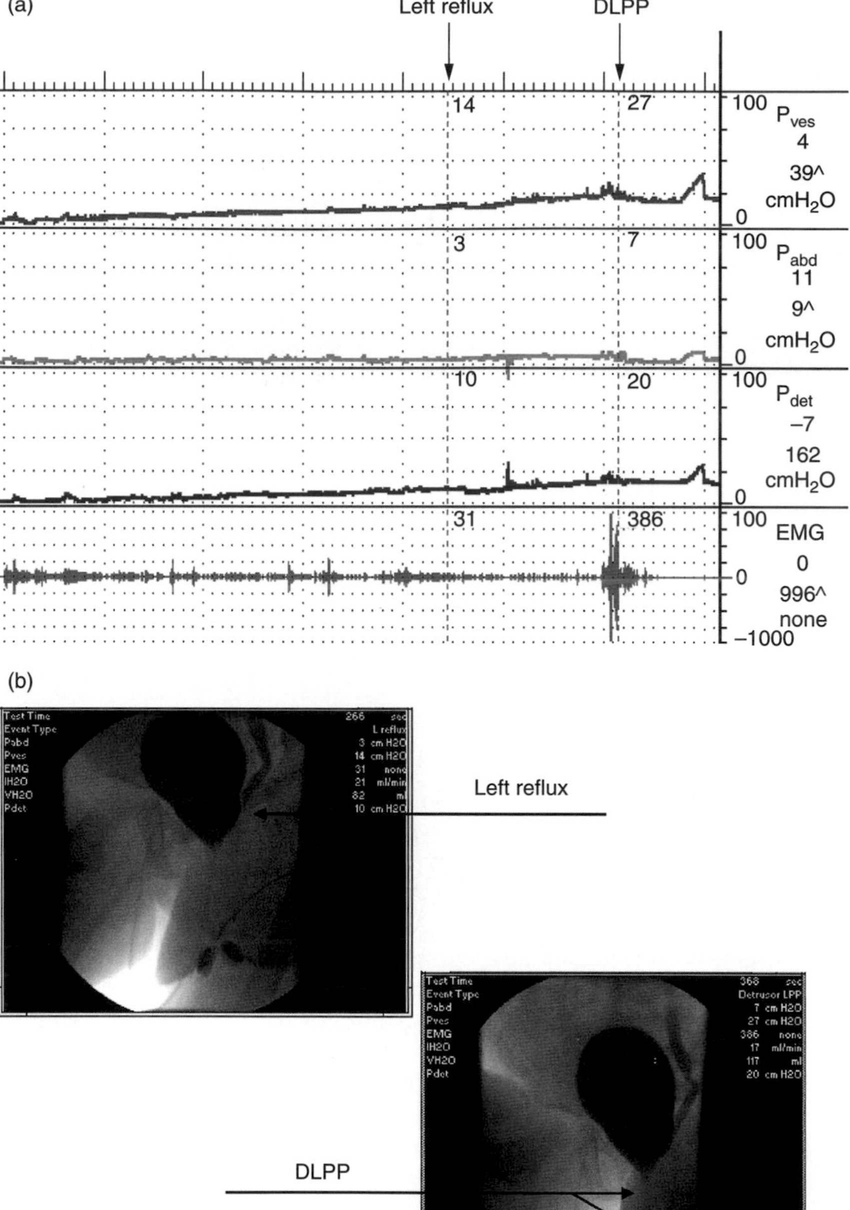

Figure 38.9
Videourodynamic study in a 3-year-old boy with myelomeningocele who is on anticholinergic medication but remains wet between catheterizations. There is mild left hydronephrosis on renal ultrasound. P_{ves}, total vesical pressure; P_{det}, detrusor pressure; P_{abd}, abdominal pressure. EMG, electromyography. This study shows that leakage occurs as a result of impaired compliance: bladder leak point pressure (DLPP) = 20 cmH_2O. Video portion shows left vesicoureteral reflux occurring at a relatively low detrusor pressure of 10 cmH_2O (upper left arrow), and confirms the DLPP of 20 cmH_2O (lower right arrow).

urinary tract can be 'silent'. Patients without a history of neurologic disease whose urologic evaluation is suspicious for neurogenic LUT dysfunction should be evaluated for occult neurologic disease.

References

1. Wein AJ. Classification of neurogenic voiding dysfunction. J Urol 1981; 125: 605.
2. Gades NM, Jacobson DJ, Girman CJ et al. Prevalence of conditions potentially associated with lower urinary tract symptoms in men. BJU Int 2005; 95: 549–53.
3. Ku JA, Jung TYL, Park JK et al. Risk factors for urinary stone formation in men with spinal cord injury: a 17-year follow-up study. BJU Int 2006; 97(4): 790–3.
4. Bunts RC. Management of urological complications in 100 paraplegics. J Urol 1958; 79: 733–6.
5. Bejany BE, Lockhart JL, Rhamy RK. Malignant vesical tumors following spinal cord injury. J Urol 1987; 138: 1390–2.
6. Bickel A, Culkin J, Wheeler J. Bladder cancer in spinal cord injury patients. J Urol 1991; 146: 1240–1.
7. Broecker BH, Klein FA, Hackler RH. Cancer of the bladder in spinal cord injury patients. J Urol 1981; 125: 196–7.
8. Abrams P, Cardozo L, Fall M et al. The standardization of terminology of lower urinary tract function. Neurourol Urodyn 2002; 21: 167–78.
9. Nitti VW. Cystometry and abdominal pressure monitoring. In: Nitti VW, ed. Practical Urodynamics. Philadelphia: WB Saunders, 1998: 38–51.

10. Toppercer A, Tetreault JP. Compliance of the bladder: an attempt to establish normal values. Urology 1979; 14: 204.
11. Gilmour RF, Churchill BM, Steckler RE et al. A new technique for dynamic analysis of bladder compliance. J Urol 1993; 150: 1200.
12. McGuire EM, Woodside JR, Borden TA. Prognostic value of urodynamic testing in myelodysplastic children. J Urol 1981; 126: 205.
13. Churchill BM, Gilmour PE, Williot P. Urodynamics. Ped Clin NA 1987; 34: 1133.
14. McGuire EJ, Fitzpatrick CC, Wan J et al. Clinical assessment of urethral sphincter function. J Urol 1993; 150: 1452–4.
15. McGuire EJ, Cespedes RD, O'Connell HE. Leak point pressures. Urol Clin N Am 1996; 23: 253–62.
16. Abrams PH, Griffiths DJ. Assessment of prostate obstruction from urodynamic measurements and from residual urine. Br J Urol 1979; 51: 129–34.
17. Schafer W. Principles and clinical application of advanced urodynamic analysis of voiding function. Urol Clin N Am 1990; 17: 553–66.
18. Abrams P. Bladder outlet obstruction index, bladder contractility index and bladder voiding efficiency; three simple indices to define bladder voiding function. BJU Int 1999; 84: 14–15.
19. Blaivas JG, Groutz A. Bladder outlet obstruction nomogram for women with lower urinary tract symptomatology. Neurourol Urodyn 2000; 19: 553–64.
20. Lemack GE, Zimmern PE. Pressure flow analysis may aid in identifying women with outflow obstruction. J Urol 2000; 163(6): 1823–8.
21. Blaivas JG, Singa HP, Zayed AAH, Labib KB. Detrusor-external sphincter dyssynergia. J Urol 1981; 125: 541–4.
22. Blaivas JG, Singa HP, Zayed AAH, Labib KB. Detrusor-external sphincter dyssynergia: a detailed EMG study. J Urol 1981; 125: 545–8.
23. Blavais JG. Videourodynamic studies. In: Nitti VW, ed. Practical Urodynamics. Philadelphia: WB Saunders, 1998: 78–93.
24. Watanabe T, Chancellor MB, Rivas DA. Neurogenic voiding dysfunction. In: Nitti VW, ed. Practical Urodynamics. Philadelphia: WB Saunders, 1998: 142–55.

39

Advanced urodynamics

Derek J Griffiths

Introduction: the variability of urodynamic measurements

Urodynamics is the study of lower urinary tract (LUT) function by any appropriate method.[1] Its purpose as usually stated is to reproduce LUT symptoms under controlled and measurable conditions so that their causes can be identified. In practice, however, there are only weak correlations between symptoms and urodynamic findings.[2] The reasons for this weak association include the intrinsic variability of urodynamic parameters,[2] not only from one subject to another but also within a single subject.

Since urodynamics is the study of urinary tract function, and since even carefully measured urodynamic parameters are variable, then the function of the LUT must be intrinsically variable. The origin, meaning, and control of this variability are the main focus of this chapter. One obvious inference is that the lower urinary tract is not – as might be naively assumed – a mechanical system with fixed biomechanical parameters that can be measured unambiguously. The variability of urodynamic parameters such as cystometric bladder capacity should not be considered an annoying artifact or a disadvantage of clinical urodynamics. On the contrary, it contains information about the working of the lower urinary tract and its control system.

There are many examples of urodynamic variability. At the 2005 ICS annual meeting, for example, it was reported[3] that voiding intervals and warning times measured during ambulatory urodynamics are not reproducible markers of treatment outcome. Thus even ambulatory urodynamics, believed by its proponents to be the gold standard of urodynamic measurement, is variable. A key urodynamic finding is the observation of detrusor overactivity (DO), believed to underlie the symptoms of the overactive bladder complex. Yet DO is intrinsically variable; Figure 39.1 indicates, for men with lower urinary tract symptoms (LUTS), how the proportion that shows DO diminishes in each repeated urodynamic study, implying that there is not just random variability but that the probability of manifesting DO diminishes systematically, by almost 50% from the first to the third study.[4] Other studies of DO in children and adults have shown similar behavior.[2,5] The bladder volumes corresponding to given sensations (e.g. normal desire to void) show similar systematic changes (increases) from one test to the next, by 30–50 cmH_2O, as well as random intrasubject variations that are even greater.[2] This type of within-subject variability leads to differences between measurements in different subjects, and ultimately to differences between results obtained in different centers. For example, the average bladder volume at *first sensation of filling* in healthy subjects in one center (350 ml)[6] is greater than the volume at *strong desire to void* (294 ml) in another.[7]

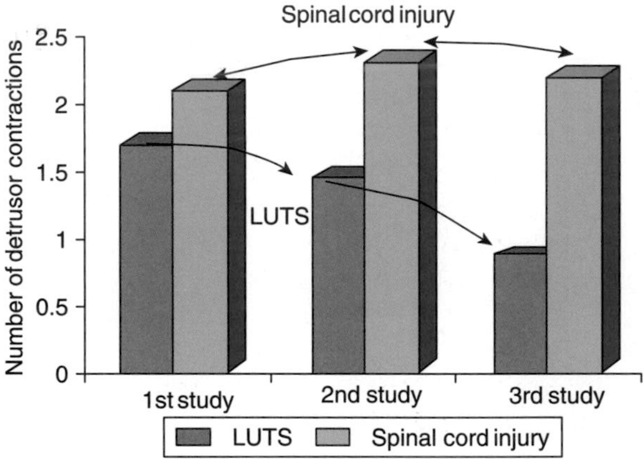

Figure 39.1
For men presenting with lower urinary tract symptoms (LUTS) but no overt neurologic defect, the proportion showing detrusor overactivity falls in each successive urodynamic study (yellow bars). For spinal cord injured patients the proportion is higher and remains almost unchanged in successive studies (blue bars). Data from reference 4.

To understand the origin of the variability it helps to remember the function of the LUT. There are two phases, storage and voiding of urine. The system is in the storage phase for the majority of the time, but urination is periodically necessary to maintain homeostasis. It must occur, and yet has to be accommodated to the social and emotional life of the individual, the more so because urination is not just elimination of waste. Urination has sexual and social aspects, such as marking of territory and establishing dominance, which are prominent in other mammals and present even in humans.[8,9] For this reason, urination is bound up with the emotions. It is the link between LUT behavior and emotion that makes urodynamics difficult to carry out in such a way that it mimics daily life. The accommodation of LUT behavior to other aspects of life implies that LUT behavior, and therefore urodynamics, must be intrinsically variable.

Accordingly the bladder control system is set up so as to ensure that voiding indeed occurs, but not *automatically*. Bladder filling generates a series of increasingly unpleasant but normal sensations (first sensation of filling, first desire to void, strong desire to void),[1] which drive the individual to empty the bladder (so maintaining homeostasis[10]) but do not normally trigger voiding. The time and place of voiding are normally under voluntary control, meaning that the moment of voiding can be postponed or advanced within certain limits. Thus the purpose of voluntary control is to take advantage of intrinsic variability, which depends on the circumstances and associated emotions of the individual, and may be influenced by memories of past bladder experiences, good or bad.

It would be expected that variability of this sort should originate where the emotions, memory, and voluntary control are situated – in the brain. In fact there is urodynamic evidence that this is so. The variability of urodynamic findings among patients with spinal cord injury is less pronounced than among subjects with an intact nervous system. Figure 39.1, for example, shows that in spinal cord injury patients the probability of observing DO in successive cystometries does not decrease with repetition,[4] as it does in patients with intact CNS. The inference is that the systematic decrease seen in LUTS patients (Figure 39.1) is not generated peripherally by accommodation of the bladder itself to repeated filling, but represents gradual habituation of the supraspinal bladder control system to the unusual or even frightening circumstances of a urodynamic test.

Thus the variability that affects even the best urodynamic measurements is not an artifact that should be eliminated. Just as heart rate variability is a sign that the cardiac control system is working, so variability of the storage/voiding cycle is a sign that CNS control of the bladder is operating as it should. Indeed, heart rate variability is governed by part of the brain – the anterior cingulate gyrus[11] – which is also closely involved in bladder control, as we shall see below.

From a practical point of view, variability of bladder storage/voiding function is harder to study than heart rate variability because the bladder operates several thousand times more slowly than the heart. Bladder function variability is governed, however, by the control system, and so a possible approach is to investigate the mechanisms of control, and classify their abnormalities, expecting that this will lead to new diagnoses and ultimately to new treatments. We thus need to consider the neural control of the LUT, and the role of voluntary control, as well as how these might be measured.

Control system

Figure 39.2 is a sketch of the subcortical control system, based primarily on a long series of observations in the cat.[12–14] In the storage phase the bladder (detrusor) is relaxed and the striated urethral sphincter contracts tonically under the influence of discharges from the sacral nucleus of Onuf. The urethral contraction is maintained by a sacral reflex,[15] although the pontine L-region, postulated to be a continence center, may also be involved.[16] As the bladder fills, afferent signals to the sacral cord increase in intensity. Secondary afferents ascend through the spinal cord and synapse in the midbrain periaqueductal gray (PAG). If there were no voluntary control and the system were automatic, the voiding reflex would be expected to work as follows. When the afferent signals reaching the PAG became strong enough to reach a threshold level, they would trigger efferents to the pontine micturition center (PMC). Excitation of the PMC would initiate descending efferent output to the sacral cord where it would both excite detrusor contraction and, via an inhibitory interneuron,[12] produce urethral relaxation, so that voiding occurred. The timing of this process is such that urethral relaxation precedes detrusor contraction by about 2 s, just as in normal voiding.[13] Because it involves both the peripheral organs and the pons and midbrain, this is often called the long-loop voiding reflex.

The process just described would lead to automatic voiding – incontinence. Normally, therefore, a more complicated process must occur. During urine storage the PMC (and thus the voiding reflex) is believed to be tonically inhibited by the higher parts of the brain (Figure 39.2).[17,18] Afferents synapsing in the PAG do not trigger voiding but lead first to sensation. When sensation is felt, a decision has to be made whether to void or not. Most often it will be not to void, but when time and place are right the voluntary decision to void may be taken. In that case a motor output signal is sent to the PAG, inhibition of the PMC is temporarily interrupted, and the voiding reflex is then triggered just as in the automatic case. For continence, the

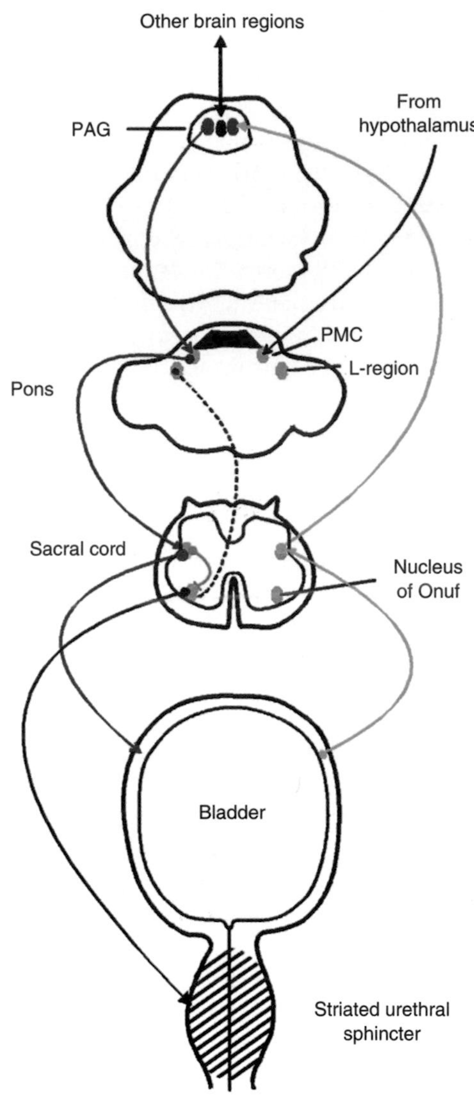

Figure 39.2
The long-loop voiding reflex that forms the basic subcortical neural control system. In the storage phase the striated urethral sphincter contracts tonically under the influence of discharges from the nucleus of Onuf, possibly reinforced by the pontine L-region (dotted pathway). The PAG is tonically inhibited by higher brain regions, preventing excitation of the PMC. As the bladder fills, increasing afferent signals ascend via the green pathway to the PAG. If a threshold is exceeded (or if inhibition by higher regions is interrupted), the PAG is triggered and excites the PMC, which in turn excites sacral parasympathetic neurons and the detrusor muscle itself (blue pathway). Just prior to detectable bladder contraction, the urethral sphincter relaxes under input from inhibitory interneurons at sacral level (gold pathway), so that voiding can be accomplished. There is also direct input to the PMC from the emotional nervous system (the hypothalamus), which is probably inhibitory during the phase of urine storage. PAG, periaqueductal gray; PMC, pontine micturition center.

essence of this process is the ability to make the decision to void or not, which clearly depends on more than just the afferent signals from the bladder. It has been suggested that, to void, a 'safe' signal to the PMC is required from the hypothalamus[12] (see Figure 39.2). Urodynamicists and continence advisors know that circumstances such as the sight of one's own front door or garage door, the sound of running water, or anxiety (e.g. before a difficult examination) affect the decision to void. Such cortical and emotional factors, or factors related to the social interaction between urodynamicist and patient, are ignored in conventional urodynamic examination. They may even be harnessed to work against the desired result, by preventing reproduction of the patient's everyday circumstances and thus preventing the patient from revealing his or her usual symptomatic behavior. It is quite typical, for example, to examine female voiding in the standing position, because it is more convenient for making X-ray pictures. Yet to ask a woman to 'please void normally' in the standing position, exposed to view on a raised platform, surrounded by other people and strange apparatus, with catheters in the urethra and rectum, is obviously absurd. The difference between how they void under these circumstances and how they would void in their own homes is part of the variability we are investigating, and clearly it is due to cortical, emotional, and social influences. Variability in these factors leads to variable urodynamics.

One solution to the problem would be to control such factors, but another would be to measure them and incorporate them in urodynamic investigations. Since they involve cortical input and states of mind the obvious approach is to examine brain activity at the same time as a standard urodynamic investigation. That is, to expand what is measured in urodynamics to include the control system as well as the peripheral organs. In the past, clinical and neurophysiologic observations (see, for example, references 13,15, and 19–21) as well as low-resolution brain scanning by single photon emission computed tomography (SPECT),[22] have yielded considerable information about cerebral control, but brain imaging methods have recently been much improved. The first modern wave of bladder-related studies[23–27] used positron emission tomography (PET) to examine brain responses to bladder events such as withholding urine or voiding. PET is invasive (it requires injection of a radioactive substance), and rather slow – changes can be measured over periods from a few minutes up to an hour or longer. A second wave of studies[28–31] has used functional magnetic resonance imaging (fMRI), which is noninvasive and less expensive. It can make measurements of whole-brain activity over periods as short as one or two seconds, so that in principle it can follow bladder events such as detrusor contraction. It has reasonably good spatial resolution also (about 3 mm). However, the fMRI signal is noisy and requires averaging of frequently repeated measurements to obtain reliable results. It has an unstable baseline and cannot be used to reliably follow long-term changes (over more than a minute or two) without special measures. In addition, the measuring space contains a very strong magnetic field, unsuitable for conventional urodynamic equipment, so that special precautions have to be taken to make urodynamic measurements. (Many of the studies performed so far did not in fact perform simultaneous urodynamics.) Moreover, lying in a scanner with limited social or sensory input is far from the situation in daily life, which makes it difficult to study the bladder's usual behavior. Finally, both PET and fMRI basically measure regional blood flow which, although related to neuronal activity, is unable to distinguish inhibitory from excitatory activity.

In spite of these difficulties, progress has been made in understanding brain control of the bladder. At an anatomic level, studies based on different paradigms for influencing brain activity show activation clustering in certain brain regions, as shown in Figure 39.3a–e. In reality, many other regions are also involved, but the principal observations can be broadly summarized in a simple model, shown in Figure 39.4. It includes the PAG, the PMC, the insula, the anterior cingulate gyrus, and the (pre)frontal cortex. The functional behavior of this anatomic system is not yet entirely clear, but hints provided by neuroanatomic and neurophysiologic observations, by clinical observations of incontinence in trauma and demented patients, and by knowledge of other organ systems, as well as by the PET and fMRI observations themselves, suggest a coherent, though still somewhat speculative account of how control is exercised over the bladder and urethra.

Imaging the cerebral control of the LUT

Useful reviews of this topic have been provided by one of the most active groups in the field.[32–34] The very first PET studies of brain activity related to bladder events[23,24] showed that two regions of the simple model shown in Figure 39.4 are closely involved in voluntary voiding – the PMC and the medial frontal or prefrontal cortex. When the decision to void was made and voluntary voiding was attempted, the PMC was activated in subjects who voided successfully (Figure 39.3e), but not in those who tried but failed to void. These observations support the concept that excitation of the long-loop voiding reflex (probably by removal of inhibition) is necessary for voiding. In addition, among subjects who were able to void in the scanner there was activation of the medial frontal lobe (Figure 39.3c), particularly on the right side, while in those who tried but failed to void the frontal-lobe activation was less intense and slightly shifted. It is tempting to relate medial frontal lobe activity to the voluntary decision to void, since executive function is believed to be located in this area of the brain, while frontal-lobe lesions frequently lead to incontinence (inability to control voiding).[19,21]

Much of the urodynamic variability that we are interested in is related to the storage phase of LUT function. Storage occupies far more time than voiding, while functional disorders of storage are common and lead to a troublesome triad of overactive bladder symptoms – urgency, frequency, and urge incontinence. Measurements made during urine storage are probably more important for understanding loss of bladder control than those made during voiding. Figure 39.5 is an example of real fMRI measurements of brain responses to bladder infusion (filling). Some of the landmarks of the simple model are marked on it. Most responses are bilateral but there is slight evidence from this and other observations[24] that, during storage as during voiding, the right side of the brain is more strongly involved than the left. In interpreting maps like Figure 39.5, it is important to remember that the observed activity may be excitatory or inhibitory. PET observations have suggested that some regions display decreased activation when the bladder is full[24] or when there is a strong desire to void,[26] suggesting inhibition. On general grounds, a complicated network like that controlling the bladder is unlikely to operate in a stable manner unless many of its interconnections are inhibitory. Thus many of the responses shown in Figure 39.5 are likely to be inhibitory.

Such measurements suggest the model of bladder control described in the caption to Figure 39.4. After synapsing in the PAG, afferent signals pass on to the insula, where sensation is mapped. The anterior cingulate gyrus monitors the situation and controls the PMC via the PAG. When bladder sensation or social life demands it, the (pre)frontal cortex is accessed and the decision to void (or not) is taken. If voiding is desired, the tonic inhibition of the PMC is interrupted, perhaps by the anterior cingulate gyrus, and voiding occurs. The thalamus is probably an important relay station for communication among these various regions (see Figure 39.5).

This picture is consistent with knowledge of other visceral organ systems. Typically, visceral sensation is registered in the insula, which can be interrogated to learn the internal condition of the body[35,36] – in this case, the degree of bladder filling. It would thus be expected that normal bladder sensations such as desire to void would be mapped in the insula. Supporting this concept, insular responses to bladder filling become stronger as the bladder becomes more distended and sensation correspondingly stronger (Figure 39.6). With stronger sensation the peak insular response also seems to shift anteriorly, consistent with the general principle that unpleasant sensations are mapped

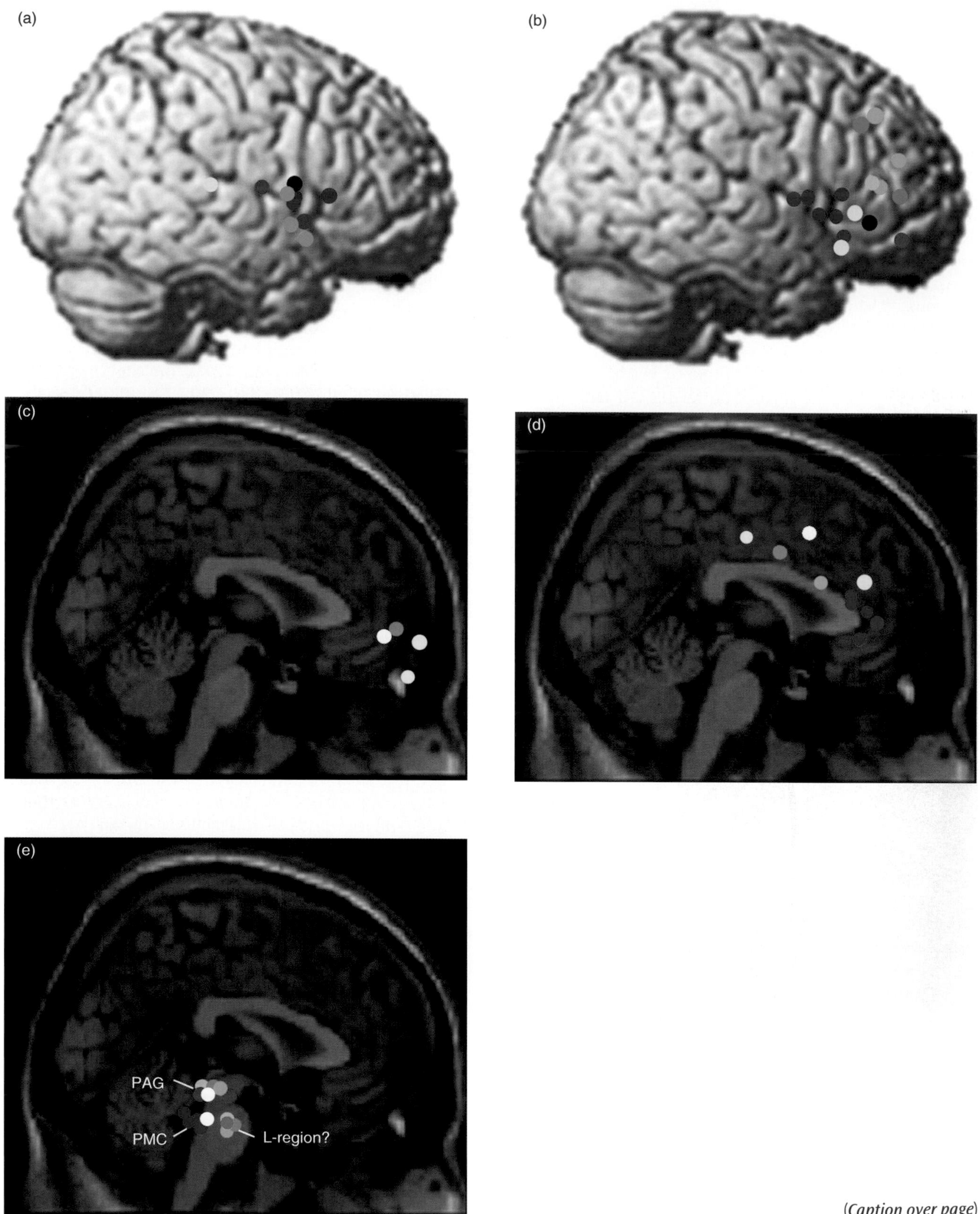

(*Caption over page*)

Figure 39.3
Brain regions activated by different bladder paradigms, showing locations of peak activation (dots). More lateral activations (both right and left) are projected on the right lateral surface of standard MNI brain; more medial on a sagittal section. (a) Regions reported as insula, during storage or withholding of urine, form a cluster near the expected location. *Red*[23,24] *(included voiding, so storage phase difficult to interpret); blue*[25] *(included voiding); magenta;*[27] *dark green;*[44] *black;*[31] *yellow*[45] *(used SPECT, so poor spatial resolution).*
(b) Lateral frontal responses during storage, withholding, or bladder filling, cluster just anterior to the insula with a few responses in anterior and superior parts of the frontal cortex. *Red*[23,24] *(included voiding); blue*[25] *(included voiding); magenta;*[28] *cyan;*[46] *green*[26] *yellow*[45] *(used SPECT, so poor spatial resolution); black;*[31] *dark green*[47] *(response to chronic sacral nerve stimulation, intended to improve withholding).* (c) Medial frontal activation during withholding or urine storage is reported infrequently. *Dark green*[47] *(response to acute sacral nerve stimulation, intended to improve withholding); yellow*[45] *(used SPECT, so poor spatial resolution); white*[31] *(region with abnormally weak response to bladder filling in urge incontinence).* (d) Regions reported as anterior cingulate gyrus (ACG) during storage or withholding form a trail from dorsal to ventral parts of this large region, suggesting that different paradigms activate different ACG areas, which are known to have different functions.[40] *Red*[23,24] *(regions with decreased response during withholding); green*[26] *(increased response with full bladder); dark green*[26] *(decreased response with increasing sensation); blue;*[27] *white;*[31] *yellow*[45] *(used SPECT, so poor spatial resolution).* (e) Brainstem and midbrain region activations reported during storage and voiding seem to cluster in three regions corresponding to pontine micturition center (PMC), periaqueductal gray (PAG), and possibly the L-region (see Figure 39.2). The paradigms used to obtain these results were very varied. *Red*[23,24] *(PMC activated during voiding); blue*[25] *(PMC during voiding); white*[31] *(PAG and PMC during bladder filling); green*[26] *(PAG and possibly L-region response with increasing volume); magenta*[27] *(PAG during storage); dark green*[44] *(PAG and possibly L-region during imagined urge to void); orange*[29] *(possibly L-region with relaxation and contraction of pelvic floor as if inhibiting imaginary voiding).*

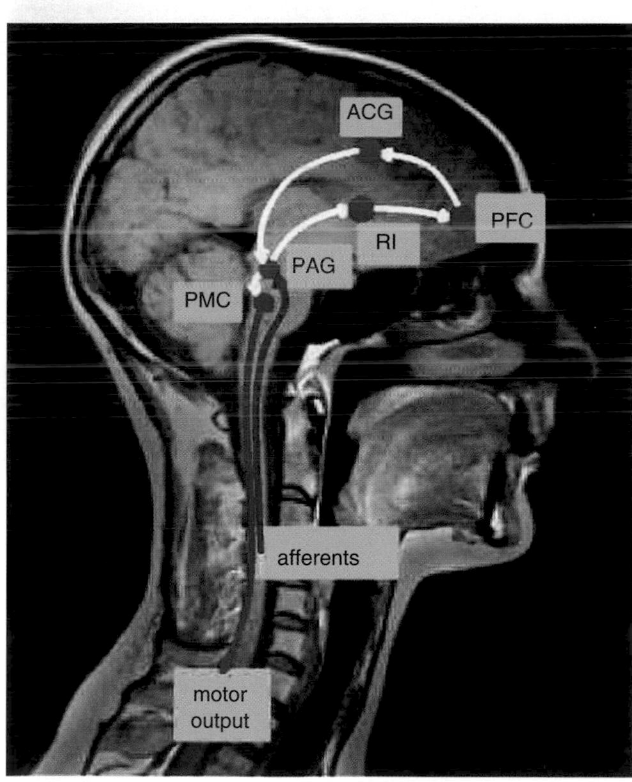

Figure 39.4
A simple working model of normal cortical control provides more detail about the 'other brain regions' shown in Figure 39.2. Among many regions involved, the five shown here seem to be important. The anatomy of the regions is well understood and some interconnections are reasonably well established, but their suggested functions are hypothetical. Afferents from the sacral cord synapse in the PAG, and are passed to the insula (predominantly on the right), where visceral sensations are mapped. The lateral parts of the prefrontal cortex are also involved. The ACG monitors the situation and sends regulatory signals (inhibitory during the storage phase) to the PAG and PMC. To initiate voluntary voiding the frontal cortex takes the decision, inhibition from the ACG is interrupted, the PMC (and therefore the long-loop reflex) is activated, and voiding takes place. PMC, pontine micturition centre; PAG, periaqueductal gray; RI, right insula; PFC, prefrontal cortex; ACG, anterior cingulate gyrus.

more anteriorly in the insula.[10] Responses in other parts of the brain, for example the anterior cingulate gyrus, also increase to a moderate extent with increasing bladder filling, but overall responses are quite similar at large and small volumes. The perifornical region of the hypothalamus, one of the few parts of the brain with direct monosynaptic connection to the PMC,[37] also responds strongly to bladder infusion (Figure 39.6c), suggesting that it may provide direct inhibition of the PMC during storage. Removal of the inhibition would correspond to the 'safe' signal mentioned above. Such a hypothalamic input to the PMC would also allow direct modulation of bladder behavior by the emotions, and would be one source of the observed urodynamic variability.

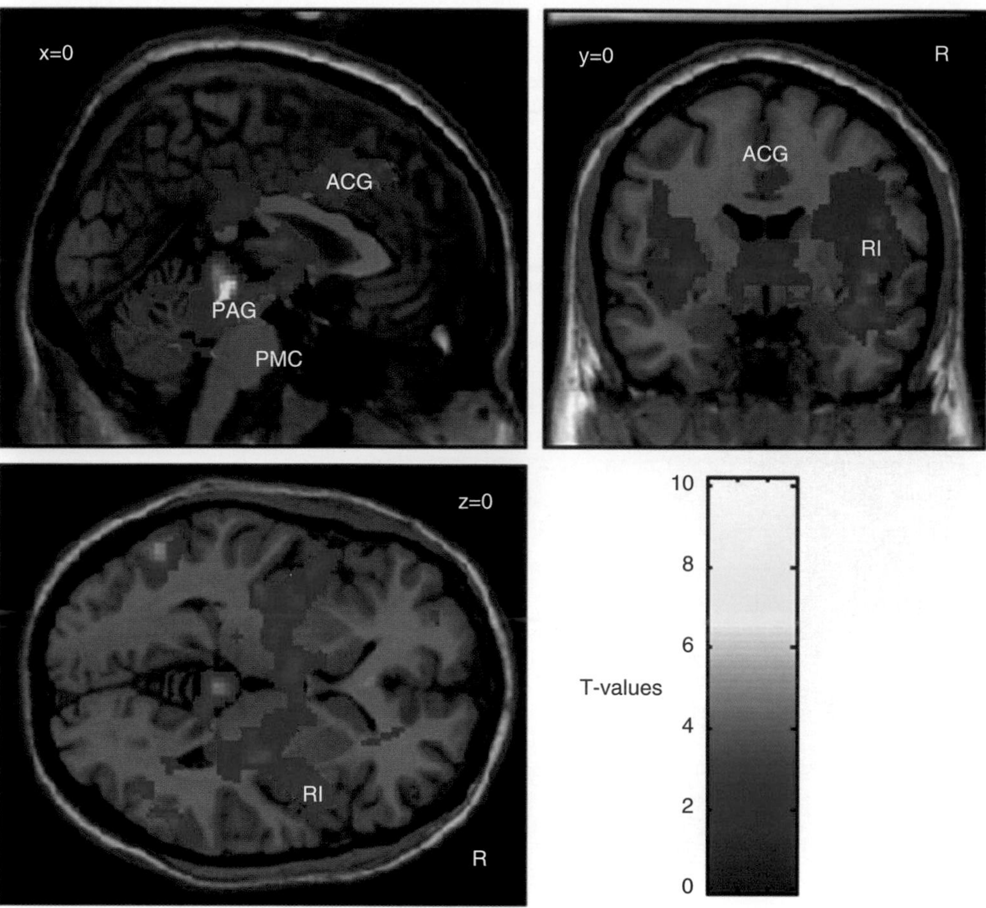

Figure 39.5
Brain responses to bladder filling measured by fMRI in a group of 6 normal females with a small volume in the bladder and mild bladder sensation. These are three sections through a 3-dimensional map showing the statistical significance of responses to repetitive infusion and withdrawal. The map is thresholded at a liberal significance level ($p < 0.05$, uncorrected for multiple comparisons) in order not to miss any important regions. The three sections (sagittal, coronal, and axial) are made through the origin of standard MNI coordinates on the midline near the anterior commissure. Some landmarks of the simple model are marked. Although strongly activated, the PAG appears misplaced posteriorly. The midline region between the right and left insulae and rostral to the PAG is the thalamus, a relay station omitted from the simple model. PAG, periaqueductal gray.

Another area of the brain, the lateral part of the frontal cortex close to the insula, also responds to bladder filling (Figures 39.3b and 39.6c),[38] but the medial part that is so important during voiding displays little observable activity during storage (Figure 39.3c). This suggests that bladder control during the storage phase is mainly exercised without intervention from the conscious decision-making parts of the frontal cortex, and indeed this must be so since otherwise much of one's waking life would be devoted to making decisions about bladder control.

The anterior cingulate gyrus is a large area believed to be responsible for monitoring of overall responses and for autonomic and emotional arousal.[11,39,40] Exactly which part is activated seems to be strongly dependent on the paradigm used to elicit it (Figure 39.3d). In subjects with normal bladder control it is not very strongly activated at either smaller or larger bladder volumes, presumably because nothing threatens the normal inhibition of the voiding reflex. In subjects with urge incontinence, however, even outside any episode of DO, part of the anterior cingulate gyrus responds very strongly to bladder filling when bladder sensation is already strong (Figure 39.7). This is accompanied by widespread and exaggerated activation of other regions, apparently representing recruitment of accessory pathways (including regions omitted from the simple model) in an attempt to maintain bladder control by more strongly inhibiting the voiding reflex. This brain state, with the anterior cingulate gyrus on 'red alert' and many pathways recruited, occurs prior to any manifestation of actual DO, and may represent

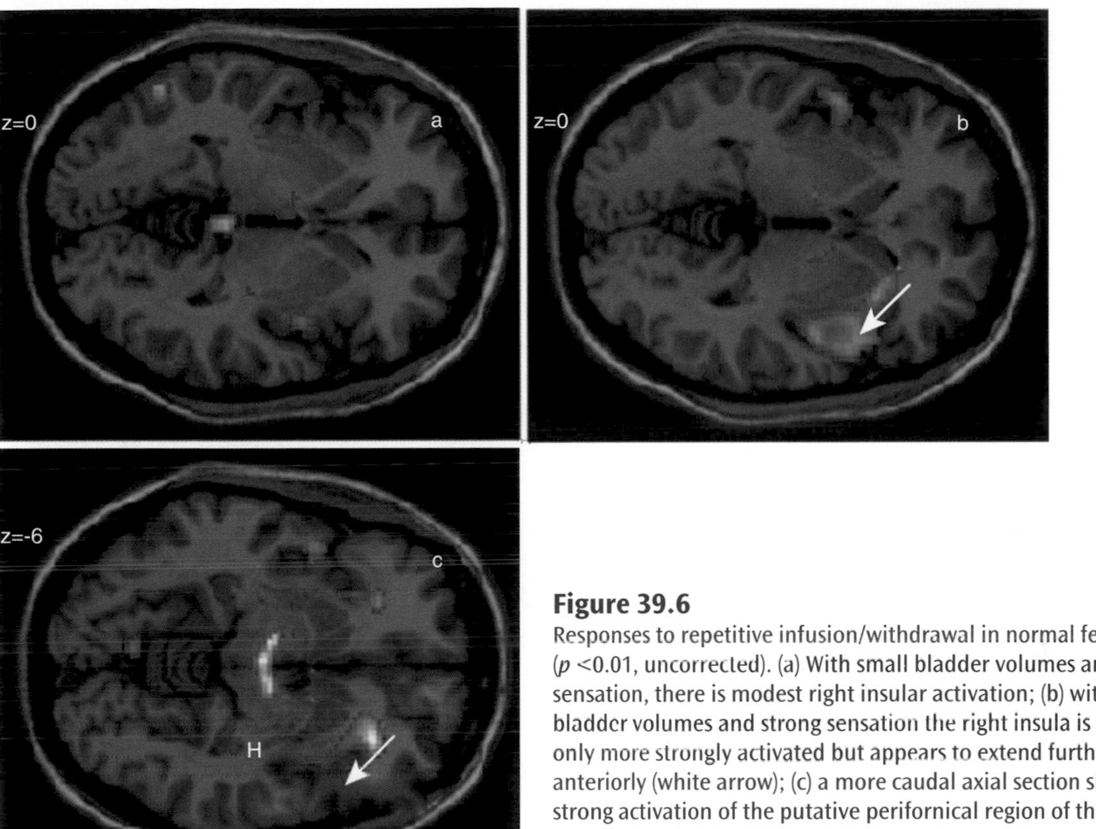

Figure 39.6
Responses to repetitive infusion/withdrawal in normal females ($p < 0.01$, uncorrected). (a) With small bladder volumes and mild sensation, there is modest right insular activation; (b) with large bladder volumes and strong sensation the right insula is not only more strongly activated but appears to extend further anteriorly (white arrow); (c) a more caudal axial section shows strong activation of the putative perifornical region of the hypothalamus (H) with large bladder volume and strong sensation.

the sensation of urgency, which has otherwise proved difficult to define.[1,41] There is some suggestion (requiring confirmation[38]) that, if DO occurs, anterior cingulate gyrus and accompanying activations decrease somewhat, suggesting that it is failure to maintain adequate inhibition that allows DO to develop.

Thus brain responses to bladder filling are abnormal in urge-incontinent individuals, even when there is no overt DO, and they appear to represent urgency. These abnormal responses, however, seem to be a reaction to threatened loss of bladder control; they do not indicate why control might be precarious in the first place. Some observations in urge-incontinent subjects suggest that, prior to any urgency, insular response to bladder filling may be weaker than normal.[31] This result – unexpected because it is generally believed that sensation is stronger in urge incontinence – may indicate that the brain is paying insufficient attention to afferent (sensory) feedback about the state of the bladder. Without adequate feedback the operation of any control system is inevitably compromised.[34,42]

Consistent with this postulate that inadequate afferent feedback and/or reduced sensation play a causal role in urge incontinence, insular responses[38] and the corresponding clinically measured bladder sensations[43] both become weaker in elderly people with normal bladder control. Declining feedback may make them gradually more susceptible to development of the urge incontinence that becomes so common and troublesome in later life. Similarly, early observations in frail elderly people showed that poor bladder control was often accompanied by reduced sensation of bladder filling, which led to severe urge incontinence.[22] There was evidence also that this type of incontinence was associated with brain disease, because it was often accompanied by cognitive impairment and reduced frontal cortical perfusion (measured by SPECT).[22] Even in relatively young urge-incontinent subjects there is some fMRI evidence for an abnormally weak response to bladder filling in the inferior part of the prefrontal cortex (the orbitofrontal cortex) (Figure 39.8),[31] suggesting that a defect in the capability to make decisions about voiding might be causally related to the incontinence. Although superficially attractive, this postulate has to contend with the observation that frontal-lobe responses to bladder filling are normally quite weak in any case, probably because (as suggested above) only the decision to void is taken there, and not the decision *not* to void.

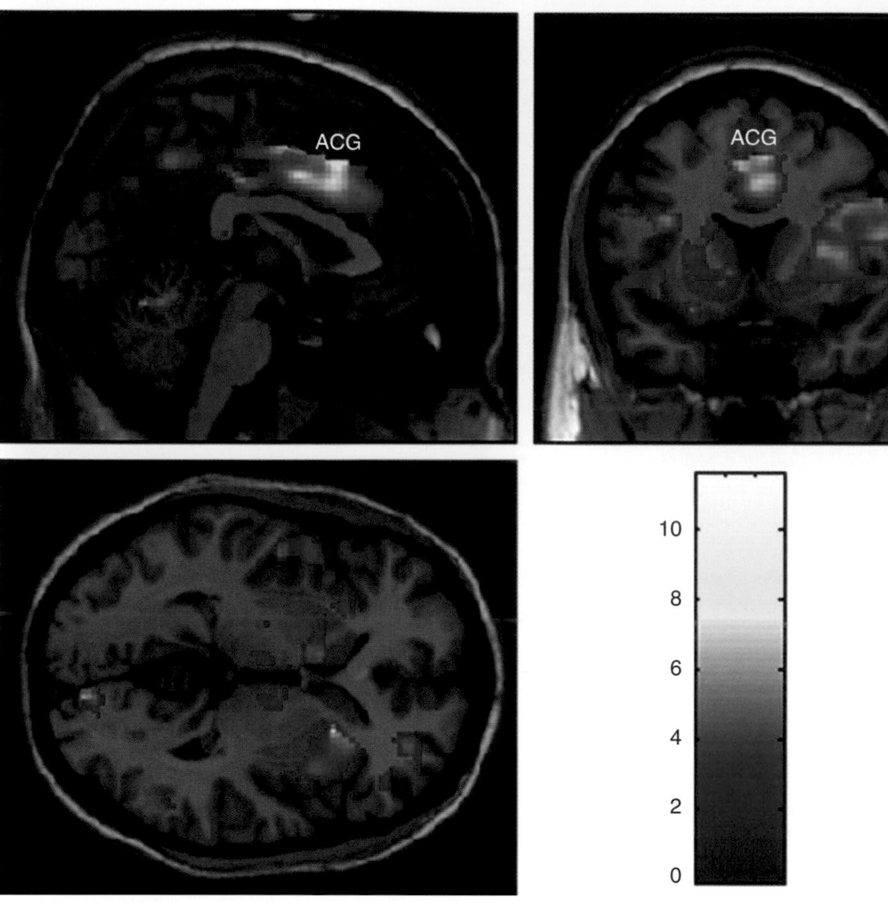

Figure 39.7
In female subjects with urge incontinence the anterior cingulate gyrus (ACG) responds very strongly to bladder filling when the bladder is full and sensation is strong (probably representing urgency but without concurrent detrusor overactivity). Other sections (not shown) reveal widespread and exaggerated activity in many brain regions.

Advanced urodynamics: the current position

It seems that we stand on the brink of a new understanding of how the LUT is controlled by the brain, and how changes in the cerebral control system influence bladder behavior and contribute to the measurement variability which has plagued the field of urodynamics for so long. We shall come to view this variability as a normal consequence of changes in the emotional state of the patient, as influenced by cortical input, social interaction with the staff, and memory of previous bladder-related events. Even without brain scanning or other high-tech methods, we may be able deliberately to alter this emotional state, by changing the circumstances of our examinations (for example by playing standardized videos during urodynamic testing), so as to observe and interpret the resulting variability of LUT behavior. We shall probably conclude that much variability is normal, and that lack of variability is a marker of abnormal (inadequate) cerebral control.

At present however, advanced urodynamics is still a research topic. The anatomic outlines of the brain/bladder control system are fairly clear, but how it operates is still a topic of very active research. We are able to make observations in small groups of subjects, but observations in individual subjects are not yet reliable enough to be of diagnostic value. Nor are the conditions under which brain scanning is performed at all ideal: they are far from daily life and this must influence the observations, just as it influences conventional urodynamics. Thus improvements in technique are required before functional brain scanning can become clinically useful.

The observations made so far suggest that in the future we shall be able to recognize the patterns of brain activity corresponding to various bladder sensations. In fact, functional brain scanning will almost certainly lead to a new classification of bladder sensation, allowing us for the first time to properly distinguish normal sensations of desire to void from other sensations such as urgency, and both of these from the various bladder pain syndromes[1] and from bladder-related anxiety. These distinctions will be of great value in a field where reliable diagnoses have until now been elusive.

The pattern of brain activity that corresponds to urgency seems to be a reaction to poor bladder control

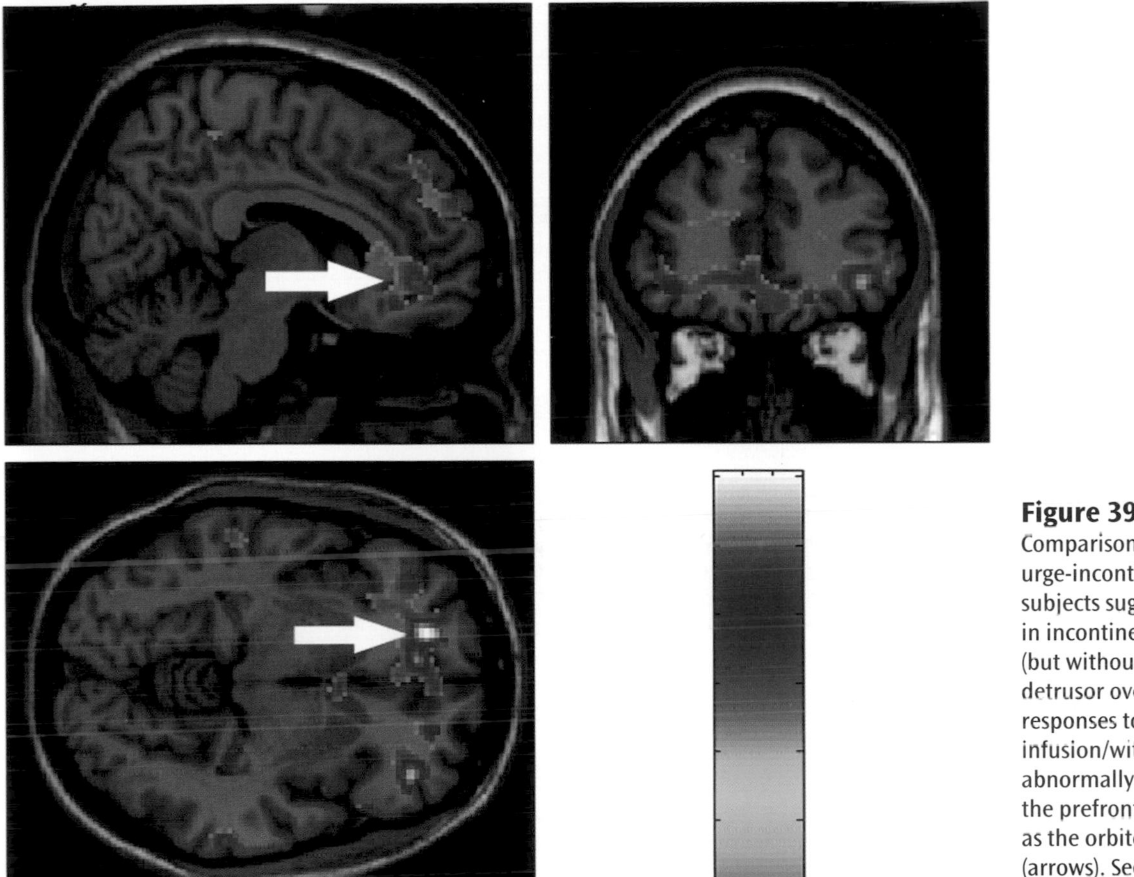

Figure 39.8
Comparison between urge-incontinent and normal subjects suggests that, in incontinent subjects (but without concurrent detrusor overactivity), responses to rapid infusion/withdrawal are abnormally weak in part of the prefrontal cortex known as the orbitofrontal cortex (arrows). See also Figure 39.3c.

rather than a cause, leaving open the possibility that there are many potential causal factors in urge incontinence and 'idiopathic' detrusor overactivity; separately or in combination they all lead to a similar reaction – urgency – that is the key characteristic of the overactive bladder syndrome. 'Advanced' urodynamics has so far not clearly identified any of these potential causes in the brain, but there are hints that reduced bladder afferents (or insufficient attention to these afferents) or reduced frontal cortical function may play a causal role in some subtypes of urge incontinence. Clearly a rich field of research is about to open up, with enormous promise of more accurate diagnoses and ultimately better treatment of the common and troublesome disorders of LUT control.

Acknowledgments

The work on which this chapter is based was supported by grants RO3AG25166, RO1AG020629, and T32AG021885 from the US Public Health Service and by the University of Pittsburgh Competitive Medical Research Fund. I am grateful to the staff of the Geriatric Continence Unit and the UPMC Magnetic Resonance Research Center for their help, and especially to Neil Resnick, Werner Schaefer, Stasa Tadic, and Mary Alyce Riley. The data analysis on which Figure 39.3 is based was performed by Stasa D Tadic, and the grid used to prepare the figure was kindly provided by Dr Stuart Derbyshire of Birmingham University, UK.

References

1. Abrams P, Cardozo L, Fall M et al. The standardisation of terminology of lower urinary tract function: report from the Standardisation Sub-committee of the International Continence Society. Neurourol Urodyn 2002; 21(2): 167–78.
2. Griffiths D, Kondo A, Bauer S et al. Dynamic testing. In: Abrams P, Cardozo L, Khoury S, Wein A, eds. Incontinence: 3rd International Consultation on Incontinence. Plymouth, UK: Health Publication Ltd, 2005: 585–673.
3. Chaliha C, Jeffery S, Lamba A, Khan M, Khullar V. Voiding intervals and warning times – are they a reproducible marker? Neurourol Urodyn 2005; 24(5–6): abstract #85.
4. Ockrim J, Laniado ME, Khoubehi B et al. Variability of detrusor overactivity on repeated filling cystometry in men with urge symptoms: comparison with spinal cord injury patients. BJU Int 2005; 95(4): 587–90.

5. Griffiths D, Scholtmeijer RJ. Detrusor instability in children. Neurourol Urodyn 1982; 1: 187–92.
6. Sorensen S, Gregersen H, Sorensen SM. Long term reproducibility of urodynamic investigations in healthy fertile females. Scand J Urol Nephrol 1988; 114: 35–41.
7. van Waalwijk van Doorn ES, Remmers A, Janknegt RA. Conventional and extramural ambulatory urodynamic testing of the lower urinary tract in female volunteers. J Urol 1992; 147(5): 1319–25; discussion 26.
8. Ralls K. Mammalian scent marking. Science 1971; 171: 443–9.
9. Smith PS. Incontinence in children. In: First International Conference on the Prevention of Incontinence 1997. Danesfield House, UK, 1997.
10. Craig AD. A new view of pain as a homeostatic emotion. Trends Neurosci 2003; 26(6): 303–7.
11. Critchley HD, Mathias CJ, Josephs O et al. Human cingulate cortex and autonomic control: converging neuroimaging and clinical evidence. Brain 2003; 126: 2139–52.
12. Blok BF, Holstege G. The neuronal control of micturition and its relation to the emotional motor system. Progr Brain Res 1996; 107: 113–26.
13. Holstege G, Griffiths D, de Wall H, Dalm E. Anatomical and physiological observations on supraspinal control of bladder and urethral sphincter muscles in the cat. J Comp Neurol 1986; 250(4): 449–61.
14. Holstege G. Micturition and the soul. J Comp Neurol 2005; 493: 15–20.
15. DeGroat WC, Booth AM, Yoshimura N. Neurophysiology of micturition and its modification in animal models of human disease. In: Maggi CA, ed. The Autonomic Nervous System, Vol 3. Nervous Control of the Urogenital System. London: Harwood Academic Publishers, 1993: 227–90.
16. Blok BF, Holstege G. The central nervous system control of micturition in cats and humans. Behav Brain Res 1998; 92(2): 119–25.
17. Torrens M. Human physiology. In: Torrens M, Morrison FB, eds. The Physiology of the Lower Urinary Tract. Berlin, Heidelberg: Springer-Verlag, 1987: 333–50.
18. Morrison J, Steers WD, Brading A et al. Neurophysiology and neuropharmacology. In: Abrams P, Cardozo L, Khoury S, Wein A, eds. Incontinence: 2nd International Consultation on Incontinence. Plymouth, UK: Plymbridge Distributors Ltd, 2002: 83–163.
19. Andrew J, Nathan PW. Lesions of the anterior frontal lobes and disturbances of micturition and defecation. Brain 1964; 87: 233–62.
20. Barrington FJF. The component reflexes of micturition in the cat. Part III. Brain 1941; 64: 239–43.
21. Sakakibara R, Hattori T, Yasuda K, Yamanishi T. Micturition disturbance after acute hemispheric stroke: analysis of the lesion site by CT and MRI. J Neurol Sci 1996; 137: 47–56.
22. Griffiths DJ, McCracken PN, Harrison GM, Moore KN. Urinary incontinence in the elderly: the brain factor. Scand J Urol Nephrol 1994; 157: 83–8.
23. Blok BF, Sturms LM, Holstege G. Brain activation during micturition in women. Brain 1998; 121(Pt 11): 2033–42.
24. Blok BF, Willemsen AT, Holstege G. A PET study on brain control of micturition in humans. Brain 1997; 120(Pt 1): 111–21.
25. Nour S, Svarer C, Kristensen JK, Paulson OB, Law I. Cerebral activation during micturition in normal men. Brain 2000; 123(Pt 4): 781–9.
26. Athwal BS, Berkley KJ, Hussain I et al. Brain responses to changes in bladder volume and urge to void in healthy men. Brain 2001; 124(Pt 2): 369–77.
27. Matsuura S, Kakizaki H, Mitsui T et al. Human brain region response to distention or cold stimulation of the bladder: a positron emission tomography study. J Urol 2002; 168(5): 2035–9.
28. Kuhtz-Buschbeck JP, Van der Horst C, Wolff S et al. Activation of the supplementary motor area (SMA) during voluntary pelvic floor muscle contractions – an fMRI study. Neuroimage 2007; 35: 449–57.
29. Seseke S, Baudewig J, Kallenberg K et al. Voluntary pelvic floor muscle control – an fMRI study. Neuroimage 2006; 31: 1399–407.
30. Zhang H, Reitz A, Kollias S et al. An fMRI study of the role of suprapontine brain structures in the voluntary voiding control induced by pelvic floor contraction. Neuroimage 2005; 24: 174–80.
31. Griffiths D, Derbyshire S, Stenger A, Resnick N. Brain control of normal and overactive bladder. J Urol 2005; 174: 1862–7.
32. Kavia RB, Dasgupta R, Fowler CJ. Functional imaging and the central control of the bladder. J Comp Neurol 2005; 493: 27–32.
33. DasGupta R, Kavia RB, Fowler CJ. Cerebral mechanisms and voiding dysfunction. BJU Int 2007; 99: 731–4.
34. Fowler CJ. Integrated control of lower urinary tract – clinical perspective. Br J Pharmacol 2006; 147(Suppl 2): S14–24.
35. Craig AD. Interoception: the sense of the physiological condition of the body. Curr Opin Neurobiol 2003; 13(4): 500–5.
36. Damasio A. Feelings of emotion and the self. Ann NY Acad Sci 2003; 1001: 253–61.
37. Kuipers R, Mouton LJ, Holstege G. Afferent projections to the pontine micturition center in the cat. J Comp Neurol 2006; 494: 36–53.
38. Griffiths D, Tadic SD, Schaefer W, Resnick NM. Cerebral control of the bladder in normal and urge-incontinent women. Neuroimage 2007; 37: 1–7.
39. Kerns JG, Cohen JD, MacDonald AW et al. Anterior cingulate conflict monitoring and adjustments in control. Science 2004; 303(5660): 1023–6.
40. Bush G, Luu P, Posner M. Cognitive and emotional influences in anterior cingulate cortex. Trends Cogn Sci 2000; 4: 215–22.
41. Abrams P, Blaivas JG, Stanton S, Andersen JT. The standardisation of terminology of lower urinary tract function. Neurourol Urodyn 1988; 7: 403–26.
42. Andersson KE. Mechanisms of disease: central nervous system involvement in overactive bladder syndrome. Nat Clin Pract Urol 2004; 1: 103–8.
43. Pfisterer M, Griffiths D, Schaefer W, Resnick N. The effect of age on lower urinary tract function: a study in women. J Am Geriatr Soc 2006: 405–12.
44. Kuhtz-Buschbeck JP, van der Horst C, Pott C et al. Cortical representation of the urge to void: a functional magnetic resonance imaging study. J Urol 2005; 174: 1477–81.
45. Yin Y, Shuke N, Okizaki A et al. Cerebral activation during withholding urine with full bladder in healthy men using 99mTc-HMPAO SPECT. J Nucl Med 2006; 47(7): 1093–8.
46. Di Gangi Herms AMR, Veit R, Reisenauer C et al. Functional imaging of stress urinary incontinence. NeuroImage 2006; 29: 267–75.
47. Blok BFM, Groen J, Bosch JLHR, Veltman DJ, Lammersma AA. Different brain effects during chronic and acute sacral modulation in urge incontinent patients with implanted neurostimulators. BJU Int 2006; 08: 1238–43.

40

Normal urodynamic parameters in children

Diego Barriéras and Steven P Lapointe

Introduction

Urodynamic examination yields invaluable information about lower urinary tract function in infants and children. First developed in adults, the techniques have been used in children extensively, using the same terminology and definitions as in adult urodynamics. The computers and devices used for evaluation of lower urinary tract function in children are similar to those in adults, with appropriate catheter sizes according to age and urethral caliber. Litvak et al[1] published a large series of urethral calibrations that gives an excellent range of appropriate catheter size to use in boys, measured in French (Table 40.1). Immergut et al[2] measured urethral size at different ages in girls (Table 40.2). Also, the urodynamic units may be adapted to incorporate special software designed to facilitate biofeedback training in children. Most importantly, these types of investigation are best performed by physicians, nurses, or physical therapists who are specialized in the care of children. The urodynamic team has to handle the child with care and patience, keeping a playful mood, distracting the child's attention from the surrounding environment, and following the pace set by the child to alleviate the pressure of performance, so reducing apprehension. This ensures that the results obtained are reliable and minimally influenced by the effect of the immediate environment on the child. A center dedicated to children's care can accomplish this more easily, but with appropriate attention to these differences, children can be accommodated in an adult-oriented facility. In this chapter we will cover the normal urodynamic evaluation of children.

Before the urodynamic evaluation

When evaluating a child with suspected lower urinary tract dysfunction, a detailed history should be obtained. The past medical history, especially previous urinary tract

Table 40.1 *Calibre of the urethral meatus in boys, according to age*

Age (years)	Size (French)	*n* (%)	Size (French)	*n* (%)
<1	6	22/160 (14)	10	138/160 (86)
1	6	10/63 (14)	10	53/63 (86)
2	6	17/109 (16)	12	92/109 (84)
3	6	13/93 (14)	12	80/93 (86)
4	8	13/83 (8)	12	70/83 (84)
5	8	10/111 (9)	12	92/111 (83)
6	8	8/87 (9)	12	61/87 (82)
7	8	4/56 (9)	12	43/56 (77)
8	8	5/61 (8)	12	41/61 (67)
9	8	4/60 (7)	12	40/60 (67)
10	8	3/50 (6)	12	37/50 (74)
11	8–10	2/45 (4)	14	36/45 (80)
12	8–10	2/40 (5)	14	28/40 (69)

Table 40.2 *Urethral calibre in girls, according to age*

Age (years)	Patients (*n*)	Mean size (French)
<2	15	14
4	18	15
6	23	15
8	25	16
10	16	19
12	6	21
14	7	23
16	9	25
18–20	6	26

Table 40.3 *Advantages and disadvantages of uroflowmetry in children*

Advantages	Disadvantages
Simple to perform	Not etiologic
Simple equipment	Less reproducible than in adults
Noninvasive	Children need to be toilet trained
Physiologic	
Can be repeated	
Low cost	

surgery or disease, and neurologic status are relevant. The present medical history should include details about urinary tract infection, trauma, voiding pattern, incontinence, urgency, frequency, and urinary stream appearance. Bowel habits should be noted. To complete the history, we have found that recording a voiding diary and a stool diary gives objective data that, coupled with the history, will allow better clarification of the lower urinary tract dysfunction. These diaries can be repeated in the follow-up to monitor improvement, and this also involves the child and his parents. Physical exam should include abdominal, genitalia, and lumbosacral spine exam, and a brief neurologic exam of the lower limbs. This complete evaluation will facilitate the choice of the appropriate urodynamic exam. In pediatrics, uroflowmetry with or without electromyography (EMG) of the pelvic floor is the most frequent exam used. A full urodynamic evaluation is done in specific situations. The next part of the chapter will cover uroflowmetry with EMG and residual volume measurement. The last part of the chapter will cover full urodynamic evaluation in children.

Uroflowmetry with EMG and postvoid residual volume

Because of the invasive and stressful nature of a complete urodynamics exam in children, uroflowmetry with EMG using surface electrodes should be performed as an initial investigation of lower urinary tract dysfunction, except for children who present with diagnosed conditions such as spinal dysraphism or posterior valves and imperforate anus. Uroflowmetry has been popularized as a study of lower urinary tract obstruction, mainly for benign prostatic hyperplasia.[3,4] Although the firsts reports on the use of uroflowmetry in children date back to the 1950s,[5] it had become a widespread tool by the 1980s.[6–9] Williot et al coupled measurement of uroflowmetry to postvoid residual volume assessment using biplanar ultrasound.[9] They stated that the combination of dynamic flow analysis and accurate bladder residual volume assessment proved to be a simple yet comprehensive appraisal of the physiology of the lower urinary tract. Residual volume measurement can also be accomplished with urethral catheterization, although this would negate the noninvasive nature of uroflowmetry with EMG and residual volume assessment. These studies have several advantages that make them almost ideal for the pediatric population (Table 40.3). They are noninvasive, physiologic, and can be repeated as frequently as necessary.

In 1981 Barrett and Wein[10] advocated EMG of the pelvic floor to determine proper relaxation of the pelvic floor muscles before and during the voiding phase of the uroflowmetry. Since then, this study has gained widespread use and is most often done using surface electrodes as opposed to needle electrodes, which are rarely used in pediatrics due to their invasive nature. Although the recording is not as precise with surface electrodes, it provides valuable information about pelvic floor activity. The relationship between uroflowmetry and pelvic floor activity can indicate the etiology of dysfunctional voiding illustrated by bladder sphincter dysynergia.

Indication for uroflowmetry/EMG/postvoid residual volume

Uroflowmetry has multiple applications in children of both sexes. It can be used in any clinical situation with suspected lower urinary tract dysfunction, even though it is not a highly specific diagnostic tool.[11] It has semiologic value and gives important information as a screening

Table 40.4 *Indications for uroflowmetry and EMG in children*

- Urgency, frequency syndrome
- Urinary tract infection
- Incontinence (except isolated night-time incontinence)
- Dysfunctional voiding syndrome
- Non-neurogenic neurogenic bladder (Hinman/Allen syndrome)
- Vesicoureteric reflux before and after surgical correction
- Neurogenic bladder
- Infravesical obstruction (urethral valves, urethral or meatal stenosis)
- Follow-up in hypospadias surgery and other urethral reconstruction
- Biofeedback method for bladder retraining (coupled with EMG)

method, helping diagnosis and/or leading to more elaborate testing (full urodynamics), particularly in evaluating voiding dysfunction and urinary tract infection. The studies can be used as a follow-up tool to assess the result of surgical treatment, especially after hypospadias repair and other urethral surgeries (epispadias, urethral stenosis, etc.), or in long-term follow-up of posterior urethral valve surgery. It is also very useful in following medical treatment, especially in bladder retraining for dysfunctional voiding and non-neurogenic neurogenic bladder.[12,13] In comparing multiple studies in the same patient, it is important to recognize that uroflowmetry in children is not as reproducible as in adults.[11,12] Consequently, the trend analysis of multiple studies has more value.

Current indications for performing uroflowmetry and EMG are listed in Table 40.4.

Normal uroflowmetry and EMG

The combination of uroflowmetry and residual volume with pelvic floor EMG estimate gives rise to a number of parameters, as is the case in adults. Figure 40.1 is a schematic representation of normal uroflowmetry, with the different variables identified. In Figure 40.2, normal uroflowmetry with EMG and residual volume assessment is presented. This recording of a 6-year-old child, shows the almost bell-shaped curve with a 23 ml/s maximal flow rate, the pelvic floor relaxation just before the flow recording, and its contraction at the end of voiding. A more detailed interpretation of the test is discussed later. Normal values for uroflowmetry are given in Table 40.5.

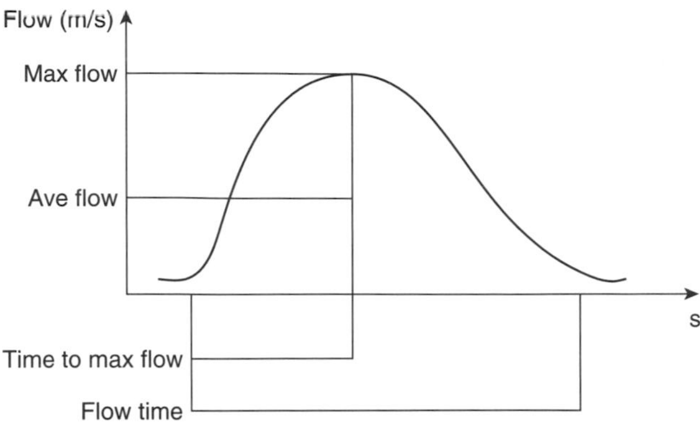

Figure 40.1
Normal uroflowmetry parameters.

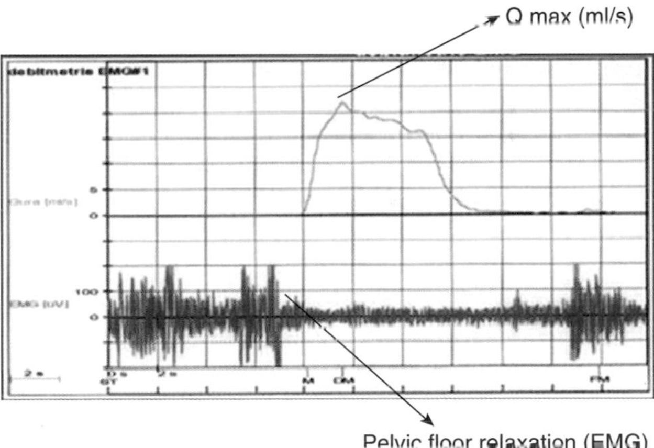

Figure 40.2
Uroflowmetry combined with pelvic floor EMG in a normal child.

Technical aspects and pitfalls

To obtain optimal results from uroflowmetry, the voiding condition should be as close to normal as possible. This is true in adults and even more important in children.[7,8] Children, especially under the age of 6, differ from older children and adults in the sense that they are usually less motivated, less patient, more apprehensive, and have limited understanding of what is going to happen.[8] The postvoid residual volume can be determined by ultrasound using a model that considers the bladder to be a rectangular box. This equipment is readily available and cost-effective. Using a sagittal and a transverse view, two measures of bladder diameter are taken, and from these the volume in milliliters is generated. This technique is simple, noninvasive (vs catheterization), accurate, and reproducible.[19] It should be noted that it has a slight tendency to overestimate the residual volume when compared to urethral catheterization.[11] Finally, like any ultrasonic technique it is operator-dependent, but this technique is easy to learn for those involved in urodynamic testing.

Table 40.5

Urodynamic characteristic	Normal value in children
Uroflow	Maximal flow rate = square root of the voided volume[8]
Bladder capacity (ml)	Houle et al:[26] 16 (age (years)) + 70
	Koff:[24] (age (years) +2) × 30
	Kaefer et al:[25] (2 × age (years) + 2) × 30 (child < 2 years old) (age (years) divided by 2 + 6) × 30 (child > 2 years old)
	Hjämåls :[8] 30 + (age (years) × 30)
Uninhibited contractions	Any appreciable detrusor contraction
Bladder compliance	> 10 ml/cmH_2O[27]
Voiding pressures	Infant male: median 100 cmH_2O[21]
	Infant female: median 70 cmH_2O[21]
	1–3 years old child male: 70 cmH_2O[8]
	1–3 years old child female: 60 cmH_2O[30]
	7 years and older: similar to adult
Postvoid residual	Infant: 1 void / 4 hour complete, median PVR 4–5 ml
(limited reliability)	up to 2 years old: 4–5 ml[23]
	3 years old and up: 0 ml

Interpretation of uroflowmetry

The availability of nomograms for analysis of uroflow data has been helpful in providing 'relative' data for size and weight, while recognizing that their absolute interpretation can be misleading.[6,13–16] However, there are general principles that guide the interpretation of the uroflowmetry data in children. As in adults, the results obtained are an integration of detrusor contractility and urethral resistance.[7] We believe that the shape of the flow curve is the most important feature of uroflowmetry, followed by maximal flow rate. Interestingly, the shape of the normal flow curve in children is the same as in adults and is a bell shape curve (Figures 40.1, 40.2, and 40.3a) in more than 90% of normal children, even if the voided volume is under 100 ml.[7,13,14,17] With low or high voided volumes the shape of the curve has a tendency toward a more plateau appearance.

There are three other frequently encountered shapes. The staccato shape (Figure 40.3b) is indicative of either abnormal sphincter relaxation, and may be a reflection of dysfunctional voiding as in the non-neurogenic neurogenic bladder, unsustained bladder contraction, or abdominal straining. Children with dysfunctional voiding often benefit from bladder retraining, in which case uroflowmetry, nomograms, and especially developed computer programs and games can be used as a method of biofeedback.[18] An example of staccato flow curve secondary to bladder sphincter dysynergia is shown in Figure 40.3c. A plateau-shaped curve (Figure 40.3d) may be normal but can indicate infravesical obstruction, especially if associated with a low maximal and average flow rates. In such a case, depending on history and physical examination, further diagnostic tests may be indicated. For example, a voiding cystogram would permit identification of posterior urethral valves that sometimes present at an older age. It should also be noted that, after hypospadias surgery, the uroflowmetry results obtained are those of a plateau type curve with low maximal and average flow rates. The physician should only be concerned when there is a trend towards worsening over successive studies.[19] Figure 40.3e illustrates an example of a plateau-shaped curve post-hypospadias surgery. Of note is a low average and peak flow rate coupled with normal sphincter relaxation. A tower-shaped curve (Figure 40.3f) is usually associated with a high maximal flow rate and is believed to reflect dysfunctional voiding. It is more frequently encountered in girls and is often referred to as 'supervoiders'. It is associated with relaxation of the pelvic floor after the beginning of the bladder contraction causing an explosive flow curve. In Figure 40.3g, a 10-year-old girl with symptoms of low frequency voiding and urge incontinence exemplifies the tower-shaped curve, typical of voiding postponement.

One has to be critical when looking at these results. Artifacts, mostly caused by misdirection of the stream, will change the shape of the curve and thus the numbers generated,[7] especially in children.

The maximal and average flow rates closely correlate with voided volume, which is dependent on the age and size of the child. Again, the nomograms are helpful as references,

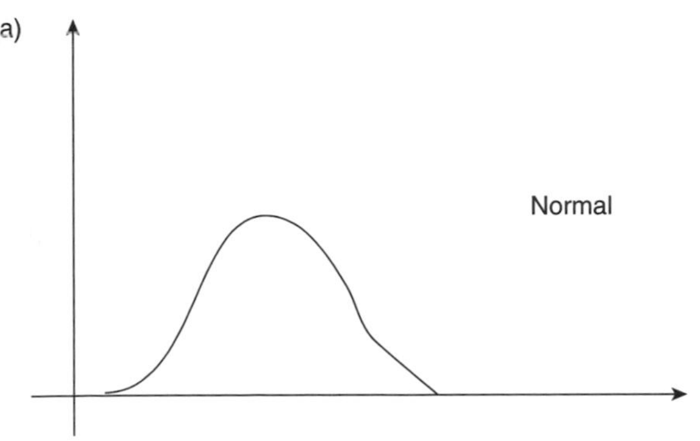

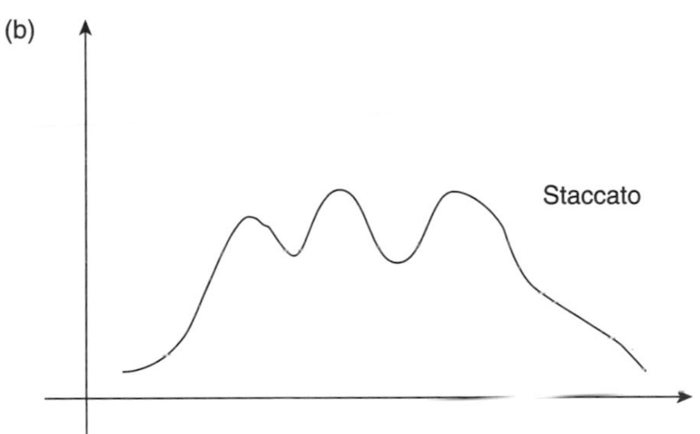

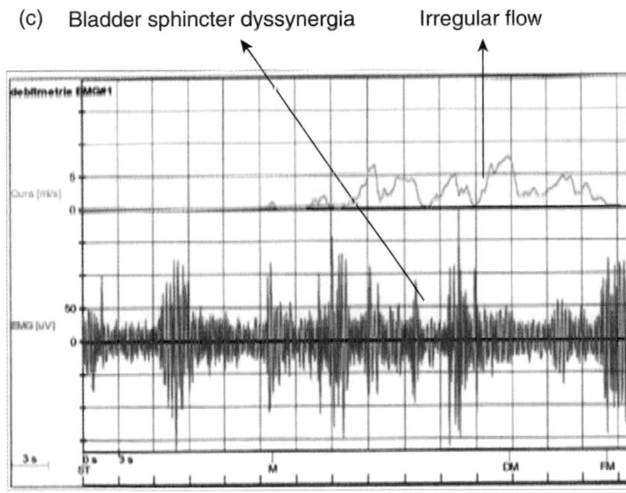

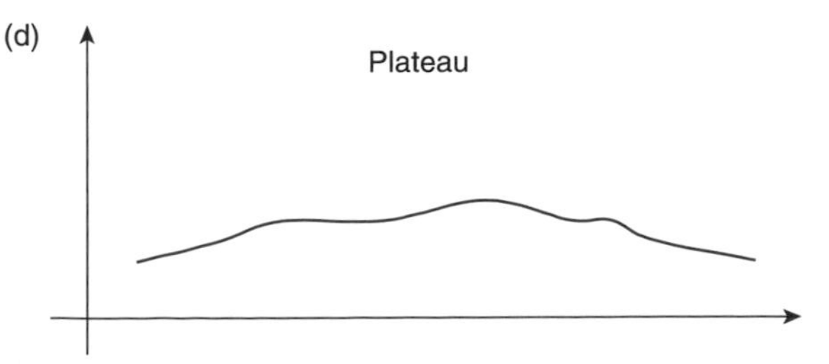

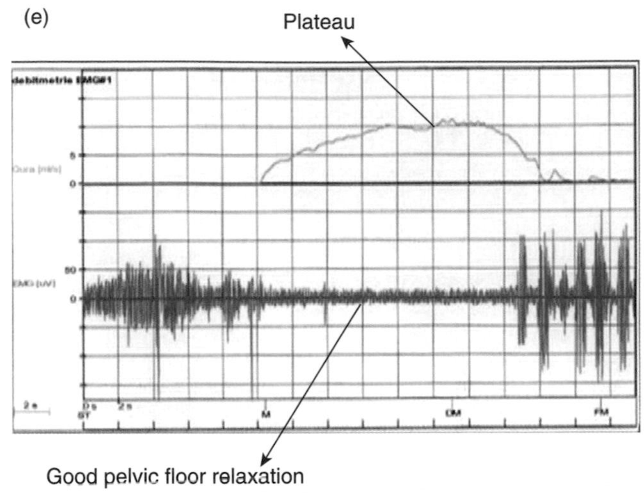

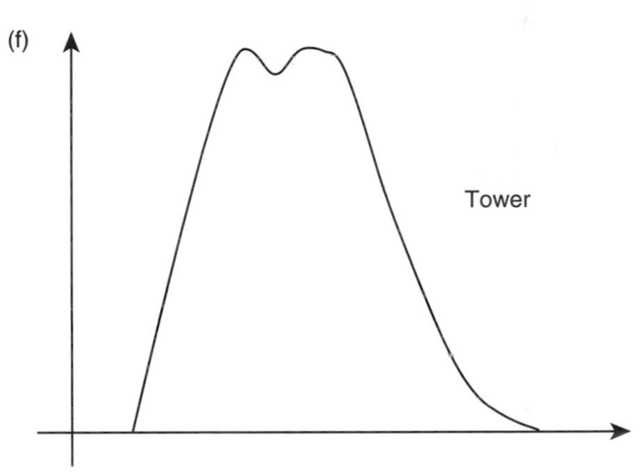

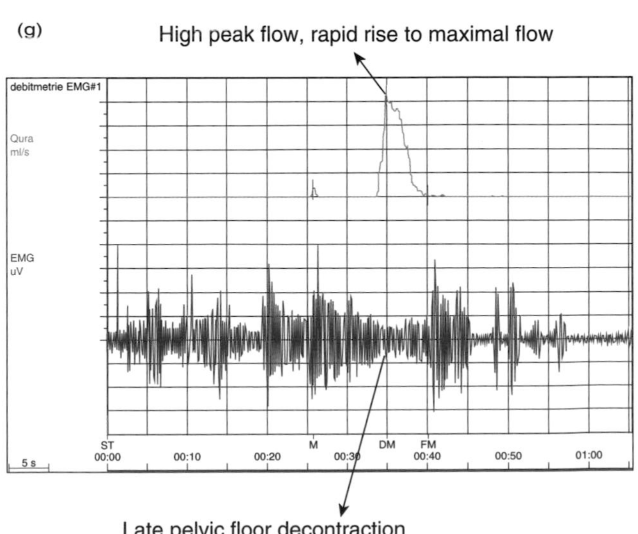

Figure 40.3
Normal and abnormal uroflowmetry curves.

and should be available in the laboratory.[6,13,14,20] From a practical standpoint, the maximal flow rate has more value than the average flow rate and has a linear relationship with the voided volume.[8] The maximal flow rate should equal the square root of the voided volume.[8] For example, with a voided volume of 100 ml the maximal expected flow rate should be 10 ml/s and with a voided volume of 225 ml it should be 15 ml/s. Most often when these values are low, they are associated with a plateau-shaped curve.

Interpretation of EMG recordings and postvoid residual volume

The residual volume estimate may provide conflicting results after uroflowmetry. There is no absolute truth when analyzing postvoid residual volume in children, particularly in view of their fear and anxiety. We believe, however, that as a screening tool a normal flow rate coupled with a complete emptying (0 ml) excludes the likelihood of serious underlying abnormalities.[4,9,16] On the contrary, defining what is a clinically significant residual volume is difficult in the face of an anxious child, and its value as a single diagnostic measure, grading of severity, or prognosis of urologic abnormality is poor. With young children, an isolated postvoid residual volume measure without symptoms may merely reflect the child's apprehension. We would not ascribe any significance to it. Thus, we routinely use simultaneous EMG recordings with perineal patch electrodes to further discriminate normal children from patients with abnormal voiding pattern, due to dysfunctional voiding or to underlying unrecognized neurogenic bladder. Normal pelvic floor activity on EMG tracing should cease almost completely just preceding the recording of the flow, and resume activity at the end of the flow. Abnormal activity during flow recording may be indicative of bladder sphincter dyssynergia secondary to dysfunctional voiding or neurogenic bladder. Also, abnormal pelvic floor activity will usually be related to an abnormal flow rate curve. Normal and abnormal voiding patterns are presented in Figure 40.3.

Treatment and further evaluation are then tailored according to the findings. If a child with no anatomic anomalies presents with supportive symptoms, high residual volume, or dyssynergia on cutaneous EMG recording, we would proceed with bladder and bowel management programs. Should the latter fail, despite simultaneous bladder-oriented pharmacotherapy, we would proceed with complete urodynamic studies. If a child presents with anatomic abnormalities during evaluation and an abnormal uroflowmetry/EMG, then we would proceed directly towards full urodynamic evaluation.

In summary, the noninvasive nature of uroflowmetry with EMG and postvoid residual assessment by ultrasound makes them ideal in screening and follow-up of children. Their relative simplicity and ease of performance add to their wide application. The results of these studies are not highly specific but, when interpreted in the light of the clinical history, physical findings, and other diagnostic studies, they yield significant information relevant to establishing a diagnosis, especially in dysfunctional voiding or the Hinman/Allen syndrome, and to elaborating a treatment plan and following its results, particularly during feedback bladder retraining and following hypospadias surgery.

Complete urodynamics

Some children require more extensive urodynamic studies. Indications include an abnormal curve pattern or dyssynergia on cutaneous EMG and flow rate seen in children with daytime urinary incontinence, and chronic or recurrent bacteriuria that is refractory to bladder retraining and constipation management. Clear indications for complete urodynamics as the initial test include patients with suspected infravesical obstruction such as posterior valves, overt or suspected neurogenic bladder dysfunction, and failed vesicoureteral reflux management.

Only a few studies have looked at normal urodynamics in children. Sillen et al[21] have evaluated bladder function in healthy neonates and infants using free voiding studies with a 4-hour voiding observation and subsequent urodynamic studies. They showed that voiding in the healthy neonate is characterized by small, frequent voids of varying volume. Thirty percent of the cases presented an interrupted voiding pattern, which seemed to be an immature phenomenon since it was seen in 60% of preterm neonates and disappeared completely before the age of toilet training. They theorized that there exists a physiologic detrusor sphincter dyssynergia (DSD), which may also explain the frequent postvoid residual observed in the young.[22,23] Along with the small caliber of the urethra, this can also explain the observed high voiding pressure. Such DSD seems to resolve by the age of toilet training. Signs of bladder instability were rarely observed on cystometric evaluation of their patient population, but rather some hyperactivity, as patients exhibited premature voiding contractions after only a few milliliters of filling with leakage of urine. Characteristics of the normal neonate micturition thus include physiologic DSD, low bladder capacity, and high voiding pressure, associated with some detrusor hyperactivity. These findings are challenging the concept that neonates simply display a voiding reflux and that regulation of micturition in neonates involves higher neuronal pathways.

Another study from Sweden evaluated urodynamics in normal infants and children.[18] One of the most important statements of this study was that a tense and apprehensive child will not produce reliable urodynamic data. Studies should be done in an appropriate setting with an experienced urodynamicist. Their study showed that inhibition of the detrusor improves during the first 5 years of life. Development of a normal voiding pattern evolves as adequate proprioception of the bladder improves, allowing the child to have a better control of micturition. To this maturational process we should add the new concept of improvement of physiologic DSD with age, as suggested by the study of Sillen.[21]

Bladder capacity

There have been numerous publications on the subject of normal bladder capacity. Hjämlås observed that most urodynamic variables are age-dependent.[8] Normal bladder capacity can be fairly well assessed by the formula 30 + (age in years × 30). Other formulas to evaluate bladder capacity have been described, including Koff's formula (age + 2) × 30,[24] and the estimation by Kaefer et al[25] of bladder capacity using 2 × age (years) + 2 = capacity (ounces) for children less than 2 years old, and age (years) divided by 2 + 6 = capacity (ounces) for those 2 years old or older. The most urodynamically sound formula, however, was described by Houle et al.[26] These authors evaluated 69 normal children, and measured total bladder capacity (ml), full resting pressure (cmH_2O), and the volume (ml) and percentage of the total bladder capacity stored at detrusor pressures of less than 10, 20, 30, and 35 cmH_2O. According to their results, the minimal acceptable total bladder capacity for age can be estimated by 16(age) + 70 in ml, which was derived using criteria for safe storage characteristics of the bladder in children. This formula has the advantage of being based on urodynamic criteria and is the one that the authors use in their clinical practice. It should be noted that the volumes derived from this formula are higher then the volumes at which patients would void in their usual environment.

Bladder compliance

Normal compliance in children has been established somewhat arbitrarily. The minimally acceptable value for bladder compliance during bladder filling has been arbitrarily set at 10 ml/cmH_2O.[27] Values above this level can be considered normal. Other researches have further stratified compliance as being poor <10 ml/cmH_2O, moderate between 10 and 20 ml/cmH_2O and mild loss between 21 and 30 ml/cmH_2O.[28] However, the clinical relevance of such classification has yet to be determined.

It is important to remember that, as observed in adults, compliance may be influenced by the rate of bladder filling, which should be at a rate corresponding to 10% of the expected bladder capacity per minute. Some advocate the use of a warm infusion solution during the filling phase in order to obtain more reliable and physiologic results. Chin-Peuckert et al nicely demonstrated, in a prospective randomized study, that a solution at room temperature rendered similar results to a warm infusion solution.[29] Compliance should be evaluated at regular intervals during cystometric recording (25–50–75%) as opposed to only at final capacity, since loss in compliance that occur early in the filling phase puts the upper tract at higher risk than changes noted only near the end of the cystometric curve.[27]

Uninhibited bladder contractions are recorded in the same way as in the adult, i.e. any appreciable detrusor contraction, especially if it causes urine leakage or urgency. (Since this chapter discusses only normal urodynamics in children, detrusor leak-point pressure and abdominal leak-point pressure will not be discussed, as they do not occur in a normal child.)

Voiding pressures

Hjälmås, in his study,[8] described intravesical pressures that are lower in girls than in boys, and lower in infants than in older children, but otherwise intravesical pressure does not vary with age. However, he mentioned that bladder pressure recordings represent the most important source of error when examining children. He strongly emphasized that the examination has to be performed in a kind, friendly, and relaxed atmosphere. Standards of voiding pressure in normal individuals have been reported. Less reliable pressure measurements have been obtained in infants, with a median of more than 100 cmH_2O in males and 60–70 cmH_2O in females.[21] In children 1 to 3 years of age, voiding pressure can be 70 cmH_2O in males[8] and 60 cmH_2O in females.[30] After the age of 7, values tend to normalize to those of adults.

Postvoid residual volume

Postvoid residual urine has been studied, but to date only a few studies have presented significant data as to what represent normal postvoid residual urine. It is recognized that infants do not empty their bladder at each void,[23] but they seem to empty their bladder completely at least once during a 4-hour observation period.[21] Residual urine using a 4-hour observational protocol has been reported to be minimal (4–5 ml) from the infant stage up to age 2.[23,31] Residual urine should be 0 ml at 3 years and older.[31] Caution should be used when postvoid residual is considered as a significant factor in diagnosis, as many children may present fear and anxiety at the time of observation. A summary of normal urodynamic values in children is presented in Table 40.5.

Conclusion

Urodynamic evaluation of children differs from adults mostly in the widespread use of noninvasive exams that included uroflowmetry with or without EMG, and postvoid residual volume. We have seen that normal values in a child differ from an adult, and that they change with the stage of development. Although full urodynamic testing is more invasive, there are many indications that render this exam invaluable and necessary. Again, both age and size of the child influence interpretation and normal values. Overall, these exams play a major role in the evaluation of voiding abnormalities in children of all ages.

References

1. Litvak AS, Morris JA, McRoberts JW. Normal size of the urethral meatus in boys. J Urol 1977; 13(5): 471.
2. Immergut M, Culp D, Flocks RH. The urethral caliber in normal female children. J Urol 1967; 97(4): 963–5.
3. Gleason DM, Lattimer JK. The pressure flow study: a method for measuring bladder neck resistance. J Urol 1962; 827: 844.
4. Abrams PH, Griffith DJ. The assessment of prostatic obstruction from urodynamics measurements and from residual urine. Br J Urol 1979; 51: 129.
5. Scott RJ, McIlhaney JS. The voiding rates in normal children. J Urol 1959; 82: 224.
6. Churchill BM, Gilmour RF, Williot P. Urodynamics. Pediatr Clin North Am 1987; 34(5): 1133–57.
7. Jorgensen JB, Jensen KM. Uroflowmetry. Urol Clin North Am 1996; 23(2): 237–42.
8. Hjälmås K. Urodynamics in normal infants and children. Scand J Urol Nephrol Suppl 1988; 114: 20–7.
9. Williot P, McLorie GA, Gilmour RF, Churchill BM. Accuracy of bladder volume determinations in children using a suprapubic ultrasonic bi-planar technique. J Urol 1989; 141(4): 900–2.
10. Barrett DM, Wein AJ. Flow evaluation and simultaneous external sphincter electromyography in clinical urodynamics. J Urol 1981; 125(4): 538–41.
11. Meunier P, Mollard P, Nemoz-Behncke C, Genet JP. [Urodynamic exploration in functional micturition disorders in children.] Arch Pediatr 1995; 2(5): 483–91.
12. Ewalt DH, Bauer SB. Pediatric neurourology. Urol Clin North Am 1996; 23(3): 501–9.
13. Segura CG. Urine flow in children: a study of flow chart parameters based on 1361 uroflowmetry tests. J Urol 1997; 157: 1426.
14. Jensen KM, Nielsen KK, Jensen H, Pedersen OS, Krarup T. Urinary flow studies in normal kindergarten- and schoolchildren. Scand J Urol Nephrol 1983; 17(1): 11–21.
15. Gaum LD, Wese FX, Liu TP et al. Age related flow rate nomograms in a normal pediatric population. Acta Urol Belg 1989; 57(2): 457–66.
16. Wese FX, Gaum LD, Liu TP et al. Body surface related flow rate nomograms in a normal pediatric population. Acta Urol Belg 1989; 57(2): 467–74.
17. Bower WF, Kwok B, Yeung CK. Variability in normative urine flow rates. J Urol 2004; 171(6 Pt 2): 2657–9.
18. Herndon CD, Decambre M, McKenna PH. Interactive computer games for treatment of pelvic floor dysfunction. J Urol 2001; 166(5): 1893–8.
19. Jayanthi VR, McLorie GA, Khoury AE, Churchill BM. Functional characteristics of the reconstructed neourethra after island flap urethroplasty. J Urol 1995; 153(5): 1657–9.
20. Farhane S, Saidi R, Fredj N et al. Uroflowmetry in children: prospective study of normal parameters. Progr Urol 2006; 16(5): 598–601.
21. Sillen U. Bladder function in healthy neonates and its development during infancy. J Urol 2001; 166(6): 2376–81.
22. Roberts DS, Rendell B. Postmicturition residual bladder volumes in healthy babies. Arch Dis Child 1989; 64(6): 825–8.
23. Sillen U, Solsnes E, Hellstrom AL, Sandberg K. The voiding pattern of healthy preterm neonates. J Urol 2000; 163(1): 278–81.
24. Koff SA. Estimating bladder capacity in children. Urology 1983; 21(3): 248.
25. Kaefer M, Zurakowski D, Bauer SB et al. Estimating normal bladder capacity in children. J Urol 1997; 158(6): 2261–4.
26. Houle AM, Gilmour RF, Churchill BM, Gaumond M, Bissonnette B. What volume can a child normally store in the bladder at a safe pressure? J Urol 1993; 149(3): 561–4.
27. Gilmour RF, Churchill BM, Steckler RE et al. A new technique for dynamic analysis of bladder compliance. J Urol 1993; 150(4): 1200–3.
28. Horowitz M, Combs AJ, Shapiro E. Urodynamics in pediatric urology. In: Nitty VW, ed. Practical Urodynamics. Philadelphia: WB Saunders, 1998.
29. Chin-Peuckert L, Rennick JE, Jednak R, Capolicchio JP, Salle JL. Should warm infusion solution be used for urodynamic studies in children? A prospective randomized study. J Urol 2004; 172(4 Pt 2): 1657–61; discussion 1661.
30. Wen JG, Tong EC. Cystometry in infant and children with apparent voiding symptoms. Br J Urol 1998; 81: 468.
31. Jansson UB, Hanson M, Hanson E, Hellstrom AL, Sillen U. Voiding pattern in healthy children 0 to 3 years old: a longitudinal study. J Urol 2000; 164(6): 2050–4.

41

Urodynamics in infants and children

Ulla Sillén and Kate Abrahamsson

Introduction

Urodynamics in infants and children is basically the same procedure as in adults and shares the same techniques and objectives. There is, however, one fundamental difference: *the patient is a child*. Essentially, this means two things. First, a child harbors intuitive fear for any unknown procedure but is, at the same time, largely unresponsive to rational argumentation about the nature of and the need for the examination. Second, the child is a growing individual, increasing in weight 20-fold from infancy to puberty. This means that for children there exists no single set of 'normal' urodynamic variables but rather a continuum of each variable, depending on and correlating to the age and the body size of the individual.

This chapter will concentrate on those two aspects: first, on how to prepare, inform, reassure, encourage, and comfort the child before and during the urodynamic examination; second, how to report the expected range of 'normal' values for urodynamic variables from infancy to adolescence.

Historical notes on urodynamics in infants and children

It is hard to understand why bladder function in children did not receive any attention from medical scientists until the mid-20th century. Before that time, it seems to have been understood, without a trace of critical thinking, that almost all children had bladders that worked perfectly well, regarding both storage and evacuation of urine. If a functional disturbance such as incontinence was indeed noted, traditional wisdom suggested that it was due to psychologic problems within the child and/or the family. In contrast, we are now aware that non-neurogenic bladder-sphincter dysfunction in children is caused by delayed maturation (most often genetically determined) of the central nervous system (CNS) bladder control. Psychologic problems in an incontinent child are a consequence of the bladder dysfunction, not the other way round, with few exceptions.

From 1959 onwards, the first urodynamic studies on normal and pathologic bladder function in infants and children came into print.[1–9] A rapidly increasing number of studies followed, once it became clear that at age 7 years as many as 10% of children have non-neurogenic disturbance of bladder/sphincter function. Knowledge surfaced that bladder dysfunction plays a major role not only for urinary incontinence but also, even more importantly, for the creation and persistence of vesicoureteral reflux (VUR) and urinary tract infection (UTI), with the accompanying risk for deterioration of renal function.[10] Children with *neurogenic* bladder dysfunction (NBD) due to myelodysplasia and other disorders of the CNS were exposed to the same risk to an even larger degree. Surprisingly, however, this fact did not become obvious until the late 1960s, when it was finally understood that the devastating UTIs and the frequent progress of bacterial resistance during antibiotic therapy in myelomeningocele children was caused by inadequate bladder emptying, leaving postvoid residual behind. Regular and low-pressure bladder evacuation with the aid of clean intermittent catheterization (CIC), introduced by Jack Lapides in 1972, led to a dramatic reduction in the rate and severity of UTIs in this patient group and even resulted in disappearance of reflux in many patients.[11]

Development of bladder function

The normal development of lower urinary tract function from infancy to adolescence has to be reviewed before describing the urodynamic procedures and techniques used in children and what results to expect. This is necessary in order to understand the dynamic nature of the urodynamic variables in the growing individual.

Bladder function during infancy has previously been regarded as automatic, with voiding induced by a constant volume in the bladder[12] and without cerebral influence. During the last decade it has been shown convincingly that the brain is already involved in the voiding reflex from birth. This is best illustrated by the finding that in the majority of cases newborn babies wake up or show signs of arousal before voiding.[13,14] This means that the reflex pathway connection to the cerebral cortex is anatomically already developed in this age group; however, voiding is neither conscious nor voluntary – the infant is only disturbed by the signal. Both maturation and probably training are needed for the voidings to be conscious and voluntary.

Neonates and infants void at varying bladder volumes during infancy and this is contrary to the belief that the voiding reflex is a simple spinal reflex elicited by a constant bladder volume. This has been shown in free voiding studies of both pre-term[15] and full-term infants[13] in whom bladder volume initiating voiding varies from 30% to 100% of functional bladder capacity. The reason for this variation is unknown, but the bladder volume initiating micturition is higher after a period of sleep.

The infant's voiding is also characterized by a physiologic form of detrusor-sphincter dyscoordination, which has been shown in free voiding studies as interrupted voidings and increase in postvoid residual urine (Figure 41.1).[16] This phenomenon has also been observed in urodynamic studies as an intermittent increase in the electromyographic (EMG) activity of the pelvic floor during voiding, concomitant with fluctuations in voiding detrusor pressure (Figure 41.2).[14,17] A longitudinal study of free voidings from birth to age 3 years revealed that the suggested dyscoordination disappears successively, and is not seen after potty-training age.[13] Another important observation in the study by Jansson et al[13] is the increase in postvoid residual urine during the first couple of years of life. The reason for the incomplete emptying in infancy is probably the physiologic form of dyscoordination discussed above, with interruption of the urine stream before the bladder is empty. However, with the acquisition of continence the residual volume decreased in this group of healthy children and the ability to empty the bladder was complete at the age of 3.

In the longitudinal study of free voidings by Jansson et al[13] it was also observed that bladder capacity was almost unchanged during the first two years of life but showed a steep increase at the time the child gets dry (see Figure 41.6). A similar accelerated increase in bladder capacity which is age related has also been noted in other studies.[12,18] This increased bladder capacity has been considered as a prerequisite for both day and night-time continence. Conversely, continence during the night has been considered to be obtained only after achievement of day dryness.[19,20] The reason for this increase in bladder capacity has previously only been discussed in terms of general maturation.

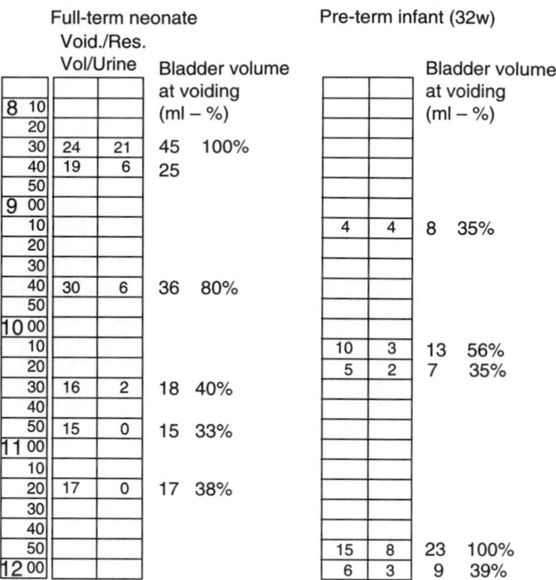

Figure 41.1
Four-hour voiding observation in a full-term neonate and a pre-term infant (gestation age 32 weeks) showing varying bladder volumes initiating voiding (the sum of voided volume and residual urine). The volumes vary between 33% and 100% of the highest volume in the bladder (= the bladder capacity) during the observation. Note the interrupted voiding seen once in the full-term and twice in the pre-term infant.

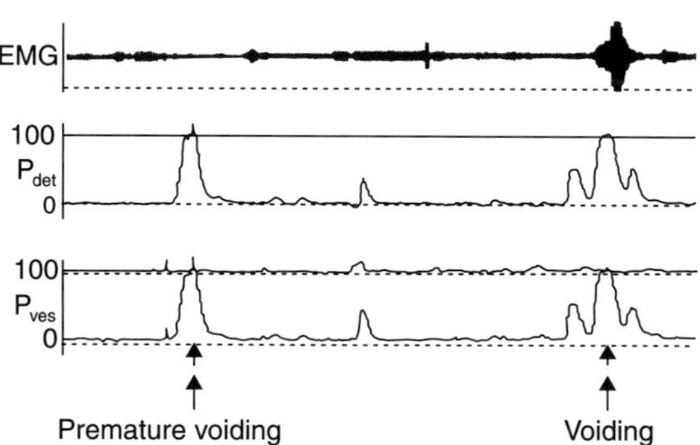

Figure 41.2
Cystometric recording in a non-refluxing newborn sibling of a child with vesicoureteral reflux (VUR). Note the premature voiding contraction after infusion of 5 ml with leakage of urine. Voiding after a total filling of 30 ml of saline shows an increase of electromyographic (EMG) activity of the pelvic floor and concomitant fluctuation in detrusor voiding pressure.

Acquisition of bladder control

Development of bladder control was earlier supposed to begin at 1 year of age and often to be fully developed by age 4.5 years. It was described by Muellner as 'a maturation which could not be influenced by training'. Another factor which was considered important was the doubling of bladder capacity between 2 and 4.5 years of age.[12,21] These statements about maturation, combined with the improvement in the quality of disposable napkins, have contributed to a more liberal view about what age potty-training should be started. In fact, during the last decades, potty-training has been regarded as unnecessary due to the belief that physical maturation should dictate when a child becomes dry. It is quite clear from other areas, however, that training can accelerate maturation.

Potty-training was instituted early before the era of disposable napkins. Some authors have reported bladder control much earlier than nowadays,[19,20] whereas others have not been able to show such a connection.[22]

If bladder control only means to void on the potty when the child is put there by the parent regularly or when the child indicates a need to void, it can be obtained early. The degree of maturation needed for such basic training is probably already present during the first year of life.[23] The goal of potty-training, to obtain full social bladder control, cannot be achieved solely with the early potty-training discussed above. The prerequisites for success are influenced both by physical maturation and the child's interest in this task as well as by support from adults, routines, and parental expectations. Most children may stay dry in their usual milieu around the age of 2. However, the child has to reach at least 3.5–4 years of age to become mature enough to be able to cope with every aspect of their own toileting (including taking off and putting on clothes, flushing the toilet, closing the door, etc.).

The markedly improved emptying after potty-training, discussed above, is very interesting, since it is something that can be used in the treatment of incomplete emptying in this age group, through institution of potty training earlier than what is common.

Indications for urodynamics in children

The indications for urodynamics in infants and children are the same as for adults: namely, suspicion of neurogenic or non-neurogenic bladder dysfunction or structural outflow obstruction. Thus, they include neurogenic bladder, gross vesicoureteral reflux (particularly in infants), recurrent UTIs, uroflow/residual measurement suggesting infravesical obstruction, and urinary incontinence (including nocturnal enuresis) that has been refractory to conventional treatment (urotherapy and drugs) for at least 1 year.

Neurogenic bladder dysfunction, whether suspected or established, is the most important of these indications. It should be said up front that cystometry in a patient with neurogenic bladder has to be repeated regularly during the patient's lifetime. In a child, cystometry should be performed at least once yearly because neurogenic bladder in the child is a dynamic disorder that is prone to change and then most often deterioration. The common cause is tethering of the spinal cord, which occurs in 75% of myelomeningoceles and in 100% of lipomyelomeningoceles.[24]

Age-related aspects

The investigation must be adapted to the child's needs!

In urology textbooks in the past, it could be read that 'cystometry cannot be performed in children younger than 7 years of age'. In one circumstance this statement was true: namely, when a young child was referred to a urodynamic laboratory that was used to examine adult patients only. Nonprepared children who hesitated to enter the laboratory and thereby upset the time schedule were looked upon as disturbing and irrational patients – which children certainly are if not treated according to their own needs! Children *are* irrational, sensitive, and skeptical towards all kinds of medical technology. Thus their need for information, patience, and loving care cannot be emphasized too much. The stress felt by a tense child during a urodynamic examination may very well generate results suggesting bladder dysfunction (overactive bladder and/or sphincter) even if that same child in a safe and relaxed mood would have shown completely normal urodynamic findings.

Ideally, the child should be prepared for what will be coming by being shown around the laboratory the day before the examination and given a summary in everyday language of what is going to happen (Figure 41.3). Several of these children have already undergone voiding cystography and may have unpleasant memories of the catheterization, so this topic has to be touched upon with great care.

During the examination, the child is handled in a relaxed and patient way. Even young children should be handled with respect for their personal integrity. As much as possible, the procedure should be performed 'as in play'. A video with popular cartoons has been a great asset in our laboratory and has helped children to overlook frightening equipment in the room (Figure 41.4). However, nothing can substitute for an experienced nurse or laboratory assistant who loves to take care of children.[25,26]

Sedation

Exceptionally, when a child expresses outspoken anxiety for the procedure, in particular the catheterization, sedation with midazolam may be an option.[27] We have no experience with using midazolam (Dormicum®, Roche) in urodynamic studies but have used the drug for several years when performing voiding cystourethrography (VCUG).[28] In these

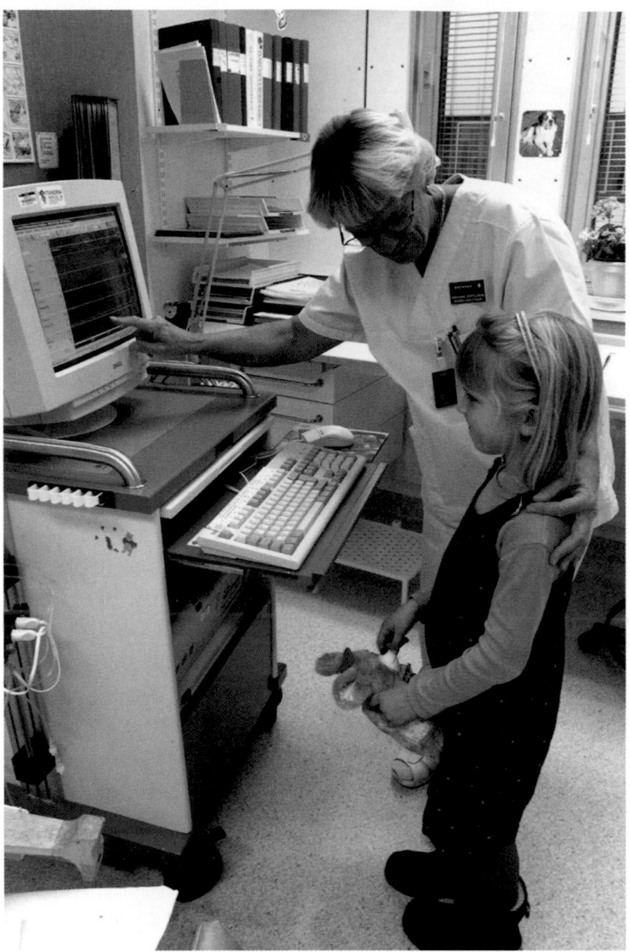

Figure 41.3
Child familiarizing herself with the urodynamic laboratory while receiving information from the laboratory assistant the day before the actual investigation.

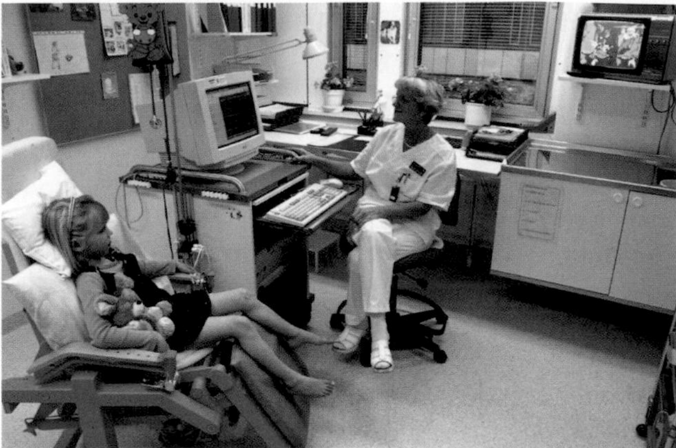

Figure 41.4
Cystometry is not necessarily a distressful experience, especially when an interesting video is running.

studies the drug does not seem to affect bladder/sphincter function in any way. The sedation is satisfactory and side-effects very rare. The drug company only offers Dormicum for intravenous use. However, in our practise, we use the intravenous preparation for oral or rectal administration and have noticed the same sedative efficacy without added side-effects. For *oral administration,* Dormicum 5 mg/ml is used in the dosage 0.3–0.5 mg per kg body weight, max 7.5 mg, mixed in a small amount of juice or cola. Effective sedation occurs within 15–30 min and the duration of sedation is 30–50 min. Dormicum 1 mg/ml is used for *rectal administration* in the dosage 0.2–0.3 mg per kg body weight, max 5 mg. Effective sedation occurs within 10–20 min and duration of sedation is 30–50 min. Observe that pulse oximeter, suction apparatus, and equipment for ventilation should be at hand. If the child falls asleep, secure free airways. The child should be supervised for at least 1 h 30 min before leaving for home.[28] Midazolam for sedation of a child going through a urodynamic investigation may be a good option in the future once placebo-controlled, randomized studies have been performed.

Age

Infants below 1 year of age pose very few problems during urodynamic investigation. They are simply too young to be afraid of the procedure. The most problematic age group are children aged 2–4 years who are old enough to feel scared but too young to understand the reasons for the examination.

Children with neurogenic bladder generally accept the urodynamic investigation without many problems. A majority of these children are treated with CIC and it is easier for them to accept and for the staff to perform the procedure than is the case for children with intact lower urinary tract sensation.

Urodynamic methodology

Noninvasive urodynamics

Uroflow

Measurement of the urinary flow rate, including assessment of the shape of the flow curve, is a very useful investigative tool in children with non-neurogenic bladder/sphincter dysfunction but has a very limited value in neurogenic bladder patients. The simple reason is that a child with neurogenic bladder is only exceptionally able to perform a formal micturition.

Postvoid residual urine (assessed with ultrasound)

This procedure is mandatory and should be repeated frequently in all children with neurogenic bladder. In infants and small children, who are not treated with CIC, the 4-hour voiding observation is used to investigate emptying ability.[16] The child uses a napkin during the test and voidings are indicated by a gossip strip or a light signal. Voided volume is measured by weighing the napkin after each voiding and postvoid residual urine is checked by ultrasonography. Since postvoid residual urine varies also in healthy babies with complete emptying only occasionally, the investigation has to include a 4-hour period and not only isolated voidings.

Postvoid residual urine should also be checked in patients on CIC to make sure that the catheterization is performed in a correct and efficient way. Some children tend to withdraw the catheter too early. Others may get a dislocation of the bladder when growing up, necessitating a change of body position during CIC in order to achieve complete emptying. Another reason for postvoid residual urine could be a trabeculated detrusor due to bad compliance by the patient in the CIC regimen and anticholinergic treatment, a phenomenon sometimes seen during puberty.

Pad test

To estimate and follow urinary leakage between voidings or catheterizations during daily activity, the pad test is the most appropriate investigation, including hourly change of pads that are weighed to get the leakage volume. When combined with a 3-hour interval change of pads at home, the most reliable results will be produced.[29] The leakage volume and frequency are important parameters to follow at least once a year, since changes can indicate tethering. The test is also important as an indicator of the efficacy of treatment with anticholinergic medication.

Pelvic electromyography using cutaneous electrodes

Pelvic EMG for registration of pelvic floor activity during cystometry will sometimes detect neuromuscular activity even in patients with neurogenic bladder, but it will be difficult or impossible to find out from which portion of the pelvic floor muscles the signals emanate.

Invasive urodynamics: traditional cystometry

Invasive urodynamics is synonymous with cystometry (with the possible addition of EMG using needle electrodes).

Frequently asked questions (FAQs) regarding cystometric techniques

At which points of time should infants and children with neurogenic bladder dysfunction be examined with cystometry? The literature provides strong evidence that CIC in congenital NBD should be started as soon as possible in infancy,[30,31] because there is an obvious risk of deterioration of bladder function already in infancy as well as later in childhood.[32,33] Frequent and regular follow-up of bladder function (cystometry at least once a year) is mandatory, in particular during the first 6 years of life.[34]

Gas or fluid filling of the bladder? Gas should not be used.

Fluid-filled or transducer tip catheters for pressure measurement? For obvious reasons, transducer tip catheters must be used for natural fill (ambulatory) cystometry. When traditional cystometry is performed in the laboratory, a fluid-filled pressure measurement system is still the standard.

Transurethral or suprapubic catheters? Double-lumen transurethral catheters are ideal for infants and children with neurogenic bladder. Most of these patients have limited or absent urethral sensation. Moreover, the possible obstruction caused by the transurethral catheter is of minor importance in this patient group, since it is hardly ever possible to perform a formal pressure–flow measurement.

What filling rate should be used? The rate at which fluid is instilled in the bladder influences bladder wall dynamics, thus capacity, intravesical pressure, and compliance.[35] High filling rates create an artificial situation, with continuous pressure rise. Therefore, filling rates have to be standardized and not allowed to exceed physiologic filling rates during maximal diuresis. The recommended rate is 1/20 (5%) of the patient's expected bladder capacity per minute, since in a healthy individual the bladder will be filled to capacity in 20 min during maximal diuresis. The patient's expected bladder capacity can be assessed from a diary in which the parents note the CIC volumes for a couple of days. The largest volume should be chosen excluding the first morning voiding. Alternatively (particularly in severe incontinence with small CIC volumes), the expected bladder capacity in children 3 years of age and above can be calculated from the simple rule-of-thumb equation:

$$\text{Expected bladder capacity (ml)} = 30 + (\text{age in years} \times 30)$$ [25]

An alternative rule of thumb is that 1% of the body weight approximately predicts a child's bladder capacity. A 3-year-old would be expected to have a bladder capacity around 120 ml, so a filling rate of 6 ml/min should be used.

When to stop filling in a patient unable to feel a desire to void? This is the common situation in patients with NBD. The infusion should be finished when any of the following occurs:

1. strong urgency
2. micturition
3. feeling of discomfort
4. high basic detrusor pressure (>40 cmH_2O)
5. large infused volume (>150% of the expected bladder capacity unless the CIC diary has shown larger volumes at CIC)
6. rate of urinary leakage ≥ rate of infusion.

How many filling cycles are needed? In non-neurogenic cases, two. Even if the child seems to be at ease during the examination, the first filling is experienced by the child as more stressful than the following ones. Detrusor and/or sphincter overactivity is therefore more commonly seen during the first filling. The second filling will already reflect the urodynamic status of the bladder in a reliable way. Additional fillings do not need to be done because they produce similar findings to the second one.[9] However, in children with neurogenic bladder a single filling may be sufficient because lower urinary tract sensation is impaired and psychologic mechanisms hardly influence bladder/sphincter function.

When is the bladder cooling test (BCT, formerly Bors ice water test) indicated in the urodynamic investigation of infants and children with established or suspected NBD? In every case, as a general rule. It has been shown that neurologically normal infants and children exhibit a positive bladder cooling test (BCT) during the first 4 years of life, whereas the test is negative in children older than 6 years.[36] In infants and children with NBD, a negative BCT before age 4 demonstrates a lesion of the sacral reflex arch, whereas a positive BCT in children older than 6 years indicates a lesion of inhibiting suprasacral spinal pathways.[37] The BCT is performed after finishing the traditional cystometry. The reactivity of the detrusor is first checked with body-warm saline infused rapidly in an amount corresponding to one-third of the cystometric bladder capacity. If this infusion does not elicit any significant detrusor contraction, the bladder is emptied and the same amount (one-third of bladder capacity) of cold (4–8 °C) saline is infused rapidly. A positive test is defined as a detrusor contraction within 1 min with detrusor pressure >30 cmH_2O.

How to measure leak-point pressure – and what is its value? The ideal way of measuring leak-point pressure (LPP) is to note the detrusor pressure at the moment when leakage of urine is observed, during cystometry. This means that the laboratory assistant would have to monitor the patient's genital area continuously, which is seldom possible. Instead, the flowmeter is often used to indicate leakage; but it is then important to make adjustments for the time delay between pressure registration and the flowmeter deflection, in particular when leakage occurs in connection with a phasic detrusor contraction. It is assumed that LPP >40 cmH_2O in children with NBD suggests an increased risk for development of renal damage. This assumption makes sense, because maintained *intravesical* pressure above 30–40 cmH_2O is certainly associated with an increased incidence of VUR and upper tract dilatation.[38] Thus, an assessment of LPP should be routinely included in the urodynamic evaluation of a child with NBD.

What is the role of electromyography in the urodynamic evaluation of children with neurogenic bladder dysfunction? 'Quantitative' EMG using perineal surface electrodes (Ag/AgCl) will not always produce clinically valuable information in this patient group.

How should intra-abdominal pressure be measured? The intrarectal pressure is easily accessible with a catheter passed through the anus. This fact – together with a solid chunk of urodynamic tradition – and, additionally, the invasive nature of the two first-mentioned options, helps to propagate intrarectal pressure as the standard for assessing perivesical pressure. The rectal catheter should be open-ended and continuously and slowly (3 ml/h) perfused with saline to prevent blocking by feces. It is important to check pressure transmission by asking the patient to strain or cough or by applying pressure on the suprapubic area. Be aware that the rectal catheter will sometimes transmit pressure peaks generated by spontaneous rectal contractions, something that may result in false-negative detrusor pressure readings. Thus, detrusor pressure calculated as intravesical minus intrarectal pressure is not always a reliable urodynamic variable.

Invasive urodynamics: videocystometry

Performing cystometry and fluoroscopic monitoring of the bladder and urethra at the same time no doubt increases the diagnostic accuracy of the urodynamic procedure, e.g. by allowing determination of bladder pressure at the moment when VUR occurs. The combined examination is also of value in patients with high-grade VUR where a common problem is to decide how much of the infused volume corresponds to bladder capacity and how much is stored in the refluxing systems. It can thus be said that some clinical questions will not be possible to answer without concurrent use of cystometry and X-ray. Therefore, videocystometry has become a standard urodynamic procedure for children with NBD (and other diagnoses) in many centers. However, videocystometry has its disadvantages. The most important of these is that videocystometry makes the examination even more complex by introducing additional machinery face to face to the (possibly) bewildered child. Even well-prepared and cooperative children may have difficulties in adapting to a highly sophisticated procedure. Since the child patient needs significant modification of the cystometric techniques compared to the adult, it can be questioned whether increasing the level of investigative sophistication is the right way to go.

Invasive urodynamics: natural fill (ambulatory) cystometry

Natural fill cystometry differs from traditional laboratory cystometry by (1) allowing the patient to be mobile, i.e. not restricting him to the laboratory chair, and (2) using the patient's own diuresis as the filling medium of the bladder. In both adults and children significant differences have been found between values obtained by artificial and natural filling urodynamics, respectively. Especially, steeper pressure rise and larger voided volumes were observed during and after artificial filling, whereas voiding pressures were found to be higher after natural filling. The natural fill cystometry also seems to be more sensitive in detecting detrusor instability than the traditional, artificial filling method.[39] The lower incidence of detrusor instability and the greater voided volumes found on traditional cystometry probably reflect an inhibition of detrusor function because of the relatively fast artificial filling.

In neurogenic bladders in adults, important differences were noted between conventional and natural fill cystometry. High increases in pressure registered during artificial filling, interpreted as low compliance of the bladder wall, were not reproduced during natural fill cystometry but rather replaced by phasic detrusor activity. Natural filling disclosed a combination of greater residual urine volumes, greater resting pressures, and greater phasic activity in patients with upper tract dilatation.[40]

In infants and children, results obtained by conventional cystometry and natural fill cystometry have shown the same differences as in adults regarding both non-neurogenic and neurogenic bladder dysfunction. The two methods were compared in a group of 17 children (mean age 6.8 years) with various urologic disorders.[41] As in adults, the natural fill study yielded lower voided volumes, a less steep pressure rise on filling, and higher detrusor pressures during micturition. Additionally, natural fill urodynamics revealed detrusor overactivity in more patients than did the conventional cystometry.

The studies cited recorded bladder and rectal pressure for time periods ranging between 4 and 6 hours. In a study from our institution[42] we took full advantage of the ambulatory, natural fill method by extending the recording time to a mean of 20 hours. It was thus possible to compare the bladder behavior between day and night, which yielded interesting results. Also, the small patients were truly ambulatory since they were carrying the recording device in a backpack. There was no disruption of the child's normal activities and the children seemed almost completely unaware that they were subjected to a sophisticated investigation of their bladder function. Sixteen boys aged 1.4–6 years (mean age 3.4) with endoscopically resected posterior urethral valves (at a mean age of 3.6 months) were studied. All the boys had detrusor instability in the daytime but the bladders became stable during sleeping hours. At natural fill cystometry, voiding detrusor pressure was higher and functional bladder capacity much lower during the day than at night. Dissimilarities noted between natural fill and conventional cystometry were the same as found in all other studies.

A couple of studies have compared natural fill with conventional cystometry in children with neurogenic bladder. In 2 of 11 children with myelodysplasia (mean age 10 years) more phasic detrusor activity and higher pressure amplitudes were found during 6 h of natural fill cystometry.[43] In another study of 20 children (age 6–11 years) with neurogenic bladder, natural fill cystometry (mean duration 12 hours) discovered detrusor overactivity in 45% of the children in contrast to traditional cystometry in the same children where half had been judged to have normal bladder function and the other half low-compliance bladders.[44]

In conclusion, natural fill cystometry in infants, children, and adults shows a lower pressure rise during filling, a higher incidence of detrusor overactivity, a higher detrusor pressure on micturition, and a lower voided volume than is found at conventional cystometry. It cannot be excluded that 'low compliance neurogenic bladder' might sometimes turn out to be an investigational artifact due to the unphysiologic high rate of artificial bladder filling, since studies in both children and adults have shown the rapid rise of pressure during artificial filling being replaced by phasic detrusor overactivity.[40,44] Natural fill urodynamics does not use artificial filling, and it causes minimal psychologic trauma, especially important for the pediatric patient, so it no doubt delivers the more authentic reflection of true bladder physiology. However, data on natural fill cystometry in children with neurogenic bladder are still sparse, and, before replacing traditional with natural fill urodynamics, additional studies are needed. In particular, it will be necessary to find out how decreased distensibility of the bladder wall is presenting itself in the natural fill studies. Increase of basal detrusor pressure above 20–30 cmH_2O is seldom seen during natural fill but has been interpreted as an important sign of poor compliance when seen in traditional cystometry and found to be associated with dilatation of the upper tracts and deterioration of renal function. Since the rapid rise of basal detrusor pressure may be looked upon as a significant finding, it is still too early to appoint natural fill urodynamics to be the future golden standard in the investigation of neurogenic bladders in children, even if the possibility remains that natural fill may lead to profound reassessment of the urodynamic neurogenic pathophysiology.

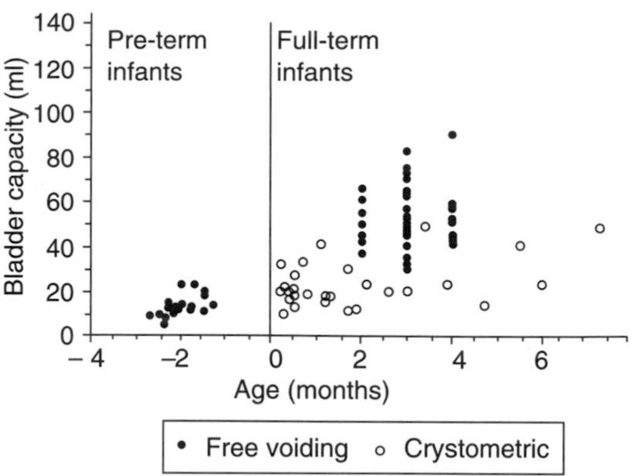

Figure 41.5
Age vs bladder capacity as measured in free voiding studies in both pre-term[15] and full-term[13] infants, and at cystometry in full-term infants.[17]

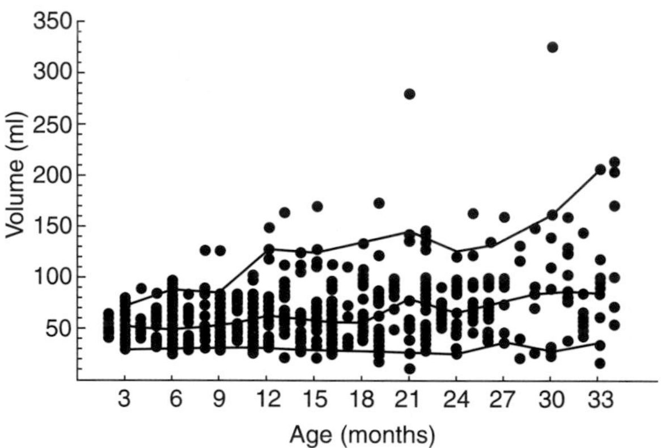

Figure 41.6
Bladder capacity vs age in a longitudinal study of free voidings in infants and children aged 0–3 years, investigated every 3rd month. The lines indicate the 5th, 50th, and 95th percentiles.[13]

Evaluation of urodynamic results

What are we looking for?

As in adult urodynamics, *the four Cs:*

- capacity (of the bladder reservoir)
- contractility (of the detrusor and sphincter)
- compliance (of the bladder wall)
- continence.

And, in addition:

- lower urinary tract sensation
- evacuation (as reflected by absence or presence of postvoid residual).

Normal urodynamic variables in infants and children

In infants and children, it goes without saying that normal values differ widely from the adult ones; and that, in growing individuals, variables such as bladder capacity vary according to the age and size of the child.

Bladder capacity

Increase of bladder capacity is not linear to age or weight during the first years of life. There are two periods when the increase is accelerated. The first is during the first months of life. In free voiding studies of pre-term infants in gestation week 32, median bladder capacity was 12 ml[15] (Figure 41.5) and in similar studies of full-term babies 3 months of age median capacity was 52 ml[13] (Figure 41.6). The capacity is almost unchanged at 1 and 2 years of age (67 and 68 ml, respectively). At 3 years of age, on the other hand, the median capacity is 123 ml, meaning a doubling during the third year of life (see Figure 41.6).[13]

The first step in increase of bladder capacity is thus around birth and is a four-fold increase, which should be compared with the increase in body weight, which is only three-fold. The second step is at the age of toilet-training when gaining control over voidings. The main stimulant for this second increase in bladder capacity can be suggested to be due to the fact that the child starts to get dry at night, which means higher overnight bladder volumes. Indications for such a connection are the finding that high overnight bladder volumes have been shown to be responsible for development of high bladder capacity in patients with VUR[45] and also in boys with posterior urethral valves.[42] Overnight bladder volume has also been shown to be the determinant for functional bladder capacity in healthy children after potty-training.[46]

The relationship between free voiding and cystometric capacity changes during the first years of life. In the neonatal period, cystometric capacity[17] is lower as compared to free voiding capacity[13] (see Figure 41.5), whereas after the infant year the opposite is seen. This can be partly attributed to the fact that older children postpone voiding at cystometry due to fear of voiding with a catheter in the bladder and of the unfamiliar situation of the assessment. This fear cannot be expected in the neonatal child and voiding is thus not postponed for this reason. Another possible explanation for the low cystometric capacity in the neonatal period might be the overactivity suggested by Bachelard et al, shown as an ease to induce detrusor contractions prematurely in catheter investigations.[17]

Even if development of bladder capacity during the first years of life is not linear, we suggest that a linear formula is used for calculation of expected bladder capacity for age as a simple rule of thumb. We have chosen to use:

$$\text{Expected bladder capacity (ml)} = 30 + (\text{age in years} \times 30)^{25}$$

since this linear increase in capacity is very similar to the nonlinear increase in capacity as described by Jansson et al[13] investigating children longitudinally from birth to age 3 years in free voiding studies (see Figure 41.6).

According to the International Continence Society (ICS), the term 'functional bladder capacity' should no longer be used because of difficulties of definition, and it should be replaced with 'voided volume'. Children void widely different volumes during the same day, sometimes when they feel a desire to void but quite often because their mothers tell them to go to the toilet.[46] The common way to decide a child's bladder capacity is to keep a voiding diary (frequency–volume chart) for 2 days and select the largest voiding volume, excluding the first morning voidings that rather represent nocturnal bladder capacity. For children on CIC, the same method is used to define the child's approximate bladder volume.

Measured capacity less than 65% of the calculated value is believed to denote a bladder which is *small for age*, whereas a measured volume that is more than 150% of the calculated value may denote a bladder that is *large for age*.[25]

Detrusor contractility

Storage phase. It has been shown during recent years that instability is rarely seen in infants,[14,17] which is contrary to the earlier concept of instability as a normal phenomenon in this age group.[9] The lack of unstable contractions during filling has been shown in natural fill cystometry,[14] which is an investigation that is sensitive when it comes to identification of instability. This lack of instability during filling has also been observed in standard cystometric investigations of healthy infants, including a study of siblings of children with reflux.[17]

In infants with bladder dysfunction, on the other hand, instability during filling is common, such as those with posterior urethral valves[42] and neurogenic bladder.[32] Therefore, instability can probably be used to diagnose bladder dysfunction in this age group just like in older children.

During the first months of life, on the other hand, there seems to be another form of overactivity, which was observed in 20% of the children as an isolated detrusor contraction after only a few milliliters of filling at cystometry and, with leakage of urine, looked at as a premature voiding contraction.[17] Bladder capacity in these age groups urodynamically registered was also low,[17] and was much lower than that seen after free voidings.[13] These findings taken together indicate that the voiding reflex can easily be elicited in this age group, in the cystometric investigations, by a catheter in the bladder and infusion of saline (see Figure 41.2). This overactivity vanishes after a few months and, simultaneously, bladder capacity increases. The phenomenon does not seem to have anything to do with instability, since instability is seldom seen in infants,[14,17] but can rather be looked upon as an immature behavior of the detrusor muscle.[47,48]

Voiding phase. Voiding detrusor pressure is probably higher during early infancy compared to that seen in older children. Bachelard et al[17] and Wen and Tong[49] investigated infants considered to have normal lower urinary tract with conventional cystometry using a urethral catheter. The pressure levels registered in these studies were very different; median 127 vs mean 75 cmH_2O. One explanation of the different results may be the age of the infants studied, which was median 1 month and 6 months, respectively. Yeung et al also found high voiding pressure levels in small infants.[41] However, it should be noted that they used natural fill cystometry, which gives higher pressure levels than standard cystometry.

Female infants have significantly lower pressures at voiding compared with males and only slightly higher than those of older girls (Table 41.1).

This difference in voiding detrusor pressure between males and females must be attributed to the difference in anatomy, with the long narrow urethra in male infants allowing higher outflow resistance and inducing higher voiding pressure. Thus, the standards for voiding pressure in healthy infants are imprecise and can be a median of more than 100 cmH_2O in males and 60–70 cmH_2O in

Table 41.1 *Voiding detrusor pressure in infants*

References	Mean voiding detrusor pressure (cmH_2O) Males	Females
Yeung et al[41]	117	75
Bachelard et al[17]	127	72
Wen and Tong[49]	75	60

females (see Table 41.1). In children 1–3 years of age median voiding pressures have been reported to be 70 cmH_2O in males[9] and 60 in females.[49]

High voiding pressure in infants is correlated with low bladder capacity. This further explains the above-described differences in voiding pressure levels in the studies by Wen and Tong[49] and Bachelard et al.[17] In the latter study, the infants were younger and thus had lower capacity.

Any discernible peak in the detrusor pressure recording during the filling phase is a pathologic finding, but in order to avoid recording artifacts it may be prudent to allow only for peaks with a duration of >10 s and amplitude of >10 cmH_2O. In neurogenic bladder urodynamics, one should keep in mind that traditional cystometry seems to suppress phasic detrusor activity and exaggerate the rise of basic pressure (giving the impression of low compliance) compared with natural fill cystometry.[40,44]

Variables to register. Variables to register comprise the following:

- Number of phasic contractions and their duration and amplitude together with the infused volume when they occurred. Note subjective reaction, if any.
- Basic detrusor pressure at start and end of filling (excluding a possible sharp terminal rise of pressure). Avoid including phasic contractions.
- Detrusor pressure at start of significant leakage (LPP) and the infused volume when leakage occurred.
- Absence or presence of a coordinated detrusor micturition contraction. In the case of a micturition contraction, any detrusor pressure above 100 cmH_2O is to be regarded as pathologic in children, denoting outflow obstruction or detrusor overactivity, or both. In infant boys, higher values may be normal.

Bladder cooling test. Variables to register are:

- outcome: positive (detrusor contraction >30 cmH_2O) or negative (≤30 cmH_2O)
- maximal detrusor pressure, registered in cmH_2O.

Sphincter contractility

In children with neurogenic bladders, EMG registration will not always produce any information about urethral sphincter activity. When the EMG recording seems unreliable, indirect evidence will have to do. Leak point pressure >40 cmH_2O denotes either neurogenic sphincter overactivity or a sphincter with intact innervation. Likewise, the finding of intravesical pressures well above 40 cmH_2O without any detectable leakage of urine suggests detrusor-sphincter dyssynergia or, alternatively, a normal sphincter contracting to prevent leakage (guarding reflex).

Compliance of the bladder wall

The concept of compliance characterizes the distensibility of the bladder wall during the reservoir phase. A subnormal compliance value denotes increase of bladder wall stiffness due to change of wall structure or a tonic detrusor contraction and is a risk factor for development of upper tract damage. Compliance is expressed as the volume (ml) that the bladder can accommodate with a resulting pressure increase of 1 cmH_2O. It is calculated from a middle segment of the detrusor pressure registration up to 30 cmH_2O, avoiding phasic contractions. A 'normal' value for compliance in adults has not been validated but it is generally felt that it should be more than 20 ml/cmH_2O, e.g. that basic pressure increase up to an adult bladder volume of 400 ml should be 20 cmH_2O or less from empty to full bladder. But we will encounter problems trying to apply this value of compliance to the wide range of bladder volumes in children. For example, a child with a bladder capacity of 100 ml (which would be normal in a 3-year-old child) and a 20 cmH_2O pressure increase from empty to full bladder will give a compliance value of 5 ml/cmH_2O, a value which would be clearly pathologic in an adult. An adjustment must be done to make values comparable between children and adults. It has been suggested that the lowest acceptable value of compliance in a child should be 1/20 (5%) of the child's normal capacity per cmH_2O, a calculation that would be compatible with the lowest limit of 'normal' compliance, 20 ml/cmH_2O, in adults. Then, a compliance of 5 ml/cmH_2O at a bladder capacity of 100 ml would be within the normal range.

Safe capacity. Instead of calculating compliance in order to characterize the reservoir properties of the bladder wall, we use the concept of 'safe capacity' at our institution. The bladder volumes at 20 cmH_2O and 30 cmH_2O base line detrusor pressure are registered. The 20 cmH_2O value stands for a truly safe and the 30 cmH_2O a borderline value for compliance at reservoir capacity.

Continence

Cystometry of a child is not only a laboratory investigation but also allows for a careful and prolonged clinical observation of the child. In addition to the urodynamic results produced by the cystometry, this observation provides important information regarding the child's reactions to bladder filling and, not least, in which situations and at which bladder volumes leakage of urine can be noted.

Lower urinary tract sensation

From age 4 onwards, it is possible to extend the clinical observation during cystometry by asking the child whether he feels the catheter being introduced and if he experiences any sensation from the bladder during filling. Some degree of urethral sensation is not seldom present in children with neurogenic bladder, whereas bladder sensation is most often absent or very weak. Discomfort or pain at end filling when the bladder has become filled to capacity is probably elicited from functional sensory nerve endings in the peritoneum partly covering the bladder. When the child signals discomfort (in small children seldom verbally, but rather by being anxious, crying, or moving restlessly), infusion should be discontinued. The cystometry protocol should include the soft data obtained regarding sensation.

Bladder evacuation

Infants do not empty the bladder at every voiding,[13,15,16,49,50,51] but, characteristically one voiding during 4 hours is complete, according to results from the 4-hour observations. This is seen both in pre-term infants (gestation week 32)[15] and neonates, and during the first years of life.[13] The residual urine during 4 hours is more or less constant from the neonatal period until just before the age of 2 years; median 4–5 ml.[13,15,16] During the third year, when gaining control over voidings, on the other hand, the emptying of the bladder becomes complete, so that the median residual urine is 0 ml.[13]

In healthy children above 3–4 years of age, the bladder empties completely at each voiding. Five milliliters in postvoid residual may be accepted due to the unavoidable time delay from the end of voiding until the bladder can be examined with ultrasound; 5–20 ml is borderline and is an indication for repeating the ultrasound. In schoolgirls treated for bacteriuria, recurrence was significantly more common in those with postvoid residual urine greater than 5 ml.[52] In children with NBD, assessing postvoid residual urine by aspiring through the bladder catheter may not always yield reliable results due to the common dislocation of the base of the neurogenic bladder, so a check with ultrasound is strongly recommended. Ultrasound to determine residual urine should also be performed frequently on all children on CIC for the same reason.

Conclusions

The free voiding pattern in the neonatal period is characterized by small, frequent voidings (one voiding per hour) with volumes that vary intra-individually and leave residual urine most of the time. The incomplete emptying is suggested to be due to a physiologic form of dyscoordination. Towards potty-training age the emptying improves, and, at that time (third year), the bladder capacity also doubles. Voiding during quiet sleep is rarely seen, even in the neonatal infant, meaning that the child shows signs of arousal at voiding.

Bladder instability is rarely seen in urodynamic studies of young infants, although premature voiding contractions are seen in the neonatal period, with leakage of urine after only a few milliliters of filling. This latter increased reactivity of the detrusor muscle is also suggested to be responsible for the cystometric small bladder capacity in this age group and the high voiding pressure levels.

Classification of neurogenic bladder dysfunction in infants and children

A classification of neurogenic bladder in spina bifida children was suggested by van Gool.[53] As can be seen in Table 41.2, a simple but clinically useful classification can be created from the urodynamic data. Detrusor and sphincter are classified as underactive or overactive, so the neurogenic dysfunction can be categorized in four main groups. Two of these display underactive sphincter with incontinence as the major clinical problem, and the two others have overactive sphincter with outflow obstruction and deficient bladder emptying as their

Table 41.2 *Four patterns of bladder-sphincter dysfunction in children with myelomeningocele*[53]

	Detrusor		
Sphincter	Underactive	Overactive	Clinical correlate
Underactive	35	10	Incontinence
Overactive	13	42	Outflow obstruction

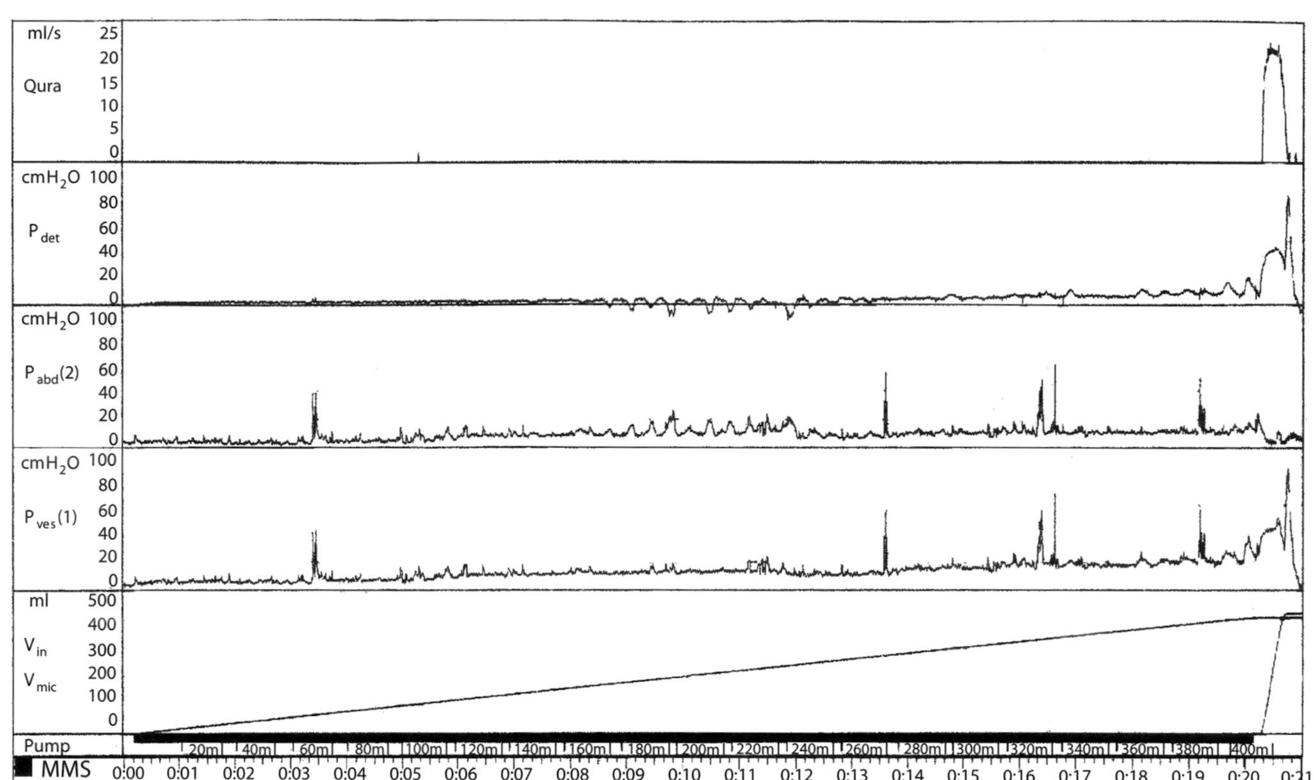

Figure 41.7
Normal cystometry in a 4-year-old boy with high thoracolumbar myelomeningocele.

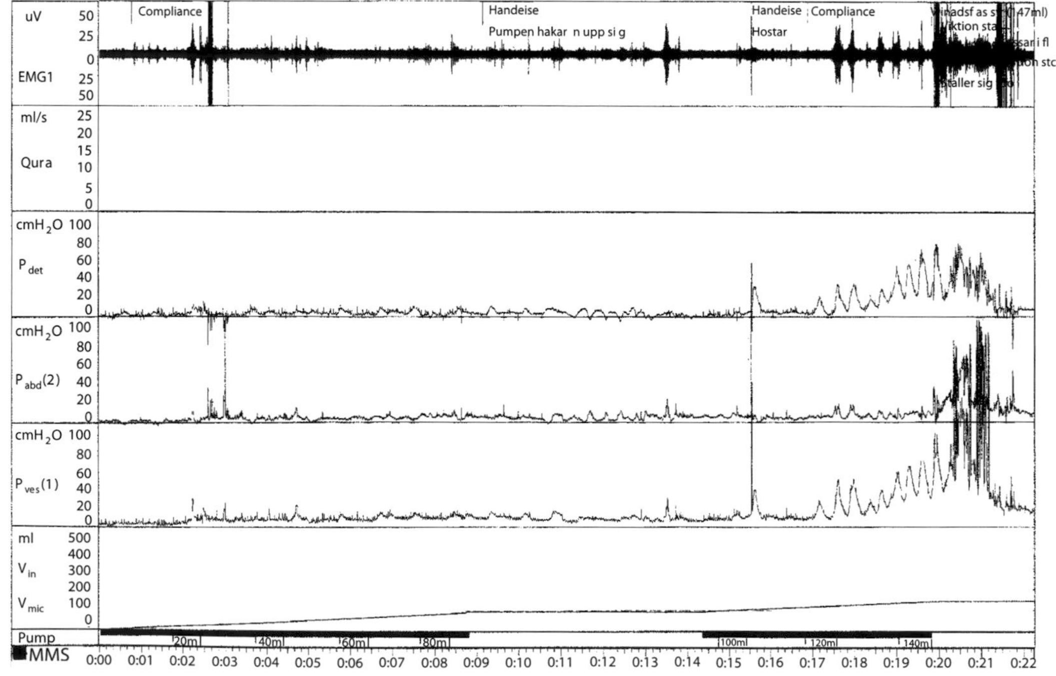

Figure 41.8
Normal compliance, discrete detrusor overactivity, and micturition contraction forcefully counteracted by sphincter contraction, thus pronounced dyssynergia, in a 4-year-old boy with lumbosacral myelomeningocele.

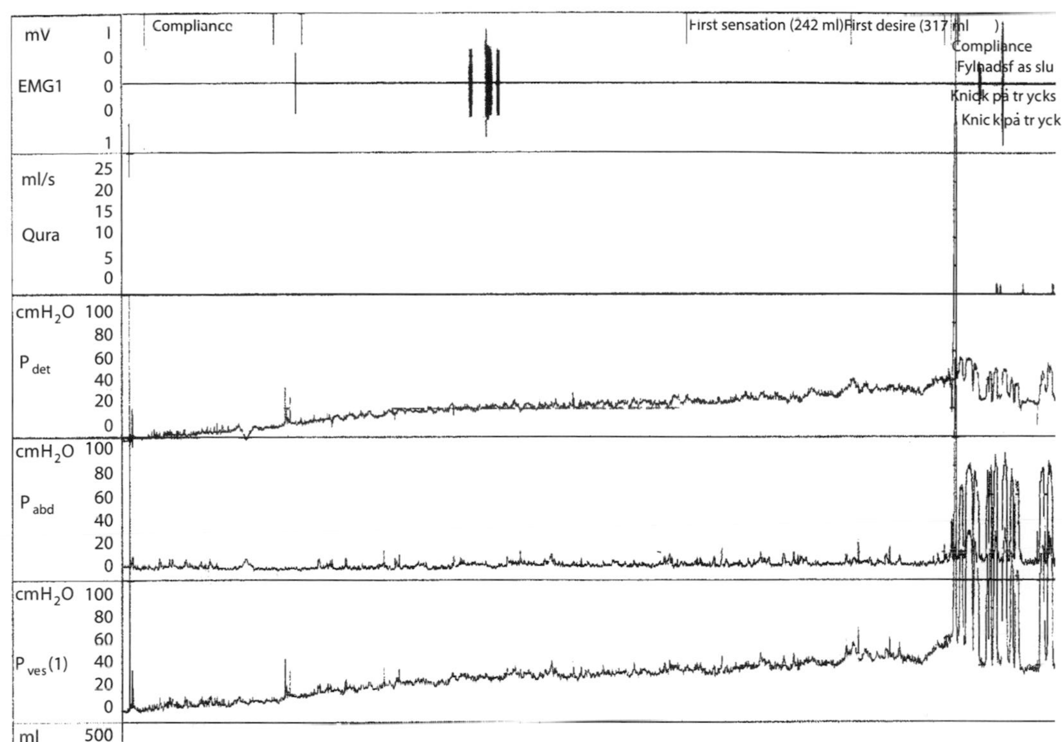

Figure 41.9
Detrusor underactivity, low bladder wall compliance, and poor effect of straining, suggesting sphincter overactivity, in a 4-year-old boy with lumbosacral myelomeningocele.

main clinical characteristics. It should be added, however, that about 5% of children with myelomeningocele display normal bladder function at cystometry, in particular those who have their spinal cord anomaly in a high position (cervical, thoracic, or high thoracolumbar) (Figure 41.7).

Examples of common urodynamic patterns in neurogenic bladder dysfunction in children

The most ominous urodynamic pattern, threatening the integrity of the kidneys, is dyssynergia between detrusor and sphincter. The micturition detrusor contraction is counteracted by sphincter contractions, leading to poor evacuation of the bladder, as seen in a 4-year-old boy with lumbosacral myelomeningocele (Figure 41.8).

Almost equally dangerous for the renal health is the pattern with an underactive or paretic detrusor, low compliant bladder wall, and overactive sphincter (Figure 41.9). The child attempts, without much success, to empty the bladder by forceful contractions of the abdominal muscles. As in the previous case, a regular, carefully performed CIC program is absolutely essential in order to avoid UTIs, reflux, and renal damage in this 4-year-old boy with lumbosacral myelomeningocele.

The pattern is often not as clear-cut as in the two previous cases. In the next example, the detrusor is overactive and there is borderline compliance (Figure 41.10). The sphincter may also be somewhat overactive, as judged from the EMG; but, on the other hand, there are several small micturitions and a larger one at the end of the registration. This patient, with lumbosacral myelomeningocele, is only 9 months old, so there may remain an element of physiologic immaturity in the urodynamic pattern.

The final example, a 5-year-old girl with lumbosacral myelomeningocele (Figure 41.11), depicts the beneficial effect on detrusor overactivity that is often attained with the use of detrusor-relaxing drugs (in this case, oxybutynin 5 mg twice daily administered intravesically). As can be seen, both phasic and tonic (compliance!) detrusor contractility normalizes.

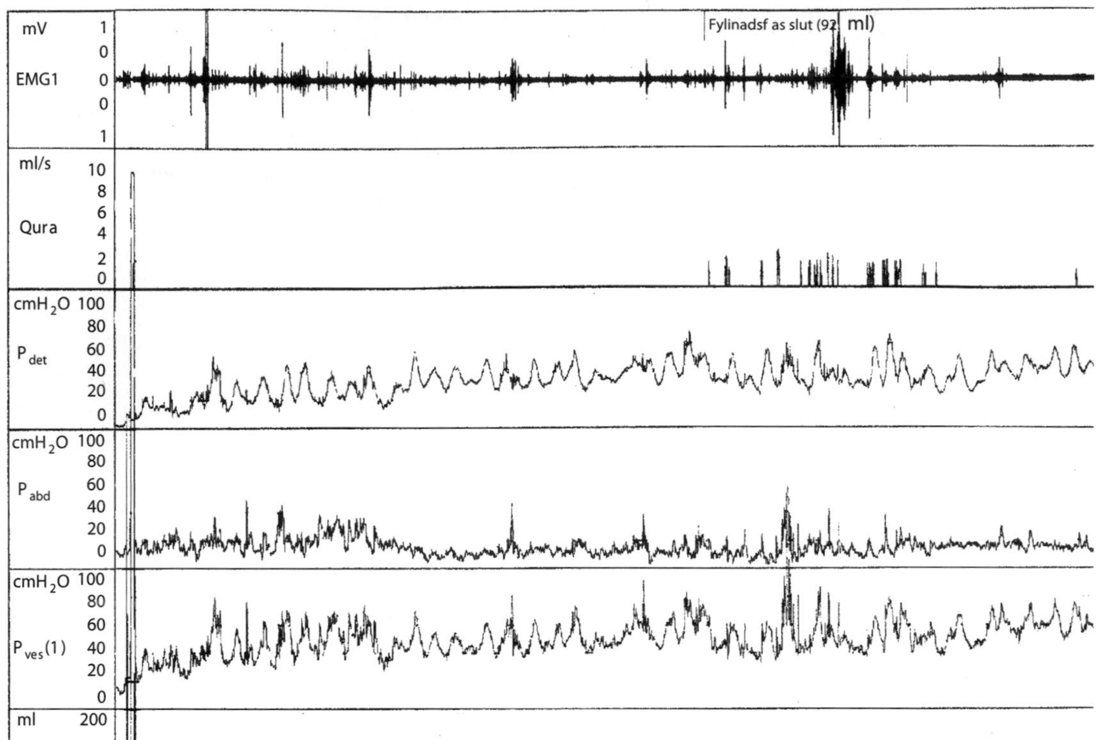

Figure 41.10
Detrusor overactivity and borderline bladder wall compliance in a 9-month-old boy with lumbosacral myelomeningocele. Electromyography (EMG) indicates an overactive pelvic floor, but there are frequent mini-micturitions and a larger one at the end of the registration ('START MIKT').

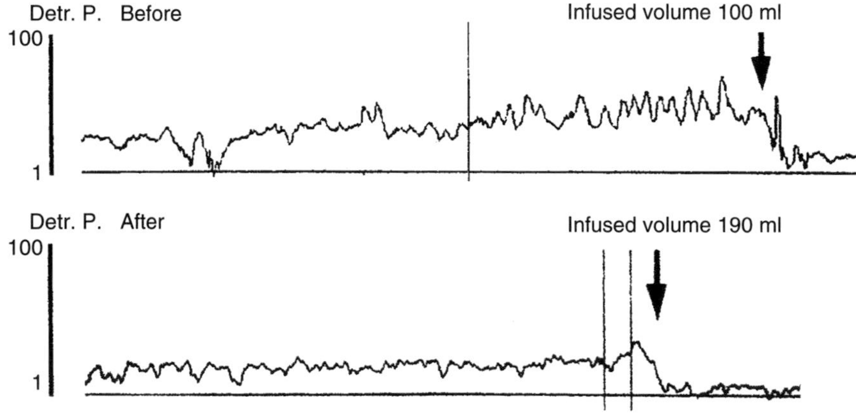

Figure 41.11
Intravesical oxybutynin may efficiently inhibit detrusor overactivity in a 5-year-old girl with lumbosacral myelomeningocele. Detrusor pressure and compliance become normal and capacity nearly doubles after intravesical instillation of 5 mg of oxybutynin.

References

1. Scott R Jr, McIlhaney JS. The voiding rates in normal male children. J Urol 1959; 82: 244.
2. Zatz LM. Combined physiologic and radiologic studies of bladder function in female children with recurrent urinary tract infections. Invest Urol 1965; 3: 278.
3. Whitaker J, Johnston GS. Estimation of urinary outflow resistance in children: simultaneous measurement of bladder pressure, flow rate and exit pressure. Invest Urol 1969; 7: 127.
4. Palm L, Nielsen OH. Evaluation of bladder function in children. J Pediatr Surg 1967; 2: 529.
5. Starfield B. Functional bladder capacity in enuretic and non-enuretic children. J Pediatr 1967; 70: 777.

6. Gierup HJW. Micturition studies in infants and children. Intravesical pressure, urinary flow and urethral resistance in boys without infravesical obstruction. Scand J Urol Nephrol 1970; 3: 217.
7. Kroigaard N. The lower urinary tract in infancy and childhood. Micturition cinematography with simultaneous pressure–flow measurement. Acta Radiol 1970; 300(Suppl): 3–175.
8. O'Donnell B, O'Connor TP. Bladder function in infants and children. Br J Urol 1971; 43: 25.
9. Hjalmas K. Micturition in infants and children with normal lower urinary tract. A urodynamic study. Scand J Urol Nephrol 1976; 37(Suppl).
10. Gool JD van, Kuijter RH, Donckerwolcke RA et al. Bladder-sphincter dysfunction, urinary infection and vesico-ureteral reflux with special reference to cognitive bladder training. Contrib Nephrol 1985; 39: 190.
11. Lindehall B, Claesson I, Hjalmas K, Jodal U. Effect of clean intermittent catheterisation on radiological appearance of the upper urinary tract in children with myelomeningocele. Br J Urol 1991; 67: 415–19.
12. Muellner SR. Development of urinary control in children. JAMA 1960; 172: 1256–60.
13. Jansson UB, Hanson M, Hanson E et al. Voiding pattern in healthy children 0 to 3 years old: a longitudinal study. J Urol 2000; 164: 2050–4.
14. Yeung C, Godley M, Ho C et al. Some new insights into bladder function in infancy. Br J Urol 1995; 76: 235–40.
15. Sillén U, Sölsnes E, Hellström A-L, Sandberg K. The voiding pattern of healthy preterm neonates. J Urol 2000; 163: 278.
16. Holmdahl G, Hanson E, Hanson M et al. Four-hour voiding observation in healthy infants. J Urol 1996; 156: 1809–12.
17. Bachelard M, Sillén U, Hansson S et al. Urodynamic pattern in asymptomatic infants: siblings of children with vesicoureteral reflux. J Urol 1999; 162: 1733.
18. Zerin M, Chen E, Ritchey M, Bloom D. Bladder capacity as measured at voiding cystourethrography in children: relationship to toilet training and frequency of micturition. J Urol 1993; 187: 803.
19. Bakker E, Wyndaele JJ. Change in the toilet-training of children during the last 60 years: the cause of an increase in lower urinary tract dysfunction? BJU Int 2000; 86: 248.
20. Brazelton TB. A child-oriented approach to toilet training. Pediatrics 1962; 29: 121.
21. Klackenberg G. A prospective longitudinal study of children. Data on psychic health and development up to 8 years of age. Acta Paediatr Scand Suppl 1971; 224: 1–239.
22. Largo R, Molinari L, von Siebenthal K, Wolfensberge U. Does a profound change in toilet-training affect development of bowel and bladder control? Dev Med Child Neurol 1996; 38: 1106–16.
23. Marten W, deVries MD, deVries PNP. Cultural relativity of toilet training readiness: a perspective from East Africa. Pediatrics 1977; 60: 170–7.
24. Shurtleff DB. 44 years experience with management of myelomeningocele: presidential address, Society for Research into Hydrocephalus and Spina Bifida. Eur J Pediatr Surg 2000; 10 (Suppl 1): 5–8.
25. Hjälmås K. Urodynamics in normal infants and children. Scand J Urol Nephrol 1988; 114(Suppl): 20–7.
26. Swithinbank L, O'Brien M, Frank D et al. The role of paediatric urodynamics revisited. Neurourol Urodyn 2002; 21: 439–40.
27. Bozkurt P, Kilic N, Kaya G et al. The effects of intranasal midazolam on urodynamic studies in children. Br J Urol 1996; 78: 282–6.
28. Stokland E, Andreasson S, Jacobsson B, Jodal U, Ljung B. Sedation with midazolam for voiding cystourethrography in children: a randomized double-blind study. Pediatr Radiol 2003; 33(4): 247–9.
29. Hellström AL, Andersen K, Hjälmås K, Jodal U. Pad test in children with incontinence. Scand J Urol Nephrol 1986; 20: 47–50
30. Tanikaze S, Sugita Y. Cystometric examination for neurogenic bladder of neonates and infants. Hinyokika Kiyo 1991; 37: 1403–5.
31. Agarwal SK, McLorie GA, Grewal D et al. Urodynamic correlates or resolution of reflux in meningomyelocele patients. J Urol 1997; 158: 580–2.
32. Sillén U, Hanson E, Hermansson G et al. Development of the urodynamic pattern in infants with myelomeningocele. Br J Urol 1996; 78: 596–601.
33. Bauer SB. The argument for early assessment and treatment of infants with spina bifida. Dialog Pediatr Urol 2000; 23(11): 2–3.
34. Tarcan T, Bauer S, Olmedo E et al. Long-term follow up of newborns with myelodysplasia and normal urodynamic findings: is follow up necessary? J Urol 2001; 165: 564–7.
35. Klevmark B. Natural pressure-volume curves and conventional cystometry. Scand J Urol Nephrol 1999; (Suppl 201): 1–4.
36. Geirsson G, Lindstrom S, Fall M et al. Positive bladder cooling test in neurologically normal young children. J Urol 1994; 151: 446–8.
37. Gladh G, Lindstrom S. Outcome of the bladder cooling test in children with neurogenic bladder dysfunction. J Urol 1999; 161: 254–8.
38. Flood HD, Ritchey ML, Bloom DA et al. Outcome of reflux in children with myelodysplasia managed by bladder pressure monitoring. J Urol 1994; 152: 1574–7.
39. Robertson A, Griffiths C, Ramsden P, Neal D. Bladder function in healthy volunteers: ambulatory monitoring and conventional urodynamic studies. Br J Urol 1994; 73: 242–9.
40. Webb RJ, Griffiths CJ, Ramsden PD, Neal DE. Ambulatory monitoring of bladder pressure in low compliance neurogenic bladder dysfunction. J Urol 1992; 148: 1477–81.
41. Yeung C, Godley M, Duffy P, Ransley P. Natural filling cystometry in infants and children. Br J Urol 1995; 75: 531–7.
42. Holmdahl G, Sillen U, Bertilsson M et al. Natural filling cystometry in small boys with posterior urethral valves: unstable bladders become stable during sleep. J Urol 1997; 158: 1017–21.
43. De Gennaro M, Capitanucci ML, Silveri M et al. Continuous (6 hour) urodynamic monitoring in children with neuropathic bladder. Eur J Pediatr Surg 1996; 6(Suppl 1). 21–4.
44. Zermann DH, Lindner H, Huschke T, Schubert J. Diagnostic value of natural fill cystometry in neurogenic bladder in children. Eur Urol 1997; 32: 223–8.
45. Sillén U, Hellström A-L, Sölsnes E, Jansson U-B. Control of voidings means better emptying of the bladder in children with congenital dilating VUR. BJU Int 2000; 85(Suppl 4): 13.
46. Mattsson SH. Voiding frequency, volumes and intervals in healthy school children. Scand J Urol Nephrol 1994; 28: 1–11.
47. Sugaya K, de Groat WC. Influence of temperature on activity of the isolated whole bladder preparation of neonatal and adult rats. Am J Physiol Regul Integr Comp Physiol 2000; 278: 238.
48. Zderic SA, Sillén U, Liu G-H et al. Developmental aspects of bladder contractile function: evidence for an intracellular calcium pool. J Urol 1993; 150: 623.
49. Wen JG, Tong EC. Cystometry in infants and children with no apparent voiding symptoms. Br J Urol 1998; 81: 468.
50. Roberts DS, Rendell B. Postmicturition residual bladder volumes in healthy babies. Arch Dis Child 1989; 64: 825–8.
51. Gladh G, Persson D, Mattsson S, Lindstrom S. Voiding patterns in healthy newborns. Neurourol Urodyn 2000; 19: 177–84.
52. Lindberg U, Bjure J, Haugstvedt S, Jodal U. Asymptomatic bacteriuria in schoolgirls. III. Relation between residual urine volume and recurrence. Acta Paediatr Scand 1975; 64: 437–40.
53. Van Gool J. Spina bifida and neurogenic bladder dysfunction: a urodynamic study. Thesis. Utrecht: Uitgeverij Impress, 1986: 154.

42

Normal urodynamic parameters in adults

Lysanne Campeau, Tala AL Afraa, and Jacques Corcos

Introduction

Urodynamic studies play an important role in the evaluation and diagnosis of lower urinary tract dysfunction. Evaluation can be undertaken in a noninvasive manner, with a voiding diary, a pad test, and free flow rate, or in an invasive manner, by cystometry, pressure flow assessment, and urethral pressure profiling. The normality of urodynamic parameters in a healthy population is found in ranges rather than in precise values. As some tests are invasive, most published data are derived from patients and not from healthy volunteers. Furthermore, urodynamic investigations may be considered as nonphysiologic tests because of the introduction of several artificial factors, such as urethral catheterization, a filling rate that is different from the usual physiologic rate, and the immobile position of patients during evaluation.[1,2] With the help of clinical data and abnormal pathologic values, it is, however, possible to define some 'normality' for most of the different parameters measured by urodynamics, and, therefore, to establish reference values for clinicians.

Pad test

The pad test is a diagnostic tool that assesses the degree of incontinence in patients in a semi-objective manner. Pad weight gain in nonmenstruating women can be attributed mainly to urine, but also to perspiration and vaginal discharges.

The short-term pad test

The short-term pad test is a standardized, objective way of assessing incontinence, lasting 15 minutes to 2 hours and including a standardized, provocative evaluation. It is often used in office practice because of its convenient nature. As described by Abrams et al, the test requires the intake of a fixed amount of fluid. The pad is weighed before and after the 1-hour period in the office. Specific activities are performed in this time frame, such as walking, standing, coughing, running, and bending forward.[3] When this test was performed in 50 healthy women with self-reported normal urinary control, Sutherst et al determined that the pad weight gain after 1 hour ranged from 0 to 2.1 g, with a mean of 0.26 g.[4] Versi and Cardozo recorded a mean value of 0.39 g with an upper 99% confidence limit (99% CL) of 1.4 g of normal weight gain during 1 hour.[5] The International Continence Society (ICS) has defined a cut-off of 1 g to distinguish continent from incontinent women.[6] Test–retest repeatability in healthy controls has not been analyzed, but different studies have examined correlation coefficients between the results in women performing the same test twice. They found a coefficient varying between 0.68 and 0.97. The results will vary if the test is performed with a standardized volume in the bladder.[7,8]

The long-term pad test

The long-term pad test requires patients to wear pads for 24 or 48 hours during regular everyday activities and in their usual surroundings. Patients are instructed to record the frequency and amount of fluid intake as well as the episodes of micturition and incontinence. At the end of the test, the pad is weighed. Studies have assessed weight gain in self-reported continent women in the 24-hour pad test. Lose et al discerned that median weight gain was 4 g/24 hours, with an upper 99% CL of 8 g/24 hours.[9] Mouritsen et al[10] and Versi et al[11] tested 24 young nursing and physiotherapy students and recorded a mean pad weight gain of 7.1 g/48 hours (upper 95% CL of 14 g). Ryhammer et al. evaluated the 24-hour pad test in continent women with a mean age of 50 years and reported a mean pad weight test result of 3.1 g/24 hours.[9,12] Test–retest repeatability was also investigated by the same authors, who observed a difference of up to 4 g per 24 hours in 95% of the cases. Karantanis et al discerned a mean pad weight gain of 0.3 g/24 hours (upper 95% CL of 0.4 g) in 120 participants

Table 42.1 *Voiding diary of healthy volunteers as reported in the literature*

	Pauwels et al[32]	De Wachter and Wyndaele[72]	Kassis and Schick[73]	Pfisterer et al[74]	Normal range
No of volunteers	32 women	15 women	33 women	24 women	
Mean age	49	21	40	50.2	
Daytime frequency	6.45	7.24 ± 2.27	5.63 ± 1.26	5.7	6–7
No of nocturia	0.07	0.07 ± 2.25	0.08 ± 0.16	0.2	0–1
Mean voided volume during day (ml)	289 ± 278	231 ± 128	237 ± 67	1045	200–250
Mean voided volume during night (ml)	450 ± 189	300 ± 50	379 ± 132	438	300–400
Mean voided volume in 24 hours (ml)	1962			1442	1400–1800

with a mean age of 48 years.[13] They did not detect any significant difference between premenopausal and postmenopausal women. A total of 14 men were tested, and their results were 2 times lower than those obtained in women (0.5 vs 0.25 g), indicating that vaginal secretions account for half of the weight gain.[13]

In summary, the short-term pad test has a mean value of approximately 0.3 g, while the long-term pad test has an average value varying between 3 and 4 g per 24 hours. (For more details, see Chapter 35.)

Voiding diary

To objectively measure subjective complaints of lower urinary tract symptoms, patients are asked to complete a voiding diary. The most commonly used is the frequency–volume chart, which provides maximum information to physicians. It records the number and timing of incontinence and micturition episodes along with the amount of urine voided.[14]

Women

These parameters have been studied in normal, healthy subjects without any urinary symptoms. Most investigations have dealt with women. Kassis and Schick evaluated a group of 33 asymptomatic women who volunteered to complete a frequency–volume chart over 7 days.[15] Daytime frequency was about 6 times (5.63 ± 1.26), and mean total voided volume (VV) per 24 hours was 1473 (±386) ml. Mean VV was 237 (±67) ml during the day, and 379 (±132) ml during the night. Voiding frequency at night was 0.08 (±0.16) with a night/day diuresis ratio of 0.81 (±0.30).[15] Huang et al analyzed the 3-day voiding diary of 68 healthy Taiwanese women. Their total daily voiding frequency was 7.34 (±1.63) times with a night-time voiding frequency of 0.25 (±0.31), the 24-hour VV was 1634 (±652) ml, and the night-time to whole day urine volume ratio was 0.24. Mean VV for each void was 225 (±81) ml.[16] Boedker et al reported comparable findings in a subset of 123 women with regard to voiding frequency (5.7), total daily VV (1350 ml), and mean VV (380 ml).[17] Fitzgerald and Brubaker presented results from an interesting study looking at the variability of 24-hour voiding diary parameters among 137 asymptomatic women. Subjects voided a median of 8 times per 24 hours in the first diary, and 7 times in the second diary. Total 24-hour voided urine volume was 1580 ml in the first and 1485 ml in the second diary. Also, mean VV was 195 ml in the first and 197 ml in the second diary.[18]

A larger investigation by Van Haarst et al recruited 1152 asymptomatic subjects aged over 20 years to complete a 24-hour frequency–volume chart.[19] They observed a 24-hour frequency decline in women of older decades, ranging from 6.9 in the third decade to 8.2 in the sixth decade. The frequency of nocturia increased with age, from 0.7 in the third decade to 1.4 in women aged more than 70 years. Mean VV decreased from 274 to 240 ml, and 24-hour VV was 1762 ml.[19]

In summary, normal voiding frequency varies between 5 and 8 times per 24 hours with total urine volume between 1350 and 1800 ml. Mean VV ranges approximately between 200 and 350 ml (Table 42.1).

Men

In the previously-cited study by Boedker et al, the same parameters were examined in 102 healthy men aged between 14 and 69 years.[17] The median frequency of micturition was 5.6, total VV was 1450 ml, and median bladder capacity was 400 ml. Two hundred and eighty-four asymptomatic males participated in an investigation by Latini et al, where they were asked to complete the IPSS (International Prostate

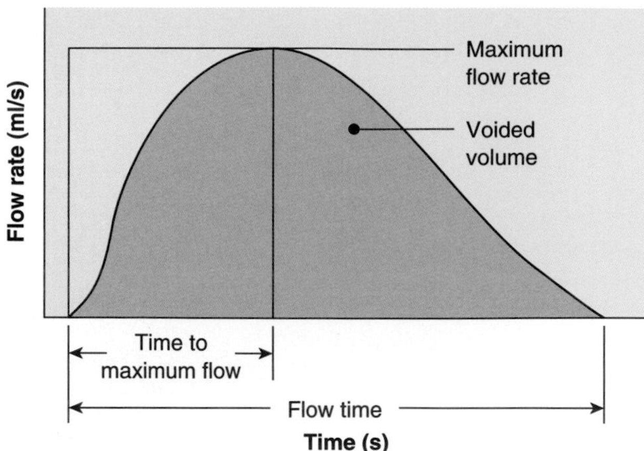

Figure 42.1
The normal shape of the flow rate curve with frequently measured parameters. Produced with permission from reference 19a.

Symptom Score) and a 24-hour voiding diary.[20] Subjects voided a median of 7 times in 24 hours, with a total urine volume of 1650 ml; mean VV was 237 ml.[20]

Van Haarst et al determined that there was a linear rise with age in 24-hour voiding frequency and nocturia in men, ranging respectively from 6.0 and 0.5 in men in the third decade to 8.5 and 1.6 in men aged over 70 years. Mean VV decreased from 313 to 209 ml, and mean 24-hour VV was 1718 ml.[19]

To summarize, men void at a frequency between 5 and 7 times per day with a mean volume per void of between 200 and 350 ml. The average 24-hour VV ranges approximately between 1450 and 1700 ml. For more details on voiding diaries, see Chapter 34.

Flowmetry and postvoid residual volume

Flowmetry is the test that evaluates several parameters that vary considerably with gender and age, such as maximal flow rate (Q_{max}), average flow rate (Q_{ave}), and voided volume (VV) (Figure 42.1 and Table 42.2).

Women

Haylen et al constructed the Liverpool nomograms based on the maximum and average flow rates of normal volunteers.[21] Their study included 331 males (average age 49 years) and 249 women (average age 32 years). In women, age and parity did not influence flow rates. Different parameters were reported by Pfisterer et al in a group of 24 pre-, peri-, and postmenopausal, healthy female volunteers who underwent uroflowmetry.[22] The Q_{max} was 25, 32, and 23 ml/s, respectively. VV was 225, 335, and 264 ml, respectively. PVR in all groups was below 20 ml. In an interesting study, Unsal and Cimentepe assessed differences in flowmetry in various positions among 72 healthy male and female volunteers.[23] In the 36 women of this group (mean age 32 years), Q_{max} values were 28.09 (±0.66) ml/s in the sitting and 27.98 (±0.59) ml/s in the crouching position. Q_{ave} was 18.26 (±0.36) ml/s in the sitting and 17.31 (±0.35) ml/s in the crouching position. Mean VV and PVR values were 331.8 (±13.28) ml and 11.82 (±0.99) ml in the sitting position, and 326.9 (±12.87) ml and 12.79 (±1.07) ml in the crouching position, respectively.

A group of 140 healthy Thai subjects was divided into two subgroups according to age (18–30 years and 50–60 years).[24] Women had a higher Q_{max} (32.5 ± 10.0 vs 27.8 ± 8.0 ml/s) and Q_{ave} (23.5 ± 8.1 vs 19.8 ± 5.8 ml/s) than men. PVR was less than 50 ml in all subjects. In summary, Q_{ave} in women ranges from 17 to 24 ml/s, and Q_{max} ranges from 23 to 33 ml/s, depending on age. Regardless of age, PVR should not exceed 50 ml in asymptomatic women.

Men

We completed a study of uroflowmetry parameters in 31 male, asymptomatic, middle-aged urologists.[25] Q_{max} and Q_{ave} were, respectively, 20.5 ml/s (SD = 3.9) and 14.3 ml/s

Table 42.2 *Normal range of uroflowmetry parameters*

	Wyndaele[2]		Jensen et al[75] n = 13 males Mean age 61 years	Pfisterer et al[74] n = 24 women Mean age 50 years
	Male	Female		
Voided volume (ml)	337.7	337.5	210	264
Q_{max} (ml/s)	24.4	30.5	15.7	26
Q_{ave} (ml/s)	13.6	21.5	7.8	
Flow time (s)	26	26	25	
Residual urine (ml)	19	19	20	20

(SD = 3.0). VV was 331.9 ml (SD = 94.8) with a voiding time of 32.7 s (SD = 15.5). Unsal and Cimentepe assessed uroflowmetry parameters in 36 young males (mean age 30 years). Q_{max} and Q_{ave} respectively varied between 23.28 and 24.29 ml/s, and between 15.56 and 15.81 ml/s. Mean VV and PVR values ranged between 297.5 and 309.9 ml, and between 12.92 and 14.02 ml, respectively.[23] Schmidt et al conducted ambulatory urodynamic studies on 39 asymptomatic male volunteers with a mean age of 25.8 years.[26] The men were divided into two groups according to water consumption: group 1 with a water consumption of 30 ml/kg daily, and group 2 with a water consumption of 60 ml/kg daily. There were no significant differences between the two groups in Q_{max} (24.4 ± 1.3 to 25.2 ± 1.8 ml/s) or VV (286 ± 20 to 329 ± 15 ml). Haylen et al demonstrated that men showed a decline of 1.0 to 1.6 ml/s/10 years in maximum urine flow rate and a decrease of 0.6 to 1.0 ml/s/10 years in average urine flow rate.[21]

Tong evaluated uroflowmetry in a group of 20 males aged over 60 years and recorded values of Q_{max} between 24.2 and 27.1 ml/s and of Q_{ave} between 14.9 and 17.2 ml/s.[27] VV varied between 338 and 532 ml. Jorgensen et al reported, in a group of asymptomatic men, that median Q_{max} decreased from 18.5 ml/s at age 50 years to 6.5 ml/s at age 80 years.[28]

To summarize, Q_{ave} in men ranges between 14.3 and 17.2 ml/s, and Q_{max} ranges between 20.5 and 27.1 ml/s. The latter values seem to decrease with age. VV varies between 250 and 550 ml, and PVR is less than 15 ml.

Cystometry during the filling phase

During the filling phase, abdominal and bladder pressures are recorded via rectal and urethral catheters, respectively, whereas detrusor pressure is calculated by subtracting abdominal pressure from bladder pressure. Baseline abdominal and bladder pressures are 5–20 cmH_2O in the supine position, 15–40 cmH_2O in the sitting position, and 30–50 cmH_2O in the standing position.[29] Detrusor pressure in an empty bladder varies between 0 and 10 cmH_2O in 90% of cases. Normal abdominal pressure is 37 ± 7 cmH_2O during filling and 35 ± 9 cmH_2O during voiding. Normal detrusor pressure during bladder filling should be less than 25 cmH_2O.[30] Several parameters are recorded during the filling phase, including bladder sensation, compliance, detrusor function, maximum cystometric bladder capacity, and urethral sphincter activity (Figure 42.2 and Table 42.3).

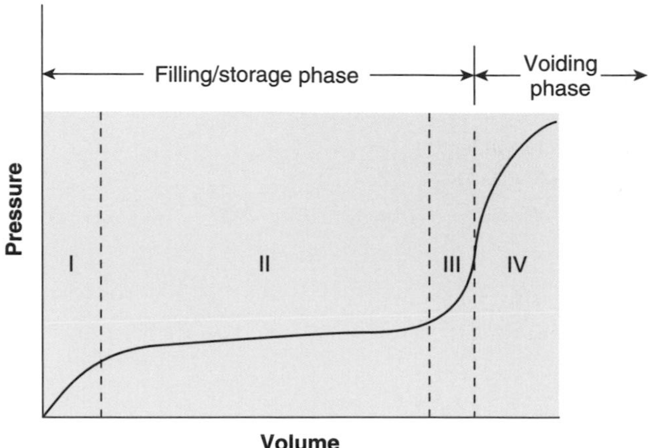

Figure 42.2
The normal cystometrogram curve has four phases: (I) an initial pressure rise to achieve resting bladder pressure; (II) the tonus limb, which reflects the viscoelastic properties of the bladder wall; (III) bladder wall structures achieving maximal elongation and pressure rise caused by additional filling (this phase should not be encountered during cystometry); and (IV) the voiding phase, representing bladder contractility. Reproduced with permission from reference 19a.

Table 42.3 *Normal reported cystometric parameters during filling in both males and females*

Parameter	Wyndaele[2,31]	Pfisterer et al[74]	Normal range
No of volunteers	38	24	
Mean age	24	50.2	
First sensation (ml)	253	107	100–250
First desire to void (ml)	326	188	200–330
Strong desire to void (ml)	563	372	350–560
Bladder compliance (ml/cmH_2O)			
Men	56.1		
Women	70.9	119	≥50
Detrusor activity	Stable		Stable
MCC (ml)			450–550
Men	552		
Women	453	580	

MCC, maximum cystometric capacity.

Table 42.4 *Normal bladder compliance[76] (Reproduced with permission)*

Definition	Comment
Compliance index:[77] Volume (ml)/detrusor pressure (in cmH_2O) at bladder capacity	Normal = 20 to 100 (with bladder capacity > 650 ml) Low = ≤20 High = >100
Compliance:[78] Volume (ml)/1 cm H_2O	Normal = 30 to 55 Capacity = 300–500 ml
Compliance:[79] Detrusor pressure (cmH_2O)/100 ml	Normal = ≤10 Low = ≥10
Compliance: detrusor pressure at capacity minus detrusor pressure at empty bladder	Normal = ≤ 20 cmH_2O

Sensation

Wyndaele studied bladder sensations in 38 normal volunteers by cystometry.[31] He described three patterns of normal bladder sensation: the first sensation was bladder filling, the first desire, and then the strong desire to void. The latter sensation was equivalent to cystometric bladder capacity. The first sensation occurred at 40% (253 ml) of bladder capacity, while the first desire occurred at 60% (326 ml) of bladder capacity, which was about 563 ml. Furthermore, he reported that the volumes in all three types of sensation were smaller in women. Also, bladder sensation could be assessed by measurement of the electrical sensory threshold (EST). Normal EST should be less than 15 mA.[32]

Compliance

Normal bladder compliance values are between 30 and 100 ml/cm. They are higher in women than in men.[2] Low normal bladder compliance values are below 30 ml/cm[33] (see Table 42.4).

Detrusor stability during filling

During bladder filling, the absence of involuntary detrusor contractions is considered to be normal and is defined as a stable detrusor.[2,32] Uninhibited detrusor contractions occurred in 10–18% of asymptomatic volunteers, but should be evaluated further because they may indicate an underlying pathology.[31,34]

Maximum cystometric capacity

Normal cystometric bladder capacity can vary widely, but is normally between 300 and 550 ml, with higher values in men than in women.[2]

Leak-point pressure

Detrusor leak-point pressure

Leak-point pressure (LPP) is the value where bladder pressure leakage occurs. The rise in bladder pressure can be secondary to a rise in detrusor pressure that is related to detrusor overactivity or impaired compliance. The value assessed is, therefore, referred to as detrusor leak-point pressure (DLPP). This value is of great importance because detrusor pressure at leakage reflects the resistance the urethra can offer to the bladder mainly by the action of the striated sphincter. A high DLPP is of clinical relevance as it can jeopardize upper urinary tract function. McGuire et al followed the clinical urodynamic progress of 42 myelodysplastic children and found that those with a DLPP of 40 cmH_2O or more developed upper tract damage if not treated.[35]

Patients with normal detrusor compliance and without overactivity or outlet resistance will not experience a rise in detrusor pressure to dangerous levels. Detrusor pressure will rise at the initiation of voiding and decrease thereafter when the sphincter relaxes and the bladder empties. Therefore, abnormal detrusor pressure values will be seen in patients suffering from neurogenic bladder dysfunction (e.g. detrusor-sphincter dysynergia, or DSD), but also in patients with infravesical obstruction.[36]

Abdominal leak-point pressure

Increased abdominal pressure can also be elicited by a rise in abdominal pressure (with the Valsalva maneuver or during coughing). Abdominal leak-point pressure (ALPP) measures the ability of the urethra to resist abdominal pressure as an expulsive force, in the absence of detrusor

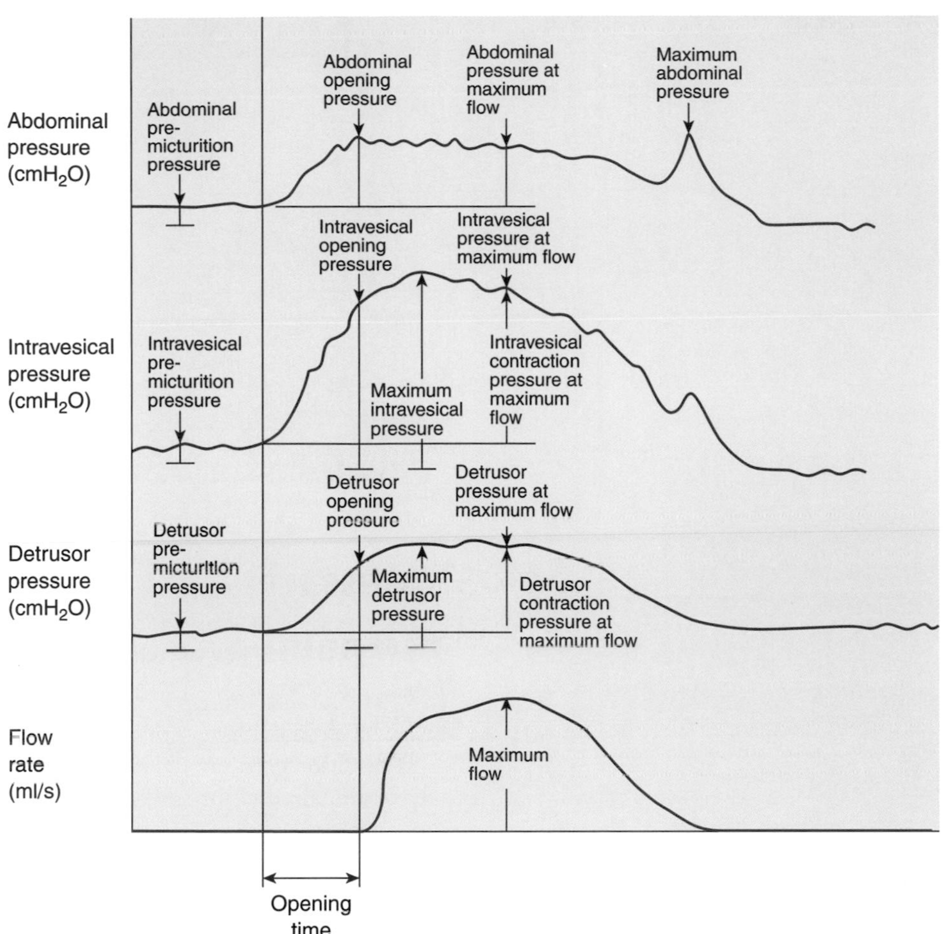

Figure 42.3
Pressure–flow study diagram labeled with frequently measured parameters and recommended terminology. Reproduced with permission from reference 19a.

contraction. This test assesses the severity of stress urinary incontinence (SUI) and may be useful in detecting intrinsic sphincter deficiency (ISD). In normal individuals, no abdominal pressure increase should cause incontinence. Therefore, there is no 'normal ALPP'. However, studies have tried to determine a cut-off between patients with or without ISD. Using videourodynamics, McGuire et al determined that 80% of women with Valsalva leak-point pressure (VLPP) below 60 cmH_2O had type III SUI.[37] They also demonstrated that VLPP values higher than 90 cmH_2O can rule out ISD. In fact, in women suffering from SUI without genital prolapse, a high ALPP of 100 cmH_2O or more is usually associated with urethral hypermobility. Those with values of between 60 and 100 cmH_2O have features of both ISD and hypermobility.[36]

Pressure–flow in men

A pressure–flow (P/Q) study simultaneously measures detrusor pressure and flow rate during voiding. P/Q assessment is considered to be the gold standard for quantifying and grading bladder outlet obstruction (BOO) and detrusor contractility.[38–43] P/Q data can be plotted on pressure–flow nomograms to classify patients as being either obstructed or not obstructed, and, at the same time, to grade the severity of obstruction. Different types of nomograms have been developed. The most commonly used in clinical practice are the Abrams–Griffiths (AG) nomogram, the Schafer nomogram, the urethral resistance factor (URA), and the ICS nomogram.[40] These nomograms have a good prognostic value in predicting the outcome after prostatectomy.[44–46] During P/Q assessment, several parameters are recorded, including opening detrusor pressure ($P_{det.open}$), maximum detrusor pressure ($P_{det.max}$), detrusor pressure at maximum flow ($P_{det.Q_{max}}$), minimum detrusor pressure during voiding ($P_{det.min.void}$), Q_{max}, VV, and PVR (Figure 42.3). In normal patients, P/Q shows low pressure generating high flow, which indicates that there is no obstruction and that detrusor function is normal.[47] Normal $P_{det.Q_{max}}$ in men ranges between 47 and 58 cmH_2O.[26]

Walker et al analyzed P/Q data on 24 asymptomatic volunteers with a mean age of 62.5 years.[48] They found that 14 of the volunteers (58%) fell in the nonobstructed zone according to the ICS nomogram and had grade 0–1 for the Schafer nomogram, correlating with an absence of

Table 42.5 *Normal reported P/Q parameters in men*

	Wyndaele[2]	Schmidt et al[26] (group 1)	Walker et al[48]	Normal range
$P_{det.open}$ (cmH_2O)		51.2 ± 3.2	43.7 ± 17	40-50
$P_{det.min.void}$ (cmH_2O)			32.5 ± 23	30
$P_{det.max}$ (cmH_2O)		58.9 ± 4.5		60
$P_{det.Q_{max}}$ (cmH_2O)	47.9	47.8 ± 2.2	49.4 ± 26	50
Maximum contractility		15.4 ± 1.4		15
Q_{max} (ml/s)	16.6	24.4 ± 1.4	17.9 ± 17	16–25
Voided volume (ml)	541.3	286 ± 20	254 ± 121	250–550
PVR (ml)	19.7		15.1 ± 21	15–20
BOOI			17 ± 35	≤17
LinPURR				Grade 0–I
URA				≤20
BCI				100–150

$P_{det.open}$, opening detrusor pressure; $P_{det.min.void}$, minimal voiding detrusor pressure; $P_{det.max}$, maximum detrusor pressure during voiding; $P_{det\cdot Q_{max}}$, detrusor pressure at maximum flow; Q_{max}, maximum flow rate; PVR, postvoid residual urine; BOOI, bladder contractility index; LinPURR, linear passive urethral resistance relation; URA, urethral resistance factor; BCI, bladder contractility index.

obstruction. The AG number was −11 ± 11.7 (Q_{max} 23 ± 5.3 ml/s and PVR 14.5 ± 17 ml).

Schmidt et al undertook ambulatory urodynamic and P/Q measurements of 39 asymptomatic male volunteers (mean age 25.8 years) divided into two groups according to water consumption regimens per day: 30 ml/kg/day in group 1 and 60 ml/kg/day in group 2. They observed that $P_{det.max}$ occurred before the onset of urine flow. Furthermore, both detrusor pressure and detrusor contractility increased with augmented water consumption and urine production.[26] Wyndaele attempted to define what can be considered as normal parameters by urodynamic study in 38 healthy adult volunteers (28 men and 10 women) with a mean age of 24 years. Free flow rate, water cystometry, and P/Q assessment were undertaken for all of them. Micturition bladder pressure was higher in men than in women, reflecting higher outflow resistance in men, but detrusor pressure was not statistically different between the sexes. Flow time was significantly longer and maximum flow rate was significantly lower during P/Q evaluation than during free flow rate measurement in both sexes. There was no residual urine at all in the majority of volunteers, but 6 men and 3 women had less than 50 ml residual[2] (Table 42.5).

The AG nomogram

The AG nomogram was described by Abrams and Griffiths in 1979. It can be calculated from two parameters generating P/Q data: $P_{det.Q_{max}}$ and Q_{max}. Both are plotted on a graph which separates patients into three categories: obstructed, equivocal, and unobstructed.[38–40] The ICS recommended this type of nomogram to diagnose BOO in older men.[49] Lim and Abrams introduced the AG number, now known as the bladder outlet obstruction index (BOOI), which can be calculated by the following equation: AG number = $P_{det.Q_{max}} - (2*Q_{max})$.[38,40] According to the BOOI, the ICS nomogram can be divided into three zones. A BOOI greater than 40 indicates obstruction, between 20 and 40 is within an equivocal zone, and below 20 rules out obstruction. The latter category suggests that patients are potentially normal or that their symptoms are secondary to detrusor hypocontractility[40] (Figure 42.4).

Linear passive urethral resistance relation

On Schafer's P/Q diagram, BOO can be classified into seven categories: 0–I = normal or no obstruction, II = mild, III–IV = moderate, and V–VI = severe obstruction. Furthermore, the zone where $P_{det.Q_{max}}$ falls can characterize detrusor muscle strength (strong, normal, weak, or very weak). Linear passive urethral resistance relation (linPURR) was introduced later on by Schafer in 1990 by manually drawing a straight line between the minimal urethral opening pressure (P_{muo}) and $P_{det.Q_{max}}$. According to the linPURR nomogram, men with P_{muo} less than 20 cmH_2O and $P_{det.Q_{max}}$ more than 20 cmH_2O have normal

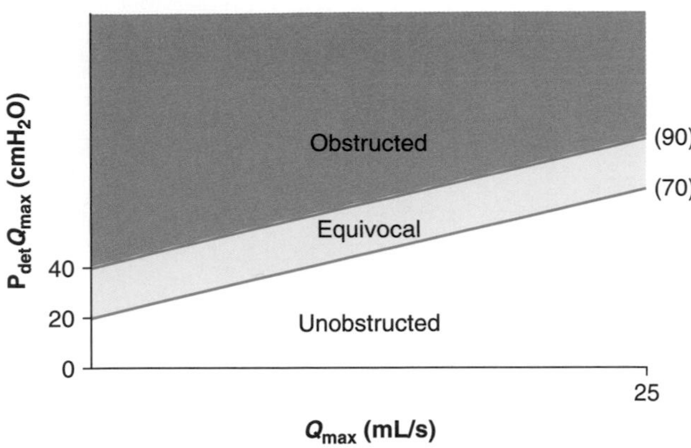

Figure 42.4
Provisional International Continence Society nomogram for analysis of voiding divides patients into three classes according to the bladder outlet obstruction index (BOOI) = ($P_{detQ_{max}} - 2Q_{max}$). Reproduced with permission from reference 19a.

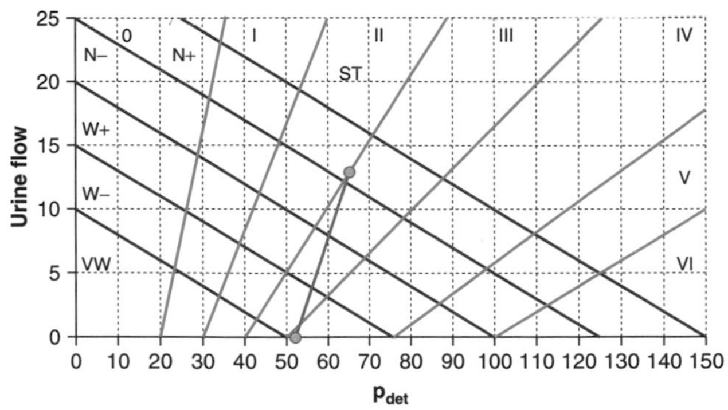

Figure 42.5
Schafer nomogram. The plot indicates that the patient has a grade III severity of obstruction and that the patient has normal detrusor contractility. Reproduced with permission from reference 19a.

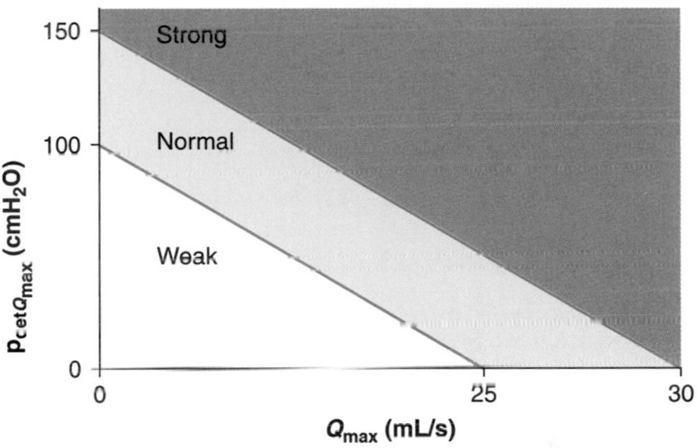

Figure 42.6
Bladder contractility nomogram divides patients into three categories according to the bladder contractility index ($P_{detQ_{max}} + 5Q_{max}$). Reproduced with permission from reference 19a.

detrusor function and no obstruction.[42,50] The upper normal limit for voiding detrusor pressure is 33 cmH_2O[42] (Figure 42.5).

Urethral resistance factor

The urethral resistance factor (URA) can be calculated from any simultaneous pressure and flow values during voiding. It should remain constant throughout voiding regardless of the values used for calculation. Patients with URA greater than 29 cmH_2O are classified as obstructed, those with URA between 21 and 29 cmH_2O are equivocal, and those with URA below 21 cmH_2O are unobstructed or normal.[51–53]

Detrusor contractility

Detrusor contractility is derived from parameters such as the maximal pressure and amplitude slope during isovolumetric detrusor contraction as well as the duration of contraction. Detrusor contractility increases with the severity of outlet obstruction.[33] Schafer's nomogram obtains the bladder contractility index (BCI) with the following formula: BCI = $P_{det.Q_{max}} + 5Q_{max}$. If the BCI is more than 150, the detrusor is considered strong, between 100 and 150, it is normal, and below 100, it is weak. Detrusor contractility can also be assessed by the linPURR nomogram[42] (Figure 42.6). Furthermore, it can be evaluated by estimating bladder voiding efficiency (BVE) according to the formula: BVE = (VV/total capacity)* 100; 75% and above is considered to be normal.[40] The BOOI and the BCI can also be calculated from the composite nomogram suggested by Abrams[40] (Figure 42.7). This nomogram is a combination of the ICS nomogram and the bladder contractility nomogram, classifying patients into 9 zones and 6 groups according to the BOOI and the BCI. Patients in zones 1 and 2 are considered normal.[40]

Pressure–flow in women

Blaivas and Groutz studied 50 women with BOO (mean age 65 years) and 20 normal controls (mean age 67 years) by videourodynamic assessment.[54] The pressure–flow (P/Q) parameters recorded in the control group were: free Q_{max} 24.4 ± 8.8 ml/s, Q_{max} 13.3 ± 6.3 ml/s, $P_{det.Q_{max}}$ 17.9 ± 7.5 cmH_2O, $P_{det.max}$ 22.2 ± 9.2 cmH_2O, VV 312 ± 131 ml, and PVR 103 ± 100 ml. These authors described a nomogram which can be used to diagnose BOO in women

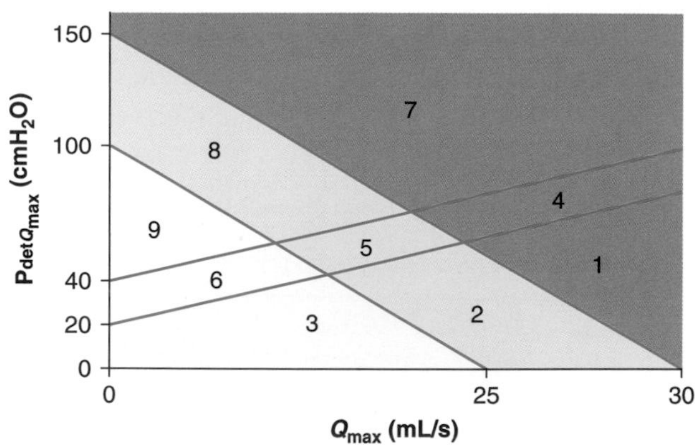

Figure 42.7
The composite nomogram allows categorization of patients into nine zones and therefore six groups according to the bladder outlet obstruction index and the bladder contractility index. Reproduced with permission from reference 19a.

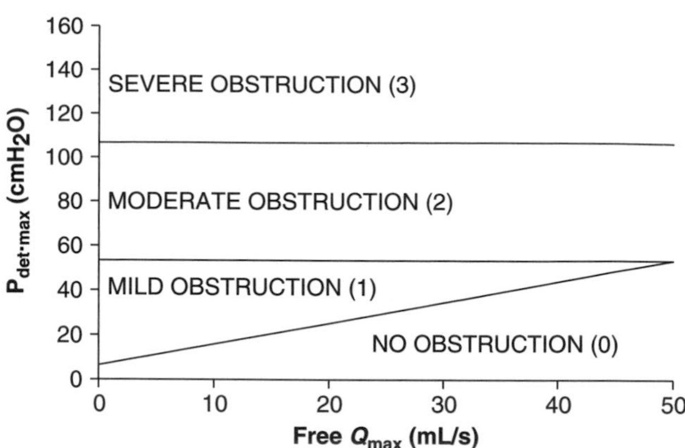

Figure 42.8
Bladder outlet obstruction nomogram for women. Reproduced with permission from reference 54.

(Figure 42.8). Two parameters are needed to construct this nomogram: free Q_{max} and $P_{det.max}$. Free Q_{max} was preferred to Q_{max} during P/Q because $P_{det.Q_{max}}$ and Q_{max} cannot be evaluated if the patient does not void during the test. The Blaivas nomogram consists of four zones which classify patients into four categories: zone 0 (normal or no obstruction), zone 1 (mild obstruction), zone 2 (moderate obstruction), and zone 3 (severe obstruction).[54] Defreitas et al investigated 169 females with BOO and 20 asymptomatic volunteers by P/Q assessment.[55] They reported normal Q_{max} and $P_{det.Q_{max}}$ as 16 ml/s and 24 cmH_2O, respectively, in the asymptomatic group. The cut-off values to detect BOO for $P_{det.Q_{max}}$ and Q_{max} were 25 cmH_2O and 12 ml/s, respectively, with sensitivity, specificity, and accuracy of 68%.[55] Chassagne et al obtained similar results earlier on. Q_{max} <15 ml/s and $P_{det.Q_{max}}$ >20 cmH_2O are reasonable P/Q parameters to diagnose female BOO.[56] Brostrom et al undertook a cystometry and P/Q study in 30 normal female volunteers with a mean age of 52 years.[57] Two sets of measurements were recorded in all. They found that, between two repeated measurements, there was a statistically significant increase in first desire to void (171 ml and 205 ml) and normal desire to void (284 ml and 351 ml) with a decrease in bladder opening pressure, whereas no change was noted in maximum cystometric capacity (572 ml and 570 ml). Other parameters are listed in Table 42.6.

Urethral pressure profile

The urethral pressure profile (UPP) is a urodynamic test that quantifies the occlusive pressure generated by active and passive structures of the urethra, and allows the evaluation of urethral competence. UPP can be measured when the bladder is empty (resting UPP), during coughing or straining (stress UPP), or during the voiding phase (voiding UPP). Urethral pressure rises in 'normal' healthy individuals with increasing bladder volume. This is the so-called 'guarding reflex'. It also rises in the erect position. However, continuous recording of maximal urethral pressure (MUP) has shown variations and oscillations between 10 and 25 cmH_2O.[14] Maximum urethral closure pressure (MUCP) above 20 cmH_2O is considered hypotonic, whereas MUCP values above 75 cmH_2O for women and 90 cmH_2O for men are deemed hypertonic. Sorensen et al analyzed urethral pressure variations in 10 healthy fertile female volunteers (mean age 32 years) and 12 healthy postmenopausal volunteers (mean age 58.7 years).[58] In the fertile group, they observed that mean maximum urethral pressure (mMUP) and mean maximum urethral closure pressure (mMUCP) had median values of 66.5 and 60 cmH_2O, respectively. Postmenopausal women had significantly lower mMUP and mMUCP: 55.5 and 43.5 cmH_2O, respectively. Van Geelen et al studied 27 nulliparous healthy women between the ages of 19 and 35 years and found mMUP of 98 ± 17 cmH_2O in the supine position, with mean urethral closure pressure of 84 ± 18 cmH_2O.[59] Pfisterer et al examined bladder function parameters in pre-, peri, and postmenopausal continent women, discerning mMUCP values of 94, 74, and 42 cmH_2O and functional urethral lengths of 3.3, 3.3, and 3.5 cm, respectively.[22]

Stress UPP measures the rise in intra-abdominal pressure transmitted to the proximal urethra. In normal women without urethral hypermobility, the increase in intravesical pressure and in proximal urethral pressure should be similar. If this is not the case, different pathologies may be postulated. The pressure transmission ratio is a different parameter, recording the increment of urethral pressure with stress as a percentage of intravesical

Table 42.6 *Normal reported P/Q parameters in women*

	Brostrom et al[57]	Blaivas and Groutz[54]	Pfisterer et al[74]	Defreitas et al[55]	Chassagne et al[56]	Normal range
No of patients	30	50	24	20	124	
Mean age	52	64.4	50.2			
Q_{max} (ml/s)	25	13.3	22	12	15	12–25
Q_{ave} (ml/s)	12					12
TQ (s)	67					60–70
$P_{det.open}$ (cmH_2O)	22					22
$P_{det \cdot Q_{max}}$ (cmH_2O)	30	17.9	27	24	20	18–30
$P_{det.max}$ (cmH_2O)	46	22.2	44			22–46
Voided volume (ml)	651	312	264			250–650

Q_{max}, maximum flow rate; Q_{ave}, average flow rate; TQ, flow time; $P_{det.open}$, opening detrusor pressure; $P_{det \cdot Q_{max}}$, detrusor pressure at maximum flow; $P_{det.max}$, maximum detrusor pressure during voiding.

pressure elevation. In normal women, this value should exceed 100.[60]

Kinesiologic EMG of the pelvic floor and sphincter

Kinesiologic measurements are recorded during urodynamic study to assess the integrity of perineal muscle innervation. They can be taken with the application of electrodes. The most commonly used are surface and concentric needle electrodes. Concentric needle electrodes offer a more precise technique, but surface electrodes are more convenient and comfortable for patients, all the while providing an excellent signal source for EMG if placed appropriately after proper skin preparation.[61]

At the beginning of cystometry and during bladder filling, baseline EMG activity of the external urethral sphincter (EUS) has a low frequency and amplitude if the patient is completely relaxed in the supine position. When the bulbocavernosus reflex test is done by squeezing the glans of the penis or clitoris, EMG activity at the EUS level is increased, indicating that the sacral reflex arc is intact.

Furthermore, when intra-abdominal pressure rises during coughing, sneezing, or straining, the EUS contracts and EMG activity is amplified. This condition should be differentiated from DSD by asking the patient to not hold urine.

Normally, EMG activity from the EUS at rest is low. It intensifies as fluid volume in the bladder grows, during bladder filling, due to EUS contraction. It is known as the guarding reflex, as already mentioned in relation to UPP. During voiding, EMG activity disappears completely for a few seconds before detrusor contraction starts. Once the bladder is empty, EMG activity resumes.[61–63]

Neurourologic tests in clinical practice

Electrophysiologic tests are complementary imaging studies of sacral dysfunction. They explore the urogenital region and are useful in evaluating incontinence, erectile dysfunction, and anorectal dysfunction. They give significant information when a lower motor neuron lesion is present.[64] Action potentials generated during sphincter activity can be recorded with specialized needle electrodes inserted in the muscle (Table 42.7).[65]

Concentric needle EMG of the pelvic floor and sphincter muscle

Concentric needle EMG (CNEMG) is the method of choice to evaluate muscle innervation because a wider range of information from several striated muscles can be assessed.[64] EMG of the external anal sphincter (EAS) is the most practical test to study the lower sacral nerves.[65–67] CNEMG of the pelvic floor and EAS muscle allows the quantitative analysis of motor unit potentials (MUPs) and qualitative assessment of interference patterns (IPs).[64] MUP measurement includes amplitude, duration, area, number of phases and turns, rise time, duration of negative peaks, and mean frequency of firing.[68] IP investigation comprises the number of turns/s, amplitude/turn, percent activity, number of short segments, and envelope vs

Table 42.7 *Normative data for sacral reflex measurement in men as reported in the literature (modified from Podnar[80])*

	Number	Muscle examined	Mean ± SD	Author
Single electrical stimulation				
Reflex latency (ms)		EUS		
	14	• Needle	33 ± 3.9	Vodusek et al[81]
	19	• surface	27.9 ± 5.4	Desai et al[82]
		BC		
	60	• Needle	32.3 ± 3.9	Vodusek et al[81]
	12	• Surface	30.7 ± 4.2	Perretti et al[83]
		EAS		
	14	• Needle	35.3 ± 4.6	Vodusek et al[81]
	19	• surface	28.1 ± 5.7	Desai et al[82]
	49	Penilo-cavernosus reflex	29.88 ± 5.65	Podnar[80]
Sensory threshold (mA)	40	Penilo-cavernosus reflex	7.8 ± 2.73	Podnar[80]
Mechanical stimulation				
Reflex latency (ms)	42	Penilo-cavernosus	28.16 ± 5.8	Podnar[80]
	22	bulbocavernosus muscle	left: 31.6 ± 4.5 right: 31.6 ± 3.8	Amarenco et al[70]
	18	EUS	39.1 ± 4	Dykstra et al[84]

EUS, external urethral sphincter; BC, bulbocavernosus muscle; EAS, external anal sphincter.

percent activity.[69] During relaxation, MUP activity is low, and IP values are equal to zero. During contraction, both activities are increased.[69] There is no significant effect of gender and age on MUP/IP.[69]

Single-fiber EMG

Single-fiber EMG (SFEMG) records the action potential of a single muscle fiber. In normal muscles, SFEMG quantifies potentials from 1–3 single muscle fibers belonging to the same motor unit. It is a useful test to diagnose lower motor neuron lesions and non-neurogenic urinary retention.[65]

Sacral reflexes

The aim of this test is to assess the sacral reflex arc. Electrical, mechanical, or magnetic stimulation can be applied to the penis or clitoris to elicit sacral reflexes.[65,70,71] Such studies are useful to detect damage to myelin and axons within the peripheral sacral reflex arc.[65] For more details on electrophysiologic evaluation, see Chapter 43.

Summary

Urodynamic tests are useful tools to evaluate lower urinary tract dysfunction. They are gold standard tests for the diagnosis of BOO and urinary incontinence. Urodynamic evaluation is a good predictor of outcome after therapeutic interventions. Urodynamic normality in healthy populations is not well known and illustrates a wide variety of data and patterns. Several important parameters, such as age, sex, and body mass index, affect urodynamic values, rendering it more challenging to define precise, normal values derived from tests performed on patients.

Mathematic models and simulation may help in the future to generate more data on normality, but additional studies on healthy volunteers must be encouraged before then to gather more information.

Acknowledgment

The authors thank Dr Erik Schick for his help and advice in writing this chapter.

References

1. Robertson AS, Griffiths CJ, Ramsden PD, Neal DE. Bladder function in healthy volunteers: ambulatory monitoring and conventional urodynamic studies. Br J Urol 1994; 73(3): 242–9.
2. Wyndaele JJ. Normality in urodynamics studied in healthy adults. J Urol 1999; 161(3): 899–902.
3. Abrams P, Blaivas JG, Stanton SL, Andersen JT. The standardisation of terminology of lower urinary tract function. The International Continence Society Committee on Standardisation of Terminology. Scand J Urol Nephrol 1988; 114(Suppl): 5–19.
4. Sutherst J, Brown M, Shawer M. Assessing the severity of urinary incontinence in women by weighing perineal pads. Lancet 1981; 1: 1128–30.

5. Versi E, Cardozo LD. Perineal pad weighing versus videographic analysis in genuine stress incontinence. Br J Obstet Gynaecol 1986; 93: 364–6.
6. Abrams P, Cardozo LD, Fall M et al. The standardisation of terminology of lower urinary tract function: Report from the standardisation sub-committee of the International Continence Society. Neurourol Urodyn 2002; 21(2): 167–78.
7. Klarskov P, Hald T. Reproducibility and reliability of urinary incontinence assessment with a 60 min test. Scand J Urol Nephrol 1984; 18(4): 293–8.
8. Jorgensen L, Lose G, Andersen JT. One-hour pad-weighing test for objective assessment of female urinary incontinence. Obstet Gynecol 1987; 69(1): 39–42.
9. Lose G, Jorgensen L, Thunedborg P. 24-hour home pad weighing test versus 1-hour ward test in the assessment of mild stress incontinence. Acta Obstet Gynecol Scand 1989; 68(3): 211–15.
10. Mouritsen L, Berild G, Hertz J. Comparison of different methods for quantification of urinary leakage in incontinent women. Neurourol Urodyn 1989; 8: 579–87.
11. Versi E, Orrego G, Hardy E et al. Evaluation of the home pad test in the investigation of female urinary incontinence. Br J Obstet Gynaecol 1996; 103(2): 162–7.
12. Ryhammer AM, Laurberg S, Hermann AP. Test–retest repeatability of anorectal physiology tests in healthy volunteers. Dis Colon Rectum 1997; 40(3): 287–92.
13. Karantanis E, O'Sullivan R, Moore KH. The 24-hour pad test in continent women and men: normal values and cyclical alterations. Br J Obstet Gynaecol 2003; 110: 567–71.
14. Jolivet-Tremblay M, Schink E. The voiding diary. In: Corcos J, Schick E, eds. The urinary sphincter. New York: Marcel Dekker, 2001: 262.
15. Kassis A, Schick E. Frequency–volume chart pattern in a healthy female population. Br J Urol 1993; 72: 708–10.
16. Huang Y-H, Lin ATL, Chen K-K, Chang LS. Voiding pattern of healthy Taiwanese women. Urol Int 2007; 77(4): 322–6.
17. Boedker A, Lendorf A, H-Nielsen A, Glahn B. Micturition pattern assessed by the frequency/volume chart in a healthy population of men and women. Neurourol Urodyn 1989; 8: 421–2.
18. Fitzgerald MP, Brubaker L. Variability of 24-hour voiding diary variables among asymptomatic women. J Urol 2003; 169: 207–9.
19. Van Haarst EP, Heldeweg EA, Newling DW, Schlatmann TJ. The 24-h frequency–volume chart in adults reporting no voiding complaints: defining reference values and analysing variables. BJU Int 2004; 93: 1257–61.
19a. Wein AJ, Kavoussi LR, Novick AC et al (eds). Campbell-Walsh Urology edition, 9th edition. Philadelphia: WB Saunders, 2006: 1986–2010.
20. Latini JM, Mueller E, Lux MM, Fitzgerald MP, Kreder KJ. Voiding frequency in a sample of asymptomatic American men. J Urol 2004; 172: 980–4.
21. Haylen BT, Ashby D, Sutherst J, Frazer MI, West CR. Maximum and average urine flow rates in normal male and female populations – the Liverpool nomograms. Br J Urol 1989; 64: 30–8.
22. Pfisterer MH, Griffiths DJ, Rosenberg L, Schaefer W, Resnick NM. Parameters of bladder function in pre-, peri- and postmenopausal continent women without detrusor overactiity. Neurourol Urodyn 2007; 26: 356–61.
23. Unsal A, Cimentepe E. Voiding postion does not affect uroflowmetric parameters and post-void residual urine volume in healthy volunteers. Scand J Urol Nephrol 2004; 38(6): 469–71.
24. Suebnukanwattana T, Lohsiriwat S, Chaikomin R, Tantiwongse A, Soontrapa S. Uroflowmetry in normal Thai subjects. J Med Assoc Thailand 2003; 86(4): 353–60.
25. Cohen DH, Steinberg JR, Rossignol M, Heaton J, Corcos J. Normal variation and influence of stress, caffeine intake and sexual activity on uroflowmetry parameters of a middle-aged asymptomatic cohort of volunteer male urologists. Neurourol Urodyn 2002; 21(5): 491–4.
26. Schmidt F, Shin P, Jorgensen TM, Djurhuus JC, Constantinou CE. Urodynamic patterns of normal male micturition: influence of water consumption on urine production and detrusor function. J Urol 2002; 168(4 Pt 1): 1458–63.
27. Tong YC. The effect of psychological motivation on volumes voided during uroflowmetry in healthy aged male volunteers. Neurourol Urodyn 2006; 25(1): 8–12.
28. Jorgensen JB, Jensen KM, Bille-Brahe NE, Morgensen P. Uroflowmetry in asymptomatic elderly males. Br J Urol 1986; 58(4): 390–5.
29. Schafer W, Abrams P, Liao L et al. Good urodynamic practices: uroflowmetry, filling cystometry, and pressure–flow studies. Neurourol Urodyn 2002; 21(3): 261–74.
30. Abrams PH, Dunn M, George N. Urodynamic findings in chronic retention of urine and their relevance to results of surgery. Br Med J 1978; 2(6147): 1258–60.
31. Wyndaele JJ. The normal pattern of perception of bladder filling during cystometry studied in 38 young healthy volunteers. J Urol 1998; 160(2): 479–81.
32. Pauwels E, De WS, Wyndaele JJ. Normality of bladder filling studied in symptom-free middle-aged women. J Urol 2004; 171(4): 1567–70.
33. Sullivan MP, Yalla SV. Detrusor contractility and compliance characteristics in adult male patients with obstructive and nonobstructive voiding dysfunction. J Urol 1996; 155(6): 1995–2000.
34. Ouslander J, Leach G, Abelson S et al. Simple versus multichannel cystometry in the evaluation of bladder function in an incontinent geriatric population. J Urol 1988; 140(6): 1482–6.
35. McGuire EJ, Woodside JR, Borden TA, Weiss RM. Prognostic value of urodynamic testing in myelodysplastic patients. J Urol 1981; 126: 205–9.
36. McGuire EJ, Cespedes RD, O'Connell HE. Leak-point pressures. Urol Clin North Am 1996; 23(2): 253–62.
37. McGuire EJ, Fitzpatrick CC, Wan J et al. Clinical assessment of urethral sphincter function. J Urol 1993; 150: 1452–4.
38. Lim CS, Abrams P. The Abrams-Griffiths nomogram. World J Urol 1995; 13(1): 34–9.
39. Abrams P, Torrens M. Urine flow studies. Urol Clin North Am 1979; 6(1): 71–9.
40. Abrams P. Bladder outlet obstruction index, bladder contractility index and bladder voiding efficiency: three simple indices to define bladder voiding function. BJU Int 1999; 84(1): 14–5.
41. Griffiths DJ. Pressure–flow studies of micturition. Urol Clin North Am 1996; 23(2): 279–97.
42. Schafer W. Analysis of bladder-outlet function with the linearized passive urethral resistance relation, linPURR, and a disease-specific approach for grading obstruction: from complex to simple. World J Urol 1995; 13(1): 47–58.
43. Eri LM, Wessel N, Tysland O, Berge V. Comparative study of pressure–flow parameters. Neurourol Urodyn 2002; 21(3): 186–93.
44. Bruskewitz R, Jensen KM, Iversen P, Madsen PO. The relevance of minimum urethral resistance in prostatism. J Urol 1983; 129(4): 769–71.
45. Jensen KM, Jorgensen JB, Mogensen P. Urodynamics in prostatism. II. Prognostic value of pressure–flow study combined with stop-flow test. Scand J Urol Nephrol Suppl 1988; 114: 72–7.
46. Javle P, Jenkins SA, Machin DG, Parsons KF. Grading of benign prostatic obstruction can predict the outcome of transurethral prostatectomy. J Urol 1998; 160(5): 1713–7.
47. Gotoh M, Yoshikawa Y, Kondo AS et al. Prognostic value of pressure–flow study in surgical treatment of benign prostatic obstruction. World J Urol 1999; 17(5): 274–8.
48. Walker RM, Romano G, Davies AH et al. Pressure flow study data in a group of asymptomatic male control patients 45 years old or older. J Urol 2001; 165(2): 683–7.
49. Griffiths D, Hofner K, van MR et al. Standardization of terminology of lower urinary tract function: pressure–flow studies of voiding, urethral resistance, and urethral obstruction. International Continence Society Subcommittee on Standardization of

Terminology of Pressure–Flow Studies. Neurourol Urodyn 1997; 16(1): 1–18.

50. Schafer W. Principles and clinical application of advanced urodynamic analysis of voiding function. Urol Clin North Am 1990; 17(3): 553–66.
51. Eckhardt MD, van Venrooij GE, Boon TA. Urethral resistance factor (URA) versus Schafer's obstruction grade and Abrams–Griffiths (AG) number in the diagnosis of obstructive benign prostatic hyperplasia. Neurourol Urodyn 2001; 20(2): 175–85.
52. Rollema HJ, van MR. Improved indication and followup in transurethral resection of the prostate using the computer program CLIM: a prospective study. J Urol 1992; 148(1): 111–5.
53. van MR, Kranse M. Analysis of pressure-flow data in terms of computer-derived urethral resistance parameters. World J Urol 1995; 13(1): 40–6.
54. Blaivas JG, Groutz A. Bladder outlet obstruction nomogram for women with lower urinary tract symptomatology. Neurourol Urodyn 2000; 19(5): 553–64.
55. Defreitas GA, Zimmern PE, Lemack GE, Shariat SF. Refining diagnosis of anatomic female bladder outlet obstruction: comparison of pressure–flow study parameters in clinically obstructed women with those of normal controls. Urology 2004; 64(4): 675–9.
56. Chassagne S, Bernier PA, Haab F et al. Proposed cutoff values to define bladder outlet obstruction in women. Urology 1998; 51(3): 408–11.
57. Brostrom S, Jennum P, Lose G. Short-term reproducibility of cystometry and pressure-flow micturition studies in healthy women. Neurourol Urodyn 2002; 21(5): 457–60.
58. Sorensen S, Waechter PB, Constantinou CE et al. Urethral pressure and pressure variations in healthy fertile and postmenopausal women with reference to the female sex hormones. J Urol 1991; 146: 1434–40.
59. Van Geelen JM, Doesburg WH, Thomas CMG, Martin CB. Urodynamic studies in the normal menstrual cycle: the relationship between hormonal changes during the menstrual cycle and the urethral pressure profile. Am J Obstet Gynecol 1981; 141(4): 384–92.
60. Steele GS, Sullivan MP, Yalla SV. Urethral pressure profilometry: vesicourethral pressure measurements under resting and voiding conditions. In: Nitti VW, ed. Practical Urodynamics. Philadelphia: WB Sanders, 1998: 108–30.
61. O'Donnell P, Beck C, Doyle R, Eubanks C. Surface electrodes in perineal electromyography. Urology 1988; 32(4): 375–9.
62. Blaivas JG, Sinha HP, Zayed AA, Labib KB. Detrusor-external sphincter dyssynergia: a detailed electromyographic study. J Urol 1981; 125(4): 545–8.
63. Blaivas JG, Sinha HP, Zayed AA, Labib KB. Detrusor-external sphincter dyssynergia. J Urol 1981; 125(4): 542–4.
64. Podnar S, Vodusek DB. Protocol for clinical neurophysiologic examination of the pelvic floor. Neurourol Urodyn 2001; 20(6): 669–82.
65. Podnar S. Neurophysiology of the neurogenic lower urinary tract disorders. Clin Neurophysiol 2007; 118(7): 1423–37.
66. Podnar S, Rodi Z, Lukanovic A, Trsinar B, Vodusek DB. Standardization of anal sphincter EMG: technique of needle examination. Muscle Nerve 1999; 22(3): 400–3.
67. Podnar S. Electrodiagnosis of the anorectum: a review of techniques and clinical applications. Tech Coloproctol 2003; 7(2): 71–6.
68. Podnar S, Vodusek DB. Protocol for clinical neurophysiologic examination of the pelvic floor. Neurourol Urodyn 2001; 20(6): 669–82.
69. Podnar S, Mrkaic M, Vodusek DB. Standardization of anal sphincter electromyography: quantification of continuous activity during relaxation. Neurourol Urodyn 2002; 21(6): 540–5.
70. Amarenco G, Ismael SS, Bayle B, Kerdraon J. Dissociation between electrical and mechanical bulbocavernosus reflexes. Neurourol Urodyn 2003; 22(7): 676–80.
71. Podnar S, Vodusek DB, Trsinar B, Rodi Z. A method of uroneurophysiological investigation in children. Electroencephalogr Clin Neurophysiol 1997; 104(5): 389–92.
72. De Wachter S, Wyndaele JJ. Frequency–volume charts: a tool to evaluate bladder sensation. Neurourol Urodyn 2003; 22(7): 638–42.
73. Kassis A, Schick E. Frequency–volume chart pattern in a healthy female population. Br J Urol 1993; 72(5 Pt 2): 708–10.
74. Pfisterer MH, Griffiths DJ, Rosenberg L, Schaefer W, Resnick NM. Parameters of bladder function in pre-, peri-, and postmenopausal continent women without detrusor overactivity. Neurourol Urodyn 2007; 26(3): 356–61.
75. Jensen KM, Bruskewitz RC, Madsen PO. Urodynamic findings in elderly males without prostatic complaints. Urology 1984; 24(2): 211–13.
76. Tessier J, Schick E. Technique et interprétation du bilan urodynamique. In: Jacques Corcos and Erik Schick, eds. Les Vessies Neurogenes de l'Adulte. Paris: Masson, 1996: 117–30.
77. Wall LL, Norton PA, DeLancey JOL. Practical urodynamics. In: Wall LL, Norton PA, eLancey JOL, eds. Practical Urogynecology. Baltimore: Williams and Wilkins, 1993: 83.
78. Abrams PH. The practice of urodynamics. In: AR Mundy, TP Stephenson, J Wein, eds. Urodynamics. Principles, Practice and Application. Edinburgh, 1984: 76.
79. Susset JG. Cystometry. In: Krane RJ, Siroky MB, eds. Clinical Neurourology, 2nd edn. Boston: Little Brown and Co, 1991: 163–4.
80. Podnar S. Neurophysiologic studies of the penilo-cavernosus reflex: normative data. Neurourol Urodyn 2007; 26(6): 864–9.
81. Vodusek DB, Janko M, Lokar J. Direct and reflex responses in perineal muscles on electrical stimulation. J Neurol Neurosurg Psychiatry 1983; 46(1): 67–71.
82. Desai KM, Dembny K, Morgan H, Gingell JC, Prothero D. Neurophysiological investigation of diabetic impotence. Are sacral response studies of value? Br J Urol 1988; 61(1): 68–73.
83. Perretti A, Catalano A, Mirone V et al. Neurophysiologic evaluation of central-peripheral sensory and motor pudendal pathways in primary premature ejaculation. Urology 2003; 61(3): 623–8.
84. Dykstra D, Sidi A, Cameron J et al. The use of mechanical stimulation to obtain the sacral reflex latency: a new technique. J Urol 1987; 137(1): 77–9.

43

Electrophysiologic evaluation: basic principles and clinical applications

Simon Podnar and Clare J Fowler

Introduction

Electrophysiologic methods record bioelectrical potentials generated by excitable cell membranes. When applied in a clinical setting to recordings from nerves and skeletal muscle these tests are often referred to as clinical neurophysiologic studies. Clinical neurophysiologic methods are well established, and have been used in clinical practice for more than half a century.

Neurophysiologic techniques have so far been applied to the sacral nervous system mostly for research purposes, but they have also been proposed for everyday diagnostics in selected groups of patients. The WHO Consensus on Incontinence stated that 'electrophysiologic assessment is useful in selected patients with suspected peripheral nervous system lesions such as lower motor neuron (LMN) lesions, patients with multiple system atrophy (MSA), and also in women with urinary retention.'[1]

The emphasis of this text is on clinically useful and established electrophysiologic tests, which are of diagnostic value in individual patients, with neurogenic bladders. Concentric needle electromyography (CNEMG) and sacral reflex testing will be discussed in detail. Other tests, not considered to be of clinical value in the diagnosis of individual patients, will be briefly described. For more detailed description of these research-type clinical uroneurophysiologic tests, reference to other reviews is recommended.[1]

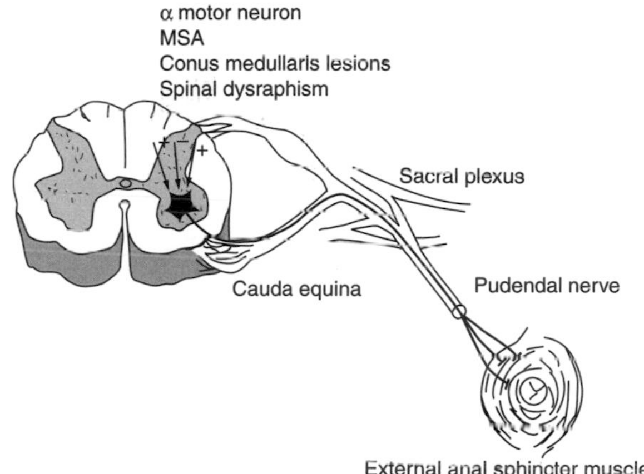

Figure 43.1
Schematic drawing of the sacral reflex arc. The sacral spinal cord, with sensory (afferent) root entering posteriorly, and motor (efferent) root leaving anteriorly, is shown. Although not shown here, below the lower end of the spinal cord (conus medullaris) lumbar and sacral spinal roots travel for several segments within the spinal canal before leaving it (cauda equina). An enlarged alpha motor neuron with facilitatory (+) and inhibitory (–) suprasegmental influences is also shown. MSA, multiple system atrophy.

Electrophysiologic tests in assessment of patients

General remarks

A particular diagnostic test should be considered in a patient when the information it may provide is expected to significantly affect further treatment and/or clarify prognosis. Clinical neurophysiologic findings consistent with the diagnosis of 'a neurogenic bladder' can be found in patients with established diagnosis of neurologic disease but in these circumstances add little to the case. However, in patients being investigated for bladder symptoms of suspected neurologic origin, neurophysiologic studies may reveal evidence of neural damage and thus point to neurologic diagnosis.[2]

Basically, in neurologic disease affecting the bladder, two main patterns of abnormalities can be found: the LMN and the upper motor neuron (UMN) pattern (see below). These are respectively due to lesions of the anterior horn cell (i.e. alpha motor neuron) spinal root, and

Table 43.1 *Unique information provided by electrophysiologic tests*

Information	Structure	Method	Finding
Integrity preserved	The lower motor neuron	CNEMG	Absent spontaneous denervation activity; continuous MUP firing during relaxation
	Lower and upper motor neuron	CNEMG	Dense IP on voluntary activation
	Sacral reflex arc	CNEMG	Dense IP on reflex activation (touch)
		Sacral reflex	Brisk response of normal latency
	Somato-sensory pathways	Pudendal SEP	Normal shape and latency of responses
Localization of lesions	Root versus plexus/nerve	CNEMG	Paravertebral denervation activity in neighboring myotomes
		SNAP	Normal (penile) SNAP with impaired (penile) skin sensation
Severity of lesions	Complete versus partial	CNEMG	Profuse spontaneous denervation activity, absent MUPs
	Severe versus moderate	Sacral reflex	Response non-elicitable
Type of lesion	Conduction block versus axonotmesis	CNEMG	Absent/sparse spontaneous denervation activity
	Axonotmesis versus neurotmesis	CNEMG	Appearance of nascent MUPs after complete muscle denervation

CNEMG, concentric needle electromyography; IP, interference pattern; MUP, motor unit potential; SEP, somatosensory evoked potentials; SNAP, sensory nerve action potential.
Normal clinical neurologic examination and appropriate electrophysiologic testing (see Method column) document preserved neural integrity – other causes for the sacral dysfunction should be sought. On the other hand, the electrophysiologic test abnormality in appropriate clinical setting supports and documents the clinical diagnosis of a neurologic lesion. The electrophysiologic studies can then often help to provide information about localization, severity, and type (mechanism) of the lesion. These factors are crucial for the assessment of prognosis.

peripheral nerve in the case of a LMN lesion (Figure 43.1) or due to damage of suprasegmental pathways in the central nervous system in the case of UMN lesions. Neurologic examination is very valuable in helping to make the distinction between these two conditions.[2] In very general terms a UMN lesion would be expected to be associated with detrusor overactivity, whereas an LMN lesion would be associated with bladder atonia (hyporreflexia), although this rule is by no means hard and fast.[3]

Electrophysiologic tests can be understood as an extension of the clinical neurologic examination. The tests are seldom useful in patients with a completely normal neurologic examination, and are helpful only in patients in whom specific neurologic lesions are suspected.[2,4] In general, neurophysiologic tests may be used to elucidate those findings summarized in Table 43.1. Some of these properties are relevant when applied to the striated muscle of the pelvic floor.

Other physiologic tests used in evaluation of bladder disorders (measurement of postvoid residual, uroflow, cystometry, etc.) are different in that they test function and, as a consequence, can be regarded as complementary to sacral electrophysiologic testing. Similarly, neurophysiologic tests are complementary to imaging studies (ultrasound, computer tomography (CT), magnetic resonance imaging (MRI), etc.) of the lower urinary tract. Neurophysiologic tests, however, have limitations (Table 43.2).

Clinical assessment before electrophysiologic evaluation

Selected patients with urinary disorders should be referred to specialists, who will perform a focused clinical examination of the lower urinary tract and anogenital region. To document and quantify patients' complaints, and obtain additional data, functional investigations (measurement of postvoid residual, uroflow, cystometry) and imaging studies might be considered. A neural lesion would be suspected, particularly in patients complaining of incomplete emptying of the bladder, or those with saddle sensory loss on clinical examination.[5] Furthermore, uroneurophysiologic evaluation would be considered in patients in whom urinary dysfunction is accompanied by bowel and sexual dysfunction.[2,5]

At the beginning of each uroneurophysiologic evaluation, a focused history of the patient's complaints must be taken, including questions about urinary, bowel, and sexual (dys)function. This is often the most valuable part of the investigation process. History of low back pain irradiating

Table 43.2 *The limitations of electrodiagnostic tests*

Limitations		Comments
Uncomfortable		Without significant risks
Difficult localization	• Multiple lesions	Proximal lesion masks distal on CNEMG, and distal lesion masks proximal on SNAP testing
	• Proximal peripheral sacral lesions	Paravertebral muscles are absent in the lower sacral segments
• Timing of investigation	• Few abnormalities before several weeks postinjury	
	• Less pronounced pathologic signs after a few months	
Tests do not reflect the function of the whole structure studied	Low correlation with function	No electrophysiologic parameter validated to measure weakness

CNEMG, concentric needle electromyography; SNAP, sensory nerve action potential.

to legs, and numbness and tingling in the saddle region, will point to a cauda equina lesion (Chapter 26). In older patients, inquiry about general movement slowness, disordered gait, tremor, and autonomic dysfunction (orthostatic hypotension, etc.) should be made to reveal extrapyramidal disorders such as Parkinson's disease (Chapters 22, 23, 24). Dissemination of neurologic symptoms in time and in neuroanatomic location (blurred vision, difficult gait, urinary and fecal urgency, etc.) suggests a diagnosis of demyelinating disease of the central nervous system (multiple sclerosis) (Chapter 27).

As a minimum, at the beginning of each electrophysiologic evaluation a brief neurologic examination should be performed, looking for signs of pyramidal (UMN) and peripheral nervous system (LMN) lesions (particularly in lower limbs), and also for extrapyramidal and cerebellar signs. Examination of the sacral region should in this setting include assessment of anal sphincter tone during rest, squeeze and relaxation (defecation attempt), sensation of touch and pinprick in the saddle area, and eliciting of the penilo-cavernosus (in men)[6] and anal reflex (bilaterally). If uroneurophysiologic tests are to be performed, a detailed explanation of the aims and methods of the electrodiagnostic evaluation should be given to the patient.

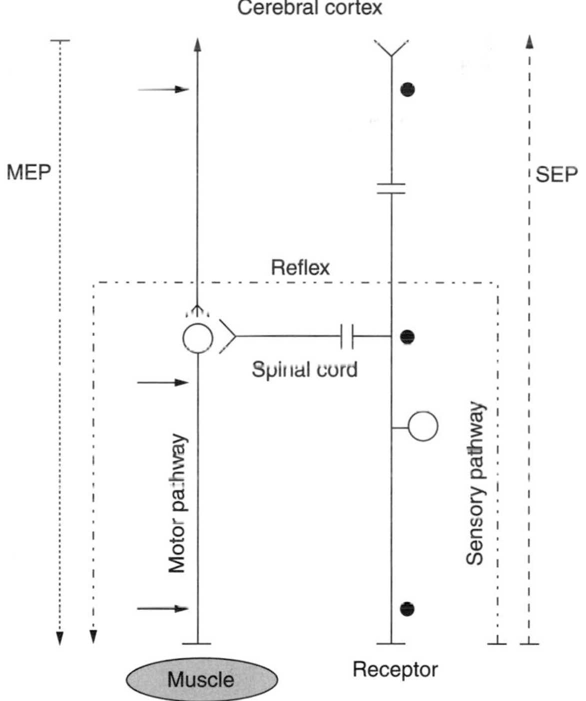

Figure 43.2
Components of the somatic sensory and somatic motor systems and the electrophysiologic tests that evaluate them. Arrows on the motor (left) side indicate different stimulation sites (from above) of motor cortex, spinal roots and peripheral nerves (terminal motor latency test). Small circles on the sensory (right) side indicate different recording sites (from below) from peripheral nerve (sensory nerve action potential – SNAP), spinal roots/cord, and somatosensory cortex. (Note that for SNAP recording both distal stimulation and proximal recording[70] or reverse[71] could be employed.) In addition, concentric needle electromyography (CNEMG) and single fiber electromyography (SFEMG) assess the lower motor neuron and muscle. Kinesiologic EMG evaluates the integrity of upper motor neuron and neurocontrol reflex arcs (Redrawn with permission from Vodušek DB.[108])

Innervation of the pelvic structures

The nervous system is divided into two motor systems (the somatic and the autonomic), and the (somato)sensory system (Figure 43.2). Within a particular anatomic system we can distinguish central and peripheral parts. The central part includes the motor and sensory pathways contained within the brain and spinal cord (the central nervous system). The central nervous system also contains, at different levels, interneuronal systems, which are important in neural 'integrative functions' (e.g. sacral spinal interneurons in the sacral reflex arc[7]).

The motor system comprises a UMN (i.e. all neurons participating in the supraspinal motor control), an LMN (innervating muscles and glands), and muscle. Cell bodies of the UMN lie in the motor cortex and other gray matter (nuclei) of the brain (including some brainstem nuclei) and connect directly or via interneurons to the LMNs of the spinal cord (and cranial motor nerve nuclei in the brainstem). The LMNs lie either in the anterior horns of the gray matter of the spinal cord (the somato-motor nuclei) or in the lateral horns of the spinal cord (the autonomic nuclei). The former innervate skeletal muscle, and the latter smooth muscle and glands.

The somatosensory system can be divided into a peripheral part (receptors and the sensory input into the spinal cord) and a central part (ascending pathways in the spinal cord and brain). Sensory fibers from the skin and those accompanying axons from alpha motor neurons are called somatic afferents. Those accompanying autonomic (parasympathetic or sympathetic) fibers are called visceral afferents.

Somatic lower motor neurons of the sacral spinal cord

Like other motor neurons, which innervate striated muscle, the alpha motor neurons of the sphincters lie in the anterior horn of the spinal cord in Onuf's nucleus. Their axons are of large diameter and myelinated to allow rapid conduction of impulses and travel to the periphery in the cauda equina, the sacral plexus, the pelvic nerves, and the pudendal nerves (Figure 43.1). Within the muscle, the motor axon tapers and then branches to innervate muscle fibers. Each motor neuron innervates a number of muscle fibers – this constitutes the motor unit (MU). The innervation of healthy muscle is such that fibers, which are part of the same MU, are unlikely to be adjacent to one another, but are scattered in a checkerboard pattern. The diameter of the muscle area innervated by each lower sacral alpha motor neuron (MU territory) is probably smaller than that of many limb or trunk muscles.

Primary sensory neuron

Sensory receptors are the most peripheral part of the somatic and autonomic sensory neurons. Receptors code mechanical or chemical stimuli into bioelectrical activity – i.e. nerve action potentials which traverse the peripheral axon (within peripheral nerves and the sacral plexus), cell body within the spinal ganglion, and the central axon of the peripheral sensory neuron (within the cauda equina). In the spinal cord the central axon branches, with segmental branches contributing in the reflex arc, and central branches (within the dorsal column) conveying sensory information to the brain. Both somatic and visceral parts of the sensory system are organized in this way.

The simplified model of the neuromuscular system includes the autonomic system, divided into the sympathetic and the parasympathetic parts.

Physiologic principles of electrophysiologic testing

An excitable membrane and transmission of traveling action potentials are characteristic of nerve and muscle cells. This bioelectrical activity is the substrate for function of the nervous tissue (i.e. transmission of information) and precedes the function of the muscle (i.e. contraction). It is this bioelectrical activity which makes possible the application of electrodiagnostic methods.

To obtain the information about the bioelectrical activity of muscle, nerve, spinal roots, spinal cord, and brain, recordings from these structures are necessary. All clinical neurophysiologic recordings are extracellular. The electrodes may be near (i.e. intramuscular needle or wire electrodes), or distant from the source of bioelectrical activity (i.e. surface electrodes applied over the skin). The spread of electrical field through tissues from the generators obeys physical laws of volume conduction.[8] From muscle, both the ongoing (spontaneous) and elicited (voluntary, reflexly, by nerve depolarization) activity can be recorded. From most of the other neural structures (nerves, spinal roots, spinal cord) spontaneous bioelectrical activity cannot be recorded in the clinical setting. To explore these structures, electrical (and less often magnetic or mechanical) stimulation is applied, and the propagated bioelectrical activity recorded at some distance along the nervous pathways. The electrophysiologic responses obtained by stimulation are 'compound action potentials' produced by simultaneous activation of populations of biological units (neurons, axons, or MUs).

Classification of electrophysiologic tests

A functional classification of the electrophysiological tests consists of (Figure 43.2):

(a) Tests evaluating the somatic motor system (electromyography, EMG; terminal motor latency measurements, and motor evoked potentials, MEP).

(b) Tests evaluating the sensory system (sensory neurography, somatosensory evoked potentials, SEP).
(c) Methods assessing reflexes (penilo/clitoro-cavernosus reflexes).
(d) Tests assessing functioning of the sympathetic (sympathetic skin response, SSR) and parasympathetic autonomic nervous systems (bladder EMG).

Uroneurophysiologic tests that are of diagnostic value in individual patients with neurogenic bladder

Electromyography

Kinesiologic electromyography

The aim of the kinesiologic EMG is to assess patterns of individual muscle activity during various maneuvers (i.e. pelvic floor muscle activity patterns during bladder filling and voiding). It is usually not called 'kinesiologic EMG', although that would be preferable to distinguish it from other types of EMG.

Various surface or intramuscular (needle or wire) electrodes can be used for recording the kinesiologic EMG signal. Bioelectrical activity will typically be sampled from a single intramuscular detection site. As the intention is not to analyze motor unit potential (MUP) parameters, the signal can be recorded with less sophisticated apparatus than required for other types of EMG, even if intramuscular electrodes are used for recording. There is no commonly accepted standardized technique. When using surface electrodes there are problems related to validity of the signal (e.g. artifacts and contamination from other muscles). In contrast, with intramuscular electrodes in large pelvic floor muscles, there are questions as to whether the whole muscle is properly represented by the measured signal. Little is known about the normal activity patterns of different pelvic floor (parts of the levator ani) and sphincter muscles, although it is generally assumed that they act in a coordinated fashion. However, differences have been demonstrated even between the intra- and peri-urethral sphincter (US) in normal women.[9] Coordinated behavior is frequently lost in abnormal conditions, as has been shown for the levator ani, the US, and the external anal sphincter (EAS).[10,11]

The normal (kinesiologic) sphincter EMG shows continuous activity of MUPs at rest, which may be increased voluntarily or reflexly. Such activity of low-threshold MUs has been recorded for up to 2 hours, and even after subjects have fallen asleep during the examination. Similar ongoing activity can also be recorded in many but not all detection sites of the levator ani,[12] and of the deeper EAS muscle.[13] The US and the EAS as well as the pubococcygeus muscles can sustain maximal voluntary activation for only about 1 minute.[12] On voiding, disappearance of all EMG activity in the US precedes detrusor contraction. In the central nervous system disorders, however, detrusor contractions may be associated with increase of sphincter EMG activity (i.e. detrusor-sphincter dyssynergia).[14,15] This can be easily demonstrated by kinesiologic EMG performed as a part of cystometric measurement. Due to significant disagreement with the voiding cystourethrogram the two methods are regarded as complementary in the diagnosis of detrusor-sphincter dyssynergia.[15]

Neurogenic incoordinated sphincter behavior has to be differentiated from voluntary contractions that may occur in poorly compliant patients. The pelvic floor muscle contractions of the so-called 'non-neurogenic voiding disorder' may be a learned abnormal behavior, and can be encountered in some women[16] and men with dysfunctional voiding.[17]

In health the pubococcygeus in woman reveals similar activity patterns to the US and the EAS at most detection sites: i.e. continuous activity at rest, some (but not invariable) increase of activity during bladder filling, and reflex increases in activity during any activation maneuver performed by the subject (talking, deep breathing, coughing). The pubococcygeus also relaxes during voiding.[12] However, in disease the patterns of activation and the coordination between the two sides may be lost.[18]

Any diagnostic value of kinesiologic EMG apart from polygraph cystometric recordings to assess detrusor/sphincter coordination has yet to be established.

The demonstration of voluntary and reflex activation of pelvic floor muscles is indirect proof of the integrity of respective neural pathways and should also be a part of a CNEMG examination, although the latter is performed primarily to diagnose an LMN lesion (see below). In contrast, kinesiologic EMG is used mainly for diagnosis of the central nervous system (i.e. UMN) lesions.

Concentric needle EMG

The aim of CNEMG testing is to differentiate abnormal from normally innervated striated muscle. Although in general EMG abnormalities are detected as a result of a host of different lesions and diseases, there are in principle only two standard manifestations which can occur: disease of the muscle fibers themselves and changes in their innervation.

The concentric needle electrode consists of a central insulated platinum wire that is inserted through a steel cannula. This type of electrode records activity from muscle tissue up to 2.5 mm from the electrode tip.[19]

For the CNEMG examination a standard EMG system, which has the facility for quantitative template-based MUP analysis (multi-MUP), is ideal.[20] The commonly used amplifier filter's setting for CNEMG is 5 Hz to 10 kHz. This must be identical to those set when reference values were compiled, and needs to be checked if MUP parameters are to be measured.

Because of easy access, sufficient muscle bulk, and relative ease of examination the subcutaneous EAS is the most practical muscle for CNEMG testing of the lower sacral segments.[21] To examine this muscle the needle is inserted about 1 cm from the anal orifice, to a depth of a 3–6 mm at a sharp angle to the skin.[22]

Both left and right EAS muscles should almost always be examined, by needle insertions into the middle of the anterior and posterior halves.[23] The needle is angled backwards and forwards in a systematic manner (through two insertion sites on each side).[24]

CNEMG examination of the EAS muscle can be divided into observation of insertion activity, observation of spontaneous denervation activity, quantitative assessment of MUPs, and qualitative assessment of interference pattern (IP). In addition, it is suggested that the number of continuously active MUPs during relaxation be observed,[13] as well as MUP recruitment on reflex and voluntary activation.[24]

In normal muscle, needle movement elicits a short burst of insertion activity, which is due to mechanical stimulation of excitable membranes. This is recorded at a gain of 50 μV per division, which is also used to record spontaneous denervation activity (sweep speed 5–10 ms/division). Absence of insertion activity with appropriately placed needle electrode[22] usually means complete muscle denervation, which is found in approximately 10% of patients with most severe cauda equina lesions.[21]

Immediately after an acute complete denervation, all MU activity ceases, and (apart from insertion activity) no electrical activity can be recorded. Ten to twenty days later insertion activity becomes more prominent and prolonged, and abnormal spontaneous activity appears in the form of short biphasic spikes (fibrillation potentials) and biphasic potentials with prominent positive deflections (positive sharp waves) (Figure 43.3a). This type of activity is referred to as 'spontaneous denervation activity' and originates from denervated single muscle fibers.

In partially denervated muscle, some MUPs remain and mingle eventually with spontaneous denervation activity. As the MUPs in sphincter muscles are also short and mostly bi- or triphasic,[25] as are fibrillation potentials, it takes considerable EMG experience to differentiate one from another. In this situation, examination of the bulbocavernosus muscle is particularly useful because, in contrast to sphincter muscles, it lacks ongoing activity of low-threshold MU during relaxation (Figure 43.3a).[24]

In longstanding partially denervated muscles, peculiar abnormal activity called simple or complex 'repetitive discharges' appears, caused by repetitive firing of groups of potentials. This activity may be provoked by needle movement, muscle contraction, etc., or may occur spontaneously. This activity may sometimes be found in USs of patients without any other evidence of neuromuscular disease, and indeed without lower urinary tract problems, although in such cases it is not prominent.[26]

A type of repetitive discharge activity, called 'decelerating bursts (DB) and complex repetitive discharges (CRD)' has been found in the external US muscles of some young women. This activity may be so abundant it is thought to cause involuntary muscle contraction and urinary retention.[27]

In contrast to limb muscles, where electrical silence is present on relaxation, in sphincter muscles some MUPs are continuously firing.[13] Additional sphincter MUPs can be activated reflexly or voluntarily, and it has been shown that there are two MUP populations with different characteristics: reflexly or voluntarily activated high-threshold MUPs, which are larger than continuously active low-threshold MUPs.[28] As a consequence, to increase accuracy of MUP analysis, for a template-based multi-MUP analysis, standardization of activity level during sampling at which 3–5 MUPs are sampled on a single muscle site is recommended.[28]

In partially denervated sphincter muscle there is a loss of MUs. To quantify this exactly, use of multi-MUP analysis was proposed.[13] By this approach the number of remaining MUs after partial denervation (e.g. in cauda equina lesions) can be estimated. Furthermore, using this technique the segmental and suprasegmental inputs, as well as the excitation level of the motor neurons within the anterior spinal horns, can be assessed. This approach was found particularly useful in patients with idiopathic fecal incontinence,[13] but has not been studied in patients with neurogenic bladders.

With direct reinnervation after complete denervation, nascent MUPs appear first, being short-duration, low-amplitude, bi- and triphasic potentials, soon becoming polyphasic, serrated, and of prolonged duration.

Changes due to collateral reinnervation are reflected by prolongation of the waveform of the MUPs (Figure 43.4), which may have small, late components (i.e. satellites). In newly formed axon sprout endplates, neuromuscular transmission is insecure, resulting in MUP instability ('jitter' and blocking of individual components).[29] Over a period of time, provided there is no further denervation, the reinnervating axonal sprouts increase in diameter so that activation of all parts of the reinnervated MU becomes nearly synchronous, which increases the amplitude and reduces the duration of the MUPs (Figure 43.4). This phenomenon may be different in sphincter muscles in ongoing degenerative disorders such as MSA, where long-duration MUPs seem to remain a prominent feature of MUs.[30] A less pronounced increase in MUP amplitude on reinnervation in sphincter muscles might also be due to a less efficient fusion of individual muscle fiber potentials in muscles with short spike components of MUPs (also in facial muscles).[31]

Several techniques are available to systematically examine individual MUPs. Of these, the recent and sophisticated

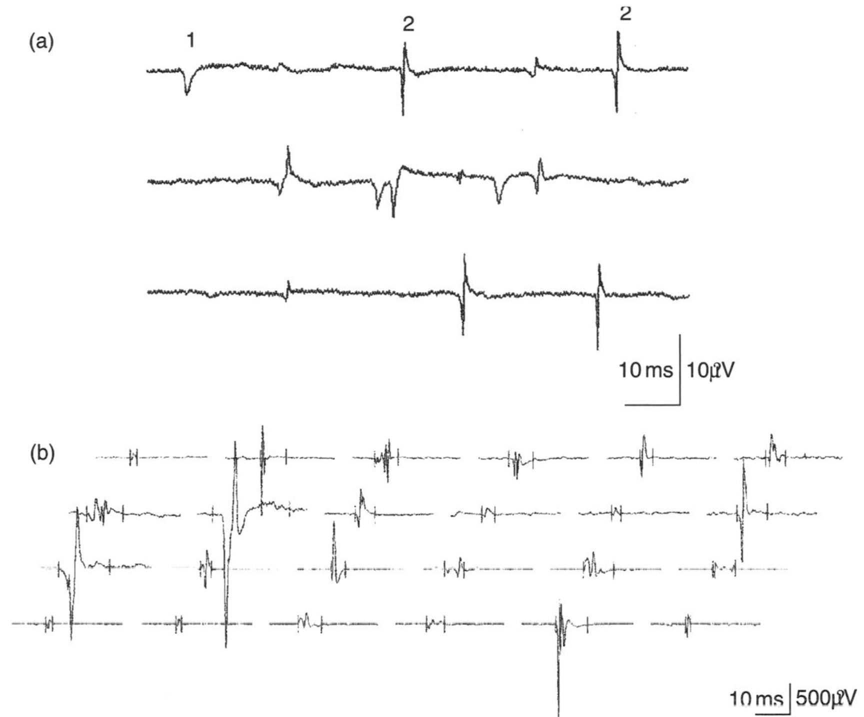

Figure 43.3
Findings of electromyographic (EMG) examination (using a standard concentric EMG needle) in a 36-year-old man after surgical decompression of the cauda equina due to central herniation of the intervertebral disc L4–L5. Patient had long-term sacral dysfunctions: atonic bladder (emptied by abdominal straining), severe constipation, and severe erectile dysfunction. (a) EMG activity during relaxation in the left bulbocavernosus muscle 2 months after surgical decompression of the cauda equina. Note distinct spontaneous denervation activity in the form of biphasic potentials with prominent positive deflections (positive sharp waves (1)) and short biphasic spikes (fibrillation potentials (2)). No motor unit potentials (MUPs) could be recruited in that muscle reflexly or voluntarily, which pointed to complete denervation of the muscle. (b) MUPs sampled (by multi-MUP analysis) from the left subcutaneous external anal sphincter (EAS) muscle during a control uroneurophysiologic examination 7 months later. Mean duration was 7.3 ms (Z = + 0.7), mean area was 808 µVms (Z = + 4.2), and the mean number of turns was 4.3 (Z = + 1.5). ('Z' value = number of SDs above or below the mean obtained in normative population.) Good reinnervation of the muscle after (probably) complete denervation pointed to a combination of neurapraxia (block in nerve transmission) and axonotmesis (degeneration of the nerve fibers with preserved continuity of nerve roots) as opposed to neurotmesis (nerve roots severed) as a mechanism of the cauda equina injury.

template-operated CNEMG techniques (e.g. 'multi-MUP' analysis) are available only on advanced EMG systems.[32,33] Multi-MUP analysis is the fastest and the easiest to apply of the quantitative MUP analysis techniques. It can be applied at continuous activity during sphincter muscle relaxation, as well as at slight to moderate levels of activation.[20] The needle must be located so that a 'crisp' sounding pattern of EMG activity can be heard over the loudspeaker, indicating that the needle electrode is near to muscle fibers. Then, during an appropriate level of EMG activity, the operator starts the analysis and the computer takes the previous (last) 4.8 s period of the signal. From that signal MUPs are automatically extracted, quantified, and sorted into up to 6 classes. MUP classes, representing consecutive discharges of a particular MUP, are then averaged and presented (Figures 43.3 and 43.4). Duration cursors are set automatically using a computer algorithm. However, after acquisition the operator has to edit the MUPs; the MUPs with an unsteady baseline (unclear beginning or end) need to be recognized and deleted. The multi-MUP technique has difficulties with highly unstable and/or polyphasic MUPs. It often fails to sample them, sorts the same MUP to several classes (recognizes it as different MUPs – duplicates), cuts prolonged MUPs into two, or distorts them by averaging.[34] Thus from each examination site up to 6 different MUPs can be obtained.[20,32]

Using multi-MUP analysis sampling of 20 MUPs (standard number in limb muscles) from each EAS muscle presents no problem in healthy controls and most patients (Figures 43.3b and 43.4b).[20] Normative data obtained from the EAS muscle by standardized EMG technique have been published.[20] Analysis made from the same taped EMG signal, using reference data for mean values and 'outliers'[35] (Figure 43.4) revealed similar sensitivity of different MUP

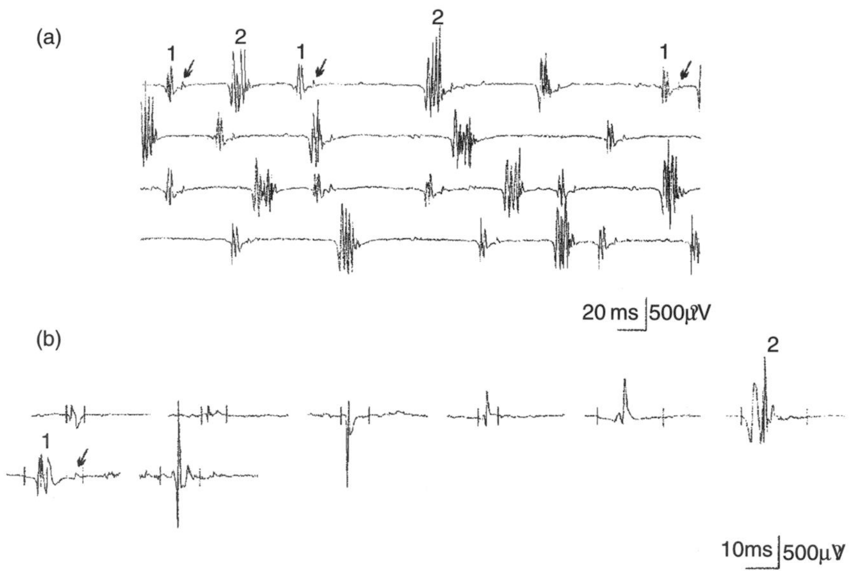

Figure 43.4
Findings of electromyographic (EMG) examination (using a standard concentric EMG needle) in a 36-year-old man with myelitis of the conus medullaris. The patient had several episodes of urinary and fecal incontinence, impaired sensation of bladder and rectum fullness, and moderate erectile dysfunction, all of which resolved spontaneously after a few months. (a) EMG activity in the right deeper external anal sphincter (EAS) muscle during voluntary activation 2 months after the beginning of the disease. Note the extremely polyphasic motor unit potentials (MUPs) of increased duration, and late potential (arrows). Consecutive firing of the same MUP slightly changed, which points to MUP instability. No spontaneous denervation activity, and no 'low threshold MUPs' continuously firing during relaxation were present. Reflex recruitment of MUPs was severely reduced but present in the same muscle. All these findings indicated subacute partial (moderately severe) denervation of the muscle. (b) During the same EMG examination only 8 MUPs needed to be sampled (by multi-MUP analysis) from the same muscle to obtain 3 MUPs with values of duration, area, and the number of turns above the upper 'outlier' limit. To declare muscle pathologic (neurogenic) using outlier criterion this number (3 out of 20 or less MUPs) is needed. Although at the same time mean values for duration, area, and the number of turns were also all pathologic (Z >2.0), they cannot be used in this situation to declare muscle neuropathic, because less than 20 MUPs were sampled. ('Z' value = number of SDs above or below the mean obtained in the normative population.) Two MUPs from (a) are also presented below. (Numbers 1 and 2). Note that averaging used by multi-MUP analysis changed the shape of unstable MUPs (reduced number of phases and turns).

analyses for detecting neuropathic changes in the EAS muscle of patients with chronic cauda equina lesions.[20]

A number of MUP parameters are used in the diagnosis of neuromuscular disease (Figure 43.5). Traditionally, MUP amplitude and duration were measured, and the number of phases was counted.[36] However, a study performed in the EAS muscle revealed that probably only the parameters of area, duration, and the number of turns are needed in MUP analysis. Other MUP parameters (amplitude, the number of phases, duration of the negative peak, thickness, size index) appear to be noncontributory, and their use might reduce the specificity of MUP analysis.[37]

In addition to continuous firing of low-threshold MUPs in sphincters, additional high-threshold MUPs[28] are recruited voluntarily and reflexly (Figure 43.4B). By such maneuvers, the amount of recruitable MUs is estimated. Normally, MUPs should intermingle to produce a dense IP on the oscilloscope screen when muscle is contracted well, and during a strong cough.

The IP can be assessed using a number of automatic quantitative analyses, the turn/amplitude analysis being the most popular.[38,39] However, quantitative IP analysis was shown to be only half as sensitive as the MUP analysis techniques in distinguishing between normal and neuropathic muscles.[20] Nevertheless, with the needle electrode in focus, qualitative assessment of IP during voluntary or reflex muscle contraction by coughing is recommended.

In summary, template based multi-MUP analysis is as sensitive as the traditional MUP analysis techniques,[20] fast (5–10 min per muscle), easy to apply, less prone to personal bias, and is a clinically useful technique.[3] In the EAS muscle its use is further facilitated by the availability of common normative data, which are unaffected by age, gender,[40] number, and characteristics of vaginal deliveries,[41] or mild chronic constipation.[42] In addition, criteria for possible, probable, and definite neuropathic changes in the EAS muscle have been proposed.[43] All these make multi-MUP analysis the technique of choice for quantitative analysis of the EAS reinnervation.

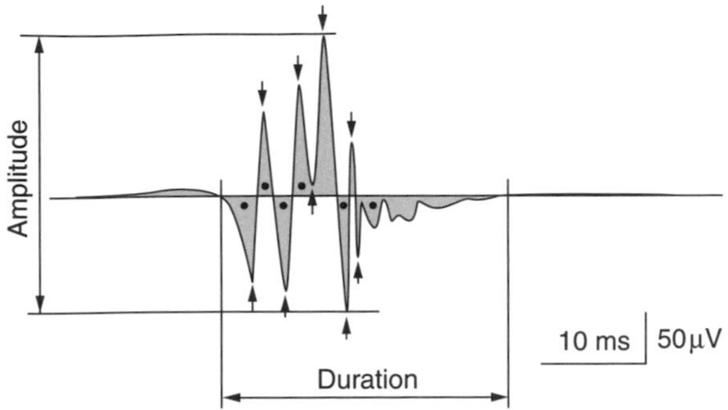

Figure 43.5
The motor unit potential (MUP) parameters. Amplitude is the voltage difference (μV) between the most positive and most negative point of the MUP trace. The MUP duration is the time (ms) between the first deflection and the point when the MUP waveform finally returns to the baseline. The number of MUP phases (small circles) is defined by the number of MUP areas (see below) alternately below and above the baseline, and can be counted as the 'number of baseline crossings plus one'. Turns (arrows) are defined as changes in direction of the MUP trace that are larger than the specified amplitude (e.g. 50 μV), but not crossing the baseline. MUP area measures the integrated surface of the MUP waveform (shaded).

Single fiber electromyography

The aim of single fiber electromyography (SFEMG) testing is similar to CNEMG – to differentiate normal from abnormal striated muscle. The SFEMG electrode has similar external proportions to a concentric needle electrode, but instead of having the recording surface at the tip, a fine insulated platinum or silver wire embedded in epoxy resin is exposed through an aperture on the side 1–5 mm behind the tip. The platinum wire forms the recording surface that has a diameter of 25 μm. It will pick up activity from within a hemispherical volume of 0.3 mm in diameter. This is very much smaller than the volume of muscle tissue from which a concentric needle electrode records, which has an uptake area of 2.5 mm diameter.[19] Because of the arrangement of muscle fibers in a normal MU, an SFEMG needle will record only 1–3 single muscle fibers from the same MU. When recording with an SFEMG needle, the amplifier filters are set so that low frequency activity is eliminated (500 Hz to 10 kHz). Thus, the contribution of each muscle fiber appears as a short biphasic positive–negative action potential.

The SFEMG parameter that reflects MU morphology is the 'fiber density', which is defined as the mean number of muscle fibers belonging to an individual MU per detection site. To assemble this data, recordings from 20 different intramuscular detection sites are necessary.[29] The normal fiber density for the EAS is below 2.0.[44]

The fiber density is increased in collaterally reinnervated muscle. The technique has been particularly applied to sphincter muscles in order to correlate increased fiber density findings to incontinence. Due to its technical characteristics, an SFEMG electrode is able to record even small changes that occur in MUs due to reinnervation, but is less suitable to detect changes due to denervation itself (i.e. abnormal insertion and spontaneous denervation activity).

The SFEMG electrode is also most suitable to record any instability of MUPs ('jitter'), although this is not routinely assessed in pelvic floor muscles for diagnostic purposes.

Single fiber electromyography versus concentric needle electromyography

Quantified CNEMG provides the same information on reinnervation changes in muscle as the SFEMG parameter of 'fiber density',[45] but, in addition, CNEMG will reveal spontaneous denervation activity. In muscle after severe partial denervation, the areas of fibrosis are silent to EMG exploration, and the results are based only on the remaining MUP activity. The remaining innervated muscle is easier to establish with CNEMG, which records from a larger volume of tissue. Furthermore, a CNEMG examination can be extended in the same diagnostic session from, for example, lumbar and upper sacral myotomes to the lower sacral myotomes, after a cauda equina lesion. A concentric electrode can also be employed at the same diagnostic session for recording evoked direct and reflex muscle responses. Use of CNEMG is the method of choice in routine examination of skeletal muscle, and is generally available in clinical neurophysiology laboratories. There has been no work which shows SFEMG use has added advantage for the evaluation of patients with neurogenic bladders.

Sacral reflexes

The term sacral reflex refers to pelvic floor muscle responses to stimulation in the sacral region. In the lower sacral segments there are two commonly clinically elicited reflexes, the anal and the penilo-cavernosus.[6] Both have the afferent and the efferent limb of their reflex arc in the pudendal nerve, and are centrally integrated at the S2 to S4 cord levels.

Electrophysiologic correlates of these and other sacral reflexes have been described, and a uniform two-part nomenclature system was proposed.[6] Measurements of reflex responses and evoked potentials, including sympathetic skin responses (SSRs), relate not only to conduction in peripheral and central neural pathways, but also to synaptic transmission within networks of central nervous system interneurons. Therefore, conduction may be influenced by factors that are not apparent from a simplified

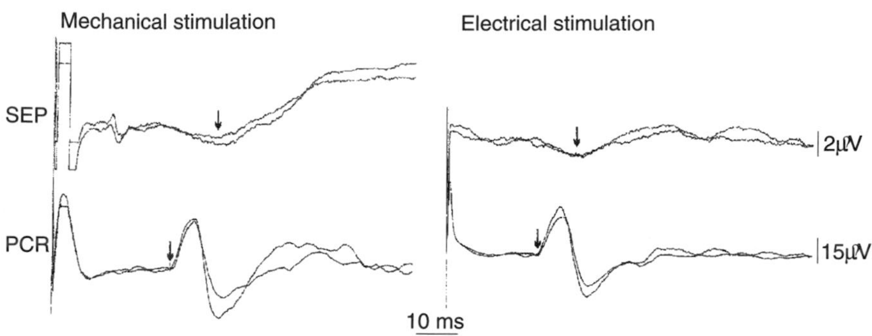

Figure 43.6
Penilo-cavernosus reflex (PCR) responses and pudendal somatosensory evoked potentials (SEP) recorded simultaneously in a 9-year-old boy (body height 140 cm), without uroneurologic abnormalities included in our normative study.[59] Responses were elicited by consecutive (left) mechanical stimulation (nonpainful squeeze of the penis by the electromechanical hammer) and (right) electrical stimulation (single 20 V stimuli over the dorsal penile nerves). Responses were detected by bifocal montage of the surface electrodes (PCR, active electrode over the external anal sphincter muscle/reference electrode over the bulbocavernosus muscle; SEP: active electrode 2 cm behind Cz/reference electrode on Fz both over the scalp according to the International 10–20 electroencephalography (EEG) System).[76] Measurements were obtained by averaging 100 responses. Latencies to the beginning of the PCR responses (arrows) were 33.4 ms and 25.2 ms; latencies to the first positive peak (P40) (arrowheads) were 47.0 ms and 36.7 ms on mechanical and electrical stimulation, respectively. Peak-to-peak amplitudes of the PCR responses were 69 μV and 63 μV; amplitude of P40 measured 2.0 μV and 1.8 μV on mechanical and electrical stimulation, respectively. Note similar amplitudes, but pronounced differences in latency measurements caused by mechanical characteristics of electromechanical hammer used in this study. Latency of the pudendal SEP on electrical stimulation in this child was already within (Z = – 1.9) normative limits for adults (41 ± 2.3 ms).[74]

anatomic model (Figure 43.1). For example, changes in the threshold, amplitude, and latency of the sacral reflex occur as a consequence of changes in the physiologic state of the bladder,[46] and differ in pathologic conditions (i.e. suprasacral spinal cord lesions).[47]

The aim of electrophysiologic testing of sacral reflexes is to assess integrity of the sacral (S2–S4) spinal reflex arc, and to evaluate excitation levels of sacral spinal cord motor neurons.

It is possible to use electrical,[48] mechanical,[49] or magnetic[50] stimulation. Whereas the latter two modalities have only been applied to the penis and clitoris, electrical stimulation can be applied at various sites: to the dorsal penile/clitoral nerve, perianally, and (using a catheter-mounted ring electrode) at the bladder neck/proximal urethra.[6,51,52] In clinical practice, electrical and mechanical stimulation of the penis or clitoris are usually used (Figure 43.6), so this will be discussed in some detail.

The sacral reflex evoked on the dorsal penile or the clitoral nerve stimulation was shown to be a complex response, often comprising two components (Figure 43.7). The first component has a latency of about 33 ms. It is stable, does not habituate, and, based on the variability of single motor neuron latency reflex discharges, is thought to be an oligosynaptic reflex.[7] The second component has a similar latency to the sacral reflexes evoked by stimulation perianally or from the proximal urethra.[6] The variability of single motor neuron reflex responses within this component is much larger, as is typical for a polysynaptic reflex.[7] The second component is not always demonstrable as a discrete response. Double electrical stimuli may be used to facilitate the reflex response if both components cannot be elicited using single electrical pulses.[53]

Sacral reflex responses recorded with needle or wire electrodes can be analyzed separately for each side of the EAS or each bulbocavernosus muscle (Figure 43.7). Using unilateral dorsal penile nerve blocks, the existence of two unilateral sacral reflex arcs has been demonstrated.[54] Thus, by detection from the left and right bulbocavernosus (and probably also the EAS) muscles separate testing of both sacral reflex arcs can be performed. Sensitivity of the test can be increased also by use of the inter-side latency difference (normative limits in case of simultaneous bilateral detection: <3.6 ms).[55] This is important, because in cases of unilateral (e.g. sacral plexopathy, pudendal neuropathy) or asymmetric lesions (e.g. cauda equina), which are common, a healthy sacral reflex arc may obscure a pathologic one. In the authors' laboratories testing of penilo and clitoro-cavernosus reflex on electrical stimulation is performed in conjunction with a CNEMG if no brisk reflex response is present on mechanical stimulation of the perianal/perineal region and recording from the EAS muscle.[24]

Standardization of the technique has been proposed.[1] It was recommended that surface stimulation electrodes be placed on the penis/clitoris, and 10 single, 0.2 ms long stimuli be applied at supramaximal intensity at time intervals of 2 s (= 0.5 Hz). Recording is by concentric needle or surface electrodes placed into/over the EAS, or bulbocavernosus

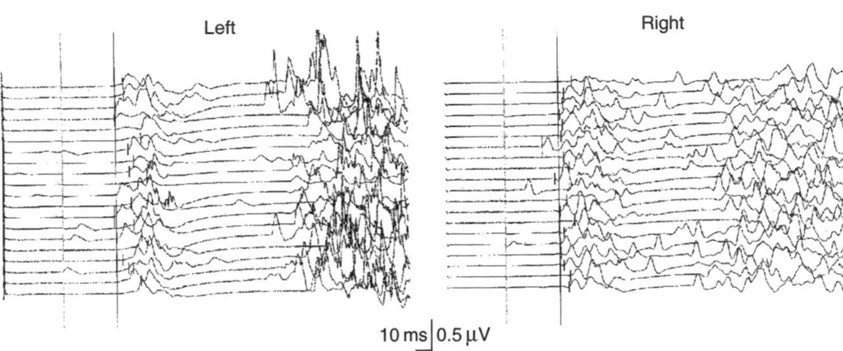

Figure 43.7
Findings of uroneurophysiologic examination in a 32-year-old man 2 months after traumatic fracture of pubic bones and urethral rupture. After surgical repair of urethra the patient continued to leak urine and complained of moderate erectile dysfunction. His bowel function was normal. On concentric needle electromyography (CNEMG) during relaxation some spontaneous denervation activity was detected in the left, but not the right bulbocavernosus muscle. On reflex and voluntary activation, normal motor unit potentials (MUPs) were recruited. In addition, normal penilo-cavernosus reflex (PCR) responses were elicited by electrical stimulation (single 80 mA stimuli over dorsal penile nerves), and CNEMG electrode detection in the left and right bulbocavernosus muscles. Left and right latency of the first component of the PCR: 29 ms (marked by solid vertical line). Note also the second component of the PCR. Electrophysiologic examination thus confirmed integrity of the neural structures, and revealed only very slight axonal damage to the left pudendal nerve, which was thought unlikely to be the cause of his prominent urinary incontinence. Instead it seemed likely that was due to direct damage to the bladder neck, urethra, or possibly urethral sphincter or its terminal innervation. Similarly, erectile dysfunction was most probably caused by local injury, and not by more proximal nervous lesion.

muscle in men, using filters: 10 Hz – 10 kHz; sweep speed: 10 ms/div; and gain: 50–1000 μV/div. Onset latency is the only parameter measured.[1]

The penilo/clitoro-cavernosus reflex has been said to be of value in patients with cauda equina and other LMN lesions, although it is recognized that a reflex with a normal latency does not exclude the possibility of an axonal lesion in its reflex arc (Figure 43.7). The sensitivity and specificity of sacral reflex responses in patients with conditions associated with neurogenic bladders are not known. In diabetics the nerve conduction studies performed in limbs are more sensitive in revealing peripheral neuropathy than sacral reflex latencies.[56] Abnormally short reflex latency of the sacral reflex has been claimed to suggest either the abnormally low position of conus medullaris in the tethered cord syndrome[57] or a suprasacral cord lesion.[58] Mechanical stimulation has been used to elicit sacral reflex in both sexes[49] and has been found to be a robust technique. Either a standard commercially available reflex hammer or a customized electromechanical hammer can be employed. Such stimulation is painless and can be used in children.[59] The latency of the mechanically elicited penilo/clitoro-cavernosus reflex is similar to the electrically elicited one (Figure 43.6).[59]

Responses of the bulbocavernosus muscle after mechanical suprapubic stimulation (pubo-cavernosus) have also been described.[60] It was hypothesized that this is a polysynaptic reflex elicited by the stimulation of the bladder wall tensoreceptors, which could be involved in pathogenesis of detrusor-sphincter dyssynergia in some patients with neurogenic bladders.[60] Penilo/clitoro-cavernosus reflex testing can be a useful adjunct in the 'diagnostic battery', with CNEMG exploration of the pelvic floor muscles being the most important test. Electrophysiologic assessment of sacral reflexes is a more quantitative, sensitive, and reproducible way of assessing the S2–S4 reflex arcs than any of the clinical methods.[61] Results, however, should be interpreted with caution, always mindful of the clinical context.

Uroneurophysiologic tests that are not of diagnostic value in individual patients with neurogenic bladders

Neurophysiology of the sacral motor system

Motor nerve conduction studies

Recording of the muscle response (compound motor action potential, CMAP)[62] on electrical stimulation of its motor nerve is the routine method of electrophysiologic evaluation of limb nerves. By stimulating the nerve at two levels, motor nerve conduction velocity can be calculated, which distinguishes between lesions of myelin and axons causing motor weakness. For this purpose, however, the technique requires access to the nerve at two well-separated points for stimulation and measurement of the distance between them, a requirement which cannot be easily met in the pelvis. Thus the only electrophysiologic parameter of motor conduction that can be measured also in the pelvic floor is the pudendal nerve terminal motor latency (PNTML).

Latency measures conduction of the fastest fibers only, and gives little or no information about the loss of biological units generating electrical currents (axons, etc.), which is the determinant of functional importance. However, latencies depend less on irrelevant biological and technical factors, and are therefore more robust measurements than amplitudes. On the other hand, the amplitude of the compound potential correlates with the number of activated biological units. (A conduction block and pathologic dispersion of conduction velocities within a neural pathway also affect amplitudes.) Amplitudes are thus the more relevant physiologic parameter, but CMAP amplitudes of the EAS, US, or other pelvic floor muscles on stimulation of the pudendal nerves have unfortunately not yet proved contributory.

PNTML is usually measured by stimulation with a special surface electrode assembly fixed on a gloved index finger – the 'St Mark's electrode'.[63] This consists of a bipolar stimulating electrode fixed to the tip of the gloved finger with the recording electrode pair placed 8 cm proximally on the base of the finger. The finger is inserted into the rectum, and the pudendal nerve stimulated close to the ischial spine. The response is recorded from the EAS muscle. Using this stimulator, the PNTML for the anal sphincter MEP is typically around 2 ms.

Prolongation of the PNTML measured by the St Mark's electrode was found in a variety of patient groups, and was taken as a sign of damage to the pudendal nerve. This has led to the term 'pudendal neuropathy', equating a prolongation of PNTML with pelvic floor denervation. This, however, is mistaken, as prolongation of latency is a poor measure of denervation, as already explained. What type of abnormality this latency prolongation indicates is unclear as there have not been any relevant morphologic studies. Furthermore, delays of PNTML in patient groups, even when present, were short – approxiamtely 0.1–0.3 ms – and it is unlikely that these represent a functionally relevant change.

In practice, the PNTML is unhelpful for diagnosis in individual patients with sacral dysfunction.[64,65] Elicitability of a compound motor action potential in pelvic floor muscles (using the perianal stimulation) may be helpful in patients with combined UMN and LMN lesions in whom no MUP activity can be recorded. In this situation the presence of compound motor action potential rules out complete (axonal) LMN lesion.

Anterior sacral root (cauda equina) stimulation

Transcutaneous stimulation of deeply situated nervous tissue became possible with the development of special electrical and magnetic stimulators. When applied over the spine at the exit from the vertebral canal, spinal roots can be stimulated and there have been reports of these techniques applied to the sacral roots.[61,66]

Electrical or magnetic stimulation depolarizes underlying neural structures in a nonselective fashion, and concomitant activation of several muscles innervated by lumbosacral segments occurs. It has been shown that responses from gluteal muscles may contaminate attempts to record from the sphincters and lead to error.[67] Thus, surface recordings from sphincter muscles are inadvisable.

Recording of MEP with magnetic stimulation has been less successful than with electrical stimulation, and there are often large stimulus artifacts. Positioning of the ground electrode between the recording electrodes and the stimulating coil may decrease the artifact.[68]

Demonstrating the presence of a perineal MEP on stimulation over the lumbosacral spine, recorded with a CNEMG electrode, may occasionally be helpful, but an absent response has to be evaluated with caution. The clinical value of the test has yet to be established.

Assessment of central motor pathways

Using the same magnetic or electrical stimulation it has been shown to be possible to stimulate the motor cortex and record a response from the pelvic floor. Magnetic stimulation is not painful and cortical electrical stimulation is nowadays only used for intraoperative monitoring. The aim of these techniques is to assess conduction in the central motor pathways.

By electrical stimulation over the motor cortex of healthy subjects, MEPs in the EAS, the US, and the bulbocavernosus muscles were reported.[66] When no facilitatory maneuver is used, mean latencies are 20–30 ms, but slight voluntary contraction of the sphincter and pelvic floor muscles shortens mean latencies to 17–27 ms.[66] By subtracting the latency of the MEPs obtained by stimulation over the scalp, and also that obtained by stimulation at the L1 level, a central conduction time of approximately 16 ms without, and 13 ms with, facilitation was obtained for pelvic floor and sphincter muscles.[66]

Substantially longer central conduction times in patients with multiple sclerosis and spinal cord lesions as compared to healthy controls have been found,[69] but as all those patients had clinically recognizable spinal cord disease, the diagnostic contribution of the technique remains doubtful.

A well-formed sphincter MEP with a normal latency in a patient with a functional disorder or a medicolegal case may occasionally be helpful, but otherwise there is no established clinical use for this type of testing.

Neurophysiology of the sacral sensory system

Electroneurography of the dorsal penile nerve

Electroneurography of the dorsal penile nerve has been used to assess sensory nerve conduction of lower sacral segments. By placing a pair of stimulating electrodes across the penile glans and a pair of recording electrodes across the base of penis a sensory nerve action potential (SNAP) can be recorded (with an amplitude of about 10 μV). The sensory conduction velocity of the dorsal penile nerve has been reported as 27 m/s. The method was claimed to be helpful in diagnosing neurogenic erectile dysfunction as a consequence of sensory neuropathy,[70] but the problems of measuring the conduction distance posed considerable practical difficulties and the test is now rarely used. More practical seems to be the method of stimulating the pudendal nerve by the St Mark's electrode transrectally, and recording from the penis.[71]

A theoretically normal amplitude SNAP of the dorsal penile nerves in an insensitive penis distinguishes a lesion of sensory pathways proximal to the dorsal spinal ganglion (central pathways, cauda equina) from a lesion of and distal to the ganglion (sacral plexus, pudendal nerves).

Electroneurography of dorsal sacral roots

SNAPs on stimulation of the dorsal penile and clitoral nerves may be recorded intraoperatively when the sacral roots are exposed. This has been found helpful in preserving roots relevant for perineal sensation in spastic children undergoing dorsal rhizotomy and possibly decreasing the incidence of postoperative voiding dysfunction.[72]

At the level of lower thoracic and upper lumbar vertebrae a low amplitude (<1 μV) spinal SEP can be recorded with surface electrodes. It is a monophasic, negative potential with a mean peak latency of about 12.5 ms,[73] and is probably due to postsynaptic activity in the spinal cord. Responses using surface electrodes are often unrecordable in obese healthy men[65] and in many women.

With epidural electrodes sacral root potentials on stimulation of the dorsal penile nerve could only be recorded in 13, and cord potentials in 9 out of 22 subjects; latencies of these spinal SEPs were 11.9 ± 1.8 ms,[73] substantiating the results obtained by surface recording.[74]

No use of such recordings out of the operating room has been established.

Pudendal somatosensory evoked potentials

The pudendal SEP is easily recorded following electrical stimulation of the dorsal penile or clitoral nerve.[75] This response is, as a rule, of highest amplitude at the central recording site (Cz – 2 cm: Fz of the International 10–20 electroencephalography (EEG) System)[76] and is highly reproducible (Figure 43.6). Amplitudes of the P40 measure 0.5–12 μV. The first positive peak at 41 ± 2.3 ms (called P1 or P40) is usually clearly defined in healthy subjects using a stimulus 2–4 times stronger than the sensory threshold current strength.[74] Later, negative (at around 55 ms) and then further positive waves occur, which are quite variable in amplitude and expression, but have no known clinical relevance.

Pudendal SEP recordings on penile/clitoral stimulation are sometimes useful in patients with sensory loss in the lower sacral dermatomes and brisk penilo-cavernosus reflex on clinical examination such that an UMN lesion is suspected.[24] Pudendal SEPs were recorded in patients with neurogenic bladder dysfunction due to multiple sclerosis, but it is now known that in this clinical situation the tibial cerebral SEPs are more often abnormal than the pudendal SEPs; only in exceptional cases are the pudendal SEPs abnormal but the tibial SEPs normal, suggesting an isolated conus involvement.[77] Pudendal SEPs were also measured in patients with neurogenic bladder due to spinal cord lesions and diabetes.[78] Pathologic pudendal SEPs seemed to predict poor surgical outcomes after resection of a tight filum terminale.[79]

A study which looked at the value of the pudendal SEP for detecting relevant neurologic disease, when investigating urogenital symptoms, found it to be of lesser value than a clinical examination looking for signs of spinal cord disease in the lower limbs (i.e. hyperreflexia and extensor plantar responses).[80] There may, however, be circumstances such as when a patient is complaining of loss of bladder or vaginal sensation that it is reassuring to be able to record a normal pudendal SEP. The method as such is valid and robust, but its clinical value, particularly in the investigation of neurogenic bladder, is minor.

Cerebral somatosensory evoked potentials on stimulation of the bladder and urethra

These responses are claimed to be more relevant to neurogenic bladder dysfunction than the pudendal SEP, as the Aδ sensory afferents from bladder and proximal urethra, which convey impulses from these regions, accompany the autonomic fibers in the pelvic nerves (see above).

Cerebral SEP can be obtained on stimulation of the bladder urothelium. When making such measurements, it is of the utmost importance to use bipolar stimulation in the bladder or proximal urethra, because otherwise somatic afferents are depolarized due to spread of electrical current. Cerebral SEPs on bipolar intravesical stimulation have been shown to have maximum amplitude over the midline (Cz – 2 cm: Fz), but were of low amplitude (1 μV and less) and variable configuration, making it difficult to identify the response in some control subjects. The typical latency of the most prominent negative potential (N1) is about 100 ms.[52, 81]

The clinical usefulness of such recordings has not been established.

Autonomic nervous system tests

All of the neurophysiologic methods for evaluation of the neurogenic bladder discussed so far assess the thicker myelinated fibers only, whereas it is the autonomic nervous system, the parasympathetic part in particular, which is the most relevant for bladder function. Although in most instances local involvement of the sacral nervous system (such as due to trauma or compression, etc.) will usually involve both somatic and autonomic fibers together, there are some local pathologic conditions that cause isolated lesions of the autonomic nervous system, such as mesorectal excision of carcinoma[82] or prostatectomy.[83] In addition, several types of peripheral neuropathy preferentially affect thin autonomic fibers. Methods assessing the parasympathetic and sympathetic systems directly would thus be very helpful. Information on parasympathetic bladder innervation can to some extent be obtained by cystometry, which, however, is a test of overall organ function and usually cannot locate the lesion. Although not strictly an electrophysiologic test, thermal sensory testing was found useful in assessment of the thin sensory nerve fibers from sacral segments,[83] which are often affected concomitantly with thin autonomic fibers.

Sympathetic skin response and other tests of thoracolumbar sympathetic function

The sympathetic nervous system mediates sweat gland activity in the skin. On stressful stimulation a potential shift can be recorded with surface electrodes from the skin of palms and soles, and has been reported to be a useful parameter in assessment of neuropathy involving unmyelinated nerve fibers. The sympathetic skin response (SSR) can also be recorded from perineal skin and the penis. The SSR is a reflex that consists of myelinated sensory fibers, a complex central integrative mechanism, and a sympathetic efferent limb (with postganglionic nonmyelinated C fibers).[84] The stimulus used in clinical practice is usually an electrical pulse delivered to the upper or lower limb (to mixed nerves), but the genital organs can also be stimulated. The latencies of SSR on the penis following stimulation of a median nerve at the wrist have been reported as between 1.5[85] and 2.3 s[86] and could be obtained in all normal subjects, but with a large variability. The responses rapidly habituate, and depend on a number of endogenous and exogenous factors, including skin temperature, which should be above 28 °C. Only an absent SSR can be taken as abnormal. SSR can also be recorded on bladder/urethra stimulation,[87] which in addition to central sympathetic pathways, also tests thin afferent fibers from the pelvic viscera.

In men another approach to test lumbosacral sympathetic function is neurophysiologic measurement of the dartos reflex obtained on cutaneous stimulation of the thigh. The dartos muscle is a sympathetically innervated dermal layer within the scrotum, distinct from the somatically innervated cremasteric muscle. A reliable and reproducible dartos reflex (i.e. scrotal skin contraction) of latency approximately 5 s was demonstrated in healthy men.[88]

The SSR might be useful in the assessment of neuropathies involving unmyelinated nerve fibers,[89] and in the assessment of thoracolumbar sympathetic.[87] The utility of SSR in bladder/urethra stimulation[87] and the dartos reflex[88] has not yet been established.

Bladder smooth muscle electromyography

Although information on sacral parasympathetic function can, to some extent, be obtained by cystometry, this cannot directly demonstrate the neuropathic etiology of the bladder dysfunction. Neurophysiologic tests of sacral parasympathetic nerve function, such as detrusor EMG, would, in principle, constitute the most definitive indicator of neurogenic bladder involvement. However, such studies are confronted with problems in discriminating between the very small extracellular membrane potential changes in bladder muscle cells and the large electromechanical artifact caused by electrode movement as the tissue contracts. In what is currently the only study performed in humans, surface electrodes were placed on the abdominal skin, and bipolar signals were recorded in horizontal, vertical, and diagonal directions. It was claimed that voiding was accompanied by a slow voltage change that could be distinguished from striated muscle activity. Activity was related to bladder emptying and to the detrusor pressure.[90] However, further studies to improve and validate these tests are expected to clarify their place in research and clinical practice.

Patient groups with neurogenic bladders in whom uroneurophysiologic tests are of clinical value

Parkinsonism

Neuropathic changes can be recorded in sphincter muscles of patients with multiple system atrophy (MSA).[14,30,91,92] MSA is a progressive neurodegenerative disease, which is often (particularly in its early stages) mistaken for Parkinson's disease. Urinary incontinence in both genders, and erectile dysfunction in men, are early features of the condition, often present for some years before the onset of typical neurologic features.[93] Autonomic failure causing postural hypotension and cerebellar ataxia causing unsteadiness and clumsiness may be additional features. The disease is usually (in 80% of patients) unresponsive to antiparkinsonian treatment. As a part of the neurodegenerative process, loss of motor neurons occurs in Onuf's nucleus so that partial but progressive denervation of the sphincter and the bulbocavernosus muscles occurs,[14] and recorded MUPs show changes of chronic reinnervation.[14,30,91,92]

Sphincter EMG has been demonstrated to be of value in distinguishing between idiopathic Parkinson's disease and MSA,[14,30,91,92] but may not be sensitive in the early phase of the disease,[14,94] and not specific after 5 years of parkinsonism.[91] The changes of chronic reinnervation may be found in other parkinsonian syndromes such as progressive supranuclear palsy (PSP),[95] in which neuronal loss in Onuf's nucleus was also demonstrated histologically.[96] In contrast to earlier citations, one study failed to demonstrate significant differences between two small groups of MSA and Parkinson disease patients,[97] but this may have been a consequence of excluding late components from MUP duration due to the automated method of analyis.[34]

Kinesiologic EMG performed during urodynamics can also be valuable in Parkinson's disease[14] and MSA[98] patients, documenting loss of coordination between detrusor and US muscles ('detrusor-sphincter dyssynergia').

Unilateral needle EMG of the subcutaneous EAS muscle, including quantitative MUP analysis,[14,30,91,92] is clearly indicated in patients with suspected MSA,[24] particularly in its early stages when the diagnosis is unclear.[91] If the test is normal, but the diagnosis remains unclear, it might be of value to repeat the test later.[14,94]

Cauda equina and conus medullaris lesions and spinal dysraphisms

Lesions to the cauda equina and/or conus medullaris are an important cause of pelvic floor dysfunction. Usually the neural tissue damage is caused by compression within the spinal canal due to disc protrusion, spinal fractures, epidural hematomas, tumors, congenital malformations, etc.[3] Unfortunately accidental damage to the cauda equina may occur during surgical interventions, mainly due to spinal stenosis.

Patient presentation depends very much on the etiology of the lesion. In cases of disc protrusion, spinal fractures, and epidural hematomas, presentation is often dramatic. Acute severe back pain radiating to the legs, associated with numbness and tingling in the saddle region, is noted first. Urinary retention with overflow incontinence and, later, severe constipation follow. When damage is due to disc protrusion there is often a history of previous back pain with sciatica, in spinal fractures a history of trauma, and in epidural hematomas a history of coagulation disorder, anticoagulation therapy, or recent spinal surgery can usually be obtained. With tumors, the presentation of the cauda equina lesion is much more insidious.

After detailed clinical examination of the perineal region (with particular emphasis on saddle sensation), CNEMG of the EAS muscle (and sometimes the bulbocavernosus muscle – see below) and electrophysiologic evaluation of the penilo/clitoro-cavernosus reflex (when absent clinically) need to be considered.[24]

Generally stated, detection of pathologic spontaneous activity by CNEMG has good sensitivity and specificity to reveal moderate and severe partial denervation, and complete denervation, of pelvic floor muscles 3 weeks or more after injury to the cauda equina and/or conus medullaris (Figure 43.3A). Traumatic lesions to the lumbosacral spine or particularly to the pelvis are probably the only acquired condition where complete denervation of the perineal muscles can be observed.[21] Most other lesions will, by contrast, cause partial denervation. CNEMG of the bulbocavernosus muscles is of particular importance a few weeks after partial denervation in the lower sacral myotomes to detect spontaneous denervation activity.[24]

CNEMG (MUP analysis) can show changes of reinnervation, which appear months after injury.[20] Following a cauda equina lesion, the MUPs are likely to be prolonged and polyphasic, and other MUP parameters are also increased (Figures 43.3b and 43.4b).[20] Similar marked changes are seen in patients with lumbosacral myelomeningocele. EMG was found to contribute to the prediction of functional outcome in children with spina bifida.[99]

Penilo/clitoro-cavernosus reflex is useful in the evaluation of subjects with cauda equina and/or conus medullaris lesions to assess the integrity of the reflex arc. In patients with a tethered cord syndrome, measurement of sacral reflex latency can be of additional value, as a very short reflex latency in this clinical situation supports the possibility of the abnormally low position of the conus medullaris.[57] Although in patients with a normal position of conus medullaris urodynamic studies better predicted occurence of a tight filum terminale, pathologic pudendal SEPs correlated with poor surgical outcomes.[79]

Electrophysiologic assessment is useful to determine the sequels of the lesion, and in insidious cases for reaching the diagnosis.

Sacral plexus and pudendal nerve lesions

Neurologic lesions located in the sacral plexus and pudendal nerves are less common than lesions of the cauda equina or conus medullaris. They can be caused by pelvic fractures, hip surgery, complicated deliveries, malignant infiltration, local radiotherapy, and the use of orthopedic traction tables. They are more often unilateral. In principle, one can distinguish between such a lesion and a cauda equina or conus medullaris lesion by unilateral absence of dorsal penile SNAP, and absent spontaneous denervation activity in the paravertebral muscles. However, both of these tests are difficult to perform (due to difficult unilateral dorsal penile/clitoral nerve stimulation, and absent paravertebral muscles in the lower sacral segments, respectively), so localization of the lesion will usually be made clinically, or in case of extensive sacral plexus lesions by examination of the first sacral and lower lumbar segments.

Urinary retention in women

For many years it was said that isolated urinary retention in young women was due either to psychogenic factors or was the first symptom of multiple sclerosis. However, CNEMG in this group has demonstrated that many such patients have profuse complex repetitive discharges (CRDs) and decelerating burst (DB) activity in the US muscle.[100]

Why this activity should occur is not known, but in the syndrome described by one of the authors, it was associated with polycystic ovaries.[101] Most commonly, the initial episode of urinary retention is precipitated by a gynecologic surgical procedure using general anesthesia, at the mean age of 28, and the condition does not progress to a general neurologic disorder.[102] It was shown that this pathologic spontaneous activity endures during micturition and may cause interrupted flow.[16] The disorder of sphincter relaxation appears to lead to secondary changes in detrusor function – either instability or failure of contractility. A recent study showed that Fowler's syndrome was the commonest cause of urinary retention in a series of 297 women.[103]

Because CNEMG will detect both changes of denervation and reinnervation as occur with a cauda equina lesion (see above), as well as this peculiar abnormal spontaneous activity, it can be argued that this test is mandatory in women with urinary retention.[16,100] It should certainly be carried out before stigmatizing a woman as having 'psychogenic urinary retention'.

Patient groups with neurogenic bladders in whom uroneurophysiologic tests are of research interest

Uroneurophysiologic techniques have been important in research, and substantiated hypotheses that a proportion of patients with sacral dysfunction, such as stress urinary and idiopathic fecal incontinence, have involvement of the nervous system,[62,104] established the function of the sacral nervous system in patients with suprasacral spinal cord injury,[105] and revealed consequences of particular surgeries.[106] However, in individual patients from these groups, uroneurophysiologic tests are unlikely to be contributory.

Generalized peripheral neuropathies

Generalized peripheral neuropathies, particularly those that affect thin nerve fibers, can also cause neurogenic bladder. Most important causes of such neuropathies are diabetes mellitus and acute inflammatory demyelinizing polyneuropathy (AIDP or Guillain–Barré syndrome). Most of these neuropathies are length-dependent, with longer fibers first and more severely affected. As a consequence, electrophysiologic tests applied on distal lower limb nerves will usually be more sensitive than when applied to nerves that innervate the perineal area/pelvic floor (see above).[56]

Diseases of the central nervous system

Kinesiologic tests, performed as part of cystometric measurements, are often useful in patients with CNS signs having diagnosis of neurogenic bladder. Electrodiagnostic tests of conduction performed in patients with 'central lesions' are only very occasionally indicated. PSEPs were found to provide information of diagnostic relevance in the initial diagnostic evaluation of patients with multiple sclerosis, and were also suggested as a screening test for cystometric evaluation in this population.[107] CNEMG is not indicated in 'central lesions' unless segmental spinal cord (conus medullaris) involvement[77] is suspected (see above).[1]

Conclusion

Several electrophysiologic tests have been proposed for evaluation of the sacral nervous system. Although all tests mentioned in this chapter continue to be of research interest, it is the CNEMG in particular which is of definite value in the everyday routine diagnostic evaluation of selected groups of patients with pelvic floor dysfunction, atypical parkinsonism, and traumatic spinal and pelvic lesions, as well as of young women with urinary retention.

It is expected that new computer-assisted techniques of CNEMG analysis will improve the usefulness of the test as a diagnostic method to reveal neuropathic pelvic floor muscle involvement.

Further research into and experience with other discussed neurophysiologic tests will reveal their contribution to the clinical assessment of individual patients, which is presently unknown. However, tests that have been available for about 30 years are unlikely to prove of high utility in clinical practice.

References

1. Vodušek DB, Amarenco G, Batra A et al. Clinical neurophysiology. In: Abrams P, Cardozo L, Khoury S, Wein A, eds. Incontinence. Volume 1, Basics & Evaluation. Plymouth (UK): Health Publication, 2005: 675–706.
2. Fowler CJ. Neurologist's clinical and investigative approach to patients with bladder, bowel and sexual dysfunction. In: Fowler CJ, Sakakibara R, Frohman EM, Steward JD, eds. Neurologic Bladder, Bowel and Sexual Dysfunction. Amsterdam: Elsevier Science, 2001: 1–6.
3. Podnar S, Trsinar B, Vodusek DB. Bladder dysfunction in patients with cauda equina lesions. Neurourol Urodyn 2006; 25: 23–31.
4. Podnar S. Critical reappraisal of referrals to electromyography and nerve conduction studies. Eur J Neurol 2005; 12: 150–5.
5. Podnar S. Which patients need referral for anal sphincter electromyography? Muscle Nerve 2006; 33: 278–82.
6. Podnar S. Nomenclature of the electrophysiologically tested sacral reflexes. Neurourol Urodyn 2006; 25: 95–7.
7. Vodusek DB, Janko M. The bulbocavernosus reflex. A single motor neuron study. Brain 1990; 113: 813–20.
8. Dumitru D, Jewett DL. Far-field potentials. Muscle Nerve 1993; 16: 237–54.
9. Chantraine A, de Leval J, Depireux P. Adult female intra- and peri-urethral sphincter-electromyographic study. Neurourol Urodyn 1990; 9: 139–44.
10. Mathers SE, Kempster PA, Swash M, Lees AJ. Constipation and paradoxical puborectalis contraction in anismus and Parkinson's disease: a dystonic phenomenon? J Neurol Neurosurg Psychiatry 1988; 51: 1503–7.
11. Nordling J, Meyhoff HH. Dissociation of urethral and anal sphincter activity in neurogenic bladder dysfunction. J Urol 1979; 122: 352–6.
12. Deindl FM, Vodusek DB, Hesse U, Schussler B. Activity patterns of pubococcygeal muscles in nulliparous continent women. Br J Urol 1993; 72: 46–51.
13. Podnar S, Mrkaic M, Vodusek DB. Standardization of anal sphincter electromyography: quantification of continuous activity during relaxation. Neurourol Urodyn 2002; 21: 540–5.
14. Stocchi F, Carbone A, Inghilleri M et al. Urodynamic and neurophysiological evaluation in Parkinson's disease and multiple system atrophy. J Neurol Neurosurg Psychiatry 1997; 62: 507–11.
15. De EJ, Patel CY, Tharian B et al. Diagnostic discordance of electromyography (EMG) versus voiding cystourethrogram (VCUG) for detrusor-external sphincter dyssynergy (DESD). Neurourol Urodyn 2005; 24: 616–21.
16. Deindl FM, Vodusek DB, Bischoff C, Hofmann R, Hartung R. Dysfunctional voiding in women: which muscles are responsible? Br J Urol 1998; 82: 814–9.
17. Groutz A, Blaivas JG, Pies C, Sassone AM. Learned voiding dysfunction (non-neurogenic, neurogenic bladder) among adults. Neurourol Urodyn 2001; 20: 259–68.
18. Deindl FM, Vodusek DB, Hesse U, Schussler B. Pelvic floor activity patterns: comparison of nulliparous continent and parous urinary stress incontinent women. A kinesiological EMG study. Br J Urol 1994; 73: 413–7.
19. Nandedkar SD, Sanders DB, Stalberg EV, Andreassen S. Simulation of concentric needle EMG motor unit action potentials. Muscle Nerve 1988; 11: 151–9.
20. Podnar S, Vodusek DB, Stalberg E. Comparison of quantitative techniques in anal sphincter electromyography. Muscle Nerve 2002; 25: 83–92.
21. Podnar S. Electromyography of the anal sphincter: which muscle to examine? Muscle Nerve 2003; 28: 377–9.
22. Podnar S, Rodi Z, Lukanovic A, Trsinar B, Vodusek DB. Standardization of anal sphincter EMG: technique of needle examination. Muscle Nerve 1999; 22: 400–3.
23. Podnar S. Bilateral vs. unilateral electromyographic examination of the external anal sphincter muscle. Neurophysiol Clin 2004; 34: 153–7.
24. Podnar S, Vodusek DB. Protocol for clinical neurophysiologic examination of the pelvic floor. Neurourol Urodyn 2001; 20: 669–82.
25. Podnar S, Zalewska E, Hausmanowa-Petrusewicz I. Evaluation of the complexity of motor unit potentials in anal sphincter electromyography. Clin Neurophysiol 2005; 116: 948–56.
26. FitzGerald MP, Blazek B, Brubaker L. Complex repetitive discharges during urethral sphincter EMG: clinical correlates. Neurourol Urodyn 2000; 19: 577–83.
27. Fowler CJ, Kirby RS, Harrison MJ. Decelerating burst and complex repetitive discharges in the striated muscle of the urethral sphincter, associated with urinary retention in women. J Neurol Neurosurg Psychiatry 1985; 48: 1004–9.
28. Podnar S, Vodusek DB. Standardisation of anal sphincter EMG: high and low threshold motor units. Clin Neurophysiol 1999; 110: 1488–91.
29. Stalberg E, Trontelj JV. Single Fiber Electromyography: Studies in Healthy and Diseased Muscle. New York: Raven Press, 1994.
30. Palace J, Chandiramani VA, Fowler CJ. Value of sphincter electromyography in the diagnosis of multiple system atrophy. Muscle Nerve 1997; 20: 1396–403.
31. Stalberg E. The Kugelberg Lecture. Neurophysiological studies of collateral reinnervation in man. Suppl Clin Neurophysiol 2000; 53: 3–8.
32. Stalberg E, Falck B, Sonoo M, Stalberg S, Astrom M. Multi-MUP EMG analysis – a two year experience in daily clinical work. Electroencephalogr Clin Neurophysiol 1995; 97: 145–54.
33. Nandedkar SD, Barkhaus PE, Charles A. Multi-motor unit action potential analysis (MMA). Muscle Nerve 1995; 18: 1155–66.

34. Podnar S, Fowler CJ. Sphincter electromyography in diagnosis of multiple system atrophy: technical issues. Muscle Nerve 2004; 29: 151–6.
35. Stalberg E, Bischoff C, Falck B. Outliers, a way to detect abnormality in quantitative EMG. Muscle Nerve 1994; 17: 392–9.
36. Buchthal F. An Introduction to Electromyography. Oslo: JW Capelen, 1957.
37. Podnar S, Mrkaic M. Predictive power of motor unit potential parameters in anal sphincter electromyography. Muscle Nerve 2002; 26: 389–94.
38. Nandedkar SD, Sanders DB, Stalberg EV. Automatic analysis of the electromyographic interference pattern. Part II: Findings in control subjects and in some neuromuscular diseases. Muscle Nerve 1986; 9: 491–500.
39. Stalberg E, Chu J, Bril V et al. Automatic analysis of the EMG interference pattern. Electroencephalogr Clin Neurophysiol 1983; 56: 672–81.
40. Podnar S, Vodusek DB, Stalberg E. Standardization of anal sphincter electromyography: normative data. Clin Neurophysiol 2000; 111: 2200–7.
41. Podnar S, Lukanovic A, Vodusek DB. Anal sphincter electromyography after vaginal delivery: neuropathic insufficiency or normal wear and tear? Neurourol Urodyn 2000; 19: 249–57.
42. Podnar S, Vodusek DB. Standardization of anal sphincter electromyography: effect of chronic constipation. Muscle Nerve 2000; 23: 1748–51.
43. Podnar S. Criteria for neuropathic abnormality in quantitative anal sphincter electromyography. Muscle Nerve 2004; 30: 596–601.
44. Jameson JS, Chia YW, Kamm MA et al. Effect of age, sex and parity on anorectal function. Br J Surg 1994; 81: 1689–92.
45. Rodi Z, Denislic M, Vodusek DB. External anal sphincter electromyography in the differential diagnosis of parkinsonism. J Neurol Neurosurg Psychiatry 1996; 60: 460–1.
46. Kaiho Y, Namima T, Uchi K et al. Electromyographic study of the striated urethral sphincter by using the bulbocavernosus reflex: study on change of sacral reflex activity caused by bladder filling. Nippon Hinyokika Gakkai Zasshi 2000; 91: 715–22.
47. Sethi RK, Bauer SB, Dyro FM, Krarup C. Modulation of the bulbocavernosus reflex during voiding: loss of inhibition in upper motor neuron lesions. Muscle Nerve 1989; 12: 892–7.
48. Ertekin C, Reel F. Bulbocavernosus reflex in normal men and in patients with neurogenic bladder and/or impotence. J Neurol Sci 1976; 28: 1–15.
49. Dykstra D, Sidi A, Cameron J et al. The use of mechanical stimulation to obtain the sacral reflex latency: a new technique. J Urol 1987; 137: 77–9.
50. Loening-Baucke V, Read NW, Yamada T, Barker AT. Evaluation of the motor and sensory components of the pudendal nerve. Electroencephalogr Clin Neurophysiol 1994; 93: 35–41.
51. Basinski C, Fuller E, Brizendine EJ, Benson JT. Bladder–anal reflex. Neurourol Urodyn 2003; 22: 683–6.
52. Hansen MV, Ertekin C, Larsson LE. Cerebral evoked potentials after stimulation of the posterior urethra in man. Electroencephalogr Clin Neurophysiol 1990; 77: 52–8.
53. Rodi Z, Vodusek DB. The sacral reflex studies: single versus double pulse stimulation. Neurourol Urodyn 1995; 14: 496.
54. Amarenco G, Kerdraon J. Clinical value of ipsi- and contralateral sacral reflex latency measurement: a normative data study in man. Neurourol Urodyn 2000; 19: 565–76.
55. Amarenco G, Ismael SS, Bayle B, Kerdraon J. Dissociation between electrical and mechanical bulbocavernosus reflexes. Neurourol Urodyn 2003; 22: 676–80.
56. Hecht MJ, Neundorfer B, Kiesewetter F, Hilz MJ. Neuropathy is a major contributing factor to diabetic erectile dysfunction. Neurol Res 2001; 23: 651–4.
57. Hanson P, Rigaux P, Gilliard C, Biset E. Sacral reflex latencies in tethered cord syndrome. Am J Phys Med Rehabil 1993; 72: 39–43.
58. Bilkey WJ, Awad EA, Smith AD. Clinical application of sacral reflex latency. J Urol 1983; 129: 1187–9.
59. Podnar S, Vodusek DB, Trsinar B, Rodi Z. A method of uroneurophysiological investigation in children. Electroencephalogr Clin Neurophysiol 1997; 104: 389–92.
60. Amarenco G, Bayle B, Ismael SS, Kerdraon J. Bulbocavernosus muscle responses after suprapubic stimulation: analysis and measurement of suprapubic bulbocavernosus reflex latency. Neurourol Urodyn 2002; 21: 210–13.
61. Opsomer RJ, Caramia MD, Zarola F, Pesce F, Rossini PM. Neurophysiological evaluation of central-peripheral sensory and motor pudendal fibres. Electroencephalogr Clin Neurophysiol 1989; 74: 260–70.
62. Anon. AAEE glossary of terms in clinical electromyography. Muscle Nerve 1987; 10: G1–60.
63. Kiff ES, Swash M. Normal proximal and delayed distal conduction in the pudendal nerves of patients with idiopathic (neurogenic) faecal incontinence. J Neurol Neurosurg Psychiatry 1984; 47: 820–3.
64. Osterberg A, Edebol Eeg-Olofsson K, Graf W. Results of surgical treatment for faecal incontinence. Br J Surg 2000; 87: 1546–52.
65. Suilleabhain CB, Horgan AF, McEnroe L et al. The relationship of pudendal nerve terminal motor latency to squeeze pressure in patients with idiopathic fecal incontinence. Dis Colon Rectum 2001; 44: 666–71.
66. Brostrom S. Motor evoked potentials from the pelvic floor. Neurourol Urodyn 2003; 22: 620–37.
67. Vodusek DB, Zidar J. Perineal motor evoked responses. Neurourol Urodyn 1988; 7: 236.
68. Lefaucheur JP. Intrarectal ground electrode improves the reliability of motor evoked potentials recorded in the anal sphincter. Muscle Nerve 2005; 32: 110–12.
69. Eardley I, Nagendran K, Lecky B et al. Neurophysiology of the striated urethral sphincter in multiple sclerosis. Br J Urol 1991; 68: 81–8.
70. Bradley WE, Lin JT, Johnson B. Measurement of the conduction velocity of the dorsal nerve of the penis. J Urol 1984; 131: 1127–9.
71. Amarenco G, Kerdraon J. Pudendal nerve terminal sensitive latency: technique and normal values. J Urol 1999; 161: 103–6.
72. Deletis V, Vodusek DB, Abbott R, Epstein FJ, Turndorf H. Intraoperative monitoring of the dorsal sacral roots: minimizing the risk of iatrogenic micturition disorders. Neurosurgery 1992; 30: 72–5.
73. Ertekin C, Mungan B. Sacral spinal cord and root potentials evoked by the stimulation of the dorsal nerve of penis and cord conduction delay for the bulbocavernosus reflex. Neurourol Urodyn 1993; 12: 9–22.
74. Vodusek DB. Pudendal SEP and bulbocavernosus reflex in women. Electroencephalogr Clin Neurophysiol 1990; 77: 134–6.
75. Haldeman S, Bradley WE, Bhatia N. Evoked responses from the pudendal nerve. J Urol 1982; 128: 974–80.
76. Guerit J, Opsomer R. Bit-mapped imaging of somatosensory evoked potentials after stimulation of the posterior tibial nerves and dorsal nerve of the penis/clitoris. Electroencephalogr Clin Neurophysiol 1991; 80: 228.
77. Rodi Z, Vodusek DB, Denislic M. Clinical uro-neurophysiological investigation in multiple sclerosis. Eur J Neurol 1996; 3: 574–80.
78. Curt A, Rodic B, Schurch B, Dietz V. Recovery of bladder function in patients with acute spinal cord injury: significance of ASIA scores and somatosensory evoked potentials. Spinal Cord 1997; 35: 368–73.
79. Selcuki M, Coskun K. Management of tight filum terminale syndrome with special emphasis on normal level conus medullaris (NLCM). Surg Neurol 1998; 50: 318–22; discussion 322.
80. Delodovici ML, Fowler CJ. Clinical value of the pudendal somatosensory evoked potential. Electroencephalogr Clin Neurophysiol 1995; 96: 509–15.

81. Ganzer H, Madersbacher H, Rumpl E. Cortical evoked potentials by stimulation of the vesicourethral junction: clinical value and neurophysiological considerations. J Urol 1991; 146: 118–23.
82. Pietrangeli A, Bove L, Innocenti P et al. Neurophysiological evaluation of sexual dysfunction in patients operated for colorectal cancer. Clin Auton Res 1998; 8: 353–7.
83. Lefaucheur JP, Yiou R, Salomon L, Chopin DK, Abbou CC. Assessment of penile small nerve fiber damage after transurethral resection of the prostate by measurement of penile thermal sensation. J Urol 2000; 164: 1416–9.
84. Arunodaya GR, Taly AB. Sympathetic skin response: a decade later. J Neurol Sci 1995; 129: 81–9.
85. Opsomer RJ, Pesce F, Abi Aad A. Electrophysiologic testing of motor sympathetic pathways: normative data and clinical contribution in neurourological disorders. Neurourol Urodyn 1993; 12: 336–8.
86. Daffertshofer M, Linden D, Syren M, Junemann KP, Berlit P. Assessment of local sympathetic function in patients with erectile dysfunction. Int J Impot Res 1994; 6: 213–25.
87. Schmid DM, Reitz A, Curt A, Hauri D, Schurch B. Urethral evoked sympathetic skin responses and viscerosensory evoked potentials as diagnostic tools to evaluate urogenital autonomic afferent innervation in spinal cord injured patients. J Urol 2004; 171: 1156–60.
88. Yilmaz U, Yang CC, Berger RE. Dartos reflex: a sympathetically mediated scrotal reflex. Muscle Nerve 2006; 33: 363–8.
89. Ertekin C, Ertekin N, Mutlu S, Almis S, Akcam A. Skin potentials (SP) recorded from the extremities and genital regions in normal and impotent subjects. Acta Neurol Scand 1987; 76: 28–36.
90. Kinder MV, van Waalwijk van Doorn ES, Gommer ED, Janknegt RA. A non-invasive method for bladder electromyography in humans. Arch Physiol Biochem 1998; 106: 2–11.
91. Libelius R, Johansson F. Quantitative electromyography of the external anal sphincter in Parkinson's disease and multiple system atrophy. Muscle Nerve 2000; 23: 1250–6.
92. Tison F, Arne P, Sourgen C, Chrysostome V, Yeklef F. The value of external anal sphincter electromyography for the diagnosis of multiple system atrophy. Mov Disord 2000; 15: 1148–57.
93. Beck RO, Betts CD, Fowler CJ. Genitourinary dysfunction in multiple system atrophy: clinical features and treatment in 62 cases. J Urol 1994; 151: 1336–41.
94. Yamamoto T, Sakakibara R, Uchiyama T et al. When is Onuf's nucleus involved in multiple system atrophy? A sphincter electromyography study. J Neurol Neurosurg Psychiatry 2005; 76: 1645–8.
95. Valldeoriola F, Valls Sole J, Tolosa ES, Marti MJ. Striated anal sphincter denervation in patients with progressive supranuclear palsy. Mov Disord 1995; 10: 550–5.
96. Scaravilli T, Pramstaller PP, Salerno A et al. Neuronal loss in Onuf's nucleus in three patients with progressive supranuclear palsy. Ann Neurol 2000; 48: 97–101.
97. Giladi N, Simon ES, Korczyn AD et al. Anal sphincter EMG does not distinguish between multiple system atrophy and Parkinson's disease. Muscle Nerve 2000; 23: 731–4.
98. Sakakibara R, Hattori T, Uchiyama T et al. Urinary dysfunction and orthostatic hypotension in multiple system atrophy: which is the more common and earlier manifestation? J Neurol Neurosurg Psychiatry 2000; 68: 25.
99. Tsai PY, Cha RC, Yang TF et al. Electromyographic evaluation in children with spina bifida. Zhonghua Yi Xue Za Zhi (Taipei) 2001; 64: 509–15.
100. Fowler CJ, Kirby RS. Electromyography of urethral sphincter in women with urinary retention. Lancet 1986; 1: 1455–7.
101. Fowler CJ, Christmas TJ, Chapple CR et al. Abnormal electromyographic activity of the urethral sphincter, voiding dysfunction, and polycystic ovaries: a new syndrome? Br Med J 1988; 297: 1436–8.
102. Swinn MJ, Wiseman OJ, Lowe E, Fowler CJ. The cause and natural history of isolated urinary retention in young women. J Urol 2002; 167: 151–6.
103. Kavia RB, Datta SN, Dasgupta R, Elneil S, Fowler CJ. Urinary retention in women: its causes and management. BJU Int 2006; 97: 281–7.
104. Snooks SJ, Barnes PR, Swash M, Henry MM. Damage to the innervation of the pelvic floor musculature in chronic constipation. Gastroenterology 1985; 89: 977–81.
105. Koldewijn EL, Van Kerrebroeck PE, Bemelmans BL et al. Use of sacral reflex latency measurements in the evaluation of neural function of spinal cord injury patients: a comparison of neuro-urophysiological testing and urodynamic investigations. J Urol 1994; 152: 463–7.
106. Liu S, Christmas TJ, Nagendran K, Kirby RS. Sphincter electromyography in patients after radical prostatectomy and cystoprostatectomy. Br J Urol 1992; 69: 397–403.
107. Sau G, Siracusano S, Aiello I et al. The usefulness of the somatosensory evoked potentials of the pudendal nerve in diagnosis of probable multiple sclerosis. Spinal Cord 1999; 37: 258–63.
108. Vodusek DB. Evoked potential testing. Urol Clin North Am 1996; 23: 427–46.

44

Practical guide to diagnosis and follow-up of patients with neurogenic bladder dysfunction

Erik Schick and Jacques Corcos

Introduction

Many traumatic, congenital, tumoral, or degenerative neurological pathologies have direct consequences on vesicourethral function. Imaging techniques will give information on the anatomic and morphologic status of the urinary tract. Endoscopy will provide further information, such as mucosal appearance, small tumors, urethral stenosis, the degree of prostatic enlargement, bladder stone(s) and urethrovesical mobility in females. Urodynamics is the only diagnostic tool that allows functional evaluation of the urinary tract. It does not replace any of the other diagnostic modalities, but rather complements them. It plays a major role in therapeutic decisions and during follow-up.

Urological surveillance of patients with neurogenic bladder dysfunction in different countries has been described by only a few authors,[1–4] mainly in spinal cord injured patients. In the United States,[1] most physicians (85%) favor yearly renal ultrasound for routine surveillance of the upper urinary tract, and urodynamic studies (65%) for the evaluation of the lower urinary tract. In the United Kingdom and Eire,[2] upper urinary tract screening and urodynamics are performed from annually to every 3 years by the majority of physicians. In Japan,[3] surveillance of the urinary tract is performed on a yearly basis by almost half (46.2%) of the 333 physicians involved in the surveillance and management of spinal cord injured patients who responded to a nationwide questionnaire. The great majority (71.8%) preferred abdominal ultrasound for the upper urinary tract. In Canada,[4] 80% of urologists who treated patients with neurogenic bladder dysfunction favored yearly renal ultrasound and urodynamic studies. Table 44.1 summarizes these practice patterns. It should be noted that all authors emphasize the need for clear guidelines in this domain.

Table 44.1 *Variation in practice patterns in the urological surveillance of patients with neurogenic bladder dysfunction in five different countries*

Country	Upper tract (% of responders in agreement)	Lower tract (% of responders in agreement)
United States	Yearly ultrasound (85%)	Yearly videourodynamics (65%)
United Kingdom and Eire	Ultrasound: 1–3 years	Ultrasound: 1–3 years
Japan	Yearly renal ultrasound (71.8%)	Yearly cystometry (52.3%)
Canada	Yearly ultrasound (80%)	Yearly urodynamics (80%)

Neurogenic bladder dysfunction after trauma

Traumatic injury to the central nervous system (cerebral or spinal) is often followed by the so-called spinal shock phase (see also Chapter 16). The bladder is areflexic during this phase, which may last from 2 weeks up to 8 weeks,[5,6] but sometimes up to 1 year.[7,8] Complete urodynamic evaluation during this period is useless.[9] Intermittent catheterization is the best treatment modality.

In the case of an incomplete spinal cord lesion, the reappearance of bladder sensation will indicate the end of the

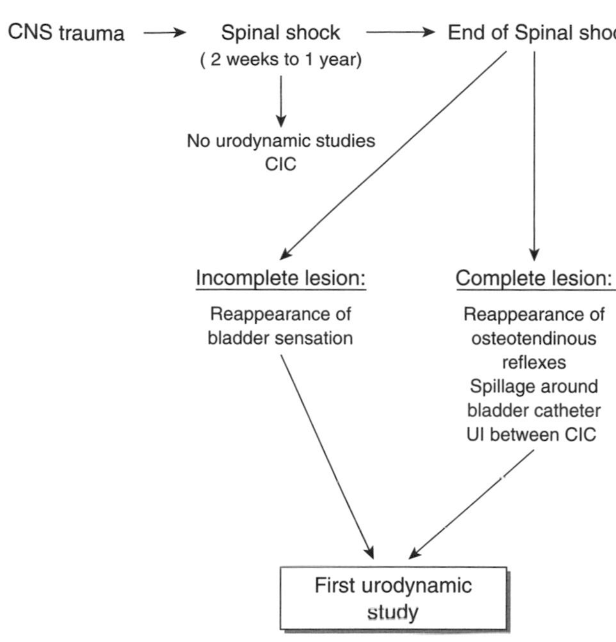

Figure 44.1
Initial evaluation and management of patients with central nervous system trauma. CNS: central nervous system; CIC: clean intermittent cathaterization; UI: urinary incontinence.

spinal shock phase. In the case of a complete lesion, the reappearance of osteotendinous reflexes, urine spillage around the urethral catheter if it was left in place, and incontinence episodes between intermittent catheterizations will suggest the presence of some kind of bladder activity. The first urodynamic evaluation is made at this time (Figure 44.1).

The site of the neurologic lesion will give some indication as to the type of neurogenic bladder function to expect. Lesions above T7 result in hyperreflexic bladder, whereas lesions at T11 or below result in areflexic bladder. Lesions between T8 and T10 constitute the 'gray zone', and can result either in hyperreflexic or areflexic bladder.[8] Vesico-sphincteric dyssynergia is more difficult to predict because only two-thirds of hyperreflexic bladders will be accompanied by dyssynergic voiding.[9]

Neurogenic bladder dysfunction after non-traumatic neurologic pathology

Usually, the urologist will see these patients with a well-defined neurologic diagnosis when urinary symptoms

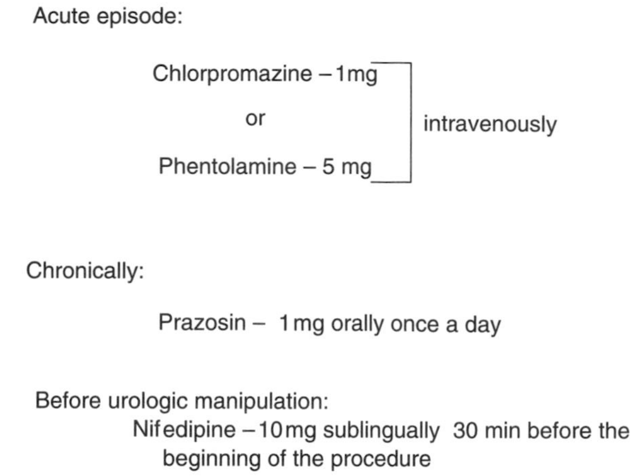

Figure 44.2
Treatment of autonomic dysreflexia.

are already present. In this case, immediate urodynamic evaluation is indicated, together with other diagnostic modalities such as urine culture, ultrasonographic imaging of the upper urinary tract, and free flowmetry, if possible.

Autonomic dysreflexia

Autonomic dysreflexia is an exaggerated sympathetic response to afferent stimulation when spinal cord injury (SCI) is at the level of T6 or above (see also Chapter 15). Acute, life threatening autonomic dysreflexic episodes can be controlled by chlorpromazine (1 mg) or phentolamine (5 mg), given intravenously.[10] On a long-term basis, chronic α adrenergic blockade in small doses, such as prazosin (1 mg daily), will be helpful.[11] Our practice is to administer nifedipine (10 mg), a calcium channel blocking agent, sublingually to patients with a potential risk of developing acute autonomic dysreflexia during urologic manipulations (e.g. endoscopy, urodynamics), 30 min before these procedures (Figure 44.2).

Renal surveillance

In a follow-up study by Donelly et al of paraplegics from World War II, renal disease was the most common cause of death in the first 20 years after the injury, accounting for 40% of all deaths.[12] More recently, in a series of 406 consecutive SCI patients followed for 15 years, Webb et al[13] reported a death rate of 0.5% (2/406) secondary from renal complications. This highlights the importance of dedicated follow-up to significantly reduce kidney-related mortality in these patients.

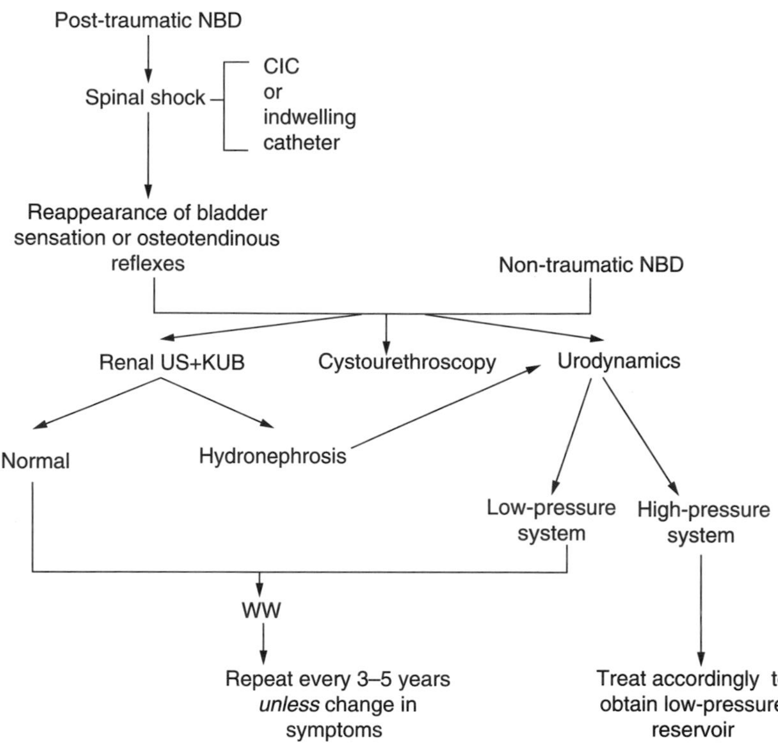

Figure 44.3
Diagnosis and follow-up of patients with neurogenic bladder dysfunction. US, ultrasound; CIC, clean intermittent catheterization; KUB, plain abdominal X-ray; NBD, neurogenic bladder dysfunction; WW, watchful waiting.

Renal ultrasound[14] combined with plain radiography of the abdomen[15] tends to replace intravenous pyelography (IVP) in upper urinary tract evaluation.[16] Color flow Doppler sonography could eventually replace retrograde cystography in the detection of vesicoureteral reflux. Papadaki et al[17] reported that color Doppler ultrasonography diagnosed all grade IV and V, 87.5% of grade III, 83.3% of grade II, and 57.4% of grade I refluxes. There were 6 false-positive and 5 false-negative findings among 187 SCI adults.

In many major SCI centers, radionuclide renograms are used for routine follow-up of renal function, instead of IVP.[10] A study by Phillips et al[18] showed that a decline in effective plasma flow was the best predictor for therapeutic intervention.

It has been our practice to obtain a renal ultrasonogram and a plain abdominal X-ray in all patients with neurogenic bladder dysfunction as part of their initial evaluation, together with urodynamic studies. The results of the latter give information on pressure conditions in the bladder. With a high-pressure system, the upper urinary tract is at high risk for deterioration, and upper tract monitoring should be more frequent (every 6–12 months). In the case of a low-pressure system, this danger is only relative, and we undertake renal ultrasound study approximately every 3–5 years if no change in clinical symptoms suggests modification of the bladder's pressure status. However, if clinical symptoms change, ultrasonography of the kidneys and urodynamic studies are repeated promptly. Figure 44.3 summarizes, in a schematic way, our initial evaluation and follow-up of patients with neurogenic bladder dysfunction.

Urodynamics

Urodynamics are cornerstones in the diagnosis and management of neurogenic bladder dysfunction. In this respect, the main parameters that require special attention are high detrusor pressure during the filling or storage phase of he bladder (decreased bladder wall compliance and/or sustained detrusor contraction), and detrusor-external sphincter dyssynergia during micturition. (The problem of compliance has been detailed in Chapter 13 and that of detrusor-sphincter dyscoordination in Chapter 14.) Well-conducted, multichannel (video)urodynamic evaluation will highlight these conditions and consequently allow the initiation of appropriate therapeutic measures that should ultimately transform a high-pressure system to a low-pressure system.

Endoscopy

Cystourethroscopy is an essential part of the initial evaluation of all patients with neurogenic bladder dysfunction.

It allows visualization of anatomic urethral occlusion, especially in the male. It should be emphasized that there is a fundamental difference between occlusion and obstruction. Urethral occlusion means a more or less pronounced change in urethral caliber, such as a fibrotic stricture. This can be diagnosed endoscopically. In contrast, obstruction is a dynamic concept, which, from the hydrodynamic point of view and simplified to some extent,[19] essentially means a 'high-pressure–low-flow' relationship. This can be diagnosed by urodynamics. Benign prostatic enlargement illustrates the relationship between the two concepts. Endoscopically, one can observe a protrusion of the lateral lobes of the prostate into the urethral lumen, joining each other on the midline. From this picture, however, it is not possible to extrapolate how the detrusor will contract, and how the urethra will relax to allow voiding to take place. In other words, one cannot estimate to what extent this prostatic enlargement will interfere with flow and be responsible for an eventual obstruction.

In the female, the best chance to visualize stress incontinence is to ask the patient to cough when the bladder has reached its cystometric capacity, at the end of the cystoscopic examination. Also, the best condition to evaluate the bladder neck hypermobility is when the bladder is completely empty.

In both sexes, bladder wall trabeculation suggests an overactive bldder, rather than outlet obstruction (see also Chapter 36).

References

1. Razdan S, Leboeuf L, Meinbach DS, Weinstein D, Gousse AE. Current practice patterns in the urologic surveillance and management of patients with spinal cord injury. Urology 2003; 61: 893–6.
2. Bycroft J, Hamid R, Bywater H, Patki P, Shah J. Variation in urological practice amongst spinal injuries unites in the UK and Eire. Neurourol Urodyn 2004; 23: 252–6.
3. Kitahara S, Iwatsubo E, Yasuda K et al. Practice patterns of Japanese physicians in urologic surveillance and management of spinal cord injury patients. Spinal Cord 2006; 44: 362–8.
4. Blok BF, Karsenty G, Corcos J. Urological surveillance and management of patients with neurogenic bladder: results of a survey among practicing urologists in Canada. Can J Urol 2006; 13: 3239–43.
5. Light JK, Faganel J, Beric A. Detrusor areflexia in suprasacral spinal cord injuries. J Urol 1985; 134: 295–7.
6. Chancellor MB, Kiilholma P. Urodynamic evaluation of patients following spinal cord injury. Semin Urol 1992; 10: 83–94.
7. Wheeler JS Jr, Walter JW. Acute urologic management of the patient with spinal cord injury: initial hospitalisation. Urol Clin N Am 1993; 20: 403–11.
8. Perlow DL, Diokno AC. Predicting lower urinary tract dysfunctions in patients with spinal cord injury. Urology 1981; 18: 531–5.
9. Chancellor MB. Urodynamic evaluation after spinal cord injury. Phys Med Rehab Clin N Am 1993; 4: 273–98.
10. Chancellor MB, Blaivas JG. Spinal cord injury. In: Chancellor MB, Blaivas JG, eds. Practical neurourology. Boston: Butterworth-Heinemann, 1995: 99–118.
11. McGuire EJ. Immediate management of the inability to void. In: Parsons FK, Fitzpatrick JM, eds. Practical Urology in Spinal Cord Injury. London: Springer Verlag, 1991: 5–10.
12. Donelly J, Hackler RH, Bunts RC. Present urologic status of the World War II paraplegic: 25-year follow-up. Comparison with status of the 20-year Korean War paraplegic and the 5-year Vietnam paraplegic. J Urol 1972; 108: 558–62.
13. Webb DR, Fitzpatrick JM, O'Flynn JD. A 15-year follow-up of 406 consecutive spinal cord injuries. Br J Urol 1984; 56: 614–17.
14. Bodley R. Imaging in chronic spinal cord injury – indications and benefits. Eur J Radiol 2002; 42: 135–53.
15. Morcos SK, Thomas DG. A comparison of real-time ultrasonography with intravenous urography in the follow-up of patients with spinal cord injury. Clin Radiol 1988; 39: 49–50.
16. Chagnon S, Vallée C, Laissy JP, Blery M. Ultrasonographic evaluation of the urinary tract in patients with spinal cord injuries. Systematic comparison with intravenous urography in 50 cases. J Radiol (Paris) 1985; 66: 801–6.
17. Papdaki PJ, Vlychou MK, Zavras GM et al. Investigation of vesicoureteral reflux with colour Doppler sonography in adult patients with spinal cord injury. Eur Radiol 2002; 12: 366–70.
18. Phillips JP, Jadvar H, Sullivan G et al. Effect of radionuclide renograms on treatment of patients with spinal cord injury. Am J Roentgenol 1997; 169: 1045–7.
20. Kranse R, van Mastrigt R. Relative bladder outlet obstruction. J Urol 2002; 168: 565–70.

Part V

Classification

45

Classification of lower urinary tract dysfunction

Anders Mattiasson

Introduction

A system of classification lives only as long as it is generally perceived to correspond to the reality it is intended to describe. The need to revise it is thus present on a continuous basis. The current classification system for disorders and terminology in the lower urinary tract[1–3] needs to be revised.[4] The new approach described herein does not represent any generally accepted system, but rather is a proposal for a new manner in which to view the reality. It is rooted in disorder/illness processes and injuries being described in terms of structure and function and not, as previously (and presently), primarily in terms of consequential effects such as symptoms. Actually, we should be speaking of lower urinary tract disorders. Dysfunction in fact describes only one half of the structure + function pair. We should also be quite aware that a classification that we use as researchers due to, among other things, pedagogical reasons, must ultimately be separated from the one which we in the capacity of caregivers use in contact with, for example, the patients.

In this chapter the general classification of lower urinary tract disorders comprises the subject matter, and thus does not specifically deal with the present system for classification of neurogenic disorders, since this is presented in Parts II and III. A consistent and uniform way of looking at things comprises the basis of a functioning classification system. What one chooses as the basis for the system is in fact of crucial significance. In most of the other fields of medicine, illnesses and injuries are described in pathophysiologic terms. So the case ought to be the same on the part of the lower urinary tract. Hence, it is difficult to maintain a system that is based upon a description of the circumstances for the genesis of different forms of urinary incontinence. In certain cases it is the patient's subjective experiences that are the point of departure, such as with urge and so-called overactive bladder, whereas physical exertion or stress is the point of departure in other cases. Instead, it is more constructive to describe how the tissues and organs are engaged on different levels in terms of structure and function (S + F) right down to the cell and molecular biology level, and to then describe what the consequences are that give rise to symptoms and difficulties and other conceivable consequential effects.[4] This can be illustrated as in Figure 45.1.

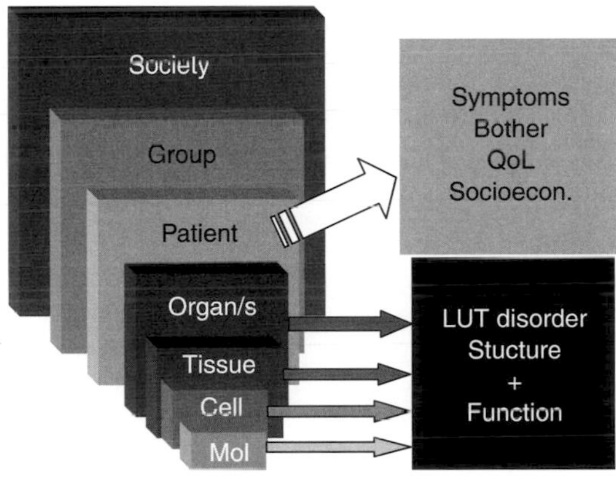

Figure 45.1
Lower urinary tract disorders are best described in pathophysiologic terms of structure and function. Symptoms and bother are secondary phenomena, and therefore not as suitable for the primary classification. QoL, quality of life; Socioecon., socioeconomics; Mol, molecule.

By deciding to use S + F as a basis for a classification system, a decision has been made once and for all as far as it concerns this system precisely. All divisions and categorizations must then, in its continuation, also fit in with each other in the holistic spirit described above. Structure and function are different ways of regarding and expressing the same thing. Complete covariance can be presumed to exist in a well-balanced situation. Structural changes do not occur without altered functionality and vice versa.

This is how the situation appears in a simple system (Figure 45.2). When multiple tissues and multiple organs are connected together, as in the lower urinary tract, new

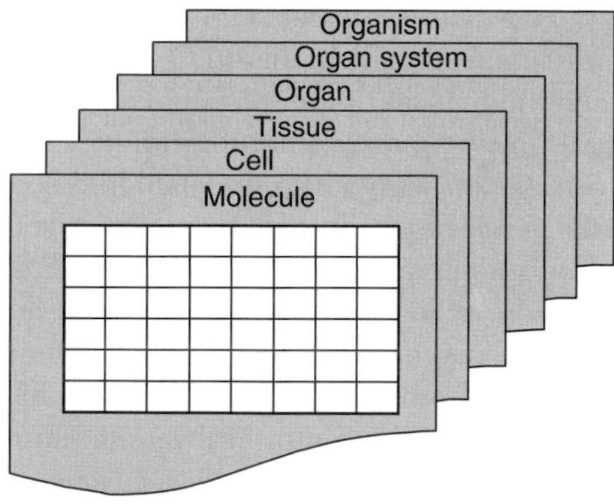

Figure 45.2
All levels and all parts of the lower urinary tract and its innervation can be included in one matrix.

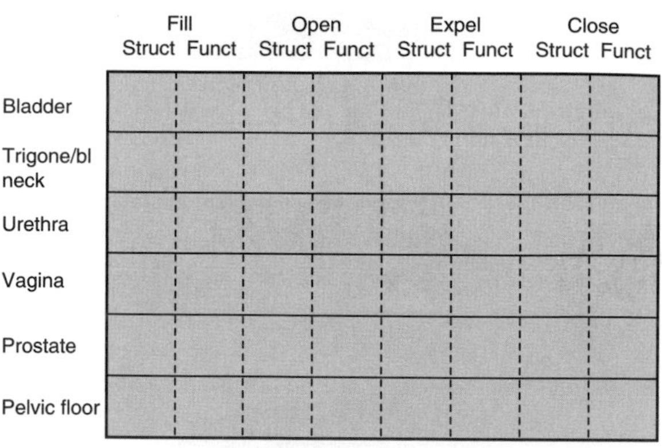

Figure 45.3
When all parts of the lower urinary tract and the whole micturition cycle are characterized regarding both structure and function, the result will be a complete recognition pattern.

conditions arise, where the different parts come to influence each other. In reality, they are all part of a balanced situation intended to fulfill the task of storing and evacuating urine, and an imbalance in one of the parts inexorably comes to have an effect on the other component parts. The lower urinary tract acts as a single functional unit.

All of the different parts of the micturition cycle and the different components of the lower urinary tract cannot, however, be included in a fully comprehensive classification system without them being represented at all levels. This is especially important as the lower urinary tract contains within itself functions that are diametrically opposed in every individual part, i.e. in a part of the micturition cycle optimized for storage and in a different part for emptying. In such a case it is important to capture all these parts as well as the transition forms between them. Hence not only should the bladder, trigone/bladder neck, and urethra be included but also the vagina, prostate, pelvic floor, as well as all the different types of supporting structures. Vessels and nerves have not been mentioned, but are included of course, and strictly speaking the parts of the nervous system involved must also be included in order to form a whole (Figure 45.3).

The micturition cycle

The classification and thus the description of lower urinary tract disturbances is directly dependent on where one finds oneself in the micturition cycle. Due to the filling and discharge functions being so intimately intertwined, it is often difficult to distinguish which signals are related to what parts of the urinary tract. For example, during filling of the bladder, activity including detrusor contractions can arise too early. This is in fact activity that is characteristic of

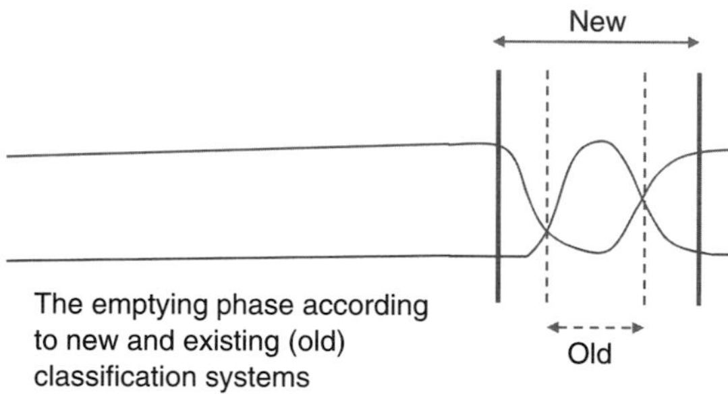

Figure 45.4
When the pressure changes of the bladder and the urethra before and after the expulsion of urine are both included in the emptying phase, this also means that the storage and the emptying phases of the micturition cycle have been redefined.

emptying that appears here during filling. How should this be classified – as storage-related or emptying-related? To do this, the initial point of departure must be fixed. Since the functional status of the lower urinary tract changes in step with the filling and emptying, we must have multiple well-defined points of departure. These actually differ from one another, and collectively represent the entire micturition cycle. The activity that belongs in the different phases can be represented graphically with a simple sketch (Figure 45.4) that depicts the pressure conditions in the bladder and urethra during the different parts of the micturition cycle.

It is logical to make a new division of the micturition cycle in such a manner that the emptying also encompasses the short transitions between storage and evacuation. It is of course precisely at their beginning and ending, respectively, that the storage pattern is broken. The commencement of micturition concerns the direct preparations for

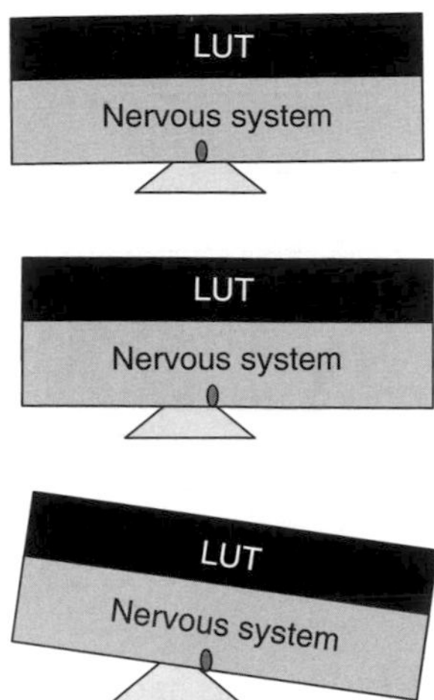

Figure 45.5
The lower urinary tract (LUT) and the nervous system are balancing each other. All parts influence each other. The system becomes more labile with increasing filling of the bladder (triangle). A disturbance can be balanced out, i.e. a disorder can be present without causing any symptoms.

emptying, such as the pressure drop in the urethra that takes place during the flow of urine itself. This also applies for the cessation of micturition when the pressure conditions are restored after the flow has ended. The entire storage phase is then governed by a picture that in itself is dynamic, but which in terms of pressure is essentially constant. It is an important and critical point in the micturition cycle when diametrically opposed functions, in contrast to those that have been prevailing, normally for a number of hours, need to be established in order to perform the emptying. The storage-to-emptying turning point is quite important and it has been proposed that it be given an identity of its own, namely the 'SE turn'.

The balance between the lower urinary tract and the nervous system

The lower urinary tract and the parts of the nervous system involved in the micturition cycle balance each other in a purposeful manner independently of the functional phase (Figure 45.5). They are so intimately associated that they can be regarded as the partners in a marriage, i.e. a unit in which both parts are needed to a similar degree. In the classification system that is based upon structure and function, no distinction is drawn between the lower urinary tract and the nervous structures involved.

During the storage phase, an adjustment occurs in the bladder wall for the increasing volume without any appreciable rise in pressure. Nevertheless, the afferent input increases and gradually increasing activity can be read in, for example, the external sphincter in step with the filling of the bladder. Continence is preserved at the bladder neck level, i.e. a low-pressure system for closure. In connection with exertion, activation of the pelvic floor and compression of the urethra become significant factors in the maintenance of continence. Somatic and adrenergic innervation of striated and smooth musculature are the most influential neuromuscular mechanisms of the closure function. The afferent nerve activity gradually seems to increase with the filling of the bladder, whereas efferent cholinergic innervation via the pelvic nerves is regarded as being inhibited during the bladder's filling phase.

A special situation exists in the lower urinary tract in the manner in which mechanisms are activated to guarantee the shutting off of the outflow and urethra, and thus continence, at the same rate as which a preparedness is also built up to be able to open up precisely these structures instantaneously. One cannot rule out the possibility that the activation of the continence-preserving external urethral sphincter leads to an activation of afferent pathways which have an inhibitory effect in the spinal cord and on the pelvic nerves. When the contraction in the sphincter is voluntarily released on command from higher centers, inhibitory influence that prevents the activation of the micturition reflex disappears, and activation with accompanying opening of the outflow tract can occur. With such an arrangement, the apparently paradoxical arrangement with the simultaneous building up of activity that promotes both filling and emptying would appear to be both possible and easily explained.

Upon initiation of emptying, a significant change occurs in the nervous and muscular activity. The outflow tract and the urethra must be opened and bladder contraction initiated. Positive feedback must be established and maintained all the way to complete bladder emptying. In order to cause the opening of the intermediate segment and the external sphincter, the stimulation of the smooth and striated muscle contraction that participates in the closure is minimized, i.e. adrenergic and somatic nervous activity is inhibited. At the same time, a contraction probably occurs of certain muscle fibers in order for the funneling of the outflow tract to be able to take place. In addition, relaxation-mediating substances are released to ensure an open outflow tract and the least possible resistance. The bladder contraction is certainly effectuated primarily under cholinergic influence; however, other substances do seem to be of significance, particularly with functional disorders. We also know that altered activity in C fibers in the bladder is significant in the process of increased activation of the entire system that takes place as a preparation for emptying. This is perhaps also significant for normal functioning, even though the perception has long been that the C fibers are normally tacit.

This switching between diametrically different functional states has spawned the 'on-and-off' concept. For individual structures and functions, it works well for describing a course of events. However, the whole is comprised of a number of on-and-off pairs, which do not operate in step with each other; hence, the designation ceases to be appropriate. When one adds that simultaneously exciting and inhibiting influences on nerves and/or muscles seem to be typical for different parts of the lower urinary tract during both filling and emptying, one understands why on-and-off can only be used to describe the occurrence of reciprocity in itself, not the course of events in the lower urinary tract.

It is possible to say, as shown in Figure 45.5, that the degree of instability in the system increases with an increasing degree of bladder filling. Under normal circumstances the system is of course in balance; however, in the event of illness/injury the main focus is displaced, albeit with retained balance, i.e. without any signs of any disorder. It is thus not always the case that this imbalance is synonymous with symptoms presenting themselves. For example, with a bladder outlet obstruction, reduced detrusor functionality can arise secondarily to the outlet obstruction without the individual experiencing any symptoms. The same applies of course with other types of disruptions. When the disease process proceeds or when the system is provoked, e.g. through an increasing degree of bladder filling, an imbalance arises.

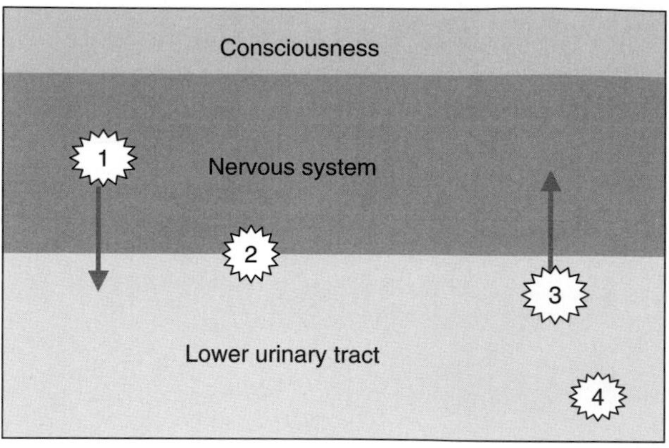

Figure 45.6
Different types of lower urinary tract disorders and their relation to the nervous system (see also Figure 45.7).

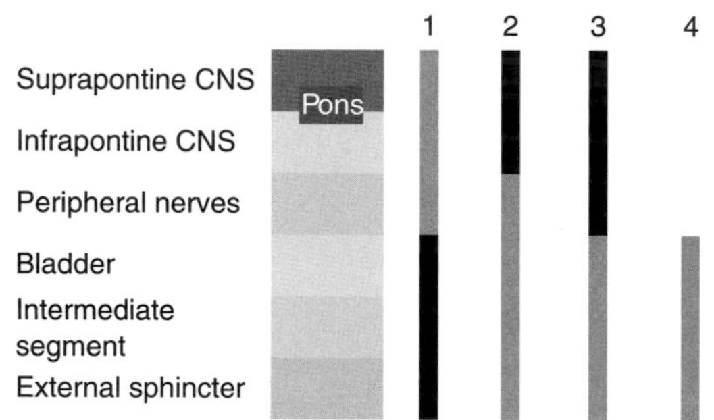

Figure 45.7
Different types of lower urinary tract disorders and their relation to the nervous system (see also Figure 45.6).
Light bars refer to primary site of disorder/lesion, dark bars to secondary involvement. 1, primary neurogenic;
2, partly neurogenic, primary; 3, secondarily neurogenic;
4, non-neurogenic, LUT.

Classification according to involvement of the nervous system

In principle it can be said that all disruptions that give rise to symptoms have a neurogenic component. The center for the perception of the illness/injury is, of course, also involved, since it is located in the same nervous system on a slightly higher level, and there, among other things, it contains the consciousness (Figure 45.6).

If the disorder/injury has its origin purely in the nervous system (1), the disruption can be regarded as primarily neurogenic; however, as soon as the lower urinary tract becomes involved it then contains both a neurogenic as well as a LUT component. The situation is the same with disorders and injuries that engage the lower urinary tract itself, i.e. most often they are both neurogenic and LUT primarily at the same time, i.e. partly neurogenic and partly LUT.

Partly neurogenic disorders usually involve a loss – e.g. neuromuscular injuries with female disorders – whereas secondary neurogenic usually means compensation – e.g. with BPH and outlet obstruction.

Disorder, consequences, and comorbidity

Primary LUT disorders can thus be non-neurogenic or partly neurogenic. Those that are partly neurogenic encompass a pathophysiologic process/lesion which probably rarely stops with this, but rather due to the presence of the disease process changes will appear both in it and in the tissues/organ that is affected, in this case the lower urinary tract. Precisely because the lower urinary tract is so closeknit functionally and morphologically, processes which injure a part of it will often ultimately also damage the whole. Figure 45.8 shows how different

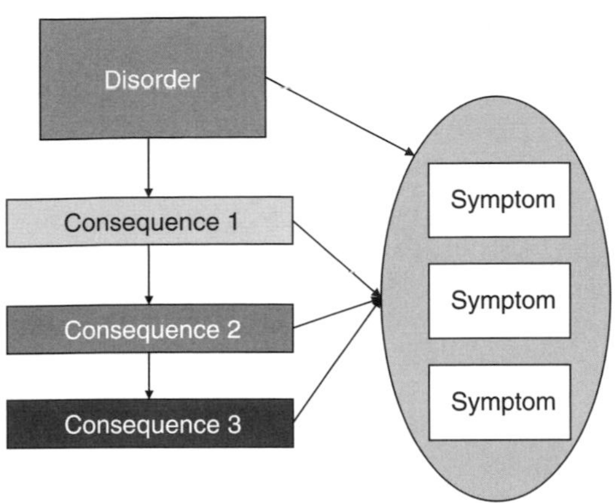

Figure 45.8
In a given clinical situation it is often unclear from what part of the pathophysiologic process that symptoms emanate.

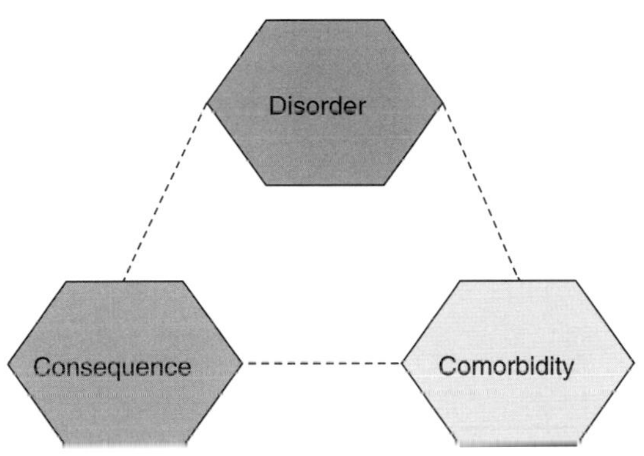

Figure 45.9
The interdependence of the disorder, its consequences, and the influence from other disease processes.

factors can be related in an entire chain, and that an individual symptom can be difficult to connect clinically to a certain factor.

Complicating factors are often logically intertwined with the disorder, even if the link may be latent. With comorbidity, the situation is, however, slightly different. Many of the changes which engage the organism as a whole, or of other organ systems, can affect the lower urinary tract and either initiate dysfunctional conditions on their own, or in conjunction with other causes, or affect a previously existing illness process (Figure 45.9). An example of a situation where difficulties can exist in reading what contributes to an illness picture is an outflow obstruction with BPH as well as simultaneous metabolic factors, possibly with an influence on the autonomous innervation of the lower urinary tract.

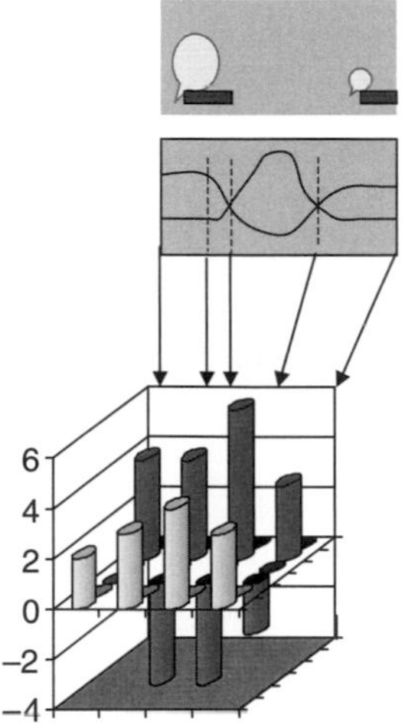

Figure 45.10
A simulated three-dimensional recognition pattern can reflect the influence of the disorder and its consequences, i.e. the impact on the lower urinary tract in different parts of the micturition cycle. Arbitrary scale.

Patterns of recognition

In theory, one can collect information on structure and functionality as measurements of different types in all parts of the lower urinary tract during all parts of the micturition cycle (Figure 45.10).

By illustrating this graphically on a simulated three-dimensional display, different disorder conditions are recognizable by their distinctive features, i.e. as patterns of recognition. Information on completely normal individuals of both genders and at different ages would serve as a reference. An example of a pattern of recognition is shown in Figure 45.10. At present it is not possible to work with such an abundance of detail; however, the largest and most important of the parts must represent the whole. It then is advantageous to seek to attain a degree of representation for different levels in the lower urinary tract and its functions. To include the bladder and external sphincter seems quite natural, but so does including the parts that play a central role in the pressure-changing phases, i.e. the trigone, bladder neck, and proximal urethra. Since we do not know precisely the details of the functional contributions of these structures to low-pressure shutting during storage and funneling as well as pressure decreases during emptying, we can amalgamate them into an intermediate segment with intermediate functionality.

Figure 45.11 illustrates three parts – the external sphincter, the intermediate segment, and the bladder – for a normal man (a) and woman (c) as well as during emptying with the unisex picture A′C′. Figure 45.11b shows how the prostate has a negative influence on the dynamics of the intermediate segment and also how the lumen is restricted

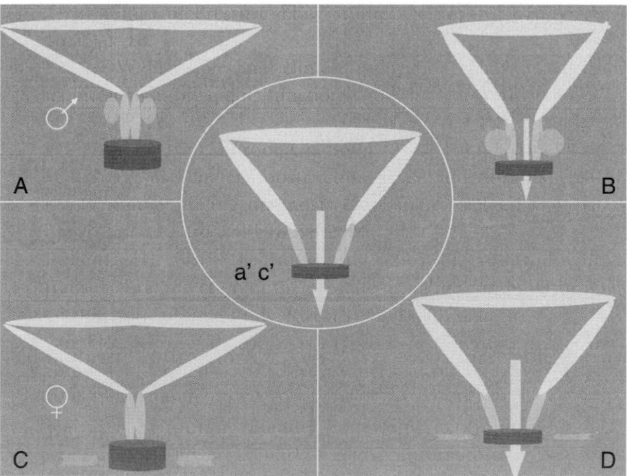

Figure 45.11
A simplified, reduced model of the lower urinary tract, introducing the intermediate segment. Three essential components – the bladder, the intermediate segment, and the external sphincter – of the lower urinary tract in both men and women are in this model. To this can be added the pelvic floor in the female and the prostate in the male. Further explanations are given in the text.

by adenomas with a reduced flow of urine as a consequence, whereas Figure 45.11d shows how it can appear with incontinent women, i.e. with a higher flow than normal.

A harmonic micturition cycle?

Lower urinary tract functionality in women with incontinence appears to be characterized by diminished outflow resistance and more efficient emptying than normal, whereas increased resistance and more difficult emptying as well as a changed voiding pattern seem to be typical for men with an outlet obstruction. One could say that it is easier for women to trigger emptying as a consequence of the decline in neuromuscular functionality, whereas for men it is easier to trigger and more difficult to empty due to the appearance of an obstruction. Even if both men and women show altered innervation as an element of these changes, the synchronization between the different component parts is still preserved. With such harmonic disorders the fundamental pattern of the micturition cycle is actually preserved. Even if overactivity, obstructions, or dislocations – via, for example, provocations – occur, the synchronization still continues to be maintained.

However, with disharmonic conditions, this pattern is broken such that simultaneously occurring activities in different parts of the lower urinary tract functionally oppose each other, resulting for example in an unsettled filling phase or more difficult emptying with an obstruction. This is first and foremost characteristic of many primarily neurogenic disturbances. With central neurogenic disruptions, the picture is dominated by mass motor behavior, dyssynergy, and overactivity. With peripheral neurogenic and mixed disruptions there is usually a lower degree of activity, synergy more often than not, and both overactivity and underactivity are common occurrences. Disharmonic disruptions can arise without any form of micturition reflex, with pathologic reflexes, and range to being with normal reflexes. The activity can thus at times arise unexpectedly during a part of the micturition cycle where it should normally not occur, such as overactivity. If this is synchronized with other parts so that the result, for example, becomes a premature micturition reflex, then it has a completely different clinical significance than if it were to appear to be unsynchronized and a bladder contraction takes place for a discharge that does not participate in the opening up, or which even actively shuts, as with detrusor-sphincter dyssynergy. Harmonic and disharmonic disruptions can thus be designated as synchronous or asynchronous.

By far the most disruptions that are not primarily neurogenic are characterized by overactivity. Even if sensory overactivity is important, it is the efferent motor overactivity that receives most of our attention. We prefer to view the bladder during filling and the urethra and outlet during emptying as being passive; then we contrast our perception of the functional condition with the conspicuous activity that they both show during emptying and filling, respectively. This is a way of looking at it that leads to errors in terms of classification. The bladder is characterized, like the outlet and urethra, by both activity and passivity simultaneously during both filling and emptying. To then attribute to solely the more obvious and visible parts of these many different activities the epithet 'active' or 'overactive' does not lead to a firm foundation for classification: that not only excitation and contraction but also an inhibitory nervous influence can be designated to be an activity is in a way easy to comprehend.

Time-related changes

As mentioned above, when a disorder process finds a foothold, completely regardless of whether it is spreading itself or not, it leads to changes in other parts of the lower urinary tract by affecting the balance. As time goes on, this imbalance grows if new balancing factors do not counterbalance the changes. Step by step those parts which are situated at the levels above the illness/injury become involved. Usually it is chronic conditions with a time scale spanning decades (Figure 45.12).

Trophic-structural changes are the rule, and are usually most pronounced in individuals who have higher degrees of obstruction and/or overactivity.[5] With women, it primarily involves, simply put, what is being lost; with men,

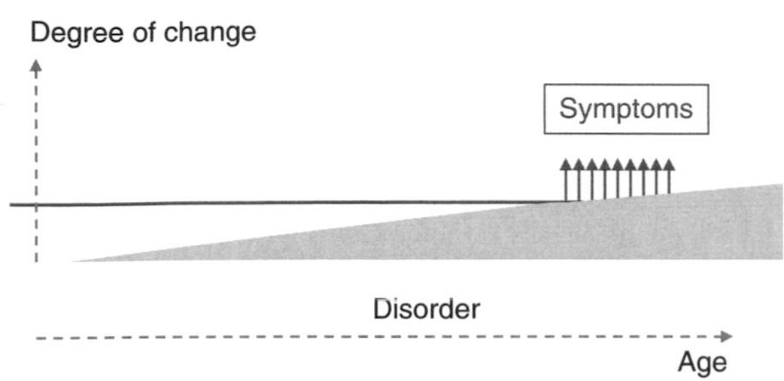

Figure 45.12
Nonmalignant disorders of the lower urinary tract often develop slowly over considerable periods of time.

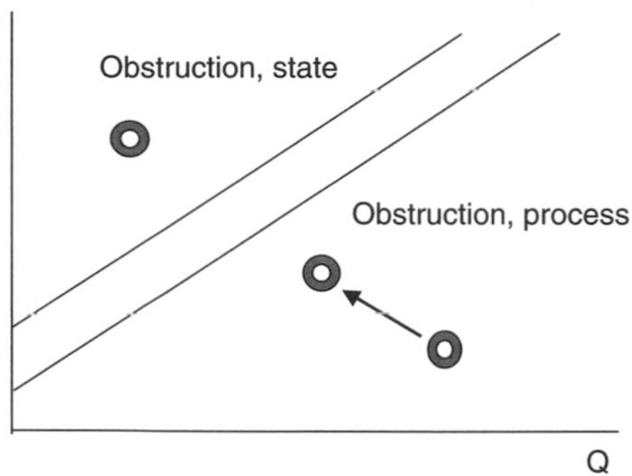

Figure 45.13
Obstruction is presently defined as illustrated in the upper left part of this nomogram from the International Continence Society (ICS). Obstruction can, however, also be a process over time, with a change in the direction of recognized obstruction.

what is being added; and with neurogenic disturbances, what is being reorganized. So, in addition to effects on the dynamics of the intermediate segment, a mechanical effect on the lumen of the urethra, and a certain flow limitation, a changed prostate also has effects on the bladder and therewith the nervous system. If no progress occurs in the primary process, growth in the secondarily arising changes will probably still occur. When remedying a problem in the lower urinary tract it is thus important that one can take hold of the problem by the root: i.e. don't treat problems that are related to the influence of the bladder first of all, but remedy the negative influence of the prostate on the urethra and the intermediate segment as the first priority. Although this is probably self-evident, it nevertheless deserves to be mentioned in this context.

The process that leads to female incontinence, and which probably often has begun with trauma in connection with childbirth, is chronic and progressive in its nature, bringing, e.g., post-polio syndrome to mind. Functional disturbances in the lower urinary tract are nearly always chronic conditions that cannot always be reversed, just compensated for, and naturally in the best case can even be prevented. Changes conditioned by the age of the organism must also be added to the pathophysiologic process.

Bladder outlet obstruction

Bladder outlet obstruction (BOO) usually develops slowly, i.e. over many years.[5,6] It is much more common among men and mainly involves an impediment in the bladder neck and/or prostate.[7] An altered micturition pattern typically occurs, both with regard to the distribution of the instances of micturition during the day as well as to the characteristics of the individual instance of emptying in terms of how quickly and efficiently the emptying is initiated and carried out. We can also see how a pattern in the development of the obstruction picture grows over time as being to a large extent dependent upon the reaction to the impediment, i.e. the lower urinary tract above the impediment and the nervous system reacting to the occurrence of a downstream obstruction to emptying.[8] The outflow resistance may be constant, but the reaction may become variable over time. Using current obstruction classification techniques, a clear discrepancy exists between the symptom picture that the patient reports and the findings of examinations we make with, for example, urodynamics in the form of pressure–flow measurements,[9,10] probably because our formula for obstruction is far too simplified. Factors that are related to an elevated urethral resistance ought to be complemented with a number of additional factors, as set out below.

The development of an obstruction usually involves successively more difficult emptying. The point in time of establishment is difficult to determine, as is obvious in an illustration of obstruction as a process besides the static condition we use for classification of obstruction today (Figure 45.13). In the typical case, an obstruction is a progressive process, and the development itself of an impediment is part of this process, i.e. a part of the obstruction; therefore, we must also include these circumstances in the new equation in order to describe impediments to evacuation of the bladder.

The obstruction can be characterized in different ways, depending upon where in the development cycle of the reaction to this change one finds oneself (Figure 45.14). Obstruction is not only equal to an increased urethral resistance, as with prostate adenoma or the like, but also changes in the level of the bladder neck, which in such cases can either be isolated or occur together with, for example, BPH (Figure 45.15).

An obstruction below the external sphincter as with, for example, a urethral stricture gives a different clinical picture than the one which appears when the bladder outflow and external sphincter are engaged. With a stricture, features of irritative symptoms such as urgency, etc., are

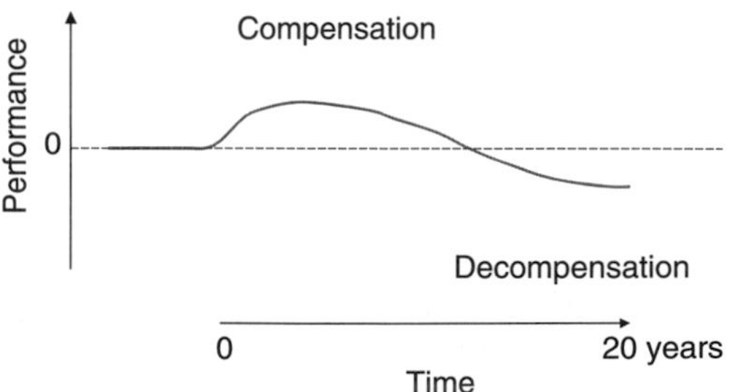

Figure 45.14
Given a certain increased, but over time unchanged, urethral outlet resistance, changes that are induced in the bladder, the nervous system, and in vessels can contribute to compensation with detrusor pressure increase during contraction, etc., in an early phase. One of the consequences of this changed function and the following remodeling of the bladder wall will be a decreased performance at comparable levels later during this process, and thus a decompensation.

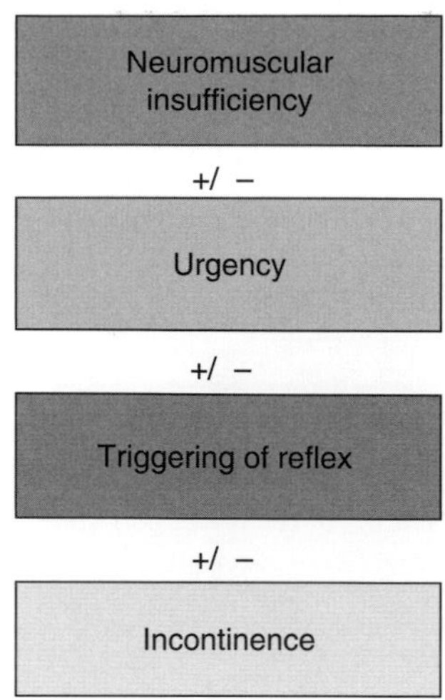

Figure 45.16
A neuromuscular insufficiency in the lower urinary tract might be present in many more women than those being incontinent. Urgency, overactivity, and incontinence might or might not be present. The relation between different types of female incontinence might be better understood.

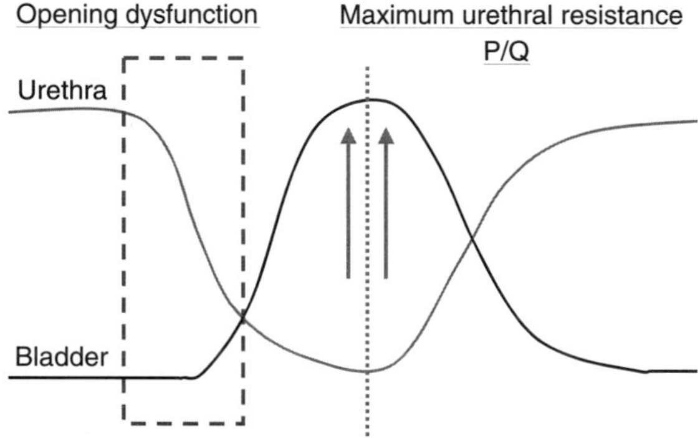

Figure 45.15
The increased detrusor pressure and the decreased urinary flow rate (not shown) used to reflect an outlet obstruction is only representing the moment of maximum performance, which means that an impediment of the opening function might only be caught and classified as an obstruction when we have included any hindrance to the emptying phase (shown as 'New' in Figure 45.4) in our definition of obstruction.

seldom seen, whereas this is common with more proximal obstructive processes.

Female incontinence

That the relationships between different female incontinence groups using the currently prevailing classification system, which of course builds upon the stress, urge, mixed, and overactivity terminology, have not become clearer over the years is certainly related to an insufficient knowledge of the structure and functionality of the underlying disorder processes, and thus the possibility of making comparisons.[11]

Neuromuscular insufficiency, triggering of normal or pathologic reflex activity with or without sensations of urgency, and possible occurrences of incontinence can be described with the simple schedule illustrated in Figure 45.16. More detailed investigations of the different groups, particularly of the urethra and the pelvic floor, have in recent years only managed to move the different incontinence groups closer to each other.[12,13] Changes which they share include a weakness in the musculature of the urethra, pelvic floor, and vaginal wall, which should have a closing effect during stress, and a – possibly of reactive origin – faster establishment of the opening phase and more effective emptying pattern during micturition. A swift activation of emptying seems to be present, which involves a lowering of the pressure in the urethra. This pattern seems to be just as common in incontinent women without urgency, i.e. those that must be classified under stress incontinence using the current terminology.

What could such observations then mean for the classification of disorder(s) eventually leading to female incontinence? One cannot rule out that such opening activity comprises one, and perhaps the foremost, of the least common denominators for different types of female incontinence.[14] Stress incontinence would then not only be composed of a passive component with insufficient closure due to imperfect contraction during stress but also have an active component in the form of a relaxation, a pressure drop, and opening of the urethra in the same situations.

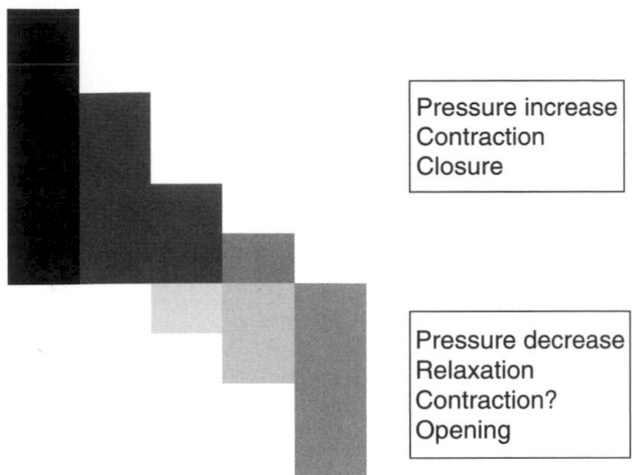

Figure 45.17
The ability to increase the urethral pressure during squeeze seems to also prevent pressure fall and urethral relaxation, whereas incontinent women who often have a reduced ability to increase the intraurethral pressure also present with a urethral relaxation. (Reproduced with permission from Teleman et al.[13])

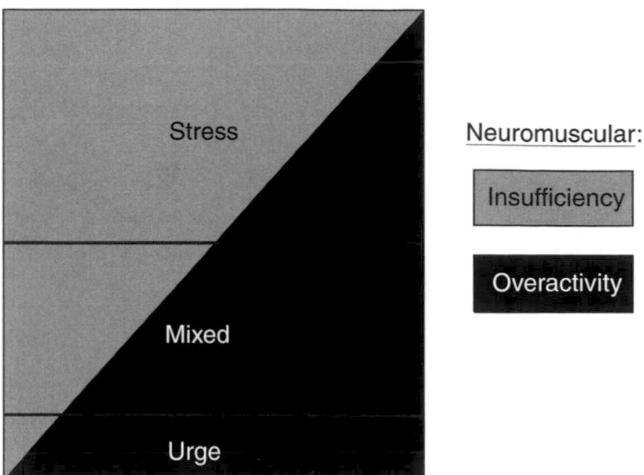

Figure 45.18
A combination of neuromuscular insufficiency and overactive behavior of the lower urinary tract could be a better way than stress, urge, and mixed to describe the condition giving rise to incontinence in women.

Such easily triggered relaxation activity that is associated with urgency would become classified in our present system as overactive bladder or mixed and urge incontinence, depending upon whether the leakage needs to be triggered with physical exertion and whether urge sensations are present or not. In contrast, using the pathophysiologic process for classification would in its functional part instead be characterized by a loss of the functionality in closing abilities of the musculature and reveal the penetration of a relaxation-mediating component in a manner that is illustrated by a movement from left to right in Figure 45.17.

To bring together a new model that builds upon the simultaneous occurrence of neuromuscular insufficiency and an increased tendency for activation of emptying-encouraging mechanisms with the traditional stress, mixed, and urge model would give a result that looks like Figure 45.18.

Increased lower urinary tract activity

There are many different types of overactivity.[15] All possible nervous activity and a set of different transmitters or so-called neuromodulators can play important roles in the generation of overactivity. Solely afferent overactivity with a sensory experience connected to it does exist. Solely efferent overactivity is somewhat more difficult to imagine; however, we certainly all believe that it is possible that purely efferential mechanisms can have an influence on, for example, reflex arches and cause overactivity to arise. Combinations are common. Afferent overactivity is probably driving the process in by far the most cases. It is worthwile to remember that a lower urinary tract that is disconnected from a functional context, i.e. without the passage of urine, does not make a nuisance of itself if complicating factors such as infections do not arise.

One often speaks of the significance of neurogenic and myogenic factors. It is important to map out both nerves and muscles; however, without the presence and contribution of both, there will not be much coordinated activity. Isolated myogenic activity with tonus and tension effects on the walls of the lower urinary tract can be found despite this.

Significant trophic changes are often a part of the pathophysiologic process in functional lower urinary tract disorders. This is quite natural since structure and functionality go hand-in-hand. At the same time, it is worth noting that the prerequisites for pliability in this case seem particularly large, as nerves and muscles appear to interact: e.g. through the production and influence of nerve-stimulating growth factors.

Since the pattern of overactivity with a pressure drop in the urethra which immediately precedes the rise in bladder pressure is the same as what one sees at the onset of micturition, it appears reasonable to presume that the sequence of events is the same in both situations (Figure 45.19). If such is the case, then one can also characterize the overactivity as LUT instead of detrusor, since all parts of the lower urinary tract seem to be engaged. In addition, it is certainly more precise to call overactivity of this type emptying-related instead of filling-related, as is currently the case with the classification of symptoms related to so-called overactive bladder (Figure 45.20).

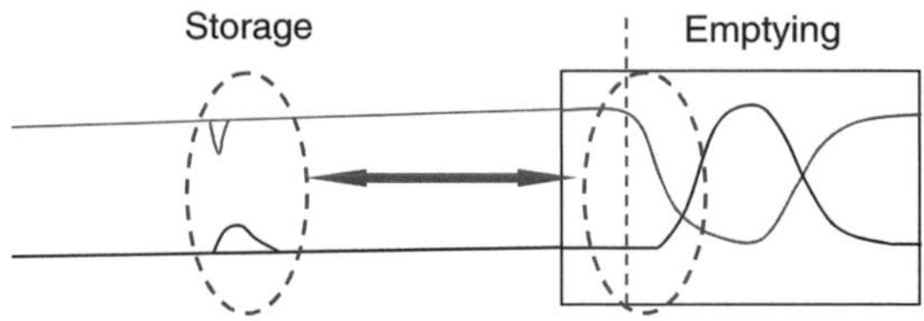

Figure 45.19 The same sequence of events with a urethral pressure fall that precedes the detrusor pressure increase is found in both overactivity and at the start of a normal micturition cycle. It seems reasonable to see this overactivity as emptying-related in nature rather than storage-related.

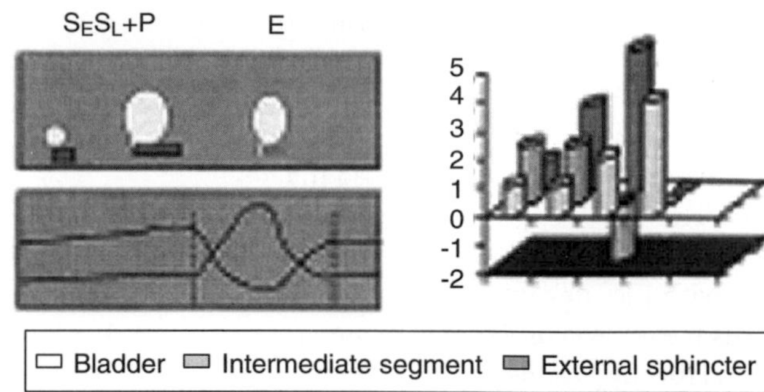

Figure 45.21
A simplified pattern of recognition can be based on a reduced number of observations, and thus provide a framework for clinical use. SE, storage, early; SL, storage, late; p, provocation; E, emptying. Arbitrary scale.

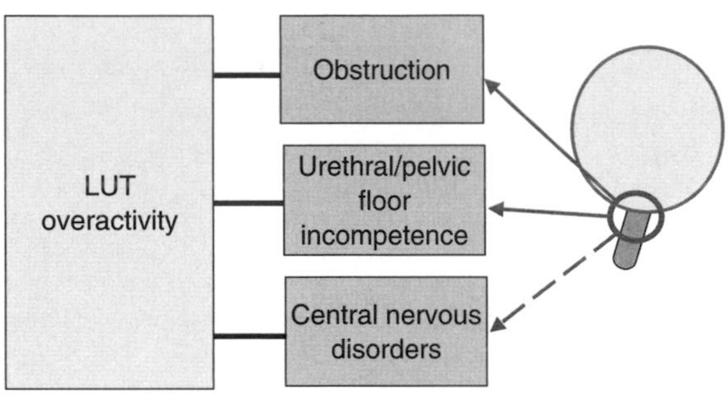

Figure 45.20
The proximal urethra is a probable trigger zone for LUT overactivity in both men and women. Another zone comprises the bladder.

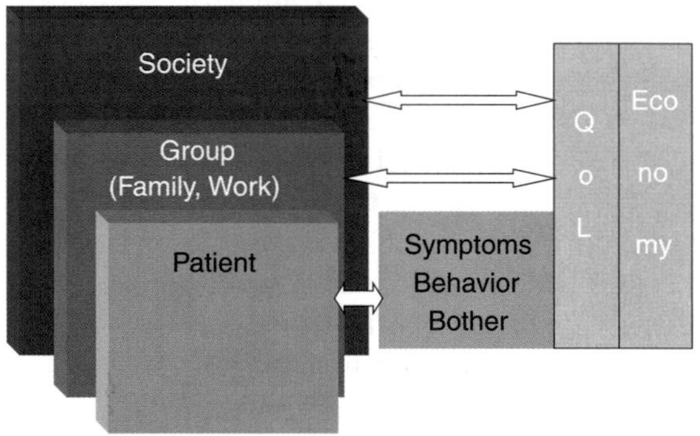

Figure 45.22
Important consequences of the patient's disorder are symptoms, behavior, bother, consequences for quality of life (QoL), and the socioeconomic situation. With increasing consequences, an increased interest should be expected from different groups and from society at large.

A simplified structure and function based classification of lower urinary tract disorders

Since it is not possible to map out all parts of every patient, there is a strong desire to be able to limit one's observations with respect to structure and functionality to a reasonable number. A simplified model that allows this should be able to include observations from the bladder and the outlet/urethra at an early point during bladder filling, at a late point in the filling phase, and with a provocation at the latter or both, as well as also having observations relating to the emptying of the bladder. With this, we must be able to move the focus from the bladder to also encompassing the outlet, urethra, prostate/pelvic floor, as well as including an evaluation of nervous functions as a part of our routine status. In doing so, we will be able to see the pathophysiologic process and the disorder or injury as forming a basis for our classification. The symptom picture and other consequences should be added in order to describe manifestations which the patient experiences of the changes that have arisen. In a simplified model we cannot handle anything other than those structures and functions that we regard as being most essential in the micturition cycle. Among these, we count the bladder and the external sphincter, and then we should include the function that is responsible for shutting and opening at the bladder neck level and in the proximal urethra. Along these lines we probably would include the trigone, bladder neck, with men the preprostatic urethra, smooth musculature in the proximal urethra, and the mucous membrane in this area. It is more practical to regard these in their interrelationships and quite simply call them the intermediate segment and the intermediate function (Figure 45.11).

How comprehensive in the sense of how widespread and how intensive a change is and how large an engagement it creates in the surrounding tissues and structures is important to include in a good classification. In addition, one should have a picture of whether afferent and efferent innervation in the three different fundamental parts displays normal characteristics or whether signs of altered innervation/functionality exist. This appears to be knowledge of increasing importance. Placing an extra emphasis on nerves and nervous activity is in line with the fundamental classification model, which proceeds from the neurogenic component in a disruption of the LUT. How this should be carried out and the means by which one should procure this information are of course important questions, but are not covered here. After sufficient experience has been built up, one can probably content oneself with a few of the parameters mentioned. A simplified pattern of recognition could then look like Figure 45.21 in its basic structure.

Consequences of disorders

The symptoms and the difficulties that an individual feels and experiences are of course completely central for how one should regard the illness/injury. However, they are consequences of what has been incurred, and thus are secondary to their nature in a classification context (Figure 45.22). That the quality of life is affected to a significant degree by disruptions to the functionality of the lower urinary tract is clear, and likewise that the financial consequences for both the individual and society are most often significant. Their mutual interrelationship can be illustrated by Figure 45.22. A number of different confirming instruments has already been prepared in order to estimate the scope and significance of these consequences, and continued developmental work will provide us with still better measuring instruments.

References

1. Abrams P, Blaivas JG, Stanton SL, Andersen JT. The standardisation of terminology of lower urinary tract function. Scand J Urol Nephrol Suppl 1988; 114(5): 5–19.
2. Abrams P, Cardozo L, Fall M et al. The standardisation of terminology of lower urinary tract function: report from the Standardisation Sub-committee of the International Continence Society. Neurourol Urodyn 2002; 21(2): 167–78.
3. Blaivas JG, Appell RA, Fantl JA et al. Definition and classification of urinary incontinence: recommendations of the Urodynamic Society. Neurourol Urodyn 1997; 16: 149–51.
4. Mattiasson A. Characterisation of lower urinary tract disorders: a new view. Neurourol Urodyn 2001; 20: 601–21.
5. Hald T, Brading AF, Horn T et al. Pathophysiology of the urinary bladder in obstruction and ageing. In: Denis, Griffiths, Khoury, et al, eds. Proceedings of the 4th International Consultation on Benign Prostatic Hyperplasia (BPH), 1997: 129–78.
6. Patel M, Tewari A, Furman J. Prostatic obstruction and effects or the urinary tract. In: Narayan P, ed. Benign Prostatic Hyperplasia. Edinburgh: Churchill Livingstone, 2000: 139–50.
7. Abrams P, Griffiths D. The assessment of prostatic obstruction from urodynamic measurements and from residual urine. Br J Urol 1979; 51: 129–34.
8. Griffiths D, Höfner K, van Mastrigt R et al. Standardisation of terminology of lower urinary tract function: pressure–flow studies of voiding, urethral resistance, and urethral obstruction. Neurourol Urodyn 1997; 16: 1–18.
9. Bates P, Bradley WE, Glen E et al. Third report on the standardisation of terminology of lower urinary tract function. Procedures related to the evaluation of micturition: pressure flow relationships, residual urine: Br J Urol 1980; 52: 348–59; Euro Urol 6: 170–71; Acta Urol Jpn 27: 1566–8; Scand J Urol Nephrol 1981; 12: 191–3
10. Bates P, Bradley WE, Glen E et al. Fourth report on the standardisation of terminology of lower urinary tract function. Terminology related to neuromuscular dysfunction of lower urinary tract. Br J Urol 1981; 52: 233–5; Urology 17: 618–20; Scand J Urol Nephrol 15: 169–71; Acta Urol Jpn 27: 1568–71.
11. Koelbl H, Mostwin J, Boiteeux JP et al. Pathophysiology. In: Abrams, Cardozo, Khoury, Wein, eds. Proceedings from the 2nd International Consultation on Incontinence, 2001: 202–41.
12. Petros PE, Ulmsten UI. An integral theory and its method for the diagnosis and management of female urinary incontinence. Scand J Nephrol Suppl 1993; 153: 1–93.
13. Teleman P, Gunnarsson M, Lidfeldt J et al. Urodynamic characterisation of women with naïve urinary incontinence – a population based study in subjectively incontinent and healthy 53–63 years old women. Eur Urol 2002; 42: 583–9.
14. Mattiasson A, Teleman P. Abnormal urethral motor function is common in female stress, mixed, and urge incontinence. Neurourol Urodyn 2006; 25: 703–8.
15. Fall M, Geirsson G, Lindström S. Toward a new classification of overactive bladders. Neurourol Urodyn 1995; 14: 635.

Part VI

Treatment

46

Conservative treatment

Jean-Jacques Wyndaele

Introduction

Conservative treatment is the most applied treatment modality in neurogenic bladder. The reasons for this are clear: most conservative therapeutic methods are cheap, available to the vast majority of patients around the world, and, within the limits of proper application, complications are rare.

In this chapter we will give an overview of most techniques used in conservative treatment, including behavioral techniques, physiotherapy, and catheterization.

Behavioral techniques

The philosophy behind behavioral techniques is that one can only have a reasonable chance of acquiring a balanced bladder if daily life adjustments are made to the new situation of the lower urinary tract function caused by the neuropathy. Adjustments can be:

- Scheduled voiding or catheterization at fixed times during the day when sensation is pathologic.
- Voiding several times consecutively in order to lower a residual.
- Increasing the voiding interval to treat frequency. This includes 'bladder drill', aimed at retraining the bladder to hold more urine and inhibit inappropriate detrusor contractions during the filling phase of the micturition cycle.
- Adapting drinking habits, which includes balanced spread of fluid intake and advice on avoiding caffeinated beverages and identifying individual bladder irritants.
- Making the toilet more accessible and improving the patient's mobility.
- Changing drug intake if this influences diuresis and/or bladder function.
- Treatment of other physical or psychologic problems such as constipation and depression.[1]

Hadley divided scheduling regimens into four conceptual categories: bladder training, habit retraining, timed voiding, and prompted voiding.[2]

Keeping a voiding diary can offer information on functional bladder capacity, leakage, and sensation, which are important data for adjusting treatment and for a better understanding by patient and physician. Keeping a voiding diary can also have a therapeutic effect and, by itself, can lead to greater comfort.[3]

Behavioral adaptation and advice is important in all patients.

Physiotherapy

Detrusor overactivity from defective central inhibition or increased detrusor afferent activity can be improved by reinforcing inhibitory pathways. In the storage phase a number of detrusor inhibitory reflexes have been described as emanating from the detrusor via the sympathetic nerves and from the pelvic floor and external urethral sphincter via pudendal afferents.[4] The latter reflex implies that the resting tone in the pelvic floor and external urethral sphincter (supplied by branches of the pudendal nerve: S2–4) has an inhibitory effect on the detrusor. Furthermore, active contraction of these muscle fibers is said to enhance this inhibitory effect. Consequently, pelvic floor training should benefit those patients with weak pelvic musculature. The nerve roots of S2–4 are also involved in some muscles of the lower limb, and there is evidence that activation of S2–4 myotomes may have an inhibitory effect on the detrusor. These muscles include the gluteus maximus, the plantar flexors, and some small muscles of the foot. Hence, one can observe young children activating these myotomes, standing on tiptoes to suppress urgency, and there is no reason why adults cannot use this 'trick'.[5,6]

The sacral dermatomes include the saddle area and the back of the thighs and legs. In particular, the anus, clitoris, and glans penis are well supplied with sensory nerves, and activation of these afferents can inhibit the detrusor.[6] Centrally, when these afferents are activated by electrical stimulation, they have at least two effects: (1) by provoking the inhibitory sympathetic neurons to the ganglia and the detrusor, and (2) by providing central inhibition of the preganglionic bladder motor neurons through a direct route in the sacral cord. Some young girls have been observed to 'curtsy' to control urgency. The pressure of the heel on the perineum presumably activates the sacral dermatomes, in addition to possibly elevating the bladder neck and supporting the proximal urethra. When learning bladder drill for urgency and urge incontinence, patients can be taught to sit down (on a rolled-up towel is best) and press on/squeeze the clitoris/glans penis and so activate the appropriate dermatomes. This reduces urgency, inhibits/reduces unwanted bladder contractions, and helps the patient to defer voiding, aiming to increase the functional bladder capacity. The daily use of transcutaneous electrical nerve stimulation (TENS) over S2–4 dermatomes has also been shown to have a beneficial effect on reducing urgency and urge incontinence. Self-adhesive electrodes delivering 2 Hz stimulation placed bilaterally over S3 in 40 children showed 67.5% response.[7] Sacral stimulation at 10 Hz over S3 in 71 adults with chronic sensory urgency, detrusor instability, or detrusor hyperreflexia during urodynamics showed a significant improvement in cystometric volumes with a concomitant reduction in detrusor pressure compared with pre-stimulation cystometry.[8] TENS applied over the peroneal or posterior tibial nerve is another option for activating sacral afferents.

Event-driven electrical stimulation of the dorsal penile/clitoral nerve has been used in multiple sclerosis[9] and in spinal cord injured patients[10] in an experimental setting and, in both instances, gave promising results. Interestingly, during the decrease of detrusor pressure the radial arterial pressure also decreased immediately and significantly in patients with cervical cord injury.[11]

There is abundant evidence to support the use of maximal electrical stimulation to activate the detrusor inhibitory reflexes from the anal and vaginal regions using electrodes specially designed for this purpose. Optimum electrical parameters include low-frequency (5–10 Hz) alternating rectangular pulses at maximum intensity. This activates the sympathetic inhibitory system to the bladder and the central inhibitory pathway to parasympathetic motor neurons, which have all been shown to operate at low frequencies.[12] In a group of 74 patients with detrusor instability and urge incontinence treated with maximal electrical stimulation, 51 were subjectively cured or significantly improved. Objectively, a significant decrease in frequency and significant increase in bladder volume were demonstrated.[13] A further study by Eriksen et al[14] demonstrated initial clinical and urodynamic cures in 50% of 48 women suffering from idiopathic detrusor instability following seven 20-min treatments of maximal stimulation using a vaginal and an anal electrode simultaneously. In addition, a significant improvement was observed in a further 33%. At 1-year follow-up, a persisting therapeutic effect was found in 77% and no serious side-effects were reported. Also, maximal stimulation on the thigh muscles gave such an effect.[15] A study on electrical stimulation of sacral dermatomes in multiple sclerosis patients with neurogenic detrusor overactivity could not demonstrate any acute effects during urodynamics.[16]

Detrusor hypoactivity may also respond to physiotherapy in the form of techniques to facilitate detrusor activity. Activation of stretch receptors in the bladder wall can instigate a detrusor contraction, and so pressing or tapping over the bladder may set off a detrusor contraction. Likewise, bending forward and straining may help to initiate detrusor activity. However, suprapubic tapping and straining are risky techniques, as described below. Bladder emptying may be further enhanced by ensuring relaxation of the pelvic floor.

Furthermore, using maximal electrical stimulation of the pelvic floor muscles, Plevnik et al[17] treated 6 patients with spinal cord lesions from C5 to T4, all demonstrating detrusor-sphincter dyssynergia, in whom urinary retention developed. After two to four 20-min treatments over 4 weeks, using vaginal or anal electrodes and monophasic square pulses of 1 ms, frequency of 20 Hz and 50–90 mA, a reduction in maximal urethral pressure was reported. In addition, uninhibited detrusor contractions were reduced in 4 patients and reflex voiding by tapping was successful in all patients.

Intravesical transurethral bladder stimulation is used to rehabilitate the neurogenic bladder.[18] Its therapeutic goals are to achieve a sensation of bladder filling, to initiate a detrusor contraction, and to achieve conscious urinary control. The procedure combines direct stimulation of the bladder receptors with visual feedback using patient observance of cystometric pressure changes. The effects are technique-dependent.[19]

Several other techniques of pelvic floor physiotherapy can be successfully used in patients with neurogenic bladder: biofeedback and relaxation can have indications in patients with partly preserved voluntary and/or sensory function. One randomized pilot study compared pelvic floor muscle training, electromyographic biofeedback, and neuromuscular electrical stimulation for bladder dysfunction in patients with multiple sclerosis. It showed that combination of all these techniques was most successful in the reduction of urinary symptoms.[20]

Intravesical biofeedback has been used successfully to improve the sensation of bladder fullness and control of involuntary contractions.[21]

Triggered reflex voiding is much less applied than a decade ago, but nevertheless it is still used. Bladder reflex triggering comprises various maneuvers performed by the patient in order to elicit reflex detrusor contractions by exteroceptive stimuli.[22] The pathophysiologic background is unphysiologic in suprasacral lesions for which the technique is mostly used: it comprises C-fiber activation, bladder contraction involuntary and not sustained, detrusor-striated sphincter dyssynergia or detrusor-bladder neck dyssynergia, and autonomic dysreflexia.[23] Only in the minority of patients will triggering lead to balanced voiding. Complications such as infection,[24,25] upper urinary tract alterations/deterioration, and incontinence are frequent. If applied, patients should be encouraged to find the best individual trigger zone and points: suprapubic tapping, thigh scratching, squeezing the glans penis and the scrotal skin, pulling on the crines pubis, as well as anal/rectal manipulation may be effective.[26]

Suprapubic tapping must be stopped in most patients when micturition starts, permitting the fast-reacting striated sphincter to relax, whereas the slowly reacting detrusor may still remain in contraction. As soon as micturition stops, tapping has to be applied again.

Drugs or surgery may be necessary to decrease outflow resistance and to improve reflex incontinence. Videourodynamics are strongly advised to find out if the urodynamic situation is safe. Triggered voiding is contraindicated in cases of:

- inadequate detrusor contraction
- unbalanced voiding
- vesico-uretero-renal reflux
- reflux in the seminal vesicles or in the vas
- uncontrollable AD
- persistence of recurrent urinary tract infections.

Bladder expression comprises various maneuvers aimed at increasing intravesical pressure in order to enable/facilitate bladder emptying. The most commonly used are the Valsalva (abdominal straining) and the Credé (manual compression of the lower abdomen) maneuvers. Bladder expression has been recommended for a long time for patients with so-called lower motor neuron lesions, resulting in a combination of an underactive detrusor with an underactive sphincter or with an incompetent urethral closure mechanism of other origin. Clinical experience has shown that by using Valsalva or Credé maneuvers many patients are able to empty their bladders, albeit mostly incompletely. Urodynamics/videourodynamics have demonstrated that, despite high intravesical pressures during straining, the urinary flow may be very poor due to an inability to open the bladder neck, or to a mechanical obstruction at the level of the striated external sphincter by bending and compression of the urethra. Moreover, Clarke and Thomas[27] showed in flaccid male paraplegics that the major component of urethral resistance is a constant, adrenergically innervated muscular resistance in the external sphincter region.

With increasing time, more than 40% of the patients on straining show influx into the prostate and the seminal vesicles, and complications due to the high pressures such as reflux to the upper urinary tract. Measures to facilitate bladder expression can be the use of α-blockers, but they usually cause or increase urinary stress incontinence.

Contraindications are:

- sphincter hyperreflexia and detrusor-sphincter dyssynergia
- vesico-uretero-renal reflux
- reflux into the male adnexa
- hernias
- hemorrhoids
- urethral pathology
- symptomatic urinary tract infections.

Some patients use the anal sphincter stretch described by Low and Donovan[28] with success.

Intermittent catheterization and intermittent self-catheterization

Intermittent catheterization (IC) and intermittent self-catheterization (ISC) have become widely used in the last 40 years. Many studies show good results and limited complications, leading to a better prognosis and a better quality of life in many patients with neurologic bladder[29–31] (Table 46.1).

IC and ISC are nowadays considered as the methods of choice for the management of neurologic bladder dysfunction.[23]

Results depend on the techniques used, which involve the types of catheters and lubricants, the catheter manipulation and introduction, and the rules needed for a short-term and long-term successful application.

Many types of catheters are used, made of different material. Some are packed in a sheet/bag, others are reusable.[32] Some have a urethral introducer that permits bypassing the colonized 1.5 cm of the distal urethra and which resulted in a significant lower infection rate in hospitalized men with spinal cord injury.[33] Studies comparing materials in a randomized controlled way are scarce. Lundgren et al[34] found, in the rabbit, that a high osmolality

Table 46.1 *Outcome of continence study*

Authors	Number of patients	Follow–up	Adjunctive treatment	Result of continence
Iwatsubo et al[143]	60 spinal cord lesions		Overdistention during shock phase	100% continent
Kornhuber and Schultz[145]	197 multiple sclerosis			Continence improved with elimination of residual urine
Kuhn et al[146]	22 spinal cord lesions	5 years	No	Continence did not change
Lindehall et al[147]	26 meningomyeloceles	7.5–12 years		24/26 better
Madersbacher and Weissteiner[141]	12 f	2–4 years		50% dry; other 50% some grade of incontinence
McGuire and Savastano[144]	22 f	2–11 years	Surgery 27%	Continent 73%
Vaidyanathan et al[149]	7 spinal cord lesions	14–30 months	Bladder relaxant drugs intravesically	84% dry, 3 dampness at awakening
Waller etal[148]	30 spinal cord lesions	5–9 years	6 anticholinergics	22 dry, 8 incontinent
Wyndaele et al[142]	30 (18 m, 12 f)	3–30 months	6 anticholinergic, 1 colocystoplasty	73% continent + 13% improvement
Wyndaele and Maes[99]	75 (69 neurogenic)	1.5–12 years	38 anticholinergics	47 dry, 22 seldom wet, 6 wet at least once a day

f, female; m, male.

is important in hydrophilic catheters with regard to removing friction and urethral trauma. Waller et al[35] had the same experience in men. Wyndaele et al[36] evaluated the use of a hydrophilic catheter in 39 male patients with neurogenic bladder using conventional catheters over a long period. The hydrophilic catheter proved as easy to use but was better tolerated. Satisfaction was better, especially in patients who experienced problems with conventional catheters. Some patients were unsatisfied for reasons of practical use or for economical reasons. Two studies were published about the use of the SpeediCath set. In a comparison of 29 men, Actreen showed better results with the Speedicath Catheterization set.[37] A prospective randomized parallel comparative trial showed a beneficial effect on urinary tract infection when Speedicath was compared with uncoated polyvinyl chloride catheters in 123 male traumatic spinal cord injured patients.[38] Vapnek et al[39] made a prospective randomized trial of the LoFric hydrophilic coated catheter versus a conventional plastic catheter in 62 male patients with neurogenic bladder. They found the use of LoFric resulted in less hematuria and a significant decrease in the incidence of urinary tract infection. They propose its use especially in patients with a history of difficult catheterization, urethral trauma, or a high rate of urinary tract infection. The reuse of a silicone catheter for an average period of 4.8 years was studied in Chiangmai, Thailand, and proved suitable and safe if cleaned and applied properly.[40] A Cochrane review has dealt with catheter policies for management of long-term voiding problems in adults with neurogenic bladder disorders. Despite a comprehensive search, no evidence from randomized or quasi-randomized controlled trials was found. The Cochrane review concludes that it was not possible to draw any conclusions regarding the use of different types of catheter.[41]

Most catheters require the use of some kind of lubricant, especially in men. Lubricants are applied on the catheter or are instilled into the urethra.[42] In some countries patients use oil or merely water as a lubricant. For patients with preserved urethral sensation, a local anesthetic jelly may be needed. Catheters with a hydrophilic and self-lubricated surface need activation with tap water or sterile water.

For adults, size 10–14 F for males and size 14–16 F for females are mostly used, but a bigger size/lumen may be necessary for those with bladder augmentation or cloudy urine that results from another origin. No studies on IC compared sizes in a randomized way.

Two main techniques have been adopted: a sterile (SIC) and a clean IC (CIC). The sterile non-touch technique advocated by Guttmann and Frankel implicates the use of sterile materials handled with sterile gloves and forceps. In an intensive care unit, some advocate wearing a mask and a sterile gown as well. In some centers, during a bladder training program SIC used to be performed only by a catheter team, which has proven to obtain a very low infection rate.[43] Nowadays, the sterile technique is mostly used only during a restricted period of time and in a hospital setting. In the majority of cases a clean technique is used.

Self-catheterization is done in many different positions: supine, sitting, or standing. Female patients may use a mirror or a specially designed catheter to visualize the meatus. After a while, most women do not need these aids anymore.

The basic principles of urinary catheter introduction are well known: the catheter must be introduced in a noninfecting and atraumatic way. Noninfecting means cleaning hands, using a noninfected catheter and lubricant, and cleaning the meatal region before catheter introduction. Atraumatic requires a proper catheter size, sufficient lubrification, and gentle introduction through the urethra, sphincter area, and bladder neck.[44,45] The catheter has to be introduced until urine flows out. Urine can be drained directly in the toilet, in a urinal, plastic bag, or other reservoir. The catheter should be kept in place until urine flow stops. Then it should be pulled out slowly, while gentle Valsalva or bladder expression is done in order to completely empty residual urine. When properly done, the residual urine should be maximum 6 ml.[46] However, Jensen et al measured residual urine repeatedly with ultrasonography and found residual urine in 70% of the catheterizations in their group of 12 patients with spinal cord lesions. The residual urine could exceed 50 ml and even 100 ml.[47]

Finally, the end of the catheter should be blocked to prevent backflow of the urine or air into the bladder. Hydrophilic catheters can be left in place for a short time only to prevent suction by the urethral mucosa, which may make removal difficult.

During the rehabilitation phase, clean intermittent self-catheterization (CISC) can be taught very early to patients with good hand function.[48]

When resources are limited, catheters are reused for weeks and months: some are resterilized or cleaned by soaking in an antiseptic solution or boiling water. Microwaving to resterilize rubber catheters has also been described. Reused supplies do not seem to be related to an increased likelihood of urinary tract infection.[49,50]

The frequency of catheterization needed can depend on many factors, such as bladder volume, fluid intake, postvoid residual, and urodynamic parameters (bladder compliance, detrusor pressure). Usually it is recommended to catheterize 4–6 times a day during the acute phase after spinal cord lesion. Some patients will need to keep this frequency if IC is the only way of bladder emptying. Other patients will catheterize 1–3 times a day to check and evacuate residual urine after voiding or on a weekly basis during bladder retraining.[51] Use of a portable ultrasound device in IC has been evaluated.[52,53]

Adjunctive therapy to overcome high detrusor pressure is often needed. Anticholinergic drugs or bladder relaxants are often indicated in patients with bladder overactivity. For patients who develop a low-compliance bladder, upper tract deterioration, or severe incontinence, injection of botulinum toxin in the bladder wall or surgery as bladder augmentation may be necessary.[54,55] Where too high a diuresis is noted during the night due to diurnal variation of antidiuretic hormone, DDAVP (desmopressin) can be safely and effectively used.[56,57] Nocturnal bladder emptying has been shown to be useful and even necessary to overcome the dangerous bladder function during sleeping hours.[58,59]

In cases of catheterization difficulty at the striated sphincter, botulinum toxin injection in the sphincter can help.[60] In individuals with tetraplegia, reconstructive hand surgery can be indicated.[61] For those with poor hand function or difficulty in reaching the meatus, assistive devices might be needed.[62,63]

Education is very important. Teaching programs have been successful in nonliterate persons in developing countries and in quadriplegic patients.[64,65]

It is clear that IC can improve incontinence or make patients with neurogenic bladder continent. To achieve this, bladder capacity should be sufficient, bladder pressure kept low, urethral resistance kept high enough, and care taken to maintain a balance between fluid intake, residual urine, and frequency of catheterization.

Not all patients starting with IC continue this treatment and there are several reasons for this (Table 46.2). A main reason to stop is continuing incontinence. Main reasons to continue are continence and autonomy of the patients.[66] Bakke and Malt found that, among those who practiced IC independently, 25.8% were sometimes and 6% were always averse, especially young patients and females. Aversion seemed to be related above all to nonacceptance of their chronic disability.[67] A retrospective analysis in spinal cord injury patients showed that, of patients on CIC at discharge, 52% discontinued the method and reverted to an indwelling catheter because of dependence on caregivers, spasticity interfering with catheterization, incontinence despite anticholinergic agents, and lack of availability of external collective devices for female patients.[68]

Social and psychologic impact have been studied in children, adolescents, and their families. From a total sample of 66, no significant difference was observed in self-esteem for those successfully catheterizing. Specific challenges involved learning SC and the practical use of the technique. Concerns were leakage and being wet, and peers finding out about their continence management.[69] Results showed that CIC by carer or self-catheterization itself did not cause major emotional and behavioral problems, but the bladder problem may act as a focus that puts considerable strain on family relationships. Although most parents disliked CIC they complied with the suggested management.[70]

An open comparative study compared the impact of volume-dependent and time-dependent intermittent catheterization on financial burden and clinical outcomes. The results, in a small sample size, showed that

Table 46.2 *Reasons for stopping intermittent self-catheterization*

Authors	Catheter-free	Incontinence	Inconvenience	Infection	Physical status	Choice of patient
Bakke[156]	10%		5%	4%	3%	
Diokno et al[150]	17%	2%	2%		7%	
Hunt et al[157]	10%					
Maynard and Glass[151]	12%					6%
Sutton et al[155]		6%	6%	3%	3%	3%
Timoney and Shaw[154]		36%				
Whitelaw et al[152]	5%		5%		5%	5%
Webb et al[153]	9%		3%		2%	2%

volume-dependent IC had economic and probably also clinical advantages.[71]

The introduction of a catheter several times a day can give rise to complications. One of the most frequent complications is infection of the urinary tract (UTI). Prevalence of UTI varies widely in the literature. This is due to the various methods used for evaluation, the different techniques of IC, different frequencies of urine analysis, different criteria for infection, the administration or not of prophylaxis to the group of patients studied, and much more. Some publications give the percentage of sterile urine at between 12 and 88%.[72–77] Eleven percent prevalence for asymptomatic UTI and 53% for symptomatic bacteriuria are given in different series.[78,79] Bakke and Vollset found that in 407 patients, 252 with neurogenic bladder, during an observation period of 1 year, 24.5% of patients had nonclinical UTI, 58.6% had minor symptoms, 14.3% had more comprehensive or frequent symptoms, while 2.6% claimed major symptoms.[80]

In the acute stage of spinal cord injury (SCI), with proper management, urine can be kept sterile for 15–20 days without antibiotic prophylaxis and for 16–55 days if prophylaxis is given.[81,82] Prieto-Fingerhut et al[83] determined the effect of sterile and nonsterile IC on the incidence of UTI in 29 patients after SCI in a randomized controlled trial. With urine analysis on a weekly basis they found a 28.6% UTI incidence in the group on sterile IC, whereas a 42.4% incidence was found in the nonsterile catheterization group. The cost of antibiotics for the sterile IC group was only 43% of the cost for those on nonsterile IC. However, the cost of the sterile IC kits was 371% of the cost of the kits used by the nonsterile IC group, bringing the total cost of the sterile program to 277% of the other program. Rhame and Perkash[84] found that in 70 SCI patients in the initial rehabilitation hospitalization treated with sterile catheterization and a neomycin-polymyxin irrigant, 54% of patients developed an infection, at an overall rate of 10.3 infections per 1000 patient-days on IC. Bakke and Volset[80] found that factors that may predict the occurrence of clinical UTI in patients using clean IC were low age and high mean catheterization volume in women, low age, neurogenic bladder dysfunction, and nonself-catheterization in men, in addition to urine leakage in patients with neurogenic dysfunction and the presence of bacteriuria. If antibacterial prophylaxis was used, fewer episodes of bacteriuria were noticed, but significantly more clinical UTIs were seen. Shekelle et al reviewed the risk factors for UTI in adults with spinal cord dysfunction[85] and found increased bladder residual volume to be a risk factor. Patients on IC had fewer infections than those with indwelling catheters.

In order to diagnose UTI, it should be recommended that the urine be obtained by catheterization.[86] The frequency of examining urine samples differs greatly between studies: daily use of a dipslide technique during the acute phase after SCI, once a week during the subacute phase, and monthly or a few times a year in long-term care.[87–89]

If a urine culture reveals more than 10^4 colony-forming units (cfu)/ml, this indicates significant bacteriuria. Pyuria alone is not considered reliable in patients with neurogenic bladder.[90,91] The bacteria found are mostly *Escherichia coli*, *Proteus*, *Citrobacter*, *Pseudomonas*, *Klebsiella*, *Staphylococcus aureus*, and *Streptococcus faecalis* in short-term cases, while the same bacteria plus *Acinetobacter* are found in the long-term IC patients.[92,93] *E. coli* is considered the dominant species.[92] The detection of *E. coli* on the periurethra corresponds, at a much higher percentage, with bacteriuria than if other bacteria are found.[94] *E. coli* isolates from patients who develop symptomatic UTI may be distinguished from bacteria recovered from patients who remain asymptomatic and possibly from normal fecal *E. coli*.[95]

Urinary sepsis is fortunately rare.[96,97] Previous treatment with an indwelling catheter represents a special risk to develop sepsis.[98] In his thesis, Wyndaele[44] found the period of 24 hours to 3 days after changing from indwelling to IC drainage when UTI was present to be dangerous for the development of sepsis.

Wyndaele and Maes[99] found several relationships between IC and UTI. If catheterization is begun by patients with recurrent or chronic UTI and urinary retention, the incidence of infection decreases and patients may become totally free of infection. If symptomatic infections occur, improper practice of IC or misuse can often be found. Chronic infection persists after IC has been started, if the cause of the chronicity remains.

To prevent UTI, a noninfecting technique is needed. But also some additional factors can play a role in infection prevention. Nursing education is important and educational intervention by a clinic nurse is a simple, cost-effective means of decreasing the risk of UTIs in individuals with SCI on IC who are identified as at risk.[100] Anderson[82] found a fivefold incidence when IC was performed 3 times a day compared with 6 times a day. Also, prevention of bladder overdistention is important.[73] Crossinfection is less if IC during hospitalization is performed by a catheter team or by the patients themselves. As residual urine plays a role in infection, attention must be made to empty the bladder completely.

Treatment of UTI is necessary if the infection is symptomatic. Waites et al[101] treated men with SCI on IC and saw susceptible organisms disappear from urine in all and significantly reduced in the perineum and urethra. However, they were replaced shortly after by resistant Gram-positive cocci. This shows the importance of reserving antibiotics for symptomatic patients only and of taking into account the data from the antibiogram. The value of nontreatment for chronic nonsymptomatic bacteriuria throughout a hospitalization has been demonstrated.[102]

With antibacterial prophylaxis, several studies have shown a lowered infection rate.[103–108] Cranberry juice has been evaluated, but the results are unclear.[109] Several studies have considered the risk of developing dangerous resistance against antibiotics when prophylaxis is given either orally or by instillation.[110–112] Galloway et al[113] state that the threat of emergence of resistant organisms, the risk to patients of side-effects of the antibiotics, the expense, and the risk to other patients from crossinfection with resistant organisms are strong arguments against prophylactic antibacterials. Therefore, it would seem logical to use antibacterial prophylaxis only for a short time, such as during the initial stage of IC. It does seem to be less indicated for long-term use, although it can help specific patients to lower the rate of symptomatic infections for which no well-defined cause is found.

Urethritis and epididymo-orchitis have been reported in several case series (Table 46.3). With a long-term indwelling catheter, a larger prevalence is seen. Genital infections can lower fertility in SCI patients.[114] If IC is used to empty the neurogenic bladder, better sperm quality and better pregnancy rates have been found than with indwelling catheterization.[115,116]

Prostatitis can be a cause of recurrent UTI: either acute or chronic, it is difficult to diagnose in patients with neurogenic bladder, and special tests have been developed for this.[117,118] The overall incidence was previously thought to be around 5–18%, but 33% may be a more realistic figure.[119]

Urethral bleeding is frequently seen in new patients and occurs regularly in one-third on a long-term basis.[120] Trauma of the urethra, especially in men, can cause false passages and meatal stenosis, but the incidence is rare (see Table 46.3). The incidence of urethral strictures increases with a longer follow-up, with most events occurring after 5 years of IC.[99] Former treatment with an indwelling catheter causes more complications. Urethral changes were also documented in SCI men on IC for an average of 5 years, using one single reusable silicone catheter for an average of 3 years.[121] IC technique and catheter type are claimed to be important factors.[122,123] Urethral trauma with false passages in neurogenic patients on CIC can be treated successfully with 5 days of antibiotics and 6 weeks of indwelling catheter. The false passage will also disappear on cystoscopy and IC can be safely restarted.[124]

Other complications such as hydronephrosis, vesicoureteral reflux, and bladder cancer seem to relate rather to infection, bladder trabeculation, detrusor pressure, or neuropathy than to IC itself.[125]

Bladder calculi caused by the introduction of pubic hair,[126,127] loss of the catheter in the bladder,[128] bladder perforation, and bladder necrosis[129] have been case reports on rare complications of IC. In a retrospective study in 140 male patients with SCI, epididymo-orchitis occurred in 27.9% over a period of 17 years. Clean intermittent catheterization was an independent risk factor and urethral stricture a contributing factor.[130] A positive case report introduces the history of a patient with SCI performing intermittent self-catheterization with 27 years' complication-free follow-up.[131]

A higher incidence of depression has been shown in patients with neurogenic bladder after SCI than in the normal population. Depression is closely related to gender (female patients had a 3.8-fold higher risk) and the ability to perform self-catheterization (if impossible, the patients had a 4.6-fold higher risk).[132]

And what if IC or ISC is not possible? There can be several reasons for this: bad hand function and no relative to perform the catheterization, unwillingness of the patient, cost, lack of knowledge from carers, persistent incontinence, general bad condition, or difficulty to reach the meatus. In many cases these problems may be overcome with proper treatment. However, in some cases an indwelling catheter will be used.

Table 46.3 *Literature data on genitourinary complications in patients on intermittent catheterization*

Author	Total no. of patients	Urethritis	Meatal stricture	Epididymitis	Urethral stricture
Bakke[156]	407 (206 m)	1%		1%	
Hellstrom et al[163]	41 (26 m)			3	
Kuhn et al[146]	22 (11 m)		1		1
Labat et al[162]	68 (48 m)	9 m		3	
Lapides et al[158]	100 (34 m)	2 m	–	–	–
Lapides et al[159]	218 (90 m)	2 m	–	2	
Maynard and Diokno[161]	28 (m?)			4 (1 with infected penile prosthesis)	
Maynard and Glass[151]	34 (m?)			3	2
Orikasa et al[160]	26 (13 m)			1	
Perkash and Giroux[165]	50 m			5	
Perrouin-Verbe et al[66]	159 (113 m)			10% short term, 28% long term	5.3%
Thirumavalan and Ransley[164]				12%	
Waller et al[148]	30 SCI (26 m)			2	4
Webb et al[153]				2%	
Wyndaele et al[142]	30 (18 m)	2 m		2	
Wyndaele and Maes[99]	75 (33 m)		3	6	7

m, male, SCI, spinal cord injury.

Transurethral and suprapubic catheters

Transurethral and suprapubic catheters have been used for a long time. The dangers of the techniques have been well documented and the complications are well known. If they are used, it is very important to stick to good rules of management:

- Catheter size 12–14.
- Place the catheter properly with the balloon in the bladder. It is important to be especially careful in the presence of a spastic sphincter.
- Control the outflow regularly to avoid overdistention.
- Change the catheter regularly several times a week in an acute situation, every 10 days if possible, and every 4–6 weeks in a chronic patient who has few complications.
- Anticholinergic drugs may be important in patients with bladder neurogenic overactivity.
- Antibacterial drugs should not be used to prevent or to treat an asymptomatic infection of the urine. With an indwelling catheter, the prevalence of infection is 100% if the catheter is used for more than a couple of weeks. In the case of symptomatic infection, treatment is necessary.
- There is no general agreement on clamping of the catheter. In cases of severe incontinence unsuccessfully treated with drugs, a continuous outflow is not the only conservative possibility.
- Complications are frequent. The transurethral catheter can cause acute septic episodes, urethral trauma and bleeding, false passages, strictures, diverticuli and fistuli of the urethra, bladder stones, squamous cell bladder carcinoma, epididymo-orchitis, and prostatitis. With application of good treatment rules, many of these conditions can be largely avoided.
- The presence of an indwelling catheter should be known to all who take care of the patient: occupational therapist (OT), physiotherapist (PT), and of course the nursing staff.

Recent studies have also shown a very much higher complication rate in patients on indwelling catheter than in those on intermittent catheterization. Pyelonephritis, epididymo-orchitis and urosepsis were significantly more prevalent in the group with an indwelling catheter.[133] In addition, stone formation was higher in SCI patients independent of age, sex, and level of injury. There was no difference between suprapubic and transurethral indwelling catheters.[134] Another study found a higher risk in urethral indwelling than in suprapubic catheter.[135]

Insertion of a suprapubic catheter is not without risk. Intraoperative complications of 10% and 30-day complication of 19% have been described. A mortality rate of 1.8% was found in 219 patients with this treatment.[136]

An interesting study evaluated the long-term safety of the contemporary balloon catheter retrospectively. The contemporary balloon catheter consists of a reusable catheter self-inserted by the patient every night before sleeping and then removed in the next morning. The incidence of febrile episodes was 0.57 times/100 months, the second lowest when different treatment options were compared. The use in the long term does seem to be safe.[137]

Screening for bladder malignancy in patients with neuropathic bladder and a chronic indwelling catheter by cystoscopy and biopsy is commonly performed. In a retrospective analysis of screening biopsies in 36 patients with neuropathic bladder and a chronic indwelling catheter, who had undergone yearly screening from 5 years after catheter insertion, no tumors were ever identified. However, histologic findings were frequently abnormal, of which the most common were active chronic cystitis and squamous metaplasia. This study reinforces the increasing body of evidence suggesting that screening cystoscopy and biopsy in this group of patients is not valid.[138]

Appliances (condom catheters, penile clamps)

Their use aims at collecting leaking urine into a device, thus preventing urinary spilling and giving better hygienic control, better control of unpleasant odor, and a better quality of life. A condom catheter is indicated in all male patients with urinary incontinence provided that there is no skin/penile lesion, and intravesical pressures during storage and voiding phase are urodynamically proven to be safe.

No absolute contraindications for such appliances seem to exist.

Condom catheters are not invasive and permit us to avoid most of the complications related to indwelling catheters. Old versions were reusable external collecting devices that fitted rather loosely around the penis. They are still preferred by a few paralysed patients who have been accustomed to them for a long time, especially those with a retractile penis.

The actual types are thin conical-shaped sheaths made of different sorts of material. They fit over the shaft of the penis, fixed with some type of glue or occlusive strip. The tips are open and connected with the tube of a urinary collecting device. In recent years special condoms and special devices allowing urethral catheterization without removing the condom have been manufactured.

While the advantages of condom catheters over indwelling catheters and incontinence pads are evident, they are not without problems and complications, sometimes severe:

- Fixation to the skin can be difficult with a smaller and/or retractile penis and/or abundant pubic fat. The problem can be partly overcome by using the proper size and proper fixation glue/strip. A penile prosthesis can be a solution in the case of a retractile small penis.
- Obstruction of urine flow is a rather common problem, due to twisting or kinking of the tip of the condom or the collecting tube. To prevent this, most of the currently available condom catheters are reinforced at the tip.
- Lesions of the penis can be secondary to mechanical damage to the skin from an excessively tight condom worn for a prolonged time. One way of prevention is to discontinue the use of the condom during part of the day or night. Another source of skin lesion is allergy to the material of the condom, usually to latex. Such an allergy is not uncommon, i.e. in myelomeningocele patients. The use of a latex-free condom is the solution.
- Urinary tract infection.

Newman and Price[139] found bacteriuria in more than 50% of patients using a condom catheter. One of the few factors correlated with increased risk for UTI was less than daily change of the condom.

Penile clamps are not recommended for patients with neuropathic voiding dysfunction, because of the danger of skin and urethral lesions.[23]

Underlying disease

Underlying disease and life expectancy should be considered for the selection of bladder management in patients with neoplastic spinal cord compression. In patients with curatively treated disease, a full bladder rehabilitation program is recommended, while in patients with malignant disease and palliative care, a suprapubic catheter might be the treatment of choice.[140]

References

1. Wyndaele JJ. Les techniques comportementales. In: Corcos J, Schick E, eds. Les Vessies Neurogènes de l'Adulte. Paris: Masson, 1996: 197–202.
2. Hadley EC. Bladder training and related therapies for urinary incontinence in older people. JAMA 1986; 256: 372–9.

3. Dowd T, Kolcaba K, Steiner R. Using cognitive strategies to enhance bladder control and comfort. Holist Nurs Pract 2000; 14: 91–103.
4. Mahoney DT, Laferte RO, Blais DJ. Integral storage and voiding reflexes; a neurophysiologic concept of continence and micturition. Urology 1980; 9: 95–106.
5. Shafik A. Study of the response of the urinary bladder to stimulation of the cervix uteri and clitoris – 'the genitovesical reflex': an experimental study. Int Urogynecol J 1995; 6: 41–6.
6. Laycock J. What can the specialist physiotherapist do? In: Wyndaele JJ, Laycock J, eds. Multidisciplinary Conservative Treatment for the Neurogenic Bladder. Wokingham: Incare, 2002: 14–18.
7. Hoebeke P, De Paepe H, Renson C et al. Transcutaneous neuromodulation in non-neuropathic bladder sphincter dysfunction in children: preliminary results. Neurourol Urodyn 1999; 18(4): 263–4.
8. Walsh IK, Keane PF, Johnston SR et al. Non-invasive antidromic sacral neurostimulation to enhance bladder storage. Neurourol Urodyn 1999; 18(4): 380.
9. Fjorback MV, Rijkhoff N, Petersen T, Nohr M, Sinkjaer T. Event driven electrical stimulation of the dorsal penile/clitoral nerve for management of neurogenic detrusor overactivity in multiple sclerosis. Neurourol Urodyn 2006; 25(4): 349–55
10. Hansen J, Media S, Nohr M et al. Treatment of neurogenic detrusor overactivity in spinal cord injured patients by conditional electrical stimulation. J Urol 2005; 173(6): 2035–9.
11. Lee YH, Creasey GH, Lim H et al. Detrusor and blood pressure responses to dorsal penile nerve stimulation during hyperreflexic contraction of the bladder in patients with cervical cord injury. Arch Phys Med Rehabil 2003; 84(1): 136–40.
12. Lindstrom S, Fall M, Carlsson C-A et al. The neurophysiological basis of bladder inhibition in response to intravaginal electrical stimulation. J Urol 1983; 129: 405–10.
13. Fossberg E, Sorensen S, Ruutu M et al. Maximal electrical stimulation in the treatment of unstable detrusor and urge incontinence. Eur Urol 1990; 18: 120–3.
14. Eriksen BC, Bergmann S, Eik-Ness SH. Maximal electrostimulation of the pelvic floor in female idiopathic detrusor instability and urge incontinence. Neurourol Urodyn 1989; 8: 219–30.
15. Okada N, Igawa A, Ogawa A, Nishizawa O. Transcutaneous electrical stimulation of thigh muscles in the treatment of detrusor overactivity. Br J Urol 1998; 81: 560–4.
16. Fjorback MV, Van Rey FS, Rijkhoff NJ et al. Electrical stimulation of sacral dermatomes in multiple sclerosis patients with neurogenic detrusor overactivity. Neurourol Urodyn 2007; 26: 525–30.
17. Plevnik S, Homan G, Vrtacnik P. Short-term maximal electrical stimulation for urinary retention. Urol 1984; 24: 521–3.
18. Katona F. Stages of vegetative afferentation in reorganization of bladder control during intravesical electrotherapy. Urol Int 1975; 30: 192–203.
19. De Wachter S, Wyndaele JJ. Quest for standardization of electrical sensory testing in the lower urinary tract: the influence of technique related factors on bladder electrical thresholds. Neurourol Urodyn 2002; 21: 1–6.
20. McClurg D, Ashe RG, Marshall K, Lowe-Strong AS. Comparison of pelvic floor muscle training, electromyography biofeedback, and neuromuscular electrical stimulation for bladder dysfunction in people with multiple sclerosis: a randomized pilot study. Neurourol Urodyn 2006; 25(4): 337–48.
21. Wyndaele JJ, Hoekx L, Vermandel A. Bladder biofeedback for the treatment of refractory sensory urgency in adults. Eur Urol 1997; 32: 429–32.
22. Andersen JT, Blaivas JG, Cardozo L, Thuroff J. Lower urinary tract rehabilitation techniques: seventh report on the standardisation of terminology of lower urinary tract function. Neurourol Urodyn 11: 593–603.
23. Madersbacher H, Wyndaele JJ, Igawa Y et al. Conservative management in the neuropathic patient. In: Abrams P, Khoury S, Wein A, eds. Incontinence. Health Publication, 1999: 775–812.
24. Stover SL, Lloyd LK, Waites KB, Jackson AB. Neurogenic urinary infection. Neurolog Clin 1991; 9: 741–55.
25. Lloyd LK, Kuhlemeier KV, Stover SL. Initial bladder management in spinal cord injury: does it make a difference? J Urol 1986; 135: 523–6.
26. Rossier A, Bors E. Detrusor response to perineal and rectal stimulation in patients with spinal cord injuries. Urol Int 1964; 10: 181–90.
27. Clarke SJ, Thomas DG. Characteristics of the urethral pressure profile in flaccid male paraplegics. Br J Urol 1981; 53: 157–61.
28. Low AI, Donovan WD. The use and mechanism of anal sphincter stretch in the reflex bladder. Br J Urol 1981; 53: 430–2.
29. Guttmann L, Frankel H. The value of intermittent catheterization in the early management of traumatic paraplegia and tetraplegia. Paraplegia 1966; 4: 63–83.
30. Lapides J, Diokno A, Silber S, Lowe B. Clean intermittent self-catheterization in the treatment of urinary tract disease. J Urol 1972; 107: 458–61.
31. Maynard FM, Diokno A. Clean intermittent catheterization for spinal cord injured patients. J Urol 1982; 128: 477–80.
32. Wu Y, Hamilton BB, Boyink MA, Nanninga JB. Re-usable catheter for longterm intermittent catheterization. Arch Phys Med Rehab 1981; 62: 39–42.
33. Bennett CJ, Young MN, Razi SS et al. The effect of urethral introducer tip catheters on the incidence of urinary tract infection outcomes in spinal cord injured patients. J Urol 1997; 158: 519–21.
34. Lundgren J, Bengtsson O, Israelsson A et al. The importance of osmolality for intermittent catheterization of the urethra. Spinal Cord 2000; 38: 45–50.
35. Waller L, Telander M, Sullivan L. The importance of osmolality in hydrophilic urethral catheters – a crossover study. Spinal Cord 1998; 36: 368–9.
36. Wyndaele JJ, De Ridder D, Everaert K et al. Evaluation of the use of Urocath-Gel catheters for intermittent self catheterization by male patients using conventional catheters for a long time. Spinal Cord 2000; 38: 97–9.
37. Leriche A, Charvier K, Bonniaud V et al. Comparative study of the acceptability of the SpeediCath set and Actreen set catheterization sets in patients performing self-catheterization. Prog Urol 2006; 16(3): 347–51.
38. De Ridder DJ, Everaert K, Fernandez LG et al. Intermittent catheterisation with hydrophilic-coated catheters (SpeediCath) reduces the risk of clinical urinary tract infection in spinal cord injured patients: a prospective randomised parallel comparative trial. Eur Urol 2005; 48(6): 991–5.
39. Vapnek JM, Maynard FM, Kim J. A prospective randomized trial of the LoFric hydrophilic coated catheter versus conventional plastic catheter for clean intermittent catheterization. J Urol 2003; 169(3): 994–8.
40. Kovindha A, Mai WN, Madersbacher H. Reused silicone catheter for clean intermittent catheterization (CIC): is it safe for spinal cord-injured (SCI) men? Spinal Cord 2004; 42(11): 638–42.
41. Jamison J, Maguire S, McCann J. Catheter policies for management of long term voiding problems in adults with neurogenic bladder disorders. Cochrane Database Syst Rev 2004; (2): CD004375.
42. Hedlund H, Hjelmas K, Jonsson O et al. Hydrophilic versus noncoated catheters for intermittent catheterization. Scand J Urol Nephrol 2001; 35: 49–53.
43. Lindan R, Bellomy V. The use of intermittent catheterization in a bladder training program, preliminary report. J Chron Dis 1971; 24: 727–35.
44. Wyndaele JJ. Early urological treatment of patients with an acute spinal cord injury. Thesis Doctor in Biomedical Science, State University of Ghent, 1983.
45. Corcos J. Traitements non médicamenteux des vessies neurogènes. In: Corcos J, Schick E, eds. Les Vessies Neurogènes de l'Adulte. Paris: Masson, 1996: 173–87.

46. Stribrna J, Fabian F. The problem of residual urine after catheterization. Acta Univ Carol Med 1961; 7: 931–43.
47. Jensen AE, Hjeltnes N, Berstad J, Stanghelle JK. Residual urine following intermittent catheterisation in patients with spinal cord injuries. Paraplegia 1995; 33: 693–6.
48. Wyndaele JJ, De Taeye N. Early intermittent selfcatheterization after spinal cord injury. Paraplegia 1990; 28: 76–80.
49. Champion VL. Clean technique for intermittent self-catheterization. Nurs Res 1976; 25: 13–18.
50. Silbar E, Cicmanec J, Burke B, Bracken RB. Microwave sterilization. Method for home sterilization of urinary catheter. J Urol 1980; 141: 88–90.
51. Opitz JL. Bladder retraining: an organized program. Mayo Clin Proc 1976; 51: 367–72.
52. Anton HA, Chambers K, Clifton J, Tasaka J. Clinical utility of a portable ultrasound device in intermittent catheterization. Arch Phys Med Rehab 1998; 79: 172–5.
53. De Ridder D, Van Poppel H, Baert L, Binard J. From time dependent intermittent selfcatheterisation to volume dependent selfcatheterisation in multiple sclerosis using the PCI 5000 Bladdermanager. Spinal Cord 1997; 35: 613–16.
54. Schurch B, Stöhrer M, Kramer G et al. Botulinum-A toxin for treating detrusor hyperreflexia in spinal cord injured patients: a new alternative to anticholinergic drugs? Preliminary results. J Urol 2000; 164: 692–7.
55. Mast P, Hoebeke P, Wyndaele JJ et al. Experience with augmentation cystoplasty. A review. Paraplegia 1995; 33: 560–4.
56. Kilinc S, Akman MN, Levendoglu F, Ozker R. Diurnal variation of antidiuretic hormone and urinary output in spinal cord injury. Spinal Cord 1999; 37: 332–5.
57. Chancellor MB, Rivas DA, Staas WE Jr. DDAVP in the urological management of the difficult neurogenic bladder in spinal cord injury: preliminary report. J Am Paraplegia Soc 1994; 17: 165–7.
58. Koff SA, Gigax MR, Jayanthi VR. Nocturnal bladder emptying: a simple technique for reversing urinary tract deterioration in children with neurogenic bladder. J Urol 2005; 174: 1629–31.
59. Canon S, Alpert S, Koff SA. Nocturnal bladder emptying for reversing urinary tract deterioration due to neurogenic bladder. Curr Urol Rep 2007; 8(1): 60–5.
60. Wheeler JS Jr, Walter JS, Chintam RS, Rao S. Botulinum toxin injections for voiding dysfunction following SCI. J Spinal Cord Med 1998; 21: 227–9.
61. Kiyono Y, Hashizume C, Ohtsuka K, Igawa Y. Improvement of urological-management abilities in individuals with tetraplegia by reconstructive hand surgery. Spinal Cord 2000; 38: 541–5.
62. Bakke A, Vollset SE. Risk factors for bacteriuria and clinical urinary tract infection in patients treated with clean intermittent catheterization. J Urol 1993; 149: 527–31.
63. Adler US, Kirshblum SC. A new assistive device for intermittent self-catheterization in men with tetraplegia. J Spinal Cord Med 2003; 26(2): 155–8.
64. Parmar S, Baltej S, Vaidynanathan S. Teaching the procedure of clean intermittent catheterization. Paraplegia 1993; 31: 298–302.
65. Sutton G, Shah S, Hill V. Clean intermittent self-catheterization for quadriplegic patients – a five year follow up. Paraplegia 1991; 29: 542–9.
66. Perrouin-Verbe B, Labat JJ, Richard I et al. Clean intermittent catheterization from the acute period in spinal cord injury patients. Longterm evaluation of urethral and genital tolerance. Paraplegia 1995; 33: 619–24.
67. Bakke A, Malt UF. Psychological predictors of symptoms of urinary tract infection and bacteriuria in patients treated with clean intermittent catheterization: a prospective 7 year study. Eur Urol 1998; 34: 30–6.
68. Yavuzer G, Gok H, Tuncer S et al. Compliance with bladder management in spinal cord injury patients. Spinal Cord 2000; 38: 762–5.
69. Edwards M, Borzyskowski M, Cox A, Badcock J. Neuropathic bladder and intermittent catheterization: social and psychological impact on children and adolescents. Dev Med Child Neurol 2004; 46(3): 168–77.
70. Borzyskowski M, Cox A, Edwards M, Owen A. Neuropathic bladder and intermittent catheterization: social and psychological impact on families. Dev Med Child Neurol 2004; 46(3): 160–7.
71. Polliack T, Bluvshtein V, Philo O et al. Clinical and economic consequences of volume- or time-dependent intermittent catheterization in patients with spinal cord lesions and neuropathic bladder. Spinal Cord 2005; 43(10): 615–19.
72. Pearman JW. Prevention of urinary tract infection following spinal cord injury. Paraplegia 1971; 9: 95–104.
73. Lapides J, Diokno AC, Lowe BS, Kalish MD. Follow-up on unsterile intermittent self-catheterization. J Urol 1974; 111: 184–7.
74. Donovan W, Stolov W, Clowers D, Clowers M. Bacteriuria during intermittent catheterization following spinal cord injury. Arch Phys Med Rehab 1978; 59: 351–7.
75. Maynard F, Diokno A. Urinary infection and complications during clean intermittent catheterization following spinal cord injury. J Urol 1984; 132: 943–6.
76. Murray K, Lewis P, Blannin J, Shepherd A. Clean intermittent self-catheterization in the management of adult lower urinary tract dysfunction. Br J Urol 1984; 56: 379–80.
77. Wyndaele JJ. Clean intermittent self-catheterization in the prevention of lower urinary tract infections. In: Van Kerrebroeck PH, Debruyne F, eds. Dysfunction of the Lower Urinary Tract: Present Achievements and Future Perspectives. Bussum: Medicom, 1990: 187–95.
78. Sutton G, Shah S, Hill V. Clean intermittent self-catheterization for quadriplegic patients – a five year follow up. Paraplegia 1991; 29: 542–9.
79. Whitelaw S, Hamonds J, Tregallas R. Clean intermittent self-catheterization in the elderly. Br J Urol 1987; 60: 125–7.
80. Bakke A, Vollset SE. Risk factors for bacteriuria and clinical urinary tract infection in patients treated with clean intermittent catheterization. J Urol 1993; 149: 527–31.
81. Ott R, Rosier AB. The importance of intermittent catheterization in bladder re-education of acute spinal cord lesions. In: Proc Eighteenth Vet Admin Spinal Cord Injury Conf 1971; 18: 139–48.
82. Anderson RU. Prophylaxis of bacteriuria during intermittent catheterization of the acute neurogenic bladder. J Urol 1980; 123: 364–6.
83. Prieto-Fingerhut T, Banovac K, Lynne CM. A study comparing sterile and nonsterile urethral catheterization in patients with spinal cord injury. Rehab Nurs 1997; 22: 299–302.
84. Rhame FS, Perkash I. Urinary tract infections occurring in recent spinal cord injury patients on intermittent catheterization. J Urol 1979; 122: 669–73.
85. Shekelle PG, Morton SC, Clark KA et al. Systematic review of risk factors for urinary tract infection in adults, with spinal cord dysfunction. J Spinal Cord Med 1999; 22: 258–72.
86. Barnes D, Timoney A, Moulas G et al. Correlation of bacteriological flora of the urethra, glans and perineum with organisms causing urinary tract infection in the spinal injuries male patient. Paraplegia 1992; 30: 851–4.
87. King RB, Carlson CE, Mervine J et al. Clean and sterile intermittent catheterization methods in hospitalized patients with spinal cord injury. Arch Phys Med Rehab 1992; 73(9): 798–802.
88. Darouiche R, Cadle R, Zenon G 3rd et al. Progression from asymptomatic to symptomatic urinary tract infection in patients with SCI: a preliminary study. J Am Parapleg Soc 1993; 16: 219–24.
89. National Institute on Disability and Rehabilitation Research Consensus Statement Jan 27–29, 1992. The prevention and management of urinary tract infections among people with spinal cord injuries. J Am Parapleg Soc 1992; 15: 194–204.
90. Gribble MJ, Puterman ML, McCallum NM. Pyuria: its relationship to bacteriuria in spinal cord injured patients on intermittent catheterization. Arch Phys Med Rehab 1989; 70: 376–9.

91. Menon EB, Tan ES. Pyuria: index of infection in patients with spinal cord injuries. Br J Urol 1992; 69: 141–6.
92. Noll F, Russe O, Kling E, Botel U, Schreiter F. Intermittent catheterisation versus percutaneous suprapubic cystostomy in the early management of traumatic spinal cord lesions. Paraplegia 1988; 26: 4–9.
93. Yadav A, Vaidyanathan S, Panigraphi D. Clean intermittent catheterization for the neuropathic bladder. Paraplegia 1993; 31: 380.
94. Schlager TA, Hendley JO, Wilson RA et al. Correlation of periurethral bacterial flora with bacteriuria and urinary tract infection in children with neurogenic bladder receiving intermittent catheterization. Clin Infect Dis 1999; 28: 346–50.
95. Hull RA, Rudy DC, Wieser IE, Donovan WH. Virulence factors of *Escherichia coli* isolates from patients with symptomatic and asymptomatic bacteriuria and neuropathic bladders due to spinal cord and brain injuries. J Clin Microbiol 1998; 36: 115–17.
96. McGuire EJ, Diddel G, Wagner F Jr. Balanced bladder function in spinal cord injury patients. J Urol 1977; 118: 626–8.
97. Sperling KB. Intermittent catheterization to obtain catheter-free bladder in spinal cord injury. Arch Phys Med Rehab 1978; 59: 4–8.
98. Barkin M, Dolfin D, Herschorn S et al. The urological care of the spinal cord injury patient. J Urol 1983; 129: 335–9.
99. Wyndaele JJ, Maes D. Clean intermittent self-catheterization: a 12 year follow up. J Urol 1990; 143: 906–8.
100. Barber DB, Woodard FL, Rogers SJ, Able AC. The efficacy of nursing education as an intervention in the treatment of recurrent urinary tract infections in individuals with spinal cord injury. SCI Nurs 1999; 16: 54–6.
101. Waites KB, Canupp KC, Brookings ES, DeVivo MJ. Effect of oral ciprofloxacin on bacterial flora of perineum, urethra, and lower urinary tract in men with spinal cord injury. J Spinal Cord Med 1999; 22: 192–8.
102. Lewis RI, Carrion HM, Lockhart JL, Politano VA. Significance of symptomatic bacteriuria in neurogenic bladder disease. Urology 1984; 23: 343–7.
103. Pearman JW. The value of kanamycin-colistin bladder instillations in reducing bacteriuria during intermittent catheterization of patients with acute spinal cord injury. Br J Urol 1979; 51: 367–74.
104. Haldorson AM, Keys TF, Maker MD, Opitz JL. Nonvalue of neomycin instillation after intermittent urinary catheterization. Antimicrob Agents Chemother 1978; 14: 368–70.
105. Murphy FJ, Zelman S, Mau W. Ascorbic acid as urinary acidifying agent. II: Its adjunctive role in chronic urinary infection. J Urol 1965; 94: 300–3.
106. Stover SL, Fleming WC. Recurrent bacteriuria in complete spinal cord injury patients on external condom drainage. Arch Phys Med Rehab 1980; 61: 178–81.
107. Johnson HW, Anderson JD, Chambers GK et al. A short-term study of nitrofurantoin prophylaxis in children managed with clean intermittent catheterization. Pediatrics 1994; 93: 752–5.
108. Kevorkian CG, Merritt JL, Ilstrup DM. Methenamine mandelate with acidification: an effective urinary antiseptic in patients with neurogenic bladder. Mayo Clin Proc 1984; 59: 523–9.
109. Jepson RG, Mihaljevic L, Craig J. Cranberries for preventing urinary tract infections. Cochrane Database Syst Rev 2000; (2): CD001321.
110. Dollfus P, Molé P. The treatment of the paralysed bladder after spinal cord injury in the accident unit of Colmar. Paraplegia 1969; 7: 204–5.
111. Vivian JM, Bors E. Experience with intermittent catheterization in the southwest regional system for treatment of spinal injury. Paraplegia 1974; 12: 158–66.
112. Pearman JW, Bailey M, Riley LP. Bladder instillations of trisdine compared with catheter introducer for reduction of bacteriuria during intermittent catheterization of patients with acute spinal cord trauma. Br J Urol 1991; 67: 483–90.
113. Galloway A, Green HT, Windsor JJ et al. Serial concentrations of C-reactive protein as an indicator of urinary tract infection in patients with spinal injury. J Clin Pathol 1986; 39: 851–5.
114. Allas T, Colleu D, Le Lannon D. Fonction génitale chez l'homme paraplégique. Aspects immunologiques. Presse Med 1986; 29: 2119.
115. Ohl DA, Denil J, Fitzgerald-Shelton K et al. Fertility of spinal cord injured males: effect of genitourinary infection and bladder management on results of electroejaculation. J Am Parapleg Soc 1992; 15: 53–9.
116. Rutkowski SB, Middleton JW, Truman G et al. The influence of bladder management on fertility in spinal cord injured males. Paraplegia 1995; 33: 263–6.
117. Kuhlemeier KV, Lloyd LK, Stover SL. Localization of upper and lower urinary tract infections in patients with neurogenic bladders. SCI Dig 1982: 336–42.
118. Wyndaele JJ. Chronic prostatitis in spinal cord injury patients. Paraplegia 1985; 23: 164–9.
119. Cukier J, Maury M, Vacant J, Mlle Lucet. L'infection de l'appareil urinaire chez le paraplégique adulte. Nouv Presse Med 1976; 24: 1531–2.
120. Webb R, Lawson A, Neal D. Clean intermittent self-catheterization in 172 adults. Br J Urol 1990; 65: 20–3.
121. Kovindha A, Na W, Madersbacher H. Radiological abnormalities in spinal cord injured men using clean intermittent catheterization with a re-usable silicone catheter in developing country. Poster 86 presented during the Annual Scientific Meeting of IMSOP, Sydney, 2000: 112 [Abstract].
122. Mandal AK, Vaidaynathan S. Management of urethral stricture in patients practising clean intermittent catheterization. Int Urol Nephrol 1993; 25: 395–9.
123. Vaidyanathan S, Soni BM, Dundas S, Krishnan KR. Urethral cytology in spinal cord injury patient performing intermittent catheterisation. Paraplegia 1994; 32: 493–500.
124. Michielsen D, Wyndaele JJ. Management of false passages in patients practising clean intermittent self catheterisation. Spinal Cord 1999; 37: 201–3.
125. Damanski M. Vesico-ureteric reflux in paraplegics. Br J Surg 1965; 52: 168–77.
126. Solomon MH, Foff SA, Diokno AC. Bladder calculi complicating intermittent catheterization. J Urol 1980; 124: 140–1.
127. Amendola MA, Sonda LP, Diokno AC, Vidyasagar M. Bladder calculi complicating intermittent clean catheterization. Am J Roentgenol 1983; 141: 751–3.
128. Morgan JDT, Weston PMT. The disappearing catheter – a complication of intermittent self-catheterization. Br J Urol 1990; 65: 113–14.
129. Reisman EM, Preminger GM. Bladder perforation secondary to clean intermittent catheterization. J Urol 1989; 142: 1316–17.
130. Ku JH, Jung TY, Lee JK, Park WH, Shim HB. Influence of bladder management on epididymo-orchitis in patients with spinal cord injury: clean intermittent catheterization is a risk factor for epididymo-orchitis. Spinal Cord 2006; 44: 165–9.
131. Mizuno K, Tsuji T, Kimura A et al. Twenty-seven years of complication-free life with clean intermittent self-catheterization in a patient with spinal cord injury: a case report. Arch Phys Med Rehabil 2004; 85(10): 1705–7.
132. Oh SJ, Shin HI, Paik NJ, Yoo T, Ku JH. Depressive symptoms of patients using clean intermittent catheterization for neurogenic bladder secondary to spinal cord injury. Spinal Cord 2006; 44(12): 757–62.
133. Turi MH, Hanif S, Fasih Q, Shaikh MA. Proportion of complications in patients practicing clean intermittent self-catheterization (CISC) vs indwelling catheter. J Pak Med Assoc 2006; 56(9): 401–4.
134. Ord J, Lunn D, Reynard J. Bladder management and risk of bladder stone formation in spinal cord injured patients. J Urol 2003; 170 (5): 1734–7

135. Ahluwalia RS, Johal N, Kouriefs C et al. The surgical risk of suprapubic catheter insertion and long-term sequelae. Ann R Coll Surg Engl 2006; 88(2): 210–13.
136. Ku JH, Jung TY, Lee JK, Park WH, Shim HB. Risk factors for urinary stone formation in men with spinal cord injury: a 17 year follow-up study. BJU Int 2006; 97(4): 790–3.
137. Ozawa H, Uematsu K, Ohmori H et al. Long-term usefulness and safety of the contemporary balloon catheter. Nippon Hinyokika Gakkai Zasshi 2005; 96(5): 541–7.
138. Hamid R, Bycroft J, Arya M, Shah PJ. Screening cystoscopy and biopsy in patients with neuropathic bladder and chronic suprapubic indwelling catheters: is it valid? J Urol 2003; 170(2Pt 1): 425–7.
139. Newman E, Price M. External catheters: hazards and benefits of their use by men with spinal cord lesions. Arch Phys Med Rehab 1985; 66: 310–13.
140. Reitz A, Haferkamp A, Wagener N, Gerner HJ, Hohenfellner M. Neurogenic bladder dysfunction in patients with neoplastic spinal cord compression: adaptation of the bladder management strategy to the underlying disease. Neurorehabilitation 2006; 21(1): 65–9.
141. Madersbacher H, Weissteiner G. Intermittent self-catheterization, an alternative in the treatment of neurogenic urinary incontinence in women. Eur Urol 1977; 3: 82–4.
142. Wyndaele JJ, Oosterlinck W, De Sy W Clean intermittent self-catheterization in the chronical management of the neurogenic bladder. Eur Urol 1980; 6: 107–10.
143. Iwatsubo E, Komine S, Yamashita H et al. Over-distension therapy of the bladder in paraplegic patients using self-catheterisation: a preliminary study. Paraplegia 1984; 22: 201–15.
144. McGuire EJ, Savastano J. Comparative urological outcome in women with spinal cord injury. J Urol 1986; 135: 730–1.
145. Kornhuber HH, Schutz A. Efficient treatment of neurogenic bladder disorders in multiple sclerosis with initial intermittent catheterization and ultrasound-controlled training. Eur Neurol 1990; 30: 260–7.
146. Kuhn W, Rist M, Zach GA. Intermittent urethral self-catheterisation: long term results (bacteriological evolution, continence, acceptance, complications). Paraplegia 1991; 29: 222–32.
147. Lindehall B, Moller A, Hjalmas K, Jodal U. Long-term intermittent catheterization: the experience of teenagers and young adults with myelomeningcele. J Urol 1994; 152: 187–9.
148. Waller L, Jonsson O, Norlén L, Sullivan L. Clean intermittent catheterization in spinal cord injury patients: long-term followup of a hydrophilic low friction technique. J Urol 1995; 153: 345–8.
149. Vaidyanathan S, Soni BM, Brown E et al. Effect of intermittent urethral catheterization and oxybutynen bladder instillation on urinary continence status and quality of life in a selected group of spinal cord injury patients with neuropathic bladder dysfunction. Spinal Cord 1998; 36: 409–14.
150. Diokno AC, Sonda LP, Hollander JB, Lapides J. Fate of patients started on clean intermittent self-catheterization 10 years ago. J Urol 1983; 129: 1120–2.
151. Maynard FM, Glass J. Management of the neuropathic bladder by clean intermittent catheterization: 5 year outcomes. Paraplegia 1987; 25: 106–10.
152. Whitelaw S, Hamonds J, Tregallas R. Clean intermittent self-catheterization in the elderly. Br J Urol 1987; 60: 125–7.
153. Webb R, Lawson A, Neal D. Clean intermittent self-catheterization in 172 adults. Br J Urol 1990; 65: 20–3.
154. Timoney AG, Shaw PJ. Urological outcome in female patients with spinal cord injury: the effectiveness of intermittent catheterization. Paraplegia 1990; 28: 556–63.
155. Sutton G, Shah S, Hill V. Clean intermittent self-catheterization for quadriplegic patients a five year follow up. Paraplegia 1991; 29: 542–9.
156. Bakke A. Clean intermittent catheterization – physical and psychological complications. Scand J Urol Nephrol Suppl 1993; 150: 1–69.
157. Hunt GM, Oakeshott P, Whitacker RH. Intermittent catheterization: simple, safe and effective but underused. BMJ 1996; 312: 103–7
158. Lapides J, Diokno AC, Lowe BS, Kalish MD. Follow-up on unsterile intermittent self-catheterization. J Urol 1974; 111: 184–7.
159. Lapides J, Diokno AC, Gould FR, Lowe BS. Further observations on self-catheterization. J Urol 1976; 116: 169–72.
160. Orikasa S, Koyanagi T, Motomura M et al. Experience with non-sterile intermittent selfcatheterization. J Urol 1976; 115: 141–2.
161. Maynard FM, Diokno A. Clean intermittent catheterization for spinal cord injured patients. J Urol 1982; 128: 477–80.
162. Labat JJ, Perrouin-Verbe B, Lanoiselée JM et al. L'autosondage intermittent propre dans la réeducation des blesses medullaires et de la queue de cheval II. Ann Réadapt Méd Phys 1985; 28: 125–36.
163. Hellstrom P, Tammela T, Lukkarinen O, Kontturi M. Efficacy and safety of clean intermittent catheterization in adults. Eur Urol 1991; 20: 117–21.
164. Thirumavalan VS, Ransley PG. Epididymitis in children and adolescents on clean intermittent catheterization. Eur Urol 1992; 22: 53–6.
165. Perkash I, Giroux J. Clean intermittent catheterization in spinal cord injury patients: a followup study. J Urol 1993; 149: 1068–71.

47

Management of neurogenic bladder with suprapubic cystostomy

Andrew Feifer and Jacques Corcos

Introduction

The management of neurogenic bladder dysfunction continues to be controversial to this day. With the introduction of clean intermittent catheterization (CIC) in the 1970s,[1] and widespread usage of anticholinergic medication, we have witnessed an important decline in both lower and upper urinary tract deterioration. CIC has revolutionized the management of neuropathic lower urinary tract dysfunction, it is now considered the gold-standard approach. However, this strategy of bladder management can present a significant difficulty to patients who are either unable to perform the maneuver themselves or who lack the support network necessary for others to aid with this technique. This is particularly relevant to patients with poor upper extremity dexterity, as well as the presence of detrusor bladder sphincter dysinergia.[2] In addition, patients with extensive urethral damage or with progression of their disease rendering other strategies impractical are additionally appropriate candidates for alternate management options.

Although well-defined surgical and medical management options for neurologic-related bladder dysfunction aside from CIC are available,[3] debate continues to linger regarding the optimal manner in which to prevent lower and upper urinary tract deterioration while minimizing treatment-related morbidity. The following discussion will highlight the evidence supporting and negating the use of suprapubic catheterization (SPC) for long-term management of the neuropathic. Other modalities are beyond the scope of this discussion.

Suprapubic cystostomy: technique and clinical implications

The technical aspects of SPC placement have been widely described using a variety of methods.[4,5] The open suprapubic cystostomy under general and spinal anesthesia remains the definitive gold-standard approach; however, several cost-effective minimally invasive alternatives have been described. Percutaneous puncture of the bladder, initially utilizing a 22 G fine spinal needle, followed by skin incision, suprapubic trocar, and 16 F silastic catheter, has been widely successful in the appropriately selected patient.[6] Further modifications of this technique have included the use of peel-away introducers,[7,8] as well as tract balloon dilatation.[9] Further use of fluoroscopy and ultrasound[10] to ensure optimal catheter placement, and the absence of intervening gastrointestinal structures, has been advocated by several authors.[11,12] Alagiri and Seidmon described a percutaneous endoscopic approach with the use of a flexible cystoscope, especially effective in obese patients.[13] Contraindications to this procedure include uncorrected coagulopathy and previous lower abdominal or pelvic surgery. Complications associated with closed SPC are reportedly low (1.6%), as demonstrated by the classical series of Flock et al in 1978.[14] Bowel injury,[15,16] significant bleeding,[17] and prostatic, vaginal, or rectal injury from caudal trocar placement have been described.[18] In sum, careful patient selection and utilization of either fluoroscopy or ultrasound, with or without endoscopic guidance, can serve as an effective alternative to open cystostomy. The open approach should be considered in complicated cases, based on the surgeon's risk assessment.

Suprapubic cystostomy: the evidence

Although CIC is the most frequent bladder management strategy after spinal injury,[19] several important limitations are well known, and, importantly, several studies have demonstrated poor overall compliance with CIC.[20] Although SPC is not considered to be the ideal means for micturitional management, and has been overshadowed by

CIC as a first-line management strategy, this modality has been used extensively and successfully in several clinical settings, including as a treatment for continued urinary incontinence in females.[21] SPC has likewise been used with success in the early treatment of spinal cord lesions.[22] Despite the purported benefits and convenience of SPC, early studies demonstrating accelerated renal deterioration[23–26] relegated it to a second-line management option. Long-term complications associated with indwelling urinary catheters are well reported elsewhere,[27] with studies demonstrating proportionately more renal and other urologic complications with long-term (>10 years) than short-term (removed just after injury) use. An important study by Hackler[28] ($n = 31$) also claimed that patients managed with SPC alone were at increased risk for bladder spasticity and bladder contracture, and thus were more likely to develop upper urinary tract deterioration. This study compared long-term Foley catheterization (>20 years) with SPC (8 years) and external appliance (Texas catheter) (>20 years). Results demonstrated a statistically significant increase in caliectesis, and a decrease in renal function in the SPC group compared to others. Although the incidence of hydronephrosis was higher in the Foley catheterization group, the incidence of de-novo reflux was higher in the SPC group, mainly grade I. Interestingly, only 6 patients were managed with long-term anticholinergic medication, and, of the 6 patients, 4 did not demonstrate deteriorating renal function. In the current climate of standard, effective, anticholinergic pharmacotherapy, it is difficult to determine the modern-day applicability of these results. Sheriff et al[29] recommended catheter clamping and anticholinergics for this purpose. McGuire and colleagues[30] reported a poorer outcome in women with an indwelling urethral catheter (both transurethral and SPC) than in those on CIC after 2 to 12 years. They demonstrated a 54% rate of change in pyelography in the indwelling group as opposed to none in the CIC group.

Risk of primary bladder neoplasia

An important concern with indwelling catheterization, whether transurethral or suprapubic, is the long-term risk of squamous cell bladder neoplasia (SCC). The reported incidence of SCC associated with chronic indwelling urinary catheters is 2.3–10%.[31,32] Although precise long-term consequences of SPC have yet to be completely elucidated, there appears to be an 8% risk of SCC after 25 years of catheterization.[33] The pathogenesis of this condition has been described as being secondary to chronic urothelial irritation and inflammation leading to metaplasia and neoplasia. Inherent in bladder management strategies consisting of indwelling catheters is the necessity for life-long surveillance cystoscopy and upper tract imaging.

Recent analysis and publications

Despite earlier evidence indicating a poor success rate with SPC, recent studies highlighting SPC as the primary modality have demonstrated otherwise. Talbot et al[34] were the first to report a relatively benign course for spinal cord injured patients managed with indwelling catheters (SPC and urethral). Barnes et al[35] described 40 SPC-managed neurogenic bladders with 66-month follow-up data. Poor compliance with CIC, poor dexterity, as well as desire to be independent of care attendants were the most common indications for SPC placement. Results demonstrated that catheter-related complications were relatively common, with a 38% rate of catheter blockage, recurrent urinary tract infections at 23%, and a 13% catheter misplacement rate. Nevertheless, the authors point to a high patient satisfaction as a strong point in their analysis. Continued urethral leakage, particularly in those with lower spinal lesions, was the factor most associated with poor overall satisfaction. Additionally, in a subgroup of patients managed by SP catheters for longer than 24 months, no deterioration of renal function was identified aside from two patients who were not adequately medicated with anticholinergic therapy, and who did not adhere to their regimen of intermittent catheter clamping. Furthermore, the authors demonstrated that daily clamping of the catheter to preserve bladder function led to maintenance of capacity, the absence of new reflux, as well as a trend to lower overall mean detrusor pressure.

Further evidence by Nomura et al[36] surfaced when they looked at 118 patients with neurogenic bladders managed by an SPC. The indications for SPC in this patient population were similar to other series: failure of CIC in 53%, severe urethral damage in 35%, worsening of the original disease in 13%, as well as various other individual indications. Their results demonstrated frequent bladder complications, with a 25% rate of bladder calculus and 10% persistent urethral leak. By using the Kaplan–Meir technique, the estimated stone-free rates at 5 and 10 years were 77% and 64% respectively. A modest rate of cystitis was observed, with no flare-ups documented secondary to the SPC procedure. Deterioration of renal function was observed in 5/118 patients, although the authors state that the upper tract stone burden for these 5 particular patients was significant, and was likely the primary factor responsible for their decline in renal function. Further subgroup analysis involved urine pH analysis in the patients who formed bladder calculus, denoting a statistically higher urinary pH value in stone formers compared to stone-free patients. Furthermore, the average urinary pH of the 118 patients was 7.24, and dividing cases into those with lower and higher values than 7.24 revealed predicted stone-free rates of 92% (>7.24) and 71% (<7.24). The authors also

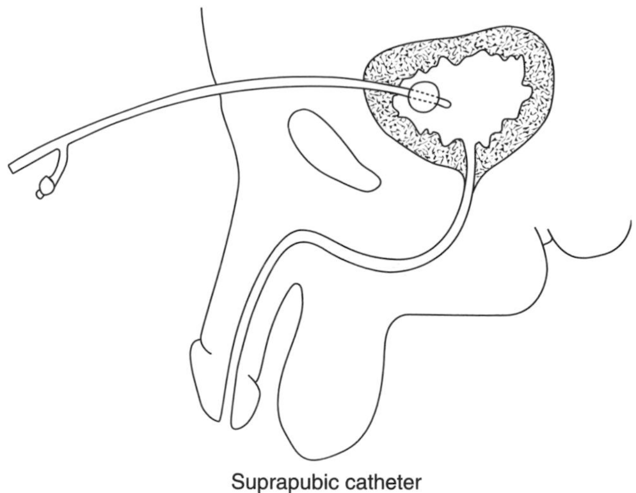

Figure 47.1
Suprapubic cystostomy.

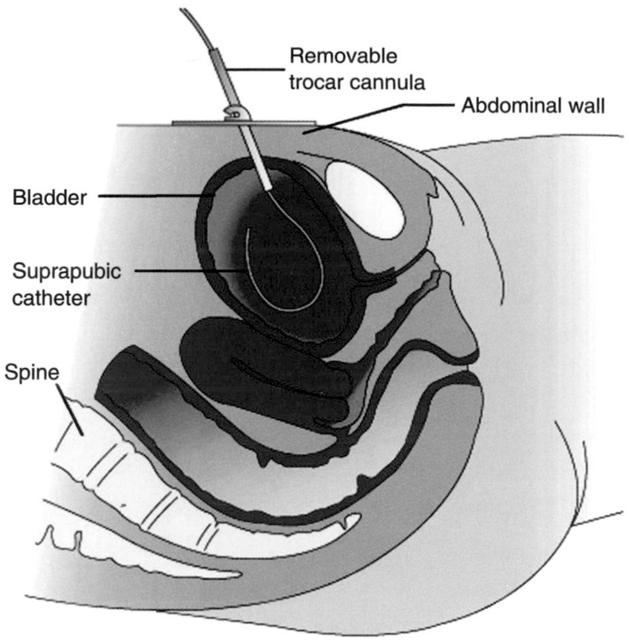

Figure 47.2
Suprapubic cystostomy in female patient.

mention high rates of *Pseudomonas* and *Staphylococcus* colonization of the epidermis.

Several studies have retrospectively compared SPC to CIC. In a study by Mitsui et al,[37] which involved 61 patients, half were managed with CIC and the other half by SPC. There were no significant differences in renal deterioration between the two groups, noted by hydronephrosis, reflux, or overall renal failure. Aside from a statistically significant difference in the incidence of bladder stone formation (65% vs 30%), favoring the SPC group, there were no other significant differences in lower urinary tract complications. The satisfaction questionnaire utilized in this study, although nonvalidated, revealed no statistical differences in satisfaction with either modality. Chao et al published a similar comparison,[38] in which they looked at different bladder management strategies. This study involved 73 patients with spinal injuries, 42 of whom were managed without indwelling catheterization, and 32 with transurethral catheters and SPC. There were no recorded statistically significant differences in renal function or renal complications between these groups. The exception was a higher incidence of calectesis and scarring in the SPC group, demonstrated by follow-up pyelography. The authors also state that of the 6 patients who developed bladder cancer during the follow-up period (3 in the SPC group and three in the CIC group). Only 1/3 patients in the SPC group with bladder cancer had squamous cell carcinoma. Based on the comparable side-effect profile as well as impressive patient satisfaction, these authors recommended SPC in patients who have failed other modalities, but advocated routine cystoscopy and upper tract imaging. Mitsui et al,[37] who also reported no incidence of SCC of the bladder despite a 21-year follow-up in several patients, also advocated frequent catheter changes and bladder irrigation as part of a routine follow-up strategy.

Dewire and colleagues[39] challenged the dogma of avoided indwelling bladder drainage when they reported on a series of 57 spinal trauma patients who were managed with or without indwelling catheter, all with 10-year follow-up. Of the 57 patients, only 5 were managed with an SPC, and 27 with a transurethral catheter, the rest were managed via CIC or other methods. Although little differentiation was made between the SPC and urethral catheter groups, there were no statistical differences between groups for both lower urinary tract complications or the rate of renal deterioration via the Kaplan–Meir technique. Despite the retrospective nature of this study and the absence of specific protocols dictating the management specifics of indwelling catheters, the strong follow-up statistics support further investigation and follow-up for patients managed with indwelling catheters. A classical review by Linden et al[40] clearly supports the role for established multidisciplinary catheter teams for spinal cord trauma patients, as their report clearly demonstrates the improved outcome and lower complication profile when regular bladder care is practiced.

In 1995, McDiarmid and colleagues[41] retrospectively reviewed their long-term SPC data in 44 patients with a 150-month follow-up (12.5 years). The authors advocated

Table 47.1 *Suprapubic cystostomy for neuropathic bladder: current litterature review*

Author	*n*	Mean follow-up (months)	SCys (%)	Bladder stone (%)	CB (%)	OM (%)	New onset reflux (%)	SCC (%)	Renal deterioration (%)
McDiarmid et al[41]	44	150	23 (47)	18 (41)	16 (36)	0	0	0	0
Hackler[28]	62	96	–	11 (18)	–	–	35 (57)	–	61
Mitsui et al[37]	34	80	4 (12)	22 (65)	–	0	0	–	0
Barnes et al[35]	40	23	–	–	–	0	3 (7.5)	–	0
Ahluwali et al[44]	219	50	21		25	10	–	–	–
Weld and Dmochowski [42]	36	30	–	–	–	–	6 (17)	–	25
Nomura et al[36]	118	50	10%	25%	–	–	–	–	5 (4.2)

SCys, symptomatic cystitis; CB, catheter blockage; OM, operative, procedural morbidity; SCC, sqaumous cell carcinoma of the bladder.

a vigorous bladder hygiene program involving both community nursing and bimonthly SPC changes with bladder washing consisting of dilute chlorohexidine. The patients investigated were quadriplegics who could not perform CIC. The results demonstrated no evidence of renal deterioration or de-novo reflux. Only 17 of 44 patients in this series received anticholinergic therapy, and, unfortunately, bladder pressures were not routinely measured. The most common complication reported was uncomplicated and untreated cystitis (51%). Bladder stones were documented in 41% of patients, and three patients presented with renal stones. Catheter blockage (36%) was the other significant complication, and this was treated with oral acidification of the urine, progressive use of larger French catheters (22 F), as well as frequent bladder irrigation. The authors stated that, due to the relatively short follow-up compared to other contemporary series, the absence of both upper and lower urinary tract deterioration, reflux, and squamous cell bladder cancer in this series could be deceiving.

Weld and Dmochowski[42] reported on a retrospective review of 316 postspinal cord injury patients managed with transurethral catheterization (114), CIC (92), and SPC (36). Complications developed in 53% of transurethral catheterized patients, 44.4% of patients with SPC, and 27.2% of patients managed with CIC. The higher rates of complications, both renal and lower urinary tract, were attributed to a significant difference in bladder compliance in the catheter-dependent group. The emphasis on urodynamic pressure in chronically catheterized patients, and its impact on upper tract deterioration, was underscored by the work of Jamil et al,[43] who reported on the urodynamics of 30 patients with SCI over 14.3 years, whose bladders were managed with an indwelling urethral catheter. They found that the indwelling catheters were not always associated with low intravesical pressure: detrusor contractions causing intravesical pressure rises greater than 40 cmH_2O for up to 4.5 minutes were observed in 11/30 patients. Renal scarring was observed in 9 patients and, of these, 6 were in the subgroup with pathologic bladder contractions whereas only 5 of 21 patients with normal kidneys had elevated detrusor pressures.

The most recent and largest retrospective analysis, by Ahluwali et al,[44] examined 219 patients with SPC catheters over 50 months. Their described rate of symptomatic cystitis was 21%, and the rate of catheter blockage was 25%, with operative morbidity and mortality rates of 10% and 1.8%, respectively. Overall, their patient cohort had a satisfaction rating of 71%, in a nonvalidated questionnaire.

Future directions

The existing controversy regarding the management of the neurogenic bladder takes origin from the aforementioned studies, which, although they are commendable and form the basis of current management strategy, are in need of modernization with fresh prospective analyses. Although classical series revealed higher complication rates with SPC compared to CIC, recent retrospective series have tended to demonstrate acceptable results. Although it is accepted that chronic catheterization, including SPC, can lead to elevated complication profiles in susceptible patients, new investigations are necessary to record the impact of full cholinergic blockade and vigorous bladder management strategies.

Conclusions

As such, for spinal cord injured patients who are either unable or unwilling to participate in a CIC program, SPC can be offered as a second-line therapy, with routine cystoscopy and upper tract surveillance forming the backbone of this strategy. Maximizing the independence of SCI patients, as well as allowing degrees of sexual expression, are often paramount, and are valid reasons to choose SPC. Reliance on a multidisciplinary team for bladder maintenance can also diminish the risk of lower tract dysfunction, including bladder calculi, infection, or blocked catheters. Anticholinergic medication as well as a possible role for periodic bladder volume maintenance via periodic catheter clamping should also be considered. Simple maneuvers such as changing the catheter with a full bladder as well as the utilization of larger French catheters will also serve to decrease immediate complications. If these criteria are employed, SPC can serve as a viable option for carefully selected patients in whom CIC is not an option.

References

1. Lapides J, Dlokno AC, Silber SJ, Lowe BS. Clean intermittent self catheterization in the treatment of urinary tract disease. J Urol 1972; 107: 458.
2. Light JK, Beric A, Wise PG. Predictive criteria for failed sphincterotomy in spinal cord injury patients. J Urol 1987; 138: 1201.
3. Dikono AC, Sonda LP, Hollander JB et al. Fate of patients started on clean intermittent self-catheterization therapy 10 years ago. J Orol 1983; 129: 1120.
4. Gottesman JE, Flanagan MJ. Suprapubic cystostomy: a simplified technique. Urology 1978; 11: 478–9.
5. Klimberg I, Wehle M. Percutaneous placement of suprapubic cystostomy tube. Urology 1985; 26: 178–9.
6. Hodgkinson CP, Hodari AA. Trocar suprapubic cystostomy for postoperative bladder drainage in the female. Am J Obstet Gynecol 1966; 96: 773–81.
7. O'Brien WM. Percutaneous placement of a suprapubic tube with peel away sheath introducer. Urol 1991; 145: 1015–6.
8. O'Brien WM, Pahira JJ. Percutaneous placement of suprapubic tube using peelaway sheath introducer. Urology 1988; 31: 524–5.
9. Chin JL, Short TWD. Percutaneous suprapubic cystostomy using balloon dilation. Urology 1990; 35: 261–2.

10. Aguilera P, Choi T. Ultrasonography-guided suprapubic cystostomy catheter placement in the emergency department (abstract). Ann Emerg Med 2002; 40: S75.
11. Michael J, Lee MJ, Papanicolaou N et al. Fluoroscopically guided percutaneous suprapubic cystostomy for long-term bladder drainage: an alternative to surgical cystostomy. Radiology 1993; 188: 787–9.
12. Mond DJ, Lee WJ. Fluoroscopically guided suprapubic cystostomy in complex urologic cases. J Vasc Interven Radiol 1994; 5: 911–4.
13. Alagiri M, Seidmon J. Percutaneous endoscopic cystostomy for bladder localization and exact placement of a suprapubic tube. J Urol 1998; 159: 963–4.
14. Flock WD, Lityak AS, McRoberts JW. Evaluation of closed suprapubic cystostomy. Urology 1978; 11: 40–2.
15. Morse RM, Spirnak JP, Resnick MI. Iatrogenic colon and rectal injuries associated with urological intervention: report of 14 patients. J Urol 1988; 140: 101–3.
16. Noller KL, Pratt JH, Symmonds RE. Bowel perforation with a suprapubic cystostomy: report of two cases. Obstet Gynaecol 1976; 48: 67–9.
17. Lawrentchuk N, Lee D, Marriott P, Russell JM. Suprapubic stab cystostomy: a safer technique. Urology 2003; 62: 932–4.
18. Stine RJ, Avila JA, Lemons MF et al. Diagnostic and therapeutic urologic procedures. Emerg Med Clin North Am 1988; 6: 547–78.
19. Stover SL, Fine PR, eds. Spinal Cord Injury: The Facts and Figures. Birmingham: University of Alabama at Birmingham, 1986.
20. Timoney AG, Shaw PJR. Urological outcome in female patients with spinal cord injury: the effectiveness of intermittent catheterization. Paraplegia 1990; 28: 556–63.
21. Feneley RCL. The management of female incontinence by suprapubic catheterization with or without urethral closure. Br J Urol 1983; 55: 203–7.
22. Peatfield RC, Burt AA, Smith PH. Suprapubic catheterization after a spinal cord injury: a follow-up report. Paraplegia 21: 220–6.
23. Bunts RC. Management of urologic complications in 1000 paraplegics. J Urol 1958; 79: 733–41.
24. Bors E, Comar AE. Neurological Urology. Baltimore University Park Press, 1971: 242.
25. Guttman L. Spinal Cord Injuries. Oxford: Blackwell Scientific Publications, 1973: 361.
26. Ross JC. Diversion of the urine in the neurogenic bladder. Br J Urol 1967; 39: 708–11.
27. Jacobs SC, Kaufman JM. Complications of permanent bladder drainage in spinal cord patients. J Urol 1978; 119: 740.
28. Hackler RH. Long-term suprapubic cystostomy drainage in spinal cord injury patients. Br J Urol 1982; 54: 120–1.
29. Sheriff MKM, Foley S, Macfarlane J et al. Long-term suprapubic catheterization: clinical outcome and satisfaction survey. Spinal Cord 1998; 36: 171–6.
30. McGuire EJ, Savastano J. Urodynamic findings and clinical status following vesical denervation procedures for control of continence. J Urol 1984; 132: 87–92.
31. Kaufman JM, Fam B, Jacobs SC et al. Bladder cancer and squamous metaplasia in spinal cord injury patients. J Urol 1977; 118: 967, 1390, 19876.
32. Bejany DE, Lockhart JL, Rahmy RK. Malignant vessical tumors following spinal cord injury. J Urol 138.
33. Locke JR, Hill DE, Walger Y. Incidence of squamous cell carcinoma in patients with long-term catheter drainage. J Urol 1985; 133: 1034–5.
34. Talbot HS, Mahony EM, Jaffee SR. The effects of prolonged urethral catheterization: I. Persistence of normal renal structure and function. J Urol 1959; 81: 138–43.
35. Barnes DG, Shaw AG, Timoney AG, Tsokos N. Management of the neuropathic bladder by suprapubic catheterization. Br J Urol 1993; 72: 169–72.
36. Nomura A, Ishido T, Teranishi JI, Makiyama K. Long term analysis of suprapubic cystostomy drainage in patients with neurogenic bladder. Urol Int 2000; 65: 185–9.
37. Mitsui T, Minami K, Furuno T, Morita H, Koyanagi T. Is the suprapubic cystostomy an optimal urinary management in high quadriplegics? A comparison study of suprapubic cystostomy and clean intermittent catheterization. Eur Urol 2000; 38: 434–8.
38. Chao R, Clowers D, Mayo ME. Fate of upper urinary tracts in patients with indwelling catheters after spinal cord injury. Urology 1993; 42(3): 259–62.
39. Dewire DM, Owens RS, Anderson GA, Gottlieb MS, Lepor H. A comparison of the urological complications associated with long-term management of quadriplegics with and without chronic indwelling urinary catheters. J Urol 1992; 147: 1069–72.
40. Linden R, Jeffler E, Freehafer AA. The team approach to urinary bladder management in spinal cord injury patients: a 26-year retrospective look at the Highland View Urinary Catheter Care Team. Paraplegia 1990; 28: 314–7.
41. McDiarmid SA, Arnold EP, Palmer NB, Anthony A. Management of spinal cord injured patients by indwelling suprapubic catheterization. J Urol 1995; 154: 492–4.
42. Weld KJ, Dmochowski RR. Effect of bladder management on urological complications in spinal cord injured patients. J Urol 2000; 163(3): 768–72.
43. Jamil F, Williamson M, Ahmed YS et al. Natural fill urodynamics in chronically catheterized patients with spinal cord injury. BJU Int 1999; 83: 396–9.
44. Ahluwali RS, Johal N, Kouriefs C et al. The surgical risk of suprapubic catheterization and long-term sequelae. Ann R Coll Surg Engl 2006; 88: 210–3.

48

Systemic and intrathecal pharmacologic treatment

Tag Keun Yoo, Dae Kyung Kim, and Michael B Chancellor

Introduction

The principal causes of urinary incontinence in patients with neurogenic bladder are neurogenic detrusor overactivity (DO) and/or incompetence of urethral closing function. Thus, to improve urinary incontinence, the treatment should aim at decreasing detrusor activity, increasing bladder capacity, and/or increasing bladder outlet resistance. Pharmacologic therapy has been particularly helpful in patients with relatively mild degrees of neurogenic bladder dysfunction. Patients with more profound neurogenic bladder disturbances may require pharmacologic treatment to augment other forms of management such as intermittent catheterization. The two most commonly used classes of agents are anticholinergics and α-adrenergic blockers (Table 48.1). Intravesical pharmacologic therapy is discussed in Chapter 49.

Table 48.1 *Systemic drugs for incontinence due to neurogenic detrusor overactivity and/or low compliant detrusor*

Bladder relaxant drugs:
- Propantheline
- Oxybutynin
- Tolterodine
- Propiverine
- Trospium
- Flavoxate
- Solifenacin
- Tricyclic antidepressants

Drugs for incontinence due to neurogenic sphincter deficiency:
- Alpha-adrenergic agonists
- Estrogens
- Tricyclic antidepressants

Drugs for facilitating bladder emptying:
- Alpha-adrenergic blockers
- Cholinergics

Drugs for incontinence due to neurogenic detrusor overactivity and/or low-compliant detrusor

Bladder relaxant drugs

Anticholinergic agents are the most commonly used pharmaceuticals in the management of neurogenic bladder. Anticholinergic agents are employed to suppress neurogenic DO. Although there is an abundance of drugs available for the treatment of neurogenic DO, for many of them, efficacy is estimated based on preliminary open studies rather than on controlled clinical trials.[1] However, drug effects in individual patients may be practically important.

General indications of pharmacologic treatment in neurogenic DO are:

1. to improve or eliminate reflex incontinence
2. to eliminate or prevent a high intravesical pressure situation
3. to enhance the efficacy of intermittent catheterization (IC), triggered voiding, and indwelling catheters.

Neurogenic DO due to spinal cord injury (SCI) is mostly associated with a functional outflow obstruction due to detrusor-sphincter dyssynergia (DSD). For the most part, pharmacotherapy in the patients with SCI is used to completely suppress reflex detrusor activity and facilitate IC. Bladder relaxant drugs decrease detrusor contractility also during voiding. With this situation, residual urine increases and must then be assisted or accomplished by IC.

Propantheline

Propantheline bromide is an antimuscarinic drug, which is nonselective for muscarinic receptor subtypes. Despite its success in uncontrolled case series, no adequate controlled study of this drug for neurogenic DO is available.[1,2] The usual adult oral dosage is 7.5–30 mg three to four times daily, although higher doses are often necessary.[3]

Oxybutynin

Oxybutynin hydrochloride is a moderately potent antimuscarinic agent with a pronounced muscle relaxant activity and local anesthetic activity as well.[1,3–5] When given orally, oxybutynin acts mainly as an antimuscarinic.

Several double-blind controlled studies have shown its efficacy for neurogenic DO.[6–11] The overall rate of good results (more than 50% symptomatic improvement) was 61–86% with 5 mg three times per day. Side-effects were noted in all studies and severity increased with dosage. The overall incidence of possible side-effects was 12.5–68%. Most of them are related to antimuscarinic action, with dry mouth as the most common complaint.

A once-a-day controlled-release formulation of oxybutynin, oxybutynin XL (Ditropan XL®), was developed. This controlled-release oxybutynin has less impact on saliva output than conventional immediate-release oxybutynin,[12] and clinical trials have also demonstrated the improvement in the dry mouth rate of oxybutynin XL.[13] Randomized, controlled clinical trials comparing the efficacy and safety of oxybutynin XL with conventional, immediate-release oxybutynin in patients with overactive bladder demonstrated that the urge urinary incontinence episodes declined log-linearly, and no significant difference was observed between the two formulations.[14,15]

Experience with oxybutynin in neurogenic bladder patients

O'Leary et al evaluated the effects and tolerability of extended-release oxybutynin chloride on the voiding and catheterization frequency of a population of multiple sclerosis (MS) patients with neurogenic bladder.[16] This was a 12-week prospective dose titration study of extended release oxybutynin (oxybutynin XL). Multiple sclerosis patients were recruited for this study from the MS clinic within the university. Entry criteria included a postvoid residual (PVR) of <200 ml (in the noncatheterized subjects). These tests were repeated at 6 and 12 weeks. After a 7-day washout period, patients recorded episodes of voiding or catheterization and incontinence for 3 consecutive days. Patients received initial doses of 10 mg oxybutynin XL in the first week. Doses were escalated to weekly or biweekly intervals to a maximum of 30 mg/day. Twenty patients completed the study: the mean age was 46.3 years (range 24–61 years), and 75% of the patients were women. Subjects reported clinical improvement with decreased urinary frequency and incontinence episodes after dosing was escalated to 30 mg. Seventeen patients chose a final effective dose greater than 10 mg, with 13 patients taking at least 20 mg/day at the end of the study. There were no serious adverse events during the course of the study.

For the SCI patients with defined neurogenic DO, O'Leary et al evaluated the urodynamic changes with extended-release oxybutynin chloride in a 12-week prospective dose titration study.[17] After a 7-day washout period, patients were evaluated by videourodynamic study and then treatment at a dose of 10 mg was initiated. Doses were increased in weekly intervals to a maximum of 30 mg/day. Ten patients (mean age 49 years) with complete or incomplete SCI were enrolled and reported clinical improvement, with decreased urinary frequency and incontinence episodes after dosing was escalated to 30 mg. All patients chose a final effective dose greater than 10 mg with 4 patients taking 30 mg/day. Mean cystometric bladder capacity increased by 274 ml to 380 ml ($p = 0.008$). No patient had serious adverse events.

Tolterodine

Tolterodine is a new competitive muscarinic receptor antagonist.[18,19] Several randomized, and double-blind controlled studies in patients with overactive bladder have demonstrated its beneficial effect.[20–28] Jonas et al reported on a randomized, double-blind, placebo-controlled study of tolterodine including urodynamic analysis in a total of 242 patients:[20] 2 mg twice daily was significantly more effective than placebo in increasing maximum cystometric bladder capacity and volume at first contraction after 4 weeks' treatment.

The better tolerability profile of tolterodine compared with oxybutynin has been confirmed in another randomized study on DO.[23] Tolterodine (2 mg twice daily) appears to be as effective as oxybutynin (5 mg three times daily), but is much better tolerated, especially in regard to dry mouth. In a meta-analysis of a four multicenter prospective trials of 1120 patients, moderate to severe dry mouth was reported in 6% of patients receiving the placebo, 4% of patients receiving 1 mg twice daily tolterodine, 17% of patients receiving 2 mg twice daily tolterodine, and 60% of those patients receiving conventional 5 mg three times daily oxybutynin.[21] The other randomized controlled trial of tolterodine by Malone-Lee et al demonstrated superior tolerability and comparable efficacy to oxybutynin in individuals 50 years old or older with overactive bladder.[26]

A comparative study between controlled-release oxybutynin (oxybutynin XL) and immediate-release tolterodine (tolterodine IR) was published:[28] 378 patients were randomized to receive either oxybutynin XL 10 mg ($n = 185$) or tolterodine IR 4 mg (2 mg twice daily) ($n = 193$). The populations were evenly matched with respect to demographics. Oxybutynin XL reduced the number of weekly episodes of urge incontinence from 25.6 to 6.1 instances. Tolterodine IR decreased the number of weekly episodes from 24.1 to 7.8 instances. Oxybutynin XL demonstrated better efficacy ($p = 0.03$) compared with tolterodine IR. Dry mouth and central nervous system side-effects were similar for oxybutynin XL and tolterodine IR.

The safety profile of tolterodine extended release (ER; 4 mg once daily) appears to be better than tolterodine IR. Van Kerrebroeck et al reported a comparative study of the efficacy and safety of tolterodine extended release (ER; 4 mg once daily), tolterodine immediate release (IR; 2 mg twice daily), as well as placebo in 1529 adult patients with overactive bladder.[27] The primary efficacy variable was the change in mean number of incontinence episodes per week, which decreased 53% from baseline in the tolterodine ER group, 45% with tolterodine IR, and 28% in the placebo group. Tolterodine ER and IR provided a similar significant reduction in incontinence episodes vs placebo. Post-hoc analysis of the data using median values, based on a rationale of skewed data distribution, demonstrated improved efficacy of tolterodine ER vs IR. Dry mouth was significantly lower with tolterodine ER than with tolterodine IR (23% tolterodine ER, 31% tolterodine IR, and 8% placebo). The incidence of other side-effects was similar to placebo in the tolterodine ER and tolterodine IR groups.

Tolterodine also proved to be effective in patients with neurogenic DO. Ethans et al compared efficacy and safety of tolterodine with placebo in patients with neurogenic DO in a prospective, randomized, double-blind, and crossover trial.[29] Ten patients with neurogenic DO due to SCI or multiple sclerosis who used intermittent catheterization participated. They found that tolterodine, 2 mg twice daily, was superior to placebo in enhancing catheterization volumes ($p < 0.0005$) and reducing incontinence ($p < 0.001$), but was comparable in cystometric bladder capacity. Incidence of dry mouth was comparable between tolterodine, 2 mg twice daily, and placebo. The authors concluded that tolterodine at the recommended dosage of 2 mg twice daily improved incontinence and bladder volumes compared with placebo, and without significant dry mouth.

An interesting study of tolterodine use in pediatric patients with neurogenic bladder has also been published.[30] The authors investigated the effects of tolterodine over a 5-year follow-up period. Of the 43 patients evaluated, 30 (70%) took their medication consistently and 13 (30%) sporadically. The mean bladder capacity was 354.7 ml in the first group but only 214.7 ml in the noncompliant group ($p < 0.001$). The mean maximal detrusor pressure decreased from 42.2 to 33.6 cmH_2O in the compliant group ($p < 0.001$) and from 49.7 to 46.4 cmH_2O in the noncompliant group ($p = 0.21$). Dry mouth (11/13) and dizziness (7/13) were common in the noncompliant group, whereas only 5/30 reported dry mouth in the compliant group. They concluded that use of tolterodine over a long follow-up period is effective and tolerable.

To have maximal benefits from tolterodine, dosage can be safely increased in some patients with neurogenic bladder. Horstmann et al used double dose tolterodine ER in 21 patients with neurogenic DO.[31] Sixteen patients significantly decreased their incontinence episodes from 8–12 to 0–2 episodes during the doubled treatment. The reflex volume increased from 202 ± 68 to 332 ± 50 ml ($p < 0.001$). Cystometric capacity increased from 290 ± 56 to 453 ± 63 ml ($p < 0.001$). One patient had to stop the medication because of intolerable side-effects and five patients did not experience satisfactory benefit. They concluded that the increased dosage of tolterodine was an effective treatment in patients with neurogenic bladder.

Propiverine

Propiverine hydrochloride is a benzylic acid derivative with musculotropic (calcium antagonistic) activity and moderate antimuscarinic effects.[32] Several randomized, double-blind, controlled clinical studies of this drug in patients with neurogenic DO have been reported.[33,34] In a placebo-controlled, double-blind, randomized, prospective, multicenter trial, Stöhrer et al evaluated the efficacy and tolerability of propiverine (15 mg three times daily for 14 days) as compared to placebo in 113 patients suffering from neurogenic DO caused by SCI.[33] The majority of patients practiced IC for bladder emptying. The maximum cystometric bladder capacity increased significantly in the propiverine group, on average by 104 ml. Sixty-three percent of the patients expressed a subjective improvement in their symptoms under propiverine in comparison to only 23% of the placebo group.

Madersbacher et al, in a placebo-controlled, multicenter study, demonstrated that propiverine is a safe and effective drug in the treatment of neurogenic DO. It is as effective as oxybutynin, but the incidence of dry mouth and its severity is less with propiverine (15 mg, three times daily) than with oxybutynin (5 mg twice daily).[34]

Another multicenter study on adult patients with neurogenic DO was published by Stöhrer et al.[35] They compared the efficacy and tolerability of propiverine and oxybutynin in 131 patients of 18 years or more with neurogenic DO. The maximum cystometric capacity and maximum detrusor pressure during the filling phase were significantly improved in both groups and no significant differences resulted between treatment groups. Dry mouth, the most frequent adverse event, was reported significantly less (47.1% versus 67.2%; $p = 0.02$) in the propiverine compared to the oxybutynin group.

Schulte-Baukloh et al conducted a prospective analysis of the urodynamic effects of propiverine hydrochloride in 20 children with neurogenic DO.[36] Before and after a twice-daily propiverine hydrochloride regimen, reflex volume (RV), maximum detrusor pressure (MDP), maximum cystometric bladder capacity (MCBC), and bladder compliance (BC) were determined urodynamically. After 3–6 months, the mean RV increased from 103.8 to 174.5 ml ($p < 0.005$), MDP decreased from 52.5 to 40.1 cmH_2O ($p < 0.05$), MCBC increased from 166 to 231.9 ml ($p < 0.005$), and BC improved from 11.2 to 30.6 ml/cmH_2O ($p < 0.01$), with propiverine treatment. The incontinence score (scale 0–3) improved from 2.4 to 1.6 ($p < 0.05$). Propiverine was well tolerated, although some children were given higher doses than recommended.

Trospium

Trospium is a quaternary ammonium derivative with mainly antimuscarinic action and has no selectivity for muscarinic receptor subtypes. It is expected to cross the blood–brain barrier to a limited extent and therefore seems to have no negative effects on cognitive function.

In a placebo-controlled, double-blind study in 61 patients with spinal DO, significant improvements in maximum cystometric capacity and maximum detrusor pressure were demonstrated with 20 mg of trospium twice daily for 3 weeks compared with placebo.[37] Few side-effects were noted, compared with placebo. Madersbacher et al compared the clinical efficacy and tolerance of trospium (20 mg twice daily) and oxybutynin (5 mg three times daily) in a randomized, double-blind, urodynamically controlled, multicenter trial in 95 patients with spinal cord injuries and DO.[38] They found that the two drugs are equal in their effects on DO (increase of the cystometric bladder capacity by 30% and decrease of the maximum detrusor pressure by 30%), but trospium has fewer severe side-effects (incidence of severe dry mouth 5% with trospium vs 25% with oxybutynin).[38]

Recently, Menarini et al conducted a double-blind study to discover whether dose escalation of oral trospium is safe and superior to standard dosing in patients with neurogenic DO.[39] They concluded that generally, in patients with neurogenic DO, daily doses of 45 mg trospium chloride can be considered as being the standard dose, and dose adjustment might not usually be necessary. However, increased daily doses of up to 135 mg appear to be safe when prescribed in individual patients less responsive to the drug.

Flavoxate

Flavoxate hydrochloride has a direct inhibitory action on detrusor smooth muscle *in vitro*. Early clinical trials with flavoxate have shown favorable effects in patients with neurogenic DO.[40,41] Several randomized controlled studies have shown that the drug has essentially no effects on DO.[10,42,43]

Solifenacin

Solifenacin succinate (YM905, (+)-(1S,3′R)-quinuclidin-3′-yl 1-phenyl-1,2,3,4-tetrahydroisoquinoline-2-carboxylate monosuccinate) is an orally active muscarinic M_3-receptor antagonist. Even though it has been suggested that M_2 receptors might directly contribute to detrusor contraction in certain disease states, the M_3 receptors are thought to be the most important ones in detrusor contraction.

The efficacy and tolerability of solifenacin in the treatment of patients with overactive bladder (OAB) have been evaluated and proved in many multinational prospective trials.[44–46] Chapple et al conducted the first double-blind multinational trials.[44] Compared with placebo, mean micturitions per 24 hours were significantly reduced with solifenacin 10 mg and 5 mg, and tolterodine. Solifenacin was well tolerated, and incidences of dry mouth were 4.9% with placebo, 14.0% with solifenacin 5 mg, 21.3% with 10 mg, and 18.6% with tolterodine 2 mg twice daily.

Another randomized, double-blind, placebo-controlled trial of the 12-week once daily solifenacin succinate in patients with overactive bladder was conducted.[45] The primary efficacy variable was change in mean number of micturitions per 24 hours. Secondary efficacy variables were changes in mean number of urgency, nocturia, and incontinence episodes per 24 hours, and mean volume voided per micturition. Compared with changes obtained with placebo (−1.59), micturitions per 24 hours were statistically significantly decreased with solifenacin 5 mg (−2.37, $p = 0.0018$) and solifenacin 10 mg (−2.81, $p = 0.0001$). A statistically significant decrease was observed in the number of incontinence episodes with both solifenacin doses (5 mg, $p = 0.002$ and 10 mg, $p = 0.016$). Of patients reporting incontinence at baseline, half of them achieved continence after treatment with solifenacin. Episodes of nocturia were statistically significantly decreased in patients treated with solifenacin 10 mg (−0.71, −38.5%) versus placebo (−0.52, −16.4%, p = 0.036). Episodes of urgency were statistically significantly reduced with both solifenacin doses. Mean volume voided per micturition was statistically significantly increased with both solifenacin doses (p = 0.0001). Dry mouth was reported in 7.7% of patients receiving solifenacin 5 mg and 23% receiving solifenacin 10 mg (vs 2.3% with placebo).

The STAR trial, a prospective, double-blind, double-dummy, two-arm, parallel-group, 12-week study, compared the efficacy and tolerability of solifenacin succinate and extended release tolterodine in patients with OAB.[46] The efficacy and safety of solifenacin 5 or 10 mg and tolterodine extended release (ER) 4 mg once daily were compared in OAB patients. After 4 weeks of treatment, patients had the option to request a dose increase but were dummied throughout, as approved product labeling only allowed an increase for those on solifenacin. As a result, solifenacin, with a flexible dosing regimen, showed a greater efficacy than tolterodine in decreasing urgency episodes, incontinence, urge incontinence, and pad usage, and increasing the volume voided per micturition. More solifenacin treated patients became continent and reported improvements in perception of bladder condition assessments. The majority of side-effects were mild to moderate in nature, and discontinuations were comparable and low in both groups.

Even though there is much evidence for the efficacy and safety of solifenacin for the treatment of OAB/DO, few data are present in the field of neurogenic DO. There is only one experimental animal study by Suzuki et al.[47] This group observed the effects of solifenacin succinate on DO in conscious cerebral infarcted rats. The effects of solifenacin, tolterodine, and propiverine on DO in cerebral infarcted rats were examined. Evaluation was done under conscious conditions using cystometry one day after middle cerebral artery occlusion. Cystometric examination revealed decreases in bladder capacity and voided volume, an increase in residual volume, and no change in micturition pressure. None of the three drugs affected residual volume or micturition pressure. In summary, solifenacin may improve DO without causing urinary retention in cerebral infarcted rats.

Tricyclic antidepressants

Many clinicians have found tricyclic antidepressants, particularly imipramine hydrochloride, to be useful agents for facilitating urine storage, both by decreasing bladder contractility and by increasing outlet resistance.[3,48] However, no sufficiently controlled trials of tricyclic antidepressants in terms of neurogenic DO have been reported. Nevertheless, in some developing countries tricyclic antidepressants are the only bladder relaxant substances that people can afford. The down side with tricyclic antidepressants is the narrow safety profile and side-effects. The potential hazard of serious cardiovascular toxic effect should be taken into consideration.[1] Combination therapy using anticholinergics and imipramine may have synergistic benefits with a low level of evidence.

Drugs for incontinence due to neurogenic sphincter deficiency

Even though the levels of evidence are low, α-adrenergic agonists,[49–51] estrogens,[52] β-adrenergic agonists,[53] and tricyclic antidepressants[54] have been used to increase outlet resistance. No adequately designed controlled studies of any of these drugs for treating neuropathic sphincter deficiency have been published. In certain selected cases of mild to moderate stress incontinence, a beneficial effect may be obtained.[1]

Drugs for facilitating bladder emptying

Alpha-adrenergic blockers

Alpha adrenoceptors have been reported to be predominantly present in the bladder base, posterior urethra, and prostate. Alpha-blockers have been reported to be useful in neurogenic bladder by decreasing urethral resistance during voiding. A multicenter, placebo-controlled, double-blind trial of urapidil – an α-blocker on neurogenic bladder dysfunction – by means of a pressure–flow study demonstrated significant improvement of straining and of the sum of urinary symptom scores, which was associated with a significant improvement of urodynamic parameters (decreases in the pressure at maximum flow rate and the minimum urethral resistance) over the placebo.[55,56]

Doxazosin therapy was reported to decrease leak-point pressure of 2 pediatric patients with neuropathic bladder secondary to myelomeningocele, and it was tolerable.[57]

Alpha-adrenergic blockade also helps to prevent excess sweating secondary to spinal cord autonomic dysreflexia. Sweat glands, primarily responsible for thermoregulatory factors, are innervated by postganglionic cholinergic neurons of the sympathetic system. Alpha-receptor blockade inhibits this postsynaptic neuronal uptake of norepinephrine (noradrenaline) and reduces neurologic sweating.[58]

Cholinergics

In general, bethanechol chloride seems to be of limited benefit for acontractile detrusor and for elevated residual urine volume. Elevated residual volume is often due to sphincter dyssynergia. It would be inappropriate to potentially increase detrusor pressure when there is concurrent DSD.[59]

Therapy for sphincter dyssynergia

In patients with sufficient manual dexterity, the most reasonable treatment option is to abolish the involuntary detrusor contractions (to insure continence) and then to institute intermittent self-catheterization (in order to empty the bladder).[60,61] Treatment options include catheterization (either intermittent or continuous), external sphincterotomy, pharmacologic therapy, urinary diversion, biofeedback, functional electrical stimulation, and several new minimally invasive alternatives to external sphincterotomy (Table 48.2).

Unfortunately, there is no class of pharmacologic agents that will selectively relax the striated musculature of the pelvic floor. Several different drugs have been used to treat detrusor external sphincter dyssynergia (DESD), including the benzodiazepines, dantrolene, baclofen, and α-adrenergic blocking agents.[62–64] Baclofen and diazepam exert their actions predominantly within the central nervous system, whereas dantrolene acts directly on skeletal muscle. Although these drugs are capable of providing variable relief of muscle spasticity, their efficacy is far from complete, and troublesome muscle weakness, adverse effects on gait, and a variety of other side-effects minimize their overall usefulness.[62]

Alpha-adrenergic antagonists have been extensively used for DESD. The rationale for their use is their proven efficacy on internal urinary sphincter (bladder neck and prostate) smooth muscle obstruction. Unfortunately, there is no good clinical study to support the use of alpha blockade for DESD. In addition, there is a report of preliminary success using oral clonidine in 4 of 5 patients with DESD.[65] Continuous intrathecal baclofen infusion has been shown to be effective in diminishing DESD in up to 40% of patients with DESD.[66]

Table 48.2 *Therapy of detrusor-external sphincter dyssynergia*

Conventional surgery:
- External sphincterotomy

Pharmacologic:
- Baclofen (oral or intrathecal)
- Dantrolene
- Benzodiazepine
- Possibly α-adrenergic blockade
- Possibly clonidine

Minimally invasive techniques:
- Sphincter stent
- Balloon sphincter dilatation
- Laser sphincterotomy
- Botulinum toxin injection

Circumventing the problem:
- Intermittent catheterization
- Indwelling catheterization (urethral or suprapubic)
- Urinary diversion

Alpha-adrenergic blockade

Although most researchers would agree that alpha blockers exert their favorable effects on voiding dysfunction primarily by affecting the smooth muscle of the bladder neck and proximal urethra, there are suggestions that they may affect striated sphincter tone as well.[67] Other data suggest that they may exert some effects on the symptoms of voiding dysfunction by decreasing bladder contractility. Alpha antagonists have been shown to be clinically effective in relieving internal sphincter obstruction by their effect on the bladder neck and prostate.[68,69] Whether the striated external urinary sphincter receives sympathetic innervation remains controversial. Most of the research has been carried out only in laboratory animals, where both the presence and absence of alpha receptors have been reported at the external sphincter level.[70–72] Clinical correlation of the effects of α-antagonists on the striated external urinary sphincter during micturition is lacking. Most clinical studies have based their conclusions on effects on the passive urethral pressure profile.[73,74]

The SCI male, with both neurogenic vesical dysfunction and DESD, offers an ideal opportunity to study the interrelationship between the function of the bladder and both the internal and external urinary sphincters.[75] The effect of α-adrenergic innervation and its clinical significance on the two sphincters is more readily apparent in such patients.

Mobley treated 37 patients with neurogenic bladder with phenoxybenzamine and noted 78% success.[76] Unfortunately, no objective data – including urodynamic parameters, length of follow-up, or indications of improvement – were specified. Whitfield et al found a significant decrease in the UPP with alpha blockade in 25 patients with neurogenic vesical dysfunction.[77] However, actual voiding pressure was not reported.

Using intravenous phentolamine, Awad et al noted a significant decrease in pressure along the entire length of the urethra in both sexes, including the peak pressure zone.[78] Olsson et al proposed that a constant state of sympathetic tonus to the internal sphincter exists, and that inhibition of this tonus during micturition results in bladder neck opening.[79]

Research providing evidence against a clinically significant effect of a sympathetic antagonist on the external sphincter includes a report by McGuire et al.[80] They reported on 9 patients with neurogenic bladders and severe autonomic dysreflexia who demonstrated dramatic improvement with phenoxybenzamine. The urethral resistance was unassociated with spasticity of the striated muscle and was abolished by administration of phenoxybenzamine. This documents abnormal urethral smooth muscle activity in SCI patients but fails to demonstrate a sympathetic effect on the external sphincter musculature.

Rossier et al used a pudendal block plus phentolamine to study the effect on the external sphincter.[81] The authors concluded that there was no significant sympathetic innervation of striated muscle in humans. Pudendal nerve blocks have demonstrated sphincter dyssynergia to be mediated through the pudendal nerves via spinal reflex arcs. Phentolamine effects on bladder activity suggest that blockade of α-adrenergic receptors inhibits primarily the transmission in vesical and/or pelvic parasympathetic ganglia, and acts only secondarily through direct depression of the vesical smooth muscle. Their neuropharmacologic results raise strong doubts as to the existence of clinically significant sympathetic innervation of the striated urethral muscle in humans.

Terazosin, a selective α_1-blocker, was examined in 15 normotensive SCI patients.[59] DESD without obstruction of the bladder neck or prostate was documented using videourodynamic evaluation in all patients. Urodynamic testing was performed both before and after treatment was initiated with terazosin (5 mg nightly). Voiding pressure before and during terazosin therapy averaged 92 ± 17 and 88 ± 27 cmH_2O, respectively ($p = 0.48$). After subsequent external sphincterotomy or sphincter stent placement, the voiding pressure was reduced to 38 ± 15 cmH_2O ($p < 0.001$). Nine other patients suffered from persistent voiding symptoms after previous sphincterotomy. Each was subsequently treated with oral terazosin. Of 5 patients who improved with this treatment, urodynamic parameters demonstrated obstruction only at the bladder neck, with no evidence of obstruction at the level of the external sphincter. The 4 patients who failed to improve were documented to have an open bladder neck but obstruction at the level of the external sphincter. This study supports that α_1 sympathetic blockade has no effect on external sphincter function and does not significantly relieve functional obstruction caused by DESD. Also noted was that terazosin is helpful in diagnosing and treating internal sphincter (bladder neck and prostate) obstruction, especially in patients who have persistent voiding symptoms after external sphincterotomy.

Bennett et al conducted another terazosin study in 60 spinal cord injured male patients with DESD.[82] Mean age was 37 years (range 15–70 years) and the patients received terazosin for a 90-day period. Videourodynamic findings were compared with the pretreatment values. Of the 60 patients, 35 completed the study. According to response to treatment, a responders group (group A, $n = 17$) and a nonresponders group (group B, $n = 18$) were identified. Though the bladder capacity and PVR did not change significantly in either group, there was a significant decrease in the maximum detrusor pressure, from a mean of 105.3 to 73.9 cmH_2O, and in maximum urethral pressure gradient (MUPG), from a mean of 84.7 to 54.1 cmH_2O in group A. The time since injury was significantly longer in group A than in group B. They concluded that terazosin in a dose of 10 mg/day was well tolerated and effective in reducing bladder outlet obstruction in many spinal cord injured patients, and they recommended that terazosin should be considered a first-line treatment of vesicosphincter dyssynergia (VSD) prior to contemplating surgery.

Patients demonstrating clinical improvement with terazosin therapy, despite no urodynamic verification of improvement in DESD, may be responding to treatment of autonomic dysreflexia symptoms.[83,84] The patients may feel better because of diminished autonomic dysreflexia activity, despite ongoing DESD.[85] Another reason for clinical improvement without resolution of DESD may be an undiagnosed functional obstruction at the level of the urethral smooth musculature, which should improve with α_1 blockade, rather than true DESD.

Baclofen

Baclofen depresses monosynaptic and polysynaptic excitation of motor neurons and interneurons in the spinal cord and possibly functions as a glycine and gamma-aminobutyric acid (GABA) agonist.[62] GABA has been identified as the major inhibitory transmitter in the spinal cord.[86]

Baclofen has been found useful in the treatment of skeletal spasticity attributable to a variety of causes, especially multiple sclerosis and traumatic spinal cord lesions.[62] Hacken and Krucker found intravenous, but not oral, baclofen effective for patients with detrusor-sphincter dyssynergia, with the side-effects of weakness and dizziness common.[64]

Leyson et al studied high-dose oral baclofen in 25 SCI patients.[87] They concluded that baclofen was helpful in decreasing the resting urethral pressure at the level of the sphincter. Residual urine decreased in 73% of their cases. However, only 20% of the patients demonstrated a reduction in intravesical pressure at high doses of between 140 and 160 mg daily. The safety of long-term oral baclofen is also of significant concern. This study verified the very limited role, if any, that baclofen may have in the treatment of DESD.

Florante et al reported that 73% of their patients with voiding dysfunction caused by acute and chronic SCI had lower striated sphincter responses and decreased residual urine volumes after oral baclofen treatment.[88] However, a very high daily dose of 120 mg was used. The potential side-effects of baclofen include drowsiness, insomnia, rash, pruritus, dizziness, and weakness. The drug may impair the ability to walk or stand, and is not recommended for the management of spasticity resulting from cerebral lesions or disease. Sudden withdrawal has been shown to provoke hallucinations, anxiety, and tachycardia; hallucinations during treatment, which have been responsive to reductions in dosage, have also been reported.[89,90]

Baclofen may be used with an alpha blocker as a combination therapy. In 21 female DSD patients, including 2 with newly diagnosed multiple sclerosis, Kilicarslan et al used baclofen and doxazosin together.[91] Urodynamic studies were performed in all symptomatic patients, and consisted of the measurement of postmicturition residuals, urethral pressure profilometry, and EMG cystometry according to the criteria of the International Continence Society. All patients were treated with baclofen 15 mg/day and doxazosin 4 mg/day. Seven patients received tolterodine 4 mg/day in addition to baclofen and doxazosin because of DO. They found that treatment with combined baclofen and doxazosin appeared to be effective in the female patients with DSD.

Benzodiazepines

Few references are available that provide valuable data on the use of any of the diazepines in the treatment of DESD. The benzodiazepines potentiate the action of GABA at both presynaptic and postsynaptic sites in the brain and spinal cord.[92,93] We have not found the recommended oral doses of diazepam to be effective in controling DESD. Anecdotal improvement may simply be attributable to the anti-anxiety effect of the drug.

Beta-adrenergic agonists

Beta-adrenergic agonists, especially those with prominent beta characteristics, are able to produce relaxation of slow-twitch skeletal muscles.[79] Gosling et al have reported that a portion of the external urethral sphincter comprising the outermost urethral wall consists exclusively of slow-twitch fibers, whereas the striated muscle fibers of the levator ani contain both fast- and slow-twitch fibers.[94] This type of action may account, at least in part, for the decrease in urethral profile parameters seen with terbutaline. There is no clinical evidence of successful treatment of DESD with β-adrenergic agonists.

Dantrolene

Dantrolene sodium exerts its effects by a direct peripheral relaxation action on skeletal muscle.[62,92] Dantrolene has been shown to dissociate excitation–contraction coupling in the sarcoplasmic reticulum of muscle.[62] Hackler et al reported improvement in voiding function in approximately half of their patients with DESD treated with dantrolene.[63]

However, dosages significantly above the recommended daily maximum were required, whereas significant side-effects, especially weakness, were common. Harris and Benson reported that the generalized weakness which dantrolene may induce is often significant enough to compromise its therapeutic effects.[95] Other potential side-effects include euphoria, dizziness, diarrhea, and hepatotoxicity. Fatal hepatitis has been reported in approximately 0.1–0.2% of patients treated with the drug for 60 days or longer, whereas symptomatic hepatitis may occur in 0.5% of patients treated for more than 60 days; chemical abnormalities of liver function are noted in approximately 1%.[96]

Drugs to increase bladder pressure

Modalities that have been tried to increase intravesical pressure to achieve bladder emptying such as suprapubic percussion, Credé's maneuver, and use of bethanechol chloride are not effective and may potentially be detrimental.[68] Increasing the detrusor pressure without simultaneously relaxing the outlet is associated with upper urinary tract morbidity and can aggravate autonomic dysreflexia.[97]

Intrathecal baclofen pump

The use of an intrathecal baclofen pump has also received some attention in the treatment of DESD.[60] These pumps were implanted for severe spasticity and some of the patients experienced improvement in bladder and sphincter functions. Nanninga et al reported their experience in 7 patients for relief of severe spasticity.[98] Six patients demonstrated an increase in bladder capacity and 4 were able to perform IC and remain dry. A slight decrease in maximum intravesical pressure was seen in all the patients. Talalla et al noted an inconsistent effect of intrathecal baclofen on urethral pressure in 6 SCI patients.[99] Two patients had significant reduction in maximum urethral and maximum detrusor pressures. Side-effects included half of the patients noticing that reflex erections were reduced or abolished for at least 24 hours following intrathecal baclofen. The authors reported that this side-effect has deterred other patients from considering this treatment modality.

With 10 patients with severe spasticity due to spinal cord pathology, a prospective, blinded study was performed to examine the effects of acute bolus and chronic continuous intrathecal baclofen on genitourinary function.[100] Symptom questionnaires and urodynamic studies were performed after a bolus dose of baclofen and 6 to 12 months after continuous intrathecal baclofen. Uninhibited bladder contractions were eliminated in all patients with irritative voiding and urge incontinence. Of 3 patients with an indwelling urethral catheter for incontinence due to neurogenic DO, 1 was converted to intermittent self-catheterization. A 72% increase in capacity and 16% improvement in compliance were observed in subjects without cervical spinal cord pathology. DESD was abolished in 40% of the patients. The authors suggested continuous intrathecal baclofen might be a good option for the patients with neurogenic bladder who have decreased bladder compliance and neurogenic DO not controlled by oral medication.

Long-term clinical, electrophysiologic, and urodynamic effects of chronic intrathecal baclofen infusion were proved for treatment of spinal spasticity.[101] Mertens et al followed 17 patients after chronic intrathecal baclofen infusion using an implanted programmable pump. Nine tetraparetics, seven paraplegics, and one paraparetic were enrolled and regularly followed for 5 to 69 months (mean 37.5 months). Due to reduction of hypertonia, spasms, and pain related to contractures, all patients experienced significant amelioration of quality of life. Neurogenic pain improved in 3 cases, and various degrees of motor improvement were detected in patients whose motor functions were partially preserved. Chronic baclofen infusion increased the flexion reflex threshold and reduced the amplitude very significantly in all our patients. In half of the patients with spastic neurogenic bladder, intrathecal baclofen produced a decrease of detrusor hypertonia and hyperactivity, with reduction of leakage and increase in functional bladder capacity.

Future perspectives in new drug development for neurogenic bladder and new therapeutic strategies in neurourology

During the past few years, research in neurourology has stimulated the development of new therapeutic approaches for incontinence, including the intravesical administration of afferent neurotoxins such as capsaicin and resiniferatoxin. What are the research priorities for the future? It will be important to focus on the development of neuropharmacologic agents that can suppress the unique components of abnormal bladder reflex mechanisms and thereby act selectively to decrease symptoms without altering normal voiding function. To end this chapter, we would like to speculate on a few areas of research with new and better treatment of neuropathic urinary incontinence.

New drug development for neurogenic bladder

Bladder-specific K^+ channel openers. Can truly bladder smooth muscle or afferent neuron-specific potassium channel openers be developed. This treatment may alleviate the overactive and sensitive bladder without any dry mouth.

Intravesical vanilloid treatment. Can the clinical utility of intravesical resiniferatoxin be perfected so that the preferred therapy for neurogenic bladder is a simple outpatient 30 min instillation of 30 ml resiniferatoxin that will last 3 months without systemic side-effects?

Anticholinergic drugs. Can the pharmaceutical companies develop a truly bladder-specific and effective anticholinergic drug with no dry mouth?

Tachykinin antagonists. These substances are appealing in that they may be effective without increasing residual urine volumes. Can clinically useful and safe NK antagonists be developed?

Calcium mobilization and calcium signal modulating agents: Calcium homeostasis in muscle cells is a critical requirement for normal contractile function. Alterations in intracellular calcium metabolism would be expected to lead to urethral sphincter and bladder dysfunction. These would be new targets for the restoration of lower urinary tract function.

New therapeutic strategies in neurourology

Beyond the horizon of nearterm advancement, we predict a brave new paradigm in neurourology. What has already started is the evolution of unstoppable forces of change in medicine that include pharmacogenomics, tissue engineering, and gene therapy. These will change how we practice urology and gynecology.

Pharmacogenomics. Medicine will be tailored to the genetic make-up of each individual. Through microarray gene chip technology, we will know how a patient metabolizes medications and the patient's receptor(s) profile and allergy risk. These factors can be screened against a list of medications prior to therapy. A physician will then be able to always prescribe the best drug for each patient without the risk of allergic reaction.

Tissue engineering. Rapid advances are being made feasible in tissue and organ reconstruction using autologous tissue and stem cells. We envisage a day, in the not too distant future, when stress incontinence is cured not with a cadaver ligament and metal screws into the bones but rather with a minimally-invasive injection of stem cells that will not only bulk up the deficient sphincter but also actually improve the sphincter's contractility and function.

Gene therapy. Diabetic neurogenic bladder and visceral pain may be cured with one or more injections of a gene vector that the physician will inject into the bladder or urethra. Injection of a nerve growth factor via a herpes virus vector into the bladder of a diabetic may restore bladder sensation and innervation. Can the introduction of a virus that expresses the production of endorphin that is site- and nerve-specific help alleviate pelvic visceral pain, regardless of the cause?

References

1. Andersson K-E. Current concepts in treatment of disorders of micturition. Drugs 1988; 35: 477.
2. Blaivas JG, Labib KB, Michalik J, Zayed AAH. Cystometric response to propantheline in detrusor hyperreflexia: therapeutic implications. J Urol 1980; 124: 259.
3. Wein AJ. Neuromuscular dysfunction of the lower urinary tract and its treatment. In: Walsh, Retik, Vaughan, Wein AJ, eds. Campbell's Urology, 7th edn. 1997: 953–1006.
4. Anderson GF, Fredericks CM. Characterization of the oxybutynin antagonism of drug-induced spasms in detrusor. Pharmacology 1972; 15: 31.
5. Yarker YE, Goa KL, Fitton A. Oxybutynin. A review of its pharmacodynamic and pharmacokinetic properties, and its therapeutic use in detrusor instability. Drugs Aging 1995; 6(3): 243.
6. Thompson IM, Lauvetz R. Oxybutynin in bladder spasm, neurogenic bladder, and enuresis. Urology 1976; 8: 452.
7. Hehir M, Fitzpatrick JM. Oxybutynin and prevention of urinary incontinence in spinal bifida. Eur Urol 1985; 11(4): 254.
8. Gajewski JB, Awad SA. Oxybutynin versus propantheline in patients with multiple sclerosis and detrusor hyperreflexia. J Urol 1986; 135(5): 966.
9. Koyanagi T, Maru A et al. Clinical evaluation of oxybutynin hydrochloride (KL007 tablets) for the treatment of neurogenic bladder and unstable bladder: a parallel double-blind controlled study with placebo. Nishi Nihon Hinyouki 1986; 48: 1050. [in Japanese]
10. Zeegers AGM, Kiesswetter H, Kramer AEJ, Jonas U. Conservative therapy of frequency, urgency and urge incontinence: a double blind clinical trial of flavoxate hydrochloride, oxybutynin chloride, emepronium bromide and placebo. World J Urol 1987; 5: 57.
11. Thüroff JW, Bunke B, Ebner A et al. Ramdomized, double-blind, multicenter trial on treatment of frequency, urgency and urge incontinence related to detrusor hyperactivity: oxybutynin versus propantheline versus placebo. J Urol 1991; 145: 813.
12. Chancellor MB, Appell RA, Sathyan G, Gupta SK. A comparison of the effects on saliva output of oxybutynin chloride and tolterodine tartrate. Clin Ther 2001; 23: 753–60.
13. Siddiqui MA, Perry CM, Scott LJ. Oxybutynin extended-release: a review of its use in the management of overactive bladder. Drugs. 2004; 64: 885–912.
14. Birns J, Lukkari E, Malone-Lee JG. A randomized controlled trial comparing the efficacy of controlled-release oxybutynin tablets (10 mg once daily) with conventional oxybutynin tablets (5 mg twice daily) in patients whose symptoms were stabilized on 5 mg twice daily of oxybutynin. BJU Int 2000; 85: 793–8.
15. Versi E, Appell R, Mobley D et al. Dry mouth with conventional and controlled-release oxybutynin in urinary incontinence. The Ditropan XL Study Group. Obstet Gynecol 2000; 95: 718.
16. O'Leary M, Erickson JR, Smith CP et al. Effect of controlled release oxybutynin on neurogenic bladder function in spinal cord injury. J Spinal Cord Med 2003; 26: 159–62.
17. O'Leary M, Erickson JR, Smith CP et al. Effect of controlled-release oxybutynin on neurogenic bladder function in spinal cord injury. J Spinal Cord Med 2003; 26: 159–62.
18. Nilvebrant L, Andersson K-E, Gillberg P-G et al. Tolterodine – a new bladder selective antimuscarinic agent. Eur J Pharmacol 1997; 327: 195.
19. Nilvebrant L, Hallen B, Larsson G. Tolterodine – a new bladder selective muscarinic receptor antagonist: preclinical pharmacological and clinical data. Life Sci 1997; 60: 1129.
20. Jonas U, Hofner K, Madersbacher H, Holmdahl TH. Efficacy and safety of two doses of tolterodine versus placebo in patients with detrusor overactivity and symptoms of frequency, urge incontinence, and urgency: urodynamic evaluation. The International Study Group. World J Urol 1997; 15: 144.
21. Appell RA. Clinical efficacy and safety of tolterodine in the treatment of overactive bladder: a pooled analysis. Urology 1997; 50: 90–6.
22. Rentzhog L, Stanton SL, Cardozo L et al. Efficacy and safety of tolterodine in patients with detrusor instability: a dose-ranging study. Br J Urol 1998; 81: 42.
23. Abrams P, Freeman R, Anderstrom C, Mattiasson A. Tolterodine, a new antimuscarinic agent: as effective but better tolerated than oxybutynin in patients with an overactive bladder. Br J Urol 1998; 81: 801.
24. Van Kerrebroeck PE, Amarenco G, Thuroff JW et al. Dose-ranging study of tolterodine in patients with detrusor hyperreflexia. Neurourol Urodyn 1998; 17: 499.
25. Goessl C, Sauter T, Michael T et al. Efficacy and tolerability of tolterodine in children with detrusor hyperreflexia. Urology 2000; 55: 414.
26. Malone-Lee J, Shaffu B, Anand C, Powell C. Tolterodine: superior tolerability than and comparable efficacy to oxybutynin in individuals 50 years old or older with overactive bladder: a randomized controlled trial. J Urol 2001; 165: 1452.
27. Van Kerrebroeck P, Kreder K, Jonas U et al. Tolterodine once-daily: superior efficacy and tolerability in the treatment of the overactive bladder. Urology 2001; 57: 414.
28. Appell RA, Sand P, Dmochowski R et al. Prospective randomized controlled trial of extended-release oxybutynin chloride and tolterodine tartrate in the treatment of overactive bladder: results of the OBJECT Study. Mayo Clin Proc 2001; 76: 358.
29. Ethans KD, Nance PW, Bard RJ, Casey AR, Schryvers OI. Efficacy and safety of tolterodine in people with neurogenic detrusor overactivity. J Spinal Cord Med 2004; 27: 214–18.
30. Christoph F, Moschkowitsch A, Kempkensteffen C et al. Long-term efficacy of tolterodine and patient compliance in pediatric patients with neurogenic detrusor overactivity. Urol Int 2007; 79: 55–9 .
31. Horstmann M, Schaefer T, Aguilar Y, Stenzl A, Sievert KD. Neurogenic bladder treatment by doubling the recommended antimuscarinic dosage. Neurourol Urodyn 2006; 25: 441–5.

32. Tokuno H, Chowdhury JU, Tomita T. Inhibitory effects of propiverine on rat and guinea-pig urinary bladder muscle. Naunyn Schmiedeberg's Arch Pharmacol 1993; 348: 659.
33. Stöhrer M, Madersbacher H, Richter R et al. Efficacy and safety of propiverine in SCI-patients suffering from detrusor hyperreflexia – a double-blind, placebo-controlled clinical trial. Spinal Cord 1999; 37: 196.
34. Madersbacher H, Halaska M, Voigt R et al. A placebo-controlled, multicentre study comparing the tolerability and efficacy of propiverine and oxybutynin in patients with urgency and urge incontinence. BJU Int 1999; 84: 646.
35. Stöhrer M, Mürtz G, Kramer G et al. Propiverine Investigator Group. Propiverine compared to oxybutynin in neurogenic detrusor overactivity – results of a randomized, double-blind, multicenter clinical study. Eur Urol 2007; 51: 235–42.
36. Schulte-Baukloh H, Mürtz G, Henne T et al. Urodynamic effects of propiverine hydrochloride in children with neurogenic detrusor overactivity: a prospective analysis. BJU Int 2006; 97: 355–8.
37. Stöhrer M, Bauer P, Giannetti BM et al. Effects of trospium chloride on urodynamic parameters in patients with detrusor hyperreflexia due to spinal cord injuries. A multicentre placebo-controlled double-blind trial. Urol Int 1991; 47: 138.
38. Madersbacher H, Stöhrer M, Richter R et al. Trospium chloride versus oxybutynin: a randomized, double-blind, multicentre trial in the treatment of detrusor hyperreflexia. Br J Urol 1995; 75: 452.
39. Menarini M, Del Popolo G, Di Benedetto P et al. TcP128-Study Group. Trospium chloride in patients with neurogenic detrusor overactivity: is dose titration of benefit to the patients? Int J Clin Pharmacol Ther 2006; 44: 623–32.
40. Kohler FP, Morales PA. Cystometric evaluation of flavoxate hydrochloride in normal and neurogenic bladder. J Urol 1968; 100: 729.
41. Pedersen E, Bjarnason EV, Hansen P-H. The effect of flavoxate on neurogenic bladder dysfunction. Acta Neurol Scand 1972; 48: 487.
42. Robinson JM, Brocklehurst JC. Emepronium bromide and flavoxate hydrochloride in the treatment of urinary incontinence associated with detrusor instability in elderly women. Br J Urol 1983; 55: 371.
43. Chapple CR, Parkhouse H, Gardener C, Milroy EJ. Double blind, placebo-controlled, crossover study of flavoxate in the treatment of idiopathic detrusor instability. Br J Urol 1990; 66: 491.
44. Chapple CR, Araño P, Bosch JL et al. Solifenacin appears effective and well tolerated in patients with symptomatic idiopathic detrusor overactivity in a placebo- and tolterodine-controlled phase 2 dose-finding study. BJU Int 2004; 93: 71–7.
45. Cardozo L, Lisec M, Millard R et al. Randomized, double-blind placebo controlled trial of the once daily antimuscarinic agent solifenacin succinate in patients with overactive bladder. J Urol 2004; 172: 1919–24.
46. Chapple CR, Martinez-Garcia R, Selvaggi L et al. for the STAR study group. A comparison of the efficacy and tolerability of solifenacin succinate and extended release tolterodine at treating overactive bladder syndrome: results of the STAR trial. Eur Urol 2005; 48: 464–70.
47. Suzuki M, Ohtake A, Yoshino T et al. Effects of solifenacin succinate (YM905) on detrusor overactivity in conscious cerebral infarcted rats. Eur J Pharmacol 2005; 512: 61–6.
48. Barrett D, Wein AJ. Voiding dysfunction diagnosis, classification and management. In: Gillenwater JY, Grayhack JT, Howards SS, Duckett JW, eds. Adult and Pediatric Urology, 2nd edn. St Louis: Mosby-Year Book, 1991: 1001–99.
49. Diokno AC, Taub M. Ephedrine in treatment of urinary incontinence. Urology 1975; 5: 624.
50. Awad SA, Downie JW, Kiriluta HG. Alpha-adrenergic agents in urinary disorders of the proximal urethra, part I: sphincteric incontinence. Br J Urol 1978; 50: 332.
51. Bauer S. An approach to neurogenic bladder: an overview: Probl Urol 1994; 8: 441.
52. Beisland HO, Fossberg E, Sander S. On incompetent urethral closure mechanism: treatment with estriol and phenylpropanolamine. Scand J Urol Nephrol 1981; 60(Suppl): 67.
53. Gleason D, Reilly R, Bottaccini M, Pierce MJ. The urethral continence zone and its relation to stress incontinence. J Urol 1974; 112: 81.
54. Gilja I, Radej M, Kovacic M, Parazajders J. Conservative treatment of female stress incontinence with imipramine. J Urol 1984; 132: 909–11.
55. Yasuda K, Yamanishi T, Homma Y et al. The effect of urapidil on neurogenic bladder: a placebo controlled double-blind study. J Urol 1996; 156: 1125.
56. Yamanishi T, Yasuda K, Kawabe K et al. A multicenter placebo-controlled, double-blind trial of urapidil, an α-blocker, on neurogenic bladder dysfunction. Eur Urol 1999; 35: 45.
57. Austin PF, Homsy YL, Masel JL et al. alpha-Adrenergic blockade in children with neuropathic and nonneuropathic voiding dysfunction. J Urol 1999; 162: 1064–7.
58. Chancellor MB, Erhard MJ, Hirsch IH, Staas WE. Prospective evaluation of terazosin for the treatment of autonomic dysreflexia. J Urol 1994; 151: 111–13.
59. Chancellor MB, Erhard MJ, Rivas DA. Clinical effect of alpha-1 antagonism by terazosin on external and internal urinary sphincter. J Am Parapleg Soc 1993; 16: 207–14.
60. Lapides J, Diokno AC, Silber SJ, Lowe BS. Clean intermittent self-catheterization in the treatment of urinary tract disease. J Urol 1972; 107: 7458–61.
61. Maynard FM, Diokno AC. Clean intermittent catheterization for spinal cord injury patients. J Urol 1982; 128: 477–80.
62. Cedarbaum JM, Schleifer LS. Drugs for Parkinson's disease, spasticity, and acute muscle spasms. In: Gilman AG, Rail TW, Nies AS, Taylor P, eds. Goodman and Gilman's The Pharmacological Basis of Therapeutics, 8th edn. New York: Pergamon, 1990: 463–84.
63. Hackler RH, Broecker BH, Klein FA, Brady SM. A clinical experience with dantrolene sodium for external urinary sphincter hypertonicity in spinal cord injured patients. J Urol 1980; 124: 78-81.
64. Hacken HJ, Krucker V. Clinical and laboratory assessment of the efficacy of baclofen on urethral sphincter spasticity in patients with traumatic paraplegia. Eur Urol 1977; 3: 237–40.
65. Herman RM, Wainberg MC. Clonidine inhibits vesico-sphincter reflexes in patients with spinal cord lesions. Arch Phys Med Rehab 1991; 72: 539–45.
66. Steers WD, Meythaler JM, Haworth C et al. Effects of acute bolus and chronic continuous intrathecal baclofen on genitourinary dysfunction due to spinal cord pathology. J Urol 1992; 148: 1849–55.
67. Hacken HJ. Clinical and urodynamic assessment of alpha adrenolytic therapy in patients with neurogenic bladder function. Paraplegia 1980; 18: 229.
68. Caine M. The present role of alpha-adrenergic blockers in the treatment of benign prostatic hypertrophy. J Urol 1986; 136: 1.
69. Lepor J, Gup DI, Baumann M, Shapiro E. Laboratory assessment of terazosin and alpha-1 blockade in prostatic hyperplasia. Urology 1988; (Suppl)32: 21.
70. Elbadawi A, Schenk EA. A new theory of the innervation of bladder musculature. Part 4: Innervation of the vesicourethral junction and external urethral sphincter. J Urol 1974; 111: 613.
71. Awad SA, Downie JW. Sympathetic dyssynergia in the region of the external sphincter. A possible source of lower urinary tract obstruction. J Urol 1977; 118: 636–40.
72. Dixon JS, Gosling JA. Light and electron microscopic observation on noradrenergic nerves and striated muscle cells of the guinea pig urethra. Am J Anat 1977; 149: 121.
73. Awad SA, Downie JW. Relative contributions of smooth and striated muscles to canine urethral pressure profile. Br J Urol 1976; 48: 347–54.
74. Yalla SV, Rossier AB, Fam B. Dyssynergic vesicourethral responses during bladder rehabilitation in spinal cord injury patients: effects of suprapubic percussion, credé method and bethanechol chloride. J Urol 1976; 115: 575.

75. Kaplan SA, Chancellor MB, Blaivas JG. Bladder and sphincter behavior in patients with spinal cord lesions. J Urol 1991; 46: 113–17.
76. Mobley DF. Phenoxybenzamine in the management of neurogenic vesical dysfunction. J Urol 1976; 116: 737–8.
77. Whitfield HN, Doyle PT, Mayo ME, Poopalasingham N. The effect of adrenergic blocking drugs on outflow resistance. Br J Urol 1976; 47: 823–7.
78. Awad SA, Downie JW, Lywood DW et al. Sympathetic activity in the proximal urethra in patients with urinary obstruction. J Urol 1976; 115: 545–547.
79. Olsson AT, Swanberg E, Svedinger L. Effects of beta adrenoceptor agonists on airway smooth muscle and on slow contracting skeletal muscle: in vitro and in vivo results compared. Acta Pharmacol Toxicol 1979; 44: 272.
80. McGuire EJ, Wagner F, Weiss RM. Treatment of autonomic dysreflexia with phenoxybenzamine. J Urol 1976; 115: 53–5.
81. Rossier AB, Fam BA, Lee IY et al. Role of striated and smooth muscle components in the urethral pressure profile in the traumatic neurogenic bladder: a neuropharmacological and urodynamic study. Preliminary report. J Urol 1982; 128: 529–35.
82. Bennett JK, Foote J, El-Leithy TR et al. Terazosin for vesicosphincter dyssynergia in spinal cord-injured male patients. Mol Urol 2000; 4: 415–20.
83. Sizemore GW, Winternitz WW Autonomic hyper-reflexia-suppression with alpha-adrenergic blocking agents. N Engl J Med 1970; 282: 795.
84. Scott MB, Morrow JW. Phenoxybenzamine in neurogenic bladder dysfunction after spinal cord injury. II. Autonomic dysreflexia. J Urol 1978; 119: 483–4.
85. Chancellor MB, Karasick S, Erhard MJ et al. Intraurethral wire mesh prosthesis placement in the external urinary sphincter of spinal cord injured men. Radiology 1993; 187: 551.
86. Bloom FE. Neurohumoral transmission and the central nervous system. In: Gilman AG, Rail TW, Nies AS, Taylor P, eds. Goodman and Gilman's The Pharmacological Basis of Therapeutics, 8th edn. New York: Pergamon, 1990: 244–68.
87. Leyson JFJ, Martin BF, Sporer A. Baclofen in the treatment of detrusor-sphincter dyssynergia in spinal cord injury patients. J Urol 1980; 124: 82–4.
88. Florante J, Leyson J, Martin F, Sporer A. Baclofen in the treatment of detrusor-sphincter dyssynergia in spinal cord injury patients. J Urol 1980; 124: 82–4.
89. Roy CW, Wakefield IR. Baclofen pseudopsychosis: case report. Paraplegia 1986; 24: 318.
90. Rivas DA, Chancellor MB, Hill K, Friedman M. Neurologic manifestations of baclofen withdrawal. J Urol 1993; 150: 1903–5.
91. Kilicarslan H, Ayan S, Vuruskan H, Gokce G, Gultekin EY. Treatment of detrusor sphincter dyssynergia with baclofen and doxazosin. Int Urol Nephrol 2006; 38: 537–41.
92. Davidoff RA. Antispasticity drugs: mechanisms of action. Ann Neurol 1985; 17: 107.
93. Lader M. Clinical pharmacology of benzodiazepines. Ann Rev Med 1987; 38: 19.
94. Gosling JA, Dixon JS, Critchley HOD et al. A comparative study of the human external sphincter and periurethral levator ani muscles. Br J Urol 1981; 153: 35.
95. Harris JD, Benson GS. Effect of dantrolene on canine bladder contractility. Urology 1980; 16: 229.
96. Ward A, Chaffman MO, Sorkin EM. Dantrolene. A review of its pharmacodynamic and pharmacokinetic properties and therapeutic use in malignant hyperthermia, the neuroleptic syndrome and an update of its use in muscle spasticity. Drugs 1986; 32: 130.
97. McGuire EJ, Woodside JR, Borden TA, Weiss RM. The prognostic significance of urodynamic testing in myelodysplastic patients. J Urol 1981; 126: 205–9.
98. Nanninga JB, Frost F, Penn R. Effect of intrathecal baclofen on bladder and sphincter function. J Urol 1989; 142: 101–5.
99. Talalla A, Grundy D, Macdonell R. The effect of intrathecal baclofen on the lower urinary tract in paraplegia. Paraplegia 1990; 8: 420–7.
100. Steers WD, Meythaler JM, Haworth C, Herrell D, Park TS. Effects of acute bolus and chronic continuous intrathecal baclofen on genitourinary dysfunction due to spinal cord pathology. J Urol 1992; 148(6): 1849–55.
101. Mertens P, Parise M, Garcia Larrea L et al. Long-term clinical, electrophysiological and urodynamic effects of chronic intrathecal baclofen infusion for treatment of spinal spasticity. Acta Neurochir Suppl 1995; 64: 17–25.

49

Intravesical pharmacologic treatment for neurogenic detrusor overactivity

Brigitte Schurch

Summary

Overactive bladder and urgency are common conditions generally treated with oral anticholinergic medication. Despite the development of new antimuscarinergic substances, many patients are refractory to or cannot tolerate the oral therapy due to severe side-effects. Intravesical instillation therapy can provide an alternative method to manage detrusor overactivity. However, the use of intravesical drugs is limited due to short-term efficacy and the need of daily intermittent catheterization. Sustained-retention drug delivery systems and liposomes are under development to provide less cumbersome treatment methods. Intravesical capsaicin and resiniferatoxin affect the afferent C-fiber innervation of the bladder, leading to a decrease in detrusor overactivity and also an increased bladder capacity. Botulinum toxin type A injections into the detrusor have been shown to increase bladder capacity and to decrease detrusor overactivity for a mean duration of 9 months.

Introduction

Overactive bladder (OAB) with or without detrusor overactivity is most commonly treated with oral anticholinergic drugs. However, their relatively frequent side-effects such as dry mouth, constipation, accommodation disturbances, and dizziness, and their limited efficacy, restrict their use to a minority of patients. In a review, Chui et al demonstrated that only 20% of the patients are still under anticholinergic drugs after 12 months, despite the introduction of new selective M_3 antagonists and slow-release forms.[1] Even if the compliance to the treatment is better in neurogenic patients, tolerance is poor, particularly because of dry mouth and severe constipation. Intravesical therapy represents a valuable option for patients resistant or intolerant to oral anticholinergic therapy. In this chapter I will give an overview of the substances currently used for intravesical treatment of detrusor overactivity and their efficacy and limits.

Intravesical oxybutynin, lidocaine, nociceptin/orphanin FQ, and atropine

Oxybutynin is a tertiary amine that combines antimuscarinergic, spasmolytic, and local anesthetic effects. Since the first use of the intravesical application by Brendler et al,[2] there have been over a hundred peer review articles reporting successes of intravesical oxybutynin to treat OAB and detrusor hyperreflexia. The main findings were, at least at short-term follow-up, an improvement in OAB symptoms, including a decreased number of incontinence episodes, an increase in maximum bladder capacity, and a decrease of the detrusor overactivity in the urodynamic recordings. Side-effects were observed less frequently compared to oral administration. Despite the assumption that intravesical oxybutynin only acts on the urothelium, and therefore causes fewer and less severe side-effects, pharmacologic studies have shown that the effect of intravesical oxybutynin is mainly related to its systemic absorption.[3] After intravesical oxybutynin application, concentrations 100 times higher than after oral administration have been found in the serum, although the patients suffered from fewer side-effects. The reason for this is related to a difference in metabolism of the substance. The majority of the side-effects, especially on the salivary gland, are produced by the oxybutynin metabolite desethyloxybutynin, which is produced not only by first-pass metabolism in the liver but also by direct cytochrome P450 metabolism in the gut wall.[3] By intravesical application, first-pass metabolism in the liver and gut wall metabolism are proportionally reduced and a reduced ratio of metabolite to parent compound is subsequently found in the systemic circulation.[4] This means one can achieve greater efficacy on the bladder with fewer side-effects, especially dry mouth. Beside its action on the efferent parasympathetic innervation of the detrusor, there is increasing evidence that oxybutynin administrated intravesically also has a local anesthetic effect on the C-fibers.[5] Accordingly, the effect of intravesical oxybutynin on detrusor overactivity is attributed today to its dual effect on the afferent as well as the efferent nerve endings in the detrusor. There is currently no standard instillation protocol concerning the use of intravesical oxybutynin for OAB. The doses vary between 5 and 30 mg, diluted in 30–40 ml saline.[6–8] In addition, the instillation frequency is not standardized and varies between 1 and 3 times/day.

The intravesical application of lidocaine to treat OAB is not well documented – there are only three published studies. A randomized, but not placebo-controlled, study on the effect of intravesical lidocaine for treating detrusor overactivity was reported by Enzelsberger et al.[9] The main clinical findings were a reduced desire to void, diminution of the symptoms of detrusor overactivity, and a reduction in urinary incontinence. In 50% of the patients the detrusor overactivity disappeared on the urodynamic tracings. The maximum bladder capacity increased by about 41% after a 15 minute instillation of 20 ml lidocaine 4%. No side-effects were observed.

Lazzeri et al recently studied the feasibility, safety, and efficacy of the daily intravesical instillation of 1 mg of the endogenous peptide nociceptin/orphanin FQ (N/OFQ) in a selected group of patients who performed clean intermittent catheterization for neurogenic detrusor overactivity (NDO).[10] N/OFQ, where F and Q represent the first and last amino acids, respectively, phenylalanine (F) and glutamine (Q), is a heptadecapeptide that exerts several physiologic actions at both the central and the peripheral level by activating a specific G-protein-coupled receptor called the nociceptin orphan peptide (NOP) receptor. Among the various actions elicited by N/OFQ, such as antinociceptive effects, stimulation of food intake, inhibition of anxiety, bradycardia, and hypotension, animal studies have demonstrated that it exerts a robust inhibitory effect on the micturition reflex in the rat.[11] A total of 18 patients with NDO and incontinence on clean intermittent catheterization were prospectively randomized to receive 1 mg N/OFQ in 10 ml saline or placebo (saline) at the first catheterization for 10 days. Mean daily urine leakage episodes significantly decreased from 2.18 at baseline to 0.94 during N/OFQ treatment, while no significant changes were reported in the placebo group. The total mean voiding diary bladder capacity significantly increased in patients receiving N/OFQ, while it remained unchanged in patients receiving placebo. The urodynamic parameters recorded during the study showed an increase in cystometric capacity and a decrease in maximum bladder pressure compared to baseline only in patients assigned to the N/OFQ group. These findings support the use of N/OFQ peptide receptor agonist as an innovative approach for controling neurogenic detrusor overactivity incontinence.

Fader et al[12] tested the efficacy and side-effect profiles of intravesical atropine compared to oxybutynin immediate release (IR) when used by individuals with multiple sclerosis. They performed a study to determine the most effective dose of atropine. Eight participants used increasing doses of intravesical atropine (2 to 6 mg in 20 ml Nacl 0.9%) during a 12-day period. Bladder diary data showed that the instillation of 6 mg atropine 4 times daily was most effective for increasing bladder capacity (voided/catheter volumes). Afterwards they performed a randomized, double-blind crossover trial. Participants received 14 days of treatment with oral oxybutynin IR 5 mg twice daily (range 2.5 twice to 5 mg 4 times daily) or with intravesical atropine, followed by 14 days of alternative treatment. Participants recorded a bladder diary and rated side-effects and quality of life. The primary outcome variable was bladder capacity. A total of 57 participants with multiple sclerosis completed the study. Average change in bladder capacity was higher in the atropine arm. The mean change in bladder capacity was 55.5 ± 67.2 ml with oxybutynin, the mean change with atropine was 79.6 ± 89.6 ml, and the mean difference between the arms was 24.1 ml ($p = 0.053$). Changes in incontinence events and voiding frequency were not statistically different between the arms. Changes in total side-effect and dry mouth scores were significantly better in the atropine treatment arm. These findings suggest that intravesical atropine is as effective as oxybutynin IR for increasing bladder capacity, and that it is probably better with fewer antimuscarinic side-effects.

Vanilloids

The vanilloids capsaicin (CAP) and resiniferatoxin (RTX) activate nociceptive sensory nerves through binding to an ion channel discovered by Caterina and associates and known as vanilloid receptor subtype 1 (VR1).[13] This receptor is a nonselective cation channel and is activated by increasing temperature within the noxious range and by protons, suggesting that it functions as a transducer of painful thermal stimuli and acidity *in vivo*. When activated, the channel opens, allowing an influx of calcium and sodium ions that depolarize the nociceptive afferent terminals, initiating a nerve impulse that travels through the dorsal root ganglion into the central nervous system. Noxious temperature uses the same elements, which explains why the mouth feels hot when eating chili peppers.[14] Previously called the capsaicin receptor, VR1 has been localized in the spinal cord, dorsal root ganglia, and visceral organs including bladder, urethra, and colon. Activation of VR1 results in spike-like currents,[15] that selectively excite and subsequently desensitize C-fibers. Capsaicin desensitization is defined as a long-lasting, reversible suppression of sensory neuron activity.[16] How fast and for how long the desensitization develops is related to the dose and time of exposure to capsaicin and the interval between consecutive doses.[17,18] The transient increase in intracellular concentration of calcium ions also leads to activation of intracellular enzymes, peptide transmitter release, and neuronal degeneration.

The rationale for intravesical instillation of vanilloids in urology is based on the underlying involvement of C-fibers in pathogenic conditions such as hypersensitive and hyperreflexic bladder. In the healthy human bladder, C-fibers carry the response to noxious stimuli but they are not implicated in the normal voiding reflex. After spinal cord injury, major neuroplasticity appears within bladder afferents in several mammalian species, including man. C-fiber bladder afferents proliferate within the urothelium and become sensitive to bladder distention. These changes lead to the emergence of a new C-fiber-mediated voiding reflex, which is strongly involved in detrusor hyperreflexia.[19] The ability to improve detrusor hyperreflexia by chemical defunctionalization of C-fibers in bladder afferents with intravesical vanilloids has been widely demonstrated in humans and animals.

Since the first report of Fowler et al,[20] several clinical studies, including one placebo controlled-trial,[21] have shown that a single instillation of a 100 ml solution of 1 nM CAP diluted in 30% ethanol is beneficial for clinical and urodynamic symptoms due to hyperactive bladder in spinal cord injured patients.[21–24] The clinical benefit lasts about 6 months. Unfortunately, such intravesical CAP administration is limited by poor immediate tolerability and is responsible for quasi-systematic transitory side-effects (suprapubic pain, worsening detrusor hyperreflexia, and hematuria). The alcoholic solvent may be a major factor in the poor tolerability of alcoholic CAP instillation, as suggested by the result of one placebo-controlled study showing that side-effects appeared to be the same after intravesical instillation of CAP diluted in 30% ethanol as after instillation of ethanol alone.[21]

RTX is a sensory antagonist approximately a thousand times more potent than capsaicin. Although RTX mimics most capsaicin actions it has also a unique pharmocologic effect,[25] such as the desensitization without prior excitation of the pulmonary chemoreflex pathways.[26] RTX induces slowly activating, persistent currents in dorsal root ganglion neurons as measured under patch clamp conditions.[15,27,28] These sustained currents prefer desensitization to excitation (the change in membrane potential is not sufficient to cause action potential formation, although the rising intracellular calcium level can activate biochemical pathways leading to desensitization) which is in accord with the general pharmacologic profile of RTX. Cruz and associates[24,29] instilled 50–100 nM RTX, dissolved in 100 ml solution of 10% alcohol, for 30 minutes in 7 neurologically impaired patients with detrusor hyperreflexia. The only symptoms were itching or mild discomfort evoked in 4 patients during the first minutes of treatment. In 5 of the 7 patients, urinary frequency decreased by 33 to 58%, and this effect was detected as soon as the first day after treatment. Three patients, who prior to treatment were incontinent, became dry most days following treatment. Improvement was sustained for up to 3 months. Four patients had urodynamic improvement with a rise in maximum cystometric capacity increasing from 50 to 900% of pretreatment measures. Lazzeri and colleagues[30] reported using intravesical RTX (10 nM) in 8 normal patients and 7 patients with OABs. In normal subjects, RTX did not decrease the volume required to elicit the first desire to void and did not produce warm or burning sensations at the suprapubic or urethral level during infusion. However, in patients with OAB the mean capacity increased from 175 ± 36 ml to 281 ± 93 ml ($p < 0.01$) immediately after instillation, but was not significantly increased after 4 weeks (217 ± 87 ml). RTX has also been reported to be helpful in patients who did not improve after capsaicin. Lazzeri et al[31] presented data on 7 SCI patients with detrusor hyperreflexia treated with RTX. These patients were reported to have failed intravesical capsaicin therapy. All 7 patients received 30 ml of 10 nM RTX for 30 minutes. Fifteen days after RTX, mean cystometric capacity significantly increased from 188 ± 21 ml to 399 ± 120 ml ($p < 0.01$), and remained increased 4 weeks later (402 ± 71 ml, $p < 0.01$).

Groups comparing RTX in saline or 10% ethanol with CAP in 30% ethanol found better tolerability of RTX.[24,31–33] The difference in tolerability of the two vanilloids (CAP vs RTX) was usually attributed to the differential pungency of the two agents. Nevertheless, because we know the role of the solvent in the irritative effect on bladder mucosa, it is reasonable to assume that differential effects could be related to the use of different vectors. From a technical point of view, the choice of the solvent is limited because of the poor hydrosolubility of CAP, imposing the use of an alcoholic, lipidic, or glucidic vector. The safety of the lipidic solution could be imperfect because of the difficulty of completely eliminating it from the bladder. On the contrary, a glucidic solution may represent a safe and valuable alternative to the alcoholic vector.[34] de Seze et al compared the efficacy and tolerability of intravesical instillations of CAP and RTX using a glucidic solvent for CAP and the 10% ethanol solvent for RTX in a controlled, randomized, double-blind study in patients with severe urinary incontinence due to spinal cord injury.[35] On day 30, clinical and urodynamic improvement was found in 78% and 83%, respectively, of patients treated with CAP vs 80% and 60% of patients treated with RTX. No significant difference between the two groups was observed. The benefit remained in two-thirds of both groups on day 90. There were no differences in regard to incidence, nature, or duration of side-effects in CAP vs RTX treated patients. These results once more strongly argue for the importance of accounting the role of vanilloid solute when interpreting efficacy and tolerance of vesical vanilloid instillation in detrusor hyperreflexia cases. They suggest that a glucidic solution is a valuable solvent for CAP instillation.[35]

The long-term safety of vanilloid agents, particularly concerning mutagenic and carcinogenic effects on the bladder wall, is not perfectly known. The use of CAP in ethanol solvent seems not to cause morphologic changes in the bladder urothelium in patients receiving repeat instillation for as long as 5 years. To our knowledge, the long-term safety of RTX remains unproven. Furthermore, RTX belongs to the family of tumor-promoting phorbol esters, strengthening the need to ensure the safety of RTX before extending its therapeutic applications.

Sustained bladder drug delivery and liposomes

Sustained intravesical delivery of drugs can ensure the continuous presence of a constant level of the drug in the bladder without the need for intermittent catheterization. It is also plausible to expect increased efficacy with increased duration of direct contact between the drug and the abnormal urothelium.[36]

A simple and sensible approach for sustained intravesical drug delivery is prolonged infusion into the bladder. This technique has often been applied to achieve slow and sustained release of drugs inside the bladder. Prolonged instillation of RTX was demonstrated as a feasible procedure for treating interstitial cystitis.[37] RTX was infused through a suprapubic 5 F mono-pigtail catheter for 10 days at a flow rate of 25 ml/h with the help of an infusion pump. Patients were evaluated 30 days after the end of infusion and after 3 months. A 30% decrease in frequency and a three-fold reduction in nocturia was observed, with a significant reduction in pelvic pain for at least 6 months after the end of infusion.

Formation of a drug depot inside the bladder appears to be an attractive option over prolonged infusion. Aqueous solutions of polyethylene glycol-β-[DLlactic acid-co-glycolic acid]-β-ethylene glycol (PEG-PLGA-PEG) triblock copolymers form a free-flowing solution at room temperature and become a viscous gel at a body temperature of 37°C.[38] The triblock copolymer was used for sustaining the residence time of hydrophobic drugs in rat bladder after its instillation at room temperature. Rats were instilled with either a 0.02% solution of fluorescein isothiocyanate (FITC) or the same amount of FITC in a 30% dispersion of thermosensitive [poly(ethylene glycol)-poly[lactic acid-co-glycolic acid]-poly(ethylene glycol)] (PEG-PLGA-PEG) polymer in a 0.1 M phosphate buffer. After instillation, rats were kept in metabolic cages for urine collection. Fluorescence emanating from FITC was measured in the urine at various time points up to 24 hours after instillation.

In addition, a rat model of cyclophosphamide-induced cystitis was chosen for the efficacy study using misoprostol as a model drug entrapped in the thermosensitive hydrogel in place of FITC. Efficacy of the hydrogel containing misoprostol was compared against rat groups instilled with saline, hydrogel, and misoprostol independently. Prolonged drug exposure to the bladder afforded by hydrogel was evident from the time course of FITC elimination in the urine and by the green fluorescence of FITC seen at the bladder surface when isolated 24 hours after instillation. Rats instilled with free FITC voided almost all of the fluorescence in the urine within the first 8 hours, whereas rats instilled with hydrogel-encapsulated FITC showed sustained release up to 24 hours after instillation. Rats with cyclophosphamide-induced cystitis and which were instilled with misoprostol, a synthetic PGE_1 analog, showed significantly reduced frequency of urine voiding as compared to the control group instilled with saline.[39] Accordingly, this study showed that the PEG-PLGA-PEG polymer could be used as a viable sustained drug delivery system for intravesical therapy

Liposomes were first studied in England in 1961 by Bangham,[40] and, since then, they have become a versatile tool of study in biology, biochemistry, and medicine. Liposomes are artificial spherical vesicles consisting of an aqueous core enclosed in one or more phospholipid layers; they are used as drug carriers and are loaded with a great variety of molecules such as small drug molecules, proteins, nucleotides, and even plasmids.[41] Previously, liposomes were shown to improve the aqueous solubility of hydrophobic drugs such as paclitaxel (Taxol) and amphotericin. A report discussed the use of liposomes as vehicles for capsaicin and evaluated their potential as a vehicle for intravesical delivery in rats.[42] Liposomes were able to deliver capsaicin with an efficacy similar to that of ethanolic saline, but toxicity to the bladder was drastically reduced. For more information on sustained drug delivery systems and liposomes see also Giannatonni et al[43] and Tyagi et al.[39,44]

Botulinum toxin

Botulinum toxin is the strongest naturally occurring lethal neurotoxin known. It is produced by the anerobic, rod-shaped gram-positive bacteria *Clostridium botulinum*. Botulinum toxin binds rapidly and tightly to the intramuscular nerve terminals and causes a prolonged local effect when injected directly into a muscle. It causes flaccid paralysis in the skeletal muscle by blocking the presynaptic acetylcholine release. There are seven distinct but structurally similar types of botulinum toxin, namely A, B, C, D, E, F, and G.[45] Of these, types A and B have been used widely with a beneficial clinical effect in many neuromuscular disorders.[46–48] After intramuscular injection the heavy chain binds to the presynaptic motor terminal and enters the cell by endocytosis. The disulfide bond linking the two botulinum toxin chains (heavy chain and light chain) is broken, and the light chain is translocated out of the endocytotic vesicle into the cytoplasm. The process of exocytosis of acetylcholine is complicated, requiring the participation of several proteins, and each serotype of the toxin works by enzymatic cleavage of one or more of these proteins. Types A, C, and E cleave the 25 kD synaptosomal associated protein SNAP-25, types B, D, F, and G cleave a synaptobrevin vesicle associated membrane protein, and type C cleaves syntaxin (see Table 49.1). In smooth muscle, botulinum toxin has been proved to trigger the release of nitric oxide that diffuses out of the endothelial cell into smooth muscle, causing the relaxation.[49]

Treatment of human detrusor overactivity (DO) with intradetrusor injections of botulinum toxin type A (BoNT/A) was introduced on the basis that it would block presynaptic release of acetylcholine, similar to its mechanism of action in skeletal muscle.[50,51] The hypothesis of the trial was based on the study of Dickson and Shevky, suggesting that parasympathetic action may be blocked by BoNT/A.[52] Disorders of the parasympathetic autonomic nervous system such as achalasia and hyperhydrosis have been successfully treated with BoNT/A injections.[53] A marked loss of contraction in a rat bladder after acute botulinum poisoning, with a decrease in acetylcholine release on motor nerve stimulation, was observed by Carpenter.[54]

However, there is increasing evidence that BoNT/A may also affect sensory nerve fibers and afferent signaling mechanisms that have an important role in the pathophysiology of DO. Studies on guinea pig[55] and rat[56] bladder strips have shown that BoNT/A is able to impair both acetylcholine and ATP release from urothelium. Moreover, BoNT/A has been shown to inhibit efferent nerve mediated bladder contraction, presumably by blocking neurotransmitter release from peripheral afferent nerve terminals.[56] These bladder afferent neurons have several types of receptors, namely vanilloids, purinergic (P2X), neurokinins, and receptors for nerve growth factor (NGF). An immunohistochemical study focused on the effect of BoNT/A on human bladder afferent mechanisms by studying the sensory receptors P2X3 and TRPV1. The density of P2X3-immunoreactive and TRPV1-immunoreactive fibers was decreased significantly after botulinum toxin injection, and it was argued that decreased levels of sensory receptors P2X3 and/or TRPV1 may contribute to the clinical effect of the toxin in detrusor overactivity.[57] In support of a possible BoNT/A-induced phenotypic change of bladder afferents, levels of neurotrophic growth factor (NGF) in bladders of patients with NDO were reported to be reduced significantly after BoNT/A treatment.[58]

Table 49.1 *Intracellular substrates for different types of botulinum toxins (BTXs)*

BTX serotype	Substrate
BTX-A	SNAP-25
BTX-B	VAMP/synaptobrevin
BTX-C	Synataxin
BTX-D	VAMP/synaptobrevin/cellubrevin
BTX-E	SNAP-25
BTX-F	VAMP/synaptobrevin/cellubrevin
BTX-G	Unknown

SNAP-25, synaptosal associated protein 25; VAMP, vesicle associated membrane protein.

The effect of injecting BoNT/A into the human detrusor muscle in spinal cord injured patients was first reported by our group in a nonrandomized prospective study.[50,51] The patients with spinal cord injury selected for this first clinical study had severe NDO and suffered from incontinence resistant to anticholinergic drugs. One of the main inclusion criteria was that patients had to be able to perform intermittent self-catheterization, as it was the voiding method after treatment. Patients with low bladder compliance due to organic detrusor muscle changes or fibrosis were excluded. Using a rigid cystoscope, 200–400 units of BoNT/A (Botox®, Allergan, Irvine, CA) were injected into the detrusor muscle, sparing the trigone (see Figures 49.1 and 49.2). The reason for sparing the trigone was to avoid a vesicorenal reflux and, at the time of the conducted study, the lack of knowledge about the effect of BoNT/A on the adrenergic nerves and on the release of nociceptive neuropeptides. In total, 19 of the 21 treated patients could be regularly observed over a period of 9 months by clinical and urodynamic checks. Six weeks' follow-up after injection showed a significant increase in the reflex volume and in the maximum cystometric bladder capacity. There was also a significant decrease in the maximum detrusor voiding pressure. At the 36-week follow-up, ongoing improvement was evident. The amount of anticholinergics could be reduced or even completely abolished. Continence was restored in all but two patients and patient satisfaction was high. The European group increased the study sample to 200 patients, with the same result profile.[59]

A more recent multicenter, randomized, placebo-controlled 24-week study examining the effect of two different doses of BoNT/A (200 and 300 units Botox®, Allergan, Irvine, CA) injected into the detrusor to treat NDO has confirmed the efficacy and safety of this treatment.[60] Out of the recruited 59 patients, 57 completed the study. The mean reduction in urinary incontinence (UI) was about 50% at all post-treatment time points in the BoNT/A groups, and zero in the placebo group ($p < 0.05$).

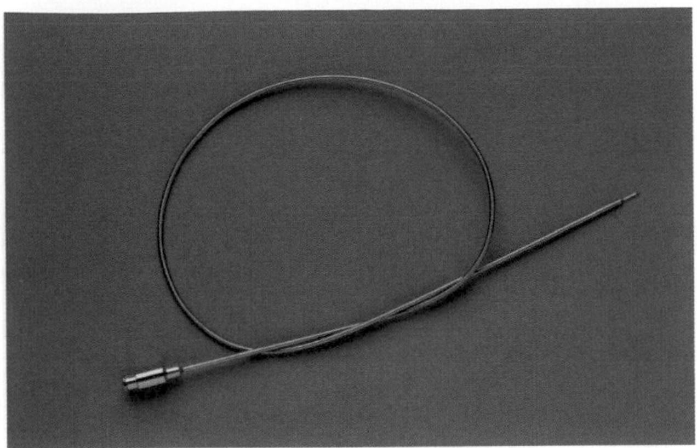

Figure 49.1
Flexible injection needle for detrusor muscle injection (Storz®, French scale 8, length: 50 cm).

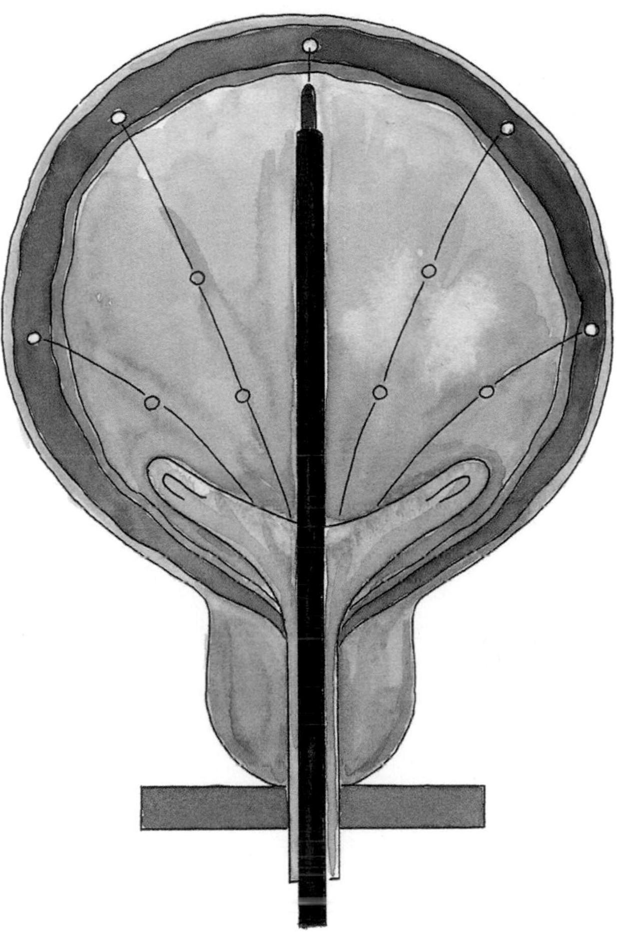

Figure 49.2
Detrusor mapping.

Overall, 29 patients (49.2%) reported no UI episodes for at least one week in the post-treatment period, of whom 24 (82.8%) were in the BoNT/A treatment group. Significant changes in key urodynamic parameters compared to baseline were observed in each BoNT/A group at all time points after treatment, which was not the case for the placebo group ($p < 0.05$). There were robust improvements in the mean change from baseline in incontinence-quality of life (I-QOL) total scores in patients treated with BoNT/A at all post-treatment time points ($p < 0.002$), which were maintained throughout the 24 study weeks. Treatment with 200 units appeared to work as well as 300 units, regarding all outcome parameters (clinical and urodynamic). However, no definitive conclusion can be drawn regarding the best dose to be used for NDO as the study was not powered to compare 200 and 300 units. Moreover, differences between the two doses might have been seen if the study had been extended to 36 weeks.

Recently, Patki et al reported on the first prospective assessment of intradetrusor injection of the English toxin type A as a treatment of drug-resistant NDO in spinal cord injury patients.[61] One thousand units of Dysport® (Ipsen Ltd, Berkshire, UK) were cystoscopically injected (30 injection sites) into the detrusor in 37 patients with drug-resistant NDO as a day case procedure. Maximum cystometric capacity (MCC), maximum detrusor pressure (MDP), continence, and anticholinergic requirements were used as outcome parameters. An International Consultation on Incontinence Questionaire (ICIQ) questionnaire was used to assess quality of life pre- and postinjection. The mean follow-up was 7 months. MCC increased from a mean of 259 ml to 521.5 ml. MDP decreased from a mean of 54.3 to 24.4 cmH_2O. Incontinence and NDO were abolished in 82% and 76% of the patients, respectively. Eighty-six percent of the patients were able to stop or reduce anticholinergics, with a similar number of patients scoring favorably on ICIQ. The mean period of improvement was 9 months. Acceptable failure rates with 24% persistence of NDO and 18% persistence of incontinence were observed. Other groups have also reported a positive effect of BoNT/A injection into the detrusor to treat NDO.[33,62–67]

About 10% of children with myelomeningocele (MMC) and NDO are nonresponders to anticholinergic medication and/or suffer from side-effects from anticholinergic drugs, even if administered intravesically.[68] There is increasing evidence that botulinum toxin is a new, highly effective second-line treatment for MMC children with NDO. Only four prospective studies have evaluated the efficacy of BoNT/A injection in the pediatric neurogenic population and NDO. Schulte-Baukloh and colleagues injected 20 children with NDO and MMC with 12 U/kg (maximum 300 U) Botox® (Allergan, Irvine, CA). Urodynamic follow-up at 2 and 4 weeks following treatment revealed significant increases in mean maximum bladder capacity (35% increase) as well as significant decreases in maximum detrusor pressure (41% decrease).[69,70] However, while significant increases in maximum bladder capacity were demonstrated up to 6 months after treatment, no significant difference in maximum detrusor pressure was seen at 3- and 6-month follow-up. A more recent pediatric study with longer follow-up in 15 patients (mean age 5.8 years) supported earlier studies by demonstrating an increase in maximal bladder capacity of 118% ($p < 0.001$) and a 46% decrease in mean maximal detrusor pressure ($p < 0.001$) following BoNT/A injection.[71] Corcos et al evaluated 20 children with MMC and NDO.[72] The results showed a somewhat less convincing effect than the one from Schulte-Baukloh[67] and Ricabonna.[71] The lower dose they used might be a reason for this lower efficacy. The clinical effects of BoNT/A in MMC children with NDO lasted on average 6–10.5 months, and were similar after repeated injection.[71–73] None of these studies reported side-effects related to the toxin or to the injection procedure.

The preliminary results of these prospective studies on NDO are overwhelming, especially considering the fact that, in all these studies, the included patients were difficult cases for conservative treatment. This treatment option seems to establish its indication in cases where anticholinergic medication fails or is intolerable and self-intermittent catheterization can be performed by the patient. This new therapeutic approach also appears to be a valuable alternative to surgery.

For patients suffering from NDO and incontinence who have preserved some normal voiding function and do not want to catheterize, such as multiple sclerosis patients or very incomplete spinal cord injury patients, combined injection into the detrusor and into the external sphincter has been emphasized.[74] In our experience in 20 multiple sclerosis patients suffering from NDO and incontinence who did not want to catheterize, a reduction of the dose to 100 units improved NDO and incontinence without increasing residual volume, as long as the patients did not have major detrusor-sphincter dyssynergia and high residual volume before treatment. Randomized controlled studies or studies aiming to compare the two techniques are required to define which is the best technique for this population.

Conclusion

Intravesical therapy represents a valuable alternative for patients suffering from NDO who are resistant or intolerant to oral anticholinergic drugs. Substances of a short working duration, such as oxybutynin, lidocaine, and N/OFQ, have the major drawback of requiring intermittent self-catheterization at least 1–4 times a day according to the substance use. Sustained bladder drug delivery and liposomes might solve the problem of intermittent catheterization in the future, however these techniques are still in the experimental testing phase. Vanilloid substances might improve NDO and incontinence without increasing residual volume. Unfortunately intravesical CAP administration is limited by poor immediate tolerability; this might be overcome by replacing the usual solvent, ethanol, by a glucidic solution. RTX is 1000 times more potent than capsaicin with a reduced purgutive effect. Unfortunately, dosage studies have been cancelled due to the instability of the substance in the recipient. Moreover, the long-term safety of vanilloid agents, particularly relating to mutagenic and carcinogenic effects on the bladder wall, is not yet fully established. The use of ethanolic CAP seems not to cause morphologic changes in the bladder urothelium in patients receiving repeated instillations for as long as 5 years. To our knowledge, the long-term safety of RTX remains unproven. Furthermore, RTX belongs to the family of tumor-promoting phorbol esters, strengthening the need to ensure the safety of RTX before extending its therapeutic applications. The efficiency of botulinum toxin in the treatment of neurogenic bladder has been demonstrated in evidence-based medicine level 1 and 2 studies. Using the standard technique and a dose of 300 units Botox®, the patients have to catheterize themselves to empty their bladder. This might be a problem if most of the normal voiding function is still present, as in multiple sclerosis patients. Even with good hand function the patients will tend to refuse the treatment. It is possible that changing the technique to injecting the detrusor together with the external urethral sphincter, or reducing the dose to 100 units Botox®, will achieve equally good results, without increasing the residual volume and without the necessity to catheterize. More studies are necessary to clarify this point.

References

1. Chui M, Williamson T, Arciniega J, Thompson C, Benecke H. Patient persistency with medications for overactive bladder. Value Health 2004; 7: 366.
2. Brendler CB, Radebaugh LC, Mohler JL. Topical oxybutynin chloride for relaxation of dysfunctional bladders. J Urol 1989; 141(6): 1350–2.
3. Massad CA, Kogan BA, Trigo-Rocha FE. The pharmacokinetics of intravesical and oral oxybutynin chloride. J Urol 1992; 148(2 Pt 2): 595–7.
4. Buyse G, Waldeck K, Verpoorten C et al. Intravesical oxybutynin for neurogenic bladder dysfunction: less systemic side effects due to reduced first pass metabolism. J Urol 1998; 160(3 Pt 1): 892–6.
5. De Wachter S, Wyndaele JJ. Intravesical oxybutynin: a local anesthetic effect on bladder C afferents. J Urol 2003; 169(5): 1892–5.
6. Enzelsberger H, Helmer H, Kurz C. Intravesical instillation of oxybutynin in women with idiopathic detrusor instability: a randomised trial. Br J Obstet Gynaecol 1995; 102(11): 929–30.
7. Evans R. Intravesical therapy for overactive bladder. Curr Urol Rep 2005; 6: 429–33.
8. Abrams P, Cardozo L, Fall M et al. The standardisation of terminology of lower urinary tract function: report from the Standardisation Sub-committee of the International Continence Society. Neurourol Urodyn 2002; 21(2): 167–78.
9. Enzelsberger H, Schatten C, Kurz C. [Comparison of emepronium bromide with intravesical administration of lidocaine gel in women with urge incontinence.] Geburtshilfe Frauenheilkd 1991; 51(1): 54–7.

10. Lazzeri M, Calo G, Spinelli M et al. Daily intravesical instillation of 1 mg nociceptin/orphanin FQ for the control of neurogenic detrusor overactivity: a multicenter, placebo controlled, randomized exploratory study. J Urol 2006; 176(5): 2098–102.
11. Lecci A, Giuliani S, Meini S, Maggi CA. Nociceptin and the micturition reflex. Peptides 2000; 21(7): 1007–21.
12. Fader M, Glickman S, Haggar V et al. Intravesical atropine compared to oral oxybutynin for neurogenic detrusor overactivity: a double-blind, randomized crossover trial. J Urol 2007; 177(1): 208–13; discussion 213.
13. Caterina MJ, Schumacher MA, Tominaga M et al. The capsaicin receptor: a heat-activated ion channel in the pain pathway. Nature 1997; 389(6653): 816–24.
14. Clapham DE. Some like it hot: spicing up ion channels. Nature 1997; 389(6653): 783–4.
15. Liu L, Simon SA. Capsaicin-induced currents with distinct desensitization and Ca^{2+} dependence in rat trigeminal ganglion cells. J Neurophysiol 1996; 75(4): 1503–14.
16. Craft RM, Cohen SM, Porreca F. Long-lasting desensitization of bladder afferents following intravesical resiniferatoxin and capsaicin in the rat. Pain 1995; 61(2): 317–23.
17. Kawatani M, Whitney T, Booth AM, de Groat WC. Excitatory effect of substance P in parasympathetic ganglia of cat urinary bladder. Am J Physiol 1989; 257(6 Pt 2): R1450–6.
18. Szallasi A, Jonassohn M, Acs G et al. The stimulation of capsaicin-sensitive neurones in a vanilloid receptor-mediated fashion by pungent terpenoids possessing an unsaturated 1,4-dialdehyde moiety. Br J Pharmacol 1996; 119(2): 283–90.
19. de Groat WC. Mechanisms underlying the recovery of lower urinary tract function following spinal cord injury. Paraplegia 1995; 33(9): 493–505.
20. Fowler CJ, Jewkes D, McDonald WI, Lynn B, de Groat WC. Intravesical capsaicin for neurogenic bladder dysfunction. Lancet 1992; 339(8803): 1239.
21. de Seze M, Wiart L, Joseph PA et al. Capsaicin and neurogenic detrusor hyperreflexia: a double-blind placebo-controlled study in 20 patients with spinal cord lesions. Neurourol Urodyn 1998; 17(5): 513–23.
22. Fowler CJ, Beck RO, Gerrard S, Betts CD, Fowler CG. Intravesical capsaicin for treatment of detrusor hyperreflexia. J Neurol Neurosurg Psychiatry 1994; 57(2): 169–73.
23. De Ridder D, Chandiramani V, Dasgupta P et al. Intravesical capsaicin as a treatment for refractory detrusor hyperreflexia: a dual center study with long-term followup. J Urol 1997; 158(6): 2087–92.
24. Cruz F, Guimaraes M, Silva C, Reis M. Suppression of bladder hyperreflexia by intravesical resiniferatoxin. Lancet 1997; 350(9078): 640–1.
25. Szallasi A, Blumberg PM. Resiniferatoxin, a phorbol-related diterpene, acts as an ultrapotent analog of capsaicin, the irritant constituent in red pepper. Neuroscience 1989; 30(2): 515–20.
26. Szolcsanyi J. Effect of capsaicin, resiniferatoxin and piperine on ethanol-induced gastric ulcer of the rat. Acta Physiol Hung 1990; 75(Suppl): 267–8.
27. Liu L, Simon SA. A rapid capsaicin-activated current in rat trigeminal ganglion neurons. Proc Natl Acad Sci USA 1994; 91(2): 738–41.
28. Oh U, Hwang SW, Kim D. Capsaicin activates a nonselective cation channel in cultured neonatal rat dorsal root ganglion neurons. J Neurosci 1996; 16(5): 1659–67.
29. Cruz F. Desensitization of bladder sensory fibers by intravesical capsaicin or capsaicin analogs. A new strategy for treatment of urge incontinence in patients with spinal detrusor hyperreflexia or bladder hypersensitivity disorders. Int Urogynecol J Pelvic Floor Dysfunct 1998; 9(4): 214–20.
30. Lazzeri M, Beneforti P, Turini D. Urodynamic effects of intravesical resiniferatoxin in humans: preliminary results in stable and unstable detrusor. J Urol 1997; 158(6): 2093–6.
31. Lazzeri M, Spinelli M, Beneforti P, Zanollo A, Turini D. Intravesical resiniferatoxin for the treatment of detrusor hyperreflexia refractory to capsaicin in patients with chronic spinal cord diseases. Scand J Urol Nephrol 1998; 32(5): 331–4.
32. Silva C, Rio ME, Cruz F. Desensitization of bladder sensory fibers by intravesical resiniferatoxin, a capsaicin analog: long-term results for the treatment of detrusor hyperreflexia. Eur Urol 2000; 38(4): 444–52.
33. Giannantoni A, Di Stasi SM, Stephen RL et al. Intravesical capsaicin versus resiniferatoxin in patients with detrusor hyperreflexia: a prospective randomized study. J Urol 2002; 167(4): 1710–14.
34. Irie T, Uekama K. Pharmaceutical applications of cyclodextrins. III. Toxicological issues and safety evaluation. J Pharm Sci 1997; 86(2): 147–62.
35. de Seze M, Wiart L, de Seze MP et al. Intravesical capsaicin versus resiniferatoxin for the treatment of detrusor hyperreflexia in spinal cord injured patients: a double-blind, randomized, controlled study. J Urol 2004; 171(1): 251–5.
36. Frangos DN, Killion JJ, Fan D et al. The development of liposomes containing interferon alpha for the intravesical therapy of human superficial bladder cancer. J Urol 1990; 143(6): 1252–6.
37. Lazzeri M, Spinelli M, Beneforti P et al. Intravesical infusion of resiniferatoxin by a temporary in situ drug delivery system to treat interstitial cystitis: a pilot study. Eur Urol 2004; 45(1): 98–102.
38. Ronneberger B, Kao WJ, Anderson JM, Kissel T. In vivo biocompatibility study of ABA triblock copolymers consisting of poly(L-lactic-co-glycolic acid) A blocks attached to central poly(oxyethylene) B blocks. J Biomed Mater Res 1996; 30(1): 31–40.
39. Tyagi P, Li Z, Chancellor M et al. Sustained intravesical drug delivery using thermosensitive hydrogel. Pharm Res 2004; 21(5): 832–7.
40. Bangham AD. A correlation between surface charge and coagulant action of phospholipids. Nature 1961; 192: 1197–8.
41. Johnson JW, Nayar R, Killion JJ, von Eschenbach AC, Fidler IJ. Binding of liposomes to human bladder tumor epithelial cell lines: implications for an intravesical drug delivery system for the treatment of bladder cancer. Sel Cancer Ther 1989; 5(4): 147–55.
42. Tyagi P, Chancellor MB, Li Z et al. Urodynamic and immunohistochemical evaluation of intravesical capsaicin delivery using thermosensitive hydrogel and liposomes. J Urol 2004; 171(1): 483–9.
43. Giannantoni A, Di Stasi SM, Chancellor MB, Costantini E, Porena M. New frontiers in intravesical therapies and drug delivery. Eur Urol 2006; 50(6): 1183–93; discussion 1193.
44. Tyagi P, Tyagi S, Kaufman J, Huang L, de Miguel F. Local drug delivery to bladder using technology innovations. Urol Clin North Am 2006; 33(4): 519–30.
45. Simpson LL. Molecular pharmacology of botulinum toxin and tetanus toxin. Annu Rev Pharmacol Toxicol 1986; 26: 427–53.
46. Brashear A, Lew MF, Dykstra DD et al. Safety and efficacy of NeuroBloc (botulinum toxin type B) in type A-responsive cervical dystonia. Neurology 1999; 53(7): 1439–46.
47. Brin MF, Lew MF, Adler CH et al. Safety and efficacy of NeuroBloc (botulinum toxin type B) in type A-resistant cervical dystonia. Neurology 1999; 53(7): 1431–8.
48. Sloop RR, Cole BA, Escutin RO. Human response to botulinum toxin injection: type B compared with type A. Neurology 1997; 49(1): 189–94.
49. Coffield JA, R.V C, Simpson LL. The site and mechanism of action of botulinum neurotoxin. In: Jankovic J, Hallet M, eds. Therapy With Botulinum Toxin. New York: Marcel Dekker, 1994: 3–13.
50. Schurch B, Schmid DM, Stohrer M. Treatment of neurogenic incontinence with botulinum toxin A. N Engl J Med 2000; 342(9): 665.
51. Schurch B, Stohrer M, Kramer G et al. Botulinum-A toxin for treating detrusor hyperreflexia in spinal cord injured patients: a new alternative to anticholinergic drugs? Preliminary results. J Urol 2000; 164(3 Pt 1): 692–7.
52. Dickson EC, Shevky R. Studies on manner in which the toxin of clostridium botulinum acts upon the body. I. The effect upon the autonomic nervous system. J Exp Med 1923; 37: 711–31.

53. Annese V, Basciani M, Borrelli O et al. Intrasphincteric injection of botulinum toxin is effective in long-term treatment of esophageal achalasia. Muscle Nerve 1998; 21(11): 1540–2.
54. Carpenter FG. Motor responses of the response of the urinary bladder and skeletal muscle in botulinum toxin intoxicated rats. J Physiol 1967; 1988: 1–11.
55. MacKenzie I, Burnstock G, Dolly JO. The effects of purified botulinum neurotoxin type A on cholinergic, adrenergic and non-adrenergic, atropine-resistant autonomic neuromuscular transmission. Neuroscience 1982; 7(4): 997–1006.
56. Smith CP, Franks ME, McNeil BK et al. Effect of botulinum toxin A on the autonomic nervous system of the rat lower urinary tract. J Urol 2003; 169(5): 1896–900.
57. Apostolidis A, Popat R, Yiangou Y et al. Decreased sensory receptors P2X3 and TRPV1 in suburothelial nerve fibers following intradetrusor injections of botulinum toxin for human detrusor overactivity. J Urol 2005; 174(3): 977–82; discussion 982–3.
58. Giannantoni A, Di Stasi SM, Nardicchi V et al. Botulinum-A toxin injections into the detrusor muscle decrease nerve growth factor bladder tissue levels in patients with neurogenic detrusor overactivity. J Urol 2006; 175(6): 2341–4.
59. Reitz A, von Tobel J, Stöhrer M et al. European experience of 184 cases treated with botulinum-A toxin injections into the detrusor muscle for neurogenic incontinence. Neurourol Urodyn 2002; 21(4): 427–8.
60. Schurch B, de Seze M, Denys P et al. Botulinum toxin type a is a safe and effective treatment for neurogenic urinary incontinence: results of a single treatment, randomized, placebo controlled 6-month study. J Urol 2005; 174(1): 196–200.
61. Patki PS, Hamid R, Arumugam K, Shah PJ, Craggs M. Botulinum-A toxin (Dysport) in the treatment of drug resistant neurogenic detrusor overactivity following traumatic spinal cord injury. BJU Int 2006; 98: 77–82.
62. Del Popolo G, Li Marzi V, Panariello G, Lombardi G. English botulinum toxin-A in the treatment of neurogenic detrusor overactivity. Neurourol Urodyn 2003; 22(5): 498.
63. Giannantoni A, Merini E, Di Stasi SM et al. New therapeutic option for refractory neurogenic detrusor overactivity. Minerva Urol Nephrol 2004; 56: 78–87.
64. Kuo HC. Urodynamic evidence of effectiveness of botulinum A toxin injection in treatment of detrusor overactivity refractory to anticholinergic agents. Urology 2004; 63(5): 868–72.
65. Kennely M, Kang J. Botulinum-A toxin injection into the detrusor as a treatment for refractory detrusor hypperreflexia. Top Spinal Cord Inj Rehabil 2003; 8: 46–53.
66. Hajebrahimi S, Altaweel W, Cadoret J, Cohen E, Corcos J. Efficacy of botulinum-A toxin in adults with neurogenic overactive bladder: initial results. Can J Urol 2005; 12(1): 2543–6.
67. Klaphajone J, Kitisomprayoonkul W, Sriplakit S. Botulinum toxin type A injections for treating neurogenic detrusor overactivity combined with low-compliance bladder in patients with spinal cord lesions. Arch Phys Med Rehabil 2005; 86(11): 2114–18.
68. Hernandez RD, Hurwitz RS, Foote JE, Zimmern PE, Leach GE. Nonsurgical management of threatened upper urinary tracts and incontinence in children with myelomeningocele. J Urol 1994; 152(5 Pt 1): 1582–5.
69. Schulte-Baukloh H, Michael T, Schobert J, Stolze T, Knispel HH. Efficacy of botulinum-a toxin in children with detrusor hyperreflexia due to myelomeningocele: preliminary results. Urology 2002; 59(3): 325–7; discussion 327–8.
70. Schulte-Baukloh H, Michael T, Sturzebecher B, Knispel HH. Botulinum-a toxin detrusor injection as a novel approach in the treatment of bladder spasticity in children with neurogenic bladder. Eur Urol 2003; 44(1): 139–43.
71. Riccabona M, Koen M, Schindler M et al. Botulinum-A toxin injection into the detrusor: a safe alternative in the treatment of children with myelomeningocele with detrusor hyperreflexia. J Urol 2004; 171(2 Pt 1): 845–8; discussion 848.
72. Corcos J, Al-Taweed W, Robichaud C. Botulinum toxin as an alternative treatment to bladder augmentation in children with neurogenic bladder due to myelomeningocele. J Urol 2004; 171: 181 (abstract).
73. Schulte-Baukloh H, Knispel HH, Stolze T et al. Repeated botulinum-A toxin injections in treatment of children with neurogenic detrusor overactivity. Urology 2005; 66(4): 865–70; discussion 870.
74. Schulte-Baukloh H, Weiss C, Stolze T et al. Botulinum-A toxin detrusor and sphincter injection in treatment of overactive bladder syndrome: objective outcome and patient satisfaction. Eur Urol 2005; 48(6): 984–90; discussion 990.

50

Transdermal oxybutynin administration

G Willy Davila

Introduction

Overactive bladder (OAB) is a chronic condition characterized by symptoms of urinary urgency, frequency, and nocturia, with or without urge incontinence, caused by involuntary contractions of the detrusor smooth muscle during bladder filling. It it estimated to affect approximately 34 million individuals in the United States, mostly women, and can have a markedly negative impact on quality of life. Long-term therapy for OAB is generally required to maintain symptomatic relief. Bladder training and other nonpharmacologic interventions may be effective in many cases, but lack of patient motivation and poor compliance restrict the long-term effectiveness of these approaches.[1,2] The mainstay of treatment for OAB is therefore pharmacologic therapy with antimuscarinic drugs. Unfortunately, they are limited in their clinical utility because of their propensity to induce dose-limiting side-effects, such as dry mouth, constipation, and sedation, thereby reducing patient compliance.

Oxybutynin, the primary antimuscarinic drug used to treat the symptoms of OAB, has been available for oral administration for more than 25 years. Although other drugs have now reached the market, oxybutynin remains a favorable treatment option.

The mechanism of action of oxybutynin, a cholinergic muscarinic receptor antagonist, is to competitively inhibit the binding of acetylcholine at postganglionic cholinergic receptor sites in the bladder smooth muscle. Oxybutynin also independently relaxes bladder smooth muscle and has local anesthetic properties.[3] Following oral administration, oxybutynin is extensively metabolized to the active compound *N*-desethyloxybutynin (*N*-DEO). *N*-DEO plasma levels have been associated with anticholinergic side-effects. With the development of a controlled-release oral formulation, and now with transdermal delivery, metabolism is reduced, efficacy is maintained, and side-effects are decreased. The contributions of the parent compound to efficacy and the metabolite to anticholinergic side-effects are becoming increasingly clear as more clinical experience is gained with improved delivery systems. The therapeutic effectiveness of oxybutynin is dose-related and occurs in conjunction with improvement in urodynamic parameters. Oxybutynin reduces the number of impulses reaching the detrusor muscle, thereby delaying the initial desire to void and increasing bladder capacity.[4]

As higher oral doses of oxybutynin are administered to achieve efficacy, dry mouth becomes more pronounced; therefore, alternative routes of administration have been tried. Intravesical therapy was found to alter the pharmacokinetic properties – a significantly lower concentration of the primary metabolite, N-DEO, reaches the systemic circulation, resulting in fewer anticholinergic side-effects.[5] Instillation of oxybutynin directly into the bladder is clinically effective and in most cases causes minimal or no dry mouth.[6] Because this route of administration is impractical, it is currently used only in special clinical circumstances.[7]

Recently, an oxybutynin transdermal delivery system (Oxytrol™, Watson Pharmaceuticals, Inc, Salt Lake City, Utah)[8] has been shown to provide continuous delivery of oxybutynin over 96 h, by way of a matrix-type delivery system applied to the patient's skin. This route of administration alters the pharmacokinetic profile of oxybutynin, thereby minimizing anticholinergic side-effects without compromising clinical efficacy.[9]

Transdermal drug delivery

Background

Transdermal drug administration for the pharmacologic treatment of systemic conditions has the known advantage of avoidance of presystemic gastrointestinal and hepatic 'first-pass' metabolism, which allows administration of lower doses to achieve similar plasma concentrations. Other advantages include avoidance of gastrointestinal interactions, consistent drug release over a prolonged period of time, ease of patient compliance, and utility

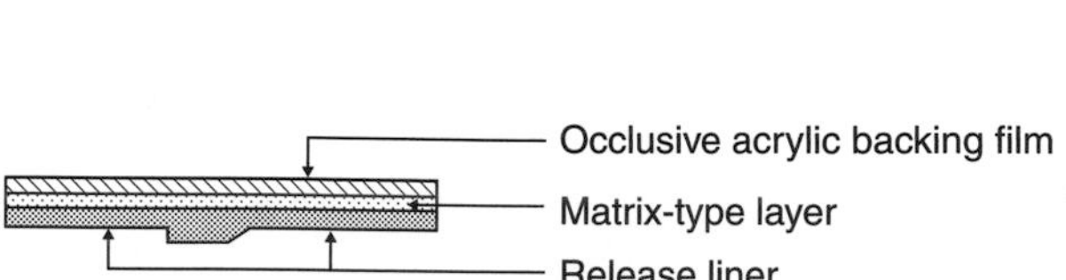

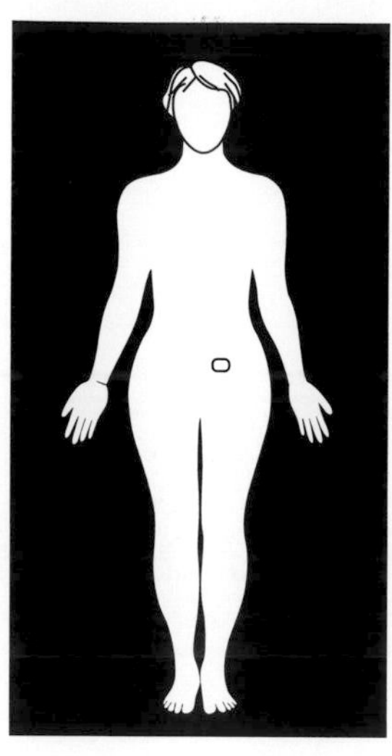

Figure 50.1
A cross-section of the matrix-type oxybutynin TDS (transdermal system). Placement of the oxybutynin TDS on the lower abdominal skin region.

when oral or parenteral drug administration is not ideal. Transdermal application systems are currently in use for the treatment of angina pectoris, chronic pain syndromes, and motion sickness; to provide hormone replacement therapy and contraception; and for assistance with smoking cessation.

Transdermal systems (TDSs) vary in the technology used for delivering drugs across the stratum corneum (first layer of skin) and in their dosing frequencies. For example, the first marketed transdermal delivery system employed both a drug reservoir and rate-controlling semipermeable membrane and required daily dosing. Subsequently, hormone replacement therapy with estradiol has been administered for $3^1/_2$ to 7 days using a matrix-type TDS to women with symptoms associated with menopause.

Transdermal drug therapy for the overactive bladder

The currently available oxybutynin TDS is a matrix-type system requiring twice-weekly dosing. It is composed of three layers (Figure 50.1), as follows:

- The first layer is a backing film that provides the occlusion required for drug absorption.
- The second layer is the basis of the matrix technology and contains:
  a thin film of acrylic adhesive, which enables the system to attach to the skin oxybutynin dissolved in an acrylic adhesive glycerol triacetate (triacetin, USP), a nonalcoholic permeation enhancer that improves the ability of the drug to penetrate the skin.
- The third layer is a release liner that is peeled off for application.

The design of the matrix-type delivery system allows a controlled rate of drug absorption by means of a chemical method of enhancing skin permeation. Flux enhancers, or chemical penetration enhancers, improve permeation of the drug through the dermal layer, thereby allowing for diffusion into the systemic circulation.[10]

Pharmacokinetic advantage

The oxybutynin TDS has a significant pharmacokinetic advantage over oral oxybutynin, as it avoids presystemic metabolism of the parent compound. Presystemic metabolism refers to the metabolism of the parent compound, prior to entering the systemic circulation, by the CYP450 enzyme system in the gastrointestinal tract and liver following oral administration. With transdermal oxybutynin administration, the avoidance of presystemic metabolism lowers the extent to which the primary metabolite, N-DEO, becomes available to the systemic circulation, thus resulting in fewer anticholinergic side-effects, such as dry mouth, constipation, and drowsiness.

Steady and predictable diffusion of oxybutynin across the stratum corneum has been demonstrated.[9] In studies of human subjects, it has been shown that a 39 cm^2 TDS containing 36 mg of drug will deliver an average dose of 3.9 mg/day and result in average plasma concentrations of oxybutynin of about 4 ng/ml during twice-weekly application (Figure 50.2). In human subjects, the application of oxybutynin TDS to three distinct skin sites – the buttock, hip, and abdomen – showed the same absorption profile.[11]

Bioavailability studies in human subjects showed that after the application of the first oxybutynin TDS, the parent compound becomes available to target tissues within 2 h, peaks at about 24 h, and is sustained at a steady level for over 96 h. Steady-state concentrations are reached with the second application.[9]

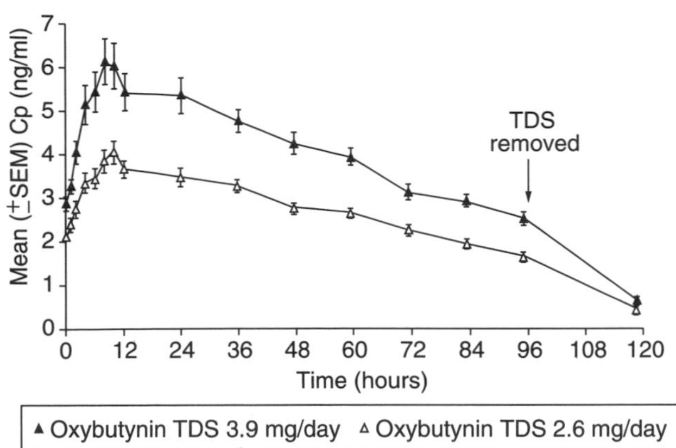

Figure 50.2
Plasma concentrations (Cp) were measured (SEM = standard error of the mean) following the subject's third application. The oxybutynin TDS (transdermal system) was removed after 96 hours.

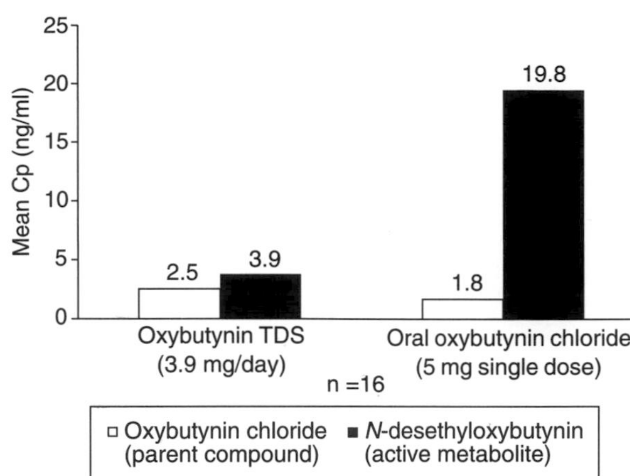

Figure 50.3
Mean plasma concentrations (Cp) were measured after a single 96-hour application of oxybutynin TDS 3.9 mg/day and a single 5 mg oral dose of oxybutynin chloride in 16 healthy subjects.

In patients with OAB, plasma concentrations showed a linear relationship between the dose of oxybutynin TDS and plasma concentrations of both the parent compound, oxybutynin, and the active metabolite, *N*-DEO. This occurred from the lower (1.3 mg/day) to the upper (5.2 mg/day) dose studied.[12]

To show the alteration in first-pass hepatic and gastrointestinal metabolism of the parent oxybutynin compound during transdermal delivery, 16 human subjects participated in a study in which the plasma concentrations of the active metabolite and parent compound were measured following both oral and transdermal drug administration.[13] In the oral oxybutynin group, the average plasma concentration for *N*-DEO was 19.8 ng/ml and for the parent compound was 1.8 ng/ml, a ratio of approximately 10:1. In the oxybutynin TDS group, average plasma concentrations for *N*-DEO, the active metabolite, and the parent compound were 3.9 and 2.5 ng/ml, respectively, a ratio of approximately 1.2:1, showing the contrast of transdermally to orally administered oxybutynin in pharmacokinetic properties (Figure 50.3).

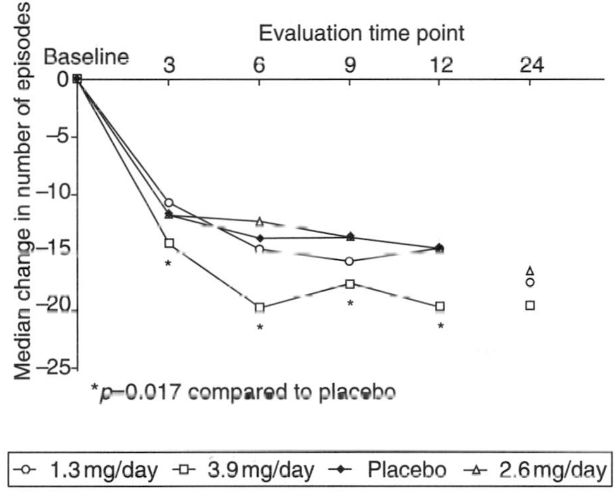

Figure 50.4
Patients taking oxybutynin TDS 3.9 mg/day had a significant decrease in the number of urinary incontinence episodes per week from baseline (BL) to end point.

Clinical efficacy in the overactive bladder

The efficacy of oxybutynin TDS in the treatment of OAB was demonstrated in two clinical trials. The pivotal trial enrolled 520 patients and consisted of a 12-week, double-blind, placebo-controlled initial phase in which three doses of oxybutynin TDS (1.3, 2.6, and 3.9 mg/day) were compared with placebo. For patients receiving oxybutynin TDS 3.9 mg/day, the median number of episodes of urinary incontinence decreased from 31 per week at baseline to 12 per week at end point (Figure 50.4), showing significance ($p = 0.017$) in the end-point change from baseline comparison to placebo (−19 vs −14.5, respectively). A supportive efficacy end point, the mean daily urinary frequency, decreased by 2.3 urinations per day from a baseline of 12 and was significant ($p = 0.046$) in comparison to placebo (−2.3 vs −1.7, respectively). In addition, the measured urinary voided volume increased significantly and quality of life scores improved in the group receiving oxybutynin TDS 3.9 mg/day.[14] Patients in all TDS treatment groups then entered a 12-week, open-label, dose-titration period and again experienced reductions in the number of urinary incontinence episodes per week.

In an earlier 6-week, dose-identification trial, 76 patients who had previously responded to treatment with oral

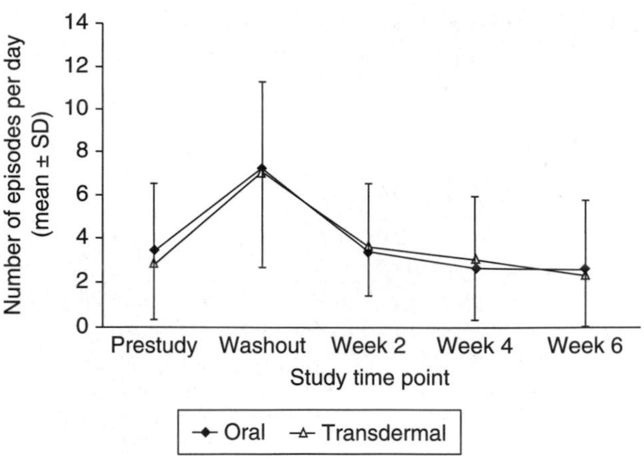

Figure 50.5
Incontinence episodes (mean ± SD) in 72 patients receiving titrated doses of both oral and transdermal oxybutynin during 6 weeks of treatment.

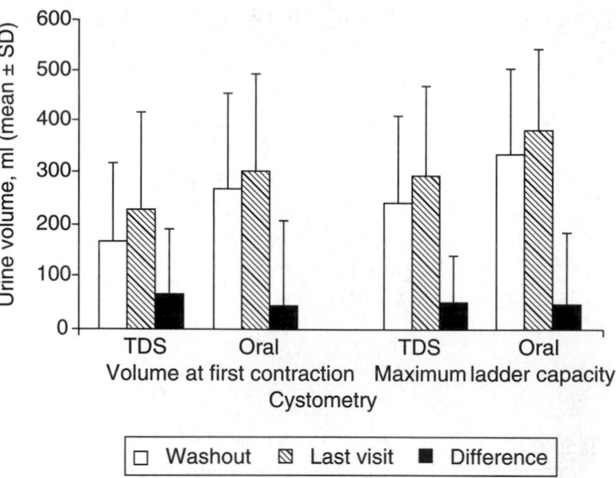

Figure 50.6
Bladder volume at first contraction and maximum bladder capacity in patients receiving TDS ($n = 33$) and oral ($n = 30$) oxybutynin in patients at washout and after 6 weeks of treatment. Patients received titrated doses of oxybutynin between time points.

oxybutynin were randomized to active treatment with either TDS or oral immediate-release oxybutynin. Dosages were titrated for each group, according to anticholinergic side-effects at weeks 2 and 4. Mean daily incontinence episodes were reduced from washout to end of treatment by approximately 5 in both groups ($p < 0.0001$), with no significant difference between transdermal and oral therapy (Figure 50.5). After 6 weeks of treatment, daily incontinence episodes were reduced to 2.4 ± 2.4 in the transdermal group and 2.6 ± 3.3 in the oral group.[12] A total of 8 patients in the TDS group and 10 patients in the oral group were continent on completion of the study.

Cystometry was performed before and at the end of treatment (Figure 50.6). Bladder volume (mean ± SD) at first detrusor contraction increased by 66 ± 126 ml for the transdermal group ($p = 0.005$) and 45 ± 163 ml in the oral group ($p = 0.1428$). Maximum bladder capacity (mean ± SD) increased by 53 ± 8 and 51 ± 138 ml in the transdermal ($p = 0.0011$) and the oral ($p = 0.0538$) groups, respectively.[12]

Side-effect profile

The improved anticholinergic side-effect profile of oxybutynin TDS over oral oxybutynin is the most important clinical consequence of this novel route of oxybutynin administration.

In the pivotal trial of 520 patients who received either TDS oxybutynin in doses of 1.3 mg/day, 2.6 mg/day, or 3.9 mg/day, or placebo, the overall frequency of dry mouth was 7.0% for the oxybutynin TDS group and 8.3% for placebo. Constipation, which can be especially troublesome in older patients, occurred in only 3% of subjects receiving either TDS oxybutynin or placebo. The incidence of dizziness and somnolence was similar to that of the placebo group.[14] The most common adverse event of TDS oxybutynin is a skin reaction at the application site – generally pruritus (16.8%) or erythema (5.6%). In all clinical trials for patients treated with the largest available patch, 3.9 mg/day of TDS oxybutynin ($n = 331$), application site reaction occurred in 14.8% of patients and was mostly mild or moderate in severity and completely reversible.[14]

A review of published clinical trial reports, such as the OBJECT study, shows the incidence of anticholinergic side-effects for oral oxybutynin formulations to be higher than reported in the TDS oxybutynin pivotal clinical trial (Table 50.1).

Dose escalation and occurrence of dry mouth

The first clinical trial of oxybutynin TDS ($n = 76$) was designed to determine the dose limitation in patients with OAB, based on tolerability of anticholinergic side-effects in two parallel groups taking either oral or TDS oxybutynin. Patients entered the trial based on their pre-study dose of oral oxybutynin at one of three TDS dose levels – 2.6, 3.9, or 5.2 mg/day – and had their dose increased every 2 weeks to the maximum of 5.2 mg/day, according to their tolerance of dry mouth. At the 6-week study visit, 68% of the patients receiving oxybutynin TDS had titrated to the maximal dose of 5.2 mg/day compared

Table 50.1 *Incidence of dry mouth for orally administered anticholinergic drugs*

Published clinical trials	OXY (%)	OXYer (%)	TOL (%)	OXYTDS (%)	PLA (%)
Appell et al:[15]					
OXYer, 10 mg/d		28.1	33.2		
TOL, 2 mg bid					
Davila et al:[12]					
OXY TDS, 2.6–5.2 mg od	94[b]			38[b]	
OXY, 10–20 mg od					
Dmochowski et al:[14]					
OXYTDS, 3.9 mg od				9.6	8.3
PLA					
Tapp et al:[16]					
OXY, 5 mg qid	29				10
PLA					
Thuroff et al:[17]					
OXY, 5 mg tid	48				12
PLA					
Birns et al:[18]					
OXY, 5 mg bid	16.7	22.6			
OXYer, 10 mg, od					
Versi et al:[19]	7 (5 mg)	4 (5 mg)			
OXY, 5–20 mg[a]	26 (10 mg)	9 (10 mg)			
OXYer, 5–20 mg[a]	39 (15 mg)	19 (15 mg)			
	45 (20 mg)	40 (20 mg)			
Anderson et al:[20]					
OXY, 5 mg od-qid[a]	87	68			
OXYer, 5–30 mg od[a]					
Burgio et al:[21]					
OXY, 2.5 mg od to 5 mg tid[a]	96.9				

[a] Titrated doses.
[b] At maximum tolerated dose.
OXY, oxybutynin; TOL, tolterodine; TDS, transdermal system; PLA, placebo; er, extended-release formulation; od, daily; bid, twice daily; tid, three times daily; qid, four times daily.

with 32% of patients taking oral oxybutynin.[12] No patient using the oxybutynin TDS had intolerable dry mouth; 62% did not report any dry mouth; and only 11% had moderate, tolerable dry mouth at the final visit.[12] This low incidence of dry mouth, the major anticholinergic side-effect of oxybutynin, contrasts with incidences of 9% intolerable and 59% moderate but tolerable for oral oxybutynin.

Convenience and quality of life

Patients may exercise, shower, or bathe with the TDS in place. The translucent nature of the oxybutynin TDS improves the esthetic acceptability to the patient. The quality of life (QoL) Incontinence Impact Questionnaire showed a significant improvement ($p < 0.05$) compared with that of placebo (Figure 50.7).

Advances in transdermal technology have achieved a reduction in patch size as well as the development of a transdermal gel delivery system. In pre-clinical studies, adequate therapeutic plasma levels of oxybutynin have been obtained that compare well with other delivery methods. Phase 2 trials are currently under way to evaluate a gel-delivery system which utilizes a pre-measured dose of oxybutynin applied to the skin (likely arms) on a daily basis. Convenience and ease of use are expected to be the major positive attributes of this new system.

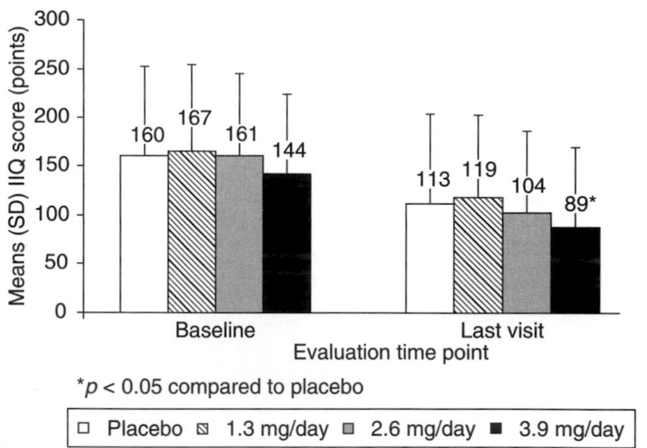

Figure 50.7
Patients with oxybutynin TDS reported improved quality of life on the Incontinence Impact Questionnaire (IIQ) during the double-blind treatment period. Numerical values are in inverse relation to quality of life.

Community-based studies

Since FDA approval and marketing of Oxytrol in 2000, experience has demonstrated specific groups of patients who may benefit from transdermal delivery. The Multicenter Assessment of Transdermal Therapy in Overactive Bladder with Oxybutynin (MATRIX) is an open-label, 6-month, randomized, prospective multicenter community-based trial of OAB subjects. They were randomized to TDS oxybutynin alone versus TDS oxybutynin plus additional educational materials. A total of 2878 subjects were recruited at 327 centers, with 13% being male. Significant improvements in QoL, as reported on the King's Health Questionnaire (KHQ) and Beck Depression Inventory-II (BDI-II), were noted at termination of the study. One of the initial data analyses evaluated sexual function in OAB subjects, and noted that therapy decreased coital incontinence, and improved interest in sex as well as personal relationships with partners.[22] More data analysis is expected as specific subject subgroups are evaluated in this large community trial.

Discussion

Transdermal delivery is a novel approach for the administration of oxybutynin to patients with OAB. Although oxybutynin has a long-established history of efficacy in reducing the number of episodes of urge incontinence, a large percentage of patients discontinue oral oxybutynin because of intolerable anticholinergic side-effects, dry mouth in particular. Because side-effects are dose-related, it has not been possible for most patients to tolerate higher, more therapeutically effective doses. The TDS was developed to minimize anticholinergic side-effects by modifying the metabolism and plasma concentration profile of oxybutynin.

By avoiding presystemic gastrointestinal and hepatic metabolism, transdermal delivery of oxybutynin reduces the incidence of anticholinergic side-effects, specifically dry mouth, while maintaining its efficacy in controling the symptoms of OAB. The incidence of dry mouth is dose-related, and reported to be 7.0% overall for oxybutynin TDS – similar to placebo (8.3%).

In conclusion, the pharmacokinetic changes that result from transdermal administration of oxybutynin make it possible to achieve higher plasma levels of oxybutynin with much lower dosing compared to oral administration. Dosing of oxybutynin can thus be optimized without intolerable anticholinergic side-effects. The TDS offers a convenient, efficacious, and well-tolerated route of administering oxybutynin to patients with symptoms of OAB.

References

1. Frewen W. Role of bladder training in the treatment of the unstable bladder in the female. Urol Clin N Am 1979; 6: 273–7.
2. Oldenburg B, Millard RJ. Predictors of long term outcome following a bladder re-training programme. J Psychosom Res 1986; 30: 691–8.
3. Rovner ES, Wein AJ. Modern pharmacotherapy of urge urinary incontinence in the USA: tolterodine and oxybutynin. BJU Int 2000; 86: 44–54.
4. United States Pharmacopeial Convention. Oxybutynin: systemic. In: United States Pharmacopeial Convention, ed. Drug Information for the Health Care Professional. Englewood, CO: Micromedex, 2001: 2300–2.
5. Buyse G, Waldeck K, Verpoorten C et al. Intravesical oxybutynin for neurogenic bladder dysfunction: less systemic side effects due to reduced first pass metabolism. J Urol 1998; 160: 892–6.
6. Dmochowski RR, Appell RA. Advancements in pharmacologic management of the overactive bladder. Urology 2000; 56: 41–9.
7. Madersbacher H, Jilg G. Control of detrusor hyperreflexia by the intravesical instillation of oxybutynin hydrochloride. Paraplegia 1991; 29: 84–90.
8. Watson Pharmaceuticals I. Data on File, Oxytrol™ NDA 21–351, 2001.
9. Zobrist RH, Thomas H, Sanders SW. Pharmacokinetics and metabolism of transdermally administered oxybutynin. Clin Pharmacol Ther 2002: P94. [Abstract]
10. Ranade VV. Drug delivery systems: 6. Transdermal drug delivery. J Clin Pharmacol 1991; 31: 401–18.
11. Sanders SW, Thomas H, Zobrist RH. Population pharmacokinetics of transdermally administered oxybutynin. Clin Pharmacol Ther 2002: P34. [Abstract]
12. Davila GW, Daugherty CA, Sanders SW. A short-term, multicenter, randomized double-blind dose titration study of the efficacy and anticholinergic side effects of transdermal compared to immediate release oral oxybutynin treatment of patients with urge urinary incontinence. J Urol 2001; 166: 140–5.

13. Zobrist RH, Schmid B, Feick A et al. Pharmacokinetics of the R- and S-enantiomers of oxybutynin and N-desethyloxybutynin following oral and transdermal administration of the racemate in health volunteers. Pharm Res 2001; 18: 1029–34.
14. Dmochowski RR, Davila GW, Zinner NR et al. Efficacy and safety of transdermal oxybutynin in patients with urge and mixed urinary incontinence. J Urol 2002; 168: 580–6.
15. Appell RA, Sand P, Dmochowski R et al. Prospective randomized controlled trial of extended-release oxybutynin chloride and tolterodine tartrate in the treatment of overactive bladder: results of the OBJECT Study. Mayo Clin Proc 2001; 76: 358–63.
16. Tapp AJ, Cardozo LD, Versi E, Cooper D. The treatment of detrusor instability in post-menopausal women with oxybutynin chloride: a double blind placebo controlled study. Br J Obstet Gynaecol 1990; 97: 521–6.
17. Thuroff JW, Bunke B, Ebner A et al. Randomized, double-blind, multicenter trial on treatment of frequency, urgency and incontinence related to detrusor hyperactivity: oxybutynin versus propantheline versus placebo. J Urol 1991; 145: 813–16.
18. Birns J, Lukkari E, Malone-Lee JG. A randomized controlled trial comparing the efficacy of controlled-release oxybutynin tablets (10 mg once daily) with conventional oxybutynin tablets (5 mg twice daily) in patients whose symptoms were stabilized on 5 mg twice daily of oxybutynin. BJU Int 2000; 85: 793–8.
19. Versi E, Appell R, Mobley D et al. Dry mouth with conventional and controlled-release oxybutynin in urinary incontinence. Obstet Gynecol 2000; 95: 718–21.
20. Anderson RU, Mobley D, Blank B et al. Once daily controlled versus immediate release oxybutynin chloride for urge urinary incontinence. J Urol 1999; 161: 1809–12.
21. Burgio KL, Locher JL, Goode PS et al. Behavioral vs drug treatment for urge urinary incontinence in older women: a randomized controlled trial. JAMA 1998; 280: 1995–2000.
22. Sand PK, Goldberg RP, Dmochowski RR, McIlwain M, Dahl NV. The impact of the overactive bladder syndrome on sexual function: a preliminary report from the Multicenter Assessment of Transdermal Therapy in Overactive Bladder with Oxybutynin trial. Am J Obstet Gynecol 2006; 195: 1730–5.

51

Management of autonomic dysreflexia

Guy Breault, Waleed Altaweel, and Jacques Corcos

Introduction

Autonomic dysreflexia (AD) is a complication commonly found in patients with spinal cord injury (SCI) at T6 or above. AD is the result of an uncontrolled sympathetic response secondary to a noxious stimulus. In consequence, this phenomenon is a medical emergency that can result in severe complications and can even be life-threatening. The incidence of AD for SCIs above T6 is between 50 and 70%.[1–3] It is important that all healthcare providers are familiar with the signs and symptoms at presentation, and are able to identify the potential causes of AD. They should also know how to manage acute episodes of AD. Successful management of patients with AD begins with its prevention through patient and family education. Identification and avoidance of noxious stimuli can often be managed by adequate bladder, bowel, and skin care.

Diagnosis of AD

In the case of any patient with SCI at T6 or above, a high level of suspicion for AD should always be present. Patients with SCI at T6 or above usually have normal systolic blood pressure of 90–110 mmHg. AD may present with a sudden increase in both systolic and diastolic blood pressure of 20–40 mmHg over baseline, associated with bradycardia. An elevation of systolic blood pressure of 15–20 mmHg in adolescents or more than 15 mmHg above baseline in children is significant and may also suggest AD.[4,5] Pounding headache, profuse sweating above the level of the lesion, piloerection or goose bumps, flushing, blurred vision, spots in the patient's visual field, nasal congestion, and anxiety are also other classic signs and symptoms of AD. Besides bradycardia, other cardiac abnormalities that might be encountered are atrial fibrillation, premature ventricular contraction, and atrioventricular conduction anomalies. In subacute AD presentation, the patient may present with minimal or absent signs and symptoms of AD, despite elevated blood pressure. Because of cognitive and verbal communication impairments, SCI patients might have difficulty disclosing their symptoms when AD presents. If AD signs and symptoms are present but the patient has normal blood pressure, he or she should be referred to an appropriate consultant, depending on the symptoms.[5]

Acute treatment of AD

Early recognition of signs and symptoms of AD at presentation is the major key to immediate and appropriate treatment of this urgent and life-threatening condition. Late recognition or inappropriate management can result in severe hypertension and complications such as cerebral or subarachnoid hemorrhage, seizures, arrhythmia, coma, and even death.[6–10]

Life-saving measures

Typical signs and symptoms suggestive of AD associated with a significant elevation in mean blood pressure indicate the need for prompt management (Table 51.1). The first step is to place the patient upright in the seated position, with his legs down. This maneuver should provoke an orthostatic drop in blood pressure by allowing pooling in the lower extremities. Additional pooling in the abdomen and lower extremities can be achieved by loosening or removing any tight clothing or constrictive devices.[5]

SCI patients might exhibit significant and rapid fluctuations in blood pressure during an AD episode due to impaired autonomic regulation; therefore it should be monitored closely, every 2 to 5 minutes, and until the patient has stabilized.[4,5,11,12]

Table 51.1 *Acute management of AD*

Intervention	Rationale
1. Seat the patient upright and lower the legs	May allow pooling of blood in the lower extremities
2. Loosen clothing or constrictive devices	May allow pooling of blood in the abdomen and lower extremities
3. Monitor blood pressure every 2–5 min	Blood pressure may fluctuate rapidly during an AD episode
4. If no indwelling urinary catheter is present, catheterize the patient	Bladder distention is the most common cause of AD
5. If the patient has an indwelling urinary catheter, check it for obstruction and irrigate the catheter (which may need to be changed)	Bladder distention is the most common cause of AD
6. If systolic blood pressure is elevated to or above 150 mmHg, consider pharmacological management	The risk of adverse sequelae increases when systolic blood pressure exceeds 150 mmHg
7. If symptoms persist, suspect fecal impaction	Fecal impaction is the second most common cause of AD
8. If symptoms persist, check for other less frequent causes	Many other precipitating factors may be the trigger, and appropriate treatment should resolve the AD episode
9. Consider admission or referral if symptoms persist or no precipitants are found	The patient is at risk of further episodes if no precipitant is found, and appropriate evaluation and treatment should be undertaken
10. Monitor the patient's symptoms and blood pressure for at least 2 hours after AD resolution	AD may resolve because of medication and not because of resolution of the underlying cause

Eliminating the cause of AD

The next step is the elimination of the trigger. Since bladder distention is the most common cause of AD, an indwelling urethral catheter must be placed in the bladder if one is not already present.[3] Catheterization itself can exacerbate AD, therefore intraurethral lidocaine (lignocaine) jelly 2% should be generously applied at least 2 minutes before every attempt to insert or change a urethral catheter, in order to decrease sensory input and relax the urinary sphincter.[5] If the patient already has an indwelling urethral catheter, the catheter and tubing system should be checked for obstruction or kinks. Irrigation of the catheter with 10 to 15 ml of warm saline may help if obstruction of the catheter is suspected. Both large volumes and cold irrigation solutions should be avoided because they can also exacerbate the AD. Irrigation should also be limited to 5 to 10 ml for children under 2 years of age and to 10 to 15 ml in older children.[5] Irrigation with lidocaine solution may help decrease sensory input from the bladder. Other provocative triggers that should be avoided are bladder distention and suprapubic percussion, because they can worsen the condition. The catheter might needed to be changed if a previous attempt to relieve the obstructed catheter has failed to decompress the bladder. A catheter with a coudé tip may be considered if catheterization is difficult or associated with bladder neck obstruction.

After adequate bladder catheterization, it is important to monitor the patient's blood pressure, because a sudden decompression of the bladder will eliminate the noxious stimulus and the blood pressure will normalize. However, hypotension might occur after resolution of the trigger, especially if the patient has been given antihypertensive medication.[5]

If blood pressure remains elevated after bladder catheterization fecal impaction should be suspected, since it is the second most common cause of AD. Appropriate precautions should be taken before disimpaction, because additional stimulation could further exacerbate AD. Gentle disimpaction can be done after introducing intrarectal lidocaine jelly 2% for at least 2 minutes before checking for stool impaction. If AD worsens during rectal manipulation, the manual evacuation should be stopped and rechecked after 20 minutes.[5]

If the precipitating trigger has still not been identified, a thorough exploration for the cause must be initiated. The blood pressure should be monitored for at least 2 hours after resolution of the symptoms of an AD episode, and the patient should be instructed to monitor his or her symptoms to identify a possible recurrence.[5]

Pharmacotherapy to lower blood pressure

Pharmaceutical treatment for refractory high blood pressure should be considered when the blood pressure is above 150 mmHg in adults, 140 mmHg in adolescents, 130 mmHg in children aged 6–12 years, or 120 mmHg in children under 5 years.[5] Appropriate-sized blood pressure cuffs are necessary when measuring blood pressure in children and adolescents. Antihypertensive medication should preferably have a rapid onset and short duration of action. Nifedipine or nitrates are the most commonly used medications during an acute attack. Nifedipine 10 mg, bitten and swallowed (rather than sublingually, S/L) in the immediate-release form, is the preferred method of administration. The treatment can be repeated in 30 minutes if the elevated blood pressure persists. Extreme caution should be exercised in the elderly or in patients with coronary artery disease, as it has been reported that nifedipine can cause hypotension and reflex tachycardia in individuals without SCI.[5,11–14] Application of 2.5 cm of Nitropast 2% (nitroglycerin ointment) on the skin above the level of the lesion can be very useful. An advantage is that the paste can be easily removed when the hypertension subsides, reducing the chances of subsequent hypotension. An intravenous sodium nitroprusside drip may be required if the hypertension is refractory to the initial medical treatment.[5] Another medication that can be used to treat acute AD is phenoxybenzamine, an α-receptor blocker, given orally at a dose of 10 mg. It has been shown that phenoxybenzamine causes relaxation of the internal sphincter and can control the symptoms. Tamsulosin, an α-receptor blocker, although it might be helpful in reducing the frequency and severity of AD, is not recommended in the acute treatment of AD.[15] Prazosin is another alternative for the management of hypertensive emergencies in AD. A pilot study has shown that captopril 25 mg S/L is safe and effective in treating patients with hypertension from AD. Both prazosin and captopril act within 30 minutes, achieve therapeutic levels within 1 to 3 hours, and have a half-life of 2 to 4 hours. Glyceryl trinitrate can be administered in an appropriately-monitored setting for rapid blood pressure control. Hydralazine, 5 mg iv or 5–20 mg im, is another alternative to maintain low blood pressure.[5,15–19]

Erectile dysfunction in SCI patients is often treated with sildenafil. Nitrates are contraindicated in patients taking sildenafil. The resulting blood pressure drop may be significant and dangerous. If sildenafil has been used within the last 24 hours, another short-acting antihypertensive medication should be given. On the other hand, if the patient receives nitrates, he should be instructed not to take sildenafil for at least 24 hours.

Managing secondary hypotension

After removal of the trigger responsible for AD, or with pharmaceutical treatment of elevated blood pressure, the blood pressure should be monitored closely for possible hypotension. If hypotension ensues, the patient should be placed lying down with the legs elevated. Volume repletion with intravenous fluids and the administration of an adrenergic agonist can also be considered if the hypotension is symptomatic or refractory.

Prevention and prophylactic treatment of AD

Education and conservative management

The primary goal in the management of AD is the prevention of acute crisis. Structured education and support for all patients and their families is an important aspect in the management of SCI, together with an appropriate follow-up by healthcare professionals with expertise in the management of those patients. To be most effective, the support should be introduced as soon as possible to prevent the occurrence of complications. An acute episode of AD is most often triggered by a noxious stimulus that can be easily identified and abolished. Special consideration of the genitourinary system is very important since bladder distention is responsible for the acute event in around 75 to 85% of cases. After bladder distention, the next most common noxious stimulus responsible for acute AD is bowel distention due to fecal impaction, which may be encountered in up to 20% of AD patients. Other urinary tract precipitants that may be encountered are acute urinary retention, urinary tract infection, bladder calculi, urethral distention, testicular torsion, and instrumentation. Other possible triggers of AD are bowel distention, anorectal distention, hemorrhoids, anal fissures, and other gastrointestinal precipitants; pressure ulcers, ingrown toenails and other skin pathology, fracture of long bones, labor, and delivery are amoung the less frequent triggers. Documentation of previous AD episodes is also very important and should include signs and symptoms at presentation, the trigger responsible for the acute event, and the treatment instituted. Blood pressure documentation and the response to treatment may also be helpful in the management of subsequent AD episodes.[5]

Pharmaceutical treatment

In patients with recurrent acute episodes of AD, an α-adrenoceptor blocker may help to suppress dysreflexic symptoms; a nightly dose of terazosin 5 mg or tamsulosin 0.8 mg may reduce the frequency, severity, and bother of AD.[15,19] Even if pharmaceutical treatment is helpful in some patients, it does not eliminate the need for appropriate care to the genitourinary, gastrointestinal, and other systems to eliminate avoidable triggers.

Acute AD may be precipitated by surgical, cystoscopic, urodynamic, and radiologic procedures. Therefore, if the patient is known to have recurrent acute AD episodes, prophylactic pharmaceutical management with nifedipine 10 mg or nitropast 2% can be given shortly before the procedure. Prophylactic treatment of chronic patients with an α-adrenoceptor blocker or premedication before a urologic procedure does not eliminate the need for careful monitoring during the procedure.[5,7,11,12,15,19]

Anesthetic considerations in AD

Most AD episodes are triggered by a urologic manipulation or surgery. For that reason, a multidisciplinary preoperative evaluation should include anesthesia assessment and determination of the level of injury with the history of dysreflexic episodes. Anesthetic techniques for controling AD include topical application for cystoscopy, general anesthesia, and spinal and epidural anesthesia. Lidocaine jelly may decrease the sensation and relax the sphincter during cystoscopy, but bladder distention may trigger an AD episode despite local anesthesia. Spinal anesthesia has been reported to give excellent control for the prevention of an AD episode, and has also been recommended in acute AD refractory to medical management.[20–29] Nifedipine may be given prophylactically 30 to 60 minutes prior to surgery when a procedure is performed under general anesthesia.[20] Some anesthetics found to be effective for the treatment of AD are halothane, isoflurane, and enflurane. When a dysreflexic episode occurs during a procedure in a patient under general anesthesia, the first step is to increase the depth of anesthesia.[20] In patients known to have had a previous AD episode, or at high risk for a dysreflexic event, intraoperative and postoperative cardiac monitoring is warranted since AD may occur up to a few days after surgery.

AD treatment during pregnancy and labor

AD is a common complication of pregnancy in SCI. Prevention remains the most important factor in AD management to avoid morbidity and mortality in patients or their fetus.

During labor and delivery, the risk of AD in patients with lesions at or above T6 is 85 to 90%.[21] SCI patients should be monitored for urinary tract infections, fecal impaction, and blood pressure during both gestation and labor. AD during pregnancy has the same pathophysiology and requires the same type of management as in nonpregnant patients. In some patients, a classic episode of AD may be the only clue to the onset of labor. An important differential diagnosis to an AD episode during pregnancy in SCI women is pre-eclampsia. Unlike pre-eclampsia, blood pressure elevation and other classic symptoms of AD occur during uterine contractions and resolve with relaxation of the uterus.[21] Anesthetic jelly should always be used to reduce stimulation for any manipulation, including before vaginal examinations, urinary catheterizations, or rectal manipulation. Bladder catheter drainage should be initiated and monitored frequently to avoid obstruction during labor. It has also been proposed that monitoring during labor and delivery should ideally include an intra-arterial catheter for continuous blood pressure reading, telemetry for continuous cardiac rhythm monitoring, and constant electronic fetal monitoring to identify fetal distress.[22,23]

A complete anesthesia consultation should be undertaken prior to labor. AD control in labor without epidural block is unsatisfactory.[24] Epidural anesthesia interrupts the reflex arc from the uterus to the cardiovascular system via the spinal cord and is thought to prevent the triggering of AD. Prophylactic placement of an epidural catheter at 37 weeks of gestation has been described as an option, but early placement of an epidural catheter is usually done at the first sign of labor.[25] A combination of bupivacaine and fentanyl has been reported in cases of successful deliveries in women with spinal cord lesions.[25] Since AD may occur up to 48 hours after delivery, maintenance of epidural anesthesia for that period is usually recommended.[27] Oral nifedipine, intravenous hydralazine, or trimethaphan has been suggested to control extremely high blood pressure in this population during labor. Intravenous nitroprusside is generally not recommended during pregnancy or labor because of elevated fetal cyanide levels. Ganglionic-blocking agents with a short duration of action, such as a 0.1% solution of trimethaphan in 5% dextrose by intravenous drip, can be administered in refractory AD cases during labor that are not adequately controlled by regional anesthesia.[29]

Conclusion

AD is a medical emergency often related to urologic, gastrointestinal, or gynecologic problems or manipulations. Its management starts primarily with its prevention, but healthcare providers should be informed of this pathology to promptly recognize and treat it. Physicians must be aware of the simple procedures and treatment cascade that can be undertaken to avoid the possibly devastating consequences of acute AD. Pregnancy and anesthesia have to be considered as precipitating factors supporting preventive and aggressive management.

References

1. Shergill I, Arya M, Hamid R. The importance of autonomic dysreflexia to the urologist. Br J Urol Int 2004; 93: 923–6.
2. Karlsson AK. Autonomic dysreflexia. Spinal Cord 1999; 37: 383–91.
3. Lindan R, Joiner E, Freehafer AA et al. Incidence and clinical features of autonomic dysreflexia in patients with spinal cord injury. Paraplegia 1980; 18: 285–93.
4. Blackmer J. Rehabilitation medicine: 1. Autonomic dysreflexia. Can Med Assoc J 2003; 169: 931–5.
5. Paralyzed Veterans of America/Consortium for Spinal Cord Medicine. Acute Management of Autonomic Dysreflexia: Individuals with Spinal Cord Injury Presenting to Health Care Facilities, 2nd edn. Washington, DC: Paralyzed Veterans of America (PVA) 2001: 29.
6. Kursh ED, Freehafer A, Persky L. Complication of autonomic dysreflexia. J Urol 1977; 118: 70–2.
7. Eltorai 1, Kim R, Vulpe M et al. Fatal cerebral hemorrhage due to autonomic dysreflexia in a tetraplegic patient. Case report and review. Paraplegia 1992; 30: 355–60.
8. Pine ZM, Miller SD, Alonso JA. Atrial fibrillation associated with autonomic dysreflexia. Am J Phys Med Rehabil 1991; 70: 271–3.
9. Vallès M, Benito J, Portell E. Cerebral hemorrhage due to autonomic dysreflexia in a spinal cord injury patient. Spinal Cord 2005; 43: 738–40.
10. Pan SL, Wang YH, Lin HL et al. Intracerebral hemorrhage secondary to autonomic dysreflexia in a young person with incomplete C8 tetraplegia: a case report. Arch Phys Med Rehabil 2005; 86: 591–3.
11. Braddom KL, Rocco JF. Autonomic dysreflexia. A survey of current treatment. Am J Phys Med Rehab 1991; 70: 234–41.
12. Dykstra DD, Sidi AA, Anderson LC. The effect of nifedipine on cystoscopy-induced autonomic hyperreflexia in patients with spinal cord injuries. J Urol 1987; 138(5): 1155–7.
13. Thyberg M, Ertzgaard P, Gylling M. Effect of nifedipine on cystometry-induced elevation of blood pressure in patients with a reflex urinary bladder after a high level spinal cord injury. Paraplegia 1994; 32: 308–13.
14. Grossman E, Messerli FH, Grodzicki T. Should a moratorium be placed on sublingual nifedipine capsule given for hypertensive emergencies and pseudo-emergencies? JAMA 1996; 276: 1328–31.
15. Abrams P, Amarenco G, Bakke A et al. Tamsulosin: efficacy and safety in patients with neurogenic lower urinary tract dysfunction due to suprasacral spinal cord injury. J Urol 2003; 170: 1242–51.
16. Scott MB, Morrow JW. Phenoxybenzamine in neurogenic bladder dysfunction after spinal cord injury. II. Autonomic dysreflexia. J Urol 1978; 119: 483–4.
17. McGuire J, Wagner FM, Weiss RM. Treatment of autonomic dysreflexia with phenoxybenzamine. J Urol 1976; 115: 53–5.
18. Esmail Z, Shalansky K, Sunderji R et al. Evaluation of captopril for the management of hypertension in autonomic dysreflexia: a pilot study. Arch Phys Med Rehabil 2002; 83: 604–8.
19. Vaidyanathan S, Soni BM, Sett P et al. Pathophysiology of autonomic dysreflexia: long-term treatment with terazosin in adult and paediatric spinal cord injury patients manifesting recurrent dysreflexia episodes. Spinal Cord 1998; 36: 761–70.
20. Hambly P, Martin B. Anaesthesia for chronic spinal cord lesions. Anaesthesia 1998; 53: 273–89.
21. Burns AS, Jackson AB. Gynecologic and reproductive issues in women with spinal cord injury. Phys Med Rehabil Clin North Am 2001; 12: 183–99.
22. Greenspoon JS, Paul RH. Paraplegia and quadriplegia. Special consideration during pregnancy and labor and delivery. Am J Obstet Gynecol 1986; 155: 738–41.
23. Cross LL, Meythaler JM, Tuel SM, Cross AL. Pregnancy, labor and delivery post spinal cord injury. Paraplegia 1992; 30: 890–902.
24. Burns R, Clark VA. Epidural anaesthesia for caesarean section in a patient with quadriplegia and autonomic hyperrreflexia. Int J Obstet Anesth 2004; 13: 120–3.
25. Kobayashi A, Mizobe T, Tojo H. Autonomic hyperreflexia during labour. Can J Anaesth 1995; 42: 1134–6.
26. Gunaydin B, Akcali D, Alkan M. Epidural anaesthesia for Caesarean section in a patient with Devic's syndrome. Anaesthesia 2001; 56: 565–7.
27. Murphy B, McGuire G, Peng P. Treatment of autonomic hyperreflexia in a quadriplegic patient by epidural anesthesia in the postoperative period. Anesth Analg 1999; 879: 148–9.
28. Colachis SC 3rd. Autonomic hyperreflexia with spinal cord injury. J Am Paraplegic Soc 1992; 15: 171–86.
29. Tabsh K, Brinkman CR 3rd, Reff RA. Autonomic dysreflexia in pregnancy. Obstet Gynecol 1982; 60: 119–22.

52

Peripheral electrical stimulation

Magnus Fall and Sivert Lindström

General background

Important prerequisites for continence are intactness of the vesicourethral supportive structures and of the smooth and the striated muscles of the urethra, the latter being composed of the intramural striated sphincter and the paraurethral components of the pelvic floor muscles. Most striated muscles of the body are composed of three motor unit types, one with slowly contracting muscle fibers and two with fast contraction properties.[1] The intramural urethral sphincter is special in being composed of slow fibers only, whereas the paraurethral striated muscles have varying numbers of all three types. The three motor unit types differ with respect to their maximal force development, fusion frequency – that is the activation frequency for a smooth sustained contraction – and resistance to fatigue. The slow units develop little force but are resistant to fatigue. Their fusion frequency is about 10 Hz. The fastest units can produce 10–20 times more contraction force but fatigue rapidly. Their fusion frequency is around 40–50 Hz. The intermediate fast units are somewhat weaker but considerably more fatigue-resistant. It follows that the intramural striated sphincter can generate a well-sustained but rather limited increase in urethral pressure. The main function of this muscle seems to be to accomplish urethral closure during bladder filling at rest, when there is little physical stress. In more provocative situations, when the intra-abdominal pressure suddenly increases, e.g. lifting, coughing, and running (when most women with stress urinary incontinence leak), the fast motor units of the paraurethral pelvic floor muscles provide a rapidly induced, strong closing force upon the urethra. This contraction is in fact governed by the central motor program during self-generated increases of the intra-abdominal pressure, thereby allowing these muscles to contract in advance of the pressure rise. They are also promptly reflexly engaged by pressure increases from the outside caused by a sudden push towards the abdominal wall, but in this situation the contraction lags behind the pressure increase. The pressures generated by the pelvic floor muscles upon the urethra clearly exceed the maximal detrusor or intra-abdominal pressures in intact subjects. Thus, there is normally a reliable safety margin.

Bladder filling is detected by mechanoreceptors in the bladder wall. These receptors respond both to passive distention and to active contraction of the detrusor.[2] The afferent signals are transmitted, mainly via the pelvic nerves, to the spinal cord, and ascend bilaterally in the dorsolateral white matter. The information eventually reaches the cerebral cortex in the medial region of its somatosensory area[3,4] and gives rise to the sensation of bladder filling and urgency. The afferent signal also influences neurons in Barrington's micturition center in the upper pons.[5] When appropriately activated, descending neurons in this center drive preganglionic bladder pelvic neurons in the sacral cord, and thereby induce a micturition contraction. Once initiated, the micturition reflex is self-sustained by a positive feedback mechanism. The reflex detrusor contraction generates an increased bladder pressure and an enhanced activation of bladder mechanoreceptors. This afference, in turn, reinforces the activation of the pontine micturition center and the pelvic motor output to the bladder, resulting in a further increase in bladder pressure and mechanoreceptor afference. When urine enters the urethra, the reflex is further enhanced by activation of urethral receptors.[6] Normally, this positive feedback mechanism ascertains a complete emptying of the bladder during micturition. As long as there is any fluid left in the lumen, the intravesical pressure will be maintained above the threshold for the mechanoreceptors, which will provide a continuous drive for the detrusor.

A drawback with this arrangement is that the reflex system may easily become unstable. Any stimulus that elicits a small burst of impulses in mechanoreceptor afferents may trigger a micturition reflex. To prevent this from happening during the filling phase, the micturition reflex pathway is controlled by several inhibitory mechanisms at spinal and supraspinal levels.[7] The micturition reflex has normally an all-or-nothing character. The pelvic efferents to the bladder are silent during the filling phase but, due to the positive feedback system, they fire maximally during micturition contractions.

Activation of continence reflexes by electrical stimulation

Penile,[8] clitoris,[9] and vaginal electrical stimulation[10,11] activates the motor fibers to the pelvic floor and the intramural urethral sphincter, either directly or by reflex mechanisms, or both.[10–13] At these sites of stimulation, further reflexes are evoked with the afferent limb in the pudendal nerve and with three concomitant central actions: activation of hypogastic inhibitory fibers to the bladder; central inhibition of the pelvic outflow to the bladder; and central inhibition of the ascending afferent pathway from the bladder.[4,12,14] This reflex is silent at rest and seems to be designed to prevent bladder contractions during coitus. Anal stimulation[15,16] inhibits the bladder in a similar fashion by a reflex with its afferent limb in pelvic nerve branches to the anal region,[17] a reflex designed to inhibit the bladder during defecation. Thus, perineal methods for electrical stimulation utilize natural reflexes that are silent during normal, everyday life but capable of sustained bladder inhibition when evoked by continuous or intermittent electrical stimulation.

It is generally believed that in the normal situation, bladder inhibition follows pelvic floor contraction and that bladder inhibition elicited by electrical stimulation would result from pelvic floor activation.[14] However, in animal experimental studies it has been demonstrated that there is rather activation of specific inhibitory pudendal afferents. Lindström et al[12] showed that complete relaxation of the pelvic floor by succinylcholine did not abolish the inhibitory effect of stimulation. Subsequently, it has been demonstrated that there are separate systems for bladder and urethral sphincter activation. Patients with so-called uninhibited overactive bladder exhibit a characteristic dysfunction with an uninhibitable micturition contraction associated with an uninhibitable sphincter relaxation. However, in 21% of patients a dissociation was demonstrated, those patients not being able to inhibit detrusor overactivity although able to perform sphincter activation voluntarily, indicating separate systems to control detrusor activation and striated muscle activation.[18] In experiments in cats, Blok and Holstege[19] described separate centers for micturition (M-region pontine center) and storage (L-region pontine center). The M region excites bladder muscle through projections to its motoneurons and inhibits the urethral sphincter through γ-aminobutyric acid (GABA) interneurons, which inhibits the sphincter. The L region acts independently and excites the sphincter motoneurons. In the brain a network of regions seem to be involved in the normal control, including the periaqueductal gray, thalamus, insula, anterior cingulae, and prefrontal cortex, all of them possible targets for activity evoked by peripheral electrical stimulation.

The nervous system is equipped with multiple mechanisms to inhibit bladder activity in specific situations. During running or walking such a mechanism is activated. It can also be elicited artificially by electrical stimulation; one site is at the posterior tibial nerve – this is also the traditional Chinese bladder acupuncture point, that can be stimulated mechanically or electrically. In human experiments it has been demonstrated that symptoms can be decreased, the first involuntary detrusor contraction delayed, and maximum cystometric capacity increased during percutaneous posterior tibial nerve electrical stimulation.[20–24.]

The therapeutic effects of functional electrical stimulation (FES), on the bladder as well as the sphincter mechanism, depend on artificial activation of nerves. The first requirement for an effect is that the stimulation intensity is high enough to evoke an activity in the relevant nerves. The threshold intensity varies inversely with the fiber diameter, distance between the nerves and the stimulating electrodes, and the pulse configuration. Large myelinated fibers, like efferents to the pelvic floor, have the lowest threshold. Anogenital cutaneous afferents involved in bladder inhibition and pelvic floor muscle reflexes (bulbocavernosus reflex) have intermediate values, whereas afferents responsible for pain sensation have the highest. In practice the distance between the electrode and nerve fiber is more important. Thus, all external electrodes induce skin or mucosal sensations at much lower intensities than pelvic floor contractions by direct stimulation of the motor fibers. For the same reason, the difference between the detection threshold and pain effects is quite narrow, with the maximal tolerance level reached at intensities about 1.5–2 times the detection threshold.[25,26] In routine practice, this is a significant problem since the ability to motivate the patient to accept a high stimulation intensity is a prerequisite for and an important limitation of a good result.[27,28] A stronger effect may be obtained in selected cases by direct stimulation of the pudendal nerve trunk by means of needle electrodes;[26] however, it is an invasive and thereby more unpleasant treatment. From experimental studies it is clear that the tolerance level is well below that required for maximal bladder inhibition or pelvic floor contraction. It follows that proper electrode design that permits positioning of the electrodes close to the relevant nerves is mandatory to achieve good clinical response.

Any pulse configuration would do for nerve activation, provided the stimulators can generate high enough intensities (in mA or V). Short square-wave pulses (0.2–0.5 ms) are most effective, however, in terms of charge transfer for a given biological effect.[29] To minimize electrochemical reactions at the electrode–mucosa interphase, it is preferable to use biphasic or polarity alternating pulses.

Stimulation frequency is another crucial factor. Due to the contractile properties of the fast and slow motor units, a high stimulation frequency, 50–100 Hz, is required for maximal urethral closure. The bladder inhibitory reflex systems operate at much lower frequencies. Maximal inhibition via the sympathetic route is obtained at about 5 Hz, and 5–10 Hz is also the best frequency for central inhibition of the pelvic outflow to the bladder. Since the lower frequency may be unpleasant, 10 Hz stimulation has been recommended as a practical compromise. In clinical experiments in women with detrusor overactivity, cystometric registrations and isobaric volume recordings were performed to document effects during intravaginal electrical stimulation.[30] With these procedures it was easy to demonstrate an abolishment of phasic detrusor contractions and an increase in bladder volume during stimulation, an effect most evident at low-frequency stimulation (10 Hz). Vereecken et al[31] and Vodusek et al[32] observed similar effects but did not see any difference in the degree of bladder inhibition at stimulation frequencies between 5 and 20 Hz. All frequencies in that range do elicit bladder inhibition and it is quite plausible that different clinical conditions, like idiopathic phasic detrusor overactivity vs detrusor overactivity in spinal cord injury, may require somewhat different technique for an optimal response. Detrusor inhibition has likewise been demonstrated by anal[16] or penile surface[8] electrodes. The frequency characteristics are similar for reflexes elicited from anal or genital stimulation. Engagement of larger pudendal nerve branches or selective stimulation of clitoris or penile nerve branches has been found to optimize the effect. It has been suggested that the effect on the bladder can be further improved if the pudendal nerve stimulation is calibrated by electrophysiologic monitoring of the 'maximal motor response'.[33]

In trials without drugs, adequate urethral closure was obtained at 20–50 Hz, the lower frequency being a good compromise for patients with mixed stress and urge incontinence. Muscle fatigue is an important problem. When using FES for incontinence, intermittent trains of impulses have been found to reduce this problem.[34,35] Another factor to consider is the long-term effect of chronic stimulation on the pelvic floor muscles. As one effect, it has been proposed that chronic stimulation increases the relative number of slow-twitch fibers in the paraurethral muscles,[36] since it has previously been found for leg muscles that long-lasting slow stimulation may transform intermediate fast motor units to such with mainly slow properties.[37] Slow and intermediate motor units are also recruited first in reflex activation of the motor pool. Intermittent high-frequency stimulation would, if anything, be expected to have the opposite effect, though. To improve urethral closure at sudden increases of the intra-abdominal pressure, stronger fast-twitch fibers would be desirable, not the opposite.

A clinically most significant result of peripheral electrical stimulation is the carry-over or re-education effect: in some patients there is long-term remission of symptoms after repeated electrical stimulation,[10,38–40] sometimes lasting for years.[41] The physiologic basis of this seemingly curative effect of stimulation is not yet fully explained, but no doubt involves modulation of central nervous activity. A change of peripheral receptor activity after chronic stimulation has been suggested, too,[42,43] which may contribute to a normalization of micturition pattern. Jiang,[44] during anogenital electrical stimulation in the rat, demonstrated that 5 min stimulation at 10 Hz induced a prolonged increase in the micturition threshold volume, which was maintained for 40 min, presumably involving modulation of synaptic transmission in the central micturition pathway. When intravesical electrical stimulation (IVES) was used, the opposite result was achieved: i.e. prolonged enhancement of the micturition reflex. In further experiments, the specific antagonist CPPene was used to block central glutaminergic receptors of the NMDA type. The IVES-induced decrease in micturition threshold was blocked by prior administration of CPPene. This finding indicates that the IVES-induced modulation of the micturition reflex is due to an enhanced excitatory synaptic transmission in the central micturition reflex pathway.[45] Similar modulation of the inhibitory, central mechanisms during electrical stimulation at relevant sites seems quite likely. A further plausible mechanism is that continence reflexes, once upgraded by artificial electrical stimulation, will be maintained when micturition is normalized, providing the chance of natural daily voiding and withholding training sessions.

A further possibility is that chronic stimulation can improve the central motor programs for activation of the relevant striated muscles, in analogy with the stimulation-induced re-education in urge incontinence. Stimulation may also improve the reinervation of partly denervated muscle fibers by enhancing sprouting of surviving motor axons. Activation in animal experiments has been observed to promote the development of large motor units with many muscle fibers.[46] In line with these observations, Schmidt et al[47] and Fall, Hjälmås, and Lindehall (unpublished work) observed an improvement of stress incontinence in children and youngsters with myelomeningocele and partly denervated pelvic floor.

It is worth remembering that electrical pelvic floor stimulation involves the coordinated bladder and urethral function. When treating bladder overactivity, an effect on the sphincter mechanism may be as significant for the patient. It is not an unusual observation that, during ongoing treatment, the patients may still experience urgency and frequency of urination but have regained control of the sphincter. They can thereby postpone voiding, an effect of utmost importance for their ability to resume normal activities of daily life.

Table 52.1 *Requirements of a stimulator for clinical use*
Adequate electrode design
Sufficient and adjustable stimulation intensity
Short pulse width (range 0.2–0.5 ms)
Biphasic pulses
Variability of stimulation frequency (range 10–50 Hz), depending on clinical demands
Continuous or intermittent stimulation, depending on clinical demands

Clinical techniques of electrical stimulation

There are two main options for clinical treatment. *Long-term stimulation* implies chronic stimulation at low intensity and requires several hours of treatment per day during several months. This modality was first used by Caldwell et al,[38] who implanted electrodes into the pelvic floor muscles and connected them to a radiolinked stimulator activated from an outside antenna. It was subsequently found that external electrodes yielded similar good results. Different shapes of vaginal and anal electrodes have been tried on a long-term basis. Advantages of long-term external stimulation are that hospital attention is not required and treatment is cheap and self-controlled by the patient. A disadvantage is that the procedure demands patient persistence. Many patients also find the different devices uncomfortable to wear for a prolonged period of time. Still, in earlier series, excellent results of up to 90% of patients being cured or markedly improved by treatment have been described.[16,41] Most patients using this mode of treatment prefer to use the device during sleep at night. Unfortunately, because of the slow progress of technical development and marketing, most of the devices for long-term treatment have gone out of the market.

A different approach was presented by Godec et al.[48] Using anal plug electrodes and needle electrodes inserted into the levator ani muscle, they applied a 15–20 min continuous train of pulses at high intensity, so-called *acute maximal stimulation.* The applications were repeated up to 10 times in the outpatient clinic. Plevnik and Janez[49] and Kralj[50] used a modified technique with only surface electrodes and obtained a successful result in more than 50% of patients. Acute maximal stimulation may be preferable as treatment in urge incontinence owing to an overactive bladder. High-amplitude stimulation induces a more pronounced bladder inhibition and fewer stimulation sessions are required for a curative effect.[12,33] A limiting factor for maximal stimulation by means of external electrodes is that the effective range up to the maximum tolerable level is rather narrow.[25] A stronger effect may be obtained in selected cases by direct stimulation of the pudendal nerve trunk by means of needle electrodes,[26] however this is an invasive and thereby more unpleasant treatment. A further development of this principle is percutaneous implantation of a rechargeable, miniaturized stimulator close to the pudendal nerve at Alcock's canal. The preliminary results of this treatment are promising.[51,52]

Presently, a combined approach of clinical and home high-intensity stimulation by means of vaginal and anal electrodes and a personal stimulator *(home maximal stimulation)* seems to be the most popular alternative.[53] Percutaneous tibial nerve stimulation, another minimally invasive technique, has been on trial in patients with overactive bladder and non-obstructive urinary retention,[23] with a positive response noted in about 60% of patients. This modality of electrical stimulation is technically more complicated and yields lower overall results than so-called pelvic floor electrical stimulation, but may be an option in patients with special requirements.

Up to half of the patients regain permanent control (re-education) of the bladder and/or the urethral sphincters after a period of long-term or a sequence of maximal electrical stimulation.[16,41,49,50,53–55] In some patients only a temporary improvement may be achieved, and recurrence of symptoms is encountered after a few weeks or months. In these cases, repeated sessions of treatment usually restore control. However, very frequent periods of treatment or daily stimulation are demanding and not readily accepted by all patients. In such a situation, implantation of a sacral root or pudendal nerve stimulator may be a better solution (see Chapter 54). It has also to be realized that patient selection and precise applications of techniques have a determining role for the results. When put into routine practice, the results may differ dramatically to those obtained in prospective studies since factors decisive for an optimal result are no longer well controlled.[16,26–28,41,54]

The problem of randomized controlled trials and functional electrical stimulation

In today's era of evidence-based medicine no treatment is fully accepted if active treatment is not superior to placebo, and one problem with FES is the relative lack of randomized controlled studies (RCTs). FES requires the sensation of stimulation to be effective so it has been difficult to design a study with a genuine placebo equivalent, i.e. electrical stimulation producing the sensation of stimulation with no other effect as a control arm. A nonfunctioning stimulator as control is too easy for the patient to reveal and thus is not an ideal placebo. In an early trial, this method was tested, but the study was not completed because of dropouts in the group having non-functioning stimulation devices.[56] Subsequently, however, successful trials have been presented using this principle,[57–59] and a statistically significant effect on stress urinary incontinence was found compared to the groups wearing a device without stimulation. Yamanishi et al[60] treated patients with detrusor overactivity with 15 min stimulation twice daily for 4 weeks, which is comparably a low quantity of stimulation. Still, subjective improvement in the active arm compared with inactive treatment was accomplished, as well as increase of cystometric capacity. Other reports have been contradictory, such as the one by Luber and Wolde-Tsadik[61] treating patients with genuine stress incontinence twice daily for 3 months, with no difference between active and control groups. Further attempts to determine the efficacy of various electrostimulation methods have included comparative, randomized protocols, electrical stimulation being compared to biofeedback, pelvic floor exercises, vaginal cones, and behavior training, with varying results.[62–65]

Control studies are important to determine the 'real' efficacy of varying FES modalities for different diagnoses. They are also desirable to get acceptance of the methods by health insurance authorities. In the report of the International Consultation on Incontinence, electrical stimulation was claimed to have an insufficient evidence base depending on the limited number of positive RCTs. It has to be remembered that control studies also include problems; the placebo effect in LUTS is subject to large variability, influenced by multiple factors difficult to control;[66] weaknesses and pitfalls accompany all techniques. Too much emphasis on RCTs, disregarding extensive experience presented in open studies, may lead to a shortsighted abandonment of further experimentation and development of techniques, and includes the risk that a useful and harmless option for treatment of stress incontinence and detrusor overactivity is disregarded. Designing studies of electrical stimulation also entails other risks and problems. If treatment is applied with suboptimal techique, an effect may be overlooked and researchers may be disencouraged to continue further trials.

Electrical stimulation in various neurogenic lower urinary tract dysfunctions

Established indications are ***stress urinary incontinence*** caused by pelvic floor insufficiency, the efficacy of FES being similar to that of pelvic floor exercises. It has been demonstrated that female stress incontinence depends not only on a defect of the urethral supporting structures but also on partial damage of the innervation to the pelvic floor muscle complex caused by delivery or other traumatic insults.[67] Up to 75% of patients referred for surgery of their stress incontinence may be sufficiently improved by FES so that an operation becomes unnecessary.[16,41,50] Some patients using pelvic floor exercises have defective perception and cannot recognize the relevant muscles, making training inefficient or impossible. By means of intravaginal stimulation, muscle identification may be possible, and a combined treatment may reinforce their training. In stress incontinence, long-term stimulation at 20–50 Hz is recommended.

The standard therapy of an ***overactive bladder*** is anticholinergic drug treatment, however limited in usefulness because of more or less pronounced side-effects owing to general effects on the receptor systems. FES circumvents this problem by acting directly on the micturition reflex mechanism. Urge incontinence due to detrusor overactivity (DO) is an ideal indication for electrical stimulation.[29,40,41,49,53–55] Detrusor overactivity is a typical feature of suprasacral spinal cord lesion as well as supraspinal neuropathy. There is an ongoing debate on the etiology and pathogenesis of detrusor overactivity in patients with so-called idiopathic DO. When making a thorough examination, however, subtle neurologic signs may frequently be revealed, mainly affecting the lower extremities,[68] which indicate that we are dealing with a neurogenic bladder disorder. Another feature of DO relevant for the application of electrical stimulation is that different functional subtypes may be identified. The ***uninhibited overactive bladder*** subtype[69] according to The International Continence Society's terminology standard now to be denominated ***terminal detrusor overactivity***[70] responds fairly well to maximal stimulation at 10 Hz, few other methods being useful. The results are even better in subjects with ***phasic detrusor instability***,[69,70] many of whom attain the unique re-education effect, too. In mixed incontinence, an individual assessment is mandatory. If stress urinary incontinence dominates, surgery is usually preferred, but electrical stimulation at 10–20 Hz may be contemplated as an alternative. When DO dominates, electrical stimulation is the therapy of choice, either as repeated maximal stimulation or as self-administrated home-maximal stimulation at 10 Hz.

Detrusor overactivity may be a severe symptomatic distress in spinal cord injury with ***spinal detrusor hyperreflexia***. In cases refractory to anticholinergic drugs, penile electrical stimulation has been demonstrated to reduce hyperreflexic contractions and urinary leaks.[31,32] Kirkham[71] utilized penile electrical stimulation in a physiologic study to modulate DO in a homogeneous series of subjects with spinal cord injury. Optimal inhibition of detrusor contraction required currents at least twice the pudendo-anal reflex, irrespective of pulse width, and was achieved with stimulation frequencies between 15 and 20 Hz. Repetitive stimulation resulted in increasing filling volumes before contraction with slow post-stimulation return to the baseline volume, indicating not only acute but also prolonged modulation of detrusor inhibitory mechanisms. No doubt, this option of treatment warrants further exploration in this group of patients.

In patients refractory to noninvasive procedures, other techniques are justified, e.g. perineally inserted or implanted electrodes for direct stimulation of the pudendal main nerve trunk.[26,72] Another option is percutaneous stimulation of the sacral nerves, a successful test being followed by implantation of a stimulator for chronic use. Other attempts to improve the efficacy of electrical stimulation for bladder control include conditional stimulation of, e.g., dorsal penile/clitoral nerves triggered by detrusor pressure increase in patients with spinal cord lesions.[73–76] This seems to be a promising technique, although so far not adapted to the clinical setting.

Acknowledgment

This work was supported by the Swedish Research Council (Project No K2004-73X-15058-01A) and Sahlgrenska University Hospital project number ALF Gbg-2887.

References

1. Burke RE, Levine DN, Tsairis P, Zajac FE 3rd. Physiological types and histochemical profiles in motor units of the cat gastrocnemius. J Physiol 1973; 234(3): 723–48.
2. Iggo A. Tension receptors in the stomach and the urinary bladder. J Physiol 1955; 128: 593–607.
3. Badr G, Fall M, Carlsson C-A et al. Cortical evoked potentials obtained after stimulation of the lower urinary tract. J Urol 1984; 131: 306–9.
4. Jiang C-H, Lindström S, Mazières L. Segmental inhibitory control of ascending sensory information from bladder mechanoreceptors in cat. Neurourol Urodyn 1991; 10: 286–8.
5. Barrington FJF. The relation of the hind-brain to micturition. Brain 1921; 44: 23–53.
6. Barrington FJF. The nervous mechanism of micturition. Q J Exp Physiol 1914; 8: 33–71.
7. Lindström S, Fall M, Carlsson C-A, Erlandson B-E. Rhythmic activity in pelvic afferents to the bladder: an experimental study in the cat with reference to the clinical condition 'unstable bladder'. Urol Int 1984; 39: 272–9.
8. Nakamura M, Sakurai T. Bladder inhibition by penile electrical stimulation. Br J Urol 1984; 56: 413–15.
9. Madersbacher H, Kiss G, Mair D. Transcutaneous electrostimulation of the pudendal nerve for treatment of detrusor overactivity. Neurourol Urodyn 1995; 14: 501–2.
10. Alexander S, Rowan D, Millar W, Scott R. Treatment of urinary incontinence by electric pessary. A report of 18 patients. Br J Urol 1970; 42: 184–90.
11. Fall M, Erlandson B-E, Carlsson C-A, Lindström S. The effect of intravaginal electrical stimulation of the feline urethra and urinary bladder. Neuronal mechanisms. Scand J Urol Nephrol 1978; 44(Suppl): 19.
12. Lindström S, Fall M, Carlsson C-A, Erlandson B-E. The neurophysiological basis of bladder inhibition in response to intravaginal electrical stimulation. J Urol 1983; 129: 40.
13. Trontelj TV, Janko M, Godec C et al. Electrical stimulation for urinary incontinence: a neurophysiological study. Urol Int 1974; 29: 213.
14. Teague CT, Merrill DC. Electric pelvic floor stimulation. Mechanism of action. Invest Urol 1977; 15: 65–9.
15. Glen E. Effective and safe control of incontinence by the intra-anal plug electrode. Br J Surg 1967; 54: 802.
16. Eriksen BC, Bergmann S, Mjolnerod OK. Effect of anal electrostimulation with the 'Incontan' device in women with urinary incontinence. Br J Obstet Gynaecol 1987; 94: 147–56.
17. Lindström S, Sudsuang R. Functionally specific bladder reflexes from pelvic and pudendal nerve branches: an experimental study in the cat. Neurourol Urodyn 1989; 8: 392–3.
18. Geirsson G, Fall M, Lindström S. Cystometric classification of bladder overactivity: assessment of a new system in 501 patients. Int Urogyn J 1993; 4: 186–93.
19. Blok BF, Holstege G. Two pontine micturition centers in the cat are not interconnected directly: implications for the central organisation of micturition. J Comp Neurol 1999; 403: 209–18.
20. Amarenco G, Ismael SS, Even-Schneider A et al. Urodynamic effect of acute transcutaneous posterior tibial nerve stimulation in overactive bladder. J Urol 2003; 169(6): 2210–15.
21 McGuire EJ, Zhang SC, Horwinski ER, Lytton B. Treatment of motor and sensory detrusor instability by electrical stimulation. J Urol 1983; 129(1): 78–9.
22. van Balken MR, Vandoninck V, Gisolf KW et al. Posterior tibial nerve stimulation as neuromodulative treatment of lower urinary tract dysfunction. J Urol 2001; 166(3): 914–18.
23. van Balken MR, Vandoninck V, Messelink BJ et al. Percutaneous tibial nerve stimulation as neuromodulative treatment of chronic pelvic pain. Eur Urol 2003; 43(2): 158–63.
24. van Balken MR, Vergunst H, Bemelmans BL. Prognostic factors for successful percutaneous tibial nerve stimulation. Eur Urol 2006; 49(2): 360–5.
25. Ohlsson BL. Effects of some different pulse parameters on the perception of intravaginal and intraanal electrical stimulation. Med Biol Eng Comput 1988; 26: 503–5.
26. Ohlsson BL, Fall M, Frankenberg-Sommar S. Effects of external and direct pudendal nerve maximal electrical stimulation in the treatment of the uninhibited overactive bladder. Br J Urol 1989; 64: 374–80.
27. Geirsson G, Fall M. Maximal functional electrical stimulation in routine practice. Neurourol Urodyn 1997; 16(6): 559–65.
28. Fehrling M, Fall M, Peeker R. Maximal functional electrical stimulation as a single treatment: is it cost-effective? Scand J Urol Nephrol 2007; 41(2): 132–7.
29. Fall M, Lindstrom S. Electrical stimulation. A physiologic approach to the treatment of urinary incontinence. Urol Clin North Am 1991; 18(2): 393–407.
30. Fall M, Erlandson B-E, Sundin T, Waagstein F. Intravaginal electrical stimulation. Clinical experiments on bladder inhibition. Scand J Urol Nephrol 1978; 44(Suppl): 41–7.
31. Vereecken RL, Das J, Grisar P. Electrical sphincter stimulation in the treatment of detrusor hyperreflexia of paraplegics. Neurourol Urodyn 1984; 3: 145–54.
32. Vodusek DB, Light JK, Libby JM. Detrusor inhibition induced by stimulation of pudendal nerve afferents. Neurourol Urodyn 1986; 5: 381–9.
33. Vodusek DB, Plevnik S, Vrtacnik P et al. Detrusor inhibition on selective pudendal nerve stimulation in the perineum. Neurourol Urodyn 1988; 6: 389–93.
34. Collins CD. Intermittent electrical stimulation. Urol Int 1974; 29: 221.
35. Rottembourg JL, Ghoneim MA, Fretin J, Susset JG. Study on the efficiency of electric stimulation of the pelvic floor. Invest Urol 1976; 13: 354–8.
36. Bazeed MA, Thuroff JW, Schmidt RA et al. Effect of chronic electrostimulation of the sacral roots on the striated urethral sphincter. J Urol 1982; 128: 1357–62.

37. Ridge RM, Betz WJ. The effect of selective, chronic stimulation on motor unit size in developing rat muscle. J Neurosci 1984; 4: 2614–20.
38. Caldwell KP, Cook PJ, Flack FC, James ED. Stress incontinence in females: report on 31 cases treated by electrical implant. J Obstet Gynaecol Br Common 1968; 75: 777–80.
39. Eriksen BC, Erik-Nes SH. Long-term electrostimulation of the pelvic floor: primary therapy in female stress incontinence? Urol Int 1989; 44: 90–5.
40. Fall M, Erlandson B-E, Nilson AE, Sundin T. Long-term intravaginal electrical stimulation in urge and stress incontinence. Scand J Urol Nephrol 1978; 44(Suppl): 55–63.
41. Fall M. Does electrostimulation cure urinary incontinence? J Urol 1984; 131: 664–7.
42. Janez J, Plevnik F, Korosec L et al. Changes in detrusor receptor activity after electric pelvic floor stimulation. In: Proc Int Cont Soc XIth Meeting, Lund, Sweden, 1981: 22.
43. Ishigooka M, Hashimoto T, Sasagawa I, Nakada T. Reduction in norepinephrine content of the rabbit urinary bladder by alpha-2 adrenergic antagonist after electrical pelvic floor stimulation. J Urol 1994; 151: 774–5.
44. Jiang CH. Prolonged modulation of the micturition reflex by electrical stimulation. Thesis, Linköping University Medical Dissertations No 582. Faculty of Health Sciences. Sweden: Linköping University, 1999.
45. Jiang C-H. Modulation of the micturition reflex pathway by intravesical electrical stimulation: an experimental study in the rat. Neurourol Urodyn 1998; 17: 543–53.
46. Salmons S, Vrbova G. The influence of activity on some contractile characteristics of mammalian fast and slow muscles. J Physiol 1969; 201: 535–49.
47. Schmidt RA, Kogan BA, Tanagho EA. Neuroprostheses in the management of incontinence in myelomeningocele patients. J Urol 1990; 143: 779–82.
48. Godec C, Cass AS, Ayala GF. Bladder inhibition with functional electrical stimulation. Urology 1975; 6: 663–6.
49. Plevnik S, Janez J. Maximal electrical stimulation for urinary incontinence: report of 98 cases. Urology 1979; 14: 638–45.
50. Kralj B. Treatment of female urinary incontinence by stimulators of the pelvic floor muscles. Artif Org 1981; 5(Suppl): 609–12.
51. Schulman J, Mobley J, Wolfe J et al. Battery powered BION FES network. Conf Proc IEEE Eng Med Biol Soc 2004; 6: 4283–6.
52. Groen J, Amiel C, Bosch JL. Chronic pudendal nerve neuromodulation in women with idiopathic refractory detrusor overactivity incontinence: results of a pilot study with a novel minimally invasive implantable mini-stimulator. Neurourol Urodyn 2005; 24(3): 226–30.
53. Plevnik S, Janez J, Vrtacnik P et al. Short-term electrical stimulation: home treatment for urinary incontinence. World J Urol 1986; 4: 24–6.
54. Eriksen BC, Bergmann S, Erik-Nes SH. Maximal electrostimulation of the pelvic floor in female idiopathic detrusor instability and urge incontinence. Neurourol Urodyn 1989; 8: 219.
55. Primus G, Kramer G. Maximal external electrical stimulation for treatment of neurogenic or non-neurogenic urgency and/or urge incontinence. Neurourol Urodyn 1996; 15: 187–94.
56. Shepherd AM, Blannin JP, Winder A. The English experience of intravaginal electrical stimulation in urinary incontinence a double blind trial. Proc International Continence Society's 15th Annual Meeting, London, 1985: 224–5.
57. Abel I, Ottesen B, Fischer-Rasmussen W, Lose G. Maximal electrical stimulation of the pelvic floor in the treatment of urge incontinence: a placebo controlled study. Neurourol Urodyn 1996; 15: 283–4.
58. Sand PK, Richardson DA, Staskin DR et al. Pelvic floor electrical stimulation in the treatment of genuine stress incontinence: a multicenter, placebo-controlled trial. Am J Obstet Gynecol 1995; 173: 72–9.
59. Yamanishi T, Yasuda K, Hattori T et al. Pelvic floor electrical stimulation in the treatment of stress incontinence: a placebo-controlled double-blind trial. Neurourol Urodyn 1996; 15: 397.
60. Yamanishi T, Yasuda K, Sakakibara R et al. Randomized, double-blind study of electrical stimulation for urinary incontinence due to detrusor overactivity. Urology 2000; 55: 353–7.
61. Luber KM, Wolde-Tsadik G. Efficacy of functional electrical stimulation in treating genuine stress incontinence: a randomized clinical trial. Neurourol Urodyn 1997; 16: 543–51.
62. Bo K, Talseth T, Holme I. Single blind, randomised controlled trial of pelvic floor exercises, electrical stimulation, vaginal cones, and no treatment in management of genuine stress incontinence in women. BMJ 1999; 318(7182): 487–93.
63. Goode PS, Burgio KL, Locher JL et al. Effect of behavioral training with or without pelvic floor electrical stimulation on stress incontinence in women: a randomized controlled trial. JAMA 2003; 290(3): 345–52.
64. Wang AC, Wang YY, Chen MC. Single-blind, randomized trial of pelvic floor muscle training, biofeedback-assisted pelvic floor muscle training, and electrical stimulation in the management of overactive bladder. Urology 2004; 63(1): 61–6.
65. McClurg D, Ashe RG, Marshall K, Lowe-Strong AS. Comparison of pelvic floor muscle training, electromyography biofeedback, and neuromuscular electrical stimulation for bladder dysfunction in people with multiple sclerosis: a randomized pilot study. Neurourol Urodyn 2006; 25(4): 337–48.
66. van Leeuwen JH, Castro R, Busse M, Bemelmans BL. The placebo effect in the pharmacologic treatment of patients with lower urinary tract symptoms. Eur Urol 2006; 50(3): 440–52.
67. Allen RE, Hosker GL, Smith AR, Warrell DW. Pelvic floor damage and childbirth: a neurophysiological study. Br J Obstet Gynaecol 1990; 97: 770–9.
68. Ahlberg J, Edlund C, Wikkelsö C, Rosengren L, Fall M. Neurological signs are common in patients with urodynamically verified 'idiopathic' bladder overactivity. Neurourol Urodyn 2002; 21: 65–70.
69. Fall M, Geirsson G, Lindström S. Toward a new classification of overactive bladders. Neurourol Urodyn 1995; 14: 635–46.
70. Abrams P, Cardozo L, Fall M et al. The standardisation of terminology of lower urinary tract function: report from the Standardisation Sub-committee of the International Continence Society. Neurourol Urodyn 2002; 21(2): 167–78.
71. Kirkham AP, Shah NC, Knight SL et al. The acute effects of continuous and conditional neuromodulation on the bladder in spinal cord injury. Spinal cord 2001; 39(8): 420–8.
72. Janez J, Plevnik S, Vrtacnik P. Maximal electrical stimulation in patients with lower motor neuron lesion. Proc Int Cont Soc XIIth Annual Meeting, Leiden, The Netherlands, 1982: 115–18.
73. Dalmose AL, Rijkhoff NJ, Kirkeby HJ et al. Conditional stimulation of the dorsal penile/clitoral nerve may increase cystometric capacity in patients with spinal cord injury. Neurourol Urodyn 2003; 22(2): 130–7.
74. Hansen J, Media S, Nohr M et al. Treatment of neurogenic detrusor overactivity in spinal cord injured patients by conditional electrical stimulation. J Urol 2005; 173(6): 2035–9.
75. Fjorback MV, Rijkhoff N, Petersen T, Nohr M, Sinkjaer T. Event driven electrical stimulation of the dorsal penile/clitoral nerve for management of neurogenic detrusor overactivity in multiple sclerosis. Neurourol Urodyn 2006; 25(4): 349–55.
76. Wenzel BJ, Boggs JW, Gustafson KJ, Grill WM. Closed loop electrical control of urinary continence. J Urol 2006; 175(4): 1559–63.

53

Emptying the neurogenic bladder by electrical stimulation

Graham H Creasey

Principles

Electrical stimulation has been investigated for many years for the purpose of restoring function to the neurogenic bladder, whose functions of micturition and continence may be impaired by either paralysis or hyperreflexia of the detrusor and/or sphincter mechanisms. Ideally, the functions of both emptying and storage should be restored. This would require coordinated contraction of the detrusor and relaxation of the sphincter mechanism for voiding, alternating with relaxation of the detrusor and adequate contraction of the sphincters for continence.

Electrical stimulation is usually thought of as producing muscle contraction, but there are also ways of using it to prevent contraction or produce relaxation. Reflex contraction or relaxation of muscle may be produced by stimulating sensory nerves. When stimulation is applied in this way, modifying activity in the central nervous system, it is sometimes called neuromodulation; this is discussed in other chapters in this volume. When stimulation is applied directly to efferent nerves to improve function by producing contraction of muscles it is sometimes called functional neuromuscular stimulation or functional electrical stimulation. This chapter describes such stimulation of sacral efferent nerves to produce emptying of the neurogenic bladder. This process clearly requires that efferent nerves to the bladder be intact, specifically the preganglionic parasympathetic efferents from the sacral segments of the cord which run via the sacral anterior nerve roots, sacral nerves, and pelvic plexus. It is therefore applicable to patients with lesions of the spinal cord above the sacral segments, who can now derive considerable clinical benefit from electrical stimulation to produce safe and effective bladder emptying. Restoration of continence to the neurogenic bladder by electrical stimulation is still under investigation, and chemical or surgical methods are still needed in many cases.

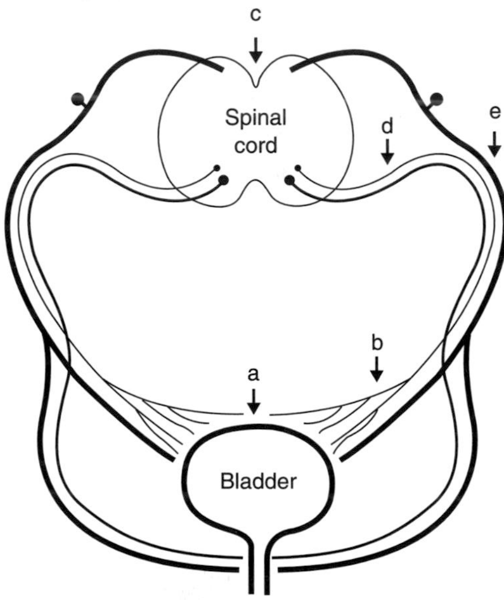

Figure 53.1
Potential sites of stimulation: (a) bladder wall; (b) pelvic nerves; (c) conus medullaris; (d) sacral anterior roots intradurally; (e) sacral nerves extradurally.

Location of stimulation

A variety of sites of stimulation have been used in patients with suprasacral spinal cord injury or disease, with electrodes on the bladder wall, the pelvic splanchnic nerves, the conus medullaris, the sacral anterior roots, or the mixed sacral nerves. In practice only the latter two sites have reached clinical significance (Figure 53.1)

Electrodes on the bladder wall produced poor results, probably for several reasons including breakage of electrodes with bladder movement, the difficulty of recruiting enough of the detrusor muscle, and the stimulation of afferents producing unwanted reflexes.[1,2] If these problems could be solved it might be useful to stimulate postganglionic parasympathetic neurons in the bladder wall for patients whose preganglionic neurons have been damaged by injuries to the sacral segments of the spinal cord or the cauda equina; such patients do not gain bladder function from electrical stimulation at present.

The pelvic splanchnic nerves appear to be a theoretically desirable site but surgical access is difficult and it may be difficult to avoid stimulating sympathetic fibers to the bladder neck and afferent fibers. Good results were claimed in a few patients but little has been published on this route.[3,4]

Stimulation of the conus medullaris was developed by Nashold et al.[5] A laminectomy from T12 to L2 was performed and a pair of electrodes inserted into the gray matter of the conus medullaris at the spinal level giving the highest bladder pressures on electrical stimulation of the dorsal surface of the conus. Nashold reported a good result in 16 of 27 patients followed for 3 to 10 years; however, the technique has not gained wide acceptance, perhaps because of the difficulty of identifying a location in the cord which could produce coordinated micturition. The availability of microelectrodes mounted on arrays of small silicon probes which can be inserted into the central nervous system may allow further research into this technique.

Stimulation of the sacral anterior roots was developed by Brindley and colleagues.[6,7] This site has the advantage that these roots do not usually contain sensory neurons, so direct activation of reflexes rarely occurs. The sacral anterior roots do, however, contain efferent neurons to both detrusor and external urethral sphincter. The lower motor neurons to the sphincter have a lower threshold for electrical activation than the parasympathetic efferent neurons to the detrusor, so it is possible to activate the sphincter without the bladder, but not usually the bladder without the sphincter. It used to be thought that attempts to produce voiding would therefore be ineffective and possibly dangerous, by causing co-contraction of detrusor and sphincter. However, Brindley made use of the fact that the smooth muscle of the detrusor contracts and relaxes much more slowly than the striated muscle of the external urethral sphincter. Stimulation in bursts of a few seconds, separated by longer gaps, builds up a sustained pressure in the bladder while allowing the external sphincter to relax rapidly between the bursts, causing urine to flow during these gaps.[8] Careful long-term clinical follow-up has shown that the brief co-contraction of the sphincter during the bursts does not cause bladder trabeculation or upper tract damage, and effective emptying of the bladder can be produced.

Sensory nerves in the end organs can nevertheless respond to muscle activity, and this may produce reflex contraction, or failure to relax, at the sphincter even during the gaps between stimulation, a condition resembling detrusor-sphincter dyssynergia, which can hinder the flow of urine in some patients.[9] Sauerwein developed the addition of posterior sacral rhizotomy to this stimulation, carrying out both procedures simultaneously at the level of the cauda equina.[10] This has the great advantage of reducing not only reflex contraction of the sphincter but also reflex contraction of the bladder, increasing bladder capacity and compliance, protecting the upper tracts from back pressure, and abolishing reflex incontinence. It also abolishes autonomic dysreflexia triggered from contraction of the bladder or lower bowel. It does, however, have other disadvantages discussed below.

If posterior sacral rhizotomy is performed, similar function can be obtained by applying bursts of stimulation to the mixed sacral nerves whose afferent connections to the cord have been divided. Electrodes and cables can thus be implanted extradurally in the sacral spinal canal. The rhizotomy is still best performed intradurally where it is easier to separate sensory from motor roots. It is easiest to separate these where they diverge to enter the conus medullaris and the sensory roots can be divided with little handling of the motor roots. The combination of extradural electrodes and intradural rhizotomy at the conus was developed by Sarrias et al and is sometimes called the Barcelona technique.[11] However, this involves a second laminectomy at the level of the conus. If there has been a previous spinal fracture or internal fixation at the thoracolumbar junction it is probably safer not to risk destabilizing the spine at this level and to carry out the rhizotomy in the cauda equina. This can be done conveniently at the lower end of the dural sac through the same laminectomy used for implanting extradural electrodes (Figure 53.2).

Methods

Surgery

General anesthesia should be carried out without anticholinergic medication, which could reduce bladder contraction, and preferably without long-acting skeletal muscle relaxants so that lower limb muscle responses can be used to assist in identifying nerves. Laminectomy is carried out according to the technique selected from Table 53.1. After opening the dura, sensory roots are distinguished from motor roots by intraoperative stimulation using hook electrodes while recording bladder pressure via a urethral catheter. Under general anesthesia sensory roots do not produce bladder contraction, though they may produce reflex contraction of the lower limbs and reflex rises in blood pressure which can be rapid. It is therefore advisable to monitor blood pressure intra-arterially. After division of posterior roots, usually S2–S5 bilaterally, electrodes are implanted on the nerves or roots that produce bladder pressure on stimulation, usually S3–4. Electrodes may also be implanted on S2, even if these roots do not produce

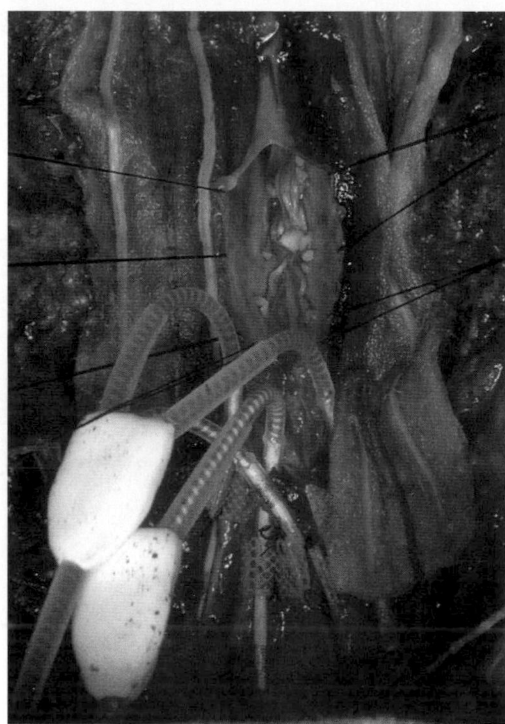

Figure 53.2
Alternative site of posterior rhizotomy with extradural electrodes. The lower end of the dural sac is shown held open with stay sutures to display the divided posterior roots; the electrodes have been attached to the sacral nerves caudal to the end of the dural sac.

bladder pressure, for the purpose of producing penile erection. The cables from the electrodes are passed subcutaneously through a cannula, usually to a temporary pocket in the flank. After repositioning the patient, they can be passed subcutaneously to the front of the body, where they are attached to a stimulator implanted in a subcutaneous pocket over the lower chest or abdomen. Detailed instructions are given in Brindley's *Notes for Surgeons and Physicians*, available from the manufacturer.[12]

Equipment

This includes implanted components, external components, and equipment used during surgery. Implantable intradural and extradural electrodes are shown in Figure 53.3. Cables from the electrodes are connected via plugs and sockets to an implantable receiver (Figure 53.4). A 3-channel receiver is typically used if S2–4 are to be stimulated individually with intradural electrodes, while a 2-channel receiver can be used if S3 and S4 are stimulated by the same channel as is often done with extradural electrodes.

The implantable components contain no batteries but are powered and controlled by radio transmission from an external controller programmed by the clinician and operated by the user. Analog and digital versions of the controller are available; their batteries can be charged weekly.

During surgery, hook electrodes connected to a battery-powered nerve stimulator are used for identification of nerves. Medical grade silicone adhesive is used to seal the connections between plugs and sockets.

The equipment is approved by the US Food and Drug Administration as a Humanitarian Use Device and in Europe is CE Marked under the requirements of the Active Implantable Medical Device Directive 90/385/EEC.

Preoperative investigation

It is essential to know that the parasympathetic efferent fibers from the sacral cord to the bladder are capable of producing bladder contraction. This may be tested by cystometry, in which it is desirable to see a reflex bladder contraction of at least 35 cm water in a woman and 50 cm water in a man.[12] Anticholinergics may need to be stopped several days before this procedure, in which case it may be necessary to prepare the patient for increased incontinence and autonomic dysreflexia. The presence of other sacral reflexes such as the anocutaneous reflex, bulbocavernosus reflex, or ankle tendon reflexes and a history of reflex erection help to confirm function of the sacral segments of the cord.

It is also desirable to confirm adequate bladder capacity and exclude severe fibrosis of the bladder wall. This can usually be determined from the patient's history, particularly when using anticholinergics, but in case of doubt can be confirmed by repeating cystometry under spinal anesthesia.

It is of course desirable to document urinary tract function thoroughly, as well as penile erection and bowel function. The appearance of the bladder neck on videocystometry

Table 53.1 *Potential sites of surgery; criteria for selecting a site are given under Discussion*

	Electrodes	Posterior rhizotomy	Laminectomies
Classical technique	Intradural	Mid cauda equina	L3–5
Barcelona technique	Extradural	Conus medullaris	S1–3 and T12–L1
Alternative technique	Extradural	Low cauda equina	S1–3

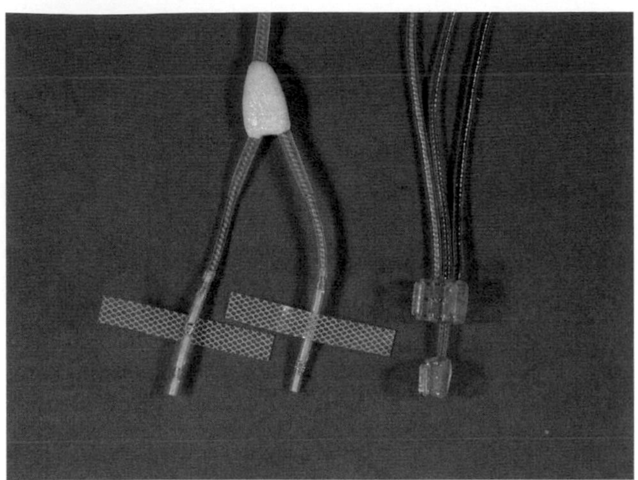

Figure 53.3
Electrodes. On the right is shown an array of intradural electrodes, with three cables corresponding to S2, S3, and S4. On the left is shown a pair of extradural electrodes, for application to left and right sacral nerves at a given segmental level, with a common lead. Three pairs of extradural electrodes may be implanted for S2–S4 but more commonly the S3 and S4 nerves are stimulated together, allowing two pairs to be used.

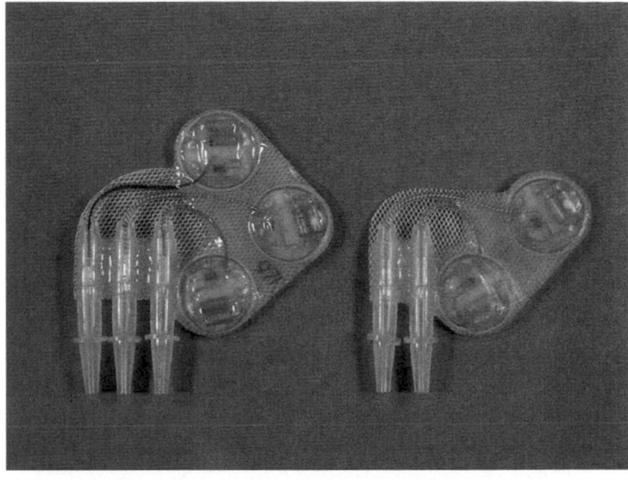

Figure 53.4
Receivers. On the left is shown a 3-channel receiver and on the right a 2-channel receiver. During implantation, cables from the electrodes are attached to the receivers using plugs and sockets located within the vertical tubular structures.

probably has prognostic value for stress incontinence, as described below.[13] Bladder diverticula are not necessarily a contraindication but may result in some persistence of urinary tract infection. Ureteric reflux or hydronephrosis is not necessarily a contraindication and may be a strong indication for posterior rhizotomy. If a subject has a suprapubic catheter it is probably preferable to revert to urethral catheterization before surgery to allow adequate closure of the stoma before generating bladder pressure with the stimulator. Prior bladder augmentation, if successful, abolishes the ability of the bladder to generate pressure and therefore renders the patient unsuitable.

Imaging of the lumbosacral spine can be used to exclude structural abnormalities. Separation of the spinal roots intradurally can be complicated by adhesions due to previous subarachnoid hemorrhage (such as from a bullet or stab wound), spinal meningitis, or myelography with an oily contrast medium,[12] and magnetic resonance imaging (particularly with gadolinium enhancement) may aid in the preoperative detection of these adhesions[14] as well as confirming the position of the conus medullaris.

Postoperative management

Extradural electrodes may be tested and brought into use on the first postoperative day. Cystometry and clinical examination should show that rhizotomy is effective; on the rare occasion that bladder reflexes persist it is easier to return to surgery and complete the rhizotomy before the wound is healed. It is wise to check residual volumes after stimulator-driven voiding for the first few days and adjust the stimulator if necessary with urodynamic monitoring of voiding pressure and flow rate. Many patients may have a high fluid output initially as a result of intravenous fluids or the habit of a high fluid intake, so it may be necessary to void frequently until this is adjusted. Overdistention of the bladder can result in poor contractility and the need to revert to catheterization until the bladder recovers.

Some surgeons prefer to postpone the use of intradural electrodes for a few days after surgery to reduce the risk of leakage of cerebrospinal fluid along the cables, but the implant should be tested within 3–4 days; reduced responses at one week, particularly of somatic muscles, may indicate nerve damage due to handling at operation. The patient can, however, be reassured that the motor responses seen in the first week are likely to return.[12]

Delay in the use of the stimulator can contribute to postoperative constipation, but thereafter regular use of the stimulator usually improves bowel function, though patients may take a few weeks to adjust to a new bowel habit. Initial follow-up by telephone is helpful and thereafter follow-up is recommended at 3 months and annually.

Results

This technique has been used in several thousand patients, primarily in Europe, where the intradural technique has been predominant, with others in North America, the Far East, New Zealand, and Australia. The device is made in England and is commercially available in over 20 countries. Reports have been published from many single-center studies,[10,13,15–22] as well as multicenter studies[23–26] and surveys.[27,28] The stimulator was the subject of conferences at Le Mans, France, in 1989,[29] Halifax, Nova Scotia, in 1992,[30] Innsbruck, Austria, in 1996 and Sydney, Australia, in 2000.

Micturition

The majority of subjects with the stimulator use it routinely for producing micturition at home 4–6 times per day. Of the 184 patients reported by van Kerrebroeck et al, 157 (85%) used the stimulator alone; a further 4 required a subsequent sphincterotomy in order to use it and a further 8 combined its use with intermittent catheterization; 7.6% did not use it for various reasons.[27] Residual volume in the bladder following implant-driven micturition was reduced in 151 patients (89% of users) to less than 30 ml, and in 95% of users to less than 60 ml. No user had a residual greater than 200 ml.

Urine infection

A substantial decrease in urinary tract infection is one of the main benefits of the technique, and has been reported by many groups following the use of the implant.[15,17,23,27,29,31] The reduction in residual volume is probably the main reason for this, together with greatly reduced use of intermittent or indwelling catheterization. As a result, antibiotic use is also greatly reduced.

Continence of urine

Reflex incontinence due to spinal reflexes is abolished by posterior sacral rhizotomy from S2–5. Some female patients have reported that incontinence can return temporarily if they have a urinary tract infection; this is probably a local reflex as a result of inflammation of the bladder wall, as it always improves following eradication of the infection.

Stress incontinence may persist following surgery in 10–15% of patients, particularly in those who have had previous sphincterotomy or bladder neck resection. MacDonagh et al reported that the state of the bladder neck on videourodynamics prior to sacral rhizotomy appeared to have a bearing on subsequent continence. All patients in their series with a closed bladder neck preoperatively became continent, except one who had had two previous sphincterotomies; another patient with previous sphincterotomy but a closed bladder neck prior to rhizotomy became continent. However, 3 out of 4 patients with an open bladder neck preoperatively had some degree of incontinence. Pre- or postoperative sphincterotomy appeared to be less of a risk to continence than bladder neck resection.[13] Of 41 early users followed up for 5–13 years, 35 reported continence day and night; of the 6 who were not continent, 4 had had previous bladder neck resections; some of these patients had not had posterior rhizotomy.[32] Stress incontinence may also occur *de novo* in a few patients; this is probably in those with an open bladder neck whose continence has been maintained preoperatively by hyper-reflexia of the external urethral sphincter; abolition of this hyper-reflexia may then result in stress incontinence.

Most paraplegic patients dispense with urine collection devices, but some tetraplegic patients wear a condom and legbag because of their limited hand function.

Urodynamics

Bladder capacity

Posterior rhizotomy dramatically increases bladder capacity by abolishing detrusor hyper-reflexia; urodynamic filling of the areflexic bladder is best limited to under 400 ml, to avoid stretching of the detrusor. MacDonagh et al showed that functional bladder capacity increased by at least 140 ml and an average of 404 ml (range 140–680 ml) in all patients who had posterior rhizotomy, an increase that was stastistically significant at the level of $p < 0.00001$.[13] Van Kerrebroeck et al, who took particular care not to overdistend the bladder postoperatively, showed in patients who had had posterior rhizotomy an average increase in cystometric capacity of 332 ml ($p < 0.001$).[33]

Bladder compliance

Since compliance is volume-dependent, it is desirable to compare it at the same volumes pre- and postoperatively; Van Kerrebroeck et al used the maximal preoperative cystometric capacity of each patient as this volume, and found that patients who had undergone posterior rhizotomy had a statistically significant increase in compliance from 8 to 53 ml/cmH_2O. The postoperative compliance at 500 ml was over 50 ml/cmH_2O in 12 of 13 patients.[33]

Detrusor pressure

Detrusor pressure can be controlled by programming the external controller, and fluctuates with bursts of stimulation. Pressures in the bladder during electrically activated micturition have been reported by several authors. Cardozo et al reported that the maximum voiding pressure was, on average, 55 cmH_2O with a range of 22–82 cmH_2O.[34] Arnold et al recorded a mean peak pressure of 88 cmH_2O and mean trough pressure of 40 cmH_2O, and concluded that this did not appear to be harmful.[15] Madersbacher et al reported a mean peak pressure of 71 cmH_2O (range 55–90 cmH_2O) and noted that post-stimulus voiding did not appear to induce detrusor hypertrophy.[17] In the first 50 patients to receive the implant, bladder trabeculation was reported to have decreased in 13 patients when followed up at 1–9 years, and no patient in this group showed evidence of increased trabeculation.[32] Van Kerrebroeck et al recorded a mean peak voiding pressure of 89 cmH_2O.[33] It is likely that voiding pressure is less significant for the upper tracts than storage pressure, which is usually reduced by posterior rhizotomy.

Upper tracts

The improvements in bladder capacity and compliance which follow posterior rhizotomy reduce the risk of upper tract damage and can result in improvement in pre-existing ureteric reflux or hydronephrosis.[10] In a multicenter review of 184 patients, reflux was present in 9 patients before the operation. After implantation it was improved or abolished in 7 of these and persisted in 2. No patient in this group developed reflux with the use of the stimulator.[27] Eight of the 184 subjects showed upper tract dilatation preoperatively. Of these, the dilatation improved in 7 and deteriorated in 1. No patient in this series developed upper tract dilatation *de novo* after implantation of the stimulator.[27]

Pain

Stimulation is never painful in patients with complete spinal cord injury and almost never in patients who undergo posterior rhizotomy. Intradural stimulation of anterior roots would usually be expected to be painless, even without rhizotomy, since these roots are usually purely motor. However, among the first 50 patients, implanted over 20 years ago, all of whom had intradural implants but not all of whom had rhizotomy, 3 were unable to use the implant because of pain on stimulation, and 4 others found use of the stimulator to some extent painful. All these patients had preserved pain sensitivity in the sacral dermatomes preoperatively.[35] It may be that current can sometimes spread from the intradural electrodes to activate nearby sensory roots, but a few patients have continued to experience pain on stimulation in spite of a thorough sacral posterior rhizotomy. This led to the belief that some anterior roots can contain sensory fibers, which has been confirmed experimentally.[36] A modified implant with a larger number of channels has been developed for use in such patients, to allow more selective stimulation of individual roots.[12] Extradural stimulation of mixed sacral nerves would be unacceptably painful if pain sensitivity was present in the sacral dermatomes and rhizotomy was not performed.

Autonomic dysreflexia

The symptoms of autonomic dysreflexia associated with contraction of the bladder or lower bowel are greatly reduced by posterior rhizotomy. Slight rises in blood pressure may occur with stimulation in rhizotomized patients, perhaps as a result of somatic muscle contraction in the sacral segments, or the presence of afferent nerves in anterior roots, but these are not sufficient to prevent use of the device.[37] If rhizotomy were not performed, extradural stimulation of mixed sacral nerves would be likely to cause significant blood pressure rises, at least in patients with cervical and upper thoracic lesions.

Nerve damage

Accidental damage to motor nerve fibers at the time of operation is less likely to occur with extradural electrodes than intradural, because of the greater surgical handling of anterior roots in the latter procedure and the lack of supporting fibrous tissue intradurally. It is dependent on surgical care and experience. It can be most sensitively detected by testing for any loss of skeletal muscle responses to the use of the stimulator during the first postoperative week, and may also become evident as a temporary loss of bladder response. It usually takes the form of neuropraxia or axonotmesis and is therefore temporary, but bladder responses may take from 2 to 6 months to return as the axons regrow, thus delaying the use of the implant for micturition.

Some patients have now been using the stimulator for 20 years or more without apparent deterioration in nerve function. The histologic appearance of stimulated nerves was reported as normal in the case of 2 patients who died (one by suicide and one from myocardial infarction) after using the implant for 3 and 5 years, respectively.[31]

Leakage of cerebrospinal fluid

Early intradural implants sometimes had leakage of cerebrospinal fluid along the cables passing through the dura. The implant has since been modified by the addition of a grommet to seal the cables to the dura, and the incidence of this complication appears to have been greatly reduced. It is rarely a problem with extradural electrodes, even though the dura may have been opened in the vicinity of the cables to perform rhizotomy.

Implant infection

Infection of the implants has been rare, particularly since a technique of coating them with antibiotics was introduced in 1982. Rushton et al reported in 1989 that one out of 104 coated implants had become infected, and in this case infection appeared to have been introduced at a subsequent operation to close a leak of cerebrospinal fluid.[38] Brindley reported a 1% infection rate for the first 500 implants.[28] The infection rate for a variety of similar implants has been shown to be significantly reduced by antibiotic coating, but not by systemic perioperative antibiotics.[38] Nevertheless, many surgeons use systemic perioperative antibiotic prophylaxis aimed at both Gram-positive and Gram-negative organisms.

If the receiver becomes infected and this is detected promptly before infection has spread along the cables, it is sometimes possible to divide the cables at a sterile location in the flank and remove the receiver, leaving the electrodes in place. If the infection has spread along the cables to the electrodes it is necessary to remove all the implanted components. In either case, vigorous treatment with antibiotics followed by a waiting period of at least 6 months is advisable before reimplanting a stimulator.

Implant reliability

The implanted components have proved to be remarkably reliable. A survey of the first 500 implants showed that faults occurred on average once every 19.2 implant-years.[39] The commonest site for faults has been in cables, which are sometimes mechanically damaged by movement. Repair or replacement of the device is usually possible, often with minor surgery, and special equipment is available from the manufacturer to facilitate repairs.[12]

Failures in the external transmitter have been more common and have primarily been due to breaks in the antenna lead, but do not require reoperation.

Penile erection

In about 60% of patients, sustained full erection sufficient for coitus can be produced by stimulation of S2, although not all of these patients use it for coitus.[23] In many of the remaining 40% of patients a partial erection is produced and this may be useful when attaching a condom for urine drainage. Some centers have reported less success with erection when using extradural electrodes; these require higher levels of stimulation to pass equivalent current through the epineurium, and some patients have had extradural electrodes implanted only on S3 and S4 nerves, but not on the S2 nerves which typically produce erection.

Bowel function

Stimulation, primarily of S3, produces contraction of the lower bowel as far proximal as the splenic flexure, reduces constipation, and increases the frequency of defecation, probably by enhancing colonic motility.[40–43] By careful adjustment of the Finetech stimulator, MacDonagh et al were able to produce defecation routinely with the stimulator alone in 6 of 12 patients, and to reduce the time spent each week in bowel emptying from 2.5 hours to half an hour.[44]

Costs

A prospective three-center study in the Netherlands collected the actual costs of hospital care, self-care, and travel expenses associated with bladder function of 52 patients before and after the procedure and through 2 years of follow-up. A model of the long-term costs indicated a break-even point of approximately 8 years, after which the procedure resulted in reduced costs.[25] In the USA a retrospective study of costs of bladder and bowel care in 12 patients using structured interviews by a life-care planner indicated a break-even point of 5 years; the lower figure may be related to a shorter length of postoperative hospitalization in the North American patients.[45]

Discussion

Selection of patients

Patients with complete spinal cord injury above the conus medullaris and inefficient reflex micturition may be considered at any time after the first few months of injury, particularly if they have complications such as frequent or chronic urine infection, reflex incontinence resistant to medication, or autonomic dysreflexia triggered by bladder or bowel.

In patients with incomplete injuries

1. it is wise to wait until 2 years after injury to allow any recovery to occur
2. it is necessary to determine whether the implant is likely to be painful

3. it is particularly important to weigh the advantages of posterior rhizotomy against any loss of function which it may cause.

Some patients with multiple sclerosis are suitable, subject to the reservations above. A few adult patients with suprasacral meningomyelocele may also be suitable, but the growth of young children might displace the electrodes if implanted in them. Betz and colleagues have investigated the use of extensible leads, and have implanted stimulators in patients as young as 14 after evaluation of their skeletal maturity.[46,47] Children with spinal cord injury have a significant risk of developing scoliosis during adolescence, so it may be worth waiting until this is unlikely, or combining implantation with spinal instrumentation if that is needed.

In assigning priorities the following generalizations may be of use:

- Patients with complete spinal cord lesions are more straightforward to investigate and treat by this technique than patients with incomplete lesions.
- Women with reflex incontinence have more to gain than men, because of the lack of satisfactory urine collecting devices for females and the fact that they have less to lose from posterior rhizotomy.
- Patients with recurrent infection have more to gain than those without. Those with persistently high reflex bladder pressures endangering renal function or with autonomic dysreflexia triggered by bladder or bowel are likely to benefit from posterior rhizotomy; this operation provides the opportunity to implant a stimulator which then provides them with a preferable alternative to intermittent catheterization.
- Men with poor or absent reflex erection have more to gain and less to lose than those whose reflex erections already suffice for coitus.
- Paraplegic men are more likely to benefit from continence, while some tetraplegic men may continue to wear a condom and legbag, at least during the day, because of difficulty in handling urine bottles and clothing.

Selection of surgical technique

Each of the techniques described above can produce excellent results in the hands of a careful surgeon who performs the operation sufficiently often to maintain skill.

The classical technique, implanting intradural electrodes and performing the rhizotomy at the level of the cauda, has the advantage of a single laminectomy. There is a slight risk of cerebrospinal fluid leakage along the cables, and if the cables later break at the site of exit through the dura they are difficult to repair at this site; extradural electrodes can be added to restore function. If the rhizotomy at the cauda later proves to be incomplete it can be revised at the conus.

The Barcelona technique, implanting extradural electrodes and performing intradural rhizotomy at the conus, has the advantage that it is easier to distinguish sensory from motor roots at the conus and little handling of the motor roots is necessary; in addition, the sacral nerves extradurally have a fibrous covering continuous with the dura and are more robust than the intradural anterior roots. It is therefore probably less likely that the motor neurons will be damaged by intraoperative handling, at least in the hands of a new operator. Extradural electrodes may be the only type possible if there is severe intradural arachnoiditis. If the rhizotomy at the conus proves to be incomplete it can be revised within a few days at the same site or later at the cauda, provided that intrathecal bleeding has not led to arachnoiditis.

The alternative technique, implanting extradural electrodes and performing rhizotomy at the lower end of the cauda, combines the advantages of a single laminectomy with those of the Barcelona technique, and avoids any risk of destabilizing the spine at the thoracolumbar junction if there has been a previous fracture or internal fixation at that level. It is slightly more difficult to identify all the posterior roots in the cauda than at the conus, so there may be a slightly higher incidence of incomplete rhizotomy.

Extradural separation of sensory and motor fibers is difficult and may damage the nerves, and is rarely performed.[48]

Detrusor-sphincter dyssynergia

Many of the complications of the neurogenic bladder are due to co-contraction of the external urethral sphincter or its failure to relax, and many forms of electrical stimulation produce contraction of the sphincter in addition to the detrusor. Several approaches to reducing sphincter contraction during electrical stimulation have been investigated. Tanagho et al used a variety of surgical procedures such as pudendal neurotomy, levatorotomy, pudendal nerve stimulation, and increasingly extensive posterior rhizotomy,[49] but effective voiding was only produced in about one-third of subjects.

Brindley and Craggs suggested the use of anodal block to prevent propagation of action potentials in the large somatic axons to the external sphincter while allowing propagation in the small parasympathetic fibers to the detrusor.[50] They demonstrated the principle experimentally and early models of the Brindley stimulator included the option of a triangular waveform for this purpose. This option was later omitted when clinical follow-up showed that post-stimulus voiding was safe and effective for voiding, at least when combined with posterior rhizotomy.

In our laboratory we showed in chronically spinalized dogs that anodal block could be used to produce contraction of the bladder with little contraction of the external urethral sphincter. However, voiding was still hindered by reflex activation of urethral muscle unless posterior rhizotomy was performed.[51,52]

High-frequency stimulation can also be applied selectively to large axons to produce either fatigue or block, while allowing smaller axons and their muscles to be activated. This has been applied by implants in chronically spinalized dogs in Montreal.[53] Although voiding pressures were not significantly different with selective stimulation, the urethral pressures were much lower and voiding was produced with low residual volumes without evidence of reflux over a 6-month period in these animals.

The role of posterior rhizotomy

Division of all the posterior roots from S2 to S5 can produce substantial benefits to a patient with a neurogenic bladder; it can also have some significant disadvantages and has therefore been a subject of some debate.

During the early 1980s sacral anterior root implants, using intradural electrodes to stimulate motor nerves, were often done without deliberate rhizotomy, though posterior roots may have been damaged accidentally in some cases.[35] Most of these patients had useful function, though some may have had persisting autonomic dysreflexia and some needed subsequent sphincterotomy.

Tanagho et al reported extradural implants on 22 patients, most of whom had other procedures to reduce outlet resistance; with increasing experience he commented that 'more extensive dorsal rhizotomy is essential to achieve good voiding'.[49]

Talalla et al placed electrodes extradurally in 7 patients without posterior rhizotomy or pudendal neurectomy and, although initial results were promising,[54] they subsequently concluded that this combination was not effective.[9]

Kirkham et al recently implanted extradural electrodes without rhizotomy in 5 patients with spinal cord injury. Reflex bladder contraction was preserved and could be inhibited by using the electrodes to stimulate only afferent neurons in the sacral nerves, but voiding was hindered in several patients, probably by reflex contraction of the sphincter.[55]

The major advantages of posterior rhizotomy are

1. A great increase in bladder compliance and capacity (except in the few cases where poor compliance is due to fibrosis), thereby protecting the upper tracts from ureteric reflux and hydronephrosis.
2. The abolition of uninhibited reflex bladder contractions, thereby reducing reflex incontinence and the need for anticholinergic medication and its side-effects.
3. The abolition of reflex contraction of the sphincter, thereby reducing detrusor-sphincter dyssynergia.
4. The abolition of autonomic dysreflexia triggered from the bladder or rectum.

The disadvantages of posterior rhizotomy include:

1. The loss of perineal sensation if present.
2. The loss of reflex erection and reflex ejaculation if present, although these are not always functional after spinal cord injury. Some patients are capable of a modified form of orgasm by stimulating the sacral dermatomes after spinal cord injury, and this too would be abolished by sacral rhizotomy. Erection is commonly produced by the implant and even more effectively by injection of papaverine or prostaglandins into the corpora cavernosa. Seminal emission can now be produced from a high proportion of spinal cord injured men by rectal probe electrostimulation, even after rhizotomy, and the procedure does not damage the implant.
3. The loss of reflex micturition and reflex defecation. The micturition produced by the implant is usually much more effective than reflex micturition, but if the implant is not used for any reason a patient will have to resort to intermittent or indwelling catheterization. Similarly, a patient with rhizotomy who uses the implant will generally become less constipated, but will be more constipated if the implant is not used.

A decision about posterior rhizotomy should therefore be made in each case. Brindley suggests the following policy:

- In women with complete lesions, who have less to lose, and much to gain from continence, complete posterior rhizotomy is usually advised.
- In men with complete lesions and without useful reflex erection or ejaculation, the same policy may be followed, but if useful reflexes or sensation are present the advantages and disadvantages of rhizotomy should be discussed more thoroughly with the patient.

The advantages of the combined procedure are such that implantation of the stimulator is now rarely performed without posterior rhizotomy, and this practice is likely to continue until a suitable alternative to surgical rhizotomy is found.

References

1. Bradley W, Timm G, Chou S. A decade of experience with electronic simulation of the micturition reflex. Urol Int 1971; 26: 283–303.
2. Halverstadt D, Parry W. Electronic stimulation of the human bladder: nine years later. J Urol 1975; 113: 341–4.

3. Burghele T. Electrostimulation of the neurogenic urinary bladder. In: Lutzmeyer Wea, ed. Urodynamics. Upper and Lower Urinary Tract. Berlin: Springer-Verlag, 1973: 319–22.
4. Kaeckenbeeck B. [Electrostimulation of the bladder in paraplegia. Method of Burghele-Ichim-Demetrescu.] Acta Urol Belg 1979; 47: 139–40.
5. Nashold BS Jr, Friedman H, Grimes J. Electrical stimulation of the conus medullaris to control the bladder in the paraplegic patient. A 10-year review. Appl Neurophysiol 1981; 44: 225–32.
6. Brindley GS. An implant to empty the bladder or close the urethra. J Neurol Neurosurg Psychiatry 1977; 40: 358–69.
7. Brindley GS, Polkey CE, Rushton DN. Sacral anterior root stimulators for bladder control in paraplegia. Paraplegia 1982; 20: 365–81.
8. Brindley GS. Emptying the bladder by stimulating sacral ventral roots. J Physiol 1974; 237: 15P–16P.
9. Talalla A, Bloom J. Sacral electrical stimulation for bladder control. In: Illis LS, ed. Functional Stimulation (Spinal Cord Dysfunction, III). Oxford: Oxford University Press, 1992: 206–18.
10. Sauerwein D. [Surgical treatment of spastic bladder paralysis in paraplegic patients. Sacral deafferentation with implantation of a sacral anterior root stimulator.] Urologe A 1990; 29: 196–203.
11. Sarrias M, Sarrias F, Borau A. The 'Barcelona' technique. Neurourol Urodyn 1993; 12: 495–6.
12. Brindley G. The Finetech–Brindley Bladder Controller: Notes for Surgeons and Physicians. Welwyn Garden City, Herts AL7 1AU, England: Finetech Medical Ltd, 1998.
13. MacDonagh RP, Forster DMC, Thomas DG. Urinary continence in spinal injury patients following complete sacral posterior rhizotomy. Br J Urol 1990; 66: 618–22.
14. Delamarter RB, Ross JS, Masaryk TJ, Modic MT, Bohlman HH. Diagnosis of lumbar arachnoiditis by magnetic resonance imaging. Spine 1990; 15: 304–10.
15. Arnold E, Gowland S, MacFarlane M, Bean A, Utley W. Sacral anterior root stimulation of the bladder in paraplegics. Aust NZJ Surg 1986; 56: 319–24.
16. Herlant M, Colombel P. Electrostimulation intra-durale des racines sacrees anterieures chez les paraplegiques. Historique, resultats, indications. Annales de Réadaptation et de Médecine physique 1986; 29: 405–11.
17. Madersbacher H, Fischer J, Ebner A. Anterior sacral root stimulator (Brindley): experiences especially in women with neurogenic urinary incontinence. Neurourol Urodyn 1988; 7: 593–601.
18. Robinson L, Grant A, Weston P et al. Experience with the Brindley anterior sacral root stimulator. Br J Urol 1988; 62: 553–7.
19. Nordling J, Hald T, Kristensen JK, Schmidt K, Gjerris F. [An implantable radio-controlled sacral nerve root stimulator for control of urination.] Ugeskr Laeger 1988; 150: 978–80.
20. Borau A, Vidal J, Sarrias F et al. Electro-estimulación de las raices sacras anteriores para el control esfinteriano en el lesionado medular. Médula Espinal 1995; 1: 128–33.
21. Schurch B, rodic B, Jeanmonod D. Posterior sacral rhizotomy and intradural anterior sacral root stimulation for treatment of the spastic bladder in spinal cord injured patients. J Urol 1997; 157: 610–14.
22. van der Aa HE, Alleman E, Nene A, Snoek G. Sacral anterior root stimulation for bladder control: clinical results. Arch Physiol Biochem 1999; 107: 248–56.
23. Egon G, Barat M, Colombel P et al. Implantation of anterior sacral root stimulators combined with posterior sacral rhizotomy in spinal injury patients. World J Urol 1998; 16: 342–9.
24. Van Kerrebroeck PEV, van der Aa HE, Bosch JLHR et al. Sacral rhizotomies and electrical bladder stimulation in spinal cord injury: clinical and urodynamic analysis. Eur Urol 1997; 31: 263–71.
25. Wielink G, Essink-Bot ML, Van Kerrebroeck PEV, Rutten FFH. Sacral rhizotomies and electrical bladder stimulation in spinal cord injury: cost-effectiveness and quality of life analysis. Eur Urol 1997; 31: 441–6.
26. Creasey G, Grill J, Korsten M et al. An implantable neuroprosthesis for restoring bladder and bowel control to patients with spinal cord injuries: a multi-center trial. Arch Phys Med Rehab 2001; 82: 1512–19.
27. Van Kerrebroeck P, Koldewijn E, Debruyne F. Worldwide experience with the Finetech–Brindley sacral anterior root stimulator. Neurourol Urodyn 1993; 12: 497–503.
28. Brindley GS. The first 500 patients with sacral anterior root stimulator implants: general description. Paraplegia 1994; 32: 795–805.
29. Colombel P, Egon G. [Electrostimulation of the anterior sacral nerve roots. An International Congress – Le Mans – 24–25 November 1989.] Ann Urol Paris 1991; 25: 48–52.
30. Brindley GS. History of the sacral anterior root stimulator, 1969–1982. Neurourol Urodyn 1993; 12: 481–3.
31. Brindley GS, Rushton DN. Long-term follow-up of patients with sacral anterior root stimulator implants. Paraplegia 1990; 28: 469–75.
32. Brindley GS. Sacral anterior root stimulators for bladder control in paraplegia: the first 50 cases. J Neurol Neurosurg Psychiatr 1986; 49: 1104–14.
33. Van Kerrebroeck P, Koldewijn E, Wijkstra H, Debruyne F. Urodynamic evaluation before and after intradural posterior rhizotomies and implantation of the Finetech–Brindley anterior sacral root stimulator. Urodinamica 1992; 1: 7–16.
34. Cardozo L, Krishnan KR, Polkey CE, Rushton DN, Brindley GS. Urodynamic observations on patients with sacral anterior root stimulators. Paraplegia 1984; 22: 201–9.
35. Brindley G, Polkey C, Rushton D, Cardozo L. Sacral anterior root stimulators for bladder control in paraplegia: the first 50 cases. J Neurol Neurosurg Psychiatr 1986; 49: 1104–14.
36. Schalow G. Efferent and afferent fibres in human sacral ventral nerve roots: basic research and clinical implications. Electromyogr Clin Neurophysiol 1989; 29: 33–53.
37. Schurch B, Knapp PA, Jeanmonod D, Rodic B, Rossier AB. Does sacral posterior rhizotomy suppress autonomic hyper-reflexia in patients with spinal cord injury? Br J Urol 1998; 81: 73–82.
38. Rushton DN, Brindley GS, Polkey CE, Browning GV. Implant infections and antibiotic-impregnated silicone rubber coating. J Neurol Neurosurg Psychiatry 1989; 52: 223–9.
39. Brindley GS. The first 500 sacral anterior root stimulators: implant failures and their repair. Paraplegia 1995; 33: 5–9.
40. Varma JS, Binnie N, Smith AN, Creasey GH, Edmond P. Differential effects of sacral anterior root stimulation on anal sphincter and colorectal motility in spinally injured man. Br J Surg 1986; 73. 478–82.
41. Binnie N, Smith A, Creasey G, Edmond P. Motility effects of electrical anterior sacral nerve root stimulation of the parasympathetic supply of the left colon and anorectum in paraplegic subjects. J Gastrointest Mot 1990; 2: 12–17.
42. Binnie N, Smith A, Creasey G, Edmond P. The effects of electrical anterior sacral nerve root stimulation on pelvic floor function in paraplegic subjects. J Gastrointest Mot 1991; 3: 39–45.
43. Binnie NR, Smith AN, Creasey GH, Edmond P. Constipation associated with chronic spinal cord injury: the effect of pelvic parasympathetic stimulation by the Brindley stimulator. Paraplegia 1991; 29: 463–9.
44. MacDonagh RP, Sun WM, Smallwood R, Forster D, Read NW. Control of defecation in patients with spinal injuries by stimulation of sacral anterior nerve roots. B Med J 1990; 300: 1494–7.
45. Creasey G, Dahlberg J. Economic consequences of an implanted neural prosthesis for bladder and bowel management. Arch Phys Med Rehab 2001; 82: 1520–5.
46. Akers JM, Smith BT, Betz RR. Implantable electrode lead in a growing limb. IEEE Trans Rehab Eng 1999; 7: 35–45.
47. Merenda LA, Spoltore TA, Betz RR. Progressive treatment options for children with spinal cord injury. SCI Nurs 2000; 17: 102–9.
48. Sauerwein D, Ingunza W, Fischer J et al. Extradural implantation of sacral anterior root stimulators. J Neurol Neurosurg Psychiatry 1990; 50: 681–4.
49. Tanagho EA, Schmidt RA, Orvis BR. Neural stimulation for control of voiding dysfunction: a preliminary report in 22 patients with serious neuropathic voiding disorders. J Urol 1989; 142: 340–5.

50. Brindley GS, Craggs MD. A technique for anodally blocking large nerve fibres through chronically implanted electrodes. J Neurol Neurosurg Psychiatry 1980; 43: 1083–90.
51. Grunewald V, Bhadra N, Creasey GH, Mortimer JT. Functional conditions of micturition induced by selective sacral anterior root stimulation: experimental results in a canine animal model. World J Urol 1998; 16: 329–36.
52. Bhadra N, Grunewald V, Creasey G, Mortimer JT. Selective suppression of sphincter activation during sacral anterior nerve root stimulation. Neurourol Urodyn 2002; 21: 55–64.
53. Abdel-Gawad M, Boyer S, Sawan M, Elhilali MM. Reduction of bladder outlet resistance by selective stimulation of the ventral sacral root using high frequency blockade: a chronic study in spinal cord transected dogs. J Urol 2001; 166: 728–33.
54. Talalla A, Bloom JW, Nguyen Q. Successful intraspinal extradural sacral nerve stimulation for bladder emptying in a victim of traumatic spinal cord transection. Neurosurgery 1986; 19: 955–61.
55. Kirkham AP, Knight SL, Craggs MD, Casey AT, Shah PJ. Neuromodulation through sacral nerve roots 2 to 4 with a Finetech–Brindley sacral posterior and anterior root stimulator. Spinal Cord 2002; 40: 272–81.

54

Central neuromodulation

Philip EV Van Kerrebroeck

Introduction

A multitude of neurological disorders can affect the bladder and although the incidence of lower urinary tract dysfunction is different among the various neurological entities, an important percentage of patients develop voiding dysfunction.[1] Incontinence and poor evacuation of urine with residual urine and recurrent urinary tract infections can cause important morbidity. In patients with spinal cord injury the lack of ability to control the storing and evacuation function of the bladder is one of the most prominent aspects of their handicap.

Besides these bladder problems with a proven neurological basis, a vast group of patients suffers from lower urinary tract dysfunction without an evident neurological cause. These are patients with different forms of so-called idiopathic dysfunctional voiding.

Therapeutic modalities are pharmacological treatment, eventually in combination with clean intermittent catheterization. Lifelong continuation of this therapy, however, is a major issue mainly because of side-effects. Furthermore, in most patients, especially in females, incontinence remains a problem even with maximal pharmacological treatment. The failure of pharmacological manipulation has led to the development of surgical approaches such as augmentation cystoplasty, sphincteric incisions, and artificial sphincter implantation. However, a considerable number of patients with neurogenic bladder dysfunction continue to have significant urological problems although maximal classical therapy is applied. Therefore the use of electrical stimulation to control storage and evacuation of urine has become an important tool in the urological treatment of voiding dysfunction.

The aim of electrical stimulation for voiding dysfunction is to treat incontinence due to a lack of activity in the striated muscles of the urethral closure mechanism by improvement of the contraction of the sphincter mechanism or to overcome incontinence due to detrusor hyperactivity by reduction of detrusor contractions. Furthermore, electrical stimulation can be used to permit evacuation of a paraplegic bladder by provocation of detrusor contractions or to control micturition in the hyperreflex bladder by a combination of dampening of spontaneous reflex excitability and controlled activation of the detrusor.

These aims can be fulfilled by stimulation of the efferent nerves to the lower urinary tract or by modulation of reflex activity as a consequence of stimulation of afferent nerves. Different modalities to apply electrical current to the lower urinary tract are available. Surface electrodes can be used as nonimplantable devices.[2] Insertable plugs in the anal canal or the vagina are applied to treat incontinence.[3–5] Intravesical electrostimulation is performed in children with meningomyelocele.[6–8] Implantable prostheses are available to induce bladder contraction in order to evacuate urine in paraplegic bladders or to control detrusor contraction in hyperreflexic bladders.[9–11] Another type of prosthesis permits the modulation of symptomatic voiding dysfunction such as urge incontinence, urgency/frequency syndrome, and retention.[12,13]

Electrical stimulation for chronic lower urinary tract dysfunction

Chronic lower urinary tract dysfunction, such as urge incontinence, urgency/frequency syndrome, and bladder evacuation problems, presents a challenge. Most patients are initially treated conservatively with bladder retraining, pelvic floor exercises, and biofeedback. In the majority, this regimen will be supplemented with drugs. However, about 40% of patients with these forms of lower urinary tract dysfunction do not achieve an acceptable condition with these forms of treatment and remain a therapeutic problem. Alternative procedures with variable success rates such as bladder transection, transvesical phenol injection of the pelvic plexus, augmentation cystoplasty, and even urinary diversion are being advocated.

During recent decades, functional electrical stimulation has gained interest in the treatment of this type of lower urinary tract dysfunction. Different stimulation sites, such as the vagina or the anus, have been reported to be successful. Since the 1960s, transcutaneous neurostimulation applied to the third or fourth sacral foramen has been tried as a method of controlling functional lower urinary tract disorders.[14] Unilateral sacral segmental stimulation with a permanent electrode at the level of the sacral foramen S3 or S4 (sacral neuromodulation) can offer an alternative nondestructive mode of treatment for patients presenting with voiding dysfunction and chronic pelvic pain refractory to conservative measures. Since 1981 a clinical trial has been underway to evaluate the effectiveness of this method. Since that time, experience has been gathered in the evaluation, surgery, and follow-up of patients presenting with voiding dysfunction and pelvic pain who have been treated with sacral foramen electrode implants.[15] The goal of such treatment is to relieve the symptoms by rebalancing micturition control.

The mode of action of this so-called sacral neuromodulation is still unclear but it has been hypothesized that the electrical current modulates reflex pathways involved in the filling and evacuation phase of the micturition cycle.[16] Stimulation of Aδ myelinated fibers of the sacral roots S3 and S4 decreases the spastic behavior of the pelvic floor and enhances the tone of the urethral sphincter. The threshold for the somatic component of the spinal nerve that innervates the pelvic floor is lower than that for the autonomic component to the bladder. Therefore, simultaneous bladder contraction is avoided during stimulation. In many subjects the primary voiding dysfunction appears to begin with unstable urethral activity, which activates the voiding reflexes, leading to detrusor instability and the associated urgency, frequency, and incontinence. The inhibitory effect of the enhanced urethral sphincter tone suppresses detrusor instability and stabilizes detrusor activity.

Ideal candidates for neuromodulation are patients presenting with urge incontinence, urinary urgency/frequency, and evacuation problems. Patients who have failed numerous other therapies should not be excluded from neuromodulation as they often show an excellent response to this technique.

Sacral neuromodulation is planned as a long-term treatment, but patients are first tested by means of a temporary trial stimulation for 3–7 days. This trial stimulation consists of two steps. The first phase is the acute testing, followed by the so-called subchronic phase. During an outpatient procedure and under local anesthesia, one of the sacral foramina, preferably the third one, is punctured with a 20-gauge hollow needle. The proximal and distal tip of the needle is not isolated and allows electrical stimulation.

Typical responses to stimulation of each nerve level are seen at both the local (perineum) and distant (foot and toe) sites. S3 stimulation produces a contraction of the levator muscles (bellows-like contraction) as well as detrusor and urethral sphincter contraction. Signs of S3 stimulation in the lower extremities include plantar flexion of the great toe. Subjectively, patients report a pulling sensation in the rectum during S3 stimulation, with variable sensations being perceived in the scrotum and the tip of the penis by men or the labia and vagina in women. S4 stimulation results in a contraction of the levator ani muscle (bellows-like contraction), with no activity being noted in the foot or leg. The sacral root at either site with the best clinical (subjective) or urodynamic response is selected and the intensity of the current adapted to the sensation of stimulation.

Through the needle a temporary electrode is placed and the needle is removed. This electrode remains in the vicinity of the sacral root selected and passes through the sacral foramen, subcutaneous tissue, and the skin. When the acute motoric responses with stimulation are confirmed, the electrode is connected to an external stimulator. Then starts the subchronic phase of the trial stimulation. Patients will check the effect for 3–7 days based on voiding diaries. Urodynamic examination is a possible other control of the effect.

Patients with a good clinical and preferably urodynamic result can be candidates for a permanent implant. This implant consists of a surgically implanted electrode with four contact points (Pisces quad lead Model 3886, Medtronic Inc., Minneapolis, Minnesota, USA) connected to a pacemaker (Interstim stimulator, Medtronic Interstim, Tolchenau, Switzerland).

Implantation is performed under general anesthesia. After a midline incision over the sacrum, the fascia overlying the foramina at one side of the sacrum is opened, giving access to the foramen selected. Acute stimulation with a needle will be repeated in order to confirm the motoric responses. The permanent electrode is positioned in the foramen with the four contact points in the neighborhood of the sacral nerve. The electrode is fixed to the posterior wall of the sacral with nonresorbable sutures and passed subcutaneously to an incision in one of the flanks. After closure of the wounds, the patient is placed in a lateral position. A subcutaneous pocket is created lateral of the umbilicus. The flank wound is opened and the electrode is connected with the pulse generator using a connection cable that is passed subcutaneously to an abdominal pocket. The pacemaker is fixed to the rectus fascia. Recently an alternative technique has been presented in which a gluteal pocket is created to receive the pulse generator. This method has the advantage that the surgery can be performed in one position. Furthermore, morbidity, especially pain at the implant side, seems to be reduced.

Generally, low amplitudes (1.5 to 5.5 V, 210 μs pulse duration at 10 to 15 cycles/s) are sufficient for stimulation of the somatic nerve fibers. With these parameters, no dyssynergia of the bladder and striated urethral musculature is induced even when voiding is initiated with the stimulator on.

Previous reports indicate an overall success rate of 60–75% at initial trial stimulation.[15] Of the patients selected after subchronic trial stimulation who underwent permanent implantation, up to 83% have derived major benefit from the definitive procedure.[17] This effect appears to be durable, as evidenced by the late results. However, about 20% of patients who respond well on trial stimulation fail to reproduce the same result after chronic stimulation. Based on clinical parameters it appears that patients with detrusor overactivity and urethral instability have the best result.[18]

The results of a multinational, multicenter clinical trial of this method have been presented.[19] In a group of 155 patients with therapy-resistant urge incontinence, 98 (63%) reacted sufficiently on the temporary trial stimulation. Of these, 38 were followed for 1 year with a successful outcome in 30 (79%).

Similar multicenter, multinational studies in patients with urgency/frequency and chronic voiding problems have been published with similar results.[20,21] Also, with long-term follow-up, results seem to be persistent over time.[22] However after permanent implantation about 20% of patients with initially favorable PNE test results fail to respond for yet unknown reasons. Further research to indicate additional parameters that may be used as reliable predictors of success is necessary.

Neuromodulation seems to be an effective treatment modality in patients with various forms of lower urinary tract dysfunction. This technique is a valuable addition to our treatment options when conservative measures fail.

References

1. Wein AJ, Raezer DM, Benson GS. Management of neurogenic bladder dysfunction in the adult. Urology 1976; 8: 432–43.
2. Bradley WE, Timm GW, Chou SN. A decade of experience with electronic stimulation of the micturition reflex. Urol Int 1971; 26: 283–302.
3. Godec C, Cass AS, Ayala GF. Electrical stimulation for incontinence. Technique, selection and results. Urology 1976; 7: 388–97.
4. Merrill DC. The treatment of detrusor incontinence by electrical stimulation. J Urol 1979; 122: 515–17.
5. Fall M. Does electrostimulation cure urinary incontinence? J Urol 1984; 131: 664–7.
6. Katona F. Stages of vegetative afferentiation in reorganization of bladder control during intravesical electrotherapy. Urol Int 1975; 30: 192–203.
7. Seiferth J, Heising J, Larkamp H. Experiences and critical comments on the temporary intravesical electrostimulation of neurogenic bladder in spina bifida children. Urol Int 1978; 33: 279–84.
8. Madersbacher H, Pauer W, Reiner E. Rehabilitation of micturition by transurethral electrostimulation of the bladder in patients with incomplete spinal cord lesions. Paraplegia 1982; 20: 191–5.
9. Caldwell KP, Flack FC, Broad AF. Urinary incontinence following spinal injury treated by electronic implant. Lancet 1965; 39: 846–7.
10. Brindley GS, Polkey CE, Rushton DN, Cardozo L. Sacral anterior root stimulators for bladder control in paraplegia: the first 50 cases. J Neurol Neurosurg Psychiatry 1986; 49: 1104–14.
11. Tanagho EA, Schmidt RA, Orvis BR. Neural stimulation for control of voiding dysfunction: a preliminary report in 22 patients with serious neuropathic voiding disorders. J Urol 1989; 142: 340–5.
12. Markland C, Merrill D, Chou S, Bradley W. Sacral nerve root stimulation: a clinical test of detrusor innervation. J Urol 1972; 107: 772–6.
13. Schmidt RA. Advances in genitourinary neurostimulation. Neurosurgery 1986; 18: 1041–4.
14. Habib HN. Experiences and recent contributions in sacral nerve stimulation for both human and animal. Br J Urol 1967; 39: 73–83.
15. Schmidt RA. Applications of neurostimulation in urology. Neurourol Urodyn 1988; 7: 585.
16. Thon WF, Baskin LS, Jonas U et al. Neuromodulation of voiding dysfunction and pelvic pain. World J Urol 1991; 9: 38.
17. Bosch JLHR, Groen J. Sacral (S3) segmental nerve stimulation as a treatment for urge incontinence in patients with detrusor instability: results of chronic electrical stimulation using an implantable neural prosthesis. J Urol 1995; 154: 504–7.
18. Koldewijn EL, Rosier PF, Meuleman EJ et al. Predictors of success with neuromodulation in lower urinary tract dysfunction: results of trial stimulation in 100 patients. J Urol 1994; 152: 2071–5.
19. Janknegt RA, Van Kerrebroeck PhEV, Lycklama à Nijeholt AA et al. Sacral nervemodulation for urge incontinence: a multinational, multicenter randomized study. J Urol 1997; 157(4): 1237.
20. Hassouna MM, Siegel SW, Nyeholt AA et al. Sacral neuromodulation in the treatment of urgency-frequency symptoms: a multicenter study on efficacy and safety. J Urol 2000; 163(6): 1849–54.
21. Jonas U, Fowler CJ, Chancellor MB et al. Efficacy of sacral nerve stimulation for urinary retention: results 18 months after implantation. J Urol 2001; 165: 15–19.
22. Bosch JL, Groen J. Sacral nerve neuromodulation in the treatment of patients with refractory motor urge incontinence: long-term results of a prospective longitudinal study. J Urol 2000; 163(4): 1219–22.

55

Intravesical electrical stimulation of the bladder

Helmut G Madersbacher, Ferenc Katona, and Marianne Berényi

Background

Already in 1887 the Danish surgeon Saxtorph et al[1] described intravesical electrical stimulation (IVES) for the atonic bladder by inserting a transurethral catheter with a metal stylet in it and with a neutral electrode on the lower abdomen. In 1899 two Viennese surgeons, Frankl-Hochwart and Zuckerkandl,[2] stated that intravesical electrotherapy was more effective in inducing detrusor contractions than external faradization.

Intravesical electrotherapy with various types of direct electric current was started and practiced from 1957 in Budapest, Hungary, by Katona.[3] It was used in adults to treat neurogenic bladder and rectum following spinal cord injury, operation for spinal tumor, herniated disc, kyphosis, and paralytic states of the gastrointestinal tract, as well as myelomeningocele (MMC) in children.[4–8] Electroencephalography (EEG) studies revealed that intravesical electric stimulation of the bladder activated the urge to void simultaneously with vegetative orientation.[9] This was demonstrated in animal experiments. Clinical observations revealed that selected control stimuli with cooled saline evoked no bladder contractions, and no urge to void. On the other hand, local anesthesia of the bladder abolished the effect of stimulation.[10]

Smooth and striated muscles with a network-like nervous system first appeared in the Cambrian period in the protomedusae and other primitive crinoid coelenterates. Currently 9000 species belong to the Crinoidea phylum. Medusae accumulate seawater under their umbrella, which is formed by smooth muscle cells with cross-striped muscle cells at the periphery. Medusae achieve rapid motion by expelling stored seawater. Thus, accumulation of fluid and its evacuation in a spray directed by a local network of nerve cells is a very old function. Katona[11] demonstrated, in *in-vivo* experiments, that Cnidaria responds to drugs and electrical stimulation in a very similar way to the bladder. Electrical stimulation with direct interrupted quadrangular or exponential current changed tentacle movements in Hydra or umbrella activity in Medusae. The addition of lidocaine (lignocaine) to sea water abolished all actions of the electric current.

Ebner et al[12] demonstrated in cat experiments that intravesical electrostimulation (IVES) activates the mechanoreceptors within the bladder wall. Further basic research was undertaken by Jiang et al,[13] who demonstrated that IVES at low frequencies (20 Hz) had a better modulatory effect than at higher frequencies. Jiang[14] proved, in animal experiments, that IVES induced modulation of the micturition reflex due to an enhanced excitatory synaptic transmission in the central micturition reflex pathway. The observed modulation may account for the clinical benefit of IVES treatment.

The afferent stimuli induced by IVES travel along afferent pathways from the lower urinary tract to the corresponding cerebral structures. This 'vegetative afferention' results in the sensation of bladder filling/urge to void, with subsequent enhancement of active contractions and possibly also voluntary control over the detrusor (Figure 55.1).

Colombo et al[15] demonstrated that intravesical electrostimulation also induces electrical changes on higher micturition centers, measured by EEG. The evaluation of viscerosensory cortical evoked potentials after transurethral electrical stimulation has been proved to be useful in determining whether a patient is suitable for IVES or not.[16]

Technique

It is essential to emphasize that IVES can be equally applied to diagnostic and therapeutic purposes.

The technique involves a catheter, with a stimulation electrode (cathode) in it, being introduced intro the bladder and connected to a stimulator. Saline (0.9%) is used as the current leading medium within the bladder. The anode (neutral) electrode (14 × 9 cm) is attached to the skin in an area with preserved sensation, usually in the lower abdomen or the arm (Figure 55.2). According to Ebner et al,[12] the following stimulation parameters have proved to be most effective in the animal experiment: pulse width, 2 ms; frequency, 20 Hz; and current, 1–10 mA (Figure 55.3). Some researches use square unipolar pulses for continuous

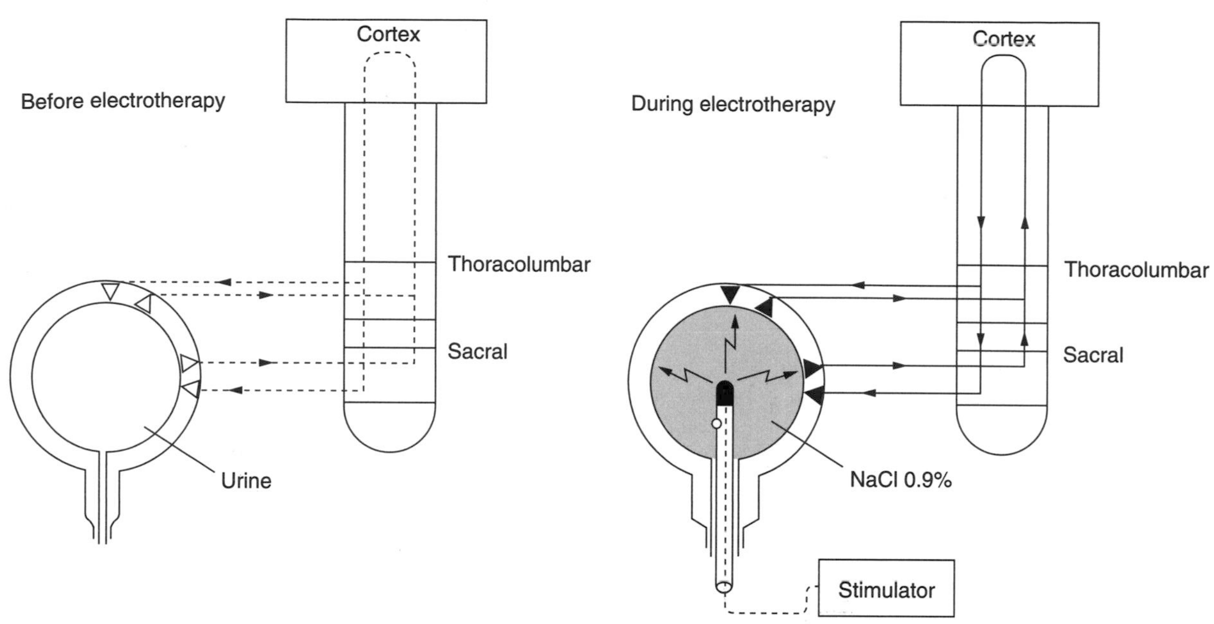

Figure 55.1
Intravesical electrostimulation activates the mechanoreceptors within the bladder wall, thus increasing the efferent input from the bladder and consequently the efferent output to the bladder. (Reproduced with permission from Ebner et al.[4])

stimulation,[17] whereas others use intermittent stimulation with bursts and gaps that can be varied (1–10 s) along with the rise time and the time of the plateau within the burst. With intermittent electrostimulation, each therapy session takes 60–90 min, on a daily basis, 5 days a week, until the maximum response is reached. For patients who have never experienced the urge to void – e.g. children with myelomeningocele or children who have lost this ability – IVES is combined with a biofeedback training: on a water manometer attached to the system the patient is able to observe the change in the detrusor pressure (Figure 55.4). This way he is able to realize that the sensation experienced is caused by a bladder contraction. This external feedback also facilitates achievement of voluntary control.

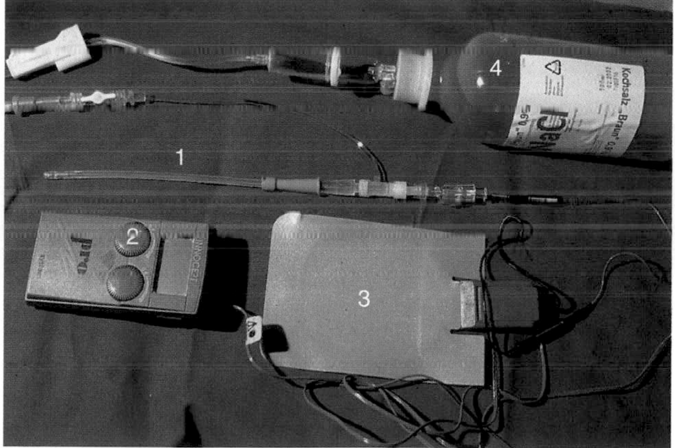

Figure 55.2
IVES armamentarium: 1, Disposable catheter with the electrode in it; 2, battery-operated stimulator; 3, neutral electrode; 4, saline (0.9%).

Results

The results presented are based on 41 studies: nine are basic research papers (animal experiments and clinical research), one is a randomized controlled trial, there are two reviews with an editorial, one pro and one contra IVES, and the others are case series.

IVES of the bladder is still a controversial therapy for patients with neurogenic detrusor dysfunction, although basic research during the last decade has evidenced the mechanism of its action and its efficacy.[12,16] At least, in animal experiments, optimal parameters have been determined.[12,18]

The controversy about the value of IVES for detrusor rehabilitation is also reflected in an editorial, in which Kaplan[19] reported favorable results in 288 children who received at least one series (20 outpatient sessions, 90 min long): 87% of patients had control and voided or catheterized with sensations or had improved bladder compliance. Eighteen percent had gained full control, they voided

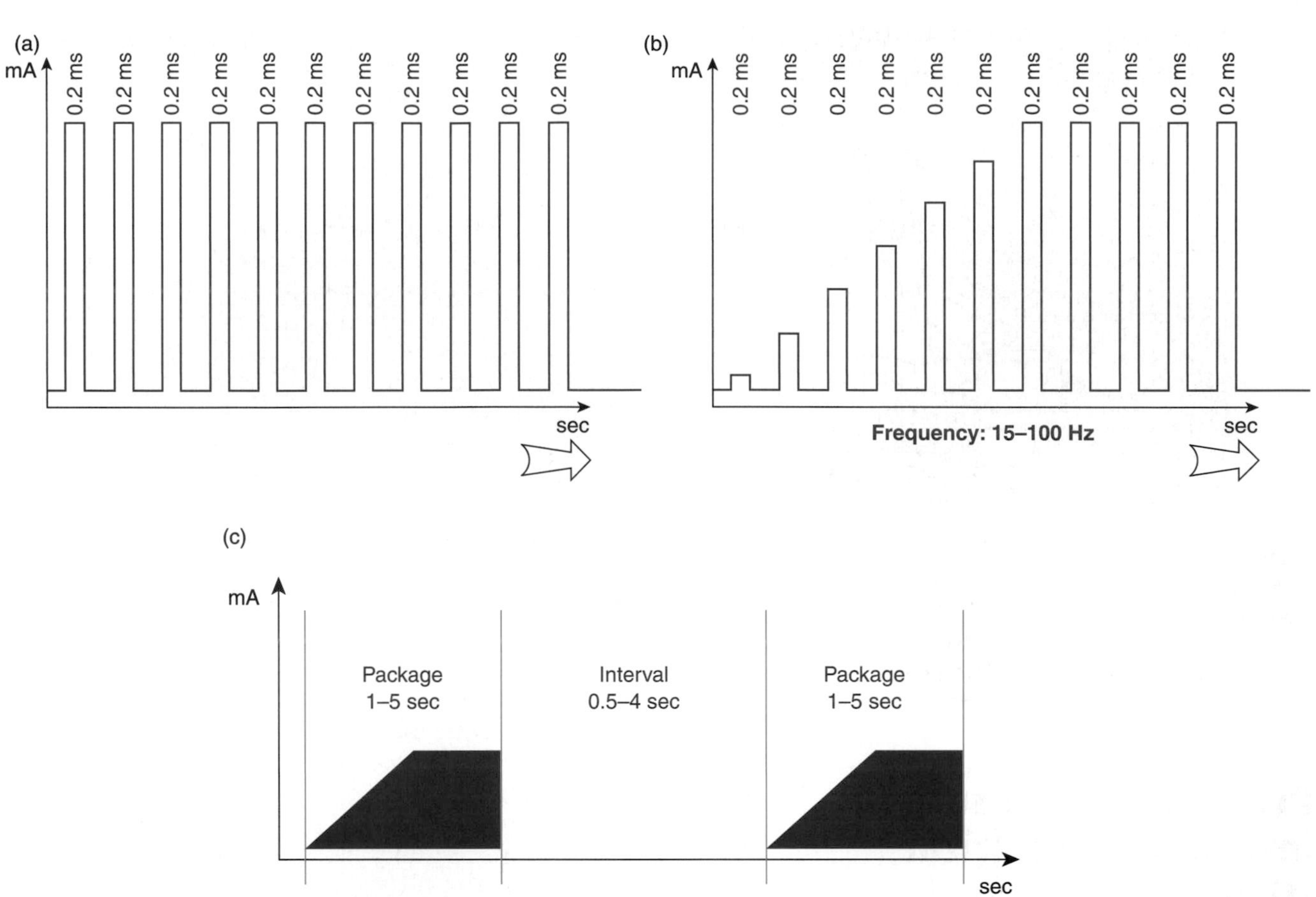

Figure 55.3
The applied electric parameters: the widths of individual rectangular currents (left side), the composition of exponential trains (right side), and the composition of packages with changeable intervals (below).

synergistically and were continent, whereas before they were either voiding poorly and incontinent or used clean intermittent catheterization and were more or less dry. Forty-four percent voided with sensation and were in biofeedback to try and gain control. Finally, in 13% the treatment failed, but the patients maintained their condition. Moreover, the results seen in an 'early' group were followed up 10 years later. As long as no intervening neurosurgical insult occurred, less than 3% of cases needed to return for a tune-up to maintain their 'healthy bladder'. The average number of daily sessions to achieve these results was 47. According to Katona,[8] from 1958 to 1991 in adults and MMC children better results were published, with an average of 80 sessions in 802 patients (Table 55.1).

In contrast, the results reported by Decter[20] were less favorable. In 25 patients during a 5-year period with, all together, 938 sessions of stimulation, bladder capacity increased greater than 20% with regard to the age-adjusted and end-filling bladder pressure and showed clinically significant decreases in 28% of patients. In response to a questionnaire, 56% of parents noted a subjective improvement in their children's bladder functions. However, the urodynamic improvements achieved after IVES did not significantly alter the daily voiding routine in these children.[21]

The only randomized controlled prospective clinical trial[22] could not find differences between active and sham treatment; however, only 15 sessions were performed at first and another 15 sessions of IVES were applied after a 3-month hiatus. Moreover, the inclusion criteria were not defined.

Other studies are either individual case-controlled studies (*Level of evidence 3B*) or case series (*Level of evidence 4*). They cannot be compared due to different or non-defined inclusion criteria, different technique details (different time of electrostimulation, varying follow-ups), and because some had only a small number of patients included.[23–39] Gladh[17] presented the results of 44 children (mean age 10.5 years), 20 of them with neurogenic bladder dysfunction: with a mean follow-up of 2.5 years, 64% had their bladder emptying normalized, 11 of 15 children on clean intermittent catheterization (CIC) had terminated catheterization, 8 of them with neurogenic bladder dysfunction, 7 children had no remaining benefit of the treatment.

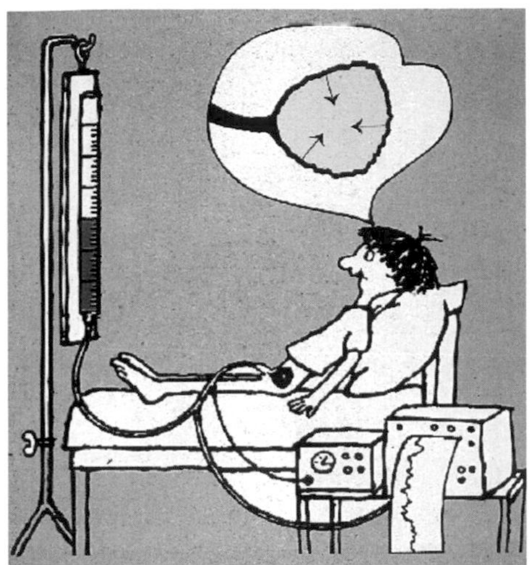

Figure 55.4
With intravesical electrostimulation a feedback training is mediated by enabling the patient to observe the change of the detrusor pressure on a water manometer: the patient is able to realize when a detrusor contraction takes place.

Prerequisites for successful intravesical electrical stimulation

The most important condition for a treatment is a correct diagnosis with the help of electric stimulation (Figure 55.5).

None of the research really focused on the inclusion criteria. According to the basic research, only those with some intact afferent fibers from the bladder to the cortex and those with spinal cord lesions, with the presence of pain sensation in the sacral dermatomes S3 and S4, can benefit from IVES. According to Nathan and Smith,[40] the pathways of bladder proprioception and for pain lie close together. The value of viscerosensoric cortical evoked potentials from the bladder neck was demonstrated by Kiss et al.[16] A precise indication seems to be one prerequisite for a good result. Regarding children with myelomeningocele, one must also take into account that myelomeningocele bladders at birth may have a threefold increase in connective tissue compared to normal controls.[41] According to clinical experience, a significant decrease of receptors tempers the enthusiasm for IVES in this particular group of patients, though the cases are individually very different.

Implications for practice

Basically, intravesical electrotherapy is able to improve neurogenic bladder dysfunction, primarily by stimulating Aδ mechanoafferents inducing bladder sensation and the urge to void and consequently increasing the efferent output with improvement of micturition and conscious control. Therefore, IVES is the only available option to induce/improve bladder sensation and to enhance the micturition reflex in incomplete central or peripheral nerve damage. However, proper indication is crucial and this type of therapy should only be applied in those with intact afferent fibers between the bladder and the cortex if possible, proved by the evaluation of viscerosensoric cortical evoked potentials. If these premises are respected, IVES is effective.

IVES is safe; no side-effects have been reported, beyond an occasional urinary infection. The question of cost-effectiveness was raised by Kaplan,[19] who stated that the most commonly used alternative for these patients is bladder augmentation, which is 'miles apart in terms of cost, discomfort and short- and long-term complications'.

One benefit of IVES was noted by most of the authors: improved sensation documents satisfactory long-term results. The patients with successful IVES get great satisfaction from knowing when their bladder is full and when it is time to catheterize or to void. Moreover, even without direct bowel stimulation, patients noted significant improvement in the warning of bowel fullness and gained greater control for their bowel movements.

Table 55.1 *Results of 802 patients treated with IVES in the National Institute of Neurosurgery, Budapest*

Basic disease	No of patients	Normalized	Improved	Unchanged
Spinal trauma	177	111	43	23
Spinal tunor (p.op.)	247	156	59	32
Prolapsed disc (p.op.)	162	102	39	21
Spina bifida (children)	186	117	45	24
Others (spinal meningitis)	30	19	7	4
No	802	505	193	104
%	100	63	24	13

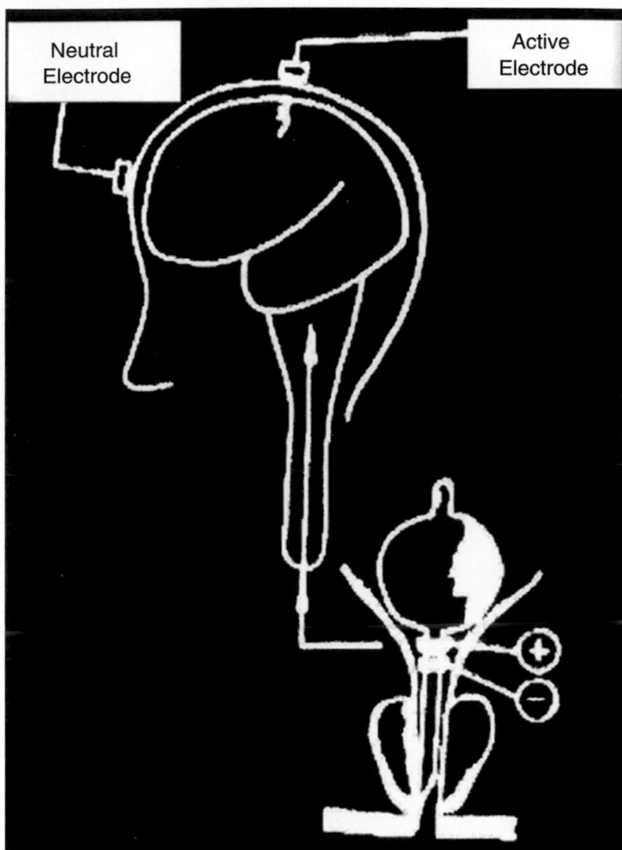

Figure 55.5
Testing of cortico-evoked potentials from the bladder neck.[16]

IVES can only be effective with certain prerequisites, the most important being that at least some afferent fibers between the bladder and the CNS are intact and the detrusor is able to contract. The method is safe, and no real complications have been reported.

Therapeutic recommendations

- The interrelation of diagnosis and treatment decides the appropriate parameters, individualized for each patients.
- IVES is able to improve neurogenic bladder dysfunction, primarily by stimulating Aδ mechanoreceptor afferents inducing bladder sensation and the urge to void and, consequently, increasing the efferent output with improvement of micturition and conscious control.
- IVES is the only available option to induce/improve bladder sensation and to enhance the micturition reflex in patients with incomplete central or peripheral nerve damage.
- Indication is crucial and IVES should only be applied if afferent fibers between the bladder and the cortex are still intact and if the detrusor muscle is still able to contract.
- If these premises are respected, IVES is effective.
- The ideal indication is the neuropathic – underactive, hyposensitive, and hypocontractile – detrusor.

Conclusions

IVES differs from all other electric stimulation methods in the direct administration of various types of interrupted DC current directly to the sensory input of the bladder, to its intramural receptor, and the afferent transport system to the brain in a noninvasive way. Its aim is to reactivate the normal physiologic control of the bladder by the patient. This is the reason why it cannot be applied in complete trans-section of the spinal cord. The pressure receptors of the bladder are the sensory 'organs' which transform electricity to a bioelectric stimulus and propagate it through afferent sensory axons to the central nervous system. The fact that, in a significant number of patients, sooner or later, IVES can activate the urge to void proves that even the cortex is affected and that selective conscious voluntary bladder control can be reached. This is the ultimate goal of the therapy.

In summary:

- Basic research during the last decade has proved the underlying working concept.
- The results reported in the literature are controversial, mainly because of different inclusion and exclusion criteria.
- In the only sham-controlled study the treatment period is too short and the inclusion and exclusion criteria are not really defined.
- The alternative may be either life-long intermittent catheterization or bladder augmentation. In this regards, IVES is cost-effective.
- It is worthwhile to apply intravesical electrostimulation, bearing in mind inclusion and exclusion criteria, especially when trying to verify functioning afferent fibers between the bladder and the cortex.

Further research

There is definitely a need for placebo/(sham)-controlled prospective studies, with clear inclusion and exclusion criteria and clear definitions of the aims. De Wachter and Wyndaele (personal communication, 2001) demonstrated in animal experiments and models that the position of the stimulating electrode, as well as the amount of saline within the bladder, may be crucial for the effects, as has already been demonstrated in patients.[8] Additional research is needed to clarify this aspect of IVES.

References

1. Saxtorph MH. Stricture ureathrae – fistula perineae – retentio urinae. Clinisk Chirurgi Copenhagen: Gyldendalske Fortlag 1878: 265–80.
2. Pankel vL, Zackerkandl O. In: Hrsg. H Senator: Die Erkrankungen der Blase. Wien: Alfred Höbler Verlag, 1809: 101.
3. Katona F. Electrical stimulation in the diagnosis and therapy of bladder paralysis. Elektromos ingerlés a hólyagbénulasok diagnosztikajaban és therapiajaban. Orv Hetil 1958; 8–9: 277–80.
4. Katona F, Benyo 1, Lang 1. Über intraluminaere Elektrotherapie von verschiedenen paralytischen Zustaenden des gastrointestinalen Traktes mit Quadrangulaerstrom. Zbl Chir 1959; 84: 24.
5. Katona F, Benyo 1, Lang 1. Erfahrungen mit der Anwendung von Quadranregulaeren Strom bei direkten Elektrotherapie des dynamischen Ileus und der akuten postoperativen Darmparese. Wien Klin. Wochenschr 1959; 71: 918.
6. Katona F. Intravesicale elektrotherapie bei Myelodysplasiebedingster Laehmungsblase. Kinderrchirurgie 1973; 13: 114–17.
7. Katona F, Berényi M. Intravesical, transurethral electrotherapy in meningomyelocele patients. Acta Paediatr Acad Sci Hung 1973; 16: 363–74.
8. Katona F. Basic principles and results in intravesical electric stimulation. Urodinamica 1992; 1: 57–64.
9. Katona F, Pasztor E, Tomka I. Untersuchungen über die kortikale Afferentation der Harnblasentaetigkeit. Acta Physiol Acad Sci Hung 1961; 28(Suppl).
10. Katona F. Stages of vegetative afferentation in reorganisation of bladder control during intravesical electrotherapy. Urol Int 1975; 30: 192–203.
11. Katona F. Induced rhythms and dysrhythmias of smooth muscle motility. In: Adam G, ed. Neurobiology of Invetebrates. Akademia Kiado, Budapest 1973: 319–26.
12. Ebner A, Jiang CH, Lindström S. Intravesical electrical stimulation – an experimental analysis of the mechanism of action. J Urol 1992; 148: 920–4.
13. Jiang Ch, Linström S, Mazéries L. Segmental inhibitory control of ascending sensory information from bladder mechanoreceptors in cat. Neurourol Urodyn 1991; 10: 286–8.
14. Jiang CH. Modulation of the micturition reflex pathway by intravesical electrical stimulation: an experimental study in the cat. Neurourol Urodyn 1998; 17(5): 543–53.
15. Colombo T, Wieselman G, Pichler Zalaudek K et al. Central nervous system control of micturition in patients with bladder dysfunctions in competition with healthy control probands. An electrophysiological study. Urologe A 2000; 39(2): 160–5.
16. Kiss G, Madersbacher H, Poewe W. Cortical evoked potentials of the vesicourethral junction – a predictor for the outcome of intravesical electrostimulation in patients with sensory and motor detrusor dysfunction. World J Urol 1998; 16(5): 308–12.
17. Gladh G. Intravesical electrical stimulation in children with micturition dysfunction. Proc ICS 2002, Heidelberg, 2002: 22. (Abstract)
18. Buyle S. Wyndaele JJ, D Hauwets K et al. Optimal parameters for transurethral intravesical electrostimulation determined in an experiment in the rat. Eur Urol 1998; 33(5): 507–10.
19. Kaplan WE. Intravesical electrical stimulation of the bladder: Pro Editorial. Urology 2000; 56(1): 2: 4.
20. Decter PM. Intravesical electrical stimulation of the bladder: Contra Editorial. Urology 2000; 56(1): 2–4.
21. Decter PM, Snyder P, Laudermilch C. Transurethral electrical bladder stimulation: a follow-up report. J Urol 1994; 152: 812–14.
22. Boone TB, Roehrborn CG, Hurt G. Transurethral intravesical electrotherapy for neurogenic bladder dysfunction in children with myelodysplasia: a prospective, randomized clinical trial. J Urol 1992; 148: 550–4.
23. Eckstein HG, Katona F. Treatment of neuropathic bladder by transurethral electrical stimulation. Lancet 1974; 1: 780–1.
24. Nicholas IL, Eckstein HG. Endovesical electrotherapy in treatment of urinary incontinence in spina bifida patients. Lancet 1975; 2: 1276–7.
25. Denes J, Leb J. Electrostimulation of the neuropathic bladder. J Pediatr Surg 1975; 10(2): 245–7.
26. Janneck C. Electrostimulation of the bladder and the anal sphincter – a new way to treat the neurogenic bladder. Prog Pediatric Surg 1976; 9: 119–39.
27. Seiferth J, Heisiog J, Larkamp H. Intravesical electrostimulation of the neurogenic bladder in spina bifida children. Urol Int 1978; 33(5): 279–84.
28. Seiferth J, Larkamp H, Heising J. Experiences with temporary intravesical electrostimulation of the neurogenic bladder in spina bifida children. Urologe A 1978; 17(5): 353–4.
29. Schwock G, Tischer W. The influence of intravesical electrostimulation on the urinary bladder in animals. Z Kinderchir 1981; 32(2): 161–6.
30. Madersbacher H, Pauer W, Reiner E et al. Rehabilitation of micturition in patients with incomplete spinal cord lesions by transurethral electrostimulation of the bladder. Eur Urol 1982; 8: 111–16.
31. Kaplan WE, Richards I. Intravesical bladder stimulation in myelodysplasia. J Urol 1988; 140: 1282–4.
32. Madersbacher H. Intravesical electrical stimulation for the rehabilitation of the neuropathic bladder. Paraplegiea 1990; 28: 349–52.
33. Lyne CJ, Bellinger ME. Early experience with transurethral electrical bladder stimulation. J Urol 1993; 15: 697–9.
34. Kölle D, Madersbacher H, Kiss G, Mair D. Intravesical electrostimulation for treatment of bladder dysfunction. Initial experience after gynecological operations. Gynakol Geburstshilflische Rundsch 1995; 35(4): 221–5.
35. Cheng EY, Richards I, Kaplan WE. Use of bladder stimulation in high risk patients. J Urol 1996; 156: 479–752
36. Cheng EY, Richards I, Balcom A et al. Bladder stimulation therapy improves bladder compliance: results from a multi-institutional trial. J Urol 1996; 156: 761–4.
37. Primus G, Trammer H. Intravesical electrostimulation in detrusor hypocontractility. Wien Klin Wochensch 1993; 105(19): 556–7.
38. Kroll P, Jankowski A, Martynski M. Electrostimulation in treatment of neurogenic and non-neurogenic voiding dysfunction. Wiad Lek 1998; 51(Suppl 3): 92–7.
39. Pugach JL, Salvin L, Stenhardt GE. Intravesical electrostimulation in pediatric patients with spinal cord defects. J Urol 2000; 164: 965–8.
40. Nathan PW, Smith MC. The centripetal pathway from the bladder and urethra within the spinal cord. J Neurol Neurosurg Psychiatry 1951; 14: 262–80.
41. Shapiro E, Beckh M, Periman E, Lepor H. Bladder wall abnormalities in myelodysplastic bladders, a computer assisted morphometric analysis. J Urol 1991; 145(5): 1024–9.

56

Surgery to improve reservoir function

Manfred Stöhrer and Jürgen Pannek

Introduction

Compensated bladder storage is a function that is decisive for the quality of life and life expectancy of patients with neurogenic lower urinary tract dysfunction. It is characterized by low-pressure storage with physiologic storage pressure at an adequate volume as the maximum value. Storage pressure should not increase significantly before filling volume reaches 300 ml. The volume at which pressure increase occurs is defined as the reflex volume.[1] A high reflex volume is the key to continence and protection of the upper urinary tract. If this condition cannot be achieved by medical treatment, a number of surgical interventions are available. Electrical stimulation and intestinal replacement are described elsewhere. The surgical procedures outlined here are effective for the majority of patients and are minimally invasive.

Two prerequisites are fundamental: intact detrusor musculature (no fibrosis) and satisfactory management of bladder emptying, preferably by intermittent catheterization. Should detrusor elasticity be impaired by morphologic conditions, (partial) bladder replacement is the only option. These changes, caused by tissue scarring, are the result of 'mismanagement' over several years. When the patient is treated correctly, this pathology will seldom occur.

In principle, to normalize the detrusor muscle its nervous supply can be altered by chemical receptor blockers, such as botulinum A toxin, which is the simplest and most promising method of ensuring compensated storage.[2,3]

For nonresponders or when the effect is unsatisfactory, detrusor myectomy (partial autoaugmentation) is a possible alternative.[4,5] Some authors have expanded this simple intervention, with the use of omentum or gastrointestinal components to cover the mucosa at the site of the muscular defect after surgery.[6–9]

Should these procedures fail, clam cystoplasty offers a compromise before embarking on extensive enterocystoplasty.[10] All three methods can help patients with both complete or incomplete lesions. Recently, bladder augmentation by tissue engineering techniques has been described.[11] Available for high and complete lesions, deafferentation by transection of the S2–S4 vertebral roots is an additional procedure to completely block detrusor overactivity.[12] In these cases, alternative emptying (preferably by intermittent catheterization) is necessary too, unless sacral root electrostimulation is applied.[13,14] The establishment of a somatic–CNS–autonomic reflex pathway by a microanastomosis from the L5 ventral root to the S3 ventral root has been introduced as an experimental approach.[15]

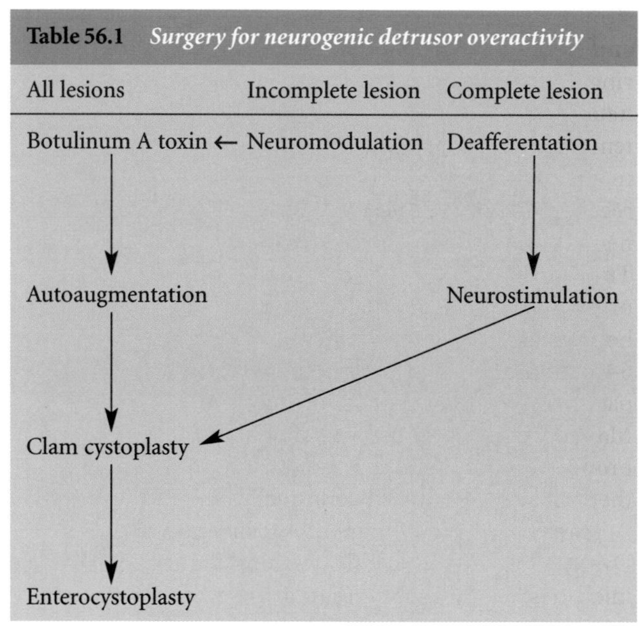

Table 56.1 *Surgery for neurogenic detrusor overactivity*

Table 56.1 presents an overview of the surgical options that could improve storage function in patients with neurogenic detrusor overactivity.

Botulinum A toxin injections in the detrusor

Botulinum A toxin has been known for many years to be not only one of the most potent venoms but also a very effective drug for the suppression of chronic muscular spasticity. It has been applied since 1980 to spastic striated muscles in many neurologic and orthopedic domains.[16,17] Esthetic plastic surgeons use it much more extensively.[18] In urology, it was injected initially in the external sphincter to treat detrusor-sphincter dyssynergia.[19] In 1998, detrusor injections were given to patients with neurogenic lower urinary tract dysfunction in Germany and Switzerland. The first results were published in 1999.[2,3]

Mode of action

Botulinum toxin has several subtypes. Subtype A is the most effective: a product of *Clostridium botulinum*, it is a strong natural venom. The molecule is composed of light and heavy nucleic acid chains connected by a disulfide ring. It blocks presynaptic nerve endings at the cholinergic neuron and prevents acetylcholine secretion, leading to temporary chemical denervation and loss of nerve activity in the target organ. The process is reversible by nerve regeneration, as new nerve endings will sprout from the neuron and reconstitute connections to the target organ. The time course of this process is dependent on the target organ type and is individually variable; it takes roughly between 3 and 4 months in the urethral sphincter, and 6–14 months in the detrusor. The average efficacy period in patients studied after detrusor injection is 10–12 months. Maximal efficacy is observed after about 2 weeks, remains pronounced until about 3 months after the injection, and then subsides slowly and continually.

Three varieties of botulinum A toxin are available: Botox®, Dysport®, and Xeomin®. Concerning the use for detrusor injections, no data about Xeomin are available. Comparing Botox and Dysport, the efficacy ratio between these two products is about 1:3. Dysport demonstrates greater dispersion. It thus appears rational to use a lower dilution to avoid its dispersion into the circulation. This mechanism may explain the isolated cases of generalized muscle weakness described in the literature.[20] We have not observed this effect in our patients who have been treated with Botox.

Indication

Botulinum A toxin injections into the detrusor are indicated when anticholinergic medication is not effective or not tolerated. As this procedure is the least invasive of all available options in these cases, it should be the method of first choice when conservative treatment fails. Its fundamental prerequisite is an effective bladder emptying after the treatment. Our experience shows that aseptic intermittent catheterization is preferred. When the detrusor overactivity is enhanced by acute urinary tract infection, the action of the toxin is insufficient to suppress it, and episodes of reflex incontinence may occur.

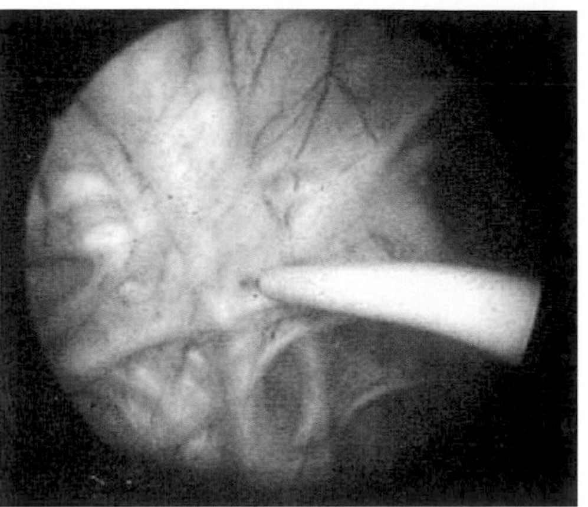

Figure 56.1
Botulinum A toxin injection in detrusor trabecule.

Method of application

Botox 300 IU (or Dysport 750–1000 IU) are given for the treatment of neurogenic detrusor overactivity. The agent is dissolved in 15 ml saline and injected in 0.5 ml aliquots through a standard endoscopic needle (30 injection sites) over the entire muscle. For children, the dosage is reduced in relation to body weight. The injections are administered preferably in visible muscular structures (trabecules) (Figure 56.1). The trigone and ureteric orifices are spared to prevent possible reflux. Thus, 10 IU Botox are injected at each site. An indwelling catheter is placed for 24 h. Antibiotic prophylaxis is started preoperatively and continued for 1 week. After removal of the indwelling catheter the patient practices intermittent catheterization – most patients adopt this routine before treatment. Peroperative anticholinergic treatment is continued during the first postoperative week and then, if possible, discontinued completely.

Results

In our center, 141 patients were treated from early 1998 until October 2002: 222 treatment sessions were performed, including multiple treatments. The underlying condition was traumatic spinal cord lesion in the majority of patients, with small groups suffering from multiple sclerosis or myelomeningocele. Patients with low bladder compliance caused by structural changes in the detrusor wall (fibrosis) secondary to neurologic disease were excluded from this treatment. Patients at risk from autonomic dysreflexia or who preserved their bladder sensation were treated under local or general anesthesia.

The condition of these patients and of those who were evaluated in cooperation with the center in Zurich was checked by videourodynamics preoperatively and at 12 and

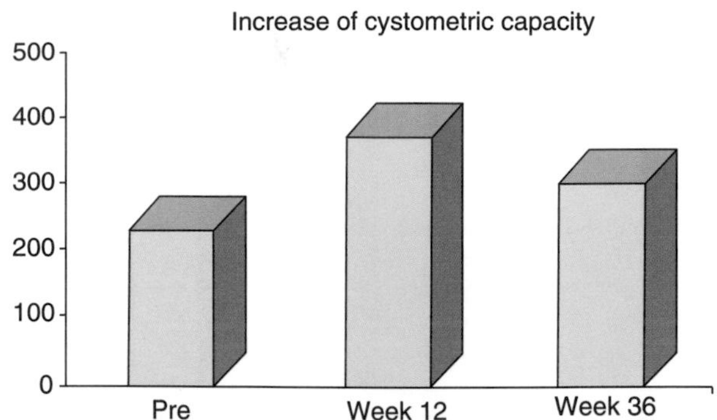

Figure 56.2
Increase of cystometric capacity at 12 and 36 weeks after botulinum treatment.

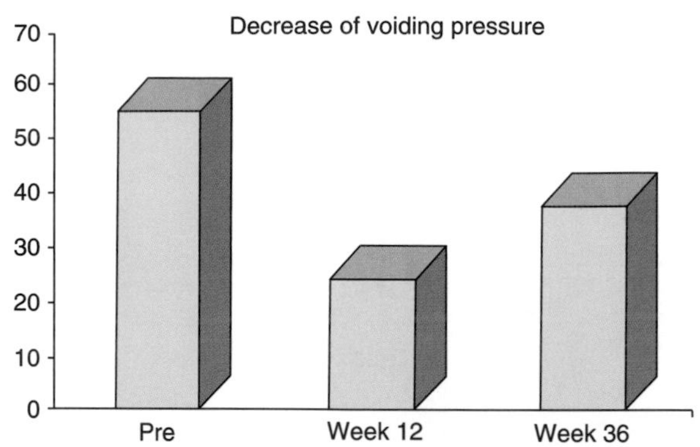

Figure 56.4
Decrease of voiding pressure at 12 and 36 weeks after botulinum treatment.

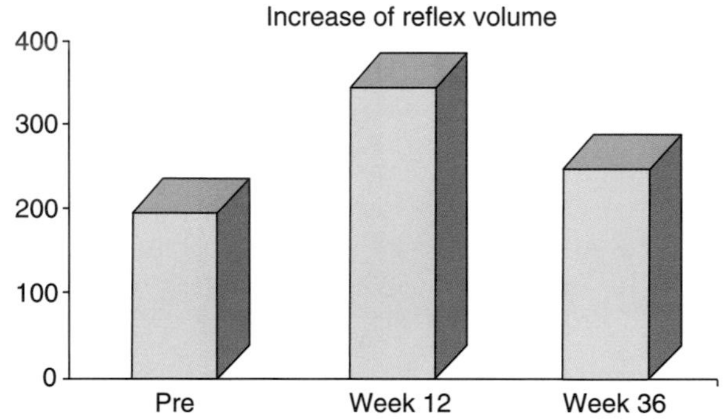

Figure 56.3
Increase of reflex volume at 12 and 36 weeks after botulinum treatment.

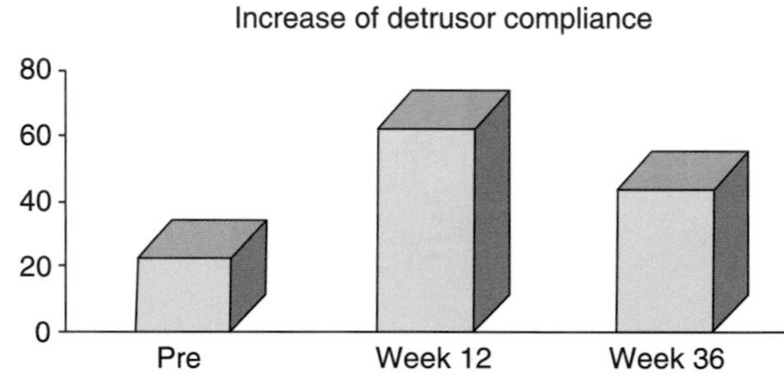

Figure 56.5
Increase of detrusor compliance at 12 and 36 weeks after botulinum treatment.

36 weeks postoperatively. The parameters studied were reflex volume, maximal voiding detrusor pressure, cystometric bladder capacity, detrusor compliance, and continence status (Figures 56.2–56.5). Patient satisfaction and the post-treatment dosage of anticholinergics were also recorded. Significant improvement of all parameters was achieved in nearly all patients (95%). Reflex volume and cystometric capacity showed considerable amelioration after 6 weeks and most responders (>90%) were continent, unless urinary tract infection was present. Spontaneous voiding was eliminated, and thus the residual was equal to the capacity. Treatment was successful, even in children. The condition of many patients with pre-existing autonomic dysreflexia improved significantly. It was not known why 5% of patients did not respond to botulinum A toxin injections, although immunity caused against the toxin by the presence of antibodies after earlier contact with it might be one reason.

Blocked nerve endings regenerate slowly – after 36 weeks, the condition of patients had deteriorated in comparison to that at 6 weeks, but was still significantly better than preoperatively. The mean efficacy period in our patients was 10–12 months. These results have been confirmed in a European multicenter study comprising over 200 patients.

Repeated botulinum A treatment sessions did not result in any loss of efficacy. In our patients, 51 had two injection sessions, 21 had three, 6 had four, and 3 had five, and increased toxin tolerance was not found.

Botox or Dysport application led to essentially similar outcomes, but generalized muscle weakness was observed in three patients after Dysport application. As discussed above, dispersion and dilution could have been determining factors here; thus, we decided to reduce the dilution volume to 7.5 ml when using Dysport. Whether this will diminish or prevent the occurrence of these generalized adverse effects is still an open question.

In summary, detrusor injections of botulinum A toxin represent an effective treatment for neurogenic detrusor overactivity. Because this therapy has not been approved by the medical authorities in most countries, its use should be

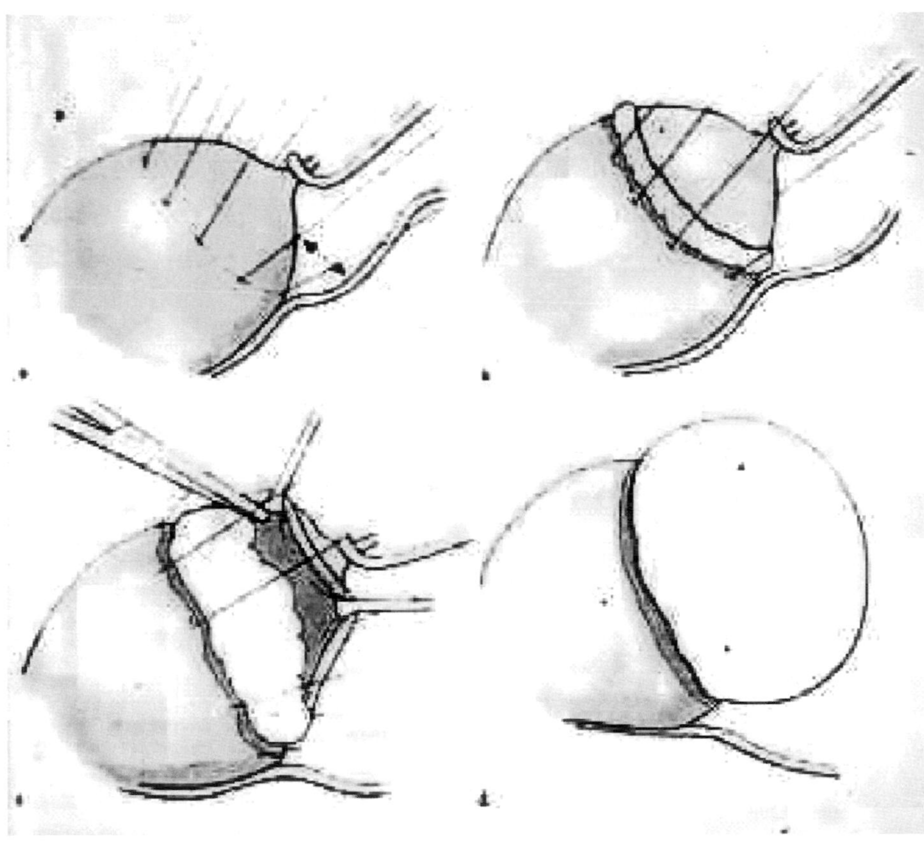

Figure 56.6
The autoaugmentation procedure (side view).

considered only with the appropriate precautions and documentation.

Recent literature

This procedure[2,3] has raised much interest since its introduction, but, apart from conference reports, the number of publications in the literature is still sparse. Its mechanism of action has been studied in rats[21] and preliminary trials have confirmed its efficacy also in myelomeningocele children.[22] Moreover, a first randomized, placebo-controlled, double-blind study has been presented, demonstrating the efficacy and clinical usefulness of the substance over a 6-month period.[23]

Partial detrusor myectomy (autoaugmentation)

The basis of this therapy is partial removal of the overactive detrusor without compromising the underlying mucosa. It decreases storage pressure and increases bladder capacity. The essential advantage of the procedure is its low invasivity and abstinence from covering the defect with intestinal tissue sections. This option remains available when later, more invasive procedures might become necessary.

Indication

Aggressive detrusor overactivity that is refractory to conservative treatment and that also does not respond to botulinum A toxin can be corrected by autoaugmentation. After this treatment, intermittent catheterization is compulsory. The functional transformation caused by the procedure needs time to be expressed. This period is at least 1 year, and the procedure is contraindicated if enough time is not available due to the patient's condition. Degenerative changes in the detrusor musculature, causing a reduction of anesthetic bladder capacity, are also a contraindication.

Method

The bladder anterior wall and dome are approached, and the peritoneum is freed from the bladder until about halfway down the bladder posterior wall. The bladder is filled to about 200 ml, and a circular section of the detrusor muscle with a radius of about 4 cm around the urachus is resected. The mucosa is left intact (Figures 56.6 and 56.7). The diverticulum created in this way will reduce

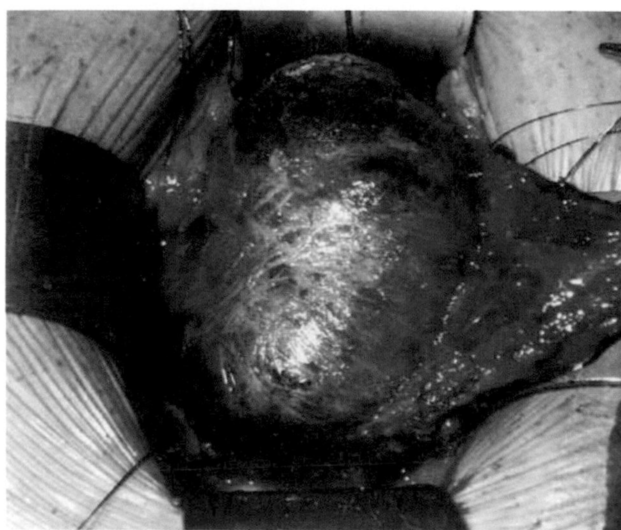

Figure 56.7
Surgical view during the autoaugmentation procedure.

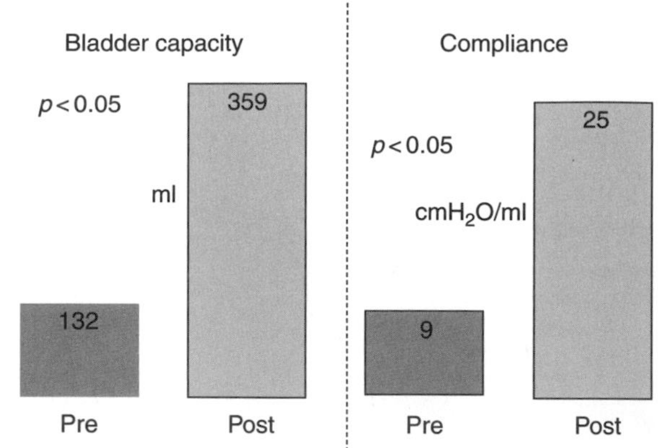

Figure 56.8
Bladder capacity and detrusor compliance after autoaugmentation.

storage pressure and improve bladder capacity after a period of 1–2 years. An indwelling catheter is left for 2 days when the mucosa has not been perforated during the procedure. When mucosal perforation has occurred, the indwelling catheter is placed for a maximum of 2 weeks and is clamped intermittently for 3–4 days, putting a low-grade load on the diverticulum.[5,24] In a few patients, ancillary injection with botulinum A toxin to accelerate the process of functional transformation has shown partial success.

In 1989, Cartwright and Snow published a paper on a similar procedure in dogs and in a child.[4] Also in 1989, we performed this for the first time in a man with an incomplete spinal cord lesion. Cartwright and Snow attached the bladder to the iliopsoas, whereas we only do the simple resection. This simpler approach produces good results. The peritoneum remains closed, and covering of the defect is unnecessary.

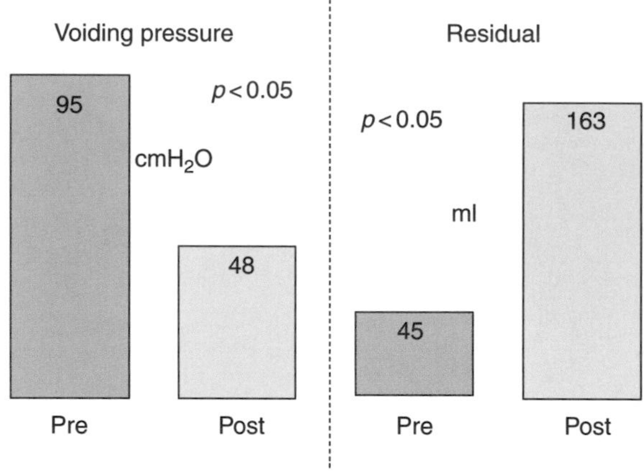

Figure 56.9
Voiding pressure and residual after autoaugmentation.

Results

From 1989 to October 2002 we treated 93 patients by this method. After the introduction of botulinum A toxin injections for the same indication, the number of autoaugmentations declined considerably, but nonresponders to botulinum A toxin are good candidates for autoaugmentation. The efficacy of this procedure has been documented by videourodynamics, preoperatively, 6–12 weeks and 1 year postoperatively, and at 1–2-year intervals thereafter. Its outcome parameters are improvement of incontinence, bladder compliance, maximum detrusor pressure during voiding, cystometric capacity, residual urine, reduced use of anticholinergics, and patient satisfaction. All parameters are significantly ameliorated after a mean follow-up period of over 6½ years in about two-thirds of patients (Figures 56.8 and 56.9). Patients who have been lost to follow-up are rated as nonresponders. The patient population consists mainly of complete and incomplete spinal cord lesions, plus multiple sclerosis and myelomeningocele. The interval between surgery and a satisfactorily improved functional condition was 3 months to 2 years (Figures 56.10 and 56.11). One woman who received an artificial sphincter after autoaugmentation and thus lost the opportunity for overflow incontinence suffered a bladder rupture at 600 ml capacity. Her condition was resolved by surgery without any sequelae. Four patients submitted to further procedures with intestinal replacement.

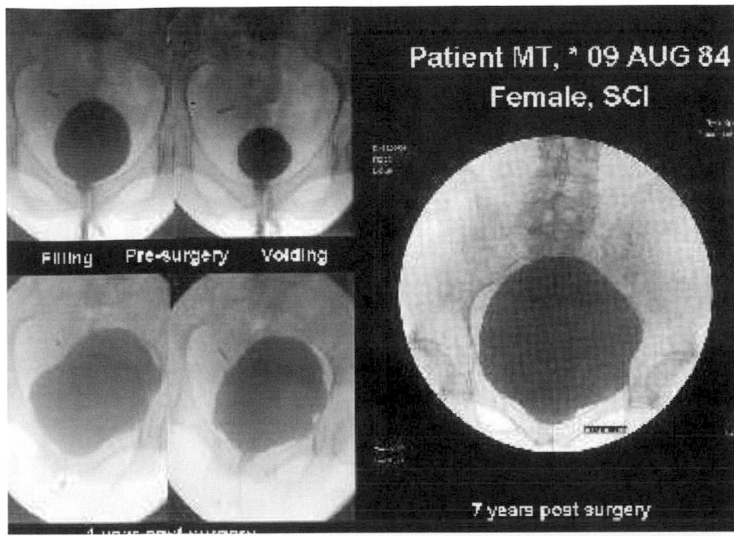

Figure 56.10
X-ray views of female patient pre, and 1 and 7 years postautoaugmentation.

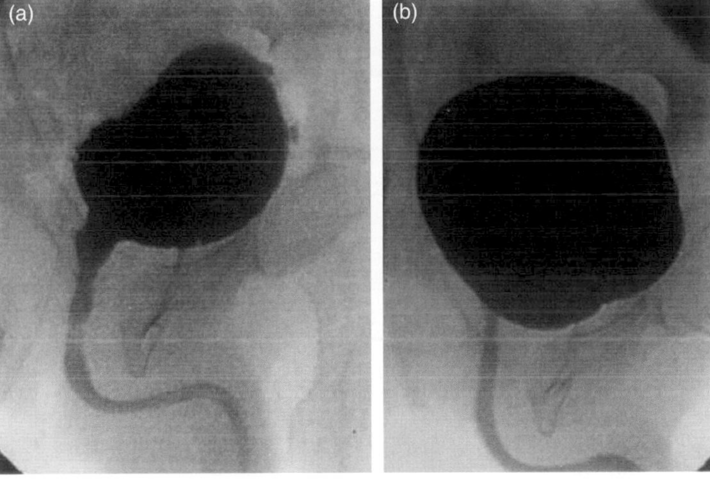

Figure 56.11
X-ray views of male patient pre (a) and 5 months after (b) autoaugmentation.

It is of the utmost importance to realize that functional improvement does not occur immediately after treatment, but may take a long time. One of our patients had already elected for intestinal augmentation, but after 2 years a positive result was obtained. Published modifications of the method, including covering the defect with omentum or intestinal sections, have not produced better outcomes. One major advantage of this uncomplicated procedure is that the peritoneum is not opened. Based on my 13 years of experience, I thus see no need to change it.

Recent literature

In a review comparing enterocystoplasty and detrusor myectomy,[25] it is stated that: 'For most clinical indications detrusor myectomy has offered comparable success or significant improvement in bladder function without incurring the significant complication rate of enterocystoplasty.' Another review[26] attests that: 'The principle of urothelial preservation, introduced by autoaugmentation, is very promising in the effort to create a compliant urinary reservoir without metabolic disturbance and without the risk of cancer.' In a review comparing Ingelman–Sundberg bladder denervation, detrusor myectomy, and augmentation cystoplasty,[27] it is argued that augmentation cystoplasty has the highest success rate but a 'much higher likelihood of early and late post-operative complications' and, thus, the less invasive methods should be favored if feasible. Two long-term follow-up studies on children[28,29] underscore the contraindication of hypertonic/poorly compliant bladders.

In this author's view, the use of backing tissue to cover the detrusor defect[29–31] does not contribute to improvement of the clinical result. The procedure, as presented in this chapter, offers fast repair of nearly inevitable mucosal perforations. This is probably the reason why a laparoscopic access for this surgery has not become established.[32,33]

Clam cystoplasty

This relatively simple bladder augmentation with only slight peroperative risks inserts an intestinal segment in the bladder defect that is made by incision of the posterior bladder wall.[10] The results so far are good,[34,35] but the procedure is far more invasive than autoaugmentation and might induce late complications from bowel use.

S2–S4 Deafferentation

Another option to achieve a low-pressure bladder without intestinal patches is the intradural bilateral transection of the S2–S4 dorsal roots. Unlike the methods described above, this procedure is indicated only in patients with complete spinal cord lesions. Moreover, it is mandatory to exclude patients with a fibrotic low-compliance bladder. The transection causes complete detrusor acontractility – the bladder must be emptied by intermittent catheterization. As many of these patients have high-level lesions, the required dexterity is often unavailable. In those cases, combination with sacral electrostimulation (e.g. Brindley stimulator) is feasible. The ventral root stimulator can be implanted either intra- or extradurally. The patient can use an external, hand-held device for voluntary initiation of voiding, defecation, and penile erections. Whereas the overwhelming majority of the implants is effective for bladder and bowel control, results for erectile function are less satisfying.[13,36] In order to avoid detrusor-spincter dyssynergia, a so-called 'post-stimulus voiding' is used.[14] By this technique, utilizing the different refractory times of the nerves supplying the bladder and the sphincter, the maximum bladder contraction occurs only after the sphincter contraction decreases. Improvement of the technique might enhance the quality of stimulated voiding.[37] Deafferentation is also an option for patients with pronounced spasticity or dysreflexia who are able to handle intermittent catheterization. Patients must be informed about the adverse effects on their sexual functions (demise of lubrification, loss of reflex erection).

Future research

Lately, two new techniques have been introduced for the surgical treatment of neurogenic bladder dysfunction.

Atala and coworkers developed a technique to avoid the use of bowel segments for bladder augmentation. Urothelial and bladder muscle cells obtained from a biopsy were grown in culture, and seeded on a biodegradable bladder-shaped scaffold. About 7 weeks after the biopsy, the autologous engineered bladder constructs were used for reconstruction and implanted either with or without an omental wrap. Follow-up range was 22–61 months (mean 46 months). The volume and compliance increase was greatest in the composite engineered bladders with an omental wrap. The engineered bladder biopsies showed an adequate structure and phenotype.[11] Despite several obstacles, this technique may possibly be helpful to avoid the use of bowel segments in selected patients in the future.

Xiao and his colleagues studied the possibilties of bladder reinnervation. After various experiments, they developed a way to establish a somatic-autonomic reflex pathway. Following animal experiments, patients with complete spinal cord injury underwent ventral root micro-anastomosis, usually between the L5 and S2/3 roots. With this technique, they claimed to control hyperreflexic bladder and detrusor-spincter dyssynergia in patients with suprasacral lesions. Encouraged by their preliminary results, they constructed artificial somatic-autonomic reflex pathways (skin–CNS–bladder reflex) in patients with hyperreflexic bladders and acontractile bladders, and in patients with spina bifida. Success rates up to 87%, regarding continence and voluntary emptying by skin stimulation, have been reported.[23] However, a longer follow-up period and reproduction of the results by other centers are mandatory before this technique might be considered as a surgical treatment option in these patients.

Conclusion

The procedures described in this chapter are sufficient to achieve compensated storage in the vast majority of patients. More complicated interventions, necessary for nonresponders, are described in other chapters of this book.

References

1. Stöhrer M, Goepel M, Kondo A et al. The standardization of terminology in neurogenic lower urinary tract dysfunction with suggestions for diagnostic procedures. Neurourol Urodyn 1999; 18: 139–58.
2. Stöhrer M, Schurch B, Kramer G et al. Botulinum-A toxin in the treatment of detrusor hyperreflexia in spinal cord injury: a new alternative to medical and surgical procedures? Neurourol Urodyn 1999; 18: 401–2.
3. Schurch B, Stöhrer M, Kramer G et al. Botulinum A-toxin for treating detrusor hyperreflexia in spinal cord injured patients: a new alternative to anticholinergic drugs? Preliminary results. J Urol 2000; 164: 692–7.
4. Cartwright PC, Snow BW. Bladder auto-augmentation: early clinical experience. J Urol 1989; 142: 505–8.
5. Stöhrer M, Kramer G, Goepel M et al. Bladder autoaugmentation in adult patients with neurogenic voiding dysfunction. Spinal Cord 1997; 35: 456–62.
6. Dewan PA, Stefanek W. Autoaugmentation gastrocystoplasty: early clinical results. Br J Urol 1994, 74: 460–4.

7. Nguyen DH, Mitchell ME, Horowitz M et al. Demucosalized augmentation gastrocystoplasty with bladder autoaugmentation in pediatric patients. J Urol 1996; 156: 206–9.
8. Carr MC, Docimo SG, Mitchell ME. Bladder augmentation with urothelial preservation. J Urol 1999; 162: 1133–6.
9. Perovic SV, Djordjevic ML, Kekic ZK, Vukadinovic VM. Bladder autoaugmentation with rectus muscle backing. J Urol 2002; 168: 1877–80.
10. Mast P, Hoebeke P, Wyndaele JJ et al. Experience with augmentation cystoplasty. A review. Paraplegia 1995; 33: 560–4.
11. Atala A, Bauer SB, Soker S, Yoo JJ, Retik AB. Tissue-engineered autologous bladders for patients needing cystoplasty. Lancet 2006; 367(9518): 1241–6.
12. Diokno AC, Vinson RK, McGillicuddy J. Treatment of the severe uninhibited neurogenic bladder by selective sacral rhizotomy. J Urol 1977; 118: 299–301.
13. Sauerwein HD. The use of nerve deafferentation and stimulation in the paraplegic female patient. In: Raz S, ed. Female Urology. Philadelphia: WB Saunders, 1996: 656–64.
14. Van Kerrebroeck PE, Koldewijn EL, Debruyne FM. Worldwide experience with the Finetech–Brindley sacral anterior root stimulator. Neurourol Urodyn 1993; 12: 497–503.
15. Xiao CG. Reinnervation for neurogenic bladder: historic review and introduction of a somatic-autonomic reflex pathway procedure for patients with spinal cord injury or spina bifida. Eur Urol 2006; 49: 22–8.
16. National Institutes of Health. Clinical use of botulinum toxin. National Institutes of Health Consensus Development Conference Statement, Nov 12–14, 1990. Arch Neurol 1991; 48: 1294–8.
17. Jankovic J, Schwartz KS. Longitudinal experience with botulinum toxin injections for treatment of blepharospasm and cervical dystonia. Neurology 1993; 43: 834–6.
18. Bulstrode NW, Grobbelaar AO. Long-term prospective follow up of botulinum toxin treatment for facial rhytides. Aesthetic Plast Surg 2002; 26: 356–9
19. Schurch B, Hauri D, Rodic B et al. Botulinum-A toxin as a treatment of detrusor-sphincter dyssynergia; a prospective study in 24 spinal cord injury patients. J Urol 1996; 155: 1023–9.
20. Wyndaele JJ, Van Dromme SA. Muscular weakness as side effect of botulinum toxin injection for neurogenic detrusor overactivity. Spinal Cord 2002; 40: 599–600.
21. Smith CP, Somogyi GT, Chancellor AM. Emerging role of botulinum toxin in the treatment of neurogenic and non-neurogenic voiding dysfunction. Curr Urol Rep 2002; 3: 382–7.
22. Schulte-Baukloh H, Michael T, Schobert J et al. Efficacy of botulinum-A toxin in children with detrusor hyperreflexia due to myelomeningocele: preliminary results. Urology 2002; 59: 325–7.
23. Schurch B, de Seze M, Denys P et al. Botox Detrusor Hyperreflexia Study Team. Botulinum toxin type a is a safe and effective treatment for neurogenic urinary incontinence: results of a single treatment, randomized, placebo controlled 6-month study. J Urol 2005; 174: 196–200.
24. Stöhrer M, Kramer A, Goepel M et al. Bladder auto-augmentation an alternative for enterocystoplasty: preliminary results. Neurourol Urodyn 1995; 14: 11–23.
25. Leng WW, Blalock HJ, Fredriksson WH et al. Enterocystoplasty or detrusor myectomy? Comparison of indications and outcomes for bladder augmentation. J Urol 1999; 161: 758–63.
26. Cranidis A, Nestoridis G. Bladder augmentation. Int Urogynecol J Pelvic Floor Dysfunct 2000; 11: 33–40.
27. Westney OL, McGuire EJ. Surgical procedures for the treatment of urge incontinence. Tech Urol 2001; 7: 126–32.
28. Marte A, Di Meglio D, Cotrufo AM et al. A long-term follow-up of autoaugmentation in myelodysplastic children. BJU Int 2002; 89: 928–31.
29. Carr MC, Docimo SG, Mitchell ME. Bladder augmentation with urothelial preservation. J Urol 1999; 162: 1133–6.
30. Oge O, Tekgul S, Ergen A, Kendi S. Urothelium-preserving augmentation cystoplasty covered with a peritoneal flap. BJU Int 2000; 85: 802–5.
31. Perovic SV, Djordjevic ML, Kekic ZK, Vukadinovic VM. Bladder autoaugmentation with rectus muscle backing. J Urol 2002; 168: 1877–80.
32. McDougall EM, Clayman RV, Figenshau RS, Pearle MS. Laparoscopic retropubic auto-augmentation of the bladder. J Urol 1995; 153: 123–6.
33. Siracusano S, Trombetta C, Liguori G et al. Laparoscopic bladder auto-augmentation in an incomplete traumatic spinal cord injury. Spinal Cord 2000; 38: 59–61.
34. Chartier-Kastler EJ, Mongiat-Artus P, Bitker MO et al. Long-term results of augmentation cystoplasty in spinal cord injured patients. Spinal Cord 2000; 38: 490–4.
35. Arikan N, Turkolmez K, Budak M, Gogus O. Outcome of augmentation sigmoidoplasty in children with neurogenic bladder. Urol Int 2000; 64: 82–5.
36. Kutzenberger J, Pannek J, Stohrer M. Neurourology. Current developments and therapeutic strategies. Urologe A 2006; 45: 158–66.
37. Schumacher S, Bross S, Scheepe JR et al. Restoration of bladder function in spastic neuropathic bladder using sacral deafferentation and different techniques of neurostimulation. Adv Exp Med Biol 1999; 462: 303–9.

57

Surgery to improve bladder outlet function

Ginger Isom-Batz, Gina Defreitas, and Philippe Zimmern

Introduction

The bladder outlet in patients with neurogenic voiding dysfunction is subject to two main abnormalities: outlet underactivity, leading to urine leakage with increased intra-abdominal pressure; and nonrelaxing urethral sphincter obstruction, resulting in reduced urine flow at the time of bladder emptying.[1] This chapter is therefore divided into two sections: surgical treatment of the underactive or incompetent bladder outlet and surgical treatment of the nonrelaxing or hyperactive bladder outlet (detrusor-sphincter dyssynergia or DSD). Procedures currently used to alleviate sphincteric deficiency in the neurogenic bladder population are injection of urethral bulking agents, slings, artificial urethral sphincters, bladder neck reconstruction procedures, and bladder neck closure. The surgical options currently available for the treatment of intractable DSD are sphincterotomy, insertion of a temporary or permanent urethral stent, balloon dilatation of the external sphincter, botulinum A toxin injection into the external sphincter, and use of a chronic indwelling catheter. The choice of surgical treatment depends on a number of factors, the most important of which are sex of the patient, the patient's comorbidities and functional status, the severity of urine leakage, whether or not the patient has had previous anti-incontinence procedures, patient and caregiver preferences, and, last but not least, the experience and expertise of the surgeon.

This chapter will focus on indications, surgical techniques, results, and complications of the various treatment options currently employed to treat bladder outlet pathology in the neurogenic bladder population. Literature dealing with the use of these surgical procedures in patients with non-neurogenic voiding dysfunction will not be discussed. Definitions and urodynamic terminology will conform to the recommendations published in the most recent report of the standardization subcommittee of the International Continence Society.[1]

Surgical management of the incompetent bladder outlet

Urethral bulking agents

Introduction

The first use of an injectable substance to treat urinary incontinence dates back to 1938 when Murless instilled sodium murrhate into the anterior vaginal wall.[1] Since then, a number of advancements have been made in agent composition, patient selection, and injection technique. Agents that have been employed for urethral injection include autologous fat, polytetrafluoroethylene (polytef, Teflon), bovine collagen (Contigen), and pyrolytic carbon-coated zirconium oxide beads (Durasphere). In 1984, Lewis et al performed periurethral Teflon injections in female patients with neurogenic bladder on intermittent catheterization and noted a favorable result on continence.[2] Subsequently, several investigators have published data on the use of urethral bulking agents to treat urinary incontinence in patients with neurogenic voiding dysfunction. Although the bulk of the literature deals with children, adults with neuropathic bladder have been addressed in a few case series. Since the majority of experience has been accrued with glutaraldehyde cross-linked bovine collagen, and it is currently the most widely used bulking agent for the treatment of urinary incontinence, this section will focus on the results obtained with this substance. The Food and Drug Administration (FDA), secondary to problems with granuloma formation and particle migration, has not approved Teflon for the treatment of urinary incontinence.[3] To date there have not been any studies published dealing with the use of autologous fat or Durasphere in patients with neurogenic bladder dysfunction.

The use of bulking agents to treat incontinence has several advantages. Delivery is minimally invasive, relatively

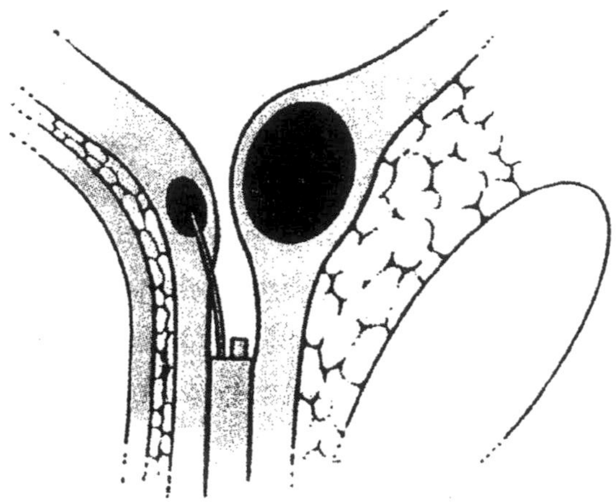

Figure 57.1
Correct placement of periurethral collagen. Injection should be at the proximal urethra in the submucosal plane. (Reproduced with permission from Functional Reconstruction of the Urinary Tract and Gynaeco-urology, 1st edn, 2002.)

easy to learn, and entails low morbidity. Furthermore, treatment with injectable substances does not jeopardize the performance and efficacy of other anti-incontinence procedures later on. The liabilities of this technology stem from a lack of durability and poorer effectiveness when compared to other, albeit more invasive, treatment modalities. This disadvantage often leads to repeat injections, which can elevate the cost of a procedure already known to be expensive.[4]

Collagen biocompatibility, durability, and allergenicity

The collagen used for urethral injection is harvested from bovine corium, which is treated to decrease its antigenicity, and then cross-linked with glutaraldehyde to improve its durability and resistance to degradation by host collagenase.[5] Comprised of 95% type I collagen and 5% type III collagen, it is marketed under the trade names Contigen, Zyderm, and Zyplast (Bard Corp, Atlanta, GA and Collagen Corp, Palo Alto, CA). Bovine collagen has weak antigenicity in humans with 1–3% of patients having a positive skin test.[5] Concerns over developing an autoimmune response to human collagen after injection with bovine collagen appear to be unfounded, since no direct relation between collagen injection and autoimmune disease has been demonstrated in clinical practice.[6] The product is not latex-free, and for this reason, the manufacturer package insert states that a positive skin test may be more prevalent in myelomeningocele patients; however, no literature or experimental data exist to substantiate this finding.

Bovine collagen was approved by the FDA for treatment of intrinsic sphincter deficiency in 1993. Since then, no reports of local or distant migration in animals or humans have surfaced. The host inflammatory response is mild and little granuloma formation occurs. The substance is supposed to undergo gradual degradation over the course of 3–19 months and becomes a matrix for host collagen deposition and neovascularization.[7] Three-dimensional ultrasonographic imaging of the urethra,[8] however, has found persistence of bovine collagen in the tissues up to 4 years postinjection,[9] indicating that resorption of this substance may be slower and more variable than was previously proposed.[10]

Mechanism of action

In the neuropathic urethra, sphincteric deficiency is caused by denervation of the musculature of the bladder neck, proximal urethra, external sphincter, and pelvic floor.[13] Collagen and other injectable agents theoretically work by increasing the length of bladder neck and proximal urethral mucosa apposition, thereby improving the efficiency of compression of the sphincter mechanism in response to increases in intra-abdominal pressure.[11,12] McGuire et al have determined that injectable agents exert their mechanism of action by increasing the Valsalva leak-point pressure (VLPP), but not the detrusor leak-point pressure (DLPP) or voiding pressure.[13] This finding has been substantiated by several other authors including Bomalaski et al, who found that in neurogenic bladder patients who experience clinical improvement with collagen injections, the VLPP increased an average of 26 cmH_2O, compared with an increase of only 8 cmH_2O in patients who were not helped by the treatment.[4]

Urethral bulking agents are not thought to increase bladder outlet resistance and, therefore, the pressure at which the bladder empties. For this reason, they are postulated to have an advantage in the treatment of neurogenic incontinence over slings and artificial sphincters, which may cause elevated detrusor pressures and upper tract deterioration.[14,15] So far, there have been no reports of renal compromise related to the use of injectable agents. Chernoff et al, however, have reported significant postoperative urodynamic changes in 3 children with neurogenic bladder who were treated with transurethral collagen injections with decreased compliance and appearance of a DLPP where none had previously existed. These investigators warn of possible bladder decompensation in patients with small-capacity, low-compliance bladders who undergo injection of urethral bulking agents.[16]

Delivery methods

There are three methods for the injection of bulking agents in the treatment of stress urinary incontinence:

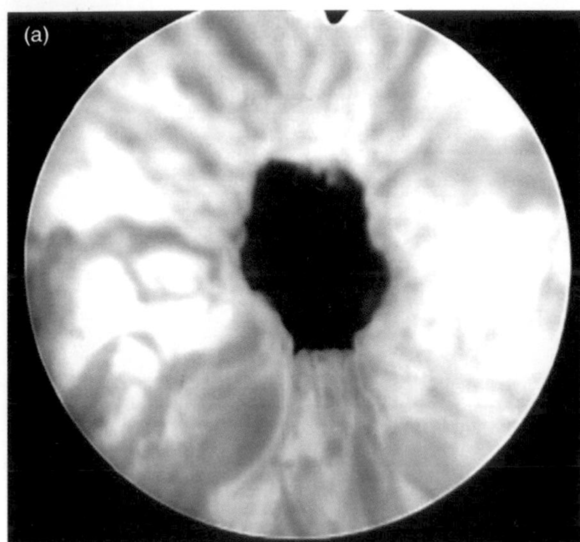

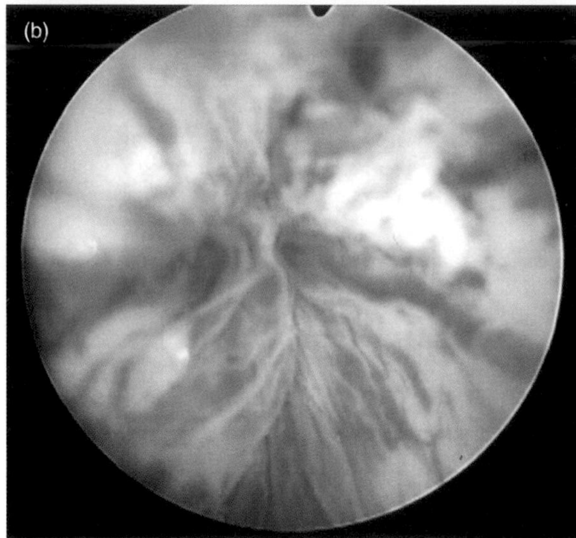

Figure 57.2
(a) Intraoperative cystoscopic view of open proximal urethra before collagen injection. (b) Intraoperative cystoscopic view of properly coapted proximal urethra after collagen injection.

periurethral, transurethral, and antegrade.[17] Before the use of collagen, 0.1 ml of skin test collagen must be injected subcutaneously into the volar surface of the forearm and observed for 4 weeks to rule out sensitivity. If the test is negative, then collagen injections can proceed. The skin test must be readministered prior to any repeat collagen treatments. Prior to injection, all patients should have a negative urine culture and receive perioperative antibiotics to prevent urosepsis post-procedure. This is especially important for the neurogenic bladder population, in whom urinary tract infections (UTIs) and bacteriuria are common. Children require a general anesthetic, but most adults, especially if they are insensate below the waist secondary to neurologic pathology, can tolerate the injection under local anesthetic or intravenous sedation. Some urologists prefer to inject all patients under general anesthetic in order to have better control over placement of the submucosal blebs. The patient is placed in the dorsal lithotomy position no matter which method of injection is used.

Periurethral technique. This method is often used in women. The urethra is injected with 2% lidocaine (lignocaine) jelly, and 1% lidocaine is injected periurethrally at 3 and 9 o'clock. A 20-gauge spinal needle is inserted at the 3 o'clock position and advanced under cystoscopic vision within the submucosal space toward the urethral lumen just distal to the bladder neck and proximal urethra. The bulking agent is slowly injected with the needle bevel facing the lumen until a mucosal bleb is raised. This process is repeated on the opposite side at 9 o'clock until the cystoscopic appearance of the lumen resembles that of lateral prostatic lobes meeting in the midline.

Transurethral technique. Although preferred for males, this method is often used in females as well. It requires a 21–24F cystoscope that can accommodate a 5F working element. A zero, 12, or 30 degree lens can be used.[18] The cystoscope is placed in the urethral lumen just proximal to the external sphincter and a needle delivery system (often 20-gauge) is placed through the working port of the cystoscope. The submucosal space is entered at 3 or 9 o'clock with the needle bevel pointing towards the urethral lumen. The bulking material is slowly injected until a sufficient bleb is raised. The process is repeated on the opposite side or anywhere else necessary to achieve good coaptation. Care should be taken to avoid more than one puncture at any single injection site in order to minimize extrusion. As with the periurethral technique, the cystoscope should not be advanced past the injection sites, because this can result in compression or extrusion of material and loss of the mucosal bleb.

Antegrade technique. This approach was developed in an attempt to achieve better closure of the bladder neck in males with scarred, noncompliant urethras post-prostatectomy. It can also be used in children or adults with previous bladder neck reconstruction in whom the urethral passage may not be wide enough or compliant enough to accommodate a cystoscope of the caliber needed to employ the needle delivery system. It can be done under general anesthetic, intravenous sedation, or spinal anesthesia. The bladder is distended with irrigation fluid and a suprapubic cystotomy is performed under cystoscopic guidance, then dilated to allow placement of a sheath large enough to accommodate the cystoscope. Antegrade cystoscopy is performed and the material is injected submucosally around the bladder neck until coaptation occurs. A suprapubic tube is left in postoperatively for 24–72 hours.

Postoperative care

Patients are discharged once they are able to void. If they go into retention, they can be taught intermittent catheterization with a small-caliber catheter. Some investigators place narrow-lumen urethral catheters for 24–72 hours post-procedure.[19] If the patient was performing intermittent catheterization preoperatively, he can usually resume catheterization with an 8–12F tube the same day of the procedure with little fear of significant molding of the material.[11,14]

Indications and patient selection

The role of injectable agents for the treatment of urinary incontinence in the neurogenic bladder population remains hard to define. Perhaps this is because there are no randomized controlled trials comparing one treatment modality with another in this subset of patients, and the literature mainly consists of case series comprised of small numbers and short follow-up. In examining these data, however, a few patterns emerge.

It is often said that the ideal candidate for urethral collagen injection has a stable, compliant, good capacity bladder with low VLPP.[14,16] Many investigators believe that detrusor overactivity or decreased compliance should be treated with anticholinergics and/or augmentation cystoplasty before attempting to treat an incompetent outlet with bulking agents.[14,20] Perez et al, however, in their series of 32 patients with neurogenic bladder, found that the presence of detrusor overactivity and decreased compliance did not adversely affect the clinical outcome.[21]

In addition to its role in leakage prevention, injection of collagen into the bladder neck and proximal urethra has also been used to provide outlet resistance in order to increase the bladder capacity of children with exstrophy-epispadias complex prior to bladder neck reconstruction.[22] Although this technique has been successful in a small number of patients, not every author has found this to be the case.[16]

Many investigators regard urethral bulking agents as adjuncts to other forms of treatment, but do not believe them capable of providing a durable cure for incontinence in the majority of patients with neurogenic voiding dysfunction when used as the sole source of intervention.[15,19,23] This is particularly true in the subset of children with exstrophy-epispadias complex who have undergone bladder neck reconstruction yet remain incontinent. Many of these patients were rendered dry or experienced substantial improvement after collagen injection.[14,19,21,22] Bomalaski et al, in their study of 40 children with neurogenic bladder, found statistically greater improvement in continence and postoperative satisfaction in the exstrophy-epispadias group than in the myelomeningocele group.[4]

Groups of investigators in Canada have determined that preoperative urodynamic data could not predict the clinical result of collagen injection.[14,20] Chernoff et al, however, in their series of 11 children, found that a preoperative VLLP of greater than 45 cmH_2O was predictive of injection failure.[16] A patulous bladder neck was thought to be a positive predictor of success by Kim et al, whose series of patients undergoing collagen injection contained 8 children with neurogenic bladder, 4 of whom had this finding on examination and were dry postinjection. These authors speculated that this cystoscopic feature, although indicative of a severely incompetent bladder outlet, may be a sign of more pliable, less-scarred tissue which would allow for optimal injection and, therefore, improved long-term treatment success.[24]

Contraindications to the use of injectable collagen for the treatment of urinary incontinence are known collagen sensitivity (a positive skin test), untreated detrusor overactivity, and untreated urinary tract infection. Scarring secondary to previous surgery or radiation treatment may decrease retention of collagen in tissue, thus contributing to its relatively poor efficacy.[11,19]

Results

Analysis of the studies published in the last 10 years on treatment of urinary incontinence with collagen injection reveals that the benefits derived from this agent by patients with neuropathic voiding dysfunction are comparable to those seen in the non-neurogenic incontinence population (Table 57.1). The proportion of patients rendered dry ranges from 20 to 50% in the majority of studies, although cure rates as low as 5% have been reported. The improvement rate, which is often the only outcome stated, ranges anywhere from 15 to 76%. The data are difficult to interpret and compare, since there is no standard definition of cure and improvement, and these terms are not always clearly delineated within the methodology of each study.

Most patients received between 1 and 4 injections, with the majority of responders having had only 1 or 2 treatments before assessment of clinical efficacy was made. The total volume of collagen injected ranged from 0.4 to 55 ml, with a total of less than 10 ml typically administered by most authors. In our experience, continence is rarely attained if a trial of 1 or 2 injections fails to achieve any improvement. We have employed three-dimensional ultrasound (3DUS) of the urethra as an objective outcome measure to aid in the decision as to whether or not to offer repeat collagen injection to patients who have failed to experience clinical improvement.[8,9] A treatment algorithm based on clinical outcome and 3DUS findings can be helpful in determining if additional collagen injections might be beneficial.[10] The administration of further collagen may be costly and delay more effective treatment. If a patient has poor retention of collagen or has some loss of an initially good result, reinjection may be an option. If a patient has good retention of collagen, yet still has symptoms, they will likely do better with another form of therapy.

Table 57.1 *Results of glutaraldehyde cross linked collages in patients with neurogernic incontinence*

Investigator	Year and patient population	Number of patients	Mean follow-up (months)	Mean amount collagen (ml)	Results	Complications	Comments
Capozza et al[22]	1995 pediatric	25–9NB, 16 EE	Range 9–36; no mean given	3 range 2.1–4.5	76% improved 9/9 NB, 10/16 EE	None	EEC patients had prior NB reconstruction
Bennett et al[11]	1995 adult	11–5 MMC, 5 SCI, 1 SC tumor	24 range 12–32	Females – 55 Males – 56	28% cured 36% improved	1 transient difficulty catheterizing	Series contained 9 men, 2 women
Ben-Chaim et al[19]	1995 3 adults, 16 children	19 – all EE	26 range 9–84	4 range 0.4–12	53% improved	1 UTI/epididymo-orchitis, 1 bladder perforation	15 patients had prior NB reconstruction
Perez et al[21]	1996 pediatric	32–24 MMC, 7 EE, 1 sacral teratoma	10 range 3–19	10 MMC, 7.5 EE range 3.5–17	MMC – 20% dry, 28% improved EEC – 43% dry, 14% improved	1 urosepsis, 2 transient worsening of incontinence	3/7 EEC patients had undergone previous NB reconstruction
Bomalaski et al[4]	1996 pediatric	40–25 MMC, 12 EE, rest non-neurogenic	25.2 range 3–75.6	10.2 range 2.5–22.5	22% cure, 54% improved Statistically significant decrease in pad use, dry interval, incontinence grade	None	8 patients followed for 4.5 years had overall cure/improvement of 86% Greater success with EE than with MMC
Leonard et al[14]	1996 pediatric	18–10 MMC, 6 EE	15 range 5–21	5 range 2.4–13	MMC – 3/6 cured, 2 improved EE – 2 cured, 2 improved	None	4 patients had ileocystoplasty, 7 had NB reconstruction, 4 had epispadias repair
Chernoff et al[16]	1997 pediatric	11–7 MMC, lSCI, 2EE, l urogenital sinus defect	14.4 range 4–20	Maximum injected 15 ml	36% dry, 18% improved	None	4 patients had previous ileocystoplasty, 3 had NB reconstruction
Sundaram et al[23]	1997 pediatric	20–12 MMC, 4 EE, 4 other neurogenic bladder causes	15.2 range 9–23	7.3 range 3–18	5% dry, 25% improved, 10 had transient improvement	None	2 patients had prior NB reconstruction
Kassouf et al[20]	2001 pediatric	20 – all MMC	50.4	6.3 range 2–13	10% dry, 15% improved, 14 had transient improvement	None	80% on CIC, all had stable bladder preoperation

CIC, clean intermittent catheterization; EEC, MMC, myelomeningocele; EE, exstrophy-epispadias complex; SCI, spinal cord injury; NB, neurogenic bladder.

Table 57.2 *Advantages and disadvantages of fascial bladder neck sling and artificial urinary sphincter (AUS)*

Surgical option	Advantages	Disadvantages
Bladder neck sling	1. No foreign body insertion 2. 'Pop-off' valve – allows leakage to occur at high intravesical pressure, protecting upper tracts 3. No concern with contamination of surgical field and infection seeding when performing a concomitant bladder augmentation	1. Majority of patients must catheterize to empty bladder 2. Less efficacious in males than females
AUS	1. Highly effective even for severe outlet incompetence 2. No 'pop-off' valve – may lead to upper tract deterioration in patients with poor preoperative compliance and high intravesical pressures 3. Allows some patients to void spontaneously without need for catheterization	1. Risk of revision for mechanical failure 2. Risk of infection and erosion

Although most studies reported moderate treatment efficacy with follow-up of 1–6.3 years, some investigators found collagen to be disappointing in terms of treatment outcome. In 20 children with neurogenic stress incontinence, Sundaram et al reported only 30% improvement in leakage status postcollagen injection, while the rest experienced transient improvement lasting an average of 52 days.[23] In children with myelomeningocele on intermittent catheterization, Kassouf et al found that only one-quarter of patients had a durable treatment response, with the rest failing at 3 months.[20] Suboptimal outcomes have been attributed in part to disruption of the collagen blebs by catheterization shortly after injection, but Sundaram et al did not find any difference in the outcome between patients on intermittent catheterization and those who voided spontaneously.[23]

Complications have been few and minor, consisting of UTI, urosepsis, epididymo-orchitis, transient difficulty with catheterization, and temporary worsening of urinary incontinence.[11,19,21] One patient sustained a bladder perforation requiring laparotomy and operative repair 3 days after injection which was felt by the investigators to be secondary to overfilling at the time of the procedure and subsequent difficulty emptying the bladder completely.[19]

Conclusion

In summary, treatment of stress urinary incontinence with glutaraldehyde cross-linked bovine collagen in the neurogenic bladder population has been demonstrated to be safe and variably successful, with follow-up extending past 5 years. Almost all the literature, however, deals with children, and very few data exist for adults with spinal cord injury or other acquired forms of neuropathic voiding dysfunction. Children with exstrophy-epispadias who have had previous bladder neck reconstruction have been found to be suitable candidates for collagen injection, as have patients with myelomeningocele. The relative efficacy of injectable agents, coupled with their minimally invasive nature and ease of administration, has continued to fuel the search for novel substances. Animal and human studies examining the feasibility of submucosal injection of autologous ear chondrocytes and autologous muscle-derived cells are currently underway in an attempt to find more durable, more biocompatible, and less allergenic alternatives to bovine collagen.[25,26] The ideal injectable agent has not yet been devised.

Bladder neck slings and wraps

Introduction

The fascial sling and the artificial urethral sphincter (AUS) are the two most commonly employed surgical treatments for patients with urinary incontinence secondary to neurogenic outlet incompetence. The pros and cons of bladder neck sling and artificial urethral sphincter are listed in Table 57.2. The issue of how much tension to place on the fascial sling is not as problematic in the neurogenic bladder population as it is in patients with stress urinary incontinence (SUI), since retention in a patient with neurogenic bladder who already performs intermittent catheterization (IC) is usually a treatment goal rather than a complication. Furthermore, the incidence of tension-induced erosion is low when autologous fascia is utilized as the sling material. Unfortunately, long-term experience with the bladder neck sling in the neurogenic bladder population is seldom reported, with most case series documenting mean follow-up times of less than 4 years. It is thus unknown whether or not the fascial sling in young women with myelomeningocele may be disrupted by pregnancy and childbirth.[27]

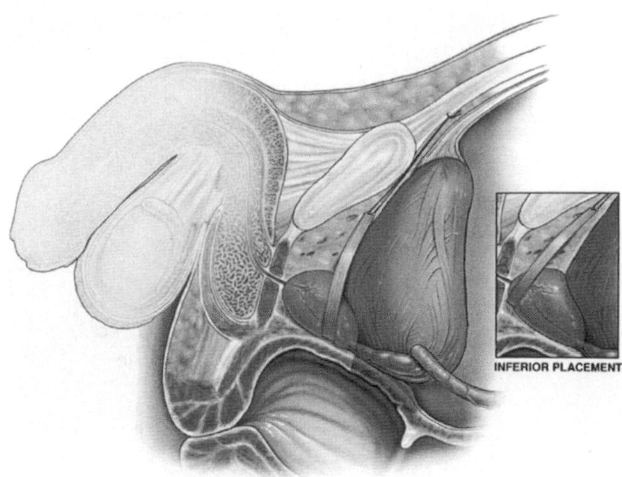

Figure 57.3
Placement of rectus fascia sling in a male patient. Sling is placed at the bladder neck posterior to the seminal vesicles.

Indications and patient selection

The ideal candidate for this procedure is a female patient with bladder outlet incompetence, preserved urethral length, and a well-managed bladder on IC.

Whether or not to perform enterocystoplasty in addition to a procedure to occlude the bladder outlet is a complex decision based on preoperative urodynamic and radiographic assessment. Bladder augmentation alone may be sufficient to cure incontinence in some neurogenic bladder patients despite low outlet resistance,[28] particularly in male children who have the potential for increased outlet competence with pubertal prostate growth. Conversely, supporting the bladder neck with a sling may be enough to abolish leakage if the preoperative urodynamic assessment, performed with some form of bladder outlet occlusion, shows a stable bladder with sufficient capacity and normal compliance.[29] Whether or not to perform both procedures together, or to do one before the other, is somewhat controversial. In general, a cystogram showing a wide open bladder neck and a VLPP less than 30 cmH_2O are indications of intrinsic sphincter deficiency, in which case a procedure to improve bladder outlet competence is recommended. Adherence to these guidelines, however, cannot always predict the patient's postoperative status. As Kreder and Webster demonstrated, a bladder neck sling may cause de-novo detrusor overactivity (DO) or decreased bladder capacity and compliance if performed without enterocystoplasty, despite a preoperative urodynamic work-up documenting normal detrusor parameters.[29] To avoid subjecting the patient to a second operation, some investigators have advocated the routine performance of concomitant enterocystoplasty and rectus fascial sling in all patients with neurogenic incontinence[30,31] One such proponent of this practice, Decter, found that the rate of postoperative leakage was higher in patients who did not undergo bladder augmentation along with bladder neck sling compared with patients who had both procedures.[31] The downside of this systematic approach, however, is that even though it saves some patients the morbidity of a second surgery, it may needlessly subject some others to the risks of enterocystoplasty.

Surgical techniques

Prior to undergoing a bladder neck sling, patients must have a negative urine culture. Perioperative broad-spectrum antibiotics are administered and, if a bladder augmentation is performed, they are continued postoperatively for a few days.

A bowel preparation should be considered in all patients undergoing concomitant enterocystoplasty. When performing both a sling and a bladder augmentation, the fascial harvest and bladder neck dissection are usually performed prior to the augmentation. Once the augmentation is completed, the fascial sling is positioned and secured in place.

A midline incision provides the best exposure if an enterocystoplasty is also to be done, but a Pfannenstiel incision can be employed, staying extraperitoneal, if only a sling is required.[32] The bladder neck dissection is often done via the abdominal incision, but a transvaginal or combined transabdominal–transvaginal approach can be employed in adult women, and has even been accomplished in adolescent girls with the help of a mediolateral episiotomy.[33] In the transabdominal dissection, the endopelvic fascia is incised bilaterally, the bladder neck and proximal urethra are freed circumferentially, and a Penrose drain is placed around the bladder neck. A finger in the vagina, or the rectum in males, can aid in the posterior dissection.[32] Some surgeons prefer just to clear a tunnel beneath the bladder neck rather than mobilizing around it completely.[30] In males, the dissection is identical to that performed for AUS bladder neck cuff placement, in that a plane is entered posterior to the bladder neck but anterior to the seminal vesicles.[34] The transvaginal dissection, if employed, is approached via a vertical midline or inverted U incision in the anterior vaginal wall. The incision should extend from 1.5 cm proximal to the urethral meatus to 1 cm proximal to the bladder neck, which is identified with the aid of the balloon of a urethral Foley catheter. The vaginal mucosa is dissected off the underlying periurethral fascia to expose the urethrovesical junction. After perforating the endopelvic fascia, the retropubic space is entered on either side of the bladder neck using a combination of sharp and blunt dissection. This dissection allows a ligature carrier to be passed safely from the suprapubic region to the vaginal area under fingertip guidance.

A strip of autologous rectus fascia 1.5–2 cm in width and 6–10 cm in length is usually employed, although fascia lata

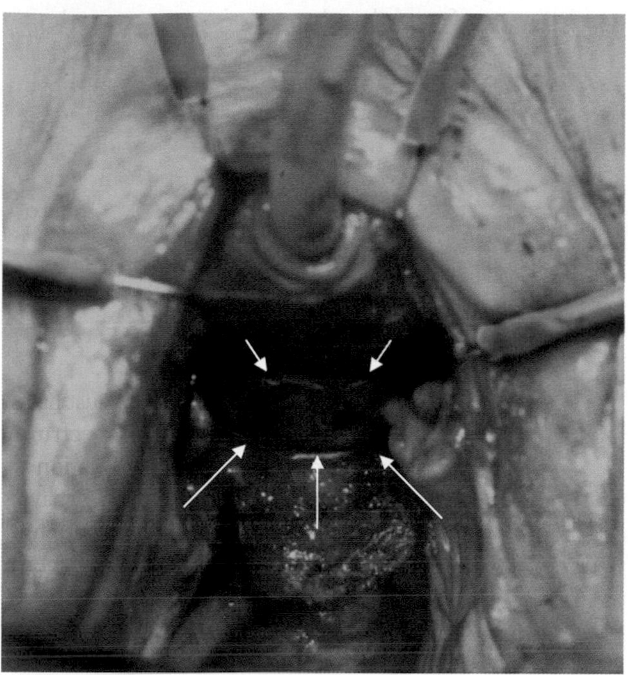

Figure 57.4
Correct placement of rectus fascia sling at the proximal urethra in a female patient (arrows indicate superior and inferior edges of the rectus sling).

may also be used. Marlex slings have also been placed, but the likelihood of infection and erosion is increased compared to autologous fascia.[34] The rectus fascia can be harvested transversely or longitudinally as a free graft, or one end of the fascial strip may be left attached to the anterior abdominal wall as a pedicle and secured to the opposite rectus sheath. In males, the sling is usually placed around the bladder neck and superior aspect of the prostate, although some surgeons place it around the distal prostatic urethra, where coaptation may be easier to achieve.[35] In females, the fascial strip is positioned around the bladder neck and proximal urethra. The sling is often sutured to the lateral edges of the bladder neck with absorbable suture to prevent rolling and displacement that may cause excessive urethral angulation or compression. If employing a free fascial graft, a zero or number one polypropylene stitch is passed through each end of the graft before the sling is positioned around the bladder neck. When the operation is done transvaginally, the sutures are brought out through the lower anterior abdominal wall using a ligature carrier passed through the retropubic space into the vaginal incision under fingertip guidance. The sutures are then tied down suprapubically at the end of the procedure. Some investigators have used Gortex bolsters or pledgets to prevent suture pull-through,[27,33] but this is not essential. Alternatively, the edges of fascia can be secured to Cooper's ligament[4] or the symphysis pubis.[31]

Several techniques have been recommended to optimize sling tension. In patients with neurogenic bladder on IC there is little concern with causing retention, but one should avoid tying the sutures too tightly to prevent urethral erosion and atrophy.[36] Elder describes filling the bladder with saline via a suprapubic tube and increasing tension on the sling until urethral leakage no longer occurs with manual bladder compression.[27] Other authors have tied the sutures so that no further movement of a Foley balloon at the bladder neck occurs, or so that 1 or 2 fingers can be placed between the knots and the fascia.[33] The sling sutures can also be tightened under cystoscopic control until the bladder neck appears closed.[31,32] Decter has suggested that, because of the prostate bulk, more tension needs to be applied to the sutures in males than in females to achieve adequate urethral elevation and compression.[31] The surgeon should ensure that catheterization can be performed before finalizing sling tension.[30]

Some surgeons leave a suprapubic tube and urethral Foley catheter in postoperatively, remove the Foley catheter within 1–2 weeks, and then the suprapubic tube once catheterization can be performed with no difficulties. Others leave just a suprapubic tube, which is removed after 1–3 weeks, depending on whether or not an enterocystoplasty was also performed.

Wrap procedures in which a pedicle of bladder detrusor, a strip of rectus fascia, a distally based rectus/pyramidalis myofascial flap, or a strip of soft polyprolene mesh is used to encircle the bladder neck completely have been employed by various authors in order to provide circumferential compression, tapering, and suspension of the bladder outlet.[35,37–39] In some cases, one end of the wrap is secured to the anterior abdominal wall fascia in order to elevate the bladder neck.[37,39] It has been theorized that catheterization may be easier with the bladder neck wrap than with the sling, since the suspending force is evenly distributed around the bladder neck, thereby avoiding urethral kinking.[35,38]

Some investigators, in addition to placing a sling support beneath the bladder neck, have tapered it to improve urethral coaptation and reduce sling tension, in an attempt to decrease the likelihood of erosion.[34] Techniques which have been described include excising a full-thickness diamond of tissue along the anterior aspect of the bladder neck and reapproximating the edges of mucosa and detrusor muscle with absorbable sutures, or, alternatively, excising full-thickness wedges of anterior bladder neck and prostate from the edges of a vertical midline incision extending to the level of the verumontanum, and tapering it over a 16F catheter.[32,34]

Results and complications

The literature on bladder neck slings to treat neurogenic urinary incontinence consists largely of case series, made up of pediatric or a mixture of pediatric and adult patients (Table 57.3). Mean follow-up ranges from 9 months to 4.5 years. Published success rates depend on the definition of

Table 57.3 *Results of fascial slings and wraps in patients with neurogenic bladder outlet incompetence*

Study	Year and patient population	Number and type of patients	Mean follow-up (months)	Surgical technique	Results	Other surgical procedures
Elder[27]	1990 adult and pediatric M and F	14: 10 F, 4 M all MMC	12 range 7–27	Periurethral or periprostatic RF sling, tied on abdominal wall	85.7% dry 1 nocturnal enuresis only	12 concomitant bladder augmentations
Herschorn and Radomski[34]	1992 adult M	13: 10 MMC, 3 SCI	34.3 range 5.5–49	2 Marlex, 11 RF pedicle sutured to opposite rectus sheath, BN tapering	69.2% dry	All had concomitant augmentations
Decter[31]	1993 adult and pediatric M and F	10: 6 F, 4 M 8 MMC, 2 SA	26.4	RF sling in 5, fascia lata in 5, symphyseal fixation	67% with augmentation dry, 25% without augmentation dry	6 concomitant bladder augmentations
Chancellor et al[119]	1993 adult F	14: neurogenic, patulous urethras	24 range 6–60	RF pedicle sling sutured to opposite abdominal wall	100% dry	5 concomitant augmentations, 5 cutaneous urostomy
Gormley et al[33]	1994 F adolescents	15: 8 MMC, 2 SA, 1 imperforate anus, 3 BN trauma	54 range 6–102	RF sling, combined abdominal and vaginal dissection, tied over abdominal wall	84.6% dry (2 redos using larger piece of RF) 1 using 1 pad/day	2 concomitant augmentations, 5 prior bladder outlet procedures
Walker et al[32]	1995 adult and pediatric M and F	17: 9 F, 8 M 10 MMC, 3 sacral lipoma, 4 other	16.2	RF sling, some with bladder neck tapering	94.1% dry 1 has some SUI	11 concomitant augmentations, 9 prior BN procedures
Kakizaki et al[36]	1995 adult and pediatric mostly M	13: 10 M, 3 F 8 MMC, 2 pelvic surgery, 1 SCI, 2 non-neurogenic patients	36 range 4–63	Sling of RF in 8, fascia lata in 5; BN placement in 11, bulbous urethra in 2; tied over abdominal wall	69.2% dry 23% improved	9 concomitant bladder augmentations
Kurzrock et al[35]	1996 pediatric M and F	24: 9 F, 15 M all MMC	Range 9–14	Bladder wall pedicle wrap suspended to pubic symphysis	100% F dry 66.7% M dry	6 prior augmentations, 1 prior RF sling
Fontaine et al[30]	1997 adult F	21: 9 MMC, 8 SCI, 3 SA, 1 sacral lipoma	28.6 range 6–60	RF sling done transabdominally, sutured to Cooper's	85.7% dry day and night 95.2% dry day only	All had concomitant bladder augmentation
Barthold et al[37]	1999 pediatric mostly F	27: 20 F, 7 M 21 MMC, 2 SA, 4 other	Wrap 43.2 sling 25.2	10 RF slings, 18 RF wraps, both secured to anterior abdominal wall	Wrap 28% dry, sling 50% dry ($p > 0.05$) 14.3% M dry, 50% F dry ($p = 0.02$)	19 concomitant, 1 prior, 2 subsequent augmentations, 17 Mitrofanofts
Austin et al[40]	2001 Pediatric M and F	18: 10 M, 8 F 16 MMC, 2 SCI	21.2 range 6–57	RF sling tied over anterior abdominal wall	78% dry, 2 dry with repeat sling	4 concomitant, 2 prior augmentations
Mingin et al[38]	2002 pediatric and adult M and F	37: 14 M, 23F 36 neurogenic, 1 traumatic	48 range 6–120	Distally based rectus/pyramidalis myofascial flap wrapped around BN and sewn to contralateral RF	92% (34) dry 2 M failures, 1 F failure	33 concomitant augmentations, 9 Mitrofanoft stomas, 5 reimplantations
Rutman et al [39]	2005 adult F	Neurologic/congenital diseases, multiple prior anti-incontinence procedures	12 months range 6–37	Soft polypropylene mesh wrap secured to anterior abdominal wall	20% failures 80% improved or cured	91% concomitant urethrolysis, 20% concomitant prolapse repair

MMC, myelomeningocele; SCI, spinal cord injury; SA,sacral agenesis; M, male; F, female; RF, rectus fascia; BN, bladder neck; SUI, stress urinary incontinence.

dryness used by the author. Continence has been described as no leakage occurring in between intermittent catheterization intervals of 3–4 hours or more, wearing less than 1 pad per day, or dry during the daytime only, with no consideration given to nocturnal incontinence. Most investigators report overall continence rates greater than 70%, with women faring better (85%) than men (69%) in some studies.[30,31,33–35] Kurzrock et al suggest that this discrepancy in sling effectiveness between the sexes may be because the prostate makes it more difficult to close and elevate the proximal urethra.[35] Fascial bladder neck wraps have not been found to be any more effective at preventing urinary leakage than slings.[35,37,38]

Complications specific to the rectus fascia sling are relatively rare and include sling breakdown resulting in postoperative leakage as a result of fascial breakage or suture pullout and urethral erosion.[31,32] The urethra may become angulated, resulting in difficulty with catheterization or retraction of the meatus into the vaginal introitus.[32] Care needs to be taken when passing a cystoscope via the urethra post-sling insertion. Elder[27] and Barthold et al[37] have described cases in which patients who were initially dry after surgery became incontinent after the performance of transurethral instrumentation. Bladder perforation may occur in patients with augmented bladders and bladder neck slings who are not compliant with IC, or in whom catheterization has become difficult.[30,37,40] Other reported complications are incisional hernia, de-novo DO, retroperitoneal hematoma, and bladder neck contracture when the outlet is tapered along with sling insertion.[32,34]

Conclusion

The rectus fascia bladder neck sling has been shown to be a versatile and valuable addition to the armamentarium of the reconstructive surgeon. Despite its lower rate of success in males with neurogenic incontinence, the lack of requirement for foreign materials and relative ease of implantation make it an attractive option for treatment of the incompetent reservoir outlet in a wide variety of patients. The long-term durability of the bladder neck sling, however, is still unknown. This is an important consideration, particularly for children, in whom the procedure may have to last decades. Many authors speculate that with growth the sling should maintain its functional obstruction of the bladder outlet, but longer follow-up is required.

Artificial urinary sphincters

Introduction

Ever since the first published clinical report in 1973 by Scott, the AUS has been used extensively to treat sphincteric incontinence.[41] High rates of efficacy and patient satisfaction, but also substantial revision rates secondary to mechanical failure as well as problems with infection and erosion resulting in sphincter removal have been reported. The high initial cost of the device, compounded with the cost of replacing components when they malfunction or wear out, makes it an expensive treatment option. Despite its availability since the 1970s, concerns have also been raised regarding silicone shedding, particularly in children, since the long-term sequelae of silicone migration is unknown.[42] There have been relatively few large series of AUS use in neurogenic patients, and there are no controlled trials comparing its efficacy to that of fascial slings or bladder neck reconstruction.

History and design evolution

The AUS 800 represents the culmination of a number of design modifications which have occurred since 1975 when the patent for the original device, the AMS 721, was issued to American Medical Systems (Minnetonka, Minnesota). This early model operated on the hydraulic principle still employed by the modern AUS, but there was no way to control the occlusive force applied to the urethra and the large number of components made it difficult to implant.[43] In 1980, the AMS 721 was altered to overcome these problems by streamlining the design and incorporating a pressure-regulating balloon reservoir, which was then marketed as the AMS 761. The AMS 742, 791, and 792 represented further design simplifications and introduced the concept of delayed activation in order to allow for tissue healing. With these devices, a second surgical procedure was needed to activate the pump.[43]

In 1982, the AMS 800 was introduced and is the only AUS currently available on the market.[44] Like its predecessors, it consists of three components: a cuff which fits around the urethra or bladder neck; a balloon fluid reservoir which is implanted in the abdomen; and a pump which is implanted in the scrotum or labia to control activation. The cuff is composed of an outer layer of Dacron (polyethylene terephthalate) monofilament backing an inner silicone shell, and is available in sizes ranging from 4 to 11 cm with 0.5 cm increments. Three different balloon reservoirs are available with plateau pressures of 51–60 cmH_2O, 61–70 cmH_2O, and 71–80 cmH_2O. The pump and reservoir are also made of silicone and are connected to each other and the pump by kink-resistant color-coded tubing. The sphincter is implanted fully primed with isotonic radiopaque fluid or normal saline in its deactivated state. The device is activated a few weeks later by sharply squeezing the bulb of the pump. This maneuver allows fluid to exit the reservoir and enter the hollow cuff, thereby occluding the urethra or bladder neck lumen. When the patient wishes to void, he pumps the bulb to direct fluid

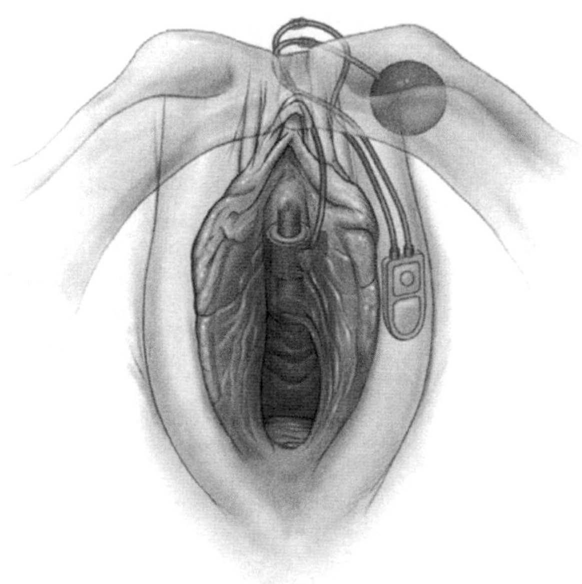

Figure 57.5
Placement of the AMS-800 in a female patient. (Reproduced with permission from The Urinary Sphincter, Chapter 34, Fig. 5.)

out of the cuff and back into the reservoir. Fluid moves back into the cuff, closing it automatically within 3–5 min. Should urethral or bladder instrumentation be necessary, the unit can be locked or deactivated by pressing a button on the pump.

In 1988, a cuff with Dacron backing that was narrower than the silicone surface facing the urethra (narrow-backed cuff) was incorporated into the AMS 800 design along with alterations in the manufacturing process used to make the reservoir. These modifications improved durability and decreased urethral pressure atrophy.[45] There have been no further changes to the AMS 800 design.

Indications and patient selection

All patients in whom an AUS is being considered should undergo preoperative urodynamic testing to document the severity and mechanism of incontinence and to assess bladder function. Determination of detrusor parameters may require bladder neck occlusion with a Foley catheter balloon during the filling phase.[46] As for the fascial sling, the ideal candidate for an AUS should have a stable bladder with good compliance and capacity as well as a good emptying. Elevated detrusor pressures can lead to upper tract deterioration once the outlet is occluded by the sphincter cuff. De Badiola et al compared the preoperative and postoperative urodynamic parameters of 23 pediatric patients who received an AUS for neurogenic sphincteric incompetence. Patients with filling pressures of less than 50 cmH_2O with preoperative bladder capacities greater than or equal to 60% of that expected for age, and/or a preoperative compliance greater than 2 ml/cmH_2O, were less likely to require subsequent augmentation for persistent incontinence and upper tract changes.[47] The average time to cystoplasty in patients who developed high intravesical pressures after AUS implantation was 14 months.[47]

Many authors advocate an AUS as primary treatment for patients who can void spontaneously.[48] Patients, however, should be informed that IC may have to be performed in the future, particularly if they receive a bladder augmentation or, in men, if prostatic growth later in life produces outlet obstruction. The AUS has also been employed as secondary treatment for patients who have failed other forms of bladder outlet surgery. Aliabadi and Gonzalez described 15 patients who had failed multiple urethral and bladder neck surgeries and were salvaged with an AUS, resulting in an overall continence rate of 73%.[49]

The optimal timing for US insertion in the pediatric population with neurogenic incontinence is controversial. Kryger et al found no difference in the number of AUS removals, continence rate, revision rate, augmentation rate, or number of complications in patients who received an AUS before age 11 compared to those placed later in life. AUS insertion, in fact, may be easier in prepubertal patients secondary to the shallower pelvis and lesser degree of periurethral venous plexus engorgement. Revisions for retraction of the pump in the scrotum were uncommon, occurring only in 1 of their 25 patients.[48] Levesque et al also found no increase in the rate of AUS revision post-puberty, with a follow-up of 12.1 years.[50]

Although Fulford et al[44] have reported a cuff erosion rate of 44% in females, and Levesque et al[50] found a higher rate of erosion in girls who had previous bladder neck surgery, other investigators have not. Salisz and Diokno described successful AUS insertion in women despite intraoperative injuries to the vagina, bladder, or urethra. Their technique involved closing the injury primarily, placing the cuff within a different plane of dissection around the bladder neck, and delaying sphincter activation for a minimum of 6 weeks.[51]

Surgical technique

AUS insertion can be performed under general or spinal anesthesia. The cuff is usually placed around the bladder neck in women and children and around the bulbar urethra in males. The dorsal lithotomy position is favored in order to access the perineum for bulbar urethral placement, or to place a finger in the vagina to aid in transabdominal dissection of the bladder neck. The urine should be sterile before surgery and the skin should be free of dermatitis or candidiasis. Broad-spectrum perioperative intravenous antibiotics are administered. Strict sterile precautions are followed in the operating room and many

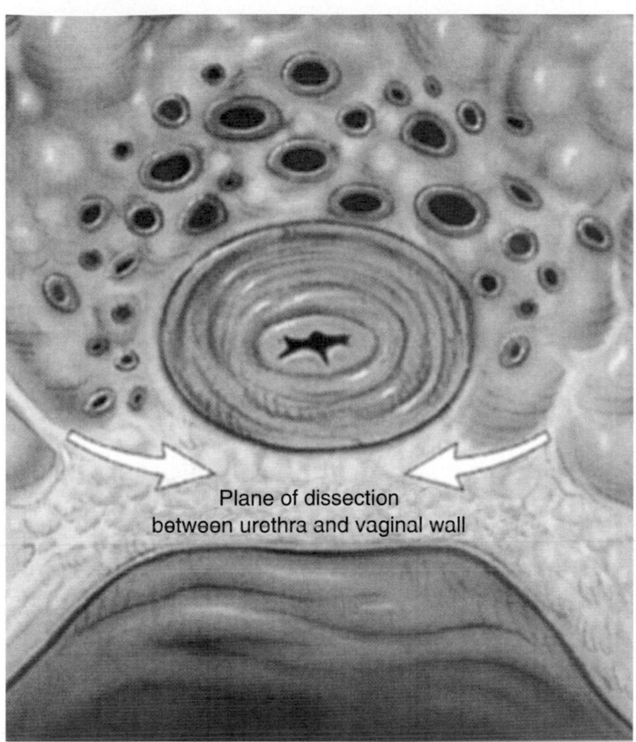

Figure 57.6
Transvaginal view of urethra and anterior vaginal wall to show dissection plane between the vagina and urethra/bladder neck.

surgeons prepare the patient with a 10–15 min antiseptic soap scrub before painting the abdomen and perineum with an antiseptic solution. Once the patient has been draped, a Foley catheter is inserted into the bladder.

Dissection of the bladder neck proceeds in much the same fashion as for placement of a fascial sling (see earlier). A 2 cm wide window behind the bladder neck is adequate for cuff placement, and a right-angled clamp is used to pass the measuring device around the bladder neck. Bladder neck cuff sizes range from 6 to 11 cm in diameter. Limited injuries to the bladder or vagina can be repaired primarily, but rectal injuries require abortion of the procedure. Once the appropriate-sized cuff is placed around the bladder neck, the cuff tubing is brought out through the rectus fascia via a separate stab incision superior to the pubis. The reservoir is placed in the retropubic space with its tubing penetrating the rectus fascia near the cuff tubing. A 71–80 cmH_2O balloon is often used for bladder neck occlusion. The reservoir can also be inserted into the peritoneal cavity, a location preferred by some to permit better balloon expansion.[43]

The anterior rectus sheath is closed and the balloon reservoir is filled with 22 ml of normal saline or an iso-osmotic contrast solution for postoperative X-ray imaging of the AUS. The pump mechanism is placed subcutaneously in the most dependent part of the scrotum or the labia. This space is created by passing a long curved Kelly clamp or sponge forceps from the lower edge of the suprapubic incision into the hemiscrotum or labium. The site of pump placement depends on whether the patient is left- or right-handed. A Babcock clamp can be placed around the pump tubing to prevent it from riding up while the components are being assembled. All tubing must be cleared of bubbles and blood clots before being connected. Straight or right-angled connectors can be used and secured with the quick-connect system or hand-tied with 2–0 or 3–0 polypropylene sutures in revision cases. The device should be cycled intraoperatively to make sure the cuff inflates and deflates properly. Some surgeons perform this maneuver while visualizing the cuff directly with flexible cystoscopy. Others perform perfusion sphincterometry to confirm proper sphincter function, to exclude unsuspected urethral injury, and to determine the refill time of the device.[52] All AUS components and incisions are irrigated copiously with antibiotic solution throughout the procedure. Before closing the incision, the AUS is deactivated by squeezing the button on the pump before it refills completely.

Placement of the cuff around the bulbar urethra begins by making a vertical incision in the perineum with its midpoint at the lower edge of the ischeal tuberosities. A Lonestar or Turner–Warwick retractor is recommended for better exposure. After incising the bulbocavernosus muscle along its midline, the bulbar urethra is mobilized circumferentially for a distance of 2–3 cm. If the urethra is injured, then the procedure should be terminated and the Foley catheter left indwelling after the injury is repaired with fine absorbable suture. A measuring device is passed around the urethra and the appropriate-sized cuff is placed. Most adult male patients will be fitted a 4.5 cm cuff, but sizes of 4 and 5 cm are also available. The cuff tubing and tab are oriented laterally so that neither one abuts the base of the penis, which can be uncomfortable postoperatively. The reservoir is placed in the retropubic space through a separate abdominal incision. The operation proceeds as described above.

Relatively, a transscrotal technique of cuff placement has been popularized.[53] After an upper transverse scrotal incision is made, the tunica albuginea of both corpora cavernosa are exposed, and the bulbar urethra is dissected free circumferentially. The cuff sizer is used to measure urethral circumference, then the occlusive cuff is placed around the urethra in standard fashion. The pressure-regulating balloon is placed similar to a penile implant reservoir. The transversalis fascia is pierced immediately above the pubic bone and the pressure-regulating balloon is placed within the retropubic space. A subdartos pouch is created for the pump. This approach is especially helpful in revision surgery.

To circumvent retention secondary to edema, a catheter is usually left in the bladder overnight and removed the next morning. Patients are discharged on oral antibiotics for 10–14 days after completing 24–48 hours of intravenous therapy. Patients should avoid heavy lifting, straining, and intercourse for 4–6 weeks. The AUS is activated in the clinic 4–6 weeks after its insertion and the patient is instructed in its use. Patients should inform medical personnel that they have an AUS when entering the hospital for surgery or any other procedure that may involve bladder catheterization, since the cuff should be deactivated beforehand to avoid damage to the device and the urethra. Patients should also carry the AUS information card provided by the manufacturer and obtain a Medicalert bracelet in case of accident or injury.

Results and complications

In patients with neurogenic sphincteric incontinence, the AUS has been reported to result in continence rates of 59–92%, revision rates of 27–57%, and removal rates of 19–41% (Table 57.4).[48,50,54–59] Perioperative and immediate postoperative complications include bladder neck, urethral, and rectal perforations, UTIs, wound infections, and scrotal hematomas.[54,55] In the long term, mechanical problems are the most common reason for revision surgery and include tubing kinks, fluid loss secondary to pump, reservoir, or cuff leaks, pump migration, pump dysfunction, and connector separation.[45,56,57,59] Nonmechanical complications consist of urethral atrophy, infection, erosion, and elevated bladder storage pressures which can result in reflux, hydronephrosis, and renal insufficiency.[45,50,54] In the Mayo Clinic series of 323 AUS patients, 26 of whom had myelomeningocele, both types of complications were shown to decrease after 1988 with incorporation of the narrow-backed cuff and improved manufacturing process: the rate of mechanical failure fell from 21 to 7.5% and the nonmechanical failure rate dropped from 17 to 9%.[45]

Infection, one of the most dreaded complications, results in sphincter removal, and accounts for 4–5% of most series.[43] Proposed mechanisms include contamination during the procedure, exposure of the AUS to chronically infected urine, and hematogenous spread of bacteria with seeding of the device.[61] The presence of an infection is often indicated by skin erythema, induration at the pump or reservoir site, erosion of the cuff through the urethra, or erosion of the pump through the scrotal or labial skin. Microorganisms recovered from infected AUS include *Staphylococcus epidermidis*, β-streptococcus, *Bacteroides fragilis*, *Escherichia coli*, *Pseudomonas*, and diphtheroid species.[61–63] A pseudocapsule made of myofibroblasts surrounds the silicone parts of the AUS and may confer protection against bacteria, which can be liberated into the bloodstream at the time of cystoplasty or with systemic infections.[62] The infection rate does not appear to increase in patients who catheterize compared to those who void spontaneously or who empty their bladders using the Credé maneuver.[62] Some investigators have found a definite increase in the occurrence of infection when cystoplasty is performed concomitantly with AUS insertion.[50,55] Holmes et al found an increased incidence of infection to be associated with prior bladder neck surgery in the neurogenic bladder population and recommended performing the AUS insertion before doing the augmentation in patients who have this risk factor.[61] Miller et al performed simultaneous bladder augmentation and AUS insertion using a variety of different bowel segments and found a 6.9% infection rate (2/29 patients). They suggested performing gastrocystoplasty along with AUS insertion since there were no infections associated with the use of stomach in their series.[63]

Erosion rates range from 6 to 31% in contemporary neurogenic bladder series and are the major cause of sphincter removal. Erosion can occur secondary to infection, ischemia from high cuff pressures, devascularization from prior surgery or radiation, and traumatic catheterization.[44,54,61] Factors which increase the likelihood of erosion include prior bladder neck surgery, placement of the cuff around the bulbar urethra in children, and placement of the cuff around the bowel used to form a neobladder.[44,54,59] Guralnick et al described AUS cuff placement through a dissection plane deep to the tunica albuginea of the corporal bodies in 31 men who experienced erosion or atrophy at the original cuff site. They were able to salvage continence in 84% of cases, but there was the potential for postoperative deterioration of erectile function.[64]

Patients who receive an AUS must undergo long-term urologic follow-up with urodynamic bladder monitoring and serial upper tract imaging to detect the onset of upper tract deterioration. High intravesical pressure requires the institution of anticholinergic medications, or, if this fails, augmentation. Hydronephrosis or reflux is usually refractory to medical management and indicates a need for cystoplasty. The proportion of AUS recipients with neurogenic bladder who ultimately require augmentation cystoplasty ranges from 4 to 42%.[49,54,56,59] Patients who are noncompliant with surveillance protocols may develop upper tract damage. A number of authors have described the occurrence of chronic renal failure in patients with incontinence of neurologic etiology who received an AUS and were then lost to follow-up for long periods of time.[45,49,57]

Conclusions

When it was first marketed in the early 1970s, the AUS represented a major advancement in the treatment of patients with severe incontinence secondary to sphincteric deficiency. The device has undergone many design modifications since its first inception, all of which have served to increase its efficacy and lower its complication rate. Erosion and infection rates are low in well-selected patients. The possibility of requiring repeat surgery for

Table 57.4 *Results of artificial urinary sphincter insertion for the treatment of incontinence in patients with neurogenic bladder*

Study	Year	Patient population	Type and location of sphincter	Mean follow-up time	Results	Complications
Bellioli et al[57]	1992	Adolescents 37: 35 male, 2 female 33 MMC, 3 SA, 1 pelvic surgery	2 AMS 792, 35 AMS 800 33 BN, 4 BU	4.5 years range 1–8.5	59% dry day and night 90% dry day only	2 upper tract deteriorations 38% reoperation rate for mechanical problems 1 infection, 1 BN perforation 1 scrotal hematoma
Gonzalez et al[56]	1995	Pediatric 19 males all neurogenic	11 AMS 800 8 AMS 721 or 792 all BN placement	8 years	84.2% continent 73.8% catheterizing	36.8% postoperative augmentation rate 1 renal loss 10% new hydro
Levesque et al[50]	1996	Adult and pediatric Most with MMC 36:22 male, 14 female before 1985 After 1985 18 children	Before 1985: 6 AMS 792, 18 AMS 292, 12 AMS 300 After 1985: all AMS 800 All BN placement	13.7 years	Mean survival time 12.1 years 82% dry 64% catheterizing 59% continent	6 developed renal failure 42% required postoperative augmentation
Singh and Thomas[55]	1996	Mostly adult 90: 75 male, 15 female 65 MMC, 19 SCI, 5 SA, 1 sacral angioma	82 AMS 800 8 AMS 792 BU and BN	4 years range 1–10	92% continent 79% with detrusor overactivity required augmentation 78% catheterizing	28% reoperation rate 6 infections, 7 erosions, 8 system failures, 2 pump failures, 1 cut tube, 1 rectal perforation, 1 bladder perforation
Simeoni et al[54]	1996	Pediatric 107: 74 male, 33 female 92 MMC	AMS 800 98 BN, 9 BU	61 months minimum of 12	41% continent with no revisions 21% augmentation rate	Immediate: 4 UTI, 2 wound infection, 3 scrotal hematoma, 3 urinary fistula, 2 retention 25% removal rate 59% revision rate 13% erosion rate
Fulford et al[44]	1997	Adult and pediatric 61: 43 male, 18 female 34 neurogenic, 15 post-radiation prostatectomy, 12 other	Combination of AMS 791, 792, and 800 BU and BN placement	10–15 years	75% functioning	49 with 1 or more revision 13% continent with original AUS *in situ* 31% erosion rate, 2/3 in 1st year after placement
Elliot and Barrett[45]	1998	Adult 323: 313 male, 10 female 70 neurogenic	All AMS 800 139 without narrow cuff backing 184 with narrow cuff backing 272 BU, 51 BN	68.8 months range 18–153	Males 27% reoperation Rate, females: 60% reoperation rate 90.4% functioning at 5 years, 72% no reoperation at 5 years	Mechanical failure: 21% pre-cuff, 7.6% post-cuff Non-mechanical failure: 17% pre-cuff, 9% post-cuff
Kryger et al[48]	2001	Pediatric 32: 25 male, 7 female Group 1 – insertion before age 11 (21) Group 2 – insertion after age 11 (11)	AMS 800–21 Pre-AMS 800–11	1 year	Group 1–54% intact, all dry Group 2–64% intact, 86% dry 15.4 years No statistical significant difference between groups	56% revision rate Group 1–43% removed: 4 infection, 5 erosion Group 2–36% removed: 1 infection, 3 erosions
Castera et al[59]	2001	Pediatric 49: 39 male, 10 female 38 MMC, 7 exstrophy, 4 trauma	All AMS 800 29 BN 20 BU	7.5 years range 2–11	67% dry: 86% dry with no prior surgery, 37.5% dry with prior BN surgery	20% erosion, 4% infection, 12% mechanical failure
Spiess et al[58]	2002	Pediatric 30 males with MMC	All AMS 800	6.5 years	63% dry, 20% slightly wet	Only 8.3% lasted > 100 months, mean lifetime 4.9 years
Pereira[60]	2006	Adolescents 35: 13 F, 22 M MM 27, SA 4, 4 other	All AMS 800, BN, 13 also had augment	5.5 years (range 4–11)	91.4% dry	8.6% BN erosions, 20% mechanical failure, 7 with worsened bladder function

MMC,myelomeningocele; SA, sacral agenesis; SCI, spinal cord injury; BN, bladder neck; BU, bulbar urethra; UTI, urinary tract infection.

mechanical failure is high, as is the cost of these revisions, but the AUS will, no doubt, continue to be utilized in the treatment of urinary incontinence.

Bladder neck reconstruction

Introduction

In 1908, Young described a technique for increasing bladder outlet resistance by narrowing the urethra and bladder neck lumen to the size of a silver probe.[65] Since this first description of bladder neck reconstruction was published, there have been many modifications to the surgical procedure. At first, reconfiguring the bladder outlet to increase its resistance was thought to be contraindicated in the neurogenic bladder population because of the subsequent necessity for IC.[66] Many investigators, however, have found this technique to be a viable alternative to bladder neck sling, AUS, or urinary diversion in patients with neurologic lesions who require treatment for severe sphincteric incompetence provided that the patient and/or caregiver is capable of performing IC and is compliant with this routine. These procedures are technically challenging and a successful outcome is highly dependent on the operative experience of the surgeon.

The main types of bladder neck reconstruction that have been utilized in the neurogenic bladder population are the Kropp anterior bladder wall flap valve and the Salle anterior bladder wall flip-flap. The Young–Dees–Leadbetter posterior bladder wall flap is primarily used for the treatment of bladder exstrophy, but has been reported in patients with neurogenic sphincteric deficiency. The Tanagho and Smith bladder neck reconstruction, which is mostly of historic interest, has been described in patients with post-prostatectomy incontinence and will not be covered in this section.[66,67] The majority of the literature deals with the pediatric population, since it is in this age group that urologic intervention is first sought. The Kropp and Salle procedures work on the flap valve principle popularized by Mitrofanoff. As the bladder fills with urine, increases in intravesical pressure are transmitted to the valve constructed from anterior bladder wall, thereby increasing leak-point threshold and preventing incontinence.[68] The Young–Dees–Leadbetter reconstruction prevents urine leakage by increasing bladder neck and urethral length and decreasing their caliber, two maneuvers which result in an increase in outlet resistance.[65]

Young–Dees–Leadbetter procedure

The Young–Dees–Leadbetter bladder neck reconstruction, as it was first described by Leadbetter in 1964, involves lengthening the urethra and creating a new bladder neck using a flap of posterior bladder wall which incorporates the trigone. The ureters are reimplanted 3–4 cm superiorly so that the trigonal muscle can be utilized. The posterior bladder wall is not mobilized in order to keep the blood and nervous supply intact, thereby helping to prevent slough and denervation of the bladder wall flap. The vertical midline cystotomy which was made to reimplant the ureters is carried into the urethra, and longitudinal lateral incisions are made on either side of the urethra and bladder neck. These incisions begin at the apex of the midline urethral incision and extend along the bladder base through the old ureteric orifice sites and 1–2 cm beyond them on the posterior bladder wall.

The resulting lateral bladder flaps are denuded of mucosa to leave a posterior strip of bladder 1.5 cm wide and 3 cm long.[69] These flaps are then folded over on each other using an 8–10F urethral catheter as a guide to caliber and closed in two layers. The mucosal layer is closed with interrupted fine absorbable suture and the muscle layer is opposed in an overlapping fashion using a fine running suture of absorbable material. The bladder neck closure is completed in layers: mucosa, muscle, and serosa. The end result is a urethra which is lengthened by 4–5 cm. The dog ears of bladder that remain are incorporated into the bladder wall closure, since resection of these segments can result in a substantial decrease in bladder capacity.[65] A urethral catheter and suprapubic tube are often placed, although some surgeons prefer to forgo urethral stenting. If employed, the urethral Foley catheter is removed within 3–4 weeks and the suprapubic tube is discontinued once the patient is able to empty the bladder by voiding or intermittent catheterization.

Placement of a silicone sheath around the bladder neck reconstruction to facilitate the insertion of an artificial urethral sphincter cuff later on if required was advocated by Mitchell et al in 1985. These authors, however, later abandoned this practice upon experiencing a 67% erosion rate at a mean of 4 years after operation.[70] Ransley's group, however, has reported a lower erosion rate of 14% after decreasing the thickness of the silicone sheath and interposing omentum between the sheath and the bladder neck.[70,71]

Kropp bladder neck reconstruction

The Kropp procedure was first described by Kropp and Aangwafo in 1986. It lengthens the urethra by attaching it to a tube of bladder muscle which is implanted into the posterior bladder wall through a submucosal tunnel to create a one-way flap valve that allows a catheter to be passed but prevents urine from leaking out. A rectangular flap 5–7 cm × 2–2.5 cm is outlined on the anterior bladder wall with stay sutures. This flap is left attached to the bladder neck and the bladder is separated completely from the bladder neck. The anterior wall flap is rolled into a tube over a 10–12F Foley catheter and sutured together with 4–0 chromic catgut. A submucosal tunnel is developed between the ureteric orifices, and the tube is pulled through this tunnel. The bladder is drawn back down to the bladder neck and sutured with absorbable sutures. The ostia of the new urethra is

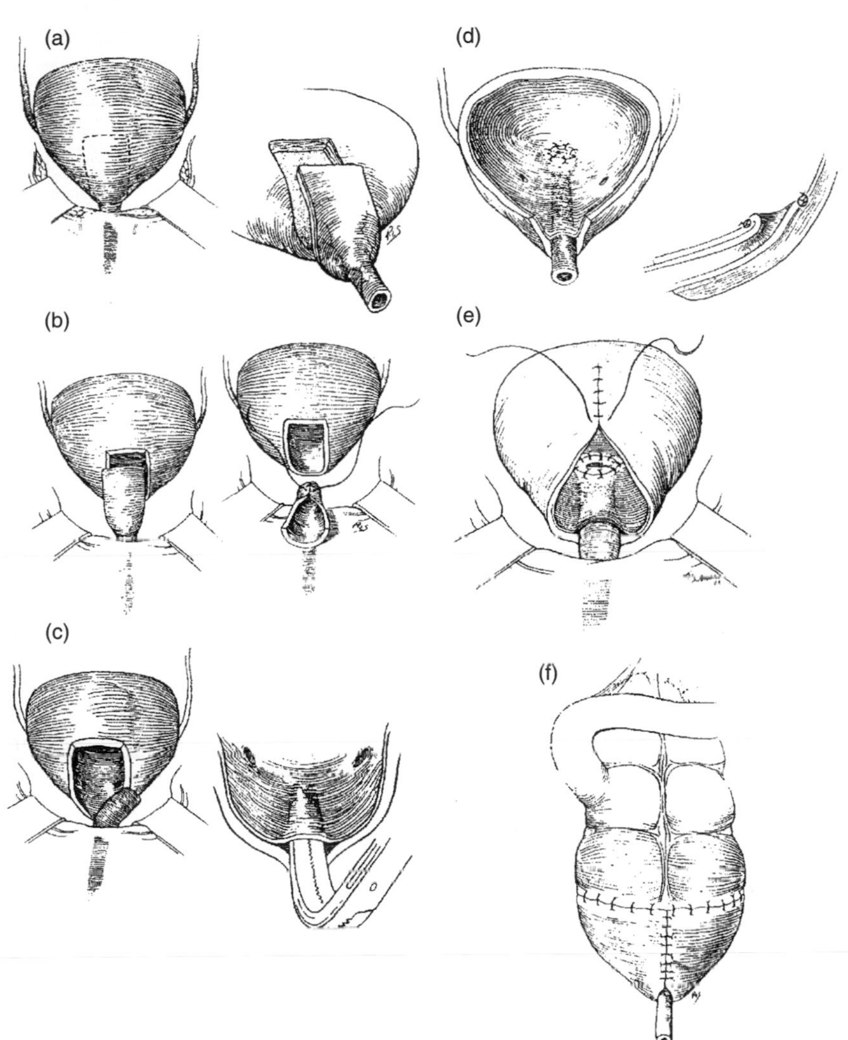

Figure 57.7
Kropp anterior flap-valve bladder neck reconstruction. (Reproduced with permission from Kropp and Angwolfo, J Urol 1986; 135: 533–6.)

sutured to the posterior bladder wall. This method can also be accomplished using a posterior strip of bladder, which is tunneled into the anterior bladder wall.[72]

Two modifications to the Kropp bladder neck reconstruction were described by Belman and Kaplan and subsequently adopted widely by other surgeons, including the originator of the Kropp procedure.[73] These alterations involve leaving the bladder neck attached to the bladder and making a groove in the posterior bladder wall into which the tube is laid, then suturing the epithelium over the tube rather than creating a submucosal tunnel.[74] Mollard et al demuscularized the bladder tube, leaving only mucosa to tunnel in some cases, and reimplanted one of the ureters cephalad to make more room to tunnel the tube in the posterior bladder wall.[68]

Pippi Salle bladder neck reconstruction

In 1994, Pippi Salle described his own version of the anterior wall flap valve in 15 dogs and 6 children with myelomeningocele. The Salle bladder neck reconstruction is a modification of the Kropp design in which the urethra is lengthened with an anterior bladder wall flap 4–5 cm × 1–1.7 cm, which is sutured to the posterior wall in an onlay fashion. In the original description, the ureters are reimplanted superiorly using the Cohen cross-trigonal technique. A border of mucosa 0.1 cm wide is removed from the flap to obtain separate nonoverlapping suture lines. The edges of the posterior bladder wall are then sewn over the lengthened urethra to create a flap valve. A urethral catheter is left in for 2–3 weeks.[75] In 1997 Salle and colleagues described a number of modifications to the original technique. The first involved making two longitudinal incisions in the trigonal mucosa to better expose the muscle for suturing to the exposed muscle edges of the anterior wall flap, then suturing the lateral edges of posterior wall mucosa over the flap to help prevent leakage of urine and fistula formation. The second modification was to widen the base of the flap to improve its blood supply but to leave the distal tip narrow to attain the correct lumen size when fashioning the neourethra. In some cases, a superior extension of mucosa was taken with the anterior wall flap and

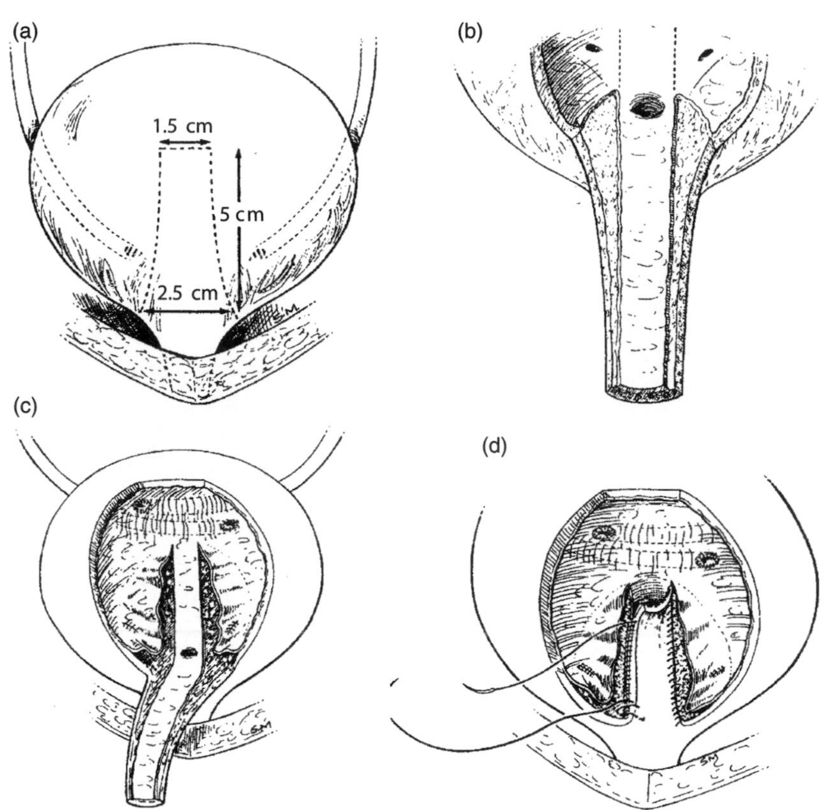

Figure 57.8
Pippi Salle flip-flap bladder reconstruction. (Reproduced with permission from Pippi-Salle, J Urol 1994; 152: 803–6.)

folded back over the intravesical urethra to cover it and prevent fistula formation. Lastly, the authors described the creation of a lateral anterior wall flap in 4 patients who had a midline scar in the anterior bladder wall from previous surgery. Ureteric reimplantations were not performed routinely in this later series.[76]

Indications and patient selection

All patients being considered for bladder neck reconstruction should undergo urodynamic assessment and voiding cystourethrogram to document the mechanism of incontinence and the degree of urethral incompetence. The filling phase should be carried out with a Foley balloon occluding the bladder outlet to determine bladder capacity, stability, and compliance.[43] Cystoscopy may aid in assessing the characteristics of the bladder wall and outlet before surgery. The urodynamic prerequisites for bladder neck reconstruction are similar to those for the AUS or bladder neck sling: a stable, adequate capacity bladder (see above). The majority of authors recommend the concomitant performance of bladder augmentation, since increasing outlet resistance will often lead to elevated storage pressures and the use of bladder wall to reconstruct the outlet can significantly decrease bladder capacity.[77,78]

Although bladder neck reconstruction can be performed as a salvage procedure for patients who have failed bladder neck sling or AUS insertion,[79] many authors advocate considering it as a primary option in patients who have total incontinence secondary to a patulous, wide-open bladder neck, since compromised blood supply from previous surgery will decrease the success of the operation.[74] Bladder neck reconstruction in general is not suitable for the correction of mild stress urinary incontinence, since it has a significant complication rate.

The Young–Dees–Leadbetter bladder neck reconstruction is mainly employed in the treatment of anatomic bladder outlet defects encountered in the exstrophy-epispadias complex; there have been few reports of its use in patients with neurogenic bladder. Continence rates are not as high in patients with neuropathic outlet incompetence as they are in the exstrophy population, and some investigators have documented better results in females than in males.[80]

The Kropp procedure was specifically designed for the treatment of neurogenic incontinence and functions on the assumption that all patients will need to catheterize to empty the bladder. It is often performed as a last resort to achieve continence before AUS insertion. Mollard et al[68] and Snodgrass[78] prefer to use the Kropp procedure as first-line bladder outlet management in females and reserve the AUS for males, with the rationale that lengthening the urethra in boys may make it more difficult for them to perform IC. Waters et al, however, in a review of catheterization problems in patients who had had Kropp reconstruction, found that the problem was experienced by equal numbers of boys and girls.[73] The Salle technique has been employed with equal success in patients with incontinence secondary to neurogenic bladder and exstrophy-epispadias complex.[75,76,81,82]

Results and complications

The Young–Dees–Leadbetter procedure and its numerous modifications have produced continence rates up to 60–80% when performed in the exstrophy population.[83,84] Published series employing this technique in neurogenic bladder patients are small, but success has been reported to be lower, with continence rates of 50–60% over a follow-up period of greater than 5 years.[80,85,86] Complications have included UTIs, de-novo vesicoureteral reflux (VUR), urethral and bladder neck fistulas, SUI, difficulty catheterizing, and bladder neck strictures, particularly in patients who have had previous bladder neck surgery.[80,84]

The Kropp bladder neck reconstruction has enjoyed continence rates of 80–94%, but this has been tempered by difficult catheterization rates of 10–44% (Table 57.5).[68,72–74,77,78] This problem is thought to occur secondary to the tube being compressed as it passes through the submucosal tunnel, or the suture line running along the back wall of the tube causing formation of an elevated scar.[72,75] An overdistended bladder resulting from delay in catheterization can also compress the valve, making it difficult to pass a drainage tube.[77] In later series, investigators have noted a decrease in the occurrence of catheterization problems when the urethral catheter was left in 4–5 weeks after bladder neck reconstruction.[74] In most cases, this situation is alleviated by passing a catheter under cystoscopic guidance and leaving it in for a few weeks, then having the patient resume catheterization.[73] Other patients who have trouble passing a catheter require bladder neck dilatation or endoscopic resection of the roof of the neourethra. Occasionally, open revision of the flap valve is required.[72,77] Snodgrass has described the performance of an appendicovesicostomy concomitant to the Kropp procedure as a means of providing an alternative route of bladder drainage should the patient be unable to catheterize via the reconstructed bladder outlet.[78]

Other complications encountered with the Kropp technique include pyelonephritis, peritonitis secondary to bladder perforation, de-novo VUR, and fistula formation between the valve and the bladder resulting in incontinence. The Kropp procedure is highly effective at increasing bladder neck resistance and can result in the attainment of a VLPP of greater than 60 cmH_2O in many patients.[74] This high level of continence, coupled with the possibility of difficult catheterization in a patient who may also have an enterocystoplasty, can result in perforation of the augmented portion of the bladder, with subsequent peritonitis, cases of which have culminated in death.[77] New-onset VUR is thought to be a consequence of elevated intravesical pressures as a result of increased outlet resistance, disruption of the trigonal musculature when tunneling the tube, or VUR which was present preoperatively but was not observed on cystourethrogram.[76,78] A small proportion of patients who develop de-novo VUR fail to resolve it spontaneously and require ureteric reimplantation. Fistulas can occur at areas of devascularization along suture lines or as a consequence of traumatic instrumentation or catheterization and usually require open revision of the flap valve in order to achieve continence.

The Salle anterior bladder wall flap has continence rates which are slightly lower than the Kropp procedure, but does not have the high incidence of catheterization difficulty which has plagued the other technique. The occurrence of fistulas between the flap valve and bladder is a problem particularly noted with the Salle procedure and catheterization problems were experienced by some of the exstrophy patients in the later series published by Pippi Salle et al (Table 57.6).[75,76]

Conclusion

In summary, bladder neck reconstruction is one of the earliest surgical treatments devised for treating urinary incontinence secondary to an incompetent bladder neck and proximal urethra. All these procedures, while they have the advantage of utilizing the patient's own tissue, are technically challenging and are associated with a number of complications, some of which may require numerous surgical revisions. Bladder neck reconstruction should not be performed in patients who have mild degrees of urinary incontinence that may be cured by urethral collagen injections or a fascial sling. Bladder neck reconstruction should be reserved for patients with severe outlet incompetence and should only be performed by an experienced surgeon. Despite the availability of the AUS and popularity of the fascial sling, bladder neck reconstruction in its many forms continues to have a role in the treatment of patients with neurogenic bladder and exstrophy-epispadias complex who suffer from total urinary incontinence.

Bladder neck closure

Introduction

Bladder neck closure is considered a last-resort procedure.[87] It is indicated in patients with outlet incompetence who have failed multiple anti-incontinence procedures, patients who are poor surgical candidates and cannot tolerate lengthy, complex reconstructive procedures, and in patients with destroyed urethras which cannot be rebuilt.[88] Closure of the bladder neck can be combined with a

Table 57.5 *Results of Kropp bladder neck reconstruction in patients with neurogenic incontinence*

Procedure	Study	Year	Patients	Follow-up time	Concomitant surgeries	Results	Complications
Kropp	Kropp and Angwafo[72]	1986	Pediatric 7 male, 6 female 13MMC	8–36 months	6 augments, 2 reimplants, 2 undiversions	92% dry	4/6 IC problems 4 de-novoVUR
Kropp	Belman and Kaplan[74]	1989	Pediatric 18: 16 MMC, 2 SA, 10 male	Not stated	14 augments	78% dry, 4 hours	44% IC problems 4 de-novoVUR, 1 pyelonephritis
Kropp	Nill et al[77]	1990	Pediatric and Adult 24: MMC and MS 14 female	1.5–7 years	19 reoperations to perform bladder augmentation	83% dry	46% IC problems 1 vesicocutaneous fistula, 5 reoperations on valve, 9 peritonitis, 8 bladder stones, 10 de-novoVUR
Kropp	Mollard et al[68]	1990	Pediatric 16 girls 15 MMC, 1 other	Not stated	6 augments, 7 reimplants	81% dry	12.5% IC problems 2 valve failures
Kropp (Belman and Kaplan modifications)	Snodgrass[78]	1997	Pediatric 23: 13 male all MMC	Mean 27 months range 3–72	20 augments	91% dry	17% IC problems all in males, 2 valve fistulas, 50% de-novo VUR

MMC, myelomeningocele; SA, sacral agenesis; IC, intermittent catheterization; VUR, vesicoureteric reflux.

Table 57.6 *Results of Salle and Young–Dees–Leadbetter bladder neck reconstruction in patients with neurogenic incontinence*

Procedure	Study	Year	Patients	Follow-up time	Concomitant surgery	Results	Complications
Salle	Pippi Salle et al[75]	1994	Pediatric 6: 3 males All with MMC	Mean 16.8 months range 7–24	Not stated	4/6 (67%) dry	1 flap fistula, 1 re-operation to narrow flap, 1 de-novo VUR, 1 pyelo
Salle	Rink et al[82]	1994	Pediatric 3 MMC females	12–15 months	Cohen reimplants 2 augments	2/3 dry, 1 noctural leakage	None
Salle	Mouriquand et al[81]	1995	Pediatric 8 girls: 7 MMC, 1 other	Mean 6.7 months range 2–18	6 augments	38% dry day and night 88% dry during day	1 flap fistula, 1 bladder calculi
Salle	Pippi Salle et al[76]	1997	Pediatric 17: 13 neurogenic, 4 EE	Mean 25.6 months range 9–49	Not stated	70% dry 9/13 neurogenic dry, 3/4 EE dry	2 flap fistulas, 2 IC problems (all in EEC), 12% de-novo VUR
Young–Dees–Leadbetter vs AUS	Sidi et al[85]	1987	Pediatric 11 BN reconstruction: 9 female 16 AUS: all male 17 MMC, 6 SA, 4 other	BNR Mean 3.2 years range 1–5 AUS Mean 5.7 years range 1–12	BNR: 64% dry AUS: 69% dry	BNR reoperation rate 0.8/patient AUS reoperation rate 1.5/patient	BNR: 9 augments AUS: 2 augments
Young–Dees–Leadbetter	Donnahoo et al[80]	1999	Pediatric 38: 25 female 32 MMC, 3 SA, 13 other	Mean 9 years range 1–17	8 silicone sheath placements, 36 reimplants, 22 augments	50% dry 12.5% partially dry 63% girls vs 25% boys dry with primary bladder neck reconstruction	10.5% IC problems 62.5% silicone sheath erosion, 14% perforation of augmented bladder

MMC, myelomeningocele; SA, sacral agenesis; EE, exstrophy-epispadias; IC, intermittent catheterization; VUR, vesicoureteric reflux; AUS, artificial urethral sphincter, BNR, bladder neck reconstruction catheterizable cutaneous stoma or a chronic indwelling suprapubic tube depending on the constitutional and functional status of the patient.

In female spinal cord injury patients who have been managed with a chronic indwelling Foley catheter, bladder neck closure and suprapubic tube insertion can improve quality of life by eliminating leakage of urine alongside the tube, which can cause chronic skin breakdown, and facilitate return to sexual activity by eliminating the urethral catheter.[89,90]

The disadvantages of bladder neck closure are its irreversibility; its abolishment of the pop-off valve, which necessitates long-term monitoring of the upper tracts to prevent occult renal deterioration;[91] and unpredictable effects on potency and ejaculation when performed in young males.[87] Patients who are managed with bladder neck closure and a chronic suprapubic tube must undergo surveillance cystoscopy in order to monitor for the formation of bladder calculi and squamous neoplasia.[88] There is also a persistent risk of infection secondary to the indwelling catheter.[89]

Transposition of the female urethra to the suprapubic area to form a continent catheterizable stoma has been described, but it is not suitable for obese patients or patients with a significant amount of periurethral scarring secondary to previous surgical procedures or years of chronic indwelling urethral Foley management.[88,89,91] Reconstruction using vaginal wall or bowel has also been attempted in females with destroyed urethras, but the success rate with these procedures is low.[92] Alternatively, a tight fascial sling can be used to achieve a functional bladder neck closure, provided that the patient has a urethral length of at least 1.5–2 cm.[90]

Surgical technique

Bladder neck closure can be performed via the transabdominal or transvaginal route. In the transabdominal approach, a transverse suprapubic incision or vertical midline incision is made and the bladder neck is mobilized. In males, the bladder is transected just cranial to the prostate after ligating the superficial dorsal venous complex and dissecting the neurovascular bundles away. The prostate is usually left intact in order to preserve fertility and antegrade ejaculation. In cases of urethral stricture or prostatorectal fistula which compromise drainage of prostatic secretions and act as a nidus of infection, the prostate is removed to avoid abscess formation. In females the bladder is transected at the vesicourethral junction once the deep dorsal vein has been ligated. Intravenous indigo carmine or ureteric catheters are used to help identify the ureteric orifices. The bladder is mobilized posteriorly to the level of the ureteric orifices. A sponge stick in the vagina can aid in identifying the correct plane of dissection.

Once the posterior and inferior aspects of the bladder have been mobilized out of its dependent position in the pelvis, the bladder neck opening is closed ventrally in two layers: mucosa and muscle with serosa. A suprapubic tube is placed and brought out through a separate stab incision before closing the bladder neck completely, and if the bladder closure is to be combined with a continent catheterizable stoma it is constructed and attached to the bladder at this stage. The urethral stump is closed dorsally in two layers and an omental flap is mobilized and placed between the closed urethral stump and the bladder neck closure to prevent fistula formation.[87,89] A drain is usually left in the space of Retzius. Postoperatively, anticholinergics are administered to prevent bladder spasms. Reid et al have described a different technique of bladder neck closure which involved denuding the bladder neck mucosa through a midline cystotomy, excising a cuff of bladder neck, then closing the denuded muscle with a purse string suture.[93]

The transvaginal approach is typically employed in females with urethral destruction secondary to chronic indwelling Foley catheter drainage who are to be managed with bladder neck closure and suprapubic tube placement. The patient is placed in the dorsal lithotomy position and a suprapubic tube is placed using a Lowsley retractor. This technique is employed to circumvent the difficulty inherent in distending a small contracted bladder with an incompetent outlet.

The patient is placed in the Trendelenburg position to displace the bowels cephalad and the curved Lowsley retractor is inserted into the urethra and pointed towards the anterior abdominal wall 1–2 cm above the pubic symphysis. A small fascial incision is made over the tip of the retractor, which is pushed out through the skin incision. The tip of a large-bore Foley catheter is grasped in its jaws and pulled back into the bladder. Intravesical placement of the catheter can be confirmed by irrigation of the tube or cystoscopic inspection.[94]

An incision circumscribing the urethral opening is extended into an inverted U incision on the anterior vaginal wall. The endopelvic fascia is pierced on either side of the bladder neck in order to free it up completely from the pubic bone and the pubourethral ligaments are transected. Intravenous indigo carmine is given to visualize the ureteric orifices. The scarred urethra, if present, is excised and the bladder neck closed in two layers: first in the vertical, and then in the horizontal direction. The second suture line should contain tissue from the bladder neck to the anterior wall located behind the symphysis to transfer the closed bladder neck to the retropubic space and remove it from a dependent position. The integrity of the closure is checked by filling the bladder through the suprapubic tube. A Martius flap is interposed between the bladder neck and anterior vaginal wall to help prevent vesicovaginal fistula formation and the vaginal wall flap is closed over the Martius flap as a third layer. A vaginal pack containing

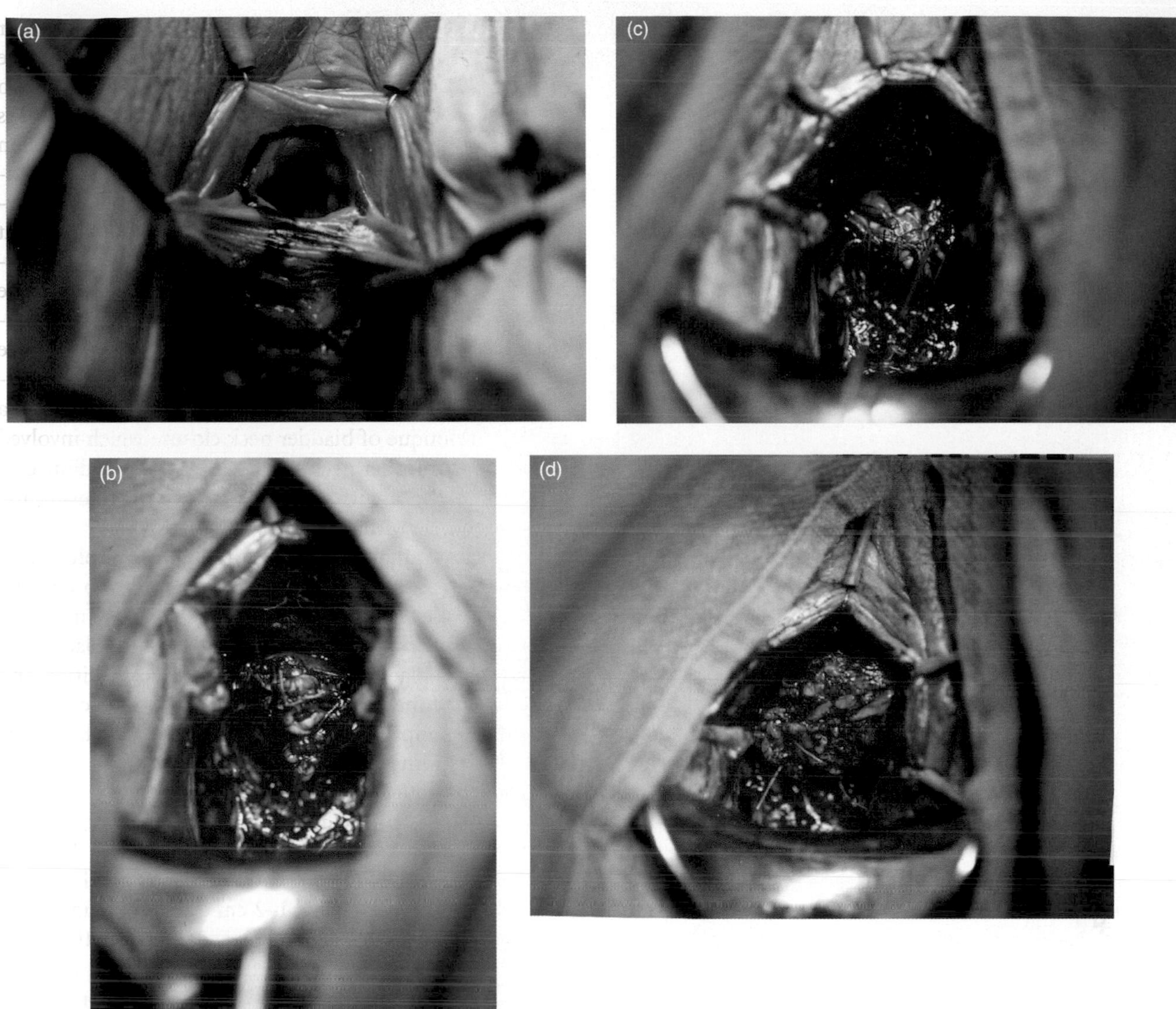

Figure 57.9
Transvaginal bladder neck closure. (a) Creation of anterior vaginal wall flap. Destroyed urethra is circumscribed. (b) Bladder neck is mobilized and urethral reminant excised. First tension-free layer of bladder neck closure. (c) Transversal second layer closure to protect against a secondary vesicovaginal fistula. (d) Placement of Martius flap tunneled beneath labia minora. (Reproduced with permission from Glenn's Urologic Surgery, 5th edn, 1998, Chapter 49, Figs 49.1–49.4.)

antibiotic solution is left in for 24 hours,[88] and anticholinergics are administered to prevent bladder spasms.

Bladder neck closure is highly effective at treating incontinence secondary to an incompetent bladder outlet. Continence rates of 75–100% have been reported in the literature, with mean follow-up times ranging from 1.5 to 3 years.[87–92,95,96] The main technical complication is bladder neck fistulization with continued leakage of urine, which has been reported to occur in 6–25% of cases.[89,93–96] The rate of fistulization is low in series which adhere to the following surgical principles: mobilization of the bladder from its dependent position in the pelvis, closure of the bladder neck and urethral stump in multiple layers without tension, and interposition of well-vascularized tissue such as omentum or a labial fat pad between the urethra and bladder neck. No adverse effect on potency or ejaculation was noted by Hoebeke et al, who performed the procedure in nine young males.

Tissue engineering

Recently, there has been increased interest and success in identifying techniques to regenerate viable smooth muscle cells for use in the GU tract, particularly in the internal urethral sphincter to enhance coaptation and contraction of the urethra. Jack et al[97] found that the lipoaspirate in patients undergoing liposuction could be processed to yield a pluripotent population of cells. After injection into the GU tract of rats, they found the processed lipoaspirate cells remained viable at 12 weeks and had incorporated into the recipient smooth muscle cells. They demonstrated *in-vivo* expression of alpha-smooth muscle actin, an early marker of smooth muscle differentiation. They concluded that these cells may provide a feasible and cost-effective cell source for urinary tract reconstruction.

Surgical treatment of the hyperactive bladder outlet

Introduction

For several years it has been recognized that detrusor-external sphincter dyssynergia (DESD), a common condition in patients with suprasacral spinal cord lesions, is associated with elevated intravesical pressure, which can result in substantial morbidity and mortality. DESD is defined as a detrusor contraction concurrent with an involuntary contraction of the urethral and/or periurethral striated muscle during voiding.[98] During urodynamic assessment, DESD is denoted by an increase in electromyographic activity of the sphincter or pelvic muscles associated with an involuntary detrusor contraction. On voiding cystourethrogram or videourodynamic assessment, dilation of the bladder neck due to a contracted external sphincter is observed during bladder emptying.[99] The condition leads to a complication rate in excess of 50%, resulting in urosepsis, hydronephrosis, nephrolithiasis, and vesicoureteric reflux, all of which can terminate in renal insufficiency and, eventually, dialysis.[100,101] DESD is also associated with autonomic dysreflexia, particularly in patients with injuries above the T5 spinal cord level. Since its description by Emmett et al in 1948, sphincterotomy has been recommended to treat DESD in a subset of spinal cord injured males who are at risk for renal damage.[102] By incising the external sphincter to render it incompetent, one can transform intermittent incontinence into continuous incontinence, which can be managed with a condom catheter drainage device.[103] Sphincterotomy is irreversible and has been associated with intraoperative bleeding and erectile dysfunction. A reduction in long-term efficacy has also been observed which may require repeat external sphincter or bladder neck incision.[104] Long-term use of a condom catheter can lead to skin ulceration, urethrocutaneous fistula, and penile retraction.[104] Despite these drawbacks, sphincterotomy is still considered the gold standard to which other treatments for DESD are compared.

A urethral stent was first used by Milroy et al in 1988 to treat stricture disease.[105] Subsequently, it has been employed in benign prostatic hyperplasia (BPH) therapy and as an alternative to sphincterotomy in patients with DESD. Most of the experience with external sphincter stenting has been with the Urolume prosthesis (American Medical Systems, Minnetonka, Minnesota), a nonmagnetic superalloy woven into a mesh cylinder which is inserted endoscopically across the external sphincter to hold it open.[106] The geometry and elasticity of the stent material exerts a radial force which maintains its position within the urethral lumen until epithelialization occurs.[107] Other urethral stents which have been used to circumvent DESD include the Ultraflex (Boston Scientific Corp, Boston, MA), which is made of a single elastalloy wire, and the Memokath (Engineers and Doctors A/S, Homback, Denmark), a coil made of thermosensitive titanium/nickel alloy. Sphincteric stenting has several advantages over sphincterotomy. It is an easier and quicker procedure that is associated with shorter hospital stay and cost.[107] Unlike sphincterotomy, stent insertion is potentially reversible, a characteristic which appeals to spinal cord injured patients still hoping for a cure.[99,106] Furthermore, sphincteric stents are not associated with diminished erectile ability or significant blood loss.[99] Despite these advantages, insertion of a stent across the external sphincter raises some legitimate concerns. The stent is a foreign body which is placed in contact with urine, resulting in encrustation.[99] Difficult removal of the Urolume stent occasionally resulting in urethral injury has also been reported.[108,109]

Among the latest developments, balloon dilation and botulinum toxin A have been considered to treat DESD. Since the first report, there has been no further interest with balloon dilation, whereas a large body of literature has already been released concerning botulinum toxin, and will be reviewed later in the chapter.

Indications and patient selection

Both sphincterotomy and urethral stents are employed in the treatment of DESD in male spinal cord injured patients with DO refractory to anticholinergics and IC, or in those unable or unwilling to carry out this conservative treatment.[100] Sphincteric stents have been used not only as primary treatment for DESD but also for patients who have failed previous sphincterotomy.[99,110] Relative contraindications to stenting include patients who are known to be recurrent stone formers, patients who have had previous bladder neck (BN) incisions or TURP (transurethral rejection of the prostate), and patients who have an artificial urinary sphincter.[99,110,112] Chancellor et al, in the North American Multicenter Urolume Trial, found that a

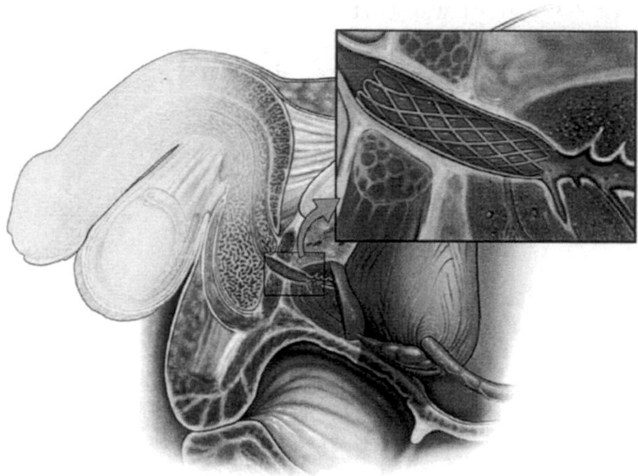

Figure 57.10
Sagittal view of male pelvis to show placement of urethral stent across external sphincter.

wide-open bladder neck secondary to previous bladder neck or prostatic surgery predisposed patients to stent migration.[99] McInerney and colleagues placed stents in 3 men with spinal cord injuries and DESD who had artificial urinary sphincters.[110] The voiding parameters of these men were not improved, and, due to perineal discomfort, one stent was eventually removed with great difficulty.

The Memokath stent has been found to be easier to remove than the Urolume device and has been advocated as a short-term treatment option for DESD. This stent may be used as an alternative to an indwelling catheter in recent spinal cord injured patients who are likely to regain enough upper extremity function to be able to perform self-catheterization, or for patients who would like to try condom catheter drainage before committing themselves to Urolume or sphincterotomy.[112] Men who are undergoing electroejaculation may also benefit from the Memokath, since the device can be easily removed and replaced later on.[112]

Sphincterotomy or sphincteric stenting with condom catheter drainage is preferable to a chronic indwelling Foley catheter, which is still often used as the management of last resort in quadriplegic patients who do not have the manual dexterity or caregiver support to perform IC or change a condom catheter. Chronic indwelling catheters are associated with recurrent urosepsis, bladder calculi, and squamous cell carcinoma in this patient population.[113]

Sphincterotomy techniques

Before proceeding with incision of the external sphincter, the patient should have a negative urine culture. The patient is placed in the dorsal lithotomy position and perioperative intravenous antibiotic prophylaxis is administered. The type of anesthesia required depends on the amount of sensation and severity of autonomic dysreflexia experienced by the individual. Intravenous sedation with or without calcium channel or alpha-antagonist prophylaxis for hypertensive crisis may be all that is needed.

Sphincterotomy is usually performed under endoscopic video control with a 24F resectoscope and Collins knife or loop electrocautery attachment. A cut is made anteriorly at the 12 o'clock or 11 o'clock position away from the neurovascular bundles to minimize the risk of bleeding and erectile dysfunction. The incision is taken from the prostatic urethra just proximal to the verumontanum to the proximal bulbar urethra. The cut must extend through the muscle fibers of the sphincter to the level of the corpus spongiosum tissue of the proximal bulb.[114] Hemostasis is attained with the electrocautery, and a 22F three-way Foley catheter is placed in the bladder. Continuous bladder irrigation is run for 24–48 hours to prevent clot retention and the patient is discharged once the urine is clear. The catheter is removed 4–7 days after the procedure and a condom catheter is applied to the penis for bladder drainage.

Sphincterotomy performed with the Nd:YAG contact laser has been described as an alternative to electrocautery.[115,116] A chisel or round-tip probe is deployed through the instrument port of a 21 or 23F cystoscope with a 30 degree lens. The sphincterotomy is performed anteriorly, as with electrocautery, with the probe tip in contact with the tissue to be vaporized. Repeated passes are made over the area until the required depth is attained. Cutting tissue requires settings of 25–50 W and hemostasis is achieved with lower energy settings of 15–25 W. Laser sphincterotomy may take a longer time than conventional electrocautery, especially if there is a large amount of scarring from previous surgery.[116]

Whether or not to perform bladder neck incision concomitant with sphincterotomy to optimize bladder emptying is somewhat controversial. Some investigators state that the bladder neck should not be incised immediately, as there is often delayed relaxation of the bladder outlet after sphincterotomy, and performing a bladder neck incision will result in complete incontinence with continuous urine leakage.[104] Other surgeons cut the bladder neck in addition to the external sphincter when preoperative urodynamics demonstrate bladder neck obstruction.[114,115] In their series of laser sphincterotomies, Perkash[115] performed concomitant laser bladder neck incisions at 3 and 9 o'clock, whereas Rivas et al[116] cut the bladder neck in the midline at 6 o'clock.

Results and complications of sphincterotomy

The results of some contemporary series of spinal cord patients treated with sphincterotomy are listed in Table 57.7. Incising the external sphincter results in statistically significant

Table 57.7 *Contemporary results of sphincterotomy in the treatment of detrusor-external sphincter dyssynergia*

Study	Year	Number and type of patients	Type of sphincterotomy	Mean follow-up (months)	Previous surgery	Results	Complications
Rivas et al[116]	1995	22 SCI males 14 quads 8 paras	Nd:YAG contact laser (round probe)	14 range 3–20	7% previous electrocautery sphincterotomy	18 successful Decreased voiding pressure and PVR ($p < 0.01$)	13.6% repeat sphincterotomy 1 skin ulceration, 1 urethrocutaneous fistula
Vapneck et al[114]	1994	16 SCI males 13 quads 3 paras	14 electrocautery 1 open 1 cold knife	39 range 3–96		50% success 8/16 still used condom drainage	5 repeat sphinc terotomy, 1 spinal headache, 1 urosepsis/ADR Long term: 3 recurrent UTIs, 2 penile skin problems, 2 ADR, 1 combo of above
Perkash	1996	76 SCI males 32% – bladder neck stenosis or BPH 32% bulbar strictures 54% quads 46% paras	Nd:YAG contact laser (chisel tip probe) Sphincterotomy ± bladder neck/ prostatic incisions	27 range 16–41	56% previous electrocautery sphincterotomy	Decreased voiding pressure ($p < 0.0003$), decreased ADR	Overall 11.8% 7 repeat sphincterotomy 2 blood loss >100 ml
Fontaine et al[103]	1996	92 SCI males 47 quads 45 paras	Electrocautery	20.6		Objective improvement in 83.7% Subjectively improved in 73%, ADR resolution in 93.2%, decreased PVR ($p < 0.001$)	Overall 10.6% 8.1% repeat sphincterotomy 4 hematurias 1 transfusion 4 de-novo ADR 2 bacteremia

SCI, spinal cord injury; ADR, autonomic dysreflexia; PVR, post-void residual; quad, quadraplegic; para, paraplegic; BPH, benign prostatic hyperplasia.

decreases in maximum detrusor pressure, postvoid residual, and the occurrence of autonomic dysreflexia. Bladder capacity is usually maintained. Complications include bleeding, clot retention, urosepsis, erectile dysfunction, and sphincterotomy failure secondary to urethral scarring. Making the incision anteriorly at 12 or 11 o'clock, rather than posterolaterally, has lowered the likelihood of damage to the urethral blood supply and cavernous body innervation, resulting in decreased rates of clot retention and erectile dysfunction compared with older series.[114,116] The need for repeat sphincterotomy secondary to scarring and stenosis of the external sphincter is usually evident within 12 months of having the procedure, but can occur years later.[104] Repeat sphincterotomy rates range from 9%, when the laser is employed, to 31%, with the use of conventional electrocautery.[114,116] Other complications said to be decreased with laser sphincterotomy compared to electrocautery are severe bleeding and erectile dysfunction. In the absence of a prospective randomized trial, there is no conclusive proof of the superiority of laser to electrocautery. The post-void residual often persists after incising the external sphincter, but many authors do not consider this finding an indication of treatment failure unless the patient continues to have recurrent UTIs due to urinary stasis.[103,114] Treatment failure despite a technically perfect sphincterotomy occurs in 10–50% of men treated for DESD. Reasons for failure include problems fitting the condom catheter as well as detrusor areflexia, which can result in poor bladder emptying despite an incompetent bladder outlet.[103,114,117]

Sphincteric stenting techniques

As with sphincterotomy, the patient is placed in the dorsal lithotomy position and is given perioperative antibiotic coverage. The Urolume device is packaged in a preloaded 24F cystoscopic insertion tool that accommodates a zero degree urethroscope. The Urolume comes in lengths of 2, 2.5, and 3 cm. The Ultraflex device comes in 2–5 cm lengths with 0.5 cm increments. The 3 cm length is usually adequate for two-thirds of patients being treated for DESD,[118] and, with the 5 cm Ultraflex prosthesis, only 10% of patients were found to need placement of a second stent.[119,120] If required, however, more than one device can be placed in order to span the entire external sphincter. Temporary suprapubic drainage is established intraoperatively to ensure good visibility and postoperative bladder drainage. Under direct vision, the insertion tool is introduced into the urethra and advanced to the level of the verumontanum, then released. The stent usually retracts 1–2 mm after deployment, and this should be accounted for when deciding on the position to release the device.[115,116] The stent should cover the caudal half of the verumontanum, leaving the ejaculatory ducts unblocked. The distal end should extend at least 5 mm into the bulbar urethra, well beyond the distal aspect of the external sphincter. If placement is incorrect, the Urolume can be moved or removed with endoscopic forceps. The Ultraflex can be pulled back using a suture located on its distal end which is removed after confirmation of proper placement.[119,120] When needed, a second stent should be placed overlapping the first by approximately 5 mm to completely bridge the sphincteric area.[121]

The Memokath stent is also inserted under direct vision mounted on a flexible or rigid cystoscope. Intraoperative fluoroscopy is used after filling the bladder with 200 ml of dilute contrast to monitor for distal movement that may occur with removal of the scope after stent deployment.[117] Once the stent is positioned correctly within the urethral lumen, saline warmed to 50°C is instilled into the device to cause expansion. Irrigation of the stent with cold saline (< 10°C) renders it soft for easy removal with alligator forceps.[122]

Postoperative oral antibiotics are usually continued for 10–14 days.[99,116] A condom catheter is used to drain the bladder postoperatively. The patient can be discharged within 24 hours. A pelvic X-ray is recommended to confirm proper position of the prosthesis before discharge. The suprapubic tube can be removed a few days later once adequate bladder emptying via the condom catheter is documented. Urethral catheterization should be avoided for at least 3 months to avoid displacement of the stent before epithelialization occurs.

Stent removal can be accomplished under intravenous sedation or general anesthesia. The resectoscope on low cutting current is used to remove all epithelium overlying the stent. The prosthesis is then grasped with alligator forceps and pulled through the scope or pushed into the bladder and removed through the scope obturator.[108,118] The stent may unravel into individual wires and may need to be removed piece-by-piece. When the stent begins to separate, more than one procedure may be required in order to remove the prosthesis completely.[121] Fluoroscopy or a pelvic X-ray should be obtained to ensure complete stent removal.

Results and complications of sphincteric stenting

Several series examining the performance of urethral stents in the treatment of DESD have found statistically significant decreases in voiding pressure, postvoid residual, and autonomic dysreflexia with no change in bladder capacity (see Table 57.8).[99,107,119] In a prospective nonrandomized trial comparing sphincterotomy to the Urolume stent, Rivas et al found no statistically significant differences in treatment outcomes between these two modalities.[107] The stent, however, was associated with a significantly shorter operative time, decreased length of hospital stay, and less

Table 57.8 *Results of urethral stents for the treatment of detrusor-external sphincter dyssynergia*

Study	Year	Number and type of patients	Type of stent	Mean follow-up (months)	Previous surgery	Results	Complications
Rivas et al[107]	1994	26 had stent, 20 sphincterotomy	Urolume vs sphincterotomy Patients selected treatment	Range 6–20		Shorter OR time, hospitalization time, lower blood loss, no difference in decrease in PVR, voiding pressure, or capacity	Stents – 15.4% migration, 2 BNO Sphincterotomy – 2 transfusions, 2 repeat ORs, 1 erectile dysfunction
Sauerwein et al[121]	1995	51 SCI males	Urolume (see above)	Range 12–36	All had sphincterotomy, 22 BNI, 18 TURBN	All had lowered ADR and voiding pressures, increased compliance	25.5% initial ADR, 9.8% migration, 5.9% explantation, 1 poor emptying
McFarlane et al[111]	1996	11 SCI males	Wallstent (American Medical Systems, UK) now Urolume	69.6 range 36–89		36.4% success – decreased PVR, maximum detrusor pressure	1 urosepsis at insertion, 5 BNO, 2 explantations, 1 recurrent UTI, 1 encrustation
Shaw et al[112]	1997	14 SCI males	Memokath (see above)	Maximum 24		50% success – decreased PVR, hydro, ADR	42.9% migration 1 mucosal hyperplasia, 1 recurrent UTI
Low and McRae[117]	1998	24 SCI males	Memokath (Engineers and Doctors A/S, Hornback, Denmark)	16 range 2–24	13 had 1 or more sphincterotomies 4 TURP, 4 other	29.1% success – decreased PVR, ADR, and UTIs	20.8% migration 25% recurrent UTIs, 12.5% de-novo ADR, 16.7% poor emptying, 4.1% encrustation
Chancellor et al[122]	1999	160 males 100 SCIs, 8 MS, 1 spinal vascular accident, 1 SC tumor	Urolume (American Medical Systems, Minnetonka, Minnesota)	60	46 had 1 or more sphincterotomies 11 TURP, 11 TURBN, 4 BNI	Significantly decreased voiding pressure, PVR, ADR, hydro, UTIs	15% explanted 28.7% migration 33% hematuria 26.3% BNO 2 urosepsis
Chartier-Kestler et al[119]	2000	40 males 30 SCI, 6 MS, 4 other	Ultraflex (Boston Scientific Corp., Boston, MA)	16.9	5–1 or more sphincterotomies 4 TUIP, 2 TURP, 3 VIU	Decreased PVR, decreased ADR in 63.1%	1 explantation for UTIs, 2 BNOs\ transient hematuria
Denys et al[120]	2004	39 SCI, 9 spinal cord diseases	Ultraflex	22	5 sphincterotomies, 7 TURP, 3 BNI	Decreased UTIs, reduced peak detrusor pressure, decreased residual, 90.8% mean epithelialization	2 explantations for UTI, 1 for pain, 21.7% less than 1 cm stent migration, 21% had BNO with BNI performed at 1 year

SCI, spinal cord injury; PVR, post-void residual; ADR, autonomic dysreflexia; BNO, bladder neck obstruction; UTI, urinary tract infection; BPH, benign prostatic hyperplasia; TURP transurethral resection of the prostate; BNI, bladder neck incision; TURBN, transurethral resection of bladder neck contracture.

blood loss when compared to sphincterotomy. Long-term complications that have been found to occur with the Urolume include epithelial hyperplasia, stent encrustation, stent migration, urethral obstruction, secondary bladder neck obstruction, and difficult stent removal.[99,105,108,111] The Memokath device is associated with a high rate of migration, recurrent UTIs, and calcification, making it more suitable for the short-term treatment of DESD.[107,117]

Urothelial hyperplasia first occurs during growth of urethral mucosa over the stent, and usually resolves by the time the stent is completely covered, a process which can take anywhere from 3 months to 1 year.[99] Incorporation of the device into the urethral wall lowers the likelihood of stone formation, infection, and migration.[105,119] Epithelial hyperplasia can lead to stent obstruction in 5% of cases, which can be remedied with endoscopic resection.[99] Calcific encrustation may occur at the ends of the Urolume device, which are the last areas to become epithelialized.[107]

Stent migration is the most common reason for stent removal and can usually be diagnosed by cystoscopy or a pelvic X-ray. The most recent report of the North American Multicenter Urolume Trial found a 28.7% rate of stent migration, with approximately 40% of cases occurring within the first 3 months after insertion.[99] Reasons for stent migration include previous bladder neck or prostatic surgery, previous sphincterotomy, urethral catheterization before epithelialization took place, and dislodgement during stool disimpaction or patient transfers.[99,108] Wilson et al, in a review of stent failures, discovered urethral obstruction in one patient who had had tandem stents placed, secondary to one stent telescoping on the other more proximal stent.[108] The long-term rate of secondary bladder neck obstruction is 26.3% with the Urolume endoprosthesis,[99] and is thought to be a result of bladder neck dyssynergia masked by the presence of DESD.[111] If conservative management with alpha-blockade fails, then bladder neck incision or resection can be performed.

Despite several large series detailing the ease with which the Urolume can be removed even when completely epithelialized, many investigators have reported cases of stent explantation which were difficult and tedious.[107,108] Despite following the manufacturer's directions for prosthesis removal, the stent has been known to disintegrate and unravel, requiring piecemeal removal of each individual wire in a time-consuming process. Wilson et al described two cases of challenging stent removal, one of which required making a perineal incision, and the other resulting in avulsion of the urethral mucosa.[108]

Balloon dilatation of the external urethral sphincter

The concept of dilating the urethra with a balloon in order to treat high intravesical pressure was first described by Bloom et al, who employed this technique to lower the leak-point pressures of 18 children with myelomeningocele.[123] Since then, Chancellor et al have compared the short-term results of balloon dilatation of the external sphincter to sphincterotomy and stent insertion in the treatment of spinal cord injured men with DESD. All three modalities were found to be equivalent in terms of decreasing voiding pressure, postvoid residual, and autonomic dysreflexia at a mean follow-up time of 15 months. Complications occurring in 20 cases of balloon dilatation were blood transfusion (1), recurrent sphincteric obstruction (3), and bulbar urethral stricture (1).[109]

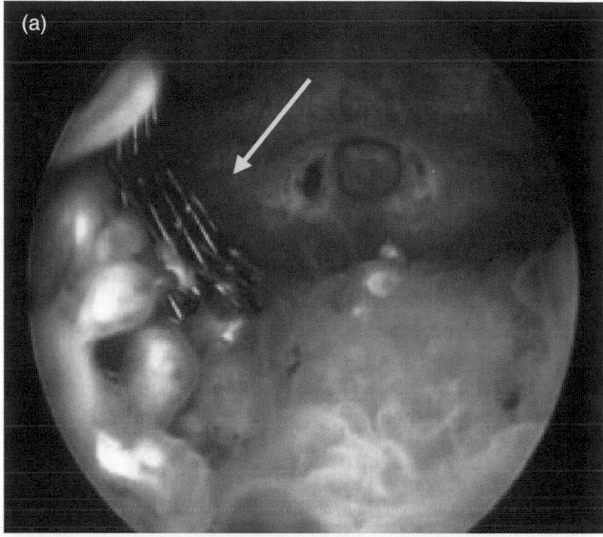

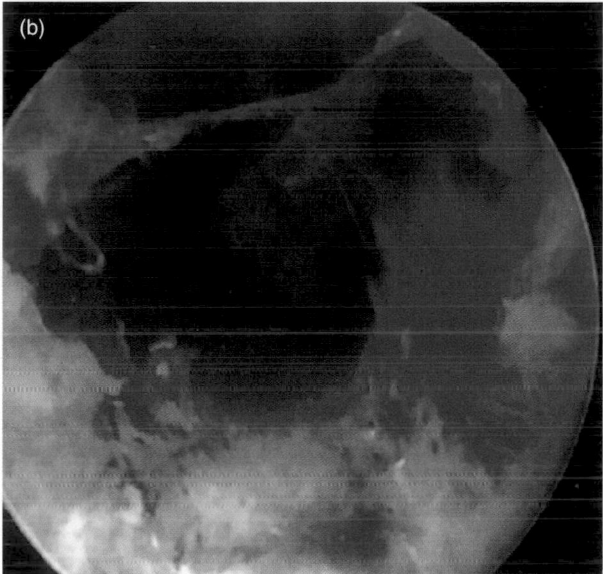

Figure 57.11
Urethral avulsion (a) stent exposed on right side (arrow); (b) after stent removal.

Botulinum toxin A injection into the external urethral sphincter

The following technique was described by Smith et al.[124] Between 100 and 200 U of botulinum toxin A (BTX-A) are mixed with 4 ml of saline just before injection. The vial should not be shaken. A rigid cystoscope and a standard cystoscopic collagen injection needle are used to inject BTX-A deeply into the external sphincter at the 3, 6, 9, and 12-o'clock positions in equal aliquots. These injections should be directed deeper than collagen injections to target the nerve terminals innervating the skeletal muscle.

Results and complications of botulinum toxin for the external sphincter

Smith et al[124] reported that, of 68 patients with either multiple sclerosis or spinal cord injury undergoing this procedure, 32 had follow-up of at least 6 months. The mean postvoid residual urine volume decreased from 250 to 88 ml after the procedure, and maximal voiding pressures decreased. Retention requiring catheterization decreased by 80%, and patients experienced decreased urinary tract infection rates. Four percent of patients noted either worsening or new-onset stress urinary incontinence. Phelan et al performed a prospective study on 21 patients, with follow-up ranging from 3 to 16 months.[125] Following urethral injection of Botox, voiding pressures decreased an average of 38%. Sixty-seven percent of patients reported improvement in voiding patterns. No complications or side-effects were noted. In another study, Schurch et al treated 24 patients with spinal cord injuries and DESD with BTX-A injection.[126] Significant improvement in DESD was noted in 88%, with decreased postvoid residuals in most. The effects lasted 3 to 9 months, with no adverse events reported. Since the muscle-relaxing properties of the toxin are time- and dose-related, repeated injections will likely be necessary.

Conclusion

In summary, treatment of the male neurogenic bladder patient with refractory DESD continues to be challenging. Sphincterotomy and urethral stents will undoubtedly continue to be used in the management of these difficult cases. While there are now several different surgical options to choose from in addition to sphincterotomy, none of these treatment modalities has been shown to be superior to another with respect to efficacy, and each is fraught with its own unique liabilities and complications. Hopefully, future technical advances in the construction and composition of urethral stents will decrease their rate of migration and improve the ease of explantation. There has been little interest in balloon dilation. However, botulinum toxin injection is being performed more often, with promising results and few side-effects. Long-term studies are needed to determine whether this technique will become a viable option for the treatment of DESD.

Conclusions

The surgeon endeavoring to treat a patient with urinary incontinence secondary to neuropathic bladder outlet incompetence has a number of surgical options at his disposal. Injectable agents are often employed in female patients with mild degrees of incontinence, patients who leak small amounts postbladder neck sling or reconstruction, and patients who are not operative candidates or who are reluctant to undergo open surgery. The sling and AUS are commonly used when a more durable, long-term solution for incontinence is required. Because slings may be more successful in females than in males, some surgeons prefer to use slings as their first-line treatment in females and AUS as their primary treatment in males with neurogenic sphincteric incompetence. Reluctance to utilize the AUS in females stems from concerns of cuff erosion. The fascial sling may be preferable to the AUS in patients who do not wish to have a foreign body implanted or who, because of their comorbidities or surgical history, are at high risk for cuff erosion or infection of the device. Bladder neck reconstruction techniques are still performed at some specialized centers with experience in treating myelomeningocele and exstrophy-epispadias patients, but their popularity is waning secondary to high complication rates, especially in patients who have already undergone bladder neck surgery. Bladder neck closure is a suitable option for select patients who have failed multiple surgical attempts to increase outlet resistance or who have poor functional and constitutional status.

Sphincterotomy and urethral stents have both been shown to be effective at treating DESD. As some recent reports have illustrated, however, the currently available urethral stents may not be as easily removed or as complication-free as was once thought. Choice of treatment option is often guided by what the patient perceives as the irreversibility of sphincterotomy compared to urethral stenting and botulinum toxin injection.

References

1. Murless BC. The injection treatment of stress incontinence. J Obstet Gynaecol 1938; 45: 67–73.
2. Lewis RI, Lockhart JL, Politano VA. Periurethral polytetrafluroethylene injections in incontinent female subjects. J Urol 1984; 131: 459–62.
3. Malizia AA Jr, Reiman HM, Myers RP et al. Migration and granulomatous reaction after periurethral injection of Polytef (Teflon). JAMA 1984; 251: 3277–81.

4. Bomalaski MD, Bloom DA, McGuire EJ, Panzi A. Glutaraldehyde cross-linked collagen in the treatment of urinary incontinence in children. J Urol 1996; 155: 699–702.
5. Kryger JV, Gonzalez R, Barthold JS. Surgical management of urinary incontinence in children with neurogenic sphincteric incompetence. J Urol 2000; 163: 256–63.
6. Cooperman L, Micheli D. The immunogenicity of injectable collagen II. A retrospective review of 72 tested and treated patients. J Am Acad Dermatol 1984; 10: 647–51.
7. Leonard MP, Carring DA, Epstein JI. Local tissue reaction to the subureteral injection of glutaraldehyde cross-linked bovine collagen in humans. J Urol 1990; 143: 1209.
8. Poon CI, Zimmern PE. Role of three-dimensional ultrasound in assessment of women undergoing urethral bulking agent therapy. Curr Opin Obst Gynecol 2004; 16: 411–17.
9. Defreitas GA, Wilson TS, Zimmern PE, Forte TB. Three dimensional ultrasonography: an objective outcome tool to assess collagen distribution in women with stress urinary incontinence. Urology 2003; 62(2): 232–6.
10. Poon CI, Zimmern PE, Wilson TS, Defreitas GA, Foreman MR. Three-dimensional ultrasonography to assess long-term durability of periurethral collagen in women with stress urinary incontinence due to intrinsic sphincter deficiency. Urology 2005; 65: 60–4.
11. Bennett JK, Green BG, Foote JE, Gray M. Collagen injections for intrinsic sphincter deficiency in the neuropathic urethra. Paraplegia 1995; 33: 697–700.
12. Wan J, McGuire EJ, Bloom DA, Ritchey ML. The treatment of urinary incontinence in children using glutaraldehyde cross-linked collagen. J Urol 1992; 148: 127–30.
13. McGuire EJ, Fitzpatrick CC, Wan J et al. Clinical assessment of urethral sphincteric function. J Urol 1993; 150: 1452–4.
14. Leonard MP, Decter A, Mix LW et al. Treatment of urinary incontinence in children by endoscopically directed bladder neck injection of collagen. J Urol 1996; 156: 637–41.
15. McGuire EJ, Apell RA. Transurethral collagen injection for urinary incontinence. Urology 1994; 43: 413–15.
16. Chernoff A, Horowitz M, Combs A et al. Periurethral collagen injection for the treatment of urinary incontinence in children. J Urol 1997; 157: 2303–5.
17. Kershen RT, Atala A. New advances in injectable therapies for the treatment of incontinence and vesicoureteral reflux. Urol Clin N Am 1999; 26: 81–94.
18. Nataluk EA, Assimos DG, Kroov RL. Collagen injections for treatment of urinary incontinence secondary to intrinsic sphincter deficiency. J Endourol 1995; 9: 403–6.
19. Ben-Chaim J, Jeffs RD, Peppas DS, Gearhart JP. Submucosal bladder neck injections of glutaraldehyde cross-linked bovine collagen for the treatment of urinary incontinence in patients with the exstrophy/epispadias complex. J Urol 1995; 154: 862–4.
20. Kasouff W, Capolicchio G, Berardinucci G, Corcos J. Collagen injection for treatment of urinary incontinence in children. J Urol 2001; 165: 1666–8.
21. Perez LM, Smith EA, Parrot TS et al. Submucosal bladder neck injection of bovine dermal collagen for stress urinary incontinence in the pediatric population. J Urol 1996; 156: 633–6.
22. Capozza N, Caione P, De Gennaro M et al. Endoscopic treatment of vesico-ureteric reflux and urinary incontinence: technical problems in the pediatric patient. Br J Urol 1995; 75: 538–42.
23. Sundaram CP, Reinberg Y, Aliabadi HA. Failure to obtain durable results with collagen implantation in children with urinary incontinence. J Urol 1997; 157: 2306–7.
24. Kim YH, Kattan MW, Boone TB. Correlation of urodynamic results and urethral coaptation with success after transurethral collagen injection. Urology 1997; 50: 941–8.
25. Bent AE, Tutrone RT, McLennan MT et al. Treatment of intrinsic sphincter deficiency using autologous ear chondrocytes as a bulking agent. Neurourol Urodyn 2001; 20: 157–65.
26. Yokoyama T, Yoshimura N, Dhir R et al. Persistence and survival of autologous muscle derived cells versus bovine collagen as potential treatment of stress urinary incontinence. J Urol 2001; 165: 271–6.
27. Elder JS. Periurethral and puboprostatic sling repair for incontinence in patients with myelodysplasia. J Urol 1990; 144: 434–7.
28. Raz S, McGuire EJ, Ehrlich RM et al. Fascial sling to correct male neurogenic sphincter incompetence: the McGuire/Raz approach. J Urol 1988; 139: 528–31.
29. Kreder KJ, Webster G. Management of the bladder outlet in patients requiring enterocystoplasty. J Urol 1992; 147: 38–41.
30. Fontaine E, Bendaya S, Desert JF et al. Combined modified rectus fascial sling and augmentation ileocystoplasty for neurogenic incontinence in women. J Urol 1997; 157: 109–12.
31. Decter RM. Use of the fascial sling for neurogenic incontinence: lessons learned. J Urol 1993; 150: 683–6.
32. Walker RD, Flack CE, Hawkins-Lee B et al. Rectus fascial wrap: early results of a modification of the rectus fascial sling. J Urol 1995; 154: 771–4.
33. Gormley EA, Bloom DA, McGuire EJ, Ritchey ML. Pubovaginal slings for the management of urinary incontinence in female adolescents. J Urol 1994; 152: 822–5.
34. Herschorn S, Radomski SB. Fascial slings and bladder neck tapering in the treatment of male neurogenic incontinence. J Urol 1992; 147: 1073–5.
35. Kurzrock EA, Lowe P, Hardy BE. Bladder wall pedicle wraparound sling for neurogenic urinary incontinence in children. J Urol 1996; 155: 305–8.
36. Kakizaki H, Shibata T, Shinno Y et al. Fascial sling for the management of urinary incontinence due to sphincter incompetence. J Urol 1995; 153: 644–7.
37. Barthold JS, Rodriguez E, Freedman AL et al. Results of the rectus fascial sling and wrap procedures for the treatment of neurogenic sphincteric incontinence. J Urol 1999; 161: 272–4.
38. Mingin GC, Youngren K, Stock JA, Hanna MK. The rectus myofascial wrap in the management of urethral sphincter incompetence. BJU Int 2002; 90: 550–3.
39. Rutman MP, Deng DY, Shah SM, Raz S, Rodriguez LV. Spiral sling salvage anti-incontinence surgery in female patients with a non-functional urethra: technique and initial results. J Urol 2006; 175(5): 1794–8.
40. Austin PF, Westney L, Leng WW et al. Advantages of rectus fascial slings for urinary incontinence in children with neuropathic bladders. J Urol 2001; 165: 2369–72.
41. Scott FB, Bradley WE, Timm GW. Treatment of urinary incontinence by an implantable prosthetic device. Urology 1973; 1: 252–9.
42. Reinberg Y, Manivel JC, Gonzalez R. Silicone shedding from artificial urinary sphincter in children. J Urol 1993; 150: 694–6.
43. Hajivassiliou CA. The development and evolution of artificial urethral sphincters. J Med Eng Technol 1998; 22: 154–9.
44. Fulford SCV, Sutton C, Bales G et al. The fate of the 'modern' artificial urinary sphincter with a follow-up of more than 10 years. Br J Urol 1997; 79: 713–16.
45. Elliot DS, Barrett DM. Mayo Clinic long-term analysis of the functional durability of the AMS 800 artificial sphincter: a review of 323 cases. J Urol 1998; 159: 1206–8.
46. Woodside JR, McGuire EJ. Technique for detection of detrusor hypertonia in the presence of urethral sphincteric incompetence. J Urol 1982; 127: 740–3.
47. De Badiola FIP, Castro-Diaz D, Hart-Austin C, Gonzalez R. Influence of preoperative bladder capacity and compliance on the outcome of artificial sphincter implantation in patients with neurogenic sphincter incompetence. J Urol 1992; 148: 1483–95.
48. Kryger JV, Lerverson G, Gonzalez R. Long-term results of artificial urinary sphincters in children are independent of age at implantation. J Urol 2001; 165: 2377–9.
49. Aliabadi H, Gonzalez R. Success of the artificial sphincter after failed surgery for incontinence. J Urol 1990; 143: 987–90.

50. Levesque PE, Bauer SB, Atala A et al. Ten year experience with the artificial urinary sphincter in children. J Urol 1996; 156: 625–8.
51. Salisz JA, Diokno AC. The management of injuries to the urethra, bladder or vagina encountered during the difficult placement of the artificial urinary sphincter in the female patient. J Urol 1992; 148: 1528–30.
52. Leach GE, Raz S. Perfusion sphincterometry. Method of intraoperative evaluation of artificial urethral sphincter function. Urology 1983; 21: 312–14.
53. Wilson SK, Delk JR, Henry GD, Siegel AL. New surgical technique for sphincter urinary control system using upper transverse scrotal incision. J Urol 2003; 169: 261–4.
54. Simeoni J, Guys JM, Mollard P et al. Artificial urinary sphincter implantation for neurogenic bladder: a multi-institutional study in 107 children. Br J Urol 1996; 78: 287–93.
55. Singh G, Thomas DG. Artificial urinary sphincter in patients with neurogenic bladder dysfunction. Br J Urol 1996; 77: 252–5.
56. Gonzalez R, Merino FG, Vaughn M. Long-term results of the artificial urinary sphincter in male patients with neurogenic bladder. J Urol 1995; 154: 769–70.
57. Bellioli G, Campobasso P, Mercurella A. Neuropathic urinary incontinence in pediatric patients: management with artificial sphincter. J Ped Surg 1992; 27: 1461–4.
58. Spiess PE, Capolicchio JP, Kiruluta G et al. Is an artificial sphincter the best choice for incontinent boys with spina bifida? Review of our long term experience with the AS-800 artificial sphincter. Can J Urol 2002; 9: 1486–91.
59. Castera R, Podesta ML, Ruarte A et al. 10-year experience with artificial urinary sphincter in children and adolescents. J Urol 2001; 165: 2373–6.
60. Periera PL, Ariba IS, Urrutia MJM, Romero RL, Monroe EJ. Artificial urinary sphincter: 11-year experience in adolescents with congenital neuropathic bladder. Eur Urol 2006; 50: 1096–101.
61. Holmes NM, Kogan BA, Baskin LS. Placement of artificial urinary sphincter in children and simultaneous gastrocystoplasty. J Urol 2001; 165: 2366–8.
62. Light K, Lapin S, Vohra S. Combined use of bowel and the artificial urinary sphincter in reconstruction of the lower urinary tract: infectious complications. J Urol 1995; 153: 331–3.
63. Miller EA, Mayo M, Kwan D, Mitchell M. Simultaneous augmentation cystoplasty and artificial urinary sphincter placement: infection rates and voiding mechanisms. J Urol 1998; 160: 750–3.
64. Guralnick ML, Miller E, Toh KL, Webster GD. Transcorporal artificial urinary sphincter cuff placement in cases requiring revision for erosion and urethral atrophy. J Urol 2002; 167: 2075–9.
65. Leadbetter GW. Surgical correction of total urinary incontinence. J Urol 1964; 91: 261–6.
66. Tanagho EA. Bladder neck reconstruction for total urinary incontinence: 10 years experience. J Urol 1981; 125: 321–6.
67. Tanagho EA, Smith DA, Meyers FH, Fisher R. Mechanism of urinary continence II. Technique for surgical correction of incontinence. J Urol 1969; 101: 305–13.
68. Mollard P, Mouriquand P, Joubert P. Urethral lengthening for neurogenic urinary incontinence (Kropp's procedure): results of 16 cases. J Urol 1990; 143: 95–7.
69. Ferrer FA, Tadros YE, Gearhart J. Modified Young–Dees–Leadbetter bladder neck reconstruction: new concepts about old ideas. Urology 2001; 58: 791–6.
70. Kropp BP, Rink RC, Adams MC et al. Bladder outlet reconstruction: fate of the silicone sheath. J Urol 1993; 150: 703–6.
71. Hollowell JG, Ransley PG. Surgical management of incontinence in bladder extrophy. Br J Urol 1991; 68: 543–8.
72. Kropp KA, Angwafo FF. Urethral lengthening and reimplantation for neurogenic incontinence in children. J Urol 1986; 135: 533–6.
73. Waters PR, Chehade NC, Kropp KA. Urethral lengthening and reimplantation: incidence and management of catheterization problems. J Urol 1997; 158: 1053–6.
74. Belman AB, Kaplan GW. Experience with the Kropp antiincontinence procedure. J Urol 1989; 141: 1160–2.
75. Pippi Salle JL, Fraga JCS, Amarante A et al. Urethral lengthening with anterior bladder wall flap for urinary incontinence: a new approach. J Urol 1994; 152: 803–6.
76. Pippi Salle JL, McLorie GA, Bagli DJ, Khoury AE. Urethral lengthening with anterior bladder wall flap (Pippi Salle procedure): modifications and extended indications of the technique. J Urol 1997; 158: 585–90.
77. Nill TG, Peller PA, Kropp KA. Management of urinary incontinence by bladder tube urethral lengthening and submucosal reimplantation. J Urol 1990; 144: 559–63.
78. Snodgrass WA. Simplified Kropp procedure for incontinence. J Urol 1997; 158: 1049–52.
79. Gearhart JP, Canning DA, Jeffs RD. Failed bladder neck preconstruction: options for management. J Urol 1991; 146: 1082–4.
80. Donnahoo KK, Rink RC, Cain MP, Casale AJ. The Young–Dees–Leadbetter bladder neck repair for neurogenic incontinence. J Urol 1999; 161: 1946–9.
81. Mouriquand PDE, Phillips SN, White J et al. The Kropp-onlay procedure (Pippi Salle procedure): a simplification of the technique of urethral lengthening. Preliminary results in eight patients. Br J Urol 1995; 75: 656–62.
82. Rink RC, Adams MC, Keating MA. The flip-flap technique to lengthen the urethra (Salle procedure) for treatment of neurogenic urinary incontinence. J Urol 1994; 152: 799–802.
83. Lepor H, Jeffs RD. Primary bladder closure and bladder neck reconstruction in classical bladder extrophy. J Urol 1983; 130: 1142–5.
84. Leadbetter GW. Surgical reconstruction for complete urinary incontinence: a 10 to 22-year followup. J Urol 1985; 133: 205–6.
85. Sidi AM, Reinberg Y, Gonzalez R. Comparison of artificial sphincter implantation and bladder neck reconstruction in patients with neurogenic urinary incontinence. J Urol 1987; 138: 1120–22.
86. Rink RC, Mitchell M. Bladder neck reconstruction in the incontinent child: bladder neck/urethral reconstruction in the neuropathic bladder. Dial Ped Urol 1987; 10: 5.
87. Hoebeke P, De Kuyper P, Goeminne H et al. Bladder neck closure for treating pediatric incontinence. Eur Urol 2000; 38: 453–6.
88. Zimmern PE, Hadley HR, Leach GE, Raz S. Transvaginal closure of the bladder neck and placement of a suprapubic catheter for destroyed urethra after long-term indwelling catheterization. J Urol 1985; 134: 554–7.
89. Syme RRA. Bladder neck closure for neurogenic incontinence. Aust NZ J Surg 1981; 2: 197–200.
90. Chancellor MB, Erhard MJ, Kilholma PJ et al. Functional urethral closure with pubovaginal sling for destroyed female urethra after long-term urethral catheterization. Urology 1994; 43: 499–505.
91. Das S, Amar AD. Abdominal transposition of the female urethra. J Urol 1986; 135: 373–5.
92. Litwiller SE, Zimmern PE. Closure of bladder neck in the male and female. In: Graham SD, Glen JF, eds. Glenn's Urologic Surgery, 5th edn. Wolters Kluwer, 1998: 407–14.
93. Reid R, Schneider K, Fruchtman B. Closure of the bladder neck in patients undergoing continent vesicostomy for urinary incontinence. J Urol 1978; 120: 40–2.
94. Zeidman EJ, Chiang H, Alarcon A, Raz S. Suprapubic cystotomy using the Lowsley retractor. Urology 1988; 32: 54.
95. Hensle TW, Kirsch AJ, Kennedy WA, Reiley EA. Bladder neck closure in association with continent urinary diversion. J Urol 1995; 154: 883–5.
96. Jayanathi VR, Churchill BM, McLorie GA, Khoury AE. Concomitant bladder neck closure and Mitrofanoff diversion for the management of intractable urinary incontinence. J Urol 1995; 154: 886–8.
97. Jack GS, Almeida FG, Zhang R et al. Processed lipoaspirate cells for tissue engineering of the lower urinary tract: implications for the treatment of stress urinary incontinence and bladder reconstruction. J Urol 2005; 174: 2041–5.

98. Abrams P, Cardozo L, Fall M et al. The standardization of terminology of lower urinary tract function: report from the standardization sub-committee of the International Continence Society. Neurourol Urodyn 2002; 21: 167–78.
99. Chancellor MB, Gajewski J, Ackman CF. Long-term followup of the North American Multicenter Urolume Trial for the treatment of external detrusor-sphincter dyssynergia. J Urol 1999; 161: 1545–50.
100. Kaplan SA, Chancellor MB, Blaivas JG. Bladder and sphincter behavior in patients with spinal cord lesions. J Urol 1991; 146: 113.
101. McGuire EJ, Brady S. Detrusor-sphincter dyssynergia. J Urol 1979; 121: 774.
102. Emmett J, Paut R, Dunn J. Role of the external urethral sphincter in the normal bladder and cord bladder. J Urol 1948; 59: 439–54.
103. Fontaine E, Hajari M, Rhein F et al. Reappraisal of endoscopic sphincterotomy for post-traumatic neurogenic bladder: a prospective study. J Urol 1996: 155: 277–80.
104. Noll F, Sauerwein D, Stohrer M. Transurethral sphincterotomy in quadraplegic patients: long term follow up. Neurourol Urodyn 1995; 14: 351–8.
105. Milroy EJG, Chapple CR, Cooper JE et al. A new treatment for urethral strictures. Lancet 1988; 1(8600): 1424–7.
106. Chancellor MB, Rivas DA, Abdill CK et al. Prospective comparison of external sphincter balloon dilatation and prosthesis placement with external sphincterotomy in spinal cord injured men. Arch Phys Med Rehab 1994; 75: 297–305.
107. Rivas DA, Chancellor MB, Bagley D. Prospective comparison of external sphincter prosthesis placement and external sphincterotomy in men with spinal cord injury. J Endourol 1994; 8: 89–93.
108. Shaw PJR, Milroy EJG, Timoney AG et al. Permanent external striated sphincter stents in patients with spinal injuries. Br J Urol 1990; 66: 297–302.
109. Wilson TS, Lemack GE, Dmochowski RR. Urolume stents: lessons learned. J Urol 2002; 167: 2477–80.
110. McInerney PD, Vanner TF, Harris SAB, Stephenson TP. Permanent urethral stents for detrusor sphincter dyssynergia. Br J Urol 1991; 67: 291–4.
111. McFarlane JP, Foley SJ, Shah PJR. Long-term outcome of permanent urethral stents in the treatment of detrusor-sphincter dyssynergia. Br J Urol 1996; 78: 729–32.
112. Shah NC, Foley SJ, Edhem I, Shah PJR. Use of Memokath temporary urethral stent in treatment of detrusor-sphincter dyssynergia. J Endourol 1997; 11: 485–8.
113. Watanabe T, Rivas DA, Smith R et al. The effect of urinary tract reconstruction on neurologically impaired women previously treated with an indwelling urethral catheter. J Urol 1996; 156: 1926–8.
114. Vapnek JM, Couillard DR, Stone AR. Is sphincterotomy the best management of the spinal cord injured bladder? J Urol 1994; 151: 961–4.
115. Perkash I. Contact laser sphincterotomy: further experience and longer follow-up. Spinal Cord 1996; 34: 227–33.
116. Rivas DA, Chancellor MB, Staas WE, Gomella LG. Contact neodymium: yttrium-aluminum-garnet laser ablation of the external sphincterin spinal cord injured: men with detrusor sphincter dyssynergia. Urology 1995; 45: 1028–31.
117. Low AI, McRae PJ. Use of the Memokath for detrusor-sphincter dyssynergia after spinal cord injury: a cautionary tale. Spinal Cord 1998; 36: 39–44.
118. Chancellor MB, Karusick S, Erhard MJ et al. Placement of a wire mesh prosthesis in the external urinary sphincter of men with spinal cord injuries. Radiology 1993; 187: 551–5.
119. Chartier-Kastler EJ, Bussel TB, Chancellor MB, Denys P. A urethral stent for the treatment of detrusor-striated sphincter dyssynergia. BJU Int 2000; 86: 52–7.
120. Denys P, Thiry-Escudie I, Ayoub N et al. Urethral stent for the treatment of detrusor-sphincter dyssynergia: evaluation of the clinical, urodynamic, endoscopic and radiological efficacy after more than 1 year. J Urol 2004; 172: 605–7.
121. Sauerwein D, Gross AJ, Kutzenberger J, Ringert RH. Wallstents in patients with detrusor-sphincter dyssynergia. J Urol 1995; 154: 495–7.
122. Chancellor MB, Rivas DA, Linsenmeyer T et al. Multicenter trial in North America of Urolume urinary sphincter prosthesis. J Urol 1994; 152: 924–30.
123. Bloom DA, Knechtel JM, McGuire EJ. Urethral dilation improves bladder compliance in children with myelomeningocele and high leak point pressures. J Urol 1990; 144: 430–3.
124. Smith CP, Nishiguchi J, O'Leary M, Yoshimura N, Chancellor M. Single-institution experience in 110 patients with botulinum toxin a injection into bladder or urethra. Urology 2005; 65: 37–41.
125. Phelan MW, Franks M, Somogyi GT et al. Botulinum toxin urethral sphincter injection to restore bladder emptying in men and women with voiding dysfunction. J Urol 2001; 165: 1107–10.
126. Schurch B, Hauri D, Rodic B et al. Botulinum A toxin as a treatment of detrusor-sphincter dyssynergia: a prospective study in 24 spinal cord injury patients. J Urol 1996; 155: 1023–9.

58

Urinary diversion

Greg G Bailly and Sender Herschorn

Introduction

The goals of urologic management of neurogenic bladder dysfunction are to achieve and maintain low-pressure urinary storage and voiding, with preservation of the upper urinary tract and achievement of urinary continence. Long-term management has been facilitated by the widespread acceptance of clean self-intermittent catheterization (CIC).[1] The introduction of new medications over the past few years has also contributed to management. The vast majority of patients with neurogenic bladder dysfunction can be managed without resorting to urinary diversion. However, there continues to be patients who are unwilling or unable to perform self-catheterization or to be intermittently catheterized. There are others who, despite appropriate management, are unable to maintain low-pressure urinary storage and voiding and/or continence. It is these patients who may benefit from lower urinary tract reconstruction and urinary diversion rather than resort to indwelling Foley catheters.

Patients with neurogenic bladder dysfunction are followed regularly with clinical evaluation, laboratory testing with serum creatinine and urine cultures, upper tract imaging (usually ultrasound), and urodynamic studies. The storage and voiding problems are usually addressed with a combination of CIC and various medications. Males with spinal cord injuries are frequently managed with condom drainage with or without CIC. However, outlet-relaxing procedures, such as transurethral sphincterotomy[2] or Urolume stent,[3] are occasionally needed in suprasacral cord injury patients with high detrusor pressures and sphincter dyssynergia.

Neurogenic bladders in women may be harder to manage. Urethral CIC may be difficult for wheelchair-bound women and incontinence between CICs may also be more difficult to contain.

The aim of long-term follow-up of patients with neurogenic bladder disease is to prevent any changes that may lead to upper tract compromise. The complications of high intravesical pressures are well described and include upper tract dilatation, reflux, stones, pyelonephritis, and renal failure.[2,4] In addition, the patients may present with clinical symptoms. Changes in overall health can often be the first sign that the bladder may not be functioning satisfactorily. Worsening of incontinence, recurrent urinary tract infections, autonomic dysreflexia, suprapubic or back pain, as well as changes in the neurologic status of some patients, often indicate an alteration in lower urinary tract. These important clues can direct the urologist toward the appropriate investigations.

An outline of management of neurogenic bladder in relation to urinary diversion is shown in Figure 58.1. Urinary diversion, although frequently employed in the past for the treatment of neurogenic bladder dysfunction, is now only required in special circumstances. The commonly accepted indications include hydronephrosis that may be accompanied by progressive renal deterioration secondary to ureteral obstruction from a thick-walled bladder or intractable ureterovesical reflux, recurrent episodes of urosepsis, and persistent storage or emptying failure when CIC is impossible.[5] If, in the opinion of the urologist, the upper tract deterioration and/or storage problem cannot be managed with bladder augmentation surgery alone then urinary diversion may be indicated. Another reason for diversion is when urethral CIC is not feasible.

Unmanageable incontinence, while not life-threatening, may lead to skin breakdown, persistent infection, social isolation, and negative psychologic impact on patients. When procedures such as bulking agents, slings, artificial sphincters, and augmentation cystoplasty are unsuccessful or contraindicated, and/or urethral CIC is not possible, urinary diversion may be considered. Often the diversion is as an alternative to an indwelling catheter. Although there have been no randomized prospective long-term trials, patients with indwelling catheters have more morbidity, such as infectious complications, calculi, and radiographic abnormalities, than those managed with CIC.[6,7] Although a long-term Foley catheter may be convenient, safe, and effective for some patients, urinary diversion may be a reasonable option. The various types of diversions will be discussed in this chapter.

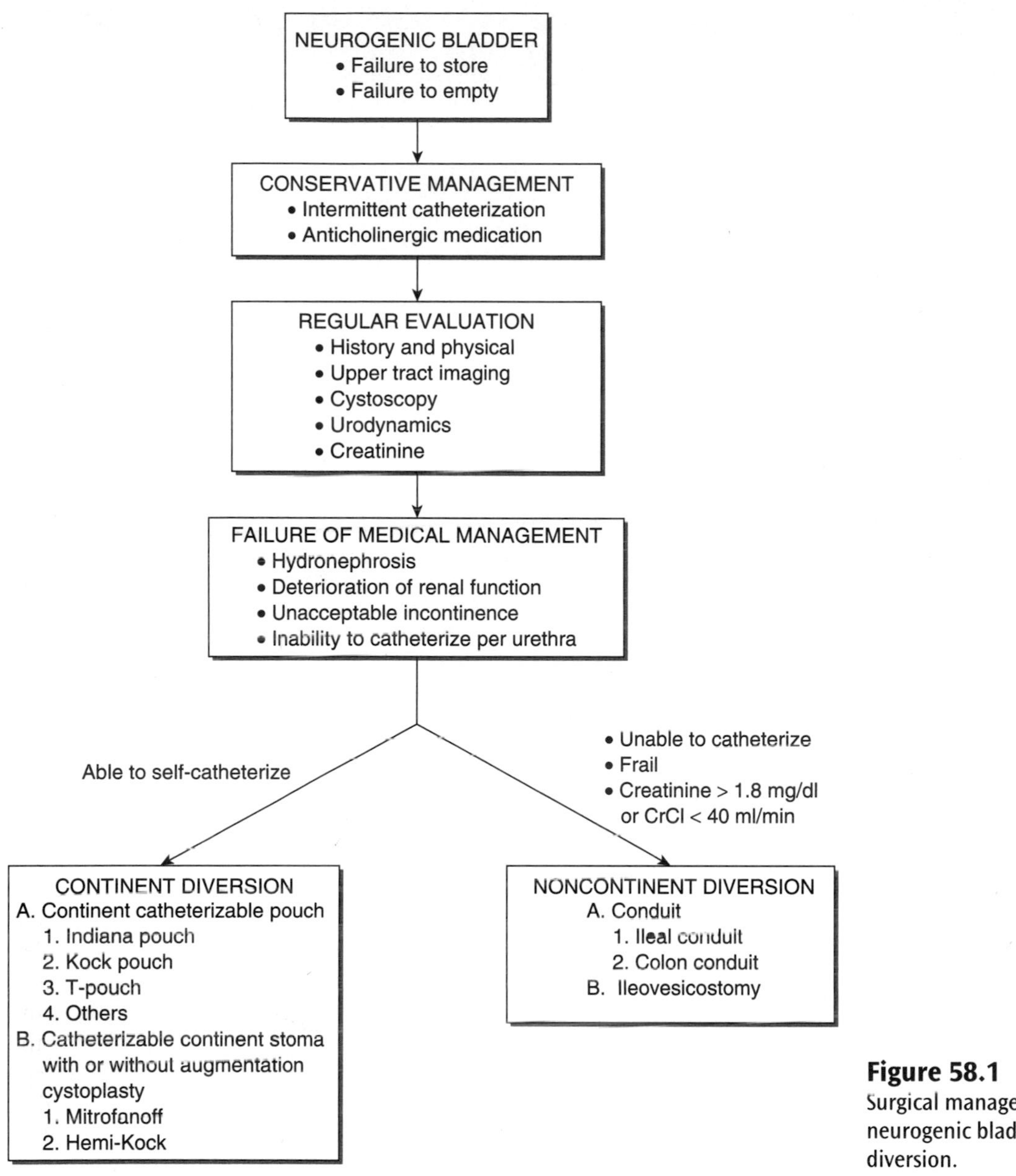

Figure 58.1
Surgical management of patients with neurogenic bladders requiring urinary diversion.

The choice of urinary diversion: patient considerations

The selection of urinary diversion procedure is largely based on the surgeon's opinion and experience, as well as his or her understanding of each individual patient's medical condition. Several important patient characteristics are considered when choosing an appropriate form of diversion (Figure 58.1). Although continent urinary diversion is considered appropriate in selected patients, these procedures are technically more challenging and are associated with higher short-term and long-term complication rates than those operations that employ an incontinent technique.[8] The patient's ability to perform self-catheterization must be evaluated as it significantly impacts on whether to construct a noncontinent or continent form of urinary diversion. Patients who cannot adequately perform self-catheterization of an abdominal stoma because of underlying neurologic disease or poor manual dexterity are not well suited for continent forms of diversion. Patients with multiple sclerosis or quadraplegia, and very frail or mentally impaired persons may at some time in their lives require the care of members of the family or supportive workers, and should be viewed as poor candidates for any kind of continent diversion.

If manual dexterity is sufficient for catheterization, other medical conditions may exclude a patient from undergoing a continent diversion. Elderly, debilitated patients with other significant medical co-morbidities are generally not good candidates for continent diversion. In addition to poor outcomes, these patients have higher perioperative risks. Although surgical techniques have improved over the past two decades, continent diversions often take longer to perform and have increased potential for complications compared to noncontinent diversion, and therefore proper patient selection is paramount to successful outcome.

Renal insufficiency is a relative contraindication to continent forms of diversion.[9–11] Continent diversion allows longer exposure time of urine to mucosa, subsequently increasing the risk of developing electrolyte disturbances, particularly in the patient with renal insufficiency. As a general rule, patients with a preoperative creatinine of greater than 1.8 mg/dl should undergo a noncontinent form of diversion.[10] A patient with borderline renal function should have a creatinine clearance calculated. A minimal creatinine clearance of 40 ml/min should be documented before the patient is deemed an appropriate candidate for a continent diversion.[12] Hepatic function must also be evaluated. Significant hepatic dysfunction increases the risk of developing hyperammonemia if the liver is unable to adequately process the ammonium chloride that may be produced by bacterial growth in the retained urine of a pouch.[9]

Once the patient has been assessed and more information is available on the above factors, it is important that the surgeon works with the patient and family/caregivers, without needlessly forcing the patient into one decision or the other. The patient's mental status may reflect the willingness and motivation to comply with self-care and follow-up. Speaking to other patients with various forms of diversions often helps the patient better realize the expectations of surgery. The Internet may also provide valuable information on different forms of diversion. The surgeon must inform the patient of all potential risks and benefits of each type of diversion. Clearly, the surgeon's experience and opinion, based on a review of the literature, is crucial in protecting the patient from inappropriate or unrealistic expectations. Ultimately the decision is made on an individual basis with input from patient, care-giver, and physician.

General principles of surgery

Preoperative preparation

Extensive history and physical examination are required to ascertain any risk factors that may affect bowel segment selection. These include previous surgery, regional enteritis, ulcerative colitis, diverticulitis, intraperitoneal malignancy, and prior bowel resection. The patient should be seen by the enterostomal therapist to have appropriate marking of the stoma site. The spot should be marked carefully with ink and then the skin etched when the patient is anaesthetized.

Bowel preparation

The patient usually receives mechanical bowel preparation prior to surgery, in an attempt to reduce the amount of feces. An antibiotic bowel preparation is used to reduce the bacterial count. Bowel preparation has been shown to decrease the rates of wound infection, intraperitoneal abscesses, and anastomotic dehiscence rate.[13,14] The true benefit of mechanical bowel preparation is poorly defined in the literature. Although it reduces the total number of bacteria, the change in concentration of bacteria may remain unchanged. Despite this, most urologic, colon, and rectal surgeons in North America routinely prescribe mechanical bowel preparations.[15,16] The type of preparation varies from center to center, but usually includes either fleet oral sodium phosphate, polyethylene glycol electrolyte (PEG) solution (GoLYTELY or NuLYTELY, Braintree Laboratories, Braintree, Massachusetts), or magnesium citrate. PEG requires administration of large volumes (approximately 4 litres) of fluid, but is extremely safe in most cases since there is virtually no net absorption of ions or water in the gut.

Oral sodium phosphate, that is Fleet Phospho-Soda (CB Fleet Co, Lynchburg, Virginia), has replaced PEG at many centers, largely because it appears to be better tolerated by patients.[16] This compound acts as an osmotic cathartic, causing large volumes of water to be translocated into the bowel, which results in diarrhea and bowel cleansing. Two 45 ml doses are usually ingested 4 hours apart the night before surgery.[17] At least three 8-ounce glasses of water should be consumed after each dose, with as much clear liquid as possible until midnight. When compared with PEG, Phospho-soda has been shown to be better tolerated and equally effective as judged by the surgeon, with similar wound infection rates.[18] Patients appear to prefer Phospho- soda to PEG as well.[19,20] It is, however, absolutely contraindicated in patients with renal insufficiency, symptomatic congestive heart failure, or liver failure with ascites.[15] Most clinical studies also exclude patients with a creatinine greater than 2 mg/dl.[18,19]

Antibiotic coverage

Preoperative antibiotic coverage for elective bowel surgery continues to be an issue of controversy. Similar to our understanding of the benefits of a mechanical preparation for urinary diversion, urologists tend to use prophylactic antibiotics based on information extrapolated from the abundance of data from the colorectal surgery literature. Even so, the literature is not clear on what to give and how to give it, and no clear consistent recommendations exist. In an extensive review of the use of antibiotic and mechanical preparations in urologic diversion surgery, Ferguson et al recommended 1 g of oral-based neomycin and 1 g metronidazole at 5 and 11 pm the night before surgery.[15] The use of antibiotics administered intravenously within an hour prior to making the skin incision is less controversial. The Centers for Disease Control (CDC) recommend a second-generation cephalosporin, such as cefoxitin or cefotetan, over a first-generation cephalosporin such as cefazolin for surgery of the rectum or colon.[21] Additional doses may be required during the surgery based on the half-life of the antibiotic, or if blood loss exceeds 1 liter. The benefit of continued prophylactic antibiotics during the postoperative period is unproven. The CDC recommends that prophylactic antibiotics should not be continued for more than 24 hours.[22]

The disadvantages of antibiotic use include postoperative increase in the incidence of diarrhea, pseudomembranous colitis, and, with prolonged use, the potential for malabsorption of protein, carbohydrate, and fat.[23]

Surgical principles

Intestinal anastomosis

Because urinary diversion is dependent on reconstructing various segments of bowel, it is important to understand certain basic principles of intestinal surgery. Much of the morbidity and mortality associated with urinary diversion in the immediate postoperative period relates to intestinal complications.[24] The fundamental principles of intestinal anastomoses include adequate mobilization, maintenance of blood supply, apposition of serosa to serosa of the two bowel segments, and creation of a watertight and tensionless anastomotic line. Various methods of performing the enteroenterostomy are well described.[23] Sutures or staples can be used with similar complication rates.[23]

Ureterointestinal anastomoses

Many different types of ureterointestinal anastomoses have been used in urinary diversion surgery, but all should follow basic surgical principles. Only as much ureter as necessary should be mobilized to result in a tensionless anastomosis. Periadventitial tissue should remain to ensure adequate blood supply. The anastomosis with the intestine should be performed with fine (4-0 or 5-0) delayed absorbable sutures, with the creation of a watertight mucosa to mucosa apposition. At our center, we attempt to retroperitonealize the anastomoses.

The issue of antirefluxing ureteric anastomoses is controversial. While some experimental literature indicates a benefit, the results of clinical studies of colonic conduits with antirefluxing anastomoses are equivocal. Deterioration of the upper tracts for ileal and colon conduits has been reported in 10 to 60% of the patients.[23] In one series, 49% of the upper tracts showed changes after conduit diversion, 16% of which had a blood urea nitrogen increase of 10 mg/dl or more.[25] However, deterioration of the upper tracts is usually a consequence of either infection or stones, or less commonly obstruction at the ureteral intestinal anastomosis.[23] In a prospective randomized comparison of ileal and colonic conduits into which one ureter was implanted with and the other without the antireflux technique, renal scarring was more prominent on the refluxing side.[26] However, split renal function test data for separate glomerular filtration rate (GFRs) showed no difference after 10 years.[26] These findings do not support the use of nonrefluxing ureterointestinal anstomoses for conduits. The final decision often rests with the surgeon's preference. At our center, we use refluxing anastomoses (Bricker or Wallace technique) for ileal conduits (Figures 58.2 and 58.3).

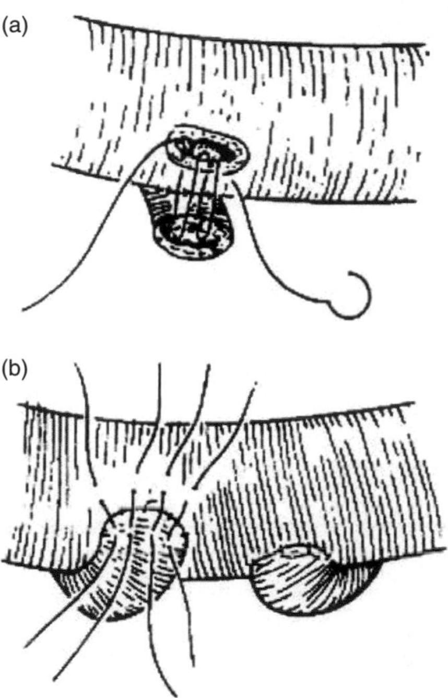

Figure 58.2
Bricker ureterointestinal anastomosis. (a) A full thickness serosa and mucosal plug is removed from the bowel. Interrupted 5-0 delayed absorbable suture approximates the ureter to the full thickness of the bowel mucosa and serosa. (b) A supportive suture layer can be added from the adventitia of the ureter to the serosa of the bowel. (Reproduced with permission from McDougal WS. Use of intestinal segments and urinary diversion. In Walsh PC, Retik AB, Vaughan ED et al, eds. Campbell's Urology, 8th edn. Philidelphia: WB Saunders, 2002: 3766.[55])

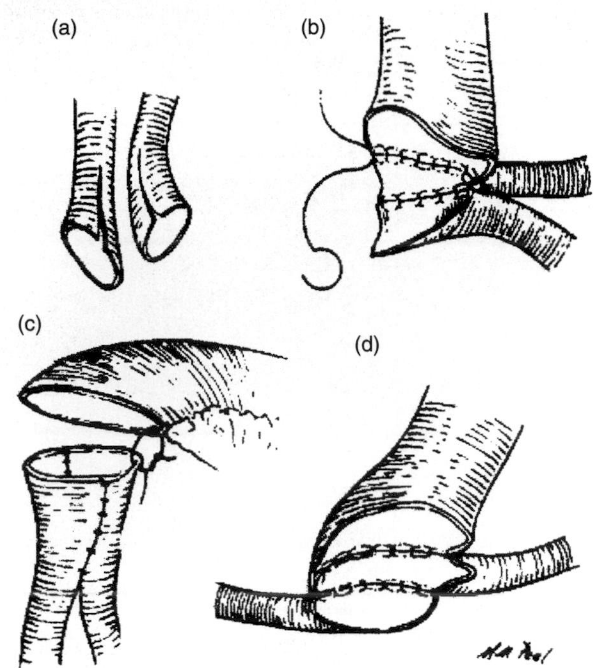

Figure 58.3
Wallace ureterointestinal anastomosis. (a) Both ureters are spatulated and are laid adjacent to each other. (b) The apex of one ureter is sutured to the apex of the other ureter. The medial walls of both ureters are then sutured together with interrupted or running 5-0 delayed absorbable suture. The lateral walls are then sutured to the bowel. (c) A 'Y-type' variant of above. (d) The 'head-to-tail' variant. (Reproduced with permission from McDougal WS. Use of intestinal segments and urinary diversion. In Walsh PC, Retik AB, Vaughan ED et al, eds. Campbell's Urology, 8th edn. Philidelphia: WB Saunders, 2002: 3766.[55])

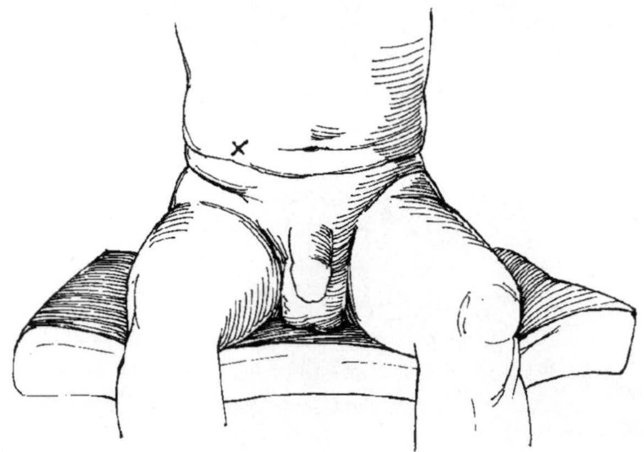

Figure 58.4
The stoma site is selected and marked on the surface of the abdomen where the skin is not rolled into folds while the patient is either sitting or standing. (Reproduced with permission from Hinman F Jr. Atlas of Urologic Surgery. Philadelphia: WB Saunders, 1998: 647.[27])

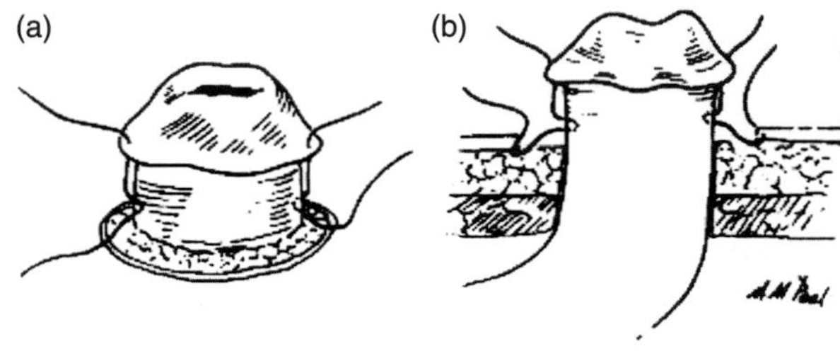

Figure 58.5
(a and b) Rosebud stoma: 5–6 cm of intestine is brought through the abdominal wall. The open bowel is sutured to the skin with four quadrant sutures of 3-0 delayed absorbable sutures that pass through the skin edge, then catch the adventitia of the bowel well below the level of the skin, and finally go through the mucosal edge, thus everting the stoma. Additional sutures are placed through the skin and bowel edge between the quadrant sutures to close the gap. (Reproduced with permission from McDougal WS. Use of intestinal segments and urinary diversion. In Walsh PC, Retik AB, Vaughan ED et al, eds. Campbell's Urology, 8th edn. Philidelphia: WB Saunders, 2002: 3760.[55])

The ureterointestinal anastomoses of continent reservoirs are usually nonrefluxing.[27] Depending upon which continent reservoir is chosen, the nonrefluxing mechanism can be constructed from intussuscepted bowel segments made by forming a flap valve in the intestinal wall, by tunnel implantation of the ureters, or by providing a long proximal loop.[27] The type of urinary diversion usually dictates which method of ureterointestinal anastomosis is chosen.

The stoma

For many patients, the stoma is a very important aspect of the surgery. Much of the success of a stoma can be dependent on appropriate selection of the stomal site. A noncontinent stomal site should accommodate a collection device that does not leak, while maintaining patient comfort when wearing clothes. It should meet these requirements in the standing, sitting, and supine position (Figure 58.4). Though commonly located in the right lower quadrant, the stoma may be positioned in other locations if body habitus creates a problem, as is sometimes seen in patients with neurogenic bladders. A commonly used stoma for an incontinent conduit is the nipple, sometimes called the rosebud, described by Brooke in 1954[28] (Figure 58.5). It is usually created as the last step in the conduit construction.

The location of the catheterizing stoma of the continent diversions is often placed in the lower quadrant of the abdomen through the rectus bulge and below the 'bikini line', or at the umbilicus. The umbilicus is the preferred location for someone in a wheelchair because of easier access, and occasionally it is placed even higher than the umbilicus due to body habitus.

Diversions

Noncontinent urinary diversion

The first attempt at using isolated segment of bowel for urinary diversion was reported in 1908 by Verhoogen, who described a technique to divert urine into an isolated segment of ileum and ascending colon.[29] Construction of the ileal loop conduit was first reported by Seiffert in 1935.[30] However, his procedure lacked effective means to collect and store urine. It was not until Bricker reported his technique that the ileal conduit became an acceptable method of urinary diversion.[31] This generally refers to the ileal conduit, although various forms of conduits can be constructed from colon or jejunum. An alternative form of noncontinent diversion to the conduit is an ileovesicostomy.

The conduits

Ileal conduit

Background

Since 1950, the Bricker ileal conduit has been the standard for noncontinent urinary diversion.[31] Still today, the ileal conduit remains the most popular form of urinary diversion.[32] It is the most straightforward of the diversionary procedures to construct, with overall fewer complications than rival continent diversions.[32] It is the most appropriate urinary diversion in elderly, debilitated patients and in those who lack the hand–eye coordination or manual dexterity for self-catheterization, or the motivation to care for a continent pouch.

Technique

Little has changed since Bricker described his technique of the ileal conduit in 1950.[31] Blood supply is based on the superior mesenteric artery (SMA). The jejunal and ileal branches of the SMA anastomose to form arcades of vessels, which can be easily transilluminated through the mesentery during the operation for preservation of the blood supply to the conduit.

A lower vertical midline incision is made from the symphysis pubis to the umbilicus or beyond. The ureters are identified and transected approximately 3 or 4 cm above the bladder. The left ureter is brought under the sigmoid colon through the sigmoid mesentery to the right side, taking care to avoid damage to both the sigmoid and ureteral blood supply. The ileum is inspected to insure healthy disease-free tissue. About 15–20 cm from the ileocecal valve, a 15–20 cm segment of ileum is selected, a length that will extend from the sacral promontory to the abdominal wall without tension. Two windows are constructed in the mesentery, with care taken to keep the base of the mesentery as wide as possible to prevent ischemia of the segment. The distal window usually measures 10–15 cm, and the proximal window can be much shorter at 3–5 cm. The bowel is transected, and the disconnected ileal segment is placed inferior to the remaining bowel segments. The bowel is reanastomosed using staplers or a standard two-layer closure. The mesenteric trap is closed. The ureteroileal anastomoses are performed either separately as with the Bricker technique, or cojoined as in the Wallace technique, at the proximal end of the loop. The final step is the creation of the stoma (Figure 58.6).

Colon conduit

Background

A colon conduit may be chosen when there are functional or anatomic factors that preclude the use of ileum. It has a larger diameter than ileum and can usually be easily mobilized into any portion of the abdomen or pelvis. The three types of colon conduits are transverse, sigmoid, and ileocecal, each having specific indications with advantages and disadvantages. The transverse colon is used when one wants to be sure that the segment of conduit employed has not been irradiated in individuals who have received extensive pelvic irradiation. It is also an excellent segment when an intestinal pyelostomy needs to be performed. The sigmoid conduit is a good choice in patients undergoing a pelvic exenteration who will have a colostomy. An ileocecal conduit has the advantage of providing a long segment of ileum when long segments of ureter need replacement, as well as the advantage of providing colon for the stoma. Because of its large lumen, stomal stenosis is rare. It is also used in situations in which free reflux of urine from the conduit to the upper tracts is thought to be undesirable. Contraindications to the use of transverse, sigmoid, and ileocecal conduits include the presence of inflammatory large bowel disease and severe chronic diarrhea.

Ileal vesicostomy

The concept of ileal vesicostomy arose from the successful management of pediatric neurogenic bladders by the creation of a vesicostomy. It is an alternative to an ileal conduit in some patients. It avoids the complications of ureterointestinal anastomosis, while maintaining the native ureteral antireflux mechanism. The addition of a small segment of ileum from the bladder to the abdominal wall acts to maintain low pressure in the bladder. The ileal segment is often referred to as a 'chimney', the distal end which is brought up

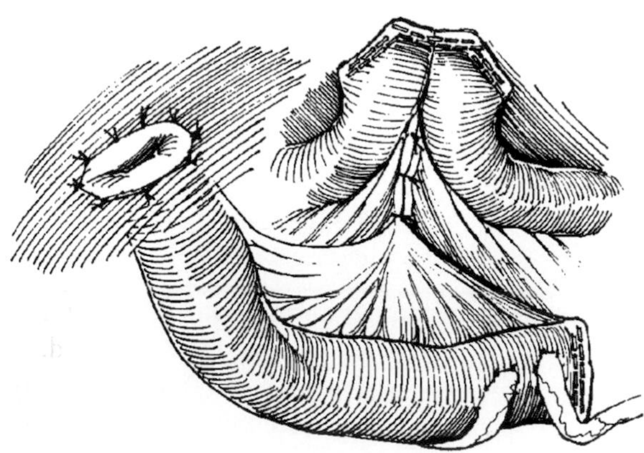

Figure 58.6
The ileal conduit at completion. (Reproduced with permission from Hinman F Jr. Atlas of Urologic Surgery. Philadelphia: WB Saunders, 1998: 654.[27])

to the abdominal wall and a rosebud stoma fashioned. It is important to use as short a segment of ileum as possible and to avoid a circular anastomosis between the ileum and the bladder. Redundancy of bowel may inhibit urinary flow and lead to electrolyte disturbances.[33] Theoretically, this results in a low-pressure reservoir that, if indicated at a later date, can be converted back to normal anatomy.

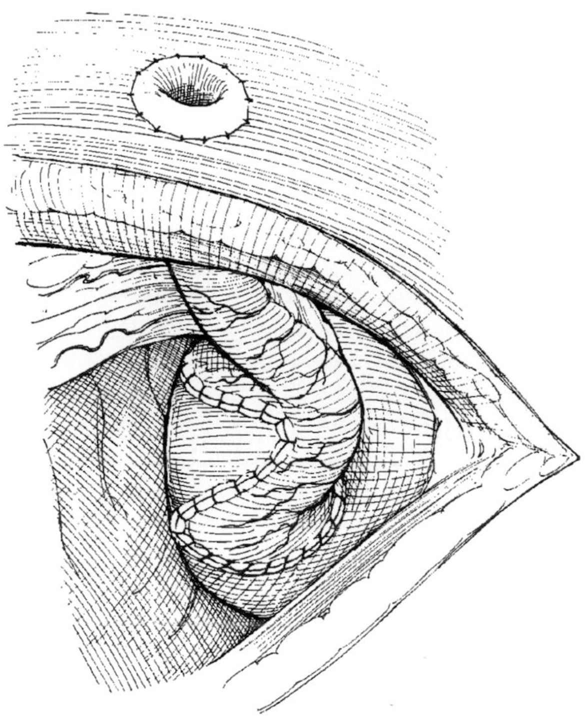

Figure 58.7
The ileovesicostomy. (Reproduced with permission from Hinman F Jr. Atlas of Urologic Surgery. Philadelphia: WB Saunders, 1998: 641.[27])

Technique

With the patient in the supine position, a lower midline incision is usually adequate. A 10–15 cm ileal segment is isolated, depending on what length is required to bridge the gap between the abdominal wall and bladder dome, leaving approximately 20 cm of terminal ileum and the ileocecal valve intact. The bowel reanastomosis is performed according to the surgeon's choice. The bladder is mobilized from the pelvic wall by dividing its lateral attachments, and the bladder dome is generously opened transversely. The proximal ileal segment is spatulated approximately 4–6 cm along its antimesenteric border, and anastomosed to the open bladder with 2-0 absorbable suture. The distal taubularized segment is brought out to the abdominal wall at a predetermined site and a stoma is created, as in the ileal conduit (Figure 58.7). A Foley catheter is left indwelling and exits through the stoma. An ileovesicostomy cystogram is performed 3 weeks postoperatively to ensure adequate healing of the suture line, and, if there is no leak, the catheter is removed.[33]

Continent urinary diversion

Background

Continent urinary diversion includes any reservoir subserved by a catheterizable efferent mechanism other than the native urethra and bladder neck.[34] Continent urinary diversion is used in patients with malignancy who require cystectomy and/or urinary diversion. It may also be used for the patient with a neurogenic bladder who requires urinary diversion and wishes to remain continent, and who is deemed to be a good candidate based on factors described earlier. The surgeon must consider the patient's motivation, adaptability, coping skills, and overall dexterity before embarking on a more complex continent diversion.

If possible, we generally try to preserve the bladder, thus maintaining the ureteral antireflux mechanism while adding to the capacity of the reservoir. When this cannot be achieved due to significant bladder disease, a continent catheterizable pouch may be a better option. The following section will review the continent supravesical reservoir and the continent bladder stoma.

The continent supravesical reservoir

Continence mechanisms

Although various forms of continent diversions were attempted in the past, it was not until Kock, in 1982,

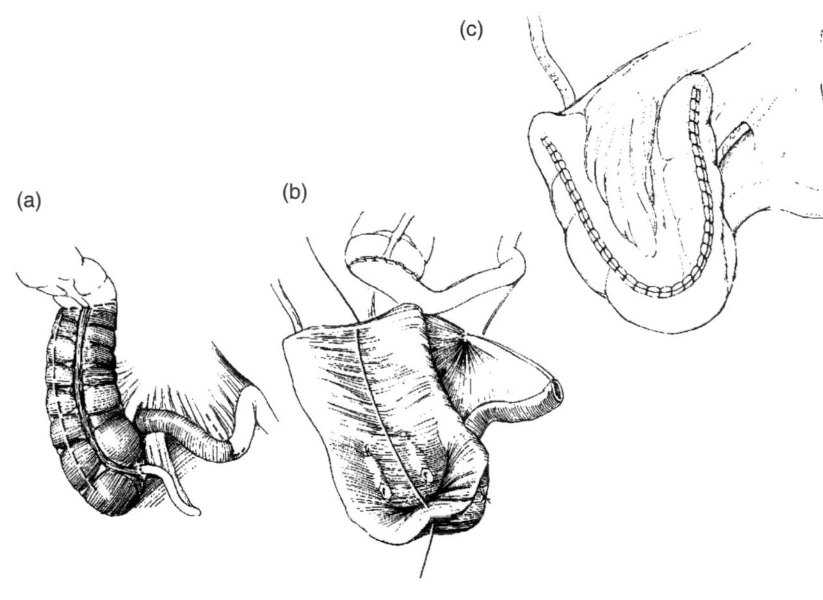

Figure 58.8
Indiana Pouch. (a) A 25–30 cm segment of cecum, ascending colon, and hepatic flexure, in addition to 8–10 cm of terminal ileum, is selected.The ascending colon is split down the antimesenteric border to within 2 cm of the caudal tip. (b) An ileocolostomy is performed using a suture technique or by a stapled method. The ureters are inserted by a submucosal technique. (c) A Malecot catheter is placed through the wall of the lowest part of the complex, in a position to allow direct exit through the abdominal wall. The U-shaped defect is closed by folding the distal portion of the colon into the proximal end and sutured into place with a running 3-0 absorbable suture. A serosal Lembert stitch with occasional lock stitches is added. The ileum is left to form the cutaneous conduit with tapering, as shown in Figure 54.9. (Reproduced with permission from Hinman F Jr. Atlas of Urologic Surgery. Philadelphia: WB Saunders, 1998: 698.[27])

reported the construction of an ileal reservoir for use in urinary diversion that renewed interest in continent diversion was generated.[35] Its use in the neurogenic bladder population requires careful evaluation of physical and mental capabilities to ensure proper patient selection.

Continent catheterizable pouches are much more surgically complex than the conduits. Perhaps the single most demanding technical aspect of a catheterizable pouch is the construction of the continence mechanism, of which four general techniques have been described.[23]

The first technique is sometimes performed for right colon pouches, and involves using the appendix or a pseudoappendiceal tube fashioned from ileum or right colon.[10]

The second type of continence mechanism used in right colon pouches is the tapered and/or imbricated terminal ileum and ileocecal valve. This involves imbrication or plication of the ileocecal valve region along with tapering of the more proximal ileum in the fashion of a neourethra.[36–39] This technique has been criticized by some because of the loss of the ileocecal valve and the consequences of more frequent bowel movements in some patients.

The third type of continence mechanism uses an intussuscepted nipple valve, or more recently, the flap valve. The creation of the nipple valve is very technically demanding, and is associated with the highest complication and reoperation rate.[36] A significant learning curve is required, and thus this technique is not meant for the surgeon who performs the occasional continent pouch. Many modifications have been made to the original Kock pouch description, because of the disappointment in long-term stability of the nipple valve in some patients. Despite the modifications, nipple valve failure can be observed in 10 to 15% of cases with the most experienced surgeons.[36] Failure may result from eversion and effacement of the intussusception and ischemic atrophy requiring a new nipple to be constructed. As well, stone formation on eroded or exposed nipples can present a problem. A group from the University of Southern California has developed a new procedure, the T pouch, which uses a much simpler procedure to create a flap valve, which results in both a continence and antireflux mechanism.[40,41]

The fourth procedure involves the construction of a hydraulic valve, as in the Benchekroun nipple.[42] This procedure has been largely abandoned because of nipple destabilization and stomal stenosis and will not be discussed.

Types of continent supravesical reservoirs

Indiana pouch

The Indiana pouch was first reported by Rowland of the University of Indiana in 1985, and has since become one of the most popular forms of continent urinary diversion.[37] It uses the right colon as a reservoir while using reinforcement of the ileocecal valve for continence and tunneled tenial ureteral implantation for antireflux (Figure 58.8). The remaining ileal limb acts as the 'neourethra', which can be tapered and brought out through the abdominal wall as a stoma (Figure 58.9). Several variations of the Indiana Pouch exist, including the Florida (Tampa) pouch[38] and the University of Miami pouch.[39]

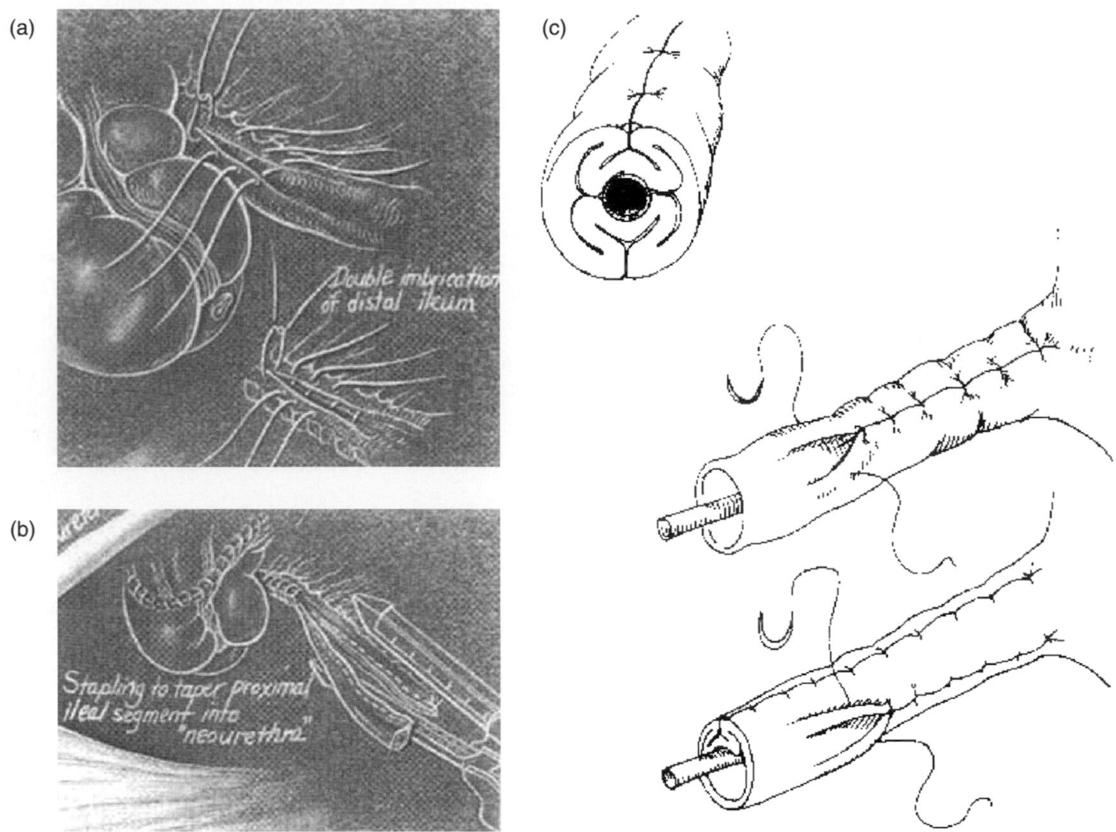

Figure 58.9
Tapering of ileal cutaneous conduit for Indiana Pouch. Apposing Lembert sutures are applied on each side of the terminal ileum. Excess ileum can also be tapered by a stapling technique. (Reproduced with permission from Benson MC, Olsson CA. Cutaneous continent urinary diversion. In Walsh PC, Retik AB, Vaughan ED et al, eds. Campbell's Urology, 8th edn. Philidelphia, WB Saunders, 2002: 3821.[36])

Kock pouch (continent ileal reservoir)

Unlike the Indiana pouch, the Kock pouch maintains the ileocecal valve, and uses only small bowel to create a low-pressure reservoir.[35] Continence of urine and prevention of reflux to the upper tracts is achieved by constructing 'nipple valves' (Figure 58.10). It has been criticized for being technically difficult and is associated with a high complication rate. As such, it has been abandoned by many urologists. However, the Kock limb (nipple valve) remains an important procedure as a means for constructing a continent catheterizable stoma, such as with the hemi-kock augmentation cystoplasty.

Other types of pouches that are used less frequently include the Mainz pouch, the UCLA pouch, the T-pouch, and the Penn pouch, none of which will be discussed here.

Continent bladder stoma

At our center, we aim to preserve the patient's native bladder if possible, thereby performing an augmentation cystoplasty and incorporating a continent bladder stoma. Preserving the bladder and avoiding the ureterointestinal anastomoses should lead to fewer complications. It is desirable for the patient to be able to visualize the opening so that the catheter tip may be directed easily and unimpeded. Two popular methods of achieving a continent catheterizable bladder stoma include the Mitrofanoff procedure and the hemi-Kock (nipple valve) with or without formal augmentation cystoplasty. Urethral continence may be addressed simultaneously if necessary, depending on its severity. This usually involves a pubourethral sling, closure of the bladder neck, or insertion of an artificial urinary sphincter.[43]

The Mitrofanoff principle

In 1980, Mitrofanoff described a continence mechanism using the appendix or ureter to create a flap valve, and at the same time a neourethral conduit to the bladder.[44,45] The appendix is mobilized on its mesenteric stalk and implanted on the bladder dome (Figures 58.11–58.13). The proximal lumen is tunneled as an antireflux mechanism. As the reservoir fills, the rise in intravesical pressure is transmitted through the epithelium and to the implanted

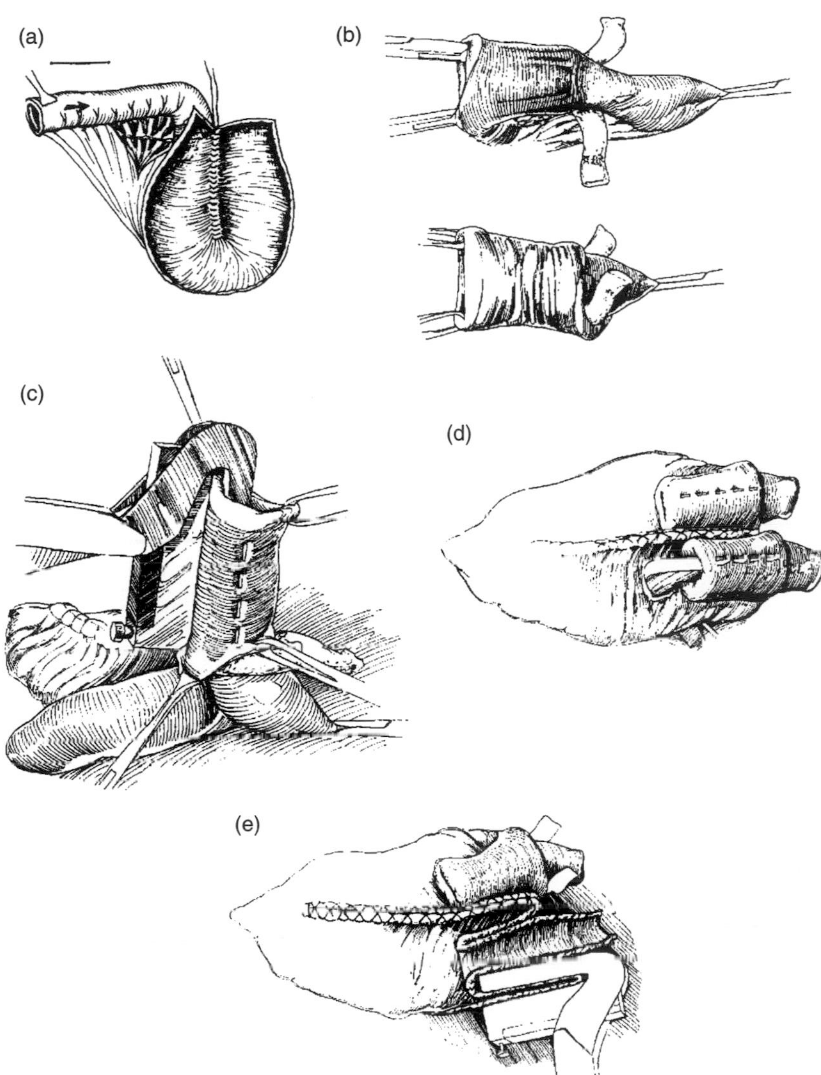

Figure 58.10
Construction of a nipple valve for the Kock Pouch. (a) A 15 cm segment of terminal ileum is isolated and opened along its antimesenteric wall. The proximal 10 cm serves as the continent intussusception and the distal 5–10 cm as the patch. The size of the patch varies according to the size of the excised segment. (b) A Babcock clamp is advanced into the terminal ileum, the full thickness of the intussuscipiens is grasped, and it is prolapsed into the pouch. (c) Three rows of 4.8 mm staples are applied to the intussuscepted nipple valve using the TA55 stapler. (d) A small buttonhole is made in the back wall of the ileal plate to allow the anvil of the TA55 stapler to be passed through and advanced into the nipple valve. A fourth row of staples is applied. The figure shows two valve mechanisms. In this instance, there would be only one. (e) The anvil of the stapler can be directed between the two leaves of the intussuscipiens and the fourth row of staples applied in this manner. The figure shows two valve mechanisms. In this instance, there would be only one.
(a) Reproduced with permission from Ghoneim MA, Kock NG, Lycke G, El-Din AB. An appliance-free, sphincter-controlled bladder substitute. J Urol 1987; 138: 1150–4;[89] (b–e) from Hinman F Jr. Atlas of Urologic Surgery. Philadelphia: WB Saunders, 1998: 688–9,[27] and Benson MC, Olsson CA. Cutaneous continent urinary diversion. In Walsh PC, Retik AB, Vaughan ED et al, eds. Campbell's Urology, 8th edn. Philidelphia: WB Saunders, 2002: 3808.[36])

conduit, coapting its lumen. This mucosal tunneling technique is very important to achieving continence.

The appendix has many advantages over methods for creating a continent catheterizable stoma.[46] The intraluminal pressure can rise nearly threefold that of the reservoir itself.[47] Perhaps the most important aspect of the flap-valve mechanism is the tunnel length to lumen ratio. Urodynamic evaluation has shown that a minimal tunnel length of 2 cm is required to achieve continence.[48] The Mitrofanoff principle can be used on native bladder, enterocystoplasty, or in a continent urinary reservoir. Because it is so reliable in preventing incontinence, it may place the patient at risk for upper tract deterioration or spontaneous rupture of the bladder or reservoir if regular catheterization is not performed. The appendix is particularly well suited for children because it is relatively longer and the abdominal wall is thinner. It also circumvents many of the secondary complications associated with using the ileocecal valve or other bowel segments.

Hemi-Kock augmentation enterocystoplasty

As an alternative to the Mitrofanoff procedure, patients may undergo a hemi-Kock ileocystoplasty with continent stoma permitting abdominal catheterization into the bladder. At our center, we have performed this procedure on various patients, including those who were wheel-chair-dependent, when urethral catheterization was difficult or impossible due to physical disability, and those who were unable to perform intermittent urethral catheterization or had a urethra that could not be rehabilitated due trauma or surgery.[49] This procedure can be performed in conjunction with an incontinence procedure, including closure of the bladder neck in select cases.

Using a low midline incision, the bladder is accessed and, in the case of an augmentation, the bladder is bivalved (clammed) in the anteroposterior direction in the midline from the bladder neck to 1 cm above the trigone. The ileal segment is measured from a point 25 to 30 cm proximal to the ileocecal valve. The next 15 cm proximal to this segment

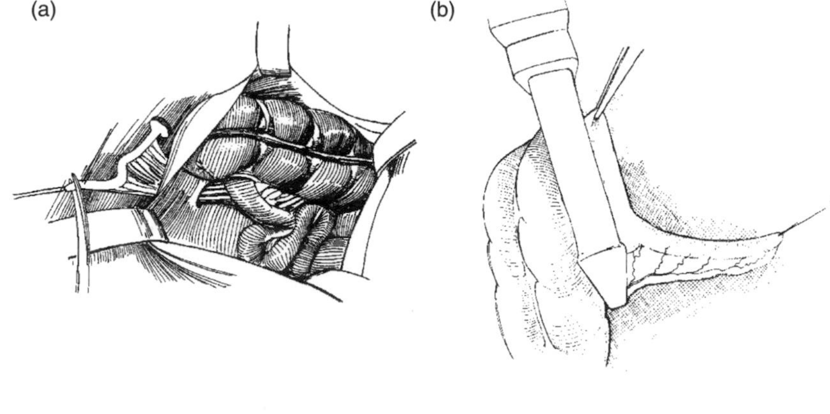

Figure 58.11
Mitrofanoff (appendicovesicostomy). (a) Stay sutures are placed at the base of the appendix, and the wall of the cecum is incised circumferentially to take a small cuff of cecum with the appendix. The appendiceal mesentery is separated a short distance from that of the cecum, preserving all of the appendiceal blood supply. The cecal defect is closed. The appendix is extraperitonealized behind the ileocecal junction. For umbilical placement of the stoma, it is not necessary to extraperitonealize the appendix. (b) For a short appendix or an obese patient, the appendix can be made longer by incorporating some of the cecal wall. (Reproduced with permission from Hinman F Jr. Atlas of Urologic Surgery. Philadelphia: WB Saunders, 1998: 709.[27])

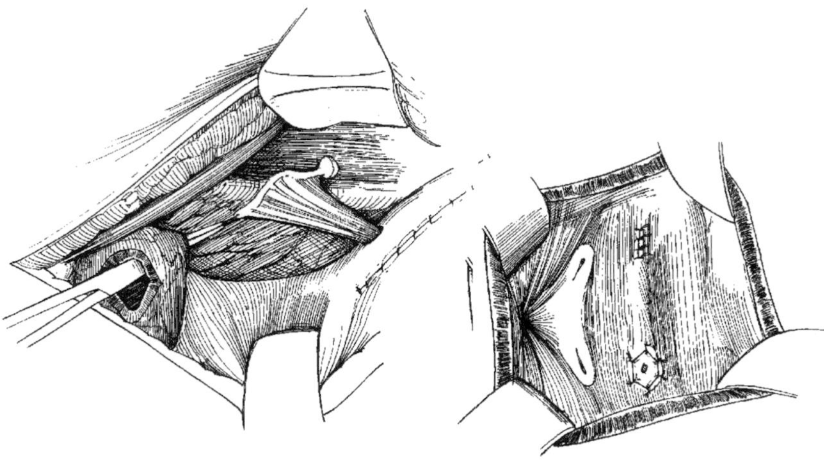

Figure 58.12
(a and b) Through a cystotomy, a submucosal tunnel is made in the posterolateral wall of the bladder, beginning well above the right ureteral orifice. The appendix tip is implanted. A bladder augmentation is usually done next. (Reproduced with permission from Hinman F Jr. Atlas of Urologic Surgery. Philadelphia: WB Saunders, 1998: 710.[27])

are for the nipple valve and the efferent limb. Up to another 45 cm are isolated on a mesenteric pedicle if an augmentation is performed. The nipple valve is constructed in the usual fashion with three lines of TA55 staples, with one line fashioning the nipple to the segment. If no augmentation is performed, the bowel segment with the nipple is approximated to the bowel incision, and the third TA55 staple line fastens the nipple directly to the bladder wall. The catheterizing limb is brought out through a hiatus in the lower abdominal wall, usually on the right side, although other sites, including the umbilicus, can be used (Figure 58.14).

In a review of 47 patients who had construction of a hemi-Kock nipple valve as a catheterizable bladder stoma, Herschorn reported that 36 were dry or had mild leakage, and 44 (94%) patients considered their surgery to be successful compared with their preoperative management at a mean follow-up of 56 months.[50] Six patients required valve revision and/or stomal hernia surgery within the first 2 years. Since the technique was modified by tapering the limb, there was a significant improvement in revision rate. Kreder et al have also reported success with using the hemi-Kock as a means of catheterizable bladder stoma.[51]

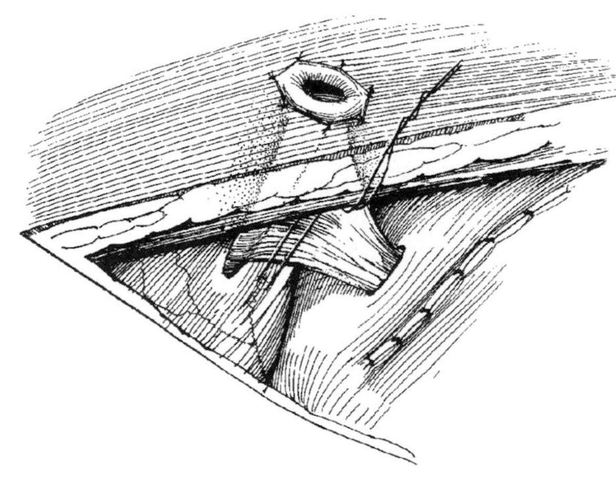

Figure 58.13
The appendiceal base is passed through an opening in the abdominal wall muscles large enough to accommodate a finger. The appendiceal opening is sutured to the skin (sometimes at the umbilicus). The bladder should be hitched to the anterior abdominal wall, and a catheter left in the appendix. (Reproduced with permission from Hinman F Jr. Atlas of Urologic Surgery. Philadelphia; WB Saunders, 1998: 710.[27])

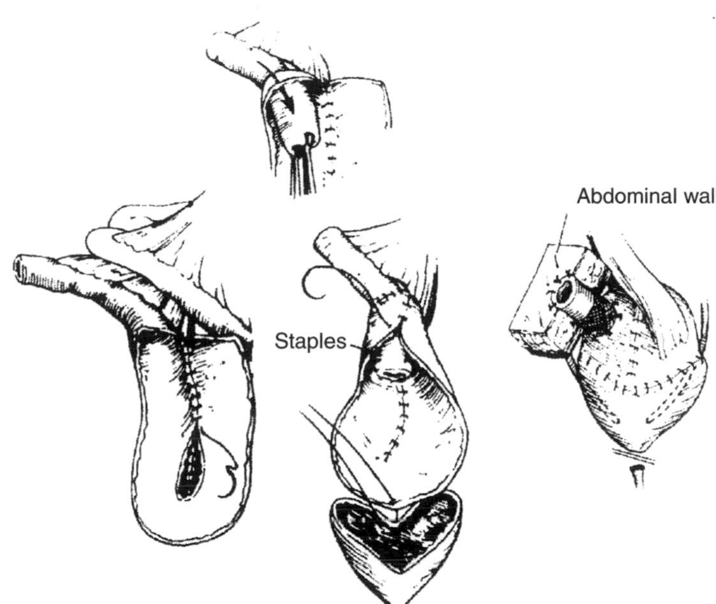

Figure 58.14
Hemi-Kock augmentation cystoplasty. (Reproduced with permission from Hinman F Jr. Atlas of Urologic Surgery. Philadelphia: WB Saunders, 1998: 732.[27])

Complications of urinary diversion

The complications associated with urinary diversion can be categorized as either technical-surgical, metabolic, or neuromechanical. Surgical complications are related to the reconstruction of the bowel and diversionary unit. Metabolic complications are the result of how the reabsorption of solutes is altered by the contact of urine with the bowel. The neuromechanical aspects involve the configuration of the reconstructed urinary reservoir and conduits and how this impacts on storage of urine.

Surgical complications

The complications associated with intestinal urinary diversion are displayed in Table 58.1. Postoperative surgical complications can also be classified as early or late. Nurmi et al reported on 144 patients with ileal conduits and found that the most common early postoperative complication was wound infection, followed by ureteroileal leakage, intestinal obstruction, intestinal fistulas, and acute pyelonephritis. Long-term complications were related to the delayed sequelae of intestinal surgery: stomal stenosis; ureteroileal stenosis; elongation; subsequent failure of the loop to propel urine adequately; and deterioration of the upper urinary tract.[52]

The complications that can occur with ureterointestinal anastomosis include leakage, stenosis, reflux in those anastomoses that were performed to prevent reflux, and pyelonephritis. Urine leakage usually presents within the first 7 to 10 days postoperatively with an incidence of 3 to 9%.[53,54] The use of soft ureteral stents reduces this incidence. Most leaks, fortunately, resolve with time and proper drainage, but they have been associated with periureteral fibrosis and scarring leading to stricture formation.[55] The incidence of ureteric stenosis is approximately 1–14%.[55] Stricture formation can occur at any time in the life of the patient, hence the importance of following patients with regular (every 1 to 2 years) upper tract imaging. Strictures can be anywhere along the ureter, as well as at the site of anastomosis. A common location is on the left ureter where it crosses over the aorta and beneath the inferior mesenteric artery. When a stricture is detected it is often treated first by endourologic or percutaneous means using balloon dilation or incision. Although these methods offer less morbidity to the patient, the long-term success rate is lower than open exploration (90% vs 50%).[56,57]

Stomal complications are the single most common problem encountered in the postoperative period after urinary diversion.[55] Early complications include bowel necrosis, bleeding, dermatitis, parastomal hernia, prolapse, obstruction, stomal retraction, and stomal stenosis. The incidence of stomal stenosis has been reported on average in 20 to 24% of patients with ileal conduits and in 10 to 20% of those with colon conduits.[55] Today, stomal stenosis has improved with proper stomal care and better fitting appliances.

Metabolic complications

Metabolic alterations are dependent on many variables including the segment of bowel used, the surface area of the bowel, the amount of time the urine is exposed to the bowel, the concentration of the solutes in the urine, renal function, and pH. When stomach is used, the patient may develop a hypochloremic, hypokalemic metabolic acidosis. In patients with normal renal function, this is usually not clinically significant. Jejunal diversions are rarely chosen because of their metabolic complications. They can cause hyponatremia, hypochloremia, hyperkalemia, and metabolic acidosis, leading to lethargy, nausea, vomiting, dehydration, weakness, and hyperthermia. This syndrome is more profound if proximal jejunum is used. Ileum and colon urinary diversion result in similar abnormalities: hyperchloremic metabolic acidosis. Abnormalities are worse in those with continent diversions than conduits, but unless renal function is impaired, their clinical significance is low. Symptoms can include easy fatigability, anorexia, weight loss, polydipsia, and lethargy. Regardless of the type of diversion, patients require regular screening of their electrolytes.[24]

Magnesium deficiency, drug intoxication, or abnormalities in ammonia metabolism are uncommon, but may lead to alteration of the sensorium. Each should be identified and treated accordingly. Drugs more likely to be problems are those that are absorbed by the gastrointestinal tract and excreted unchanged by the kidneys. This has been reported for phenytoin.[58] Methotrexate toxicity has been documented in a patient with an ileal conduit.[59] The problems with chemotherapeutic agents, in particular, the antimetabolites, are relatively rare, but caution should be given to those with continent diversions receiving chemotherapy. In this case, it is recommended that a pouch be drained during the time the toxic drugs are being administered.

Osteomalacia may occur in patients with urinary diversion secondary to a combination of persistent acidosis, vitamin D resistance, and excessive calcium loss by the kidney.[24] The degree to which each of these factors contributes to the syndrome varies from patient to patient. With this syndrome comes lethargy, joint pain, especially on the weight-bearing joints, and proximal myopathy. Serum calcium may be low or normal, and the alkaline phosphatase is usually elevated. Treatment involves correcting the acidosis and providing dietary supplements of calcium, and rarely vitamin D supplements.

Bacteruria, bacteremia, and sepsis occur with greater frequency when patients have intestinal diversions, especially in those with conduits. About three-quarters of those with conduits have bacteruria at any time, yet many of them are asymptomatic and do not require treatment for their colonization. The main indication to treat asymptomatic bacteruria is the presence of cultures dominant for *Proteus* or *Pseudomonas* Spp. It has been suggested that these organisms may contribute to upper tract damage.[24]

The majority of patients with catheterized pouches will have chronic bacteruria. Most urologists do not suggest treating asymptomatic bacteruria.[60] Patients are usually well protected from pyelonephritis from their nonrefluxing urterointestinal anastomosis. With a symptomatic pouch infection or pyelonephritis, antibiotic treatment should be administered. True pouch infections may require long courses of antibiotics, and, if frequently recurrent, we occasionally employ regular pouch instillation with antibiotics. A condition known as 'pouchitis' is manifested by pain in the region of the pouch along with increased pouch contractility.[24] The patient may experience sudden explosive discharge of urine from the continent stoma in this setting. This type of scenario usually responds to longer courses of antibiotics.

Because of the devastating consequences, these patients and caregivers must be well informed regarding urinary retention. It may occur from simply not catheterizing the stoma or occasionally when the stoma, particularly the with the nipple valve, obstructs or does not allow entrance of a catheter. This is considered a true emergency and the patient is instructed to seek attention from experienced medical personnel. It is recommended that various sizes and types of catheters are used, including the coude tip catheter. Sometimes, flexible cystoscopy is necessary. When significant manipulation of the stoma/pouch is required, we recommend leaving a catheter in for about 3 days due to edema.

There is substantial evidence that urinary intestinal diversion has a negative impact on growth and development.[61] These effects are most prominent in children who have diversions performed prior to puberty.

Most stones formed in intestinal urinary diversions are composed of calcium, magnesium, and ammonium phosphate. Patients with hyperchloremic metabolic acidosis, pre-existing pyelonephritis, and urinary tract infection with urea-splitting organisms are at the greatest risk of developing stones.[62] The major cause of calculus formation in conduits and pouches is the presence of a foreign body, such as staples or nonabsorbable sutures.

The exact risk of developing cancer in a segment of bowel that has been incorporated into the urinary tract is unknown. After bladder augmentation for benign disease, there have been 14 cases of malignancy reported in the literature.[63] In a series of 2000 patients with a maximum follow-up of 22 years, only 1 case of malignancy was reported.[64]

Neuromechanical complications

Perforation of a cutaneous continent diversion or augmentation cystoplasty with catheterizable stoma occurs infrequently. In the former, the incidence of perforation/rupture is in the range of 1–2%.[65] In a survey of 1700 patients in Scandinavia, 20 episodes of perforation occurred in 18 patients.[66] Rupture may occur from reservoir catheterization, endoscopic examination, a fall, or spontaneously. The signs and symptoms may be vague, especially in patients with neurologic disease who may not sense fullness. This possible complication should be kept in mind when these

Table 58.1 *Complications of urinary intestinal diversion*

Complications	Type of diversion	Patients (complications/*n*)	Incidence (%)
Bowel obstruction	Ileal conduit	124/1289	10
	Colon conduit	9/230	5
	Gastric conduit	2/21	10
	Continent diversion	2/250	4
Ureteral intestinal obstruction	Ileal conduit	90/1142	8
	Antireflux colon conduit	25/122	20
	Colon conduit	8/92	9
	Continent diversion	16/461	4
Urine leak	Ileal conduit	23/886	3
	Colon conduit	6/130	5
	Continent diversion	104/629	17
	Ileum colon	5/123	4
Stomal	Ileal conduit	196/806	24
stenosis or hernia	Colon conduit	45/227	20
	Continent diversion	28/310	9
Renal calculi	Ileal conduit	70/964	7
	Antireflux colon conduit	5/94	5
Pouch calculi	Continent diversion	42/317	13
Acidosis requiring treatment	Ileal conduit	46/296	16
	Antireflux colon conduit	5/94	5
	Gastric conduit	0/21	0
	Continent diversion		
	Ileum	21/263	8
	Colon or colon-ileum	17/63	27
Pyelonephritis	Ileal conduit	132/1142	12
	Antireflux colon conduit	13/96	13
	Continent diversion	15/296	5
Renal deterioration	Ileal conduit	146/808	18
	Antireflux colon conduit	15/103	15

From Dahl DM, McDougal WS. Use of intestinal segments in urinary diversion. In Wein AJ, Kavoussi LR, Novick AC et al, eds. Campbell-Walsh Urology, 9th edn. Philidelphia: WB Saunders, 2007:2534–78.[24]

Composite from the literature. Follow-up averages 5 years for ileal conduits, 3 years for colon conduits, 2 years for gastric conduits, and 2 years for continent diversions.

Data from Adams et al, 1988;[73] Althausen et al, 1978;[74] Beckley et al, 1982;[53] Boyd et al, 1989;[75] Castro and Ram, 1970;[76] Elder et al, 1979,[77] Flanigan et al, 1975;[78] Hagen-Cook and Althausen, 1979;[79] Jaffe et al, 1968;[80] Loening et al, 1982;[54] Malek et al, 1971;[81] Middleton and Hendren, 1976;[82] Pitts and Muecke, 1979;[83] Richie, 1974;[84] Schmidt et al, 1973;[85] Schwarz and Jeffs, 1975;[25] Shapiro et al, 1975;[86] Smith, 1972;[87] Sullivan et al, 1980.[88]

patients present with pain, and consideration should be given to performing enterocystography or a CT scan.

Quality of life

In addition to maintaining low-pressure urinary storage and protecting the upper tracts, urinary diversion in the patient with a neurogenic bladder aims to improve the patient's quality of life (QoL). Often this translates into providing a reliable state of urinary continence which positively impacts on the patients' lives. QoL issues in neurogenic bladder patients who have undergone urinary diversion are infrequently described in the literature. Much of what we know is extrapolated from the cancer population, which, in many ways, is an entirely different patient population. Several studies have recently shown an improved QoL in the neurogenic bladder population undergoing continent urinary diversion.[67,68]

Whether one procedure is better than another is very much based on what factors were considered when choosing which type of diversion. Newer or more complicated methods do not always result in a better QoL in these patients.[69] In a prospective study, perceived global satisfaction was found to be high with both conduit and continent cutaneous diversion; it was also noted that most patients would choose the same procedure again.[70] The most important aspect of the decision-making process is to try to tailor the medical needs and wishes of the individual patient. If this can be achieved, the discussion regarding which method offers the best QoL is superfluous.

Another important issue regarding continent versus noncontinent forms of diversion is the effect on the body image and sexuality of the patient. From the reports in the literature, the creation of a continent stoma results in an improved body image, a better QoL, and even a better sex life.[71,72]

References

1. Barkin M, Dolfin D, Herschorn S, Bharatwal N, Comisarow R. The urologic care of the spinal cord injury patient. J Urol 1983; 129(2): 335–9.
2. Madersbacher H, Scott FB. Twelve o'clock sphincterotomy: technique, indications, results. Urol Int 1975; 30(1): 75–6.
3. Chancellor MB, Gajewski J, Ackman CF et al. Long-term follow-up of the North American multicenter UroLume trial for the treatment of external detrusor-sphincter dyssynergia. J Urol 1999; 161(5): 1545–50.
4. Rivas DA, Karasick S, Chancellor MB. Cutaneous ileocystostomy (a bladder chimney) for the treatment of severe neurogenic vesical dysfunction. Paraplegia 1995; 33(9): 530–5.
5. Wein AJ. Neuromuscular dysfunction of the lower urinary tract and its management. In: Walsh PC, Wein AJ, Vaughan EDJ, Retik AB, eds. Campbell's Urology, 8th edn. Philadelphia: WB Saunders; 2002: 755–812.
6. Weld KJ, Dmochowski RR. Association of level of injury and bladder behavior in patients with post-traumatic spinal cord injury. Urology 2000; 55(4): 490–4.
7. Jamil F, Williamson M, Ahmed YS, Harrison SC. Natural-fill urodynamics in chronically catheterized patients with spinal-cord injury. BJU Int 1999; 83(4): 396–9.
8. Benson MC, McKiernan JM, Olsson CA. Cutaneous continent urinary diversion. In: AJ W, LR K, Novick AC, eds. Campbell-Walsh Urology, 9th edn. Philadelphia: WB Saunders; 2007: 2579–612.
9. Mills RD, Studer UE. Metabolic consequences of continent urinary diversion. J Urol 1999; 161(4): 1057–66.
10. Benson MC, Olsson CA. Continent urinary diversion. Urol Clin North Am 1999; 26(1): 125–47, ix.
11. Kristjansson A, Mansson W. Renal function in the setting of urinary diversion. World J Urol 2004; 22(3): 172–7.
12. Kristjansson A, Davidsson T, Mansson W. Metabolic alterations at different levels of renal function following continent urinary diversion through colonic segments. J Urol 1997; 157(6): 2099–103.
13. Irvin TT, Goligher JC. Aetiology of disruption of intestinal anastomoses. Br J Surg 1973; 60(6): 461–4.
14. Dion YM, Richards GK, Prentis JJ, Hinchey EJ. The influence of oral versus parenteral preoperative metronidazole on sepsis following colon surgery. Ann Surg 1980; 192(2): 221–6.
15. Ferguson KH, McNeil JJ, Morey AF. Mechanical and antibiotic bowel preparation for urinary diversion surgery. J Urol 2002; 167(6): 2352–6.
16. Nichols RL, Smith JW, Garcia RY, Waterman RS, Holmes JW. Current practices of preoperative bowel preparation among North American colorectal surgeons. Clin Infect Dis 1997; 24(4): 609–19.
17. Henderson JM, Barnett JL, Turgeon DK et al. Single-day, divided-dose oral sodium phosphate laxative versus intestinal lavage as preparation for colonoscopy: efficacy and patient tolerance. Gastrointest Endosc 1995; 42(3): 238–43.
18. Oliveira L, Wexner SD, Daniel N et al. Mechanical bowel preparation for elective colorectal surgery. A prospective, randomized, surgeon-blinded trial comparing sodium phosphate and polyethylene glycol-based oral lavage solutions. Dis Colon Rectum 1997; 40(5): 585–91.
19. Thomson A, Naidoo P, Crotty B. Bowel preparation for colonoscopy: a randomized prospective trial comparing sodium phosphate and polyethylene glycol in a predominantly elderly population. J Gastroenterol Hepatol 1996; 11(2): 103–7.
20. Heymann TD, Chopra K, Nunn E et al. Bowel preparation at home: prospective study of adverse effects in elderly people. BMJ 1996; 313(7059): 727–8.
21. Mangram AJ, Horan TC, Pearson ML, Silver LC, Jarvis WR. Guideline for Prevention of Surgical Site Infection, 1999. Centers for Disease Control and Prevention (CDC) Hospital Infection Control Practices Advisory Committee. Am J Infect Control 1999; 27(2): 97–132; quiz 133–4; discussion 196.
22. Rowe-Jones DC, Peel AL, Kingston RD et al. Single dose cefotaxime plus metronidazole versus three dose cefuroxime plus metronidazole as prophylaxis against wound infection in colorectal surgery: multicentre prospective randomised study. BMJ 1990; 300(6716): 18–22.
23. Dahl DM, McDougal WS. Use of intestinal segments in urinary diversion. In: Wein AJ, Kavoussi LR, Novick AC, eds. Campbell-Walsh Urology, 9th edn. Philadelphia: WB Saunders; 2007: 2534–78.
24. Mansson W, Colleen S, Stigsson L. Four methods of uretero-intestinal anastomosis in urinary conduit diversion. A comparative study of early and late complications and the influence of radiotherapy. Scand J Urol Nephrol 1979; 13(2): 191–9.
25. Schwarz GR, Jeffs RD. Ileal conduit urinary diversion in children: computer analysis of followup from 2 to 16 years. J Urol 1975; 114(2): 285–8.
26. Kristjansson A, Bajc M, Wallin L, Willner J, Mansson W. Renal function up to 16 years after conduit (refluxing or anti-reflux anastomosis) or continent urinary diversion. 2. Renal scarring and location of bacteriuria. Br J Urol 1995; 76(5): 546–50.
27. Hinman F Jr. Atlas of Urologic Surgery. Philadelphia: WB Saunders Company, 1998: 682.
28. Brooke BN. Ulcerative Colitis and Its Surgical Management. Edinburgh: Churchill Livingstone, 1954: 92.
29. Verhoogen J. Neostomie urétéro-caecale. Formation d'une nouvelle poche vésicale et d'un nouvel urètre. Assoc Fr Urol 1908; 12: 362–5.
30. Seiffert L. Die 'Darm-Siphonblase'. Arch Klin Chir 1935; 183: 569–74.
31. Bricker EM. Bladder substitution after pelvic evisceration. Surg Clin North Am 1950; 30(5): 1511–21.
32. Williams O, Vereb MJ, Libertino JA. Noncontinent urinary diversion. Urol Clin North Am 1997; 24(4): 735–44.
33. Atan A, Konety BR, Nangia A, Chancellor MB. Advantages and risks of ileovesicostomy for the management of neuropathic bladder. Urology 1999; 54(4): 636–40.
34. Kaefer M, Retik AB. The Mitrofanoff principle in continent urinary reconstruction. Urol Clin North Am 1997; 24(4): 795–811.
35. Kock NG, Nilson AE, Nilsson LO, Norlen LJ, Philipson BM. Urinary diversion via a continent ileal reservoir: clinical results in 12 patients. J Urol 1982; 128(3): 469–75.
36. Benson MC, Olsson CA. Cutaneous continent urinary diversion. In: Walsh PC, Retik AB, Vaughan EDJ, Wein AJ, eds. Campbell's Urology. Philadelphia: WB Saunders Company, 2002: 3789–834.
37. Rowland RG, Mitchell ME, Bihrle R. The cecoileal continent urinary reservoir. World J Urol 1985; 3: 185–90.
38. Lockhart JL. Remodeled right colon: an alternative urinary reservoir. J Urol 1987; 138(4): 730–4.

39. Bejany DE, Politano VA. Stapled and nonstapled tapered distal ileum for construction of a continent colonic urinary reservoir. J Urol 1988; 140(3): 491–4.
40. Stein JP, Lieskovsky G, Ginsberg DA, Bochner BH, Skinner DG. The T pouch: an orthotopic ileal neobladder incorporating a serosal lined ileal antireflux technique. J Urol 1998; 159(6): 1836–42.
41. Stein JP, Skinner DG. The craft of urologic surgery: the T pouch. Urol Clin North Am 2003; 30(3): 647–61, xi.
42. Benchekroun A. Hydraulic valve for continence and antireflux. A 17-year experience of 210 cases. Scand J Urol Nephrol Suppl 1992; 142: 66–70.
43. Leng WW, McGuire EJ. Reconstructive surgery for urinary incontinence. Urol Clin North Am 1999; 26(1): 61–80, viii.
44. Mitrofanoff P. [Trans-appendicular continent cystostomy in the management of the neurogenic bladder.] Chir Pediatr 1980; 21(4): 297–305.
45. Keating MA, Rink RC, Adams MC. Appendicovesicostomy: a useful adjunct to continent reconstruction of the bladder. J Urol 1993; 149(5): 1091–4.
46. Hinman F, Jr. Functional classification of conduits for continent diversion. J Urol 1990; 144(1): 27–30.
47. Malone RR, D'Cruz VT, Worth PHL, Woodhouse RJ. Why are continent diversions continent? J Urol 1989; 141: 303A.
48. Watson HS, Bauer SB, Peters CA et al. Comparative urodynamics of appendiceal and ureteral Mitrofanoff conduits in children. J Urol 1995; 154(2 Pt 2): 878–82.
49. Herschorn S, Thijssen AJ, Radomski SB. Experience with the hemi-Kock ileocystoplasty with a continent abdominal stoma. J Urol 1993; 149(5): 998–1001.
50. Herschorn S. Durability of the hemi-Kock continent bladder stoma. J Urol 2001; 165(5): Suppl 88.
51. Kreder K, Das AK, Webster GD. The hemi-Kock ileocystoplasty: a versatile procedure in reconstructive urology. J Urol 1992; 147(5): 1248–51.
52. Nurmi M, Puntala P, Alanen A. Evaluation of 144 cases of ileal conduits in adults. Eur Urol 1988; 15(1–2): 89–93.
53. Beckley S, Wajsman Z, Pontes JE, Murphy G. Transverse colon conduit: a method of urinary diversion after pelvic irradiation. J Urol 1982; 128(3): 464–8.
54. Loening SA, Navarre RJ, Narayana AS, Culp DA. Transverse colon conduit urinary diversion. J Urol 1982; 127(1): 37–9.
55. McDougal WS. Use of intestinal segments and urinary diversion. In: Walsh PC, Retik AB, Vaughan EDJ, Wein AJ, eds. Campbell's Urology. 8th edn. Philadelphia: WB Saunders Company, 2002: 3745–88.
56. Kramolowsky EV, Clayman RV, Weyman PJ. Endourological management of ureteroileal anastomotic strictures: is it effective? J Urol 1987; 137(3): 390–4.
57. Kramolowsky EV, Clayman RV, Weyman PJ. Management of ureterointestinal anastomotic strictures: comparison of open surgical and endourological repair. J Urol 1988; 139(6): 1195–8.
58. Savarirayan F, Dixey GM. Syncope following ureterosigmoidostomy. J Urol 1969; 101(6): 844–5.
59. Bowyer GW, Davies TW. Methotrexate toxicity associated with an ileal conduit. Br J Urol 1987; 60(6): 592.
60. Skinner DG, Lieskovsky G, Skinner EC, Boyd SD. Urinary diversion. Curr Probl Surg 1987; 24(7): 399–471.
61. Koch MO, McDougal WS, Hall MC et al. Long-term metabolic effects of urinary diversion: a comparison of myelomeningocele patients managed by clean intermittent catheterization and urinary diversion. J Urol 1992; 147(5): 1343–7.
62. Dretler SP. The pathogenesis of urinary tract calculi occurring after ileal conduit diversion. I. Clinical study. II. Conduit study. 3. Prevention. J Urol 1973; 109(2): 204–9.
63. Treiger BF, Marshall FF. Carcinogenesis and the use of intestinal segments in the urinary tract. Urol Clin North Am 1991; 18(4): 737–42.
64. Rowland RG, Regan JS. The risk of secondary malignancies in urinary reservoirs. In: Hohenfellner R, Wammack R, eds. Continent Urinary Diversion. London: Churchill Livingstone, 1992: 299–308.
65. Studer UE, Stenzl A, Mansson W, Mills R. Bladder replacement and urinary diversion. Eur Urol 2000; 38(6): 790–800.
66. Mansson W, Bakke A, Bergman B et al. Perforation of continent urinary reservoirs. Scandinavian experience. Scand J Urol Nephrol 1997; 31(6): 529–32.
67. Zommick JN, Simoneau AR, Skinner DG, Ginsberg DA. Continent lower urinary tract reconstruction in the cervical spinal cord injured population. J Urol 2003; 169(6): 2184–7.
68. Pazooki D, Edlund C, Karlsson AK et al. Continent cutaneous urinary diversion in patients with spinal cord injury. Spinal Cord 2006; 44(1): 19–23.
69. Mansson A, Mansson W. When the bladder is gone: quality of life following different types of urinary diversion. World J Urol 1999; 17(4): 211–8.
70. Hardt J, Petrak F, Filipas D, Egle UT. Adaptation to life after surgical removal of the bladder – an application of graphical Markov models for analysing longitudinal data. Stat Med 2004; 23(4): 649–66.
71. Moreno JG, Chancellor MB, Karasick S et al. Improved quality of life and sexuality with continent urinary diversion in quadriplegic women with umbilical stoma. Arch Phys Med Rehabil 1995; 76(8): 758–62.
72. Watanabe T, Rivas DA, Smith R, Staas WE Jr, Chancellor MB. The effect of urinary tract reconstruction on neurologically impaired women previously treated with an indwelling urethral catheter. J Urol 1996; 156(6): 1926–8.
73. Adams MC, Mitchell ME, Rink RC. Gastrocystoplasty: an alternative solution to the problem of urological reconstruction in the severely compromised patient. J Urol 1988; 140(5 Pt 2): 1152–6.
74. Althausen AF, Hagen-Cook K, Hendren WH 3rd. Non-refluxing colon conduit: experience with 70 cases. J Urol 1978; 120(1): 35–9.
75. Boyd SD, Schiff WM, Skinner DG et al. Prospective study of metabolic abnormalities in patient with continent Kock pouch urinary diversion. Urology 1989; 33(2): 85–8.
76. Castro JE, Ram MD. Electrolyte imbalance following ileal urinary diversion. Br J Urol 1970; 42(1). 29–32.
77. Elder DD, Moisey CU, Rees RW. A long-term follow-up of the colonic conduit operation in children. Br J Urol 1979; 51(6): 462–5.
78. Flanigan RC, Kursh ED, Persky L. Thirteen year experience with ileal loop diversion in children with myelodysplasia. Am J Surg 1975; 130(5): 535–8.
79. Hagen-Cook K, Althausen AF. Early observations on 31 adults with non-refluxing colon conduits. J Urol 1979; 121(1): 13–16.
80. Jaffe BM, Bricker EM, Butcher HR Jr. Surgical complications of ileal segment urinary diversion. Ann Surg 1968; 167(3): 367–76.
81. Malek RS, Burke EC, Deweerd JH. Ileal conduit urinary diversion in children. J Urol 1971; 105(6): 892–900.
82. Middleton AW Jr, Hendren WH. Ileal conduits in children at the Massachusetts General Hospital from 1955 to 1970. J Urol 1976; 115(5): 591–5.
83. Pitts WR Jr, Muecke EC. A 20-year experience with ileal conduits: the fate of the kidneys. J Urol 1979; 122(2): 154–7.
84. Richie JP. Intestinal loop urinary diversion in children. J Urol 1974; 111(5): 687–9.
85. Schmidt JD, Hawtrey CE, Flocks RH, Culp DA. Complications, results and problems of ileal conduit diversions. J Urol 1973; 109(2): 210–6.
86. Shapiro SR, Lebowitz R, Colodny AH. Fate of 90 children with ileal conduit urinary diversion a decade later: analysis of complications, pyelography, renal function and bacteriology. J Urol 1975; 114(2): 289–95.
87. Smith ED. Follow-up studies on 150 ileal conduits in children. J Pediatr Surg 1972; 7(1): 1–10.
88. Sullivan JW, Grabstald H, Whitmore WF Jr. Complications of ureteroileal conduit with radical cystectomy: review of 336 cases. J Urol 1980; 124(6): 797–801.

59

The trans-appendicular continent cystostomy technique (Mitrofanoff principle)

Bernard Boillot, Jacques Corcos, and Paul Mitrofanoff

Introduction

Since its brief description by Mitrofanoff in 1980, in a French pediatric journal,[1] trans-appendicular continent cystostomy has become the most frequently-used operation in patients of all ages. Surprisingly, the technique has not been formally described, although it is often mentioned in technical reference books and numerous articles.[2–8] Only Mitrofanoff's second publication in 2002[9] gave more technical details, but it was mainly oriented towards pediatrics (congenital malformations and neurologic bladders).

Initially described as an intervention 'reserved' for pediatric neurogenic bladders, this procedure has seen its indications broadened to complex cases: serious malformations of the lower urinary tract in infants and acquired urinary retention of neurologic, traumatic, or iatrogenic origin in adults. Advances in urodynamics have redefined its indications of bladder augmentation, which are now more frequent; in all these cases, the question of whether to perform a concomitant trans-appendicular cystostomy should be raised.

Thus, more than 25 years after its initial description, the Mitrofanoff technique remains topical, and we think it is important to provide technical information on an operation whose success depends on respecting both its broad principles and procedural details. After having reviewed the literature, we realized that numerous modifications and variations of the initial technique have been proposed, some of which represent significant changes of the original procedure.[7,10–14] We are describing the original technique that we still follow today in our daily practice, irrespective of patient age and pathology.

Technique

The cystostomy implantation site is chosen before the intervention, appreciating that when umbilical implantation is not possible, the right iliac site can be targeted.

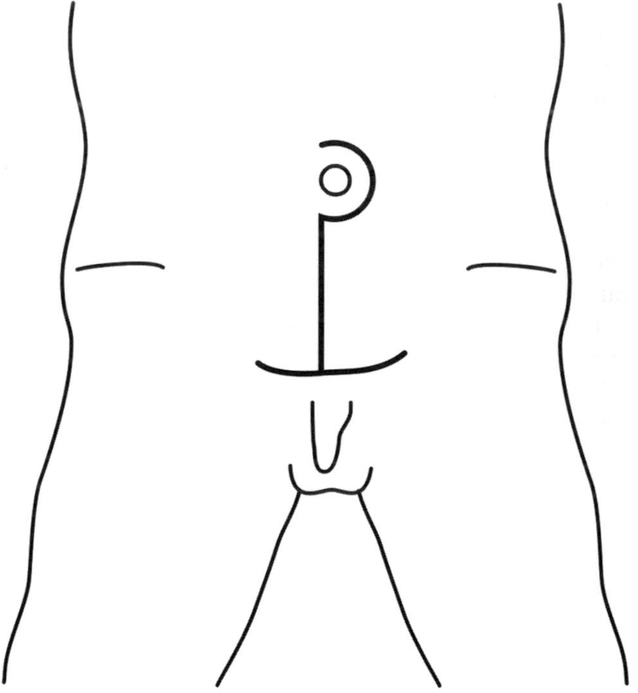

Figure 59.1
Median sub- and peri-umbilical laparotomy.

Approach

Figure 59.1 illustrates the median infra- and peri-umbilical laparotomy. To undertake umbilical cystostomy implantation, a cutaneous incision must be made at more than 10 mm from the left external edge of the umbilicus. However, the white line incision must remain medial until the umbilicus is relieved of its ligamentary attachments. The umbilical depression, freed of all its subcutaneous attachments, must be perfectly mobile. We resect the bottom so that a 20F catheter can pass through easily. It is extremely important to avoid traumatizing the umbilical skin, to limit the risk of stomal stenosis.

The abdominal cavity is explored and, if present, the ventriculo-peritoneal diversion catheter is displaced to the level of the upper abdomen.

Appendix preparation

The minimal appendix length needed is 6 cm in lean subjects but, in most cases, we prefer to deploy a 10-cm tube.

After palpation of the appendix, we dissect the mesoappendix by freeing it from the internal side of the cecum, with 4-0 absorbable ligatures (Figure 59.2a). We progress until we make it mobile without traction up to the cystostomy opening. If necessary, the cecum and right colon are mobilized medially. The ascending colon is then clamped to allow sectioning of the appendix tip and measurement of its lumen: it should admit a 14F catheter. If not, it should be recut higher until 14F catheter passage is possible.

The ceco–appendicular junction is sectioned with a cold blade and a cecal collar of 1 cm maximum diameter, which will disclose the appendix's vascularization, and facilitate stomal suturing. The cecal stump is closed by continuous stitching with an absorbable monobrin 4-0 suture, without burying it.

It may be that the appendix is too short; in this case, we eventually perform an enlargement procedure with a cecal tube modeled after a 14F catheter (Figure 59.2b). However, the vasculature of that enlargement has to be evaluated meticulously to prevent tubal stricture.

At the level of the appendicular tip resection, the mucosa is attached to the appendix wall by 4 stitches with a rapidly-absorbable 5-0 suture (Figure 59.3a). The last 3 cm of the appendix tip must be freed from the mesoappendix by bipolar cautery of the appendix; this distal part will be implanted in the bladder (Figure 59.3b).

At the end of the preparation stage, the tube must have the following characteristics:

- sufficient mobility to link the bladder with the umbilicus or right iliac fossa
- a rectilinear aspect
- a regular caliber equal to at least 14F
- a well-vascularized cecal mucosa collar for the cutaneous side of the stoma
- a well-vascularized tip despite sectioning of the mesoappendix over its last 3 cm.

The tube is then cleaned well with saline solution, intubated with a 14F catheter, and wrapped in damp compresses, making sure that the pedicle is not twisted. If we choose subperitoneal passage (possible only if the stoma is in the right iliac fossa), we create slight peritoneal scarification through which the appendix and mesoappendix are exteriorized.

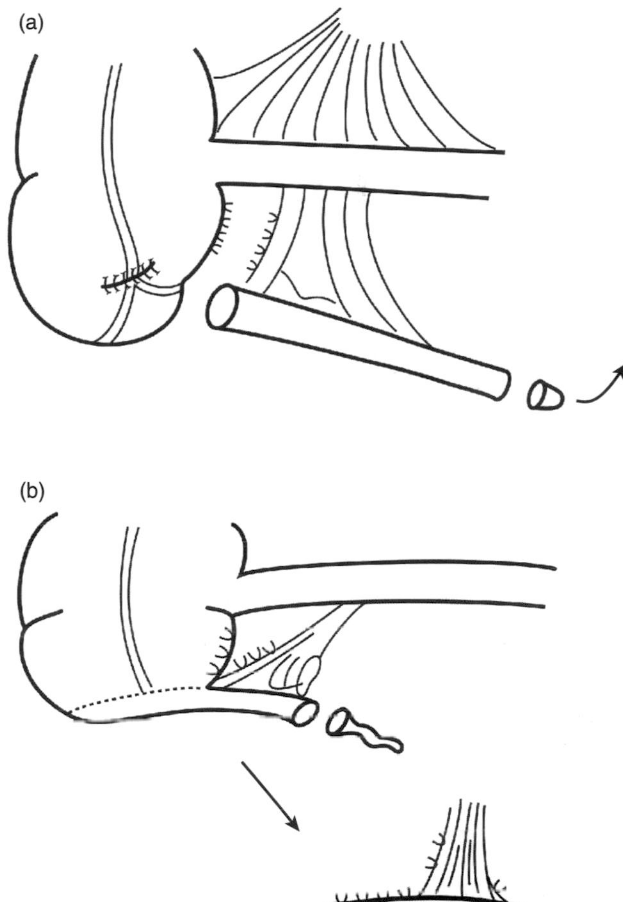

Figure 59.2
(a) The appendix tip is resected for insertion of a 14F catheter. The appendix is then mobilized with selective ligatures of the mesoappendix vessels, and a cecal collar is sectioned. (b) If the appendix is too short, and if the mesoappendix is favorable, we perform a cecoplasty to enlarge the appendix 5 to 8 cm.

Eventual preparation of the bowel for bladder enlargement and/or cecostomy

The intestinal segment chosen for bladder enlargement is isolated, prepared, and wrapped in damp compresses for the time being. It is now that a continent Malone type cecostomy is performed, if planned.

Cystostomy

The bladder is filled with saline, then opened. The type of bladder incision must allow a long enough bladder flap to

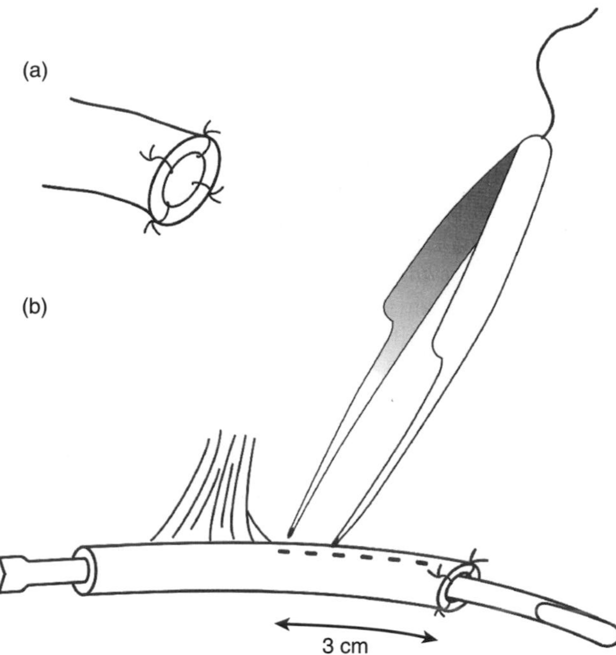

Figure 59.3
(a) After resection of the appendix tip, the mucosa is fixed to the appendix wall by 4 stitches of rapidly-absorbable 5–0 sutures. (b) At the end of preparation, the appendix conduit must be freed from the mesoappendix up to 3 cm to allow its implantation in the bladder.

be fixed to the posterior side of the anterior abdominal wall 2 cm below the level chosen for the cystostomy implant (taking its oblique trajectory into account). This flap will be the implantation site of the cystostomy tube. The bladder incision line will depend on bladder size and choices for mobilizing the right lateral side. Generally, the cystostomy is created with a very full bladder through a median line if the bladder is large (Figure 59.4a), or by a V- or Y-shaped incision with a posterior upper angle if the bladder is small (Figure 59.4b). This will create a large anterior flap. Three traction sutures, facilitating easy access to both sides of the flap, are positioned at least 15 mm from the appendix opening in the bladder. If the bladder is supple and large, it is, of course, possible to avoid the flap procedure, but, here again, placement of the three sutures framing the appendix opening in the bladder will simplify all subsequent manipulations.

Appendix implantation in the bladder

The appendicular tube is implanted into the bladder by an antireflux technique similar to the Glenn–Anderson type of uretero-vesical reimplantation.[15]

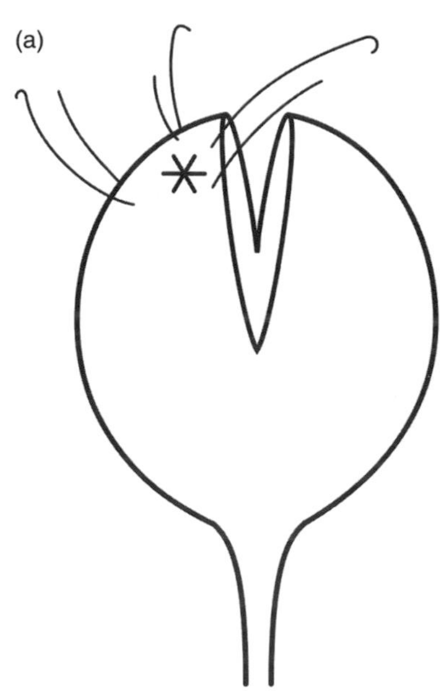

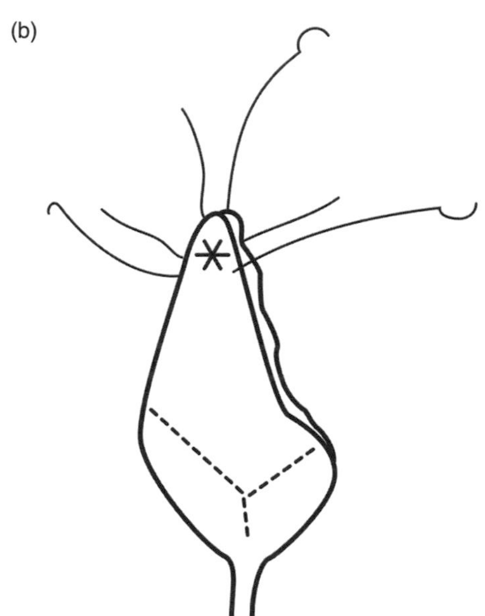

Figure 59.4
(a) If the bladder is large, it is opened along the median line, and the implantation zone is marked off with three absorbable Monobrin 2–0 sutures. (b) If the bladder is small, an inverted Y or V incision is made in such a way that a long anterior tip reaches the area chosen for the continent stoma.

The bladder tip (or the right side of the bladder in the case of a large bladder) is presented by the three triangulation sutures oriented towards 4 h, 8 h and 12 h (Figure 59.5a). The suture needles are retained. This triangulation will allow good disposition of the mesoappendix at that level. The opening for bladder penetration is made with an electric knife and should admit a 20F catheter. In the case of a bladder flap, it must be situated at least 15 mm from the sides of the tip to allow parietal anchorage without risk,

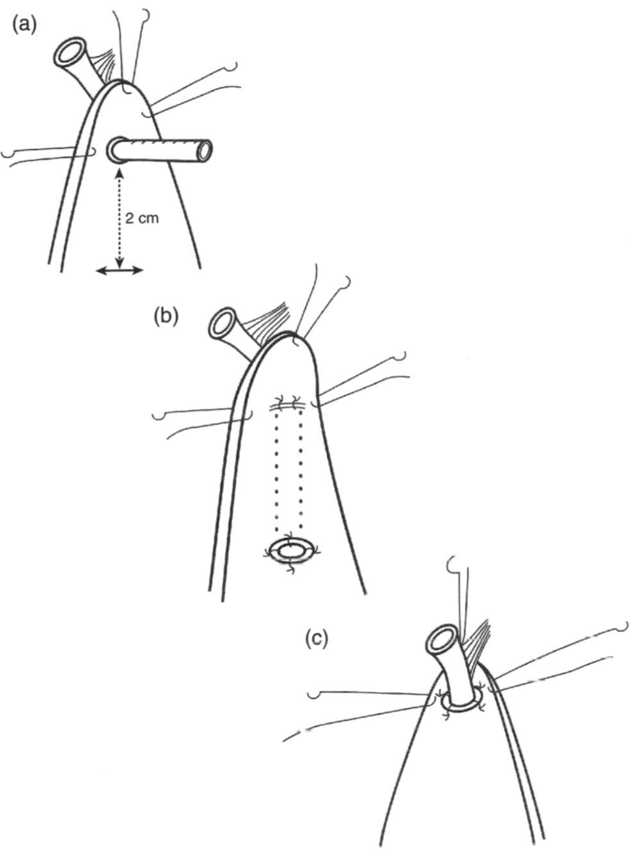

Figure 59.5
(a) The distal part of the appendix, relieved of its mesoappendix up to 3 cm, is passed through the opening situated 1 cm from the tip. (b) The appendix is positioned in the bladder submucosa for a length of at least 2 cm. (c) The appendix is lightly fixed to the bladder exterior by three stitches with absorbable 3–0 sutures.

and easy bladder closure. The part of the appendix without the mesoappendix is brought down into the bladder. A broad submucosal trajectory is created with scissors over at least 2 cm towards the bladder base (Figure 59.5b). The tube is placed in this trajectory and fixed to the bladder by five absorbable 4-0 suture stitches, of which the two that are the most external firmly hold the bladder musculature.

From here onwards, the trajectory must be rectilinear, oriented towards the bladder neck, and easy to catheterize. The mesoappendix must be placed harmoniously between the bladder and the abdominal wall. We must sometimes shorten the appendix to ensure that the whole tube is perfectly rectilinear and that there is no misalignment of its trajectory. Generally, the cecal part can be easily shortened, but if the disposition of the appendix vessels requires it, we may then have to undo the bladder implantation and shorten the tip.

When we are certain of its good positioning, the appendix is lightly fixed to the external side of the bladder to ensure the stability of its length along the antireflux trajectory (Figure 59.5c).

'Parietalization' of the bladder and cutaneous suture

The bladder segment where the appendix is implanted must be firmly fixed to the abdominal wall by 3 to 5 stitches with a slowly-absorbable 2-0 suture. A 14F catheter serves as a suture guide for bladder fitting and fixation (Figure 59.6a).

In cases of umbilical stomas, this is the time when the fitting becomes a bit more difficult, as the autostatic retractor must be loosened.

Umbilico-appendicular attachment is accomplished by 6 to 8 stitches with absorbable PDF (monofilament) 5-0 sutures, after placement of a Foley 14F catheter. The congruence of the two diameters must be perfect; if not, a spatulation must be made either on the umbilical skin or on the appendix. Then, the three triangulation suture stitches of the bladder flap are firmly fixed to the anterior abdominal wall (Figure 59.6b). The positioning of these 'parietalization' points determines whether the cystostomy trajectory is rectilinear, and whether the mesoappendix is harmoniously placed. Slight downward traction of the bladder will help in aligning the appendix (Figure 59.6c).

Several important steps have to be followed: (1) The appendix must cross the median line 1 to 3 cm below the previous umbilicus. (2) No excess appendicular length must be allowed. (3) The route being median first, we are obliged to lightly push the tube to the right side of the incision, to fix the bladder well, and also to be able to continue the operation (bladder augmentation) with a loosened retractor.

If the site chosen for the stoma is the right iliac fossa, according to patient morphotype and desire, the cutaneous V-incision will be slightly oblique, or in the case of obesity, the flap will be adapted to the abdomen shape. The bladder is fixed to the abdominal wall in the same way, and the appendix is attached to the skin by separate stitches with 5-0 absorbable sutures. Globally, this implantation site is easier to target than the umbilical option.

Bladder drainage and closure

The final part of the operation consists of closing the bladder on itself or on an intestinal segment for bladder enlargement. In general, we prefer not to install a urethral catheter as a Malécot 24F trans-vesico-parietal catheter will keep the bladder empty. A Jackson–Pratt type drain is installed in the perivesical space. Any mesenteric windows or other causes of secondary ileus must be meticulously controlled at this stage

Parietal closure

This part of the operation is difficult in the case of an umbilical cystostomy, since the median line must be closed

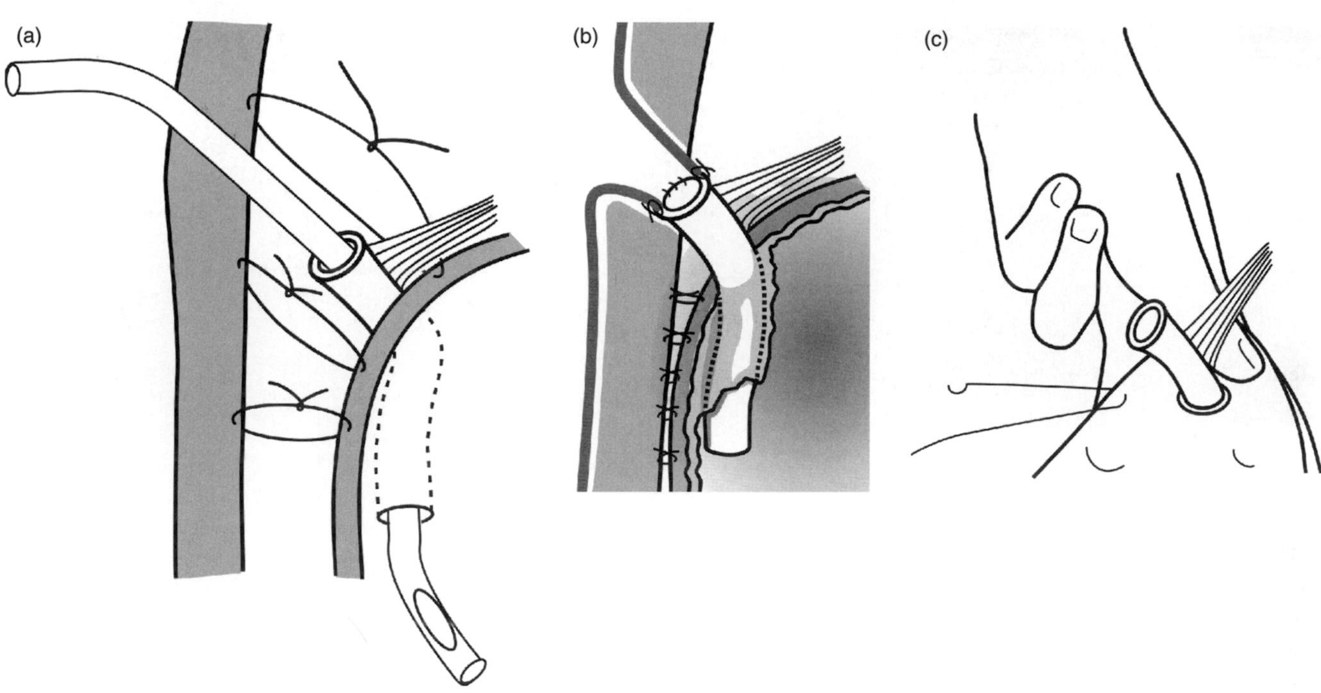

Figure 59.6
(a) The bladder and appendix are brought toward the opening under slight tension. (b) The three sutures for presentation of the bladder are fixed to the abdominal wall. The 14F catheter, which is calibrated to the suture scars, serves as a guide to assemble the appendix–bladder. (c) The three stitches are tightened and then knotted for perfect positioning of the appendix and the mesoappendix.

Table 59.1 *General principles*
Patient capable of personal control
Good knowledge of self-catheterization via the urethra
Bladder can be emptied via two continence orifices
Early and long-term treatment
Associated Malone cecostomy
Commitment of the surgeon to treat possible residual incontinence

Table 59.2 *Broad principles of cystostomy performance*
Give preference to an appendix that is usable
Keep the appendix for the bladder
Implant in the bladder (and not in an intestinal patch)
'Parietalize' the bladder and fix it to the anterior abdominal wall
Follow a rectilinear and downward trajectory to the bladder neck
Give preference to the umbilicus, except in women who could be pregnant

with slowly-absorbable, interrupted 1 PDF sutures. We ensure that neither the appendix nor the mesoappendix is stenosed.

Postoperative care

Second-generation cephalosporin is administered for antibioprophylaxis at the beginning of the operation, and continued if the intervention lasts more than 4 hours. Systemic antibiotherapy is not provided postoperatively.

The bladder is kept empty for 2 weeks with a transparietal cystostomy catheter at least equal to 20F. A closed 14F catheter is left in place in the cystostomy.

At the first follow-up visit, 4 weeks after surgery, the surgeon removes the 14F catheter and verifies the ease of catheter passage into the bladder through the Mitrofanoff and its downward orientation towards the bladder neck.

Discussion

Numerous studies and publications have been devoted to the Mitrofanoff technique of watertight cystostomy, which is considered more as 'a principle',[1,9] but very few have given details of its implementation.

The technique that we have described here is the fruit of experience of the initial author and of our centers which

Table 59.3 *Specific problems and solutions during implantation*

Appendix part	Specific problems	Prevention and solutions
External part	Stenosis	1. Large interrupted suture with a big cecal collar 2. Interposition of a cutaneous flap in an appendicular refend
Middle part	Mesoappendix constriction: • at bladder fixation points • during closure of the median incision	Always inspect the mesoappendix and color of the appendix
	Nonrectilinear trajectory (quinck) because of excessive length	Reposition the parietal mooring, shorten the appendix
Terminal part	Submucosal trajectory is too short (incontinence)	Re-do the assembly

learned from him.[16] We consider that the original technique, by its coherence, reduces the risk of complications.

On a purely technical point, we would insist on implantation of the tube in the fixed portion of the bladder, as described earlier under 'Appendix implantation in the bladder and '"Parietalization" of the bladder and cutaneous suture'. This technical aspect is probably the most frequently altered by other surgeons.[2–8,17] Appendix implantation into the mobile part of the bladder (bladder dome, lateral face, or an intestinal segment) is often suggested. Respect of this relatively difficult technical detail may, in our view, prevent major complications, such as stomal retraction and difficult catheterization. We think that tube implantation on a mobile wall carries the inconvenience of having a variable axis dependent on bladder filling, with the possibly increased risk of going down a wrong route. When the cystostomy is 'parietalized' in front and towards the bladder neck, the urethra is, as a matter of fact, in the axis of the cystostomy. This fixed position makes catheterizations and eventual endoscopic manipulations easier.

Another important technical point is the stomal implantation site. It is chosen according to criteria which will not be discussed here in detail. These criteria are particular patient anatomy and scars, the personal wishes of patients, possible future pregnancies, the risk of renal transplantation, and the potential concomitant creation of a continent Malone cecostomy. This decision, well-known in pediatric centers, is rarely proposed in adults, although its impact on quality of life is very significant.[16,18,19]

We are increasingly inclined to propose umbilical implantation, except in patients likely to be pregnant. It is theoretically contraindicated in such cases because of the surgical risk of vesicostomy injury during cesarian section performed by obstetricians not aware of its technical details. Several case reports and a few articles have dealt with the issue of delivery and bladder reconstruction.[20–23] Vaginal delivery has been shown to be possible, but no long-term follow-up has evaluated the effects on continence and prolapse. In our practice, we encourage cesarian section, considering that a neurogenic pelvic musculature may not respond to delivery trauma as well as a normal pelvis. Furthermore, experience has taught us that in 'medializing' the urinary assembly, renal transplantation can be undertaken with an acceptable level of difficulty.

The notable inconvenience of umbilical implantation relates to positioning of the stoma at the center of the abdominal incision. Space given by the incision is limited for bladder augmentation, making the procedure more difficult and a bit longer. Another frequent inconvenience encountered is the difficulty with repeated abdominal laparotomies: in our experience, in such rare cases, the problem is resolved with a catheter in the appendicular tube, filling the bladder to the maximum, making a longer incision upwards in the abdomen, and moving the aponeurotic incision a few cm left of the appendicostomy. These inconveniences do not appear to obviate the advantages of the technique, particularly in terms of continence.

Complications are not very frequent when the technique is meticulously done. Incontinence through the stomal opening rarely occurs with a scrupulously-performed technique ('parietalization' and minimum submucosal trajectory of at least 2 cm). When it does occur, endoscopic treatment of incontinence under cystoscopic guidance appears to be rarely effective.[24] Based on very limited experience with only one case, we believe, however, that endoscopic treatment inspired by the antireflux procedure, via the urethral route, can be effective and less invasive than a re-operation.

Similarly, residual incontinence through the urethra can also be improved by endoscopic treatment, by a fascial sling procedure in females, or a mesh sling procedure in males. In general, we prefer to implant a sling at the time of abdominal surgery, but in the absence of any history of stress urinary incontinence, we may decide, with the patient, to wait and see the results of bladder augmentation on continence and go with the sling only afterward, if needed. Experience with such a technique in our hands and in the literature is extremely limited.[25,26]

Stomal stenoses may occur, even with a perfectly-performed technique. It seems to be related to poor vascularization of the base of the implanted appendix and/or to traction on the stoma secondary to a too short appendix or a mobile 'montage'. Nevertheless, if dilatations are needed, the known direction and fixed submucosal trajectory make them simpler.

Conclusions

The trans-appendicular continent cystostomy technique that we have described here has proven advantages: easier catheterization, optimal continence, and the facility of possible surgical changes, which remain frequent. The choice of doing everything to implant the appendix in the bladder (and not in an intestinal patch), as well as its solid parietalization in regard to the stoma so that the trajectory is towards the bladder neck, appears to be indispensable in the success of this therapeutic option. In our experience, however, the intervention will satisfy the patient only if his/her motivation is strong, if quasi-perfect urinary continence remains the common goal of the patient and the surgical team, and if anorectal incontinence is treated efficiently to eliminate the need for diapers.

References

1. Mitrofanoff P. Cystostomie continente transappendiculaire dans le traitement des vessie neurologiques. [Trans-appendicular continent cystostomy in the management of the neurogenic bladder.] Chir Pediatr 1980; 21: 297–305. [In French]
2. Woodhouse CRJ, Malone PR, Cumming J, Reilly TM. The Mitrofanoff principle for continent urinary diversion. Br J Urol 1989; 63: 53–7.
3. Mitchell ME, Rink RC. Pediatric urinary diversion and undiversion. Pediatr Clin North Am 1987; 34: 1319–32.
4. Skinner EC, Xie HW. Urinary undiversion using the Mitrofanoff technique. In: Douglas Whitehead E, ed. Atlas of Surgical Techniques in Urology. Philadelphia: Lippincott-Raven, 1997; 118–22.
5. Turner-Warwick R, Chapple CR. The Mitrofanoff Appendix-Conduit Procedure. I: Functional Reconstruction of the Urinary Tract and Gynaeco-Urology. London: Blackwell Science, 2002: 733–5.
6. Hinman F. Appendicovesicostomy. In: Hinman F Jr, ed. Atlas of Pediatric Urologic Surgery. Philadelphia: WB Saunders, 1994: 421–5.
7. Harris CF, Cooper CS, Hutcheson JC, Snyder HM 3rd. Appendicovesicostomy: the Mitrofanoff procedure – a 15-year perspective. J Urol 2000; 163(6): 1922–6.
8. Cendron M, Gearhart JP. The Mitrofanoff principle. Technique and application in continent urinary diversion. Urol Clin North Am 1991; 18(4): 615–21.
9. Mitrofanoff P, Liard A. Continent diversions, bladder reconstruction and substitution. In: Gearhart JP, Rink RC, Mouriquand PDE, eds. Pediatric Urology. Philadelphia: WB Saunders, 2002: 947–55.
10. Hsu TH, Shortliffe LD. Laparoscopic Mitrofanoff appendicovesicostomy. Urology 2004; 64(4): 802–4.
11. Clark T, Pope JC 4th, Adams C, Wells N, Brock JW 3rd. Factors that influence outcomes of the Mitrofanoff and Malone antegrade continence enema reconstructive procedures in children. J Urol 2002; 168(4 Pt 1): 1537–40.
12. Cain MP, Casale AJ, King SJ, Rink RC. Appendicovesicostomy and newer alternatives for the Mitrofanoff procedure: results in the last 100 patients at Riley Children's Hospital. J Urol 1999; 162(5): 1749–52.
13. Bruce RG, McRoberts JW. Cecoappendicovesicostomy: conduit-lengthening technique for use in continent urinary reconstruction. Urology 1998; 52(4): 702–4.
14. Cromie WJ, Barada JH, Weingarten JL. Cecal tubularization: lengthening technique for creation of catheterizable conduit. Urology 1991; 37(1): 41–2.
15. Glenn JF, Anderson EE. Distal tunnel ureteral reimplantations. J Urol 1967; 97: 623–6.
16. Liard A, Seguier-Lipszyc E, Mathiot A, Mitrofanoff P. The Mitrofanoff procedure: 20 years later. J Urol 2001; 165(6 Pt 2): 2394–8.
17. Kaefer M, Retik AB. The Mitrofanoff principle in continent urinary reconstruction. Urol Clin North Am 1997; 24(4): 795–811.
18. Liard A, Bocquet I, Bachy B, Mitrofanoff P. Enquête sur la satisfaction des patients porteurs d'une caecostomie continente de Malone. [Survey on satisfaction of patients with Malone continent cecostomy.] Prog Urol 2002; 12(6): 1256–60. [In French]
19. Perez M, Lemelle JL, Barthelme H, Marquand D, Schmitt M. Bowel management with antegrade colonic enema using a Malone or a Monti conduit – clinical results. Eur J Pediatr Surg 2001; 11(5): 315–18.
20. Fenn N, Barrington JW, Stephenson TP. Clam enterocystoplasty and pregnacy. Br J Urol 1995; 75: 85–6.
21. Kennedy WA 2d, Hensle TW, Reiley EA, Fox HE, Haus T. Pregnancy after orthotopic continent urinary diversion. Surg Gynecol Obstet 1993; 177(4): 405–9.
22. Mundy AR. Continent urinary reconstruction and reproductive function. Scand J Urol Nephrol Suppl 1992; 142: 129.
23. Schilling A, Krawczak G, Friesen A, Kruse H. Pregnancy in a patient with an ileal substitute bladder followed by severe destabilization of the pelvic support. J Urol 1996; 55(4): 1389–90.
24. Godbole P, Bryant R, MacKinnon AE, Roberts JP. Endourethral injection of bulking agents for urinary incontinence in children. BJU Int 2003; 91(6): 536–9.
25. Austin PF, Westney OL, Leng WW, McGuire EJ, Ritchey ML. Advantages of rectus fascial slings for urinary incontinence in children with neuropathic bladders. J Urol 2001; 165(6 Pt 2): 2369–71; discussion 2371–2.
26. Hamid R, Khastgir J, Arya M, Patel HR, Shah PJ. Experience of tension-free vaginal tape for the treatment of stress incontinence in females with neuropathic bladders. Spinal Cord 2003; 41(2): 118–21.

60

Tissue engineering and cell therapies for neurogenic bladder augmentation and urinary continence restoration

René Yiou

Research in the field of cell-based therapy and tissue engineering for functional urologic disorders has advanced considerably over the past decade, allowing several recent clinical trials. Here, we review two uses of these new technologies in neurourologic disorders, namely, bladder-tissue engineering for neurogenic bladder and cell therapy for urethral rhabdosphincter insufficiency.

Bladder replacement for patients with neurogenic bladder

Hypertonic low-compliant bladder responsible for urinary incontinence or reflux in the upper urinary tract can develop during the course of several neurologic disorders.[1,2] Bladder augmentation performed to treat neurogenic bladder traditionally involves the use of intestinal segments, which can lead to complications such as urolithiasis, adhesion formation, increased intestinal mucus secretion, and metabolic disturbances.[3] Therefore, investigators have evaluated a number of other methods for increasing the size of the bladder. Many tissues have been used to create free grafts, including the skin, omentum, dura, and peritoneum. However, the results were unsatisfactory, mainly due to mechanical failure.

In recent years, attention has turned to tissue engineering as an alternative to free tissue grafts for bladder augmentation.[4–13] Promising results were obtained in various animal models of cystectomy. Acellular matrices or scaffolds made of various materials have been tested, either alone or after seeding with viable cells. The most sophisticated tissue-engineering approach involves harvesting autologous cells from the diseased organ, expanding these cells *in vitro*, and seeding them onto a matrix, which is then implanted into the donor organ (Figure 60.1). Several artifices can be used to promote vascularization of the construct, allowing the cells to grow in the shape of the scaffold. Eventually, the artificial scaffold breaks down, leaving a functionally normal organ. Three factors are known to influence the organ regeneration process: the biomaterial, which should replicate the effects of the extracellular matrix (ECM); the source of the cells that are seeded onto the biomaterial; and the environmental conditions during regeneration, which influence the development of the blood vessel and nerve supply to the construct.

Biomaterials

The biomaterial used to produce the scaffold acts as a substitute for the ECM, providing anchorage for the seeded cells, guiding their growth into the appropriate tissue architecture, and storing and releasing growth factors that are crucial to growth and repair. The main ECM components are fibrous proteins and glycosaminoglycans (GAGs), which are produced by resident cells. GAGs are carbohydrate polymers that attach to ECM proteins, forming proteoglycans. Proteoglycans have a negative charge that attracts water molecules, ensuring adequate hydration of the ECM and resident cells. ECM proteoglycans include heparan sulphate, chondroitin sulfate, and keratin sulphate. Heparan sulphate regulates a wide range of biological activities, including developmental processes and angiogenesis. Chondroitin sulfate contributes to the tensile strength of the cartilage, tendons, ligaments, and aortic walls. In addition to proteoglycans, the ECM contains hyaluronic acid, collagens, fibronectin, elastin, and laminin. Hyaluronic acid absorbs water, causing the tissue to swell and therefore to resist compression. Hyaluronic acid acts as an environmental cue that regulates cell behavior during

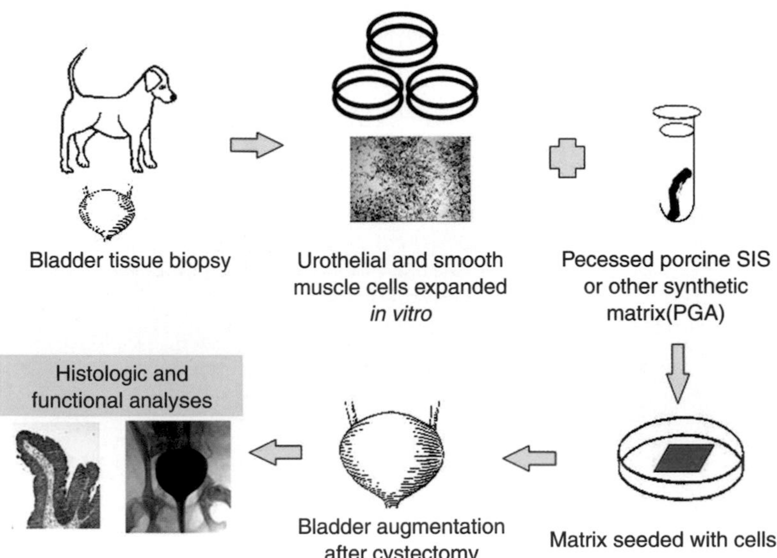

Figure 60.1
Design of bladder tissue engineering protocols. SIS, small intestinal submucosa; PGA, polyglycolic acid.

embryonic development, healing processes, inflammation, and tumor development. Collagens, the most abundant glycoproteins in the ECM, form fibrillar proteins that serve as struts to resident cells. They can be divided into several families based on their structure: fibrillar collagen is composed of collagens types I, II, III, V, and XI; fibril-associated collagen with interrupted triple helices (FACIT) is composed of types IX, XII, and XIV; short-chain collagen is composed of types VIII and X; basement membrane collagen is type IV; and other collagens include types VI, VII, and XIII. Fibronectin connects cells to collagen fibers, allowing the cells to move through the ECM. Elastins, which are produced by fibroblasts and smooth muscle cells, confer elasticity, allowing the tissue to stretch and subsequently to recover its previous shape. Laminins are proteins found in the basal lamina, where they form networks of web-like structures that resist tensile forces related to the adhesion of cells, most notably muscle cells. Integrins are cell-surface proteins that bind cells to ECM components such as fibronectin and laminin, as well as to integrin proteins on the surface of other cells.

The ideal biomaterial for tissue engineering should be biocompatible, promote cellular interactions, and enhance tissue development, thus replicating the functions of the normal ECM. The biomaterial should degrade slowly after implantation while undergoing colonization by host cells, so that it is eventually replaced by ECM components produced by the seeded or ingrowing cells. Biomaterials that have been evaluated for engineering genitourinary tissues include naturally derived materials, such as collagen and alginate; decellularized tissue matrix such as bladder submucosa and small intestinal submucosa (SIS); and synthetic polymers such as polyglycolic acid (PGA), polylactic acid (PLA), and polylactic-coglycolic acid (PLGA). The degradation products of PGA, PLA, and PLGA are nontoxic and slowly eliminated from the body.

SIS is a xenogenic, nonimmunogenic, acellular, biodegradable, collagen-rich membrane derived from the submucosal layer of the porcine small intestine. SIS has been shown to promote bladder regeneration *in vivo*[9,11,12] and to support three-dimensional growth of human bladder cells *in vitro*.[5] After implantation in the bladder, SIS is resorbed within 8 to 12 weeks and replaced by bundles of organized smooth-muscle cells.[14] The results differ, however, according to the bowel segment and to the age of the donor animal, with optimal results possibly being obtained with distal ileum from sows older than 3 years.[12] In early experiments, unseeded SIS was used to replace bladder tissue. Strips of rat bladder regenerated from SIS were capable of contracting in organ-bath studies; in addition, histology established the presence of muscarinic, purinergic, and β-adrenergic receptors, indicating sprouting of host nerves toward the scaffold.[9] In dogs, unseeded SIS promoted bladder regeneration with mucosal, smooth-muscle, and serosal layers.[11] Overall, experiments with SIS yielded promising results, although studies in dogs raised concern about possible stone formation, calcification, and graft shrinkage.[7]

Bladder augmentation with unseeded biomaterial relies on the ingrowth of smooth muscle and urothelial cells from the surrounding residual bladder tissue. There is now general agreement that urothelial cells, which have shown considerable regenerative potential *in vivo*,[15] can colonize the inner surface of the scaffold, whereas smooth muscle cells cannot if replacement of large bladder segments is required.[8,16] The lack of colonization by smooth muscle cells results in collagen deposition on the scaffold, eventually leading to scaffold shrinkage. These data suggesting a need for seeding the scaffold were confirmed by Oberpenning et al,[16] who compared seeded and unseeded PGA scaffolds used in dogs for bladder replacement after subtotal cystectomy. The seeded scaffolds were obtained by culturing autologous urothelial and smooth muscle cells from bladder biopsies and seeding them onto bladder-shaped PGA scaffolds. Identical scaffolds were used unseeded in the other group of dogs. After 11 months, the neobladders obtained using seeded PGA were histologically normal and had identical urodynamic parameters to those measured before cystectomy. In contrast, compared to precystectomy values, bladder capacity was 46% in the group treated with unseeded PGA and 22% in the cystectomy-only control group. Overall, most attempts with unseeded synthetic materials failed due to urinary stone formation and fibroblast deposition, which led eventually to bladder shrinkage. Therefore, seeding of the biomaterials with urothelial and smooth muscle cells prior to implantation is now recommended by most investigators.

Cells for bladder-tissue engineering

Bladder smooth muscle cells

An area of concern is the quality of the smooth muscle cells harvested from the neurogenic bladder for *in vitro* expansion and seeding of the biomaterial. It is unclear whether cells from diseased bladders can produce functionally normal tissue. Cultured smooth muscle cells from neurogenic bladders showed abnormal phenotypic features and gene expression profiles.[17,18] They grew more quickly, contracted less frequently, and adhered less well than smooth muscle cells from normal bladder.[17] Abnormal expression profiles were noted for up to 18 genes, including genes for fibroblast growth factor and integrin signaling.[18] In another study, however, muscles engineered from normal and diseased bladders exhibited similar phenotypes.[19] In this study, human smooth muscle cells from functionally normal bladders, exstrophic bladders, and neurogenic bladders were grown, expanded, and seeded onto polymer scaffolds, which were then implanted into athymic mice. The engineered bladders were removed subsequently for evaluation of their contractile response to various stimuli in organ-bath studies. Contractility to electrical and chemical stimulation was the same regardless of the origin of the cells. Therefore, it can be assumed that, although smooth muscle cells from neurogenic bladders may exhibit phenotypic differences compared to those from normal bladders, they remain capable of generating a normally functioning bladder *in vivo*. One possible explanation is that the regenerated muscle originates in a small subset of the seeded smooth muscle cells characterized by stem-cell capabilities, which are unaffected by the neurologic disorder.

Possible harmful effects of the cell-culturing process constitute another focus of concern when producing smooth muscle cells for bladder engineering. In recent investigations of muscle-precursor cell (myoblast) therapy for striated muscle diseases, the culture conditions and enzymatic digestion severely reduced the myogenic potential of the cells after transplantation, although vitality and function seemed normal *in vitro*.[20–26] Whether prolonged culturing of smooth muscle cells results in similar deleterious effects remains unknown.

Controversy continues to surround the relative merits of using large numbers of fully differentiated smooth muscle cells expanded by culturing, or smaller numbers of smooth muscle cell progenitors capable of proliferating and differentiating *in vivo*. A similar debate exists in the field of myoblast therapy for striated muscle diseases, as discussed later in this chapter.

Bone marrow mononuclear cells

Bone marrow mononuclear cells obtained by Ficoll-Paque density gradient separation of bone marrow aspirate constitute another source of smooth muscle cells for tissue engineering. The bone marrow mononuclear cell population contains several types of multipotent stem cells capable of differentiating into smooth muscle cells, including hematopoietic stem cells and mesenchymal stem cells. Studies comparing bone marrow cells and bladder smooth muscle cells for bladder-tissue engineering in dogs showed similar contractile responses to calcium ionophore.[4] Bone marrow cells differentiated into contractile cells expressing alpha smooth muscle actin but not desmin or myosin.

In the future, other cell sources might be investigated. The same stem-cell source might be suitable for obtaining both urothelial cells and smooth muscle cells. Adult multipotent stem cells have been isolated from the skin[27] and from fat tissue.[28] Embryonic stem cells and amniotic stem cells constitute additional promising sources of cells for bladder-tissue engineering.[29]

Vascularization and innervation of engineered bladder

Vascularization and innervation of the implanted scaffold are critical to successful tissue engineering. Tissue thicker than 0.8 mm can survive only if ingrowing blood vessels supply sufficient oxygen and nutrients to all the cells in the tissue.[30,31]

Several methods for promoting neoangiogenesis have been investigated, including omental wrap,[13] incorporation of vascular growth factor into the scaffold,[32] seeding of endothelial progenitor cells, and prevascularization of the scaffold.[4] The development of new vascular beds from endothelial cells present within tissues is enhanced by several angiogenic factors, such as vascular endothelial growth factor, fibroblast growth factor, and platelet-derived growth factor. Local, controlled delivery of these factors via incorporation into the scaffold of plasmids carrying the relevant genes may enhance blood vessel formation in the engineered tissue.[32] Injection of autologous endothelial progenitor cells constitutes another approach. The endothelial progenitor cells and mesenchymal stem cells found in bone marrow have proangiogenic properties that may hold promise for treating ischemic diseases.[33] In experimental and clinical studies, when these cells were transplanted into ischemic or infarcted foci of the myocardium, they were incorporated into sites of new vessel growth, and regional blood flow was improved. These cells might therefore enhance the development of an adequate vascular bed within engineered bladders.

Schultheiss et al described an original technique for increasing the vascular supply of decellularized porcine SIS seeded with smooth muscle cells and urothelial cells.[10] The arteriovenous pedicles were preserved during SIS preparation then injected with endothelial progenitor cells. The pedicles were then clamped for 24 hours, and the reseeded matrix was cultured under specific conditions designed to promote vessel development and re-endothelialization. After 3 weeks of cultivation, the larger vessels, as well as the intramural scaffold capillary network, were repopulated with cell monolayers expressing endothelium-specific markers. When the scaffold was implanted into the SIS-donor animal, the arterial and venous pedicles were anastomosed to the corresponding iliac vessels. After implantation, vascular perfusion remained intact, with no thrombus formation. In contrast, implanted scaffolds that were not previously seeded with endothelial progenitor cells exhibited stagnant blood flow and thrombosis within 30 minutes. This promising approach deserves further investigation.

Clinical reports of bladder augmentation using tissue engineering

In 2006, Atala and colleagues reported the first clinical trial of tissue-engineered bladders in 7 patients who had myelomeningocele with poorly compliant bladders and frequent urinary leakage as often as every 30 min despite maximal pharmacotherapy.[13] For the scaffolds, collagen matrix derived from decellularized bladder submucosa was used in the first 4 patients, and a composite of collagen and PGA in the next 3 patients. The scaffolds were seeded with autologous smooth muscle and urothelial cells. A bladder biopsy of 1–2 cm^2 was obtained from the bladder dome through a small suprapubic incision. Smooth muscle cells and urothelial cells were cultured separately for 7 weeks. Then, the smooth muscle cells were seeded on the outer surface and the urothelial cells on the inner surface of the scaffold. The scaffold was covered with omentum in 4 patients (including the 3 patients with composite scaffolds). Compared to preoperative values, mean maximum bladder capacity decreased by 30% in the 3 patients treated with collagen scaffolds and no omental wrap. A 1.22-fold increase (from 438 ml to a mean of 535 ml) was noted in the patient treated with collagen and omental wrap, suggesting a major role of the omentum in the development of an adequate vascular bed in the neobladder. In the 3 patients treated with the composite scaffold and omental wrap, mean maximum bladder capacity increased 1.58-fold and the maximum mean dry intervals during the day increased from 3.0 to 7.0 h. This pioneering study shows that tissue engineering can be used to generate bladders for patients who require cystoplasty. The beneficial effects of omental wrap emphasize the crucial role played by the vascular supply in the development of the seeded scaffold. Several questions remain open, such as the long-term fate of cultivated cells and the risk of premature senescence. In addition, recurrence of the urinary symptoms is theoretically possible, since the underlying neurologic disease remains present.

Cell therapy for urethral rhabdosphincter insufficiency

Urinary incontinence due to intrinsic urethral sphincter insufficiency develops in many central or peripheral neurologic disorders affecting the nerves that supply the urethral rhabdosphincter. In patients with severe incontinence, the treatment of reference remains the implantation of an artificial urinary sphincter.[34] Alternatively, a compressive device can be implanted or a bulking agent injected. Biologic or synthetic bulking agents investigated over the last decades include collagen, Teflon, and adipocytes.[34–37] The main goal of bulking agent injection is to increase resistance to urine flow. Results have been disappointing, however, because of particle migration or rapid resorption, indicating a need for new treatment approaches.

Cell therapy holds promise for restoring urethral tonicity and sphincter function in patients with urinary sphincter insufficiency. Several types of precursor cells have been tested to improve the tone exerted by the smooth or striated components of the urethral musculature. To augment the smooth muscle component, stem cells from bone marrow[38] or human lipoaspirate[28] injected into the urethra have been investigated in rodents. Lipoaspirate stem cells differentiated into smooth muscle cells capable of tonic contractions in this model.[28] However, urethral injection of striated muscle precursor cells (MPCs) is the most extensively studied cell therapy approach to urinary incontinence.[39–42] In rodents, improved contractility of the urethral rhabdosphincter was noted after the injection of autologous MPCs expanded in culture.[39,41] A clinical trial has been conducted using MPCs and fibroblasts suspended in collagen.[40] Here, we provide an overview of MPC-based cell therapy for skeletal muscle diseases and we discuss the biological basis for MPC transfer into the urethra to treat urinary incontinence.

Origin and function of skeletal muscle precursor cells

The cells involved in regenerating adult skeletal muscle are believed to closely resemble the cells involved in myogenesis. During embryogenesis, the somites give rise to successive waves of myoblasts, which colonize the limbs within the first 18 days after conception. These myoblasts fuse into primary myotubes, which eventually mature into myofibers. A subset of myoblasts sequestered in a quiescent state between the basal lamina and the sarcolemma, known as satellite cells, ensures muscle repair in adulthood. Satellite cells constitute the main population of MPCs. In the event of muscle injury, the satellite cells proliferate and differentiate into secondary myoblasts, which fuse into new myotubes or repair the parental myofibers (Figure 60.2). Evidence is accumulating that bone marrow stem cells may be involved in renewing the adult satellite cell population, most notably in patients who have chronic muscle diseases characterized by recurrent degeneration-regeneration cycles.[43]

Importantly, resident satellite cells can fully reconstitute the myofiber mass lost after a muscle injury, although they initially contribute less than 1% of all myonuclei.[44] The considerable myogenic potential of MPCs was emphasized by Collins et al,[21] who found that as few as seven satellite cells generated more than 100 new myofibers, each of which contained thousands of myonuclei.

Importantly, all satellite cells are not at the same stage of commitment in the myogenic lineage.[45] Therefore, the potential for producing myofibers may vary considerably. Most satellite cells express the early myogenic marker Myf5. A small subset of Myf5-negative satellite cells may serve as stem cells that renew the satellite cell compartment. This subset of so-called muscle stem cells was found in mice to express markers (sca-1) common to other stem-cell types, such as hematopoietic stem cells.[46,47] Muscle stem cells have also been found in the connective tissue surrounding each myofiber, in association with capillaries, and it is believed that they may originate from the bone marrow.[48,49]

Interestingly, the urethral rhabdosphincter of rodents, which is believed to differ in its embryologic origin from other striated muscles,[50] also contains satellite cells that can execute a standard myogenic program after injury.[51] Given that the muscle rhabdosphincter and skeletal muscle share the same regeneration process, satellite cells transferred from peripheral muscle into the rhabdosphincter may improve urethral rhabdosphincter insufficiency.

Muscle precursor cell transfer for neuromuscular disorders

Pioneering work done in the 1980s showed that MPCs transferred from normal muscle into genetically deficient muscle fused with the host myofibers, thereby supplying them with the missing gene.[52] These studies suggested that MPC injections might hold promise for treating many genetic muscular diseases, mainly Duchenne muscular dystrophy,[53] as well as heart disease.[54] However, clinical trials involving injection of a myoblast suspension into genetically deficient muscle consistently produced disappointing results.[53] Many factors contributed to the failure of this approach, including immune reactivity against allogeneic myoblasts, poor survival of cells exposed to ischemia, and limited cell migration requiring multiple injection sites for each muscle.[20,47,53,55,56] This approach has been nearly abandoned as a tool for treating genetic muscle diseases, the group of conditions for which it was initially designed. Researchers have shifted their focus to the use of autologous MPCs for treating localized muscle abnormalities. Intrinsic rhabdosphincter insufficiency is among the most promising candidates for treatment with MPC injection.

The main challenge faced by autologous MPC transfer resides in the high sensitivity of these cells to ischemia, which may impair their survival after implantation. Several solutions to this problem have been investigated. Beauchamp et al showed that the majority of MPCs died after injection into muscle, despite *in vitro* evidence of vitality, and that the tiny minority that survived exhibited stem cell characteristics.[20] These findings were confirmed by several other groups, prompting researchers to investigate new preparation methods that select MPCs exhibiting the stem cell phenotype.[46,47] However, no clinical studies of such selected MPCs are available.

Other groups investigated the impact of the cell preparation process on myoblast survival.[21–26] The few animal studies comparing injections of myoblasts with or without

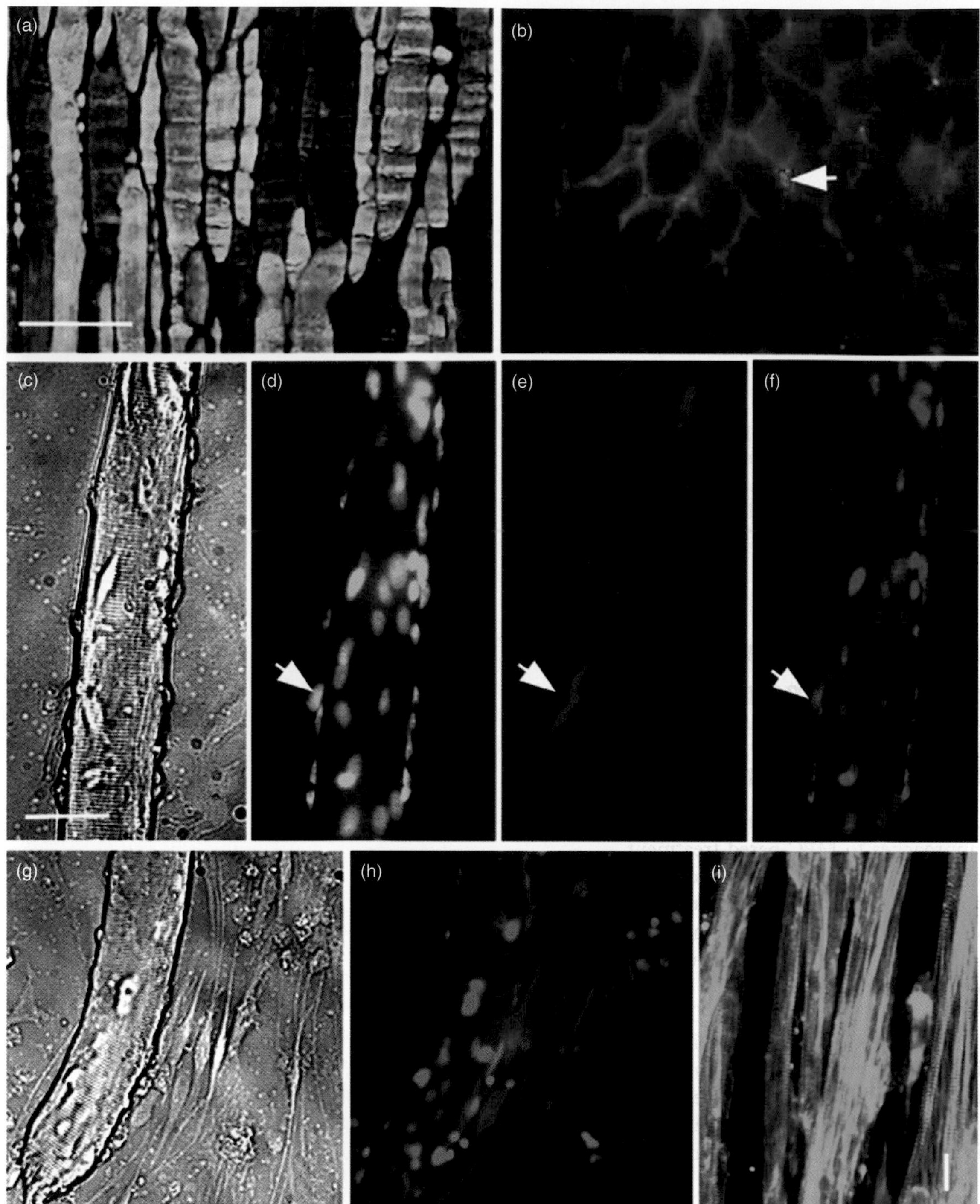

Figure 60.2
Description of satellite cells (main muscle precursor cells) and of the myogenic process using the single myofiber implant technique. (a and b) Longitudinal (a) and transverse (b) cross-section of a skeletal muscle biopsy showing organization of myofibers parallel to each other. (b) Nuclei stained with DAPI (blue). Nuclei of satellite cells (arows) are detected by immunostaining with anti-Pax7 (red). The extracellular matrix is immunostained with anti-laminine (green). Only one satellite cell can be observed on this cross-section. Resident satellite cells can fully reconstitute the myofiber mass lost after a muscle injury, although they initially contribute less than 1% of all myonuclei. (a and b) Bar = 100 μm. (c–f) One myofiber has been isolated by gentle trituration of a muscle biopsy, placed in a Petri dish and immunostained with desmin (red) to detect satellite cells. All nuclei are counterstained with DAPI (blue). One satellite cell can be detected (arrow). (f) Superposition of (d) and (e). (g and h) Twenty-four hours after plating, satellite cells (desmin, red) detach and proliferate around the parental myofiber. (I) After 2 weeks in culture the satellite cells have fused to form new myofibers (immunostaining with anti-alpha-actinine 2, green). (c–i) Bar = 20 μm.

prior culturing consistently showed deleterious effects of culture conditions. Enzymatic disaggregation of muscle biopsies was a major cause of MPC death following implantation. For instance, 150 MPCs obtained by gentle physical means was several thousand times more efficient in producing new myofibers than 10^4 MPCs dissociated by enzyme digestion.[21] MPC exposure to culture conditions may also contribute to loss of myogenic potential.[25] Montarras et al found that culturing prior to transplantation markedly reduced the regenerative efficiency of MPCs, so that culture expansion seemed to constitute an 'empty' process yielding the same amount of muscle as the number of cells from which the culture was initiated.[24] Thus, there is evidence that the myogenic potential of injected MPCs can be impaired by the cell preparation process, most notably the enzyme digestion step, and by cell culture conditions. It remains to be determined whether injecting small numbers of cells without previous cultivation is more effective than injecting large numbers of MPCs previously expanded *in vitro.*

Challenges faced by the use of muscle precursor cells to treat intrinsic urethral rhabdosphincter insufficiency

The findings reviewed above prompted the investigation of several approaches to MPC-based treatment of urethral sphincter insufficiency. (1) use of selected MPCs having the stem cell phenotype, (2) injection of large numbers of MPCs with the goal of increasing the number of surviving cells, and (3) injection of MPCs without prior cultivation. Here, we review the data obtained by several groups, including ours, about the biology of MPC transfer into the urethra for the treatment of intrinsic rhabdosphincter insufficiency. In addition to MPC survival after implantation into the sphincter, important issues include the ability of the urethra to innervate the MPC-derived myotubes and the ability of the MPCs to produce tonic activity.

Role of MPC injection in neurogenic urinary incontinence

Whether the host tissue can innervate MPC-derived myotubes is of special concern when seeking to treat intrinsic sphincter insufficiency, since this condition is often associated with chronic muscle denervation.[57] Several groups found that activated MPCs and the myofiber regeneration process promoted motoneuron sprouting.[41,58,59] For instance, following experimental muscle denervation via afferent nerve transection, myofibers and the surrounding ECM released potent neurotrophic factors, such as neuroleukin, insulin-like growth factor, and neural cell adhesion molecules, which can stimulate the sprouting of nearby nerve endings, ultimately leading to myofiber reinnervation.[59] These cytokines and growth factors represent the main mechanism for self-repair of the neuromuscular junction. Consequently, the injection of MPCs or myofibers with attached satellite cells may improve neurogenic intrinsic sphincter insufficiency by activating the sprouting of urethral nerves. We used a rat model of electrocautery-induced sphincter injury to show that the injection of autologous MPCs obtained by the myofiber explant technique led to the development of innervated and functional myotubes in the damaged area (i.e. on the side of the sphincter). Interestingly, we found that this injury irreversibly destroyed not only sphincter myofibers with their satellite cells, but also their nerve supply, resulting in the development of dense fibrosis. The regenerated myotubes were connected to newly formed nerve endings after one month, strongly suggesting that the myogenic process induced by MPC injection exerted neurotrophic effects resulting in the sprouting of residual nerves (Figure 60.3). A neurotrophic effect of MPC injection was demonstrated subsequently by Cannon et al in a model of neurogenic sphincter insufficiency induced by sciatic nerve transection.[39]

We recently described a new method of MPC transfer into the urethra, in which myofibers and their attached satellite cells, without prior tissue processing, were implanted near the bladder neck at a distance from the rhabdosphincter.[60] The satellite cells underwent activation and fusion, replacing the parent myofibers, which degenerated rapidly after implantation. A large number of myotubes exerting tonic contraction developed (Figure 60.4). Importantly, these myotubes had cholinergic receptors connected to nerve endings after one month, demonstrating connection with urethral nerves. Thus, it can be assumed that the myogenic process allows self-innervation of the new muscle in an ectopic position.

Can MPC transplantation increase urethral muscle tone?

Another important issue is whether myotubes derived from transplanted MPCs improve urethral muscle tone. In humans, the urethral rhabdosphincter is a unique muscle that participates in urinary continence by developing tonic contractions, thereby maintaining a resting urethral tone. Classically, this activity is mediated by type I myofibers, which are slow-twitch, tonic, aerobic fibers that can sustain long periods of contraction.[57,61] Type II myofibers, in contrast, are fast-twitch, chiefly anaerobic fibers that develop strong contractions but fatigue rapidly. Therefore, it was important to determine whether the phenotype of

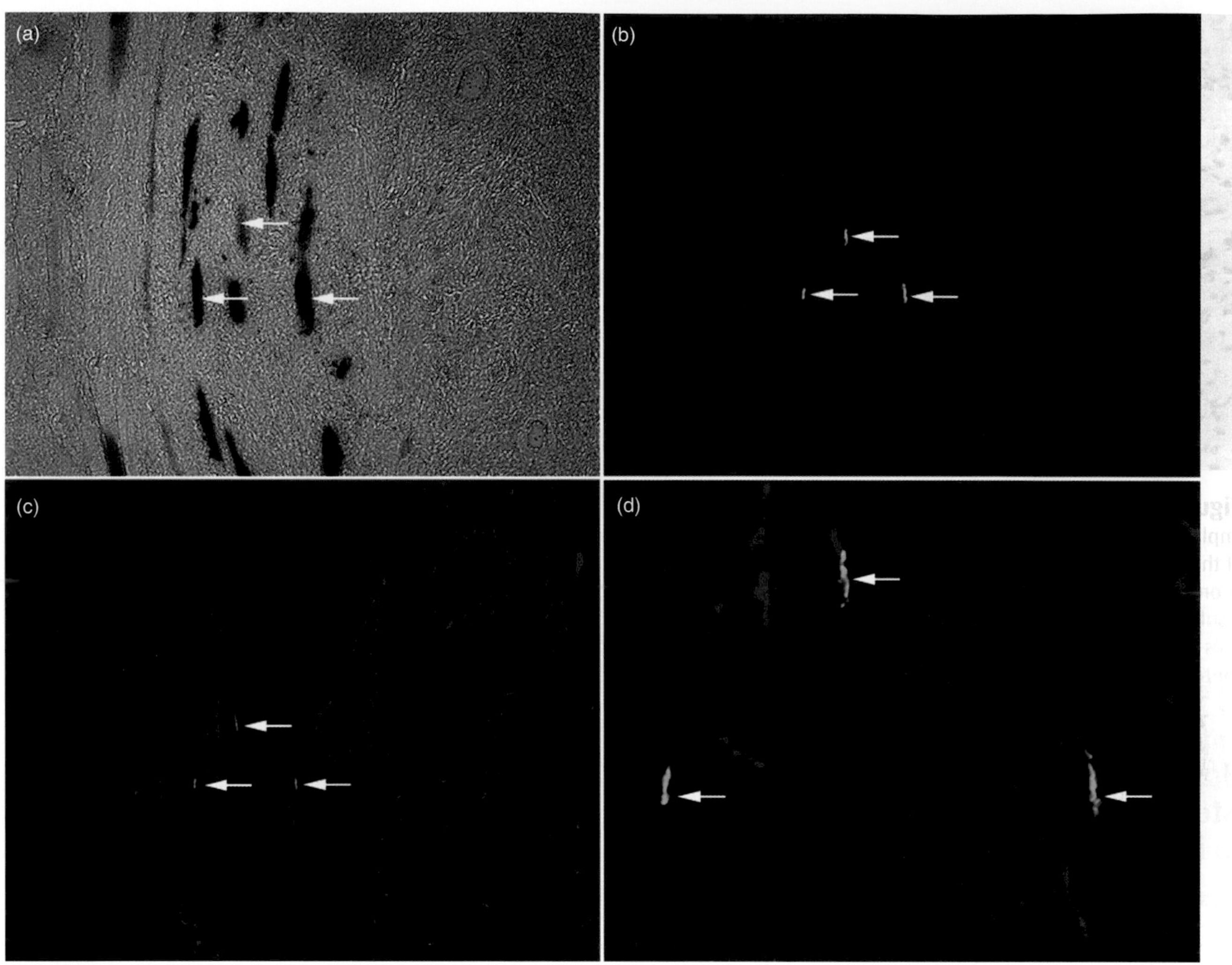

Figure 60.3
Injection of muscle precursor cells (MPCs) in an irreversibly damaged sphincter in the rat results in the formation of innervated myotubes. (a) Autologous MPCs expressing β-galactosidase differentiate into myotubes after one month and can be detected with the X-Gal solution (stained in blue). (b) Staining of the same section with bungarotoxin (green) shows the presence of acetylcholine receptors on the β-galactosidase-expressing myotubes. In this animal model, both myofibers and nerve endings were destroyed by electrocautery prior to autologous MPC grafting. (c) Immunostaining with anti-PGP9.5 (Texas Red, red) shows numerous nerve endings in the vicinity of the myotubes. (d) At a larger magnification, nerve endings reaching acetylcholine receptors can be observed. Initial magnification: ×10 (a–c) and ×40 (d).

myotubes derived from transplanted MPCs is consistent with sphincter-like muscle activity.

The development of models in large animals was required to investigate this point, since the small sphincter of rodents precludes intraurethral pressure measurements and chiefly contains type II myofibers.[62] An original porcine model developed by Zini et al[63] consists in recording urethral pressure before and after curare injection. The pig sphincter contains 52% of type I myofibers exhibiting tonic contractions. Curare specifically blocks the neuromuscular junctions of striated muscle, its effect on smooth muscle being minimal. Therefore, the comparison of urethral pressure profiles before and after curare injection provides an evaluation of the tonic contraction of functional, innervated, striated muscle. In this model, the myotubes developed after implantation of myofibers with their satellite cells exhibited tonic contractions under neural control.

These preliminary results suggest that MPCs exhibit plasticity, which allows them to adapt to their new function. Environmental factors, most notably interaction of MPCs with urethral nerves, may be critical to the terminal differentiation of the myotubes, as previously observed in cross-innervation studies of striated muscles.[64]

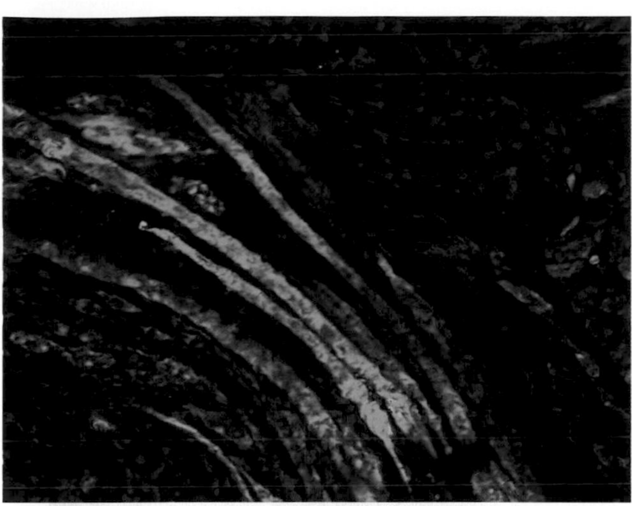

Figure 60.4
Implantation of myofibers with satellite cells in the bladder neck of the pig. Immunostaining with anti-myosin heavy chain (green) at one month shows the presence of numerous myotubes resulting from activation *in vivo* of the satellite cells. Satellite cells rapidly fuse to replace the parental myofibers. Nuclei are conterstained with DAPI (blue). Initial magnification: ×10.

How many and what type of MPCs (stem cell like vs mature) are required to improve sphincter function?

Most of the MPCs die shortly after implantation.[20] The current method of reference for delivering MPCs to diseased muscle involves isolating cells from a muscle biopsy by enzymatic digestion then expanding the cell population by cultivation. The low yield of this method has been demonstrated in the mdx mouse, the animal model for Duchenne muscular dystrophy: fewer than 3% of the injected cells survived and participated in myofiber formation.[20] The small subset of surviving cells, which eventually generated new muscle tissue, exhibited several features of hematopoietic stem cells.[20,46] This fact suggested two methods for increasing the number of surviving MPCs, namely, selection and amplification of so-called muscle stem cells, and increasing the number of injected MPCs under the assumption that the injected stem cell population would increase commensurately.

Improved sphincter function has been reported after the injection of muscle-derived stem cells obtained by the preplating technique in a model of sciatic nerve transection.[39] However, we found that muscle-derived stem cells obtained using another method (presence of the MDR receptor[46]) survived after injection but failed to form myotubes in an irreversibly injured sphincter characterized by complete myofiber destruction. When the stem cells were mixed with differentiated MPCs before injection, myotubes developed, whereas mature MPCs deprived of their stem-cell subpopulation failed to survive after injection. Taken together, these results emphasize the fact that environmental cues and/or interactions between mature and stem-cell-like MPCs are crucial to myotube development *in vivo*.

The effect of increasing the number of injected MPCs was evaluated in a porcine model under the working hypothesis that increasing the number of injected MPCs would increase the number of surviving MPCs.[65] Although the number of animals was too small (n = 5) to detect a plateau effect, which was previously reported with MPCs, a dose-dependent increase in urethral closure pressure was noted with the best results obtained with 7.8×10^7 cells (myoblasts).

We recently suggested a new approach to improving MPC survival after injection, based on the hypothesis that the MPC preparation process may cause alterations responsible for cell death after injection.[60] We developed a method in which myofibers and satellite cells are isolated then immediately implanted into the urethra. The number of injected MPCs was several thousand times smaller than with previously reported techniques. Nevertheless, a large amount of myotubes developed. Thus, attention to cell quality rather than quantity may be in order. Interestingly, various methods of MPC transfer developed in other settings are now being investigating in the field of urology.

Results of clinical trials

Recently, Strasser et al reported the first randomized clinical trial of cell therapy for urinary incontinence.[66] Sixty-three women with urinary stress incontinence were randomly allocated to treatment with transurethral ultrasonography-guided injections of autologous MPCs into the urethral sphincter and of injection of fibroblasts in collagen into the submucosa to treat atrophy (n = 42) or to endoscopic collagen injections (n = 21). After 12 months, 38 of the 42 women given cell therapy were completely continent, compared to only 2 of the 21 controls. Ultrasonographic measurements showed increased thickness and contractility of the sphincter in the cell-therapy group.

Although these results are encouraging, long-term outcomes remain to be determined, and multicenter trials in large numbers of patients are needed. The exact role played by the injected MPCs is unclear, as there was no control group given fibroblasts in collagen without MPCs. Finally, it is to be hoped that this cell therapy method will be investigated in other disorders, such as neurogenic incontinence.

Conclusion

Several cell therapy approaches designed to improve urinary sphincter tone are being investigated. MPC transplantation holds promise for the treatment of neurogenic urinary incontinence, as the cells release neurotrophic factors. However, the best method for transferring MPCs from peripheral muscle to the urinary sphincter remains to be determined. Preliminary studies in large animals and the first clinical results indicate that one or more of these emerging strategies will soon earn a place of prominence among tools used to treat urinary incontinence.

References

1. Kiddoo DA, Carr MC, Dulczak S, Canning DA. Initial management of complex urological disorders: bladder exstrophy. Urol Clin North Am 2004; 31: 417.
2. Snodgrass WT, Adams R. Initial urologic management of myelomeningocele. Urol Clin North Am 2004; 31: 427.
3. McDougal WS. Metabolic complications of urinary intestinal diversion. J Urol 1992; 147: 1199.
4. Zhang Y, Lin HK, Frimberger D, Epstein RB, Kropp BP. Growth of bone marrow stromal cells on small intestinal submucosa: an alternative cell source for tissue engineered bladder. BJU Int 2005; 96: 1120.
5. Zhang Y, Kropp BP, Moore P et al. Coculture of bladder urothelial and smooth muscle cells on small intestinal submucosa: potential applications for tissue engineering technology. J Urol 2000; 164: 928.
6. Zhang Y, Kropp BP, Lin HK, Cowan R, Cheng EY. Bladder regeneration with cell-seeded small intestinal submucosa. Tissue Eng 2004; 10: 181.
7. Zhang Y, Frimberger D, Cheng EY, Lin HK, Kropp BP. Challenges in a larger bladder replacement with cell-seeded and unseeded small intestinal submucosa grafts in a subtotal cystectomy model. BJU Int 2006; 98: 1100.
8. Yoo JJ, Meng J, Oberpenning F, Atala A. Bladder augmentation using allogenic bladder submucosa seeded with cells. Urology 1998; 51: 221.
9. Vaught JD, Kropp BP, Sawyer BD et al. Detrusor regeneration in the rat using porcine small intestinal submucosal grafts: functional innervation and receptor expression. J Urol 1996; 155: 374.
10. Schultheiss D, Gabouev AI, Cebotari S et al. Biological vascularized matrix for bladder tissue engineering: matrix preparation, reseeding technique and short-term implantation in a porcine model. J Urol 2005; 173: 276.
11. Kropp BP, Rippy MK, Badylak SF et al. Regenerative urinary bladder augmentation using small intestinal submucosa: urodynamic and histopathologic assessment in long-term canine bladder augmentations. J Urol 1996; 155: 2098.
12. Kropp BP, Cheng EY, Lin HK, Zhang Y. Reliable and reproducible bladder regeneration using unseeded distal small intestinal submucosa. J Urol 2004; 172: 1710.
13. Atala A, Bauer SB, Soker S, Yoo JJ, Retik AB. Tissue-engineered autologous bladders for patients needing cystoplasty. Lancet 2006; 367: 1241.
14. Badylak SF, Kropp B, McPherson T, Liang H, Snyder PW. Small intestional submucosa: a rapidly resorbed bioscaffold for augmentation cystoplasty in a dog model. Tissue Eng 1998; 4: 379.
15. de Boer WI, Rebel JM, Vermey M, de Jong AA, van der Kwast TH. Characterization of distinct functions for growth factors in murine transitional epithelial cells in primary organotypic culture. Exp Cell Res 1994; 214: 510.
16. Oberpenning F, Meng J, Yoo JJ, Atala A. De novo reconstitution of a functional mammalian urinary bladder by tissue engineering. Nat Biotechnol 1999; 17: 149.
17. Lin HK, Cowan R, Moore P et al. Characterization of neuropathic bladder smooth muscle cells in culture. J Urol 2004; 171: 1348.
18. Dozmorov MG, Kropp BP, Hurst RE, Cheng EY, Lin HK. Differentially expressed gene networks in cultured smooth muscle cells from normal and neuropathic bladder. J Smooth Muscle Res 2007; 43: 55.
19. Lai JY, Yoon CY, Yoo JJ, Wulf T, Atala A. Phenotypic and functional characterization of in vivo tissue engineered smooth muscle from normal and pathological bladders. J Urol 2002; 168: 1853.
20. Beauchamp JR, Morgan JE, Pagel CN, Partridge TA. Dynamics of myoblast transplantation reveal a discrete minority of precursors with stem cell-like properties as the myogenic source. J Cell Biol 1999; 144: 1113.
21. Collins CA, Olsen I, Zammit PS et al. Stem cell function, self-renewal, and behavioral heterogeneity of cells from the adult muscle satellite cell niche. Cell 2005; 122: 289.
22. Fan Y, Beilharz MW, Grounds MD. A potential alternative strategy for myoblast transfer therapy: the use of sliced muscle grafts. Cell Transplant 1996; 5: 421.
23. Fan Y, Maley M, Beilharz M, Grounds M. Rapid death of injected myoblasts in myoblast transfer therapy. Muscle Nerve 1996; 19: 853.
24. Montarras D, Morgan J, Collins C et al. Direct isolation of satellite cells for skeletal muscle regeneration. Science 2005; 309: 2064.
25. Smythe GM, Grounds MD. Exposure to tissue culture conditions can adversely affect myoblast behavior in vivo in whole muscle grafts: implications for myoblast transfer therapy. Cell Transplant 2000; 9: 379.
26. Smythe GM, Hodgetts SI, Grounds MD. Problems and solutions in myoblast transfer therapy. J Cell Mol Med 2001; 5: 33.
27. Bartsch G, Yoo JJ, De Coppi P et al. Propagation, expansion, and multilineage differentiation of human somatic stem cells from dermal progenitors. Stem Cells Dev 2005; 14: 337.
28. Jack GS, Almeida FG, Zhang R. et al. Processed lipoaspirate cells for tissue engineering of the lower urinary tract: implications for the treatment of stress urinary incontinence and bladder reconstruction. J Urol 2005; 174: 2041.
29. De Coppi P, Bartsch G Jr, Siddiqui MM et al. Isolation of amniotic stem cell lines with potential for therapy. Nat Biotechnol 2007; 25: 100.
30. Walles T, Herden T, Haverich A, Mertsching H. Influence of scaffold thickness and scaffold composition on bioartificial graft survival. Biomaterials 2003; 24: 1233.
31. Nomi M, Atala A, Coppi PD, Soker S. Principals of neovascularization for tissue engineering. Mol Aspects Med 2002; 23: 463.
32. Shea LD, Smiley E, Bonadio J, Mooney DJ. DNA delivery from polymer matrices for tissue engineering. Nat Biotechnol 1999; 17: 551.
33. Kinnaird T, Stabile E, Epstein SE, Fuchs S. Current perspectives in therapeutic myocardial angiogenesis. J Interven Cardiol 2003; 16: 289.
34. Haab F, Zimmern PE, Leach GE. Female stress urinary incontinence due to intrinsic sphincteric deficiency: recognition and management. J Urol 1996; 156: 3.
35. Haab F, Zimmern PE, Leach GE. Urinary stress incontinence due to intrinsic sphincteric deficiency: experience with fat and collagen periurethral injections. J Urol 1997; 157: 1283.
36. Wilson TS, Lemack GE, Zimmern PE. Management of intrinsic sphincteric deficiency in women. J Urol 2003; 169: 1662.
37. Hubner WA, Schlarp OM. Treatment of incontinence after prostatectomy using a new minimally invasive device: adjustable continence therapy. BJU Int 2005; 96: 587.
38. Adamiak A, Rechberger T. [Potential application of stem cells in urogynecology.] Endokrynol Pol 2005; 56: 994.
39. Cannon TW, Lee JY, Somogyi G et al. Improved sphincter contractility after allogenic muscle-derived progenitor cell injection into the denervated rat urethra. Urology 2003; 62: 958.
40. Strasser H, Marksteiner R, Margreiter E et al. [Stem cell therapy for urinary incontinence.] Urologe A 2004; 43: 1237.
41. Yiou R, Yoo JJ, Atala A. Restoration of functional motor units in a rat model of sphincter injury by muscle precursor cell autografts. Transplantation 2003; 76: 1053.
42. Peyromaure M, Sebe P, Praud C et al. Fate of implanted syngenic muscle precursor cells in striated urethral sphincter of female rats: perspectives for treatment of urinary incontinence. Urology 2004; 64: 1037.

43. Ferrari G, Cusella-De Angelis G, Coletta M et al. Muscle regeneration by bone marrow-derived myogenic progenitors. Science 1998; 279: 1528.
44. Zammit PS, Heslop L, Hudon V et al. Kinetics of myoblast proliferation show that resident satellite cells are competent to fully regenerate skeletal muscle fibers. Exp Cell Res 2002; 281: 39.
45. Beauchamp JR, Heslop L, Yu DS et al. Expression of CD34 and Myf5 defines the majority of quiescent adult skeletal muscle satellite cells. J Cell Biol 2000; 151: 1221.
46. Gussoni E, Soneoka Y, Strickland CD et al. Dystrophin expression in the mdx mouse restored by stem cell transplantation. Nature 1999; 401: 390.
47. Qu-Petersen Z, Deasy B, Jankowski R et al. Identification of a novel population of muscle stem cells in mice: potential for muscle regeneration. J Cell Biol 2002; 157: 851.
48. Tavian M, Zheng B, Oberlin EJ. et al. The vascular wall as a source of stem cells. Ann NY Acad Sci 2005; 1044: 41.
49. Dreyfus PA, Chretien F, Chazaud B et al. Adult bone marrow-derived stem cells in muscle connective tissue and satellite cell niches. Am J Pathol 2004; 164: 773.
50. Borirakchanyavat S, Baskin LS, Kogan BA, Cunha GR. Smooth and striated muscle development in the intrinsic urethral sphincter. J Urol 1997; 158: 1119.
51. Yiou R, Lefaucheur JP, Atala A. The regeneration process of the striated urethral sphincter involves activation of intrinsic satellite cells. Anat Embryol (Berl) 2003; 206: 429.
52. Partridge TA, Morgan JE, Coulton GR, Hoffman EP, Kunkel LM. Conversion of mdx myofibres from dystrophin-negative to -positive by injection of normal myoblasts. Nature 1989; 337: 176.
53. Mendell JR, Kissel JT, Amato AA et al. Myoblast transfer in the treatment of Duchenne's muscular dystrophy. N Engl J Med 1995; 333: 832.
54. Menasche P, Hagege AA, Scorsin M et al. Myoblast transplantation for heart failure. Lancet 2001; 357: 279.
55. Qu Z, Balkir L, van Deutekom JC et al. Development of approaches to improve cell survival in myoblast transfer therapy. J Cell Biol 1998; 142: 1257.
56. Urish K, Kanda Y, Huard J. Initial failure in myoblast transplantation therapy has led the way toward the isolation of muscle stem cells: potential for tissue regeneration. Curr Top Dev Biol 2005; 68: 263.
57. Hale DS, Benson JT, Brubaker L, Heidkamp MC, Russell B. Histologic analysis of needle biopsy of urethral sphincter from women with normal and stress incontinence with comparison of electromyographic findings. Am J Obstet Gynecol 1999; 180: 342.
58. van Mier P, Lichtman JW. Regenerating muscle fibers induce directional sprouting from nearby nerve terminals: studies in living mice. J Neurosci 1994; 14: 5672.
59. English AW. Cytokines, growth factors and sprouting at the neuromuscular junction. J Neurocytol 2003; 32: 943.
60. Lecoeur C, Swieb S, Zini L et al. Intraurethral transfer of satellite cells by myofiber implants results in the formation of innervated myotubes exerting tonic contractions. J Urol 2007; 178: 332.
61. Gosling JA, Dixon JS, Critchley HO, Thompson SA. A comparative study of the human external sphincter and periurethral levator ani muscles. Br J Urol 1981; 53: 35.
62. Yiou R, Delmas V, Carmeliet P et al. The pathophysiology of pelvic floor disorders: evidence from a histomorphologic study of the perineum and a mouse model of rectal prolapse. J Anat 2001; 199: 599.
63. Zini L, Lecoeur C, Swieb S et al. The striated urethral sphincter of the pig shows morphological and functional characteristics essential for the evaluation of treatments for sphincter insufficiency. J Urol 2006; 176: 2729.
64. Bacou F, Rouanet P, Barjot C et al. Expression of myosin isoforms in denervated, cross-reinnervated, and electrically stimulated rabbit muscles. Eur J Biochem 1996; 236: 539.
65. Mitterberger M, Pinggera GM, Marksteiner R et al. Functional and Histological Changes after Myoblast Injections in the Porcine Rhabdosphincter. Eur Urol 2007.
66. Strasser H, Marksteiner R, Margreiter E et al. Autologous myoblasts and fibroblasts versus collagen for treatment of stress urinary incontinence in women: a randomised controlled trial. Lancet 2007; 369: 2179.

61

Restoration of complete bladder function by neurostimulation

Michael Craggs

Introduction

During the past 30 years two key developments using implantable neuroprostheses have had a significant impact on treating and managing patients with a neurogenic bladder. The first of these was the Brindley sacral anterior root stimulator,[1] used principally for bladder emptying (see Chapter 53). The second was the sacral nerve stimulator originally developed by Tanagho and Schmidt for neuromodulating a variety of bladder dysfunctions,[2,3] including the overactive bladder and urinary retention (see Chapter 54). It is timely to consider how these two techniques, among others, may in the future be combined using emerging technologies to restore more complete control of the dysfunctional bladder in people with a suprasacral spinal cord injury (SCI).

Suprasacral lesions to the spinal cord nearly always lead to serious disruption of lower urinary tract function: impairment of voluntary sphincter control and sensation of bladder fullness, aberrant reflexes of the bladder, and an uncoordinated urinary sphincter[4] (see Chapter 30). As a consequence, bladder emptying is impaired and the result is reflex incontinence. Reflex incontinence is primarily caused by detrusor hyperreflexia, an aberrant reflex that emerges after a period of spinal shock following SCI (Figure 61.1). It is often associated with dyssynergenic contractions of the striated sphincter muscle of the urethra, preventing efficient emptying of the bladder. Persons with SCI frequently develop large residual volumes and urinary tract infections, and are prone to upper urinary tract damage and subsequent renal failure if managed incorrectly.

Medical treatment is usually by a combination of drugs for suppressing detrusor hyperreflexia and intermittent catheterization for emptying the bladder. However, the antimuscarinic drugs used to treat incontinence often have debilitating side-effects, such as constipation, dry mouth, and visual disturbance.

Emptying the bladder can also be very troublesome, especially in women for whom no reliable collection device exists (other than indwelling catheters and bags or ungainly pads), and intermittent catheterization can often introduce bladder infections. Other more radical approaches such as surgery for augmenting the bladder, sphincterotomies, cutting

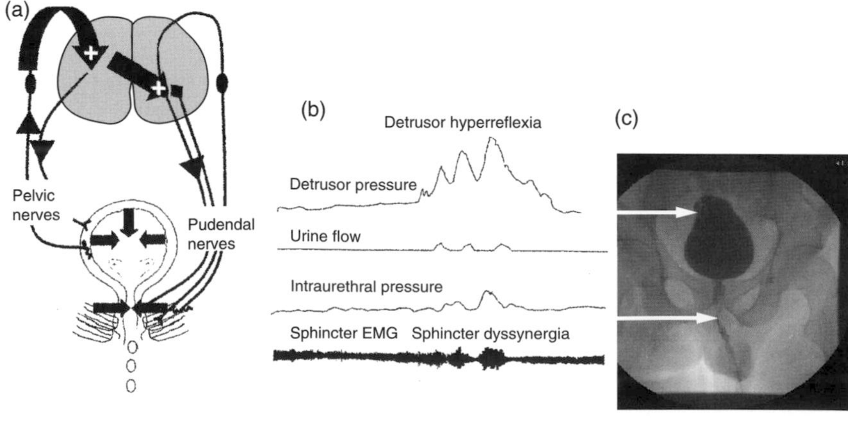

Figure 61.1
The neurogenic bladder in suprasacral spinal cord injury. (a) Aberrant pelvic reflexes causing detrusor hyperreflexia and detrusor-external sphincter dyssynergia. (b) Traces showing the high bladder pressures generated, dyssynergia of the sphincter, associated electromyography (EMG), and urine leakage during videourodynamics. (c) X-ray image shows the bladder and sphincter at the exact time of dyssynergia.

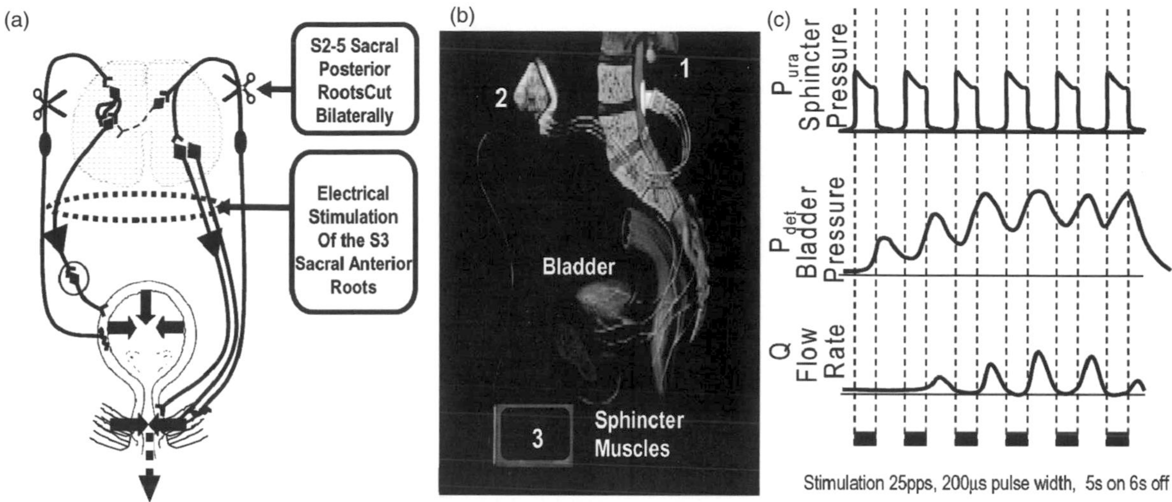

Figure 61.2
Sacral anterior root stimulation (SARS) with sacral deafferentation for bladder control. (a) The Finetech–Brindley SARS implantable stimulator uses bilaterally placed intrathecal or extradural electrodes on the S2–S4 sacral roots to activate the preganglionic parasympathetic pathway to produce efficient bladder emptying. A rhizotomy of the corresponding posterior roots (sensory) prevents detrusor hyperreflexia, dyssynergia of the sphincter, and incontinence. (b) Anatomic configuration of the Finetech–Brindley implant. (c) Bursts of stimulation activate simultaneously the striated sphincter muscle and detrusor smooth muscle. During the intervals between the bursts the sphincter relaxes rapidly to leave a low urethral resistance whilst the detrusor is still contracting slowly to a higher pressure so as to enable very efficient voiding.

posterior sacral roots to suppress hyperreflexia, or repeated injections of toxins such as botulinum toxin to paralyze the sphincter and bladder may all have destructive effects which could preclude the use of future developments, including more novel implantable neurostimulating devices.

This chapter briefly reviews some future possibilities for combining existing and emerging science and technologies[5,6] to develop an implantable neuroprosthesis capable of restoring complete control to the bladder and sphincters in SCI. Seven areas of development will be addressed:

- sacral anterior root stimulation for emptying the paralyzed bladder
- sacral nerve stimulation for suppressing detrusor hyperreflexia
- conditional neuromodulation for automatic control of reflex incontinence
- the extradural sacral posterior and anterior root stimulator implant (SPARSI)
- selective stimulation of sacral roots to prevent detrusor-sphincter dyssynergia
- differential motor and sensory stimulation of the sacral roots through a new sacral posterior and anterior intrathecal root stimulator (SPAIRS) implant
- prospects for complete restoration of bladder control by neuroprosthesis.

Sacral anterior root stimulation for emptying the paralyzed bladder

In the 1970s, Brindley and his colleagues developed an implantable device to empty the bladder and control the sphincters.[7] The prosthesis uses sacral anterior root stimulation (Finetech–Brindley SARS, Finetech Medical Limited, Welwyn Garden City, UK) to activate bladder motor pathways and produce clinically effective voiding (Figure 61.2). For reflex incontinence and sphincter dyssynergia to be overcome in these patients, the sacral sensory nerve roots from S2 to S4 have to be cut (sacral deafferentation (posterior rhizotomy)).[8]

The Finetech–Brindley device has been successfully used in many countries throughout the world.[9] The implant, when combined with sacral deafferentation, has been shown to be very effective in increasing bladder volume, promoting complete emptying of the bladder, reducing bladder infections, and significantly improving the quality of life for many patients.[10] Early in the Brindley program of sacral anterior root stimulator implants it was shown that the technique is very efficient for emptying the bladder (Figure 61.3),[11] and over many years this has proven to be significantly better than reflex voiding.

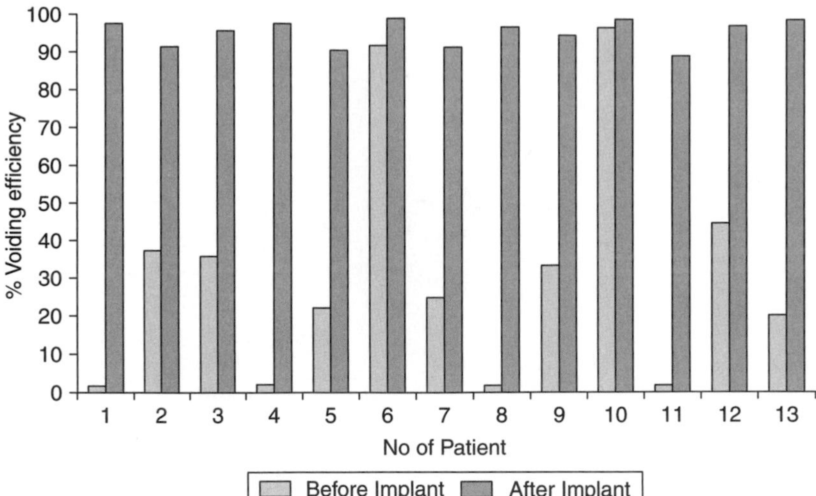

Figure 61.3
Data graphed from information in Cardozo et al[11] to show the significant benefit of using a Brindley sacral anterior root stimulator (SARS) implant to improve voiding efficiency in a group of 13 patients. Voiding efficiency (%) = $(V_v/V_v + V_r) \times 100$ (where V_v = voided volume and V_r = residual bladder volume). Reflex voiding before implantation gave an efficiency of 31% (±32) across this group of patients whereas with their SARS the efficiency was greater than 96% (±4%), giving a very significant improvement (p <0.001).

However, the need for sacral deafferentation, with the consequent loss of reflex erections, reflex ejaculation, bowel problems, and potential pelvic floor weakness, can deter many very suitable young male patients from accepting SARS. Furthermore, the hope by some patients of a 'cure' for SCI in the future using neural regeneration and repair techniques is a further obstacle to acceptance. Patients who have already suffered accidental damage to their spinal cord are understandably reluctant then to accept deliberate cutting of their sacral afferent nerve roots. Realistically, a cure for restoring autonomic functions controling bladder and bowel may take many years to perfect and, meanwhile, management has to try to give the patient the best quality of life. With good medical management of the neurogenic bladder in SCI, most patients can now expect a near normal life span and SARS can definitely help many patients, but clearly it would be much more acceptable if it did not involve further destruction of potentially useful reflexes. There may be an alternative solution to sacral deafferentation which involves stimulation of these same afferent pathways rather than cutting them to suppress reflex incontinence.

Sacral root stimulation for suppressing detrusor hyperreflexia

During the 1980s Tanagho and Schmidt developed the use of electrical stimulation of sacral nerves to treat a variety of lower urinary tract problems, including those of the neurogenic bladder[12] (see Chapter 54). Subsequently, a neuroprosthesis was developed (Interstim, Medtronic, Inc, Minneapolis, USA) which comprised an implanted pulse generator attached to a multipole electrode surgically inserted into the S3 sacral foramina for stimulating the mixed sacral nerves.[13] Such stimulation, commonly known as *neuromodulation*, has also been successfully used to increase bladder capacity in patients with an SCI.[14]

Studies using noninvasive multipulse magnetic stimulation over the sacrum to stimulate the mixed extradural sacral roots (S2–4) have demonstrated that the increase in bladder capacity is brought about by suppression of detrusor hyperreflexia in patients with SCI.[15] The mechanism for this 'neuromodulatory' action has yet to be determined in man, but one theory, based on experimental work in animals,[16] suggests that neuromodulation involves inhibitory action by pudendal afferent (sensory) nerve stimulation on pelvic nerve motor pathways to the bladder through spinal cord circuits.[17] Pudendal afferents course through S2–4 posterior (sensory) roots to the spinal cord. Evidence in support of the theory was obtained by electrically stimulating purely pudendal afferent pathways at the level of the dorsal penile[18,19] (or dorsal clitoral) nerves in patients. Dorsal penile nerve (DPN) stimulation through surface electrodes in patients with SCI produces a profound and repeatable suppression of provoked detrusor hyperreflexia when applied either continuously (preemptively) or conditionally (i.e. when bladder pressure just begins to increase)[20,21] (Figure 61.4). Furthermore, in addition to suppressing hyperreflexia, DPN stimulation can produce significant increases in bladder volume, as demonstrated in serial cystometrograms.[22] These effects depend essentially on stimulation, and diminish when stimulation is switched off. Interestingly, intermittent stimulation also appears to produce good results, although the ideal interval between bursts has yet to be determined, balancing the need to suppress every hyperreflexic contraction reliably against preserving the battery life of the stimulator.[23]

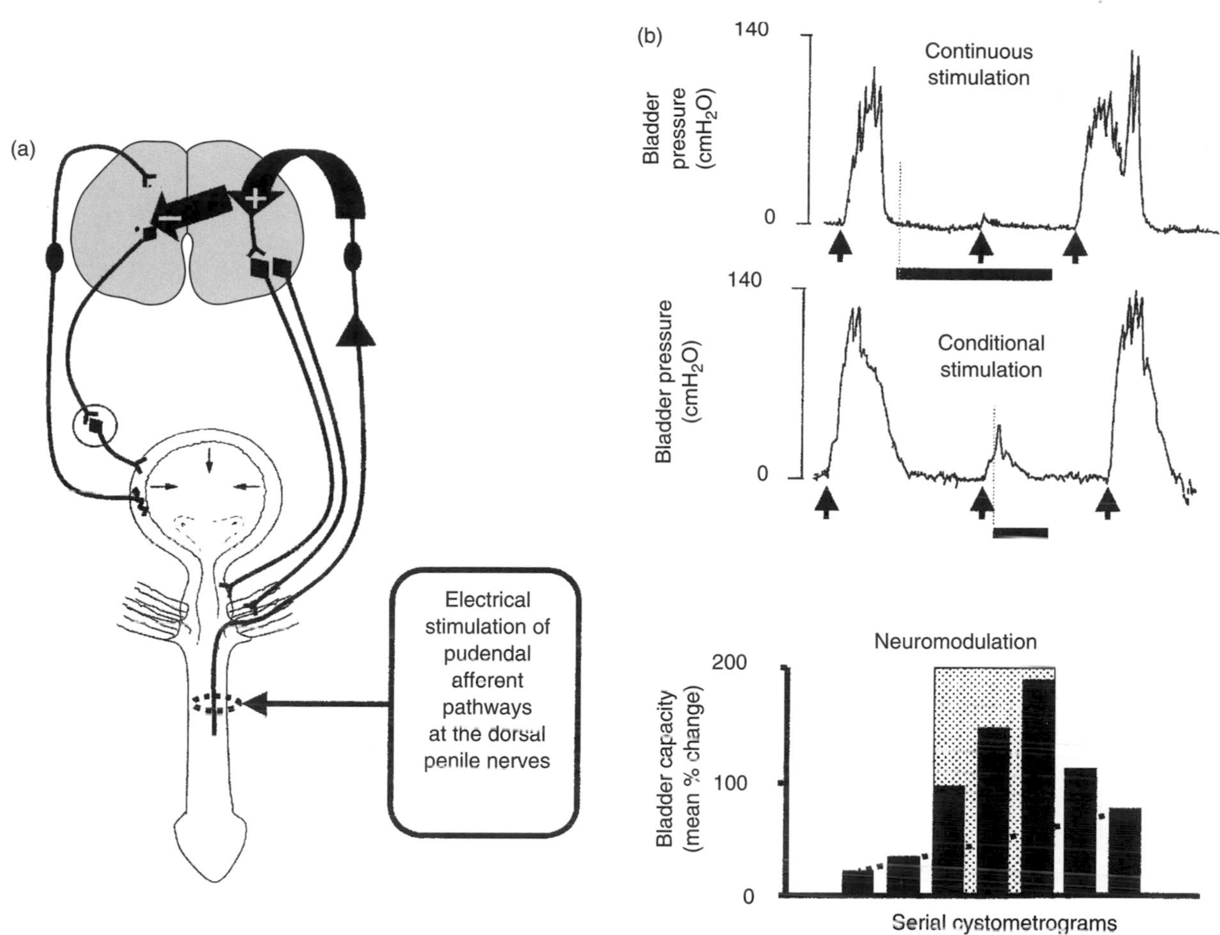

Figure 61.4
Controling detrusor hyperreflexia by noninvasive neuromodulation through pudendal afferent pathways. (a) By stimulating the dorsal penile (or clitoral) nerves with electrical pulses between 10 and 20 per second and above twice the threshold for the pudendo anal reflex, it is possible to profoundly suppress detrusor hyperreflexia. (b) The upper trace shows the effect of continuous stimulation of the dorsal penile nerves on the bladder pressure rise associated with a detrusor hyperreflexia contraction provoked at the middle arrow. Control hyperreflexic contractions provoked at the other arrows can be seen before and after stimulation. The lower trace shows the effect of applying neuromodulation conditionally (that is only when detrusor hyperreflexia just appears) in response to provocation at the middle arrow. Again, this response is flanked by control provocations. (c) Repeated cystometrograms with continuous neuromodulation (shaded area), demonstrating significant increases in bladder volume when compared to control fills. Following stimulation the bladder takes some time to restore to its smaller capacity, probably as a result of stretching of the bladder wall during the period of neuromodulation.

In a pilot study the same benefit has been shown using a Finetech–Brindley implantable device to stimulate extradural or intradural sacral roots but without deafferentation.[24] In a small group of patients with a suprasacral spinal injury, electrodes were placed bilaterally on either the mixed extradural sacral (S2–4) roots or separated anterior and posterior sacral roots (S3) intrathecally. Each patient was assessed preoperatively with DPN stimulation, as described above, to demonstrate the efficacy of neuromodulation. Preliminary results indicated that patients were able to achieve both good suppression of detrusor hyperreflexia and clinically useful increases in bladder volume (Figure 61.5).

Conditional neuromodulation for automatic control of reflex incontinence

In the implant studies described above it was also demonstrated that conditional stimulation, applied only at the onset of hyperreflexic contractions, was at least as good as continuous stimulation at increasing bladder capacity and was sometimes better. Bladder contractions were sensed by measuring intravesical pressure with a standard catheter and the pudendal afferents stimulated either at the level of the penile dorsal nerve or sacral roots to inhibit bladder

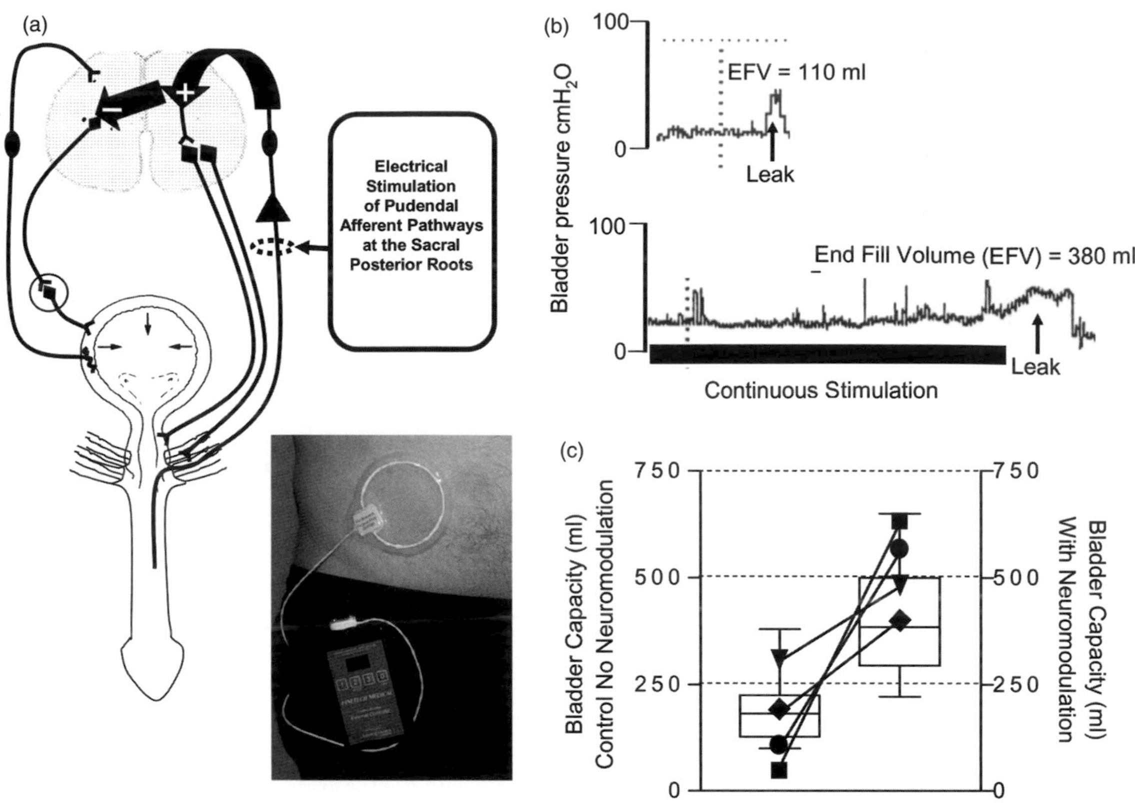

Figure 61.5

Controling detrusor hyperreflexia and increasing bladder capacity by neuromodulation through sacral posterior root stimulation. (a) A Finetech–Brindley implanted stimulator (without deafferentation) is used to apply neuromodulation bilaterally through the S3–S4 sacral roots using a semipermanent coil fixed to the skin over the implanted receiver (inset photograph.) (b) Continuous stimulation at about 15 pulses per second (240 μs pulse width) with a current level set to suppress detrusor hyperreflexia significantly increased bladder capacity over control tests (EFV = end-fill volume). (c) The graph shows box and whisker results from a group of 11 patients with SCI tested using continuous neuromodulation through the dorsal penile nerves (DPN) compared with the effect of applying neuromodulation through the posterior roots in 4 patients (solid lines with symbols) from this same group with a SPARSI implant. It can be seen that bladder capacity is markedly increased with stimulation of the roots and compares favorably with the significant group result using DPN stimulation. DPN stimulation may be a good predictor for success with a sacral nerve stimulator.

contractions (Figure 61.6).[22,24] Interestingly, a similar approach has recently been used to suppress neurogenic detrusor overactivity (detrusor hyperreflexia) in patients with multiple sclerosis.[25]

A conditional system that detects the onset of unstable bladder contractions and then suppresses them has a number of theoretic advantages. Although continuous neuromodulation is an effective and simple way to increase bladder capacity in spinally injured patients, in many situations it may not be ideal, not least because of habituation effects. Furthermore, the need for constant current delivery could shorten both battery and electrode life in a completely implanted device, and continuous stimulation of the sacral afferents may have undesirable long-term reflex effects on the anal and urethral sphincters, perhaps exacerbating any residual dyssynergia.

Hence, a device that could stimulate the sacral nerves for neuromodulation only when necessary might have considerable benefits and would have the added advantage that it could provide feedback about bladder fullness to the patient. That is, stimulating pulses associated with the conditional neuromodulation could also be applied to sensate parts of the body to warn of detrusor hyperreflexia at bladder capacity.

What sort of reliable detection system for conditional neuromodulation could be incorporated into an implant? Brindley was the first to suggest that it might be possible to monitor bladder pressure by implant and use the information to control electrical stimulation of the pudendal nerves to inhibit unstable bladder contractions. Subsequently, an implanted applanation tonometer was developed which could be sutured onto the bladder wall to record pressure. However, tests to assess its long-term performance in

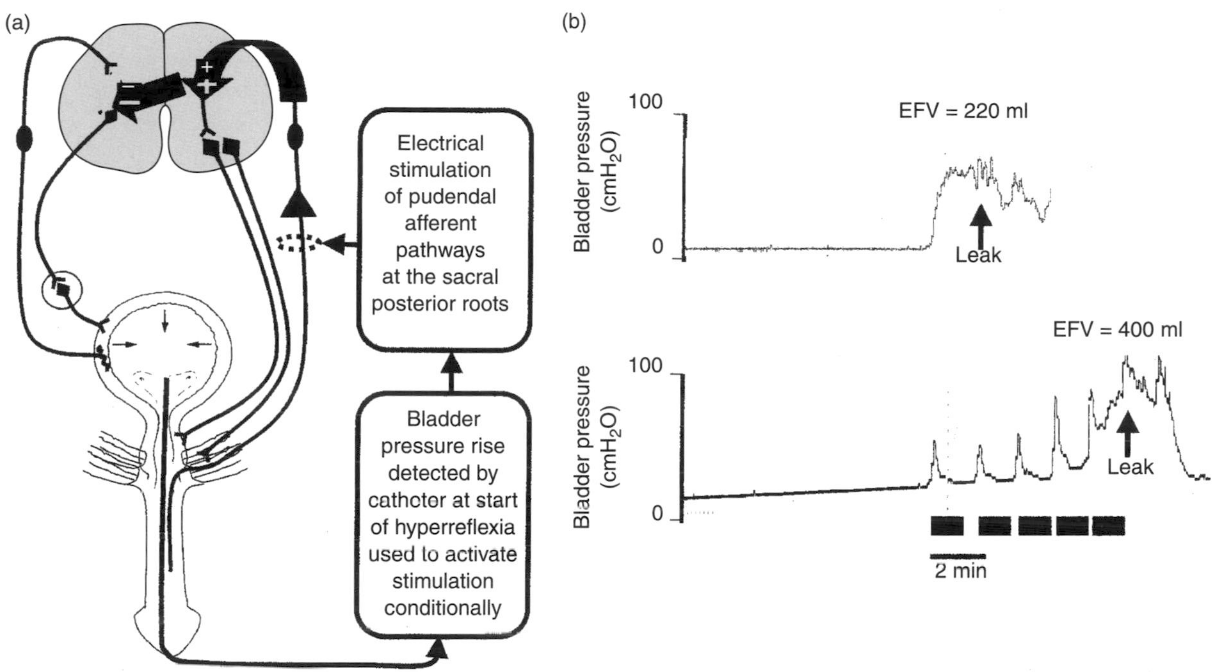

Figure 61.6
Using bladder pressure to automatically control detrusor hyperreflexia with conditional neuromodulation. (a) By measuring bladder pressure with a catheter it is possible to detect exactly when a detrusor hyperreflexic contraction begins and this can be used to activate stimulation of the sacral posterior roots to suppress the contraction automatically. The cystometrograms in this figure were obtained from a patient with an incomplete upper thoracic spinal lesion, but similar results have also been shown in patients with complete lesions. (b) The upper trace shows a cystometrogram without stimulation and a relatively low bladder capacity. The lower trace shows that when a pressure rise is detected, the applied stimulation immediately reduces the pressure, and by automatically repeating this suppression on successive detrusor hyperreflexic contractions a much larger bladder capacity can be achieved. A point is reached at this new maximum capacity when suppression is no longer possible. EFV = end-fill volume.

experimental animals were not very successful, as the device eroded or became dislodged from the bladder.[26] Further obstacles, such as infection and encrustation, preclude the immediate development and implementation of such vesical devices.

Recently it has been shown in experimental animals that it is possible to detect very small electroneurographic signals at fractional microvolt levels, using sophisticated recording techniques, from the afferents in the mixed sacral nerve roots during hyperreflexia-like bladder contractions.[27] The recorded signals could then be used to trigger stimulation of the pudendal or sacral posterior nerves to inhibit conditionally in a feedback loop those same contractions (Figure 61.7).

Some preliminary work in patients with SCI during implantation of sacral anterior root stimulators indicates that detecting bladder contractions from the sacral sensory nerves may also be possible.[28–30] However, although an implanted conditional neuromodulation device may be feasible in people with a spinal cord injury, it is likely to be considerably more complex than present devices tried in animals and will have to be very reliable. Implantable microcircuits for detecting minute neural signals in humans which could be used to activate conditional neuromodulation are now being developed for this purpose.[31]

Whether detrusor hyperreflexia is to be controlled by automatic conditional stimulation or simply by continuous neuromodulation, the interesting possibility now exists for combining the benefits of bladder emptying with control of reflex incontinence in one implantable sacral root stimulator.

The sacral posterior and anterior root stimulator implant

This new concept was developed using a single implant (Finetech–Brindley) to combine bladder emptying through sacral anterior root stimulation with posterior sacral root stimulation to prevent reflex incontinence.[32] If successful, the major advantage of SPARSI would be restoration of bladder function without the need for sacral deafferentation.

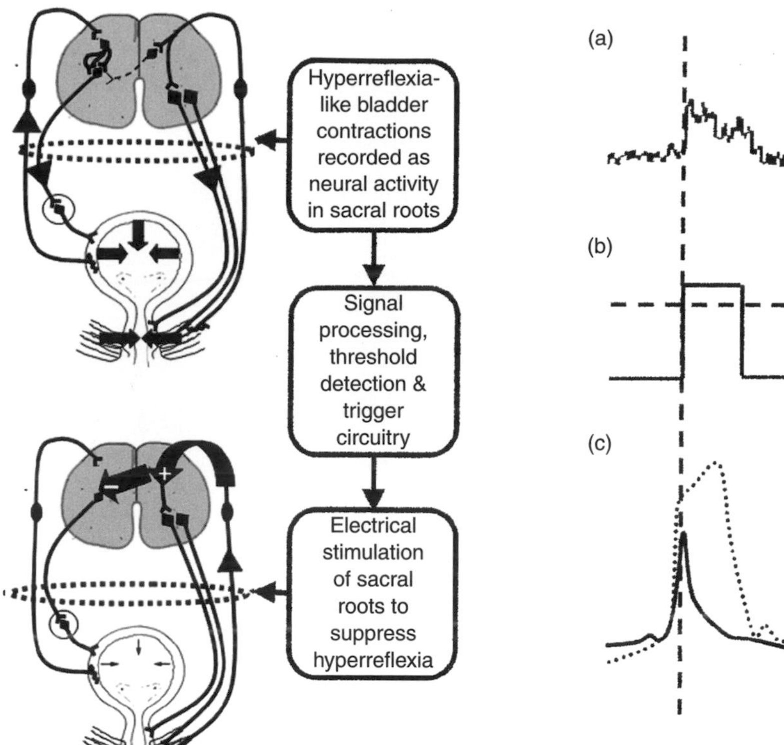

Figure 61.7
Sacral nerve activity as feedback control for conditional neuromodulation. (a) A miniature electrical signal (<0.5 μV) from the sacral nerves associated with a hyperreflexia-like contraction in an experimental animal. (b) Using special signal processing techniques it is possible to detect the changes and then activate stimulation of the sacral posterior roots for conditional neuromodulation. (c) The hyperreflexia-like contraction (dotted line) without neuromodulation is very effectively suppressed (solid line) when stimulation is applied.

In one study, 5 patients with a suprasacral spinal injury were implanted with a standard bilateral extradural Finetech–Brindley device (Figure 61.8), but without sacral deafferentation, to test the concept of SPARSI. These patients were part of the neuromodulation study described above.[24]

A significant finding in this study, reported first in 2001,[33] demonstrated that the benefits of neuromodulation by a SPARSI implant at home were comparable to the effects of oxybutynin in improving functional bladder capacity in the same patient (Figure 61.9). Furthermore, the improvement also compared favorably with the benefits of sacral deafferentation. Another interesting finding, which agrees with other studies of sacral neuromodulation for the overactive bladder (e.g. using the Medtronic sacral nerve stimulator), showed that the effects do not necessarily diminish appreciably with time, but that when stimulation is stopped symptoms such as incontinence return. With SPARSI, bladder capacity always returned to much smaller values in less than 24 h when stimulation was stopped.

Unfortunately, in this small group of patients, bladder emptying was not always very efficient despite the generation of adequate bladder pressures. The concept of SPARSI using extradural electrodes will only be successful when good bladder emptying (as in the original SARS with posterior rhizotomy) is also achieved. SARS uses post-stimulus voiding to empty the bladder efficiently so that, during the intervals between bursts of stimulation, urethral pressure is much lower than bladder pressure, allowing unimpeded urine flow. In SPARSI, where both striated sphincter and bladder reflex pathways are intact, there can be residual increases in urethral pressure as the slow bladder pressure develops in the post-stimulation gap (Figure 61.10). This is reflex detrusor-sphincter dyssynergia, and leads to urinary outflow obstruction, making emptying much less reliable (compare with Figure 61.2).

The SPARSI concept could achieve its original objective if the problems of bladder emptying could be overcome. A number of possible solutions to control detrusor-external sphincter dyssynergia are available – including pharmacotherapy (e.g. botulinum toxin), stenting, and surgery (sphincterotomy) – but ideally we should find a neurophysiologic solution which could be applied through the same stimulating implant. One possible approach which may be technically difficult to effect is selective stimulation to block sphincter activity during bladder emptying.

Selective stimulation of sacral roots to prevent detrusor-sphincter dyssynergia

Sacral anterior roots contain both the large somatic nerves to the urethral striated sphincter and the small preganglionic

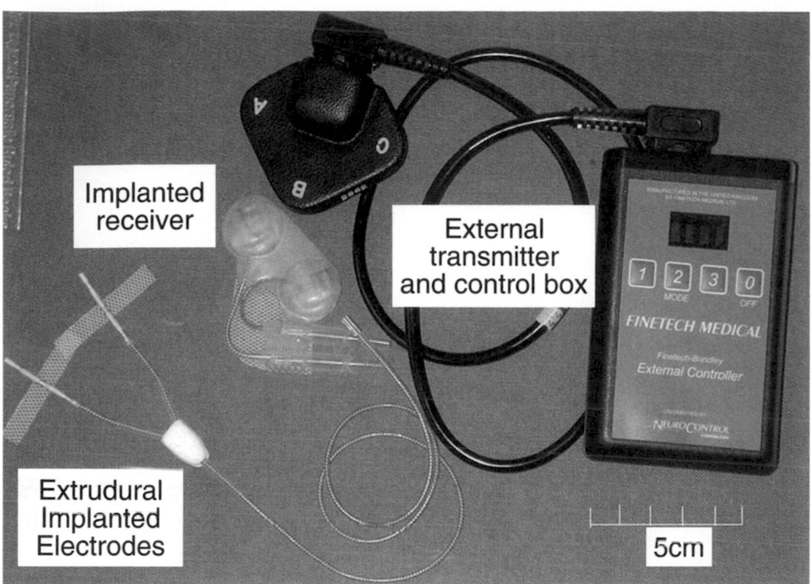

Figure 61.8
The Finetech–Brindley bladder stimulator with extradural implanted electrodes.

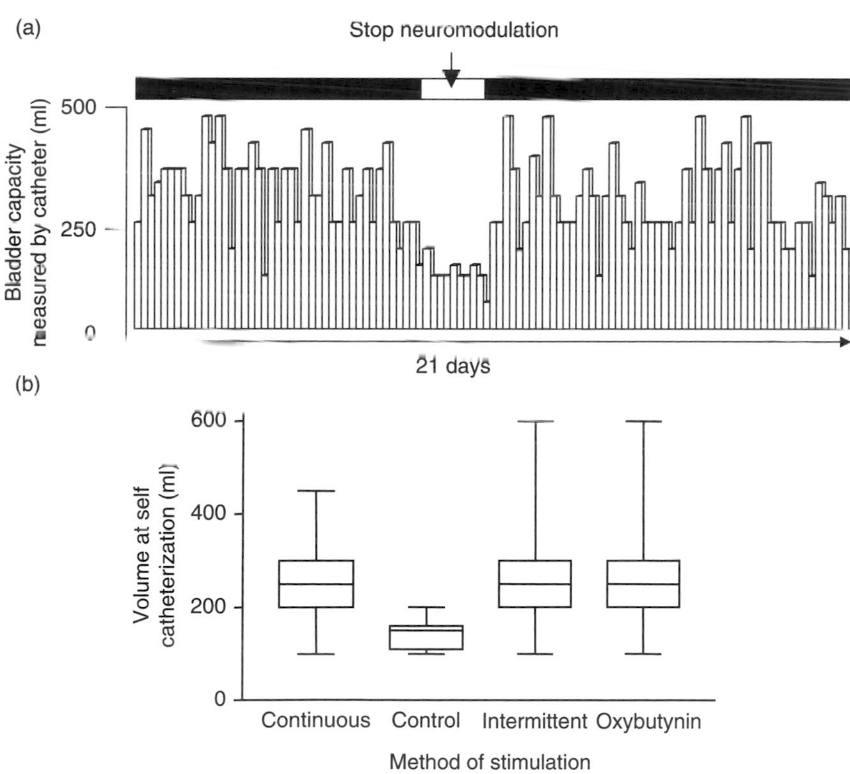

Figure 61.9
Neuromodulation through SPARSI at home. (a) A continuous set of data showing that over a 3-week period neuromodulation through the implant maintained good bladder capacity when compared to a short period during which stimulation was stopped. (b) Continuous stimulation was shown to be comparable to intermittent stimulation given on a 50 s 'on' to 50 s 'off' cycle and both gave bladder volumes statistically greater than no stimulation during a control period. An interesting finding was the near equivalence of benefit with neuromodulation alone or oxybutynin (an anticholinergic drug to block detrusor hyperreflexic contractions) alone.

parasympathetic nerves to the bladder detrusor smooth muscle. Consequently, during anterior root stimulation, bladder emptying is impaired by coactivation of these two groups of nerve fibers (see Figure 61.2). This is the reason for adopting the post-stimulus voiding technique,[34] which takes advantage of the rapid relaxation of the sphincter and slow contraction of the detrusor to achieve good bladder emptying. This type of voiding is not particularly physiologic, but it is efficient. However, in the presence of intact sacral reflexes (i.e. no rhizotomy), the dyssynergia persists in the gap between the bursts of stimulation to prevent efficient emptying as described above. For this problem to be overcome, tests have been done using a variety of techniques, including sphincter fatiguing methods and selective nerve blocking ('anode block') of sphincter motor pathways.

The principle of selective electrical stimulation relies on blocking the large nerve fibers to the striated muscles by anodal hyperpolarization. This prevents the passage of action potentials down the large nerves to the sphincter whilst permitting the flow of action potentials along the small motor

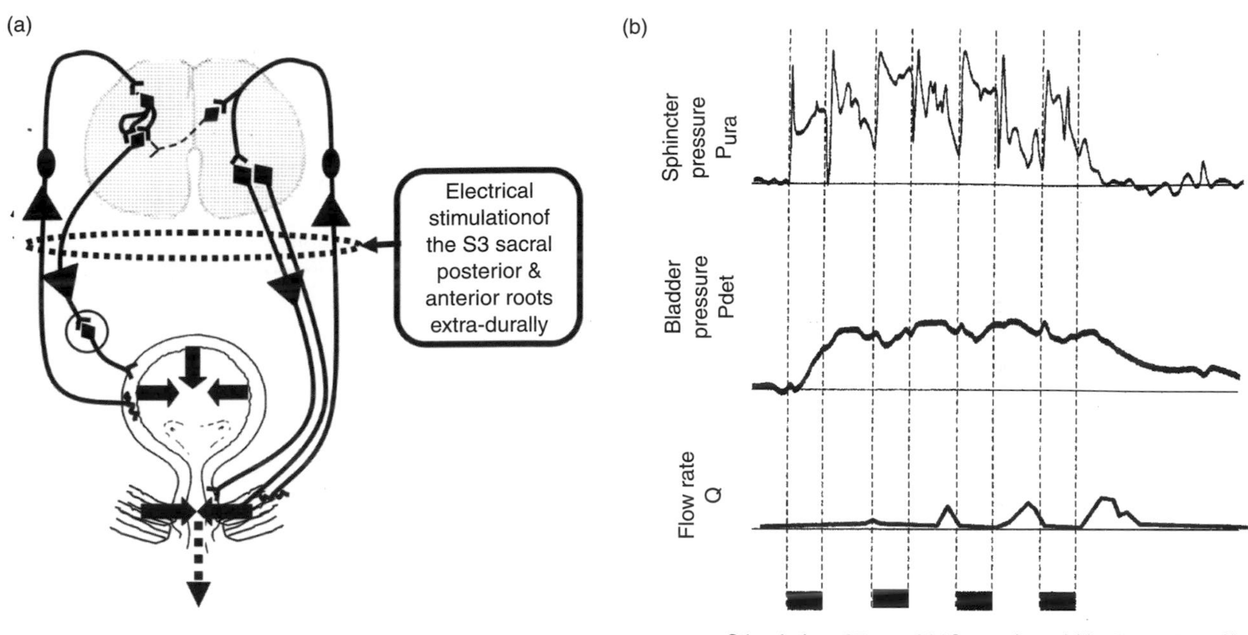

Figure 61.10
Bladder contraction through SPARSI. (a) Stimulation of the mixed sacral roots through extradural electrodes or separated roots through intrathecal electrodes activates both efferent (motor) and afferent (sensory) pathways either directly or reflexly. (b) Good bladder pressures are generated by bursts of stimulation, but voiding is very inefficient in the gaps as a result of reflex contractions of the sphincter, elevating urethral pressure above the bladder pressure (compare with the traces shown in Figure 61.2).

nerves to the bladder muscle (Figure 61.11). To prevent 'anode-break' excitation when the individual stimulating pulses in the train switch off, they must be switched off slowly.

This method of stimulation was originally shown by Brindley and Craggs to be effective in experimental animals using a specially designed chronically implanted tripolar electrode and triangular-shaped electrical pulses to stimulate the sacral anterior roots selectively.[35] The range of stimulating currents where sphincter motor potentials were blocked while bladder pressure increased was relatively small but effective. However, Brindley and Craggs did not demonstrate bladder emptying in their experiments.

Interestingly, a similar type of tripolar electrode is used in the standard intrathecal Finetech–Brindley SARS implant, so theoretically it should be possible to investigate the possibility of using this technique for actual bladder emptying in patients. However, to prevent reflex effects on all of the motor fibers to the sphincter it may be necessary to apply anode blockade to all of the sacral anterior roots simultaneously.

It has been shown that during implantation of a Finetech–Brindley SARS it is possible to demonstrate intraoperatively that an anode-blocking technique with long rectangular pulses can be used to achieve selective stimulation in anesthetized patients,[36] but again efficient bladder emptying was not demonstrated. It has been claimed that physiologic micturition (i.e. natural voiding where the sphincter relaxes during contraction of the bladder to produce a good stream of urine and complete bladder emptying) is possible using a modified Finetech–Brindley intrathecal electrode to activate the bladder in the dog.[37] Unfortunately, this study did not present data to substantiate the claim but did demonstrate a significant lowering of sphincter pressure simultaneous with good bladder pressures during sacral stimulation with quasitrapezoidal pulses.[38]

So, it remains to be seen whether such selective stimulation techniques can produce efficient voiding; the evidence from animal studies is promising,[39] but awaits a successful resolution in patients in whom we may wish to preserve all sacral reflexes. If resolved, although technically difficult, the concept of an extradural SPARSI described above may become a realistic possibility.

Sacral anterior and posterior intrathecal root stimulation implants

Following the important contribution of Sauerwein in the 1980s advocating deafferentation of the S2–S5 sacral roots to prevent detrusor hyperreflexia,[8] Brindley confirmed that this procedure also improved bladder emptying,[10] and so implantation of a Finetech–Brindley device for bladder

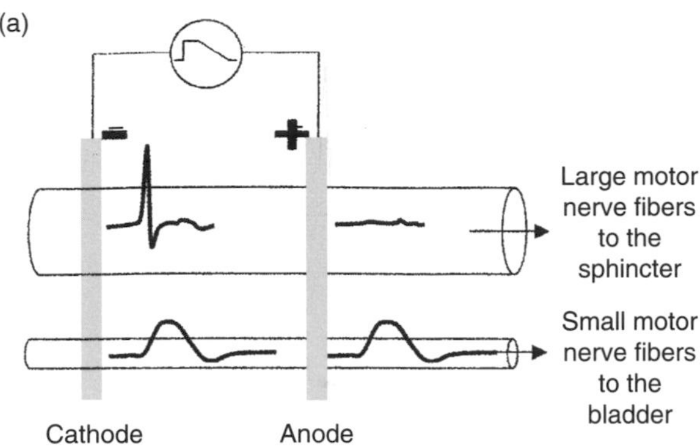

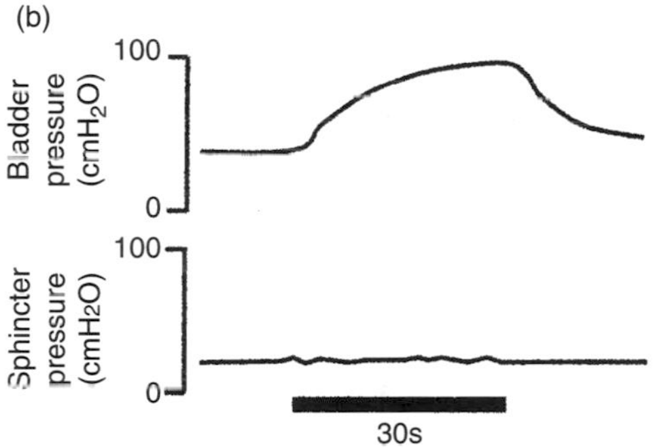

Figure 61.11
Selective blockade of the motor nerves to the sphincter.
(a) Applying triangular or quasitrapezoidal electrical pulses to groups of different diameter nerve fibers in the sacral roots it is possible to find a range of stimulating currents that block the large motor nerves to the striated sphincter at the anode electrode (anode block), while still permitting conduction down the small motor nerves to the bladder detrusor muscle.
(b) Selective anode blockade of the sphincter successfully applied while a good bladder contraction is elicited during stimulation with a train of triangular pulses at 30 pulses per second.

emptying without a rhizotomy in patients with severe detrusor-external sphincter dyssynergia has not normally been advised. Interestingly, Brindley's earlier patients[40] did not often have a rhizotomy but most achieved good emptying; of course the devices were intrathecal and there was always the possibility of iatrogenic posterior root damage, which might anyway abolish detrusor hyperreflexia in some cases. However, in more than two-thirds of these patients, sacral reflexes, including detrusor hyperreflexia, were preserved and yet the patients could empty their bladders very efficiently with their SARS implant (see Figure 61.3).

So we know that in many patients, where the posterior roots are separated from their anterior partners but not included with them on the stimulating electrodes, then efficient voiding can be achieved without reflex dyssynergia. With this knowledge a newer approach to achieving the concept of SPARSI was undertaken, but using an intrathecal implant with separated anterior and posterior roots at the level of S3, each placed on their own electrodes.[41] This implant has been named the sacral posterior and anterior intrathecal root stimulator (SPAIRS) and achieved voiding efficiencies of over 95%, much like the earlier Brindley implants without rhizotomies (Figure 61.12). Furthermore, with careful surgery to separate out the S3 posterior roots and place on their own electrodes it has enabled separate stimulation for the purpose of neuromodulation and so we may have the possibility of a viable implant to both control neurogenic detrusor overactivity and empty the bladder efficiently.

Prospects for complete restoration of bladder control by neuroprosthesis

In this chapter we have considered some old, new, and emerging developments and technologies using sacral root stimulation which together may, in the future, provide full restoration of bladder control to the neurogenic bladder (Figure 61.13).

In recent times our understanding of the neurophysiology of the lower urinary tract has advanced in ways that may lead to even more sophisticated ways of controling the neurogenic bladder, bowel, and sexual dysfunction. Of these emerging techniques currently being developed in experimental animal models is the exciting possibility of actually stimulating and recording from the nuclei of origin of the sacral motor pathways in the spinal cord. Intraspinal microsimulation, as it has become known, involves inserting fine wire electrodes into the tracts in these structures.[42–45] Interestingly, as with sacral root stimulation, the problem of controling the dyssynergia of the urethral sphincter presents as the most difficult problem to be overcome in these experimental studies. Neurophysiologic studies have shown that spinal interneurons are very much involved in the segmental coordination of the bladder and sphincters and therefore it may become possible to activate these interneuronal pathways by stimulation to obtain the synergic control necessary to empty the bladder efficiently.[46] It seems that considerable technical advances will be needed to apply microstimulation, not least the problem of keeping fine microelectrodes in close contact with the appropriate neural substrates, while at the same time preventing tethering of the spinal cord, which in itself could cause significant damage.

Whichever future development provides the best and safest solution for controlled neurostimulation it still remains that, for a significant number of patients with lower motor neuron problems, such as corda equina lesions, the possibility for restoration of pelvic function is problematic. For this important group of patients,

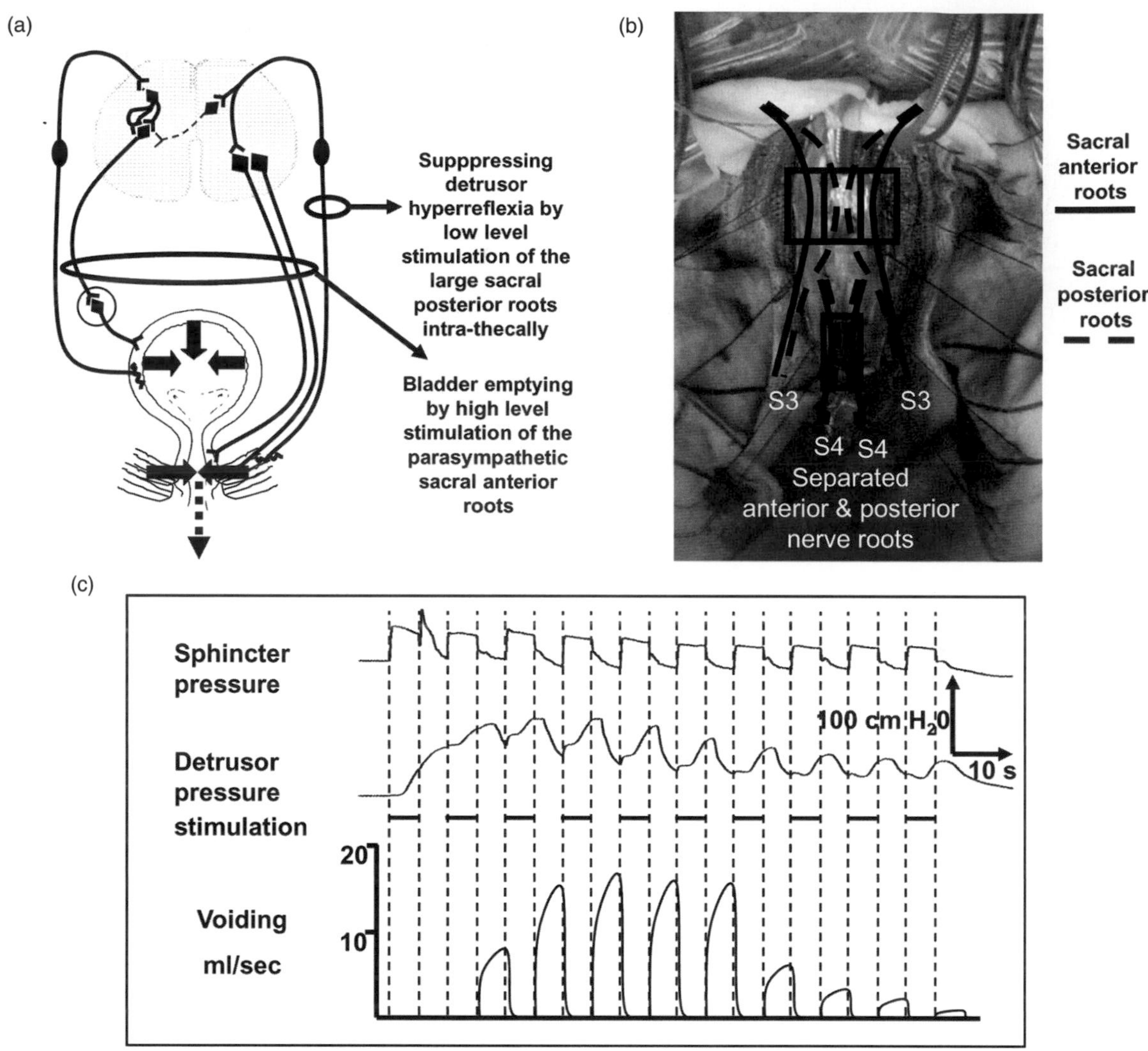

Figure 61.12
The sacral posterior and anterior intra-thecal root stimulator (SPAIRS) implant. (a) Posterior and anterior S3 sacral roots divided and placed on separate intra-thecal electrodes for neuromodulation of neurogenic detrusor overactivity and bladder empting respectively. (b) The standard Finetech–Brindley 4-slot intra-thecal electrode array at surgery superimposed over the exposed corda equine following a laminectomy involving the 4th, 5th, lumbar vertebrae and part sacrum. (c) A typical emptying of the bladder during bilateral S3 anterior root stimulation with the SPAIRS implant. (Compare with the obstructed voiding seen in Figure 61.10 using extradural S3 mixed nerve roots.) The voiding efficiency is regularly greater than 95%.

coordination of the bladder and sphincter is less important than impaired contraction, but problems of incontinence and the inability to void remain impediments to good management and quality of life. Perhaps the new surgical techniques for neural repair and regeneration of the motor pathways may offer some prospect for helping these patients.[47] There may even be a place to assist or combine neuronal repair with neurostimulation,[48] but whichever method yields opportunities, careful assessments and evaluations of the pathways controling the bladder and sphincters will be important in this regard.[49,50]

Although recovery of central afferent pathways is less likely in these repairs, any sacral reflexes that are restored may be more aberrant than in suprasacral injuries and therefore present with new and more difficult challenges to be overcome. Interestingly, some very recent experimental research in animals has been re-examining the role of the pudendal pathways and the opportunities for developing more peripheral nerve stimulating devices which can promote reflex voiding of the neurogenic bladder and minimize sphincter dyssynergia.[51,52] As with many good ideas these developments are based on physiology of the lower

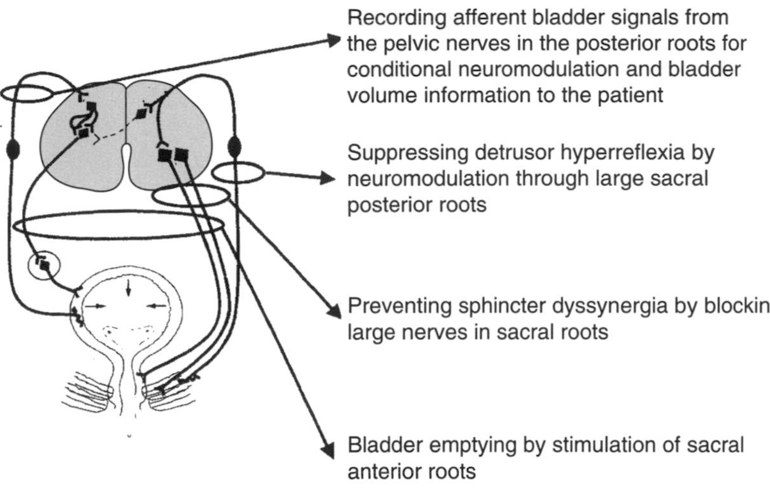

Figure 61.13
Possible techniques to overcome problems of the neurogenic bladder in SCI.

urinary tract that has been known for over 70 years and certainly since the time of Barrington.[53] Irrespective of the pathways or reflexes we fix or tap into there is no doubt that the most important need is for a system that can eliminate urinary incontinence, give socially good bladder capacity, and empty the urinary bladder efficiently.

Finally, some of the ideas presented here might be limited by current technology, but this is very likely to become realizable in the near future. Such technologic advances might include more appropriately designed and stable electrode–nerve interfaces (especially important if the electrodes are to be implanted inside the spinal cord or brain), new implantable integrated electronics capable of processing tiny signals and delivering patterned stimuli, and improved systems for transferring or using power efficiently in implants. A new range of intelligent sensor technology for detecting physiologic changes in the body is likely to emerge. The future may also see the increased use of telemetries for computerized control of implants, including the transfer of data to and from these devices to improve function.

Summary

Ultimately, it is hoped that by combining conditional neuromodulation for reflex incontinence with selective neurostimulation for bladder emptying we can completely control the neurogenic bladder without cutting any sacral sensory nerves. The big challenge will probably be to overcome the detrusor-sphincter dyssynergia resulting from the emergence of aberrant reflexes following spinal injury. By preserving all pelvic reflexes, including those for erection, ejaculation, and bowel control, as well as those essential to guard against stress incontinence, we will help to reassure people with a spinal cord injury that this technology will improve their quality of life until the time comes when neural repair becomes a realistic possibility for them.

References

1. Brindley GS, Polkey CE, Rushton DN. Sacral anterior root stimulators for bladder control in paraplegia. Paraplegia 1982; 20: 365–81.
2. Schmidt RA. Treatment of the unstable bladder. Urology 1991; 37: 28–32.
3. Tanagho EA. Concepts of neuromodulation. Neurourol Urodyn 1993; 12: 487–8.
4. Selzman AA, Hampel N. Urologic complications of spinal cord injury. Urol Clin N Am 1993; 20: 453–64.
5. Grill WM, Craggs MD, Foreman RD et al. Emerging clinical applications of electrical stimulation: opportunities for restoration of function. J Rehab Res Dev 2001; 38: 641–53.
6. Jezernik S, Craggs M, Grill WM et al. Electrical stimulation for the treatment of bladder dysfunction: current status and future possibilities. Neurol Res 2002; 24: 413–30.
7. Brindley GS. An implant to empty the bladder or close the urethra. J Neurol Neurosurg Psychiatry 1977; 43: 1083–90.
8. Sauerwein D. Funktionelle Elektrostimulation der Harnblase: Erste Erfahrungen mit sakraler Deafferentation (SDAF) und Vorderwurzelstimulation (SARS) nach Brindley in Deutschland. Vb Dtsch Ges Urol 1987; 39: 595–7.
9. van Kerrebroeck PEV. Worldwide experience with the Finetech–Brindley Sacral Anterior Root Stimulator. Neurourol Urodyn 1993; 12: 497–503.
10. Brindley GS. The first 500 patients with sacral anterior root stimulator implants: general description. Paraplegia 1994; 32: 795–805.
11. Cardozo L, Krishnan KR, Polkey CE, Rushton DN, Brindley GS. Urodynamic observations on patients with sacral anterior root stimulators. Paraplegia 1984; 22: 201–9.
12. Tanagho EA, Schmidt RA. Electrical stimulation in the clinical management of the neurogenic bladder. J Urol 1988; 140: 1331–9.
13. Schmidt RA, Jonas U, Oleson KA et al for the Sacral Nerve Stimulation Study Group. Sacral nerve stimulation for the treatment of refractory urinary urge incontinence. J Urol 1999; 162: 352–7.

14. Chartier-Kastler EJ, Bosch RJL, Perrigot M et al. Long-term results of sacral nerve stimulation (S3) for the treatment of neurogenic refractory urge incontinence related to detrusor hyperreflexia. J Urol 2000; 164: 1476–80.
15. Sheriff MKM, Shah PJR, Fowler C et al. Neuromodulation of detrusor hyperreflexia by functional magnetic stimulation of the sacral roots. Br J Urol 1996; 78: 39–46.
16. Lindström S, Fall M, Carlsson CA, Erlandson BE. The neurophysiological basis of bladder inhibition in response to intravaginal electrical stimulation. J Urol 1983; 129: 405–10.
17. Craggs MD, McFarlane JP. Neuromodulation of the lower urinary tract. Exp Physiol 1999; 84: 149–60.
18. Nakamura M, Sakurai T. Bladder inhibition by penile electrical stimulation. Br J Urol 1984; 56: 413–5.
19. Wheeler JS, Walter JS, Zaszczurynski PJ. Bladder inhibition by penile nerve stimulation in spinal cord injury patients. J Urol 1992; 147: 100–3.
20. Shah N, Edhem I, Knight SL, Craggs MD. Acute suppression of provoked detrusor hyperreflexia with detrusor sphincter dyssynergia by electrical stimulation of the dorsal penile nerves in patients with a spinal injury. Eur Urol 1998; 33(Suppl): 60.
21. Kirkham A, Knight S, Casey A et al. Conditional neuromodulation of end-fill hyperreflexia to increase bladder capacity in spinally injured patients. Neurourol Urodyn 2000; 19: 515–6.
22. Kirkham APS, Shah NC, Knight SL et al. The acute effects of continuous and conditional neuromodulation on the bladder in spinal cord injury. Spinal Cord 2001; 39: 420–8.
23. Zafirakis H, Knight SL, Shah PJR et al. Intermittent versus continuous electrical stimulation of the dorsal penile nerve on bladder capacity in spinal cord injury. Neurourol Urodyn 2002; 21: 400.
24. Kirkham APS, Knight SL, Casey ATM et al. Neuromodulation of sacral nerve roots 2 to 4 with a Fintech–Brindley sacral posterior and anterior root stimulator. Spinal Cord 2002; 40: 272–81.
25. Fjorback MV, Rijkhoff N, Petersen T, Nohr M, Sinkjaer T. Event driven electrical stimulation of the dorsal penile/clitoral nerve for management of neurogenic detrusor overactivity in multiple sclerosis. Neurourol Urodyn 2006; 25(4): 349–55.
26. Koldewijn EL, van Kerrebroeck PE, Schaafsma E et al. Bladder pressure sensors in an animal model. J Urol 1994; 151: 1376–84.
27. Jezernik S, Grill WM, Sinkjaer T. Detection and inhibition of hyperreflexia-like bladder contractions in the cat by sacral nerve root recording and electrical stimulation. Neurourol Urodyn 2001; 20: 215–30.
28. Sinkjaer T, Rijkhoff N, Haugland M et al. Electroneurographic (ENG) signals from intradural S3 dorsal sacral nerve roots in a patient with a suprasacral spinal cord injury. Proc 5th Int Functional Electrical Stimulation Soc Conf, Aalborg, Denmark, 2000: 361–4.
29. Grill WM, Creasey GH, Wu K, Takaoka Y. Detection of hyperreflexia-like increases in bladder pressure by recording of sensory nerve activity in human spinal cord injury. Abstract in Proc 5th Int Functional Electrical Stimulation Soc Conf, Aalborg, Denmark, 2000: 234.
30. Kurstjens GA, Borau A, Rodriguez A, Rijkhoff NJ, Sinkjaer T. Intraoperative recording of electroneurographic signals from cuff electrodes on extradural sacral roots in spinal cord injured patients. J Urol 2005; 174(4 Pt 1): 1482–7.
31. Donaldson N de N, Zhou L, Haugland M, Sinkjaer T. An implantable telemeter for long-term electroneurographic recordings in animals and humans. Proc 5th Int Functional Electrical Stimulation Soc Conf, Aalborg, Denmark, 2000: 378–81.
32. Craggs MD, Casey A, Shah PJR et al. SPARSI: an implant to empty the bladder and control incontinence without a posterior rhizotomy in spinal cord injury. Br J Urol Int 2000; 85(Suppl 5): 2.
33. Kirkham APS, Knight SL, Casey ATM et al. Acute and chronic use of a sacral posterior and anterior nerve root stimulator to increase bladder capacity in spinal cord injury. Proc 6th Int Functional Electrical Stimulation Soc Conf Cleveland, Ohio, USA, 2001: 172–4.
34. Jonas U, Tanagho EA. Studies on the feasibility of urinary bladder evacuation by direct spinal cord stimulation. II. Poststimulus voiding: a way to overcome outflow resistance. Invest Urol 1975; 13: 151–3.
35. Brindley GS, Craggs MD. A technique of anodally blocking large nerve fibres through chronically implanted electrodes. J Neurol Neurosurg Psychiatry 1980; 43: 1083–90.
36. Rijkhoff NJM, Wijkstra H, van Kerrebroeck PEV, Debruyne FMJ. Selective detrusor activation by electrical sacral nerve root stimulation in spinal cord injury. J Urol 1997; 157: 1504–8.
37. Seif Ch, Braun PM, Bross J et al. Selective block of urethral sphincter contraction using a modified Brindley electrode in sacral anterior root stimulation of the dog. Neurourol Urodyn 2002; 21: 502–10.
38. Fang ZP, Mortimer JT. Selective activation of small motor axons by quasitrapezoidal current pulses. IEEE Trans Biomed Engng 1991; 38: 168–74.
39. Grünewald V, Bhadra N, Creasey GH, Mortimer JT. Functional conditions of micturition induced by selective sacral anterior root stimulation. World J Urol 1998; 16: 329–36.
40. Brindley GS, Polkey CE, Rushton DN, Cardozo L. Sacral anterior root stimulators for bladder control in paraplegia: the first 50 cases. J Neurol Neurosurg Psychiatry 1986; 49: 1104–14.
41. Craggs MD, Bycroft J, Kirkham A et al. A model for combined bladder emptying and neuromodulation using independent anterior and posterior sacral nerve stimulation. Proc Int Spinal Cord Soc 2004, Athens, Greece.
42. Carter RR, McCreery DB, Woodford BJ et al. Micturition control by microstimulation of the sacral spinal cord of the cat: acute studies. IEEE Trans Rehab Engng 1995; 3: 206–14.
43. Grill WM, Bhadra N, Wang B. Bladder and urethral pressures evoked by microstimulation of the sacral spinal cord in cats. Brain Res 1999; 836: 19–30.
44. Tai C, Booth AM, de Groat WC, Roppolo JR. Colon and anal sphincter contractions evoked by microstimulation of the sacral spinal cord in cats. Brain Res 2001; 889: 38–48.
45. Tai C, Booth AM, de Groat WC, Roppolo JR. Penile erection produced by microstimulation of the sacral spinal cord of the cat. IEEE Trans Rehab Engng 1998; 6: 374–81.
46. Grill WM. Electrical activation of spinal neural circuits: application to motor system neural prostheses. Neuromodulation 2000; 3: 97–106.
47. Carlstedt T. Approaches permitting and enhancing motoneuron regeneration after spinal cord, ventral root, plexus and peripheral nerve injuries. Curr Opin Neurol 2000; 13: 683–6.
48. Grill WM, McDonald JW, Peckham PH et al. At the interface: convergence of neural regeneration and neural prostheses for restoration of function. J Rehab Res Dev 2001; 38: 633–9.
49. Craggs MD. Pelvic somato-vesiceral reflexes after spinal cord injury: measures of functional loss and partial preservation. Prog Brain Res 2006; 152: 205–19.
50. Craggs MD, Balasubramaniam AV, Chung EAL, Emanuel AV. Aberrant reflexes and function of the pelvic organs following spinal cord injury in man. Autonom Neurosci Basic Clin 2006: 126–7, 355–70.
51. Boggs JW, Wenzel BJ, Gustafson KJ, Grill WM. Frequency-dependent selection of reflexes by pudendal afferents in the cat. J Physiol 2006; 577(Pt 1): 115–26.
52. Tai C, Wang J, Wang X, de Groat WC, Roppolo JR. Bladder inhibition or voiding induced by pudendal nerve stimulation in chronic spinal cord injured cats. Neurourol Urodyn 2007; 26(4): 570–7.
53. Barrington FJF. The component reflexes of micturition in the cat. Brain 1931; 54: 177–88.

62

Neuroprotection and repair after spinal cord injury

Steven Casha

Introduction

The pathophysiology of spinal cord injury (SCI) has generated significant research interest and many attempts to limit injury (neuroprotection), improve regeneration, or to augment the function of surviving tissue (neuroaugmentation) have met with success in animal models. Several neuroprotective agents and one neuroaugmenting compound have progressed to clinical trials. Unfortunately, none have provided convincing efficacy and no standards of care have emerged. The American Association of Neurological Surgeons and Congress of Neurological Surgeons Joint Section on Disorders of the Spine and Peripheral Nerves' 2002 *Guidelines for the Management of Acute Cervical Spine and Spinal Cord Injury*[1] specifically recognized methylprednisolone and GM-1 ganglioside as options for treatment in the acute spinal cord injured patient. However, these were qualified 'without demonstrated clinical benefit' in the case of GM-1 ganglioside and with 'evidence suggesting harmful side effects is more consistent than any suggestion of clinical benefit' in the case of methylprednisolone. Tirilazad and naloxone had been studied, but without any evidence of efficacy to warrant inclusion in the guidelines.

Several possible reasons exist for the failure to translate promising animal strategies to human therapies. These include a lack of pharmacologic agents to address therapeutic mechanisms that have been successful in animals using other means (e.g. the use of RNA knockdown techniques); heterogeneity and increased variability in human SCI compared to standardized models, which makes detecting an effect more difficult, particularly when any one compound is unlikely to have a large effect given the spectrum of targetable mechanisms; animal models which do not duplicate human pathophysiology and which thus may emphasize mechanisms less prominent in humans, e.g. the lack of spinal cavitation in commonly used mouse models;[2] insensitivity of human outcome measures in some patients diluting any detectable effect, e.g. improvement in a few thoracic segments will not be reflected in lower extremity motor changes; and an inability to identify and achieve the appropriate therapeutic window which almost certainly differs between humans and animal models and for which there is generally a lack of means to correlate between species.

This chapter will attempt to summarize a wealth of animal literature aiming to identify the prominent mechanisms and approaches identified in these preclinical studies and will review the human randomized control trials in SCI to date.

Epidemiology of spinal cord injury

The annual incidence of SCI is estimated to be between 11.5 and 53.4 per million population,[3–10] and prevalence is estimated at around 700 spinal cord injured persons per million in the United States.[11] These injures are characterized by high mortality and morbidity. In those surviving to arrive at an acute care institution, mortality rates range between 4.4 and 16.7%.[5,7,10] These survivors typically experience prolonged hospitalization in acute care hospitals and rehabilitation centers.[10,12] Furthermore, the financial burden of managing these injuries both to the individual and to society is enormous. The estimated cost to the United States for care of all spinal cord injured patients in 1990 was 4 billion dollars.[10]

Patients are typically young (mean and median ages ranging in the late 20s and early 30s) and male (80–85%).[10] Approximately 45% of patients experience a complete neurologic injury with no detectable neurologic function below the level of the lesion;[13] 55% of patients are injured between C1 and C7–T1.[10] The mechanism of injury involves a traffic accident in about 50% of cases, with recreational injuries, falls, work injuries, and violence being other common causes.[10]

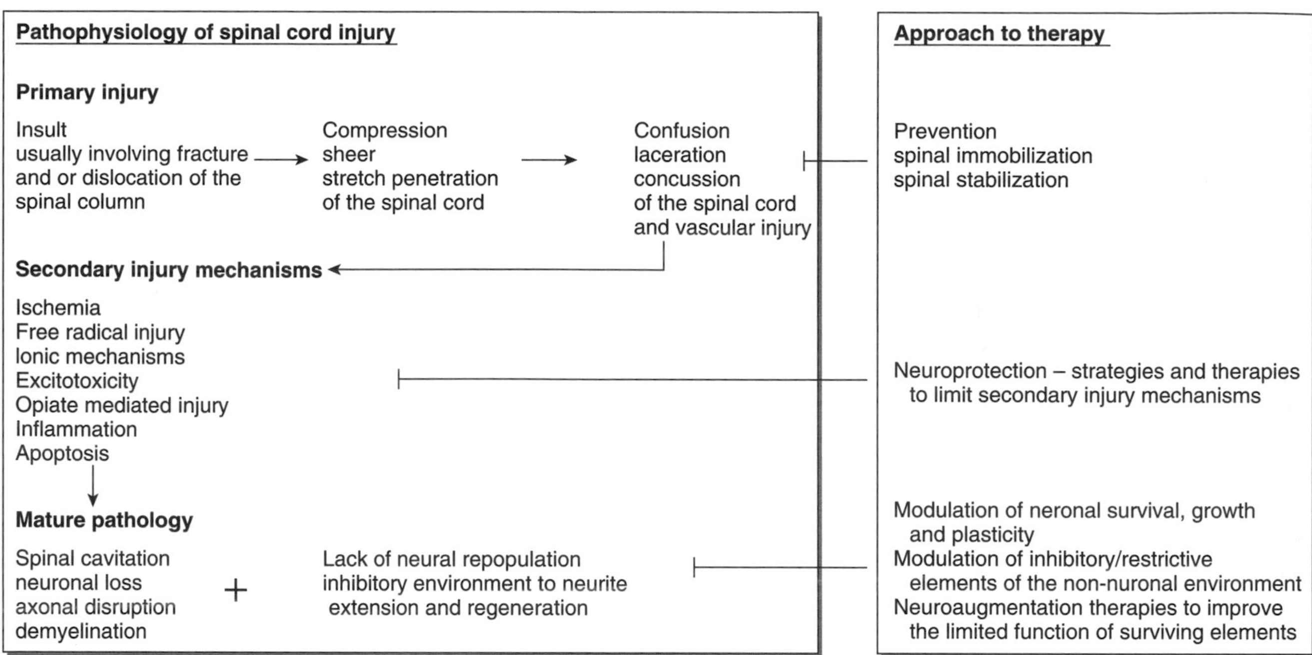

Figure 62.1
The pathophysiology of spinal cord injury

Hospital admissions of a week or longer are necessary in approximately 10% of patients with SCI every year due to complications including pressure sores, autonomic dysreflexia, pneumonia, atelectasis, deep venous thrombosis, and renal calculi.[14–16] Spasticity and pain also add significantly to neurologic disability in 25%.[14] Long-term reduced life expectancy is largely accounted for by pneumonia, pulmonary emboli, and septicemia.

Pathophysiology of spinal cord injury

The pathophysiology of SCI is commonly described in two phases: the primary and secondary injury (Figure 62.1). The primary injury refers to the mechanical perturbation of the spinal cord. This involves any combination of compression, sheer, stretch, and penetration mechanisms leading to varying degrees of contusion, laceration, and concussion. Most commonly this involves an injury of the vertebral column and results from some combination of fracture and dislocation. The secondary injury refers to a complex array of biochemical events which further the cell damage and cell death caused by the primary insult. Additionally, systemic factors promoting these secondary mechanisms, including hypotension and hypoxia, are often referred to as systemic secondary injury mechanisms.

Secondary injury mechanisms and neuroprotection

A major focus of research efforts intended to improve neurologic outcome after SCI involves secondary injury mechanisms. Amelioration of secondary injury is intended to decrease the damage caused by this phase of injury, thus preserving neural elements of the spinal cord and thus preserving neurologic function. Animal research has succeeded in elucidating a complex array of secondary injury mechanisms and has provided repeated evidence that inhibition of these processes results in improved neurologic outcome in animals.[17–34] Prominent mechanisms that have been investigated are discussed below.

Ischemia

A rapid decrease in local blood flow occurs after SCI and is sustained for about 24 hours in animals.[35] Gray matter is more vulnerable to this insult, perhaps in part due to its increased metabolic vulnerability, as evidenced by its normal increased blood flow compared to white matter, and also in part due to vascular changes which are more pronounced centrally.[36–39] Several factors contribute to vascular alterations after SCI, including vasospasm due to mechanical vascular injury, endothelial injury, and vasoactive amines; thrombosis; edema due to increased vascular permeability and cytotoxic mechanisms; impaired vascular autoregulation; impaired venous drainage; and systemic hypotension.[40–43]

While this secondary injury mechanism has not, and likely never will be the subject of high-quality randomized control studies, several studies have reported experience with blood pressure augmentation with the aim of augmenting spinal cord perfusion after injury. Vale et al treated 77 SCI patients with volume expansion and vasopressor therapy.[44] The neurologic outcome seen in these patients was notably improved over that expected from previously published outcome studies. Zach et al aggressively treated SCI with volume expansion for blood pressure maintenance.[45] They observed a correlation between earlier admission time and neurologic outcome, and concluded that early institution of medical management including blood pressure maintenance improves outcome after SCI. Tator et al compared aggressive hemodynamic and respiratory management in an intensive care setting to historical controls.[46] They observed reduced morbidity, mortality, and length of stay in those patients treated in the dedicated ICU. Similarly, Wolf et al observed improved outcome in a group of patients with SCI secondary to bilateral facet dislocation treated with an intensive protocol including maintenance of mean arterial pressure greater than 85 mmHg.[47]

In animal models of SCI the effects of hypertension and hypotension have not been consistent. Hukuda et al used hypertension and hypercarbia in an attempt to improve spinal perfusion after SCI.[48] They found a nonsignificant improvement in neurologic outcome with this approach. Dolan and Tator applied hypertension after a severe SCI in rat and showed no improvement in outcome.[49] This study, however, used an injury severity well beyond that usually studied in their model, which may have decreased sensitivity. Using a similar model with mild or moderate injury, Guha et al found that hypertension does not improve outcome and may actually exacerbate edema and hemorrhage.[50,51] Haghighi et al reported nimodepine to worsen outcome in experimental SCI, which he attributed to induced hypotension.[52]

Free radical mediated injury

Following neural trauma, several conditions promote formation of free radicals. Increased cytosolic calcium induces several free radical producing pathways, including xanthane oxidase, nitrous oxide synthetase, and the phospholipase A2–cyclooxygenase pathway.[53] Free radicals (superoxide) are also produced through the Fe^{2+}-dependent Fenton and Haber–Weiss reactions.[53] Alterations in the inner mitochondrial membrane proteins (removal, release, or inactivation) may reduce the efficiency of the electron transport chain leading to increased production of superoxide radical.[53,54] Activated inflammatory cells yield reactive oxygen species.[53] The resultant increased production of free radicals overwhelms the cell's free radical scavenging systems (e.g. superoxide dysmutases – catalases, glutathione, ascorbic acid) leading to oxidation of lipids, proteins, and nucleic acids. This in turn may lead to cell death.[55]

Several animal studies provide good evidence for the involvement of free radicals and peroxidation reactions in the pathophysiology of SCI. Studies have demonstrated increases in specific free radicals;[56–59] evidence of increased macromolecular oxidation afterwards;[57,60–62] and evidence that free radical scavenging compounds, decreased free radical production, and increased free radical scavenging are neuroprotective.[57,63–67]

Ionic mechanisms

Disruptions of homeostasis of two cations, Na^+ and Ca^{++}, appear pivotal in the pathophysiology of SCI.

A variety of Na^+ channels contribute to the maintenance of the neuronal electrochemical gradient under normal physiologic conditions and perturbations in this gradient which are responsible for signaling and the action potential. Following SCI several factors, most prominently ischemia, lead to energy depletion and decreased intracellualar ATP. This leads to a breakdown of the normal membrane electrochemical gradients and membrane depolarization. This then triggers the opening of voltagegated Na^+ channels, further exacerbating the dissipation of that gradient. Increased intracellular Na^+ has several consequences, including cell swelling and cytotoxic edema, activation of phospholipases, intracellular acidification via the Na^+/H^+ exchanger, increased intracellular Ca^{++} via reversal of a Na^+/Ca^{++} exchanger, and reverse operation of Na^+-dependent glutamate transporters exacerbating rises in extracellular glutamate and excitotoxicity. A variety of Na^+ channel blockers have been found neuroprotective in a variety of models. *In vitro* ion exchange studies have also provided neuroprotective evidence.

Many intracellular processes are calcium-dependent and, under normal physiologic conditions, intracellular calcium is tightly regulated, allowing it frequent use in cell signaling. Dramatic rises in intracellular Ca^{++} occur after SCI and may trigger a variety of intracellular pathways including proteases, nucleases, NO synthases, and phospholipases, leading to a complex cascade to cell death.[68] Evidence of the importance of Ca^{++} in SCI comes from studies demonstrating rises in intracellular Ca^{++} and studies inhibiting Ca^{++}-dependent proteases. Ca^{++} channel antagonists themselves, after SCI, have not provided clear evidence of neuroprotection.[69–73]

Excitotoxicity

It has been well established that glutamate, the predominant excitatory amino acid in the CNS, achieves elevated extracellular concentrations following SCI.[74] Furthermore, it is known that the concentrations achieved are toxic to neurons and oligodendrocytes and it is believed that the elevations in extracellular glutamate contribute to post-traumatic cell death, a process termed excitotoxicity.[75,76] This is mediated through both ionotropic and metabotropic glutamate receptors which are present on both neurons and glia.[77–79] In animal models, agents that block glutamate receptors improve functional outcomes and reduce damage to traumatized spinal cord tissue.[80–83] Several obstacles exist in translating these findings to human trials; given the ubiquity of glutamate in the CNS it is not surprising that application of these inhibitory agents results in significant undesirable side-effects which limit their application in humans.[84–86] Secondly, the rise in extracellular glutamate occurs rapidly after SCI and application of inhibitors in the hospital setting may be too late to have significant benefit. In fact, one randomized trial has been successfully completed (discussed below).

Opiate-mediated injury

Following SCI some endogenous opioids accumulate at the injury site.[87] Exogenously administered opioids exacerbate the pathology of SCI, while inhibition is neuroprotective.[88–92] The mechanism of action of opioid-mediated injury is complex and involves both opioid receptor dependent and independent mechanisms.[88,93] These effects include diminished blood flow, release of excitotoxic amino acids, phospholipid hydrolysis, and modulation of intracellular Mg^{++}.[90,94] Naloxone, an opioid antagonist, and thyrotropin-releasing hormone (TRH) have shown neuroprotective effects in animal models of SCI,[92,95–100] and have been investigated in humans as well (see below).

Inflammation

The pathophysiology of SCI includes a prominent inflammatory component. This process is similar to that seen in other tissues following injury (for review see reference 101). Key events include microglial activation, plasma protein extravasation and edema, and the sequential recruitment of neutrophils, monocytes, and lymphocytes.[101] The process is initiated by the local tissue and vascular disruption,[43,102] and includes a complex interplay between the local spinal cellular compliment, components of the clotting system, and the blood-borne inflammatory system.[101] This complex interplay is evident in the effect of some inflammatory cytokines on local cells. For example interkleukin 1-β (Il-1) stimulates proliferation and hypertrophy of astrocytes and is almost certainly involved in the development of the glial scar;[103] Il-1 and TNFα increase endothelial adhesion molecule and chemotactic factor expression, facilitating further leukocyte recruitment.[104–106] Immune cells also release factors capable of killing neurons and glia (e.g. myeloperoxidase, elastase, proteases, reactive oxygen intermediates, NO, quinolinic acid, cytokines), directly acting to further the injury.[101,107] While many studies in animals have attempted to decrease the immune response and have shown this to be neuroprotective,[101] it has become increasingly evident that different components of inflammation may also have beneficial effects at varying times following injury. For example, neuronal degeneration is enhanced following brain injury and SCI in TNF receptor (TNFR)-deficient mice, presumably due to the absence of signaling from microglial-derived TNF.[108,109] These mice also demonstrate impaired functional recovery after SCI.[110] The challenge remains to define more specific therapies to target the detrimental effects of inflammation at the appropriate time following injury while not effecting or perhaps even enhancing those processes which appear beneficial.

Apoptosis

Apoptosis has relatively recently been recognized among secondary injury mechanisms. In those studies that demonstrated apoptosis in the spinal cord after SCI,[111–119] early apoptosis, which included neurons, was followed by a delayed wave of predominantly oligodendroglial programmed cell death in degenerating white matter tracts.[113,116,117,119,120] These observations point to a longer therapeutic window for anti-apoptiotic strategies in SCI than that of therapies aimed at other secondary mechanisms.[111] Apoptosis in white matter after dorsal cordotomy or after transection suggests that glial apoptosis occurs, at least in part, as a consequence of axonal degeneration.[121,122] Likely, the loss of trophic support derived by the oligodendrocyte from the axon results in activation of programmed cell death.[123–125] However, the presence of activated microglia in contact with apoptotic oligodendrocytes after SCI suggests that this interaction may also activate cell death programs in the oligodendrocyte.[120] Secondary axonal degeneration may then follow, as is seen in models of multiple sclerosis[126] and in myelin associated glycoprotein deficiency.[127] Apoptotic cell death has also been implicated in the pathophysiology of human SCI by an autopsy study which demonstrated in-situ terminal-deoxytransferase mediated dUTP nick-end labelling (TUNEL) and caspase 3 immunohistochemistry.[119]

Inhibition of FAS-mediated apoptosis using FAS-deficient mice resulted in decreased post-traumatic apoptosis in the spinal cord as well as histologic and behavioral evidence of neuroprotection.[128] Similarly, antibody neutralization of FASL resulted in decreased apoptosis and improved locomotor function after SCI.[129]

Characterization of apoptosis has gradually revealed an enormous complex array of interrelated programmed cell death cascades. It is unlikely that a single pathway leading to apoptosis predominates in any pathologic process including SCI. Mechanisms deserving exploration include both pro-apoptotic processes, which should be inhibited, and anti-apoptotic process, which perhaps may be enhanced. It is also important to recognize that cell death may have a useful role in restricting certain processes, particularly early inflammation, thus limiting the application of strategies which broadly inhibit cell death. More focused, cell-specific inhibition may be more effective.

Neural regeneration after spinal cord injury

It has long been recognized that a fundamental difference exists between the relatively robust regenerative capacity of the peripheral nervous system and the growth-limiting environment of the central nervous system (CNS). This has led to attempts to identify and to overcome the obstacles inherent in the CNS in the hopes of re-establishing lost tissue and connections so as to restore neurologic function. These approaches have focused on identifying the properties of CNS neurons that limit their potential for extending axons centrally, as well as attempts to identify cellular and extracellular factors in the supporting glial environment that inhibit axonal regeneration. The prominent approaches are listed and discussed below.

Neurotrophic factors

Neurotrophic factors are proteins that are known to modulate neuronal survival, growth, and plasticity behaviors.[130] Some of these, when added exogenously, can promote desirable neural phenotypes after SCI. For example, brain-derived neurotrophic factor (BDNF) maintains neurons in the red nucleus, which would otherwise undergo atrophy and death, and promotes axonal regeneration.[131,132] This response is dependent on the expression of the trkB receptor, which is lost in axons after several weeks but maintained at the neuronal soma chronically.[133] Several growth factors have shown such promising effects, however it has been recognized that these molecles may have deleterious effects as well.[134] For example, homodimeric p75 receptor (i.e. absence of trk receptors) results in NGF toxicity and BDNF can induce NOS-mediated cell death.[134]

cAMP is a key second messenger for some growth factor/receptor interactions, most notably BDNF.[135] It has the potential itself for increasing the growth potential and axonal regenerative capacity of neurons.[136,137] It has been applied in combination with other strategies, which provide a more permissive extracellular environment for axonal extension, as well as alone.[138–140] These studies confirm that cAMP improves axonal extension even in the unusually suppressive CNS environment. cAMP may act through inactivation of Rho (ras homology protein) which results in disinhibition of Rho-mediated axonal growth arrest.[134–141]

The glial scar

The pathophysiology of SCI eventually leads to a glial scar which is viewed by most as a barrier to regeneration and recovery. Its cellular component is composed predominantly of reactive astrocytes with the surrounding matrix rich in proteoglycans.[142] This structure is thought to provide a physical barrier to axonal extension and, in addition, contains proteins such as chondroitin sulphate proteoglycans which inhibit axonal growth.[142] Chondroitinase ABC, which removes glycosaminoglycan side-chains from these molecules, promotes axonal extension and functional recovery after SCI.[143] In addition to being a potentially useful primary treatment in SCI, the strategy of limiting the glial scar and in reducing its inhibitory effects may be key in strategies involving cell transplant (below). In those strategies, axons that traverse a cell transplant may be inhibited from re-entering the CNS distally in part by glial scar.[144] Other proteins in the glial scar are also inhibitory to neurite growth and are expressed largely by the cellular component of the scar; these include SEMA3, ephrin-B2, and Slit proteins.[142]

Recent evidence may indicate that the glial scar also provides some important beneficial functions after injury. Targeted depletion of reactive astrocytes that undergo mitosis indicated that, after injury, this component of the glial scar serves to repair the blood–brain barrier (BBB), prevent an overwhelming inflammatory response, and limit cellular degeneration.[145,146] The role of the glial scar may be to seclude the injury site from healthy tissue, preventing the spread of tissue damage.[146]

Myelin-associated inhibitory proteins

It has long been recognized that CNS myelin is a very non-permissive substrate for neurite extension.[147] Attempts to identify the molecular components responsible for that inhibition have identified three proteins of key interest: Nogo,[148] MAG,[149] and oligodendrocyte-myelin glycoprotein.[150] All three of these bind the Nogo-66-receptor (NgR1).[134] MAG also binds NgR2. These ligands and their shared receptors therefore provide targets which may disinhibit neurite extension in a myelin envoirnment. Inhibition of Nogo using a portion of its receptor or neutralizing antiserum has shown evidence of improved axonal extension and improved functional recovery.[151,152] However, NgR1 null mice failed to show improved corticospinal regeneration following SCI, suggesting other inhibitory pathways may still exist.[134]

Cell transplant strategies

Much attention has been paid to the use of cell transplant approaches in the management of SCI. These strategies provide several potentially useful mechanistic interventions. The prominent candidate cells include stem cells, bone marrow stromal cells, fetal cells, Schwann cells, and olfactory ensheathing glia. Transplants may provide a means of diminishing the cystic cavitation seen in human SCI and through which axonal extension cannot proceed.[133] They may allow the creation of a permissive environment for axonal extension (e.g. Schwann cells and olfactory ensheathing glia), although to be successful regenerative strategies require extension into distal spinal tissue and exit from such a transplanted environment.[153] They may elaborate growth factors that can influence local neurons and axonal elements (e.g. by *ex vivo* genetic modification).[154] They may have the potential of differentiating into neurons or glia, providing the cellular elements for true regeneration (e.g. stem cells).[133] Many of these therapies are intended to be cultured, perhaps modified, and introduced into the spinal cord. Schwann cells, however, may also be transplanted as peripheral nerve grafts.[155] Animal data have provided evidence for improved axonal extension using these strategies and several of these strategies have now entered early human studies, including some reports of peripheral nerve grafts and transplantation of olfactory ensheathing glia.[133]

Human randomized control trials in spinal cord injury

This section will review those therapies that have come to randomized control trials of efficacy in human SCI. Other therapies such as cell transplant strategies that are at the phase 1 stage of human investigation (safety) are mentioned in the above discussion but will not be reviewed in detail here as most of these are ongoing unpublished trials. There have been a total of nine randomized control trials completed in this field (Table 62.1). They all address neuroprotective strategies.

Methylprednisolone and other corticosteroids

Steroids in various forms have been used in the treatment of SCI for many years; however, their role became more rigorously considered following publication of the NASCIS II study. Initial enthusiasm for an apparent positive effect of methylprednisolone in SCI has not stood up to the extensive scrutiny that ensued.[156–159] In spite of significant criticism this medication continues to be used by many, and a 2002 study suggests that most practitioners prescribe it because of peer pressure or due to fear of litigation rather than a firm belief that it is indeed efficacious.[160]

The first NASCIS study compared low- and high-dose methylprednisolone and did not include a placebo group.[161] It failed to demonstrate a difference between the doses tested. It was followed by a randomized control trial comparing a 24-hour protocol to placebo in NASCIS II.[162,163] The dose selected in NASCIS II was higher that that of the original study due to further animal work that suggested a therapeutic threshold of 30 mg/kg.[163] NASCIS II concluded that improved neurologic recovery was seen when the methylprednisolone treatment protocol was initiated within 8 hours of injury. That study was then followed by NASCIS III, which compared patients randomized to the 24-hour NASCIS II protocol to those randomized to a 48-hour protocol.[164,165] That study concluded that patients initiating therapy within 3 hours do not gain any benefit from extending treatment to 48 hours, while those initiating between 3 and 8 hours do benefit further. No benefit had been shown if initiating beyond 8 hours in NASCIS II.

Both the NASCIS II and NASCIS III trials were well designed and executed. However, closer scrutiny reveals that the primary analyses of methylprednisolone treatment effect were negative in both studies. The stated conclusions were based on post-hoc analyses which suggested a minor treatment effect on motor scores at 1 year and when therapy was initiated in the 8- and 3–8 hour-windows identified in NASCIS II and III respectively. Statistical probability was slightly greater than 0.05 for one-year motor scores in the NASCIS III 48-hour steroid group. None of the sensory scores were different between treatment groups in either study. Several concerns have arisen regarding the post-hoc analyses of NASCIS II and III. The left-sided motor scores were not published but reported 'similar' to right-sided scores. Thus half the available data were excluded. The statistical analyses failed to correct for multiple statistical comparisons and it is unclear whether the repeated measures design was considered. Over 65 methylpredisolone related t-tests were performed in NASCIS II and over 100 t-tests in NASCIS III. There was therefore a high likelihood of type I error (erroneously detecting a statistical difference that does not exist) through random chance. The rationale for an 8-hour subanalysis (NASCIC II) is unclear. It has been claimed that this subgroup was selected based on median time-to-treatment. However, by definition, 50% of patients should have initiated treatment before the median time of treatment initiation. In fact only 38% of patients (183 of 487) were included in this post-hoc analysis. The justification for the 3- and 8-hour windows in NASCIS III is similarly obscure. Finally, the outcomes lacked an assessment of function recovery meaningful to the patient's expected activities.

Table 62.1 *Human clinical trials in spinal cord injury*

Author	Year	Design	Agent	Reported result
Methylprednisolone and other corticosteroids:				
Bracken et al[161] (NASCIS I)	1984	Prospective, randomized, double-blind	Methylprednisolone	Negative
Bracken et al[162,163] (NASCIS II)	1990 1992	Prospective, randomized, double-blind	Methylprednisolone	Positive
Bracken et al[164,165] (NASCIS III)	1997 1998	Prospective, randomized, double-blind	Methylprednisolone	Positive
Otani et al[166]	1994	Prospective, randomized, no blinding	Methylprednisolone	Positive
Pointillart et al[168]	2000	Prospective, randomized, blinded	Methylprednisolone	Negative
Kiwerski[167]	1993	Retrospective, concurrent case control	Dexamethasone	Positive
Gangliosides:				
Geisler et al[176]	1991	Prospective, randomized, double-blind	GM-1 Ganglioside	Positive
Geisler et al[177]	2001	Prospective, randomized, double-blind	GM-1 Ganglioside	Negative
Opiod antagonists:				
Bracken et al[162,163] (NASCIS II)	1990 1992	Prospective, randomized, double-blind	Naloxone	Negative
Flamm et al[190]	1985	Prospective feasibility/safety study	Naloxone	N/A
Pitts et al[191]	1995	Prospective, randomized, double-blind	Thyrotropin-releasing hormone	Positive
Excitatory amino acid antagonists:				
Tadie et al[198]	1999	Prospective, randomized, double-blind	Gacyclidine	Negative
Calcium channel blockers:				
Pointillart et al[168]	2000	Prospective, randomized, blinded	Nimodipine	Negative
Antioxidants and free radical scavengeres				
Bracken et al[164,165] (NASCIS III)	1997 1998	Prospective, randomized, double-blind	Tirilazad	Positive

In addition to the NASCIS studies, Otani et al published a prospective randomized trial investigating the NASCIS II methylprednisolone dosing protocol.[166] The investigators were not blinded to treatment and the control group was allowed to receive alternate steroids at the physicians' discretion. Of 158 patients entered, 117 were analyzed. The primary outcome measures (American Spinal Injury Association (ASIA) motor and sensory scores) were not different between treatment groups. Post hoc analyses suggested that more patients improved on the NASCIS II steroid regimen compared to controls. However, in order for a greater number of steroid-treated patients to improve, the fewer control patients who also improved must have demonstrated a larger magnitude of recovery (since overall ASIA motor and sensory scores were no different between groups). Thus such post-hoc analyses become difficult to interpret in the face of a negative overall effect.

A retrospective study with concurrent case controls also suggested a benefit with corticosteroid administration.[167] This study investigated the use of dexamethasone initiated within 24 hours of injury, with the specific dose left to the discretion of the attending physicians. Length of follow-up was not specified and a new but unvalidated neurologic grading system was used for outcome assessment. This study reported that the percentage of patients improved was significantly higher in the methylprednisolone-treated group. However, there was a much higher mortality rate within the control group, suggesting a selection bias to more severely injured patients in the control arm. The magnitude of the mortality rate is also a concern and suggests that the study population may not be representative and that the results are not generalizable.

A randomized control trial designed to examine the potential therapeutic benefit of nimodipine (a calcium channel antagonist, discussed below) included a NASCIS II methylprednisolone regimen as well as a placebo group.[168] This study, which included approximately 25 patients in each group, failed to show any difference between any of four groups (placebo, nimodipine, methylprednisolone, and methylprednisolone and nimodipine) using ASIA scores and ASIA grade outcomes. However, this study was remarkable for an increase in infectious complications in the methylprednisolone group.

In summary, while well designed and executed studies have been performed they have failed to demonstrate convincingly a beneficial effect of methylprednisolone or other corticosteroids in the management of SCI. Post-hoc analyses have been used to argue a small effect on motor function in three randomized trials. However, all of these analyses contain significant flaws, rendering conclusions of efficacy dubious. These observations have led two national organizations to publish guidelines recommending methylprednisolone administration as a treatment option rather than as a standard of care or recommended treatment.[1,169] It must also be recognized that corticosteroid administration comes with increased risk of several adverse events, including pneumonia, sepsis, and steroid-induced myopathy, all of which may negatively impact outcome in SCI patients, potentially overshadowing any unproven beneficial effect.[170] In addition, the CRASH trial investigating the use of a corticosteroid regimen similar to that used in NASCIS II in the setting of closed head injury[171] demonstrated increased mortality with steroid use in that population. One must certainly recognize the possibility of an elevated mortality risk in SCI patients as well.

Gangliosides

Gangliosides are sialic acid-containing glycophosphingolipids which are found in high concentration in the outer cell membranes of central nervous system cells, especially in the vicinity of synapses. Although their exact function is unknown, they appear to play a role in neural development and plasticity. The proposed mechanisms of action of exogenously administered gangliosides include anti-excitotoxic activities, prevention of apoptosis, augmentation of neurite outgrowth, and induction of neuronal sprouting and regeneration.[172–175]

GM-1 ganglioside has been the subject of two human studies. The first study was a randomized placebo-controlled trial of 37 patients.[176] Patients were administered 100 mg of intravenous GM-1 ganglioside or placebo daily for 18 to 32 days, starting within 72 hours of injury. In addition, all patients received methylprednisolone for 72 hours. A significant difference was seen between groups using change in Frankel grades and mean ASIA motor score from baseline at one year. Furthermore, the increased recovery in the GM-1-treated group was attributed to recovery of useful strength in initially paralyzed muscle groups, rather than to strengthening of paretic muscles. There were no reported adverse events attributed to the study drug.

Based on the encouraging results of the first trial a larger prospective, multicenter, double-blind, randomized trial of GM-1 ganglioside in SCI patients was initiated.[177] Seven hundred and ninety-seven patients were enrolled; all received NASCIS II protocol methylprednisolone and were randomized to placebo, low-dose GM-1 (300 mg loading dose then 100 mg/day for 56 days), or high-dose GM-1 (600 mg loading dose then 200 mg/day for 56 days), starting at completion of the 23-hour methylprednisolone infusion. The primary outcome assessed was the proportion of patients, who improved two or more grades from baseline using the modified Benzel score at 26 weeks. Secondary outcomes included timing of recovery, ASIA motor and sensory evaluations, relative and absolute sensory levels of impairment, and assessments of bladder and bowel function. The high-dose regimen was discontinued after 180 patients where enrolled, when an interim assessment revealed a trend toward increased mortality. At the end of the study, in 760 patients the authors found no significant difference in mortality between the groups and no significant difference in the primary outcome. However, the authors also reported that there was a large, consistent, and, at some points, significant effect in the primary outcome in the subgroup of nonoperated patients. The ASIA motor, light touch, and pinprick scores showed a consistent trend in favor of GM-1, as did bladder function, bowel function, sacral sensation, and anal contraction.

In summary, these studies provide suggestive but not conclusive evidence of a positive effect on neurologic recovery after SCI with administration of GM-1 ganglioside.

Opiate antagonists

Vasospasm, post-traumatic ischemia, and infarction are known contributors to the pathophysiology of SCI.[43] In addition, human SCI may occur in the setting of polytrauma and spinal shock syndromes, which contribute to the ischemic pathophysiology. Opiate receptor antagonists and physiologic opiate antagonists improve blood pressure and survival following traumatic shock.[178] In addition, endogenous opioid peptides are released in the spinal cord after SCI.[179,180] Dynorphin decreases microcirculatory blood flow in the spinal cord and may contribute directly to neurotoxicity, possibly through the NMDA receptor.[181–183] Opiate antagonists may thus be useful in maintaining circulation and in preventing some neurotoxicity. Of these nalmefene, naloxone, and TRH are neuroprotective in animal models.[20,21,92,95,97,99,179,184–188] The latter two have been studied in humans.

Naloxone was one of the treatment arms in NASCIS II[163] and was therefore compared to methylprednisolone and placebo treatment. Comparison of naloxone (5.4 mg/kg bolus followed by a 23-hour, 4.0 mg/kg/hour infusion) and placebo failed to demonstrate a therapeutic benefit.[162,163] Post hoc analysis suggested an effect on long tract recovery when naloxone was started within 8 hours of injury, which may warrant further study.[189]

In a dose escalation phase 1 study of naloxone in SCI, 20 patients received 0.14 to 1.43 mg/kg loading followed by 20% of loading 47-hour infusion (low dose), and 9 patients received 2.7 to 5.4 mg/kg loading dose followed by 75% of loading 23-hour infusion (high dose).[190] More patients in the low-dose group had complete injuries (85% vs 44%) and initiated their treatment later (average 12.9 vs 6.6 hours). No improvement in neurologic exam or SSEPs was seen with the low-dose regimen, but in the high-dose group a small number of patients demonstrated sustained improvement of both. The observed improvements were encouraging but this study was not designed to examine efficacy. The authors were able to show that the high doses of naloxone needed to be consistent with animal data in SCI were tolerated clinically with minimal side-effects.

In one human study of TRH, 20 SCI patients were administered a 0.2 mg/kg bolus followed by 0.2 mg/kg/hour 6 hour infusion or placebo within 12 hours of injury.[191] No discernible treatment effect was found in 6 patients with complete injuries, while in 11 incompletely injured patients TRH treatment was associated with significantly higher motor and sensory recovery, and Sunnybrook Cord Injury Scale scores at 4 months. While this is a small study and should be interpreted cautiously it was nonetheless positive. Unfortunately, it has not as yet been replicated.[170]

In summary, to date three human studies have provided positive evidence which likely deserves further study. Definitive efficacy studies remain lacking, although one small randomized trial was positive.

Excitatory amino acid receptor antagonists

Receptor-mediated excitotoxicity of neurons and glia is a well-recognized secondary injury mechanism following neural injury.[17,28,75,192–195] Inhibition of excitotoxicity in animal models of SCI results in improved behavioral and histologic outcomes.[194,196,197] However, the rise in excitatory amino acids after SCI occurs early and is transient (likely complete within 2 hours), suggesting that the therapeutic window is small.[192]

To date, one human SCI study has been performed using the NMDA (*N*-methyl-D-aspartate) ionotropic glutamate receptor antagonist gacyclidine.[198] Two hundred and seventy-two patients were randomized in four groups (0.005 mg/kg, 0.01 mg/kg, or 0.02 mg/kg gacyclidine, or placebo). The doses selected were similar to those used in a safety and efficacy trial in traumatic brain-injured patients.[199] Gacyclidine was administered twice, first within 2 hours of injury followed by another administration 4 hours later. While the 1-month data showed a nonsignificant trend to better outcome in the high-dose group, there was no significant difference in ASIA or FIM scores at one year.[170,198]

Thus, strong animal data suggest that inhibition of post-traumatic excitotoxicity is likely to be efficacious in the treatment of SCI, however the therapeutic window may be very short. A single human study to date did not show efficacy.

Calcium channel blockers

Dysregulation of calcium homeostasis and cyoplasmic calcium-mediated events are common to many pathways leading to cell death.[68] Calcium channel blockers may ameliorate calcium fluxes, decreasing cell death. They may also affect vascular smooth muscle and decrease vasospasm. In animal SCI models, calcium channel blockade is neuroprotective[18,200–202] and increases post-traumatic spinal blood flow.[203,204] In a single human SCI randomized placebo-controlled trial of the calcium channel blocker nimodepine, 106 SCI patients were administered methylprednisolone (NASCIS II protocol), nimodipine (0.015 mg/kg/hour for 2 hours followed by 0.03 mg/kg/hour for 7 days), both agents, or placebo.[168,205] No difference in blinded neurologic recovery (ASIA score and grade) was found among these groups at 1 year.

Thus, cellular calcium fluxes are thought to be key regulators of cell death after neural trauma and calcium channel inhibition in animal studies has proven neuroprotective. However, to date a single study failed to reproduce this in humans.

Antioxidants and free radical scavengers

Following neural trauma, free radical mediated macromolecule peroxidation may lead to cell death.[55] Several conditions following SCI promote increased formation of free radicals and there is ample animal evidence that this is a significant targetable secondary injury event after SCI.[53,54,57,63–67]

Tirilizad mesylate is thought to act through inhibition of iron-dependent lipid peroxidation. The NASCIS III study included a 166 patient tirilazad group (2.5 mg/kg bolus infusion every 6 hours for 48 hours administered after their 30 mg/kg methylprednisolone bolus).[206] This study showed no difference in motor recovery compared to 24-hour methylprednisolone treatment.[164,165] Given the lack of convincing evidence regarding the role of methylprednisolone (as discussed above), this study does not provide evidence that tirilizad is effective in human SCI. In addition, while the predominant mechanism of action of methylprednisone is unclear, it is thought to include inhibition of peroxidation reactions (methylprednisolone is discussed in detail above).

In summary, the human data on methylprednisolone and tirilizad mesylate, which are believed to decrease peroxidation, do not support their use in the treatment of SCI.

Conclusions

A wealth of interest in the pathophysiology of SCI has identified many potential therapeutic targets in animal models. Of these, several have come to high-quality human investigations. Unfortunately, none have been proven effective in humans. Several challenges exist when translating successful strategies from animal models to human studies. However, several groups have now demonstrated an ability to coordinate and execute large trials which are well designed.

There are currently several ongoing human trials which will add to an already interesting, although largely disappointing, human literature in SCI, which to date has not established any clearly effective therapeutic options. These trials include investigations of minocycline (a tetracycline derivative which may affect several secondary injury mechanisms including apoptotic cell death and inflammation), cethrin[207] (a Rho antagonist which is believed to promote axonal regeneration), anti-Nogo-A antiserum,[170] and autologous activated macrophages[208] (thought to act through elaboration of growth factors and modulation of the inflammatory response). In addition, there is significant interest in stem cell, Schwann cell, and olfactory unsheathing glia transplantation therapies, all of which are involved in ongoing human investigations.[170]

References

1. Hadley MN, Walters BC, Grabb PA et al. Guidelines for the management of acute cervical spine and spinal cord injuries – pharmacological therapy after acute cervical spinal cord injury. Neurosurgery 2002; 50: S63–72.
2. Joshi M, Fehlings MG. Development and characterization of a novel, graded model of clip compressive spinal cord injury in the mouse: Part 1. Clip design, behavioral outcomes, and histopathology. J Neurotrauma 2002; 19: 175–90.
3. Botterell EH, Jousse AT, Kraus AS et al. A model for the future care of acute spinal cord injuries. Can J Neurol Sci 1975; 2: 361–80.
4. Gjone R, Nordlie L. Incidence of traumatic paraplegia and tetraplegia in Norway: a statistical survey of the years 1974 and 1975. Paraplegia 1978; 16: 88–93.
5. Kraus JF, Franti CE, Riggins RS, Richards D, Borhani NO. Incidence of traumatic spinal cord lesions. J Chron Dis 1975; 28: 471–92.
6. Kraus JF. A comparison of recent studies on the extent of the head and spinal cord injury problem in the United States. J Neurosurg 1980; (Suppl): S35–43.
7. Kraus JF. Injury to the head and spinal cord. The epidemiological relevance of the medical literature published from 1960 to 1978. J Neurosurg 1980; (Suppl): S3–10.
8. Kurtzke JF. Epidemiology of spinal cord injury. Exp Neurol 1975; 48: 163–236.
9. Minaire P, Castanier M, Girard R et al. Epidemiology of spinal cord injury in the Rhone-Alpes Region, France, 1970–75. Paraplegia 1978; 16: 76–87.
10. Tator CH. Epidemiology and general characteristics of the spinal cord-injured patient. In: Tator CH, Benzel EC, eds. Contemporary Management of Spinal Cord Injury: From Impact to Rehabilitation. Park Ridge: The American Association of Neurological Surgeons Publications Committee, 2000: 15–19.
11. Harvey C, Rothschild BB, Asmann AJ, Stripling T. New estimates of traumatic SCI prevalence: a survey-based approach. Paraplegia 1990; 28: 537–44.
12. Tator CH, Duncan EG, Edmonds VE, Lapczak LI, Andrews DF. Complications and costs of management of acute spinal cord injury. Paraplegia 1993; 31: 700–14.
13. Tator CH, Duncan EG, Edmonds VE, Lapczak LI, Andrews DF. Changes in epidemiology of acute spinal cord injury from 1947 to 1981. Surg Neurol 1993; 40: 207–15.
14. Johnson RL, Gerhart KA, McCray J, Menconi JC, Whiteneck GG. Secondary conditions following spinal cord injury in a population-based sample. Spinal Cord 1998; 36: 45–50.
15. Krause JS. Aging after spinal cord injury: an exploratory study. Spinal Cord 2000; 38: 77–83.
16. McKinley WO, Jackson AB, Cardenas DD, DeVivo MJ. Long-term medical complications after traumatic spinal cord injury: a regional model systems analysis. Arch Phys Med Rehabil 1999; 80: 1402–10.
17. Agrawal SK, Theriault E, Fehlings MG. Role of group I metabotropic glutamate receptors in traumatic spinal cord white matter injury. J Neurotrauma 1998; 15: 929–41.
18. Agrawal SK, Nashmi R, Fehlings MG. Role of L- and N-type calcium channels in the pathophysiology of traumatic spinal cord white matter injury. Neuroscience 2000; 99: 179–88.
19. Anghelescu N, Petrescu A, Alexandrescu I. The effect of calcium channel blockers in experimental spinal cord injury. Rom J Neurol Psychiatry 1994; 32: 101–9.
20. Faden AI, Jacobs TP, Holaday JW. Opiate antagonist improves neurologic recovery after spinal injury. Science 1981; 211: 493–4.
21. Faden AI, Sacksen I, Noble LJ. Opiate-receptor antagonist nalmefene improves neurological recovery after traumatic spinal cord injury in rats through a central mechanism. J Pharmacol Exp Ther 1988; 245: 742–8.
22. Fujimoto T, Nakamura T, Ikeda T, Takagi K. Potent protective effects of melatonin on experimental spinal cord injury. Spine 2000; 25: 769–75.
23. Kaptanoglu E, Tuncel M, Palaoglu S et al. Comparison of the effects of melatonin and methylprednisolone in experimental spinal cord injury. J Neurosurg 2000; 93: 77–84.
24. Rosenberg LJ, Teng YD, Wrathall JR. Effects of the sodium channel blocker tetrodotoxin on acute white matter pathology after experimental contusive spinal cord injury. J Neurosci 1999; 19: 6122–33.
25. Schumacher PA, Siman RG, Fehlings MG. Pretreatment with calpain inhibitor CEP-4143 inhibits calpain I activation and cytoskeletal degradation, improves neurological function, and enhances axonal survival after traumatic spinal cord injury. J Neurochem 2000; 74: 1646–55.
26. Schwartz G, Fehlings MG. Evaluation of the neuroprotective effects of sodium channel blockers after spinal cord injury: improved behavioral and neuroanatomical recovery with riluzole. J Neurosurg 2001; 94: 245–56.
27. Teng YD, Wrathall JR. Local blockade of sodium channels by tetrodotoxin ameliorates tissue loss and long-term functional deficits resulting from experimental spinal cord injury. J Neurosci 1997; 17: 4359–66.
28. Agrawal SK, Fehlings MG. Role of NMDA and non-NMDA ionotropic glutamate receptors in traumatic spinal cord axonal injury. J Neurosci 1997; 17: 1055–63.
29. Agrawal SK, Fehlings MG. The effect of the sodium channel blocker QX-314 on recovery after acute spinal cord injury. J Neurotrauma 1997; 14: 81–8.
30. Arias MJ. Effect of naloxone on functional recovery after experimental spinal cord injury in the rat. Surg Neurol 1985; 23: 440–2.
31. Baskin DS, Simpson RK Jr, Browning JL et al. The effect of long-term high-dose naloxone infusion in experimental blunt spinal cord injury. J Spinal Disord 1993; 6: 38–43.
32. Benzel EC, Khare V, Fowler MR. Effects of naloxone and nalmefene in rat spinal cord injury induced by the ventral compression technique. J Spinal Disord 1992; 5: 75–7.

33. Fehlings MG, Agrawal S. Role of sodium in the pathophysiology of secondary spinal cord injury. Spine 1995; 20: 2187–91.
34. Wrathall JR, Choiniere D, Teng YD. Dose-dependent reduction of tissue loss and functional impairment after spinal cord trauma with the AMPA/kainate antagonist NBQX. J Neurosci 1994; 14: 6598–607.
35. Rivlin AS, Tator CH. Regional spinal cord blood flow in rats after severe cord trauma. J Neurosurg 1978; 49: 844–53.
36. Balentine JD. Pathology of experimental spinal cord trauma. II. Ultrastructure of axons and myelin. Lab Invest 1978; 39: 254–66.
37. Fairholm D, Turnbull I. Microangiographic study of experimental spinal injuries in dogs and rabbits. Surg Forum 1970; 21: 453–5.
38. Hayashi N, Green BA, Gonzalez-Carvajal M, Mora J, Veraa RP. Local blood flow, oxygen tension, and oxygen consumption in the rat spinal cord. Part 1: Oxygen metabolism and neuronal function. J Neurosurg 1983; 58: 516–25.
39. Wolman L. The disturbance of circulation in traumatic paraplegia in acute and late stages: a pathological study. Paraplegia 1965; 2: 213–26.
40. Hsu CY, Hogan EL, Gadsden RH Sr et al. Vascular permeability in experimental spinal cord injury. J Neurol Sci 1985; 70: 275–82.
41. Nemecek S. Morphological evidence of microcirculatory disturbances in experimental spinal cord trauma. Adv Neurol 1978; 20: 395–405.
42. Senter HJ, Venes JL. Loss of autoregulation and posttraumatic ischemia following experimental spinal cord trauma. J Neurosurg 1979; 50: 198–206.
43. Tator CH, Fehlings MG. Review of the secondary injury theory of acute spinal cord trauma with emphasis on vascular mechanisms. J Neurosurg 1991; 75: 15–26.
44. Vale FL, Burns J, Jackson AB, Hadley MN. Combined medical and surgical treatment after acute spinal cord injury: results of a prospective pilot study to assess the merits of aggressive medical resuscitation and blood pressure management. J Neurosurg 1997; 87: 239–46.
45. Zach GA, Seiler W, Dollfus P. Treatment results of spinal cord injuries in the Swiss Paraplegic Centre of Basle. Paraplegia 1976; 14: 58–65.
46. Tator CH, Rowed DW, Schwartz ML et al. Management of acute spinal cord injuries. Can J Surg 1984; 27: 289–93, 296.
47. Wolf A, Levi L, Mirvis S et al. Operative management of bilateral facet dislocation. J Neurosurg 1991; 75: 883–90.
48. Hukuda S, Mochizuki T, Ogata M. Therapeutic trial of combined hypertension and hypercarbia on experimental acute spinal cord injury. Neurosurgery 1980; 6: 644–8.
49. Dolan EJ, Tator CH. The treatment of hypotension due to acute experimental spinal cord compression injury. Surg Neurol 1980; 13: 380–4.
50. Guha A, Tator CH, Rochon J. Spinal cord blood flow and systemic blood pressure after experimental spinal cord injury in rats. Stroke 1989; 20: 372–7.
51. Guha A, Tator CH, Smith CR, Piper I. Improvement in post-traumatic spinal cord blood flow with a combination of a calcium channel blocker and a vasopressor. J Trauma 1989; 29: 1440–7.
52. Haghighi SS, Chehrazi BB, Wagner FC Jr. Effect of nimodipine-associated hypotension on recovery from acute spinal cord injury in cats. Surg Neurol 1988; 29: 293–7.
53. Lewen A, Matz P, Chan PH. Free radical pathways in CNS injury. J Neurotrauma 2000; 17: 871–90.
54. Kowaltowski AJ, Castilho RF, Vercesi AE. Ca^{2+}-induced mitochondrial membrane permeabilization: role of coenzyme Q redox state. Am J Physiol 1995; 269: C141–7.
55. Gardner AM, Xu FH, Fady C et al. Apoptotic vs. nonapoptotic cytotoxicity induced by hydrogen peroxide. Free Radic Biol Med 1997; 22: 73–83.
56. Liu D, Ling X, Wen J, Liu J. The role of reactive nitrogen species in secondary spinal cord injury: formation of nitric oxide, peroxynitrite, and nitrated protein. J Neurochem 2000; 75: 2144–54.
57. Liu D, Li L, Augustus L. Prostaglandin release by spinal cord injury mediates production of hydroxyl radical, malondialdehyde and cell death: a site of the neuroprotective action of methylprednisolone. J Neurochem 2001; 77: 1036–47.
58. Liu D, Liu J, Wen J. Elevation of hydrogen peroxide after spinal cord injury detected by using the Fenton reaction. Free Radic Biol Med 1999; 27: 478–82.
59. Liu D, Sybert TE, Qian H, Liu J. Superoxide production after spinal injury detected by microperfusion of cytochrome c. Free Radic Biol Med 1998; 25: 298–304.
60. Leski ML, Bao F, Wu L et al. Protein and DNA oxidation in spinal injury: neurofilaments – an oxidation target. Free Radic Biol Med 2001; 30: 613–24.
61. Springer JE, Azbill RD, Mark RJ et al. 4-Hydroxynonenal, a lipid peroxidation product, rapidly accumulates following traumatic spinal cord injury and inhibits glutamate uptake. J Neurochem 1997; 68: 2469–76.
62. Barut S, Canbolat A, Bilge T et al. Lipid peroxidation in experimental spinal cord injury: time–level relationship. Neurosurg Rev 1993; 16: 53–9.
63. Kaptanoglu E, Sen S, Beskonakli E et al. Antioxidant actions and early ultrastructural findings of thiopental and propofol in experimental spinal cord injury. J Neurosurg Anesthesiol 2002; 14: 114–22.
64. Farooque M, Isaksson J, Olsson Y. Improved recovery after spinal cord injury in neuronal nitric oxide synthase-deficient mice but not in TNF-alpha-deficient mice. J Neurotrauma 2001; 18: 105–14.
65. Fujimoto T, Nakamura T, Ikeda T, Taoka Y, Takagi K. Effects of EPC-K1 on lipid peroxidation in experimental spinal cord injury. Spine 2000; 25: 24–9.
66. Katoh D, Ikata T, Katoh S, Hamada Y, Fukuzawa K. Effect of dietary vitamin C on compression injury of the spinal cord in a rat mutant unable to synthesize ascorbic acid and its correlation with that of vitamin E. Spinal Cord 1996; 34: 234–8.
67. Naftchi NE. Treatment of mammalian spinal cord injury with antioxidants. Int J Dev Neurosci 1991; 9: 113–26.
68. Tymianski M, Tator CH. Normal and abnormal calcium homeostasis in neurons: a basis for the pathophysiology of traumatic and ischemic central nervous system injury. Neurosurgery 1996; 38: 1176–95.
69. Black P, Markowitz RS, Finkelstein SD, McMonagle-Strucko K, Gillespie JA. Experimental spinal cord injury: effect of a calcium channel antagonist (nicardipine). Neurosurgery 1988; 22: 61–6.
70. Danielisova V, Chavko M. Comparative effects of the *N*-methyl-D-aspartate antagonist MK-801 and the calcium channel blocker KB-2796 on neurologic and metabolic recovery after spinal cord ischemia. Exp Neurol 1998; 149: 203–8.
71. Faden AI, Jacobs TP, Smith MT. Evaluation of the calcium channel antagonist nimodipine in experimental spinal cord ischemia. J Neurosurg 1984; 60: 796–9.
72. Haghighi SS, Stiens T, Oro JJ, Madsen R. Evaluation of the calcium channel antagonist nimodipine after experimental spinal cord injury. Surg Neurol 1993; 39: 403–8.
73. Holtz A, Nystrom B, Gerdin B. Spinal cord injury in rats: inability of nimodipine or antineutrophil serum to improve spinal cord blood flow or neurologic status. Acta Neurol Scand 1989; 79: 460–7.
74. Liu D, Thangnipon W, McAdoo DJ. Excitatory amino acids rise to toxic levels upon impact injury to the rat spinal cord. Brain Res 1991; 547: 344–8.
75. Liu D, Xu GY, Pan E, McAdoo DJ. Neurotoxicity of glutamate at the concentration released upon spinal cord injury. Neuroscience 1999; 93: 1383–9.
76. Xu GY, Hughes MG, Ye Z, Hulsebosch CE, McAdoo DJ. Concentrations of glutamate released following spinal cord injury kill oligodendrocytes in the spinal cord. Exp Neurol 2004; 187: 329–36.
77. Mills CD, Xu GY, Johnson KM, McAdoo DJ, Hulsebosch CE. AIDA reduces glutamate release and attenuates mechanical allodynia after spinal cord injury. Neuroreport 2000; 11: 3067–70.
78. Mills CD, Xu GY, McAdoo DJ, Hulsebosch CE. Involvement of metabotropic glutamate receptors in excitatory amino acid and GABA release following spinal cord injury in rat. J Neurochem 2001; 79: 835–48.

79. Agrawal SK, Fehlings MG. Role of NMDA and non-NMDA ionotropic glutamate receptors in traumatic spinal cord axonal injury. J Neurosci 1997; 17: 1055–63.
80. Wrathall JR, Teng YD, Marriott R. Delayed antagonism of AMPA/kainate receptors reduces long-term functional deficits resulting from spinal cord trauma. Exp Neurol 1997; 145: 565–73.
81. Wrathall JR, Teng YD, Choiniere D. Amelioration of functional deficits from spinal cord trauma with systemically administered NBQX, an antagonist of non-*N*-methyl-D-aspartate receptors. Exp Neurol 1996; 137: 119–26.
82. Wrathall JR, Choiniere D, Teng YD. Dose-dependent reduction of tissue loss and functional impairment after spinal cord trauma with the AMPA/kainate antagonist NBQX. J Neurosci 1994; 14: 6598–607.
83. Faden AI, Lemke M, Simon RP, Noble LJ. *N*-methyl-D-aspartate antagonist MK801 improves outcome following traumatic spinal cord injury in rats: behavioral, anatomic, and neurochemical studies. J Neurotrauma 1988; 5: 33–45.
84. Muir KW, Lees KR. Clinical experience with excitatory amino acid antagonist drugs. Stroke 1995; 26: 503–13.
85. Ellison G. Competitive and non-competitive NMDA antagonists induce similar limbic degeneration. Neuroreport 1994; 5: 2688–92.
86. Olney JW, Farber NB. NMDA antagonists as neurotherapeutic drugs, psychotogens, neurotoxins, and research tools for studying schizophrenia. Neuropsychopharmacology 1995; 13: 335–45.
87. Faden AI, Molineaux CJ, Rosenberger JG, Jacobs TP, Cox BM. Endogenous opioid immunoreactivity in rat spinal cord following traumatic injury. Ann Neurol 1985; 17: 386–90.
88. Faden AI. Opioid and nonopioid mechanisms may contribute to dynorphin's pathophysiological actions in spinal cord injury. Ann Neurol 1990; 27: 67–74.
89. Faden AI, Jacobs TP. Dynorphin-related peptides cause motor dysfunction in the rat through a non-opiate action. Br J Pharmacol 1984; 81: 271–6.
90. Long JB, Kinney RC, Malcolm DS, Graeber GM, Holaday JW. Intrathecal dynorphin A1-13 and dynorphin A3-13 reduce rat spinal cord blood flow by non-opioid mechanisms. Brain Res 1987; 436: 374–9.
91. Long JB, Petras JM, Mobley WC, Holaday JW. Neurological dysfunction after intrathecal injection of dynorphin A (1–13) in the rat. II. Nonopioid mechanisms mediate loss of motor, sensory and autonomic function. J Pharmacol Exp Ther 1988; 246: 1167–74.
92. Arias MJ. Effect of naloxone on functional recovery after experimental spinal cord injury in the rat. Surg Neurol 1985; 23: 440–2.
93. Walker JM, Moises HC, Coy DH, Baldrighi G, Akil H. Nonopiate effects of dynorphin and des-Tyr-dynorphin. Science 1982; 218: 1136–8.
94. Faden AI. Dynorphin increases extracellular levels of excitatory amino acids in the brain through a non-opioid mechanism. J Neurosci 1992; 12: 425–9.
95. Akdemir H, Pasaoglu A, Ozturk F et al. Histopathology of experimental spinal cord trauma. Comparison of treatment with TRH, naloxone, and dexamethasone. Res Exp Med (Berl) 1992; 192: 177–83.
96. Ceylan S, Ilbay K, Baykal S et al. Treatment of acute spinal cord injuries: comparison of thyrotropin-releasing hormone and nimodipine. Res Exp Med (Berl) 1992; 192: 23–33.
97. Hashimoto T, Fukuda N. Effect of thyrotropin-releasing hormone on the neurologic impairment in rats with spinal cord injury: treatment starting 24 h and 7 days after injury. Eur J Pharmacol 1991; 203: 25–32.
98. Takami K, Hashimoto T, Shino A, Fukuda N. Effect of thyrotropin-releasing hormone (TRH) in experimental spinal cord injury: a quantitative histopathologic study. Jpn J Pharmacol 1991; 57: 405–17.
99. Benzel EC, Khare V, Fowler MR. Effects of naloxone and nalmefene in rat spinal cord injury induced by the ventral compression technique. J Spinal Disord 1992; 5: 75–7.
100. Benzel EC, Lancon JA, Bairnsfather S, Kesterson L. Effect of dosage and timing of administration of naloxone on outcome in the rat ventral compression model of spinal cord injury. Neurosurgery 1990; 27: 597–601.
101. Jones TB, McDaniel EE, Popovich PG. Inflammatory-mediated injury and repair in the traumatically injured spinal cord. Curr Pharm Des 2005; 11: 1223–36.
102. Nelson E, Gertz SD, Rennels ML, Ducker TB, Blaumanis OR. Spinal cord injury. The role of vascular damage in the pathogenesis of central hemorrhagic necrosis. Arch Neurol 1977; 34: 332–3.
103. Giulian D, Woodward J, Young DG, Krebs JF, Lachman LB. Interleukin-1 injected into mammalian brain stimulates astrogliosis and neovascularization. J Neurosci 1988; 8: 2485–90.
104. Bartholdi D, Schwab ME. Expression of pro-inflammatory cytokine and chemokine mRNA upon experimental spinal cord injury in mouse: an in situ hybridization study. Eur J Neurosci 1997; 9: 1422–38.
105. Ma M, Wei T, Boring L et al. Monocyte recruitment and myelin removal are delayed following spinal cord injury in mice with CCR2 chemokine receptor deletion. J Neurosci Res 2002; 68: 691–702.
106. McTigue DM, Tani M, Krivacic K et al. Selective chemokine mRNA accumulation in the rat spinal cord after contusion injury. J Neurosci Res 1998; 53: 368–76.
107. Blight AR. Delayed demyelination and macrophage invasion: a candidate for secondary cell damage in spinal cord injury. Cent Nerv Syst Trauma 1985; 2: 299–315.
108. Bruce AJ, Boling W, Kindy MS et al. Altered neuronal and microglial responses to excitotoxic and ischemic brain injury in mice lacking TNF receptors. Nat Med 1996; 2: 788–94.
109. Liu J, Marino MW, Wong G et al. TNF is a potent anti-inflammatory cytokine in autoimmune-mediated demyelination. Nat Med 1998; 4: 78–83.
110. Kim GM, Xu J, Xu J et al. Tumor necrosis factor receptor deletion reduces nuclear factor-kappaB activation, cellular inhibitor of apoptosis protein 2 expression, and functional recovery after traumatic spinal cord injury. J Neurosci 2001; 21: 6617–25.
111. Casha SWRY, Fehlings MG. Oligodendroglial apoptosis occurs along degenerating axons and is associated with FAS and P75 expression following spinal cord injury. Neuroscience 2001; 103: 203–18.
112. Li GL, Brodin G, Farooque M et al. Apoptosis and expression of Bcl-2 after compression trauma to rat spinal cord. J Neuropathol Exp Neurol 1996; 55: 280–9.
113. Li GL, Farooque M, Holtz A, Olsson Y. Apoptosis of oligodendrocytes occurs for long distances away from the primary injury after compression trauma to rat spinal cord. Acta Neuropathol (Berl) 1999; 98: 473–80.
114. Katoh K, Ikata T, Katoh S et al. Induction and its spread of apoptosis in rat spinal cord after mechanical trauma. Neurosci Lett 1996; 216: 9–12.
115. Lou J, Lenke LG, Ludwig FJ, O'Brien MF. Apoptosis as a mechanism of neuronal cell death following acute experimental spinal cord injury. Spinal Cord 1998; 36: 683–90.
116. Crowe MJ, Bresnahan JC, Shuman SL, Masters JN, Beattie MS. Apoptosis and delayed degeneration after spinal cord injury in rats and monkeys. Nat Med 1997; 3: 73–6.
117. Liu XZ, Xu XM, Hu R et al. Neuronal and glial apoptosis after traumatic spinal cord injury. J Neurosci 1997; 17: 5395–406.
118. Yong C, Arnold PM, Zoubine MN et al. Apoptosis in cellular compartments of rat spinal cord after severe contusion injury. J Neurotrauma 1998; 15: 459–72.
119. Emery E, Aldana P, Bunge MB et al. Apoptosis after traumatic human spinal cord injury. J Neurosurg 1998; 89: 911–20.
120. Shuman SL, Bresnahan JC, Beattie MS. Apoptosis of microglia and oligodendrocytes after spinal cord contusion in rats. J Neurosci Res 1997; 50: 798–808.
121. Warden P, Bamber NI, Li H et al. Delayed glial cell death following wallerian degeneration in white matter tracts after spinal cord dorsal column cordotomy in adult rats. Exp Neurol 2001; 168: 213–24.

122. Abe Y, Yamamoto T, Sugiyama Y et al. Apoptotic cells associated with Wallerian degeneration after experimental spinal cord injury: a possible mechanism of oligodendroglial death. J Neurotrauma 1999; 16: 945–52.
123. Frost EE, Buttery PC, Milner R, ffrench-Constant C. Integrins mediate a neuronal survival signal for oligodendrocytes. Curr Biol 1999; 9: 1251–4.
124. Fernandez PA, Tang DG, Cheng L et al. Evidence that axon-derived neuregulin promotes oligodendrocyte survival in the developing rat optic nerve. Neuron 2000; 28: 81–90.
125. Flores AI, Mallon BS, Matsui T et al. Akt-mediated survival of oligodendrocytes induced by neuregulins. J Neurosci 2000; 20: 7622–30.
126. Bjartmar C, Yin X, Trapp BD. Axonal pathology in myelin disorders. J Neurocytol 1999; 28: 383–95.
127. Yin X, Crawford TO, Griffin JW et al. Myelin-associated glycoprotein is a myelin signal that modulates the caliber of myelinated axons. J Neurosci 1998; 18: 1953–62.
128. Casha S, Yu WR, Fehlings MG. FAS deficiency reduces apoptosis, spares axons and improves function after spinal cord injury. Exp Neurol 2005; 196: 390–400.
129. Demjen D, Klussmann S, Kleber S et al. Neutralization of CD95 ligand promotes regeneration and functional recovery after spinal cord injury. Nat Med 2004; 7: 7.
130. Markus A, Patel TD, Snider WD. Neurotrophic factors and axonal growth. Curr Opin Neurobiol 2002; 12: 523–31.
131. Liu Y, Himes BT, Murray M, Tessler A, Fischer I. Grafts of BDNF-producing fibroblasts rescue axotomized rubrospinal neurons and prevent their atrophy. Exp Neurol 2002; 178: 150–64.
132. Liu Y, Kim D, Himes BT et al. Transplants of fibroblasts genetically modified to express BDNF promote regeneration of adult rat rubrospinal axons and recovery of forelimb function. J Neurosci 1999; 19: 4370–87.
133. Kwon BK, Liu J, Oschipok L et al. Rubrospinal neurons fail to respond to brain-derived neurotrophic factor applied to the spinal cord injury site 2 months after cervical axotomy. Exp Neurol 2004; 189: 45–57.
134. Schwab JM, Brechtel K, Mueller CA et al. Experimental strategies to promote spinal cord regeneration – an integrative perspective. Prog Neurobiol 2006; 78: 91–116.
135. Cai D, Shen Y, De Bellard M, Tang S, Filbin MT. Prior exposure to neurotrophins blocks inhibition of axonal regeneration by MAG and myelin via a cAMP-dependent mechanism. Neuron 1999; 22: 89–101
136. Neumann S, Bradke F, Tessier-Lavigne M, Basbaum AI. Regeneration of sensory axons within the injured spinal cord induced by intraganglionic cAMP elevation. Neuron 2002; 34: 885–93.
137. Qiu J, Cai D, Dai H et al. Spinal axon regeneration induced by elevation of cyclic AMP. Neuron 2002; 34: 895–903.
138. Lu P, Yang H, Jones LL, Filbin MT, Tuszynski MH. Combinatorial therapy with neurotrophins and cAMP promotes axonal regeneration beyond sites of spinal cord injury. J Neurosci 2004; 24: 6402–9.
139. Nikulina E, Tidwell JL, Dai HN, Bregman BS, Filbin MT. The phosphodiesterase inhibitor rolipram delivered after a spinal cord lesion promotes axonal regeneration and functional recovery. Proc Natl Acad Sci USA 2004; 101: 8786–90.
140. Pearse DD, Pereira FC, Marcillo AE et al. cAMP and Schwann cells promote axonal growth and functional recovery after spinal cord injury. Nat Med 2004; 10: 610–16.
141. Yuan XB, Jin M, Xu X et al. Signalling and crosstalk of Rho GTPases in mediating axon guidance. Nat Cell Biol 2003; 5: 38–45.
142. Silver J, Miller JH. Regeneration beyond the glial scar. Nat Rev Neurosci 2004; 5: 146–56.
143. Bradbury EJ, Moon LD, Popat RJ et al. Chondroitinase ABC promotes functional recovery after spinal cord injury. Nature 2002; 416: 636–40.
144. Chau CH, Shum DK, Li H et al. Chondroitinase ABC enhances axonal regrowth through Schwann cell-seeded guidance channels after spinal cord injury. FASEB J 2004; 18: 194–6.
145. Bush TG, Puvanachandra N, Horner CH et al. Leukocyte infiltration, neuronal degeneration, and neurite outgrowth after ablation of scar-forming, reactive astrocytes in adult transgenic mice. Neuron 1999; 23: 297–308.
146. Faulkner JR, Herrmann JE, Woo MJ et al. Reactive astrocytes protect tissue and preserve function after spinal cord injury. J Neurosci 2004; 24: 2143–55.
147. Cajal R. Degeneration and Regeneration of the Nervous System. New York: Hafner Press, 1928.
148. Chen MS, Huber AB, van der Haar ME et al. Nogo-A is a myelin-associated neurite outgrowth inhibitor and an antigen for monoclonal antibody IN-1. Nature 2000; 403: 434–9.
149. McKerracher L, David S, Jackson DL et al. Identification of myelin-associated glycoprotein as a major myelin-derived inhibitor of neurite growth. Neuron 1994; 13: 805–11.
150. Wang KC, Koprivica V, Kim JA et al. Oligodendrocyte-myelin glycoprotein is a Nogo receptor ligand that inhibits neurite outgrowth. Nature 2002; 417: 941–4.
151. Fouad K, Klusman I, Schwab ME. Regenerating corticospinal fibers in the Marmoset (*Callitrix jacchus*) after spinal cord lesion and treatment with the anti-Nogo-A antibody IN-1. Eur J Neurosci 2004; 20: 2479–82.
152. Li S, Liu BP, Budel S et al. Blockade of Nogo-66, myelin-associated glycoprotein, and oligodendrocyte myelin glycoprotein by soluble Nogo-66 receptor promotes axonal sprouting and recovery after spinal injury. J Neurosci 2004; 24: 10511–20.
153. Xu XM, Chen A, Guenard V, Kleitman N, Bunge MB. Bridging Schwann cell transplants promote axonal regeneration from both the rostral and caudal stumps of transected adult rat spinal cord. J Neurocytol 1997; 26: 1–16.
154. Murray M, Kim D, Liu Y et al. Transplantation of genetically modified cells contributes to repair and recovery from spinal injury. Brain Res Brain Res Rev 2002; 40: 292–300.
155. Richardson PM, McGuinness UM, Aguayo AJ. Axons from CNS neurons regenerate into PNS grafts. Nature 1980; 284: 264–5.
156. Nesathurai S. Steroids and spinal cord injury: revisiting the NASCIS 2 and NASCIS 3 trials. J Trauma 1998; 45: 1088–93.
157. Coleman WP, Benzel D, Cahill DW et al. A critical appraisal of the reporting of the National Acute Spinal Cord Injury Studies (II and III) of methylprednisolone in acute spinal cord injury. J Spinal Disord 2000; 13: 185–99.
158. Hurlbert RJ. Methylprednisolone for acute spinal cord injury: an inappropriate standard of care. J Neurosurg 2000; 93: 1 7.
159. Short DJ, El Masry WS, Jones PW. High dose methylprednisolone in the management of acute spinal cord injury – a systematic review from a clinical perspective. Spinal Cord 2000; 38: 273–86.
160. Hurlbert RJ, Moulton R. Why do you prescribe methylprednisolone for acute spinal cord injury? A Canadian perspective and a position statement. Can J Neurol Sci 2002; 29: 236–9.
161. Bracken MB, Collins WF, Freeman DF et al. Efficacy of methylprednisolone in acute spinal cord injury. JAMA 1984; 251: 45–52.
162. Bracken MB, Shepard MJ, Collins WF Jr et al. Methylprednisolone or naloxone treatment after acute spinal cord injury: 1-year follow-up data. Results of the second National Acute Spinal Cord Injury Study. J Neurosurg 1992; 76: 23–31.
163. Bracken MB, Shepard MJ, Collins WF et al. A randomized, controlled trial of methylprednisolone or naloxone in the treatment of acute spinal-cord injury. Results of the Second National Acute Spinal Cord Injury Study. N Engl J Med 1990; 322: 1405–11.
164. Bracken MB, Shepard MJ, Holford TR et al. Administration of methylprednisolone for 24 or 48 hours or tirilazad mesylate for 48 hours in the treatment of acute spinal cord injury. Results of the Third National Acute Spinal Cord Injury Randomized Controlled Trial. National Acute Spinal Cord Injury Study. JAMA 1997; 277: 1597–604.
165. Bracken MB, Shepard MJ, Holford TR et al. Methylprednisolone or tirilazad mesylate administration after acute spinal cord injury:

1-year follow up. Results of the third National Acute Spinal Cord Injury randomized controlled trial. J Neurosurg 1998; 89: 699–706.
166. Otani K, Abe H, Kadoya S. Beneficial effect of methylprednisolone sodium succinate in the treatment of acute spinal cord injury. Sekitsui Sekizui J 1994; 7: 633–47.
167. Kiwerski JE. Application of dexamethasone in the treatment of acute spinal cord injury. Injury 1993; 24: 457–60.
168. Pointillart V, Petitjean ME, Wiart L et al. Pharmacological therapy of spinal cord injury during the acute phase. Spinal Cord 2000; 38: 71–6.
169. Hugenholtz H, Cass DE, Dvorak MF et al. High-dose methylprednisolone for acute closed spinal cord injury – only a treatment option. Can J Neurol Sci 2002; 29: 227–35.
170. Tator CH. Review of treatment trials in human spinal cord injury: issues, difficulties, and recommendations. Neurosurgery 2006; 59: 957–82; discussion 982–7.
171. Roberts I, Yates D, Sandercock P et al. Effect of intravenous corticosteroids on death within 14 days in 10008 adults with clinically significant head injury (MRC CRASH trial): randomised placebo-controlled trial. Lancet 2004; 364: 1321–8.
172. Zeller CB, Marchase RB. Gangliosides as modulators of cell function. Am J Physiol 1992; 262: C1341–55.
173. Rahmann H. Brain gangliosides and memory formation. Behav Brain Res 1995; 66: 105–116.
174. Sabel BA, Stein DG. Pharmacological treatment of central nervous system injury. Nature 1986; 323: 493.
175. Gorio A. Gangliosides as a possible treatment affecting neuronal repair processes. Adv Neurol 1988; 47: 523–30.
176. Geisler FH, Dorsey FC, Coleman WP. Recovery of motor function after spinal-cord injury – a randomized, placebo-controlled trial with GM-1 ganglioside. N Engl J Med 1991; 324: 1829–38.
177. Geisler FH, Coleman WP, Grieco G, Poonian D. The Sygen multicenter acute spinal cord injury study. Spine 2001; 26: S87–98.
178. McIntosh TK, Faden AI. Opiate antagonist in traumatic shock. Ann Emerg Med 1986; 15: 1462–5.
179. Faden AI, Jacobs TP, Mougey E, Holaday JW. Endorphins in experimental spinal injury: therapeutic effect of naloxone. Ann Neurol 1981; 10: 326–32.
180. Faden AI, Holaday JW. A role for endorphins in the pathophysiology of spinal cord injury. Adv Biochem Psychopharmacol 1981; 28: 435–46.
181. Winkler T, Sharma HS, Gordh T et al. Topical application of dynorphin A (1–17) antiserum attenuates trauma induced alterations in spinal cord evoked potentials, microvascular permeability disturbances, edema formation and cell injury. An experimental study in the rat using electrophysiological and morphological approaches. Amino Acids 2002; 23: 273–81.
182. Hauser KF, Knapp PE, Turbek CS. Structure–activity analysis of dynorphin A toxicity in spinal cord neurons: intrinsic neurotoxicity of dynorphin A and its carboxyl-terminal, nonopioid metabolites. Exp Neurol 2001; 168: 78–87.
183. Hu WH, Lee FC, Wan XS, Chen YT, Jen MF. Dynorphin neurotoxicity induced nitric oxide synthase expression in ventral horn cells of rat spinal cord. Neurosci Lett 1996; 203: 13–16.
184. Behrmann DL, Bresnahan JC, Beattie MS. A comparison of YM-14673, U-50488H, and nalmefene after spinal cord injury in the rat. Exp Neurol 1993; 119: 258–67.
185. Benzel EC, Hoffpauir GM, Thomas MM et al. Dose-dependent effects of naloxone and methylprednisolone in the ventral compression model of spinal cord injury. J Spinal Disord 1990; 3: 339–44.
186. Arias MJ. Treatment of experimental spinal cord injury with TRH, naloxone, and dexamethasone. Surg Neurol 1987; 28: 335–8.
187. Flamm ES, Young W, Demopoulos HB, DeCrescito V, Tomasula JJ. Experimental spinal cord injury: treatment with naloxone. Neurosurgery 1982; 10: 227–31.
188. Faden AI, Jacobs TP, Holaday JW. Thyrotropin-releasing hormone improves neurologic recovery after spinal trauma in cats. N Engl J Med 1981; 305: 1063–7.
189. Bracken MB, Holford TR. Effects of timing of methylprednisolone or naloxone administration on recovery of segmental and long-tract neurological function in NASCIS 2. J Neurosurg 1993; 79: 500–7.
190. Flamm ES, Young W, Collins WF et al. A phase I trial of naloxone treatment in acute spinal cord injury. J Neurosurg 1985; 63: 390–7.
191. Pitts LH, Ross A, Chase GA, Faden AI. Treatment with thyrotropin-releasing hormone (TRH) in patients with traumatic spinal cord injuries. J Neurotrauma 1995; 12: 235–43.
192. Farooque M, Hillered L, Holtz A, Olsson Y. Changes of extracellular levels of amino acids after graded compression trauma to the spinal cord: an experimental study in the rat using microdialysis. J Neurotrauma 1996; 13: 537–48.
193. Panter SS, Yum SW, Faden AI. Alteration in extracellular amino acids after traumatic spinal cord injury. Ann Neurol 1990; 27: 96–9.
194. Mills CD, Johnson KM, Hulsebosch CE. Group I metabotropic glutamate receptors in spinal cord injury: roles in neuroprotection and the development of chronic central pain. J Neurotrauma 2002; 19: 23–42.
195. Liu D. An experimental model combining microdialysis with electrophysiology, histology, and neurochemistry for studying excitotoxicity in spinal cord injury. Effect of NMDA and kainate. Mol Chem Neuropathol 1994; 23: 77–92.
196. Lang-Lazdunski L, Heurteaux C, Vaillant N, Widmann C, Lazdunski M. Riluzole prevents ischemic spinal cord injury caused by aortic crossclamping. J Thorac Cardiovasc Surg 1999; 117: 881–9.
197. Wrathall JR, Choiniere D, Teng YD. Dose-dependent reduction of tissue loss and functional impairment after spinal cord trauma with the AMPA/kainate antagonist NBQX. J Neurosci 1994; 14: 6598–607.
198. Tadie M, Gaviria M, Mathe JF et al. Early care and treatment with a neuroprotective drug, Gacyclidine, in patients with acute spinal cord injury. Rachis 2003; 15: 363–76.
199. Lepeintre JF, D'Arbigny P, Mathe JF et al. Neuroprotective effect of gacyclidine. A multicenter double-blind pilot trial in patients with acute traumatic brain injury. Neurochirurgie 2004; 50: 83–95.
200. Ross IB, Tator CH, Theriault E. Effect of nimodipine or methylprednisolone on recovery from acute experimental spinal cord injury in rats. Surg Neurol 1993; 40: 461–70.
201. Pointillart V, Gense D, Gross C et al. Effects of nimodipine on post-traumatic spinal cord ischemia in baboons. J Neurotrauma 1993; 10: 201–13.
202. De Ley G, Leybaert L. Effect of flunarizine and methylprednisolone on functional recovery after experimental spinal injury. J Neurotrauma 1993; 10: 25–35.
203. Ross IB, Tator CH. Spinal cord blood flow and evoked potential responses after treatment with nimodipine or methylprednisolone in spinal cord-injured rats. Neurosurgery 1993; 33: 470–6.
204. Guha A, Tator CH, Piper I. Effect of a calcium channel blocker on posttraumatic spinal cord blood flow. J Neurosurg 1987; 66: 423–30.
205. Petitjean ME, Pointillart V, Dixmerias F et al. Medical treatment of spinal cord injury in the acute stage. Ann Fr Anesth Reanim 1998; 17: 114–22.
206. Kavanagh RJ, Kam PC. Lazaroids: efficacy and mechanism of action of the 21-aminosteroids in neuroprotection. Br J Anaesth 2001; 86: 110–19.
207. Baptiste DC, Fehlings MG. Pharmacological approaches to repair the injured spinal cord. J Neurotrauma 2006; 23: 318–34.
208. Kigerl K, Popovich P. Drug evaluation: ProCord – a potential cell-based therapy for spinal cord injury. IDrugs 2006; 9: 354–60.

Part VII

Special considerations on meningo-myelocele

63

Neural tube defects: etiology, prevention, and prenatal diagnosis

Atsuo Kondo, Shinji Katsuragi, and Osamu Kamihira

Introduction

In 1905, Moore[1] reviewed 190 articles in the literature and collected 378 cases with spina bifida who had undergone excision of the sac. He found that the mortality rate was more than 35% in patients within the first few months of life, but 4.7% in patients over 5 years at operation. In 1932, Penfield and Cone[2] from Montreal successfully operated upon 19 of 33 children suffering from spina bifida or posterior cranium bifidum without any incidence of death. Although children with a minor degree of spinal dysraphism were surgically treated, most children with spina bifida were either inappropriately treated or simply left untreated to die, until the 1950s. In the 1960s, many such children started to survive longer, thanks to advances in shunting technology for hydrocephalus treatment, the use of antibiotics, and improvements in surgical techniques. For the next two to three decades, ileal loop conduit, reported by Bricker[3] in 1950, was extensively applied to let wet myelodysplastics dry. In the 1970s, an ethical dilemma and medical concerns were expressed with regard to whether a myelodysplastic infant should be actively treated or left untreated.[4,5] Lorber[6] proposed his criteria for selecting patients based on the degree of paralysis, head circumference, kyphosis, and associated gross congenital anomalies, and considered that continuous reassessment was vital, even after a positive treatment strategy had been selected.

In 1972, Lapides et al[7] reported clean intermittent catheterization that dramatically led to changes in treatment concepts and surgical strategies. Although ileal loop conduit was initially considered to be a panacea for those with myelodysplasia, this surgical technique was denied 25 to 30 years later because of a variety of complications such as urolithiasis, skin ulceration, and psychosomatic problems.[8] Then urinary undiversion became a topic of discussion and was recommended for restoration of the normal urinary tract and subsequent intermittent catheterization.[9,10] In the 1980s and 1990s, bladder augmentation procedures using either the ileum, colon, or sigma became the gold standard for urologists in association with antireflux surgery, the anti-incontinence sling operation, or implantation of an artificial urinary sphincter when required.[11] The majority of patients with an augmented bladder certainly required intermittent catheterization postoperatively. In 1980, Mitrofanoff[12] reported the use of the appendix as a catheterizable stoma, whose construction would have been impossible without the application of the principle of Lapides. After 10 years, Malone[13] took advantage of the Mitrofanoff procedure as an antegrade continence enema (ACE) to prevent or improve fecal incontinence.

In 1991, the Medical Research Council Vitamin Study Research Group[14] reported, based on their landmark prospective randomized controlled trial, that a periconceptional intake of 4 mg/day of folic acid reduced the incidence of neural tube defects (NTDs) in subsequent pregnancies by 72%. In 1999, a population-based intervention study was conducted in which 400 μg/day of folic acid was administered to Chinese nulliparae.[15] The outcome indicated that folic acid decreased the first occurrence of neural tube defects by 79% in northern China and 41% in southern China. In December 2000, the Ministry of Health and Welfare of Japan[16] advised young Japanese women to take 400 μg folic acid supplements daily when planning pregnancy. Currently, health agencies in many countries have officially recommended the periconceptional consumption of folic acid in the range of 400–500 μg/day by those young women capable of conceiving or who are planning to conceive.[17] Based on the analysis of 13 published reports, Wald et al stressed that the chance of an offspring developing NTDs decreases with an increase in the folic acid supplement intake and that women planning pregnancy should take 5 mg folic acid tablets daily instead of 0.4 mg.[18] Observations and epidemiologic findings continue to unmask the biochemistry, biology, and molecular genetics underlining NTDs, and have contributed to the significant progress in developing strategies for the prevention of this devastating anomaly.[19–21] Prenatal fetal screening comprising imaging tools and biochemical scanning has contributed to identifying fetal malformation that, in turn, provides exact and valuable information for the counseling of expectant parents.

Prevalence of neural tube defects

The NTD comprises myelodysplasia (myelomeningocele), anencephaly, encephalocele, craniorhachischisis, and iniencephaly, while spina bifida occulta is not included among NTDs because it is often undetectable or its relation to NTDs is uncertain. Since many patients with anencephaly and some with myelomeningocele die during early gestation, the incidence of NTDs in early embryos and their prevalence at birth are not identical. Although the prevalence of NTDs at birth varies greatly between countries and ethnic groups, it has considerably declined during the past three decades due to advancements in the refined resolution of ultrasonography for *in utero* fetal examination, the clinical availability of serum alpha-fetoprotein measurements, termination of affected pregnancies, and the wide consumption of folic acid supplements by women of childbearing age. Shurtleff[22] noted a general decline in the birth incidence of NTDs in the majority of countries worldwide. He reported that the incidence of myelomeningocele in Seattle, USA, was 0.5 per 1000 births in 1981–82, which then declined further to 0.05 per 1000 births in 2001–2. Laurence et al[23] investigated the incidence of spina bifida and anencephaly in the South Wales for 7 years from 1956 to 1962. They found that the overall incidence of the malformations was 7.89 per 1000 total births, and this value was the highest in the total population at that time. Morris and Wald[24] estimated a large decline in the birth prevalence of NTDs in England and Wales in 1999 on an assumption that the true total number of NTD pregnancies remained constant, or changed by a constant amount per year. Their analysis is shown in Figure 63.1. The prevalence of NTDs was 3.80 per 1000 live births in 1965, which steadily declined to 0.14 in 1997, i.e., a reduction of 96%. Conversely, the estimated number of terminations increased considerably from 0 per 1000 live births in 1965 to 1.50 per 1000 live births in 1997, resulting in a true prevalence of 1.64 per 1000 NTD births and terminations in 1997. It is said that the prevalence of NTDs in Poland has been persistently rather high over the last 20 years: 2.05–2.68 per 1000 newborns.[25]

The decreases in the prevalence were further reported in relation to the increased accuracy of antenatal diagnoses, folic acid supplementation, and fortification of cereals with folic acid. For instance, Rankin et al[26] studied statistical data from the Northern Congenital Abnormality Survey of the UK from 1984 to 1996. The authors found that 907 NTDs among a total number of 507 409 livebirths, stillbirths, and terminations of pregnancy during the 13 years, i.e., the total prevalence of NTDs at birth, was 1.79 per 1000 births and terminations. This prevalence, however, significantly declined by 51%, from 2.16 in 1985 to 1.44 in 1996. On the other hand, termination of pregnancy for NTDs significantly increased from 50% (35/70 cases) in 1984 to 92% (45/49 cases) in 1996. Contrary to the declining tendency of NTDs in Occidental countries, Sumiyoshi[27] reported that the prevalence of NTDs in Japan has barely altered during the past two decades. Figure 63.2 shows the prevalence of NTDs in Japan: 1.17 per 1000 live births in 1975 and 1.06 per 1000 live births in 2002. We believe that following factors are closely related to the unaltered prevalence of NTDs in Japan:

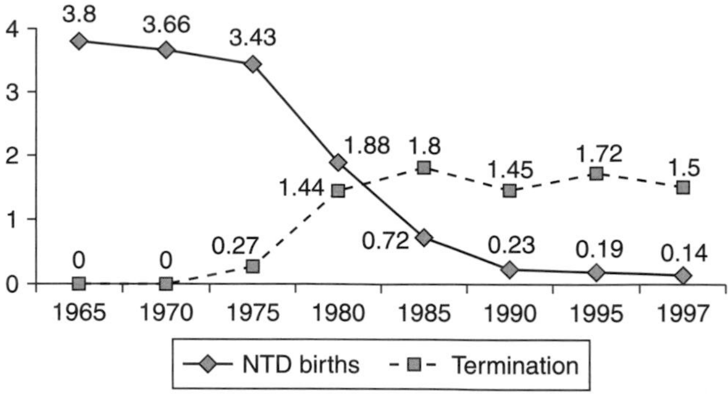

Figure 63.1
Prevalence of neural tube defects per 1000 live births significantly decreased and the number of terminations per 1000 live births significantly increased during the past 30 years in England and Wales.

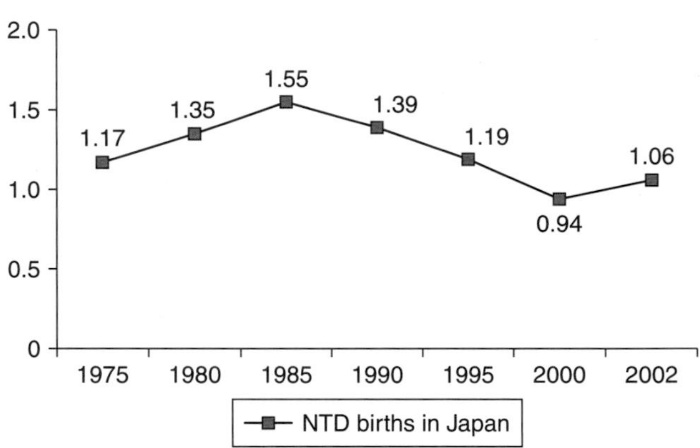

Figure 63.2
The number of births with neural tube defects per 1000 live births remained rather constant in Japan over the past 30 years.

Table 63.1 *The prevalence of spina bifida per 1,000 live births in 7 countries from 1980 to 2002*

	1980	1990	2000	2002
England & Wales	1.14	0.17	0.13	
Finland	0.17	0.23	0.26	
France	0.41	0.21	0.02	
Japan	0.25	0.36	0.49	0.56
New Zealand	1.26	0.44	0.31	
Norway	0.66	0.39	0.38	
USA (Atlanta)	0.77	0.52	0.21	

1. The systematic inability of the government to accumulate precise information on livebirths, stillbirths, and fetuses terminated.
2. The insufficient efforts of the government in presenting information on the link between folic acid and NTDs to the general public.
3. Reluctance of the Japanese public to take any supplements during pregnancy for fear of causing fetal malformation.
4. Neglect of the traditional Japanese food rich in vegetables, fish, and rice, and willingness to consume fast food/Westernized food lacking in vegetables and carbohydrates.

Sumiyoshi[27] also reported the prevalence of myelodysplasia in several developed countries, as shown in Table 63.1. In 1980, Japan ranked second among the countries with a low NTD prevalence, with Finland ranking the lowest, however, in 2000 Japan ranked first with the highest prevalence of 0.49 per 1000 live births.

Etiology of neural tube defects

The neural tube normally closes *in utero* within 4 weeks of conception, or 2 weeks after the missed menstrual period when almost 50% of women are not aware of their pregnancy. Although the causative mechanism of NTDs remains poorly understood, a combination of genetic abnormalities and environmental and nutritional factors plays a definite role in their development. An estimated 300 000 or more of spina bifida and anencephaly cases occur worldwide each year.[28,29] The fact that folic acid supplementation of 4 mg daily for women with a history of NTD-affected pregnancy resulted in the reduction of NTD[14] focused research into the genetic defects of the methyl cycle of homocysteine metabolism over the past 10 to 20 years. There is ample evidence suggesting that genetic abnormalities have a strong impact on the causation of NTD:

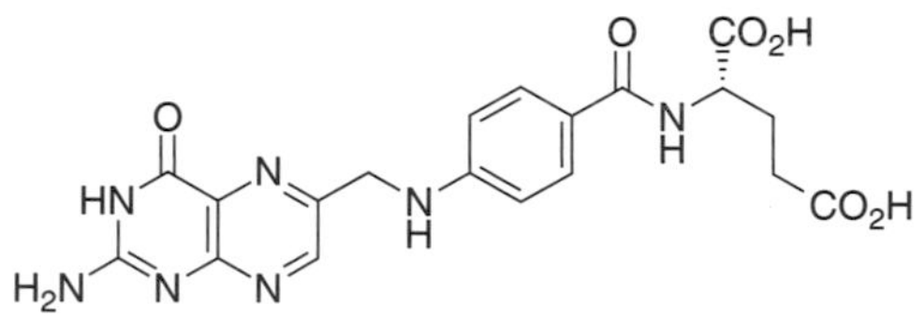

Figure 63.3
The chemical structure of folic acid.

- NTDs are related to genes encoding proteins that are directly or indirectly connected with folic acid and methionine metabolism.
- A significantly higher number of female fetuses compared to male fetuses are afflicted with NTDs.
- A significantly higher incidence of consanguinity has been indicated among the parents of NTD-afflicted babies.
- Parents who have had an affected pregnancy are at an increased risk of its recurrence: at a 3- to 5-fold higher risk than the general population.

Genetic factor: MTHFR C677T polymorphism

A common mutation in the 5,10-methylenetetrahydrohydrofolate reductase (MTHFR) gene has been identified which produces a thermolabile variant of MTHFR 677TT with a reduced enzyme activity. This mutation is identical as a risk factor common to both NTDs and adult cardiovascular diseases. Folic acid (pteroilglutamic acid), illustrated in Figure 63.3, is a water-soluble B vitamin and is involved in single-carbon transfers that are an integral part of important processes, including the synthesis of nucleotides and a variety of methylation reactions that occur in several cell compartments. The activity of the variant MTHFR is enhanced by folate, leading to a decrease in the plasma homocysteine level. Figure 63.4 briefly illustrates the folate and homocysteine metabolism. Tetrahydrofolate (THF) and 5,10-methylenetetrahydrofolate (5,10-MTHF) are methylated derivatives of folate that are consumed as diet or folate supplements. They are the donors of one-carbon groups for nucleotide synthesis. 5-Methyl-tetrahydrofolate is produced from 5,10-MTHF by the activity of MTHFR, which donates its methyl group for methionine synthesis from homocysteine. This reaction is catalyzed by methionine synthase (MS) with cobalamin (vitamin B12) as a cofactor. MS activity requires the functioning of methionine synthase reductase (MSR). Methionine is subsequently metabolized by methionine

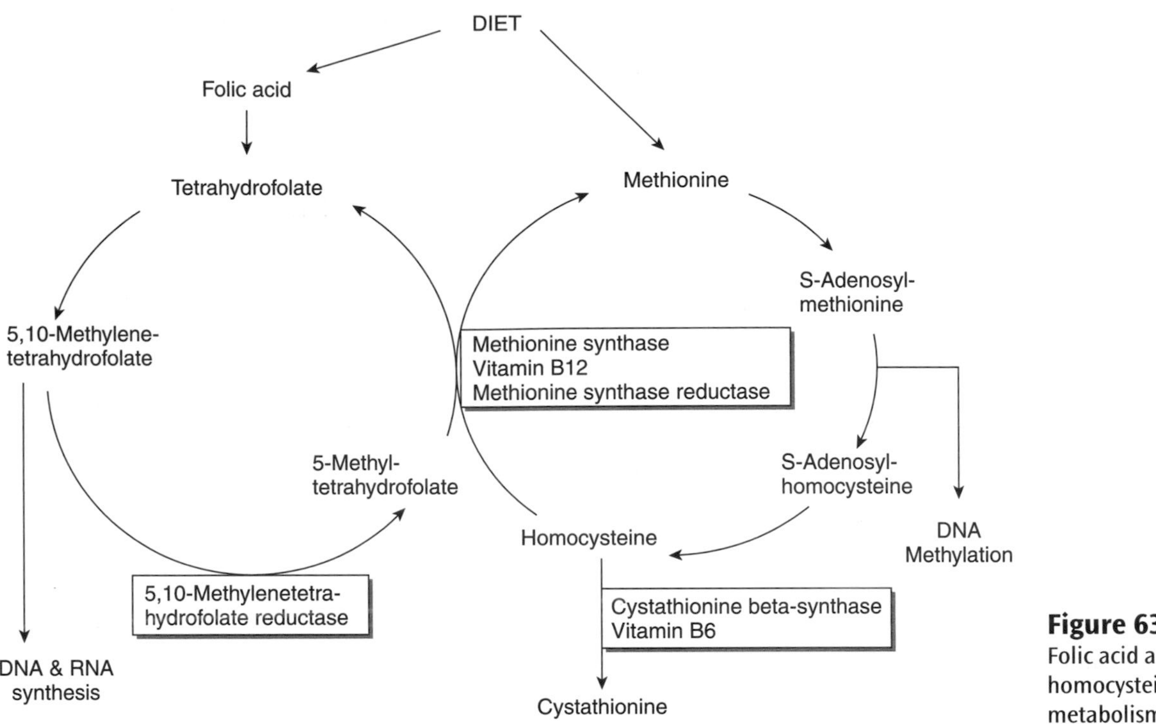

Figure 63.4
Folic acid and homocysteine-methionine metabolism.

Table 63.2 *Distribution of the MTHFR 677 genotypes among healthy subjects of different ethnic groups. Those with the TT homozygous varied from 4.0 to 16.2% who are susceptible to NTDs or other ailments and could be protected by folic acid supplementation*

Genotypes	Irish women (n=560)	Dutch subjects (n=207)	Japanese male (n=203)	Brazilian white (n=103)	Brazilian Non-white (n=149)
CC	46.8%	53.6%	33.3%	56.3%	53.7%
CT	42.3%	41.5%	50.5%	35.0%	42.3%
TT	10.9%	4.8%	16.2%	8.7%	4.0%
References	Molloy[33]	van der Put[34]	Miyake[35]	Perez[36]	Perez[36]

adenosyltransferase to form *S*-adenosylmethionine (SAM). SAM is a donor of methyl groups in transmethylation reactions and one of the products is *S*-adenosylhomocysteine (SAH), which can be used again for methionine synthesis. When homocysteine is catalyzed by cystathionine synthase (CBS) together with vitamin B6, it is metabolized to cystathionine. Thus, there are four key enzymes involved in folate and methionine-homocysteine metabolism, i.e., MTHFR, MS, MSR, and CBS.[25,30–32]

It is known that a specific thermolabile variant of MTHFR T677T causing partial enzyme deficiency is present in 4 to 16% of the normal population in different ethnic groups. Table 63.2 depicts that, among five ethnic groups,[33–36] Japanese males exhibited the highest proportion of MTHFR T677T (16.2%), followed by Irish women (10.9%), and Brazilian caucasians of both sex (8.7%). The folate pathway enzyme, MTHFR, is one of the principal means that enables cells to regulate intracellular concentrations of methionine and homocysteine and is related to the occurrence of NTDs by preventing the conversion of homocysteine to methionine. Polymorphism of C677T (C for cytosine, T for thymidine) in the MTHFR gene has been identified as a mutation that renders the enzyme thermolabile and causes it to lose its activity with an increase in temperature, thereby leading to an increase in the serum homocysteine concentration. Decreased enzyme activity is a risk factor for NTDs, cerebrovascular diseases, venous thrombosis, urogenital anomalies, oral

Table 63.3 *Distribution of the MTHFR C677T polymorphism between affected children (cases) and the control children. Significant difference in proportion of TT genotypes is observed between groups in two of three manuscripts*

Authors Cases & control	CC (wild type)	CT (heterozygous)	TT (homozygous)	*p* value
Van der Put[34]				
Cases (n=55)	40% (22)	47% (26)	13% (7)	p= 0.047
Controls (n=207)	54% (111)	42% (86)	5% (10)	
Perez[36]				
Cases (n=131)	45.0% (59)	47.3% (62)	7.6% (10)	p= 0.16
Controls (n=126)	54.0% (68)	35.7% (45)	10.3% (13)	
Kirke[38]				
Cases (n=395)	38.2% (151)	43.3% (171)	18.5% (73)	p<0.0001
Controls (n=848)	51.8% (439)	38.4% (326)	9.8% (83)	

and cleft palate, and colon cancer. In order to suppress the mutation effect, folate supplements are essential and effective, because they increase MTHFR stability. Although Parle-McDermott et al genotyped 276 complete triads (mother, father, and an affected child) and 256 controls in 2003;[37] the role of a second MTHFR polymorphism, 1298A→C, in the etiology of NTDs could not be confirmed.

Table 63.3 depicts the distribution of the MTHFR C677T polymorphism among the affected children and the controls reported in three articles, and suggests that individuals with the TT homozygous genotype, a risk factor for NTDs, may require a higher folate intake to regulate the plasma homocysteine concentration. Van der Put et al, in 1995,[34] studied the correlation between the 677C→T mutation in the MTHFR and the MTHFR activity in 55 NTD cases and 207 controls among Dutch people. Compared to subjects with the CC genotype, those with the TT homozygous genotype were associated with decreased MTHFR activity, decreased thermolability, increased plasma homocysteine concentrations, high red-cell folate (RCF) concentrations, and decreased plasma folate concentrations. The authors speculated that folate administration would benefit subjects with the TT homozygous genotype by improving the MTHFR activity and lowering the serum homocysteine level. Perez et al[36] quantified plasma homocysteine levels in relation to genotypes of MTHFR among Brazilian subjects: 131 children with and 126 children without myelodysplasia. The authors reported that the homocysteine levels were higher in case children than in the control children, irrespective of the genotype, but the proportion of the TT homozygous genotype was not statistically different between the two groups. Kirke et al[38] genotyped 395 Irish patients with NTD and 848 controls and reported that both homozygous (TT) and heterozygous (CT) genotypes showed a better correlation with lower tissue folate concentration, higher homocysteine concentration, and lower tissue enzyme activity than the wild type (CC) genotype. The authors mentioned that the combined CT and TT genotypes accounted for approximately 26% of NTD occurrence in the population, and that both genotypes of MTHFR T677T and C677T should be regarded as risk factors and as much as 50 to 60% of the population at NTD risk would benefit from food fortification.

Mills et al[39] investigated homocysteine and vitamin B12 levels in 81 pregnant women with previous NTD-afflicted children and 247 normal controls whose children were normal. Mothers of children with NTDs had significantly higher homocysteine values than the B12-matched controls (8.62 vs 7.95 μmol/l); however, the vitamin B12 level did not differ between the two groups. The authors reported that an abnormality in homocysteine metabolism related to methionine synthase is present in many women who have delivered NTD-afflicted children and that administration of both folic acid and B12 would be the most effective method to prevent NTDs. Molloy et al[33] investigated the impact of polymorphism homozygosity on the amount of RCF in 560 healthy women (242 pregnant and 318 nonpregnant) recruited in Dublin, Ireland. The RCF levels are more reliable than the serum folate concentration because they reflect the tissue folate status over the lifetime of the erythrocyte. Table 63.4 shows that the RCF level was significantly higher in pregnant and non-pregnant women with the CC wild genotype and in pregnant women with the CT heterozygous genotype than in women with the TT homozygous genotype. Miyake et al[35] studied the effects of intake of 1 mg folic acid with regard to the three MTHFR genotypes in 203 males suffering from atherosclerosis. After 3 months, the authors observed that the folic acid supplementation significantly decreased the plasma homocysteine levels and increased the folic acid concentration in all three genotype groups; nevertheless, subjects with the TT homozygous genotype experienced the largest changes in the plasma concentrations.

Chatkupt et al[40] reported that, besides the role of genotypes, there exists a genetic contribution to the occurrence

Table 63.4 *Red-cell folate (RCF) depending on C677T polymorphism in MTHFR in 242 pregnant and 318 non-pregnant women. RCF level was significantly higher in pregnant and non-pregnant women with the CC wild type and significantly higher in pregnant women with the CT heterozygous compared to women having TT homozygous type*

			RCF (µg/L)	
Genotypes	Pregnant (n=242)	No-pregnant (n=318)	Pregnant	Non-pregnant
CC	114	148	347**	347**
CT	108	129	321*	314
TT	20	41	252	284

**$p<0.01$ *$p<0.05$

of NTDs. The authors studied 72 families with familial spina bifida, including 180 patients from the USA. Since the authors observed a high proportion of families with Irish and German ancestry, a low proportion of families with African-American ancestry, and a low prevalence of spina bifida in the African-Americans, they suggested that their data could reflect different genetic susceptibilities. Smoking reduces the serum folate concentration, particularly in people with the TT homozygous genotype. McDonald and her associates[41] evaluated the effect of smoking on the serum folate and RCF concentrations in 80 pregnant women during their first or early second trimester. Of the 80 women, 40 smoked and 40 did not. They found an absence of significant difference in the dietary folate and vitamin B12 intakes between the two groups; however, the serum folate concentration was significantly lower in the smokers than in the nonsmokers ($p=0.001$) and there was a trend toward a lower RCF concentration in pregnant women who smoked ($p = 0.38$). When the serum folate concentration was compared between subjects with MTHFR 677TT and those with MTHFR 677CC or MTHFR 677CT, women who were identified with 677TT and smoked exhibited a significantly lower serum folate concentration. In 2004, Rothenberg et al[42] investigated the presence of autoantibodies in serum against folate receptors in 12 women who were or had been pregnant with an NTD-affected fetus and in 24 control women. The authors reported (1) the existence of a high affinity in the binding of autoantibodies to folate receptors in the 12 women with NTD-affected pregnancy, (2) that autoantibodies were present in the serum of 9 of these 12 case subjects and in 2 of the 20 control subjects (4 nulligravida were excluded from the statistical analysis), and (3) that the binding of autoantibodies to folate receptors blocked the cellular uptake of folate. However, they commented that additional studies are necessary to identify the frequency of folate-receptor autoantibodies in women who have complicated pregnancies and to determine whether these autoantibodies are pathologic.

Nutritional factors: folic acid deficiency

In the first half of the 20th century, folic acid was identified as one of the B vitamins that does play a significant role in the occurrence or recurrence of NTDs.[43] As early as 1933, Willis[44] reported that marmite, an autolyzed yeast product, was actively effective in treating patients with tropical macrocytic anemia in Bombay, India. Patients of both sexes responded to 30 g per day Marmite with an increase in the proportion of red blood cells and reticulocytes in the total red cell count. In 1960, Nelson[45] observed that a folic acid-deficient diet administered to experimental rats resulted in embryonic anomalies such as anemia, skeletal anomalies, anomalies of the urinary tract, and vacuolation of the lens. The author stressed that diet administration should correspond to the time when the sensitivity to the folate deficiency is the highest.

Clinical implications of folic acid deficiency have been reported since the mid 1960s in the UK. In 1964, Hibbard BM[46] from Liverpool investigated 1484 patients under obstetric care in whom folic acid deficiency was extremely common, and recognized that folic acid that governs DNA synthesis was highly demanded at the time of rapid proliferation of cells and organs, beginning at the 2-celled embryo stage up to a 2 billion-celled fetus. He concluded that folic acid deficiency resulted in megaloblastic anemia, abruptio placentae, and fetal congenital malformations and that true prophylaxis must begin before conception. In 1965, Hibbard and Smithells[47] noted a significant relationship between defective folate metabolism and mothers who gave birth to fetuses with malformation. In 1980, Smithells et al[48] recruited 438 women, who had had one or more NTD infant, and gave daily multivitamin tablets containing 0.36 mg folic acid to 178 of these women; the tablet administration was commenced at 28 days before conception and was continued up to at least the date of the second missed menstruation. The remaining 260 women were treated as controls. The authors did find a significant

Table 63.5 *Congenital anomalies developed in two groups. Prevalence of anomalies in folic acid group (800µg/day) was significantly lower than the trace-element group*

Malformations	Folic acid group (2104 women)	Trace-element group (2052 women)
Neural tube defects	0	6
Cardiovascular malformation	6	9
Cleft palate w/wo cleft lip	4	5
Down's syndrome	2	3
Exomphalos and gastroschisis	1	1
Foramina parietale permagna	0	2
Hydrocephalus	0	2
Hypospadias	1	1
Large hemangioma on the face	3	1
Limb-reduction defect	1	5
Obstructed urinary system	1	2
Postural deformity	2	0
Other malformations	7	10
Total	28 (13.3 per 1000)*	47 (22.9 per 1000)

*$p = 0.029$

difference in the recurrence rates of NTD-afflicted infants/fetuses between the two groups: 0.6% (1/178) in the supplemented group vs 5% (13/260) in the control group ($p = 0.009$). In 1981, Laurence et al[49] confirmed the effectiveness of periconceptional folic acid administration for the prevention of NTD in a rather small-sized randomized controlled trial. A total of 111 women with a history of NTD-affected pregnancies were recruited and instructed to take 4 mg folic acid tablets daily or placebo; the supplementation/placebo was started at the time contraceptive precautions were discontinued. The authors found that the recurrence rate was 0% in the supplemented group of 44 women and 9.0% in the noncompliant or placebo group of 67 women, and this difference in the recurrence rate was significant ($p = 0.05$).

In 1991, the MRC vitamin study research group[14] reported a memorable, large-scaled randomized controlled trial of folic acid in a total of 1031 women who had already had a pregnancy with an NTD. The subjects were recruited from 7 countries: UK, Hungary, Israel, Canada, USSR, France, and Australia. The women were allocated into 1 of 4 supplementation groups: supplements containing 4 mg folic acid, multivitamins without folic acid, both of these, or neither. The recurrence rate of NTD was 1.0% (5/514) in the folic acid supplementation groups and 3.5% (18/517) among those who did not take folic acid. The relative risk for the women allocated to receive folic acid was 0.28, i.e., 72% of NTDs were prevented (95% CI: 29 to 88%). A Hungarian group,[50] through a randomized trial, investigated whether daily periconceptional supplementation of 0.8 mg folic acid or trace element micronutrients without folic acid could prevent the first occurrence of NTDs among 4156 women (Table 63.5). Although the amount of folic acid administered was only one-fifth of the dose in the MRC vitamin study,[14] the outcome was as promising as expected, i.e., there were 6 cases of NTDs in the trace element supplement group and no incidence of NTDs in the folic acid supplement group ($p = 0.029$). Furthermore, the number of congenital anomalies observed in the two groups was significantly more in the trace element group (22.9 per 1000 live births) compared to the folic acid group (13.3 per 1000 live births) ($p = 0.029$). A Chinese cohort study[15] administered 400 µg of folic acid daily to women planning to conceive in the northern and southern regions and investigated the effect of periconceptional folic acid intake. The NTD occurrence rates in women not receiving folic acid were 4.8 per 1000 pregnancies in the northern region and 1.0 per 1,000 pregnancies in the southern region. Among the women with periconceptional folic acid supplementation, these rates were 1.0 per 1000 pregnancies in the northern and 0.6 per 1000 pregnancies in the southern regions. The reduction in the risk of NTD occurrence in the first pregnancy was significant in both regions, i.e., 79% in the northern and 41% in the southern region.

Table 63.6 *The risk of obesity in relation to the occurrence of NTDs. The relative risk for NTDs increases form 1.9 for women weighing 80 to 89 kg to 4.0 for women weighing 110 Kg or more in comparison with women of 50 to 59 Kg*

Pre-pregnant Weight (kg)	Case mothers with NTDs (n=604)	Control mothers with major malformations (n=1658)	Multivariate RR (95% CI)
50–59	217	625	Reference
60–69	126	453	0.8 (0.6–1.1)
70–79	93	204	1.2 (0.9–1.6)
80–89	45	65	1.9 (1.2–2.9)
90–99	19	45	1.3 (0.7–2.3)
100–109	13	14	3.1 (1.4–7.0)
>=110	13	9	4.0 (1.6–9.9)

Environmental factors such as diabetes mellitus, obesity, drugs, and smoking

Environmental factors also affect the occurrence of NTDs by modulating gene expression, and this is reflected by the varying frequencies of NTD cases. Furthermore, NTDs have been prevalent in countries or regions with a devastating economic status and compromised food supplies. Here we will discuss several teratogens.

Diabetes mellitus in pregnant mothers is a risk factor for NTDs. Becerra et al[51] studied a total of 4929 diabetic pregnant mothers and 3029 control pregnant mothers who were identified and interviewed over the telephone. The relative risks for major central nervous system malformations (spina bifida, anencephaly, encephalocele, etc.) and cardiovascular system malformations were 15.5 and 18.0, respectively, among infants of mothers with insulin-dependent diabetes mellitus. The authors stressed that strict metabolic control well before conception and educating the women about the risks of diabetes mellitus can significantly reduce the incidence of birth defects among infants of diabetic mothers.

Obesity in mothers is also a risk factor for NTDs, and the effect of extreme obesity is independent of the effects of folate intake. Werler and associates[52] collected data in a case-control surveillance program of birth defects from 1988 to 1994 (Table 63.6): 604 fetuses or infants had NTDs and 1658 fetuses or infants exhibited other major malformations within 6 months of delivery. The relative risk for NTDs increased from 1.9 for women weighing 80–89 kg to 4.0 for women weighing 110 kg or more in comparison with women of weight 50 to 59 kg. The risk of NTDs decreased by 40% with an intake of 400 µg/day or more of folate among women weighing less than 70 kg; however, no benefits were observed among heavier women.

Anti-epileptic drugs (AEDs) cross the placenta, raise the pharmacologically active concentration of the drug in the embryo or fetus, alter folate metabolism, and decrease the plasma folate or RCF concentration.[53] Although the mechanisms underlying the effects of AEDs remain to be further elucidated, several theories have been suggested for their adverse effects: liver enzyme induction by AEDs, impairment of folate absorption, competitive interaction between folate co-enzymes and drugs, and an increased demand for folate as a co-enzyme for anti-epileptic hydroxylation. Goggin and associates[54] clearly showed that all anti-epileptic drugs interfere with folate metabolism. The authors studied the effects of AEDs on the RCF levels among 200 patients with epilepsy and 72 controls. They found that the median RCF levels were significantly lower in patients treated with phenytoin (170.5 µg/l), carbamazepine (173.5 µg/l), or more than one drug (154.0 µg/l) compared to the controls (247.5 µg/l). Kaneko et al[55] prospectively analyzed 983 offspring born in Japan, Italy, and Canada and observed that the prevalence of congenital anomalies in these newborns was 9.0% when they were exposed to AEDs, but was 3.1% when they were not. The authors found that the prevalence of malformations increased with the number of drugs administered; the rate of malformation was 7.8% for one AED, 9.6% for two AEDs, 11.5% for three AEDs, 13.5% for four AEDs, and 15.4% for five AEDs. According to recent data, valproate is significantly more teratogenic than carbamazepine, and a combination of valproate and lamotrigine is particularly teratogenic.[56] In fact, the Japanese government has banned the prescription of both trimethadione and valproate to pregnant women and has cautioned that primidone should be prescribed only when its usefulness exceeds the risk of harm to the mother and fetus.

Hyperthermia is another risk factor for NTDs. An elevated body temperature was the first teratogen observed in experimental animals and was subsequently proved teratogenic in humans. Graham and associates[57] stated in their review that hyperthermia during the first trimester was significantly associated with NTDs; the sources of hyperthermia considered were febrile illness, sauna use, hot tub use, or excessive physical exercise in a hot and humid environment. In Finland, women in the early stages of pregnancy have been advised to limit their exposure to hot tubs set at 40°C to less than 10 min and to saunas set over 90°C to a maximum of 15 min. The authors suggested that hyperthermia at or above 102°F (38.9°C) for more than 24 hours in the first 4 weeks after conception may affect both brain and facial morphogenesis in the human fetus.

A variety of drugs are known to interfere with the metabolism of or prevent the absorption of folic acid. These drugs comprise sulfamethoxazole-trimethoprim (antimicrobials), methotrexate (anticancer agent), aspirin (anticoagulant), sulfadoxine-pyrimethamine (antimalarial agent), sulfasalazine (antiulcerative colitis), azathioprine (immunosuppressant), antacid, rifampicin (antituberculosis), antiepileptic drugs, and so forth.[58–60] These agents should be avoided or prescribed with caution to women of childbearing age in particular.

Vitamin A has been teratogenic in experimental animals.[61] Rothman and associates[62] reported an epidemiologic study wherein they recruited 22 748 pregnant women between weeks 15 and 20 of pregnancy and obtained information on diet, medications, and illnesses during the first trimester of pregnancy and general information about their family, medical history, and exposure to environmental agents. A total of 339 congenital anomalies (14.9/1000 live births) including 48 NTDs developed in infants born to these women. The ratio of prevalence of malformations among babies born to women who consumed > 15 000 IU of preformed vitamin A per day from food and supplements to the prevalence among the babies whose mothers consumed 5000 IU or less per day was 3.5. If a woman took vitamin A from supplements alone, then this rate increased to 4.8. Based on these observations, the authors concluded that high dietary intake of preformed vitamin A appeared to be teratogenic and it should be avoided.

Cigarette smoking during pregnancy is a causative factor for the occurrence of cleft lip or cleft palate, congenital heart defects, decrease in birth weight, placental abruption, sudden infant death syndrome (SIDS), and Down syndrome.[63–66] Although none of these reports suggested a direct linkage between cigarette smoking and NTDs, women with MTHFR 677TT who smoked were reported to have significantly lower serum folate levels,[41] and this indirectly suggests that smoking is detrimental to both the mother and her unborn child. It is noteworthy that the American Academy of Pediatrics[67] issued an important message advocating no smoking to the American public as early as 1976.

Alcohol consumption during pregnancy is significantly associated with low birth weight, cleft lip/palate, and fetal alcohol syndrome, but its relation to NTDs is as yet uncertain. Shurtleff et al[68] analyzed 621 patients with myelodysplasia and observed the heterogeneous nature of this defect; among these patients, 13 cases had suspected etiologies, leaving 608 or 98% of the cases with an unknown etiology. The authors mentioned that there were two North American Indian mothers of offspring with meningomyelocele associated with fetal alcohol syndrome, and suggested that severe alcoholism and their racial propensity might have been responsible for the NTDs in their infants.

Prevention of neural tube defects

Prepregnancy counseling is of prime importance for women who have had an affected pregnancy or who have a family history of NTDs. Periconceptional consumption of folic acid supplementation is strongly recommended and any etiologic factors such as diet, drugs, or vitamins which might disturb folic acid metabolism should be avoided. Additionally, prenatal examination[69] is essential to diagnose fetal abnormality; the findings of such an examination would provide increased options for parents and a decreased prevalence of children with major abnormalities. A larger number of parents would be able to either prepare for a baby with a disorder well in advance or consider termination of the pregnancy.

Folic acid intake and balanced diet

The neural tube normally closes within 28 days after conception and other major malformations develop within 12 weeks of gestation. Therefore, folic acid supplementation should be started from 4 weeks before to 12 weeks after conception to reduce the risk of having fetuses or newborns afflicted with major malformations. If a woman has a history of a malformed offspring she should consult her doctor, who should recommend taking 4 mg/day folic acid supplementation. Furthermore, she should avoid alcohol, drugs, and smoking; consume well-balanced meals comprising vegetables, fruits, and carbohydrates; and reduce the amount of lipids in food. The correlation between poor nutrition and occurrence of NTDs provides a powerful tool for primary prevention. Several articles from North America have reported a significant reduction in the prevalence of NTDs since the commencement of cereal grain fortification with folic acid. Presently, it is presumed that a typical American woman consumes 100 μg of folate daily through enriched grain products. In a northern Mexican state, a folic acid campaign with free distribution of folate

Table 63.7 *Dietary folate consumption and plasma folate levels were studied in five groups of women. Statistical difference was tested in comparison with healthy women group*

Five groups of women	Age/BMI	Dietary folate with 95% CI (μg/day)	Plasma folate with 95% CI (ng/ml)
Healthy women (n=61): the control	37/21.0	338 (305–370)	8.2 (7.6–8.9)
Pregnant women (n=41)	31/21.5	356 (310–402)	11.9 (7.1–16.6)
Mothers of patients with NTDs (n=66)	42/21.6	301 (273–330)	8.2 (7.1–9.4)
Patients with NTDs (n=32)	24/22.8	273 (237–308)*	7.3 (6.3–8.3)
Student nurses (n=45)	20/20.1	217 (196–238)**	6.8 (6.1–7.4)**

*$p < 0.05$ **$p < 0.01$.

to low-income women resulted in a reduction in the number of NTDs by 50%, i.e., the occurrence rates were 1.04 per 1000 live births in 1999 vs 0.58 per 1000 live births in 2001.[70] A recent national population-based case-control study in Norway identified that folic acid supplements during early pregnancy appear to reduce the risk of isolated cleft lip by approximately one-third and that other vitamins and dietary factors may provide additional benefits.[71]

Folate consumed in foods is in the form of polyglutamates and that present in supplements or fortified food is in the form of monoglutamates. To be metabolized in the body the former has to be converted to the latter form. Moreover, the bioavailability of the former is relatively low, 50%, whereas that of the latter is as high as 85%. Although the periconceptional intake of folic acid supplements and a well-balanced diet have been recommended by a number of countries, the question that arises is, are young women of child-bearing age really compliant with this recommendation? We studied the amount of dietary folate consumed and plasma folate levels in 5 groups of young and adult women from 2001 to 2002; the data of this study are depicted in Table 63.7.[72] Two hundred and forty-five women participated in this study. The recommended dietary allowance (RDA) of folic acid prior to 2004 in Japan was 200 μg/day and 400 μg/day for nonpregnant women and pregnant women, respectively. Pregnant women consumed the largest amount of folate via foods (356 μg/day) and showed the highest value of plasma folate values (11.9 ng/ml). Dietary folate was significantly lower among patients with NTDs and student nurses, and the plasma folate level was also lower in student nurses than in healthy women (the controls). With regard to the RDA, the majority of nonpregnant women studied fulfilled the RDA, but 71% of pregnant women did not. Our data suggest that the majority of the nonpregnant women appear to be eating adequately; however, the pregnant women need to change their eating habits in terms of consuming more folate-rich foods and/or folate supplements.

We analyzed the dietary records collected from a total of 332 pregnant women from 2003 to 2006 in Japan (52 women in 2003, 94 women in 2004, 104 women in 2005, and 82 women in 2006). These pregnant women voluntarily took part in this study by completing the dietary records for 3 days, and these records were then analyzed by experienced dietitians based on the 5th Standard Table of Food Composition of Japan (unpublished data). It was observed that, during 2003–2006, the consumed proportion of four micronutrients was less than 80% of the RDA of Japan for pregnant women (Figure 63.5). These deficient micronutrients were iron (RDA = 19.5 mg/day), vitamin B1 (RDA = 0.9–1.2 mg/day), folic acid (RDA = 400–440 μg/day), and dietary fibers (RDA = 17–20 g/day). Please note that the RDAs were revised in 2005 by increasing the recommended values of most nutrients. As seen in Figure 63.5, the amount of dietary iron was definitely less, only 40% of RDA, and that of dietary folic acid varied from 86% to 76%. The imbalance in nutrients may be attributed to the neglect of traditional Japanese food, increased consumption of 'fast' foods, increased consumption of soft drinks,[73] and an inappropriate dieting despite a normal body mass index in young women of childbearing age.

The effects of food fortification

Table 63.8 depicts the effect of food fortification on the occurrence of NTDs. In Ontario, Canada, the total number of NTDs (live births, stillbirths, and therapeutic abortions) decreased from 1.17 per 1000 pregnancies in 1986 to 0.86 per 1000 pregnancies in 1999.[74] In Nova Scotia, Canada, the total incidence of open NTDs (live births, stillbirths, and terminated pregnancies) decreased by 54% after food fortification.[75] In South Carolina, USA, the increased periconceptional use of folic acid supplements among women of childbearing age decreased the prevalence rate of NTDs by 50%.[76] Honein and associates[77] investigated the impact of folic acid fortification of the USA food supply on the occurrence of NTDs. Based on the number of birth certificates issued, they found that the prevalence of NTDs decreased by 19%. In 2004, Mills and Signore[78] compared the articles accumulated before and after the food fortification in the USA and Canada; similar fortification programs were instituted in each of these countries. The authors

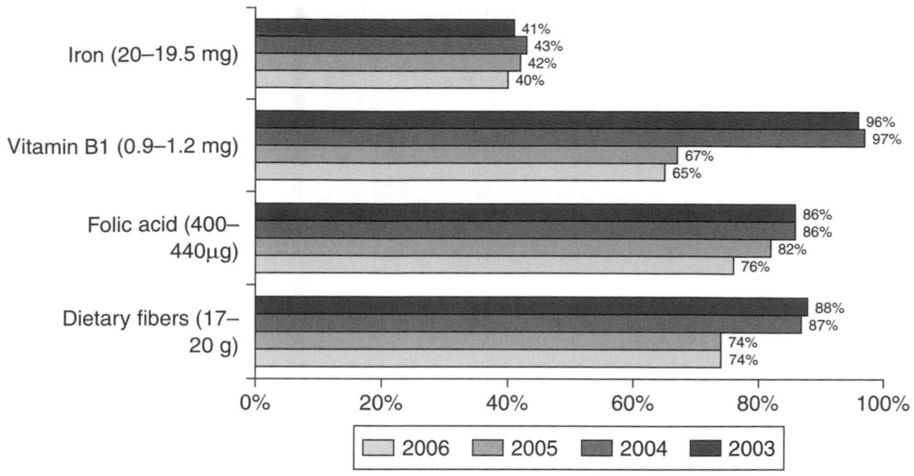

Figure 63.5
Analysis of the diet in 332 pregnant women showed that four micronutrients did not fulfill the recommended dietary allowance (RDA) which was expressed as 100%.

Table 63.8 *Reduced prevalence of NTDs after food fortification in the North America*

Location (References)	Prevalence prior to food fortification	Prevalence after food fortification	Reduction rates
Ontario, Canada (Gucciardi[74])	1.17/1000 live births, (1986)	0.86 (1999)	Reduction of 27%
Nova Scotia, Canada (Persad[75])	2.58/1000 live births, stillbirths & abortion (1991–1997)	1.17 (1998–2000)	Reduction of 54%
South Carolina, US (Stevenson[76])	1.89/1000 live births & fetal death (1992)	0.95 (1998)	Reduction of 50%
45 states & Washington DC (Honein[77])	0.378* (1995–1996)	0.305* (1998–1999)	Reduction of 19%

* Prevalence of NTDs based on birth certificates per 1000 births.

reported that the 26% decrease in NTDs calculated by the Centers for Disease Control and Prevention (CDC) was an underestimate,[79] and they estimated that the reduction in NTDs due to food fortification is in fact about 50%.

To what extent did the plasma folate concentration improve after food fortification? Cuskelly et al[80] investigated the changes in RCF concentration after folate was administered by three routes: folate-rich natural food (400 μg/day), fortified food (400 μg/day), or folic acid supplements (400 μg/day). Sixty-two young women were allocated to the three groups, and only dietary advice was given to the control group. Three months later the authors found a significant increase in the RCF concentration in the fortified food group (from 326 to 498 μg/l) and folic acid supplement group (from 351 to 492 μg/l). They criticized the recommendation of an increased intake of folate-rich food for women of childbearing age and considered it ineffective, nonbeneficial and misleading. Daly et al[81] recruited 121 women with RCF levels between 150 and 400 μg/l and assigned them to receive placebo, 100 μg, 200 μg, or 400 μg folic acid supplements daily. After 6 months, the authors found significant changes ($p < 0.001$) in the median incremental values and the median post-treatment concentrations in the three folic acid supplemented groups, but not in the placebo group: 67 μg/l and 375 μg/l, 130 μg/l and 475 μg/l, and 200 μg/l and 571 μg/l, for the 100 μg/day supplements, 200 μg/day supplements, and 400 μg/day folic acid supplement groups, respectively.

Jacques and associates[82] studied how plasma folate concentration is affected by food fortification by comparing the blood data of subjects with a mean age of 55 years. Blood samples were obtained from the 5th and 6th Framingham Offspring Study cohorts and the results were compared between them (Table 63.9). The study group comprised 248 subjects who were examined before and after food fortification. The control group of 553 subjects was examined twice before fortification, with a 3-year interval between examinations. The authors observed a significant increase in the serum folate concentration and a decrease in the total homocysteine concentration in the study group subjects who were not on folic acid supplementation, while there were no significant changes in the control group. They also found that the prevalence of low folic acid levels (< 3 ng/ml) significantly decreased from 22% to 2%, and the prevalence of high homocysteine levels (> 13 μmol/l) significantly decreased

Table 63.9 *Food fortification resulted in a significant increase in plasma foliate and a significant reduction in total homocysteine concentrations in the study group of Framingham Offspring Study cohorts. The control group visited twice with a three year interval before the fortification*

	Plasma folate (ng/ml)			Total homocysteine (ng/ml)		
Subjects	Pre-	Pre-	Post-fortification	Pre-	Pre-	Post-fortification
Study Group ($n=248$)	4.6 ng/m		10.0 ng/m**	10.1 ng/m		9.4 ng/m**
Control Group ($n=553$)	4.6	4.8		10.2		

**Comparison was done with the pre-fortification value ($p < 0.001$).

from 19% to 10%. Evans et al[83] observed a marked decrease in high maternal serum alpha-fetoprotein (MSAFP) values after introduction of folic acid fortification in bread and grains. A total of 61119 pregnant women underwent prenatal screening, and the data were categorized by multiples of the median (MoM) between two groups before (1997) and after (2000) the mandatory supplementation in the USA. They observed a 32% decrease in the patients with MoM values greater than 2.75, demonstrating a highly successful public health policy for the primary prevention of birth defects. Laurence et al[84] studied 98351 samples of serum folate concentrations measured from 1994 to 1999 in the USA. The median serum folate levels were 12.6 ng/ml in 1994, which remained stable up to 1996. However, the levels started increasing from 1997, i.e., the concentration was 14.9 ng/ml in 1997 and increased to 16.7 ng/ml in 1998. The authors suggested folic acid fortification of food as the most likely reason for the increase in the folate concentration because fortification was formally completed in January 1998.

In 2001, Wald DA and associates[85] investigated folic acid supplementation in 151 subjects with ischemic heart disease, by allocating them to either the placebo, 0.2, 0.4, 0.6, 0.8, or 1.0 mg/day folic acid supplementation groups. The authors found that the median serum homocysteine level decreased with an increase in the folic acid dose, to a maximum at 0.8 mg of folic acid per day, and the median serum homocysteine level was 2.7 μmol/l. They also found that the higher the initial serum homocysteine level, the more sensitive the response to the administered folic acid. They concluded that cereal grain fortified with folic acid is the most effective, simple, and inexpensive means of increasing folic acid consumption in the population, but that the level of fortification mandated in the USA (0.14 mg/100 g) and in the UK (0.24 mg/100 g of flour) is inadequate to reduce the homocysteine level. Wald et al[18] analyzed the preventive effect of folic acid intake based on 13 previously published articles. It was observed that the preventive effect is greater in women with low serum folate (5.0 ng/ml) than in those with a higher concentration (10.0 ng/ml) (Table 63.10). The authors commented that for young women with a typical background serum folate of 5 ng/ml, an increase of 0.4 mg/day folic acid intake would increase the serum folate concentration to 8.8 ng/ml and reduce the NTD risk by 36%, and an increase of 5 mg/day folic acid intake would increase its concentration to 52.0 ng/ml and reduce the NTD risk by 85%. The authors believed that the recommended folic acid intake of 0.4 mg/day is too low, and that an intake of 5 mg/day would be required for a woman planning a pregnancy.

On the other hand, there are some safety concerns related to large-dose folic acid supplementation, such as masking of anemia due to vitamin B12 deficiency, thus allowing the accompanying neurologic damage to progress untreated. Mills et al[86] investigated whether B12 deficiency-induced anemia could be erroneously treated with a large amount of folic acid, leading to neurologic symptoms such as confusion, paresthesias, and dementia. A total of 1573 elderly subjects (mean age 67 years) with a low vitamin B12 concentration (< 258 pmol/l) were studied. It was observed that food fortification did not cause a major increase in the masking of vitamin B12 deficiency. They concluded that vitamin B12 deficiency without anemia probably does not increase despite the current high exposure to folic acid-fortified food.

In 2007, Cole et al reported on their randomized clinical trial of the efficacy of folic acid supplements (1 mg/day), aspirin (81 or 325 mg/day) or both in preventing recurrence of colorectal adenoma.[87] They recruited 1021 patients with a recent treatment history of colorectal adenoma and followed up for 3 to 6 years with colonoscopic surveillance cycles. At a second follow-up among 607 patients, the incidence of at least 1 advanced lesion was 11.6% for folic acid and 6.9% for placebo, where statistical difference was significant ($p = 0.05$), while the incidence of at least 1 colorectal adenoma recurred evenly in both groups without significant difference ($p = 0.23$). The authors were cautious to mention that folic acid 1 mg/day does not reduce colorectal adenoma risk and that further research is needed to investigate the possibility that folic acid supplements might increase the risk of colorectal neoplasia. Their observations were actually contrary to what had been observed in animal experiments[88] and in

Table 63.10 *An expected serum folate concentration (ng/ml) and an estimated reduction in NTD risk (%) by taking folic acid supplements depicted in the first column*

Amount of folic acid intake through diet or supplements	Expected serum folate concentration & reduction in NTDs (%)	
	5.0 ng/ml*	10.0 ng/ml*
0.2 mg/day	6.9 ng/ml & 23%	11.9 ng/ml & 13%
0.4 mg/day	8.8 ng/ml & 36%	13.8 ng/ml & 23%
1.0 mg/day	14.4 ng/ml & 57%	19.4 ng/ml & 41%
3.0 mg/day	33.2 ng/ml & 78%	38.2 ng/ml & 66%
5.0 mg/day	52.0 ng/ml & 85%	57.0 ng/ml & 75%

*The initial folate levels of two groups.

Table 63.11 *Serum folate concentrations were compared between 51 epileptic mothers and the same number of the control mothers. Values of the epileptic group and 7 mothers were significantly lower than those of control mothers at 4 study periods ($p < 0.05$)*

Subjects	Pre-pregnancy	1st trimester	2nd trimester	3rd trimester
Epileptic mothers ($n=51$)	6.2 ng/ml*	4.5 ng/ml*	5.1 ng/ml*	4.3 ng/ml*
Seven epileptic mothers#	3.5*	2.3*	2.7*	3.0*
Control mothers ($n=51$)	7.4	7.2	7.2	6.3

#Seven mothers of the study group gave birth to newborns with congenital anomalies. *$p < 0.05$

epidemiological studies where a higher intake of folate was associated with a decreased risk of colorectal polyps and cancer.[132] As long as young women at the reproductive age take folate supplements for a short period of time starting 4 weeks prior to and ending 12 weeks after conception, it is safe to say that there will be no adverse effects of folic acid on fetal and maternal wellbeing and health.

One single anti-epileptic drug and folic acid supplements

Although there is no evidence indicating that folic acid supplementation decreases the risk of AED-induced NTDs, systematic supplementation of 2.5–5 mg/day of folate is strongly recommended. Hiilesmaa et al observed the outcome of drug therapy in 125 women with epilepsy in Finland.[90] Approximately 90% of the women took folate supplements at a mean dose of 500 μg/day (range 100–1000 μg/day), and 21 congenital malformations that were mild and did not include NTDs developed in 133 pregnancies. The authors recommended that the best treatment modality is to maintain the serum AED level as low as possible, prescribe 500 μg/day folic acid, prescribe one single drug as monotherapy where valproate should be preferably prohibited as the first-line treatment, and monitor the serum concentrations of AED and folate. Ogawa et al[91] clearly demonstrated that individuals who were on daily AEDs exhibited a significantly decreased serum folate concentration. The authors quantified serum folate concentrations in 51 epileptic pregnant women and 51 matched control pregnant women (Table 63.11). Of the epileptic women, 7 delivered 7 newborns with variable congenital anomalies, i.e., spina bifida, Down syndrome, cleft lip, patent ductus arteriosus, pilonidal sinus, retention testis, and strabismus. The folate concentrations of the 51 epileptic women including the 7 women were significantly lower than those of the control group at prepregnancy and throughout pregnancy periods ($p < 0.05$), thereby implying that AEDs decreased the serum folate level by suppressing the absorption of folic acid, thereby increasing the risk of congenital anomalies.

The pharmacotherapy guidelines for women of childbearing age or those planning to conceive have been reported by Tettenborn.[92] The guidelines include (1) counseling about contraception and pregnancy well before conception, (2) administering optimized monotherapy to obtain the lowest possible dose to achieve satisfactory seizure control, (3) prescribing 2.5–5 mg folic acid daily, (4) fetal monitoring with high-resolution ultrasonography before week 20 and measurement of serum alpha-fetoprotein level where amniocentesis is not routinely required, and (5) encouraging breastfeeding regardless of the treatment administered.

Awareness of folic acid

In the Netherlands, a mass media campaign started in 1995 was of great success in increasing awareness about periconceptional use of folic acid tablets. De Walle et al[93,94] reported that the proportion of pregnant women who were aware of folic acid increased from 28% before the campaign to 78% after 3 years, and that the proportion of women who used folic acid during any period of their pregnancy increased by 8% to 63%. We advocate the recommendation of Bekkers and Eskes[95] that collaboration among mass media, healthcare professionals, and governmental authorities is essential because mass media is the main source of educating the general public. The use of mass media sources such as television, radio, newspapers, and journals enables the transfer of information to not only young and/or pregnant women but also to healthcare workers. Health education programs are another means to promote the role of folic acid and the benefits of the periconceptional use of folic acid tablets. Presently, in Japan, few programs that emphasize the pivotal link between folic acid and NTDs or programs that propagate the preventive effects of folic acid on NTDs are available. Such programs should be initiated in the junior high school years, that is, much before young women conceive.

In Japan, we have been monitoring pregnant women with regard to their awareness about folic acid and folic acid supplementation, and their health-related behaviors during the past 5 years.[72] Pregnant women were randomly recruited at the Obstetrics-Gynecology clinics of 30 hospitals in Honshu or Kyushu Island; 770 women were recruited in 2002, 823 in 2003, 1467 in 2004, 1359 in 2005, and 1247 in 2006. Figure 63.6 indicates that rates of awareness regarding folic acid and rates of supplementation were initially very low (15% and 9%, respectively, in 2002); however, these rates steadily increased year after year, and, in 2006, these rates were 32% and 35%, respectively. Figure 63.7 illustrates lifestyle changes in pregnant women during the past 5 years. The proportion of pregnant women consuming well-balanced diets varied from 68% to 84%, while that of pregnant women who did not smoke or drink ranged from 91% to 97% during the past 5 years. It is reported that smoking and drinking are considerably more prevalent in their counterparts in the USA and UK; in the USA the prevalence of maternal smoking and drinking was 9–17% and 3–10%, respectively, and in the UK the prevalence of smoking and drinking during pregnancy was 17% and 61%, respectively.[96,97] Awareness about the role of periconceptional intake of folic acid was assessed in 10 groups of subjects[72] by the use of postal questionnaires from December 2002 to March 2003 in Japan (Figure 63.8). The 10 groups were as follows: group 1 comprised 500 female citizens aged 20–49 years who were randomly selected from the National Register of Komaki City; group 2, 1692 mothers who gave birth to their live children in 2001 in the Tokai district; and group 3, 250 female myelodysplastic patients aged over 18 years and 250 mothers who delivered a myelodysplastic child during the past 6 years. The subsequent 7 groups were consistent with healthcare professionals: 1858 nurses, 400 general practitioners (GPs), 400 urologists, 400 pharmacists, 147 midwives, 400 dietitians, and 400 obstetricians-gynecologists (OB/GYNs); these were randomly selected from their membership directories. The response rate ranged from 32% to 59%. Awareness varied greatly depending on the group. Less than 15% of laymen groups were aware of a linkage between folic acid and NTDs. The exception was the myelodysplastic families, 92% of whom had knowledge of the role of folic acid, that was obtained through newsletters issued from their patient association. Regarding the healthcare professionals, fewer than 30% of nurses, GPs, and urologists were aware of folic acid, while over 40% of pharmacists, midwives, dietitians, and OB/GYNs showed adequate awareness, with the highest awareness of 76% among the OB/GYNs.

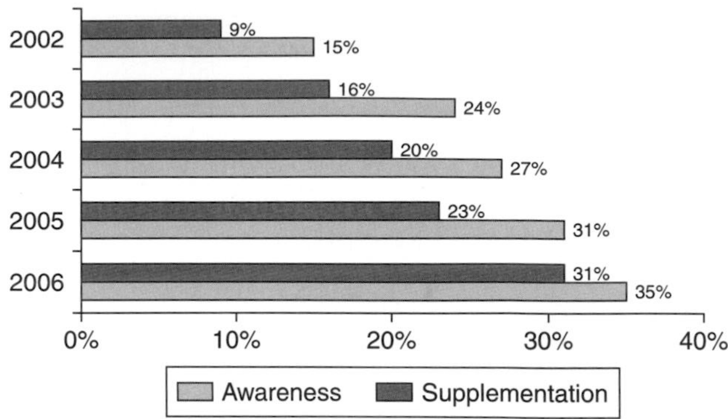

Figure 63.6
The proportion of pregnant women who were aware of the role of folic acid and took folic acid supplements increased year after year.

We extended our research in terms of the international awareness of the role of folic acid.[98] A questionnaire was dispatched to OB/GYNs and urologists residing in Japan, South Korea, Taiwan, USA/Canada, and Europe/Oceania by post or email. The questionnaire inquired about their knowledge of the role of folic acid and their views on the lifestyle of young women of childbearing age. The investigation was conducted between December 2002 and November 2004. Figure 63.9 illustrates that an average of 91% of OB/GYNs and 56% of urologists were aware of the role of folic acid, and that the proportion of urologists in Asia who knew the relationship between folic acid and NTDs was significantly lower than that of urologists in the Occident. It can be stated that the awareness among OB/GYNs is much higher than that among urologists.

AEDs have been generally prescribed by neurosurgeons, neurologists, and psychiatrists in Japan. Their knowledge on the possible adverse effects of AEDs in pregnant women (Figure 63.10) was investigated by questionnaire in 2006.[99] A total of 400 neurosurgeons, 300 neurologists, and 300

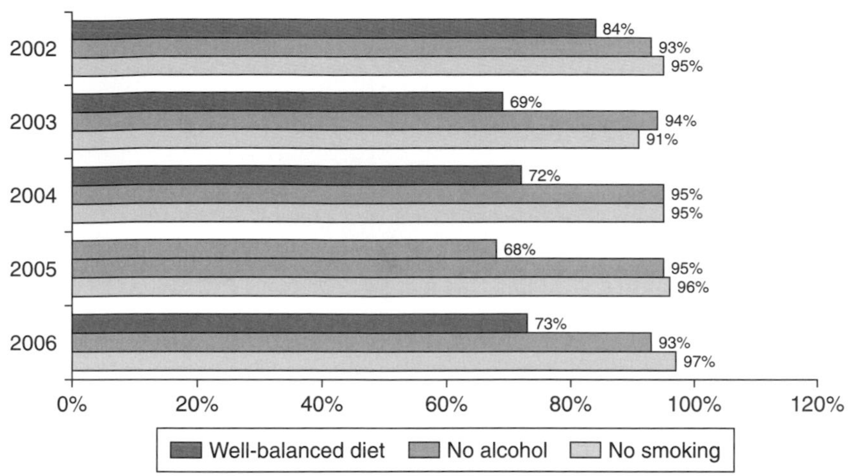

Figure 63.7
Lifestyle changes in 5666 pregnant women during the past 5 years.

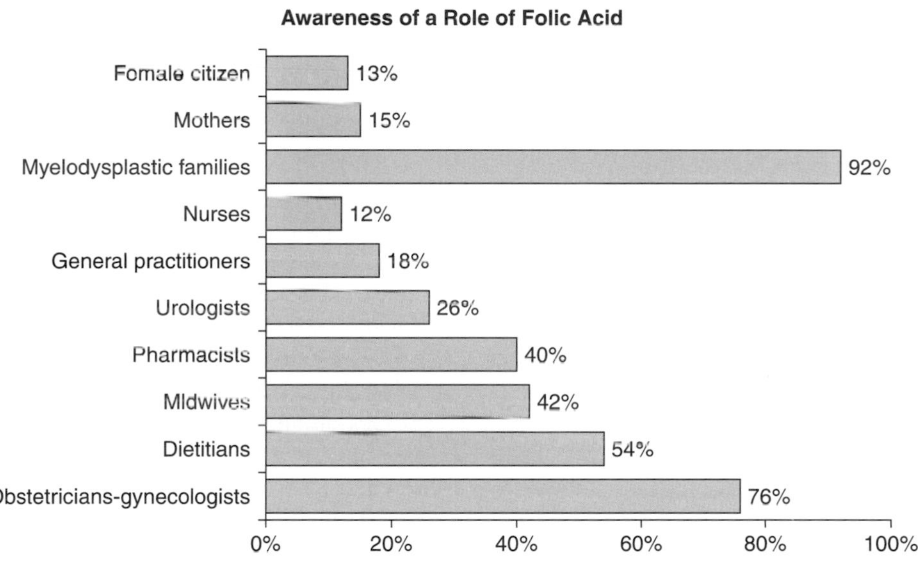

Figure 63.8
Awareness of the role of folic acid among 3 groups of laymen and 7 groups of healthcare providers. Reprinted with permission from Wiley-Blackwell (J Obstet Gynaecol Res 2005; 31: 172–7).

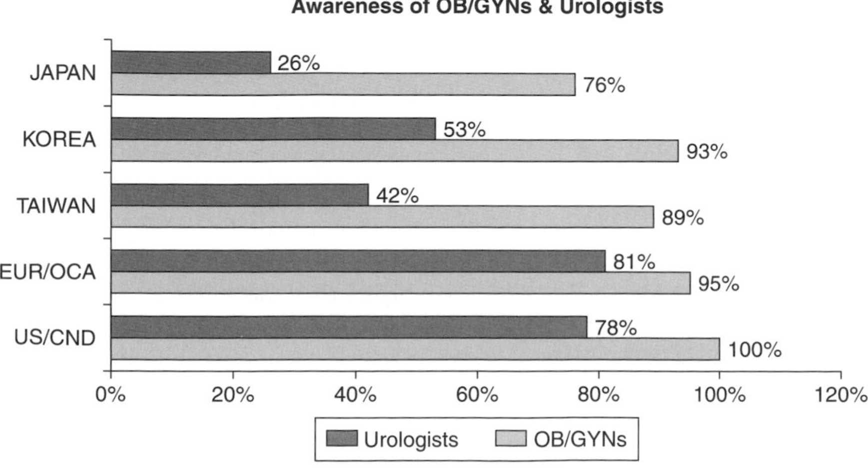

Figure 63.9
Awareness of the role of folic acid was internationally evaluated among obstetricians-gynecologists and urologists. EUR/OCA, Europe/Oceania; US/CND, The United States/Canada. Reprinted with permission from Wiley-Blackwell (J Obstet Gynaecol Res 2007; 33: 63–7).

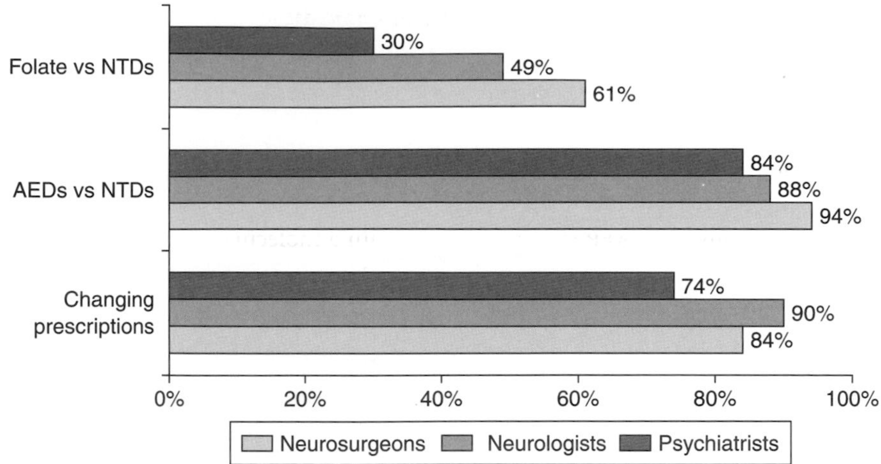

Figure 63.10
Awareness of a pivotal relationship between folic acid and neural tube defects (NTDs), and between anti-epileptic drugs (AEDs) and NTDs, and responses of neurosurgeons, neurologists, and psychiatrists when asked about the treatment of young women who plan to conceive.

psychiatrists were randomly chosen and their response rates were 31%, 43%, and 37%, respectively. An average of 47% (range 30–61%) of doctors knew the important role played by folic acid; nevertheless, 89% (range 84–94%) of the doctors correctly recognized the correlation between AEDs and congenital anomalies such as myelodysplasia. A mean of 83% (range 74–90%) of the doctors responded that they would reduce the dose of AEDs, decrease the number of AEDs, or prescribe folic acid tablets when their patient conceives or plans to conceive.

Economic benefits of fortification

The economic burden of spina bifida in the USA was calculated in 1989; at that time in the USA, 1500 infants with spina bifida were born each year and more than 1000 were expected to survive into childhood.[100] It was reported that the average annual cost for medical and surgical care for all these surviving children would approach $100 million and that an individual with typical severe spina bifida would require $250 000 as lifetime expenses, which would comprise direct (medical and surgical care, long-term care, disability management, and education) and indirect costs (survivor productivity effects and loss of parental income). In 1993, the Food and Drug Administration[101] performed a cost-benefit analysis for food fortification with folic acid at 140 μg/100 g and estimated that the net monetary benefit would be $651 to $788 million per year. Romano and associates from California[102] analyzed the economic benefit of fortifying cereal grain with folate prior to the release of the USA government fortification mandate. Under a range of assumptions about discount rates based on the aggregate cost in dollars, baseline folate intake, effectiveness of folate in preventing NTDs, threshold dose that minimizes risk, and cost of surveillance, they predicted a benefit of $94 million with low-level folate fortification (140 μg/100 g grain) and of $252 million with high-level folate fortification (350 μg/100 g grain). After 10 years, the same group of authors[103] re-evaluated the benefits of folic acid fortification, because they observed a greater decline in the NTD rates than that predicted before fortification. Their new estimate was that the annual economic benefit of $312 million to $425 million was associated with folic acid fortification together with a net reduction in the direct cost to the patients ranging from $88 million to $145 million per year. It is thus quite obvious that fortification of grain products saves $400 to $500 million each year in the USA. Governments that have not mandated food fortification with folic acid should seriously consider programs similar to those in the USA or UK in order to reduce the prevalence of infants with NTDs and to reduce the economic burden.

The practical guideline for obstetricians and gynecologists

The Society of Obstetricians and Gynaecologists of Canada recommended a practical guideline to prescribe folic acid to women of reproductive age.[104] The guidelines comprise the following points:

1. Pregnant women should be advised to maintain a healthy nutritional diet.
2. Women at no risk of NTD should be prescribed a daily multivitamin containing 0.4–1.0 mg folic acid.
3. Women at intermediate or high risk for NTD should be prescribed 4–5 mg/day folic acid; in such cases the supplement should contain folic acid alone and should not be in a multivitamin form so that the risk of excess

intake of other vitamins such as vitamin A can be avoided.

4. Signs or symptoms of vitamin B12 deficiency should be considered before initiating folic acid supplementation of doses greater than 1.0 mg/day.
5. Pregnant women should be advised to undergo serum triple marker screening at 15 to 20 weeks, ultrasound at 16 to 20 weeks, and amniocentesis after 15 weeks only when the positive screening test is present.

Prenatal diagnosis of spina bifida

In the 1970s, it became apparent that a fetus with an open NTD has increased levels of maternal serum alpha-fetoprotein (MSAFP). Since then, the combination of MSAFP and imaging examinations such as ultrasound (US) and magnetic resonance imaging (MRI) has become the major diagnostic modality for detecting NTDs.[105] In many countries, screening of MSAFP for NTDs is routinely performed during pregnancy at 16–18 weeks of gestation. In the low-risk pregnancies, MSAFP measurement can detect 80–90% of fetuses with NTDs. The result of MSAFP measurement is expressed as the multiple of the median (MoM), and cases with over 2.5 times MoM are regarded to be at risk of this anomaly. Positive findings of either MSAFP plus US or MSAFP plus MRI can be followed by amniocentesis, detailed US, or both. When amniocentesis is performed, amniotic fluid alpha-fetoprotein (AFP) and acetylcholinesterase concentrations can be used as a marker to confirm the presence of open spina bifida and to differentiate open ventral wall defects, such as gastroschisis and omphalocele, from open NTDs. Additionally, the fetal karyotype can be examined to rule out chromosomal anomalies. When spina bifida is definitely diagnosed, spontaneous leg and foot motions, leg and spine deformities, the presence of Chiari II malformation, and other physical defects should be evaluated by US.[106] Both US and MRI will easily reveal anomalies of myelomeningocele. Excellent detail and soft-tissue resolution can be obtained with MRI, but US is probably more accurate in determining the level of the defect and the termination of the neural placode; thus, the two modalities are complementary. Persson et al[107] assessed the clinical effectiveness of fetal US combined with semiquantitative measurements of the MSAFP level for the early detection of NTDs and omphalocele in 10 147 pregnancies. They reported that 8 out of 10 cases with malformations were detected when both the modalities were used simultaneously. However, if the screening was performed with either US or AFP alone, only 4 or 7 malformations were identified, respectively. In the 1990s, a new technology of three-dimensional and four-dimensional brain ultrasonography was developed; though this new technology has obvious advantages over the conventional one, the highly expensive machine prevents its introduction as a standard diagnostic procedure.[108]

Alpha-fetoprotein

AFP is a glycoprotein with a molecular weight of approximately 70 000 and is produced as early as 5 weeks' gestation by the embryonic yolk sac. The fetal liver and gastrointestinal tract become the main source of AFP production after 11 weeks of gestation.[109,110] The highest concentration of AFP is found in the fetal blood, followed by the amniotic fluid, and maternal blood. Alpha-fetoprotein is believed to enter the maternal blood by diffusion through the placental membranes and deciduas.[111] The MSAFP concentration increases throughout pregnancy, stabilizing at approximately 30 weeks' gestation; its peak level in the amniotic fluid occurs at 14 postmenstrual weeks. Because of this non-correspondence in the timing of the maximum AFP level in the maternal serum and amniotic fluid, knowledge about the accurate fetal age is indispensable.[112] In the case of an NTD-afflicted fetus, the amount of AFP transferred to the amnion from the fetal circulation also increases. Brock et al[113] first reported in 1973 that the MSAFP measurement was useful for detecting anencephaly in pregnant women. Wald et al[114] further observed that spina bifida and anencephaly could be identified based on the elevated MSAFP. The first large population-based study on MSAFP was reported from the UK in 1977; this study investigated 18 684 singleton pregnancies and 163 twin pregnancies without fetal NTDs, and 301 singleton pregnancies with fetal NTDs.[19] At 16–18 weeks of pregnancy, 88% of cases of anencephaly, 79% of cases of open spina bifida, and 3% of cases of unaffected singleton pregnancy exhibited AFP levels equal to or greater than 2–5 times the MoM. The results indicated that screening women by MSAFP measurement is effective in selecting women for US and amniocentesis.

Milunsky and Alpert[115] offered MSAFP screening to 21 000 nondiabetic and 442 diabetic pregnant women with apparently normal pregnancies. They observed that detection rates before 24 weeks of gestation were 86% (12/14) for anencephaly, 63% (5/8) for open and closed spina bifida, and 100% (1/1) for encephalocele. A raised MSAFP level was observed in 10 of the 442 diabetic women; 4 of these 10 women were carrying a fetus with an open NTD. Nevertheless, the authors expressed a strong caution against the use of MSAFP screening outside an established program coordinating the expertise of obstetricians, clinical geneticists, ultrasonographers, and laboratory staff. A cost-benefit analysis of MSAFP screening is an important issue because a large number of women are willing to undergo the test. Layde et al[116] considered the economic consequences of MSAFP screening coupled with US and amniocentesis, which were indicated in a hypothetic cohort of 100 000 pregnant women at a risk of having an affected fetus and who would elect to terminate their pregnancies if a malformed fetus were detected. The total cost of the program to screen 100 000 such women was calculated to be $2 047 000, or slightly over $20 per woman screened, and the total economic benefits exceeded $4 000 000. Prenatal screening with MSAFP is being widely employed in most developed countries, although ethical problems related to AFP screening and termination of the affected fetuses remain to be solved and have been disputed in several countries.

The relationship between the amniotic fluid AFP and the occurrence of NTDs was evaluated by the second report of the UK Collaborative Study in 1979.[117] Data on 13 105 singleton pregnancies without fetal NTDs and on 385 pregnancies with fetal NTDs were accumulated. By using different cut-off levels at different gestational ages, such as 2.5 times the median value at 13–15 weeks, 3 times at 16–18 weeks, 3.5 times at 19–21 weeks, and 4 times at 22–24 weeks, 98% of spina bifida (120/123) and 98% of anencephaly (218/222) cases exhibited positive findings, while the false positive rate was only 0.48% (61/12 804 pregnancies) in unaffected singleton pregnancies. Although the amniotic fluid AFP level exhibits a very high detection rate of NTDs, the sampling procedure is not only invasive but also harmful to some mothers and fetuses. Subsequently, amniocentesis has not prevailed as a screening technique in the low-risk group of women.

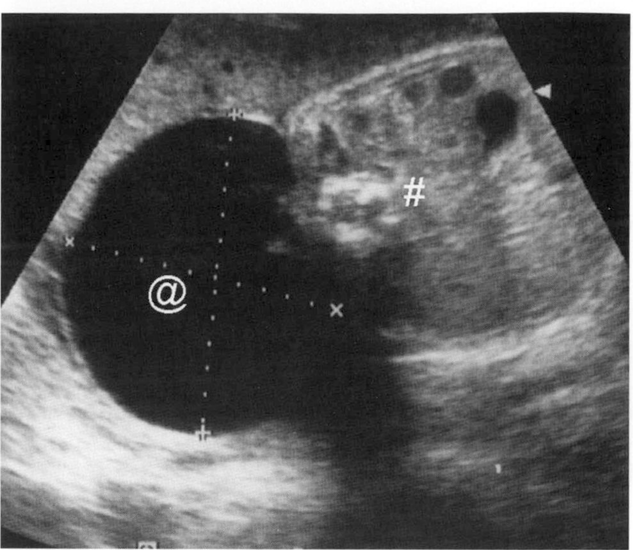

Figure 63.11
(Case 1) Transverse fetal ultrasonography of myelomeningocele at 31 weeks of gestation. A 78 mm × 68 mm ballooned cyst (@) is connected to the spine (#).

Ultrasound

It has been widely accepted that the diagnostic accuracy of US is excellent in pregnancies at a high risk of NTDs. Robbin et al[118] reported an adjunctive role of targeted sonography when elevated levels of amniotic fluid AFP (AF-AFP) were detected. From 1978 to 1990, the authors performed amniocentesis in 22 356 patients because of advanced maternal age, history of NTDs and chromosomal anomaly, and abnormal values of MSAFP. A total of 263 cases with an elevated AF-AFP of more than 2 MoM were examined by sonologists with knowledge that the patient was at increased risk for NTDs and other defects. Sonography correctly diagnosed 84 of 89 cases with anomalies (sensitivity of 94%) and identified anomalies in none of 174 patients (specificity of 100%). As for NTDs, US was powerful in depicting all the 32 cases (sensitivity and specificity are both 100%). Although amniocentesis carries a 0.7% risk of pregnancy loss, the authors believe that AF-AFP analysis followed by detailed US is highly successful for the detection of anomalous fetuses and the recognition of normal fetuses.

Since there is a definite risk related to amniocentesis, one should carefully evaluate the risk of the procedure against the additional information that would be provided. Nadel et al[119] discussed whether amniocentesis is necessary for those with elevated MSAFP by evaluating data from the Malformation Surveillance Program at Brigham and Women's Hospital. The authors found 198 pregnancies affected with spina bifida, encephalocele, gastroschisis, or omphalocele that ended in delivery or voluntary termination from 1984 to 1990. Of the 198, 51 underwent sonography between the 16th and 24th weeks of gestation at their facility with experienced sonologists with sophisticated machines, i.e., level 2 scans. All the pregnancies were correctly diagnosed in the first evaluation in comparison with clinical or autopsy findings with a sensitivity of 100% (95% confidence interval: 94 to 100%), while there were no false negative results. Since there is considerable overlap between MSAFP values in normal pregnancies and in pregnancies affected with malformations, the likelihood that a patient with an elevated level of MSAFP is carrying an affected fetus is low. The authors calculated likelihood ratios based on previous published data, and suggested that the likelihood of one of these anomalies in a fetus whose mother had, for instance, an MSAFP of 3.0 times MoM is less than 0.07% if she had normal findings with the level 2 US scan. The authors recommended that women with elevated MSAFP be assessed with the level 2 US. If the scan is normal, the parents can be counseled that the risk of an anomaly is low and can make an informed decision about whether to proceed with amniocentesis.

With fetal growth, myelomeningocele is observed as a cystic tumor attached to the spine (Figures 63.11 and 63.12), as an abnormal alignment, or as separation or defect of the vertebral arch (Figure 63.13). Establishing a

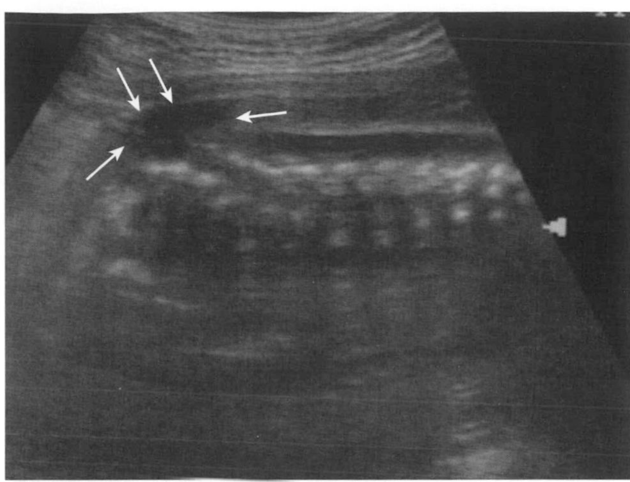

Figure 63.12
(Case 2) Sagittal spine ultrasonography in a fetus with spina bifida at 30 weeks of gestation. An echogenic cyst, indicated by arrows, is located at the caudal end of the spine.

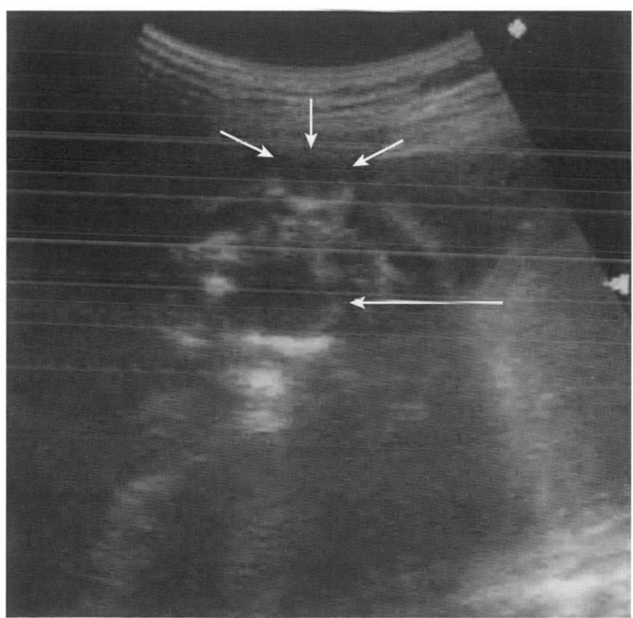

Figure 63.13
(Case 2) Transverse ultrasonography of the spine at the affected spine level. A cyst is indicated with short arrows, while a long arrow indicates the urinary bladder.

diagnosis is somewhat difficult when the fetus has myeloschisis or a small myelomeningocele. Furthermore, since the vertebral arch is not closed until 15 weeks of gestation, i.e., physiologic spina bifida, it is not easy to precisely detect spina bifida before 22 weeks' gestation. On the other hand, the observation of ventriculomegaly or microcephalus

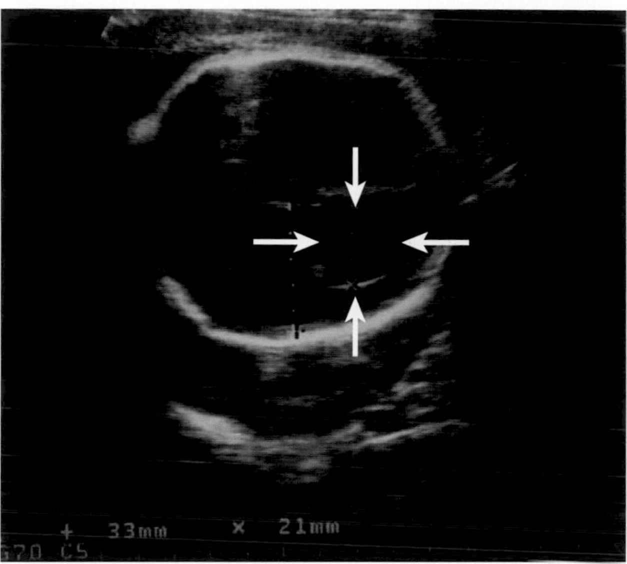

Figure 63.14
(Case 2) Fetal head ultrasonography at the biparietal diameter level. The lateral ventricle indicated with arrows is moderately dilated.

on the fetal cranium would often suggest the presence of NTDs. Figure 63.14 illustrates a fetal head sonography of the patient in Figure 63.12 at the biparietal diameter level. The lateral ventricle is moderately dilated; the ratio of the lateral ventricle width to the hemispheric width (LVW/HW) is 0.43 where the normal ratio ranged from 0.22 to 0.37 with a mean of 0.3.[120]

There are two significant cranial and cerebellar signs in spina bifida: *the lemon sign* and *the banana sign* (Figure 63.15). Nicolaides et al[121] retrospectively reviewed the records of 70 fetuses referred to their unit at 16–23 weeks of gestation, and identified two prominent imaging signs. Firstly, *the lemon sign*, presenting as scalloping of the frontal bones, was observed in all 54 cases of open spina bifida wherein images were obtained at the level of the biparietal diameter (BPD). The Arnold–Chiari II malformation observed in open spina bifida may be attributed to tethering of the spinal cord at the site of the lesion, with the downward displacement of the brain as the fetus grows. This movement reduces the contents of the cranium and leads to a decrease in the BPD and head circumference, resulting in the lemon sign. This sign is observed at the biparietal level (Figure 63.16) until 24 weeks of gestation in 90–100% of cases of open spina bifida. Secondly, *the banana sign*, presenting as the anterior curvature of the cerebellar hemispheres and obliterated cisterna magna, was observed in 12 of 21 fetuses for whom suboccipital bregmatic views were obtained. The abnormal shape of the cerebellar hemisphere resembles that of the banana. In 8 of the 21 cases the cerebellum could not be seen, and 1 case exhibited normal cerebellar hemispheres. Neither the lemon sign nor the

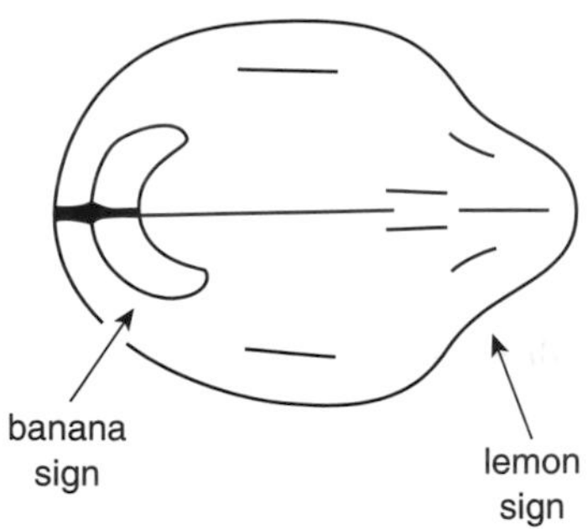

Figure 63.15
Schematic representation of the lemon sign and the banana sign. Reprinted with permission from Elsevier (The Lancet 1986; 2: 72–4).

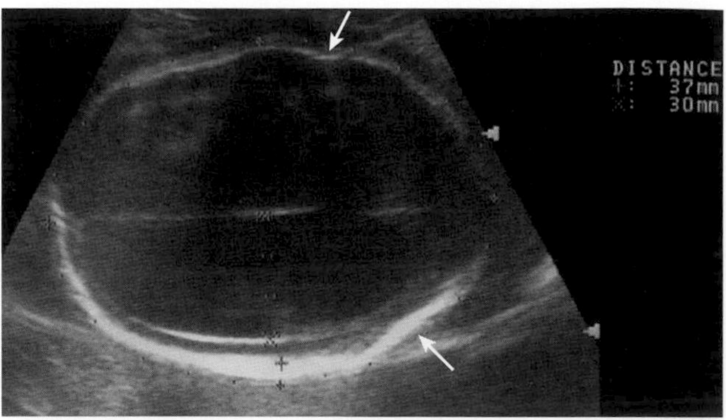

Figure 63.16
(Case 3) Head ultrasonography at the biparietal diameter level at 32 weeks of gestation in a spina bifida case. The lemon sign at the frontal bones is illustrated with two arrows.

banana sign was observed in 100 control fetuses. Because an anteriorly pointed configuration of the cerebellar hemisphere is present in Arnold–Chiari II malformation, downward traction on the cord may force the cerebellum to wrap around the brainstem, thus creating the banana sign. The presence of fetal microcephaly, ventriculomegaly, the lemon sign, the banana sign, and absent cerebellum should alert the ultrasonographer to the possibility of open spina bifida and encourage a detailed examination of NTDs.

Campbell et al[20] prospectively assessed cranial and cerebellar ultrasound markers of open spina bifida in 436 fetuses referred during 16–23 weeks' gestation. Of these, 26 fetuses (6%) had open spina bifida, 14 (3%) had major structural anomalies, and the remaining 396 (91%) were identified as normal fetuses. The authors reported that the sensitivities of the lemon sign and banana sign/absent cerebellum were 100% and 99%, respectively, and that the specificities were 99% and 100%, respectively. Benacerraf et al[122] evaluated the usefulness of the banana sign in 23 fetuses with NTDs and 38 control fetuses. They observed the banana sign in 22 of the 23 NTD-affected fetuses (96%), but none in the control fetuses. They mentioned that this sign is an indirect sign of open spina bifida in cases where the sonographic detection of NTDs is difficult. Van den Hof et al[123] evaluated the presence of the lemon and banana signs in 130 fetuses with open spina bifida and found a relationship between gestational age and the presence of these markers. The lemon sign was present in 98% of the fetuses of less than or equal to 24 weeks' gestation, but in only 13% of the fetuses of more than 24 weeks' gestation. The cerebellar abnormality was present in 95% of fetuses irrespective of their gestational age. However, the banana sign (72%) was predominant at less than 24 weeks' gestation, while the 'absence' of the cerebellum (81%) was the predominant sign at more 24 weeks' gestation.

Boyd et al[21] reported a large population-based study concerning prenatal diagnosis of spina bifida by US and biochemical screening. During a 30-month study period, 670 766 deliveries occurred in 18 congenital malformation registers from 11 European countries. An NTD was diagnosed at delivery in 542 cases, i.e., at a rate of 0.81 per 1000 deliveries. Of the 542 cases, the lesion was isolated in 84% of cases: 252 cases of spina bifida, 166 cases of anencephaly, and 35 cases of encephalocele were diagnosed prenatally (Table 63.12). The accuracy of prenatal diagnosis was 68%, 96%, and 60%, respectively. It is to be noted that the mean reduction in birth prevalence of spina bifida due to termination of pregnancy was 47%; the largest reduction was attained in France (91%) and UK (83%) centers, and the lowest reduction was found in Lithuania (6%). It is observed that routine US scans obtained at 18–22 weeks are significantly more effective than no routine US to identify anencephaly (85% vs 97%) and spina bifida (47% vs 71%), and that AFP or triple test screening is also significantly more valuable than no biochemical screening to diagnose spina bifida (52% vs 87%). The authors concluded that (1) US was an effective tool for the prenatal detection of NTDs because the detection rate of spina bifida was not as high as that of anencephaly, (2) there was a wide variation between centers with regard to the prenatal detection rate (33–100%), rate of termination of prenatally diagnosed abnormal pregnancies (17–100%), and gestational age at both diagnosis and termination of pregnancy, and (3) this variation may reflect the different policies and cultural differences between countries.

Chan et al[124] reported that the sensitivity of US screening for spina bifida increased with the level of risk in pregnancy: 60% in low-risk pregnancies, 89% in high-risk pregnancies, and 100% in women referred for the confirmation of spina bifida, and that US screening for NTDs achieved a higher level of sensitivity with an MSAFP program in place. Norem et al[125] compared the clinical value of MSAFP screening with that of US in the diagnosis of NTDs among 219 000 consecutive pregnancy outcomes. They detected 189 NTD cases, 102 of which had undergone MSAFP screening. However, the outcome of MSAFP was negative in

Table 63.12 *Isolated spina bifida was found at delivery in 252 of 542 cases with NTDs. A total of 68% of the 252 were prenatally diagnosed by ultrasonography and 47% of pregnancy was terminated*

Congenital malformation centers/Country	Prevalence per 1,000 births	Number of cases	Prenatally diagnosed (%)	Termination of pregnancy	
				n	%
Austria	0.21	6	83	1	17
Croatia	0.47	5	60	2	40
Denmark	0.68	6	50	1	17
France (2 centers)	0.37	22	80–100	20	80–100
Germany (2 centers)	0.81	15	70–80	5	20–60
Italy (3 centers)	0.21	41	60–83	28	20–78
Lithuania	0.63	63	38	4	6
Spain (2 centers)	0.48	12	63–75	6	50 & 50
The Netherlands (2 centers)	0.6	14	33–58	4	8 25
UK (2 centers)	0.52	36	96–100	30	82–88
Ukraine	0.49	22	82	17	77
Total	0.45	252	68	118	47

25 of the 102 cases (25%) and the correct diagnosis would have been missed without other screening tests. Of the 186 NTD cases diagnosed prenatally, 115 (62%) were initially detected by routine US, 69 (37%) were diagnosed by targeted US after MSAFP had indicated a higher risk for NTD, and 2 (1%) were diagnosed by pathologic examination after miscarriage. The authors concluded that routine second-trimester US was more efficient in detecting an NTD. Dashe et al[126] assessed the efficacy of MSAFP screening and standard US scan for detecting NTD in one institution. They detected 66 NTDs, 1 per 950 deliveries, and the sensitivities of MSAFP and US were 65% and 100%, respectively. The authors mentioned that standard US improved the NTD detection rate over MSAFP screening alone, and this observation was in general accord with previous reports.

Briefly, US at the second trimester is superior to MSAFP measurements in terms of identifying NTDs and should be the first-line screening tool for pregnant women.

Magnetic resonance imaging

Prenatal MRI is a useful diagnostic tool to detect the details of fetal anomalies, and its use would lead to the diagnosis of spina bifida and placental abnormalities with great accuracy.[127] In 2003, Aaronson et al[128] compared transabdominal US and fetal MRI with regard to the level of occurrence of myelomeningocele in the first 100 fetuses who underwent intrauterine myelomeningocele repair. They reported that the findings at prenatal MRI and US were equally accurate with regard to the assignment of the myelomeningocele level in a fetus. In 2000, Tortori-Donati et al[129] reviewed the neurologic features of spinal dysraphism and correlated them with clinical findings. A series of 986 patients were diagnosed and imaged with MRI at their spina bifida center over a 24-year period. They divided spinal dysraphism into open and closed forms. An open spinal dysraphism (OSD), comprising 353 children (36%), is a condition wherein the neural elements and/or their coverings are exposed through a bone defect and are not covered with skin. OSD was subdivided into two major diagnoses: myelomeningocele and myelocele. The Arnold–Chiari II malformation is always accompanied by OSD, and is a complex congenital anomaly of the hindbrain, characterized by a posterior cranial fossa that is smaller than normal, accompanied by the caudal displacement of the vermis, brainstem, and fourth ventricle. A closed spinal dysraphism (CSD), comprising 633 children (64%), is a condition wherein the neural elements and/or their coverings are covered with skin and is more heterogeneous than OSD. Some of these lesions are not clinically evident at birth, and parents with these lesions may seek medical attention when complications such as tethered cord syndrome ensue later in infancy. Physicians and surgeons should not refrain from careful examination of the children's back as this leads to a correct diagnosis. In most cases, the mass was located at the lumbosacral level and a subcutaneous mass represented 18.8% of CSD cases in their series (119 cases).

Figure 63.17 demonstrates a small cyst located at the lower lumbosacral spine in sagittal T2-weighted MRI. Figure 63.18 shows separation of the vertebral arch in the middle and myelomeningocele protruding to the body surface in transverse MRI. In 2006, Wang et al[130] assessed the use of MRI in 34 women with complicated pregnancies at

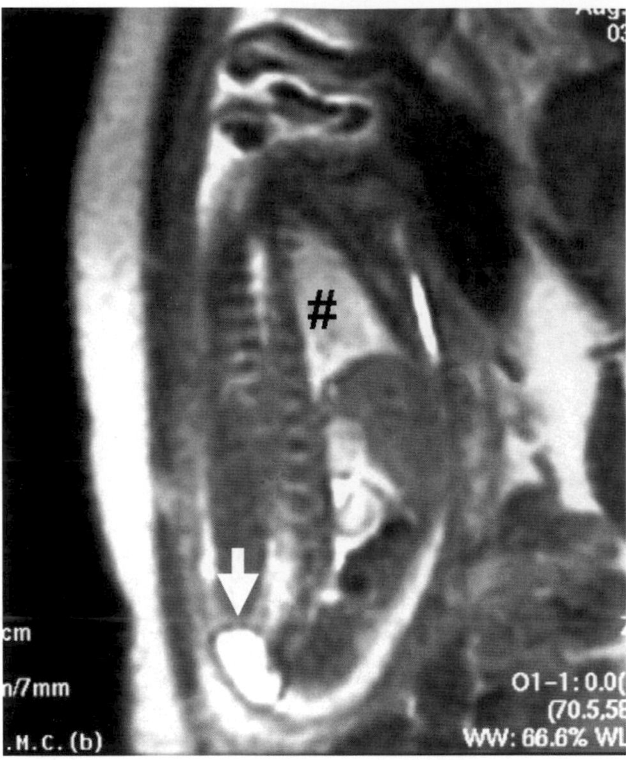

Figure 63.17
(Case 2) Sagittal T2-weighted fetal MRI at 30 weeks of gestation illustrates myelomeningocele. A cystic lesion consistent with a high signal intensity area is shown with an arrow at the sacral spine. The lung (#) is also clearly shown.

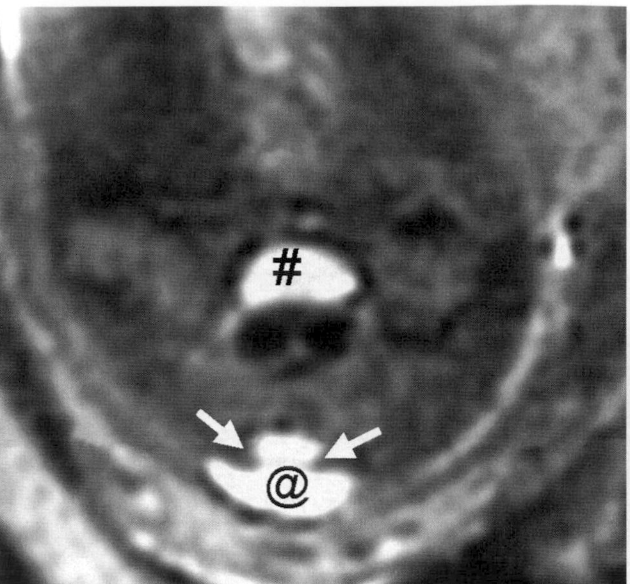

Figure 63.18
(Case 2) Transverse MRI of the fetal trunk at the affected spine level. The vertebral arch is separated (two arrows) and a cystic lesion (@) is illustrated on T2-weighted sequences. The urinary bladder (#) is shown in the middle.

a mean of 30 weeks of gestation. MRI was performed within 24 hours after US scan. The intracranial and spinal cord malformations were shown more clearly on T2-weighted MRI images than on T1-weighted images. MRI corrected the diagnosis of US in 10 cases (29%), and the diagnosis was missed in 1 case (3%). The authors considered MRI superior to US in terms of assessing the fetal central nervous system (CNS) in detail; however, in complicated pregnancies, MRI would be supplemental to US. Prenatal MRI has the advantage of better detection of associated CNS and non-CNS anomalies, which may have an impact on prognosis. Ultrafast T2-weighted sequences are useful for the prenatal detection of fetal CNS anomalies. It is important for an obstetrician to comprehend the fetal CNS condition in the uterus, and the findings thus obtained would lead to appropriate obstetric management.

From 1997 to 2004 in Miyazaki Medical College in Japan, one of us (SK) assessed the use of fetal MRI in patients with suspected hydrocephalus. There were 2042 deliveries during the period, 30 (1.5%) of which had been suspected of having hydrocephalus by US and subsequently underwent MRI examination. Of the 30 fetuses, MRI identified hydrocephalus in 24 (80%): 8 cases with Chiari II malformation with myelomeningocele, 5 cases with enphalocele, 5 cases with agenesis of corpus callosum (ACC), 2 cases with Dandy–Walker syndrome, 2 cases with stenosis of aqueductus cerebri, and 2 cases with porencephaly. Four cases suffered from agenesis of corpus callosum and the remaining 2 were normal. Postnatal MRI findings were consistent with the antenatal findings. Figure 63.19 reveals dilated lateral ventricles in T2-weighted fetal MRI, suggesting the presence of spinal dysraphism. Sagittal T2-weighted MRI (Figure 63.20) illustrates the smaller and tighter posterior cranial fossa, implying the descent of the cerebellum into the spinal cavity in Chiari II malformation together with a small cyst of the spinal canal in the sacrum.

In 2000, Simon et al[131] prospectively performed MRI tests in 73 fetuses with suspected CNS abnormalities and compared these with the available fetal US, postnatal images, and clinical examinations. They reported that 24 of 52 cases (46%) exhibited MRI findings that were different from the US findings. The referring physicians believed that MRI provided a measure of confidence that was valuable for counseling patients and for taking more informed decisions. Levine et al[132] assessed 214 fetuses using both US and MRI. US findings were normal in 69 and abnormal in 145, while MRI imaging findings changed the diagnosis in 46 of the 145 fetuses with abnormal US observations. Since therapeutic choices or management decisions often rely on an exact diagnosis, MRI is an important test for decreasing ambiguity in the counseling of expectant parents when questionable abnormalities are visualized on US but the

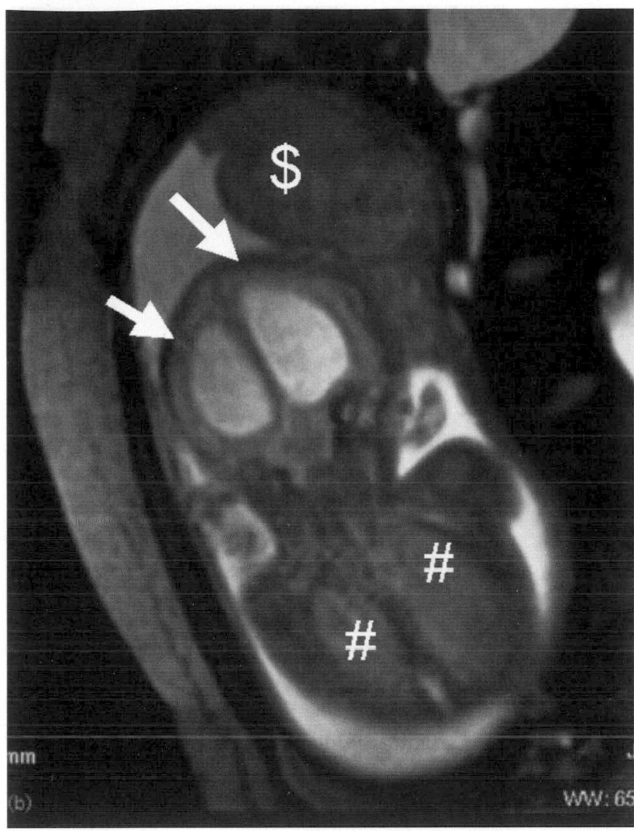

Figure 63.19
(Case 3) Dilated lateral ventricles are shown with arrows in T2-weighted sequences of MRI at 25 weeks of gestation. The lung (#) and the placenta ($) are also illustrated.

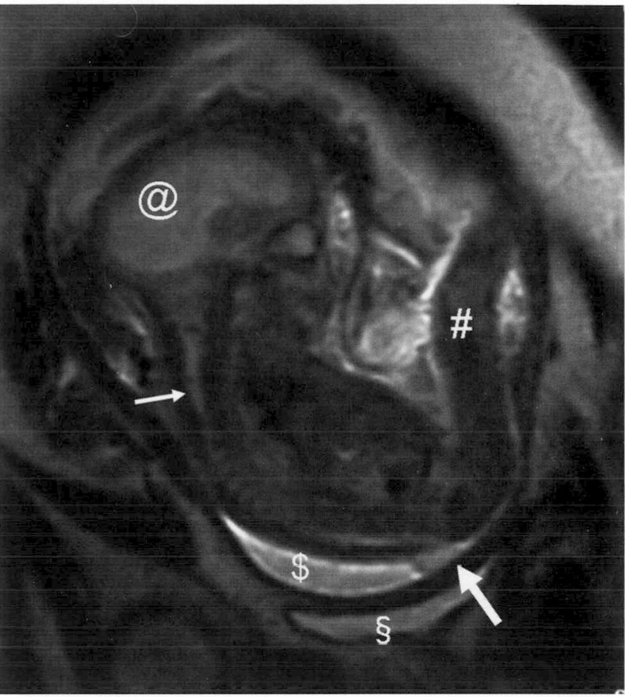

Figure 63.20
(Case 3) Sagittal T2-weighted imaging shows the dilated lateral ventricle (@), the spinal cord (small arrows), and a small cyst at the sacrum (a larger arrow). The fetal leg (#), the amniotic cavity ($), and the maternal urinary bladder (§) are also illustrated.

exact diagnosis is not obtainable. Briefly, US scan is inexpensive and remains the mainstay for diagnosis of NTDs. On the other hand, MRI of the fetal CNS is evolving as a powerful tool for obtaining additional information with which selected patients and their healthcare professionals can make decisions and execute important pregnancy managements. MRI and US are complementary, noninvasive imaging methods in the evaluation of high-risk pregnancy.

Summary

Primary prevention of NTDs by periconceptional intake of folic acid is a major public health opportunity and has a wide implication in reducing both mortality and morbidity due to congenital anomalies. Women who plan to conceive should be informed about the important role of folic acid in the development of a fetus; about avoiding exposure to environmental hazards, including a variety of medications; and about taking folic acid supplements in addition to a well-balanced diet. Once pregnancy is confirmed, conventional prenatal screening with ultrasound and MSAFP should be performed. In case of suspected fetal malformation, MRI and/or targeted US with/without amniocentesis should be indicated; the findings thus obtained should help decrease ambiguity and increase accuracy on fetal abnormalities. We totally agree with Swash[133] in the management of neural tube defects that 'prevention is better than cure'.

Acknowledgments

We are grateful to Tomoaki Ikeda, MD, for his contribution to the section on 'Prenatal diagnosis of spina bifida' and for the support of Komaki Shimin Hospital, Komaki. The present study was partly supported by Research Grants (14A–4 and 17A–6) for Nervous and Mental Disorders from the Ministry of Health, Labour and Welfare, Japan, and by grants from the Japan Spina Bifida and Hydrocephalus Research Foundation (2003 to 2006).

References

1. Moore JE. Spina bifida, with report of three hundred and eighty-five cases treated by excision. Surg Gynecol Obstet 1905; 1: 137–40.
2. Penfield W, Cone W. Spina bifida and cranium bifidum. JAMA 1932; 98: 454–61.

3. Bricker EM. Bladder substitution after pelvic evisceration. Surg Clin North Am 1950; 30: 1511–21.
4. Freeman JM. To treat or not treat: ethical dilemmas of treating the infant with a myelomeningocele. Clin Neurosurg 1973; 20: 134–46.
5. Shurtleff DB, Hayden PW, Loeser JD, Kronmal RA. Myelodysplasia: decision for death or disability. N Engl J Med 1974; 291: 1005–11.
6. Lorber J. Results of treatment of myelomeningocele. Develop Med Child Neurol 1971; 13: 279–303.
7. Lapides J, Diokno AC, Silber SJ, Lowe BS. Clean intermittent self-catheterization in the treatment of urinary tract disease. J Urol 1972; 107: 458–61.
8. Shapiro SR, Lebowitz R, Colodny AH. Fate of 90 children with ileal conduit urinary diversion a decade later: analysis of complications, pyelography, renal function and bacteriology. J Urol 1975; 114: 289–95.
9. Borden TA, Kaplan WE, McGuire EJ et al. Urinary undiversion in patients with myelodysplasia and neurogenic bladder dysfunction. Urology 1980; 18: 223–8.
10. Perlmutter AD. Experiences with urinary undiversion in children with neurogenic bladder. J Urol 1980; 123: 402–6.
11. Goldwasser B, Webster GD. Augmentation and substitution enterocystoplasty. J Urol 1986; 135: 215–24.
12. Mitrofanoff P. Cystostomie continente trans-appendiculaire dans le traitement des vessies neurologiques. Chir Pediatr 1980; 21: 297–305. [In French]
13. Malone PS, Ransley PG, Kiely EM. Preliminary report: the antegrade continence enema. Lancet 1990; 336: 1217–18.
14. MRC vitamin study research group. Prevention of neural tube defects: results of the Medical Research Council Vitamin Study. Lancet 1991; 338: 131–7.
15. Berry RJ, Li Z, Erickson JD et al. Prevention of neural-tube defects with folic acid in China. N Engl J Med 1999; 341: 1485–90.
16. Ministry of Health and Welfare of Japan. Information on promoting intake of folic acid in order to reduce children afflicted with neural tube defects among young women who are capable of becoming pregnant. A report of the Ministry of Health and Welfare, Tokyo, December 28, 2000. [In Japanese]
17. Cornel MC, Erickson JD. Comparison of national policies on periconceptional use of folic acid to prevent spina bifida and anencephaly (SBA). Teratology 1997; 55: 134–7.
18. Wald NJ, Law MR, Morris JK, Wald DS. Quantifying the effect of folic acid. Lancet 2001; 358: 2069–73.
19. Wald NJ, Cuckle H, Brock JH et al. Maternal serum-alpha-fetoprotein measurement in antenatal screening for anencephaly and spina bifida in early pregnancy. Report of UK collaborative study on alpha-fetoprotein in relation to neural-tube defects. Lancet 1977; 1: 1323–32.
20. Campbell J, Gilbert WM, Nicolaides KH, Campbell S. Ultrasound screening for spina bifida: cranial and cerebellar signs in a high-risk population. Obstet Gynecol 1987; 70: 247–50.
21. Boyd PA, Wellesley DG, De Walle HEK et al. Evaluation of the prenatal diagnosis of neural tube defects by fetal ultrasonographic examination in different centres across Europe. J Med Screen 2000; 7: 169–74.
22. Shurtleff DB. Epidemiology of neural tube defects and folic acid. Cerebrospinal Fluid Res 2004; 1: 5–8.
23. Laurence KM, Carter CO, David PA. Major central nervous system malformations in South Wales. Br J Prevent Soc Med 1967; 21: 146–60.
24. Morris JK, Wald NJ. Quantifying the decline in the birth prevalence of neural tube defects in England and Wales. J Med Screen 1999; 6: 182–5.
25. Gos M, Szpecht-Potocka A. Genetic basis of neural tube defects. II. Genes correlated with folate and methionine metabolism. J Appl Genet 2002; 43: 511–24.
26. Rankin J, Glinianaia S, Brown R, Renwick M. The changing prevalence of neural tube defects: a population-based study in the North of England, 1984–96. Paediatr Perinat Epidemiol 2000; 14: 104–10.
27. Sumiyoshi Y. Monitoring of congenital anomalies in the intractable ailments. Report of the Ministry of Health, Labour and Welfare, Japan, http://mhlw-grants.niph.go.jp (February 2007). [In Japanese]
28. Sadler TW. Mechanisms of neural tube closure and defects. MRDD Res Rev 1998; 4: 247–53.
29. Botto LD, Moore CA, Khoury MJ, Erickson JD. Neural tube defects. N Engl J Med 1999; 341: 1509–19.
30. Hall J, Solehdin F. Folic acid for the prevention of congenital anomalies. Eur J Pediatr 1998; 157: 445–50.
31. Molloy AM. Role of genetic variation in establishing nutritional requirements: folate, a case in point. World Rev Nutr Diet 2001; 89: 68–75.
32. Sharp L, Little J. Polymorphism in genes involved in folate metabolism and colorectal neoplasia. Am J Epidemiol 2004; 159: 423–43.
33. Molloy AM, Daly S, Mills JL et al. Thermolabile variant of 5,10-methylenetetrahydrofolate reductase associated with low red-cell folate: implications for folate intake recommendations. Lancet 1997; 349: 1591–3.
34. Van der Put NM, Steegers-Theunissen RPM, Frosst P et al. Mutated methylenetetrahydrofolate reductase as a risk factor for spina bifida. Lancet 1995; 346: 1070–1.
35. Miyake K, Murata M, Kikuchi H et al. Assessment of tailor-made prevention of atherosclerosis with folic acid supplementation: randomized, double-blind, placebo-controlled trials in each MTHFR C677T genotype. J Hum Genet 2005; 50: 241–8.
36. Perez ABA, D'Almeida V, Vergani N et al. Methylenetetrahydrofolate reductase (MTHFR): incidence of mutations C677T and A1298C in Brazilian population and its correlation with plasma homocysteine levels in spina bifida. Am J Med Genet 2003; 119A: 20–5.
37. Parle-McDermott A, Mills JL, Kirke PN et al. Analysis of the MTHFR 1298AC and 677CT polymorphism as risk factors for neural tube defects. J Hum Genet 2003; 48: 190–3.
38. Kirke PN, Mills JL, Molloy AM et al. Impact of the MTHFR C677T polymorphism on risk of neural tube defects: case-control study. BMJ 2004; 328: 1535–6.
39. Mills JL, McPartlin JM, Kirke PN et al. Homocysteine metabolism in pregnancies complicated by neural-tube defects. Lancet 1995; 345: 149–51.
40. Chatkupt S, Skurnick JH, Jaggi M et al. Study of genetics, epidemiology, and vitamin usage in familial spina bifida in the United States in the 1990s. Neurology 1994; 44: 65–70.
41. McDonald SD, Perkins SL, Jodouin CA, Walker MC. Folate levels in pregnant women who smoke: an important gene/environment interaction. Am J Obstet Gynecol 2002; 187: 620–5.
42. Rothenberg SP, da Costa MP, Sequeira JM et al. Autoantibodies against folate receptors in women with a pregnancy complicated by a neural-tube defect. N Engl J Med 2004; 350: 134–42.
43. Welch AD. Folic acid: discovery and the exciting first decade. Perspect Biol Med 1983; 27: 64–75.
44. Willis L. The nature of the haemopoietic factor in marmite. Lancet 1933; 1: 1283–6.
45. Nelson MM. Teratogenic effects of pteroylglutamic acid deficiency in the rat. In: Wolstenholme GEW, O'Connor CM, eds. Ciba Foundation Symposium on Congenital Malformations. Boston: Little, Brown and Co, 1960: 134–51.
46. Hibbard BM. The role of folic acid in pregnancy. J Obstet Gynaecol Br Commonwealth 1964; 71: 529–42.
47. Hibbard ED, Smithells RW. Folic acid metabolism and human embryopathy. Lancet 1965; i: 1254.
48. Smithells RW, Sheppard S, Schorah CJ et al. Possible prevention of neural-tube defects by periconceptional vitamin supplementation. Lancet 1980; i: 339–40.
49. Laurence KM, James N, Miller MH, Tennant GB, Campbell H. Double-blind randomized controlled trial of folate treatment before conception to prevent recurrence of neural-tube defects. BMJ 1981; 282: 1509–11.

50. Czeizel AE, Dudas I. Prevention of the first occurrence of neural tube defects by periconceptional vitamin supplementation. N Engl J Med 1992; 327: 1832–5.
51. Becerra JE, Khoury MJ, Cordero JF, Erickson JD. Diabetic mellitus during pregnancy and the risks for specific birth defects: a population-based case-control study. Pediatrics 1990; 85: 1–9.
52. Werler MM, Louik C, Shapiro S, Mitchell AA. Prepregnant weight in relation to risk of neural tube defects. JAMA 1996; 275: 1089–92.
53. Kaneko S. Antiepileptic drug therapy and reproductive consequences: functional and morphologic effects. Repr Toxicol 1991; 5: 179–98.
54. Goggin T, Gough H, Bussessar A et al. A comparative study of the relative effects of anticonvulsant drugs and dietary folate on the red cell folate status of patients with epilepsy. QJ Med 1987; 65(247): 911–19.
55. Kaneko S, Battino D, Andermann E et al. Congenital malformations due to antiepileptic drugs. Epilepsy Res 1999; 33: 145–58.
56. Crawford P. Best practice guideline for the management of women with epilepsy. Epilepsy 2005; 46(Suppl): 117–24.
57. Graham JM Jr, Edwards MJ, Edwards MJ. Teratogen update: gestational effects of maternal hyperthermia due to febrile illness and resultant patterns of defects in humans. Teratology 1998; 58: 209–21.
58. Russell RM, Golner BB, Krasinski SD et al. Effect of antacid and H2 receptor antagonists on the intestinal absorption of folic acid. J Lab Clin Med 1988; 112: 458–63.
59. Hernandez-Diaz S, Werler MM, Walker AM, Mitchell AA. Folic acid antagonists during pregnancy and the risk of birth defects. N Engl J Med 2000; 343: 1608–14.
60. Hernandez-Diaz S, Werler MM, Walker AM, Mitchell AA. Neural tube defects in relation to use of folic acid antagonists during pregnancy. Am J Epidemiol 2001; 153: 961–8.
61. Yasuda Y, Okamoto M, Konishi H et al. Developmental anomalies induced by all-trans retinoic acid in fetal mice: I. Macroscopic findings. Teratology 1986; 34: 37–49.
62. Rothman KJ, Moore LL, Singer MR et al. Teratogenicity of high vitamin A intake. N Engl J Med 1995; 333: 1369–73.
63. Abel EL. Smoking and pregnancy. J Psychoactive Drugs 1984; 16: 327–38.
64. Tuthill DP, Stewart JH, Coles EC, Andrews J, Cartridge PHT. Maternal cigarette smoking and pregnancy outcome. Paediatric Prenat Epidemiol 1999; 3: 245–53.
65. Hook EB, Cross PK. Maternal cigarette smoking, Down syndrome in live births, and infant race. Am J Hum Genet 1988; 42: 482–9.
66. Chun RC, Kowalski CP, Kim HM, Buchman SR. Maternal cigarette smoking during pregnancy and the risk of having a child with cleft lip/palate. Plast Reconstr Surg 2000; 105: 485–91.
67. American Academy of Pediatrics – Committee on environmental hazards. Effects of cigarette-smoking on the fetus and child. Pediatrics 1976; 57: 411–13.
68. Shurtleff D, Lemire RJ, Warkany J. Embryology, etiology, and epidemiology. In: Shurtleff DB, ed. Myelodysplasia and Extrophies. Orland: Grune & Stratton, Inc, 1986: 39–64.
69. Boyd PA, Chamberlain P, Hicks NR. 6-year experience of prenatal diagnosis in an unselected population in Oxford, UK. Lancet 1998; 352: 1577–81.
70. Villarreal LM, Perez JZV, Vazquez PA et al. Decline of neural tube defects cases after a folic acid campaign in Neuvo Leon, Mexico. Teratology 2002; 66: 249–56.
71. Wilcox AL, Lie RT, Solvoll K et al. Folic acid supplements and risk of facial clefts: national population based case-control study. BMJ 2007; 334: 464–7.
72. Kondo A, Kamihira O, Shimosuka Y et al. Awareness of the role of folic acid, dietary folate intake and plasma folate concentration in Japan. J Obstet Gynaecol Res 2005; 31: 172–7.
73. Vartanian LR, Schwartz MB, Brownell KD. Effects of soft drink consumption on nutrition and health: a systematic review and meta-analysis. Am J Public Health 2007; 97: 667–75.
74. Gucciardi E, Pietrusiak M-A, Reynolds DL, Rouleau J. Incidence of neural tube defects in Ontario, 1986–1999. CMAJ 2002; 167: 237–40.
75. Persad VL, Van den Hof MC, Dube M, Zimmer P. Incidence of open neural tube defects in Nova Scotia after folic acid fortification. CMAJ 2002; 167: 241–5.
76. Stevenson RE, Allen WP, Pai GS et al. Decline in prevalence of neural tube defects in a high-risk region of the United States. Pediatrics 2000; 106: 677–83.
77. Honein MA, Paulozzi LJ, Mathews TJ, Erickson JD, Wong L-Y C. Impact of folic acid fortification of the US food supply on the occurrence of neural tube defects. JAMA 2001; 285: 2981–6.
78. Mills JL, Signore C. Neural tube defect rates before and after food fortification with folic acid. Birth Defects Res (Part A) 2004; 70: 844–5.
79. Centers for Disease Control. Spina bifida and anencephaly before and after folic acid mandate: United States, 1995–1996 and 1999–2000. MMWR 2004; 53(17): 362–5.
80. Cuskelly GJ, McNulty H, Scott JM. Effect of increasing dietary folate on red-cell folate: implications for prevention of neural tube defects. Lancet 1996; 347: 657–9.
81. Daly S, Mills JL, Molloy AM et al. Minimum effective dose of folic acid for food fortification to prevent neural-tube defects. Lancet 1997; 350: 1666–9.
82. Jacques PF, Selhub J, Bostom AG, Wilson PWF, Rosenberg IH. The effect of folic acid fortification on plasma folate and total homocysteine concentrations. N Engl J Med 1999; 340: 1449–54.
83. Evans MI, Llurba E, Landsberger EJ, O'Briaen JE, Harrison HH. Impact of folic acid fortification in the United States: markedly diminished high maternal serum alpha-fetoprotein values. Obstet Gynecol 2004; 103: 474–9.
84. Laurence JM, Petitti DB, Watkins M, Umekubo MA. Trends in serum folate after food fortification. Lancet 1999; 354: 915–16.
85. Wald DA, Bishop L, Wald NJ et al. Randomized trial of folic acid supplementation and serum homocysteine levels. Arch Intern Med 2001; 161: 695–700.
86. Mills JL, Kohorn IV, Conley MR et al. Low vitamin B-12 concentration in patients without anemia: the effect of folic acid fortification of grain. Am J Clin Nutr 2003; 77: 1474–7.
87. Cole BF, Baron JA, Sadler RS, Haile RW, Ahnen DJ et al. Polyp prevention study group. Folic acid for the prevention of colorectal adenomas. JAMA 2007; 297: 2351–9.
88. Kim YI. Folate, colorectal carcinogenesis, and DNA methylation: lessons from animal studies. Environ Mol Mutagen 2004; 44: 10–25.
89. Giovannucci E. Epidemiologic studies of folate and colorectal neoplasia: a review. J Nutr 2002; 132: 2350S–55S.
90. Hiilesmaa VK, Teramo K, Granstrom M-L, Bardy AH. Serum folate concentrations during pregnancy in women with epilepsy: relation to antiepileptic drug concentrations, number of seizures, and fetal outcome. BMJ 1983: 287: 577–9.
91. Ogawa Y, Kaneko S, Otani K, Fukushima Y. Serum folic acid levels in epileptic mothers and their relationship to congenital malformations. Epilepsy Res 1991; 8: 75–8.
92. Tettenborn B. Management of epilepsy in women of childbearing age. CNS Drugs 2006; 20: 373–87.
93. De Walle HEK, Van der Pal KM, De Jong-van den Berg LTW et al. Periconceptional folic acid in the Netherlands in 1995. Socioeconomic difference. J Epidemiol Community Health 1998; 52: 826–7.
94. De Walle HEK, De Jong-van den Berg LTW, Cornel MC. Periconceptional folic acid intake in the northern Netherlands. Lancet 1999; 353: 1187.
95. Bekkers RLM, Eskes TKAB. Periconceptional folic acid intake in Nijmegen, Netherlands. Lancet 1999; 353: 292.
96. Department of Health, UK. Statistical work area: public health. http://www.dh.gov.uk./PublicationsAndStatistics/statistics/StatisticalWorkAreas/stasticticalpublichealth/fs/en (March 2007).

97. Phares TM, Morrow B, Lansky A et al. Surveillance for disparities in maternal health-related behaviors – selected states, pregnancy risk assessment monitoring system (PRAMS), 2000–2001. MMWR 2004; 53(SS04): 1–13.
98. Kondo A, Kamihira O, Gotoh M et al. Folic acid prevents neural tube defects: international comparison of awareness among obstetricians/gynecologists and urologists. J Obstet Gynecol Res 2007; 33: 63–7.
99. Kondo A, Kamihira O, Ozawa H, Gotoh M, Okai I. Anti-epileptic drugs and congenital anomalies: awareness among prescribing doctors. Nihon Iji-Shinpou 2006; 4281: 67–70. [In Japanese]
100. Centers for Disease Control. Economic burden of spina bifida – United States, 1980–1990. MMWR 1989; 38: 264–7.
101. Food and Drug Administration. Food standards: amendment of the standards of identity for enriched grain products to require addition of folic acid. Fed Reg 1993; 58: 53305–12.
102. Romano PS, Waitzman NJ, Scheffter RM, Pi RD. Folic acid fortification of grain: an economic analysis. Am J Public Health 1995; 85: 667–76.
103. Grosse SD, Waitzman NJ, Romano PS, Mulinare J. Reevaluating the benefits of folic acid fortification in the United States: economic analysis, regulation, and public health. Am J Public Health 2005; 95: 1917–22.
104. Wilson RD, Davies G, Desilets V et al. The use of folic acid for the prevention of neural tube defects and other congenital anomalies. J Obstet Gynaecol Can 2003; 25: 959–65.
105. Milunsky A. The prenatal diagnosis of neural tube and other congenital defects. In: Milunsky A, ed. Genetic disorders and the fetus: diagnosis, prevention and treatment. 2nd ed. New York: Plenum Press, 1986: 453–519.
106. Mitchell LE, Adzick NS, Melchionne J et al. Spina bifida. Lancet 2004; 364: 1885–95.
107. Persson PH, Kullander S, Gennser G, Grennert L, Laurell CB. Screening for fetal malformations using ultrasound and measurements of alpha-fetoprotein in maternal serum. BMJ 1983; 286: 747–9.
108. Stanojevic M, Pooh RK, Kurjak A, Kos M. Three-dimensional ultrasound assessment of the fetal and neonatal brain. Ultrasound Rev Obstet Gynecol 2003; 3: 117–30.
109. Gitlin D, Boesman M. Serum alpha-fetoprotein, albumin, and gamma-G-globulin in the human conceptus. J Clin Invest 1966; 45: 1826–38.
110. Gitlin D, Perricelli A. Synthesis of serum albumin, prealbumin, alpha-fetoprotein, alpha-1-antitrypsin and transferrin by the human yolk sac. Nature 1970; 228: 995–7.
111. Lau HL, Linkins SE. Alpha-fetoprotein. Am J Obstet Gynecol 1976; 124: 533–54.
112. Monteagudo A, Timor-Tritsch IE. Fetal neurosonography of congenital brain anomalies. In: Timor-Tritsch IE, Monteagudo A, Cohen HL, eds. Ultrasonography of the Prenatal and Neonatal Brain. 2nd ed. New York: McGraw-Hill, 2001: 151–4.
113. Brock DJ, Bolton AE, Monaghan JM. Prenatal diagnosis of anencephaly through maternal serum-alphafetoprotein measurement. Lancet 1973; 2: 923–4.
114. Wald NJ, Brock DJ, Bonnar J. Prenatal diagnosis of spina bifida and anencephaly by maternal serum-alpha-fetoprotein measurement. A control study. Lancet 1974; 1: 765–7.
115. Milunsky A, Alpert E. Results and benefits of a maternal serum alpha-fetoprotein screening program. JAMA 1984; 252: 1438–42.
116. Layde PM, von Allmen SD, Oakley GP Jr. Maternal serum alpha-fetoprotein screening: a cost-benefit analysis. Am J Public Health 1979; 69: 566–73.
117. Second report of the U.K. Collaborative study on alpha-fetoprotein in relation to neural-tube defects. Amniotic-fluid alpha-fetoprotein measurement in antenatal diagnosis of anencephaly and open spina bifida in early pregnancy. Lancet 1979; 2: 651–62.
118. Robbin M, Filly RA, Fell S et al. Elevated levels of amniotic fluid alpha-fetoprotein: sonographic evaluation. Radiology 1993; 188: 165–9.
119. Nadel AS, Green JK, Holmes LB, Frigoletto FD Jr, Benacerraf BR. Absence of need for amniocentesis in patients with elevated levels of maternal serum alpha-fetoprotein and normal ultrasonographic examinations. N Engl J Med 1990; 323: 557–61.
120. Jeanty P, Dramaix-Wilmet M, Delbeke D et al. Ultrasonic evaluation of fetal ventricular growth. Neuroradiology 1981; 21: 127–31.
121. Nicolaides KH, Campbell S, Gabbe SG, Guidetti R. Ultrasound screening for spina bifida: cranial and cerebellar signs. Lancet 1986; 2: 72–4.
122. Benacerraf BR, Stryker J, Frigoletto FD Jr. Abnormal appearance of the cerebellum, (banana sign): indirect sign of spina bifida. Radiology 1989; 171: 151–3.
123. Van den Hof MC, Nicolaides KH, Campbell J, Campbell S. Evaluation of the lemon and banana signs in one hundred thirty fetuses with open spina bifida. Am J Obstet Gynecol 1990; 162: 322–7.
124. Chan A, Robertson EF, Haan EA, Ranieri E, Keane RJ. The sensitivity of ultrasound and serum alpha-fetoprotein in population-based antenatal screening for neural tube defects. South Australia 1986–1991. Br J Obstet Gynaecol 1995; 102: 370–6.
125. Norem CT, Schoen EJ, Walton DI et al. Routine ultrasonography compared with maternal serum alpha-fetoprotein for neural tube defect screening. Obstet Gynecol 2005; 106: 747–52.
126. Dashe JS, Twickler DM, Santos-Ramos R, McIntire DD, Ramus RM. Alpha-fetoprotein detection of neural tube defects and the impact of standard ultrasound. Am J Obstet Gynecol 2006; 195: 1623–8.
127. Laifer-Narin S, Budorick NE, Simpson LL, Platt LD. Fetal magnetic resonance imaging: a review. Curr Opin Obstet Gynecol 2007; 19: 151–6.
128. Aaronson OS, Hernanz-Schulman M, Bruner JP, Reed GW, Tulipan NB. Myelomeningocele: prenatal evaluation – comparison between transabdominal US and MR imaging. Radiology 2003; 227: 839–43.
129. Tortori-Donati P, Rossi A, Cama A. Spinal dysraphism: a review of neuroradiological features with embryological correlations and proposal for a new classification. Neuroradiology 2000; 42: 471–91.
130. Wang GB, Shan RQ, Ma YX et al. Fetal central nervous system anomalies: comparison of magnetic resonance imaging and ultrasonography for diagnosis. Chin Med J 2006; 119: 1272–7.
131. Simon EM, Goldstein RB, Coakley FV et al. Fast MR imaging of fetal CNS anomalies in utero. AJNR 2000; 21: 1688–98.
132. Levine D, Barnes PD, Robertson RR, Wong G, Mehta TS. Fast MR imaging of fetal central nervous system abnormalities. Radiology 2003; 229: 51–61.
133. Swash M. Neural tube defects: prevention is better than cure. J R Soc Med 1982; 75: 689–90.

64

Initial management of meningo-myelocele children

Stuart B Bauer

First impressions

The urologic management of the newborn with myelodysplasia ideally begins shortly after the child is born and identified with a spinal abnormality. It is important to evaluate babies this early for a number of reasons. Knowing when the child voided after birth and whether or not he (she) can empty the bladder before any corrective spinal surgery is undertaken gives the clinician a clue regarding potential changes in lower urinary tract function, once surgery has been performed. Combined with a renal and bladder ultrasound, an examination of the lower extremities and a look at the anus completes this initial assessment. Unfortunately, reality is not always compatible with utopia. The children are often sequestered and then whisked off to the operating room for spinal canal closure within the first 24 hours of life. Rarely is the initial closure postponed beyond 48 hours unless there are mitigating circumstances that warrant a delay. Thus, the urologist is left with consulting on the child a variable period of time after the newborn closure of the meningocele. Consequently, one is not sure what further neurologic injury might have occurred with surgical correction. There has been only one study addressing the findings of urodynamic studies in babies performed both before and after spinal canal closure; fortunately, those investigators found only a 3.2% incidence of change following correction of the spinal defect in 30 newborns studied.[1] Whether or not this represents a true picture of what might transpire is impossible to say. Spinal shock and a transient inability to empty the bladder lasting as long as 1 month may be seen in up to 10% of newborns. Given this limitation and the unlikelihood of altering this practice in the near future, we are left with the notion that the chance of a neurologic injury, either transient or permanent, is small as a result of the newborn closure.

Practically speaking, the initial evaluation generally occurs on day 2 or 3 of life. The most important concern at this time is 'can the child empty his or her bladder and at what pressures to insure a normal upper urinary tract?' The best way to answer part one of the question is with a postvoid residual urine measurement by catheterizing the bladder immediately after the infant has leaked urine or voided spontaneously. If the residual is high (above 5 ml) a repeat measurement is undertaken following a Credé maneuver a few hours later and, if that volume is again elevated, either clean intermittent catheterization (CIC) or continuous Foley catheter drainage system is initiated. CIC is continued every 4 hours. Sometimes, the neurosurgeon has placed a Foley catheter at the time of closure, but this has not been uniformly practiced. As mentioned, spinal shock and transient detrusor areflexia following closure is a real phenomenon occurring as much as 10% of the time.[2] Therefore, adequate bladder drainage is necessary to prevent urinary infection during this critical time of postoperative spinal closure healing. Catheter drainage is maintained for several days until it is safe to transport the child to the ultrasound department and the urodynamic facility where additional investigative studies can be carried out, allowing an answer to part two of the question.

Initial comprehensive assessment

The initial comprehensive assessment (Table 64.1) begins with an examination of the lower extremities, checking muscle mass, spontaneous movements, deep tendon reflexes, sensation (both lower extremity and perineal areas), and anal tone in order to determine what are the child's sensory and motor neurologic levels. Although the correlation between neurologic level and lower urinary tract function is not a good one,[3] there are some clues to bladder and sphincter behavior that can be gleaned from this examination, i.e., a patulous anus suggests there might be a complete lower motor neuron lesion involving the urethral sphincter, whereas the presence of an anal wink (an anal muscle reaction to gently scratching the pigmented, ruggated skin adjacent to the anus) implies intact

Table 64.1 *Initial assessment*

Postvoid residual
- After a spontaneous void or Credé maneuver

Renal and bladder ultrasound
- Kidney size, appearance, collecting system dilation
- Ureteral dilation – proximal and distal
- Bladder wall thickness and residual urine volume

Urodynamic study
- Cystometrogram (compliance, contractility, leak-point pressure)
- Voiding pressure studies and ability to empty at specific pressure
- External urethral sphincter electromyography (baseline potentials, reflexes, response to voiding, or maneuvers to empty)

Neurologic examination
- Lower extremity strength, tone, reflexes, sensation, spontaneous movements
- Perineal tone and sensation

Laboratory values
- Urine culture
- Serum creatinine after 5–7 days of life

Voiding cystourethrogram
- Bladder wall characteristics
- Bladder neck appearance and pelvic floor position
- Vesicoureteral reflux
- Ability to empty

Nuclear scanning
- DMSA scan if reflux is present
- Mag 3 lasix renogram if hydronephrosis is present

sacral spinal cord function and reflexes, but with the possibility that detrusor-sphincter dyssynergia exists as well.

This is to be followed by a complete urodynamic evaluation that includes a very slow fill cystometrogram (5 ml or less per minute) using saline warmed to 37°C,[4] looking at detrusor compliance, contractility, leak-point pressure, and the ability to void at capacity and empty the bladder with respectable pressures. The normal bladder capacity at this age varies between 10 and 15 ml. Simultaneously, a small concentric needle electrode is placed in the external urethral sphincter to evaluate individual motor unit action potentials at rest, in response to various sacral stimuli, bladder filling, and emptying.[5] The most important findings are end detrusor filling pressure, leak or voiding pressure, the presence of detrusor overactivity, and the reaction of the external urethral sphincter electromyogram in response to a bladder contraction; all of these parameters determine what type of treatment or further assessment, if any, should be instituted following this study.

Although still somewhat controversial,[6–11] urodynamic testing in the newborn period provides several important advantages: (1) an understanding of the current physiology

Table 64.2 *Indications for conventional or nuclear cystography*

Ultrasound
- Hydronephrosis – either static or changing throughout exam
- Discrepancy in kidney size
- Increased bladder wall thickness

Urodynamic studies
- Poor compliance
- High pressure detrusor overactivity (> 75 cmH_2O)
- Dyssynergic sphincter activity
- High leak-point pressure with complete sphincter denervation
- Large postvoid residual

of the lower urinary tract; (2) a baseline assessment so that comparisons can be made if changes in either neurologic or urologic function take place over time; (3) a degree of predictability for urinary tract deterioration if the child is just observed; (4) a reason to intervene urologically even in infants who have a normal appearing upper urinary tract in order to prevent this deterioration from occurring; and (5) a reasonably accurate picture to counsel parents about future bladder and sexual function.[12]

Renal ultrasonography, either just before or after the urodynamic testing, is complementary to it. The size, position, and appearance of the kidneys and the collecting systems, especially the distal ureters, and the thickness of the bladder wall are images that need to be looked at in conjunction with the findings on the urodynamic study. The kidneys are normal 98% of the time. The only anomaly reported with any consistency in the newborn period has been horseshoe kidneys, but that too is rare. Historically, a voiding cystogram has been undertaken only when the images on the renal ultrasound suggest reflux or another abnormality, or the urodynamic study indicates that reflux is a strong possibility, and if present may have considerable consequences for the upper urinary tract (Table 64.2).

Although some clinicians continue to rely solely on ultrasound images and their physical examination to determine whether or not they should intervene,[11] most centers now consider urodynamic testing an integral part of the initial work-up and management of these children.[8,12,13] The reasons promulgated by the 'observers' are (1) the incidence of deterioration is small; (2) it can be reversed if treatment is instituted early enough after it occurs; (3) overall renal function is not impaired when comparing expectant to prophylactic treatment; (4) why subject the child and family to risks that might be unfounded; and (5) why subject parents to learn techniques and be even more burdened by procedures when caring for their children than they truly need to be.[10,11,14,15] However, those who espouse prophylactic therapy counter these arguments by saying that no one has

UDS Findings in 225 Myelodysplastic Newborns

- Bladder function
  - Contractile 63%
  - Acontractile – poor compliance 17%
  - Acontractile – good compliance 20%
- Sphincter innervation
  - Intact sacral reflex arc 40%
  - Partial denervation 24%
  - Complete denervation 36%
- Lower urinary tract function
  - Dyssynergy 37%
  - Synergy 26%
  - Complete denervation 36%

Figure 64.1
The types of bladder function and sphincter innervation noted in 225 newborns with myelodysplasia who underwent urodynamic testing within the first month of life over the last 25 years at our institution. Lower urinary tract function refers to the response of the sphincter to bladder filling at the time capacity was reached. Complete denervation is applied to those infants with no bioelectric activity in the sphincter during needle electromyography.

shown that CIC begun in the newborn period harms any infant, places undo hardships on parents, leads to repeated urinary infection or other potential complications from the catheterizations, or injures the urethra.[13,16] In fact, several important benefits have arisen following the initiation of this long-term prophylactic treatment: the ease in which children have taken to accepting CIC as a regular means of emptying their bladder as they grow; the ability to attain continence with less adjunctive medical and surgical measures; the earlier goal of achieving independence in self-management of the lower urinary tract, when this program is begun early in the life of the child; and the ultimate reduced need for augmentation cystoplasty, with its attendant set of complications that inevitably occur over time.[13,17]

Newborn urodynamic findings

Urodynamic studies in newborns have demonstrated surprising results when compared to findings in older children, a reflection of the changing nature of the neurologic lesion in myelodysplastic children.[18] Bladder function has been classified using the newly accepted terminology promulgated by the International Children's Continence Society:[19] contractile means that a voiding contraction occurred at capacity during a cystometrogram, whereas acontractile implies that no contraction of the bladder took place.

Sixty-three percent of 225 newborns (Figure 64.1) demonstrated a bladder contraction on cystometry, and 37% did not. Of the latter, 20% had good and 17% had poor compliance (end filling pressure defined at the time as less than 40 cmH_2O).[20] Electromyographic (EMG) assessment of the external urethral sphincter revealed an intact sacral reflex arc with normal motor unit potentials and normal responses to sacral stimuli in 40% of the children, partial denervation of the sphincter with variable sacral reflex responses in 24%, and complete denervation with no electrical activity and no responses to sacral stimulation in 36%.

Detrusor and urethral sphincter function can be further correlated to denote the reaction of the latter in response to the former. Synergy is defined as quieting of the sphincter when the bladder contracts at capacity, whereas dyssynergy or DSD implies that the urethral sphincter increases its activity in response to a bladder contraction or fails to relax as the bladder is filled to capacity. The incidence of synergy in our newborn series was 26%, DSD occurred in 37%, and complete denervation was seen in 36%.[20]

Initial treatment

Initial management is dictated by the findings on urodynamic assessment irrespective of the upper urinary tract appearance on X-ray imaging (Table 64.3).[21–24] No intervention is necessary in the child with a synergic sphincter who voids to completion with normal pressure. Similarly, no specific treatment is needed in the child with complete denervation, a low leak-point pressure, and sporadic but complete emptying. However, intervention employing CIC is considered mandatory in the child with DSD because experience has shown that expectant therapy alone often leads to a decompensated bladder with poor compliance, hydroureteronephrosis, and vesicoureteral reflux, all of which may not be completely reversible with subsequent management (Figure 64.2).[24] Besides, it has been clearly shown that augmentation cystoplasty is needed more often than not if these bladders are allowed to progress to inelasticity from the continued high bladder outlet resistance associated with DSD.[13,17] DMSA scanning has provided

Table 64.3 *Initial management*

No intervention	CIC only	CIC + anticholinergic meds
Synergic voiding with complete emptying	Dyssynergy	DSD + poor compliance
Low LPP 2° denervation fibrosis	Reflux ≥ 3	DSD + poor compliance + reflux ≥ 3

LLP, leak point pressure; Reflux grades 1–5 (international classification).

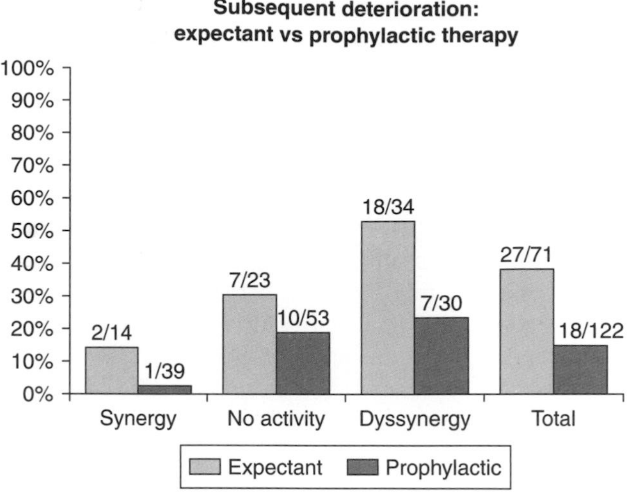

Figure 64.2
Comparison made of the response in those 225 infants followed postnatally with either expectant (71) or prophylactic (122) therapy, excluding 32 children who had deterioration of their urinary tract at the time of birth from the prenatal effects of increased bladder outlet resistance.

another, more paramount reason for intervening early, due to the irreversibility of a renal injury that can occur with high pressure reflux and urinary infection.[25]

Spinal shock following meningocele repair occurs in 3% of newborns.[26] Its presence can be readily ascertained on urodynamic testing – an underactive detrusor (unsustained or no contractility of the bladder muscle) and no reactivity of the urethral sphincter muscle to sacral stimuli despite the apparent absence of signs of denervation on sphincter electromyography. In some instances there may be complete denervation of the urethral sphincter and an adynamic detrusor but, in either case, the child is not able to empty the bladder. When CIC is initiated as a result of spinal shock, the need for catheterization is only continued until the bladder can regain its contractility and completely empty itself periodically. The time to resolution is variable, but spinal shock usually lasts no more that 2 to 4 weeks after surgery. Prophylactic antibiotics are administered for the first few weeks after initiation of the CIC program to minimize the threat of urinary infection while the parents are adjusting to the catheterization technique and emptying the bladder completely and regularly. Antibiotics are stopped once parents are comfortable with the program. This has not resulted in a subsequent increased incidence of urinary infection. When spinal shock is not the issue and DSD is noted, then CIC is begun in earnest as a permanent means of emptying the bladder to avoid the potentially hazardous effects of high voiding or leak-point pressures that lead to upper urinary tract damage and to the creation of an inelastic bladder over time.[17,27]

If the initial urodynamic study reveals poor detrusor compliance with end filling pressure exceeding 20 cmH_2O, detrusor overactivity with pressures exceeding 50 cmH_2O, or voiding pressures greater than 80 cmH_2O, anticholinergic medication is begun as an adjunct to CIC (Figure 64.3).[15,28,29] The most readily administered anticholinergic drug is oxybutynin HCl. It has been available for more than 25 years and its liquid form allows it to be easily titrated based on the child's age and/or weight. The dosing schedule used in our department is 1 mg/year of age bid to tid,

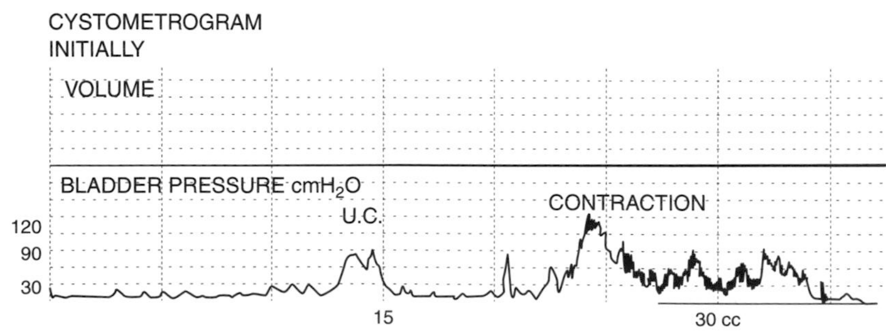

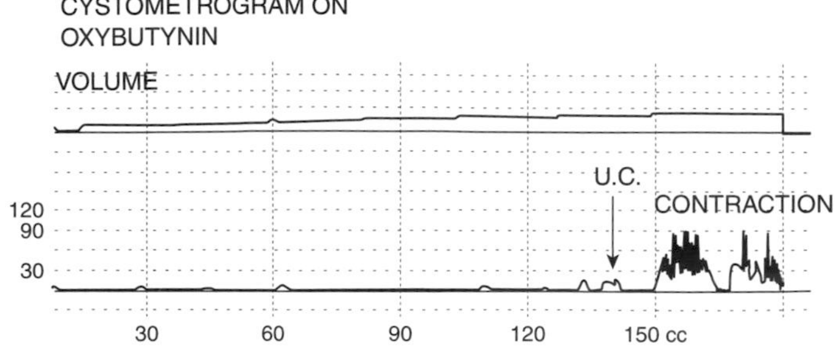

Figure 64.3
Effect of oxybutynin HCl administered orally (according to dosing noted in the text) on bladder function for infants with increased bladder outlet resistance.

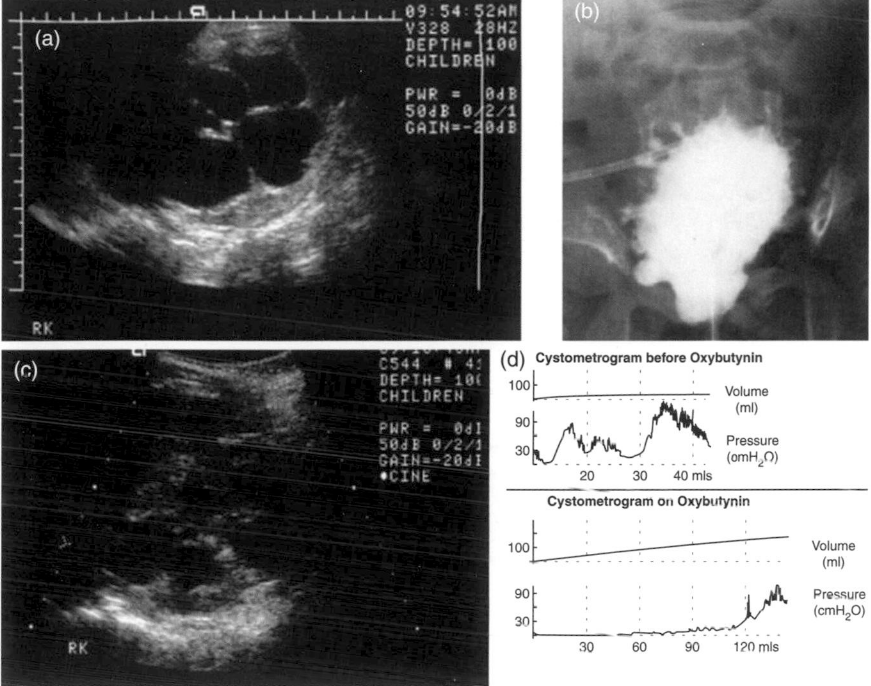

Figure 64.4
The ultrasound of the right kidney (a), the voiding cystogram (b), and the urodynamic study (d) in a 1-year-old girl with detrusor-sphincter dyssynergy. Note the effect of high filling pressures on the right kidney despite the absence of reflux. Once treatment with intermittent catheterization and oxybutynin were begun the right kidney improved (c), but did not completely resolve its hydronephrosis.

with proportionately less prescribed for children younger that 1 year (0.1 mg at birth, which is increased by 0.1 mg each 5 weeks during that first year) (Figure 64.4).[30] Side-effects with this dosing have been minimal, with facial flushing as the most likely observed symptom; no long-term sequclae have been noted affecting the gastrointestinal tract or cardiovascular system. The incidence of deterioration is small (15%) in the proactively treated children, and certainly lower than the 38% rate seen in the expectant therapy group (Figures 64.5 and 64.6).[20]

Credé voiding to empty the bladder is no longer practiced on a routine basis. It is effective in young babies when the bladder remains an abdominal organ, but it should only be used when the external urethral sphincter is not reactive to sacral stimuli.[31] With a nonreactive sphincter, there is no corresponding increase in activity or any increase in urethral resistance during this type of 'voiding' so the bladder is emptied at safe pressures. When the sphincter muscle is reactive it tightens in response to any increase in abdominal pressure causing bladder outlet resistance to increase as well (Figure 64.7). This results in higher 'voiding' pressure, to empty the bladder; thus, it is not a salutary way to empty the bladder.

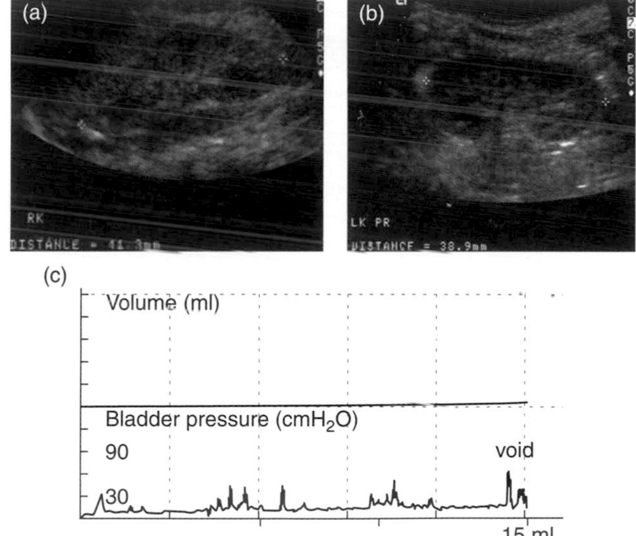

Figure 64.5
This newborn boy with a lumbar level myelodysplasia had normal kidneys (a and b) and a benign urodynamic study initially (c) with low filling and voiding pressures and complete denervation in the sphincter (not shown).

Vesicoureteral reflux

The incidence of vesicoureteral reflux varies between 3 and 5% of newborns with myelodysplasia, usually in association with poor detrusor compliance, detrusor overactivity, and/or DSD.[25,32] When voiding or nuclear cystography is performed (for the reasons cited earlier) and vesicoureteral reflux is detected, additional measures are undertaken. If CIC has not been started before this time, it is begun now. The degree and extent of any further intervention is determined in part by the grade of reflux. The international classification of

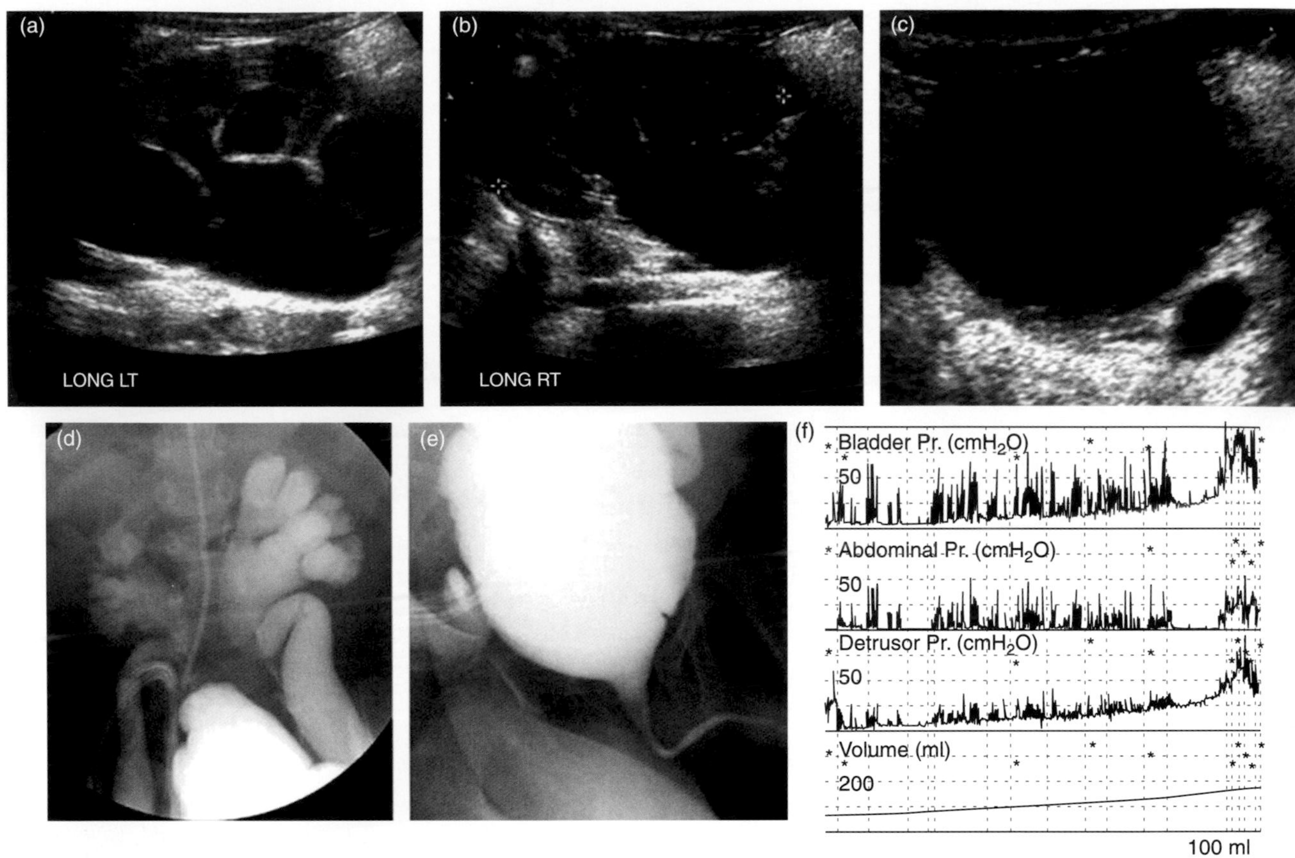

Figure 64.6
At 1 year of age the newborn boy had a urinary tract infection and his ultrasound revealed bilateral hydronephrosis (a and b) with a dilated right ureter extending down to the bladder (c). A voiding cystogram demonstrated grade 5/5 reflux bilaterally (d), narrowing in the region of the external urethral sphincter (e), and a markedly hypertonic bladder (f). His EMG revealed reinnervation of the sphincter with concomitant dyssynergy at capacity (not shown).

grades 1 through 5 is used to describe its severity. Prophylactic antibiotics are either initiated or continued on a regular basis for all reflux grades other than grade 1. A dimercaptosuccinic acid (DMSA) renal scan is obtained when the reflux is grade 3 or higher to determine the extent of parenchymal scarring. In our original series of newborns with myelodysplasia evaluated in the newborn period, vesicoureteral reflux was only seen this early after birth in those children who had DSD, suggesting that bladder outflow obstruction in the prenatal period already had a profound effect on the ureterovesical junction that led to reflux.[22] Knowing whether or not renal damage has occurred as a result of *in utero* high pressure voiding from the dyssynergy during this critical time in the development of the kidney is paramount to insuring that no further injury takes place.

If the initial cystometrogram demonstrates poor compliance, high-pressure premature contractions (above 25 cmH_2O), or high voiding pressures (≤75 cmH_2O), anticholinergic medication is started, if it has not been done so already, in an attempt to lower intravesical pressure and ultimately to effect resolution of the reflux.[23,28,32,33] The dosing of oxybutynin is as noted above, but probably should be given 3 times per day to maximize its effect.

Urine cultures need to be obtained routinely, every 3 months, as well as specifically when symptoms suggestive of an infection are present, and treated appropriately, if positive. If hydroureteronephrosis is evident on the initial imaging of the kidneys it is repeated 6 months later to see whether it has resolved. Otherwise, repeat urinary tract imaging and urodynamic studies are performed close to 1 year of age. At that time, a renal ultrasonogram, nuclear or voiding cystogram, and a cystometrogram (in conjunction with the nuclear or voiding cystogram – videourodynamics) are performed to denote (1) any changes in renal architecture and growth, (2) the continued presence of reflux and its grade, and (3) the efficacy of the anticholinergic medication being given, respectively.

If the reflux remains high grade (grade ≥3), the poorly compliant bladder has not improved with medication, or the kidneys have failed to grow or have progressive scarring on DMSA scanning and continue to exhibit hydroureteronephrosis, surgical intervention is deemed necessary.

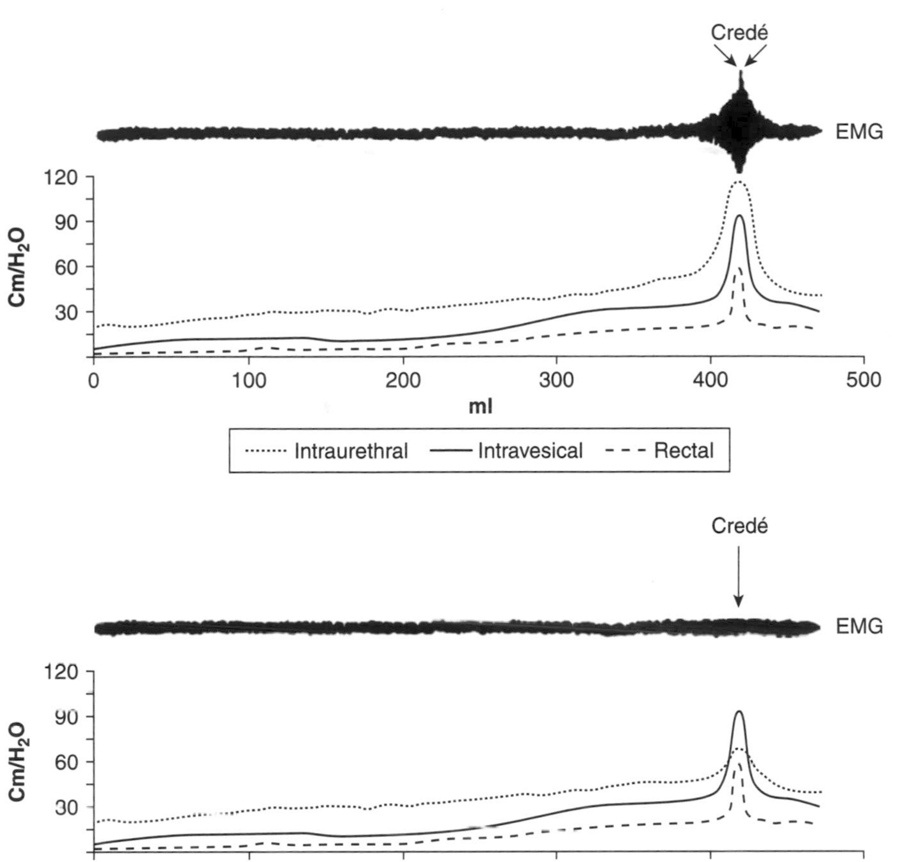

Figure 64.7
When the urethral sphincter is reactive to sacral reflexes a Credé maneuver can lead to increases in abdominal pressure and high pressure 'voiding'. However, when the sphincter is extensively denervated there is no corresponding reactivity to a Credé maneuver so bladder outlet resistance does not change and it is relatively safe to perform.

The indications for antireflux surgery are similar to those in normal children: recurrent breakthrough urinary infection despite continuous antibiotics; persistent high-grade reflux despite an improvement in detrusor compliance and/or overactivity with anticholinergic medication; failure of renal growth on serial ultrasounds; the development or progression of renal scarring on subsequent studies; and the need to perform bladder outlet surgery to improve urinary continence.[34,35] Excellent success rates for resolution of reflux with surgery have been achieved when combined with anticholinergic medication and CIC to insure low detrusor filling pressure and complete emptying.[36,37]

Agents have been developed that can be endoscopically injected into the ureteral orifice (Figure 64.8) to correct reflux, and they have become increasingly popular in recent years – thus lowering the threshold for correcting reflux in these children. Despite this, the long-term efficacy of this treatment has not been clearly established.[38,39] The risk of recurrence of reflux in the child with a neurologically impaired lower urinary tract, especially in a disease process that is dynamic, is unknown. Therefore, caution following its use cannot be overstated.

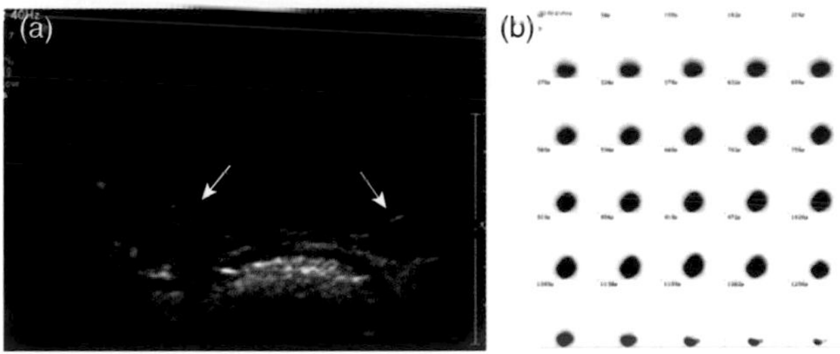

Figure 64.8
Following a Deflux injection into each ureteral orifice in the boy shown in Figure 64.6 a mound can be seen (arrows) surrounding each intramural ureter (a), while no reflux is noted during a postinjection nuclear cystogram (b).

Again, the use of Credé voiding to empty the bladder should be avoided in babies who have a reactive external urethral sphincter for the reasons cited earlier in the chapter. This is especially true for children with reflux, for the increased 'voiding' pressure generated by a reactive sphincter may lead to a more injurious effect if reflux is present.[31]

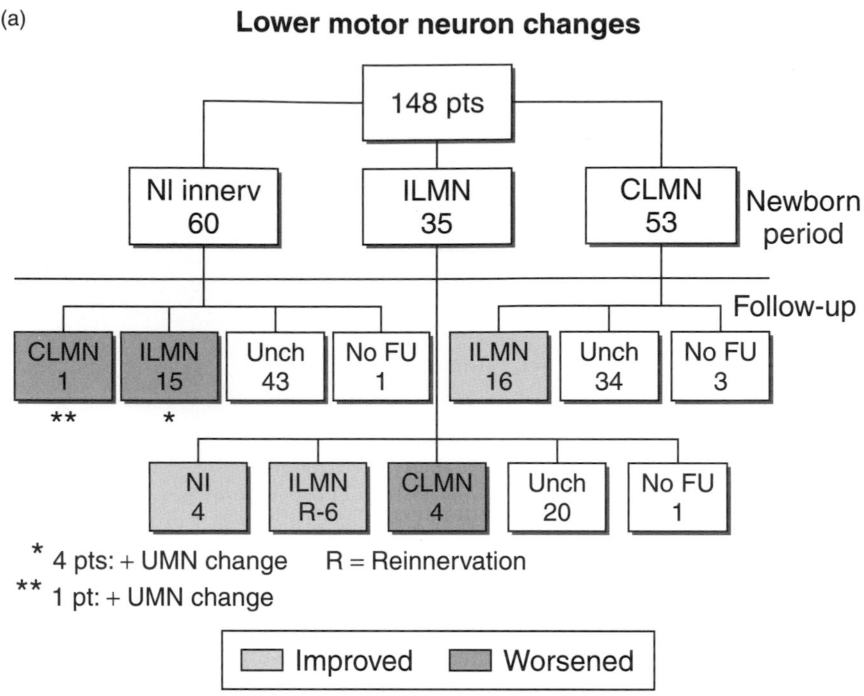

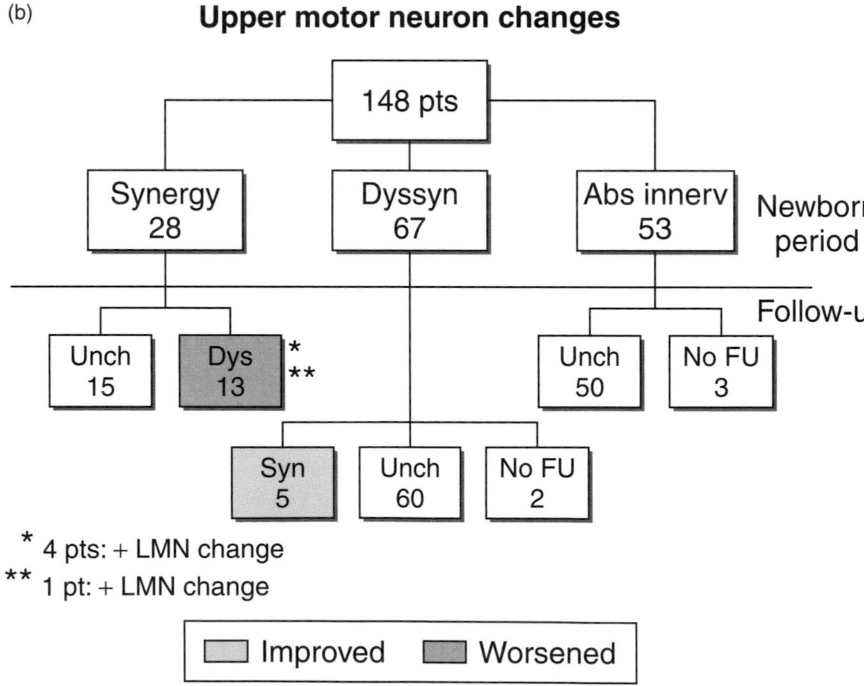

Figure 64.9
The flow chart emphasizes the changing neurologic lesion involving (a) sacral reflex and spinal cord (b) function in newborns with myelodysplasia over time. ILMN, incomplete lower motor neuron; CLMN, complete lower neuron; UMN, upper motor neuron; Nl, normal; innerv, innervation; Unch, unchanged; FU, follow-up; Dyssyn and Dys, dyssynergy; Syn, synergy LMN, lower motor neuron.

Vesicostomy drainage

Before the advent of CIC in early infancy for these children, vesicostomy drainage was frequently employed to drain the bladder in children with vesicoureteral reflux and/or hydronephrosis.[40,41] Since that time few vesicostomies have been performed, mostly in children whose parents were not able to follow a regimen of sufficiently frequent catheterizations, or who experienced urethral injury, or exhibited a poorly compliant or markedly overactive detrusor unresponsive to anticholinergic medication in the face of high-grade reflux and/or hydronephrosis.[42] It should be emphasized that this is a temporizing measure for draining the bladder and should not be considered a long-term solution. As the child approaches 3 to 4 years of age strong consideration should be given to reversing the

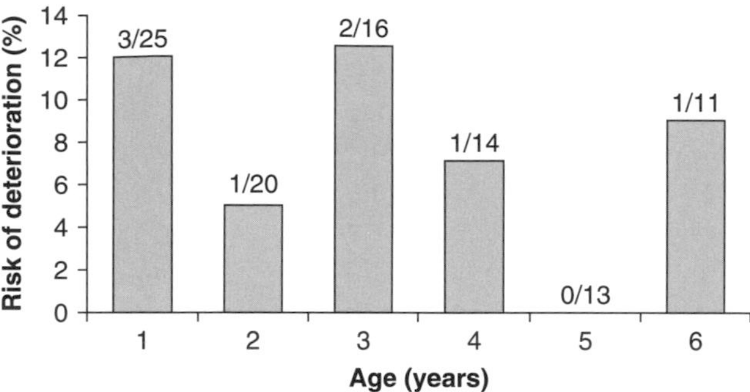

Figure 64.10
Risk of deterioration with increasing age in newborns with myelodysplasia who had normal urodynamic findings and a normal neurologic exam at birth. The denominator above each column refers to the number of infants at risk while the numerator refers to those who actually changed at that particular age, at the time the analysis was undertaken. Once a child deteriorated he/she was not included in those at risk for neurologic deterioration the following year.

process and instituting CIC and drug therapy. The continued presence or resolution of vesicoureteral reflux is difficult to assess before take-down of the vesicostomy, so a repeat cystogram is necessary shortly after closure of the stoma. Some have observed that a poorly compliant bladder may not improve with the creation and subsequent reversal of a vesicostomy. Thus, a vesicostomy may only delay the ultimate need for augmentation cystoplasty. Others have noted that it is difficult to impose CIC on a child at an older age once they have had a vesicostomy for several years. For these reasons, vesicostomy drainage should be undertaken in very specific instances. Most importantly, it is only applicable if there is no secondary ureterovesical junction obstruction.

Neurologic changes

It has become apparent over the last 20 years that the neurologic injury in myelodysplasia is not a static lesion but rather a dynamic disease process (Figure 64.9).[43] Therefore, the findings in early infancy do not always correlate with what is seen in later years on X-ray imaging and urodynamic studies. When a change occurs it is often the reason for failure of initial management. We noted a 19% incidence for changes during the first several years of life, with most of the changes occurring in the first 2 to 3 years.[44] The changes in neurologic function are not confined to children with any one level of lesion.[45,46] In fact, there is a 32% risk for deterioration subsequently when newborns have normal urodynamic findings (Figure 64.10).[47] Therefore, the clinician must remain vigilant to the possibility of its occurrence and consider repeating the urodynamic study routinely in those children with the most lower urinary tract function to lose, i.e., normal or near normal detrusor and external urethral sphincter function.

Subsequent surveillance

Depending on the findings in the early newborn period and the type of intervention, if any, subsequent surveillance is based on that initial evaluation and the potential for neurologic and/or urologic change (Table 64.1). If a child has a complete lower motor neuron lesion with no bioelectric activity in the sphincter and a good compliant bladder with low filling and leak-point pressures at capacity, little residual, and a normal renal ultrasound, he (she) can be followed expectantly. Periodic residual urine

Table 64.4 *Surveillance*

Type of lower urinary tract lesion	Complete denervation	Normal function bladder/sphincter	Good function w DSD ± DO and intervention begun
Parameter			
Residual urine	3×/yr	3×/yr	N/A
Urine culture	3×/yr	3×/yr	3×/yr
Renal ECHO	Yearly	Yearly	Yearly
Urodynamic study	age 1	Yearly till 6	To check effectiveness of therapy or yearly if substantial function is present
Cystography (see text) VCUG or nuclear	See text		Yearly to follow progress of reflux
DMSA scan for high grade reflux	biennial	biennial	biennial

DSD, detrusor sphincter dyssynergy; DO, detrusor overactivity.

measurements with urine cultures 2 to 3 times a year and yearly renal ultrasounds for the first several years after birth are all that is necessary until it is time to try and achieve continence. It is rare to find reinnervation of the external urethral sphincter producing increased bladder outlet obstruction. More likely, denervation fibrosis of this sphincter can occur, resulting in an increase in urethral resistance and leading to increased residual urine.[48] Any change in residual urine volume, incidence of urinary infection, or dilation of the collecting system warrants further investigation with repeat urodynamic studies to determine its cause, and voiding cystography or isotope renography, (depending on the new findings) to denote its consequence.

If the child has normal bladder and external urethral sphincter function with a good compliant bladder early in filling, a normal voiding contraction at capacity with normal pressure, normal or only partial denervation in the sphincter with normal sacral reflexes and detrusor-sphincter synergy, and normal kidneys on ultrasound, then a residual urine volume with urine cultures twice a year and a yearly renal ultrasound and urodynamic study are necessary to insure a stable neurologic picture. Deterioration as well as reinnervation (in those with partial denervation) is possible. The earlier it is detected, the greater the likelihood that external urethral sphincter function can be preserved or improved with secondary spinal cord untethering.

If the child has urologic and urodynamic parameters that warrant intervention, such as an overactive detrusor, a poorly compliant bladder with high leak-point pressure, detrusor-sphincter dyssynergy or a nonrelaxing sphincter at capacity, elevated residual urine after a spontaneous void, hydronephrosis, and dilated ureter(s), various treatment measures will have to be initiated. Depending on the type of intervention – medical therapy with anticholinergics, intermittent catheterization, or surgery (open or endoscopic treatment of reflux, vesicostomy) – follow-up is predicated on what has been instituted. Surveillance with urine cultures and residual urine measurements at least twice a year and renal ultrasonography yearly is usually the minimum standard of follow-up.

A repeat urodynamic study is warranted if the clinician needs to know (1) the effectiveness of anticholinergic medication that has been started, (2) why an increase in residual urine has occurred if the child has been voiding spontaneously, (3) the reason for a change in the level of continence, (4) what effect recurrent UTI has had on detrusor muscle compliance and contractility, and (5) what may have caused an increase in collecting system dilation on radiologic imaging. As noted in the reasons cited above, external urethral sphincter EMG should be repeated as part of the urodynamic study if there is an apparent change in lower extremity function, an increase in detrusor leak-point pressure and/or residual urine, a change in the level of urinary continence, or an increase in or new onset of dilation of the upper urinary tract, for these signs might suggest either reinnervation of the external urethral sphincter and/or the development of detrusor sphincter dyssynergy or loss of sphincter function when an increase in urinary incontinence occurs.

Nuclear or voiding cystography is indicated on a yearly basis to follow children with vesicoureteral reflux or if there is a change in function on the urodynamic study, dilation of the upper urinary tract on renal ultrasonography, or recurrent UTI that warrants a repeat study. Renal scintigraphy is helpful to detect any upper urinary tract deterioration in those children with recurrent UTI, persistent high-grade reflux, or deterioration in lower urinary tract function on urodynamic studies that predisposes them to kidney deterioration as well.

Measurement of serum creatinine has not been a useful tool for either initial assessment or subsequent follow-up because it is an inaccurate way to detect early changes in renal function. However, an initial serum creatinine level is helpful when juxtaposed against later measurements in those children who have repeated UTI in the face of vesicoureteral reflux and/or kidneys that do not grow with advancing age.

CONCLUSIONS

It is fascinating to muse over the changes in management of the infant with myelodysplasia during the last 30 years.[49] One could sum up the entire management philosophy of years ago into one or two phrases – watchful waiting, or urinary diversion in those with any signs of deterioration or just the presence of myelodysplasia. The advent of CIC and the development of numerous agents that modulate lower urinary tract function have altered the way these children are initially assessed and treated in a profound way. There is still some controversy whether or not proactive treatment versus careful surveillance with rapid initiation of therapy when a change takes place is the correct method of treatment. The important outcome, however, is that the children are receiving a markedly higher level of urologic care that they did in the 1960s and 1970s. Their quality of life, their overall kidney health, and their ability to integrate into and become functional members of society are clearly that much better.[25]

References

1. Kroovand RL, Bell W, Hart LJ, Benfeld KY. The effect of back closure on detrusor function in neonates with myelodysplasia. J Urol 1990; 144: 423.
2. Chiaramonte RM, Horowitz EM, Kaplan GA et al. Implications of hydronephrosis in newborns with myelodysplasia. J Urol 1986; 136: 427.
3. Bauer SB, Labib KB, Dieppa RA et al. Urodynamic evaluation in a boy with myelodysplasia and incontinence. Urology 1977; 10: 354.

4. Joseph DB. The effect of medium-fill and slow-fill cystometry on bladder pressure in infants and children with myelodysplasia. J Urol 1992; 147: 444.
5. Blaivas JG, Labib KB, Bauer SB, Retik AB. A new approach to electromyography of the external urethral sphincter. J Urol 1977; 117: 773.
6. McGuire EJ, Woodside JR, Borden TA, Weiss RM. The prognostic value of urodynamic testing in myelodysplastic patients. J Urol 1981; 126: 205.
7. Bauer SB, Hallet M, Khoshbin S et al. The predictive value of urodynamic evaluation in the newborn with myelodysplasia. JAMA 1984; 152: 650.
8. Sidi AA, Dykstra DD, Gonzalez R. The value of urodynamic testing in the management of neonates with myelodysplasia: a prospective study. J Urol 1986; 135: 90.
9. Perez LM, Khoury J, Webster GD. The value of urodynamic studies in infants less than one year old with congenital spinal dysraphism. J Urol 1992; 148: 584.
10. Teichman JMH, Scherz HC, Kim KD et al. An alternative approach to myelodysplasia management: aggressive observation and prompt intervention. J Urol 1994; 152: 807.
11. Hopps CV, Kropp KA. Preservation of renal function in children with myelomeningocele managed with basic newborn evaluation and close followup. J Urol 2003; 169: 305.
12. Bauer SB. Myelodysplasia: newborn evaluation and management. In: McLaurin RL, ed. Spina Bifida: A Multidisciplinary Approach New York: Praeger, 1984: 262–7.
13. Wu H-Y, Baskin LS, Kogan BA. Neurogenic bladder dysfunction due to myelomeningocele: neonatal versus childhood treatment. J Urol 1997; 157: 2295–7.
14. Klose AG, Sackett CK, Mesrobian H GJ. Management of children with myelodysplasia. Urologic alternatives. J Urol 1990; 144: 1446.
15. Tanaka H, Kakizaki H, Kobayashi S et al. The relevance of urethral resistance in children with myelodysplasia: its impact on upper urinary tract deterioration and the outcome of conservative management. J Urol 1999; 161: 929–32.
16. Joseph DB, Bauer SB, Colodny AH et al. Clean intermittent catheterization in infants with neurogenic bladder. Pediatrics 1989; 84: 78.
17. Kaefer M, Pabby A, Kelly M et al. Improved bladder function after prophylactic treatment of the high risk neurogenic bladder in newborns with myelomeningocele. J Urol 1999; 162: 1068–71.
18. Bauer SB. Early evaluation and management of children with spina bifida. In: King LR ed, Urologic Surgery in Neonates and Young Infants. Philadelphia: WB Saunders 1988: 252–64.
19. Neveus T, von Gontard A, Hoebeke P, Hjalmas K et al. Standardization of terminology of lower urinary tract function in children and adolescents: report from Standardization Committee of International Children's Continence Society. J Urol 2006; 176: 314.
20. Bauer SB. Neuropathic dysfunction of the lower urinary tract. In: Wein AJ, Kavoussi LR, Novick AC, Partin AW, Peters CA, eds. Campbell-Walsh Urology, 9th edn. Philadelphia: Saunders Elsevier, 2006: 3625–55.
21. van Gool JD, Dik P, de Jong TP. Bladder-sphincter dysfunction in myelomeningocele. Eur J Pediatr 2001; 160: 414–20.
22. Bauer SB. The management of spina bifida from birth onwards. In: Whitaker RH, Woodard JR eds, Paediatric Urology. London: Butterworths, 1985: 87–112.
23. Edelstein RA, Bauer SB, Kelly MD et al. The long-term urologic response of neonates with myelodysplasia treated proactively with intermittent catheterization and anticholinergic therapy. J Urol 1995; 154: 1500.
24. Dik P, van Gool JD, de Jong-de Vos van Steenwijk CC, de Jong TP. Early start therapy preserves kidney function in spina bifida patients. Eur Urol 2006; 49: 908–13.
25. Chiaramonte RM, Horowitz EM, Kaplan GA et al. Implications of hydronephrosis in newborns with myelodysplasia. J Urol 1986; 136: 427.
26. Van Gool JD, Juijten RH, Donckerwolcke RA, Kramer PP. Detrusor-sphincter dyssynergia in children with myelomeningocele: A prospective study. Z Kinderchir 1982; 37: 148.
27. Ghoniem GM, Roach MB, Lewis VH et al. The value of leak point pressure and bladder compliance in the urodynamic evaluation of myelomeningocele patients. J Urol 1990; 144: 1440.
28. Geranoitis E, Koff SA, Enrile B. Prophylactic use of clean intermittent catheterization in treatment of infants and young children with myelomeningocele and neurogenic bladder dysfunction. J Urol 1988; 139: 85.
29. Landau EH, Churchill BM, Jayanthi VR et al. The sensitivity of pressure specific bladder volume versus total bladder capacity as a measure of bladder storage dysfunction. J Urol 1994; 152: 1578.
30. Kasabian NG, Bauer SB, Dyro FM et al. The prophylactic value of clean intermittent catheterization and anticholinergic medication in newborns and infants with myelodysplasia at risk of developing urinary tract deterioration. Am J Dis Child 1992; 146: 840.
31. Barbalais GA, Klauber GT, Blaivas JG. Critical evaluation of the Credé maneuver: a urodynamic study of 207 patients. J Urol 1983; 130: 720.
32. Flood HD, Ritchey ML, Bloom DA et al. Outcome of reflux in children with myelodysplasia managed by bladder pressure monitoring. J Urol 1994; 152: 1574.
33. Agarwal SK, McLorie GA, Grewal D et al. Urodynamic correlates of resolution of reflux meningomyelocele patients. J Urol 1997; 158: 580.
34. Bauer SB, Colodny AH, Retik AB. The management of vesico-ureteral reflux in children with myelodysplasia. J Urol 1982; 128: 102.
35. Kaplan WE, Firlit CF. Management of reflux in myelodysplastic children. J Urol 1983; 129: 1195.
36. Jeffs RD, Jones P, Schillinger JF. Surgical correction of vesico-ureteral reflux in children with neurogenic bladder. J Urol 1976; 115: 449.
37. Kass EJ, Koff SA, Lapides J. Fate of vesico-ureteral reflux in children with neuropathic bladders managed by intermittent catheterization. J Urol 1981; 125: 63.
38. Schlussel R. Cystoscopic correction of reflux. Curr Urol Rep 2004; 5: 127.
39. Elder JS, Diaz M, Caldamone AA et al. Endoscopic therapy for vesicoureteral reflux: meta-analysis. I. Reflux resolution and urinary tract infection. J Urol 2006; 175: 716.
40. Duckett JW. Cutaneous vesicostomy in childhood. Urol Clin North Am 1974; 1: 485.
41. Mandell J, Bauer SB, Colodny AH, Retik AB. Cutaneous vesicostomy in infancy. J Urol 1981; 126: 92.
42. Morrisroe SN, O'Connor RC, Nanigian DK, Kurzrock EA, Stone AR. Vesicostomy revisited: the best treatment for the hostile bladder in myelodysplastic children? BJU Int 2005; 96: 397.
43. Spindel MR, Bauer SB, Dyro FM et al. The changing neuro-urologic lesion in myelodysplasia. JAMA 1987; 258: 1630.
44. Lais A, Kasabian NG, Dyro FM et al. Neurosurgical implications of continuous neuro-urological surveillance of children with myelodysplasia. J Urol 1993; 150: 1879–83.
45. Dator DP, Hatchett L, Dyro EM et al. Urodynamic dysfunction in walking myelodysplastic children. J Urol 1992; 148: 362–5.
46. Pontari MA, Keating M, Kelly MD et al. Retained sacral function in children with high level myelodysplasia. J Urol 1995; 154: 775.
47. Tarcan T, Bauer S, Olmedo E et al. Long-term follow-up of newborns with myelodysplasia and normal urodynamic findings: is it necessary? J Urol 2001; 165: 564–7.
48. Mandell J, Lebowitz RL, Hallett M, Khoshbin S, Bauer SB. Urethral narrowing in region of external sphincter: radiologic urodynamic correlations in boys with myelodysplasia. Am J Roentgenol 1980; 134: 731–5.
49. Bauer SB. The management of the myelodysplastic child: a paradigm shift. BJU Int 2003; 92: 23.

65

Intravesical electrical stimulation in newborn infants and children

Marianne Berényi, Ferenc Katona, and Helmut G Madersbacher

Introduction

Meningomyelocele (MMC) is a complex developmental malformation of the central nervous system. It usually involves the vertebral system (spina bifida), the spinal cord and nerves (meningomyelocele), the ventricular system (hydrocephalus), and the brain. The symptomatology of the defect is individually different, though similarities are frequent. The multiorgan involvement of MMC is represented by the diagnostic and therapeutic tools, such as ultrasound, MRI, valve implantation, early closure of the cele, intravesical transurethral electrostimulation, electromodulation, intermittent catheterization, implantation of artificial sphyncter, surgery on the hip and lower extremities, and physiotherapy. Life-threatening defects are hydrocephalus and/or bladder infection.

According to this concept, it is therefore the practice to follow MMC from the preoperative examination of the newborn continuously through to age 2–3 years.[1–8]

The symptoms and consequences of this complex malformation can influence each other, and the success of treatment depends on the plan, which considers the epigenetic connections. Initially, life-endangering symptoms must be attended to. Ventriculoperitoneal shunt can treat hydrocephalus and special attention must be given to bladder function.

Preoperative diagnostic methods in MMC neonates

The concept of such planning begins with a thorough and complex investigation of the MMC newborn before early closure. This extensive program includes ultrasound, special neuro-urodynamic examination of the urinary bladder, and rectodynamic examination of the rectum. This examination program assists to fulfill the task of secondary prevention according to the WHO nomenclature, because it improves the result of the early closure. Since 1984 the Department of Developmental Neurology has run a 24-hour service for this purpose. The spina bifida newborns requiring operation during the first 24 hours arrive by ambulance car directly from obstetric departments. The examination program requires neuro-imaging (brain and spinal cord), to detect the presence of hydrocephalus or other brain malformation; spinal ultrasound; bladder, ureter, and kidney ultrasound; neurourodynamics and rectodynamics; EEG; and brainstem-evoked potential. Developmental neurologic examination of elementary motor functions is designed to reveal the functional integrity of the pelvic floor and the lower extremities. This type of examination is based on stimulation of the vestibular and reticular system through the labyrinth and activates complex, sensorimotor functions such as unsupported sitting, crawling up and down on an incline, and elementary walking. This is the only way to achieve an early correct diagnosis. Tests of elementary attention, habituation, and other precognitive functions are also part of the complex preoperative examination.

Bladder configuration is examined by ultrasound. Owing to the physiologic anuria being present at 3–4 hours after birth, when the majority of preoperative examinations are performed, even in normal cases normal bladder capacity by ultrasound estimation and/or good urination in spray cannot be used, and further examinations are needed. Preoperatively no close connection can be observed between the grade of paraparesis and bladder dysfunction. Occasionally normal bladder function, no dribbling, and no retention can be observed, even in cases with very severe paraparesis, or paraplegia investigated by vestibular stimulation of the sensorimotor functions, somatosensory-evoked potential. These findings indicate the necessity of using the most careful operative technique, in order to preserve existing functions. The detailed preoperative case reports help the surgeon, who does the early covering in this respect too.

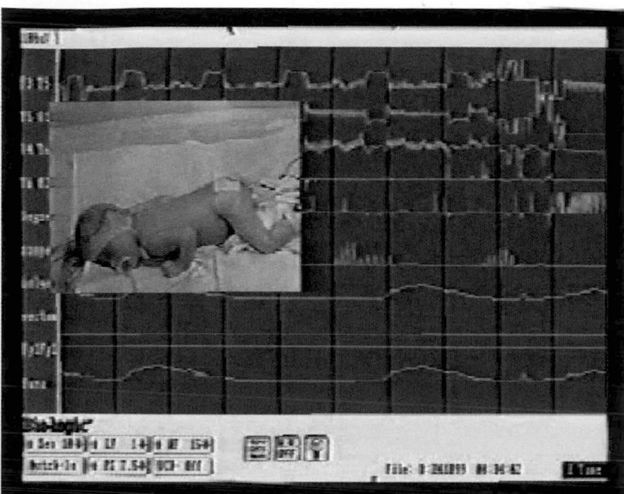

Figure 65.1
Neuro-urodynamic examination during electrical stimulation of the bladder in a neonate with sacral MMC.

In all cases so-called 'neuro-urodynamics' are performed. This consists of catheterization with a thin (K-31) catheter, with a smooth metal tip and thin cable inside (electrocatheter), to introduce sterile fluid by a slow drip (10/minute), filling the bladder to one third of its actual capacity. The electro-catheter is connected to a polygraphic recording system. A balloon catheter is introduced 4–5 cm into the rectum and also connected to the polygraph. Bladder, rectal, differential pressure, and body movement are recorded simultaneously. With electroencephalography (EEG), the activity of the brain is registered continuously during the pressure recording, and the whole procedure is recorded by video (Figure 65.1).

The first step in the examination is the recording of the spontaneous activity of the bladder following retrograde filling. Pressure changes, if any, are recorded during a 20-minute period. When no bladder function is measured, electrical stimulation is initiated. The applied electrical currents comprise interrupted direct current (DC) with a stabile 2 ms duration for each individual current, with changeable frequency, rise time, train duration and interval in a package (see Chapter 55, Figures 55.4–55.6). The positive electrode is in the bladder at the tip of the catheter and the negative one is attached firmly to the arm. The current flows from the positive electrode in the bladder to the negative electrode on the arm. Stimulation starts with the lowest intensity (0–5 mA) and is gradually increased. The highest intensity used is 8 mA. During this procedure the polygraph recordings are observed. It often happens that, after an initial recording period of 20 minutes, the initiation of electrical stimulation produces changes in bladder tone and activity and pelvic floor tone, and, occasionally, a very strong contraction appears which causes evacuation of the bladder. The type of contraction is important in the assessment of bladder function. Several types of bladder contractions can be recorded: (1) normal, (2) slow-rise, low-peak, and short-duration, (3) short-rise, normal-height, short-duration, among others.

EEG of neonates and infants often changes during the initial period of voiding, and this change becomes even more pronounced if the pressure reaches a certain level (usually around 40 cmH_2O, or more). In children, EEG shows desynchronization, while in neonates and young infants, as well as the characteristic changes of desynchronization, arousal or awakening reactions can be seen. In neonates, a very sensitive behavioral sign of alteration in either the external or internal environment is a change in nonfeeding sucking activity. To use this age-dependent specialty, the polygraphic program contains continuous recording of sucking with the help of a pacifier connected to a transducer. In neonates and young infants, strong detrusor contractions produce an immediate alteration in the sucking bursts. With the simultaneous recording of EEG and pressures from the bladder and the rectum, a new possibility arises to study the integrity of the afferent sensory processes from the urinary bladder to the central nervous system. With the aid of this complex neuro-urodynamic program, innervation of the urinary bladder can be evaluated in a more objective way. It often happens that no change in bladder pressure occurs during the first phase of pressure recording. In such cases, however, pressure waves develop later, after the start of transurethral intravesical electrostimulation. Intravesical electrical stimulation (IVES) is an important diagnostic aid which, in many cases, reveals hidden reactive capabilities of the intramural receptor systems of the bladder.

Between 1973 and 2005, 328 neonates were investigated a couple of hours following birth. Of these, 231 were operated on during the first 24 hours of life (Figures 65.2–65.4). All operated infants were re-examined after wound healing to compare pre- and postoperative data. The state and prognosis of the operated newborn was evaluated by developmental neurologic methods and neuro-urodynamics, and the type of incontinence was examined (Figures 65.5 and 65.6). The preoperative examination revealed in 73 cases normotonic, normoactive bladder, strong detrusor contraction (>40 cmH_2O), and definite signs of vegetative orientation in the EEG. In 97 cases the severity and/or the complexity of malformations (e.g. hydranencephalia) contraindicated the early closure, and this patient population has not received IVES. As the most severe cases were excluded, the treated population is consequently a selected one. Surgery saved good bladder function in 64 cases, and 161 families accepted the regularity and prolonged duration of IVES (Figure 65.2). The 161 IVES-treated infants, together with the 64 MMC infants with good bladder function, were regularly checked on a monthly basis. The Developmental Neurology Department in Budapest is responsible for the complex

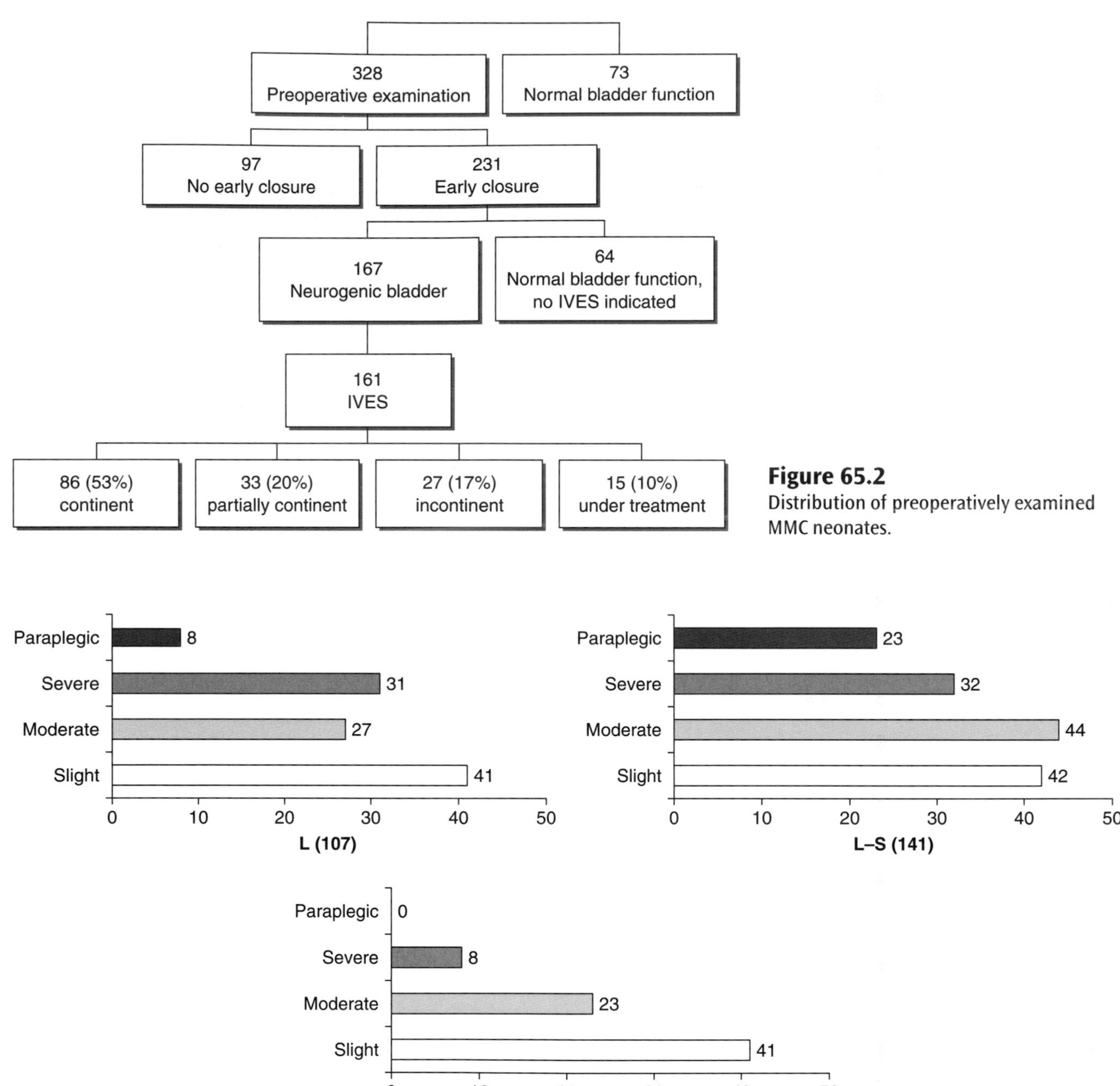

Figure 65.2
Distribution of preoperatively examined MMC neonates.

Figure 65.3
Localization of the cele and the grade of paraparesis in 328 MMC newborns before early closure.

treatment of all symptoms of MMC (i.e. paraparesis, eventual consequences of hydrocephalus, and bladder and rectal functions). These regular check-ups, including examination of bladder function in those patients who showed normal bladder function postoperatively, revealed that this good detrusor ability was sustained throughout the follow-ups, which lasted until the patients were 4 years of age.

Therapy

The aim of IVES in MMC patients is the physiologic *organization* of bladder function. In other patients the aim is *reorganization*, to give back a lost function. In MMC patients bladder innervation never developed during the embryonic and fetal period – there is nothing to reorganize. In MMC patients intramural receptors have not lost

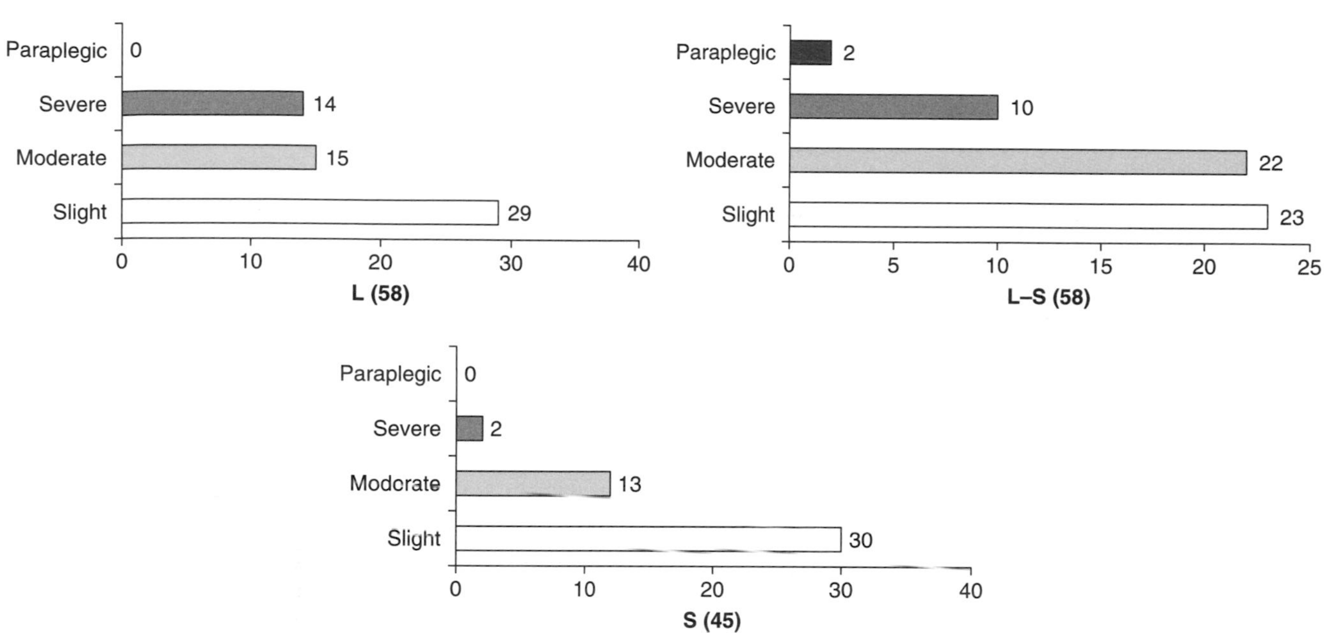

Figure 65.4
Localization of the cele and grade of paraparesis in 161 operated MMC infants at initiation of IVES.

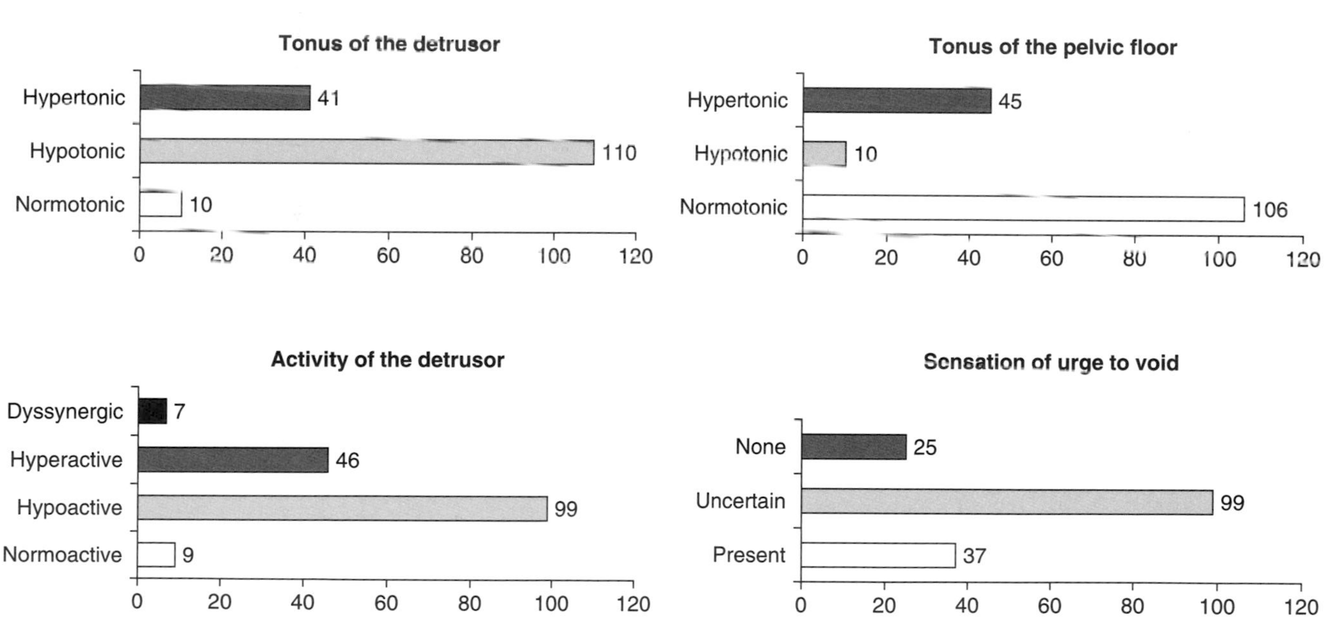

Figure 65.5
Results of neuro-urodynamics at the initiation of IVES in the treated 161 MMC patients.

contact with spinal neurons – such contacts were never built up. MMC, however, rarely presents a complete absence of neurons connecting the bladder and spinal cord. Nerve development may be seriously impaired, nevertheless a small percentage of neurons has usually reached the bladder during fetal development. The essential aim is to organize a new developmental variety of bladder innervation and achieve more satisfactory bladder function. The earlier this approach is initiated, the better are the results.[9–17]

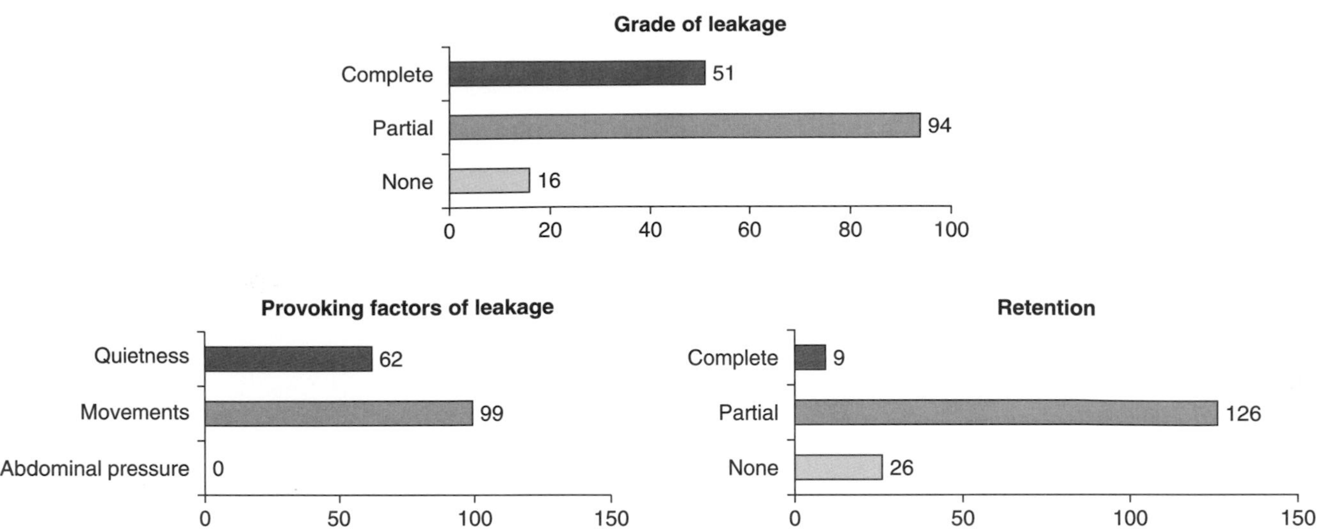

Figure 65.6
Types of abnormal voiding at the initiation of IVES in the 161 MMC patients.[19]

Infants and children

Regular intravesical, transurethral electrotherapy was applied in 161 infants.[19] The comparative results of the pre- and postoperative examinations served as parameters for the bladder electrotherapy. IVES was performed daily for 90 minutes. The diagnostic and therapeutic conditions were similar, but no polygraphic neurourodynamics was performed, only a special transistorized bladder, rectal, and average pressure recorder was used (Figures 65.7 and 65.8).

The parameters of the electric stimulation were (1) current: DC 1–10 mAs, according to type of the bladder paresis (the current is harmless); (2) wave form: repetitive 2 ms wide rectangular impulses composed of longer or shorter trains with an exponentially increasing rise time. The duration in seconds of the rise time, the length of the train, and the duration of the interval can be altered according to needs. The frequency of the individual impulses can be changed. The most effective frequency is between 70 and 90 Hz.

The aim of the therapeutic stimulation depends on the age of the patient. In infants the first goal is to reach alternating dry and wet periods, to improve detrusor contractility, and to accomplish voiding in stream with complete evacuation of the bladder without retention. The speedy disappearance of retention reduces the risk of ascending infections, upper urinary tract dilations, and reflux. The other goal is the prevention of shrinkage, extensive enlargement, or flaccidity in the bladder.[18,19] Among the aims of IVES, the prevention of dyssynergy has an important role. The stimulation at the area of the cross-striated sphincter musculature, together with activation of the hip and pelvic muscles using elementary sensorimotor functions, serves to fulfill this goal.

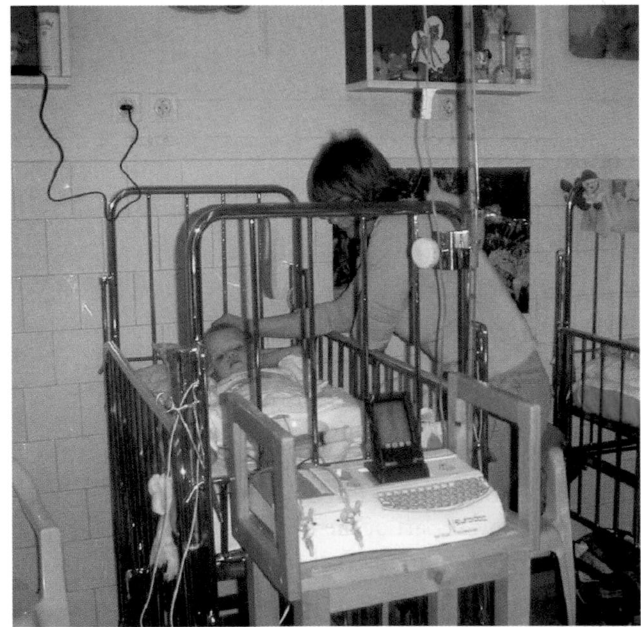

Figure 65.7
The set-up of regular IVES.

IVES is not a mechanical process using the same electric current throughout the treatment. The parameters of electrostimulation must be continuously adjusted to the changes which have already developed in the bladder function due to the treatment. Initially the intramural receptors are hyperpolarized owing to the lack of efferent impulses, which are necessary to maintain a base level of sensitivity.

tr = 1000 ms
th = 4000 ms
toff = 1000 ms
Ima = 2 mA
P = 90 Hz
tin = 90 s
td = 15 min
Peak Nr : 1
Pnul I = 2 wcm
Pmax = 9 wcm
Time = 5 s
P range : –5.. 20 wcm
EMG range : 8000

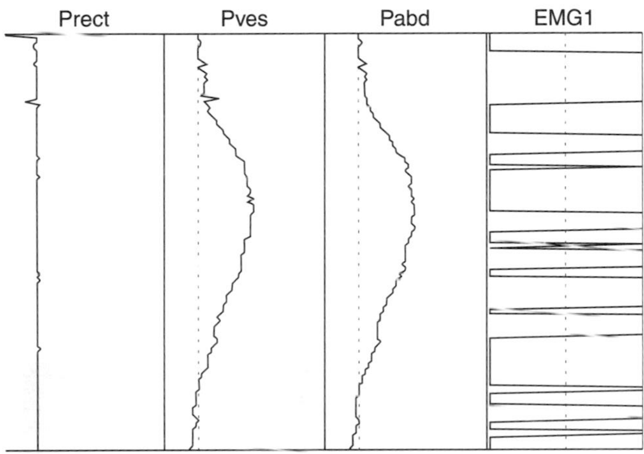

Figure 65.8
Chart of urodynamics during IVES.

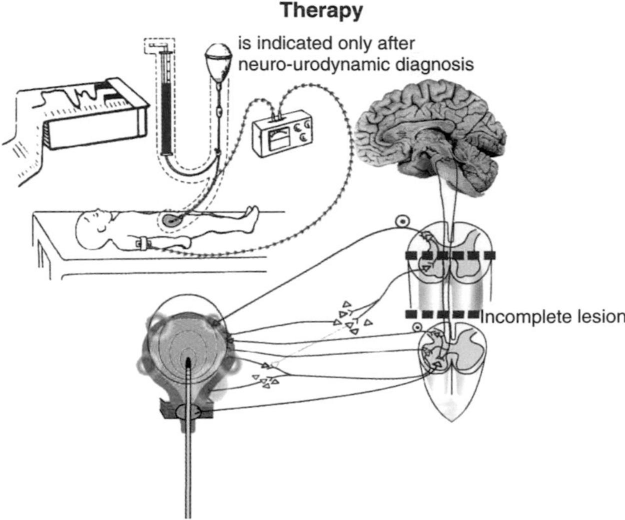

Figure 65.9
The patient (infant or child) is catheterized with an electrocatheter, and the bladder is filled with sterile, colored saline. The electric stimulus depolarizes the intramural sensory (pressure) receptors and bioelectric impulses arise. These are transported through intact sensory axons to the central nervous system in case of incomplete lesion of the spinal cord or its nerves. Cooperative children can observe the colored fluid in the manometer.

The first period of treatment is dedicated to change this state and effect depolarization of the receptors. When this new 'normal' state is achieved, the receptor system is able to transport its own stimuli through afferentation. Sometimes this is the longest part of the treatment. The first contractions may develop from local contacts among stimulated receptors and intramural motor neurons. Contractions reciprocally activate the pressure receptors. Stronger contractions with prolonged duration are activated from higher parts of the nervous system. It is not known how the new information reaches the cerebral cortex, nevertheless, in many MMC patients a real urge to void develops after several months of treatment. Patients usually indicate 'funny' sensations in their tummy, corresponding to increased pressure in the bladder, recorded manometrically. Neuro-urodynamic control shows some kind of desynchronization in the EEG record, which corresponds to vegetative orientation. When this level is reached, the next goal is to build up conscious bladder control. In infants this level correlates with the appearance of dry and wet periods, stream urination, and the disappearance of 'dripping' (Figure 65.9).

Results

The first aim of IVES is to achieve and maintain the infantile control of the bladder (i.e. stream urination, complete evacuation of the bladder without any residual, the development of dry and wet periods, prevention of dripping due to movements or crying, and strengthening of the urge to void, which at this age is not conscious. To realize this goal, regular continuous IVES was provided 5 times a week for 1.5–2 years, occasionally interrupted after the first year of life for 2–3 weeks. After this period the treatment was continued, and the patients were treated regularly on a 3-month treatment 3-month interval schedule, until three or three-and-a-half years of age. At this age, the child's level of cooperation level permits the development of voluntary control, based on the activated sensation of the urge to void. The treatment was finished when the patient reached between four and four-and-a-half years.

With cooperative children, realization of conscious bladder control starts with the help of biofeedback and regular toilet training. The first step of biofeedback happens

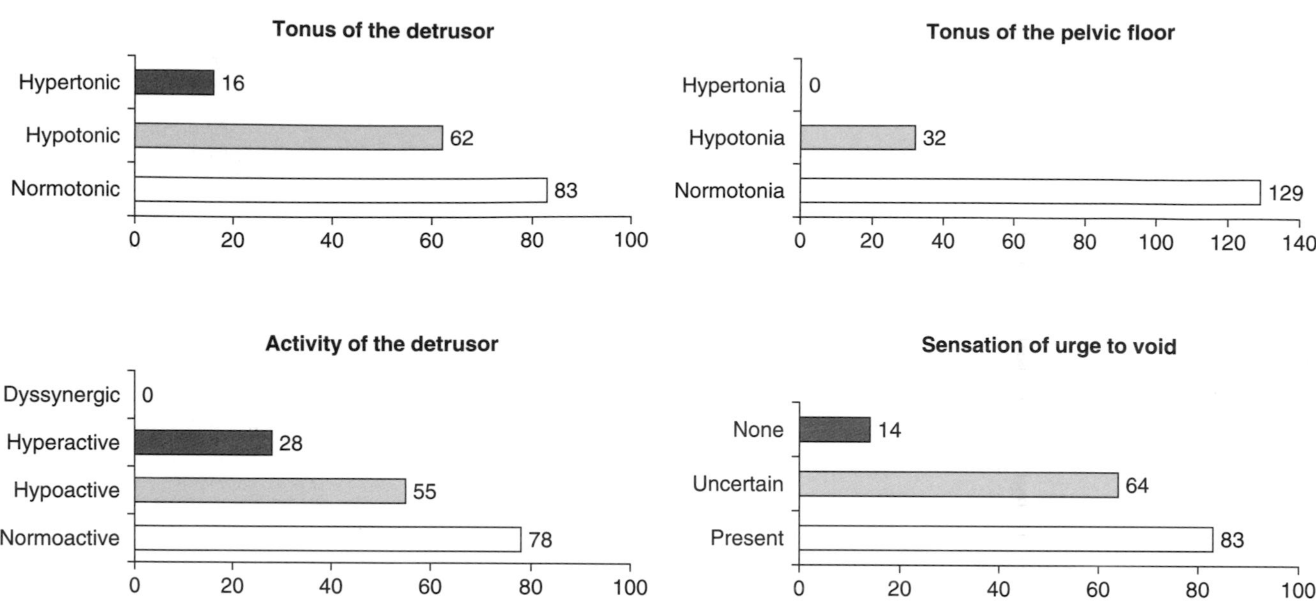

Figure 65.10
Results of neuro-urodynamics at the conclusion of IVES in the 161 MMC treated patients.

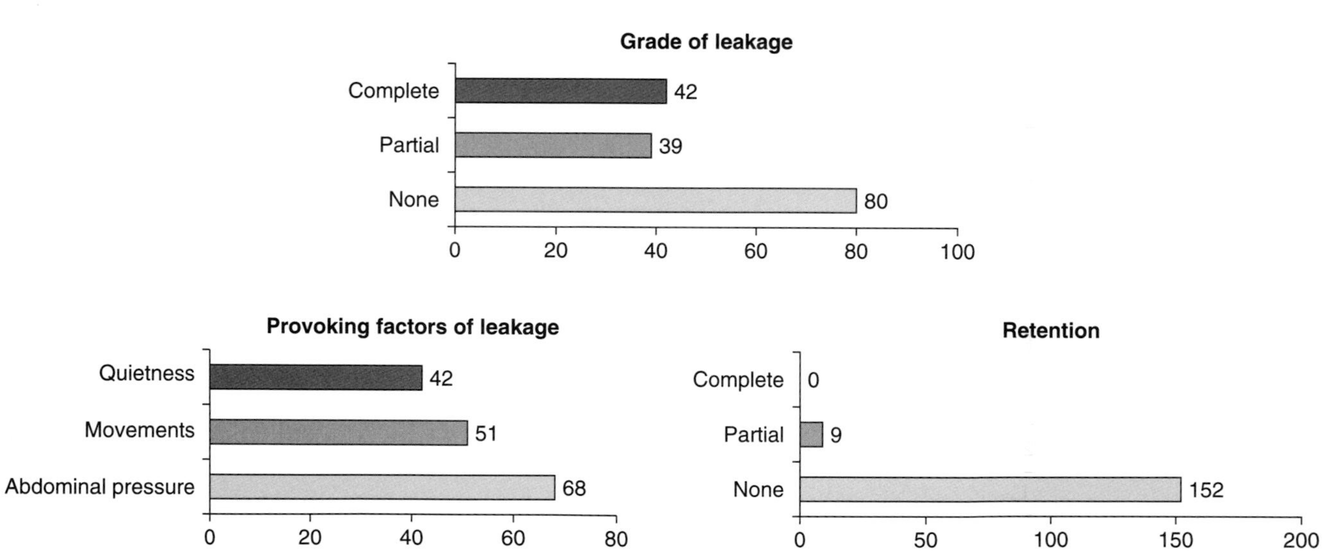

Figure 65.11
Types of abnormal voiding at the conclusion of IVES in the 161 MMC patients.

during the intravesical stimulation. The bladder, which is connected to a water manometer system, is filled with a colored sterile solution (NaCl + xantichridine). When the detrusor contracts the level of the fluid in the manometer system increases. The patient can see this elevation, and starts to sense the strange sensation simultaneously. The child is informed that the 'strange' sensation is the feeling of the urge to void and is instructed to stop fluid level elevation. With the help of IVES, the patient is gradually able to fulfill this instruction, and the regular feedback trials help him/her to learn how to do it automatically, without pelvic exertion. Later this practice follows without stimulation. In this way the MMC child may become clinically and socially continent. At the conclusion of regular IVES, those MMC children, who are considered continent are able to voluntarily control their bladder; they are familiar with the sensation of urge to void, can withhold urination, until they reach the toilet, and can urinate in stream, without

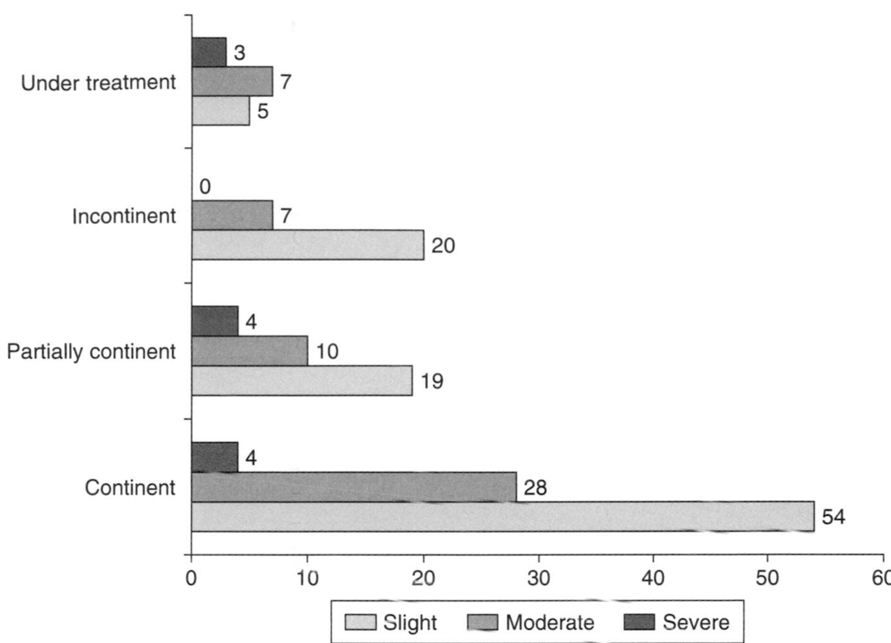

Figure 65.12
Correlation between the results of IVES and grades of paraparesis in the 161 MMC patients.

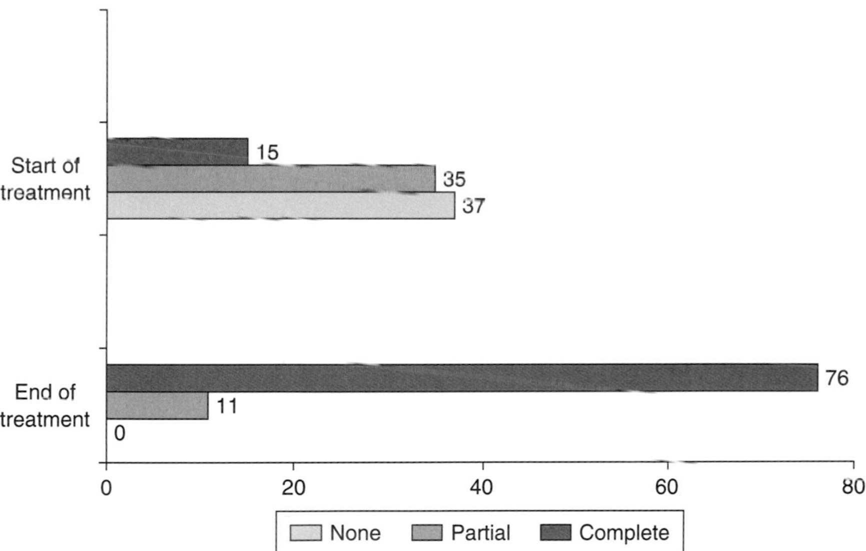

Figure 65.13
Results of intrarectal electrotherapy of 87 MMC infants with constipation.

residual, and are dry for at least 3 hours. Those who can feel the sensation of urge to void, but this sensation is occasionally not strong enough, and those who cannot withhold it for a sufficiently long time to reach the toilet, and are dry for 1.5 hours, are considered 'partially continents' (Figures 65.10–65.12).

IVES for diagnostics and IVES for therapy are strongly correlated. Changes in electric parameters and catheter positions (inside the bladder, bladder neck) must continuously correspond to actual diagnostic results during the sessions, from the beginning to the conclusion of the therapy. Regular diagnostic check-ups are made to identify the state of bladder innervation and the results compared with the state of voiding, adaptation of age-dependent requirements, and social situations (family, kindergarten).

The functional state of the pelvic floor has both direct and indirect influences on bladder function. Dyssynergy often develops and regular training of the pelvic floor muscles may offer additional help to IVES. Therapeutic training must begin immediately after wound healing. At this early age the only way to activate the pelvic floor is by the regular application of elementary sensorimotor functions, for example activated elementary crawling. This kind of training also helps to maintain the integrity of all innervated muscles (the hip and lower extremities). Later, the development of bipedal walking may help in toileting.[20,21]

Anal incontinence and constipation are frequent accompanying factors. Electrotherapy of the loose anal sphincter and the inefficient bowel motility can reduce these additional symptoms of MMC.[22,23] This therapy is performed with a different kind of electric current. The active electrode is a modified rectal tube, with a 2 cm wide silver ring running smoothly near the tip on the outer surface of the tube, and the cable inside. The duration of the stimulation is usually 15 minutes, and it is effected after bladder stimulation (Figure 65.13).

References

1. Berényi M. Complex preoperative developmental neurologic examination (including electro-urodynamics) and the transurethral intravesical electrotherapy of the bladder in meningomyelocele neonates and young infants. In: McLaurin RL, ed. Spina Bifida, Praeger, New York, London, 1986: 341–5.
2. Berényi M. Meningomyelocelés újszülöttek preoperatív neurodinamikai kivizsgálása. [Preoperative neuro-urodynamic examination of meningomyelocele neonates.] Rehabilitáció (Rehabilitation) 1998; 8: 17–21. [In Hungarian]
3. Katona F. Neue Methoden in der Sauglingsneurologie und Rehabilitation. Acta Paediatr Acad Sci Hung 1974; 15: 67–75.
4. Berényi M. The developmental treatment of the neurogenic bladder in MMC infants. Urodinamica 1992; 1: 65–70.
5. Berényi M, Katona F. Meningomyelocelés csecsemök neurogén hólyagjának korai terápiája. [Early treatment of neurogenic bladder in meningomyelocele infants.] Gyermekgyógyászat (Pediatrician) 2000; 5: 511–20. [In Hungarian]
6. Katona F, Berényi M. Intravesical transurethral electrotherapy in meningomyelocele patients. Acta Paediatr Acad Sci Hung 1975; 16: 363–74.
7. Katona F. Intravesikale Elektrotherapie bei Myelodysplasiebedingter Lahmungsblase. Z. Kinderchirurgie 1973; 13: 114–17.
8. Berényi M, Katona F. A meningomyelocelés beteg korai komplex neuroterápiája és késöbbi rehabilitációja. [Early complex neurotherapy and later rehabilitation of meningomyelocele patients.] Ideggy Szeml (Clinical Neuroscience) 2001; 54(9–10): 260–70. [In Hungarian]
9. Nicholas JL, Eckstein HB. Endovesical electrotherapy in tratment of urinary incontinence in spina bifida patients. Lancet 1975; 1276–7.
10. Fransthworth RH. Electrostimulation in the management of neurogenic bladder disorders. Br J Urol 1976; 48: 149–50.
11. Berger D, Berger K, Genton W. Endovesical transurethral electrostimulation in the rehabilitation of neurogenic bladder in children. Eur Urol 1978; 4: 33–45.
12. Seiferth J, Larkamp H, Heising J. Experiences with temporary intravesical electro-stimulation of the neurogenic bladder in spina bifida children. Urologe 1978; 17: 353–4.
13. Seiferth J, Heising J, Larkamp H. Experiences and critical comments on the temporary intravesical electrostimulation of the neurogenic bladder in spina bifida children. Urol Int 1978; 33: 279–84.
14. Madersbahcer H. Blasen (Re)habilitation bei Kindern mit neurogener Harnentleerungsstörung mittels Biofeedback unter Verwendung der transurethralen electrostimulation. Akt Urol 1984; 15: 248–53.
15. Madersbacher H, Ebner A. Die intravesikale Electrotherapie in Kombination mit Biofeedback – Eine wertvolle Hilfe zu (Re)dukation bei Kindern mit funktionellen Miktionsstörungen. Kinderurologie 1984; 340–1.
16. Kaplan WE, Richards I. Intravesical transurethral bladder stimulation. Kinderarchir 1986; 41(1): 25–7.
17. Kaplan WE, Richards TW, Richards I. Intravesical transurethral bladder stimulation to increase bladder capacity. J Urol 1989; 142: 600–2.
18. Kaplan WE, Richards I. Inravesical transurethral electrotherapy for the neurogenic bladder. J Urol 1986; 136: 243–6.
19. Cheng EZ, Richards I, Balcom A et al. Bladder stimulation therapy improves bladder compliance: results from a multi-institutional trial. Urol 1996; 156: 761–4.
20. Berényi M, Katona F. Meningomyelocelés csecsemök csípö- és alsóvégtag-parasiseinek korai neuroterápiája. [Early neurotherapy of hip and lower extremities paresis in meningomyelocele infants.] Gyermekgyógyászat 2000; 6: 596–606. [In Hungarian]
21. Berényi M. *Rehabilitáció a perifériás és a vegetatív idegrendszer kórképeiben. [Rehabilitation of peripheric and vegetative neurologic diseases.]* In: Katona F, Siegler J eds. Orvosi Rehabilitáció (Medical Rehabilitation) Medicina, Budapest 1999: 296–301. [In Hungarian]
22. Janneck C. Electric stimulation of the bladder and the anal sphincter – a new way to treat neurogenic bladder. Prog Pediatr Surg 1976; 9: 119–39.
23. Berényi M, Katona F. Az incontinentia alvi és az obstipatio korai therápiája MMC-s csecsemökben. Gyermekgyógyászat 2001; 52: 458–64.

66

Fecal incontinence management in the neurogenic bladder patient

Anthony R Stone, Paula J Wagner, and Angela DiGrande

Introduction

Bowel dysfunction often goes hand in hand with neurogenic bladder. Practitioners dealing with the bladder issues in neurogenic or neuropathic patients need to pay similar attention to bowel dysfunction. It is of little use to patients to have achieved bladder control, when fecal incontinence is still a problem. Bowel care is a quality of life issue that significantly impacts a patient's psychosocial, physical, and emotional well-being.[1] Chronic constipation, fecal impaction, and recurring fecal incontinence are also associated with significant morbidity including abdominal discomfort, nausea, vomiting, diminished appetite, urinary tract infections, skin breakdown, rectal fissures, rectal prolapse, megacolon, intestinal obstruction, VP shunt malfunction, bowel perforation, and even death. It is recognized that establishing an acceptable and effective treatment plan involves time, commitment, teamwork, and an understanding of the factors that can affect compliance and success. Patient assessment and education on bowel care need to be initiated as early as possible in the disease process.

This chapter will emphasize the management of bowel dysfunction in patients with spina bifida and after spinal cord injury. The principles outlined can, however, be applied to all neurogenic bladder patients, including those with degenerative spinal cord pathology and multiple sclerosis (MS).

Spectrum of problem

The prevalence and spectrum of bowel dysfunction depends on how this problem is defined. In spina bifida, fecal incontinence has been reported to range from as low as 28% to over 90%. Problems with defecation are consistently reported to be >85%.[2] In spinal cord injury, some degree of fecal incontinence affecting quality of life has been reported in up to 62% of patients. This prevalence depends on the level of the lesion and whether it is complete or not. Vallès et al[3] have correlated the nature of the dysfunction to the level of lesion and colonic transit time, identifying three broad patterns of behavior: lesions below T7 are characterized by constipation (86%) and occasional incontinence; lesions above T7 with preserved sacral reflexes have far less constipation, significant defecatory difficulty, and also occasional incontinence, and lesions above T7 without sacral reflexes, with not very frequent constipation (56%), have less defecatory difficulty and a greater severity of incontinence. These patterns of bowel behavior can be applied broadly to all neurogenic patients and allow a rational approach to management.

Quality of life

There are no specific measures to assess the relative quality of life (QoL) impacts of fecal incontinence and bowel difficulty on bladder problems. Although the problems faced are similar, bowel dysfunction poses specific problems to the patient, including management of accidents, use of protective garments, time required on bowel issues and additional support for a bowel program, as well as the impact of the medical issues listed above. Several tools have been developed to determine the impact of fecal incontinence on aspects of QoL. Krogh et al[4] conducted a study to develop and validate a symptom-based tool to score neurogenic bowel dysfunction. The authors were able to correlate self-reported bowel dysfunction scores with impact on QoL. Although this study focused on patients with spinal cord injury, it may have applicability to other patient populations with neurogenic bowel dysfunction.

The Fecal Incontinence Quality of Life (FIQL) tool has been shown to be valid and reliable by the American Cancer Society of Colon and Rectal Surgeons. This tool, developed for use in adults, evaluates four distinct domains: lifestyle, coping/behavior, depression/self-perception, and embarrassment. Each of the items is scored on a 5-point Likert scale.[5]

Psychosocial and developmental considerations

The spina bifida patient presents a unique illustration of the effects of bowel dysfunction, on multiple levels, across the whole lifespan. Starting in early infancy, the time and resources involved in monitoring and managing constipation, fecal impaction, and fecal incontinence can be significant. Caring for a newborn is stressful for any parent. Management of neurogenic bowel during the infant and toddler years can add to the caregiver's burden, often resulting in parental time taken away from other responsibilities. This can include spousal relationships, sibling care, social obligations, and employment. Missed time from work, frequent visits to the physician, and costly medications or supplies can drain a family's limited financial resources. The continual soiling can contribute to skin breakdown and urinary tract infections. Chronic constipation with impaction can impair the young child's appetite, potentially affecting the child's overall nutritional status and growth.

As the child moves into the preschool/school age years, the inability to be toilet trained can create barriers to entrance into the daycare, preschool, or school settings. Development of independence, self-esteem, and self-concept are all negatively impacted. The child with a poorly managed neurogenic bowel often has problems with school attendance, and lacks opportunities to develop and maintain peer relationships or engage in age-appropriate recreational and social activities. Peer relationships can be particularly stressful, as children can be quite cruel in their dealings with classmates who are different. The need to wear diapers and the smell of excrement can present an impossible situation for the young child. Many parents will 'opt out' of the traditional school setting in favor of home schooling, primarily for this reason.

As the child enters the adolescent years, peer contacts and relationships become increasingly important. Bowel incontinence can interfere with the teen's emerging sense of self, their need for independence, dating, and sexuality. Opportunities for participation in healthy recreation, higher education, and employment can also be affected. As health care professionals, we need to be proactive, looking at patients across the lifespan. Our goal is to promote regular bowel emptying and fecal continence through an individualized bowel management program, while fostering independence.

When working with children, it is important to establish a good rapport with the parents. Listening to and valuing parental concerns is key to their developing trust in the healthcare team. Patients and families may be reluctant or embarrassed to openly discuss their experiences and the impact it is having on their lives. Parents may view their child's bowel program failures as a reflection of their parenting ability. Current perceptions, past experiences, and fear of failures do affect a patient's or family's receptiveness to trying alternative management strategies. Families may be reassured to know that there may be periodic temporary set-backs. They need to be advised that each individual is unique and that no one program works well for every individual.

These factors will be just as important in the adolescent and adult patient with acquired neuropathy. Fear of bowel accidents will similarly and significantly impact the psychosocial and physical well-being of these patients.

Bowel management program

Goals

The goals of a bowel management program are (1) to control constipation, (2) allow elimination at a socially acceptable time, and (3) foster independence.[5] The bowel management program is a series of interventions aimed at achieving these goals.

Patient assessment

There are multiple factors to take into consideration in prescribing a bowel management program. These will include patient age, degree of disability, primary neurologic diagnosis, support personnel, home circumstances, patient goals, and overall motivation. This list of factors, although not exhaustive, will come in to play in the management of these patients at all times.

Bowel history

The bowel history should include the basics of bowel movement intervals, timing, amount, diameter, consistency, and what percentage of stool is deposited into the toilet or diaper. Are the stools a planned or unplanned event? The patient is asked about factors that affect their stool consistency, frequency, and incontinence. Factors that may affect frequency of defecation include fluid intake, diet, use of bulking agents, medications, activity levels, and emotional status, etc.

It is important to know who performs the bowel care. Is the patient independent? Does he/she require assistance? If so, what level or type of assistance is required? Is that assistance available when needed? Where is the toileting performed in home and out of the home? Are there bathroom access issues?

Determine what the patient has tried in the past, what has worked and what hasn't. Obtain specific information on how the past program was implemented. A bowel function and dietary log can be helpful in identifying patterns.

It also facilitates tracking of the patient's progress once an intervention is implemented.

Relevant past medical history should include achievement of developmental milestones, ability to toilet train, disorders or surgery of the gastrointestinal tract, anorectal surgery, trauma or malformations, pelvic or gynecologic surgery, pregnancies and outcomes, back surgery or trauma, neurologic disease, level of the spinal lesion, diabetes, urinary incontinence, and medication usage (prescribed, over-the-counter, herbal preparations).

In children, eliciting a bowel function history needs specific tools.[6] In general, the bowel history starts with the patient or family's description of the problem in their own words, including a list of their major defecatory problems. Current bowel management must be documented with attention placed on how this is affecting their daily life and activities. The timing of the various problems should be noted along with the patient's overall treatment goals. Level of satisfaction with their current regime is documented. Patients may not be on any formal program, or may describe long periods with no bowel accidents (accompanied by little to no stool). This 'controlled constipation' with infrequent emptying is not considered to be an appropriate bowel program.

Physical exam

The initial evaluation needs to include an assessment of the individual's knowledge, cognition, and function to determine their overall capacity to be able to learn to perform or direct a caregiver to provide for their bowel care program. The assessment should cover vital signs, growth parameters, general hygiene, developmental age, gait (where applicable), body habitus, sitting balance and tolerance, ability to transfer, upper extremity proprioception and strength, hand and arm function, spasticity, anthropometrics, and skin problems or risks.

Abdominal exam assesses palpable stool along the course of the large intestine. Note any surgical scars. Inspect the back, noting any hairy tufts or dimpling at the base of the spine or scars from previous spinal surgery. Note the position of the anus and observe the sphincter at rest as open or closed. Inspect for rectal tags, fissures, prolapse or skin breaks/rashes, or hemorrhoids. Check for anal wink. Perform digital exam for rectal sphincter tone and the ability to voluntarily contract/relax the sphincter. Note the presence and type of stool present in the rectal vault.

The neurologic exam should include muscle tone and strength, presence of extremity spasticity, cremasteric reflex, and deep tendon reflexes. If appropriate, the amount of reflex activity retained below the lesion should be assessed. If the reflex pathways are functional and can be used to initiate defecation, management will be less challenging. In addition, in such upper motor neuron type patients, the goal is to keep the stool soft/firm, with evacuation recommended at least every other day. In lower motor neuron impairment with loss of reflex activity, the bowel is areflexic (damage at or below T12). These patients will be unresponsive to digital stimulation, as the sacral reflex arc at S2–4 has been partially or completely affected by the disease or injury. The goal in this group of patients is to keep the stool soft and formed and the rectal vault empty. This assessment is relatively straightforward in the spinal cord patient, but less clearcut in spina bifida or in MS.

Diagnostics testing

Generally specific tests of bowel function are unnecessary. Unless required for the diagnosis and management of the neurologic condition, tests such as anorectal manometry, transit studies, and/or defecography rarely add to improving bowel care. An abdominal plain X-ray (kidneys, ureter and bladder view) is useful to determine the amount of stool present in the colon. It is also helpful when working with families who may not be able to visualize or comprehend the extent of the problem.

Management

A 'team' approach including the patient, caregivers, healthcare providers, community primary care physician, and, in children, the school nurse, is necessary. Developing a plan that is acceptable to the patient, family, and caregivers will improve overall compliance. Patients and families need education on all aspects of the proposed bowel care program and to have an opportunity to address their concerns. Communication is enhanced when families have a specific point of contact to discuss issues, questions, or concerns. Finding an effective treatment plan may take weeks to months. Close follow-up is important so that evaluation and adjustments to the program can be made, if needed. The plan developed will again depend on close collaboration between all parties.

Nonsurgical management

Dietary management The basic components of an effective program include a healthy, high fiber diet, plenty of fluids, some form of regular exercise and activity, a consistent daily time for toileting, and a large measure of patience. Fiber is needed for stool consistency. Typical daily dietary intake may not include an adequate source of fiber. Several over-the-counter fiber supplements are currently available; however, some may not be appropriate for use in young children. Williams et al[7] have recommended a minimum amount of dietary fiber equivalent to the child's age plus 5 g per day for children over 2 years of age. The recommended dose of fiber in the average adult patient with neurogenic bowel is 15 g/day. These are starting recommendations, from which adjustments can be made based on the quantity, frequency, and quality of the stool produced. The best sources of fiber will come from natural sources; however, dietary habits may preclude adequate daily dietary intake. Patient care pamphlets on culturally relevant dietary recommendations for sources of dietary fiber or an evaluation with the nutritionist may prove to be helpful in getting patients started.

Fluid intake is also essential to optimal stool consistency. Patients will often do better with fluid intake if specific recommendations are made regarding daily fluid requirements. Maintenance fluid requirements for age should be reviewed and incorporated into the dietary recommendations for your patient.

Physical activity and exercise Activity should be encouraged as part of the overall treatment plan. This is obviously a problem in individuals who have limited mobility and who may be socially isolated because of their disability. Regular exercise not only supports cardiovascular health, mood, and weight management, but also enhances intestinal motility. Collaboration with rehabilitation physicians, nurses, and physical therapists is essential to identify resources to optimize exercise and physical activity.

Timed toileting As described, a program of regular and scheduled emptyings is the mainstay of management and should be emphasized. Input by caregivers will be essential in initiating this and many of the following management steps. Simple Valsalva techniques may be required with this program.

Rectal stimulation and evacuation In the patients with reflexic bowel function, the defecation reflex should be triggered as part of the bowel program. Digital stimulation is the mainstay of this process, but may need to be enhanced, using suppositories, enemas, or a combination of these methods. In patients with areflexic bowel, a manual evacuation technique may be necessary.

Pharmacologic agents Prior to establishing a successful daily bowel program, the patient may require a thorough bowel 'clean-out'. This can best be accomplished with the use of oral agents to soften the stool mass. Polyethyleneglycol (PEG) has worked extremely well for this, particularly in the pediatric population. It is odorless, colorless, and tasteless, thus passing the all-important 'kid palatability' test. It can be mixed in any beverage, including water, and titrated by weight and effect. There is minimal absorption via the intestine when administered orally and it is excreted unchanged in the urine.

The clean-out regimen is generally given over a period of 5 to 7 days, as the hard stool is rehydrated. Some patients may require a longer period of time. Adequate fluid intake during clean-out is recommended for all patients. A rectal check should be performed prior to starting the program, as hard stool in the rectal vault could present blockage to the further movement of stool and initial disimpaction will be necessary. Once a thorough bowel clean-out has been achieved, the *daily maintenance* bowel-emptying regimen can be established. This may be as simple as timed toileting via Valsalva after meals, or the use of a mini enema or suppository to induce rectal emptying may be necessary. Bisacodyl suppositories or docusate sodium mini enemas are the most popular in this area. Laxatives are generally minimally helpful in long-term bowel management. Their use is often abandoned due to the unpredictability of action and the resultant increased loss of control.

Enema techniques In some situations, especially with lower motor neuron type bowel function, the bowel program will need to be supplemented with formal enemas. Various techniques have been described including pulsed irrigation evacuation (PIE) and transrectal irrigation, using a specialized stoma cone.[8,9]

Biofeedback training Specially trained physiotherapists help patients learn bowel movement techniques through biofeedback. The patient must have some sensory awareness for this to work. The process helps patients to isolate, identify, and strengthen related muscles, sense when the stool is ready to be evacuated, and contract the muscles if evacuation is inconvenient. This technique requires careful patient selection, as it requires a significant time commitment and follow-through from patients and families.[10]

Surgical management

When a patient cannot be established on a successful bowel program, surgical options may be indicated. In most cases the decision to opt for surgery will be dictated by QoL factors rather than medical indications. Since the introduction of antegrade colonic enema techniques in children, especially those with spina bifida, the QoL benefits and improved independence have been so dramatic that the decision is made very easily and at increasingly younger ages. Important factors to consider when evaluating surgical options include the patient's age, existing comorbidities, prior abdominal surgeries, presence of ventrico-peritoneal (VP) shunt or other devices, history of complications associated with surgery or anesthetic, and ability for the patient to be independent with the bowel program (or ease of burden for the caregivers).

Sacral nerve stimulation Sacral nerve stimulation (neuromodulation), similar in technique to that used for urge incontinence, has been used in spinal cord patients.[11] A significant improvement in the frequency of accidents and ability to defer defecation was observed. The indications and long-term success of this modality have not been established at this time.

Antegrade enema techniques The most dramatic improvement in bowel management, specifically in the spina bifida population, occurred with the introduction, by Malone, of the antegrade colonic enema procedure.[12]

Malone antegrade continence enema The Malone antegrade continence enema (MACE) has proved invaluable in the management of children and adults with fecal incontinence. In the neurogenic population, it has mostly been used in the spina bifida population. There are anecdotal reports of its use in lower motor neuron spinal cord injured patients also. This simple operation utilizes the appendix as a conduit to the colon. In Malone's original description the appendix was detached from the cecum on its mesentery, reversed, and reimplanted into the cecum. Subsequent techniques leave the appendix in situ and plicate the appendiceal–cecal junction. Presently, no attempt is made to reinforce this valve. The appendix is brought out to skin level and a continent catheterizable stoma is created (appendicostomy), typically located in the umbilicus.

In many cases, the MACE is accomplished at the time of surgical correction of urinary incontinence. In view of its success in managing bowel problems in this group of patients, our threshold for recommending this is quite low. Once the decision to correct the bladder dysfunction is made, many patients and/or parents will request the MACE procedure, even if their bowel programs are relatively successful. In the face of 'sluggish' bowel function, antegrade enemas are more efficient than the best 'conservative' bowel program.

Patients introduce a catheter into the stoma to administer a daily antegrade colonic enema. The wash-out effect and the simulated colonic peristalsis will empty the colon and rectum. Thus, chronic constipation is prevented and fecal incontinence dramatically improved. Overall success rates have been described in the range of 60 to 90%.[13] Retrospective studies have demonstrated a significant improvement in fecal incontinence post-procedure when compared to the patient's previous bowel care program.[14] The newly gained continence has resulted in significant improvement in all QoL domains.

Laparascopic approach The procedure can be performed laparoscopically, bringing the appendix out through an umbilical or right iliac fossa port site and suturing the opened appendix to the skin *ex vivo*.[15] The simplicity and safety of this technique have encouraged the use of this procedure in younger children, even accomplishing this prior to definitive surgical management of the urinary tract. It appears that it is easier to establish a good MACE bowel program before the onset of chronic constipation

Alternatives to appendix If the appendix has been removed, is unsuitable for use as a conduit, or the clinician may wish to use it for a Mitrofanoff construction, several alternative strategies are available. There are reports in the literature of using the terminal ileum, necessitating an ileo-tranverse anastomosis to restore intestinal continuity. Additionally, some authors have formed a Monti type bowel tube for this purpose.[16] We prefer to use a cecal flap to construct a neoappendix, as it obviates the need for an additional bowel anastomosis. An anterior cecal flap with its base at the antimesenteric border is dissected. This is rolled into a tube over a 12 or 14F catheter and then folded back over the cecum. The adjacent cecum is then embrocated over the tube to support it and form a valve.[17] This neoappendix may be brought out at the umbilicus or iliac fossa, in similar fashion to a native appendix.

Cecostomy A useful alternative to the appendix is to insert a cecostomy tube. Indications for this will be similar to those where the appendix is absent, unsuitable, or unavailable. Some surgeons use this technique primarily, feeling that the appendix is sufficiently unreliable and they would rather use this simple alternative. The cecostomy is created by mobilizing the anterior cecum and placing a 12 or 14F catheter through a small cecostomy. A purse-string suture is placed around this to prevent peritoneal soiling and the tube is brought through a right iliac fossa stab incision. The cecum should be anchored to the adjacent parietal peritoneum to support the cecum against the abdominal wall. The catheter is left in place for 6 weeks to allow the cecostomy track to mature. The catheter can then be exchanged for a cecostomy (gastrostomy) button, as a simple outpatient procedure. These buttons are then exchanged every 3–4 months.[18]

The cecostomy may be successfully placed anywhere in the colon. Patients may have had their right colons removed, may have significant adhesions, or the VP shunt may impact this decision.

A cecostomy may be accomplished percutaneously, under fluoroscopic control, using conscious sedation.[19] Placement of the catheter is performed under direct fluoroscopy. It can be completed in an outpatient setting with local anesthetics and conscious sedation. Additional benefits are that it is minimally invasive, esthetically more appealing than the traditional cecostomy tube, the tube prevents stenosis, there is a shorter recovery time and a decreased length of hospital stay, patients can swim after healing, and it is reported to be a more comfortable device. Risks associated with this procedure include the development of granulation tissue at the site, skin irritation and pressure necrosis at the site, cellulitis, and the risk of perforation and sepsis.

Pre- and postoperative antegrade enema management Good bowel preparation is required prior to all these procedures. Clearly, from a safety point of view this is essential, but many of these patients will have significant constipation. A good clean-out will make establishment of the bowel program much easier. Postoperatively, colonic irrigation is commenced as early as possible through the stenting catheter prior to commencing catheterization of the MACE or placement of the cecostomy button.

It is recommended that patients access the stoma daily. The most common solutions used to irrigate the bowel are tap water, saline, PEG, and phosphate enema. The type, volume, and frequency must be individualized for each patient. Volumes may vary from 300 to 1500 ml. We recommend starting with a smaller volume (based on the size of the patient). The goal is to evacuate the bowels daily, with no unplanned bowel movements in-between. If the patient continues to have unplanned movements, or has minimal or no result from the day's irrigation, we recommend increasing the daily volume by 50 ml increments, until the desired results are achieved. Tap water usage has been found to be safe for use. It is recommended that households requiring water softeners use bottled water for the procedure.

Patients are instructed to complete the bowel program at approximately the same time every day, typically after a meal. This takes advantage of the gastro-colic reflex. The irrigation solution can be delivered via a hanging enteral feeding bag, attached to a funnel-end urinary catheter. The irrigation solution can be run in by gravity, pumped, or pushed by syringe. The patient sits on the toilet, administers the irrigation, and waits for stool to be evacuated. Most patients report the entire process takes approximately 20–60 minutes. A padded toilet seat and arm and foot supports are recommended for patients with impaired sensation, balance, or mobility.

If a patient experiences difficulty with catheterization of the stoma, we recommend that they leave the catheter in and capped on completion of the irrigation. The catheter should be left in place for a period of 72 hours. The MACE is still accessible for use, and the catheter in place may assist in preventing stoma closure. If access difficulties persist, the stoma may require dilatation or a minor surgical revision.

Reported complications with the procedure include the risk of anesthetic, bleeding, peritonitis, bowel perforation, abscess formation, intestinal obstruction, leakage at the stoma site, stenosis of the stoma site, and superficial wound infections.[20] In our experience, the most common occurrences are stomal leaks or stenosis. Leakage may resolve if patients are instructed to make sure the catheter is inserted far enough into the tract and to 'pinch off' the irrigation tubing prior to removal from the stoma. If leakage persists, a stomal revision may be indicated. A silicone stoma plug (MACE stopper) is now available and may be useful in selected patients. Continued or recurrent fecal accidents usually reflect poor or inefficient wash-outs. Patients should be evaluated with plain X-ray and rectal exam. Management of these problems requires counseling and alteration in technique, which may include increasing the volume of irrigation or addition of PEG to the washout. Occasionally the bowel may become so impacted that complete wash-out and possibly fecal disimpaction may be required prior to recommencing the regular irrigation program.

The success of these programs, as with any of the bowel programs described, needs continued commitment by the patient and caregivers. Additionally, support by trained nursing staff is essential. Although bowel care can be significantly improved with the MACE, improvements are not 100%. Patients and families should be advised during their preoperative counseling that they will need to make a daily time commitment, that their program will require fine-tuning afterwards, and that, for some, continued problems with periodic constipation and accidents may occur

Colostomy Colostomy may be used as a last resort for treating fecal incontinence. Indications are mostly relative and will include a combination of intractable bowel issues, severe disability, and problems with care support. Very occasionally the colon may become so obtunded that bowel diversion becomes a matter of urgency. Patients who fit into this category are usually quadriplegic or have severe progressive MS. Careful selection of the stoma site should be applied as body habitus and chair bound status will impact significantly into this decision.

Summary

When faced with a patient with neurologic disease, it is essential to assess and treat all functional deficits including bowel dysfunction. This chapter outlines the management options available to improve this. In the majority of patients, the simple conservative measures outlined will suffice. Success of these will depend on a team approach including the patient, caregiver, rehabilitation nurses, social worker, physical therapist, and occupational therapist. The physician will have a relatively minor role. Surgical options are available for selected patients, specifically spina bifida children and adolescents, and a few adults with severe neurologic disability.

References

1. Correa GI, Rotter KP. Clinical evaluation and management of neurogenic bowel after spinal cord injury. Spinal Cord 2000; 38(5): 301–8.
2. Ponticelli A, Iacobelli BD, Silveri M et al. Colorectal dysfunction and faecal incontinence in children with spina bifida. Br J Urol 1998; 81(Suppl 3): 117–9.
3. Vallès M, Vidal J, Clavé P, Mearin F. Bowel dysfunction in patients with motor complete spinal cord injury: clinical, neurological, and pathophysiological associations. Am J Gastroenterol 2006; 101(10): 2290–9.

4. Krogh K, Christensen P, Sabroe S, Laurberg S. Neurogenic bowel dysfunction score. Spinal Cord 2006; 44(10): 625–31.
5. Trasanovska M, Cato-Smith AG. Quality of life measures for fecal incontinence and their use in children. J Gastroenterol Hepatol 2005; 20(6): 919–28.
6. Jinbo AK. The challenge of obtaining continence in a child with a neurogenic bowel disorder. J Wound Ostomy Cont Nurs 2004; 31(6): 336–50.
7. Williams CL, Bollella M, Wynder EL. A new recommendation for dietary fiber in childhood. Pediatrics 1995; 96(5 Pt 2): 985–8.
8. Christensen P, Kvitzau B, Krogh K, Buntzen S, Laurberg S. Neurogenic colorectal dysfunction – use of new antegrade and retrograde colonic wash-out methods. Spinal Cord 2000; 38(4): 255–61.
9. Mattsson S, Gladh G. Tap-water enema for children with myelomeningocele and neurogenic bowel dysfunction. Acta Pædiatr 2006; 95(3): 369–74.
10. Wiesel PH, Norton C, Roy AJ et al. Gut focused behavioural treatment (biofeedback) for constipation and faecal incontinence in multiple sclerosis. J Neurol Neurosurg Psychiatry 2000; 69(2): 240–3.
11. Jarrett ME, Matzel KE, Christiansen J et al. Sacral nerve stimulation for faecal incontinence in patients with previous partial spinal injury including disc prolapse. Br J Surg 2005; 92(6): 734–9.
12. Malone PS, Ransley PG, Kiely EM. Preliminary report: the antegrade continence enema. Lancet 1990; 336(8725): 1217–8.
13. Teichman JM, Zabihi N, Kraus SR, Harris JM, Barber DB. Long-term results for Malone antegrade continence enema for adults with neurogenic bowel disease. Urology 2003; 61(3): 502–6.
14. Yerkes EB, Cain MP, King S et al. The Malone antegrade continence enema procedure: quality of life and family perspective. J Urol 2003; 169(1): 320–3.
15. Van Savage JG, Yohannes P. Laparoscopic antegrade continence enema in situ appendix procedure for refractory constipation and overflow fecal incontinence in children with spina bifida. J Urol 2000; 164(3 Pt 2): 1084–7.
16. Yerkes EB, Rink RC, Cain MP, Casale AJ. Use of a Monti channel for administration of antegrade continence enemas. J Urol 2002; 168(4 Pt 2): 1883–5; discussion 1885.
17. Kurzrock EA, Karpman E, Stone AR. Colonic tubes for the antegrade continence enema: comparison of surgical technique. J Urol 2004; 172(2): 700–2.
18. Cascio S, Flett ME, De la Hunt M, Barrett AM, Jaffray B. MACE or caecostomy button for idiopathic constipation in children: a comparison of complications and outcomes. Pediatr Surg Int 2004; 20(7): 484–7.
19. Chait PG, Shlomovitz E, Connolly BL et al. Percutaneous cecostomy: updates in technique and patient care. Radiology 2003; 227(1): 246–50.
20. Graf JL, Strear C, Bratton B et al. The antegrade continence enema procedure: a review of the literature. J Pediatr Surg 1998; 33(8): 1294–6.

67

Adult meningo-myelocele

JLH Ruud Bosch

Introduction

Meningo-myelocele (MMC) and spina bifida occulta are by far the commonest causes of neurogenic bladder dysfunction in childhood, and can also be the cause of significant problems in adults, with complications such as incontinence, obstructive uropathy, vesicoureteric reflux, pyelonephritis, and subsequent renal failure. In the majority of the spina bifida cases, the lumbosacral region is involved, leading to neurogenic disturbance of urogenital, colorectal, and pelvic floor function.

The mortality of MMC patients was high before the 1940s. A change in prognosis occurred in a step-wise fashion in the second half of the 20th century. Initially, improved obstetric and neonatal care resulted in an increase of surviving MMC children by the end of the first half of the 20th century. More aggressive neurosurgical management including early closure of the neural tube defect and shunting techniques for the accompanying hydrocephalus followed this. Thereafter, many of these children received comprehensive health care. In many developed countries management and follow-up protocols were developed and delivered by multidisciplinary teams. These teams usually involved a pediatric nephrologist, neurosurgeon, orthopedic surgeon, and urologist. A much higher number of severely affected children now reach adulthood and 97% of these have urogenital problems.[1]

A new phase may have been entered since the recognition of the role of folic acid supplementation for all women of childbearing age as an important measure in the prevention of neural tube defects. In the US and in Australia a statistically significant decrease in the prevalence of neural tube defects has been noticed after enrichment of certain foods with folic acid.[2,3] Therefore it is recommended that all women of childbearing age consume 0.4 mg of folic acid daily.

An abnormality such as a meningocele that is an extension of the dural sac outside the spinal canal (usually through a posterior defect) may be seen on fetal ultrasound scanning. Although a diagnosis *in utero* by ultrasound and alpha-fetoprotein is now routinely possible, there may be very difficult management decisions to take, including the possibility of terminating the pregnancy. A more widespread use of preventive measures and the diagnosis of neural tube defects in early pregnancy will probably lead to a decrease of the number of adult patients with spina bifida within a few decades.

Urodynamic types of lower urinary tract dysfunction

Four basic types of lower urinary tract dysfunction have been identified in MMC patients. In a series of 111 children the following patterns were found:[4] an 'inactive detrusor plus inactive pelvic floor' in 32%; an 'overactive detrusor and overactive pelvic floor' were seen in 38%. A combination of 'overactive pelvic floor plus inactive detrusor' and 'inactive pelvic floor plus overactive detrusor' was found in 12% and 9%, respectively. In 10%, normal lower urinary tract function was seen. So, more than 50% of the patients either had a normal or a low-pressure detrusor. The 'classic' urodynamic pattern of the lower urinary tract in young adults with MMC was formerly described as the 'inactive detrusor plus inactive pelvic floor' or areflexive bladder with open vesical outlet.[5] This, however, was mainly a reflection of the selection and survival of the 'fittest', because these patients are at low risk for upper tract deterioration and only rarely develop vesicoureteral reflux and pyelonephritis.[4] More recently, adult patients with other urodynamic patterns are seen more frequently as well as adult patients who have undergone lower urinary tract reconstruction and those who are candidates for a kidney transplantation and need a low-pressure lower urinary tract to accept the transplant.

Patients with a so-called overactive pelvic floor or dyssynergic sphincter are particularly at risk for upper urinary tract deterioration. If untreated, approximately 70% of neonates have or will develop hydroureteronephrosis.[6]

Poor bladder compliance is another important problem in patients with abnormal detrusor function. Particularly detrimental to the function of the upper tracts and kidneys is the combination of poor compliance and a nonrelaxing or dyssynergic sphincter. If the pressures in the bladder are almost permanently above 40 cmH_2O, ureteral delivery of urine boluses to the bladder stops. Patients with an abdominal leak-point pressure above 40 cmH_2O are at risk for upper tract damage.[7]

In a comprehensive urologic evaluation of 104 patients without adequate urologic management, during a median period of 5 years (range 5 months to 33 years) before presentation to the neurourologist, Bruschini et al[8] found that, in those who had a detrusor leak-point pressure (DLPP) below 40 cmH_2O, 5.2% presented with renal scars, whereas in those who had a DLPP of 40 cmH_2O or higher, 37.8% showed scars. Stratification according to functional bladder capacity above or below 33% of the expected volume for age also showed significant differences in the risk for renal scars (10% versus 33%). The more than 7 times increased risk of upper urinary tract damage in those with a DLPP ≥40 cmH_2O is probably an underestimation of the risk because of survival bias.

Changing neurourologic lesion in meningo-myelocele patients

In the series reported by van Gool, patients with a normal bladder function all had defects limited to the sacral area that had been surgically closed.[4] However, a normal lower urinary tract function in the early years of life is no guarantee for the absence of future problems. Furthermore, the neurourologic status found at the initial postnatal examination may change in more than a third of the tested children. In one series, the urethral sphincter innervation changed in 37% during the first 3 years of life; this necessitated a second neurosurgical procedure (most often untethering of the spinal cord) in 9%.[6] These findings emphasize the importance of close urodynamic surveillance during the first 3 years of life. However, these patients should be followed closely into adult age because they remain at risk for development of the so-called tethered cord syndrome. The pathogenesis of the tethered cord syndrome is explained by traction on the lumber spinal cord between two fixation points. The upper fixation point is at the exit site of the posterior and anterior spinal nerve roots, and the lower fixation point is at the site of the tethering or the site of scar fixation from the previous neurosurgical closure. The repetitive injury to the small blood vessels due to stretching and kinking leads to a reduction of the blood supply to this section of the cord and consequent neuronal hypoxemia.[9] The alternative explanation based on the concept of 'abnormal ascent' of the spinal cord during growth of the child is wrong: during the 8th week of fetal development the spinal cord has already attained the level of L1–2.[10] The decision to neurosurgically untether the cord in patients with a normal bladder function is a difficult one, since there is no solid evidence that the function will deteriorate if the cord is not untethered; alternatively, about 11% of children with a normal bladder develop neurogenic bladder dysfunction after untethering.[11]

Principles of management of lower urinary tract dysfunction

Preservation of kidney function

The primary goal in the management of MMC patients is preservation of kidney function. To achieve this goal, the bladder should function as a low-pressure reservoir. Obstructive uropathy and high bladder pressures during a significant part of the filling phase are the most important causes of kidney failure in these patients. If, on urodynamic testing, the detrusor pressure begins to rise only above a filling volume of 300–400 ml, it is feasible for most patients to limit the high-pressure time by clean intermittent (self)-catheterization (CISC). If the compliance of the bladder is lower or if the detrusor is hyperreflexive even at relatively small volumes, the combination of anticholinergic drugs and CISC may achieve the goal of reasonable dryness and preservation of the upper tracts. However, if these measures fail, the bladder should be converted into a low-pressure reservoir; this can be achieved by several different surgical techniques, such as an augmentation cystoplasty (e.g. Clam ileocystoplasty) or autoaugmentation (detrusor myectomy).[12] In those who have a very thick bladder wall substitution cystoplasty may be more appropriate.[13] Continuation of CISC in these cases is the rule. Conversion of the lower urinary tract into a low-pressure reservoir by CISC with or without medication, augmentation, or diversion may not be able to prevent late renal failure if some kidney damage has already occurred.[14] In most adult MMC patients who come to our attention the issue of high pressures will have been taken care of at an earlier age.

Several authors have shown that the early initiation of a proactive management protocol, preferably from the day of birth on, minimizes renal damage and reduces the need for surgery. Such a protocol includes CISC and antimuscarinic therapy with the addition of profylactic antibiotics in selected patients. Dik et al have reported on 144 patients with spina bifida aperta who were started on a proactive management protocol shortly after birth.[15] Of these children, 4.2% had renal scarring after long-term follow-up.

Five of the six patients with renal scarring were started on therapy with CISC and antimuscarinic therapy several months after birth. Therefore, only 0.7% of those who started management immediately after birth developed renal scarring. At the age of 6, 77% of the children with spina bifida were dry, although 59% of those who were dry had not had a surgical intervention. Proactive treatment had resulted in a negligible loss of renal function, even though early urinary continence was included in the protocol as a treatment goal.

Kessler et al presented a retrospective study on 133 patients with MMC who were started on proactive neurourologic management as early as possible.[16] Among others, 22 of these were initially evaluated and started on the management protocol after the age of 10 years, and 67 between birth and the age of 2 years. Mean follow-up was 9 and 11 years, respectively. The upper urinary tract function was normal in 86% and 99%, respectively, at last follow-up (p = 0.012). Following failure of conservative therapy only, the proportions of patients undergoing surgical intervention with the intention to preserve or normalize the upper urinary tract function were significantly different (p = 0.0002), at 59% and 15%, respectively.

These studies show that early proactive management, ideally started immediately after birth, improves upper urinary tract function and reduces the need for surgery in MMC patients in the long term.

Urinary continence

An unsolved problem of urinary incontinence may have a serious impact on quality of life. Incontinence is multifactorial: hyperreflexia, decreased compliance, and sphincteric or pelvic floor incompetence all play a role. A comprehensive urodynamic examination can help to identify these factors and determine their relative importance in the individual patient.

Hyperreflexia can be addressed by medical treatment and both hyperreflexia and low compliance can be treated by an augmentation cystoplasty or detrusorectomy, usually in combination with CISC. More recently, the treatment of detrusor overactivity by intradetrusorial injections of botulinum-A toxin has proven to be a viable option in selected MMC patients.[17]

A poorly compliant bladder can also be treated with (auto)augmentation. When performing a bladder augmentation it is important to avoid the creation of an 'hourglass' deformity. A circular band of detrusor muscle, the so-called fundus ring, is situated in the bladder wall at a distance of about 2.5 cm from the bladder neck. If the fundus ring is not divided when clam shelling the bladder, it will contract and create the hourglass deformity. The bladder has to be opened in such a fashion that the fundus ring is divided on both ends of the opened bladder. It is preferred to bring the bladder extraperitoneally by closing the peritoneum around the vascular pedicle. Extraperitonization of the bladder seems to reduce the risk of spontaneous perforation of the bladder, a risk that is prominent in children and adolescents because of the tendency for poor compliance with CISC.

A weak outlet can be treated by the creation of a fixed outlet resistance. To achieve this, techniques like injection of bulking agents, colposuspension, or a fascial sling (puboprostatic or pubovaginal) can be employed; again, CISC is usually needed as an adjunctive measure in these situations. The artificial sphincter holds the theoretic promise of near normal voiding; however, in most patients with MMC this cannot be achieved.

Alternatively, the natural outlet can be abandoned; the bladder neck can be closed and a catheterizable stoma, using the Mitrofanoff or Monti principle, can be created with or without an augmentation cystoplasty. The catheterizable stoma of the Monti or Mitrofanoff type is prone to complications. Stomal stenosis, mostly at skin level, is a frequently occurring complication; surgical revision is often indicated. Stomal leakage of urine can be a frustrating complication: lengthening of the intravesical tunnel or reimplantation of the stoma will often be needed in such cases.

A continent urinary diversion in the form of an Indiana pouch is another alternative. The life of many MMC patients it is made easy when they do not have to transfer out of the wheelchair to catheterize.

Many surgical alternatives exist to reach urinary continence. The Kropp and Pippi-Salle procedures rely on the creation of a flap valve from the bladder neck. The Young-Dees, Tanagho, and Mitchell procedures lengthen the urethra.

The neural tube defect mainly involves the dorsal part of the spinal cord. The neurologic deficit therefore is mainly determined by a sensory defect. In fact, about 90% of the anteriorly located motor neurons are intact in MMC patients.[18] Therefore, despite the fact that the afferent parts of the sacral reflex arcs are absent or severely deficient, the efferent nerves to the sphincter and pelvic floor muscles may be responsive to electrical stimulation. Electrical stimulation of the pudendal nerve at the site of the ischial spine may improve urethral and anal sphincteric function in these patients.[19]

The reputation of the artificial urinary sphincter in MMC patients is somewhat poor, because placement of an artificial urinary sphincter (AUS) can lead to secondary changes in bladder function that may be detrimental to the upper urinary tract. Bladder overactivity or a decrease in bladder compliance may occur *de novo* after increasing the outflow resistance of the lower urinary tract by the implantation of an artificial sphincter.[20,21] In one series, 32 of 47 implanted patients who were implanted as children could be followed-up for a minimum of 10 years (mean 15.4 years). There were 13 removals (due to erosion or infection) and 19 sphincters were still intact (59.4%). Of these patients, 18 were dry and 7 of 19 voided spontaneously.

There were 0.03 revisions per patient-year and it was noted that 9 of 13 with placement after 1987 had not needed revisions. This series therefore shows that a long-term successful outcome of the AUS is possible in well-selected patients, even if the device is implanted at a young age.[20]

The main advantage of the AUS is the potential preservation of spontaneous voiding. However, in a population of patients with MMC, only 27% were able to void spontaneously and were continent after the implantation of an AUS.[21] One could therefore reason that other methods to increase the outflow resistance, such as a fascia sling procedure, would be preferable in these patients because the main advantage of the AUS, i.e. preservation of spontaneous voiding, cannot be achieved in these patients anyway.

Concerning the combination of enterocystoplasty and AUS placement, Furness et al have reviewed the literature and their own experience in 17 MMC patients.[22] Of these, 3 had the AUS placed before the augmentation and 4 had the sphincter placed after the bladder augmentation. In 10 patients the procedures were performed simultaneously. Based on the compiled literature data and their own results, they summarized that the infection rates were 14.5% and 6.8% for simultaneous and staged procedures, respectively. However, these rates were not statistically different. Only three of the reviewed papers reported rates for both the staged and the simultaneous procedures. In these papers the differences in infection rates were 40.5%, 18.2%, and 3.7%, with the simultaneous procedures always showing the higher rates. In their own series the difference was 4.3%. There are many factors that can mitigate the infection rate, but this review did not control for any of the possible factors like other simultaneous reconstructive procedures, duration of the procedure, positive preoperative urine cultures, type of bowel used, or antibiotic prophylaxis. Miller et al did not find an influence of these factors, except for type of bowel used.[23] Gastrocystoplasty was associated with a 0% infection rate. The overall AUS infection rate in their series was 6.9%. However, it was 20% excluding the gastrocystoplasties.

Other important questions in relation to the bladder augmentation are: Who needs a bladder augmentation in combination with an AUS or fascial sling procedure and are there urodynamic parameters that can predict the necessity for enterocystoplasty?

In their retrospective review, Miller et al[23] found that the average bladder compliance of those in whom an augmentation was performed was 7.8 ml/cmH_2O; in 2 patients the compliance was more than 10 ml/cmH_2O and in none of the patients was it less than 2 ml/cmH_2O.

Kronner et al[24] found that 15 of 38 MMC patients (39.5%), who were younger than 18 years at the time of the implant, subsequently required augmentation after a mean follow-up of 101 months. The mean time to augmentation was 49 (range 10–118) months. An augmentation was performed if urodynamics had worsened. Repeat urodynamic tests were performed when intractable incontinence and/or upper tract changes occurred. Before the implant of the AUS, the bladder capacity and the compliance were not significantly different between the patients who were (8.0 ± 4.8 ml/cmH_2O) and those who were not (7.0 ± 3.3 ml/cmH_2O) treated by bladder augmentation ($p = 0.45$). The authors contended that cut-off values of bladder compliance below which others have recommended simultaneous augmentation, such as bladder compliance below 2 and below 6.7 ml/cmH_2O, are inaccurate. In fact, many of their patients had a compliance below one of these cut-off values but did not need an augmentation. It should be noted, however, that the original group consisted of 80 patients; of these, 35 underwent a primary augmentation because of severely decreased compliance or capacity. So it seems that the jury is still out on this subject. Furthermore, Spiess et al reported that the long-term survival of the AUS in boys with spina bifida rarely exceeded 8 to 9 years, questioning whether the AUS is a good choice in children with neurogenic urinary incontinence.[25]

It is clear that a plethora of operative techniques exists for the above-mentioned problems. Many authors have reported the results of a particular technique; however, it remains unclear whether the results are reproducible by others. It is also unclear whether the presented techniques result in better outcomes than other surgical techniques, since up until now not a single randomized controlled study comparing two surgical techniques has been reported.

A large retrospective analysis from six centers in France, evaluating incontinence management and its outcome in spina bifida patients, yielded interesting data.[26] A total of 421 adolescent and adult patients were included. Of these, 191 (45%) had been treated conservatively only. Of the conservatively treated patients a normal voiding pattern was claimed by 21%, clean intermittent catheterization was performed by 61%, whereas 18% reported no specific bladder emptying method. The mean leakage score was 2.74, on a scale of 1 to 5, with a higher score indicating less incontinence. On the other hand, 230 patients (55%) were surgically treated. Except for 23 patients who underwent noncontinent urinary diversion, 207 were included in the evaluation of treatment and continence outcome. The mean leakage score was 3.45.

The authors gave three broad categories in which some 40 different surgical techniques and combinations of techniques/procedures to treat urinary incontinence in these patients were listed. The first category was bladder neck surgery without augmentation; the second, bladder augmentation without continent diversion; and the third, bladder augmentation with continent urinary diversion. Patients with cutaneous noncontinent diversions were not included in the continence evaluation for obvious reasons. The outcomes were summarized as follows: an AUS in both genders and a bladder neck sling or Kropp procedure in females were satisfactory as continence procedures when bladder augmentation was not indicated. In cases of bladder augmentation without continent diversion, an AUS in males and a bladder neck sling, Kropp, or Young–Dees procedure in females gave the best results. When bladder augmentation with continent urinary diversion was required, bladder neck closure has provided the best results in both genders.

Health-related quality of life in relation to incontinence and its management

Most pediatric urologists agree that incontinence may adversely affect quality of life. However, most of these patients have lived with their handicaps for their whole life and have often adapted to it in a remarkable way. Contrary to patients who have an acquired neurogenic bladder problem, they have no previous personal experience with normal function of the urinary tract. This is important to keep in mind because this notion may help to understand that those who have a comparable but congenital problem perceive the margin for improvement, which is present in patients with acquired disease, quite differently. Most of the remaining problems cannot be solved without creating new ones!

A recent study indeed did *not* confirm the assumption that urinary incontinence may have a serious impact on quality of life. Lemelle et al investigated the influence of (in)continence on health-related quality of life (HRQoL) in a cross-sectional study from six centers in France.[27] A total of 460 spina bifida patients (300 adults and 160 adolescents) were included in this study. Interestingly, adolescents with spina bifida had HRQoL scores that were higher when self-rated than when questionnaires were completed by their parents. The investigators did not find a strong relationship between incontinence and HRQoL in this population. Moreover, patients who were surgically managed for urinary or fecal incontinence did not show significantly higher scores of HRQoL. They concluded that urinary or fecal incontinence and their medical management may not play a determinant role in HRQoL of persons with spina bifida. However, many other factors affect HRQoL in these patients. A longitudinal study design is recommended to assess whether incontinence management is associated with improved HRQoL.

Undiversion and conversion

Today urinary diversion is rarely performed in children with MMC. Those who have reached adulthood and were diverted in the past might wish to become candidates for orthotopic undiversion or conversion to a continent urinary diversion such as an Indiana pouch or one of its alternatives. Although cosmetic reasons do play a role, undiversion is more indicated in those with upper tract problems in order to create a nonrefluxing low-pressure continent reservoir.

Before undiversion, patients should be evaluated with urine cultures, creatinine clearance, a renogram, CT urography, and a loop-o-gram to adequately describe function and anatomy. If orthotopic undiversion is contemplated this should be complemented by videourodynamic studies or a cystogram and retrograde ureterograms if there is no reflux.

Contraindications to undiversion include inability to perform CISC and poor kidney function. As a general rule, patients with a serum creatinine greater than 2 mg/dl (175 μmol/ml) will have difficulty in coping with the metabolic challenges posed by the use of small or large bowel for a continent reservoir.[28] In MMC patients the lean body mass is decreased and therefore the creatinine clearance is a more reliable parameter than serum creatinine: in MMC patients, a creatinine clearance cut-off of 50 ml/min would be roughly equivalent to the abovementioned values. MMC patients with an impaired anal sphincteric function will be at increased risk for fecal incontinence when intestinal function becomes (slightly) impaired due to the use of bowel segments to reconstruct the urinary tract.

In those with an efficiently working cutaneous diversion and no upper tract complications, the risks of an undiversion should be taken into account. A new anastomosis between the ureters and the bowel segment is more prone to stenosis, even if the caliber appears to be large at the time of the undiversion. Probably, the changed tissue quality and vascularity of the ureteral wall is the explanation for this observation. In one series a 22% stenosis rate was reported in a group of 48 neurogenic patients as opposed to only 6.4% in the total group of 374 patients.[29]

Those MMC patients who are wheelchair bound are not good candidates for an orthotopic undiversion because of the difficulty in performing CISC. For women it is particularly troublesome to have to catheterize through the urethra. In MMC women we often find large labia that complicate CISC via the urethra. Since most of these patients also have an increased body mass index, with increased diameters of the thighs and limited ranges of movement in the hips, it is much easier for them to be able to catheterize without having to transfer out of the wheelchair. This can be accomplished by a catheterizable stoma at an easily accessible spot on the (upper) abdomen or via the umbilicus. In wheelchair-bound male MMC patients the penis is often concealed due to the abnormal body habitus, making CISC more difficult as well as the fitting of a condom catheter.

Adult MMC patients who have previously undergone an enterocystoplasty and those who opt for an undiversion or conversion of a cutaneous stoma into a catheterizable orthotopic or heterotopic reservoir can be confronted with several complications. Urologists following adult MMC patients should be aware of these complications that include stomal stenosis, stenosis of the ureteroenteric anastomoses, reservoir perforation, mucus production in the reservoir, struvite stone formation, clinically significant urinary tract infections,[30] and metabolic problems such as acid–base disturbances, osteopenia, osmotic diarrhea, fatty diarrhea, calcium oxalate urolithiasis, and vitamin B12 deficiency.[28] Treatment of these complications is according to generally accepted guidelines not specific for MMC patients. One measure should, however, be highlighted and that is daily irrigation with normal saline that frees the reservoir of mucus and helps prevent the formation of calculi.

Pretransplant surgical preparation of the lower urinary tract is a special situation in which reconstruction, diversion, or even undiversion may be indicated. When the bladder is not reparable or usable with acceptable results, ileal conduit, continent urinary diversions, and/or bladder augmentation may be required.[31–33] Each method has its specific set of possible complications and these should be thoroughly discussed with individual patients prior to use. A native dilated ureter can be used to augment the bladder and this may be the procedure of choice in neurogenic bladder associated with grossly dilated ureters.[34]

Sexual dysfunction

Sexual dysfunction, with both genders having loss of genital sensation, is a common problem. As patients with spina bifida now have increased life expectancy this is recognized as an important quality of life issue. Theoretically, the effects on penile erection, vaginal lubrication, and orgasm are related to the level and completeness of the lesion. In reality, there is a paucity of literature about sexual function in MMC patients. Erections are claimed by about 70% of adolescent males, although most of the erections are probably reflex in nature and not in response to sexual stimuli. The occurrence of erections is positively correlated with a lower sensory level and the presence of an anocutaneous reflex.[35] Those with normal bladder function and intact sacral reflexes are likely to have normal erectile function. There are no studies on the use of oral medication, intracorporeal injections, or penile prostheses specifically on these patients. Although men with intact sacral reflexes can achieve erection and sexual intercourse they do not have any sensation in the penis. The possibility of restoration of sensation in the glans penis has recently been explored by Overgoor et al, who cut the sensory ilioinguinal nerve (L1) distally in the groin and joined it by microneurorrhaphy to the divided ipsilateral dorsal nerve of the penis (S2–4) at the base of the penis. The operation was performed in 3 patients who were 17, 18, and 21 years old and who suffered from a spinal lesion at L5, L4, and L3–L4, respectively. By 15 months postoperatively all patients had achieved excellent sensation on the operated side of the glans penis. They were unequivocally positive about the results and the penis had become more integrated into the body image.[36]

In women, pregnancy and vaginal delivery is possible, although complications related to urinary tract dysfunction and deformation of the pelvis occur frequently.[37] In the French multicenter evaluation, 5 of 230 men (2.2%) and 12 of 191 women (6.3%) had one or more children.[26]

Follow-up schedules

Although roughly 78% survive to the age of 17 years,[38] patients continue to be subject to excess morbidity and mortality into and throughout adulthood. Mortality before the age of 35 years has been reported to be 54%.[39] Therefore the issue of follow-up is an important one.

However, no guidelines that specifically address the follow-up of adolescent and adult spina bifida patients have been issued by any of the major international urologic scientific societies like AUA, EAU, ICS, and the SIU, or the International Consultation on Incontinence. Furthermore, the sections on follow-up in existing guidelines for the management of patients with neuro-urologic problems are either very short or completely absent and generally lack an evidence base.

In an attempt to overcome these deficiencies we can define four domains that are relevant for follow-up schedules in these patients:

1. Functional issues. The maintenance of kidney function is the primary goal of management. Related to kidney function is lower urinary tract function, which is defined by the following parameters: bladder pressure during the filling phase, bladder compliance, bladder contractility, urethral sphincter and bladder neck function, coordination between bladder and outflow tract, antireflux mechanism, and uretero-pelvic function.
2. Surgical and anatomic issues like stomal stenosis, stenosis of the uretero-enteric anastomoses, reservoir perforation, upper tract reflux, and incompetent continence mechanism.
3. Metabolic issues are related to the incorporation of bowel segments in the lower urinary tract and include mucus production in the reservoir, struvite stone urolithiasis, clinically significant urinary tract infections,[30] and problems such as acid–base disturbances, osteopenia, osmotic diarrhea, fatty diarrhea, calcium oxalate urolithiasis, and vitamin B12 deficiency.[28] Renal ultrasound and plain abdominal films can diagnose most urinary tract stones.
4. Sexual counseling.

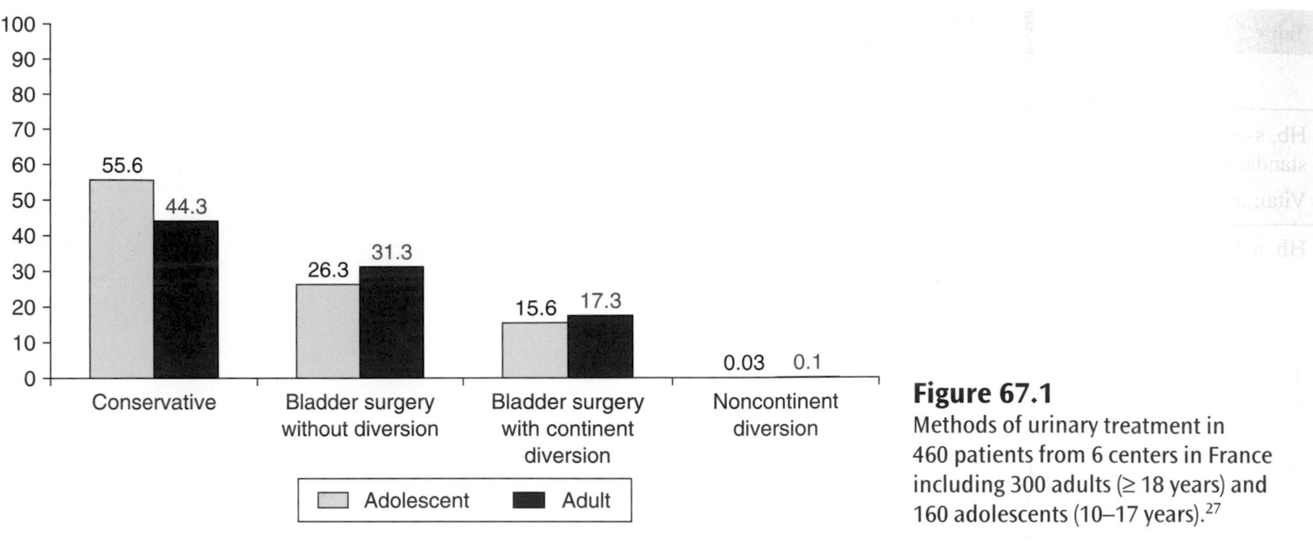

Figure 67.1
Methods of urinary treatment in 460 patients from 6 centers in France including 300 adults (≥ 18 years) and 160 adolescents (10–17 years).[27]

The French survey gives data on the relative importance of certain patient groups (Figure 67.1).[27] About 45% of adults were treated conservatively, about 30% had bladder surgery without diversion, and 17% had bladder surgery with continent diversion; less than 0.1% had a noncontinent diversion.

In *conservatively treated patients* with a *low-pressure system* and *normal renal function* who have been shown to be *symptomatically stable over a number of years*, evaluation of upper tract function and anatomy can be done every 2–3 years, unless there are reasons to suspect that motivation and IQ are suboptimal. Some form of sexual counseling can be incorporated in these follow-up visits. EAU guidelines for follow-up of neuro-urologic patients in general suggest more frequent follow-up visits (Table 67.1);[40] these guidelines, however, seem to apply more to those who have not achieved a symptomatically stable low-pressure situation. It should also be noted that renal ultrasound is inadequate for the demonstration of obstruction; however, renal isotope scans can diagnose (functional) obstruction and show the differential function of the kidneys.

In *low-pressure, symptomatically stable patients with a decreased glomerular filtration rate* (GFR), the advice of a nephrologist is sought. Dietary measures can often be taken to prevent further deterioration of renal function.

It is unclear whether regular urodynamic follow-up as suggested by EAU guidelines is necessary in stable adult patients. No evidence to support this policy in spina bifida patients is available. However, if the outflow tract needs to be manipulated (e.g. because of treatment for incontinence) in patients with a low-pressure system, a new urodynamic base line has to be established after this treatment. Furthermore, patients who have not achieved the low-pressure status should be followed more closely, approximately on a 3-monthly basis, while active conservative or surgical measures are being taken, to convert the lower urinary tract into a low-pressure one.

In *symptomatically stable patients with a low-pressure system that has been achieved by incorporating bowel in the lower urinary tract* or by some form of diversion, a more frequent follow-up is necessary, most importantly because of metabolic issues (Table 67.2). These patients should be followed regularly (initially 3-monthly and later 6-monthly) for metabolic complications. If necessary, medical treatment should be instituted. Metabolic acidosis is rare in patients with a normal renal function. When renal function is impaired, as is often the case in MMC patients, acidosis is more likely. If standard bicarbonate is less than 21 mmol/l, alkalizing therapy with sodium bicarbonate should be started. This is particularly important during growth and development. On the basis of a review of the literature on this issue, Mingin et al concluded that bladder augmentation does not affect final adult height. Initially there is metabolic acidosis, but this is corrected over time.

Table 67.1 *EAU Guidelines for follow-up of neuro-urologic patients*

2-monthly	Urinalysis (possible UTI between times can be self-checked by the patient, using dip stick)
6-monthly	Ultrasound kidney and bladder (for postvoid residual, stones, upper tract dilatation)
12-monthly	Physical examination (including blood pressure) and lab (blood)
12- to 24-monthly	Specialist examination in a neuro-urologic center, including at least a video-urodynamic study

Table 67.2 *Follow-up guidelines for patients with bowel segments incorporated in the urinary tract*

	3 m	6 m	9 m	1 yr	1.5 yr	2 yr	2.5 yr	3 yr	3.5 yr	4 yr	4.5 yr	5 yr	etc.
Hb, s-creatinine, Na, K, Cl, standard bicarbonate	x	x	x	x	x	x	x	x	x	x	x	x	x
Vitamin B12				x				x				x	x

Hb, hemoglobin; s-creatine, serum creatinine; Na, sodium; K, potassium; Cl, chloride.

Furthermore, over the long term bone mineral density decreases, although this does not seem to translate into more pathologic fractures in young adults.[41] Patients with longer segments of terminal ileum that are excluded from the gastrointestinal tract are at risk for low vitamin B12 levels; these should be checked 2-yearly and vitamin B12 should be substituted if the serum level becomes less than 200 pmol/l. These patients are also at risk for malabsorption of fat, diarrhea, and calcium oxalate urolithiasis.

In general it is more difficult to maintain a certain level of self care in MMC patients than in the average population. The importance of compliance with CISC and regular irrigation of augmented lower urinary tract with bowel or continent reservoir needs to be emphasized at every encounter with the patient. The urine of patients who have bowel segments incorporated in the urinary tract or those with urinary diversions, and those who perform intermittent catheterization, is seldom sterile, but clinical signs of infection are rare. In fact, between 2/3 and 3/4 of patients with continent diversions have bacteriuria. In case of asymptomatic bacteriuria no antibiotic therapy is necessary, except for those with pure cultures of *Proteus* or *Pseudomonas*, since those patients are more likely to develop stones and upper tract deterioration. Patients with septic complications and symptomatic UTIs should be followed on a regular basis with cultures and active management, including eradication of infectious foci, such as stones of the upper and/or lower tract and ineffective CISC. Check-ups on a 3-monthly basis, at least, may be necessary until the situation has stabilized.

A multicenter survey in clinics listed by the Spina Bifida Association of America has revealed a lack of consensus on the use of urine cultures during follow-up of spina bifida patients.[42] Of these clinics, 49% used cultures and 59% performed urinalysis on a 6–12-monthly basis. A lack of consensus on the indications for treatment became evident as well. A positive urine culture in combination with fever, flank pain, urinary pattern change, or dysuria was an indication for antibiotic treatment in more than 70% of the centers. In addition, more than 50% of the centers treated in case of chills, abdominal pain, and more than 50 WBC/hpf (white-blood cells per high-power field).

It is clear that evidence-based guidelines for the follow-up and management of adult MMC patients and neurourologic patients in general have to be defined with priority.

References

1. Durham Smith E. Urinary prognosis in spina bifida. J Urol 1972; 108: 815–17.
2. Stevenson RE, Allen WP, Pai GS et al. Decline in prevalence of neural tube defects in a high risk region of the United States. Pediatrics 2000; 106: 677–83.
3. Halliday JL, Riley M. Fortification of foods with folic acid (letter). N Engl J Med 2000; 343: 970–1.
4. Van Gool JD. Spina Bifida and Neurogenic Bladder Dysfunction: A Urodynamic Study. Impress Utrecht 1986: 219.
5. McGuire EJ, Denil J. Adult myelodysplasia. AUA Update Series 1991; 10: 298–303.
6. Spindel MR, Bauer SB, Dyro FM et al. The changing neurourologic lesion in myelodysplasia. JAMA 1987; 258: 1630–3.
7. McGuire EJ, Woodside JR, Borden TA. Upper tract deterioration in patients with myelodysplasia and detrusor hypertonia with a follow up study. J Urol 1983; 129: 873.
8. Bruschini H, Almeida FG, Srougi M. Upper and lower urinary tract evaluation of 104 patients with myelomeningocele without adequate urological management. World J Urol 2006; 24: 224–8.
9. Fujita I, Yamamoto H. An experimental study on spinal cord traction effect. Spine 1989; 14: 698–705.
10. Wilson DA, Prince JR. Imaging determination of the location of the normal conus medullaris throughout childhood. AJR 1989; 152. 1029–32.
11. Keating MA, Rink RC, Bauer SB et al. Neurourological implications of the changing approach in management of occult spinal lesions. J Urol 1988; 140: 1299–301.
12. Dik P, Tsachouridis GD, Klijn AJ, Uiterwaal CSPM, de Jong TPVM. Detrusorectomy for neuropathic bladder in patients with spinal dysraphism. J Urol 2003; 170: 1351–4.
13. Stephenson TP, Mundy AR. Treatment of the neuropathic bladder by enterocystoplasty and selective sphincterotomy or sphincter ablation and replacement. Br J Urol 1985; 57: 27–31.
14. Brem AS, Martin D, Callaghan J, Maynard J. Long term renal risk factors in children with meningomyelocele. J Pediatr 1987; 110: 51–4.
15. Dik P, Klijn AJ, van Gool JD, de Jong-de Vos van Steenwijk CC, De Jong TP. Early start to therapy preserves kidney function in spina bifida patients. Eur Urol 2006; 49: 908–13.
16. Kessler TM, Lackner J, Kiss G, Rehder P, Madersbacher H. Early proactive management improves upper urinary tract function and reduces the need for surgery in patients with myelomeningocele. Neurourol Urodyn 2006; 25: 758–62.
17. Riccabona M, Koen M, Schindler M et al. Botulinum-A toxin injection into the detrusor: a safe alternative in the treatment of children with myelomeningocele with detrusor hyperreflexia. J Urol 2004; 171(2 Pt 1): 845–8.

18. Stark GD. The nature and cause of paraplegia in myelomeningocele. Paraplegia 1972; 9: 219.
19. Schmidt RA, Kogan BA, Tanagho EA. Neuroprosthesis in the management of incontinence in myelomeningocele patients. J Urol 1990; 143: 779–82.
20. Kryger JV, Spencer Barthold J, Fleming P, Gonzales R. The outcome of artificial sphincter placement after a mean 15-year follow-up in a paediatric population. BJU Int 1999; 83: 1026–31.
21. Roth DR, Vyas PR, Kroovand RL, Perlmutter AD. Urinary tract deterioration associated with the artificial urinary sphincter. J Urol 1986; 135: 528–30.
22. Furness III PD, Franzoni DF, Decter RM. Bladder augmentation: does it predispose to prosthetic infection of simultaneously placed artificial genitourinary sphincters or in situ ventriculoperitoneal shunts? BJU Int 1999; 84: 25–9.
23. Miller EA, Mayo M, Kwan D, Mitchell M. Simultaneous augmentation cystoplasty and artificial urinary sphincter placement: infection rates and voiding mechanisms. J Urol 1998; 160: 750–3.
24. Kronner KM, Rink RC, Simmons G et al. Artificial urinary sphincter in the treatment of urinary incontinence: preoperative urodynamics do not predict the need for future bladder augmentation. J Urol 1998; 160: 1093–5.
25. Spiess PE, Capolicchio JP, Kiruluta G et al. Is an artificial sphincter the best choice for incontinent boys with spina bifida? Review of our long term experience with the AS-800 artificial sphincter. Can J Urol 2002; 9: 1486–91.
26. Lemelle JL, Guillemin F, Aubert D et al. A multicenter evaluation of urinary incontinence management and outcome in spina bifida. J Urol 2006; 175: 208–12.
27. Lemelle JL, Guillemin F, Aubert D et al. Quality of life and continence in patients with spina bifida. Qual Life Res 2006; 15: 1481–92.
28. Stamper DS, McDougal WS, McGovern FJ. Metabolic and nutritional complications. Urol Clin N Am 1997; 24: 715–22.
29. Stein R, Matani Y, Doi Y et al. Continent urinary diversion using the Mainz pouch I technique – ten years later. J Urol 1995; 153 (4 Suppl): 241A.
30. Rink RC. Bladder augmentation: options, outcomes, future. Urol Clin N Am 1999; 26: 111–23.
31. MacGregor P, Novick AC, Cunningham R et al. Renal transplantation in end stage renal disease patients with existing urinary diversion. J Urol 1986; 135: 686–8.
32. Hatch DA, Belitsky P, Barry JM et al. Fate of renal allografts transplanted in patients with urinary diversion. Transplantation 1993; 56: 838–42.
33. Dawahra M, Martin X, Tajra LC et al. Renal transplantation using continent urinary diversion: long-term follow-up. Transplant Proc 1997; 29: 159–60.
34. Koyle MA, Pfister RR, Kam I et al. Bladder reconstruction with the dilated ureter for renal transplantation. Transplant Proc 1994; 26: 35–6.
35. Diamond DA, Rickwood AMK, Thomas DG. Penile erections in myelomeningocele patients. Br J Urol 1986; 58: 434–5.
36. Overgoor ML, Kon M, Cohen-Kettenis PT et al. Neurological bypass for sensory innervation of the penis in patients with spina bifida. J Urol 2006; 176: 1086–90.
37. Richmond D, Zaharievski I, Bond A. Management of pregnancy in mothers with spina bifida. Eur J Obstet Reprod Biol 1987; 25: 341–5.
38. Mitchell LE, Adzick NS, Melchionne J et al. Spina bifida. Lancet 2004; 364: 1885–95.
39. Hunt, GM and Oakeshott P. Outcome in people with open spina bifida at age 35: prospective community based cohort study. BMJ 2003; 326: 1365–6.
40. Stöhrer M, Castro-Diaz D, Chartier-Kastler E et al. EAU Guidelines on Neurogenic Lower Urinary Tract Dysfunction. Chapter 7: Guidelines for follow-up, 2007: 53 Available at: www.uroweb.org/professional-resources/guidelines.
41. Mingin G, Maroni P, Gerharz EW, Woodhouse CRJ, Baskin LS. Linear growth after enterocystoplasty in children and adolescents: a review. World J Urol 2004; 22: 196–9.
42. Elliott SP, Villar R, Duncan B. Bacteriuria management and urological evaluation of patients with spina bifida and neurogenic bladder: a multicenter survey. J Urol 2005; 173: 217–20.

Part VIII

Synthesis of treatment

68

The vesicourethral balance

Erik Schick and Jacques Corcos

Introduction

In Chapter 70 we summarize the different treatment modalities that can be considered to correct bladder dysfunction or urethral dysfunction, independently of each other. In clinical practice, however, most patients present simultaneous alterations of reservoir and outlet functions.

The ultimate goal in neurogenic bladder management is the preservation of normal kidney function. The most important factor to achieve is to maintain the lower urinary tract at a low pressure. Ensuring regular bladder emptying, decreasing outlet resistance in patients who void spontaneously, preventing infection by eliminating foreign bodies from the urethra and/or the bladder, and treating infection when it becomes symptomatic are some of the modalities used to attain this goal. Additionally, maintaining or restoring continence will significantly increase the patient's quality of life. To avoid or minimize potential complications, these objectives have to be constantly kept in mind when dealing with the problem of neurogenic bladder dysfunction.

Vesicourethral balance and balanced bladder are by no means synonymous. The balanced bladder concept emerged after World War II and was part of the bladder rehabilitation process. It implied reflex bladder voiding and a postvoid residual urine volume of less than 100 ml. Clinicians felt safe in trying to achieve this goal. Later experience proved that the approach was not necessarily safe, because it could not prevent infection, sepsis, loss of renal function, etc. The flaw with this empirical therapy is that elevated bladder filling and emptying pressures can occur, causing silent renal damage despite low postvoid residual urine volume.[1]

The concept of vesicourethral balance helps us to understand the pathophysiologic consequences of vesicourethral dysfunction. It indicates how to modify reservoir function, outlet function, or both in order to restore normal vesicourethral function to a safe, normal, low-pressure zone. Urodynamics are essential in this respect, because they allow bladder and urethral function to be evaluated independently along with the interaction between them.

Normal vesicourethral balance

The vesicourethral unit can be compared to a balance where the bladder represents one arm, and the urethra with its sphincteric mechanism the other arm of the balance. Figure 68.1 illustrates this concept.

During the filling phase of the voiding cycle, the bladder is accommodating a progressively increasing volume. Because of normal bladder wall compliance, pressure inside the bladder remains constant, about 15–20 cmH_2O, and never exceeds 40 cmH_2O. The system is in a low-pressure state, and the upper urinary tract is safe.[2,3] During the voiding phase, the detrusor contracts, the urethral sphincteric mechanism relaxes, and there is normal vesicourethral synergia.

Under pathologic conditions, this relatively delicate balance can easily be disturbed. Bladder function can be normal or altered by some pathologic process in several ways. It may become underactive, noncontractile, or overactive, with or without impaired contractility, with or without decreased compliance. Urethral function can be normal, hypotonic (incontinence), or hypertonic (obstruction). The different combinations of these vesicourethral alterations can lead to several different clinical situations, as illustrated in Table 68.1.

The aim of any therapeutic intervention is to ensure the restoration of normal balance in the security zone – security from the point of view of the preservation of renal function.

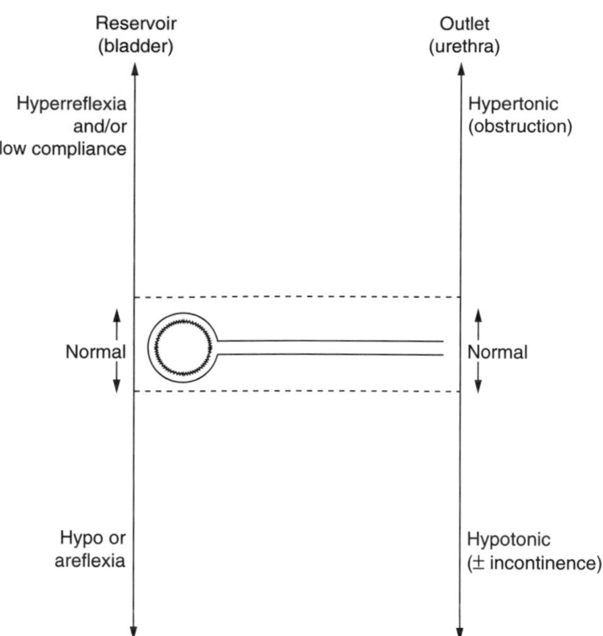

Figure 68.1
Normal vesicourethral balance. Bladder filling and micturition under normal pressure conditions, within the 'security zone' of <40 cmH_2O.

Table 68.1 *Summary of vesico-urethral balance*

Figure number	Bladder activity/compliance	Outlet
68.1	Normal	Normal
68.2a	Normal	Hypotonic
68.3a	Normal	Obstructive
68.4a	Overactive/low compliant	Normal
68.5a	Overactive/low compliant	Hypotonic
68.6a	Overactive/low compliant	Obstructive
68.7a	Underactive/noncontractile	Normal
68.8a	Underactive/noncontractile	Hypotonic
68.9a	Underactive/noncontractile	Obstructive

Alterations in vesicourethral balance

Normal bladder contractility and compliance

The hypotonic outlet

Principle:
This is characteristic of the stress incontinent patient. By simply improving outlet function, normal vesicourethral conditions in normal pressure ranges can be restored (Figure 68.2a).

Clinical example

Urodynamic tracings of a 66-year old female who consulted for urinary incontinence. Bladder capacity was normal (540 ml), without significant postvoid residual urine (10 ml). Urethral pressure profile at two consecutive withdrawals showed a hypotonic urethra: maximum urethral closure pressure = 17 cmH_2O (Figure 68.2b).

On multichannel pressure–flow study the bladder was stable. Detrusor pressure at maximum flow was 10.4

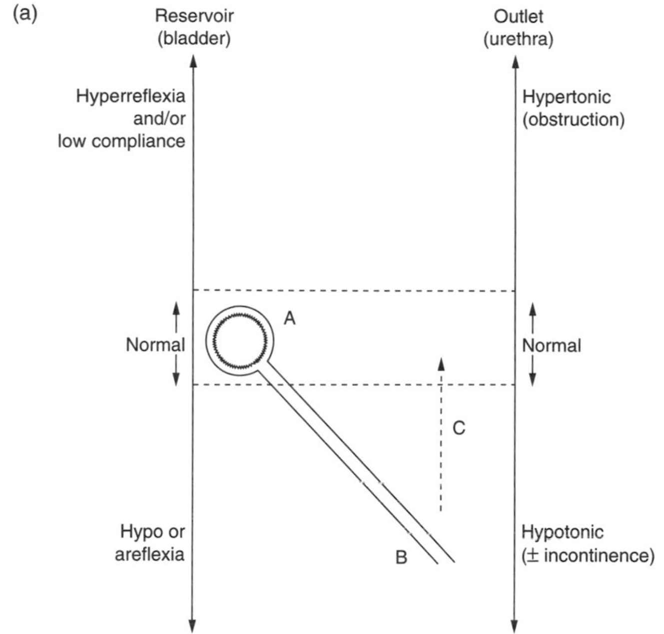

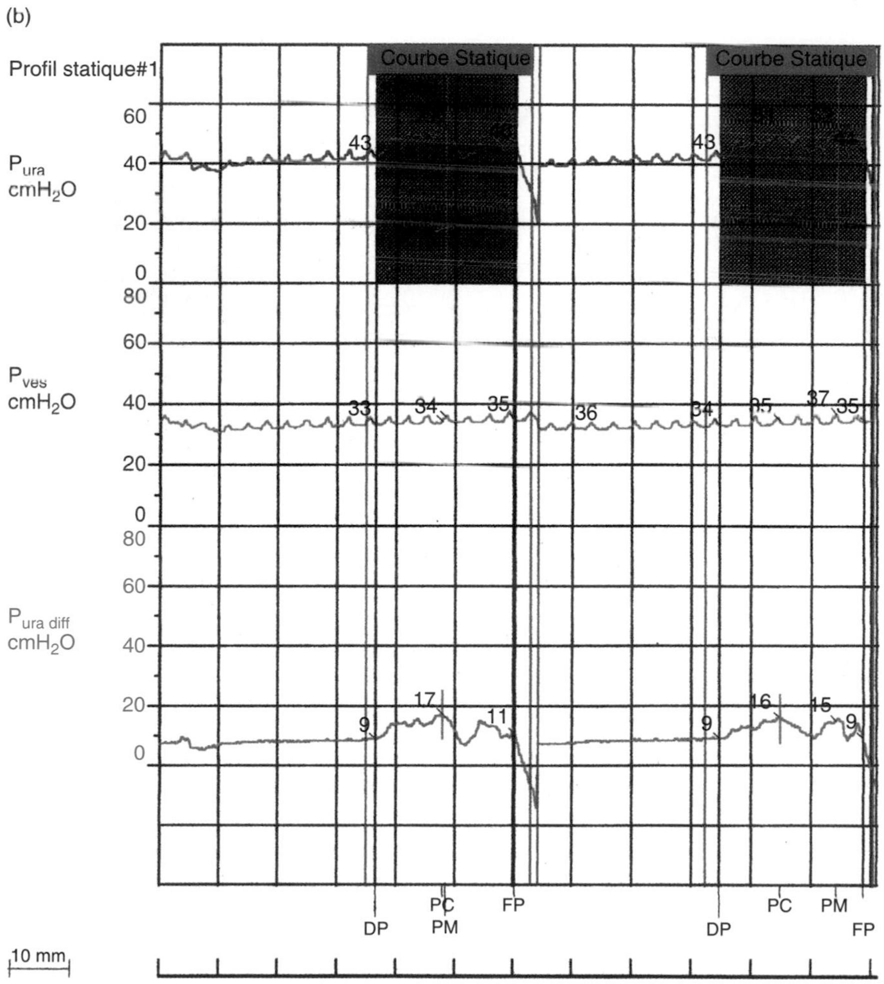

Figure 68.2 (*Continued*)

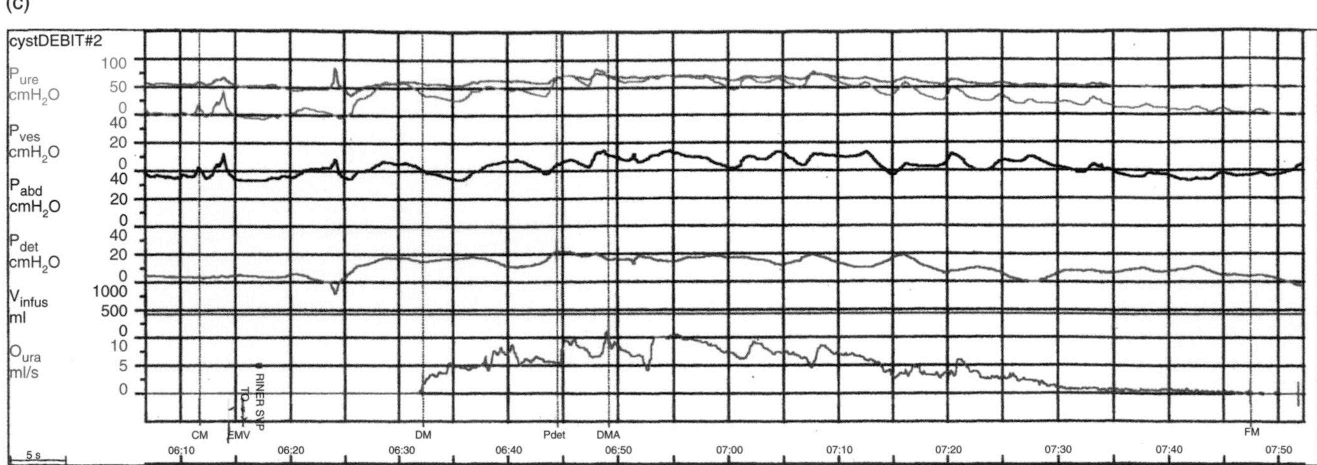

(d)

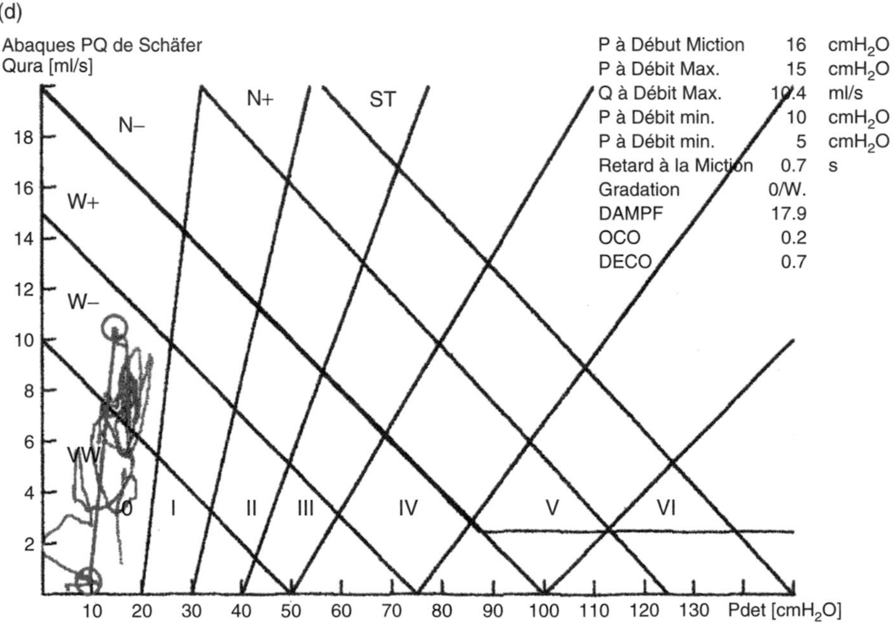

Figure 68.2
(a) The bladder is normal (a), but the urethra hypotonic (b), a condition favorable for incontinence. By increasing urethral tonicity (or improving pressure transmission conditions from the abdominal cavity to the urethra) (c), continence is re-established. Overcorrecting may induce urinary retention, as in Figure 68.3a. (b) Urethral pressure profile at 2 consecutive withdrawals (see abreviations at end of chapter). (c) Multichannel pressure flow study. (d) Schäfer's nomogram.

cmH_2O (Figure 68.2c). According to Schäfer's nomogram, bladder contractility was somewhat deficient (Figure 68.2d). This, however, is difficult to ascertain because this nomogram was not designed for females, and furthermore some female patients empty their bladder by simply relaxing their urethra.[4] No stop tests have been done to better document bladder contractility. *Conclusion* Bladder: stable with normal compliance. Urethra: hypotonic. *Treatment* increase outlet resistance.

The obstructive outlet

Principle

Benign prostatic obstruction is a good example of this situation. The treatment strategy should not be to increase bladder contractility, but rather to decrease urethral resistance (Figure 68.3a). By eliminating obstruction the system will return to normal equilibrium in the security zone.

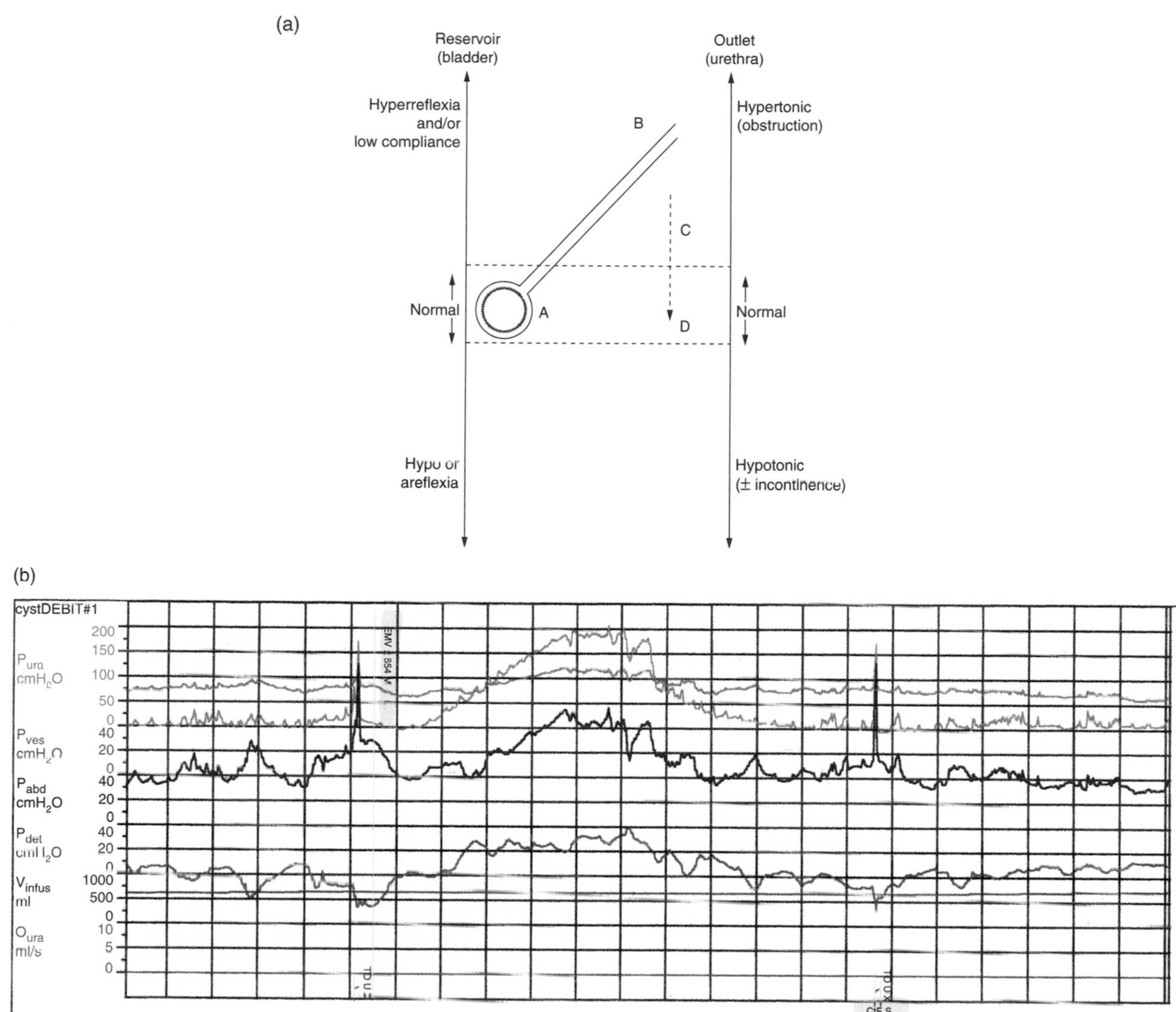

Figure 68.3
(a) The bladder is normal (A), and the urethra obstructive (B), as in benign prostatic hyperplasia or urethral stenosis. Correction of outlet conditions (C) allows the re-establishment of micturition under normal pressure conditions (D). (b) Multichannel urodynamic study of a 76-year-old man with acute urinary retention.

Clinical example:
In this 76-year old man, who consulted because of acute urinary retention, the multichannel urodynamic study demonstrated a stable and compliant bladder with increased cystometric capacity (850 ml) (Figure 68.3b). First desire to void (B1) was at 51 ml. Total bladder pressure during the entire filling phase was ± 40 cmH_2O. At voiding attempt the detrusor contracted, but no flow was initiated. The maximum detrusor pressure generated was 40 cmH_2O. *Conclusion* Bladder contractile and compliant. Urethra obstructed. *Treatment* Decrease outlet resistance. Spontaneous voiding should follow.

Overactive and/or low-compliant bladder

The normal outlet

Principle:
When the bladder is overactive and/or low compliant, but the urethra still has normal closure pressure, the patient may be incontinent. The solution to this problem is not to increase urethral closure pressure, because – although the patient will become continent – the system will be transformed to a high-pressure one, jeopardizing the integrity

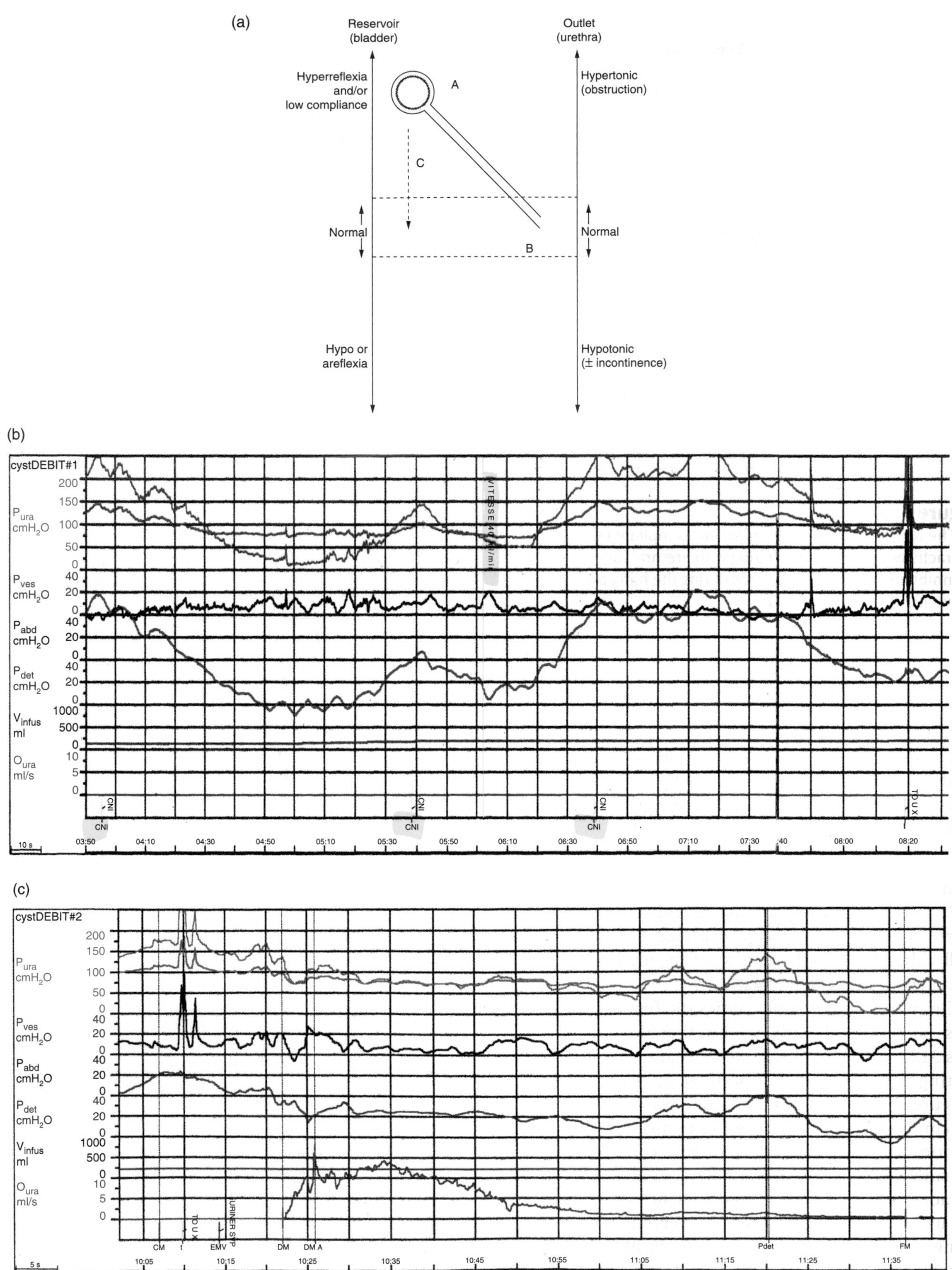
(a)
Reservoir (bladder)
Outlet (urethra)
Hyperreflexia and/or low compliance
Hypertonic (obstruction)
A
C
Normal
Normal
B
Hypo or areflexia
Hypotonic (± incontinence)
(b)
cystDEBIT#1
Pura cmH2O
Pves cmH2O
Pabd cmH2O
Pdet cmH2O
Vinfus ml
Oura ml/s
CNI
TDUX
(c)
cystDEBIT#2
CM
EMV
URINER STP
DM
DM A
Pdet
FM

Figure 68.4

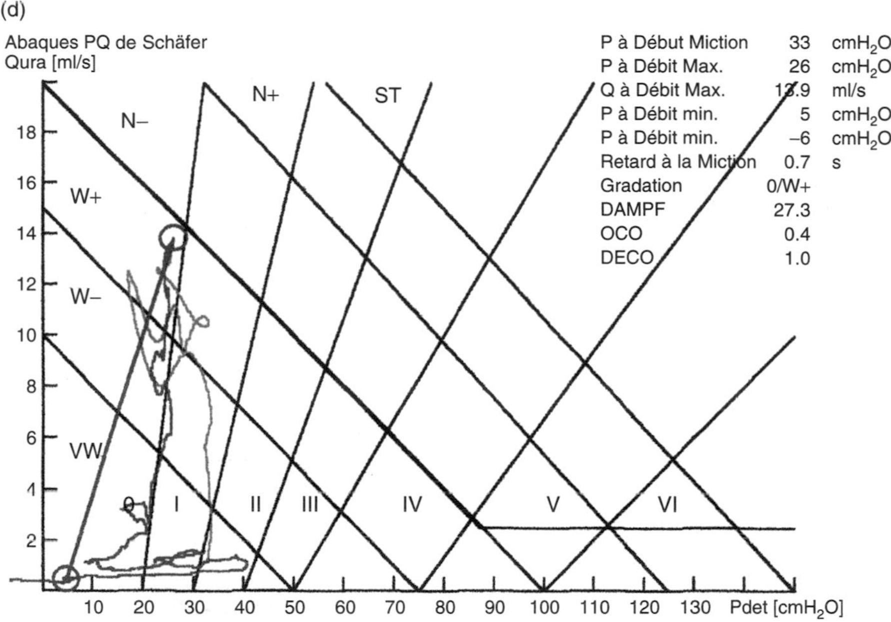

Figure 68.4
(a) The bladder is overactive and/or low compliant (A) with a normal outlet (B), predisposing to incontinence. Treatment should correct overactivity (C) without interfering with urethral function (D). Continence should be re-established. (b) Sustained, high-amplitude, uninhibited detrusor contractions during the filing phase. (c) During voiding detrusor pressure remains low. (d) Schäfer's nomogram shows no obstruction.

of the upper urinary tract. Treatment should be directed to controling overactivity or to improving bladder wall compliance. Thus, the system will be balanced in the security zone (Figure 68.4a).

Clinical example:
A 79-year-old man was investigated for nocturia and urinary incontinence. Endoscopy disclosed a marked bladder wall trabeculation and occlusion of the urethral lumen by the lateral lobes of the prostate.

On multichannel urodynamics the first desire to void was perceived at 144 ml and the bladder capacity was 328 ml. The filling phase was characterized by long-lasting uninhibited contractions of high amplitude (Figure 68.4b). The total bladder pressure was above 40 cmH_2O during the entire filling phase. During micturition the detrusor pressure was constantly below 40 cmH_2O (Figure 68.4c). Schäfer's nomogram did not demonstrate obstruction (Figure 68.4d). Postvoid residual urine was 100 ml. *Conclusion* Overactive bladder creating a high pressure system. Urethra nonobstructive. *Treatment* Control hyperactivity to create a low-pressure reservoir.

The hypotonic outlet (low urethral closure pressure)

Principle:
This clinical situation is relatively rare. With decreased outlet resistance, the patient will almost certainly be incontinent, but because of this hypotonicity a high-pressure system is unlikely to develop. Correcting urethral function alone, although continence may be established, might put the upper urinary tract in a precarious situation, as in the preceding example. Together with the improvement of urethral hypotonicity, one should also control bladder overactivity and/or compliance (Figure 68.5a).

Clinical example:
This situation was encountered in a 20-year old male with spina bifida. He consulted mainly because of complete urinary incontinence (permanent dribbling). On multichannel urodynamics, bladder sensation (B1) was abolished and cystometric capacity was 317 ml. The maximum urethral pressure was ± 100 cmH_2O, but the maximum urethral closure pressure was only 22 cmH_2O (Figure 68.5b). Because of low closure pressure the urethra was considered to be hypotonic. On multichannel urodynamics, bladder sensation (B1) was

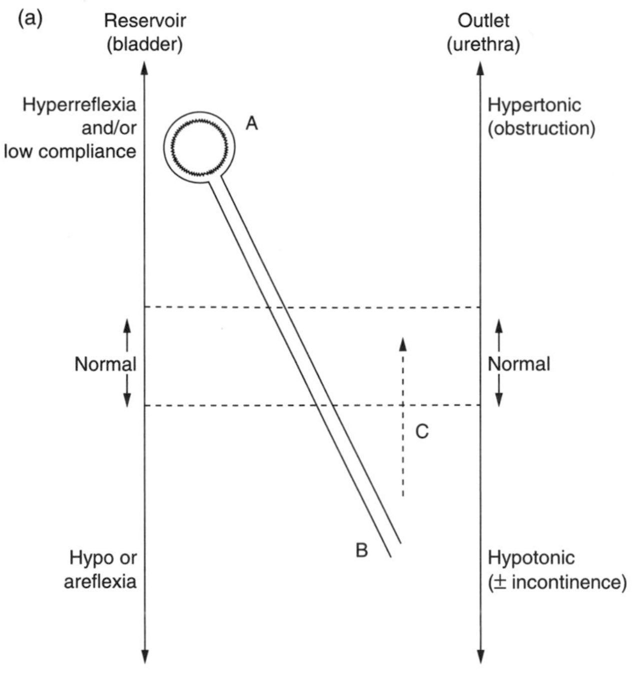

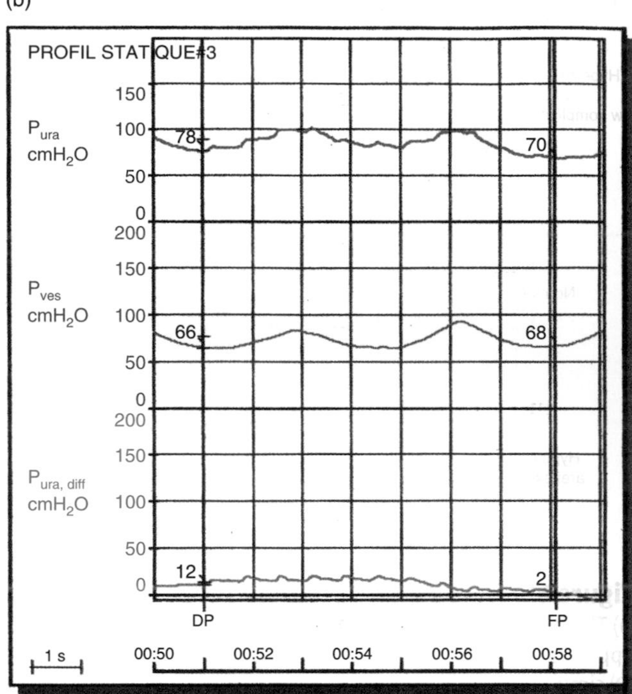

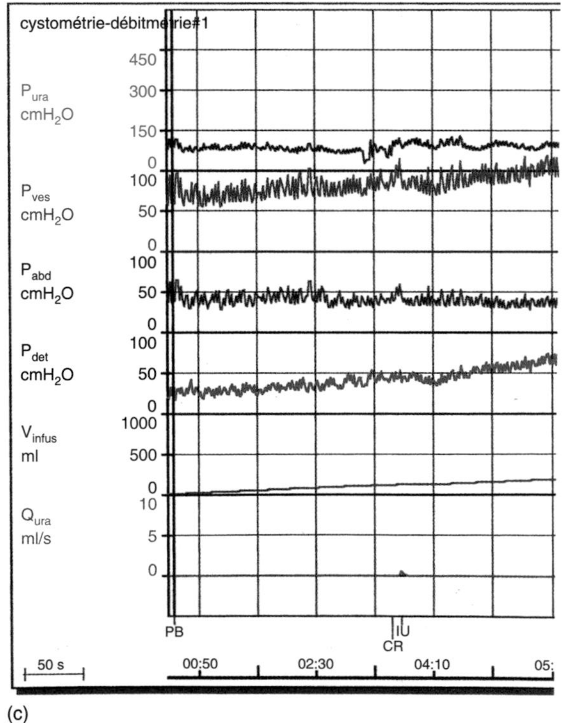

Figure 68.5
(a) The bladder is overactive and/or low compliant (A), associated with a hypotonic outlet (B). The patient will almost certainly be incontinent. Increasing urethral resistance (C) will probably not be sufficient; conditions similar to those in Figure 68.4a will be created. Detrusor overactivity should also be controlled (d) in order to reach normal vesicourethral equilibrium. (b) Urethral pressure profile at rest. (c) Multichannel urodynamics.

abolished and cystometric capacity was 317 ml. Bladder wall showed decreased compliance, no detrusor overactivity was observed. Incontinence appeared at a total intravesical pressure of ± 100 cmH_2O which corresponded to a detrusor pressure of 40 cmH_2O (Figure 68.5c). *Conclusion* Bladder noncontractile and low compliant. Urethra hypotonic. *Treatment* Start to improve bladder compliance and if, incontinence persists, increase outlet resistance secondarily.

The hypertonic (obstructed) outlet

Principle:

It is estimated that more than 50% of males with outlet obstruction will develop bladder overactivity.[5,6] Elimination of obstruction will normalize urethral function, but may expose the patient to incontinence. In a non-neurologic context, bladder overactivity will subside

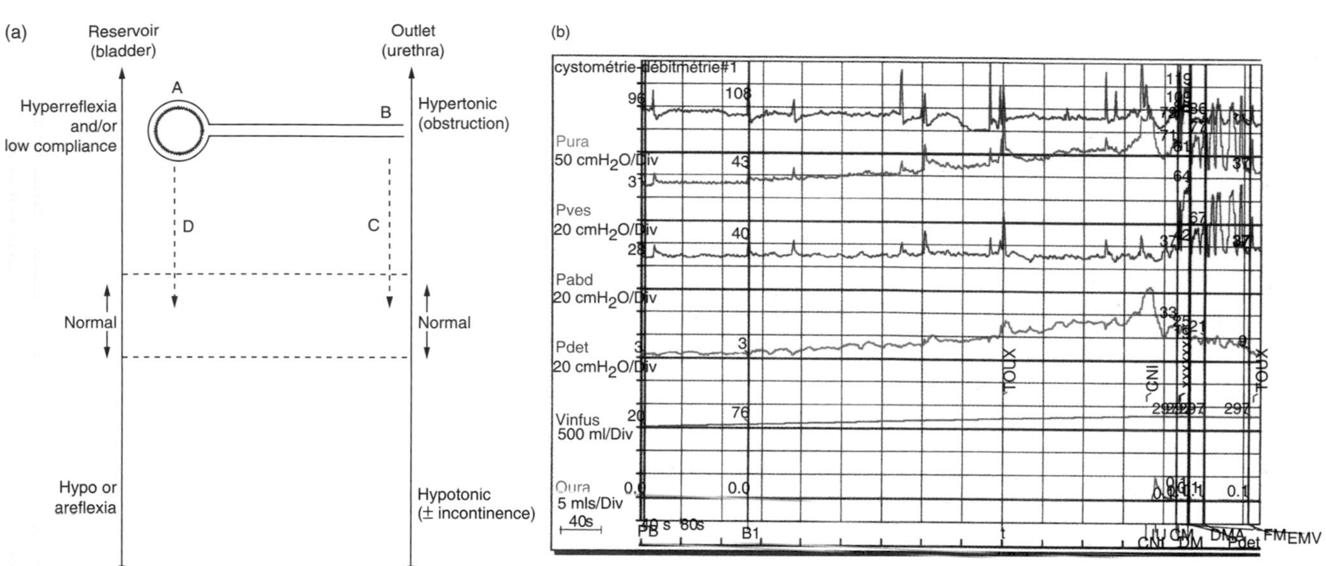

Figure 68.6
(a) The bladder is overactive and/or low compliant (A), associated with obstructed outlet (B). The patient is probably continent, but the upper tract is in real danger of decompensation. Therapeutic measures should be directed toward the urethra (C) and the bladder (D) simultaneously to establish normal balance in the security zone. (b) Multichannel urodynamic study.

spontaneously within 1 year after the removal of the obstruction in a significant proportion of patients.[7] In the neurologic patient, however, therapeutic measures should be taken to control overactivity, in conjunction with the correction of outlet function (Figure 68.6a).

Clinical example:
A clinical example of this situation is that of a 43-year-old man, quadraplegic since the age of 18. Bladder drainage was insured by condom catheter. Cystoscopy revealed grade 4 bladder wall trabeculation. Ultrasonography demonstrated bilateral uretero-hydronephrosis. Multichannel urodynamic study (Figure 68.6b) showed first desire to void at 76 ml and bladder capacity at 450 ml. Decreased compliance with uninhibited contractions. Intravesical pressure reached the critical value of 40 cmH$_2$O at 100 ml. Postvoid residual was 300 ml. Detrusor-external sphincter dyssynergia was present (not shown here). *Conclusion* Bladder: neurogenic overactive and low compliant; high-pressure system. Urethra: obstructed. *Treatment* Improve compliance and eliminate outlet obstruction.

Underactive and/or noncontractile bladder

The normal outlet

Principle:
This is the case of the patient who underwent prostatectomy for chronic urinary retention, but who is still unable to void spontaneously (Figure 68.7a).

Clinical example:
This condition can also develop spontaneously, as in this 39-year-old male who consulted because of daytime frequency and nocturia. The postvoid residual urine was 100 ml. Cystoscopy showed normal bladder. On multichannel urodynamic study (Figure 68.7b) the first desire to void (B1) was present at 116 ml and bladder capacity was measured at 504 ml. During the filling phase the total bladder pressure was ± 40 cmH$_2$O. No uninhibited contractions were seen. During micturition (Figure 68.7c) the detrusor pressure was less than 40 cmH$_2$O and the flow was irregular. The patient used Valsalva maneuver to facilitate voiding. However, at each bear-down maneuver the pelvic floor muscles contracted also, witnessed by the simultaneous increase in maximum urethral pressure. (Note that the scale for urethral pressure is different from the other pressure lines.) On Schäfer's nomogram (Figure 68.7d) there was no obstruction, but the detrusor was very weak. *Conclusion* Underactive bladder. Urethra nonobstructed. *Treatment* improve detrusor contractility.

The hypotonic outlet

Principle:
The patient may or may not be incontinent. Improving outlet function alone will almost certainly precipitate the patient into urinary retention. Every effort should be made to improve bladder contractility as well (Figure 68.8a).

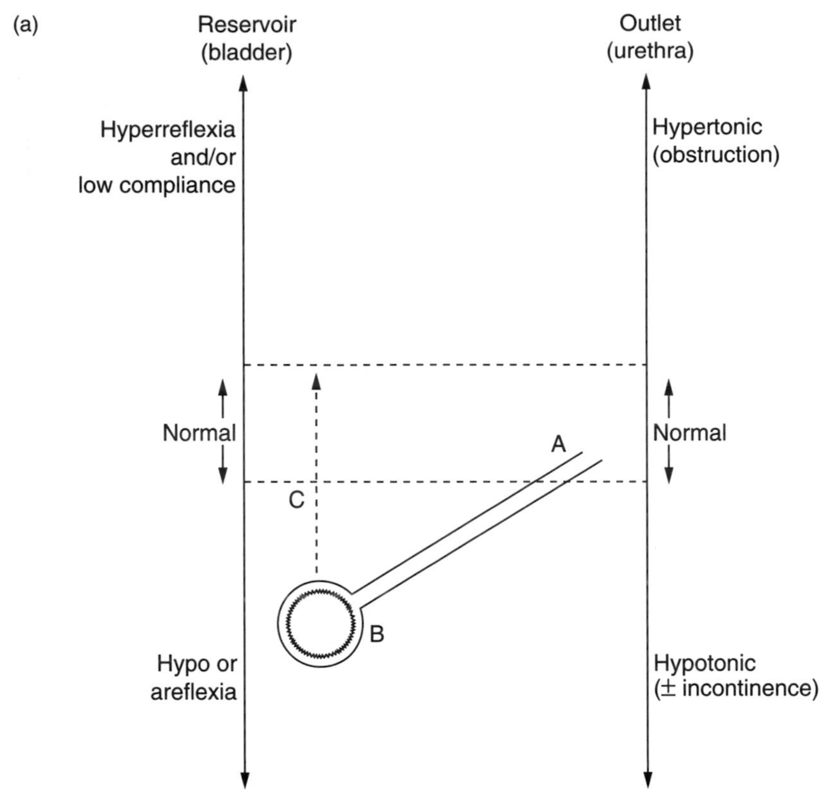
(a)
Reservoir (bladder)
Outlet (urethra)
Hyperreflexia and/or low compliance
Hypertonic (obstruction)
Normal
Normal
A
C
B
Hypo or areflexia
Hypotonic (± incontinence)

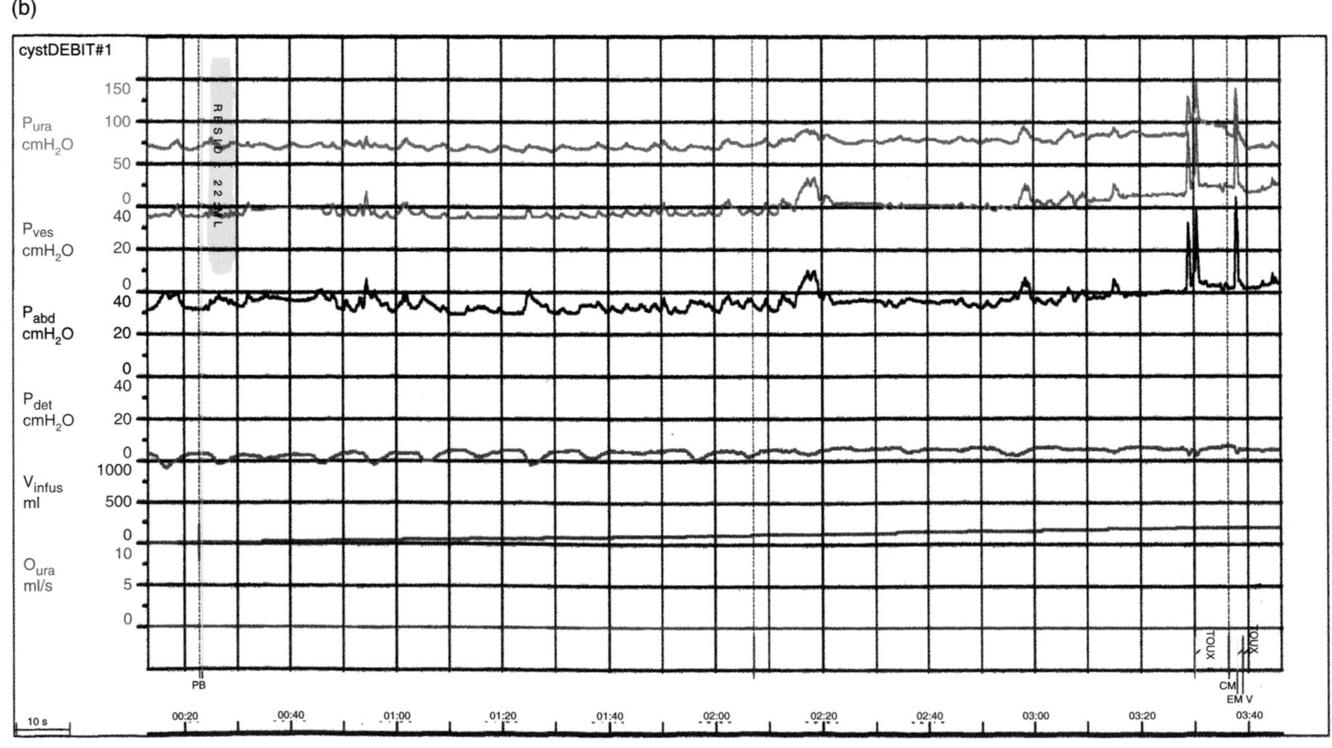
(b)
cystDEBIT#1
Pura cmH2O
Pves cmH2O
Pabd cmH2O
Pdet cmH2O
Vinfus ml
Qura ml/s
150
100
50
0
40
20
0
40
20
0
40
20
0
1000
500
0
10
5
0
PB
TOUX
TOUX
CM
EM V
10 s
00:20
00:40
01:00
01:20
01:40
02:00
02:20
02:40
03:00
03:20
03:40

Figure 68.7

(c)

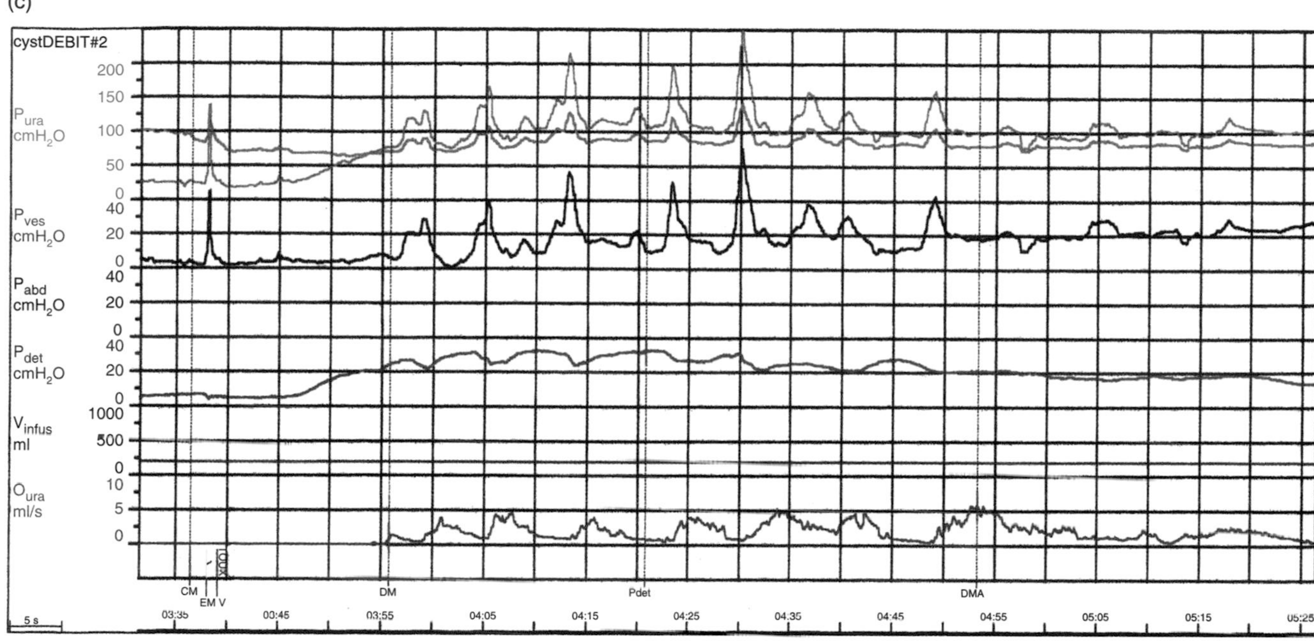

(d)

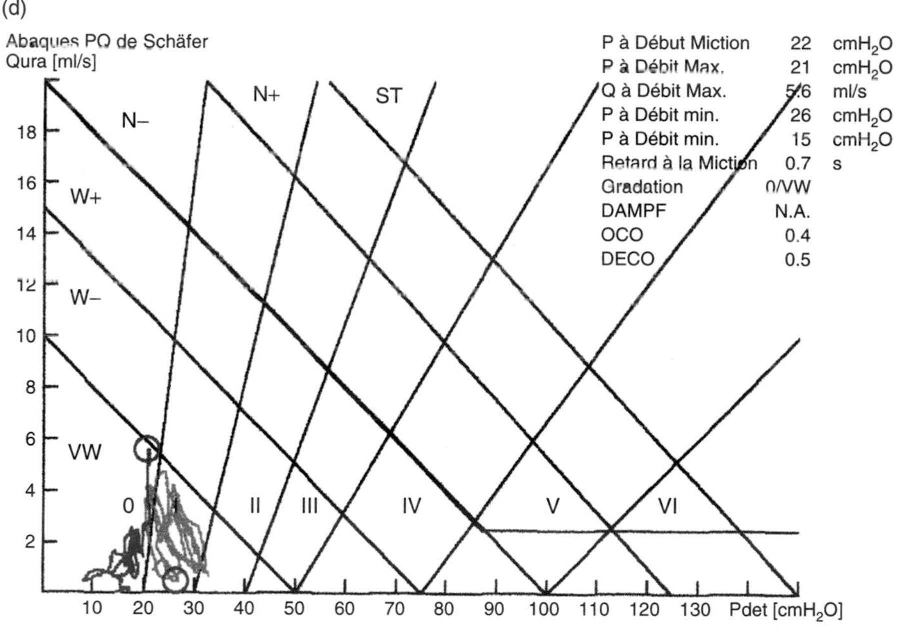

Figure 68.7

(a) The outlet is normal (A) and the bladder is underactive and/or noncontractile (B). Spontaneous voiding may be possible, but with significant postvoid residual volume. Treatment should reinforce detrusor contractility (C) without interfering with outlet conditions (A). Spontaneous voiding, within the security zone, should be re-established. (b) Filling phase shows a "flat" detrusor. (c) Voiding takes place mainly by valsalva manoeuver. (d) Schafer's nomogram shows no obstruction but a very weak detrusor.

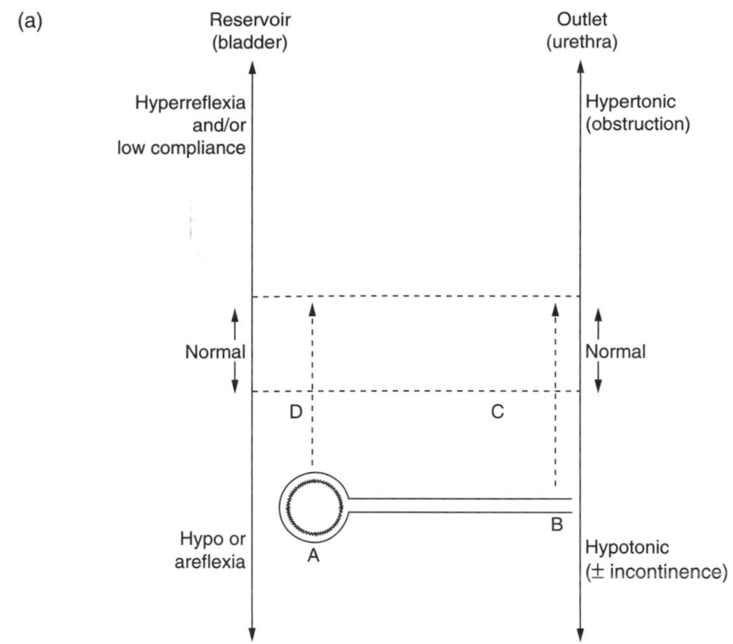
(a)
Reservoir
(bladder)
Outlet
(urethra)
Hyperreflexia
and/or
low compliance
Hypertonic
(obstruction)
Normal
Normal
D
C
B
A
Hypo or
areflexia
Hypotonic
(± incontinence)

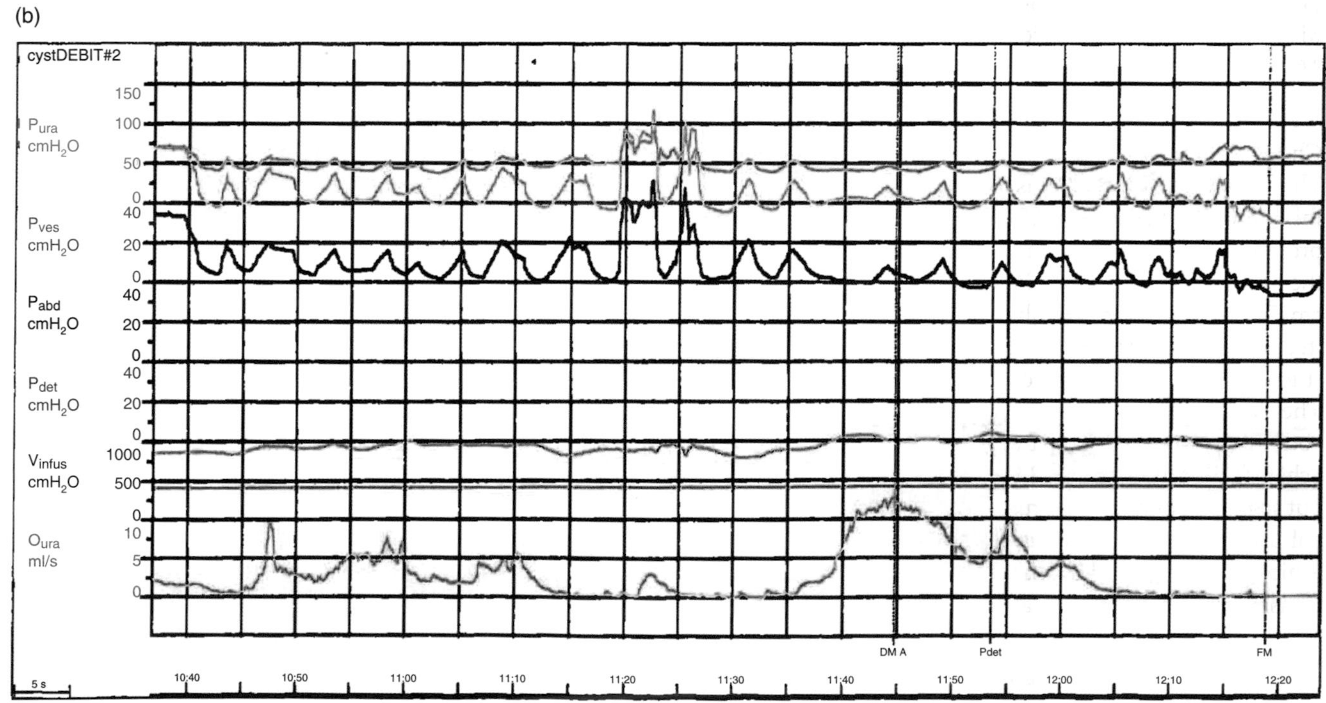
(b)
cystDEBIT#2
Pura
cmH2O
Pves
cmH2O
Pabd
cmH2O
Pdet
cmH2O
Vinfus
cmH2O
Oura
ml/s
DM A
Pdet
FM
5 s
10:40
10:50
11:00
11:10
11:20
11:30
11:40
11:50
12:00
12:10
12:20

Figure 68.8

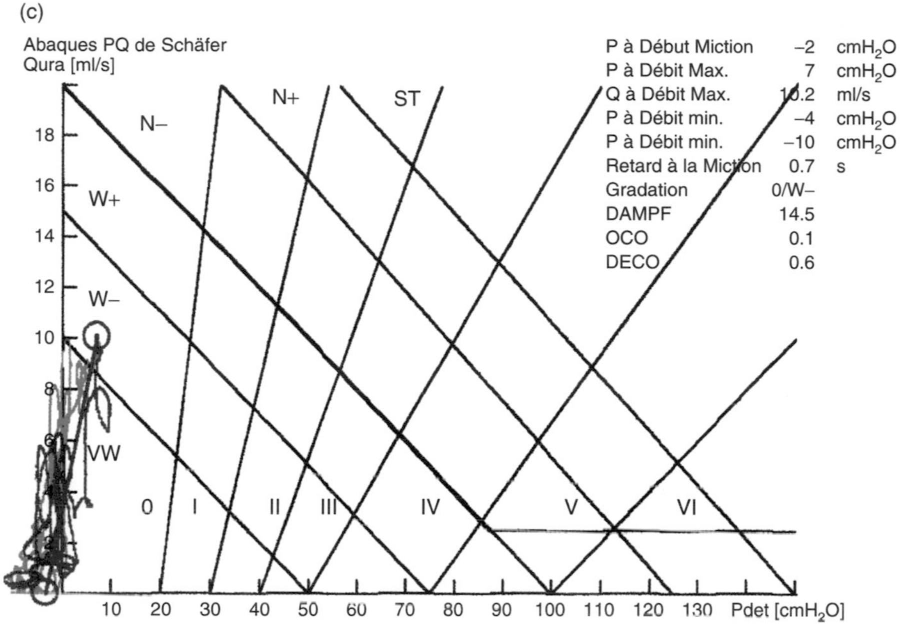

Figure 68.8
(a) Underactive and/or noncontractile bladder (A) with a hypotonic outlet (B) If the patient is continent, one might adopt a watchful waiting policy, because the system is a low-pressure one. In case of incontinence, the outlet (C) and bladder (D) should be reinforced together. If only the outlet is corrected, the patient might not void spontaneously. If bladder contractility is improved only, the patient will remain incontinent. (b) Voiding phase on the multichannel urodynamic study. (c) Schafer's nomogram suggests no obstruction and a weak detrusor.

Clinical example:
This 52-year-old female consulted because of symptoms of mixed urinary incontinence. The stress component was more pronounced than was urgency. On urethral pressure profile the MUCP was 20 cmH_2O. Cough leak-point pressure was 80 cmH_2O. During the filling phase (Figure 68.8b) no uninhibited detrusor contractions were recorded. Pressure–flow study demonstrated an almost absent detrusor contraction. The flow was irregular and interrupted and resulted from abdominal pressure, at least at the begining of micturition. Schäfer's diagram (Figure 68.8(c)) did not show obstruction, but suggested decreased detrusor contraction. Postvoid residual urine was 74 ml. *Conclusion* Underactive bladder, hypotonic and hypermobile urethra. *Treatment* Improve pressure transmission from abdominal cavity or urethra.

The obstructive outlet

Principle:
In this case, the patient will almost certainly be in urinary retention. Decreasing outlet resistance by eliminating the obstructive factor will not necessarily permit normal voiding without significant postvoid residual volume. Attempts should also be made to improve bladder contractility simultaneously (Figure 68.9a).

Clinical example:
A 69-year-old man presented with urge urinary incontinence. Postvoid residual urine was 900 ml. On multichannel urodynamic study the first desire to void was noted at 29 ml and the first uninhibited contraction at 102 ml (not shown). Bladder wall compliance was normal. The detrusor pressure at maximum flow was 57 cmH_2O, which produced a maximum flow of 4.9 ml/s. (Figure 68.9(b)) On Schäfer's nomogram the detrusor pressure on initiation of voiding was 44 cmH_2O (grade III compressive type of obstruction) (Figure 68.9c); detrusor pressure at the end of the flow was 30 cmH_2O. A moderately severe constrictive type of obstruction was present. The detrusor was somewhat weak. *Conclusion* Bladder: huge capacity, decompensated, but still contractile, within a low-pressure system. Urethra: obstructed. *Treatment* Decrease outlet resistance. (Spontaneous voiding depends on remaining bladder contractility.)

Conclusion

Normal vesicourethral balance signifies a low-pressure system with normal bladder contractility and compliance, together with no outlet obstruction, and normal urethral tone. Urodynamics allow us to determine which elements are responsible for vesicourethral dysfunction or the disruption of vesicourethral balance. Treatment is directed towards the element(s) responsible for this dysfunction and so restoring vesicourethral balance in the normal, safe pressure ranges.

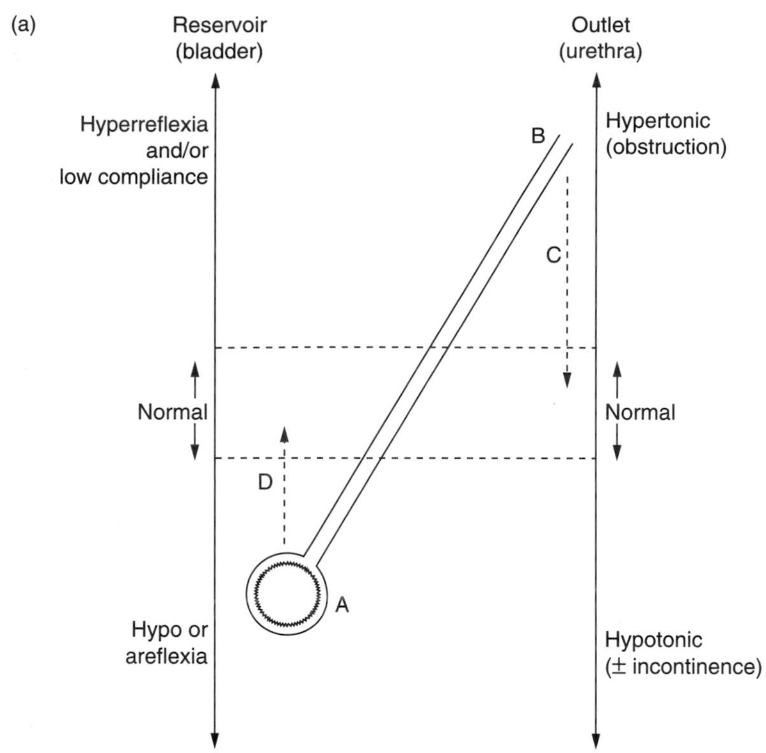
(a)
Reservoir
(bladder)
Outlet
(urethra)
Hyperreflexia
and/or
low compliance
Hypertonic
(obstruction)
B
C
Normal
Normal
D
A
Hypo or
areflexia
Hypotonic
(± incontinence)

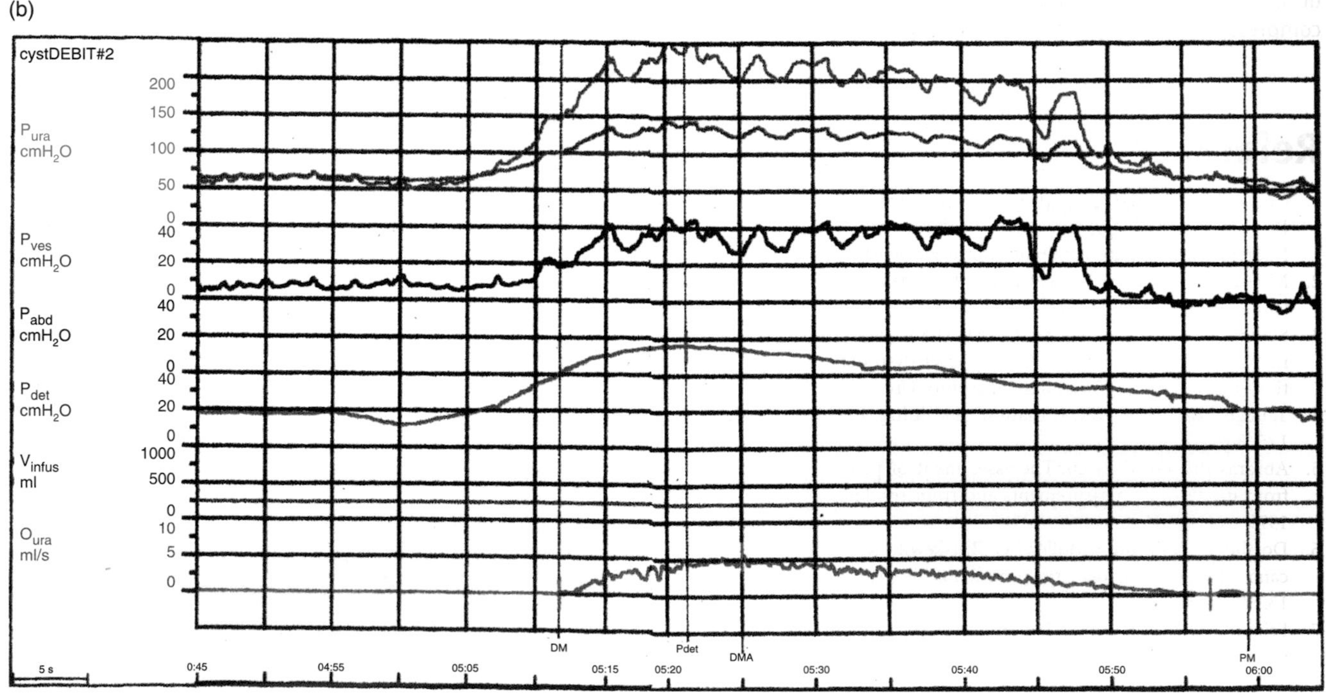
(b)
cystDEBIT#2
Pura
cmH2O
Pves
cmH2O
Pabd
cmH2O
Pdet
cmH2O
Vinfus
ml
Oura
ml/s
DM
Pdet
DMA
PM
5 s

Figure 68.9

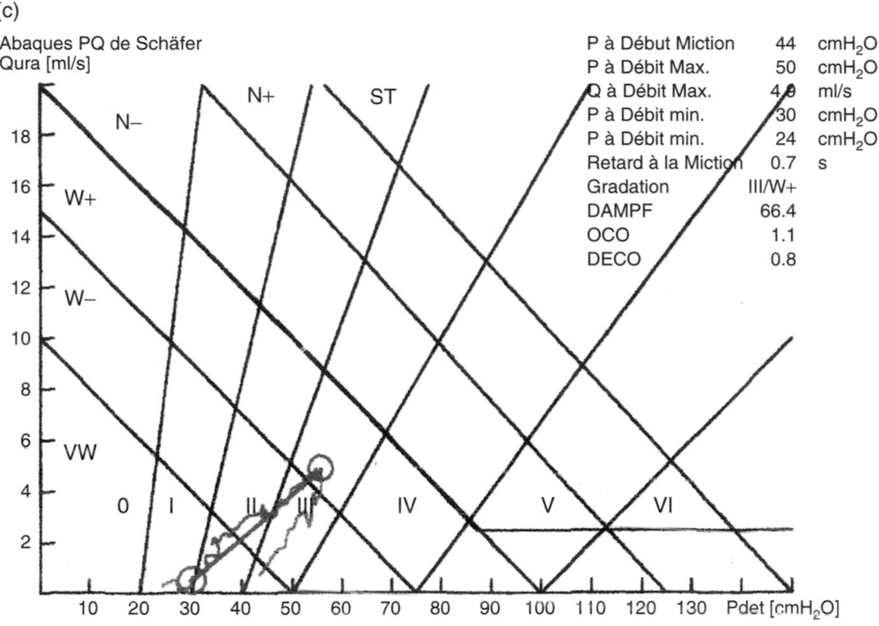

Figure 68.9
(a) Underactive and/or noncontractile bladder (A) combined with an obstructed outlet (B). No spontaneous voiding is expected. Urethral resistance must be decreased (C) and bladder contractility increased (D) to ensure normal vesicourethral balance. (b) Voiding phase during the pressure-flow study. (c) Schafer's nomogram exhibits a moderately severe constrictive obstruction, associated with a grade III compressive type obstruction, along with a somewhat weakened detrusor.

References

1. Chancellor MB, Blaivas GJ. Spinal cord injury. In: Chancellor MB, Blaivas JG, eds. Practical Neurourology: Genitourinary Complications in Neurologic Diseases. Boston: Butterworth-Heinemann, 1995: 99–118.
2. McGuire EJ, Cespedes RD, O'Connell HE. Leak point pressures. Urol Clin N Am 1996; 23: 253–62.
3. Stöhrer M, Goepel M, Kondo A et al. The standardization of terminology in neurogenic lower urinary tract dysfunction with suggestions for diagnostic procedures. Neurourol Urodyn 1999; 18: 139–58.
4. Tanagho EA, Miller ER. Initiation of voiding. Br J Urol 1970; 42: 175–83.
5. Abrams PH, Griffiths DJ. The assessment of prostatic obstruction from urodynamic measurements and from residual urine. Br J Urol 1979; 51: 129–34.
6. Dorflinger T, Frimodt-Møller PC, Bruskewitz RC et al. The significance of uninhibited detrusor contractions in prostatism. J Urol 1985; 133: 819–21.
7. Frimodt-Møller PC, Jensen KM, Iversen P et al. Analysis of presenting symptoms in prostatism. J Urol 1984; 132: 272–6.

Abbreviations

B1 = first desire to void
CNI = uninhibited contraction
CR = catheter repositioned
DM = beginning of flow
DMA = maximum flow
DP = starting point of UPP
EMV = initiate voiding
FM = end of flow
FP = end of UPP
IU = urinary incontinence
N = normal
P_{abd} = intraabdominal pressure
PB = baseline pressure
PC = maximum closing pressure
P_{det} = detrusor pressure
V_{infus} = infused volume
PM = end point of UPP
PM = maximum urethral pressure
P_{ura} = urethral pressure
$P_{ura\ diff}$ = closing pressure
P_{ves} = bladder pressure
Q_{ura} = flow curve
ST = strong
TOUX = cough
UPP = urethral pressure profile
VW = very weak
W = weak

69

Treatment alternatives for different types of neurogenic bladder dysfunction in children

Roman Jednak and Joao Luiz Pippi Salle

Introduction

Congenitally acquired lesions of spinal cord development collectively referred to as neurospinal dysraphisms are the most common cause of neurogenic bladder dysfunction in children. Abnormal bladder innervation is found in the overwhelming majority of patients with myelodysplasia, and, consequently, impaired drainage of the lower and upper urinary tract, if not managed appropriately, can be a significant cause of morbidity.

Management goals include establishing satisfactory bladder emptying, maintaining safe bladder storage pressures to prevent upper urinary tract deterioration, avoiding urinary tract infections, and, in the long term, achieving urinary continence. Fortunately, significant advances in the treatment of children with myelodysplasia have resulted in an impressive decrease in the incidence of upper urinary tract deterioration and marked improvements in the achievement of urinary continence. Naturally, this has translated into decreased morbidity and notable improvements in the quality of life for affected children.

Renal damage, nevertheless, remains a real risk and patients require careful evaluation and follow-up. It should also be emphasized that in the myelodysplastic child, the neurologic lesion and bladder dynamics can change with time. Regular urodynamic testing should be performed both in order to identify worsening parameters before upper urinary tract deterioration occurs and to appropriately select management strategies when trying to establish urinary continence.

Here we outline some of the medical and surgical alternatives available when managing the child with neurogenic bladder. The reported outcomes of various surgical techniques in the pediatric population are reviewed.

Management of the bladder

Anticholinergic medications and clean intermittent catheterization

Bladder management is tailored according to the results of urodynamic evaluation.[1–4] Management goals are the maintenance of a compliant low-pressure reservoir that can be regularly emptied in order to both protect the upper urinary tract from deterioration and achieve urinary continence.

Not all children require early clean intermittent catheterization and/or anticholinergic medications.[2,5] Children who empty the bladder effectively in association with synergic or incompetent sphincter function can be observed closely. Clean intermittent catheterization should be started in those patients with a flaccid bladder that empties poorly.[6–8] Latex catheters should be avoided in order to minimize the risk of developing a latex allergy.[9–12] Antibiotic prophylaxis need not be routinely administered in all children, but should be considered in those with documented vesicoureteral reflux.[13–15]

Catheterization is ideally performed at intervals of every 3–4 hours. Clean intermittent catheterization used in combination with an anticholinergic medication is indicated in patients with a poorly compliant or hyperreflexic bladder or in those with detrusor-sphincter dyssynergia.[16–24] Detrusor contraction is primarily mediated by the action of acetylcholine.[25,26]

Anticholinergic agents effectively increase the bladder capacity achieved prior to the onset of an uninhibited contraction, decrease the magnitude of uninhibited contractions, and produce an increase in total bladder capacity. Oxybutynin is the most commonly used anticholinergic and in children can be introduced 2–3 times per day at a dose of 0.1–0.2 mg/kg. The medication can be safely used, even in the neonatal period. The most common anticholinergic side-effects encountered in children are dry mouth, constipation, flushing of the skin, blurred vision, and hyperactivity.[27] An extended-release formulation that can be administered once daily and may produce fewer adverse effects is also available. Alternatively, intravesical instillation can also be performed. It should be remembered, however, that intravesical instillation is also associated with a similar spectrum of side-effects.[27–33] The most recent innovation in anticholinergic therapy has been the introduction of a transdermal delivery system for oxybutynin.[34–37] Transdermal delivery allows for bypassing of gastrointestinal and hepatic first-pass metabolism, thereby providing for more consistent absorption and a reduction in oxybutynin metabolite levels. As a result, lower drug dosages can be used and metabolite-related side-effects are reduced. Adult studies have shown marked improvements in urinary frequency, incontinent episodes, and nocturia, with a rate of side-effects that is lower than that associated with oral preparations.[38,39] The most common adverse event is a localized skin reaction characterized by erythema and pruritis at the site of application. Clinical studies in children have yet to be performed, but the therapeutic potential certainly looks promising.

Cutaneous vesicostomy

Occasionally, despite maximal efforts, clean intermittent catheterization and anticholinergics are unsuccessful in managing high-risk bladders, controling reflux, avoiding infections, or preventing upper urinary tract deterioration. In addition, clean intermittent catheterization may not be reliably instituted because of social or anatomic factors. In these cases, cutaneous vesicostomy is a useful and reliable form of temporary urinary diversion in neonates and infants.[40–42] The procedure involves creating a communication between the bladder and the skin of the lower abdominal wall, which allows for free and unobstructed drainage of urine (Figure 69.1).[43] Complications include prolapse, stomal stenosis, stomal eversion, stones, and peristomal dermatitis.[44,45] Anterior bladder wall stomas can allow for posterior bladder wall prolapse. The incidence of prolapse can therefore best be minimized by using a posterior portion of the bladder wall cephalad to the urachus for the vesicostomy.

Bladder augmentation

The objective of bladder augmentation is to create a low-pressure storage reservoir of sufficient capacity to preserve upper urinary tract function and maintain or establish urinary continence when maximal medical therapy is unsuccessful. Advances in surgical techniques have enabled the attainment of these goals with a high degree of reliability, and the experience with bladder enlargement has been extended to a variety of materials and techniques.[46] Most commonly, intestinal segments are selected for bladder augmentation.[47] More recent developments have focused on techniques attempting to preserve the bladder urothelium and thereby avoiding the introduction of intestinal mucosa into the urinary tract.[48–51] Irrespective of the technique used, bladder emptying is usually impaired to some degree and, consequently, most children require clean intermittent catheterization postoperatively. All patients should additionally be made aware of the risk of bladder perforation, a potentially life-threatening complication that may occur following any form of bladder augmentation.[52]

Techniques which do not preserve the urothelium

Ileo- and colocystoplasty Bladder augmentation using ileum or colon has proven to be a reliable means of increasing bladder capacity and reducing bladder pressures.[53–58] The incorporation of these intestinal segments into the urinary tract, however, is associated with a number of long-term complications.[47] Because of the young patient population typically being treated, this long-term exposure to these complications is of significant concern. Complications most commonly observed include mucus production, bacterial colonization, electrolyte imbalances, metabolic acidosis, somatic growth retardation, and vitamin B_{12} deficiency.[59–63] Other concerns are the risk of calculus formation and the development of malignancy (Table 69.1).[64–72]

Gastrocystoplasty Stomach first gained popularity as an alternative to colon or ileum in children with chronic renal failure and azotemia as a direct result of its natural acid-secreting ability, which does not worsen the metabolic acidosis.[73,74] The technique is also useful when bowel resection is not an option, as is the case with short-bowel syndrome. Mucus production is less problematic and the acidic urine may also reduce bacterial colonization and the incidence of urinary tract infections. Specific complications include intermittent hematuria, metabolic alkalosis, and the hematuria–dysuria syndrome, which is characterized by bladder or urethral pain and hematuria in the absence of infection (Table

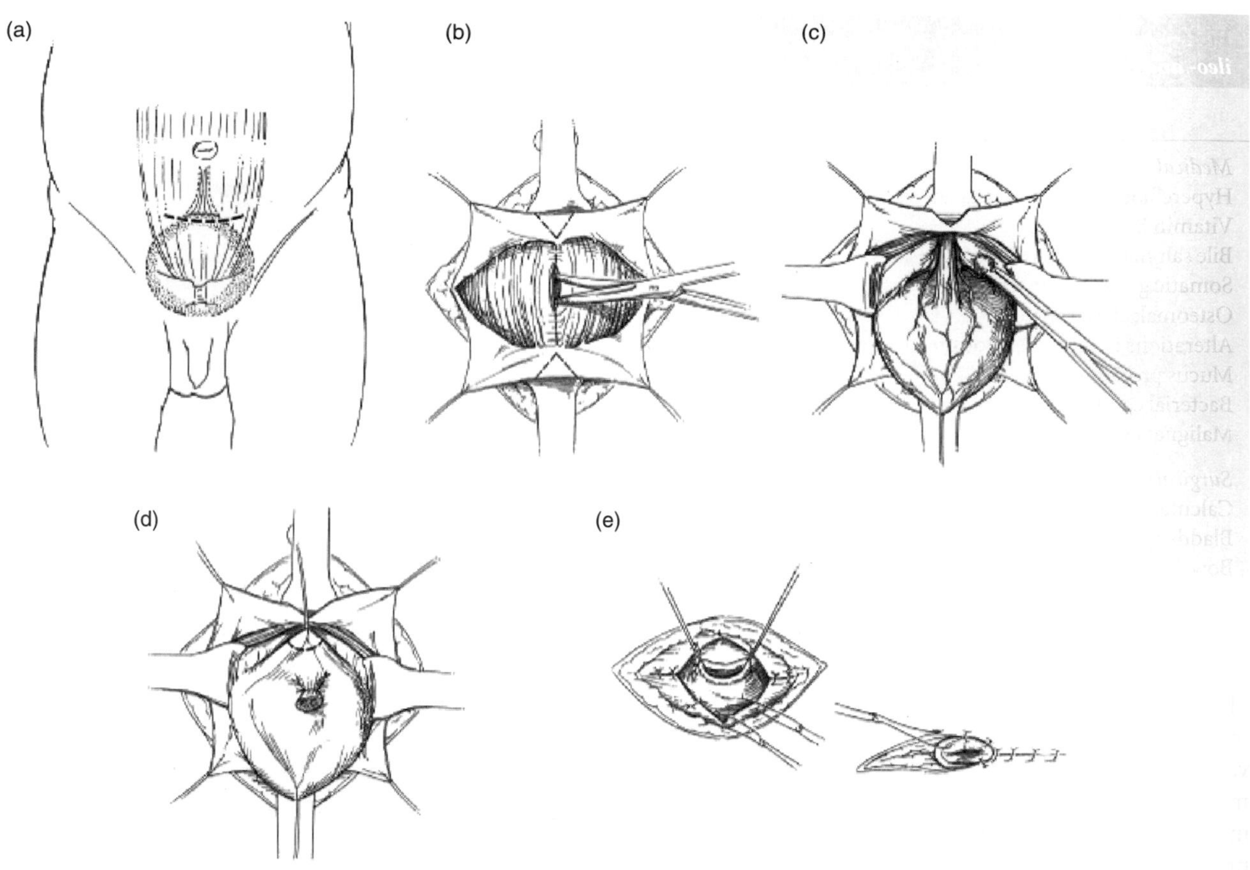

Figure 69.1
Cutaneous vesicostomy. (a) Transverse incision made midway between the umbilicus and symphysis pubis. (b) Modified Pfannenstiel approach. Fascial flaps are raised and the rectus muscles separated in the midline. (c) Urachal remnant, dome, and posterior bladder gradually accessed by progressively retracting the bladder inferiorly and sweeping away the peritoneum. (d) Site for cystostomy selected behind the ligated urachus. (e) Detrusor circumferentially anastomosed to the fascia below the cystostomy. The musosa is sutured to the skin with interrupted sutures. (From Keating MA: Incontinent urinary diversion. In: Marshall FF, ed. Textbook of Operative Urology. Philadelphia: WB Saunders, 1996, with permission Dr FF Marshall.)

69.2).[75,76] Children with incontinence or renal insufficiency/oliguria tend to experience more problems with the hematuria–dysuria syndrome. Since the hematuria–dysuria syndrome does not always respond well to histamine antagonists, this may pose a significant problem in children with normal bladder and urethral sensation. Although the majority of malignancies have been reported in patients undergoing enterocystoplasty, malignancies following gastrocystoplasty have been reported.[77–80] These patients should have careful long-term follow-up.

Techniques which preserve the urothelium

Ureterocystoplasty The dilated ureter serving a nonfunctioning kidney can occasionally be used for bladder augmentation (Figure 69.2).[81,82] Success with ureterocystoplasty has been excellent and, since the urothelium is preserved, acid–base disturbances and mucus production are not a problem.[83–85] In addition, the procedure can be performed using an exclusively extraperitoneal approach.[86] Since the procedure requires a severely dilated ureter and nonfunctioning kidney, however, its usefulness is limited to specific clinical situations. One report has proposed patient criteria for a successful ureterocystoplasty.[87] Specifically, patients without reflux and either a single or duplex collecting system can benefit from ureterocystoplasty if the ureter is at least 1.5 cm in diameter. Patients with reflux improve only if the compliance of the total system is normal or mildly noncompliant (compliance greater than 20 ml/cmH_2O).

Autoaugmentation Excision or incision of the diseased detrusor with preservation of the urothelium creates a urothelium diverticulum that serves to augment the

Table 69.1 *Long term complications associated with ileo- and colocystoplasty*

	Ileum	Colon
Medical		
Hyperchloremic metabolic acidosis	+	+
Vitamin B_{12} deficiency	+	–
Bile salt malabsorption	+	–
Somatic growth retardation	+	–
Osteomalacia/rickets	+	+
Alterations in drug metabolism	+	+
Mucus production	+	+
Bacterial colonization	+	+
Malignancy	+	+
Surgical		
Calculus formation	+	+
Bladder perforation	+	+
Bowel obstruction	+	+

bladder.[88,89] The benefits of preserving the urothelium are maintained but the reported urodynamic outcomes have varied. Some reports have described only slight improvements in bladder capacity, whereas others have noted improvements in capacity with persistently high bladder pressures.[90–92] Several series have reported poor success rates in patients with neurogenic bladder dysfunction.[93–96] The results of one such study suggest that the mechanism of action with autoaugmentation may be a direct effect on the ability of the detrusor to contract rather than augmentation of bladder volume. The authors feel that the patients most likely to benefit are those with primary detrusor instability and a high leak-point pressure.[95]

Seromuscular enterocystoplasty The complications associated with enterocystoplasty are attributable to the presence of intestinal mucosa within the urinary tract.[47,59–63] Seromuscular enterocystoplasty makes use of demucosalized segments of ileum, colon, or stomach to augment the bladder and thereby avoid the potential disadvantages of urine contact with intestinal mucosa.[49–51] The procedure can be performed with or without preservation of the urothelium. When the urothelium is preserved the detrusor is excised, leaving a urothelial diverticulum over which the seromuscular patch is then placed (Figure 69.3).[97–102] When no attempt is made to preserve the urothelium, a standard clam enterocystoplasty technique is used and the seromuscular patch is used to augment the bladder using the standard enterocystoplasty technique.[103–105]

The importance of postoperative bladder distention has consistently been stressed as essential to achieving an optimal result in all reports describing the technique.[99,102–104,106] This can be achieved by one of two methods. When the urothelium is preserved and the seromuscular patch is positioned over the exposed urothelial bubble, a Foley catheter can be left to straight drainage and positioned 20–30 cm above the level of the symphysis pubis for a period of 4–5 days.[97–100,102,106] A competent bladder outlet is important to optimize bladder distention in this case, and a concomitant bladder outlet procedure is recommended in patients with poor outlet resistance. In addition, since urothelial integrity is critical to minimizing postoperative leaks, performing concomitant procedures that violate the urothelium should be avoided.[99,102,106]

An alternative method makes use of an intravesical silicone mold that maintains the seromuscular patch in a distended state for a period of 10–14 days.[103,104] This technique can be used both when the urothelium is and is not preserved. Short-term results to date have been encouraging, with postoperative urodynamic parameters and continence rates paralleling those of standard augmentation techniques. Mucus production and electrolyte abnormalities do not appear to be a problem.

Table 69.2 *Complications associated with gastrocystoplasty*

Hyperchloremic metabolic alkalosis
Hypergastrinemia
Hematuria–dysuria syndrome
Peptic ulcer disease
Dumping syndrome

Management of the bladder outlet

Medications to increase outlet resistance

Adrenergic nerves innervate the muscular fibers of the bladder base. Alpha agonists (ephedrine, pseudoephedrine) produce an increase in bladder outlet resistance and on occasion may improve urine storage.[107–109] The results with these agents, however, are often less than satisfactory, but improvements in continence can occasionally be obtained in children with mild degrees of wetting due to sphincteric incompetence. In addition, side-effects, including hypertension, anxiety, headaches, and insomnia, may

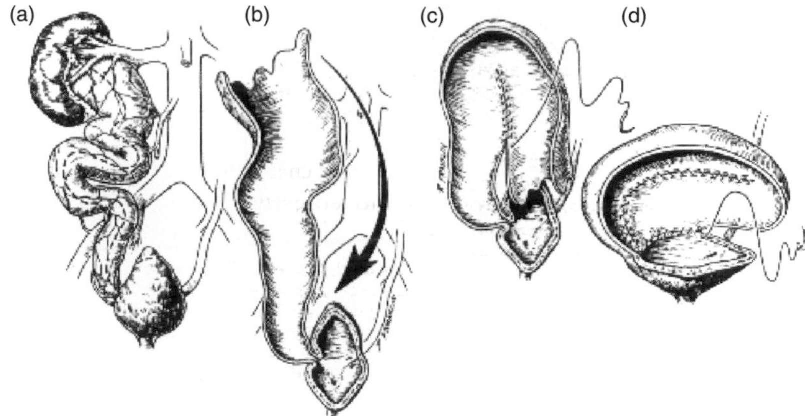

Figure 69.2
Operative stages of ureteral bladder augmentation. (a) Normal blood supply to ureter. (b) Ureteral detubularization following mobilization. (c) Reconfiguration of ureter into U-shaped patch. (d) Anastomosing ureteral patch to native bivalved bladder. (From Churchill BM et al. Ureteral bladder augmentation. J Urol 1993; 150: 716–720.)

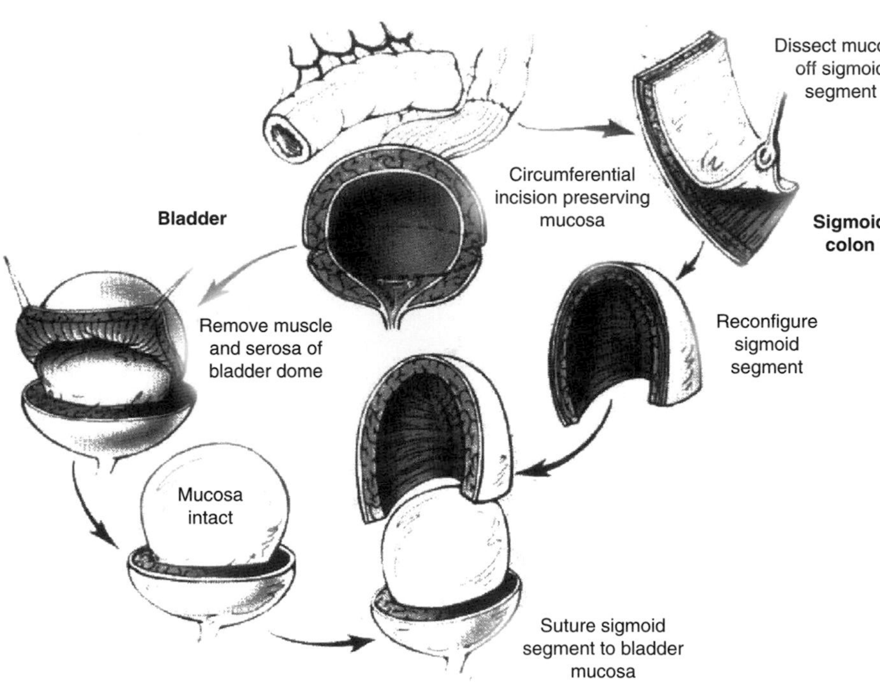

Figure 69.3
Operative technique of seromuscular colocystoplasty lined with urothelium. (Reprinted with modification from Urology 44, Buson et al, Seromuscular colocystoplasty lined with urothelium: experimental study, pp. 743–748, Copyright 1994, with permission from Elsevier Science.)

be problematic, so that the use of these agents in managing the incompetent bladder outlet remains limited.

Periurethral injection of bulking agents

Bulking agents such as collagen, Teflon, and, more recently, dextranomer/hyaluronic acid copolymer can be injected submucosally at the bladder neck to facilitate mucosal coaptation and achieve continence.[110–121] Continence rates are difficult to interpret since variable criteria have been reported to define success. In addition, some authors have failed to show a durable response with long-term follow-up.[118,121] When defined as a dry interval of 4 hours, continence rates are in the range of 5–63%. Success is often dependent on more than one injection, and as a result cost may become an important issue. Predictors of response to the injection of bulking agents are inconsistent, but at least one group has noted improved outcomes in patients with detrusor areflexia and low-pressure bladders.[117] Attempts at defining urodynamic characteristics that may serve as predictors of long-term success have been unsuccessful.[122] Importantly, collagen injection has not been found to interfere with bladder neck surgery if this is subsequently required.

Bladder neck suspension and fascial sling procedures

The use of bladder neck suspension techniques for the treatment of the pediatric neurogenic bladder has not gained widespread use. Reported continence rates achieved in girls in association with bladder augmentation have been at least 80%, with the longest period of follow-up being 30 months.

Fascial slings improve outlet resistance by compression and elevation of the urethra. Reported continence rates have varied from 40 to 100% over a follow-up period of at most 4.5 years.[123–136] The majority of patients have been girls. Attempts at improving outlet resistance have led to a number of modifications, including concomitant bladder neck tapering or circumferentially wrapping the bladder neck with rectus fascia, a rectus myofascial flap, or a strip of anterior bladder wall.[137–143] Bladder augmentation is often necessary to improve continence rates and intermittent catheterization is frequently required. Success using the procedure in boys has been reported in several series.[127,131,133–137,139,140,142,143]

Urethral lengthening procedures

The Kropp and Pippi Salle procedures create a fixed increase in bladder outlet resistance by using a portion of the anterior bladder wall to construct a one-way valve. The Kropp procedure consists of performing urethral lengthening with a tubularized segment of anterior bladder wall, which is reimplanted in the posterior intertrigonal area, creating a one-way valve mechanism similar to the antireflux mechanism procedures used for correction of vesicoureteral reflux (Figure 69.4).[144] Increases in intravesical pressures are transmitted to the submucosal urethral tube, thereby increasing closure pressure and preventing incontinence.

The procedure is technically demanding and, consequently, revisions have been proposed to facilitate creation of the submucosal tube. Mollard and colleagues described resection of the muscular layer of the distal 50% of the tube to make it more pliable and facilitate submucosal tunneling.[145] Snodgrass made use of a longitudinal bladder incision starting from the bladder neck and extending up between the ureteral orifices into which the detrusor tube was laid. Lateral mucosal flaps are then secured to either side of the tube.[146] The Pippi Salle procedure consists of fashioning an anterior bladder wall flap, which is then sutured to the posterior bladder wall in an onlay fashion. The neourethra is then covered with bladder wall and lateral mucosal flaps to fashion a submucosal tunnel (Figure 69.5).[147–149]

Both these techniques commit the patient to intermittent catheterization, which at times may be difficult.[144,147,148,150–152] Overall, more catheterization difficulties seem to be encountered with the Kropp procedure. As a result, thought should be given to performing a concomitant continent catheterizable channel to facilitate intermittent catheterization postoperatively.[153] Because bladder wall is sacrificed to lengthen the urethra, the postoperative development of low bladder capacity and poor compliance is a risk and, consequently, concomitant bladder augmentation is often required with both techniques.[146,148–151,153–155] As a result of the potential risk for upper tract deterioration should bladder storage characteristics worsen, careful radiologic and urodynamic follow-up is essential.

Reported continence rates are in the range of 77–91% for the Kropp[144–148,150,151] procedure, whereas those rates for the Pippi Salle[146,148–151,153–155] procedure are in the range of 64–94%. Outcome with the Pippi Salle procedure tends to be more favorable in girls.[154–156]

An interesting variation on the Kropp and Pippi Salle procedures has recently been described.[157] The miniature intravesical urethral lengthening procedure similarly utilizes an anterior bladder wall flap isolated in continuity with the bladder neck. The flap, which is shorter than that used for the Kropp and Pippi Salle procedures (1 × 3 cm), is then tubularized proximally and tunneled under the trigone. The remaining distal strip is then sewn to the bladder floor in an onlay fashion to complete the intravesical extension of the urethra. Continence was achieved in eight of nine patients and all except one were simultaneously augmented. The mean period of follow-up was 31 months. The authors suggest that since less bladder wall is used, this technique can be performed without concomitant bladder augmentation. It should be remembered however, that any reinforcement of the bladder outlet puts the patent at risk for loss of bladder compliance. It seems unlikely that the change in flap size will have a major impact on the need for augmentation.

The artificial urinary sphincter

The artificial urinary sphincter was first introduced in 1974 and has since undergone a number of improvements in design.[158-161] Continence is achieved by compression of the bladder neck or urethra by an inflatable cuff that can be intermittently deflated to allow for catheterization or voiding. The preferred site of placement in children is around the bladder neck. Patients who empty their bladder without the need for catheterization prior to surgery may continue to do so following sphincter placement[161–169] but, if necessary, intermittent catheterization can be instituted safely.[170–172] It is essential that bladder capacity and

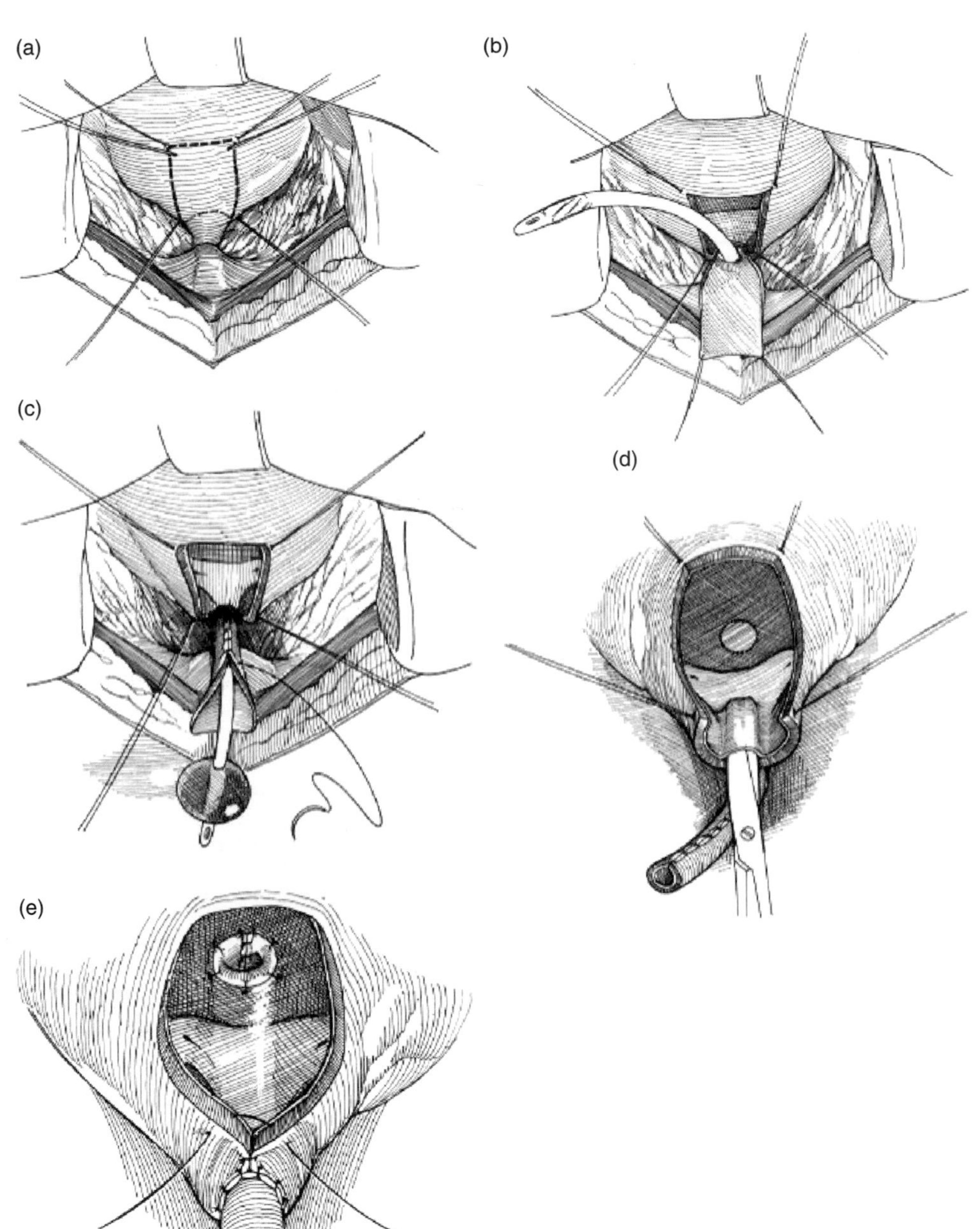

Figure 69.4
(a) An anterior bladder wall flap (5 to 7 cm × 2.5 cm wide) is outlined. (b) The junction of the trigone and the bladder neck is identified from within and the mucosa of the bladder neck separated from the urethra. (c) The anterior bladder flap is tubularized with a one-layer suture (interrupted suture in the last 2 cm). (d) A posterior trigonal tunnel (6 × 3 cm wide) is created, beginning at the bladder neck and carried upward beyond the ureteral orifices. (e) The tubularized flap is reimplanted in the posterior submucosal tunnel and the anterior bladder wall is sutured over the bladder neck at the base of the neourethra. (Reprinted from Pippi Salle JL. Urethral lengthening for urinary incontinence. In: Gearhart et al, eds. Pediatric Urology, Copyright 2001, with permission from Elsevier Science.)

compliance be evaluated prior to placing an artificial sphincter, but admittedly this may be difficult in the presence of an incompetent bladder neck.

Some centers have found that preoperative urodynamics may not accurately predict which patient will go on to require bladder augmentation[173,174] but, nevertheless, failure to recognize a clearly noncompliant bladder preoperatively may put the upper urinary tract at an unnecessary and significant risk when outlet resistance is increased. In cases where bladder augmentation is required, this can be performed concomitantly without increasing the risk of complications.[175,176]

Despite having favorable preoperative bladder dynamics some patients may develop deterioration in bladder compliance and, therefore, postoperative urodynamic studies and careful radiologic and urodynamic follow-up are essential.[163,165–169,177,178] The most common complications include mechanical failure, erosion, and infection. Both erosion and infection result in permanent failure. Revision of the device has been high in most published

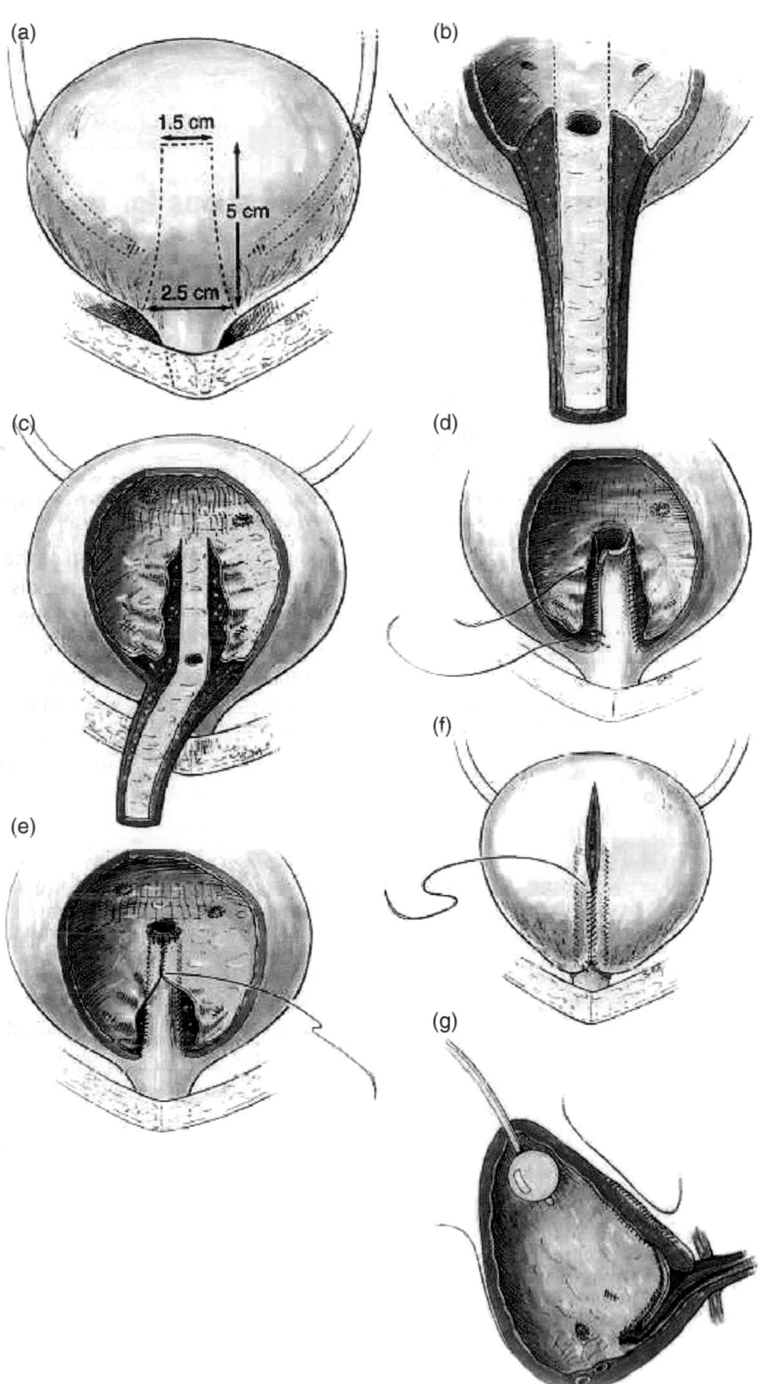

Figure 69.5
(a) Anterior bladder wall flap with a wide base to improve vascular supply. (b) The flap mucosal edges are excised from the muscle to achieve a narrow rectangular mucosal strip with a rich blood supply. This allows a nonoverlapping two-layer anastomosis. (c) Parallel incisions are made in the posterior trigonal mucosa. If reimplantation is necessary, both ureters are disconnected and reimplanted superiorly in a cross-trigonal fashion. (d) The anterior flap is dropped onto the incised posterior mucosa and sutured in two layers (mucosa–mucosal and muscle–muscular) to the posterior wall in an onlay fashion. (e) The posterior mucosa lateral to either side of the trigonal incision is mobilized from the detrusor and used to cover the neourethra. (f) The anterior bladder wall is closed in front of the intravesical urethra in a tension-free manner. Tension over the neourethra can cause impairment of the flap vascular supply. (g) Schematic lateral view of the neourethra demonstrating its intravesical position and the flap-valve mechanism when the bladder fills. (From Pippi Salle JL, et al. Modifications of and extended applications for the Pippi Salle procedure. World J Urol 1998; 16: 279–284, Spinger-Verlag publishers, with permission.)

series, but more recent reports have noted a considerable improvement in the revision rate. Given that the artificial sphincter is a mechanical device with a finite lifespan, however, it can be expected that most patients will at some time require surgery for revision. Overall, continence rates from 61% to over 95% have been reported in those children having a functional artificial urinary sphincter still in place.[163,164,166–169,179–181]

Bladder neck closure

Surgical failures following bladder neck reconstruction can be a challenge to manage. Scarring and poor tissue quality can make additional surgery difficult and prone to complications and, as a result, the surgeon may be left with limited options. The best chance for establishing continence and salvaging a favorable outcome may rely on bladder neck closure and creation of a continent catheterizable channel. A number of reports have documented a high rate of success with this procedure.[182–187] The main concern following bladder neck closure is that of fistula formation. Measures to reduce this include interposition of rectus muscle or omentum between the closed bladder neck and urethral stump.[182,183] An alternative to this involves extensive mobilization of the bladder neck posteriorly for at least 2 cm. The posterior bladder neck can then be brought anterior such that the closure lies anterior rather than inferior. Naturally, complications related to the continent catheterization channel are also a concern and not all that uncommon.[185–187] It should be remembered that closure of the bladder neck eliminates a pop-off mechanism should catheterization become impossible. As is the case with any type of bladder reconstructive procedure, it is imperative that patients comply with a regular catheterization schedule.

Conclusions

The treatment of neurogenic bladder dysfunction in children has been a major driving force behind a myriad of innovative surgical solutions; unfortunately, we must accept that none of these are perfect. It also needs to be kept in mind that the successful management of any given patient is defined by a multitude of variables and is not simply a good surgical outcome. Management goals are consistent from patient to patient, but the management strategies are not simply defined by urodynamic studies and urinary tract imaging. Often, the patient's physical limitations as well as their emotional and social needs play a critical role in determining a rational therapeutic strategy.

Before any surgical reconstruction is entertained, available medical management options should be exhausted. Bladder augmentation remains a reliable and highly successful means of dealing with the small capacity, poorly compliant, or hyperreflexic bladder. Far more controversy surrounds the management of the incompetent bladder neck, and the inherent difficulty of dealing with bladder neck incompetence underlies the variety of reconstructive techniques that has been described over the years. The most favorable management approach in a specific clinical situation is therefore often defined by surgeon preference against the background of clearly defined patient expectations. Urodynamic studies performed with a balloon catheter to occlude the bladder neck may facilitate the process.

References

1. McGuire EJ, Woodside JR, Borden TA, Weiss RM. Prognostic value of urodynamic testing in myelodysplastic patients. J Urol 1981; 126: 205–9.
2. Bauer SB, Hallett M, Khoshbin S et al. Predictive value of urodynamic evaluation in newborns with myelodysplasia. JAMA 1984; 252: 650–2.
3. Sidi AA, Peng W, Gonzalez R. The value of urodynamic testing in the management of newborns with myelodysplasia: a prospective study. J Urol 1986; 135: 90–3.
4. Wang SC, McGuire EJ, Bloom DA. A bladder pressure management system for myelodysplasia – clinical outcome. J Urol 1988; 140: 1499–502.
5. Fernandes ET, Reinberg Y, Vernier R, Gonzalez R. Neurogenic bladder dysfunction in children: review of pathophysiology and current management. J Pediatr 1994; 124: 1–7.
6. Lapides J, Diokno AC, Silber S, Lowe BS. Clean, intermittent self-catheterization in the treatment of urinary tract disease. J Urol 1972; 107: 458–61.
7. Lapides J, Diokno AC, Lowe BS, Kalish M. Followup on unsterile, intermittent self-catheterization. J Urol 1974; 111: 184–7.
8. Lapides J, Diokno AC, Gould FR, Lowe BS. Further observations on self-catheterization. J Urol 1976; 116: 169–71.
9. Slater JE, Mostello LA, Shaer C. Rubber-specific IgE in children with spina bifida. J Urol 1991; 146: 578–9.
10. Ellsworth PI, Merguerian PA, Klein RB, Rozycki AA. Evaluation and risk factors of latex allergy in spina bifida patients: is it preventable? J Urol 1993; 150: 691–3.
11. Pasquariello CA, Lowe DA, Schwartz RE. Intraoperative anaphylaxis to latex. Pediatrics 1993; 91: 983–6.
12. Nguyen DH, Burns MW, Shapiro GG et al. Intraoperative cardiovascular collapse secondary to latex allergy. J Urol 1991; 146: 571–4.
13. Kass EJ, Koff SA, Diokno AC, Lapides J. The significance of bacilluria in children on long-term intermittent catheterization. J Urol 1981; 126: 223–5.
14. Ottolini MC, Shaer CM, Rushton HG et al. Relationship of asymptomatic bacteriuria and renal scarring in children with neuropathic bladders who are practicing clean intermittent catheterization. J Pediatr 1995; 127: 368–72.
15. Schlager TA, Anderson S, Trudell J, Hendley JO. Nitrofurantoin prophylaxis for bacteriuria and urinary tract infection in children with neurogenic bladder on intermittent catheterization. J Pediatr 1998; 132: 704–8.
16. Diokno AC, Kass E, Lapides J. New approach to myelodysplasia. J Urol 1976; 116: 771–2.
17. Crooks KK, Enrile BG, Wise HA. The results of clean intermittent catheterization on the abnormal upper urinary tracts of children with myelomeningocele. Ohio State Med J 1981; 77: 377–9.
18. Perez-Marrero R, Dimmock W, Churchill BM, Hardy BE. Clean intermittent catheterization in myelomeningocele children less than 3 years old. J Urol 1982; 128: 779–81.
19. Geraniotis E, Koff SA, Enrile B. The prophylactic use of clean intermittent catheterization in the treatment of infants and young children with myelomeningocele and neurogenic bladder dysfunction. J Urol 1988; 139: 85–6.
20. Joseph DB, Bauer SB, Colodny AH et al. Clean, intermittent catheterization of infants with neurogenic bladder. Pediatrics 1989; 84: 78–82.
21. Klose AG, Sackett CK, Mesrobian H-GJ. Management of children with myelodysplasia: urological alternatives. J Urol 1990; 144: 1446–9.
22. Baskin LS, Kogan BA, Benard F. Treatment of infants with neurogenic bladder dysfunction using anticholinergic drugs and intermittent catheterisation. Br J Urol 1990; 66: 532–4.
23. Kasabian NG, Bauer SB, Dyro FM et al. The prophylactic value of clean intermittent catheterization and anticholinergic medication in newborns and infants with myelomeningocele at risk of developing urinary tract deterioration. Am J Dis Child 1992; 146: 840–3.
24. Edelstein RA, Bauer SB, Kelly MD et al. The long-term urological response of neonates with myelodysplasia treated proactively with intermittent catheterization and anticholinergic therapy. J Urol 1995; 154: 1500–4.
25. de Groat WC, Yoshimura N. Pharmacology of the lower urinary tract. Ann Rev Pharmacol Toxicol 2001; 41: 691–721.

26. Yamanishi T, Chapple CR, Chess-Williams R. Which muscarinic receptor is important in the bladder? World J Urol 2001; 19: 299–306.
27. Andersson KE, Chapple CR. Oxybutynin and the overactive bladder. World J Urol 2001; 19: 319–23.
28. Greenfield SP, Fera M. The use of intravesical oxybutynin chloride in children with neurogenic bladder. J Urol 1991; 146: 532–4.
29. Kasabian NG, Vlachiotis JD, Lais A et al. The use of intravesical oxybutynin chloride in patients with detrusor hypertonicity and detrusor hyperreflexia. J Urol 1994; 151: 944–5.
30. Kaplinsky R, Greenfield S, Wan J, Fera M. Expanded followup of intravesical oxybutynin chloride use in children with neurogenic bladder. J Urol 1996; 156: 753–6.
31. Painter KA, Vates TS, Bukowski TP et al. Long-term intravesical oxybutynin chloride therapy in children with myelodysplasia. J Urol 1996; 156: 1459–62.
32. Palmer LS, Zebold K, Firlit CF, Kaplan WE. Complications of intravesical oxybutynin chloride therapy in the pediatric myelomeningocele population. J Urol 1997; 157: 638–40.
33. Ferrara P, D'Aleo CM, Tarquini E et al. Side-effects of oral or intravesical oxybutynin chloride in children with spina bifida. BJU Int 2001; 87: 674–7.
34. Nitti VW. Transdermal therapy for overactive bladder: present and future. Rev Urol 2003; 5(Suppl 8): S31–6.
35. Starkman JS, Dmochowski RR. Management of overactive bladder with transdermal oxybutynin. Rev Urol 2006; 8: 93–103.
36. Davila GW, Starkman JS, Dmochowski RR. Transdermal oxybutynin for overactive bladder. Urol Clin N Am 2006; 33: 455–63.
37. Cartwright R, Cardozo L. Transdermal oxybutynin: sticking to the facts. Eur Urol 2007; 51: 907–14.
38. Dmochowski RR, Davila GW, Zinner NR et al. Efficacy and safety of transdermal oxybutynin in patients with urge and mixed urinary incontinence. J Urol 2002; 23: 580–6.
39. Dmochowski RR, Nitti V, Staskin D et al. Transdermal oxybutynin in the treatment of adults with overactive bladder: combined results of two randomized clinical trials. World J Urol 2005; 23: 263–70.
40. Cohen JS, Harbach LB, Kaplan GW. Cutaneous vesicostomy for temporary urinary diversion in infants with neurogenic bladder dysfunction. J Urol 1978; 119: 120–1.
41. Mandell J, Bauer SB, Colodny AH, Retik AB. Cutaneous vesicostomy in infancy. J Urol 1981; 126: 92–3.
42. Snyder HM III, Kalichman MA, Charney E, Duckett JW. Vesicostomy for neurogenic bladder with spina bifida: followup. J Urol 1983; 130: 724–6.
43. Duckett JW Jr. Cutaneous vesicostomy in childhood: the Blocksom technique. Urol Clin N Am 1974; 1: 485–95.
44. Hurwitz RS, Ehrlich RM. Complications of cutaneous vesicostomy. Urol Clin N Am 1974; 10: 503–8.
45. Duckett JW, Ziylan O. Uses and abuses of vesicostomy. AUA Update Series 1995; 14: 130–5.
46. Duel BP, Gonzalez R, Barthold JS. Alternative techniques for augmentation cystoplasty. J Urol 1999; 159: 998–1005.
47. Gough DCS. Enterocystoplasty. BJU Int 2001; 88: 739–43.
48. Ureterocystoplasty: the latest developments. BJU Int 2001; 88: 744–51.
49. Jednak R, Schmike CM, Ludwikowski B, González R. Seromuscular colocystoplasty. BJU Int 2001; 88: 752–6.
50. Close CE. Autoaugmentation gastrocystoplasty. BJU Int 2001; 88: 757–61.
51. Lima SVC, Araújo LAP, Vilar FO et al. Experience with demucosalized ileum for bladder augmentation. BJU Int 2001; 88: 762–4.
52. Shekarriz B, Upadhyay J, Demirbilek S et al. Surgical complications of bladder augmentation: comparison between various enterocystoplasties in 133 patients. Urology 2000; 55: 123–8.
53. Hendren WH, Hendren RB. Bladder augmentation: experience with 129 children and young adults. J Urol 1990; 144: 445–53.
54. Mitchell ME, Kulb TB, Backes DJ. Intestinocystoplasty in combination with clean intermittent catheterization in the management of vesical dysfunction. J Urol 1986; 136: 288–91.
55. Decter RM, Bauer SB, Mandell J et al. Small bowel augmentation in children with neurogenic bladder: an initial report of urodynamic findings. J Urol 1987; 138: 1014–6.
56. Mitchell ME, Piser JA. Intestinocystoplasty and total bladder replacement in children and young adults: followup in 129 cases. J Urol 1987; 138: 579–84.
57. Krishna A, Gough DCS, Fishwick J, Bruce J. Ileocystoplasty in children: assessing safety and success. Eur Urol 1995; 27: 62–6.
58. Wang K, Yamataka A, Morioka A et al. Complications after sigmoidocolocystoplasty: review of 100 cases at one institution. J Pediatr Surg 1999; 34: 1672–7.
59. McDougal WS. Metabolic complications of urinary intestinal diversion. J Urol 1992; 147: 1199–208.
60. Stampfer DS, McDougal WS, McGovern FJ. Metabolic and nutritional complications. Urol Clin N Am 1997; 24: 715–22.
61. Nurse DE, Mundy AR. Metabolic complications of cystoplasty. Br J Urol 1989; 63: 165–70.
62. Wagstaff KE, Woodhouse CRJ, Duffy PG, Ransley PG. Delayed linear growth in children with enterocystoplasties. Br J Urol 1992; 69: 314–7.
63. Mundy AR, Nurse DE. Calcium balance, growth and skeletal mineralisation in patients with cystoplasties. Br J Urol 1992; 69: 257–9.
64. Blyth B, Ewalt DH, Duckett JW, Snyder HM. Lithogenic properties of enterocystoplasty. J Urol 1992; 148: 575–7.
65. Palmer LS, Franco I, Kogan SJ et al. Urolithiasis in children following augmentation cystoplasty. J Urol 1993; 150: 726–9.
66. Nurse DE, McInerney PD, Thomas PJ, Mundy AR. Stones in enterocystoplasties. Br J Urol 1996; 77: 684–7.
67. Khoury AE, Salomon M, Doche R et al. Stone formation following augmentation cystoplasty: the role of intestinal mucus. J Urol 1997; 158: 1133–7.
68. Kronner KM, Casale AJ, Cain MP et al. Bladder calculi in the pediatric augmented bladder. J Urol 1998; 160: 1096–8.
69. Mathoera RB, Kok DJ, Nijman RJM. Bladder calculi in augmentation cystoplasty in children. Urology 2000; 56: 482–7.
70. Filmer RB, Spencer JR. Malignancies in bladder augmentations and intestinal conduits. J Urol 1990; 143: 671–8.
71. Trieger BFG, Marshall FF. Carcinogenesis and the use of intestinal segments in the urinary tract. Urol Clin N Am 1991; 18: 737–42.
72. Malone MJ, Izes JK, Hurley LJ. Carcinogenesis. The fate of intestinal segments used in urinary reconstruction. Urol Clin N Am 1997; 24: 723–8.
73. Adams MC, Mitchell ME, Rink RC. Gastrocystoplasty: an alternative solution to the problem of urological reconstruction in the severely compromised patient. J Urol 1988; 140: 1152–6.
74. Sheldon CA, Gilbert A, Wacksman J, Lewis AG. Gastrocystoplasty: technical and metabolic characteristics of the most versatile childhood bladder augmentation modality. J Pediatr Surg 1995; 30: 283–7.
75. Nguyen DH, Bain MA, Salmonson KL et al. The syndrome of dysuria and hematuria in pediatric urinary reconstruction with stomach. J Urol 1993; 150: 707–9.
76. Kinahan TJ, Khoury AE, McLorie GA, Churchill BM. Omeprazole in post-gastrocystoplasty metabolic alkalosis and aciduria. J Urol 1992; 147: 435–7.
77. Qui H, Kordunskaya S, Yantiss RK. Transitional cell carcinoma arising in the gastric remnant following gastrocystoplasty. Int J Surg Pathol 2003; 11: 143–7.
78. Baydar DE, Allan RW, Castellan M et al. Anaplastic signet ring cell carcinoma arising in gastrocystoplasty. Urology 2005; 65: 1226e4–6.
79. Esquena Fernandez S, Abascal JM, Tremps E et al. Gastric cancer in augmentation gastrocystoplasty. Urol Int 2005; 74: 368–70.
80. Balachandra B, Swanson PE, Upton et al. Adenocarcinoma arising in a gastrocystoplasty. J Clin Pathol 2007; 60: 85–7.

81. Bellinger MF. Ureterocystoplasty: a unique method for vesical augmentation in children. J Urol 1993; 149: 811–3.
82. Churchill BM, Aliabadi H, Landau EH et al. Ureteral bladder augmentation. J Urol 1993; 150: 716–20.
83. Landau EH, Jayanthi VR, Khoury AE et al. Bladder augmentation: ureterocystoplasty versus ileocystoplasty. J Urol 1994; 152: 716–9.
84. Nahas WC, Lucon M, Mazzucchi E et al. Clinical and urodynamic evaluation after ureterocystoplasty and kidney transplantation. J Urol 2004; 171: 1428–31.
85. Podestá M, Barros D, Herrera M et al. Ureterocystoplasty: videourodynamic assessment. J Urol 2006; 176: 1721–5.
86. Dewan PA, Nicholls EA, Goh DW. Ureterocystoplasty: an extraperitoneal urothelial bladder augmentation technique. Eur Urol 1994; 26: 85–9.
87. Husmann DA, Snodgrass WT, Koyle MA et al. Ureterocystoplasty: indications for a successful augmentation. J Urol 2004; 171: 376–80.
88. Cartwright PC, Snow BW. Bladder autoaugmentation: partial detrusor excision to augment the bladder without use of bowel. J Urol 1989; 142: 1050–3.
89. Cartwright PC, Snow BW. Bladder autoaugmentation: early clinical experience. J Urol 1989; 142: 505–8.
90. Reid C, Moorehead JD, Hadley HR. Experience with detrusorectomy procedures. J Urol 1990; 143: 331A.
91. Stothers L, Johnson H, Arnold W et al. Bladder autoaugmentation by vesicomyotomy in the pediatric neurogenic bladder. Urology 1994; 44: 110–3.
92. Skobejko-Wlodarska L, Strulak K, Nachulewicz P, Szymkiewicz C. Bladder autoaugmentation in myelodysplastic children. Br J Urol 1998; 81(Suppl 3): 114–6.
93. Swami KS, Feneley RCL, Hammonds JC, Abrams P. Detrusor myectomy for detrusor overactivity: a minimum 1-year follow-up. Br J Urol 1998; 81: 68–72.
94. Potter JM, Duffy PG, Gordon EM et al. Detrusor myotomy: a 5-year review in unstable and non-compliant bladders. BJU Int 2002; 89: 932–5.
95. Marte A, Di Meglio D, Cotrufo AM et al. A long-term follow-up of autoaugmentation in myelodysplastic children. BJU Int 2002; 89: 928–31.
96. MacNeily AE, Afshar K, Coleman GU et al. Autoaugmentation by detrusor myotomy: its lack of effectiveness in the management of congenital neuropathic bladder. J Urol 2003; 170: 1643–6.
97. Dewan PA, Stefanek W. Autoaugmentation colocystoplasty. Pediatr Surg Int 1994; 9: 526–8.
98. Dewan PA, Stefanek W. Autoaugmentation gastrocystoplasty: early clinical results. Br J Urol 1994; 74: 460–4.
99. González R, Buson H, Churphena R, Reinberg Y. Seromuscular colocystoplasty lined with urothelium: experience with 16 patients. Urology 1995; 45: 124–9.
100. Nguyen DH, Mitchell ME, Horowitz M et al. Demucosalized augmentation gastrocystoplasty with bladder autoaugmentation in pediatric patients. J Urol 1996; 156: 206–9.
101. Dayanç M, Kilciler M, Tan Ö et al. A new approach to bladder augmentation in children: seromuscular enterocystoplasty. Br J Urol 1999; 84: 103–7.
102. Jednak R, Schimke CM, Barroso U Jr et al. Further experience with seromuscular colocystoplasty lined with urothelium. J Urol 2000; 164: 2045–9.
103. Lima SVC, Araújo LAP, Vilar FO et al. Nonsecretory sigmoid cystoplasty: experimental and clinical results. J Urol 1995; 153: 1651–4.
104. Lima SVC, Araújo LAP, Montoro M et al. The use of demucosalized bowel to augment small contracted bladders. Br J Urol 1998; 82: 436–9.
105. de Badiola F, Ruiz E, Puigdevall J et al. Sigmoid cystoplasty with argon beam without mucosa. J Urol 2001; 165: 2253–5.
106. Vates TS, Smith C, Gonzalez R. Importance of early bladder distension for the success of the seromuscular colocystoplasty lined with urothelium. Pediatrics 1997; 100: 564.
107. Diokno AC, Taub M. Ephedrine in treatment of urinary incontinence. Urology 1975; 5: 624–5.
108. Raezer DM, Benson GS, Wein AJ, Duckett JW Jr. The functional approach to the management of the pediatric neuropathic bladder: a clinical study. J Urol 1977; 117: 649–54.
109. Decter RM. Pharmacologic management of the neurogenic bladder. Probl Urol 1994; 8: 373–88.
110. Vorstman B, Lockhart JL, Kaufman MR, Politano V. Polytetrafluoroethylene injection for urinary incontinence in children. J Urol 1985; 133: 248–50.
111. Wan J, McGuire EJ, Bloom DA, Ritchey ML. The treatment of urinary incontinence in children using glutaraldehyde cross-linked collagen. J Urol 1992; 148: 127–30.
112. Capozza N, Caione P, De Gennaro M et al. Endoscopic treatment of vesico-ureteric reflux and urinary incontinence: technical problems in the paediatric patient. Br J Urol 1995; 75: 538–42.
113. Leonard MP, Decter A, Mix LW et al. Treatment of urinary incontinence in children by endoscopically directed bladder neck injection of collagen. J Urol 1996; 156: 637–41.
114. Bombalski MD, Bloom DA, McGuire EJ et al. Glutaraldehyde cross-linked collagen in the treatment of urinary incontinence in children. J Urol 1996; 155: 699–702.
115. Pérez LM, Smith EA, Parrott TS et al. Submucosal bladder neck injection of bovine dermal collagen for stress urinary incontinence in the pediatric population. J Urol, Part 2, 1996; 156: 633–363.
116. Sundaram CP, Reinberg Y, Aliabadi HA. Failure to obtain durable results with collagen implantation in children with urinary incontinence. J Urol 1997; 157: 2306–7.
117. Silveri M, Capitanucci ML, Mosiello G et al. Endoscopic treatment for urinary incontinence in children with a congenital neuropathic bladder. Br J Urol 1998; 82: 694–7.
118. Kassouf W, Capolicchio G, Berardinucci G, Corcos J. Collagen injection for treatment of urinary incontinence in children. J Urol 2001; 165: 1666–8.
119. Caione P, Capozza N. Endoscopic treatment of urinary incontinence in pediatric patients: 2-year experience with dextranomer/hyaluronic acid copolymer. J Urol, Part 2, 2002; 168: 1868–71.
120. Lottmann HB, Margaryan M, Bernuy M et al. The effect of endoscopic injections of dextranomer based implants on continence and bladder capacity: a prospective study of 31 patients. J Urol 2002; 168: 1863–7.
121. Godbole P, Bryant R, MacKinnon AE et al. Endourethral injection of bulking agents for urinary incontinence in children. BJU Int 2003; 91: 536–9.
122. Kim YH, Kattan MW, Boone TB. Correlation of urodynamic results and urethral coaptation with success after transurethral collagen injection. Urology 1997; 50: 941–8.
123. Woodside JR, Borden TA. Suprapubic endoscopic vesical neck suspension for the management of urinary incontinence in myelodysplastic girls. J Urol 1986; 135: 97–9.
124. Raz S, Ehrlich RM, Zeidman EJ et al. Surgical treatment of the incontinent female patient with myelomeningocele. J Urol 1988; 139: 524–7.
125. Gearhart JP, Jeffs RD. Suprapubic bladder neck suspension for the management of urinary incontinence in the myelodysplastic girl. J Urol 1988; 140: 1296–8.
126. Freedman ER, Singh G, Donnell SC et al. Combined bladder neck suspension and augmentation cystoplasty for neuropathic incontinence in female patients. Br J Urol 1994; 73: 621–4.
127. McGuire EJ, Wang C-C, Usitalo H, Savastano J. Modified pubovaginal sling in girls with myelodysplasia. J Urol 1986; 135: 94–6.
128. Raz S, McGuire EJ, Ehrlich RM et al. Fascial sling to correct male neurogenic sphincter incompetence: the McGuire/Raz approach. J Urol 1988; 139: 528–31.
129. Bauer SB, Peters CA, Colodny AH et al. The use of rectus fascia to manage urinary incontinence. J Urol 1989; 142: 516–9.

130. Elder JS. Periurethral and puboprostatic sling repair for incontinence in patients with myelodysplasia. J Urol 1990; 144: 434–7.
131. Decter RM. Use of the fascial sling for neurogenic incontinence: lessons learned. J Urol 1993; 150: 683–6.
132. Gormley EA, Bloom DA, McGuire EJ, Ritchey ML. Pubovaginal slings for the management of urinary incontinence in female adolescents. J Urol 1994; 152: 822–5.
133. Kakizaki H, Shibata T, Shinno Y et al. Fascial sling for the management of urinary incontinence due to spincteric incompetence. J Urol 1995; 153: 648–9.
134. Pérez LM, Smith EA, Broecker BH et al. Outcome of sling cystourethropexy in the pediatric population: a critical review. J Urol 1996; 156: 642–6.
135. Dik P, van Gool JG, De Jong TPVM. Urinary continence and erectile function after bladder neck sling suspension in male patients with spinal dysraphism. BJU Int 1999; 83: 971–5.
136. Austin PF, Westney OL, Leng WW et al. Advantages of rectus fascial slings for urinary incontinence in children with neuropathic bladders. J Urol, Part 2, 2001; 165: 2369–72.
137. Herschorn S, Radomski SB. Fascial slings and bladder neck tapering in the treatment of male neurogenic incontinence. J Urol 1992; 147: 1073–5.
138. Ghoniem GM. Bladder neck wrap: a modified fascial sling in treatment of incontinence in myelomeningocele patients. Eur Urol 1994; 25: 340–2.
139. Walker RD, Flack CE, Hawkins-Lee B et al. Rectus fascial wrap: early results of a modification of the rectus fascial sling. J Urol 1995; 154: 771–4.
140. Kurzrock EA, Lowe P, Hardy BE. Bladder wall pedicle wraparound sling for neurogenic urinary incontinence in children. J Urol 1996; 155: 305–8.
141. Barthold JS, Rodriguez E, Freedman AL et al. Results of the rectus fascial sling and wrap procedures for the treatment of neurogenic sphincteric incontinence. J Urol 1999; 161: 272–4.
142. Walker RD, Erhard M, Starling J. Long-term evaluation of rectus fascial wrap in patients with spina bifida. J Urol 2000; 164: 485–6.
143. Mingin GC, Youngren K, Stock JA, Hanna MK. The rectus myofascial wrap in the management of urethral sphincter incompetence. BJU Int 2002; 90: 550–3.
144. Kropp KA, Angwafo FF. Urethral lengthening and reimplantation for neurogenic incontinence in children. J Urol 1986; 135: 533–6.
145. Mollard P, Mouriquand P, Joubert P. Urethral lengthening for neurogenic urinary incontinence (Kropp's procedure): results of 16 cases. J Urol 1990; 143: 95–7.
146. Snodgrass W. A simplified Kropp procedure for incontinence. J Urol 158: 1049–52.
147. Pippi Salle JL, de Fraga JCS, Amarante A et al. Urethral lengthening with anterior bladder wall flap for urinary incontinence: a new approach. J Urol 1994; 152: 803–6.
148. Pippi Salle JL, McLorie GA, Bagli DJ, Khoury AE. Urethral lengthening with anterior bladder wall flap (Pippi Salle procedure): modifications and extended indications of the technique. J Urol 1997; 158: 585–90.
149. Pippi Salle JL, McLorie GA, Bagli DJ, Khoury AE. Modifications of and extended indications for the Pippi Salle procedure. World J Urol 1999; 16: 279–84.
150. Belman AB, Kaplan GW. Experience with the Kropp anti-incontinence procedure. J Urol 1989; 141: 1160–2.
151. Nill TG, Peller PA, Kropp KA. Management of urinary incontinence by bladder tube urethral lengthening and submucosal reimplantation. J Urol 1990; 144: 559–63.
152. Waters PR, Chehade NC, Kropp KA. Urethral lengthening and reimplantation: incidence and management of catheterization problems. J Urol 1997; 158: 1053–6.
153. Koyle MA. The Kropp bladder neck reconstruction and its variations in the incontinent patient with neurogenic bladder. Pediatrics 1996; 98: 602.
154. Mouriquand PD, Sheard R, Phillips N et al. The Kropp-onlay procedure (Pippi Salle procedure): a simplification of the technique of urethral lengthening. Preliminary results in eight patients. Br J Urol 1995; 75: 656–62.
155. Hayes MC, Bulusu A, Terry T et al. The Pippi Salle urethral lengthening procedure; experience and outcome from three United Kingdom centres. BJU Int 1999; 84: 701–5.
156. Rink RC, Adams MC, Keating MA. The flip-flap technique to lengthen the urethra (Salle procedure) for treatment of neurogenic urinary incontinence. J Urol 1994; 152: 799–802.
157. Canales BK, Fung LCT, Elliott SP. Miniature intravesical urethral lengthening procedure for treatment of pediatric neurogenic urinary incontinence. J Urol 2006; 176: 2663–7.
158. Scott FB, Bradley WE, Timm GW. Treatment of urinary incontinence by an implantable prosthetic urinary sphincter. J Urol 1974; 112: 75–80.
159. Furlow WL, Barrett DM. The artificial urinary sphincter: experience with the AS 800 pump-control assembly for single-stage primary deactivation and activation – a preliminary report. Mayo Clin Proc 1985; 60: 255–8.
160. Light JK, Reynolds JC. Impact of the new cuff design on reliability of the AS800 artificial urinary sphincter. J Urol 1992; 147: 609–11.
161. Leo ME, Barrett DM. Success of the narrow-backed cuff design of the AMS800 artificial urinary sphincter: analysis of 144 patients. J Urol 1993; 150: 1412–4.
162. Mitchell ME, Rink RC. Experience with the artificial urinary sphincter in children and young adults. J Pediatr Surg 1983; 18: 700–6.
163. Gonzalez R, Koleilat N, Austin C, Sidi AA. The artificial sphincter AS800 in congenital urinary incontinence. J Urol 1989; 142: 512–5.
164. Bosco PJ, Bauer SB, Colodny AH et al. The long-term results of artificial sphincters in children. J Urol 1991; 146: 396–9.
165. Belloli G, Caampobasso P, Mercurella A. Neuropathic urinary incontinence in pediatric patients: management with artificial sphincter. J Pediatr Surg 1992; 27: 1461–4.
166. González R, Merino FG, Vaughn M. Long term results of the artificial urinary sphincter in male patients with neurogenic bladder. J Urol 1995; 154: 769–70.
167. Levesque PE, Bauer SB, Atala A et al. Ten-year experience with the artificial urinary sphincter in children. J Urol 1996; 156: 625–8.
168. Kryger JV, Barthold JS, Fleming P, González R. The outcome of artificial urinary sphincter placement after a mean 15-year follow-up in a paediatric population. BJU Int 1999; 83: 1026–31.
169. Hafez AT, McLorie G, Bägli D, Khoury A. A single-centre long-term outcome analysis of artificial urinary sphincter placement in children. BJU Int 2002; 89: 82–5.
170. Toh K, Diokno AC. Management of intrinsic sphincter deficiency in adolescent females with normal bladder emptying function. J Urol 2002; 168: 1150–3.
171. Diokno AC, Sonda LP. Compatibility of genitourinary prostheses and intermittent self-catheterization. J Urol 1981; 125: 659–60.
172. Barrett DM, Furlow WL. Incontinence, intermittent selfcatheterization and the artificial genitourinary sphincter. J Urol 1984; 132: 268–9.
173. de Badiola FIP, Castro-Diaz D, Hart-Austin C, Gonzalez R. Influence of preoperative bladder capacity and compliance on the outcome of artificial sphincter implantation in patients with neurogenic sphincter incompetence. J Urol 1992; 148: 1493–5.
174. Kronner KM, Rink RC, Simmons G et al. Artificial urinary sphincter in the treatment of urinary incontinence: preoperative urodynamics do not predict the need for future bladder augmentation. J Urol 1998; 160: 1093–5.

175. Strawbridge LR, Kramer SA, Castillo OA, Barrett DM. Augmentation cystoplasty and the artificial genitourinary sphincter. J Urol 1989; 142: 297–301.
176. Gonzalez R, Nguyen DH, Koleilat N, Sidi AA. Compatibility of enterocystoplasty and the artificial urinary sphincter. J Urol 1989; 142: 502–4.
177. Bauer SB, Reda EF, Colodny AH, Retik AB. Detrusor instability: a delayed complication in association with the artificial sphincter. J Urol 1986; 135: 1212–5.
178. Murray KHA, Nurse DE, Mundy AR. Detrusor behavior following implantation of the Brantley Scott artificial urinary sphincter for neuropathic incontinence. Br J Urol 1988; 61: 122–8.
179. Simeoni J, Guys JM, Mollard P et al. Artificial urinary sphincter implantation for neurogenic bladder: a multi-institutional study in 107 children. Br J Urol 1996; 78: 287–93.
180. Castera R, Podesta ML, Ruarte A et al. 10-year experience with artificial urinary sphincter in children and adolescents. J Urol 2001; 165: 2373–6.
181. Spies PE, Capolicchio JP, Kiruluta G et al. Is an artificial sphincter the best choice for incontinent boys with spina bifida? Review of our long term experience with the AS-800 artificial sphincter. Can J Urol 2002; 9: 1486–91.
182. Jayanthi VR, Churchill BM, McLorie GA et al. Concomitant bladder neck closure and Mitrofanoff diversion for the management of intractable urinary incontinence. J Urol 1995; 154: 886–8.
183. Hensle TW, Kirsch AJ, Kennedy WA II et al. Bladder neck closure in association with continent urinary diversion. J Urol 1995; 154: 883–5.
184. Khoury AE, Agarwal SK, Bägli D et al. Concomitant modified bladder neck closure and Mitrofanoff urinary diversion. J Urol 1999; 162: 1746–8.
185. Hoebeke P, De Kuyper P, Goeminne H et al. Bladder neck closure for treating pediatric incontinence. Eur Urol 2000; 38: 453–6.
186. Nguyen HT, Baskin LS. The outcome of bladder neck closure in children with severe urinary incontinence. J Urol 2003; 169: 1114–6.
187. Bergman J, Lerman SE, Kristo B et al. Outcomes of bladder neck closure for intractable urinary incontinence in patients with neurogenic bladders. J Pediatr Urol 2006; 2: 528–33.

70

Treatment alternatives for different types of neurogenic bladder dysfunction in adults: an overview

Erik Schick and Jacques Corcos

Introduction

Vesicourethral dysfunction secondary to degenerative processes, traumas, or neoplasias of the central or peripheral nervous system will most certainly have a deleterious effect on the patient's quality of life.

For centuries, the prognosis of these pathologies on patient survival was bad. We know from the Edwin Smith papyrus that as far back as 1600 BC the ancient Egyptians were aware of the relationship between the nervous system and urinary bladder function.[1] They considered spinal cord trauma as a 'disease not to treat'.[2]

Statistics on spinal cord trauma are available since World War I. The mortality rate was extremely high in those days – more than 90% – mainly due to urinary complications such as urosepsis and renal insufficiency. Dramatic improvements in prognosis came during World War II when Sir Ludwig Guttmann, in England, established specialized units to take care of these patients, and introduced the method of intermittent catheterization.[3] During the 1970s the use of urodynamics became more widespread, allowing a better understanding of the physiology and pathophysiology of the lower urinary tract. Translation of these new notions has significantly improved the prognosis of these patients.

The main goals in treating patients with neurogenic bladder dysfunction are threefold:

1. to preserve upper urinary tract integrity
2. to insure adequate continence
3. to minimize stone formation and urinary infection.

All these therapeutic goals aim to improve the patient's quality of life and prolong life expectancy.

In the ideal situation, these objectives should be attainable without the necessity of having to rely on a foreign body (i.e. a catheter) permanently installed in the urinary tract.

Therapeutic classification of vesicourethral dysfunction

Several classifications of vesicourethral dysfunction have been proposed in the literature. The latest, and probably the most original, is developed elsewhere in this book by A Matthiasson (see Chapter 45). Based mainly on Krane and Siroky's work, we have elaborated a simple and practical classification that is derived from observations obtained from urodynamic studies, and which focuses on therapeutic goals.[4]

The bladder, as a reservoir, can exhibit only three types of dysfunction:

1. underactivity or noncontractility
2. overactivity (including those with decreased contractility)
3. small capacity bladder with or without decreased compliance.

The urethra, the outlet, can be obstructive owing to an anatomic cause (e.g. stenosis, or benign prostatic hyperplasia), functional alterations (e.g. vesicosphincteric dyssynergia), or it can be hypotonic (e.g. incontinence). In clinical practice, most often, both structures function abnormally to varying degrees (Table 70.1).

Urodynamics investigation is the cornerstone of any treatment strategy in neurogenic bladder dysfunction. Nosseir et al[5] reported on a retrospective study of 80 spinal cord injured patients in whom treatment modifications were based on the urodynamic findings. Except in 3

Table 70.1 *Urodynamic classification of neurogenic bladder dysfunction*

Bladder function	Urethral function
Normal	Hypotonic
Normal	Hypertonic
Overactive[a,b]	Normal
Overactive[a,b]	Hypotonic
Underactive or noncontractile[a]	Normal
Underactive or noncontractile[a]	Hypotonic

[a] With or without decreased compliance; [b] with or without impaired contractility.

patients (3.75%), the treatment strategy had to be modified in all the other patients during the follow-up (mean: 67.3 months; range 60–103 months). Urodynamics allows us to separately evaluate the reservoir function and outlet function, as well as the coordination of these structures during micturition. A well-conducted urodynamics study should answer the questions summarized in Table 70.2.

In any kind of neurologic pathology associated with vesicourethral dysfunction, even complex situations can be logically analyzed by urodynamic evaluation, which estimates the component of the lower urinary tract that is dysfunctional and to what extent. This allows us to elaborate a logical therapeutic plan that is adapted or personalized to each patient's condition (see Chapters 68 and 69).

Altered reservoir function

As mentioned above, neurologic pathology can modify bladder function with three possible end results.

The underactive or noncontractile bladder

In this situation, the bladder cannot empty itself, or can do so only partially, leaving a high postvoid residual volume behind. Complete bladder emptying can be promoted by the following techniques.

Clean intermittent catheterization

Whenever the clinical situation permits, clean intermittent catheterization is one of the major approaches taken to ensure adequate bladder emptying. The credit goes to Lapides, who demonstrated that self-catheterization does not need to be sterile and is safe and harmless if the catheter is simply clean.[6–8] His observations, which revolutionized the management of patient bladder evacuation problems, are based on the premise that one of the mechanisms the bladder has to resist bacterial colonization is its

Table 70.2 *Expected answers from a urodynamic study*

	Questions to be answered
Bladder behavior	Overactive, underactive, noncontractile
	Wall compliance
	Volume at first desire to void (B1)
	Cystometric capacity
	Postvoid residual volume
	High- or low-pressure system
	Bladder volume at limit of high pressure
Urethral behavior	Hypertonic, hypotonic (UPP* at rest)
	'Unstable' (during the filling phase)
	Pressure transmission from the abdominal cavity (females)
Micturition	Synergic, dyssynergic
	Infravesical obstruction
	Detrusor contractility

* UPP, urethral pressure profile.

periodic and complete emptying. At the present time this is the safest bladder management method for spinal cord injured patients with underactive or noncontractile bladder in terms of urologic complications.[9]

Transurethral electrical stimulation of the detrusor

Katona et al,[10] who stimulated the bladder wall with a monopolar electrode placed in the bladder *per urethram,* proposed direct stimulation of the detrusor muscle itself. Continuous 60–100 mA current stimulates the mechanoreceptors of the bladder, provoking reflex detrusor contraction.[11] The sacral reflex arc must be intact and the patient must feel the desire to void during the sessions to successfully apply this technique. Daily stimulation sessions of 60–90 min for up to 80 days are necessary. This approach differs significantly from neurostimulation of the sacral roots, since the aim here is to rehabilitate the bladder to regain voluntary control of micturition. The 75% success rate claimed by the original investigators has been confirmed by others[12–15] (see Chapters 55 and 65).

Myoplasty of the detrusor

To decrease a large, decompensated bladder, Klarskov et al[16] suggested a partial cystectomy. It has been postulated that this will not only decrease bladder volume but also might increase the contractile efficiency of the detrusor. Hanna,[17] on the other hand, proposed 'remodeling' of the bladder, whereby a part of the bladder wall, stripped of its mucosa, covers the remaining bladder wall, much like a double-breast closure of the abdominal cavity. This would double the thickness of the detrusor, increasing its overall contractility. He operated on 11 patients (9 adults and 2 children): 10 of them have been improved.

Bladder wall strengthening by striated muscle flap

More recently, the group of Tanagho[18] demonstrated in the dog that use of the skeletal muscle, which can be stimulated, may serve to facilitate bladder emptying. Stenzl et al[19] proposed detrusor myoplasty in humans, which consists of transposing a part of the latissimus dorsi muscle around the bladder in such a way that 75% of the bladder wall will be covered by this striated muscle. This free neuromuscular flap is anastomosed to the lowest branches of the intercostal nerve and the deep epigastric vessels. After a mean follow-up of 44 months (range 18–74 months), of the 20 patients operated on, 14 were able to void spontaneously with less then 100 ml of postvoid residual urine 4 months following the operation. Additional bladder neck incision was necessary in 4 and only 2 (10%) remained on clean intermittent catheterization. No deterioration of the upper tract was observed.[20]

Tissue engineering techniques

To realize a complete bladder substitution, Stenzl and Ninkovic[21] suggested combining the above mentioned neurovascular muscle transfer with cultivated and expanded autologous urothelial cells which could be conveyed onto the muscle. No clinical data are available using this technique at the present time.

The use of acellular matrix as a bladder augmentation material is a subject of intensive experimental work,[22–30] but no clinical data are available using these different techniques either. Graft contracture and fibroproliferative reaction seem to be the major problems. Nevertheless, all these innovative approaches are promising for the future (see Chapter 60).

Pharmacologic therapy

Because motor innervation of the detrusor is mainly cholinergic, it seems logical to use this type of medication to enhance bladder emptying. Despite the theoretic advantages of this approach, very little success has been achieved in clinical practice. Awad et al[31] pointed out the importance of the agent's route of administration. They succeeded in obtaining spontaneous voiding and decreasing postvoid residual by injecting the medication subcutaneously. Comparable results were not obtained with oral administration. However, it should be noted that side-effects increased with prolonged subcutaneous treatment.

Decreasing urethral resistance

Obviously, decreasing or eliminating urethral resistance should improve bladder emptying. This will be discussed in more detail below.

Summary

The underactive or noncontractile bladder is best managed at the present time, whenever possible, by clean intermittent catheterization. Electrostimulation becomes an increasingly valuable alternative, but is still expensive. Direct electrical stimulation of the bladder wall should be attempted when the sacral reflex arc is preserved. The time-consuming nature of this approach and the relatively limited indications might prevent its widespread use, in spite of the favorable results reported in the literature. Striated muscle flap is still in its experimental phase and reserved for highly specialized centers within defined protocol

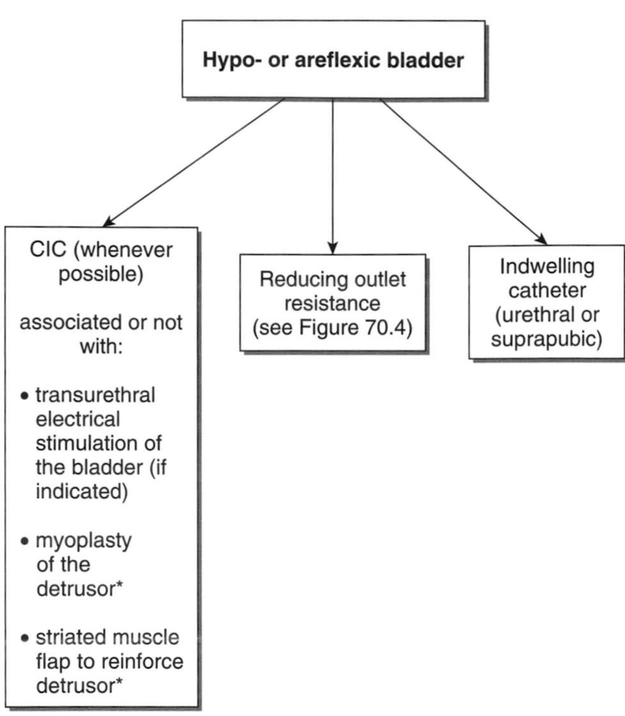

Figure 70.1
Algorithm for the treatment of underactive or noncontractile bladder. CIC, clean intermittent catheterization (see also Chapters 46 and 47).

conditions. Long-term results in a substantial number of patients are not yet available. Tissue engineering techniques are promising, but still in the research laboratory. Pharmacologic manipulation in this group of patients has limited success and, at the present, has no real indication.

The overactive bladder

The pathophysiologic consequences of bladder overactivity are threefold:

1. urinary incontinence can be provoked when the amplitude of bladder contractions exceeds urethral closure pressure
2. a low-pressure system can become a high-pressure system if the uninhibited contractions are frequent, with an amplitude over 40 cmH_2O, and/or bladder compliance decreases as a result of progressive bladder wall fibrosis
3. vesicoureteral reflux can develop as a result of overactivity.

Overactivity can be controlled by pharmacologic, electrical, and/or surgical means.

Pharmacological manipulation

Oral administration In the last decade, a large number of pharmacologic substances have been developed to control bladder overactivity. All of these substances have antimuscarinic properties, interfering with M_3 type receptors. Their overall efficacy in neurogenic overactivity is about 50%.[32] M_3-selective antimuscarinic agents have not significantly improved the efficacy, but have reduced the major side-effect of excessively dry mouth.[33] No published randomized clinical trials have been performed on the newly developed anticholinergics – Ditropan XL (oxybutynin chloride™, (Ditropan, Ditropan XL)), tolterodine™ (Detrol, Detrol LA), Darifenacine bromhydrate™ (Enablex), etc. – in the neurogenic bladder patient population. However, 15–30 mg daily doses of Ditropan XL have been found to be very effective in the overactive bladder in clinical practice.[34,35] Tropsium chloride™ (Trosec), a quaternary ammonium compound recently introduced in the United States, with high affinity to M_1, M_2, and M_3 muscarinic receptors, showed significant improvements in overactive neurogenic bladder patients. It is significantly better tolerated than immediate-release oxybutynin.[36] A recent meta-analysis of antimuscarinics on health-related quality of life did not show significant differences among antimuscarinic agents, but provided evidence that these agents improve health-related quality of life in patients with overactive bladders.[37] When the usual dosage of antimuscarinics failed, doubling the recommended doses could be efficacious[38] (see also Chapter 48).

Transcutaneous administration James and Iacovon,[39] in a pilot study, used nitroglycerin dermal patches to control bladder overactivity. They observed a reduction in diurnal and nocturnal frequency as well as a decrease in incontinence episodes per 24 hours. More recently, Davila et al[40] reported the results of a multicenter trial with transcutaneous oxybutynin. Compared with oral administration, the transdermal route had equal efficacy and a significantly improved side-effect profile in adults with urge urinary incontinence. This subject is examined in more detail in Chapter 50.

Intravesical treatment Bladder overactivity involves an intact sacral reflex arc. Intravesically administered substances can act on the efferent or on the afferent branches of this reflex arc.

Anticholinergics block the efferent part of the reflex. Brendler et al[41] used 5 mg of oxybutynin chloride in 20–30 ml of water in 10 incontinent patients. All of them became continent. Madersbacher and Jilg[42] studied oxybutynin in 13 overactive bladder patients: out of 10 of these who presented incontinence between clean intermittent catheterizations, 9 became continent. Even if the oxybutynin serum level was higher after intravesical than afteroral administration, the side-effects of anticholinergics were totally absent in the intravesical group. In patients with enterocystoplasty, the side-effects were identical to the oral group. This observation led Massad et al[43] to conclude that a hepatic metabolite of oxybutynin is probably responsible for the side-effects. In a study of 12 patients with overactive bladder, Di Stasi et al[44] found that oral oxybutynin had no effect. When administered intravesically, passive diffusion of oxybutynin significantly reduced urinary leakage, but with electromotive diffusion it caused significantly greater postvoid residual urine volume and fewer episodes of urinary leakage, together with measurable changes in urodynamic parameters: decreased duration and amplitude of uninhibited contractions as well as increased bladder wall compliance.

Multisite botulinum A toxin injection in the bladder (up to a total of 300 units) has been proposed to control overactivity. Schurch et al[45] reported their experience in 31 spinal cord injury patients. Bladder capacity and mean reflex volume increased significantly, mean maximum voiding pressure decreased, and postvoid residual volume rose. The duration of bladder paresis was at least 9 months, when repeated injections were required (see also Chapter 49).

Among substances interfering with the afferent branch of the reflex arc, one should mention capsaicin, resiniferatoxin, and Marcain (bupivacaine). Capsaicin and resiniferatoxin, both vanilloids, block neurotransmission via small demyelinized C fibers, which come into function only after spinal disruption when myelinized Aδ fibers cannot transmit information to the central nervous system. In idiopathic detrusor overactivity and in suprapontine pathology, where the C-fiber-mediated reflex does not emerge, these substances seem not to be effective.[46] A controlled trial by de Sèze et al[47] showed that capsaicin was significantly more effective than placebo for continence, frequency, urgency, and patient satisfaction. In a meta-analysis by this same group,[48] 84% of patients (97 out of 115) with detrusor overactivity presented some improvement in their symptoms when treated with intravesical capsaicin. Worldwide experience suggests that 60–100% of patients might respond favorably to this kind of therapy by decreasing or eliminating incontinence episodes between clean intermittent catheterizations for 1–9 months without systemic toxicity.[35]

At 1000-fold more potent than capsicin, resiniferatoxin is mainly interesting for the reduced local reaction that it provokes in the bladder.[49] Resiniferatoxin trials were summarized by De Ridder and Baert.[50] The results on vanilloids are updated in Chapter 49.

Local anesthetics block axonal conduction in unmyelinated nerve fibers. The clinical response is of very short duration, and no protocol has been proposed using this approach to control detrusor overactivity. An extensive review on the intravesical administration of drugs in patients with bladder overactivity has been published by Ekström.[51]

Intrathecal administration According to the experience of Steers et al,[52] intrathecal infusion of baclofen, a γ-aminobutyric acid (GABA) agonist, proved to be successful in patients with severe spasticity and bladder overactivity. In all of them, overactivity disappeared, bladder capacity increased by 72%, and bladder compliance improved in 16%. Kums and Delhaas[53] made similar observations in 9 quadriplegics. In the last decade, however, no report on this approach to treat detrusor overactivity has been found in the literature (see Chapter 48).

Neurostimulation

Neurostimulation is the term used when electrical stimulation is applied directly to a nerve fiber to achieve a desired function (sphincter contraction or detrusor relaxation). Neuromodulation is the term used when electrical stimulation is applied to indirectly modify sensory and/or motor functions of the lower urinary tract.

Neurostimulation is applied mainly in patients with complete SCI and preserved detrusor function. (It excludes patients with noncontractile bladder.) Introduced by Tanagho and Schmidt[54] and Brindley et al,[55] this technique is most often associated with bilateral sacral posterior rhizotomy to reduce overactivity and autonomic dysreflexia. The success rate is high for bladder function, but less for rectal function.[56–58] The problem of electrical stimulation of the lower urinary tract is extensively covered in Chapters 52, 53, 54, 55, and 61.

Surgery

Two main surgical procedures have been proposed in the literature to decrease detrusor overactivity and/or to manage low-compliant bladders: partial detrusorectomy (autoaugmentation) and enterocystoplasty. The ultimate goal with each procedure is to increase reservoir capacity and reduce the amplitude of detrusor contractions.

Enterocystoplasty is contemplated in patients with bladder capacity less than 300 ml under anesthesia. Most commonly, a detubularized segment of the distal ileum is used for this purpose, but a detubularized colic segment or part of the gastric wall can also be used.

Excellent long-term results were reported in about 75% of patients, with improvement in another 20%. The most frequent complications were stone formation in the reservoir (20%) and reoperation (15%) to reaugment the bladder.[59]

The main advantages of autoaugmentation over enterocystoplasty are its lower morbidity (the peritoneal cavity is not opened, the gastrointestinal tract is not violated) and, in case of failure, further intestinal substitution is not precluded. We reserve partial detrusorectomy for patients with bladder capacity over 300 ml under general anesthesia.

Detrusor myomectomy and enterocystoplasty offer comparable success or improvement[60] (see also Chapter 56).

Summary

The first step in the management of the overactive bladder should be a pharmacologic one. The oral route of administration is used most frequently. Among transdermal anticholinergic patches, oxybutynin is the only one which underwent clinical trials. It showed equal efficacy and a better side-effect profile than the traditional oral route. Intravesical capsaicin will probably be replaced by the better-tolerated resiniferatoxin, but clinical trials have been recently suspended by the sponsoring pharmaceutic companies.[46] Botulinum A toxin injections in the detrusor are promising, but must be repeated, probably on an annual basis or so. No long-term results exist. Intrathecal baclofen is not indicated at present for the treatment of overactive bladder, but one should remember that if a baclofen infusion pump is installed for other reasons (e.g. uncontrollable skeletal muscle spasticity), the patient might have some benefit from the urologic point of view as well. Neurostimulation constitutes the less-invasive surgical alternative. The still very expensive nature of this treatment modality limits its widespread use. More invasive surgical procedures include bladder autoaugmentation or enterocystoplasty, with equally good long-term results and an acceptable complication rate (Figure 70.2).

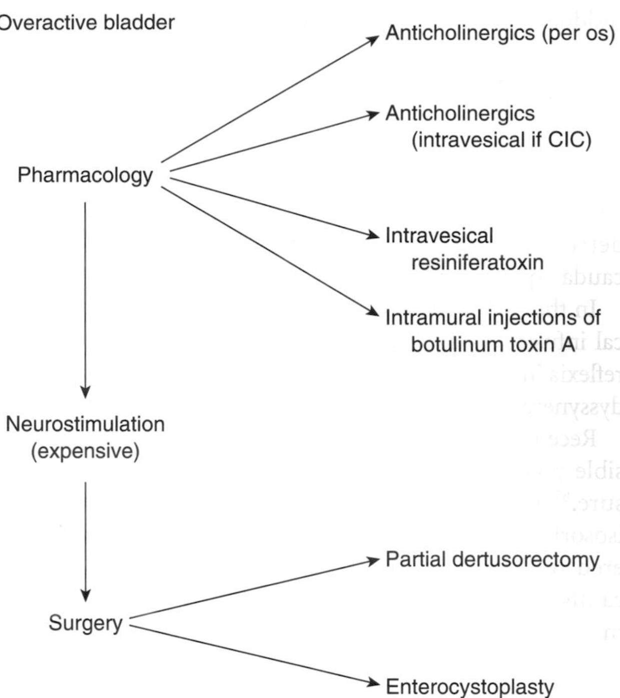

Figure 70.2
Algorithm for the treatment of overactive bladder. CIC, clean intermittent catheterization.

Altered outlet function

Infravesical obstruction

From the functional point of view, distinction should be made between occlusion and obstruction. Occlusion is a static phenomenon, as it can be observed: e.g., during a cystoscopic examination. Viewing the lateral lobes of the prostate from the verumontanum, one is looking at a static image. It is impossible to extrapolate from this observation how the proximal urethra will relax in response to detrusor contraction and to what degree urethral funneling will allow the normal passage of urine. In contrast, obstruction is a dynamic phenomenon which, in hydrodynamics, means high pressure associated with decreased flow. This can only be objectively demonstrated by urodynamics. Infravesical urethral obstruction can be anatomic (e.g. urethral stenosis or BPH) or functional (e.g. vesicosphincteric dyssynergia). The specific problem of benign prostatic hypertrophy and neurogenic bladder dysfunction is discussed in more detail elsewhere in this book (see Chapter 73). We will concentrate on functional obstructions.

The pharmacologic approach

From the theoretic point of view, alpha-blocking agents and those that might relax the striated sphincter (together with the pelvic floor) should decrease urethral resistance during micturition. This approach can be beneficial in the neurologically intact patient, but their use in the neurologic patient is less effective. It should be noted, however, that no randomized, double-blind study has demonstrated the role of these substances in the neurologic bladder.

Dykstra and Sidi[61] injected botulinum A toxin locally in the striated sphincter once a week for 3 consecutive weeks in 5 patients with proven vesicourethral dyssynergia. Electromyographic (EMG) activity in the striated sphincter was abolished after the injections, while maximum urethral closure pressure, voiding pressure, and postvoid residual all decreased. Follow-up of these patients was not provided.

Fowler et al[62] also injected botulinum A toxin in the external sphincter of 6 non-neurologic women who exhibited chronic urinary retention. None of the women improved, a failure that might be explained by the fact that these patients were neurologically normal.

Phelan et al[63] reported on the efficacy of botulinum toxin injection in the urethral sphincter of men and women with acontractile bladder. All but 1 of the 21 patients treated voided without catheterization, postvoid residual decreased by 71%, and voiding pressure by 38%. Transient incontinence was sometimes observed.[64] Indications for botulimun A toxin injection in the urethral striated sphincter include at the present time (1) neurogenic detrusor-sphincter dyssynergia (e.g., traumatic spinal cord injury, multiple sclerosis, etc.) and (2) an alternative to self-catheterization in urinary retention (e.g., detrusor underactivity,[65] surgical bladder denervation, cauda equina injuries, etc.).[66]

In the previously quoted study by Steers et al,[52] intrathecal infusion of baclofen not only abolished bladder hyperreflexia in all patients but it also eliminated vesicosphincteric dyssynergia in 40% of them.

Recently a new substance, nitric oxide, emerged as a possible pharmacologic agent that may lower urethral pressure.[67] It has been demonstrated in healthy males that isosorbide dinitrate, a nitric oxide donor, effectively lowered resting urethral pressure.[68] It also reduced significantly bladder outlet obstruction in 12 spinal cord injured men with detrusor-sphincter dyssynergia.[69]

Reversible surgical procedures

Intraurethral stents Growing experience suggests that intraurethral stents are effective in eliminating vesicosphincteric dyssynergia. According to the North American experience, 13% of the prostheses were withdrawn during the 24-month observation period.[70] The result was 11% in a European study, with a global complication rate of 38%.[71] An excellent in-depth review of the subject, including sphincterotomy and a comparison between the two treatment modalities, was presented by Rivas and Chancellor.[72]

Clinical experience with a thermo-expandable stent (Memokath®) was disappointing, mainly because of the number of complications necessitating its removal, and also because of the relatively limited 'lifetime' of the stent (21 months).[73] Long-term follow-up (12 years) with the mesh wallstent (Urolume®) suggests that it can be an alternative to sphincterotomy. The main complication with this device is bladder neck dyssynergia, which can be successfully managed by bladder neck incision.[74]

Transurethral balloon dilatation Chancellor et al[75] proposed hydraulic dilatation of the striated urethral sphincter. Their study, of 17 male patients with vesicourethral dyssynergia, demonstrated interesting results 1 year later: micturition pressure decreased significantly (83 ± 35 cmH_2O vs 37 ± 15 cmH_2O), as well as postvoid residual (163 ± 162 vs 68 ± 59 cmH_2O). One year postoperatively, 82% of the patients voided adequately. Even autonomic dysreflexia, when present, was improved. No long-term follow-up was provided.

Overdistention of the female urethra Overdistention should be very generous to rupture the helicoidal fibers of the urethra. If the bladder neck is competent, stress incontinence should not result from this approach.[76] Transurethral resection of the bladder neck in females should be avoided, as stress incontinence will most likely be its consequence.

Credé's maneuver This maneuver is more efficacious, especially in females, when the pelvic floor muscles are paralyzed. The increased abdominal pressure is dissipated in part by the flaccid pelvic floor, and lesser pressure will be exerted simultaneously on the proximal urethra. Bladder evacuation, however, is never complete with this technique.

Irreversible surgical procedures

Transurethral bladder neck/prostate incision/resection If the patient is able to void during urodynamic testing, distinction can be made between constrictive and compressive obstruction.[77] If the obstruction is constrictive in nature and there is no anatomic stenosis at the level of the anterior urethra, we prefer transurethral incision of the bladder neck, as described a number of years ago by Turner-Warwick.[78] Our incision, however, is not limited strictly to the bladder neck, but goes down to the level of the verumontanum, including the lateral lobes of the prostate as well. We observed less restenosis after incision than after resection of the bladder neck, which is contrary to the experience of others.[76]

Sphincterotomy When fluoroscopy cannot be combined with urodynamics (video-urodynamics), it is not always easy to decide when to perform sphincterotomy alone and when to combine it with bladder neck incision. Gardner et al[79] combined cystography and static urethral pressure measurements: their algorithm is illustrated in Figure 70.3. In our experience, X-ray studies are recommended, but not absolutely mandatory. When pressure–flow assessment demonstrates obstruction and maximum urethral closure pressure (MUCP) is high, transurethral surgery can include sphincterotomy as well. If MUCP is low, sphincterotomy is probably not useful.

Summary

Increased urethral resistance can be weakened by pharmacologic means, which, in the form of oral medication, is less efficacious than in the non-neurologic patient. However, it should be the first-line treatment. In case of failure, transurethral injection of botulinum A toxin can be offered. Nitric oxide donors might prove useful in the near future. Intraurethral stents are effective, but not exempt from causing morbidity and their removal after a prolonged

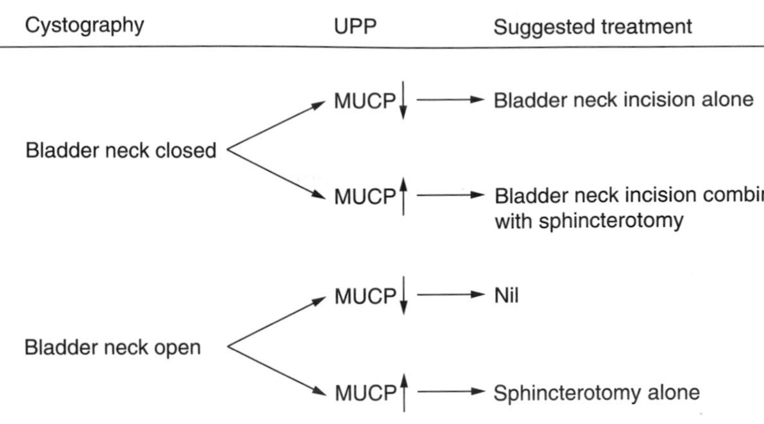

Figure 70.3
Algorithm to decrease urethral resistance. UPP, static urethral pressure profile; MUCP, maximum urethral closure pressure. (Reproduced with permission from Gardner et al[79]).

time period can be quite challenging. Balloon dilatation has never gained wide acceptance, despite the fact that it is easy to perform, relatively inexpensive, produces limited complications, and gives good results. Unfortunately, no long-term results are available with this form of therapy. Overdilation of the female urethra should not result in stress urinary incontinence. Sphincterotomy with or without bladder/prostate incision/resection, although the most invasive alternative, remains the gold standard in the management of the obstructive male urethra (Figure 70.4).

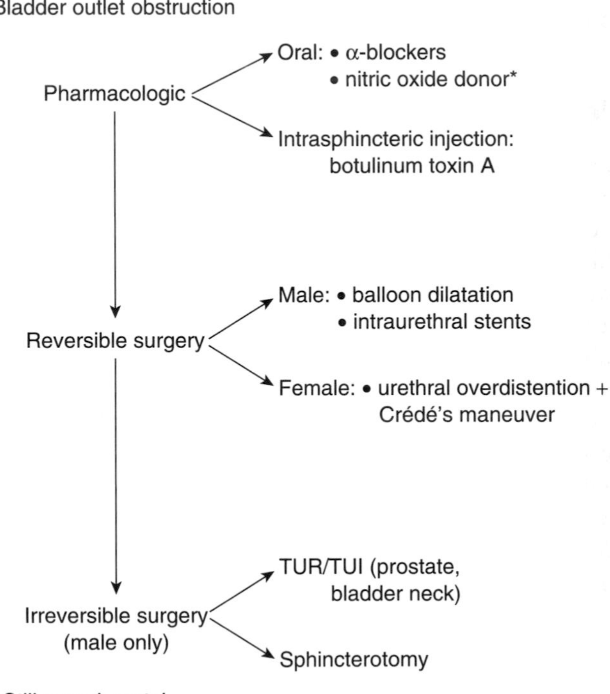

Figure 70.4
Algorithm for the treatment of functional bladder outlet obstruction. TUR, transurethral resection; TUI, transurethral incision.

The hypotonic outlet – incontinence

Urinary incontinence can result from an alteration in reservoir function (overactivity, decreased compliance, small capacity) or a sphincteric failure at the level of the urethra. How to obviate alterations in reservoir function has been discussed previously. In the following sections we will summarize the possibilities of increasing urethral resistance. It should be pointed out that the prerequisite to augmented resistance is a low-pressure bladder reservoir.

Urethropexy

When intrinsic sphincter deficiency and abdominourethral pressure transmission failure are demonstrated in patients with neurogenic bladder, urethropexy can be performed. A detailed description of the multiple techniques proposed in the literature to achieve this is beyond the scope of our chapter. At the moment, Burch urethropexy[80] is the gold standard, as modified by Tanagho.[81] After having been used mainly for the failure of previous urethropexy, and the treatment of stress urinary incontinence without bladder neck hypermobility, sling operations became more popular during the last decade, and indications have been widened. Recent studies comparing the efficacy of Burch colposuspension with suburethral slings suggest that there is probably no significant difference between these procedures as far as the cure of stress urinary incontinence is concerned.[82–86] However, a recent Cochrane Review analyzing different sling operations for urinary incontinence in women concluded that 'reliable evidence on which to judge whether or not suburethral slings are better or worse then other surgical or conservative management is currently unavailable'.[87] Different sling materials have been used, such as autologous fascia, cadaveric fascia, and a variety of artificial materials. Among the commercially available materials, the tension-free vaginal tape (TVT) technique, and more recently the transobturator tape (TOT), have gained much popularity, and have the potential to replace the traditional retropubic approach.[88] The precise indications for TVT or TOT use are not yet clearly defined in the literature.

Suburethral sling operations in neurogenic bladder dysfunction are reported mainly in children with spina bifida,[89,90] however a few cases in adult males with puboprostatic slings have also been described.[91] No long-term results are available for the recently developed devices which provide a fixed urethral compression to insure continence in the male. They may prove to be effective in the long run in mild-to-moderate incontinence.[92]

Periurethral injections

Berg was the first to report on periurethral injection of Teflon paste in the submucosa of the vesical neck to increase urethral resistance.[93] Because microparticles of this paste have been recovered from the lymphatic ganglia, liver, spleen, brain, and kidney, alternative substances have been proposed.[94] Collagen has been the most widely used substance,[95] followed by autologous fat tissue[96] and silicone microspheres (Genisphere®).[97] Pineda and Hadley published an extensive review on the subject.[98] The overall success rate in the reported series in females is between 54% and 83% for collagen and 43% and 86% for fat. In men, the overall success rate is between 36% and 100% for collagen. No series were found with fat injection in males. This treatment modality has not been studied in detail in the neurogenic population. Only a few reports reflect the experience in patients with neurogenic bladder dysfunction.[99]

Artificial urinary sphincter

Artificial urinary sphincter remains the gold standard, especially in males, for the treatment of urinary incontinence secondary to sphincter weakness. Fulford et al[100] reported on 68 patients, all of them followed for more than 10 years: 75% of them had satisfactory continence, but only 13% still retained their original device. This suggests that the lifetime of the artificial sphincter is around 10–15 years, which has been confirmed by Spiess et al,[101] who studied 30 meningomyelocele children in whom an artificial sphincter was implanted at the bladder neck or the bulbar urethra. Survival analysis of the sphincter device revealed a sharp drop after 100 months, with only 8.3% of the sphincters still functioning beyond this point. A recent long-term follow up (13 years) suggest that artificial urinary sphincter implantation remains a durable treatment also for the neurogenic bladder patient population.[102]

Urethra replacement

When the urethra is judged nonsalvageable from the functional point of view, it can be replaced by a muscular tube obtained from the detrusor. Two main surgical techniques have been described. The Young–Dees–Leadbetter technique creates a muscular tube from the trigone. This necessitates reimplantation of both ureters in an extratrigonal site. Long-term results showed perfect continence in 57% of adults and 70% of children.[103] Tanagho[104] proposed creation of the tube from the anterior bladder wall. This leaves the ureterovesical junction undisturbed. Good to excellent results were obtained in 71.5% of the 56 patients operated on (see also Chapter 57).

Supraurethral derivation

When the clinical situation is such that neither the Young–Dees–Leadbetter operation nor the Tanagho technique is feasible, supraurethral derivation might become necessary. This creates an abdominal stoma which can be continent or incontinent. It frequently implies, especially in females, the simultaneous closure of the bladder neck (see Chapter 58).

Summary

Failure of the sphincter mechanism in males is best treated by the implantation of an artificial sphincter, which might even be the first line of treatment. Pharmacologic substances are rarely effective enough in ensuring continence, and periurethral injections do not resist time. In females, suburethral slings are an interesting option, especially if the patient is on a clean intermittent catheterization regimen. In this case, the sling might even be overstretched to some extent to allow continence, bladder emptying being secured by catheterization. When complete replacement of a nonsalvageable urethra is indicated, both posterior (trigonal) and anterior bladder wall tubes give almost the same good results. It should be kept in mind, however, that these are complex surgical procedures with some degree of associated morbidity. Supraurethral derivation (continent or incontinent) should be considered as a last resort treatment (Figure 70.5).

Finally, when treating patients with neurogenic vesicourethral dysfunction, we should keep in mind the recommendation of the National Institute on Disability and Rehabilitation Research Concensus Statement,[105] which concluded: 'A common concern among people with spinal cord injuries is that physicians will alter bladder management programs without regard to lifestyle needs. Social/vocational flexibility may be more important to

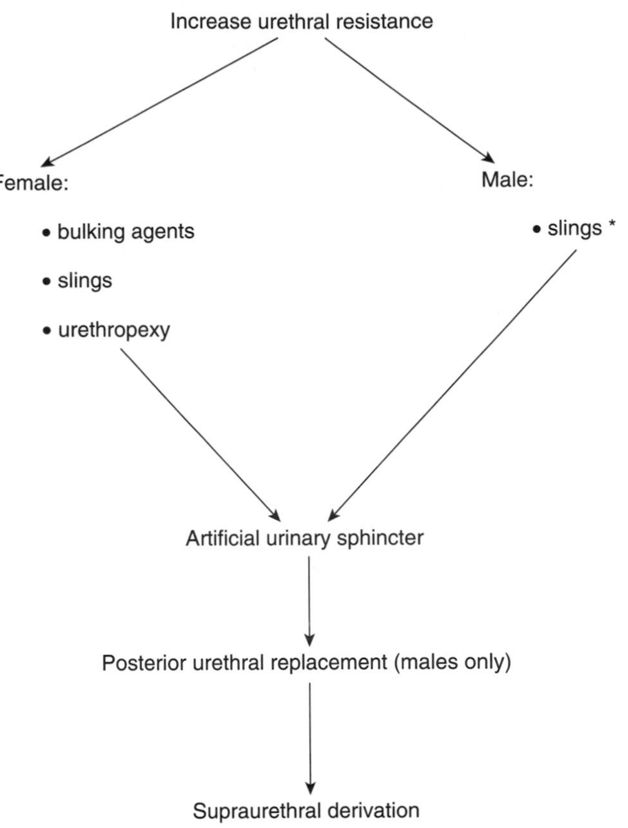

Figure 70.5
Algorithm for the hypotonic outlet – incontinence.

them than state-of-the-art bladder management programs. Future research should focus on obtaining more representative samples and investigate psycho-social-vocational implications as well as additional clinical-medical factors.'

References

1. Küss R, Grégoire W. Histoire illustrée de l'Urologie de l'Antiquité à nos Jours. Paris (France): R Dacosta, 1988.
2. Gutierrez PA, Young RR, Vulpe M. Spinal cord injury – an overview. Urol Clin N Am 1993; 20: 373–82. [Quote]
3. Guttman L, Frankel H. The value of intermittent catheterization in the early management of traumatic paraplegia and tetraplegia. Paraplegia 1966; 4: 63–84.
4. Schick E. Synthèse thérapeurique: traitement des grands types de vessies neurogènes. In: Corcos J, Schick E, eds. Les Vessies neurogènes de l'Adulte. Paris (France): Masson et Cie, 1996: 203–26.
5. Nosseir M, Hinkel A, Pannek J. Clinical usefulness of urodynamic assessment for maintanence of bladder function in patients with spinal cord injury. Neurourol Urodyn 2007; 26: 228–33.
6. Lapides J, Diokno AC, Silber SJ, Lowe BS. Clean, intermittent self-catheterization in the treatment of urinary tract disease. J Urol 1972; 107: 458–61.
7. Lapides J, Diokno AC, Lowe BS, Kalish MD. Follow-up on unsterile, intermittent self catheterization. J Urol 1974; 111: 184–7.
8. Diokno AC, Sonda P, Hollander JB, Lapides J. Fate of patients started on clean intermittent self-catheterization therapy 10 years ago. J Urol 1983; 129: 1120–2.
9. Weld KJ, Dmochowski RR. Effect of bladder management on urological complications in spinal cord injured patients. J Urol 2000; 163: 768–72.
10. Katona F, Berényi M. Intravesical transurethral electrotherapy in meningomyelocele patients. Acta Paediatr Acad Sci Hung 1975; 16: 363–74.
11. Ebner A, Jiang C, Lindström S. Intravesical electrical stimulation – an experimental analysis of the mechanism of action. J Urol 1992; 148: 920–4.
12. Madersbacher H, Hetzel H, Gottinger F, Ebner A. Rehabilitation of micturation in adults with incomplete spinal cord lesions by intravesical electrotherapy. Neurourol Urodyn 1987; 6: 230–2. [Abstract]
13. Kaplan WE, Richards I. Intravesical transurethral electrotherapy for the neurogenic bladder. J Urol 1986; 136: 243–6.
14. Decter RM, Snyder P, Rosvanis TK. Transurethral electrical bladder stimulation: initial results. J Urol 1992; 148: 651–3.
15. Lyne CJ, Bellinger MF. Early experience with transurethral electrical bladder stimulation. J Urol 1993; 150: 697–9.
16. Klarskov P, Holm-Bentzen M, Larsen S et al. Partial cystectomy for the myogenous decompensated bladder with excessive residual urine. Urodynamics, histology and 2–13 years follow-up. Scand J Urol Nephrol 1988; 22: 251–6.
17. Hanna MK. New concept in bladder remodeling. Urology 1982; 19: 6–12.
18. von Heyden B, Anthony JP, Kaula M et al. The latissimus dorsi muscle for detrusor assistance: functional recovery after nerve division and repair. J Urol 1994; 151: 1081–7.
19. Stenzl A, Strasser H, Klima G et al. Reconstruction of the lower urinary tract using autologous muscle transfer and cell seeding: current status and future perspectives. World J Urol 2000; 18: 44–50.
20. Ninkovic M, Stenzl A, Schwabegger A et al. Free neuromuscular transfer of latissimus dorsi for the treatment of bladder acontractility: II. Clinical results. J Urol 2003; 169: 1379–83.
21. Stenzl A. Ninkovic M. Autologous muscle transfer for reconstruction of the lower urinary tract. Adv Exp Med Biol 2003; 539(Pt B): 853–67.
22. Sievert KD, Fandel T, Wefer J et al. Collagen I: III ratio in canine heterologous bladder acellular matrix grafts. World J Urol 2006; 24: 101–9.
23. Cartwright LM, Shou Z, Yeger H, Farhat WA. Porcine bladder acellular matrix porosity: impact on hyaluronic acid and lyophilization. J Biomed Mater Res A 2006; 77: 180–4.
24. Brown AL, Ringuette MJ, Prestwich GD, Bagli DJ, Woodhouse KA. Effects of hyaluronan and SPARC on fibroproliferative events assessed in an in vitro bladder acellular model. Biomaterials 2006; 27: 3825–35.
25. Farhat WA, Chen J, Sherman C et al. Impact of fibrin glue and urinary bladder cell spraying on the in vivo acellular matrix cellularization: a porcine pilot study. Can J Urol 2006; 13: 3000–8.
26. Obara T, Matsuura S, Narita S et al. Bladder acellular matrix grafting regenerates urinary bladder in the spinal cord injury rat. Urology 2006; 68: 892–7.
27. Bolland F, Korossis S, Wilshaw SP et al. Development and characterization of a full-thickness acellular porcine bladder matrix for tissue engineering. Biomaterials 2007; 28: 1061–70.
28. Urakami S, Shiina H, Enokida H et al. Functional improvement in spinal cord injury-induced neurogenic bladder by bladder augmentation using bladder acellular matrix graft in the rat. World J Urol 2007; 25: 207–13.
29. Brown AL, Farhat W, Merguerian PA et al. 22 week assessment of bladder acellular matrix as a bladder augmentation material in a porcine model. Biomaterials 2002; 23: 2179–90.

30. Yokoyama T, Huard J, Pruchnic R et al. Muscle-derived cell transplantation and differentiation into lower urinary tract smooth muscle. Urology 2001; 57: 826–31.
31. Awad SA, McGinnis RH, Downie JW. The effectiveness of bethanechol chloride in lower motor neuron lesions: the importance of mode of administration. Neurourol Urodyn 1984; 3: 173–8.
32. Barrett DM, Wein AJ, Parulkar BG. Surgery for neuropathic bladder. AUA Update Series 1990; 9: 298–303.
33. Appel RA. Pharmacotherapy for overactive bladder: an evidence-based approach to selecting an antimuscarinic agent. Drugs 2006; 66: 1361–70.
34. Appel RA. Treatment of overactive bladder with once-daily extended release tolterodine or oxybutynin: the antimuscarinic clinical effectiveness trial (ACET). Curr Urol Rep 2002; 3: 343–4.
35. Elliott DS, Barrett DM. Surgical and medical management of the neurogenic bladder. AUA Update Series 2002; 21: 138–43.
36. Rovner E. Tropsium chloride in the management of overactive bladder. Drugs 2004; 64: 2433–46.
37. Khullar V, Chapple C, Gabriel Z, Dooley JA. The effects of antimuscarinics on health-related quality of life in overactive bladder: a systemic review and meta-analysis. Urology 2006; 68(2 Suppl): 38–48.
38. Horstmann M, Schaefer T, Aguilar Y, Stenzl A, Sievert KD. Neurogenic bladder treatment by doubling the recommended antimuscarinic dosage. Neurourol Urodyn 2006; 25: 441–5.
39. James MJ, Iacovon JW. The use of GNT patches in detrusor instability: a pilot study. Neurourol Urodyn 1993; 12: 399–400. [Abstract]
40. Davila GW, Daugherty CA, Sanders SW. Transdermal Oxybutynin Study Group. A short-term, multicenter, randomized double-blind dose titration study of the efficacy and anticholinergic side effects of transdermal compared to immediate release oxybutynin treatment of patients with urge urinary incontinence. J Urol 2001; 166: 140–5.
41. Brandler CB, Radebaugh LC, Mohler JL. Topical oxybutynin chloride for relaxation of dysfunctional bladders. J Urol 1989; 141: 1350–2.
42. Madersbacher H, Jilg G. Control of detrusor hyperreflexia by the intravesical installation of oxybutynin chloride. Paraplegia 1991; 29: 84–90.
43. Massad CA, Kogan BA, Trigo-Rocha FE. Pharmacokinetics of intravesical and oral oxybutynin chloride. J Urol 1992: 595–7.
44. Di Stasi SM, Giannantoni A, Navarra P et al. Intravesical oxybutynin: mode of action assessed by passive diffusion and electromotive administration with pharmacokinetics of oxybutynin and *N*-desethyl-oxybutynin. J Urol 2001; 166: 2232–6.
45. Schurch B, Stöhrer M, Kramer G et al. Botulinum-A toxin for treating detrusor hyperreflexia in spinal cord-injured parients: a new alternative to anticholinergic drugs? Preliminary results. J Urol 2000; 164: 692–7.
46. Fowler CJ. Bladder afferents and their role in overactive bladder. Urology 2002; 59(Suppl 5A): 37–42.
47. de Sèze M, Wiart L, Joseph PA et al. Capsaicin and neurogenic detrusor hyperreflexia: a double-blind placebo-controlled study in 20 patients with spinal cord lesions. Neurourol Urodyn 1998; 17: 513–23.
48. de Sèze M, Wiart L, Ferrière JM et al. Intravesical installation of capsaicin in urology: a review of the literature. Eur Urol 1999; 36: 267–77.
49. Maggi CA, Patacchini R, Tramontana M et al. Similarities and differences in the action of resiniferatoxin and capsaicin on central and peripheral endings of primary sensory neurons. Neuroscience 1990; 37: 531–9.
50. De Ridder D, Baert L. Vanilloids and the overactive bladder. BJU Int 2000; 86: 172–80.
51. Ekström B. Intravesical instillation of drugs in patients with detrusor hyperactivity. Scand J Urol Nephrol 1992; 149(Suppl): 1–67.
52. Steers WD, Meythaller JM, Haworth C et al. Effects of acute bolus and chronic continuous intrathecal Baclofen on genito-urinary dysfunction due to spinal cord pathology. J Urol 1992; 148: 1849–55.
53. Kums JJM, Delhaas EM. Intrathecal Baclofen infusion in patients with spasticity and neurogenic bladder disease. Preliminary results. World J Urol 1991; 9: 99–104.
54. Tanagho EA, Schmidt RA. Electrical stimulation in the clinical management of the neurogenic bladder. J Urol 1988; 140: 1331–9.
55. Brindley GS, Pulkey CE, Rushton DN, Cardozo L. Sacral anterior root stimulators for bladder control in paraplegia: the first 50 cases. J Neurol Neurosurg Psychiatry 1986; 49: 1104–14.
56. Chartier-Katler EJ, Denys P, Chancellor MB et al. Urodynamic monitoring during percutaneous sacral nerve neurostimulation in patients with neurogenic detrusor hyperreflexia. Neurourol Urodyn 2001; 20: 61–71.
57. Van Kerrebroeck PE, Koldewijn EL, Debruyne FM. Worldwide experience with the Finetech–Brindley sacral anterior root stimulator. Neurourol Urodyn 1993; 12: 497–503.
58. Van Kerrebrock PE. Neurostimulation. In: Corcos J, Schick E, eds. The Urinary Sphincter. New York: Marcel Dekker, 2001: 553–63.
59. Flood HD, Malhotra SJ, O'Connell HE et al. Long-term results and complications using augmentation cystoplasty in reconstructive urology. Neurourol Urodyn 1995; 14: 297–309.
60. Leng WW, Blalock HJ, Frederiksson WH et al. Enterocystoplasty or myomectomy? Comparison of indications and outcomes for bladder augmentation. J Urol 1999; 161: 758–63.
61. Dykstra DD, Sidi AA. Treatment of detrusor-sphincter dyssynergia with Botulinum A toxin: a double–blind study. Arch Phys Med Rehab 1990: 71: 24–6.
62. Fowler CJ, Betts CD, Christmas TJ et al. Botulinum toxin in the treatment of chronic urinary retention in women. Br J Urol 1992; 70: 387–9.
63. Phelan MW, Franks M, Somogyi GT et al. Botulinum toxin urethral sphincter injection to restore bladder emptying in men and women with voiding dysfunction. J Urol 2001; 164: 1107–10.
64. Boyd RN, Britton TC, Robinson RO, Borzyskowski M. Transient urinary incontinence after Botulinum A toxin. Lancet 1996; 348(9025): 481–2. [Letter]
65. Kuo HC. Effect of Botulinum toxin A in the treatment of voiding dysfunction due to detrusor underactivity. Urology 2003; 61: 550–4.
66. Karsenty G, Baazeem A, Elzayat E, Corcos J. Injection of botulinum toxin type A in the urethral sphincter to treat lower urinary tract dysfunction: a review of indications, techniques and results. Can J Urol 2006; 13: 3027–33.
67. Mamas MA, Reynard JM, Brading AF. Augmentation of nitric oxide to treat detrusor-external sphincter dyssynergia in spinal cord injury. Lancet 2001; 357(9272): 1964–7.
68. Reitz A, Bretscher S, Knapp PA et al. The effect of nitric oxide on the resting tone and the contractile behaviour of the external urethral sphincter: a functional urodynamic study in healthy humans. Eur Urol 2004; 45: 367–73.
69. Reitz A, Knapp PA, Muntener M, Schurch B. Oral nitric oxide donors: a new pharmacological approach to detrusor-sphincter dyssynergia in spinal cord injured patients. Eur Urol 2004; 45: 516–20.
70. Oesterling JE, Kaplan SA, Epstein HB et al, and The North American Urolume Study Group. The North American experience with the Urolume endoprosthesis as a treatment for benign prostatic hyperplasia. Long term results. Urology 1994; 44: 353–62.
71. Guazzone G, Montorsi F, Coulange Ch et al. A modified prostatic wallstent for healthy patients with symptomatic benign prostatic hyperplasia: a European multicenter experience. Urology 1994; 44: 364–70.
72. Rivas DA, Chancellor MB. Sphincterotomy and sphincter stent prosthesis placement. In: Corcos J, Schick E, eds. The Urinary Sphincter. New York: Marcel Dekker, 2001: 565–82.

73. Mehta SS, Tophill PR. Memokath stents for the treatment of detrusor sphincter dyssynergia (DSD) in men with spinal cord injury: the Princess Royal Spinal Injuries Unit 10-year experience. Spinal Cord 2006; 44: 1–6.
74. Hamid R, Arya M, Patel HR, Shah PJ. The mesh wallstent in the treatment of detrusor external sphincter dyssynergia in men with spinal cord injury: a 12-year follow-up. BJU Int 2003; 91: 51–3.
75. Chancellor MB, Karasick S, Strup S et al. Transurethral balloon dilation of the external urinary sphincter: effectiveness in spinal cord-injured men with detrusor-sphincter dyssynergia. Radiology 1993; 187: 557–60.
76. Parsons KF. Difficulty with voiding or acute urinary retention having previously voided satisfactorily. In: Parsons KF, Fitzpatrick JM, eds. Practical Urology in Spinal Cord Injury. London: Springer-Verlag, 1991: 27–42.
77. Schäfer W. Principles and clinical application of advanced urodynamic analysis of voiding function. Urol Clin N Am 1990; 17: 553–66.
78. Turner-Warwick R. Clinical problems associated with urodynamic abnormalities with special reference to the value of synchronous cinepressure–flow cystography and the clinical importance of detrusor function studies. In: Lutzeyer W, Melchior H, eds. Urodynamics – Upper and Lower Urinary Tract. Berlin: Springer-Verlag, 1970: 237–63.
79. Gardner BP, Parsons KF, Machin DG et al. The urological management of spinal cord damaged patients: a clinical algorithm. Paraplegia 1986; 24: 138–47.
80. Burch JC. Cooper's ligament urethrovesical suspension for stress incontinence. Nine years' experience – results, complications, technique. Am J Obstet Gynecol 1968; 100: 764–74.
81. Tanagho EA. Colpocystourethropexy: the way we do it. J Urol 1976; 116: 751–3.
82. Weber AM, Walters MD. Burch procedure compared with sling for stress urinary incontinence: a decision analysis. Obstet Gynecol 2000; 96: 867–73.
83. Culligan PJ, Goldberg RP, Sand PK. A randomized controlled trial comparing a modified Burch procedure and a suburethral sling: long-term follow-up. Int Urogynecol J Pelvic Floor Dysfunct 2003; 14: 229–33.
84. Bai SW, Sohn WH, Chung DJ, Park JH, Kim SK. Comparison of the efficacy of Burch colposuspension, pubovaginal sling, and tension-free vaginal tape for stress urinary incontinence. Int J Gynaecol Obstet 2005; 91: 246–51.
85. deTayrac R, Deffieux X, Droupy S et al. A prospective randomized trial comparing tension-free vaginal tape and transobturator suburethral tape for surgical treatment of stress urinary incontinence. Am J Obstet Gynecol 2004; 190: 602–8.
86. David-Montefiore E, Frobert JL, Grisard-Anaf M et al. Perioperative complications and pain after suburethral sling procedure for urinary stress incontinence: a French prospective randomized multicenter study comparing the retropubic and transobturator routes. Eur Urol 2006; 49: 133–8.
87. Bezerra CA, Bruschini H, Cody DJ. Traditional suburethral sling operations for urinary incontinence in women. Cochrane Database Syst Rev 2005; (3): CD001754.
88. Ulmsten U, Falconer C, Johnson P et al. A multicenter study of tensionfree vaginal tape (TVT) for surgical treatment of stress urinary incontinence. Int Urogynec J Pelvic Floor Dysfunc 1998; 9: 210–13.
89. Castellan M, Gosalbez R, Labbie A, Ibrahim E, Disandro M. Bladder neck sling for treatment of neurogenic incontinence in children with augmentation cystoplasty: long-term followup. J Urol 2005; 173: 2128–31.
90. Dik P, Klijn AJ, van Gool JD, de Jong TP. Transvaginal sling suspension of bladder neck in female patients with neurogenic sphincter incontinence. J Urol 2003; 170(2 Pt 1): 580–1.
91. Daneshmand S, Ginsberg DA, Bennet JK et al. Puboprostatic sling repair for treatment of urethral incompetence in adult neurogenic incontinence. J Urol 2003; 169: 199–202.
92. Triaca V, Twiss CO, Raz S. Urethral compression for the treatment of postprostatectomy urinary incontinence: is history repeating itself? Eur Urol 2007; 51: 304–5. [Editorial]
93. Berg S. Polytef augmentation urethroplasty. Arch Surg 1973; 107: 379–81.
94. Malizia AA, Reiman HM, Myers RP et al. Migration and granulomatous reaction after periurethral injection of polytef (Teflon). JAMA 1984; 251: 3277–81.
95. Corcos J, Fournier C. Periurethral collagen injection for the treatment of female stress urinary incontinence: 4-year follow-up results. Urology 1999; 54: 815–18.
96. Santarosa RP, Blaivas JG. Periurethral injection of autologous fat for the treatment of sphincteric incontinence. J Urol 1994; 151: 607–11.
97. Barrett DM, Ghoniem G, Bruskewitz R et al. The Genisphere: a new percutaneously placed anti-incontinence device. J Urol 1990; 141: 224A.
98. Pineda EB, Hadley HR. Urethral injection treatment for stress urinary incontinence. In: Corcos J, Schick E, eds. The Urinary Sphincter. New York: Marcel Dekker, 2001: 497–515.
99. Kassouf W, Capolechio J, Bernardinucci G, Corcos J. Collagen injection for treatment of urinary incontinence in children. J Urol 2001; 165: 1666–8.
100. Fulford SC, Sutton C, Bales G et al. The fate of the 'modern' artificial urinary sphincter with a follow-up of more than 15 years. Br J Urol 1997; 79: 713–16.
101. Spiess PE, Capolicchio JP, Kiruluta G et al. Is an artificial sphincter the best choice for incontinent boys with spina bifida? Review of our long term experience with the AS800 artificial sphincter. Can J Urol 2002; 9: 1486: 91.
102. Lai HH, Hsu EI, The BS, Butler EB, Boone TB. 13 years of experience with artificial urinary sphincter implantation at Baylor College of Medicine. J Urol 2007; 177: 1021–5.
103. Leadbetter GW Jr. Surgical reconstruction for complete urinary incontinence: a 10 to 22 year follow-up. J Urol 1985; 113: 205–6.
104. Tanagho EA. Bladder neck reconstruction for total urinary incontinence: 10 years of experience. J Urol 1981; 125: 321–6.
105. The prevention and management of urinary tract infections among people with spinal cord injuries. National Institute on Disability and Rehabilitation Research Consensus Statement. January 27–29, 1992. J Am Paraplegia Soc 1992; 15: 194–204.

Part IX

Complications

71

Complications related to neurogenic bladder dysfunction – I: infection, lithiasis, and neoplasia

Gamal Ghoniem and Mostafa Elmissiry

Infection

Definitions

- *Urinary tract infection* is an inflammatory response of the urothelium to bacterial invasion that is usually associated with bacteriuria and pyuria. It is defined by 'urine culture showing more than 10^5 bacterial colonies in 1 ml of urine'.[1]
- *Bacteriuria* is 'the presence of bacteria in the urine'. It is well known that urine is normally free of bacteria; hence, bacteruria implies that these bacteria are from the urinary tract and are not contaminants from the skin, vagina, or prepuce. Bacteruria can be symptomatic or asymptomatic. It does not necessarily mean a urinary tract infection (UTI).[1]
- *Pyuria* is 'the presence of white blood cells (WBCs) in the urine'. It is generally indicative of an inflammatory response of the urothelium to bacterial invasion. Pyuria alone is not diagnostic of infection, because it may occur from the irritative effect of a urinary catheter, especially if it is at a low level of less than or equal to 30 WBC/HPF (high power field). Bacteriuria without pyuria indicates bacterial colonization rather than infection.[2]

Incidence

UTIs are among the most common urologic complications of neurogenic bladder. It has been estimated that approximately 33% of spinal cord injury patients have bacteriuria at any time.[3] One prospective study on patients on intermittent catheterization or condom catheterization reported an incidence of febrile UTIs of 1.8 per person per year.[4] UTI is the most common cause of fever in the spinal cord injury patient;[5] the UTI can be acute or chronic, relapsing or recurrent. The term 'relapse' implies infection by the same organism, while 'recurrent' infection implies infection with a different strain of bacteria.[6]

Specimen collection for culture

In both sexes, the external urethral meatus must be exposed and cleaned by antiseptic solution. The first 50 ml of urine is passed without collection. Afterwards, approximately 50 ml of midstream urine is collected in a sterile container. The urine should be cultured as soon as possible or kept refrigerated and cultured within 24 hours.[7] To obtain a urine specimen from a patient with neurogenic bladder dysfunction (NBD), external stimulation (usually suprapubic percussion) can be used. If this is impossible, urine should be obtained by a single catheterization.

Pathogenesis

There are many risk factors that lead to the development of UTIs in patients with NBD. The 1992 National Institute on Disability and Rehabilitation Research Consensus Conference examined the problems associated with UTIs in spinal cord injury patients. Among the risk factors identified were overdistention of the bladder, elevated intravesical pressure, increased risk of urinary obstruction, vesicoureteric reflux (VUR), presence of bladder diverticulae, impaired voiding, instrumentation, and increased incidence of stones (Figures 71.1 and 71.2). Other factors that have been implicated are decreased fluid intake, poor hygiene, perineal colonization, decubiti and other evidence of local tissue trauma, and reduced host defense associated with chronic illness.[4]

The method of bladder management has a profound impact on UTI. Suprapubic catheters and indwelling urethral catheters eventually have an equivalent infection rate.[8] However, the onset of bacteruria may be delayed using a suprapubic catheter compared with a urethral catheter. Since its introduction by Lapides[66] and colleagues in 1972, clean (but not sterile) intermittent catheterization (CIC) has been shown to decrease lower tract infections by

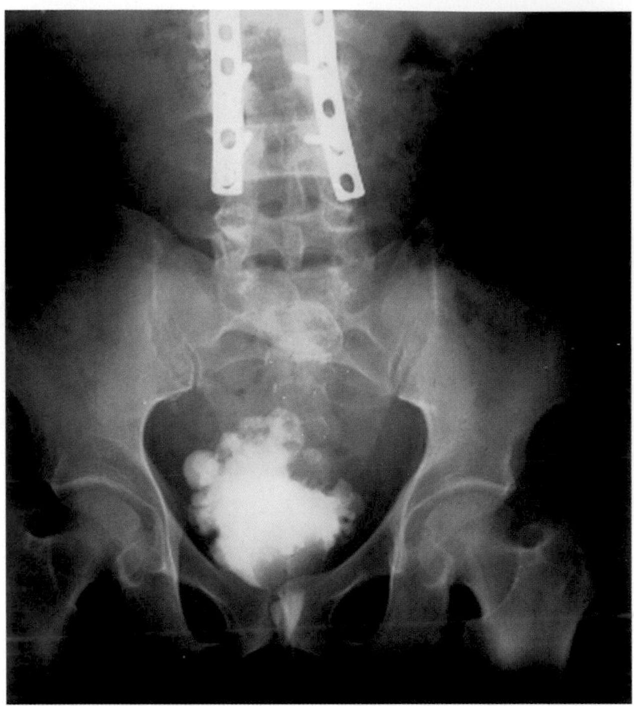

Figure 71.1
Cystogram of an 18-year-old patient with post-traumatic spinal cord injury. Classic 'Christmas tree' bladder can be seen with an indwelling urethral catheter inside it.

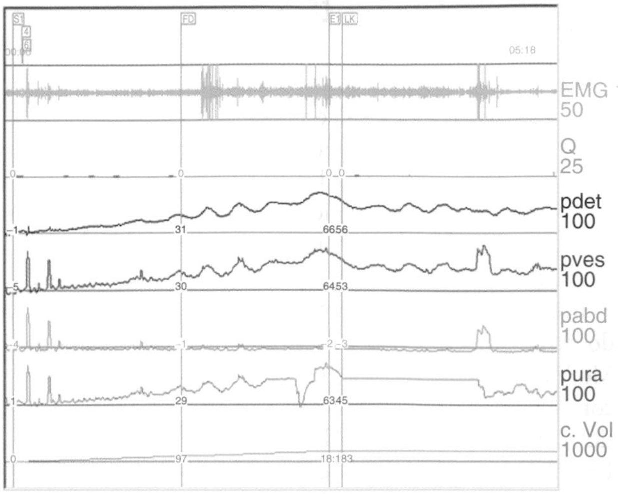

Figure 71.2
Combined pressure–flow–EMG study of a 21-year-old male with spinal cord injury. The bladder has a low capacity and low compliance with superadded detrusor overactivity (DOA). Note the high detrusor leak-point pressure (DLPP = 66 cmH_2O at a volume of 181 ml). This patient needs augmentation.

maintaining low intravesical pressure and reducing the incidence of stones.[8,9]

Bacteriology and laboratory findings

Urinalysis will show bacteriuria and pyuria. The National Institute on Disability and Rehabilitation Research Consensus Statement recommended the following criteria for the diagnosis of significant bacteriuria in spinal cord injury patients. Any detectable bacteria from indwelling or suprapubic catheter aspirates was considered significant because the vast majority of patients with an indwelling catheter and low-level bacteriuria showed an increase to greater than 10^5 cfu (colony forming unit)/ml within a short period of time. For patients on CIC, greater than or equal to 10^2 cfu/ml was considered significant. For catheter-free males, a clean voided specimen showing greater than or equal to 10^4 cfu/ml was considered significant.[10,11]

Bacteriuria in spinal cord injury patients differs from that in patients with intact spinal cords in its etiology, complexity, and antimicrobial susceptibility and is influenced by the type and duration of catheterization. *Escherichia coli* is isolated in approximately 20% of patients. *Enterococci*, *Proteus mirabilis*, and *Pseudomonas* are more common among spinal cord injury patients than patients with intact spinal cords. Other organisms that are quite often cultured *Klebsiella*, *Proteus*, *Serratia*, *Providencia*, *Staphylococcus*, and *Candida* species.[1]

The bacteria which produce urease are particularly harmful. Urease is an enzyme that causes significant alkalinization of urine, which promotes the precipitation of struvite stone (magnesium–ammonium–phosphate and calcium carbonate) in the upper and lower urinary tract. The most common organism associated with struvite calculi is *P. mirabilis*. Other organisms include *Ureaplasma urealyticum*, *Providencia stuartii*, *Yersinia enterocolitica*, and *Bacteroids corrodens*.[12,13]

Most bacteriuria in short-term catheterization is of a single organism, whereas patients catheterized for longer than a month will usually demonstrate a polymicrobial flora caused by a wide range of gram-negative and gram-positive bacterial species.[14] Such specimens commonly have two to four bacterial species, each at concentrations of 10^5 cfu/ml or more.[15] Some may have up to six to eight species at that concentration. This phenomenon is due to an incidence of new episodes of bacteriuria approximately every 2 weeks and the ability of these strains to persist for weeks and months in the catheterized urinary tract.[16] Two of the most persistent species are *E. coli* and *P. stuartii*. *P. stuartii* is rarely found outside the long-term catheterized urinary tract and may use the catheter itself as a niche.[17,18]

Lower urinary tract infections

Cystitis

Cystitis is the most common complication of neurogenic bladder. Flow of urine through the urinary tract and voiding are the primary bladder defenses against infection. Since most of the NBD patients have residual urine in their bladders, they are usually susceptible for recurrent attacks of cystitis.[19]

Because of partial or complete loss of sensation, patients do not usually experience frequency, urgency, or dysuria. More often, they complain of fever, back or abdominal discomfort, leakage between catheterizations, increased spasticity, malaise, lethargy, and/or cloudy, malodorous urine.[19] Urinalysis usually shows bacteriuria, pyuria, and hematuria. Urine culture remains the definitive test to prove infection.

Treatment is by giving the specific antibiotics. The duration of therapy is not established, but 4 to 5 days is recommended for the mildly symptomatic patient and 10 to 14 days for sicker patients. Some times, acute cystitis may cause severe bleeding requiring bladder drainage and periodic irrigation together with antibiotic therapy.[19] Recurrent UTIs may be associated with high storage pressures, and intervention to decrease storage pressure may decrease the incidence of symptomatic UTI.[20]

Urethritis

This usually occurs in patients with indwelling urethral catheters, less commonly with CIC. Occasionally, blockage of the periurethral gland by the catheter occurs and, with secondary infection, this will lead to the formation of a periurethral abscess. Acute nontreated periurethral abscess may represent a life-threatening condition when the Buck's fascia is penetrated, leading to necrosis of the subcutaneous tissue and fascia. Immediate suprapubic cystostomy is mandatory together with wide debridment of all nonviable tissues. At the same time, aggressive intravenous antibiotic therapy should be started.[21]

In a less acute or more chronic stage, the abscess may evolve in three different directions. It can drain spontaneously to the penile skin and heal without sequel. More often, however, it may drain inside the urethral lumen, creating a diverticulum that needs surgical excision otherwise recurrent periurethral abscess may develop (Figure 71.3). The last fate of the abscess is to drain simultaneously at both sides forming a urethra–cutaneous fistula, which also needs surgical excision.

Epididymitis

This is also a catheter-related infection. It is usually caused by spread of infection from the urethra or bladder which reaches the epididymis via the vas deferens in a retrograde fashion. The most common cause of epididymitis in NBD patients, therefore, is due to the organisms that cause urethritis. These include *Neisseria gonorrhea*, *E. coli*, and *Chlamydia trachomatis*.[22] Acute epididymitis is a clinical syndrome consisting of pain, swelling, and inflammation of the epididymis of less than 6 weeks. In neurologically affected patients, pain is usually absent because they do not have adequate sensation. The only clinical sign is swelling and flare. Fever may be detected in the acute stage. Treatment is by specific antibiotics according to culture results. Quinolones can be given until the result of culture appears. In rare conditions, in neglected cases, infection may reach the testicle and cause orchitis, with the eventual formation of abscess. Treatment should include abscess drainage plus strong antibiotics. Sometimes, if the testis is found damaged, orchiectomy becomes the solution.[22]

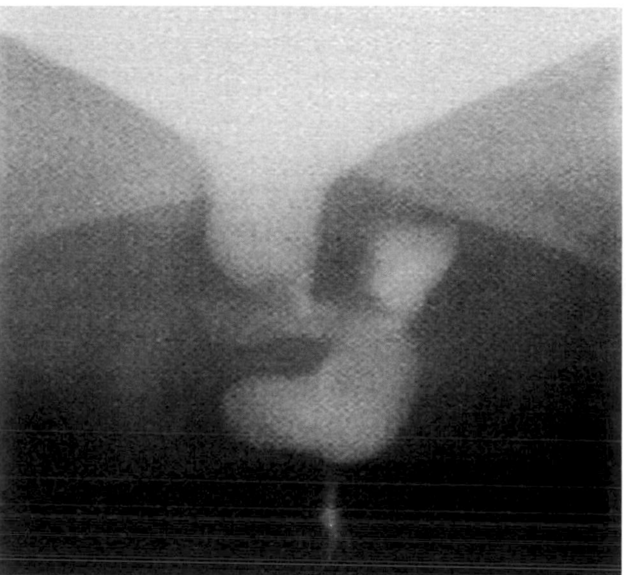

Figure 71.3
Voiding cystourethrogram (VCUG) of a 28-year-old female with urethral diverticulum developing after history of chronic indwelling catheterization. Note the saddle configuration of the diverticulum.

Prostatitis

Prostatitis is the most common urologic diagnosis in men younger than 50 years and the third most common urologic diagnosis in men older than 50 years (after BPH and prostate cancer).[23] Bacteria most often gain the prostate by infected urine refluxing into prostatic ducts.

In patients with NBD, neurophysiologic obstruction resulting in high-pressure dysfunctional flow patterns has

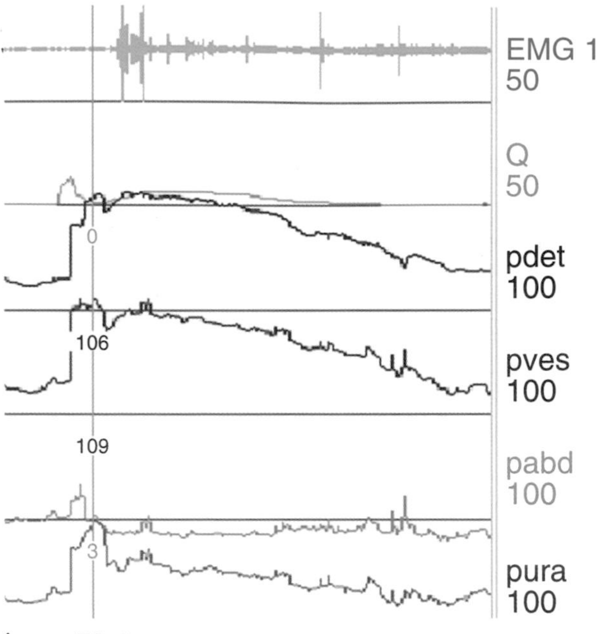

Figure 71.4
Combined pressure–flow–EMG of a 16-year-old male with type-I detrusor-sphincteric dyssynergia (DSD). Note the low urinary flow in spite of the sustained high detrusor pressure with detrusor contraction (>100 cmH_2O).

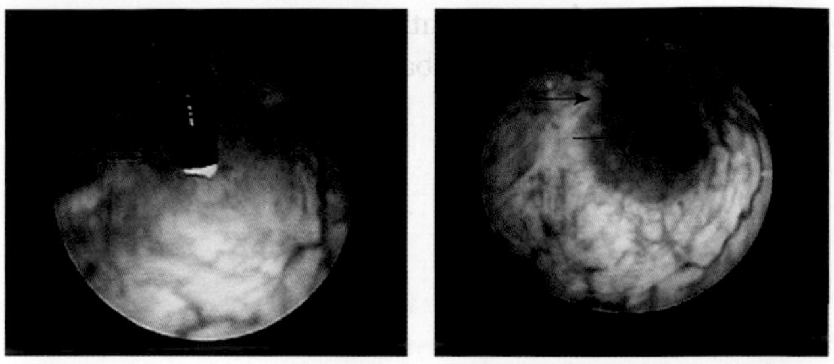

Figure 71.5
Cystoscopy of the same patient showing closed bladder neck with bladder filling (left side, black arrow). On bladder contraction, the bladder neck opens (right side, black arrow) but the external sphincter contracts at the same time (right side, blue arrow) leaving only the prostatic urethra opened.

been implicated in the pathogenesis of the prostatitis syndrome. On video-urodynamic studies, many patients with prostatitis show incomplete funneling of the bladder neck as well as vesicourethral dyssynergic patterns. This high-pressure, dysfunctional voiding may increase intraprostatic ductal reflux in susceptible individuals (Figures 71.4 and 71.5). Alternatively, this dyssynergic voiding may lead to an autonomic overstimulation of the perineal–pelvic neural system with subsequent development of a chronic neuropathic pain state.[24]

The most common cause of prostatitis is the Enterobacteriaceae family of gram-negative bacteria, commonly strains of *E. coli*, identified in 65 to 80% of infections. *Pseudomonas aeruginosa, Serratia* species, *Klebsiella* species, and *Enterobacter aerogenes* are identified in a further 10 to 15%.[25]

Bacterial prostatitis in NBD is generally chronic and asymptomatic. The most important clue in the diagnosis is a history of documented recurrent UTIs. Between 25 and 43% of patients diagnosed with chronic bacterial prostatitis were reported to have had a history of recurrent UTIs.[26] Urinalysis is usually free of pus cells. Segmented lower urinary tract cultures should be done to localize the infection in the prostate.[27] Treatment is composed mainly of antibiotics that have good diffusion power into the prostatic tissues, such as trimethoprim and fluoroquinolones. Other agents like alpha-blockers and anti-inflammatory drugs may also be used.[1]

Upper urinary tract infection (pyelonephritis)

There are two main risk factors contributing to the occurrence of pyelonephritis among NBD patients. Firstly, recurrent lower urinary tract infections may interfere with the antireflux mechanism, causing reflux of infected urine to the kidney. Secondly, functional infravesical obstruction, such as detrusor-sphincteric dyssynergia (DSD), leads to stasis of urine and high intravesical pressure, both creating a risk of reflux of an already infected urine.[21] In a study on a group of patients with DESD, Chancellor and Rivas found that over 50% of men with DESD will develop significant complications, such as VUR, upper tract deterioration, urolithiasis, urosepsis, and ureterovesical obstruction.[28]

As sensation is often absent in neurologic patients, the main clinical symptom of acute pyelonephritis is fever up to 40°C. Urinalysis shows pyuria, bacteruria, and microscopic hematuria. Blood tests may show a polymorphonuclear leukocytosis, increased erythrocyte sedimentation rate, elevated C-reactive protein levels, and elevated creatinine levels if renal impairment developed.

Acute pyelonephritis in NBD patients is considered a complicated infection and requires hospitalization. At first, the patient should be adequately hydrated, blood culture time three and urine culture should be done, and double intravenous antibiotics (ampicillin–gentamicyn) should be started until the results of cultures appear. On day 3 appropriate oral antibiotic should be started, and the duration of therapy should be 14 days.[29]

If symptoms persist beyond 72 hours, however, the possibility of perinephric or intrarenal abscesses, urinary tract abnormalities, or obstruction should be considered and radiologic investigation with ultrasonography or CT should be performed. Urine and blood cultures should be repeated at appropriate intervals, and antimicrobial therapy should be adjusted, if necessary, on the basis of susceptibility testing.[30]

Lithiasis

Incidence

Urolithiasis is a well-documented problem in patients with neurogenic voiding dysfunction. It is estimated that 10–20% of patients with spinal cord injury will have struvite stones within 10 years of injury; of these, 7% will have renal stones.[31,32] The incidence of renal calculi in myelomeningocele patients may be greater.[33] Once a kidney stone develops, there is a 34% chance of a second stone developing within the next 5 years.[34]

Risk factors

The main risk factors for stone development are recurrent UTIs, especially due to urea-splitting organisms, infravesical obstruction producing stasis, indwelling catheters, vesicoureteral reflux, hypercalciuria resulting from immobilization, and high specific gravity of urine.[35]

The patient's age and injury characteristics have an important role in determining the type of urinary stone formed. In a longitudinal cohort study, Chen et al found that the risk factors for bladder stone were younger age, neurologically complete lesion, and indwelling catheterization.[36] In a case-control study, DeVivo et al noted that patients who developed renal stones were more likely to be older, have had neurologically complete quadriplegia, and to have had a history of bladder stone.[37,38]

Stone composition

For the last few decades, most studies have reported that patients with NBD develop exclusively struvite stones composed of magnesium ammonium phosphate. This was attributed to UTI with urea-splitting organisms which render the urine pH >7.24.[39,40] Recent studies, however, reported that many patients with NBD harboring calculi have been found to have metabolic stones. Matlaga et al found that out of 32 patients with NBD who harbored urinary stones, 20 patients (62.5%) had metabolic stones while the remaining 12 (37.5%) had infection stones.[41] They related this observation to the advances in urologic care of patients with NBD, including accurate urodynamic evaluation of the detrusor and sphincteric function and greater use of CIC and bladder augmentation. These led to a significant decrease in the incidence of UTI among patients with NBD and subsequently a fall in the incidence of struvite stones among those patients.[42,43] The importance of this observation is that once a metabolically derived stone is identified, the patient should be offered further metabolic evaluation and medical and dietary therapy.[44]

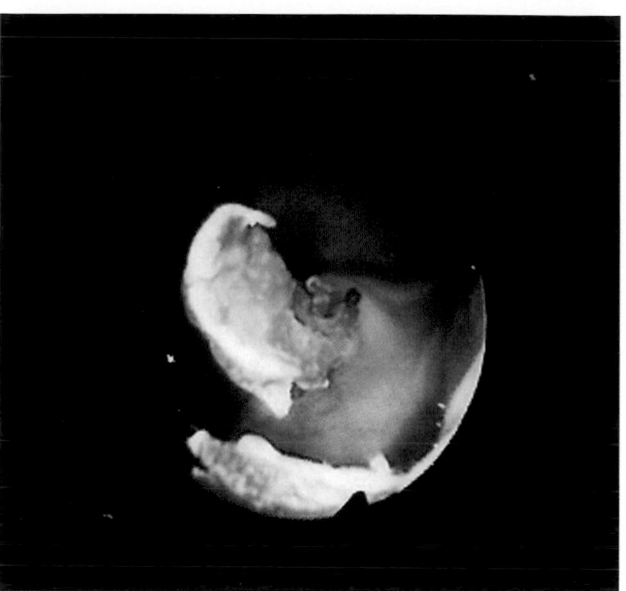

Figure 71.6
Cystoscopy of a 22-year-old male patient with a history of chronic indwelling catheter. Multiple typical eggshell-shaped stones could be seen which were formed around the balloon of the Foley's catheter.

Diagnosis

Patients with renal stones usually have non-specific symptoms including feeling unwell, abdominal discomfort, increased spasms, and autonomic dysreflexia. These vague symptoms can alert a well-informed physician, so the need for radiologic examination by plain kidney, ureter and bladder (KUB), ultrasonography, computerized tomography, and intravenous pyelography (IVP) becomes essential for diagnosis.[45]

Patients with bladder stones usually suffer from irritative symptoms, hematuria, and recurrent UTI. Again, radiologic examination is essential. Bladder stones usually start as small pieces of thin struvite calculi formed around the balloon of the Foley's catheter. These calculi may grow but they will retain the typical eggshell shape that appears in cystoscopy (Figure 71.6). Small struvite stones with a low calcium content can easily be missed on X-ray and are often incidentally discovered during cystoscopy.[46]

Treatment

Successful treatment of renal stones depends on complete elimination of the calculus, eradication of infection, and

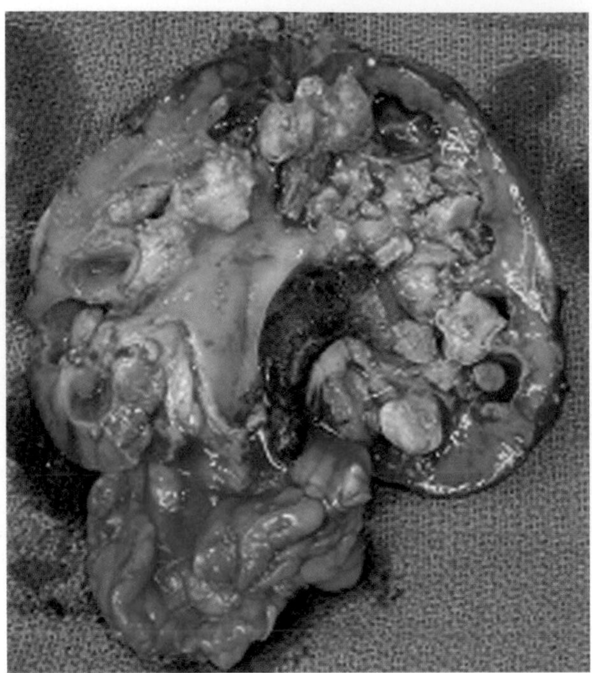

Figure 71.7
A surgical specimen from a 31-year-old patient who underwent nephrectomy for a nonfunctioning kidney harboring a stag horn stone.

removal of the obstruction. Selection of the best method of treatment should be individualized and adapted to every patient.[47]

In paraplegic and quadriplegic patients, typical extracorporeal shock wave lithotripsy (ESWL) alone is not recommended because of the difficulty in eliminating the stone fragments.[48] Furthermore, ESWL may predispose to the development of autonomic dysreflexia. Stowe et al reported on 9 out of 52 patients with NBD (17.3%) who developed autonomic dysreflexia after ESWL.[49] If ESWL is considered in these patients, it is better to be done without adding the risk of general anesthesia but with careful monitoring to avoid development of hypertension. Prophylaxis can also be done by giving 10–20 mg of nifedipine sublingually 15–20 min before the procedure.[50] The other drawback of ESWL is that it may exacerbate post-traumatic syringomyelia, presumably by reverberating the fluid within the intramedullary cavity, producing further damage to the spinal cord.[51] The recommended technique for treatment is percutaneous nephrolithotripsy (PCNL), in some selected cases with ESWL. In rare cases, patients may require surgery to remove the stones. Nephrectomy should be performed when the kidney is nonfunctioning, or if there is pyonephrosis (Figure 71.7).

Ureteric stones can be managed through ureteroscopic fragmentation and extraction. However, if the stone is big enough and remains blocked in the middle third, surgery should be considered.

Treatment of bladder stones is straightforward, because of easy access to the bladder both endoscopically and surgically. The stone can be fragmented endoscopically by mechanical forceps, holmium laser, ultrasonics, pneumatics, or electrohydraulic lithotripsy. Small fragments can then be washed out from the bladder by the Ellik evacuator. Careful monitoring of blood pressure, however, is important for fear of development of autonomic dysreflexia, which is also reported after cystolithotripsy in NBD patients.[52] Open surgery is indicated only when bladder capacity is small or the size of the stone is so big that endoscopic litholapaxy would be extremely difficult. Impacted urethral stones are rare and occur mainly with obstruction or urethral diverticulum.[53] Endoscopic treatment is by visual urethrotomy, pushing the stone into the bladder and fragmenting it. Surgery is performed in cases of a stone in a diverticulum, where diverticulectomy is used for stone removal.

Prevention

Successful prevention of urinary stones in NBD patients depends on regular positioning of the paralyzed patients, high fluid intake, early mobilization, proper treatment of UTI and prevention of subsequent infection. One of the most effective methods in prevention of struvite stone formation is the use of urinary acidifiers; these agents will decrease the urinary pH, preventing precipitation of phosphate stones and subsequently struvite stone formation. One of the most commonly used urinary acidifiers is methenamine mandelate at a dose of 4–5 g per day. It can stabilize the urinary pH at a value of 5.5, so reducing urinary saturation and crystallization of phosphates and carbonates.[54] Other examples of urinary acidifiers are 3–4 g daily of L-methionine and 3–4 g daily of ammonium chloride.[55,56]

Neoplasm

Incidence and types

It is estimated that patients with NBD are 16–28 times more susceptible to develop bladder cancer than the normal population.[57] The most common histologic type occurring in these patients is squamous cell carcinoma.[58] Bejany et al found that 81% of bladder cancer patients in spinal cord injury units harbored squamous cell carcinoma, while the other 19% had either transitional cell or mixed tumor.[59]

Risk factors

The most important risk factors for the development of bladder cancer in NBD patients are those causing chronic irritation of the bladder mucosa. These include chronic bladder infection, prolonged indwelling catheterization, and bladder stone disease. This is why squamous cell carcinoma is the most common type of malignancy among these patients.[60]

Vaidyanathan and associates hypothesized that certain histologic changes are seen more frequently in spinal cord injury patients with long-term indwelling catheters. These changes include papillary or polypoid cystitis, widespread cystitis glandularis, moderate to severe acute and chronic inflammatory changes in bladder mucosa, follicular cystitis, squamous metaplesia, and urothelial dysplasia.[61]

Screening

The screening of NBD patients with chronic indwelling catheterization is controversial. Some advocate the use of screening cystoscopy, arguing that this will detect malignant lesions in an earlier stage.[62] Others believe that cystoscopy with or without biopsy does not fulfill the necessary criteria for screening for bladder cancer in NBD patients.[63,64]

Screening cytology may be of benefit. Stonehill and colleagues studied patients with indwelling catheters for more than 5 years. Positive cytology had a sensitivity of 71% and a specificity of 97%. Based on these observations, they recommended yearly cytology in all patients with chronic indwelling catheters, followed by biopsy if it was positive.[65]

This review of the literature suggests that NBD patients with longstanding indwelling catheterization (certainly after 10 years, perhaps after 5 years post-trauma) should undergo yearly urine cytology. If it is doubtful or positive, cystoscopy and cold cup biopsy should be performed randomly, if no suspicious lesion was found. A history of bladder stone and chronic UTI should be considered as significant risk factors for the development of bladder cancer in these patients. New onset of gross hematuria should be investigated in the same way as in the neurologically normal population.

References

1. Achaeffer AJ. Infections of the urinary tract. In: Walsh PC, Retik AB, Vaughan ED, Wein AJ, eds. Campbell's Urology, 8th edn. Philadelphia: WB Saunders, 2002: 515–7.
2. Menon EB, Tan ES. Pyuria: index of infection in patients with spinal cord injuries. Br J Urol 1992; 69: 144–6.
3. Stover SL, Lioyd LK, Waites KB, Jackson AB. Urinary tract infection in spinal cord injury. Arch Phys Med Rehab 1989; 70: 47–54.
4. Waites KB, Canupp CK, Devivo MJ. Epidemiology and risk factors for urinary tract infection following spinal cord injury. Arch Phys Med Rehab 1993; 74: 691.
5. Beraldo PSS, Neves EGC, Alves CMF et al. Pyrexia in hospitalized spinal cord injury patients. Paraplegia 1993; 31: 186.
6. Ward TT, Jones SR. Genitourinary tract infections. In: Reese RE, Betts RF, eds. A Logical Approach to Infectious Diseases, 3rd edn. Boston: Little, Brown and Company, 1991: 357–89.
7. Horton JA 3rd, Kirshblum SC, Lisenmeyer TA, Johnston M, Rustagi A. Does refrigeration of urine alter culture results in hospitalized patients with neurogenic bladder? J Spinal Cord Med 1998; 21: 342–7.
8. Gilmore DS, Schick DJ, Young MN, Montgomerie JZ. Effect of external urinary collection system on colonization and urinary tract infections with *Pseudomonas* and *Klebsiella* in men with spinal cord injury. J Am Paraplegia Soc 1992; 15: 155.
9. Tambyah PA, Maki DG. Catheter-associated urinary tract infection is rarely symptomatic: a prospective study of 1,497 catheterized patients. Arch Intern Med 2000; 160: 678.
10. Cardenas DD, Hooton TM, Urinary tract infection in persons with spinal cord injury. Arch Phys Med Rehab 1995; 76: 272.
11. National Institute on Disability and Rehabilitation Research Consensus Statement. The prevention and management of urinary tract infections among people with spinal cord injury. SCI Nurs 1993; 10: 49–61.
12. Babayan RK. Urinary calculi and endourology. In: Siroky MB, Krane RJ, eds. Manual of Urology. Boston: Little, Brown and company, 1990; 123–31.
13. Silverman DE, Stamey TA. Management of infection stones: the Stanford experience. Medicine (Baltimore) 1983; 62: 44–51.
14. Edwards LE, Lock R, Powell C, Jones P. Post-catheterization urethral strictures: a clinical and experimental study. Br J Urol 1983; 55: 53.
15. Nickel JC, Olson ME, Costerton JW. In vivo coefficient of kinetic friction: study of urinary catheter biocompatibility. Urology 1987; 14: 501.
16. Gabriel MM, Mayo MS, May LL et al. In vitro evaluation of the efficacy of a silver-coated catheter. Curr Microbiol 1996; 33: 1.
17. Hockstra D. Hyaluronan-modified surfaces for medical devices. Med Device Diagn Ind 1999; 48–56.
18. Liedberg H, Lundeberg T. Silver alloy-coated catheters reduce catheter-associated bacteriuria. Br J Urol 1990; 65: 379.
19. Beraldo PSS, Neves EGC, Alves CMF et al. Pyrexia in hospitalized spinal cord injury patients. Paraplegia 1993; 31: 186.
20. Cardenas DD, Hooton TM. Urinary tract infection in persons with spinal cord injury. Arch Phys Med Rehab 1995; 76: 272.
21. Buczynski AZ: Urological complications in paraplegic and quadriplegic patients. New Med 1999; 89: 13–15.
22. Berger RE, Kessler D, Holmes KK. The etiology and manifestations of epididymitis in young men: correlations with sexual orientation. J Infect Dis 1987; 155: 1341.
23. McNaughton-Collins M, Stafford RS, O'Leary MP, Barry MJ. How common is prostatitis? A national survey of physician visits. J Urol 1998; 159: 1224–8.
24. Kaplan SA, Te AE, Jacobs BZ. Urodynamic evidence of vesical neck obstruction in men with misdiagnosed chronic nonbacterial prostatitis and the therapeutic role of endoscopic incision of the bladder neck. J Urol 1994; 152: 2063–5.
25. Weidner W, Schiefer HG, Krauss H et al. Chronic prostatitis: a thorough search for etiologically involved microorganisms in 461 patients. Infection 1991; 19: 119–25.
26. Weidner W, Ludwig M. Diagnostic management of chronic prostatitis. In: Weidner W, Madsen PO, Schiefer HG, eds. Prostatitis – Etiopathology, Diagnosis and Therapy. Berlin, Springer-Verlag, 1994; 158–74.
27. Stamey TA, Meares EMJ, Winningham DG. Chronic bacterial prostatitis and the diffusion of drugs into prostatic fluid. J Urol 1970; 103: 187–94.
28. Chancellor MB, Rivas DA. Current management of detrusor-sphincter dyssynergia. In: McGuire E, ed. Advances in Urology. Mosby, CV: St Louis, 1995: 291–324.
29. Talan DA, Stamm WE, Hooton TM et al. Comparison of ciprofloxacin (7 days) and trimethoprim-sulfamethoxazole (14 days) for acute uncomplicated pyelonephritis in women. JAMA 2000; 12: 1583.
30. Soulen MC, Fishman EK, Goldman SM et al. Bacterial renal infection: role of CT. Radiology 1989; 171: 703.

31. Chen Y, DeVivo MJ, and Roseman JM. Current trend and risk factors for kidney stones in persons with spinal cord injury: a longitudinal study. Spinal Cord 2000; 38: 346–53.
32. Takasaki E, Suzuki T, Honda M et al. Chemical compositions of 300 lower urinary tract calculi and associated disorders in the urinary tract. Urol Int 1995; 54: 89–94.
33. Nimkin K, Lebowitz RL, Share JC, Teele RL. Urolithiasis in a children's hospital from 1985 to 1990. Urol Radiol 1992; 14: 193–7.
34. Chen Y, DeVivo MJ, Stover SL, Lioyd LK. Recurrent kidney stone: a 25 year follow up study in persons with spinal cord injury. Urology 2002; 60: 228–32.
35. Ost MC, Lee BR. Urolithiasis in patients with spinal cord injuries: risk factors, management, and outcomes. Curr Opin Urol 2006; 16(2): 93–109.
36. Chen Y, DeVivo MJ, Lioyd LK. Bladder stone incidence in persons with spinal cord injury: determinants and trends, 1973–1996. Urology 2001; 58: 665–70.
37. Devivo MJ, Fine PR. Predicting renal calculus occurrence in spinal cord injury patients. Arch Phys Med Rehab 1986; 67: 722–5.
38. Hyeon KU, Jung TY, Lee JK, Park WH, Shim HB. Risk factors for urinary stone formation in men with spinal cord injury: a 17-year follow up study. BJU Int 2006; 97: 790–3.
39. Burr RG. Urinary calculi composition in patients with spinal cord lesions. Arch Phys Med Rehab 1978; 59: 84–9.
40. Nikakhter B, Vaziri ND, Khonsary F, Gordon S, Mirahmadi MD. Urolithiasis in patients with spinal cord injury. Paraplegia 1981; 19: 363–9.
41. Matlaga BR, Kim SC, Watkins SL et al. Changing composition of renal calculi in patients with neurogenic bladder. J Urol 2006; 175(5): 1716–9.
42. Donnellan SM and Bolton DM. The impact of contemporary bladder management techniques on struvite calculi associated with spinal cord injury. BJU Int 1999; 84: 280–7.
43. vanGool JD, deJong TP, Boemers TM. Effect of intermittent catheterization on urinary tract infection and incontinence in children with spina bifida. Monatsschr Kinderheilkd 1991; 193: 592–9.
44. Mardis HK, Parks JH, Muller G, Ganzel K, Coe FL. Outcome of metabolic evaluation and medical treatment for calcium nephrolithiasis in a private urological practice. J Urol 2004; 171: 85–93.
45. Vaidyanathan S, Singh G, Soni BM et al. Silent hydronephrosis/pyonephrosis due to upper urinary tract calculi in spinal cord injury patients. Spinal Cord 2000; 38: 331–8.
46. Park YI, Linsenmeyer TA. A method to minimize indwelling catheter calcification and bladder stones in individuals with spinal cord injury. J Spinal Cord Med 2001; 24: 105–8.
47. Robert M, Bennani A, Ohanna F et al. The management of upper urinary tract calculi by piezoelectric extracorporeal shock wave lithotripsy in spinal cord injury patients. Paraplegia 1995; 33: 132–5.
48. Niedrach WL, Davis RS, Tonetti FW, Cockett AT. Extracorporeal shock-wave lithotripsy in patients with spinal cord dysfunction. Urology 1991, 38: 152–6.
49. Stow DF, Bernstein JS, Madson KE, McDonald DJ, Ebert TJ. Autonomic hyperreflexia in spinal cord injured patients during extracorporeal shock wave lithotripsy. Anath Analg 1989; 68: 788–91.
50. Sugiama T, Fugelso P, Avon M. Extracorporeal shock wave lithotripsy in neurologically impaired patients. Semin Urol 1992; 10: 109–11.
51. DiLorenzo N, Maleci A, Williams BM. Severe exacerbation of post-traumatic syringomyelia after lithotripsy: case report. Paraplegia 1994; 32: 694–6.
52. Vespasiani G, Pesce F, Finazzi AE et al. Endoscopic ballistic lithotripsy in the treatment of bladder calculi in patients with neurogenic voiding dysfunction. Endourology 1996; 10: 551–4.
53. Vaidyanathan S, Singh G, Sett P, Soni BM. Complication of penile sheath drainage in a spinal cord injury patient: calculus impacting in the urethra proximal to the rim of a condom. Spinal Cord 2001; 39: 240–1.
54. Jeantet A, Thea A, Fernando U et al. Infectious nephrolithiasis: results of treatment with methenamine mandelate. Contr Nephrol 1987; 58: 233–5.
55. Jarrar K, Boedeker RH, Weidner W. Struvite stones: Long term follow up under metaphylaxis. Ann Urol 1996; 30(3): 112–17.
56. Wall I, Tieselius HG. Long term acidification of urine in patients treated for infected renal stones. Urol Int 1990; 45(4): 336–41.
57. Hess MJ, Zhan Eh, Foo DK, Yalla SV. Bladder cancer in patients with spinal cord injury. J Spinal Cord Med 2003; 26(4): 335–8.
58. van Velzen D, Kirshnan KR, Parsons KF et al. Comparative pathology of dome and trigone of urinary bladder mucosa in paraplegics and tetraplegics. Paraplegia 1995; 33: 565–72.
59. Bejany DE, Lockhart IL, Rhamy RK. Malignant vesical tumors following SCI. J Urol 1987; 138: 1390–2.
60. Groah SL, Weitzenkamp DA, Lammertse DP et al. Excess risk of bladder cancer in spinal cord injury: evidence for an association between indwelling catheter use and bladder cancer. Arch Phys Med Rehab 2002; 83: 346–51.
61. Vaidyanathan S, Mansour P, Soni BM, Singh G, Satt P. The method of bladder drainage in spinal cord injury patients may influence the histological changes in the mucosa of the neuropathic bladder – a hypothesis. BMC Urol 2002; 2: 5–11.
62. Navon JD, Soliman H, Khonsari F, Ahlering T. Screening cystoscopy and survival of SCI patients with squamous cell carcinoma of the bladder. J Urol 1997; 157: 2109–11.
63. Yang CC, Clowers TE. Screening cystoscopy in chronically catheterized SCI patients. Spinal Cord 1999; 37: 204–7.
64. Hamid R, Bycroft J, Arya M, Shah PJ. Screening cystoscopy and biopsy in patients with neuropathic bladder and chronic suprapubic indwelling catheter: is it valid? J Urol 2003; 170(2 Pt 1): 425–7.
65. Stonehill WH, Goldman HB, Dmochowski RR. The use of urine cytology for diagnosing bladder cancer in spinal cord injured patients. J Urol 1997; 157: 2112–14.
66. Lapides J, Diokno AC, Silber SJ et al. Clean intermittent self-catheterization in the treatment of urinary tract disease. J Urol 1972; 107(3): 458–16.

72

Complications related to neurogenic bladder dysfunction – II: reflux and renal insufficiency

Imre Romics, Antal Hamvas, and Attila Majoros

Introduction

After World War I, 80% of the spinal cord injury (SCI) patients died from urologic complications, mostly from urinary infection, which was untreatable at that time in the absence of antibiotics, and from secondary upper urinary tract damage.[1] Urodynamics being unknown, the accepted approach was the 'balanced bladder' method, i.e. if voiding took place with no or minimal residual urine, the patient's condition was considered satisfactory. With no information on intravesical pressures during storage and voiding, there was no way to prevent upper urinary tract damage resulting from lower tract dysfunction.[2]

Today, widespread use of antibiotics, anticholinergics, urodynamic evaluation, clean intermittent self-catheterization (CIC), and up-to-date management of urolithiasis have led to considerable improvements in life expectancy and, indeed, in the quality of life of SCI patients.

The deterioration of renal function and renal insufficiency, as its consequence, remained the most frequent late consequences of neurogenic bladder dysfunction, in spite of developments in investigations and therapy to this day. The causes of this are, primarily, the late establishment of a diagnosis, improper principles of treatment (in quite a few places, primarily in areas having improper healthcare infrastructure, for example, they apply the possibly worst solution: a permanent bladder catheter to remedy complaints in respect of voiding dysfunction of these patients), and the improper cooperation of patients. According to an epidemiologic study the neurogenic bladder dysfunction of paraplegic and meningomyelocelic (MMC) patients entails an increased risk from the point of the developing renal insufficiency when compared to the general population.[3] Urinary infections are still considered the most frequent complication in SCI patients and, without treatment, 40% of the patients will die of renal insufficiency.[4] Singhal and Mathew have found that, among the leading causes of death of spina bifida patients, renal insufficiency was the most frequent (33%).[5]

Pathophysiology of upper urinary tract damage caused by neurogenic bladder dysfunction

Abnormally high intravesical storage and/or voiding pressure may predispose to vesicoureteral reflux (VUR), urinary retention, and urinary infection, leading ultimately to renal insufficiency. The most frequent urologic abnormality associated with vesicoureteral reflux appears to be uninhibited bladder contraction. Koff et al found uninhibited detrusor contractions during the storage phase in the majority of neurologically normal children with recurrent urinary infections; nearly 50% of them had VUR, and 30% had an abnormal ureteric orifice but without VUR. Their findings were confirmed by the fact that, after reducing intravesical pressure with anticholinergic medication, 58% of urinary infections were cured without the use of antibiotics.[6]

Urinary infection in itself will increase intravesical pressure, reduce compliance, and weaken the ureterovesical junction, thus predisposing to reflux. The incidence of VUR in SCI patients varies between 17 and 25%, and can be found in 20% of neonates with MMC.[7–9] Soygur et al examined a group of children with reflux and without neurologic symptoms, noting unilateral reflux in 40.3% and bilateral reflux in 59.7%. Urodynamic evaluation revealed asymptomatic voiding dysfunction in 28% of the unilateral and in 72% of the bilateral reflux cases. This significant difference seems to indicate that bilateral reflux is caused by some (perhaps silent) voiding dysfunction, whereas unilateral reflux may be attributed in patients with intact bladder function to primary damage of the vesicoureteral junction.[10] Apart from high intravesical pressure, VUR may also be related directly to urinary infection and high-pressure bladder function. Retention, high intrapyelic pressure, and proliferation of mostly urease-producing microorganisms may lead to the formation of renal calculi, to hydronephrosis, pyonephrosis, and renal insufficiency. Intrapyelic pressure rises may cause pyelocaliceal reflux and reduce postglomerular blood flow, resulting in ischemic damage.[11] The drop in glomerular filtration rate (GFR) noticed at the end of puberty (<60 ml/min/1.73 m^2, but especially a value under 40) is a good precursor of end stage kidney failure. The pathophysiology is explained by a hyperfiltration type damage of the surviving nephrons.[12] Hypertonia and proteinuria also play a significant role in the deterioration of renal function and the development of renal insufficiency.[13] Rickwood et al did not notice hypertonia in MMC patients with unimpaired kidneys at 16 years old, however at the age of 20 they found hypertonia in 6% of all cases. In patients, in whose kidneys morphologic anomalies were seen already (renal scarring), hypertonia was found in 12% of all cases at 16 years old and 23% at 20.[14]

Gerridzen et al examined 140 SCI patients with voiding dysfunction and found detrusor hyperreflexia in 100 and areflexia in 40, with kidney damage in 16 and 7 patients, respectively. The 7 patients in the areflexic group with kidney damage showed significantly higher storage pressures (58 cmH_2O on average) than the rest of the same group (24 cmH_2O on average). In the hyperreflexic group, the 16 patients with kidney damage also showed significantly higher detrusor pressure values (115 cmH_2O on average) than the 84 patients with no renal impairment (72 cmH_2O on average). However, the pathologically high bladder pressures in this group were taken during the voiding phase.[15] High-pressure hyperreflexia was combined with detrusor-sphincter dyssynergia (DSD) in 55% of cases. In 4 of 23 patients, there was only radiographic evidence of kidney damage, 7 developed VUR, and 9 had hydronephrosis. Kidney damage from VUR was found in less than 1% of the cases.[15,16]

Dik et al performed follow-up studies on 144 children with spina bifida. In 69 cases they noticed overactive sphincter and in 61 cases overactive detrusor functions. They saw VUR in 27 cases; in 12 cases with an active and in 15 cases with an inactive sphincter. The latter fact also indicates that VUR is not necessarily a consequence of detrusor-sphincter dyssynergy (DSD). As a result of their regular control investigations, and their early treatment conserving renal function, after an average follow-up period of 81 months they noticed a drop in creatinine clearance in only 2 cases, or rather DMSA scintigraphy showed damage to the parenchyma in only 6 cases.[17]

Patients with neurogenic bladder dysfunction secondary to suprasacral lesions (injuries above the sacral micturition center) usually develop detrusor hyperreflexia with or without DSD. High-pressure values are measured during both the storage and the voiding phase, at more than 40 and 90 cmH_2O, respectively. This may be the consequence of protracted, intensive, uninhibited contractions, reduced bladder compliance, or functional (DSD) or organic (benign prostatic hyperplasia) urinary obstruction.[18–20] Therefore, the chances of upper tract damage are higher than in the case of lower motoneuron lesions (level of injury within or below the sacral micturition center). In this latter circumstance, the detrusor will be hypo- or areflexic, so that even with reduced bladder compliance, pathologically high pressure values will only appear during the storage phase. Among patients voiding spontaneously via reflex contractions and exhibiting normal pressure values, both in the storage and voiding phases, there are still a few who will show some degree of reflux or urinary retention.

Table 72.1 *Risk factors associated with kidney damage*

General risk factors:
Newborns
Old age
Immobilization
Diabetes mellitus
Immunosuppression
Polymorbidity
Neurologic risk factors:
Quadriplegia > paraplegia
Complete lesion > incomplete lesion

Linsenmeyer et al found 4 cases of VUR and 9 cases of upper tract dilatation in 84 patients voiding via reflex contraction. The only significant difference between the two groups was in the duration of the reflexly induced contractions.[21]

However, it does happen that an intially areflexic bladder decreases compliance and changes into a hyperreflexic state, which may lead to upper tract damage. This is suggested by the results of Jamil et al, who performed natural-fill urodynamics in 30 patients with indwelling catheters. Intravesical pressure rises of >40 cmH_2O were found in 11 and renal scarring in 9 patients, 6 of them from the high-pressure group.[22]

On the other hand, 'silent' voiding dysfunctions with no lower tract symptoms may also result in upper tract complications.[23,24]

Tables 72.1–72.3 summarize the risk factors that are associated with kidney damage.

Etiology of neurogenic bladder dysfunction leading to reflux and renal failure

Spinal cord injury

Spinal cord injury due to an accident, disc prolapse, acute myelitis, operation of thoracic aorta aneurysms, etc.,

Table 72.2 *Urologic abnormalities representing risk for kidney damage*
Urinary tract infection
Bladder outlet obstruction (BPH, stricture, etc.)
Urinary lithiasis
Bladder diverticulum
VUR with secondary reflux nephropathy
Foreign body in the urinary tract (catheter, urethral stent, etc.)

BPH, benign prostatic hypertrophy; VUR, vesicoureteral reflux.

Table 72.3 *Urodynamic abnormalities representing risk for kidney damage*
Decreased bladder compliance (<10 ml/cmH_2O)
LPP or storage pressure >40 cmH_2O
Reduced bladder capacity
Sustained high-pressure detrusor contraction
Voiding pressure >90 cmH_2O
DESD or detrusor-bladder neck dyssynergia
High postvoid residual (>30% of bladder capacity)

LPP, leak-point pressure; DESD, detrusor-external sphincter dyssynergia.

occurs in the United States approximately 12 000 times a year. Half of these victims end up quadriplegic, and the rest paraplegic, 53% with complete and 47% with incomplete lesions, half of the total number in the upper thoracal section above the 12th thoracic level, and 75% are male.[25] As a consequence, most SCI patients have a hyperreflexic bladder. Reports suggest a 7–32% incidence of renal lithiasis in SCI patients. Comarr and colleagues found an 8.2% incidence of renal lithiasis.[26] Hall et al examined 898 SCI patients after an average of 27 years, detecting renal calculi in 14.8%, in association with VUR in 37.7%, and without reflux in 10%.[27] Of those with renal calculi, 56.6% were on indwelling catheters. This contrasts with the 700 patients with no renal calculi, where only 28% were on indwelling catheters. They also found 261 patients with bladder stones, 17.7% of them combined with renal stones. There was no correlation with the prevalence of VUR. A review of this large population suggested three conclusions:

1. the incidence of renal calculi is significantly higher in patients with renal reflux
2. bladder stones and simultaneous reflux will not significantly increase the number of renal calculi
3. indwelling catheters significantly raise the incidence of renal and bladder stones.

The incidence of reflux among SCI patients varies from 5% to 23%.[15,16,26,27] Killorin et al reported upper tract damage in 7% of their SCI patients with areflexic bladder; 32% had hyperreflexic bladder, and there was no upper tract damage in those with normal detrusor function.[28]

Neural tube defects

Neural tube defects (spina bifida occulta, meningocele, MMC) are the most frequent reasons for bladder dysfunction in infancy. The prognosis of spina bifida is poor, however neurogenic bladder dysfunction (i.e. minor neural tube defects such as occult spinal dysraphism) does not develop in every child suffering from spina bifida. In Great Britain 60% of patients with MMC reach adulthood but the outlook for these patients is reduced. The risk of renal insufficiency is strongly associated with the sensory level. Renal failure is rare with sensory levels at or below L4 and common at or above T10.[12] In the majority of patients, the lumbar section (at the conus medullaris) is involved, resulting in an areflexic bladder and often an open bladder neck. Hydronephrosis is found in less than 10%, VUR in 16%, and bladder diverticuli in 23.5% of these newborns. Based on data in a pediatric myelodysplastic population, in 1981 McGuire et al described the correlation between storage pressure and chances of upper tract damage. He identified the so-called leak-point pressure (LPP) at which urine will leak at the urethral meatus, and showed the risk of upper tract damage to be high with LPP >40 cmH_2O, but significantly lower with LPP <40 cmH_2O. In the low LPP group, he observed no VUR and only two intravesicular diverticuli, in contrast to 68% VUR and 81% retention in the high LPP (>40 cmH_2O) group.[18] Beyond primary bladder dysfunction, age also plays a role in the development of renal insufficiency. Kidney damage was noticed in 18% of British children with neurogenic bladder before puberty, and in 30% of them following puberty.[14] As a result of early control and follow-up examinations, or rather of adequate therapy, a reduction in renal function was noticed in only 1.2–2.1% of children with MMC.[17,29]

Multiple sclerosis

Detrusor hyperreflexia is the leading anomaly in multiple sclerosis, which is often accompanied by DSD. Detrusor underactvity is rare. Lawrenson et al, in their epidemiologic study, did not detect a close correlation between multiple sclerosis and renal insufficiency compared to the normal population.[3]

Iatrogenic damage

Iatrogenic damage is associated with various perioperative complications, the most frequent of which are upper motoneuron lesions due to operations on aneurysms of the thoracic aorta or areflexic bladders resulting from peripheral neural lesions due to radical surgery of the pelvis. Both types of damage may lead to upper tract injury or deteriorated function.

Diagnosis of upper tract damage

Laboratory tests

Serum creatinine, urea nitrogen, serum bicarbonate, blood pH, urine pH, urine gravity and osmolarity, proteinuria, and cylindruria are good indicators of renal function.

Video-urodynamic examination

Storage and voiding pressure, maximum bladder capacity, bladder compliance, bladder neck condition, bladder configuration, detrusor-external sphincter or detrusor-bladder neck dyssynergia, and passive and/or active VUR are well documented with this test. It is essential for neurogenic bladders to be initially evaluated by video-urodynamics and to repeat the test at least on an annual basis (Madersbacher, personal communication), because bladder dysfunction may change later on. In myelodysplasia, for instance, areflexic bladder dysfunction is likely to change with time to hyperreflexia.[30] In other cases (e.g. control of bladder compliance in MMC), conventional urodynamics without video control may be all that is needed for follow-up.

Bauer et al proposed possibly the earliest urodynamic examination of the newborn with MMC, following the closure of the spinal defect, in order to establish bladder function or rather the sphincter's functioning. On the basis of the results obtained, and according to the risk of upper urinary tract damage, the patients were divided into three groups and the authors proposed regular urodynamic examinations.[31] Hopps et al[29] divided the patients, according to basic investigations (history, physical examination, urine culture, and renal ultrasound) performed on newborns into high- (hydronephrosis, urinary retention) and low-risk groups. In the case of high-risk patients they performed an immediate urodynamic examination and started adequate (CIC, antibiotics, anticholinergics) treatment. They closely followed up both cohorts and performed regular basic examinations (in the case of high-risk patients, they performed urodynamic examinations if needed). In cases where urinary tract infection caused fever, VUR, urinary retention, and hydronephrosis the low-risk patients were transferred to the high-risk group and later on were treated accordingly. By application of the above principles, Hopps et al were successful in retaining renal function even without the use of regular, invasive urodynamic investigations.

Urodynamic investigations performed on a routine basis also entail the risk of introducing errors. A rapid filling speed applied during cystometry may lead to an increase in LPP and a drop in compliance. It may thus lead to an unnecessary 'overtreatment'. Ultrasound has been proved to be an adequate method of follow-up in the assessment of retained renal function in children with spina bifida.[17,32]

Ultrasonography

This is the simplest and least-invasive way to gather information on vesicoureteral dilatation, nephrolithiasis, renal parenchyma thickness, and residual urine. Urine transport abnormalities, both functional (or the nonobstructive type, e.g. VUR, brimming bladder, overhydrated condition, acute pyelonephritis) and organic (or the obstructive type, e.g. stones, strictures), are easily detected using frusemide (frusemide).

The Doppler technique can define the arterial resistance index. Increased arterial resistance index values are present even before actual dilatation of the collecting system has appeared. Values of 0.7 or more are indications of obstruction. The color Doppler technique demonstrates reflux with no X-ray exposure: a transducer directed toward the ureteral orifices will image retrograde flow in the ureter as a colored jet. Virgili et al sonographed 115 SCI patients and found upper tract anomalies (vesicorenal dilatation, chronic pyelonephritis) in 21.7% of them.[33] Calenoff et al compared ultrasonography with conventional intravenous urograms in 54 SCI patients and observed that all abnormalities seen on intravenous urograms (retention in 36% and VUR in 56% of cases) can also be detected by ultrasonography. They suggested the use of ultrasonography for follow-up rather than intravenous urography.[34] Ozer et al used ultrasonography in a prospective study to screen SCI patients with no urologic symptoms and reported that upper tract abnormalities which needed therapeutic intervention were only detected in symptomatic patients. Therefore, they did not recommend ultrasonography for large-scale preventive early diagnosis in asymptomatic patients.[35] Bih et al compared ultrasonographic results before and after micturition and noted that upper tract ultrasonography performed on a full bladder was more likely to show urine transport abnormalities.[36] During the follow-up of 144 children with MMC, the ultrasound test, compared with DMSA (dimercaptosuccinyl) renal scan, failed to indicate parenchymalesion (renal scarring), a sign of reduced function, in no more than 4 cases.[17]

Intravenous urography

Intravenous urography is considered to be the gold standard for the detection of upper tract abnormalities due to neurogenic bladder dysfunction. Even if it involves X-ray exposure and possible allergic reactions to the contrast material (very rare, though, today with tri-iodides), the fact remains that this is the most reliable source of information on the morphology and, to some extent, also on the function of the upper urinary tract. In cases of renal damage, it will provide the following information: focal or diffuse atrophy of the parenchyma; dilated, bulky calices; and decreased excretion of the contrast material. In a report by Heidler, in cases of VUR, 30% of the urograms were negative, 5% showed ureteral dilatation, 25% renal scars and calyceal dilatation, 10% cortical atrophy, and 30% a nonfunctioning kidney.[20] Rutuu et al performed 206 intravenous urograms on 119 patients with neurogenic bladder dysfunction and detected 42% upper tract abnormalities, mostly delayed renal emptying. Among patients with pathologic urograms, 40% had at least one acute urinary infection episode within the last year, whereas among those with no pathologic signs in their urograms, the incidence was only 8%.[37] Rao et al compared secretory urography and ultrasonography in a prospective study of 202 asymptomatic SCI patients to assess their respective effectiveness in diagnosing upper tract damage. Hydronephrosis was detected by urography in 100% of cases vs 86% by ultrasonography; for renal stones, the detection ratios were 87 and 78%, and for signs of chronic pyelonephritis, 100 and 25%, respectively. However, the discrepancy decreased if ultrasonography was combined with plain X-rays of the abdomen.[38]

Cystography and voiding cystourethrography

Cystography at bladder capacity will show low-pressure or passive reflux, in contrast to the Valsalva maneuver, made during micturition effort, which will provide information on high-pressure or active reflux. The same results are, however, available also by video-urodynamic testing, which gives exact intravesical pressure values for storage and voiding, while imaging the bladder filled with contrast material will reveal VUR, if any (Figure 72.1). The same applies to intravenous urography (provided that all contrast material has been discharged from the kidneys). Stover et al studied the influence of retrograde cystography on excretory urograms when the former was performed immediately before the latter. They showed that iatrogenic dilatation, indistinguishable from true pathologic dilatation of the upper tract, occurred in patients with upper motor neuron lesions when intravenous urography was conducted immediately after cystography. They suggested a time delay between the two examinations to avoid this artifact.[39]

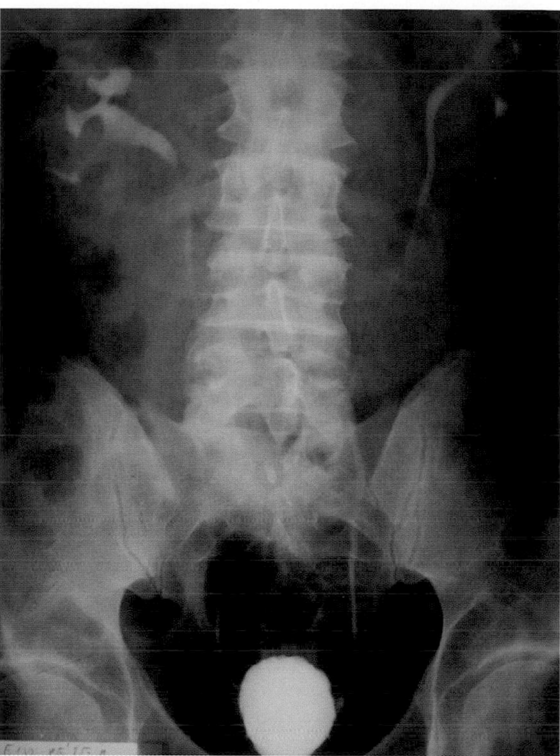

Figure 72.1
Bilateral vesico-ureteral reflux. Retrograde cystogram demonstrating bilateral vesico-ureteral reflux in a 48-year-old spinal cord injured male patient with detrusor-external sphincter dyssynergia.

Renal scintigraphy

The renal isotope technetium 99m glucoheptonate defines renal function quantitatively and also helps to differentiate obstructive from nonobstructive types of uropathy (Figure 72.2). Scintigraphy, a dynamic imaging technique, is highly sensitive in depicting minute renal lesions, but is less specific for any given renal pathology. Fabrizio et al used it with good effect in acute septic conditions of SCI patients to identify a urologic cause of the sepsis. Scintigrams localized the renal damage every time when fever was due to a urologic condition.[40] Although parenchymal lesions can be indicated in a very sensitive manner by DMSA scintigraphy, in the case of normal serum creatinine levels and normal untrasound findings its routine use in the follow-up of children with meningocele is not advised.[17]

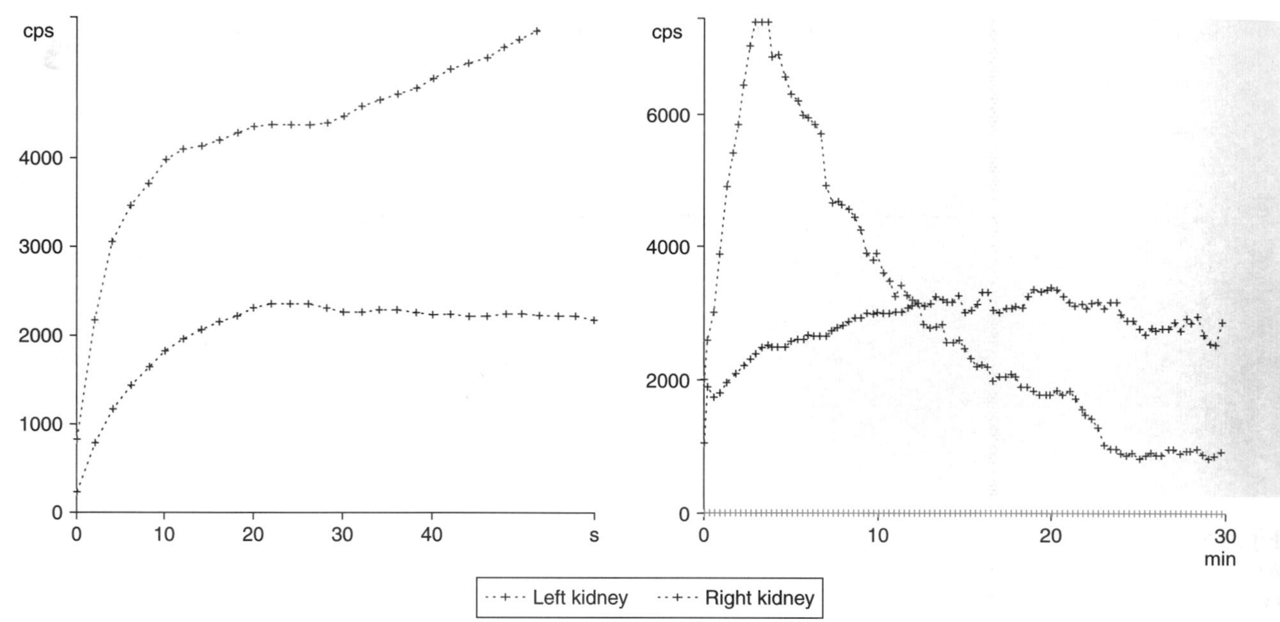

Figure 72.2
Renal scintigraphy. Neurogenic bladder dysfunction in a 30-year-old female patient with thoracic meningomyelocele. Right kidney perfusion is prolonged (left diagram) and excretion on the same side is delayed (right diagram).

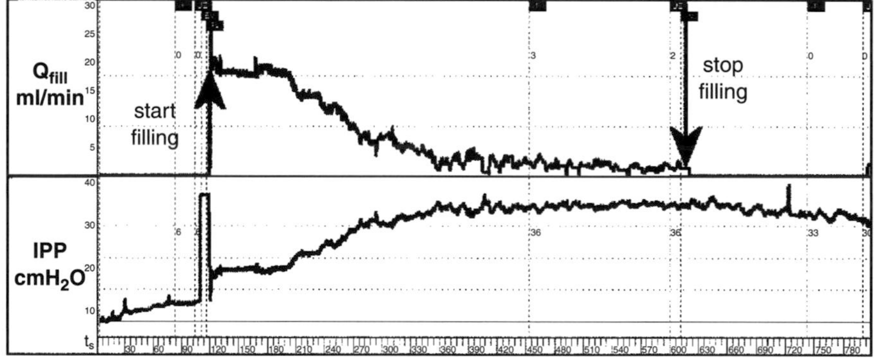

Figure 72.3
Urodynamic tracing of the upper urinary tract. Neurogenic bladder dysfunction with thickening of the bladder wall, responsible for the obstruction of the uretero-vesical junction in a 30-year-old male patient. Reaching steady state at external filling, the flow rate is reduced and intrapelvic pressure is markedly elevated. Qfill, filling rate; IPP, intrapelvic pressure.

Urodynamics of upper urinary tract

In cases when we see a dilatation of the upper urinary tract and the existence of an obstruction is uncertain, in order to quantitatively evaluate a possible dilation of the pyelon without an obstruction, or a high-pressure voiding alongside a partial obstruction, we perform a urodynamic examination of the upper urinary tract.

There is no need for an invasive intervention if, because of an obstruction, we have already placed a nephrostomic catheter. In cases like this, the catheter may be used to perform the examination. The practical benefit of this examination is the possibility of making a safe decision on removing the earlier placed percutaneous nephrostomy. In certain selected cases involving diagnostic difficulties, creation of a nephrostomy in order to perform urodynamic investigation is only minimally invasive (ultrasound-guided puncture of the kidney pyelon).

The earlier described pressure–flow studies in the upper urinary tract applied either a constant intrapyelar perfusion velocity[41] or a constant filling pressure.[42] These either record measures partly in the nonphysiologic realm, or they investigate a single pair of pressure–flow values and hence only offer static information.[41,42] In recent years, Lovász developed a dynamic examination of the correlation between flow and pressure by raising the filling pressure in several steps (Figure 72.3). He calculated the obstruction coefficient from the resulting pressure–flow curves to obtain the rate of obstruction in a quantitative form.[43]

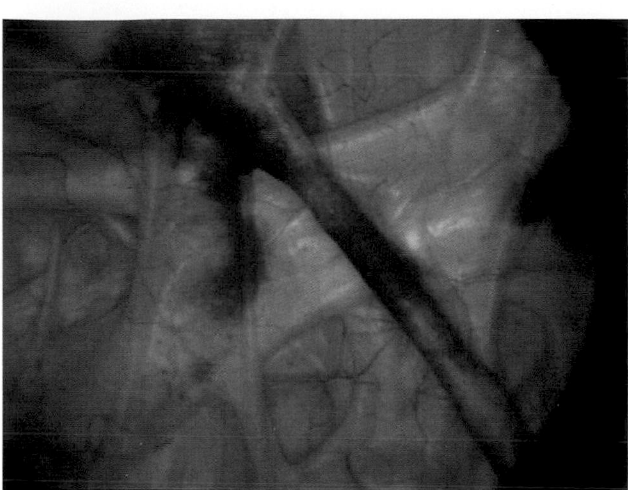

Figure 72.4
A significant degree of bladder wall trabeculation on cystoscopy may indicate bladder wall thickening.

Cystoscopy

Cystoscopy plays an important role in differentiating functional from organic lower tract obstructions in patients with upper tract abnormalities. For this group of patients, it is advisable to use a flexible cystoscope, considering the frequent occurrence of sphincter spasticity. A significant degree of bladder wall trabeculation (Figure 72.4) may represent thickening of the bladder wall and be responsible for the obstruction of the vesico-ureteral junction.

Therapy

The principal aim of neurogenic bladder dysfunction treatment is the maintenance of renal function. This requires successful and complete rehabilitation of the lower urinary tract, which means a complete and concerted neurourologic intervention. The maintenance or creation of a low-pressure reservoir with no residual urine, the control of urinary infection, and the avoidance of an indwelling catheter are all measures that will promote the main goal, which is upper tract protection. Together with the adequate control of continence, they will ensure quality of life improvement as well. Whenever possible, a program of CIC should be implemented, but this demands some manual dexterity from the patient. After a well-designed rehabilitation program, even quadriplegics may be able to use CIC, if not via the urethra, then at least via a continent abdominal stoma. Therapeutic measures may be divided into acute intervention, to avoid some imminent complication, or elective treatment, fitting into the long-term management program.

Treatment of acute conditions

Lower urinary tract drainage

In the acute phase of SCI and cerebrovascular injuries, the so-called spinal or cerebral shock that will develop is characterized by an areflexic bladder. At this stage, the main goal is to avoid overflow incontinence. The condition will improve within 2–12 weeks, but in the meantime, until CIC (operated by the patient or nursing caregiver) can be implemented, continuous bladder drainage must be assured.[30] If no contraindication exists, a suprapubic cystostomy should be done with ultrasonographic guidance. A thin 8–10F catheter is recommended. If suprapubic catheterization is not possible, an indwelling urethral catheter should be introduced for the shortest possible duration. Silicone tubes are recommended, size 14–16F for females and 12–14F for males.[44]

Upper urinary tract drainage

If, after successful lower tract drainage, upper tract dilatation still exists (bladder wall fibrosis, stricture, stone), causing renal dysfunction, then percutaneous nephrostomy must be done. When the existence of an upper urinary tract obstruction is in doubt, we clarify the issue by performing a urodynamic investigation of the upper urinary tract.

Hemodialysis

If the upper tract passage is free but renal failure persists or progresses, acute dialysis may be necessary.

Antibiotic treatment

Urinary tract infections combined with urosepsis require an antimicrobial treatment.[19]

Nephrectomy

Nephrectomy may become necessary if a septic condition (acute pyelonephritis, renal abscess, etc.) is maintained in spite of adequate drainage and appropriate antibiotics.

Conservative treatments

Spontaneous micturition

Spontaneous micturition is advisable after reflex contraction of the detrusor in response to the Credé maneuver or to various trigger mechanisms, only if intravesical pressure values are below 40 cmH_2O during the storage phase and less than 90 cmH_2O during the voiding phase, if residual urine is less than 30% of cystometric bladder capacity, and if bladder capacity is more than 200 ml. Lower tract obstruction, DSD, VUR, and reduced bladder compliance constitute contraindications for this approach. Reflex micturition usually means incontinence, and, therefore, the use of absorbent pads or, for males, urinary condoms, is indicated. However, 70% of patients using condom catheters are reported to suffer from chronic urinary infection. Skin problems are often due to allergic reactions to latex.[19,44]

Urine drainage

Drainage may be indicated in any form of bladder dysfunction: in the case of detrusor hyperreflexia, to maintain low bladder pressure (kidney protection) and continence; in the case of DSD, to eliminate the obstruction; in the case of areflexia, to eliminate any residual urine; in the case of decreased compliance, to reduce bladder pressure.

Intermittent catheterization This technique was introduced in the 1940s by Sir Ludwig Guttman to clear the bladder in SCI patients during the spinal shock phase.[45] In 1972, Lapides et al suggested CIC for patients with neurogenic bladders. Follow-up in 66 patients showed no upper tract alteration.[46] Among 85 SCI patients using CIC, Nanninga et al found 28 incidents of upper tract damage, detrusor hyperreflexia, and DSD in subjects presumed to have areflexic bladders.[47] This study emphasizes once again the importance of regular urodynamic follow-up in such patients. Three patients had sphincterotomy, 15 needed more frequent catheterization, and 10 failed to cooperate and so had to be placed on indwelling catheter drainage.[47] Mollard et al, from Paris, reported on 50 CIC cases. They found that girls and young boys accepted CIC better than did adolescent males.[48] Brem et al studied renal dysfunction and structural abnormalities in 28 children with meningocele on CIC. They reported VUR in 9 cases, renal dysfunction in 14%, and bacteriuria in 38%. They concluded that complications occurred in those patients who had small, noncompliant, trabeculated bladders.[49]

CIC has its own complications. Urinary infection is the most frequent, but urethral damage, stricture, and autonomous dysreflexia have also been noted. Kuhn et al reported a 5-year follow-up of 22 patients on CIC, with sterile urine in 23%, *Escherichia coli* infection in 36.5%, and other pathogenic bacteria *(Pseudomonas, Proteus, Klebsiella)* in another 36% of patients. They found urethral stricture in 1 patient, and autonomous dysreflexia in another. There was no upper tract damage. None of the patients was on anticholinergics, alpha-blockers, or on any continuous antibiotic prophylaxis.[50]

McGuire and Savastano compared patients on CIC for 2–12 years with those on indwelling catheters, finding significantly less acute urinary infections, bladder stones, and episodes of autonomic dysreflexia in the CIC group.[51] According to Madersbacher's experience, 20% of CIC patients had urethral complications, 40% had intermittent and 30% chronic urinary infections, whereas 30% had permanently sterile urine (Madersbacher, personal communication).

For intermittent catheterization, we may use PVC catheters with a lubricant that contains some anesthetics, or with a hydrophilic coating, size 12–14F for males and 14–16F for females. The control of fluid intake is important: no more than 2000 ml per day. In the case of a normally compliant bladder, catheterization should be repeated 4–6 times a day. However, the catheter should be passed before the amount of urine in the bladder reaches 500 ml. In the case of decreased bladder compliance, urodynamic studies will indicate at what volume the bladder pressure reaches the critical level of 40 cmH_2O. The frequency of catheterization should be adjusted, so that this critical intravesical pressure is not reached. It should also be kept in mind that the more frequent the catheterizations, the less frequent is the incidence of urinary infections, and vice versa. Antibiotic prophylaxis is not unanimously recommended: there are some physicians who would only give antibiotics in the case of acute urinary infections, whereas others advocate prophylactic administration of small doses of varied antibiotic types.[44]

Indwelling bladder catheters They are the worst solution and should only be used as a last resort. If possible, it should be a suprapubic diversion to eliminate urethral complications, particularly in males. In females, simultaneous surgical closure of the bladder neck is often required to ensure continence. Regular daily care of the catheter, together with changing it every 4 or 6 weeks (silicone catheters), is necessary. Although it seems to be a contradiction, several authors confirmed the occurrence of high bladder pressures, even in the chronically catheterized, a consequence of decreasing compliance. Jamil et al found storage pressures of more than 40 cmH_2O in 11, and renal damage in 9 of 30 patients on indwelling catheters, renal damage presenting merely in the high-pressure group.[22]

Chao et al compared the upper tract situation of 41 patients on CIC and 32 on indwelling catheters, noting a statistically higher number of renal damage and radiologic alterations in the second group.[52] The most frequent complications were ever-present urinary infection, urethral damage and strictures, urethro-cutaneous fistulae, epididymitis, and bladder stones. In a retrospective study of a large SCI population, Hall et al found a 56.6% renal stone and 62.5% bladder stone incidence in patients on indwelling catheters.[27] They recommended prophylactic administration of small doses of varied antibiotic types.

Temporary urethral stents They are an alternative to indwelling catheters. The Nissenkorn polyurethane or the Urolume endourethral Wallstent prosthesis may be placed at the level of the external sphincter under local anesthesia. According to published reports, within 6 months after placement of the stents there was no evidence of upper tract damage. Migration and secondary bladder neck obstruction were noted in 27% of patients. After a certain period of time the temporary stents were removed, and a final solution implemented. This is a less invasive and, to some extent, a more reversible solution than sphincterectomy.[53,54]

In summary, whenever possible, the best method of managing the neurogenic bladder is CIC, which will provide regular emptying of a low-pressure bladder and often insure continence as well. At the same time, it will protect the upper tract. It may be combined, if necessary, with medication (overactive bladder), sphincterotomy (DSD), artificial sphincter implantation (reduced sphincter function), or bladder augmentation cystoplasty (reduced capacity, restricted compliance that fails to respond to other conservative treatments). Even in children with a neurogenic bladder dysfunction, renal function can be retained for longer if the condition is diagnosed immediately after birth and the necessary treatments are started at the earliest opportunity. Owing to early treatment, Dik et al only noticed 6 cases of impaired renal function in the course of treating 144 children with spina bifida.[17] Indwelling urethral catheters mean permanent urinary infection and several complications; they do not necessarily entail a low-pressure reservoir and often lead to renal damage. They should only be used as a last resort; urethral stents may serve as a temporary solution.

Dietetic treatment

Avoidance of alcohol and spices and also urine acidification may help to prevent urinary infections; a low-protein diet may be indicated in renal dysfunction.

Medication

Hyperreflexia In detrusor hyperreflexia medication is targeted to eliminate, or at least to decrease, reflex contractions, to normalize high-pressure bladder dysfunction, and to improve the effectiveness of intermittent catheterization. Oral anticholinergics, spasmolytics, and mixed-action products (oxybutynin, propiverine, trospium chloride, tolterodine, solifenacin, darifenacin) are meant to increase bladder capacity and to reduce detrusor contractility, but since they have considerable side-effects (dry mouth, troubled vision, arrhythmia), they are not readily tolerated by many patients. Oxybutynin is the standard medication in the United States, but 61% of patients do not tolerate it orally, while it is ineffective in 48%. Intravesical oxybutynin solution is more easily tolerated, has fewer side-effects, and the same efficacy on the detrusor.[11,44,55] Among the antimuscarinic drugs introduced recently, darifenacin shows the greatest M_3 receptor (urinary bladder) selectivity. Thus, while being an effective treatment it has minimal side-effects (dry mouth and constipation).[56] Intravesically administered capsaicin and resiniferatoxin provide permanent receptor blockade for 2–7 months, increasing bladder compliance and intravesical pressure while protecting kidney function with no systemic side-effects (except for autonomic dysreflexia, which may occur sometimes).[44] Schurch was the first to use local injections of botulinum toxin A (BTX-A) to treat detrusor overactivity of neurogenic origin. Among patients treated with either 200 or 300 U BTX-A, 89% became continent.[57] In a systematic review of the literature, more than 600 patients with neurogenic detrusor overactivity treated with botulinum toxin have been reported.[58] The maximal cystometric capacity and the reflex volume were increased and maximal detrusor pressure during the voiding phase and the frequency of incontinent episodes were decreased. The first placebo-controlled multicenter randomized controlled trial with botulinum toxin in patients with neurogenic detrusor overactivity was also published by Schurch et al.[59] Karsenty et al found no change in efficacy or safety by decreasing the number of injection sites.[60]

Areflexia In areflexia, we may try cholinergic agents (bethanecol), but there is not much to expect from them, partly because of poor intestinal absorption and partly because they act simultaneously on the bladder, bladder neck, and urethra, so that they do not decrease outlet resistance.

Intravesical electrostimulation

This method was developed by Katona in 1959 to ameliorate bladder emptying by strengthening the detrusor reflex and simultaneously improving bladder sensation and compliance.[61]

Elective surgery

Surgical treatments cause irreversible changes. Therefore, they should only be used if other conservative treatments will not achieve a low-pressure reservoir, effective protection of the upper urinary tract, and/or continence.

Denervation techniques

Surgical or chemical interference with the nerve fibers of the pelvic plexus will increase bladder capacity, reduce reflex incontinence, and improve compliance. Injective techniques imply locally injected anesthesic agents or phenol (the latter being irreversible). The early results with phenol are generally very good, but, after a year or so, the symptoms will relapse in about 80% of patients. Also, many complications (fistulae, complete areflexia) have been reported; therefore, this technique has been virtually abandoned.[11]

Bladder transection through the entire thickness of the detrusor above the trigone will also increase bladder capacity. Early cure rates are reported to be 74%, but after 5 years the success rate goes down to 65%.[16] Intradural posterior root rhizotomy combined with the implantation of an extradural anterior root stimulator is the most frequently used method.[62,63] Rhizotomy will suppress bladder spasticity, normally low-pressure storage will be achieved, and voiding can be programmed through the anterior root nerve stimulator.

Brindley et al reported on the first 50 implantations in 1986: 60% of patients were continent. Deafferentation was not yet done routinely in every case at that time.[62] Sauerwein tried this method in 45 patients from 1986 to 1989: 95% were cured from hyperreflexia, 91% became continent, and 84% were spontaneous voiders. Postoperatively, 6 patients showed low-pressure reflux, which was corrected by antireflux surgery. No renal damage was noted.[64] Schurch et al reported that implantation of a Brindley stimulator cured reflex incontinence, while increasing bladder compliance and reducing postvoid residual urine volume from an average of 340 ml to 140 ml: VUR disappeared in 3 and was improved in 2 patients.[65] Egon et al implanted the stimulator in 93 patients, 82 of whom became continent and 83 became spontaneous voiders. Before surgery, 3 had had VUR, which disappeared after the intervention.[66]

Bladder augmentation techniques

Augmentation techniques should only be used when bladder compliance is reduced because of organic causes.

Autoaugmentation This technique is a means of partial myectomy, i.e. the detrusor muscle is excised from the upper half of the bladder, which will then dilate, forming a diverticulum. Follow-up results after 5 years show a success rate of 65%. This surgery is easier to perform than conventional intestinal augmentation, and no postoperative carcinoma is to be feared, but there is a high risk of intraoperative mucosal tear. The bladder takes a long time, almost 1 year, to expand sufficiently, so that in the meantime 45% of patients have to be put on intermittent catheterization. As a result of a lower intravesical pressure decrease than that found in intestinal augmentation, the risk of renal damage is somewhat higher.[67,68]

Enterocystoplasty This technique is indicated in patients with small bladder capacity, reduced compliance, and renal damage, or incontinence between catheterizations, should the condition be refractory to medication. Augmentation can be done either with the small or the large intestine. The patient may develop metabolic acidosis and runs the risk of intestinal carcinoma due to urine contact with the bowel mucosa. The intestine to be used must first be detubularized. In ileum augmentation, the reported success rate is 52–80%, but 20% of patients need to be put on intermittent catheterization due to increased residual urine volume.[30,67] Flood et al evaluated the results of 122 augmentation cystoplasties performed during an 8-year period on patients with reduced bladder compliance (77%), or refractory detrusor hyperreflexia/instability (23%). The clinical diagnosis in over 50% of cases was neuropathic bladder dysfunction (28% SCI, 23% myelodysplasia). They performed detubularized ileal augmentation in 67% of the patients, detubularized ileocecocystoplasty in 30%, and detubularized sigmoid in 3%. Seventy-five percent of patients were cured, and 20% improved. The reported complications included bladder stones in 21%, incontinence in 13%, and pyelonephritis in 11% of these patients. The reoperation rate was 16%.[69] Renal insufficiency is a relative contraindication for this type of surgery.

Supravesical diversion

Supravesical stomas are made if urethral catheterization is not viable, augmentation cystoplasty fails, or if there is an infiltrating bladder tumor. Incontinent stomas (ileal or colonic conduit) mean less comfort than continent stomas. Brem et al created ileal conduits in 14 children with MMC, and found ureteral reflux in all patients after the intervention, with renal dysfunction in 28% and bacteriuria in 70%.[49] Continent stomas (Mitrofanoff, Koch pouch, Mainz I, II pouch) induce fewer upper tract complications. The most important complications are stomal stenosis, catheterization difficulty, stone formation in the pouch, and incontinence (i.e. incompetence of the continent stoma).

Antireflux surgery

Reflux in neurogenic bladder dysfunction is mostly the result of high intravesical pressures, large residual urine volumes, poor bladder capacity, restricted compliance, or serious urinary infections. Antireflux surgery by itself will not be the unique solution in the majority of cases, as it does not decrease bladder pressure or improve compliance and capacity. Therefore, this type of surgery is mostly done in combination with some other surgical intervention.

The less-invasive endoscopic method to correct VUR consists of submucosal bulking agent injection at the ureteral orifice, but the reflux resolution following endoscopic therapy is lower as compared to contemporary reports of open surgical correction. It seems that Deflux (a dextranomer/hyaluronic acid copolymer) and Macroplastique (polymethysiloxane) are safer than bovine collagen and Teflon.[70] A recent meta-analysis of endoscopic therapy revealed resolution of reflux in 79% of ureters with grade I and II, 72% with grade III, and 65% with grade IV reflux after one injection of bulking agent.[71] Silveri et al administered endoscopic injections in 15 children with MMC and performed open surgery in 2. Follow-up results showed renal failure in 8 cases.[23] Casals et al pointed out that the endoscopic method is fast, simple, and repeatable.[72]

Today open surgery still remains the gold standard procedure to treat VUR.[70] The success rate of open surgery is 80–95%. The Lich–Gregoir method consists of elongating the intramural portion of the distal ureter by burying a 3–4 cm segment between the bladder mucosa and the detrusor muscle via an entirely extravesical route. A success rate of more than 98% has been claimed by Heimbach et al.[73] The Politano–Leadbetter antireflux procedure, which consists of elongating of the submucosal portion of the refluxing ureter, is probably used most widely. The Cohen method is mainly undertaken to correct bilateral reflux, with the ureters crossing each other on the midline through a submucous tunnel. Burbidge compared the results of the two latter techniques and found an equal success rate (97–98%) for both types of repairs.[74]

Sphincterotomy

This type of intervention is only indicated in males with high-pressure storage due to a DSD causing upper tract deterioration. The intervention reduces LPP theoretically to zero. The resulting incontinence may be managed by a condom catheter. Sphincterotomy is performed particularly when CIC is not possible (e.g. in quadriplegics). Upper tract abnormalities and VUR respond favorably to sphincterotomy in 70–90% of cases.[75] The 12 o'clock incision suggested by Madersbacher involves fewer complications than conventional 3 or 9 o'clock incisions (lower risk of bleeding and postoperative erectile dysfunction).[76]

Nephrectomy

Nonfunctioning kidneys with pyelonephritis or hydronephrosis, especially if they cause hypertension, should eventually be removed.

Transplantation

Following nephrectomy a patient will need regular dialysis treatments. The patient's quality of life will improve significantly if, following a successful transplantation, he becomes independent on the dialysis center once again. If the lower urinary tract is inappropriate for implantation of a donor kidney, at least 6 to 10 weeks before the transplantation a proper reconstruction (augmentatio, urinary conduit, etc.) should be performed.[77] Power et al gave an account of the greatest number of transplantations performed on spina bifida patients. They found a graft survival rate of 80.8% in 1 year, and for 5 years this number was 72.7%.[78] While other authors indicated 5% as the number of surgical complications in nonselected, normal cases, this share in the case of transplantations performed alongside urinary diversion was 12–19%.[79]

References

1. Graham SD. Present urological treatment of spinal cord injury patients. J Urol 1981; 126: 1–4.
2. Bors E. Neurogenic bladder. Urol Surg 1957; 7: 177–250.
3. Lawrenson R, Wyndaele JJ, Vlachonikolis I, Farmer C, Glickman S. Renal failure in patients with neurogenic lower urinary tract dysfunction. Neuroepidemiology 2001; 20(2): 138–43.
4. Donelly J, Hackler RH, Bunts RC. Present urologic status of the World War II paraplegic: 25-year follow-up. Comparison with status of the 20-year Korean war paraplegic and 5-year Vietnam paraplegic. J Urol 1972; 108: 558–62.
5. Singhal B, Mathew KM. Factors affecting mortality and morbidity in adult spina bifida. Eur J Pediatr Surg 1999; (Suppl 1): 31–2.
6. Koff SA, Lapides J, Piazza DH. Association of urinary tract infection and reflux with uninhibited bladder contractions and voluntary sphincteric obstruction. J Urol 1979; 122: 373–6.
7. Cosbie-Ross J. Vesico-ureteric reflux in the neurogenic bladder. Br J Surg 1965; 52: 161–7.
8. Thomas DG, Lucas MG. The urinary tract following spinal cord injury. In: Chisholm GD, Fair WR, eds. Scientific Foundations of Urology. Chicago: Year Book Medical, 1990: 289–99.
9. Light K, Bleik JP. Causes of renal deterioration in patients with meningomyelocele. Br J Urol 1977; 49: 257–60.
10. Soygur T, Arikan N, Yesilli C, Gogus O. Relationship among voiding dysfunction and vesicoureteral reflux and renal scars. Urology 1999; 54: 905–8.
11. Madersbacher H. Neurogene Harninkontinenz. In: Höfner K, Jonas U, eds. Praxisratgeber Harninkontinez. Bremen: UNI-MED Verlag AG, International Medical Publishers, 2000: 221–30.
12. Woodhouse CRJ. Myelomeningocele in young adults. BJU Int 2005; 95: 223–30.
13. Wingen AM, Fabian-Bach C, Schaefer F, Mehls O. Randomised multicentre study of a low-protein diet on the progression of chronic renal failure in children, European Study Group of Nutritional Treatment of Chronic Renal Failure in Childhood. Lancet 1997; 349: 1117–23.
14. Rickwood AMK, Hodgson J, Lonton AP, Thomas DG. Medical and surgical complications in adolescent and young adult patients with spina bifida. Health Trends 1984; 16: 91–5.
15. Gerridzen RJ, Thijssen AM, Dehoux E. Risk factors for upper tract deterioration in chronic spinal cord injury patients. J Urol 1992; 147: 416–18.
16. Mundy AR. Vesicouretheric reflux in adults. In: Whitfield HN, Hendy WF, Kirby RS, Duchet JW, eds. Textbook of Genitourinary Surgery. Oxford: Blackwell Science, 1998: 440–7.
17. Dik P, Klijn AJ, van Gool JD, de Jong-de Vos van Steenwijk CCE, de Jong TPVM. Early start to therapy preserves kidney function in spina bifida patients. Eur Urol 2006; 49: 908–13.

18. McGuire EJ, Woodside JR, Borden TA, Weiss RM. Prognostic value of urodynamic testing in myelodysplastic patients. J Urol 1981; 126: 205–9.
19. Society of German Urologists. Guideline for urological treatment of spinal cord injured patients, 1998.
20. Heidler H. Neurogene Blasenfunktionsstörungen. In: Altwein J, Rübben H, eds. Urologie. Ferdinand Enke Verlag Stuttgart, Heinz Neubert GmbH Druckerei Bayreuth, 1993: 379–94.
21. Linsenmeyer TA, Bagaria SP, Gendron B. The impact of urodynamic parameters on the upper tracts of spinal cord injured men who void reflexly. J Spin Cord Med 1998; 21: 15–20.
22. Jamil F, Williamson M, Ahmed YS, Harrison SC. Natural fill urodynamics in chronically catheterized patients with spinal cord injury. BJU Int 1999; 83: 396–9.
23. Silveri M, Capitanucci ML, Capozza N et al. Occult spinal dysraphism: neurogenic voiding dysfunction and long term urologic follow-up. Pediatr Surg Int 1997; 12: 148–50.
24. Vaidyanathan S, Singh G, Soni BM et al. Silent hydronephrosis/pyonephrosis due to upper urinary tract calculi in spinal cord injury patients. Spinal Cord 2000; 38: 661–8.
25. DeVivo MJ, Rutt RD, Black KJ et al. Trends in spinal cord injury demographics and treatment outcomes between 1973 and 1986. Arch Phys Med Rehab 1992; 73: 424–30.
26. Comarr AE, Kawaichi GK, Bors E. Renal calculosis of patients with traumatic cord lesions. J Urol 1962; 87: 647–5.
27. Hall MK, Hackler RH, Zampieri TA, Zampieri JB. Renal calculi in spinal cord-injured patient: association with reflux, bladder stones, and Foley catheter drainage. Urology 1989; 34: 126–8.
28. Killorin W, Gray M, Bennet JK, Green BG. The value of urodynamics and bladder management in predicting upper urinary tract complications in male spinal cord injury patients. Paraplegia 1992; 30: 437–41.
29. Hopps CV, Kropp KA. Preservation of renal function in children with myelomeningocele managed with basic newborn evaluation and close followup. J Urol 2003; 169: 305–8.
30. Sukin SW, Boone TB. Diagnosis and treatment of spinal cord injuries and myeloneuropathy. In: Rodney AA, ed. Voiding Dysfunction. Totowa: Humana Press, 2000: 115–39.
31. Bauer SB, Hallett M, Khoshbin S et al. Predictive value of urodynamic evaluation in newborns with myelodysplasia. JAMA 1984; 252: 650–2.
32. Lewart TJ, Kenig A, Fettich JJ et al. Sensitivity of ultrasonography in detecting renal parenchymal defects in children. Pediatr Nephrol 2003; 17: 1059–62.
33. Virgili G, Finazzi AE, Giannantoni A et al. Ultrasonography of the upper urinary tract in patients with spinal cord injury. Arch Ital Urol Androl 2000; 72: 225–7.
34. Calenoff L, Neimen HL, Kaplan PE et al. Urosonography in spinal cord injury patients. J Urol 1982; 128: 1234–7.
35. Ozer MN, Shannon SR. Renal sonography in asymptomatic persons with spinal cord injury: a cost-effectiveness analysis. Arch Phys Med Rehab 1991; 72: 35–7.
36. Bih LI, Tsai SJ, Tung LC. Sonographic diagnosis of hydronephrosis in patients with spinal cord injury: influence of bladder fullness. Arch Phys Med Rehab 1998; 79: 1557–9.
37. Ruutu M, Kivisaari A, Lehtonen T. Upper urinary tract changes in patients with spinal cord injury. Clin Radiol 1984; 35: 491–4.
38. Rao KG, Hackler RH, Woodlief RM et al. Real-time renal sonography in spinal cord injury patients: prospective comparison with excretory urography. J Urol 1986; 135: 72–7.
39. Stover SL, Witten DM, Kuhlemeier KV et al. Iatrogenic dilatation of the upper urinary tract during radiographic evaluation of patients with spinal cord injury. J Urol 1986; 135: 78–82.
40. Fabrizio MD, Chancellor MB, Rivas DA et al. The role of renal scintigraphy in the evaluation of spinal cord injury with presumed urosepsis. J Urol 1996; 156: 1730–4.
41. Whitaker RH. Methods of assessing obstruction in dilated ureters. Br J Urol 1973; 45: 15–22.
42. Vela-Navarrete R. Constant pressure flow-controlled antegrade pyelography. Eur Urol 1982; 8(5): 265–8.
43. Lovász S, Lovász L, Romics I. New variable in quantification degree of postrenal obstruction at urodynamic studies of upper urinary tract – the obstruction coefficient. Urologe 2006; 45(Suppl 1): 95.
44. Madersbacher H. Konservative Therapie der neurogenen Blasendysfunktion. Urologe 1999; 38: 24–9.
45. Guttman L, Frankel H. The value of intermittent catheterization in the early management of traumatic paraplegia and tetraplegia. Paraplegia 1966; 4: 63–5.
46. Lapides J, Diokono A, Silber S, Lowe B. Clean intermittent self-catheterisation in the treatment of urinary tract disease. J Urol 1972; 107: 458–61.
47. Nanninga JB, Wu Y, Hamilton B, Long-term intermittent catheterization in the spinal cord injury patient. J Urol 1982; 128: 760–3.
48. Mollard P, Meunier P, Berard C, Henriet M. Treatment of urinary incontinence of neurologic origin in children and adolescents. J Urol (Paris) 1984; 90: 227–36.
49. Brem AS, Martin D, Callaghan J, Maynard J. Long term renal risk factors in children with meningomyelocele. J Pediatr 1987; 110: 51–5.
50. Kuhn W, Rist M, Zaech GA. Intermittent urethral self catheterisation: long term results (bacteriological evolution, continence, acceptance, complications). Paraplegia 1991; 29: 222–32.
51. McGuire EJ, Savastano J. Comparative urological outcome in women with spinal cord injury. J Urol 1986; 135: 730–1.
52. Chao R, Clowers D, Mayo ME. Fate of upper urinary tracts in patients with indwelling catheters after spinal cord injury. Urology 1993; 42: 259–62.
53. Chartier-Kastler EJ, Thomas L, Bussel B et al. Feasibility of a temporary urethral stent through the striated sphincter in patients in the early phase (6 months) of spinal cord injury. Eur Urol 2001; 39: 326–31.
54. Rivas DA, Chancellor M. Sphincterotomy and sphincter stent prosthesis placement. In: Corcos J, Schick E, eds. The Urinary Sphincter. New York: Marcel Dekker, 2001: 565–83.
55. Szollar SM, Lee SM. Intravesical oxybutynin for spinal cord injury patients. Spinal Cord 1996; 34: 284–7.
56. Chapple C, Khullar V, Gabriel Z, Dooley JA. The effects of antimuscarinic treatments in overactive bladder: a systematic review and meta-analysis. Eur Urol 2005; 48: 5–26.
57. Schurch B, Stohrer M, Kramer G et al. Botulinum-A toxin for treating detrusor hyperreflexia in spinal cord injured patients: a new alternative to anticholinergic drugs. J Urol 2000; 164: 692–7.
58. Patel AK, Patterson JM, Chapple CR. Botulinum toxin injections for neurogenic and idiopathic detrusor overactivity: a critical analysis of results. Eur Urol 2006; 50: 684–710.
59. Schurch B, de Seze M, Denys P et al. Botulinum toxin type A is a safe and effective treatment for neurogenic urinary incontinence: results of a single treatment, randomized, placebo controlled 6-month study. J Urol 2005; 174: 196–200.
60. Karsenty G, Boy S, Reitz A et al. Botulinum toxin-A (BTA) in the treatment in neurogenic detrusor overactivity incontinence (NDOI) – a prospective randomized study to compare 30 vs. 10 injection sites. International Continence Society Annual Meeting. Montreal, Canada, 2005; Abstract No 93.
61. Katona F. Stages of vegetative afferentation in reorganisation of bladder control during electrotherapy. Urol Int 1975; 30: 192–203.
62. Brindley GS, Polkey CE, Rushton DN, Cardozo L. Sacral anterior root stimulators for bladder control in paraplegia. The first 50 cases. J Neurol Neurosurg Psychiatry 1986; 49: 1104–14.
63. Tanagho EA, Schmidt RA, Orvis BR. Neural stimulation for the control of voiding dysfunction: a preliminary report on 22 patients with serious neuropathic voiding disorders. J Urol 1989; 142: 340–5.
64. Sauerwein D. Die operativen Behandlung der spastischen Blasenlahmung bei Querschnittlahmung. Urologe A 1990; 19: 196–203.

65. Schurch B, Rodic B, Jeanmonod D. Posterior sacral rhizotomy and intradural anterior sacral root stimulation for treatment of the spastic bladder in spinal cord injured patients. J Urol 1997; 157: 610–14.
66. Egon G, Barat M, Colombel P et al. Implantation of anterior sacral root stimulators combined with posterior sacral rhizotomy in spinal injury patients. World J Urol 1998; 16: 342–9.
67. Müller SC, Chirurgische Therapie. In: Höfner K, Jonas U, eds. Praxisratgeber Harninkontinez. Bremen: UNI-MED Verlag AG, 2000: 144–77.
68. Christmas TJ, Kirby RS. Principles of management of the neurogenic bladder. In: Whitfield HN, Hendy WF, Kirby RS, Duchet JW, eds. Textbook of Genitourinary Surgery. Oxford: Blackwell Science, 1998: 918–26.
69. Flood HD, Malhotra SJ, O'Connel HE et al. Long-term results and complications using augmentation cystoplasty in reconstructive urology. Neurourol Urodyn 1995; 14: 297–309.
70. Ismaili K, Avni FE, Piepsz A et al. Vesicoureteric reflux in children. EAU-EBU Update Series, 2006; 4: 129–40.
71. Elder JS, Diaz M, Caldamone AA et al. Endoscopic therapy for vesicoureteral reflux: a meta-analysis. I. Reflux resolution and urinary tract infection. J Urol 2006; 175: 716–22.
72. Casals J, Rivero A, Rivero J. Endoscopic treatment of vesico-ureteral reflux in the neurogenic bladder. Arch Esp Urol 1997; 50: 381–7.
73. Heimbach D, Bruhl P, Mallmann R. Lich-Gregoir antireflux procedure; indications and results with 283 vesicoureteral units. Scand J Urol Nephrol 1995; 29: 311–16.
74. Burbidge KA. Ureteral reimplantation: a comparison of results with the cross trigonal and Politano–Leadbetter techniques in 120 patients. J Urol 1991; 146: 1352–3.
75. Ruutu ML, Lehtonen TA. Bladder outlet surgery in men with spinal cord injury. Scand J Urol Nephrol 1985; 19: 241–6.
76. Madersbacher H. The twelve o'clock sphincterotomy: technique, indications, results. Paraplegia 1976; 13: 261–7.
77. Müller T, Arbeiter K, Aufricht C. Renal function in meningomyelocele: risk factors, chronic renal failure, renal replacement therapy and transplantation. Curr Opin Urol 2002; 12: 479–84.
78. Power RE, O'Malley KJ, Little DM et al. Long-term follow up of cadaveric renal transplantation in patients with spina bifida. J Urol 2002; 167: 477–9.
79. Koo HP, Bunchman TE, Flynn JT et al. Renal transplantation in children with severe lower urinary tract dysfunction. J Urol 1999; 161: 210–45.

73

Benign prostatic hyperplasia and lower urinary tract symptoms in men with neurogenic bladder

Jerry G Blaivas and Ruhee Sidhu

Introduction

Lower urinary tract symptoms (LUTS) in men afflicted with neurologic diseases are usually attributed to the underlying neurologic condition and termed 'neurogenic bladder', yet this is not necessarily the case. Urologic disorders such as infection, benign prostatic hypertrophy (BPH), urolithiasis, prostate cancer, urethral stricture, and bladder cancer are probably as common in these patients as in the general population and require the same kind of diagnostic evaluation. On the other hand, because of the well-known effect of neurologic disorders on the process of micturition, neurogenic bladder is not only a confounding variable, but it may be entirely responsible for all of the patient's symptoms. For this reason, the diagnosis and treatment of men with LUTS who have underlying neurologic disease is best accomplished when there is a clear understanding of the underlying pathophysiology. This, in turn, requires knowledge about the neurophysiology of micturition and the effect of specific neurologic lesions on normal physiology.

BPH results in benign prostate enlargement (BPE) and, in some instances, this results in bladder outlet obstruction (BPO). However, not all patients with BPE have BPO and, conversely, not all patients with BPO have BPE. Further, the symptoms historically associated with BPH, termed LUTS, may be identical to those of neurogenic bladder. For this reason, it is important to determine, as far as possible, whether the symptoms are caused by the prostate, the neurologic disorder, or both, because treatment directed towards the underlying condition is usually effective while empiric therapies may not only be ineffective, but actually harmful. In our judgment, the best method to determine the underlying pathophysiology in these patients is the video-urodynamic study (VUDS). The X-ray portion of the study is particularly important because, as discussed below, the radiographic appearance of the vesical neck and the prostatic and membranous urethra may be the only clues to a neurogenic etiology of what might otherwise appear to be symptoms due to BPH.

In this chapter, we describe the diagnostic and therapeutic relationship between BPH and various causes of neurogenic bladder, including stroke, Parkinson's disease (and multisystem atrophy), multiple sclerosis, diabetes mellitus, spina bifida, and spinal cord injury.

Pathophysiology of BPH

The term BPH refers to prostatic cellular proliferation and hypertrophy that comprises both epithelial and stromal elements. It is the most common benign tumor in men and there is an increasing incidence of BPH with advancing age. The first manifestations of BPH usually begin at about age 40. By age 50 the prevalence is about 60% and it rises to 90% by age 85 (Figure 73.1).[1–4] It is no surprise, then, that a substantial number of men with neurogenic bladder have concomitant BPH.

The development of BPH is thought to be related to both aging and hormonal function. The relationship between aging and BPH has been well documented, as depicted in Figure 73.1. The hormonal milieu responsible for BPH requires a functioning hypothalamic–pituitary–testes–prostate axis; BPH does not develop in men castrated before puberty, nor in those with the genetic androgen deficiencies.[5] Luteinizing hormone-releasing hormone (LHRH) is released from the hypothalamus in response to decreased levels of circulating testosterone. LHRH results in the release of luteinizing hormone (LH) by the pituitary, which reaches the testes via the peripheral circulation. At the testis, LH binds to surface receptors on Leydig cells and stimulates the release of testosterone, which reaches the prostate where it acts as a prehormone on the prostatic epithelial cell. At this site, it is converted by the enzyme 5α-reductase to dihydrotestosterone (DHT), which binds to specific nuclear androgen receptors. DHT stimulates prostatic cell growth and proliferation, causing BPH.[6,7]

Microscopically, prostatic hyperplasia is characterized by nodules of benign adenoma in the periurethral zone of the

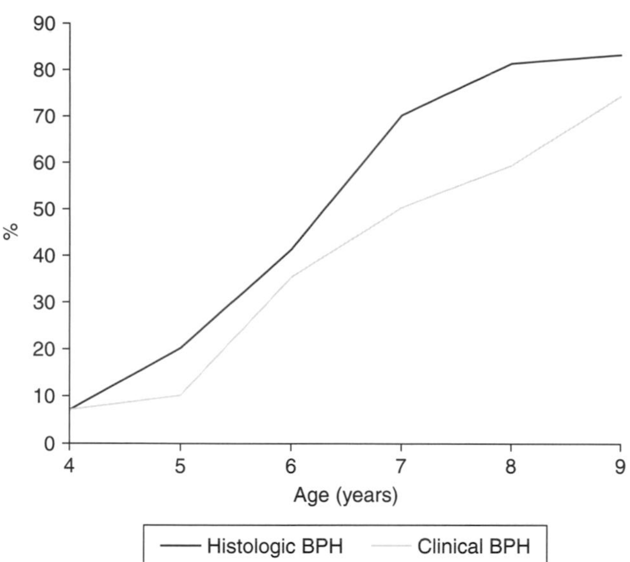

Figure 73.1
Relationship between BPH and age.

prostate. As these nodules grow and coalesce, they may encroach on the lumen of the prostatic urethra, causing prostatic obstruction.

Pathophysiology and differential diagnosis of urethral obstruction

Historically, the relationship between BPH, BPE, and BPO had a simplistic paradigm. It was thought that BPH resulted in BPE which, in turn, caused mechanical obstruction of the prostatic urethra and that it was prostatic obstruction that caused all of the symptoms associated with BPH. This theorem was underscored by the fact that, no matter what the symptoms, the majority of men undergoing transurethral prostatectomy (TURP) had satisfactory resolution of their symptoms. However, subsequent studies have shown that only about two-thirds of men with BPH actually have BPO.[8] In fact, the pathophysiology of LUTS in men with BPH is multifactorial, composed of urethral obstruction, detrusor overactivity, impaired or absent detrusor contractility, low bladder compliance, and sensory urgency (Figure 73.2).

Prostatic urethral obstruction is attributed to both mechanical and functional causes. Mechanical obstruction is caused by enlargement of the prostate gland, which results in urethral compression. Of course the only enlargement that matters is that which impinges upon the urethra. Thus, it is possible to have a very large prostate

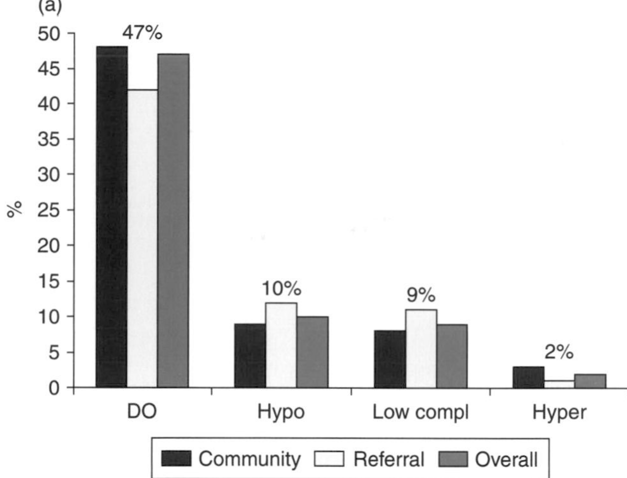

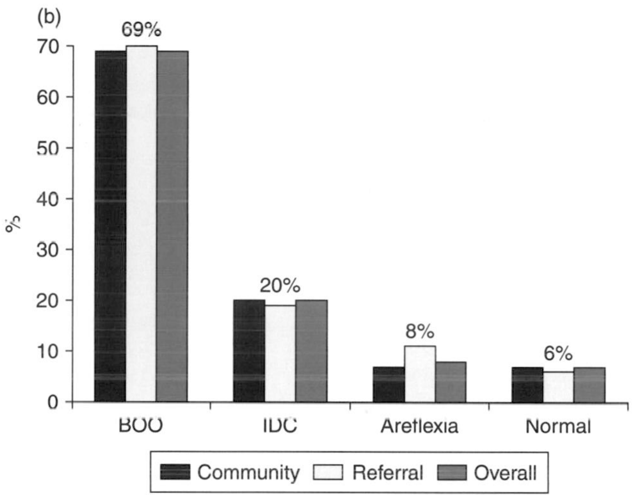

Figure 73.2
Pathophysiology of LUTS. (a) Urodynamic diagnosis during storage. DO, detrusor overactivity; Hypo, hyposensitive bladder; Hyper, hypersensitive bladder; Low compl, low bladder compliance. (b) Urodynamic diagnosis during voiding. BPO, bladder outlet obstruction; IDC, impaired detrusor contractility; Areflexia, detrusor areflexia. Adapted from Fusco et al.[8]

without urethral compression, or a very small prostate with significant obstruction. This explains why there is a poor correlation between prostatic size and the degree of obstruction.[9,10]

Functional obstruction is caused by contraction and/or failure of relaxation of the smooth muscle within the walls of the prostatic urethra. The prostate contains an abundance of α_1-adrenergic receptors that are located in the prostatic stroma. Three subtypes, and α_{1A}, α_{1B}, and α_{1C}, have been identified that are thought to modulate the contractility of

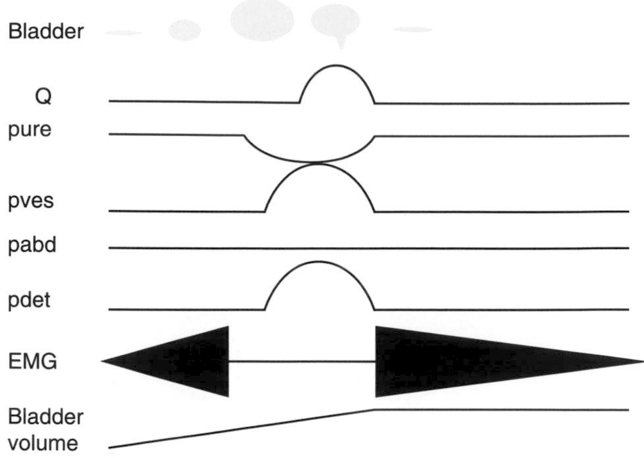

Figure 73.3
Micturition reflex – this is characterized by an orderly sequence of events: (1) relaxation of the striated muscles of the sphincter (EMG silence), (2) fall in urethral pressure, (3) rise in detrusor pressure, (4) opening of the urethra, and (5) uroflow.

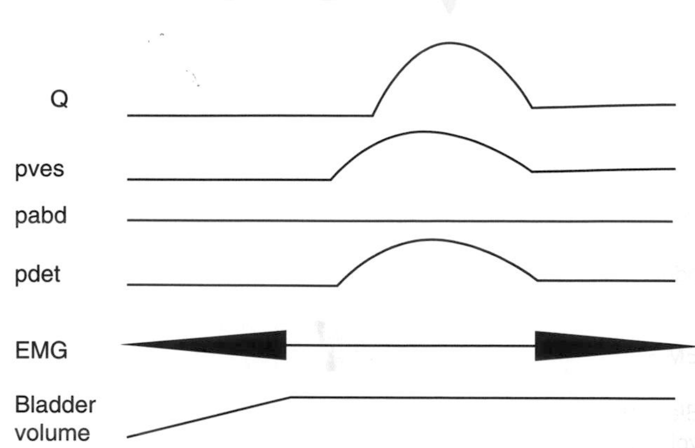

Figure 73.4
Detrusor hyperreflexia (type 4 overactive bladder) due to neurologic lesions above the brainstem that leave the pontine micturition center intact results in a normal micturition reflex that the patient cannot completely control. The patient has no awareness of the involuntary detrusor contraction and simply voids 'normally', but without control. The urodynamic tracing is identical to a normal micturition reflex.

prostatic smooth muscle. Stimulation of these receptors by norepinephrine and other α-active agents results in contraction of the smooth muscle and compression of the prostatic urethra, increasing the resistance to urinary flow.[11,12]

Effect of neurologic lesions on micturition

Neurologic disorders, independent of BPH, can cause most of the very same conditions that cause LUTS in men with BPH. In order to understand the clinical relationship between LUTS and neurologic disease, it is important to consider normal micturition and the effect of neurologic lesions on the process of micturition.

Micturition is normally accomplished by activation of the micturition reflex (Figure 73.3). The micturition reflex is integrated and modulated at numerous sites throughout the central nervous system, including the pontine mesencephalic reticular formation (pontine micturition center), parasympathetic and somatic components of the sacral spinal cord (the sacral micturition center), and the thoracolumbar sympathetics.[13–16] Neurologic lesions above the pons usually leave the 'micturition reflex' intact and, when they affect voiding at all, there is usually loss of voluntary control. In these patients micturition is physiologically normal (there is a coordinated relaxation of the sphincter during detrusor contraction), but the patient has simply lost the ability to initiate and/or prevent voiding.[13,17] The resulting incontinence is due to involuntary detrusor contractions, which is called detrusor overactivity (DO).

There is great variability in the degree of the patient's awareness, control, and concern about micturition. Some patients have either no awareness or concern and/or are unable to contract their sphincter or abort the detrusor contraction and simply void involuntarily (Figure 73.4). This pattern is also called type 4 OAB[18] and appears identical to the micturition reflex except for the absence of control. Other patients with suprapontine neurologic lesions can sense the impending onset of an involuntary detrusor contraction and are able to voluntarily contract the sphincter and abort the detrusor contraction before it starts. This pattern is called type 2 OAB (Figure 73.5). Others are aware of the involuntary detrusor contraction and can contract the striated sphincter, but this does not abort the detrusor contraction and incontinence ensues. This pattern is called type 3 OAB.

Still other patients with supraspinal neurologic lesions have both involuntary detrusor contractions and impaired detrusor contractility (Figure 73.6). Some, inexplicably, have detrusor areflexia or an acontractile detrusor. The neurophysiologic pathways responsible for this have not been elucidated.

Interruption of the neural pathways connecting the 'pontine micturition center' to the 'sacral micturition center' usually results in detrusor-external sphincter dyssynergia (DESD) or other manifestations of poor coordination of the micturition reflex, such as weak, poorly sustained detrusor contractions.[13,19] DESD is characterized by involuntary contractions of the striated musculature of the urethral sphincter during an involuntary detrusor contraction. It is seen exclusively in patients with neurologic lesions between the brainstem (pontine micturition center) and the sacral spinal cord (sacral micturition center). These include traumatic

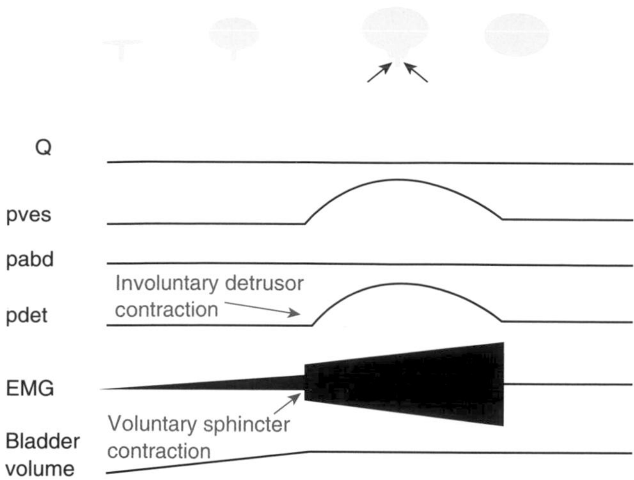

Figure 73.5
Detrusor hyperreflexia (type 2 OAB). The impending onset of an involuntary detrusor contraction is sensed by the patient, who immediately contracts the striated sphincter. This is manifested as increased EMG activity. At this point, the urethra is dilated in its proximal extent with obstruction in the distal third by the sphincter contraction (white arrows). Through a reflex mechanism, the detrusor contraction is abated and continence maintained (no flow, flat Q tracing).

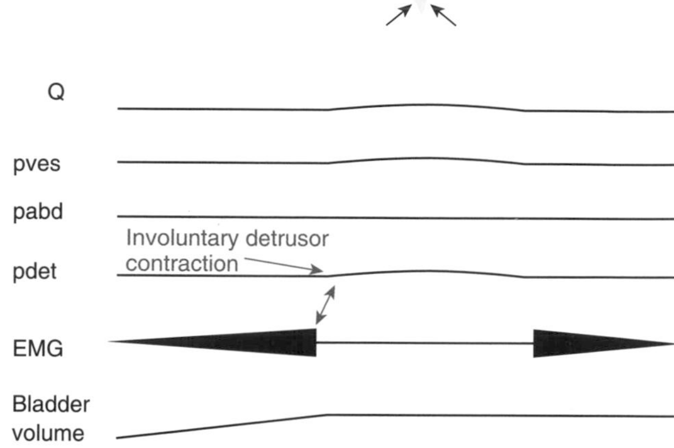

Figure 73.6
Detrusor overactivity or detrusor hyperreflexia and impaired detrusor contractiity. An involuntary detrusor contraction is heralded by a sudden and complete relaxation of the sphincter EMG (orange arrow), but the detrusor contraction is barely discernible as a subtle rise in detrusor pressure. Uroflow is low, but the urethra opens normally. The patient does not empty completely.

spinal cord injury, multiple sclerosis, myelodysplasia, and other forms of transverse myelitis.

There are three main types of DESD. In type I there is a concomitant increase in both detrusor pressure and EMG activity (Figure 73.7). At the peak of the detrusor contraction, the sphincter suddenly relaxes and unobstructed voiding occurs. Type II DESD is characterized by sporadic contractions of the external urethral sphincter throughout the detrusor contraction (Figure 73.8). In type III DESD there is a crescendo–decrescendo pattern of sphincter contraction which results in urethral obstruction throughout the entire detrusor contraction (Figure 73.9).

The diagnosis of DESD should be suspected in any patient with a neurologic lesion involving the spinal cord. Conversely, in patients without such a lesion, this diagnosis should be viewed with skepticism. In neurologically normal patients, a presumed diagnosis of DESD is almost always due to an acquired disorder of micturition characterized by a contraction of the striated sphincter in a conscious or subconscious attempt to abort micturition. The correct diagnosis is best attained by video-urodynamic evaluation with EMG monitoring. In DESD the onset of the detrusor contraction is preceded by an increase in sphincter EMG activity. In learned voiding dysfunction the sphincter EMG activity diminishes just prior to the contraction, then sporadically increases as the patient contracts and relaxes the sphincter (Figure 73.10). If EMG is unavailable, the characteristics of the urethral contractions

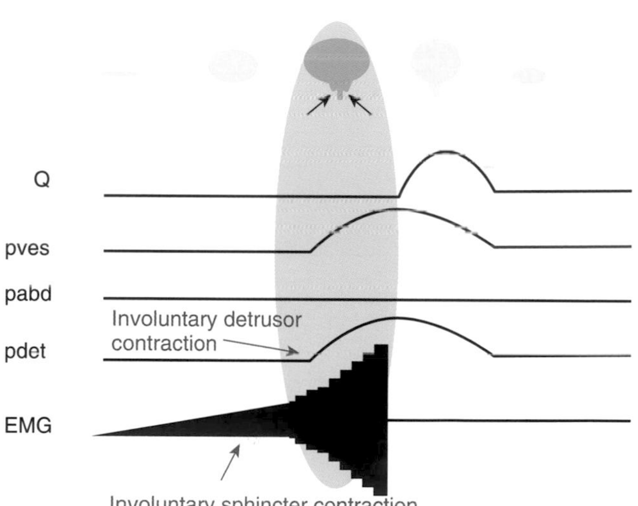

Figure 73.7
Type 1 Detrusor-external sphincter dyssynergia (DESD). The involuntary sphincter contraction precedes the involuntary detrusor contraction. At the peak of the detrusor contraction there is a sudden and complete relaxation of the striated sphincter (EMG silence) and (unobstructed) voiding ensues. During the first half of the detrusor contraction there is the classic appearance of DESD – a dilated proximal urethra and narrowed distal urethra (arrows) associated with increased EMG activity and an involuntary detrusor contraction (blue oval).

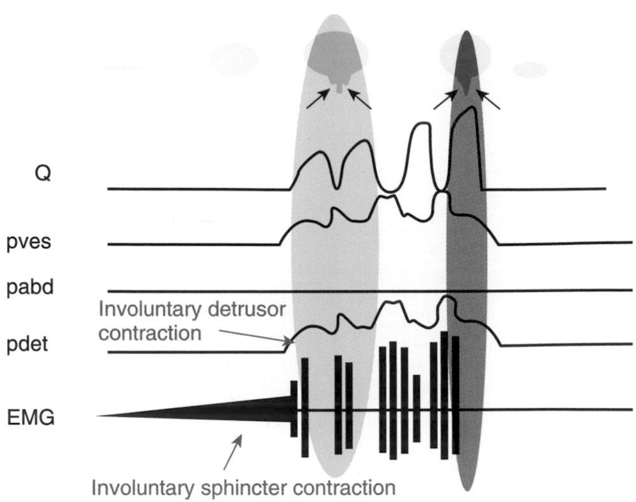

Figure 73.8
Type 2 detrusor-external sphincter dyssynergia. There are sporadic involuntary sphincter contractions throughout the involuntary detrusor contraction. During the sphincter contractions, the patient is obstructed by his own sphincter (blue oval); during sphincter relaxation, voiding is unobstructed (orange oval).

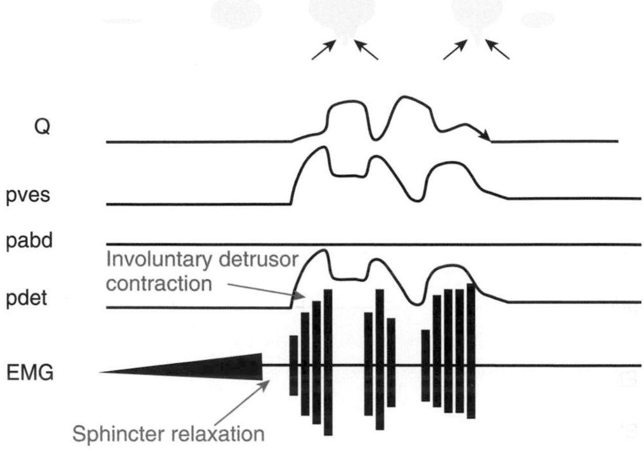

Figure 73.10
Acquired voiding dysfunction. The involuntary detrusor contraction is preceded by relaxation of the sphincter, then, in a subconscious attempt to suppress micturition, the patient has sporadic sphincter contractions that interrupt the stream. During the sphincter contractions, detrusor pressure rises and uroflow falls as the patient is obstructed by his own sphincter.

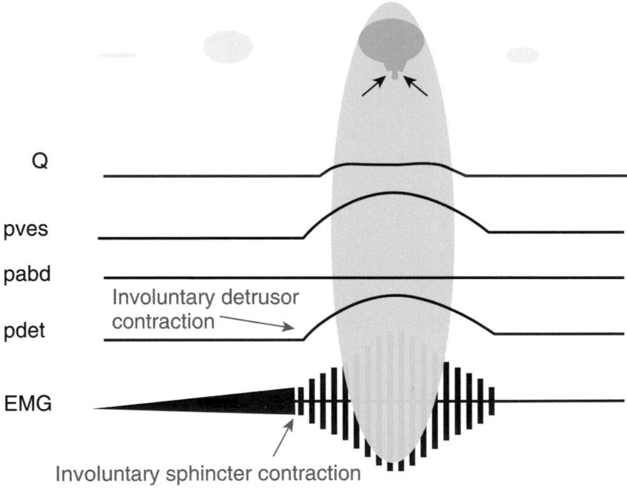

Figure 73.9
Type 3 detrusor-external sphincter dyssynergia. The involuntary sphincter contraction precedes the involuntary detrusor contraction. There is a crescendo–decrescendo pattern in EMG activity and voiding is obstructed throughout (blue oval).

seen at fluoroscopy often provide enough information for a definitive diagnosis.

Sacral neurologic lesions have a variable effect on micturition depending upon the extent to which the neurologic injury affects the parasympathetic, sympathetic, and somatic systems. In complete parasympathetic lesions the bladder is areflexic and the patient is in urinary retention (Figure 73.11). In many cases, there is also low bladder compliance (Figure 73.12). When, in addition to a parasympathetic lesion, there is also a sympathetic one, the proximal urethra loses its sphincteric function. Clinically, this results in incomplete bladder emptying (due to the acontractile detrusor) and sphincteric incontinence (due to the nonfunctioning proximal urethra), as seen in Figure 73.13.[20–22] In some patients it is difficult to determine whether the rise in P_{det} is due to low bladder compliance or a detrusor contraction. If detrusor pressure falls when bladder infusion is stopped, the rise in pressure is due to low bladder compliance; if pressure continues to rise or stays the same, it is due to a detrusor contraction (Figure 73.14).

Somatic neurologic lesions affect pudendal afferents and efferents. In addition to loss of perineal and peri-anal sensation, these lesions abolish the bulbocavernosus reflex, and impair the ability to voluntarily contract the urethral and anal sphincters. Herniated discs, diabetic neuropathy, multiple sclerosis, spinal cord injury, and tumors can cause sacral neurologic lesions. They are also commonly encountered after extensive pelvic surgery such as abdominoperineal resection of the rectum.[20–22]

Clinical evaluation and decision-making

It should be evident from the discussion above that neurogenic bladder and BPH can cause exactly the same

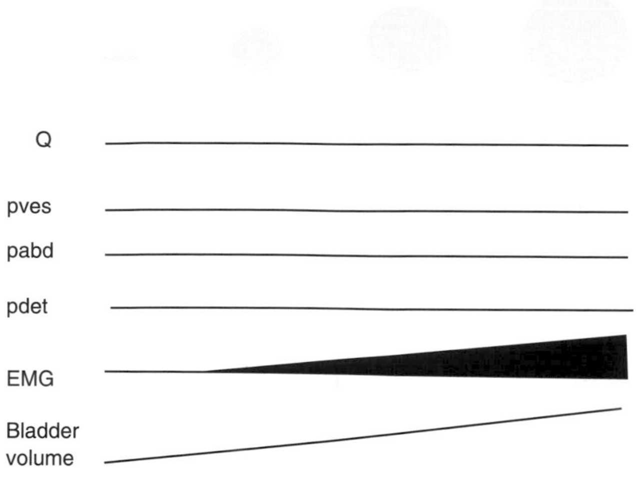

Figure 73.11
Detrusor areflexia. Despite bladder filling to a large volume, there is no detrusor contraction at all and the urethra remains closed.

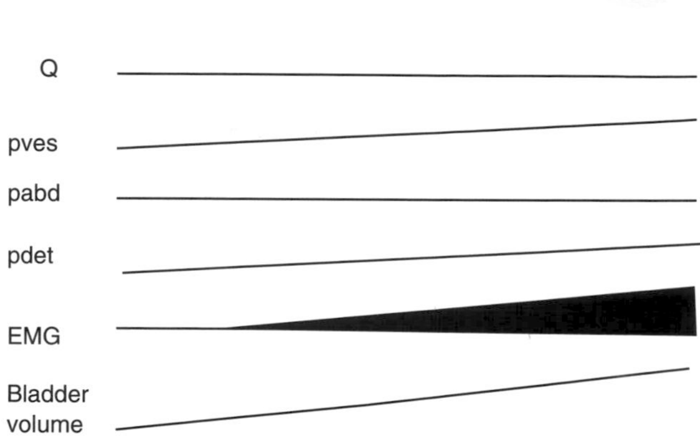

Figure 73.12 Detrusor areflexia and low bladder compliance. Despite bladder filling to a large volume, there is no detrusor contraction, but there is a steep rise in vesical and detrusor pressure (low bladder compliance). The urethra remains closed.

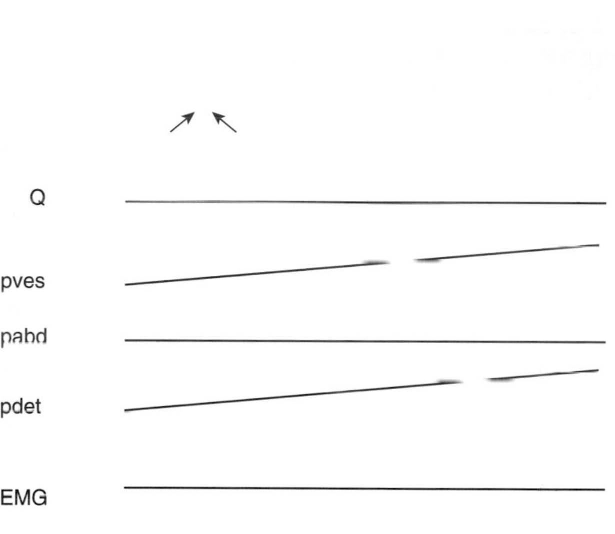

Figure 73.13
Detrusor areflexia, low bladder compliance, open bladder neck, and sphincteric incontinence due to parasympathetic and sympathetic injury. During bladder filling the bladder neck is open (arrows), there is a gradual rise in detrusor pressure, and the patient begins to void/leak with a low flow rate.

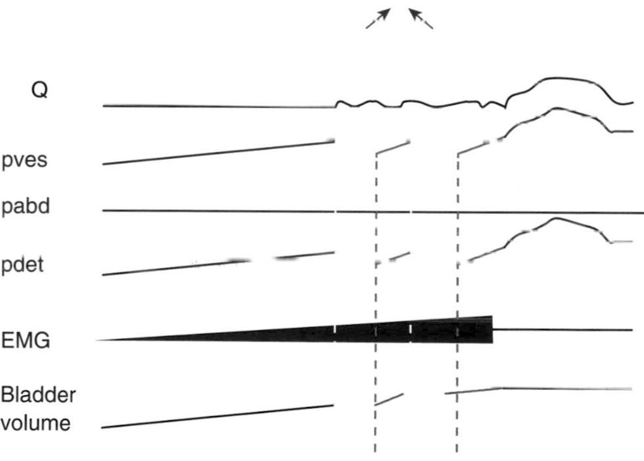

Figure 73.14 Low bladder compliance versus involuntary detrusor contraction. During bladder filling there is a gradual rise in detrusor pressure and the patient begins to void/leak with a low flow rate (arrow). Is this a detrusor contraction or low bladder compliance? There are two clues that this is low compliance. Firstly, each time the bladder infusion is stopped (dashed yellow lines), detrusor pressure falls (solid yellow lines), and when bladder infusion is started again (dashed orange lines), detrusor pressure rises (solid orange lines). Secondly, the rise in detrusor pressure is unassociated with any EMG changes. At the end of bladder filling there is complete relaxation of the striated sphincter (EMG silence), heralding the onset of an involuntary detrusor contraction (yellow arrow). The detrusor pressure continues to rise after bladder filling has stopped, confirming that detrusor contraction and not low bladder compliance is causing the pressure rise.

symptoms and underlying pathophysiology. How, then, can the clinician determine whether LUTS are due to the underlying neurologic disorder, to BPH, or both? And more importantly, do these distinctions make a difference with respect to treatment and/or prognosis? The answer to

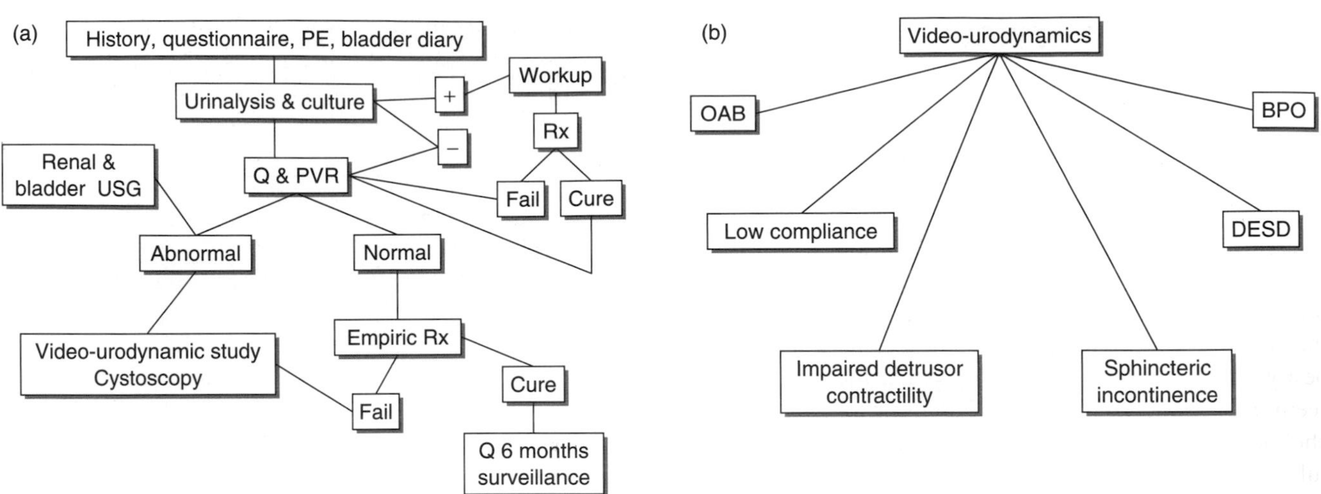

Figure 73.15
(a) Diagnostic algorithm. See text for details. (b) Diagnostic possibilities after video-urodynamic studies. See text for therapeutic options.

the latter question is a resounding yes, but the method of making such distinctions and assessing the relative contributions of BPH and neurologic disorders requires a sophisticated approach, as delineated below.

To begin with, no matter what the symptoms, we recommend that evaluation should begin with a focused history and physical examination, questionnaire, urinalysis and urine culture, bladder diary, pad test (for incontinent patients), uroflow, and measurement of postvoid residual urine. Urinary tract infection or bacteriuria should be treated with culture-specific antibiotics and the patient re-evaluated afterwards. In some patients with persistent bacteriuria or recurrent infection it is advisable to perform urodynamic evaluation and cystoscopy while the patient is taking culture-specific antibiotics.

Microscopic hematuria is not uncommon in patients with neurologic disorders and BPH and its evaluation needs to be put into context with the clinical scenario. In a newly diagnosed patient, who has not undergone urologic instrumentation (urethral catheter or cystoscopy), we recommend that a formal hematuria workup be done (cystoscopy and upper urinary tract imaging +/– urinary cytology). In patients with chronic conditions who have had prior hematuria workup, we believe that it is best to repeat the hematuria evaluation every few years if hematuria recurs. For those patients on intermittent catheterization, it is probably best to do a single hematuria workup at some point within the first 3 months or so, and periodically thereafter if the patient develops gross hematuria in the absence of infection. In our unpublished experience with thousands of patients with neurogenic bladder who are not treated with an indwelling catheter, bladder cancer has only been found in 2 patients, but, of course, bladder and upper tract stones are occasionally found. In patients with indwelling catheters (which we deplore) the incidence of bladder cancer has been reported to be about 1%.

Although it is presumed that LUTS in men has something to do with BPO and/or BPH, in fact, the relationship between the neurogenic bladder (NGB), BPH, and BPO is sufficiently muddled so that the presence or absence of prostatic enlargement has no effect whatsoever on pathophysiologic diagnosis, but, nevertheless, may have important therapeutic implications. For example, prostate size is an important consideration in the choice of surgical and minimally invasive therapies. Further, there are certain urodynamic risk factors that, untreated, are associated with a high risk of serious urinary tract infection, hydronephrosis, vesico-ureteral reflux and urolithiasis. The most serious of these is detrusor-external sphincter dyssynergia and low bladder compliance

Once the preliminary evaluation has been completed we follow the algorithm depicted in Figure 73.15. For those who fail empiric therapy, video-urodynamic evaluation remains the cornerstone of diagnosis. One caveat, though. There are some men who have low uroflow and/or large PVR who are not sufficiently bothered by symptoms to warrant treatment. We recommend that such a patient not undergo invasive urodynamic testing or cystoscopy because of the risk that it might be become the 'straw that breaks the camel's back' and cause urinary retention or infection. Rather, we recommend renal ultrasound and serum creatinine. If hydronephrosis or renal failure is found, we urge the patient to undergo the invasive testing; if not, we recommend semi-annual evaluation with creatinine, Q, PVR, and renal and bladder ultrasound (USG). In the following sections, we detail the clinical algorithm more completely based on symptoms.

Treatment overview

A detailed discussion of the treatment of BPH is beyond the scope of this chapter; rather, the focus is on understanding the goals and mechanisms by which effective therapy is accomplished. For men with BPH and neurogenic bladder the goals of therapy are threefold: (1) to ameliorate symptoms, (2) to prevent complications, and (3) to manage complications. It is important to be cognizant that symptomatic improvement does not necessarily imply improvement in the underlying condition and, in some instances, there may be asymptomatic disease progression while the patient is on seemingly effective treatment. For example, both anticholinergics and α-adrenergic blocking agents can successfully treat urgency as silent hydronephrosis develops in patients with DESD or prostatic obstruction. For this reason, it is particularly important that, in addition to treatment, a lifetime of active surveillance be ongoing in patients with risk factors such as DESD, low bladder compliance, urethral obstruction, and elevated residual urine. Although the particulars of surveillance may vary, we recommend, at the least, semi-annual evaluations comprising upper and lower urinary tract imaging (renal and bladder ultrasound) alternating with renal function studies (creatinine) and urodynamics in such high-risk patients. At the first sign of deterioration of any of these parameters, appropriate treatment should be instituted.

Treatment guidelines are depicted in more detail in the following discussions, but the goals of therapy are elucidated here. First and foremost, effective (and safe) treatment requires a clear understanding of the underlying pathophysiology. In patients with neurogenic disorders and LUTS, we deplore the indiscriminant use of empiric therapies unless they are accompanied by very careful surveillance, as delineated above, to be sure that asymptomatic complications do not occur.

Symptomatic treatment is designed simply to ameliorate symptoms. Treatment for LUTS can be broadly classified into pharmacologic and behavioral, minimally invasive, and surgical therapies. These therapies are being developed at such a rapid pace by industry, that by the time you are reading this chapter, some important new therapies may not even be listed and some listed ones may be considered obsolete. Nevertheless, for patients with prostatic obstruction, we believe that that the gold standard, currently transurethral resection of the prostate, will continue to be some form of treatment that relieves the obstruction. To date, pharmacologic and minimally invasive therapies for obstruction offer, at best, moderate improvement for the majority of patients, although they might be very effective in some.

For those with typical obstructive and irritative LUTS, α-adrenergic blocking agents are widely considered to be the first line of treatment, but their mechanism of action is not well understood. They were originally chosen because of their theoretic impact upon prostatic obstruction.[23,24] It was hypothesized that, since the prostatic stroma has an abundance of α_1-adrenergic receptors, blockade would relax the smooth muscle and reduce the degree of urethral resistance offered by the prostatic urethra. Although this does occur in some patients, it has been subsequently shown that effective symptomatic treatment can be accomplished without any amelioration of obstruction at all.[25,26] This means that the clinician cannot rely on symptoms as a proxy for urethral obstruction and mandates careful follow-up, as outlined above. Accordingly, we recommend following the algorithm depicted in Figure 73.15 for all patients with BPH and neurologic disease.

Table 73.1 *Risk factors for development of urologic complications*
Indwelling bladder catheter
Detrusor-external sphincter dyssynergia
Low bladder compliance
Prostatic obstruction
Vesico-ureteral reflux
Urolithiasis

The potential complications of neurogenic bladder and BPH include recurrent and/or persistent gross hematuria or infection, bladder and kidney stones, hydronephrosis, and renal failure. Further, in those managed by indwelling urethral catheters (which we deplore) urethral strictures may occur. In our judgment, bladder stones, hydronephrosis, and renal failure are almost always the tragic consequences of failure to insure proper surveillance and treatment; they are entirely preventable complications that are caused by underlying risk factors (Table 73.1). Of course, the responsibility of insuring high-quality care is a shared one, borne by the physician, the patient, his family, and the healthcare system. Sadly, all too often, economics, apathy, and poor patient compliance come into play, blunting our ability to provide the high-quality care that our current state of knowledge and expertise demand.

Treatment of symptoms is, of course, elective, but treatment to manage complications has strong indications. Further, urodynamic studies provide important prognostic information about the likelihood developing complications caused by low bladder compliance and detrusor-external sphincter dyssynergia, both of which portend hydronephrosis and/or vesicoureteral reflux, recurrent infections, stones, and ultimately renal failure. In our judgment, these conditions mandate treatment even in patients who are not bothered by their symptoms. When low bladder compliance is accompanied by prostatic urethral obstruction, outlet-reducing surgery is likely to prevent upper tract damage and also to reverse the low compliance.[27] For those patients in whom postoperative continence is a concern, intermittent catheterization +/– anticholinergic medications is an effective alternative. In our judgment, augmentation enterocystoplasty and/or continent urinary diversion is a better long-term solution than a chronic indwelling catheter.[28,29] Although, α-adrenergic blocking agents have been used to treat low bladder compliance, we do not believe that they are effective in most patients. Further, the role of minimally invasive therapies is not known. No matter what treatment is chosen for low bladder compliance, the importance of upper tract surveillance cannot be overemphasized. For patients with pre-existing hydronephrosis, we recommend renal ultrasound 3 months after the initiation of treatment and, if the hydronephrosis is not resolved or improved, repeat urodynamics should be done to document that the bladder compliance is normal; if not, further therapy should be instituted.

Urinary retention and voiding 'obstructive' symptoms

Urinary retention is the inability to void once bladder capacity has been reached or exceeded. At first glance, the diagnosis seems straightforward, but it is important to distinguish urinary retention from a kind of paresthesia that sometimes occurs in patients with supraspinal neurologic lesions (stroke, multiple sclerosis) and in some other patients with detrusor overactivity. Such patients confuse abnormal bladder sensations or involuntary detrusor contractions with the urge to void when, in fact, there is little urine in the bladder. Heeding the urge to void, they try to do so, but because of the low bladder volume or loss of voluntary bladder control they are unable to, and their symptom is misconstrued as being urinary retention. In either case, the correct diagnosis should be apparent when bladder volume is measured.

The sine-qua-non of the diagnosis of urinary retention, then, is the post-attempt-at-urination measure of residual urine. If residual urine is not elevated, it is important to also rule out bacterial cystitis as a treatable cause.

Treatment of the paresthesias alluded to above is accomplished when there is a clear understanding of the underlying pathophysiology and, to this end, urodynamics is indispensable. If the patient complains of urgency and urodynamics confirms type 3 or 4 detrusor overactivity (as described above), paradoxically, anticholinergics alone might be effective treatment. If type 1 or 2 detrusor overactivity is found, behavioral therapy alone might be more appropriate and, of course, combinations of the two are another option.

In the vast majority of men who complain of urinary retention the diagnosis is correctly confirmed by measurement of residual urine. Occasionally, there is a precipitating, remediable event that causes urinary retention. Alpha-adrenergic agents (that may be found in over-the-counter cough medications or nasal decongestants) cause urinary retention by causing contraction (or failure of relaxation) of prostatic smooth muscle. Antihistamines and anticholinergics may precipitate retention by a direct inhibitory effect on detrusor contractility. Acute bacterial prostatitis, prostatic infarction, and acute bladder overdistention during surgery also may cause urinary retention.

Table 73.2 *Numeric criteria for diagnosing obstruction and impaired detrusor contractility*

	$P_{det}Q_{max}$(cmH_2O)	Q_{max}(ml/s)
Obstruction	> 40	< 12
Equivocal	30–39	< 12
Impaired detrusor		
Contractility	< 30	< 12

Chronic, asymptomatic urinary retention may develop in men with neurogenic bladder as well as those with BPH. These patients remain undetected until they are finally unable to void at all, or are found to have a large bladder and/or hydronephrosis during surveillance upper tract imaging.

No matter what the presentation, when urinary retention is found, there are two major concerns: (1) Is the urinary retention due to impaired detrusor contractility, urethral obstruction, or both? (2) Is it caused by BPH,neurogenic bladder, or both? The answer to both questions is best attained by interpreting the results of video-urodynamics in perspective with neurologic diagnosis and clinical findings.

Synchronous measurement of detrusor pressure and uroflow is the most accurate means of determining the relative contributions of urethral obstruction and impaired or absent detrusor contractility to urinary retention. Without more information, it is not possible to determine whether these abnormalities are of neurologic etiology or due to BPH (or other kinds of urethral obstruction). In our judgment, nomograms are useful for grading the severity of obstruction and adequacy of detrusor contractility, but we rely on visual inspection of the detrusor pressure/uroflow curves (coupled with radiologic visualization of the urethra) for making the diagnosis. Numeric criteria for this are presented in Table 73.2. We prefer the Schaefer (Figure 73.16)[30,31] to the Abrams Griffith nomogram[32] because it defines 6 gradations of urethral obstruction. Grades 0–1 are unobstructed, 2 is equivocal, and 3–6 represent increasing degrees of obstruction. Further, it classifies detrusor contractility into 5 graded categories ranging from very weak to very strong.

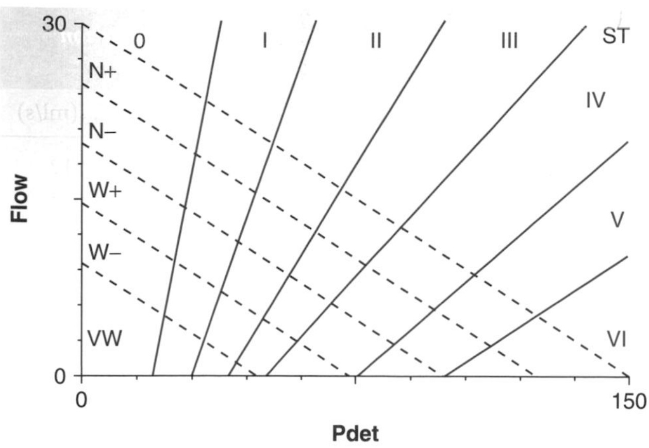

Figure 73.16
Schaefer bladder outlet obstruction and detrusor contractility nomogram.

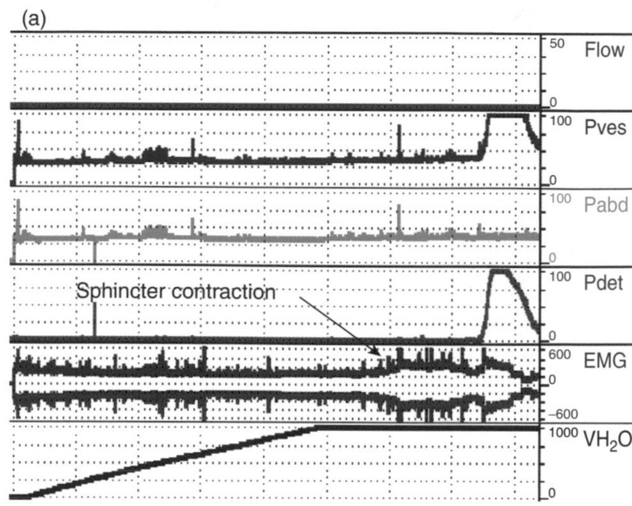

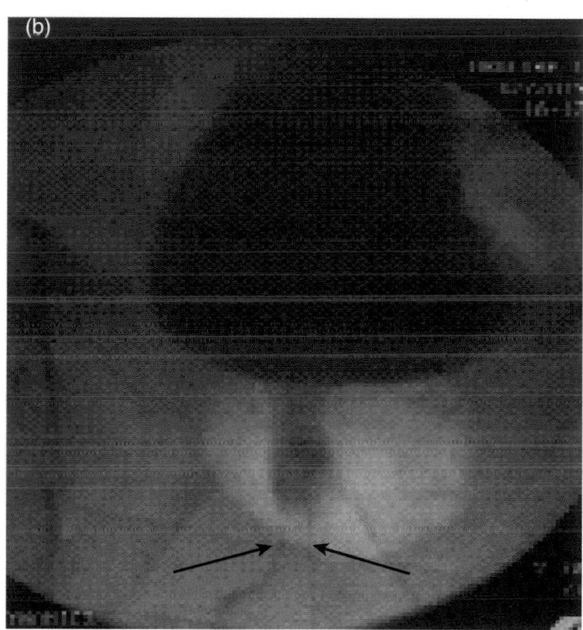

Figure 73.17
Detrusor-external sphincter dyssynergia (DESD) (a) Urodynamic tracing. This is a classic urodynamic tracing of DESD – an involuntary contraction of the striated sphincter that precedes and continues throughout the involuntary detrusor contraction. The increased EMG activity (arrow), that proxies for the sphincter contraction, begins long before the onset of the involuntary detrusor contraction. The flat line at the peak of the pves and pdet tracings is caused by a preset computer cutoff than can be switched on or off. Actual pdetmax = 115 cmH_2O. The bladder volume at which the detrusor contraction occurred (in this patient 1000 ml) is unusual. Most patients with DESD have a much smaller bladder capacity. (b) X-ray obtained at pdet max shows the classic picture of DESD – complete obstruction at the membranous urethra (arrows) and a trabeculated bladder, often with a 'Christmas tree' shape, as seen here. (Figure courtesy of Jerry G Blaivas MD.)

The detrusor pressure/uroflow data, though, cannot distinguish BPH-induced obstruction from that due to neurogenic bladder. In fact it may be impossible to make this distinction with certainty, but there are clinical and radiographic findings that favor one or the other etiology. Neurogenic urethral obstruction is almost always due to DESD and, in its usual form DESD has a characteristic appearance – dilation of the prostatic urethra and narrowing of the membranous urethra (Figure 73.17). DESD is almost always due to a neurologic lesion between the sacral and pontine micturition centers, such as spinal cord injury and multiple sclerosis (Table 73.3). Treatment of DESD takes two generic forms – relieving the obstruction (external sphincterotomy, botulinum toxin injections into the striated sphincter, or urethral stent) or bypassing the obstruction with intermittent catheterization and aborting the involuntary detrusor contractions (pharmacologic, botox injections into the bladder, enterocystoplasty). Treatments that relieve the obstruction result in incontinence, so the patient will need to use a condom catheter or other appliance.

In contradistinction to DESD, the site of obstruction due to BPH is in the prostatic urethra (Figure 73.18). In some patients, there is both prostatic obstruction and DESD. This is difficult to diagnose with certainty because the classic spinning top configuration of the prostatic urethra is not present. The diagnosis should be suspected when both the prostatic and membranous urethra are narrowed in a patient with neurologic findings that make DESD suspect (Figure 73.19). Another confounding factor is that some quadriplegic men after spinal cord injury develop secondary vesical neck obstruction that has a similar radiographic appearance (Figure 73.20).

The distinction between prostatic obstruction and DESD is more than an academic one. It has very important therapeutic and prognostic implications. The symptoms

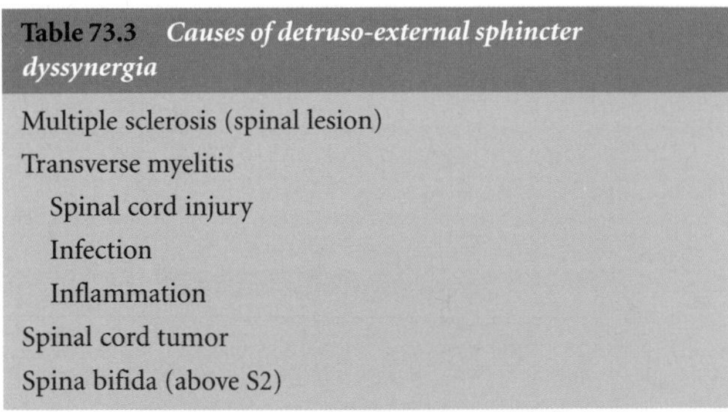

Table 73.3 *Causes of detruso-external sphincter dyssynergia*
Multiple sclerosis (spinal lesion)
Transverse myelitis
Spinal cord injury
Infection
Inflammation
Spinal cord tumor
Spina bifida (above S2)

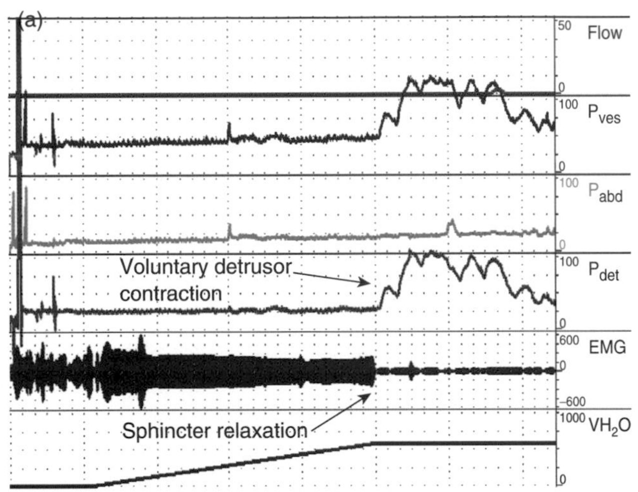

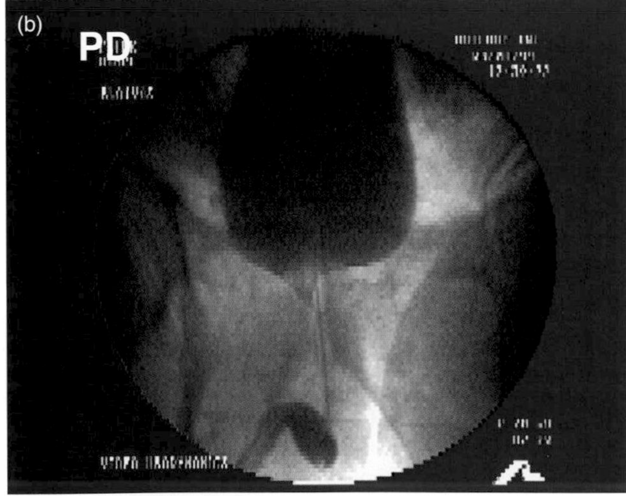

Figure 73.18
Prostatic obstruction associated with BPH. (a) Urodynamic tracing. Urethral obstruction associated with BPH. The patient is a 73-year-old neurologically normal physician with 4+ prostatic enlargement. (b) X-ray obtained at Qmax shows a markedly narrowed prostatic urethra and a filling defect at the bladder base caused by intravesical protrusion of the prostate. (Figure courtesy of Jerry G Blaivas MD.)

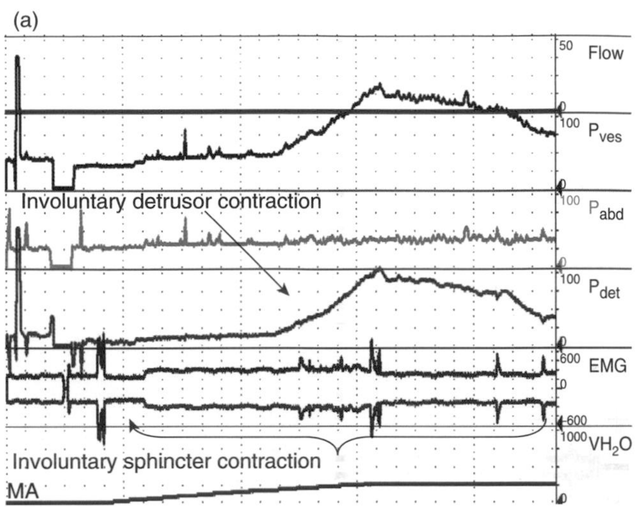

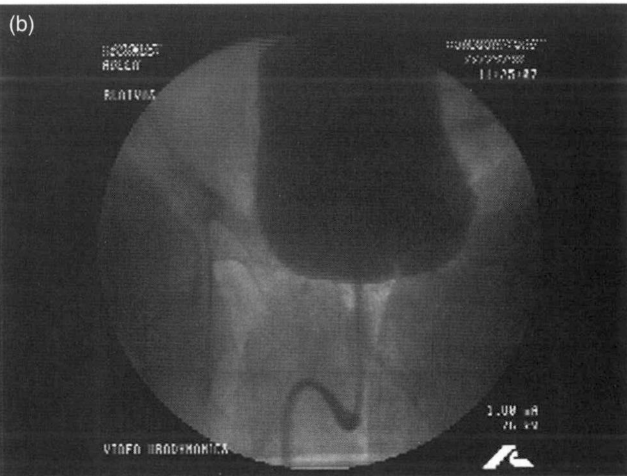

Figure 73.19
Urethral obstruction due to DESD and prostatic urethral obstruction in a 52-year-old man with spastic paraparesis owing to radiation myelitis (lymphoma). (a) Urodynamic tracing. An involuntary detrusor contraction occurred at a bladder volume of 264 ml. Q_{max} = 0.7 ml/s, P_{det} Q_{max} = 92 cmH_2O, P_{detmax} = 108 cmH_2O, voided volume = 16 ml, postvoid residual = 224 ml. (b) X-ray obtained at P_{detmax} demonstrates some contrast in the bulbar urethra and in the mid-prostatic urethra. There is narrowing of both the proximal and distal prostatic urethra, suggesting both bladder neck obstruction (from BPH) and DESD. It is impossible from this study to determine to what degree the patient's symptoms are due to prostatic obstruction versus DESD. (Figure courtesy of Jerry G Blaivas MD.)

and consequences of prostatic obstruction are, for practical purposes, cured by effective surgical treatment such as TURP and symptomatic improvement can be expected in the majority of men with pharmacologic and minimally invasive therapies (Table 73.4). These treatments are of no benefit in men with DESD.

On the other hand, surgical treatment of DESD such as external sphincterotomy can cause irreversible harm in

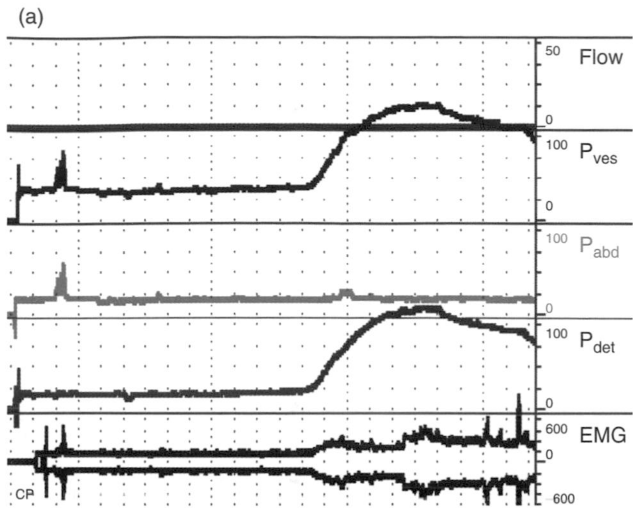

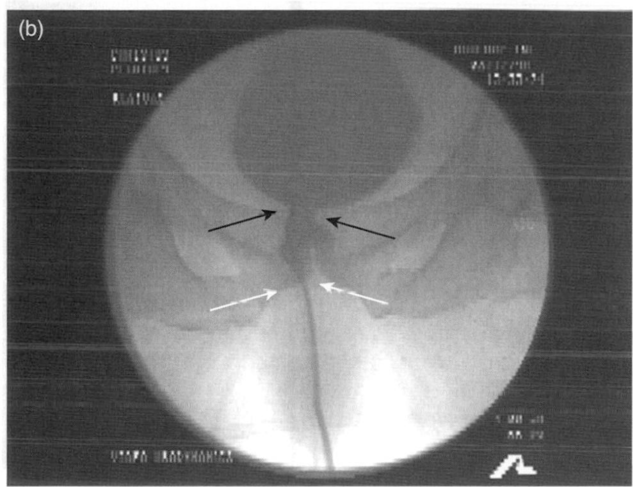

Figure 73.20
DESD and bladder neck obstruction in a 67-year-old male, paraplegic due to an arteriovenous malformation at T6. (a) Urodynamic tracing. Note that the increase in EMG activity occurs just prior to the onset of the detrusor contraction. (b) X-ray. The prostatic urethra is dilated and completely obstructed at the membranous urethra by the involuntary sphincter contraction (white arrows). In addition, though, there is narrowing of the bladder neck and proximal urethra (black arrows), suggestive of secondary bladder neck or prostatic obstruction. (Figure courtesy of Jerry G Blaivas MD.)

men with prostatic obstruction, because once the correct diagnosis is ascertained, subsequent TURP is likely to cause sphincteric incontinence.

Overactive bladder symptoms

The evaluation of overactive bladder (OAB) in men with NGB and BPH should commence with a search for remediable causes (Table 73.5). Urinary tract infection should be treated with culture-specific antibiotics and bladder stones eliminated. Thereafter, the diagnosis and treatment are best accomplished by video-urodynamic evaluation, cystoscopy, and careful attention to the clinical evaluation obtained by history, exam, bladder diary, and pad test. The video-urodynamic evaluation, though, is the cornerstone of making diagnostic and treatment decisions. During bladder filling, the type of OAB is determined (see OAB classification, above) and during the voiding phase the presence or absence of urethral obstruction and impaired detrusor contractility is observed. For those patients with urethral obstruction it is crucial to be certain whether the obstruction is prostatic or due to DESD as outlined above. Armed with this information, therapeutic decisions can be made with greater prognostic accuracy, though it often requires a sophisticated evaluation of the particulars of the clinical situation.

Table 73.4 *Treatment of prostatic obstruction*
Pharmacologic
α-adrenergic antagonists
Alfuzosin
Doxazosin
Tamsulosin
Terazosin
5 alpha reductase inhibitors
Dutasteride
Finasteride
Combination: alpha blocker + 5α-reductase inhibitor
Anticholinergics
Minimally invasive therapies
Transurethral/transrectal thermotherapy
Transurethral needle ablation
Transurethral stent
Surgical
Transurethral incision of the prostate
Transurethral resection of the prostate
Transurethral KTP laser electrovaporization
Transurethral holmium laser resection/enucleation
Open prostatectomy

Table 73.5 *Remediable causes of overactive bladder*
Urinary tract infection
Urethral obstruction
Bladder stones
Bladder cancer

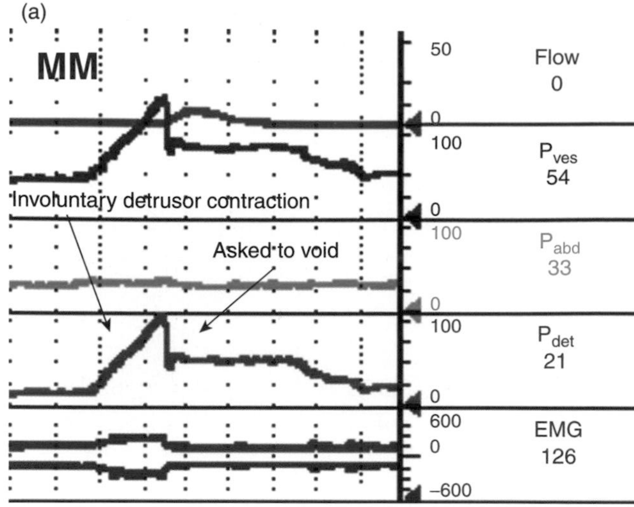

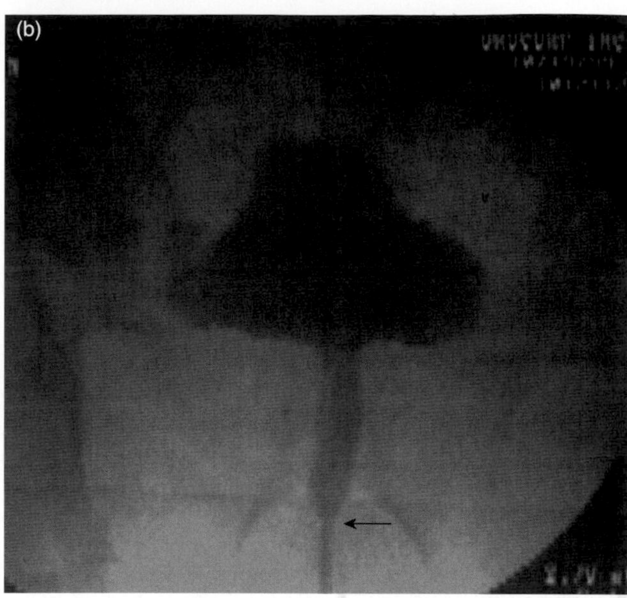

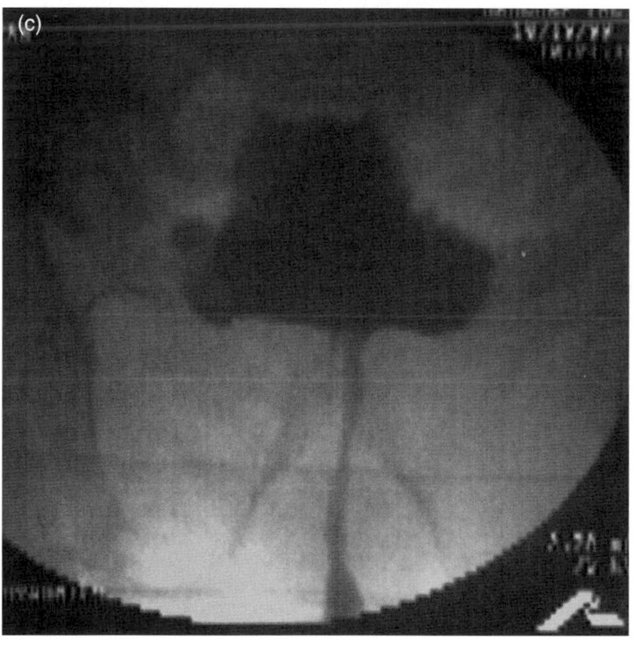

Figure 73.21
Type 3 detrusor overactivity and grade 3 prostatic obstruction in an 80-year-old man who sustained a cerebrovascular accident (CVA) (right hemiplegia) 1 year prior to this study. He developed urinary retention immediately after the stroke and was treated with a Foley catheter for 5 months and then switched to intermittent self-catheterization. On that regimen, he complained of urge incontinence. (a) Urodynamic tracing. This is a closeup of an involuntary detrusor contraction that he senses as an urge to void and contracts his sphincter to prevent incontinence. As the detrusor contracts against the closed sphincter there is a steep rise in pdet and he maintains continence. The detrusor contraction does not abate and he is then told to void, the sphincter relaxes, and he voids (pdetQmax = 55 cmH_2O; Qmax = 8 ml/s). (b) X-ray exposed while he is contracting his sphincter in an attempt to prevent incontinence shows the typical picture of DESD with obstruction at the membranous urethra (arrow). (c) X-ray exposed during voluntary micturition shows a narrowed prostatic urethra typical of prostatic obstruction associated with BPH. He underwent TURP and had resolution of his OAB symptoms and no longer needed intermittent catheterization. (Figure courtesy of Jerry G Blaivas MD.)

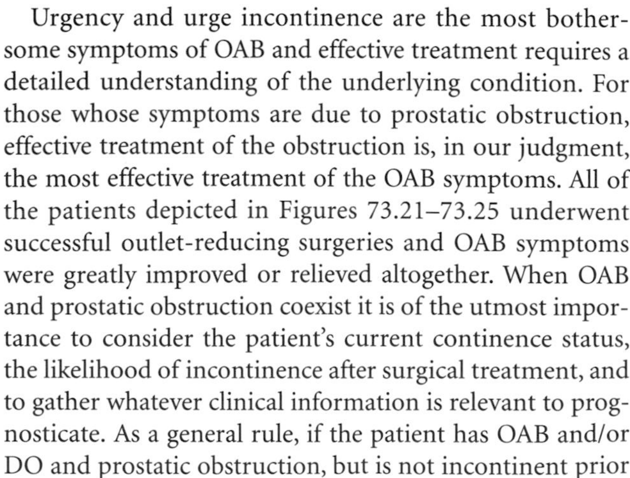

Urgency and urge incontinence are the most bothersome symptoms of OAB and effective treatment requires a detailed understanding of the underlying condition. For those whose symptoms are due to prostatic obstruction, effective treatment of the obstruction is, in our judgment, the most effective treatment of the OAB symptoms. All of the patients depicted in Figures 73.21–73.25 underwent successful outlet-reducing surgeries and OAB symptoms were greatly improved or relieved altogether. When OAB and prostatic obstruction coexist it is of the utmost importance to consider the patient's current continence status, the likelihood of incontinence after surgical treatment, and to gather whatever clinical information is relevant to prognosticate. As a general rule, if the patient has OAB and/or DO and prostatic obstruction, but is not incontinent prior to TURP, the chance of postoperative incontinence due to OAB is very low. On the other hand, if the patient already has urge incontinence, we believe the risk of persistent incontinence is much greater, but surgery is still worthwhile in suitable candidates because a substantial number will be improved. Because there is so much variability in neurologic status amongst patients, it is difficult to generalize, but the lower the OAB type (i.e. type 1 or 2), the greater the chances that OAB symptoms will be improved after outlet-reducing surgery. Nevertheless, the preoperative continence status is probably the most important predictor of postoperative continence.

When detrusor overactivity and impaired detrusor contractility coexist, effective treatment is very difficult to accomplish (Figure 73.26). There are several therapeutic

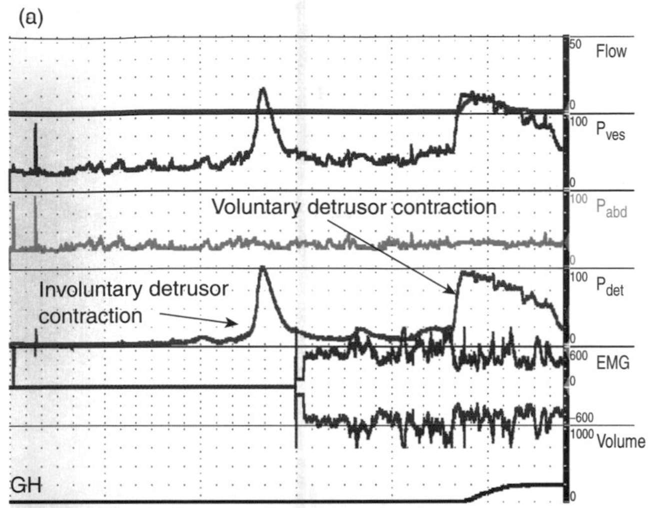

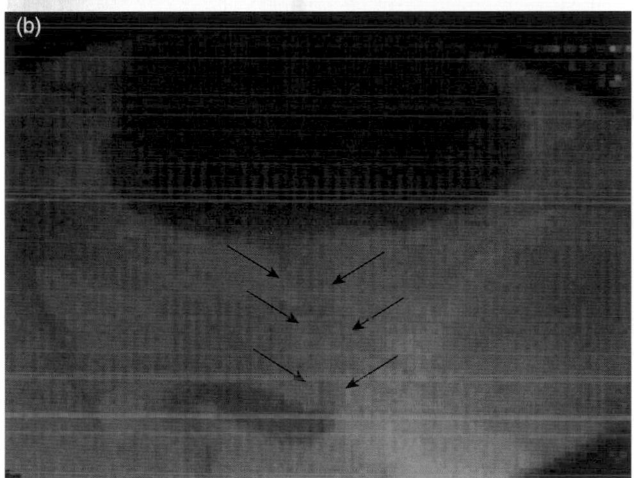

Figure 73.22
Grade 4 prostatic urethral obstruction and type 2 detrusor overactivity in a 68-year-old diabetic man with juvenile onset, type 1 insulin-dependent diabetes who complained of urinary frequency, decreased stream, urgency, and urge incontinence. After TURP his obstruction was relieved, but his OAB symptoms persisted for about 2 months and then gradually subsided. (a) Urodynamic tracing. At a bladder volume of about 150 ml, he had an involuntary detrusor contraction that he was aware of. He was able to contract his sphincter, prevent incontinence, and abort the detrusor contraction. The EMG tracing was not on at that time. The bladder was then filled until he sensed the need to void and he had a voiding of 244 ml. $P_{detQ_{max}} = 99$ cmH_2O; $Q_{max} = 10$ ml/s; PVR = 6 ml; this corresponds to Schafer grade 4 obstruction. (b) X-ray obtained at Q_{max} demonstrated diffuse narrowing of the prostatic urethra (arrows). (Figure courtesy of Jerry G Blaivas MD.)

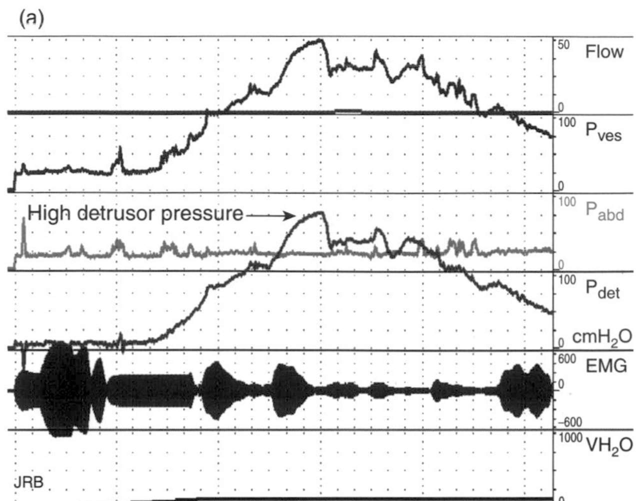

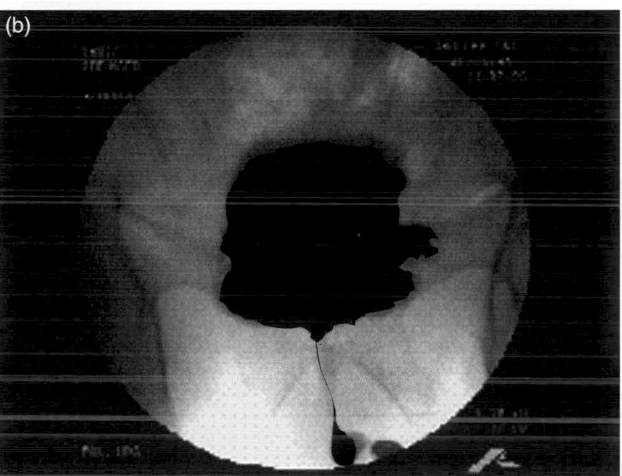

Figure 73.23
Prostatic obstruction in a 73-year-old man with Parkinson's disease. (a) Urodynamic tracing. $Q_{max} = 1$ ml/s; $P_{detQ_{max}} = 150$ cmH_2O; $P_{detmax} = 187$ cmH_2O; voided volume = 33 ml; postvoid residual = 88 ml. (b) X-ray obtained during voiding shows a heavily trabeculated bladder and narrowed prostatic urethra. (Figure courtesy of Jerry G Blaivas MD.)

approaches. The most straightforward is to attempt to abolish the involuntary detrusor contractions and add intermittent catheterization if residual urine is too high. Alternatively, since it is not possible to accurately determine whether or not the impaired detrusor contractility is the result of detrusor decompensation due to underlying prostatic obstruction, empiric outlet-reducing surgery such as TURP could be tried and, if that fails, one could revert to the first approach. Unfortunately, in many such men, intermittent catheterization is impractical because of either cognitive or physical comorbidities. In these instances, none of the options are appealing and pads, appliances, indwelling catheters, or urinary diversion must be resorted to.

As alluded to above, it may be difficult or impossible to determine with certainty whether the OAB symptoms and obstruction are due to BPH, neurogenic bladder, or both, but when the converse is true (i.e., the patient has OAB but no urethral obstruction), the problem is more straightforward (Figures 73.27 and 73.28). In these instances, treatment

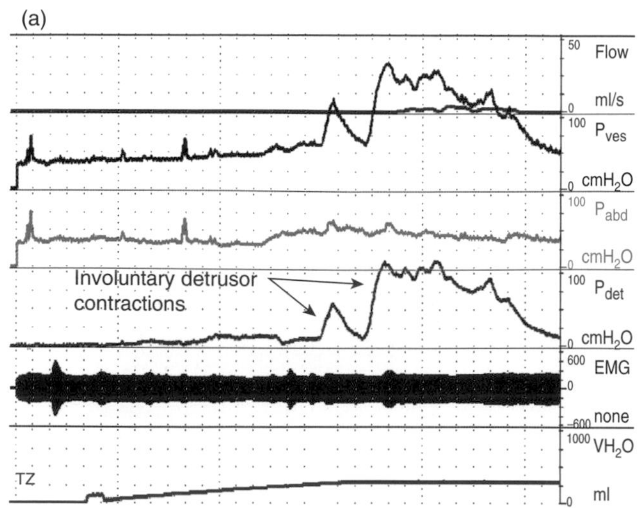

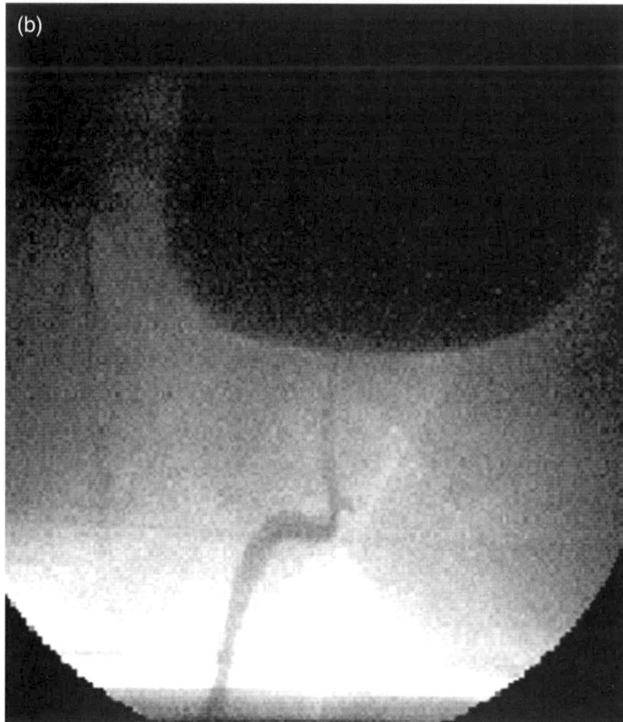

Figure 73.24
Sphincter bradykinesia and grade 5 prostatic urethral obstruction in a 65-year-old man with Parkinson's disease. He has had Parkinson's disease for about 12 years. He complains of urge incontinence most days (mostly when he's frozen, but he keeps urinary bottles everywhere at home because he won't be able to make it in time). His AUA symptom score is 20. He's had these symptoms for several years and is treated with tamsulosin and oxybutinin, but doesn't consider the symptoms bad enough to require further interventions. (a) Urodynamic tracing. There is no change in EMG activity during the involuntary detrusor contraction. This is characteristic of sphincter bradykinesia. $Q_{max} = 4.8$ ml/s; $P_{detQ_{max}} = 95$ cmH_2O; voided volume = 275 ml; postvoid residual = 30 ml. This corresponds to a Schafer grade 5 urethral obstruction. (b) X-ray obtained at Q_{max} shows a narrowed prostatic urethra consistent with prostatic obstruction. (Figure courtesy of Jerry G Blaivas MD.)

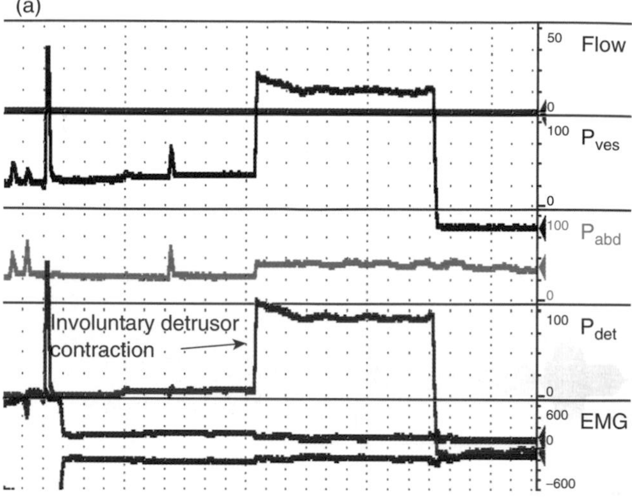

Figure 73.25
Grade 6 prostatic obstruction and type 4 OAB in an 81-year-old man with Parkinson's disease of 3 years' duration. He developed urinary retention and a prostatic stent was then placed, which failed to resolve his urinary retention. Cystoscopy revealed the proximal prostatic urethra and vesical neck to be 'filled' with what appeared to be prolapsing prostatic lobes. (a) Urodynamic tracing. $Q_{max} = 0.5$ ml/s; $P_{detQ_{max}} = 108$ cmH_2O; $P_{detmax} = 123$ cmH_2O; voided volume = 10 ml; postvoid residual = 60 ml. (b) X-ray exposed at Q_{max} shows no contrast in the urethra and grade 6 left vesicoureteral reflux. Note that the proximal margin of the stent (arrows) is about 1 cm distal to the bladder neck. At cystoscopy the tissue proximal to the stent appeared to be protruding prostatic lobes causing obstruction. (Figure courtesy of Jerry G Blaivas MD.)

should be directed at the OAB no matter how large the prostate is. Surgical treatment of the prostate, in particular, is likely to be ineffective and may even be harmful. Men with OAB due to neurogenic detrusor overactivity are best served by treatment of OAB described in the preceding section, but in men with types 3 and 4 OAB and other comorbidities, such treatment is notoriously ineffective.

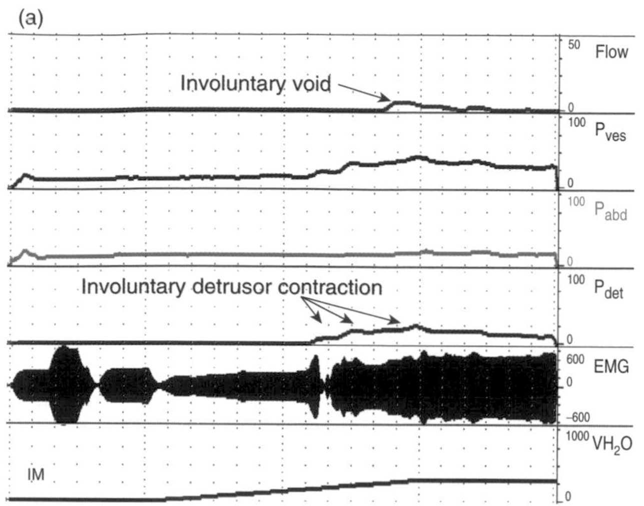

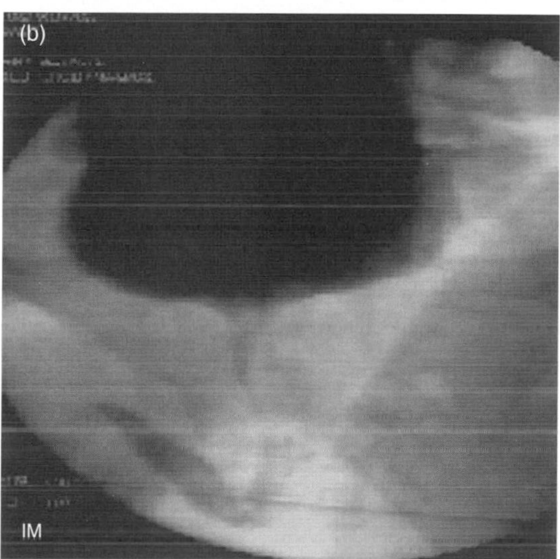

Figure 73.26
Detrusor hyperreflexia (type 3 OAB) and impaired detrusor contractility associated with CVA in an 82-year-old man who is 4 months S/P CVA that resulted in right hemiparesis. There are no cognitive deficits. He complains of urinary frequency, urgency, and urge incontinence and soaks through large pads day and night. (a) Urodynamic tracing. At a bladder volume of 269 ml there was an involuntary detrusor contraction. He perceived the contraction as urge. He contracted his sphincter and temporarily prevented incontinence, but the detrusor contraction continued and, after a short time, he voided involuntarily. Note that there is a disparity between the EMG tracing and pressure–flow curves. One would expect that when the EMG becomes silent, just after the detrusor contraction occurred, that pdet would fall and voiding ensue. Further, the EMG activity is increased throughout the detrusor contraction, but there appears to be no correlation between the increased EMG activity, uroflow, detrusor pressure, or the radiographic appearance of the urethra. When such a disparity exists, we believe that the EMG is artifact. Q_{max} = 6 ml/s; $P_{detQ_{max}}$ = 20 cmH_2O; P_{detmax} = 26 cmH_2O. According to the Schafer nomogram, this represents a very weak bladder without urethral obstruction. Voided volume = 171 ml; PVR = 101 ml. (b) X-ray obtained during voiding at Q_{max} shows poor visualization of the prostatic urethra, but the bulbar and anterior urethra are well seen. (Figure courtesy of Jerry G Blaivas MD.)

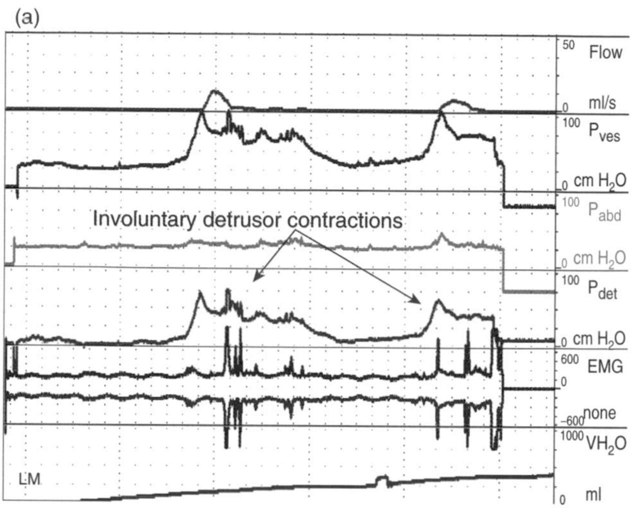

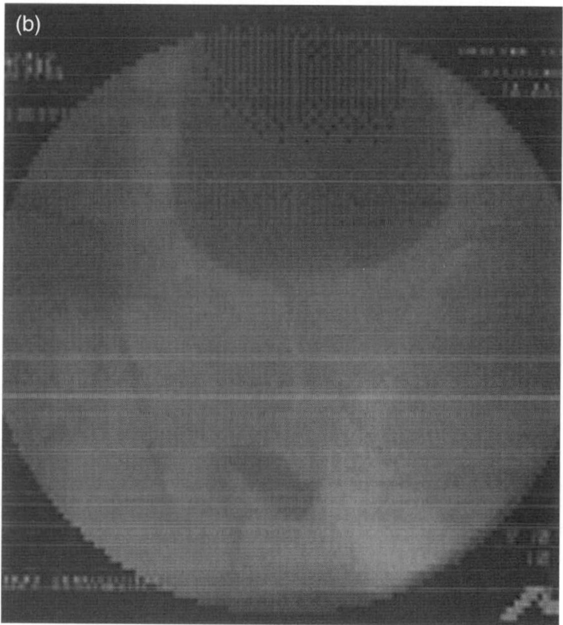

Figure 73.27
Detrusor hyperreflexia (type 4 detrusor overactivity) in a 66-year-old man 3 years after a cerebrovascular accident that that left him with left hemiparesis and incontinence. (a) Urodynamic tracing. During bladder filling there were involuntary detrusor contractions beginning at a volume of 240 ml. He perceived the contraction as urge, but was not able to contract his sphincter and he voided involuntarily. Q_{max} = 13 ml; $P_{detQ_{max}}$ = 46 cmH_2O. This corresponds to a Schafer grade 1, which is not considered to be urethral obstruction. Voided volume = 243 ml; postvoid residual = 0 ml. (b) X-ray obtained at Q_{max} shows a normal urethra in this . (Figure courtesy of Jerry G Blaivas MD.)

Incontinence

Incontinence is due to bladder abnormalities and/or sphincter abnormalities. Bladder abnormalities (detrusor overactivity or low bladder compliance) are by far the most common causes. The treatment is outlined above.

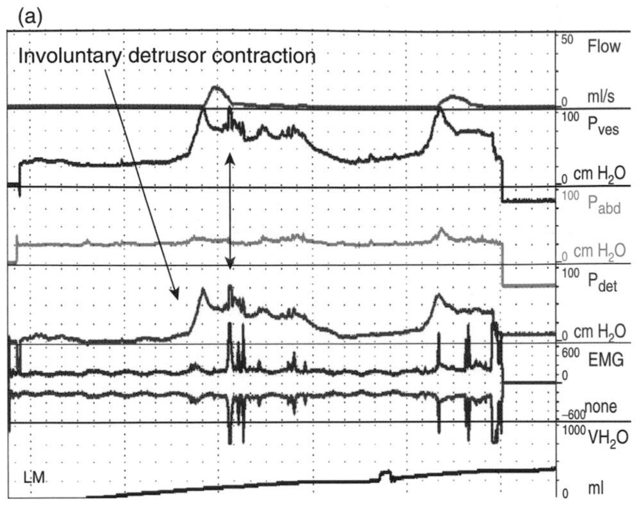

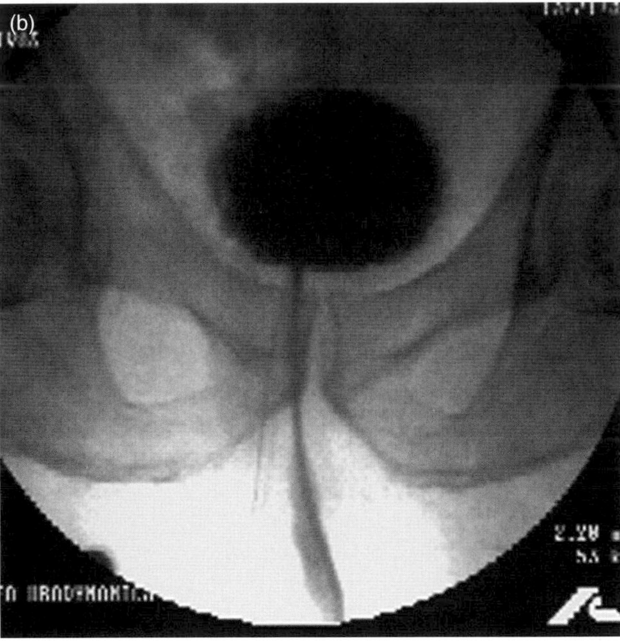

Figure 73.28

Detrusor hyperreflexia (type 4 detrusor overactivity) due to CVA. LM is a 66-year-old man 3 years S/P CVA that left him with left hemiparesis and incontinence. (a) Urodynamic tracing. During bladder filling there were spontaneous involuntary detrusor contractions beginning at a volume of 240 ml. He perceived the contractions as urge, but was not able to contract his sphincter and he voided involuntarily. After the first detrusor contraction had almost abated, when the bladder was almost empty, there was an involuntary sphincter contraction that obstructed the urethra and caused a momentary rise in detrusor pressure (arrow). The detrusor contraction continued and the remaining bladder urine was voided with a flow of only about 1 ml/s. p_{det}@Q study $Q_{max} = 13$ ml; $P_{detQ_{max}} = 46$ cmH_2O. This corresponds to a Schafer grade 2 which is not considered to be urethral obstruction. Voided volume = 243 ml; postvoid residual = 0 ml. (b) X- ray obtained near the end of micturition shows a normal caliber bulbar urethra. The prostatic urethra seems narrowed, but was wide open on earlier views that are not reproduced here. The bladder has an irregular contour consistent with coarse trabeculations. (Figure courtesy of Jerry G Blaivas MD.)

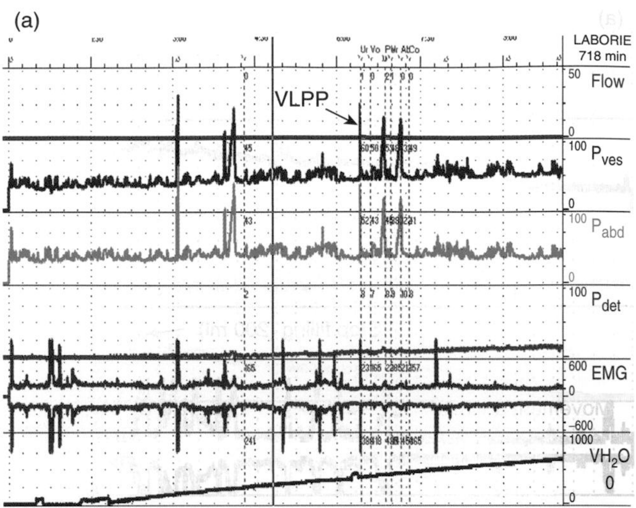

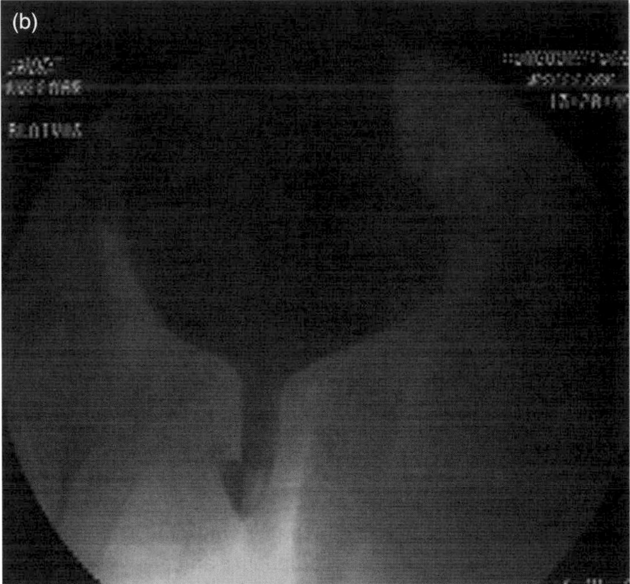

Figure 73.29

Sphincteric incontinence and detrusor areflexia in a 51-year-old man who underwent excision of a giant cell tumor of the sacrum 20 years previously. He complains of sphincteric incontinence and needs to strain to void. (a) Urodynamic tracing. The bladder is areflexic and when he strains there is overt sphincteric incontinence. (b) X-ray exposed at the VLLP (vesical leak-point pressure) shows a wide open urethra down to the midportion of the bulb. (Figure courtesy of Jerry G Blaivas MD.)

Sphincteric causes of incontinence are rare and include prior prostatic or urethral surgery and certain neurologic conditions that involve the thoracolumbar and sacral spinal cord segments. The diagnosis of sphincteric incontinence should be suspected from the history and confirmed by examination with a full bladder and/or a video-urodynamic study. Management of sphincteric incontinence depends, to a large extent, on the underlying neurologic condition and associated urodynamic abnormalities.

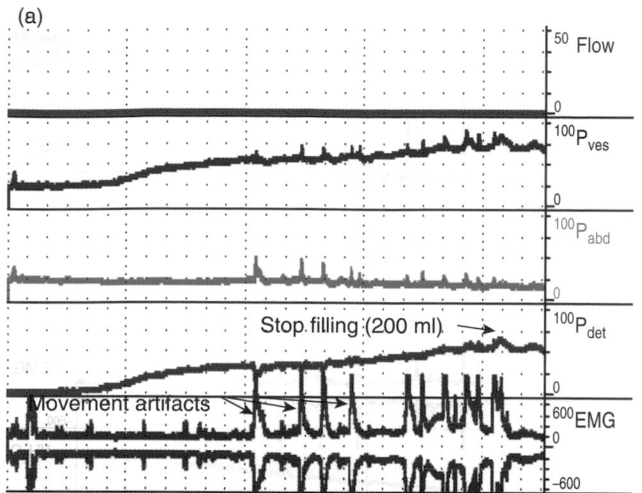

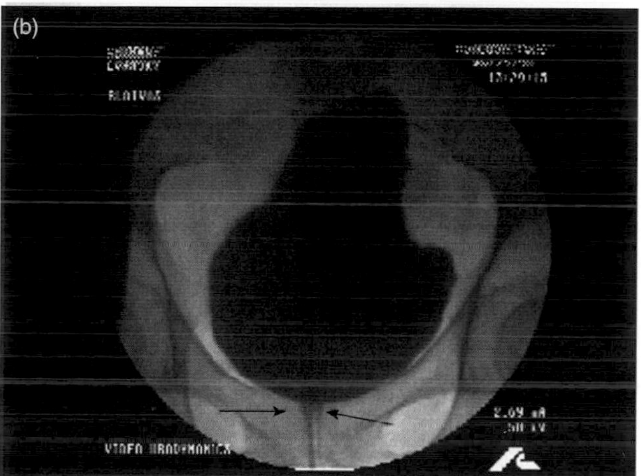

Figure 73.30
Typical urodynamic study in Shy–Drager syndrome showing detrusor areflexia, low bladder compliance and open bladder neck at rest. (a) Urodynamic tracing. During bladder filling, there is a steep rise in detrusor pressure and when filling is stopped, pdet falls, showing that this is due to low bladder compliance and not a detrusor contraction. The sporadic bursts of EMG activity are movement artifacts, as each burst is accompanied by an increase in pabd and pves. (b) X-ray shows an open bladder neck with 175 ml in the bladder (arrows). (Figure courtesy of Jerry G Blaivas MD.)

For those whose only abnormality is sphincteric incontinence (i.e., detrusor contractility is normal and there is no urethral obstruction), sphincter prosthesis is the treatment of choice. Alternatively, one may consider a male sling, but we prefer the former. Unfortunately, such patients are rarely encountered in clinical practice. More commonly, sphincteric incontinence is accompanied by detrusor areflexia (Figure 73.29). Sphincteric incontinence and detrusor areflexia are seen most commonly in patients with spinal cord tumors, anterior spinal artery occlusion, and spina bifida. In these patients, a sphincter prosthesis may ameliorate the incontinence and they may be able to void

Table 73.6 *Etiology of sphincteric incontinence*
Post-prostatectomy
Multisystem atrophy (particularly Shy–Drager syndrome)
Thoracolumbar and sacral spinal cord lesions
Spina bifida
Anterior spinal artery thrombosis
Spinal cord tumors
Trauma
Post-abdominoperineal resection of the rectum

by straining. If not, intermittent catheterization becomes necessary, but this increases the chances of erosion of the sphincter cuff. The worst pathophysiology is that which results in low bladder compliance, detrusor areflexia (or detrusor hyperreflexia), and sphincteric incontinence (Figure 73.30). These combinations are seen most often in patients with spina bifida, Shy–Drager syndrome (and other multisystmen atrophy patients), and spinal cord tumors (particularly after radiation). Treatment must take the nature of the underlying neurologic condition into account. For those with progressive degenerative disorders like multisystem atrophy, we believe that it is best to manage them very conservatively from the beginning, with timed intermittent catheterization and treatment to abolish involuntary detrusor contractions. As the disease progresses, over time, it is likely that the catheterization will require a caregiver. Alternatively, early urinary diversion may afford a better long-term life style.

Conclusion

In men with neurogenic bladder, the incidence of BPH, BPE, and BPO probably mirrors that seen in the general population. That means that the chances of these conditions coexisting with neurogenic bladder increases with advancing age and, by age 80 clinical BPH is apparent in over 60% of men. When BPH and neurogenic bladder coexist, the most reliable means of identifying the underlying pathophysiology is the video-urodynamic study. Effective treatment is best accomplished when based on the underlying cause. No matter what the treatment, though, careful long-term surveillance is important to prevent complications.

References

1. Berry SJ, Coffey DS, Walsh PC et al. The development of human benign prostatic hyperplasia with age. J Urol 1984; 132(3): 474–9.
2. Gupta A, Gupta S, Pavuk M et al. Anthropometric and metabolic factors and risk of benign prostatic hyperplasia: a prospective cohort study of Air Force veterans. Urology 2006; 68(6): 1198–205.
3. Roehrborn CG, McConnell JD. Etiology, pathophysiology, epidemiology and natural history of benign prostatic hyperplasia. In: Walsh PC, Retik AB, Vaughan ED Jr, Wein AJ, eds. Campbell's Urology. Philadelphia, PA: WB Saunders Company, 2002: 1297–330.

4. Shabbir M, Mumtaz FH. Benign prostatic hyperplasia. J R Soc Health 2004; 124(5): 222–7.
5. Geller J, Sionit L. Castration-like effects on the human prostate of a 5 alpha-reductase inhibitor, finasteride. J Cell Biochem Suppl 1992; 16H: 109–12.
6. Carson C 3rd, Rittmaster R. The role of dihydrotestosterone in benign prostatic hyperplasia. Urology 2003; 61(4 Suppl 1): 2–7.
7. Walsh PC, Hutchins GM, Ewing LL. Tissue content of dihydrotestosterone in human prostatic hyperplasia is not supranormal. J Clin Invest 1983; 72(5): 1772–7.
8. Fusco F, Groutz A, Blaivas JG et al. Videourodynamic studies in men with lower urinary tract symptoms: a comparison of community based versus referral urological practices. J Urol 2001; 166(3): 910–13.
9. Barry MJ, Cockett AT, Holtgrewe HL et al. Relationship of symptoms of prostatism to commonly used physiological and anatomical measures of the severity of benign prostatic hyperplasia. J Urol 1993; 150: 351–8.
10. Wadie BS, Badawi AM, Ghoneim MA et al. The relationship of the International Prostate Symptom Score and objective parameters for diagnosing bladder outlet obstruction. Part I: when statistics fail. J Urol 2001; 165(1): 32–4.
11. Lepor H, Gup DI, Baumann M, Sharpio E. Laboratory assessment of terazosin and alpha-1 blockade in prostatic hyperplasia. Urology 1988; 32(6 Suppl): 21–6.
12. Price DT, Schwinn HP, Lomasney JW et al. Identification, quantification, and localization of mRNA for three distinct alpha 1 adrenergic receptor subtypes in human prostate. J Urol 1993; 150(2 Pt 1): 546–51.
13. Blaivas JG. The neurophysiology of micturition: a clinical study of 550 patients. J Urol 1982; 127(5): 958–63.
14. de Groat WC. Anatomy of the central neural pathways controlling the lower urinary tract. Eur Urol 1998; 34(Suppl 1): 2–5.
15. Bradley WE, Timm GW. Physiology of micturition. Vet Clin North Am 1974; 4(3): 487–500.
16. Blaivas JG, Sinha HP, Zayed AA, Labib KB. Detrusor-external sphincter dyssynergia. J Urol 1981; 125(4): 542–4.
17. Khan Z, Hertann J, Yang WC et al. Predictive correlation of urodynamic dysfunction and brain injury after cerebrovascular accident. J Urol 1981; 126(1): 86–8.
18. Flisser AJ, Walmsley K, Blaivas JG. Urodynamic classification of patients with symptoms of overactive bladder. J Urol 2003; 169(2): 529–33.
19. Blaivas JG, Sinha HP, Zayed AAH, Labib KB. Detrusor External-sphincter dyssynergia: a detailed EMG study. J Urol 1981; 125: 545–8.
20. Blaivas JG, Barbalias GA. Characteristics of neural injury after abdominoperineal resection. J Urol 1983; 129(1): 84–7.
21. Gerstenberg TC, Nielson ML, Clausen S et al. Bladder function after abdominoperineal resection of the rectum for anorectal cancer. Urodynamic investigation before and after operation in a consecutive series. Ann Surg 1980; 191(1): 81–6.
22. Yalla SV, Andriole GL. Vesicourethral dysfunction following pelvic visceral ablative surgery. J Urol 1984; 132(3): 503–9.
23. Caine M, Pfau A, Perlberg S. The use of alpha-adrenergic blockers in benign prostatic obstruction. Br J Urol 1976; 48(4): 255–63.
24. Caine M, Raz S, Zeigler M. Adrenergic and cholinergic receptors in the human prostate, prostatic capsule and bladder neck. Br J Urol 1975; 47(2): 193–202.
25. Jensen KME, Bruskewitz R, Iversen P, Madsen PO. Predictive value of voiding pressure in benign prostatic hyperplasia. Neurourol Urodyn 1983; 2: 117–25.
26. McConnell JD. Medical management of benign prostatic hyperplasia with androgen suppression. Prostate Suppl 1990; 3: 49–59.
27. Leng WW, McGuire EJ. Obstructive uropathy induced bladder dysfunction can be reversible: bladder compliance measures before and after treatment. J Urol 2003; 169(2): 563–6.
28. Blaivas JG, Weiss JP, Desai P et al. Long-term followup of augmentation enterocystoplasty and continent diversion in patients with benign disease. J Urol 2005; 173(5): 1631–4.
29. Drinka PJ. Complications of chronic indwelling urinary catheters. J Am Med Dir Assoc 2006; 7(6): 388–92.
30. Schafer W. Principles and clinical application of advanced urodynamic analysis of voiding function. Urol Clin North Am 1990; 17(3): 553–66.
31. Schafer W. Urodynamics in benign prostatic hyperplasia (BPH). Arch Ital Urol Androl 1993; 65(6): 599–613.
32. Abrams PH, Griffiths DJ. The assessment of prostatic obstruction from urodynamic measurements and from residual urine. Br J Urol 1979; 51(2): 129–34.

Part X

Sexual dysfunction in neurologic disorders

74

Pathophysiology of male sexual dysfunction after spinal cord injury

Pierre Denys and Djamel Bensmail

Sexual function is a fundamental need in human beings. After spinal cord injury (SCI), the modification of neurologic control and its consequences on reproductive organs have been extensively described in humans. Globally, sexual satisfaction decreases but sexuality remains a major concern, specifically after the first year following the injury.[1] Moreover, recovery of sexual function is the major concern of paraplegic patients before locomotion,[2] after the acute rehabilitation phase. For these specific sequelae/complications we have to keep in mind that the majority of patients are male and young.[3] The impact of the neurologic lesion and its physiologic consequences must be balanced by the fact that the quality of life with respect to sexuality after spinal cord lesion concerns more the relationship with a partner and mental well-being rather than the preservation of sexual ability.[1,4] In clinical practice it is well known that this population have specific problems such as dissociation between sensation, erection, ejaculation, and orgasm. Such dissociation is only seen in cases of neurologic lesion. Erection can be improved by several treatments, but sensation is not modified, and furthermore the ability to ejaculate during intercourse is not improved by any of the available treatments.

Sexual behavior is under the control of a complex neural network which connects autonomic, somatic reflex pathways and cerebral control. Very little is known about the physiology and physiopathology of sexual function in animal models after a spinal lesion, which is a complicated subject with many unknowns. Historically, the approach was to characterize the sexual response to the level and extent of the injury in men and women. This gave a lot of information on the respective roles of the spinal segments (i.e. sacral, thoracolumbar) for reflexogenic, psychogenic erection and ejaculation, orgasm, and sexual response in women. However, very little is known about the dynamic neurologic process and reorganization (neuroplasticity) that might occur after a spinal lesion. This is in contrast to an extensive literature which addresses the role of neuroplasticity and neurotrophic factors in the reappearance of bladder contraction after the spinal shock phase. Modifications of afferent properties and the role of neurotrophic factors are now well described in rat and cat models of complete spinal cord lesions for the control of bladder and striated sphincter or for autonomic dysreflexia.[5] The description of a central generator of ejaculation[6] will probably change the way of thinking about modifications induced by spinal lesions, both in terms of pharmacologic regulation and the impact on the regulation of this paramount sexual function from a fertility perspective.

Impact of a lesion of the ascending and/or descending pathways on sexual function in the male

Neural circuitry controling erection and ejaculation is located within specific regions of the spinal cord,[7,8] and is described in Chapter 8 of this volume. In spinal cord injured patients, sexual behavior modifications can be induced by lesion of the spinal cord centers themselves (sacral or low thoracic) or by lesion of descending and ascending pathways controling their activities. This chapter will mainly review the impact of lesions on pathways related to the ejaculatory response.

Several supraspinal regions are involved in the regulation of the spinal centers for ejaculation and of the spinal ejaculation generator (for review see reference 9). They can be either inhibitory or excitatory and include the nucleus paragigatantocellularis (nPGi), the paraventricular nucleus of the hypothalamus (PVN), and the medial preoptic area (MPOA). The group of lumbar spinothalamic (LSt) neurons that is a candidate for the spinal ejaculation generator surrounds the central canal at the L3 and L4 level in rats, and these neurons project to the parvocellular subparafascicular thalamic nucleus.

To investigate the effect of ascending and/or descending pathways involved in the regulation of ejaculation, the location of injury must be at the midthoracic level to avoid lesions of spinal autonomic centers, and the effect of the lesions must be evaluated 30 days after injury to avoid the spinal shock phase. Early behavioral studies on rats with transections at the midthoracic level showed an enhanced erectile and depressed ejaculatory reflex.[10–12] More recently, Nout et al[13] used telemetric corpus spongiosum penis pressure monitoring. They reported that the number of full erectile episodes decreased significantly 24 days after T10 standardized lesions, but the level of pressure registered in the bulb increased during erection. Johnson and colleagues developed rodent models with chronic midthoracic incomplete partial spinal cord injury to assess the effect of descending pathways involved in ejaculation.[14–16] Spinal ejaculatory pathways are dependent on bilateral pathways from the brainstem which modulate pudendal motor reflex and pudendal nerve autonomic fiber activities. Sensory input from the dorsal nerve of the penis required to trigger ejaculation is no longer inhibited from the nPGi after unilateral incomplete lesion. This inhibition is important in the organization of rhythmic contractions of the perineal muscles during the expulsion phase of ejaculation. Chronic incomplete unilateral lesion results in new connections of the pudendal reflex inhibitory and pudendal sympathetic activation pathways across a midline below the lesion which contribute to poor coordination of the perineal muscles during the contractions that are mandatory for ejaculation. The new connections in the thoracic spinal cord may be due to reorganization of the segmental autonomic circuits. The requirement for very high intensity stimulation during penile vibratory stimulation in SCI men can be related to these modifications. Several clinical observations in the SCI population are in accordance with modifications observed in animals after high-level spinal cord injury with a loss of central synaptic efficacy of penile afferents: the inability of SCI patients to induce ejaculation during intercourse, and the high level of vibratory stimulation parameters used to obtain ejaculation which are beyond the intensity required for normal sensation in the able-bodied population.[17]

The particular case of autonomic dysreflexia

After SCI, large increases in arterial blood pressure can develop after the spinal shock phase in response to sensory input entering the spinal cord below the lesion. This acute hyperpertension is a part of SCI complications termed autonomic dysreflexia (AD). AD has been reported in 50–90% of patients with tetraplegia or high-level paraplegia.[18,19] Severe AD may result clinically in headaches, seizures, strokes, and even death. Blood pressure is normally under supraspinal control of sympathetic neurons, and a spinal cord lesion can result in the disappearance of supraspinal inhibitory control. AD occurs mainly if the injury is rostral to T6, because in this case the extensive abdominal circulation is under uninhibited spinal reflexes. Both noxious and non-noxious stimulation below the level of the lesion can induce AD. Ejaculation and penile vibratory stimulation are frequently responsible for AD and electrocardiographic anormalities, sometimes with severe consequences,[20,21] hence the need for preventive treatment during these procedures.[22,23] Rodent models of spinal cord lesions at the T2–4 level developed AD after bladder or colonic irritation, and this response increased with time after the lesion.[24,25] Within the dorsal horn after SCI the arbors of calcitonin gene-related peptide (CGRP)-immunoreactive, small-diameter, primary afferent neurons enlarge significantly,[26] and the extent of this immunoreactivity correlates with the magnitude of AD.[27] This modification of afferent arbors seems to be dependent on nerve growth factor (NGF) action.[28] Furthermore, treatment with high-affinity NGF antibody of trk A-IgG fusion protein delivered intraspinally can limit the development of afferent sprouting and the magnitude of AD.[28,29] All these elements strongly suggested an ongoing process after SCI leading via neuroplasticity. Such a process has been extensively described for the pathophysiology of neurogenic detrusor overactivity after SCI involving afferent property modifications in relation to neurotrophic factors. Such modifications involve perineal afferents which may play a role either in bladder function or in sexual function. For example, after SCI the micturition reflex switches back to a spinal reflex after the spinal shock phase. In neonates, such a reflex can be triggered by perineal afferent stimulation. This reflex reappears several weeks after SCI in rats and is used by patients who void using cutaneous stimulation to induce bladder contraction and micturition.[5,30,31] The same perineal afferents can be stimulated electrically to modulate detrusor reflux contraction.[31,32] In another words, the same afferent pathway in both SCI animals and humans can trigger various behaviors, and spinal lesions can strongly modify those actions.

Summary

Spinal cord lesions dramatically modify sexual behavior in animals and humans. Few studies have addressed the dynamic process of reorganization within the spinal cord of pathways and centers involved in sexual function. Some recent reports suggest an ongoing process of reorganization, which can be correlated with difficulty in inducing ejaculation via stimulation of perineal afferents, and with the development of AD after SCI.

References

1. Reitz A, Tobe V, Knapp PA, Schurch B. Impact of spinal cord injury on sexual health and quality of life. Int J Impot Res 2004; 16(2): 167–74.
2. Anderson KD. Targeting recovery: priorities of the spinal cord-injured population. J Neurotrauma 2004; 21(10): 1371–83.
3. Jackson AB, Dijkers M, Devivo MJ, Poczatek RB. A demographic profile of new traumatic spinal cord injuries: change and stability over 30 years. Arch Phys Med Rehab 2004; 85(11): 1740–8.
4. Phelps J, Albo M, Dunn K, Joseph A. Spinal cord injury and sexuality in married or partnered men: activities, function, needs, and predictors of sexual adjustment. Arch Sex Behav 2001; 30(6): 591–602.
5. Vizzard MA. Neurochemical plasticity and the role of neurotrophic factors in bladder reflex pathways after spinal cord injury. Prog Brain Res 2006; 152: 97–115.
6. Truitt WA, Shipley MT, Veening JG, Coolen LM. Activation of a subset of lumbar spinothalamic neurons after copulatory behavior in male but not female rats. J Neurosci 2003; 23(1): 325–31.
7. Giuliano F, Rampin O. Central neural regulation of penile erection. Neurosci Biobehav Rev 2000; 24(5): 517–33.
8. Allard J, Truitt WA, McKenna KE, Coolen LM. Spinal cord control of ejaculation. World J Urol 2005; 23(2): 119–26.
9. Coolen LM. Neural control of ejaculation. J Comp Neurol 2005; 493(1): 39–45.
10. Sachs BD, Garinello LD. Spinal pacemaker controlling sexual reflexes in male rats. Brain Res 1979; 171(1): 152–6.
11. Hart BL, Odell V. Elicitation of ejaculation and penile reflexes in spinal male rats by peripheral electric shock. Physiol Behav 1981; 26(4): 623–6.
12. Hart BL, Odell V. Effects of intermittent electric shock on penile reflexes of male rats. Behav Neural Biol 1980; 29(3): 394–8.
13. Nout YS, Schmidt MH, Tovar CA et al. Telemetric monitoring of corpus spongiosum penis pressure in conscious rats for assessment of micturition and sexual function following spinal cord contusion injury. J Neurotrauma 2005; 22(4): 429–41.
14. Johnson RD, Hubscher CH. Brainstem microstimulation differentially inhibits pudendal motoneuron reflex inputs. Neuroreport 1998; 9(2): 341–5.
15. Johnson RD. Descending pathways modulating the spinal circuitry for ejaculation: effects of chronic spinal cord injury. Prog Brain Res 2006; 152: 415–26.
16. Johnson RD, Hubscher CH. Brainstem microstimulation activates sympathetic fibers in pudendal nerve motor branch. Neuroreport 2000; 11(2): 379–82.
17. Sonksen J, Biering-Sorensen F, Kristensen JK. Ejaculation induced by penile vibratory stimulation in men with spinal cord injuries. The importance of the vibratory amplitude. Paraplegia 1994; 32(10): 651–60.
18. Giannantoni A, Di Stasi SM, Scivoletto G et al. Autonomic dysreflexia during urodynamics. Spinal Cord 1998; 36(11): 756–60.
19. Krassioukov AV, Weaver LC. Episodic hypertension due to autonomic dysreflexia in acute and chronic spinal cord-injured rats. Am J Physiol 1995; 268(5 Pt 2): H2077–83.
20. Claydon VE, Elliott SL, Sheel AW, Krassioukov A. Cardiovascular responses to vibrostimulation for sperm retrieval in men with spinal cord injury. J Spinal Cord Med 2006; 29(3): 207–16.
21. Elliott S, Krassioukov A. Malignant autonomic dysreflexia in spinal cord injured men. Spinal Cord 2006; 44(6): 386–92.
22. Brackett NL, Ferrell SM, Aballa TC et al. An analysis of 653 trials of penile vibratory stimulation in men with spinal cord injury. J Urol 1998; 159(6): 1931–4.
23. Steinberger RE, Ohl DA, Bennett CJ, McCabe M, Wang SC. Nifedipine pretreatment for autonomic dysreflexia during electroejaculation. Urology 1990; 36(3): 228–31.
24. Jacob JE, Pniak A, Weaver LC, Brown A. Autonomic dysreflexia in a mouse model of spinal cord injury. Neuroscience 2001; 108(4): 687–93.
25. Jacob JE, Gris P, Fehlings MG, Weaver LC, Brown A. Autonomic dysreflexia after spinal cord transection or compression in 129Sv, C57BL, and Wallerian degeneration slow mutant mice. Exp Neurol 2003; 183(1): 136–46.
26. Wong ST, Atkinson BA, Weaver LC. Confocal microscopic analysis reveals sprouting of primary afferent fibres in rat dorsal horn after spinal cord injury. Neurosci Lett 2000; 296(2–3): 65–8.
27. Krenz NR, Weaver LC. Changes in the morphology of sympathetic preganglionic neurons parallel the development of autonomic dysreflexia after spinal cord injury in rats. Neurosci Lett 1998; 243(1–3): 61–4.
28. Krenz NR, Meakin SO, Krassioukov AV, Weaver LC. Neutralizing intraspinal nerve growth factor blocks autonomic dysreflexia caused by spinal cord injury. J Neurosci 1999; 19(17): 7405–14.
29. Marsh DR, Wong ST, Meakin SO et al. Neutralizing intraspinal nerve growth factor with a trkA-IgG fusion protein blocks the development of autonomic dysreflexia in a clip-compression model of spinal cord injury. J Neurotrauma 2002; 19(12): 1531–41.
30. de Groat WC, Yoshimura N. Mechanisms underlying the recovery of lower urinary tract function following spinal cord injury. Prog Brain Res 2006; 152: 59–84.
31. Tai C, Wang J, Wang X, de Groat WC, Roppolo JR. Bladder inhibition or voiding induced by pudendal nerve stimulation in chronic spinal cord injured cats. Neurourol Urodyn 2007.
32. Wieder JA, Brackett NL, Lynne CM, Green JT, Aballa TC. Anesthetic block of the dorsal penile nerve inhibits vibratory-induced ejaculation in men with spinal cord injuries. Urology 2000; 55(6): 915–17.

75

Sexual dysfunction in patients with multiple sclerosis and other neurologic diseases

Dirk De Ridder

Introduction

Neurologic diseases such as multiple sclerosis (MS) have a serious impact on the patient's personal, professional, and social life. While many physicians and caregivers might focus on the treatment of the neurologic disease or its symptoms, patients themselves and their partner are confronted with an uninvited third partner in their relationship. MS will have an important impact on their relationship, their sexuality, and their sexual function, an impact that is often neglected by caregivers. Limiting the investigation and treatment of sexual dysfunction to the mechanics of sex is not always an answer to the real underlying anxiety. Addressing the psychologic needs is at least as important.

Interference with normal neurologic processes for sexuality and sexual function can happen at several neuroanatomic sites (Table 75.1). This 'primary' interference directly affects sexual functioning: erectile dysfunction, vaginal lubrification, libido, ejaculation, and orgasm. For a detailed reading on the neurology of sexual function and dysfunction we refer to other authors.[1–4]

At the secondary level, consequences of the neurologic disease that interfere with sexuality are described: fatigue, spasticity, urinary and/or fecal incontinence, cognitive dysfunction, side effects of medication, depression, etc.

At the tertiary level the social and relational consequences are situated: the role of sexual partner versus caregiver, social isolation, sexual isolation, changing expectations.

Table 75.1 *Neuroanatomic sites of sexual functioning and sexual response (adapted from Rees PM et al[4])*

Libido and orgasm	Brainstem, midbrain, cortex, pudendal nerve
Attention	Reticular system
Affection	Limbic system
Voluntary movement	Motor cortex
Cognition, emotion	Frontal and temporal cortex
Perception, sensory awareness	Parietal cortex
Reflex erection/lubrification	Sacral innervation S2–S4
Psychogenic erection/ lubrification	Spinal cord T11–L2
Ejaculation	Spinal cord L1–L3
Detumescence	Sympathetic control

MS and sexuality

Primary sexual dysfunction

The prevalence of sexual dysfunction (SD) is high in MS. MS affects people at a young age, when their sexual relationship is still quite young and their family planning is not always completed. In a minority of patients, sexual dysfunction even precedes the diagnosis of MS or is present at the time of the diagnosis, indicating that the presence of SD might help to define the diagnosis of MS.

Once MS has been diagnosed nearly 60% of men and 25% of women will have a less active sex life than before, while 87% of men and 66% of women find sexual issues to be very important. However, less than 10% of patients will discuss sexuality with their physician, which means that an active attitude must be adopted by the neurologist, urologist, and rehabilitation specialists to incorporate sexuality in the routine workup of these patients.

Zorzon et al showed that patients with MS (PwMS) reported sexual dysfunction in 73.1% of cases, compared to 39.2% of patients with chronic rheumatic diseases and 12.7% of healthy controls.[5] Male patients reported sexual dysfunction more frequently than females. Anorgasmia and hyporgasmia (37–52%), decreased vaginal lubrification (35.7–55%), and reduced libido (31–63%) are most prevalent in women. Men complained of erectile dysfunction (63.2–72%), ejaculatory and orgasmic dysfunction (50–53%), and reduced libido (39–63%).[5,6] The sexual dysfunction correlated with bladder dysfunction and with destructive lesions at the pontine level, when investigated with MRI.[7] The extent of sexual dysfunction in women correlated with high sensory thresholds at the clitoral level, but not with tibial or pudendal evoked potentials.[8,9] Patients with relapsing-remitting MS seemed to be less affected than those with primary or secondary progressive disease. Over the course of time, the number of primary SD symptoms and their severity increased. Relapses had little impact on this process, and the progression of the SD symptomatology correlated with the eventual worsening of bladder control.[10,11]

Table 75.2 *Significant correlations between sexual dysfunction and secondary influencing factors according to several authors.*

	All MS patients	Women	Men
Gender		+	++
Age	+	0	+
Age at onset of disease	+	+	+
Duration of disease	?	?	?
Primary of secondary progressive MS	+	+	+
EDSS	+	+	0
Dependency	+	+	0
Sphincter dysfunction	+	+	0
Bladder dysfunction	+	+	0
Bowel dysfunction	0	0	0
Fatigue	+	+	+
Cognition	+	+	0

+, Positive correlation; 0, no correlation; ?, conflicting data.

Secondary sexual dysfunction

Of the secondary factors fatigue was reported as the most important one (up to 40%), followed by muscle weakness, spasticity, dysesthesia, pain, or concerns about urinary and fecal continence. Fatigue was more frequently reported by women than by men.

Several authors have found significant correlations between interfering secondary symptoms and sexual dysfunction (Table 75.2).[6,12] Comparison of the studies is difficult since the definition of sexual dysfunction may vary from author to author. Some authors use the presence of one or more symptoms to define SD, while others use a validated questionnaire with several subscores for primary, secondary, and tertiary SD.[13] All authors agree that gender, fatigue, disease course, cognitive problems, and sphincter and bladder problems interfere considerably with sexuality. Conflicting data are found on the duration of the disease. Some gender differences may also exist. Men seem to be less bothered by some of these secondary factors than women. However, the number of men was invariably lower than the number of women in all studies, making these findings less robust. The degree of disability might also play a role: in severely disabled women with MS bowel dysfunction was a significant factor, while this was not the case in less disabled women.[14] Patients with advanced disease have been less investigated, but even in this group sexuality seems to be of major concern.

Tertiary sexual dysfunction

Tertiary aspects of sexual dysfunction are very important to the patient and his or her partner and family. These psychological, emotional, social, and cultural aspects may induce negative changes in self-image, self-esteem, mood, and body image, as well as depression, anxiety, and sexual aversion.

The influence of emotional aspects of MS affects sexuality in correlation with depression and anxiety scores. This influence also correlates with a lower level of education and even unemployement.[6,12] Being married is associated with complaining of more symptoms of sexual dysfunction. This may reflect a higher number of coital attempts in stable relationships than in single or divorced patients. Besides these, medical treatments of these psychologic consequences by antidepressants and anxiolytic agents might interfere with sexual function as well. The prevalence of sexual disorders in women taking antidepressants varies from 22 to 58%, with higher rates for selective serotonin-reuptake inhibitors and lower rates for bupropion. In most cases, the antidepressant cannot be stopped just for sexual dysfunction and drug holidays are not recommended either, because of the risk of withdrawal symptoms and less compliance.[15]

Practical approach to sexual dysfunction in MS

Assessment of sexual functions and sexuality should be part of the normal routine in the neurologic, urologic, gynaecologic, and rehabilitation approach to people with MS. While restoring the mechanics of the sexual function might be rather successful in some patients, secondary and tertiary factors may not be overlooked because of their huge impact on the quality of life. If needed, referral to professional counsellors, psychiatrists, psychologists, or sex therapists must be organized. The multilevel assessment of sexual dysfunction can easily be done in an open interview or by using the validated Multiple Sclerosis Intimacy and Sexuality Questionnaire (MSISQ-19).[13] Other specific questionnaires can be used for the assessment of erectile dysfunction or female sexual dysfunction as well. The diagnosis of MS does not preclude other etiologies of SD to be present as well: hypercholesterolemia, diabetes mellitus, cardiovascular disease, etc., must be investigated, as guided by the clinical need.

In men, the minimal investigation should consist of a medical and psychosexual history which can identify common causes of SD (other than MS) and reversible risk factors (e.g. smoking). The clinical examination should focus on eventual penile deformities, prostatic disease (men over 50), signs of hypogonadism, and the neurologic status. Moreover, a blood pressure measurement should be performed. Eventually laboratory tests such as a glucose-lipid profile and testosterone measurements can complete the assessment. Specialized tests such as nocturnal penile tumescence and rigidity measurements, vascular studies, electrophysiologic tests, endocrinology studies, and specialized psychodiagnostic testing are not routinely used, but should be reserved for special indications.[16] Problems at the secondary and tertiary level must be addressed as well. For the treatment of erectile dysfunction we refer to the following chapter.

In women, history-taking should focus on several issues: decrease in libido, impaired arousal, orgasmic dysfunction, pain from attempted or completed intercourse, difficulty with vaginal entry (due to fear, avoidance of muscle spasticity) and the awareness of vaginal lubrification. Fatigue as a cause for SD must be asked for specifically, while other secondary and tertiary problems are assessed. Physical examination can be very useful to asses the sensory function, reflexes, and muscle tone of the pelvic region, while it also offers gynecologic information (e.g. vaginal infection, postmenopausal changes, prolapse). Additional laboratory testing can be useful if urinary or vaginal infections are suspected. Hormonal testing for estrogen and testosterone levels can be useful in perimenopausal women or in women where estrogen or testosterone therapy is being proposed to treat libido and arousal disorders.[17,18] The treatment of female sexual dysfunction needs further study. Sildenafil citrate was proven to have only a marginal effect on vaginal lubrification and not to have an effect on orgasm.[9] Treatment of orgasmic disorders in both men and women is disappointing.[19] Increasing the sensory stimulation at the genitals by vibratory stimulation can be tried.

Besides the treatment of the physical features of SD in MS, strategies to cope with the secondary SD can be developed. For example, changing the time when a couple usually wants to have intercourse from evening to the morning can limit the effect of fatigue considerably. Adequate treatment of urinary and fecal incontinence can reduce the fear of leaking during sexual activities. Finding physical positions to allow painless and comfortable sex can be taught through specific tips, books or even videos. The development of these coping strategies and the improvement of the communication within the couple can be guided by a counsellor or specialized therapist, provided that the physician who detects the primary sexual dysfunction is open to collaboration with other specialists and is able and willing to discuss secondary and tertiary SD. Sexual rehabilitation in MS has not yet been studied properly, but initial reports are encouraging.[20,21]

It is clear that the treatment of sexual dysfunction in MS must be multimodal, taking into account the impact of the disease on different levels. To achieve this a team approach will be necessary in many cases.

Other neurologic diseases

As in MS, other neurologic diseases will be accompanied by sexual dysfunction at different levels. Progressive diseases such as Parkinson's disease and multiple system atrophy will yield a different symptomatology to nonprogressive stabilizing disorders such as craniocerebral trauma, spinal cord injury, cauda equina syndrome. The age at which some of these diseases occur will also dictate the eventual comorbidities such as diabetes, cardiovascular disease, and cognitive deterioration.

Morbus Parkinson

Parkinson patients are likely to suffer from sexual dysfunction in 35–87.5% of cases.[22,23] Especially in young-onset Parkinsonism this might lead to a serious impact on the quality of life.[24] The presence of depression (and its treatment) and unemployment are known risk factors. Patients taking dopaminergic drugs can develop compulsive sexual behavior.[25]

Patients with atypic Parkinsonism might suffer from multiple system atrophy (MSA). In these patients sexual dysfunction usually precedes the neurologic symptoms by a few years. While phosphodiesterase-5 inhibitors can successfully be used in Parkinson patients, care should be taken in MSA patients where these drugs might induce severe arterial hypotension.[26]

Stroke

Sexual dysfunction after stroke is very common. Often preexisting cardiovascular disease will have caused erectile dysfunction even before the stroke occurred. Interfering factors such as depression, impaired mobility, and the use of antihypertensive drugs must be taken into account. Depending on the site and the extent of the stroke, variable changes in sexual function can be seen. Spontaneous recovery of erectile function has been described, but sexual satisfaction does not seem to be correlated with a successful recovery of other functions.[4]

Epilepsy

Most people with epilepsy maintain normal reproductive and sexual lives. Some women develop problems with libido, arousal, and orgasm. Men with epilepsy are at risk for decreased libido and erectile dysfunction. Increased sex hormone-binding globulin levels and lower bioactive testosterone levels, particularly in association with the use of enzyme-inducing antiepileptic drugs, such as phenytoin and carbamazepine, are at the base of these problems.[27] The experience with enzyme-neutral drugs such as gabapentin and lamotigine is limited. Psychosocial factors, anxiety and stigma associated with epilepsy, can also affect the sexual life of patients with epilepsy.

References

1. Lundberg PO. Physiology of female sexual function and effect of neurological disease. In: Fowler CJ, ed. Neurology of Bladder, Bowel and Sexual Dysfunction. Oxford: Butterworth-Heinemann, 1999: 33–45.
2. Betts CD. Bladder and sexual dysfunction in multiple sclerosis. In: Fowler CJ, ed. Neurology of Bladder, Bowel and Sexual Dysfunction. Oxford: Butterworth-Heinemann, 1999: 289–98.
3. Beck RO. Physiology of male sexual function and dysfunction in neurologic disease. In: Fowler CJ, ed. Neurology of Bladder, Bowel and Sexual Dysfunction. Oxford: Butterworth-Heinemann, 1999: 47–54.
4. Rees PM, Fowler CJ, Maas CP. Sexual Dysfunction 2 – Sexual function in men and women with neurological disorders. Lancet 2007; 369: 512–25.
5. Zorzon M, Zivadinov R, Bosco A et al. Sexual dysfunction in multiple sclerosis: a case-control study. I. Frequency and comparison of groups. Mult Scler 1999; 5: 418–27.
6. Demirkiran M, Sarica Y, Uguz S, Yerdelen D, Aslan K. Multiple sclerosis patients with and without sexual dysfunction: are there any differences? Mult Scler 2006; 12: 209–14.
7. Zivadinov R, Zorzon M, Locatelli L et al. Sexual dysfunction in multiple sclerosis: a MRI, neurophysiological and urodynamic study. J Neurol Sci 2003; 210: 73–6.
8. Gruenwald I, Vardi Y, Gartman I et al. Sexual dysfunction in females with multiple sclerosis: quantitative sensory testing. Mult Scler 2007; 13: 95–105.
9. DasGupta R, Wiseman OJ, Kanabar G, Fowler CJ. Efficacy of sildenafil in the treatment of female sexual dysfunction due to multiple sclerosis. J Urol 2004; 171: 1189–93.
10. Zorzon M, Zivadinov R, Bragadin LM et al. Sexual dysfunction in multiple sclerosis: a 2-year follow-up study. J Neurol Sci 2001; 187: 1–5.
11. McCabe MP. Exacerbation of symptoms among people with multiple sclerosis: impact on sexuality and relationships over time. Arch Sex Behav 2004; 33: 593–601.
12. Zivadinov R, Zorzon M, Bosco A et al. Sexual dysfunction in multiple sclerosis: II. Correlation analysis. Mult Scler 1999; 5: 428–31.
13. Sanders AS, Foley FW, LaRocca NG, Zemon V. The Multiple Sclerosis Intimacy and Sexuality Questionnaire-19 (MSISQ-19). Sexuality Disab 2000; 18: 3–26.
14. Hulter BM, Lundberg PO. Sexual function in women with advanced multiple sclerosis. J Neurol Neurosurg Psychiatry 1995; 59: 83–6.
15. Taylor MJ, Rudkin L, Hawton K. Strategies for managing antidepressant-induced sexual dysfunction: systematic review of randomised controlled trials. J Affect Disord 2005; 88: 241–54.
16. Wespes E, Amar A, Hatzichristou K et al. Guidelines on erectile dysfunction. In: EAU Guidelines Office, ed. European Association of Urology Guidelines. EAU: Arnhem, 2006: 1–27.
17. Basson R, Althof S, Davis S et al. Summary of the recommendations on sexual dysfunctions in women. J Sex Med 2004; 1: 24–34.
18. Basson R. Sexual desire and arousal disorders in women. N Engl J Med 2007; 354: 1497–506.
19. Sipski ML, Behnegar A. Neurogenic female sexual dysfunction: a review. Clin Auton Res 2001; 11: 279–83.
20. Christopherson JM, Moore K, Foley FW, Warren KG. A comparison of written materials vs. materials and counselling for women with sexual dysfunction and multiple sclerosis. J Clin Nurs 2006; 15: 742–50.
21. Foley FW, LaRocca NG, Sanders AS, Zemon V. Rehabilitation of intimacy and sexual dysfunction in couples with multiple sclerosis. Mult Scler 2001; 7: 417–21.
22. Basson R. Sex and idiopathic Parkinson's disease. Parkinson's Dis 2001; 86: 295–300.
23. Goecker D, Rosing D, Beier KM. Influence of neurological diseases on partnership and sexuality. Particularly in view of multiple sclerosis and Parkinson's disease. Urology 2006; 45: 992–8.
24. Jacobs H, Kis B, Klein C, Vieregge P. Sexuality, in young patients with Parkinson's disease: a population-based comparison to healthy controls. Neurology 2000; 54: A374.
25. Weintraub D, Siderowf AD, Potenza MN et al. Association of dopamine agonist use with impulse control disorders in Parkinson disease. Arch Neurol 2006; 63: 969–73.
26. Hussain IF, Brady CM, Swinn MJ, Mathias CJ, Fowler CJ. Treatment of erectile dysfunction with sildenafil citrate (Viagra) in parkinsonism due to Parkinson's disease or multiple system atrophy with observations. J Neurol Neurosurg Psychiatry 2001; 71: 371–4.
27. Harden CL. Sexuality in men and women with epilepsy. CNS Spect 2006; 11: 13–8.

76

Treatment modalities for erectile dysfunction in neurologic patients

Reinier-Jacques Opsomer

Introduction

Sexual dysfunction is no longer a taboo subject, but is now clearly recognized as a potential medical disorder. The term 'impotence' has become obsolete, not only because of its pejorative connotations but also because of its oversimplification of the complexity of the male sexual function and dysfunctions. Indeed, it makes no distinction between libido, erectile, ejaculatory, and orgasmic disorders.[1]

This chapter focuses on the therapeutic modalities of erectile dysfunction (ED), a medical problem that affects a large number of men and so deserves the careful attention of both general practitioners and specialists. The first precise figures for the prevalence of ED were compiled by Feldman and coworkers in the Massachusetts Male Aging Study.[2] They estimated the prevalence of complete ED to be approximately 5% among 40 to 50-year old men, 10% of those in their 60s, 15% of those in their 70s, and more than 30% of those in their 80s.[2] Extensive epidemiologic studies have recently been undertaken all over the world confirming and extending the results of the Boston study. Porst and Sharlip summarized these epidemiologic studies in the recently published report of the Standards Committee of the International Society for Sexual Medicine.[3]

The therapeutic approach to ED has evolved dramatically over the last decade thanks to the improvement of our understanding of the physiology of erection and the development of effective drugs that can be taken 'on demand' before sexual intercourse. The best results in the treatment of ED have been observed when the problem is viewed from the perspective of the couple with a multidisciplinary approach.

ED in the neurologic population is a frequent condition, sometimes being the first symptom of the underlying disorder leading to the definitive diagnosis (e.g., multiple sclerosis and multiple system atrophy).[4] Most neurologic patients may benefit from a symptomatic (pharmacologic or nonpharmacologic) therapy for ED, adapted to their physical condition and combined with sexual counseling.

The pathophysiology of erectile function

Penile erection is a vascular event controlled by the autonomic and the somatic nervous systems. Neuroendocrine messages from the brain activate the autonomic nuclei in the spinal cord.[1] These result in:

1. dilatation of the cavernosal and helicine arteries, which significantly increases the blood flow to the penis
2. relaxation of the cavernosal smooth-muscle fibers, which opens the vascular lacunar spaces
3. expansion and filling of the lacunar spaces, which leads to the tumescence and consequently the rigidity of the penis.

In the healthy man, sexual stimulation triggers the release of nitric oxide (NO), which is produced by the endothelial cells and the nonadrenergic noncholinergic (NANC) nerve terminals. NO stimulates the enzyme guanylate cyclase in the cavernosal smooth muscle fiber leading to the production of cyclic guanosine monophosphate (cGMP), which, in turn, mediates intracellular signal transduction. Consequently, corporeal smooth muscle fibers relax, allowing the opening of the lacunar spaces[5] (Figure 76.1).

ED is defined as the persistent inability of a man to achieve and/or to maintain an erection sufficient to enable sexual performance that is satisfactory to both partners. From a 'cartesian' point of view, a subdivision of the causes of ED into organic and psychogenic etiologies is convenient but simplistic, since most patients present a mixed etiology. Table 76.1 lists the different etiologies of ED of organic origin. Patients with a primary 'mechanical-organic' problem will sooner or later develop performance anxiety. Arterial risk factors such as diabetes mellitus, hypertension, hypercholesterolemia, and smoking contribute to the development of ED. The Cologne study showed that 20% of ED patients suffer from diabetes mellitus, 30% from hypertension, and 30% are current smokers.[6] Other factors may also

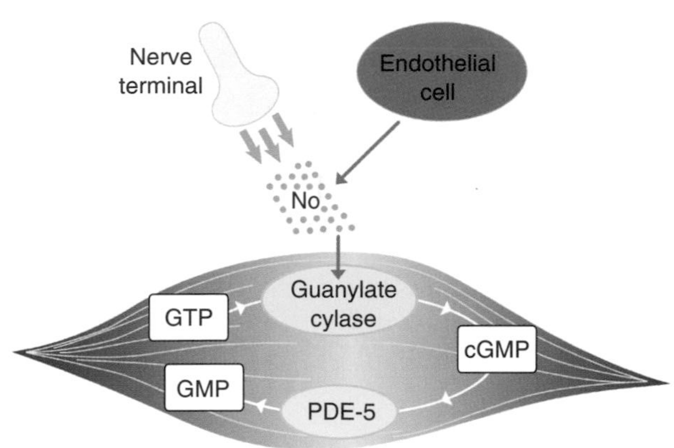

Figure 76.1
Physiology of erection at the level of the cavernosal smooth muscle fiber, nitric oxide (NO) produced by endothelial cells and nonadrenergic noncholinergic nerve fibers activates the production of cGMP. Phosphodiesterases (PDE-5) will convert cGMP into GMP.

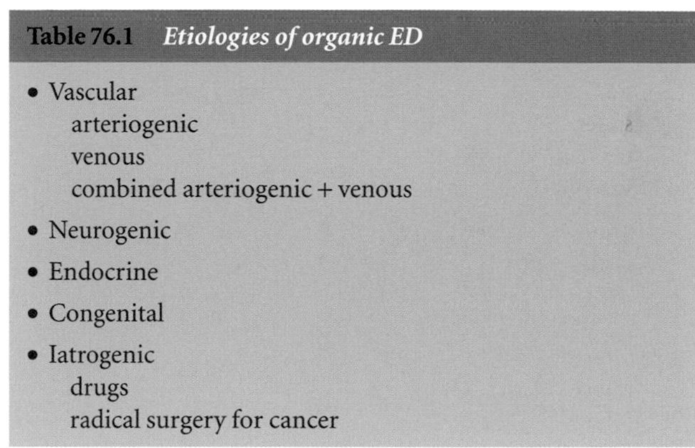

Table 76.1 *Etiologies of organic ED*

- Vascular
  - arteriogenic
  - venous
  - combined arteriogenic + venous
- Neurogenic
- Endocrine
- Congenital
- Iatrogenic
  - drugs
  - radical surgery for cancer

interfere with sexual function, such as depression, drugs, obesity, and lack of regular exercise.[7,8] Patients with an overt neurologic pathology often suffer from a sexual dysfunction: in some situations, ED is directly related to the neurologic deficit, as is the case with traumatic spinal cord disorders, but in others the relationship is unclear or dubious, as is the case with epilepsy and depression.

A full history and a thorough physical examination are mandatory to determine the cause of ED. Physical examination consists of an assessment of the external genitalia and the lower extremity pulses and a digital rectal examination of the prostatic gland in patients over 50 years old. Neurologic examination includes evaluation of the tonus of the anal sphincter and the voluntary control over the pelvic floor. The genital reflexes (bulbocavernosus reflex and anal reflex) and the lower limb reflexes (Achilles reflex and Babinski's sign) will be tested. When hormonal evaluation is indicated, the laboratory tests should be performed in the morning (between 7 and 9 o'clock).[1,9]

Theoretically, the persistence of spontaneous rigid nocturnal and/or morning erections will help to differentiate organic from psychogenic ED: a patient complaining of ED during intercourse but who has spontaneous nocturnal or morning rigid erections may be assumed to be suffering from psychogenic ED. However, the possibility of 'false positive' and 'false negative' observations has to be kept in mind, especially in neurologic patients: for example, most multiple sclerosis (MS) patients complain of ED even though they regularly have spontaneous and involuntary rigid nocturnal erections.[9,10] Furthermore, patients with a spinal cord injury frequently have spontaneous reflex erections during nursing care but develop short-lasting, nonrigid erections during sexual intercourse.

In the general population, the cornerstone of the evaluation of ED is the duplex Doppler sonogram combined with an intracavernous injection of a vasoactive agent (prostaglandin E-1, PGE 1). The test has not only diagnostic but also therapeutic value as the patient is given an intracavernosal injection of a small dose of PGE-1, a drug that is regularly proposed as a treatment, after adaptation of the dosage, to achieve a full erection. A duplex Doppler sonogram evaluates the arterial inflow (measurement of the systolic peaks), the venous outflow (measurement of the telediastolic flows), and the resistive indexes of the corpora cavernosa. Classic neurologic tests (somatosensory and motor evoked potentials and sacral reflexes) explore the somatic nervous system.[10,11] The integrity of the genitourinary autonomic nervous system will be 'approached' by testing the cardiovascular reflexes and by sympathetic skin responses.[12]

ED also has to be evaluated from the perspective of the couple. In our institution, a multidisciplinary center (*Centre de Pathologie Sexuelle Masculine*, CPSM) including urologists, gynecologists, endocrinologists, sexologists, and psychiatrists was created in 1997. The objective is to assess the different aspects of the sexual function (libido, erection, ejaculation, orgasm) from a multidisciplinary perspective by taking into account the organic, the psychologic, and the relational aspects of the sexual problem of the subject and his partner.

Treatment modalities of ED

Patients with an obvious psychogenic or relational problem will be referred to a sexologist (psychiatrist). In most cases, however, ED is mixed or multifactorial in origin, and so the urologist will frequently be consulted. In neurologic patients, only symptomatic (nonetiologic) therapeutic modalities will be proposed. The treatment of ED is stratified into 5 levels (Table 76.2). It should be emphasized that

Table 76.2 *Algorithm for the treatment of ED*
1. Oral treatment: inhibitors of type 5-phosphodiesterase sildenafil tadalafil vardenafil
2. Intraurethral injections
3. Intracavernous injections
4. Vacuum devices
5. Penile prostheses: malleable inflatable

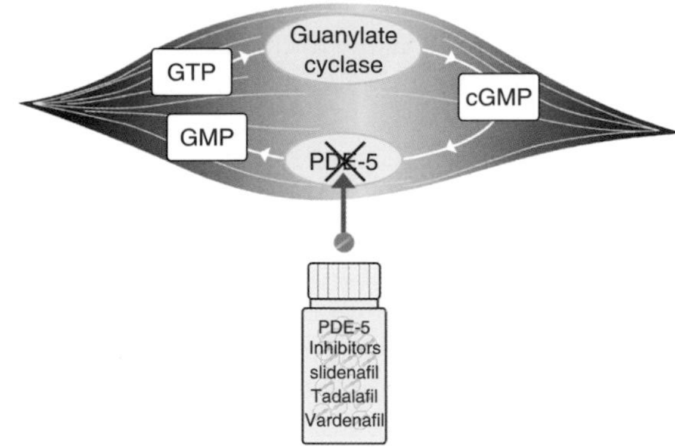

Figure 76.2
Mechanism of action of PDE-5 inhibitors. These inhibit the PDE-5 enzyme responsible for the degradation of cGMP into GMP.

in sexology, unlike other medical specialties, the treatment is selected by the patient himself, preferably in agreement with his partner, after having been informed by the clinician of the different treatment options appropriate for his situation and physical condition.

The first level of therapy consists of prescribing an oral treatment: phosphodiesterase 5 (PDE-5) inhibitors constitute the first choice. Patients who do not respond to oral pharmacotherapy and those for whom PDE-5 inhibitors are contraindicated may be candidates for intraurethral or intracavernosal injections of a vasoactive drug, such as PGE-1. The efficacy of intracavernosal injections is high, but the invasiveness of the procedure is certainly a disadvantage. The fourth-line treatment option is a vacuum device while the fifth modality is a penile prosthesis implanted surgically.

Oral pharmacologic agents

The concept of taking a pill before engaging in sexual intercourse has been popularized with the development of the first PDE-5 inhibitor. The arrival of the 'blue pill' (sildenafil citrate) on the market in 1998 launched a revolution in the minds of both doctors and patients alike and was a breakthrough in the treatment of ED. While sildenafil was being tested in cardiac patients, fortuitously, it was found that it had a positive effect on erection. Twenty years of intensive research on sildenafil led to the recognition of multiple indications for this drug, not only for ED but also for premature ejaculation, lower urinary tract symptoms, pulmonary hypertension, and other conditions.[13] Two other PDE-5 inhibitors have been available since March 2003: tadalafil and vardenafil. PDE-5 inhibitors are potent and selective inhibitors of the cGMP-specific PDE-5, which is responsible for the degradation of cGMP into GMP in the corpus cavernosum (Figure 76.2). PDE-5 inhibitors improve penile rigidity by local control mechanisms, but do not act on the central nervous system.

Sildenafil is available in three dosages: 25, 50, and 100 mg. The medication has to be taken 30 minutes before anticipated intercourse. The half-life of the drug ranges from 3 to 5 hours. It should not be taken during a heavy meal, as this may delay the time of onset of efficacy.[5,14] The period of responsiveness is approximately 8 hours.

Vardenafil is available in 3 dosages: 5, 10, and 20 mg. Like sildenafil, its half-life is about 4 to 5 hours. Interaction with food is minimal. As with sildenafil, the period of responsiveness is approximately 8 hours.

Tadalafil is available in 2 dosages: 10 and 20 mg. It has a half-life of 17.5 hours, which clearly distinguishes it from sildenafil and vardenafil. Consequently, the period of responsiveness with tadalafil is significantly longer than with the two other PDE-5 inhibitors: it extends to at least 24 hours and in certain cases up to 36 hours.[15] It offers efficacy without planning and thus reduces dependency on a pill. The advantage of the long half-life is that the patient may engage in sexual activity more than once after a single dose. Furthermore, there is no interaction between tadalafil and food intake.[14,16] These two characteristics of the drug may be expected to contribute to more spontaneity during sexual activity. On the other hand, the long half-life of tadalafil has to be taken into account in elderly and cardiac patients: indeed, the general practitioner and the ICU specialist should be aware that, in patients with cardiovascular problems, NO donors and nitrates will be contraindicated for a longer period after intake of tadalafil than with the other PDE-5 inhibitors.

The side-effects of the three PDE-5 inhibitors are mild and transient. They include flushing, nasal congestion, headache, and visual disturbances (at higher dosages). These medications, as usual, are contraindicated for subjects for whom sexual intercourse is not recommended for cardiac reasons (recent myocardial infarction, unstable angina) and for patients taking nitrates or NO donors.

PDE-5 inhibitors are effective in approximately 80% of patients, being effective for ED of psychogenic, organic, and/or mixed etiologies. They are usually less effective in peripheral neuropathies such as diabetes mellitus and after radical pelvic surgery for cancer (radical prostatectomy, cystectomy, or rectal surgery). However, after nerve-sparing radical prostatectomy, PDE-5 inhibitors are showing some encouraging results. In a large multicenter study undertaken with ED patients after nerve-sparing radical prostatectomy, the best responses were observed in patients who had undergone a bilateral nerve-sparing procedure and in the younger group.[14] PDE-5 inhibitors have been tested in spinal cord injured patients. The presence of an upper motor neuron lesion was significantly associated with therapeutic success, while lower motor neuron lesions and cauda equina patients were poor responders.[17]

Other oral drugs used but not approved for ED Trazodone, which is approved for the treatment of depression, facilitates relaxation of the cavernous smooth muscle fibers. The success rates of trazodone in placebo-controlled trials were up to 67% vs 39% for the placebo. The indication of trazodone appears to be psychogenic ED and concomitant depression. However, cases of prolonged erections associated with trazodone therapy have been reported.[18] Trazodone will therefore be prescribed with caution.

The following drugs have been tested with some 'subjective results': L-arginine, *Ginkgo biloba* extract, and Korean red ginseng.[19]

Intraurethral (transurethral) therapy

The vasoactive drug alprostadil is delivered as a pellet into the urethra by means of a specific polypropylene applicator. The pellet dissolves in the urethra, and the drug is then assumed to reach the corpus cavernosum by diffusion through the tissues. This drug is not available in several countries in Europe. An extensive review of the results in terms of clinical efficacy and safety with intraurethral therapy has been presented by Padma-Nathan et al.[20]

Intracavernosal injection therapy (IC injections)

Erection can be obtained pharmacologically by injecting a vasoactive drug directly into the corpora cavernosa. Several drugs have been tested such as papaverin, phentolamine, phenoxybenzamine, PGE-1, and a combination of several

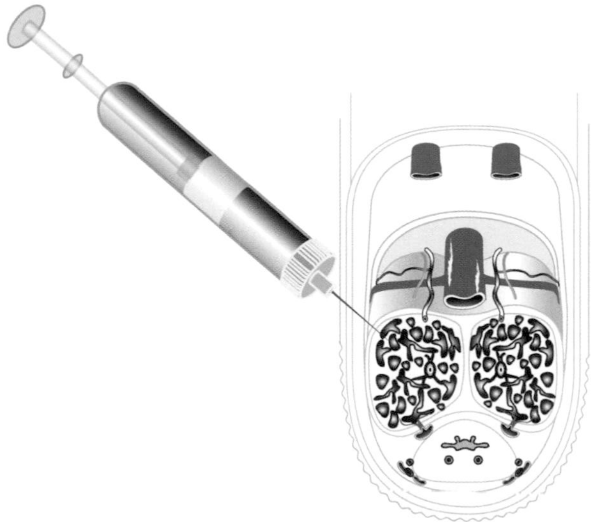

Figure 76.3
Intracavernosal injection of a vasoactive drug: principle of the method. The medication has to be injected into the lateral aspect of one of the two corpora cavernosa. Injections will be performed alternatively into the right or the left corpus cavernosum to avoid local fibrosis.

components. The compound is injected 5 to 10 minutes before sexual intercourse, the patient having been instructed by the urologist or his team on how to perform self-injections (Figure 76.3). When the patient is reluctant to inject himself (or unable to do so), the partner may be initiated to the technique. In our department, the patient who is a candidate for intracavernosal therapy is first administered a duplex Doppler sonogram with an intracavernous injection of a standard 3 μg dose of PGE-1. The test has both a diagnostic (vascular evaluation) and a therapeutic value (clinical responsiveness to the drug). IC injections are recommended for patients who do not respond to oral treatment or who may not benefit from PDE-5 inhibitors. The patient is enrolled in an injection training program: increasing dosages of PGE-1 are injected in the clinic (once a week); the nurse injects the first two doses, then the patient performs the next injection under supervision. Once he is able to inject himself, the final titration is performed at home. In this way, prolonged erections seldom occur. The patient is allowed to perform one or two injections/week. In the event of a prolonged erection, the patient is instructed to contact the urologist on duty. This happens very rarely. Spinal cord injured patients, especially those with thoracic and cervical lesions, are at risk of prolonged erections and should be given only small dosages of IC injections.[21–23]

In our institution, when a patient is admitted for a prolonged erection, initial treatment consists of a simple puncture of the corpora cavernosa to aspirate a small volume of blood in order to decompress the corpora. If need

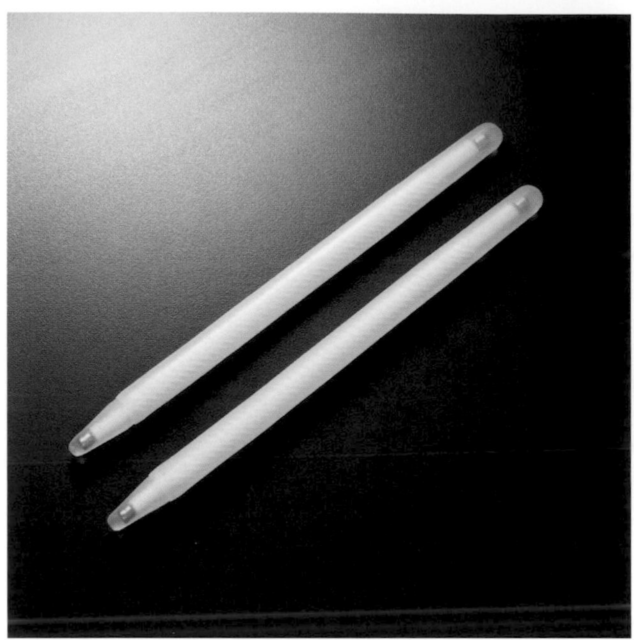

Figure 76.4
Malleable (semi-rigid) penile implant (AMS Malleable™ 650) (courtesy of American Medical Systems, Inc, Minnetonka, Minnesota, USA).

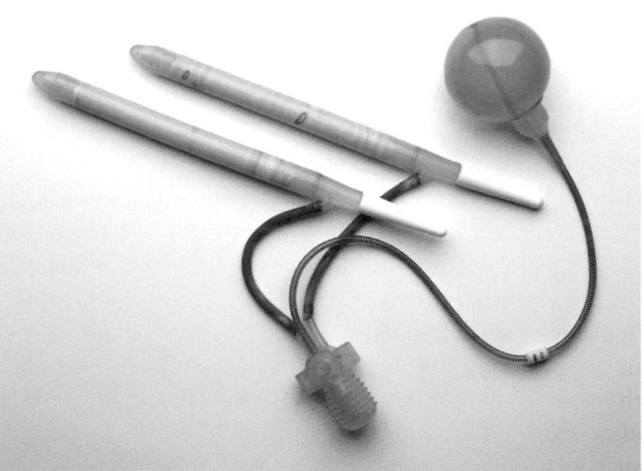

Figure 76.5
Inflatable penile implant (AMS 700 MS™ Series Penile Prosthesis) (courtesy of American Medical Systems, Inc, Minnetonka, Minnesota, USA). The implant has been impregnated with a combination of rifampicin and minocycline (InhibiZone).

be, the corpora cavernosa are irrigated using normal saline and a diluted solution of phenylephrine or other similar α-adrenergic agents under careful cardiovascular monitoring, especially in patients with a previous history of cardiovascular disease.[9,22,23] A surgical procedure (surgical shunt) is rarely requested.

Vacuum constriction devices

The vacuum constriction device consists of a cylinder, a vacuum pump, and a constrictive tension ring. The principle behind the vacuum device is to obtain an erection by inserting the penis into the cylinder and creating a negative pressure in the 'chamber'. In this way, blood is aspirated and collected in the penis and then mechanically blocked by the tension ring applied at the base of the penis. The device is recommended in elderly patients for whom pharmacotherapeutic agents are contraindicated.[24,25]

Implantation of penile prostheses

Penile prosthetic implants are an adequate alternative for patients who refuse IC injections or a vacuum device and for whom oral drugs are either ineffective or contraindicated. Two types of implants are available: malleable and inflatable prostheses (Figures 76.4 and 76.5).[25] The motivation of the partner has to be taken into account before deciding on the implantation. Montorsi conducted a multicenter study assessing the long-term reliability of three-piece AMS prostheses: at a mean follow-up of 59 months, 92.5% of the patients were still engaging in sexual intercourse with a mean frequency of 1.7 times weekly. Patient and partner satisfaction rates reached 98% and 83%, respectively.[26] Postoperative complications are rare and include mechanical malfunction, corporal cross-over, corporal and urethral perforation, infection (in 3 to 5% of the patients), erosion of the prosthesis, and glans bowing (supersonic transport deformity). Malleable prostheses may also be indicated in incontinent patients to facilitate the application and maintenance of a urine-collecting device.[27,28]

Discussion

Comprehensive studies evaluating the different therapeutic modalities of ED in specific neurologic pathologies (diabetes mellitus, MS, and spinal cord injured patients) have been published over the last few years.[29–31] All of these authors concluded that PDE-5 inhibitors have revolutionized the treatment of ED by introducing an effective noninvasive approach to the management of this 'difficult-to-treat condition' in disabled patients.[29] Basu and Ryder, in an extensive review paper, evaluated the effectiveness of the different treatments of ED in diabetic patients.[29] Ramos and Samso detailed the specific aspects of ED in spinal cord injury patients from two rehabilitation centers in Spain.[30]

Landtblom[31] published a very elegant contribution in 2006 entitled 'Treatment of erectile dysfunction in multiple sclerosis'; the author not only reviewed the pharmacologic and psychologic therapeutic options to be recommended in MS patients, but also raised a series of fundamental questions on the ethical and socioeconomic aspects of the 'modern' therapeutic approach to sexual dysfunction. ED in MS patients may be multifactorial: it may be related to the neurologic dysfunction, to psychologic factors, to side-effects of medication, or to generalized MS symptoms, such as fatigue and depression, frequently in combination. First line treatments of ED in MS patients are PDE-5 inhibitors and IC injections of PGE-1.[31]

Sexual counseling is recommended for all cases in order to help the patient and his partner deal with the functional and relational aspects of the sexual problem. The efficacy of the treatment will be greatly enhanced when the partner is closely involved in the evaluation of ED and in the selection of the adequate therapy. Sexual counseling is particularly advisable in paraplegic and tetraplegic patients: indeed in these patients, the partner is closely involved in the 'administration of the therapy' as well as in the 'general' care. Sexual assistants are available in some countries to help paraplegic or tetraplegic patients cope with their sexual difficulties. This may raise some ethical considerations.

In most countries, ED is considered to be outside the framework of general healthcare and PDE-5 inhibitors are not reimbursed. However, in Denmark, ED medication is subsidized in specific diagnostic groups, such as patients with diabetes mellitus and MS.[31]

Sexuality is one of the basic needs, and should therefore be a natural part of healthcare. Sexuality symptoms are as equally worthy of treatment as any other complaint.[31,32]

Conclusion

ED is no longer a 'hidden disorder' but is clearly recognized as a medical pathology that requires adequate diagnosis and investigations. With the development of new therapeutic options, especially oral drugs, general practitioners and specialists are encouraged to talk openly with their patients about sexual function and dysfunction(s). Oral pharmacotherapy is clearly the first-line therapeutic option for most patients. The three PDE-5 inhibitors have proven to be effective in patients with moderate or severe erectile dysfunction. Neurologic patients may benefit from these therapies provided both the indications and the contraindications have been taken into account.

References

1. Kirby RS, Holmes S, Carson C. Erectile dysfunction. In: Fast Facts. Indispensable Guides to Clinical Practice. Oxford: Health Press, 1998.
2. Feldman HA, Goldstein I, Hatzichristou DG. Impotence and its medical and psychological correlates: results of the Massachussetts Male Aging Study. J Urol 1994; 150: 54–61.
3. Porst H, Sharlip ID. History and epidemiology of male sexual dysfunction. In: Porst H, Buvat J, eds. Standard Practice in Sexual Medicine. Blackwell Publishing, 2006: 43–8.
4. Chandiramani VA, Fowler CJ. Urogenital disorders in Parkinson's disease and multiple system atrophy. In: Fowler CJ, ed. Neurology of Bladder, Bowel and Sexual Dysfunction. Boston: Butterworth-Heineman, 1999: 245–54.
5. Gresser U, Gleitter CH. Erectile dysfunction: comparison of efficacy and side effects of the PDE-5 inhibitors sildenafil, vardenafil and tadalafil. Review of the literature. Eur J Med Res 2002; 7: 435–46.
6. Braun M, Wassmer G, Klotz T et al. Epidemiology of erectile dysfunction: results of the 'Cologne Male Survey'. Int J Impot Res 2000; 12: 305–11.
7. Condra M, Surridge DH, Morales A et al. Prevalence and significance of tobacco smoking in impotence. Urology 1986; 27: 495–8.
8. Horrowitz JD, Goble AJ. Drugs and impaired male sexual function. Drugs 1979; 18(3): 206–17.
9. Carson C, Kirby RS, Goldstein I. Textbook of Erectile Dysfunction. Oxford: ISIS Medical Media, 1999.
10. Opsomer RJ. Management of male sexual dysfunction in multiple sclerosis. Sexuality Disabil 1996; 14: 57–63.
11. Opsomer RJ. Electrophysiological evaluation of genitourinary nervous pathways. In: Corcos J, Schick E, eds. The Urinary Sphincter. New York: Marcel Dekker, 2001: 423–35.
12. Opsomer RJ, Boccasena P, Traversa R, Rossini P. Sympathetic skin responses from the limbs and the genitalia: normative study and contribution to the evaluation of neurourological disorders. Electroencephal Clin Neurophysiol 1996; 101: 25–31.
13. Ghofrani HA, Osterloh IH, Grimminger F. Sildenafil: from angina to erectile dysfunction to pulmonary hypertension and beyond. Nature Reviews 2006; 5: 689–702.
14. Montorsi F, Salonia A, Deho F et al. Pharmacological management of erectile dysfunction. BJU Int Eur Urol Update Series 2003/2; 91(5): 446–54.
15. Porst H, Padma Nathan H, Giuliano F et al. Efficacy of Tadalafil for the treatment of erectile dysfunction at 24 and 36 hours after dosing: a randomized controlled trial. Urology 2003; 62: 121–6.
16. Patterson B, Bedding A, Jewell H et al. The effect of intrinsic and extrinsic factors on the pharmacokinetic properties of tadalafil (IC351). Int J Impot Res 2001; 13(Suppl 4): A120.
17. Soler JM, Prévinaire JG, Denys P, Chartier-Kastler E. Phosphodiesterase inhibitors in the treatment of erectile dysfunction in spinal cord-injured patients. Spinal Cord 2007; 45: 169–73.
18. Porst H. Oral pharmacotherapy of erectile dysfunction. In: Porst H, Buvat J, eds. Standard Practice in Sexual Medicine. Blackwell, 2006: 75–94.
19. Choi HK, Seong DH, Rha KH. Clinical efficacy of Korean red ginseng for erectile dysfunction. Int J Impot Res 1995; 7: 181–6.
20. Padma-Nathan H, Hellstrom WJ, Kaiser FE et al. Treatment of men with erectile dysfunction with transurethral alprostadil. Medicated Urethral System for Erection (MUSE) Study group. N Engl J Med 1997; 336(1): 1–7.
21. Kirby RS, Carson CC, Webster GD. Impotence: Diagnosis and Management of Male Erectile Dysfunction. Oxford: Butterworth-Heinemann, 1991.
22. Vidal J, Curcoll L, Roig T, Bagunya J. Intracavernous pharmacotherapy for management of erectile dysfunction in multiple sclerosis patients. Rev Neurol (Barc) 1995; 24(120): 269–71.
23. Gordon SA, Stage KH, Tansey KE, Lotan Y. Conservative management of priapism in acute spinal cord injury. Urology 2005; 65(6): 1195–7.
24. Opsomer RJ, Wese FX, Van Cangh PJ. Long-term results with vacuum constriction device. Proceedings of the 8th World Meeting on

Impotence Research. Bologna: Monduzzi Editore, International Proceedings Division, 1998: 271–4.
25. Sadeghi-Nejad H, Seftel AD. Vacuum devices and penile implants. In: Seftel AD, ed. Male and female sexual dysfunction. Edinburgh: Mosby, 2004: 129–43.
26. Montorsi F, Rigatti P, Carmignani G et al. AMS three-piece inflatable implants for erectile dysfunction: a long-term multi-institutional study in 200 consecutive patients. Eur Urol 2000; 37: 50–5.
27. Sohn M, Martin-Morales. Penile prosthetic surgery. In: Porst H, Buvat J, eds. Standard Practice in Sexual Medicine. Blackwell Publishing, 2006: 136–48.
28. Zermann DH, Kutzenberger J, Sauerwein D, Schubert J, Loeffler U. Penile prosthetic surgery in neurologically impaired patients: long-term follow-up. J Urol 2006; 175: 1041–4.
29. Basu A, Ryder REJ. New treatment options for erectile dysfunction in patients with diabetes mellitus. Drugs 2004; 64(23): 2667–88.
30. Ramos AS, Samso JV. Specific aspects of erectile dysfunction in spinal cord injury. Intern J Impotence Res 2004; 16: S42–5.
31 Landtblom AM. Treatment of erectile dysfunction in multiple sclerosis, Expert Rev Neurotherapeut 2006; 6(6): 931–5.
32. Maslow AH. Towards a Psychology of Being. New York: Van Nostrand Company, 1968.

77

Fertility issues in men with spinal cord injury

Nancy L Brackett and Emad Ibrahim

Introduction

Spinal cord injury (SCI) occurs most often to young men at the peak of their reproductive health. In the United States, 80% of new injuries occur to men between the ages of 16 and 45.[1] Around the world, similar statistics are found.[2–8] The most common causes of SCI are motor vehicle accidents, violence, sports-related injuries, and falls.[1] It is assumed that more men than women are injured because men engage in more risk-taking behavior that leads to injury. The actual cause for the disproportionately high percent of injured men, however, is unknown. Recent evidence suggests that sex hormones may play a role in this discrepancy, i.e., that estrogen may be neuroprotective and/or that testosterone may be neurotoxic after injury.[9,10]

Following SCI, fertility is severely impaired in men, but not in women. For example, 90% of men with SCI cannot father a child via sexual intercourse.[11] Women with SCI, however, can conceive and deliver children with nearly the same success rate as the general population.[17] Reproductive function is of great importance to men with SCI.[13,14] Regaining sexual function has been identified as the highest priority among individuals with paraplegia.[13] Most men with SCI require medical assistance to father children due to impairments in erection, ejaculation, and semen quality.[15]

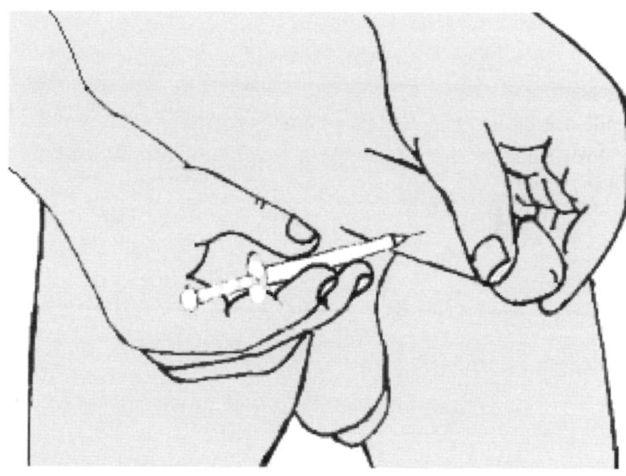

Figure 77.1
Intracavernous injections are effective remedies for erectile dysfunction in men with SCI.

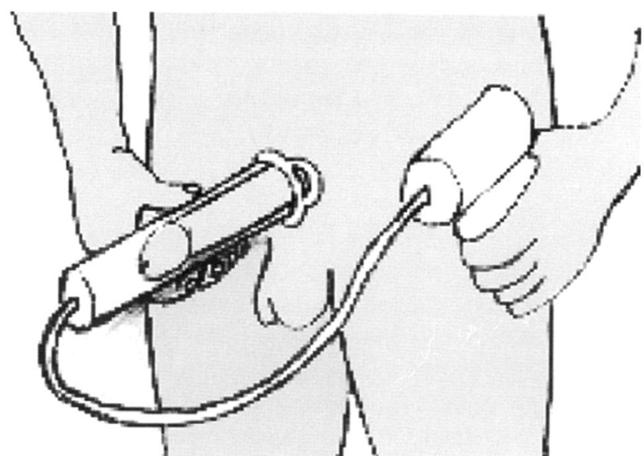

Figure 77.2
An example of a vacuum erection device, one of the available therapies for erectile dysfunction in men with SCI.

Treatments for erectile dysfunction

The same treatments used for treatment of erectile dysfunction in noninjured men are used for treatment of erectile dysfunction in men with SCI. Most men with SCI respond well to oral administration of phosphodiesterase-5 inhibitors (PDE-5 inhibitors), including Viagra (sildenafil citrate), Levitra (vardenafil HCl) and Cialis (tadalafil).[16–19] Men with SCI who do not respond well to oral PDE-5 inhibitors may respond better to medications injected into the corpus cavernosum of the penis, such as Caverject (alprostadil) or Trimix (a mixture of papaverine/regitine/prostaglandin E-1, Figure 77.1). Other therapies for erectile dysfunction include MUSE, or medicated urethral system for erections (which is a pellet of alprostadil inserted into the penile urethra), vacuum erection devices (Figure 77.2), or a surgically implanted penile prosthesis (Figure 77.3).

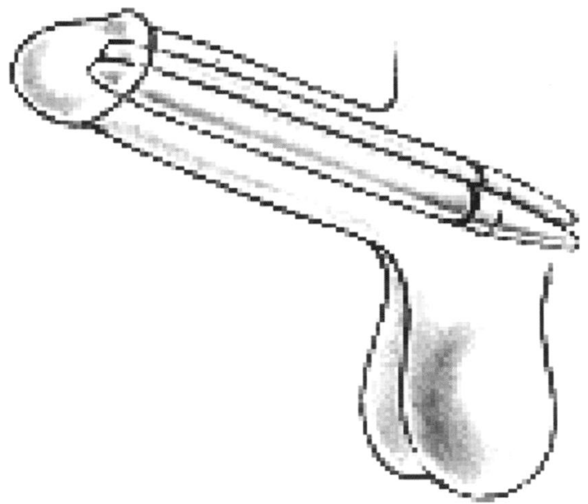

Figure 77.3
Penile implants are indicated for erectile dysfunction in some men with SCI who are unresponsive to other methods. Risks of this therapy include infection and, in nonsensate patients, inability to detect erosion of the penile implant through the skin.

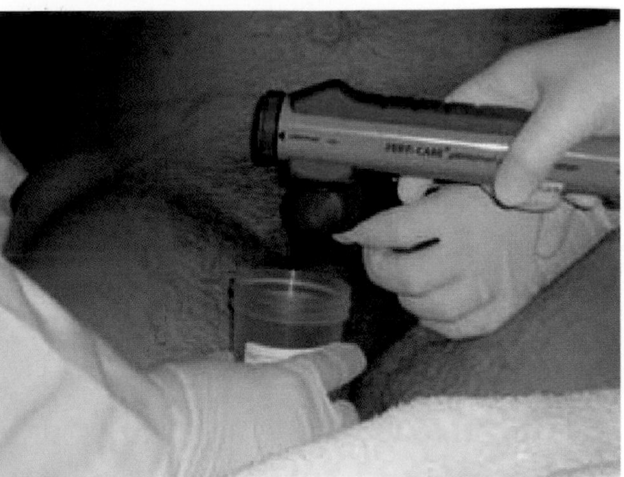

Figure 77.4
Penile vibratory stimulation is recommended as the first line of treatment for anejaculation in men with SCI.

Treatments for anejaculation

The majority of men with SCI are anejaculatory, i.e., unable to ejaculate during sexual intercourse.[20] Methods are available to improve or overcome anejaculation in men with SCI. The choice of the method depends on the purpose of the ejaculation. The primary purposes of ejaculation in men with SCI are: (1) to retrieve sperm for use in assisted reproductive technologies, or (2) for sexual pleasure. Several methods are available to retrieve sperm for assisted reproductive technologies, including penile vibratory stimulation (PVS), electroejaculation (EEJ), surgical sperm retrieval, and prostate massage.

Penile vibratory stimulation

PVS is usually recommended as the first line of treatment for anejaculation in men with SCI.[21,22] PVS involves placing a vibrator on the dorsum or frenulum of the glans penis (Figure 77.4).[23] Mechanical stimulation produced by the vibrator recruits the ejaculatory reflex to induce ejaculation.[24] This method is more effective in men with an intact ejaculatory reflex, i.e., men with a level of injury T10 or above (88% success rate) compared to men with a level of injury T11 and below (15% success rate).[25,26]

Unlike the methods of EEJ, surgical sperm retrieval, and prostate massage, PVS may be performed at home by some couples. Couples should first be evaluated in a clinic prior to trying PVS at home. The evaluation should include assessment for risk of autonomic dysreflexia, assessment for optimal stimulation parameters to induce safe ejaculation in the given patient, and demonstration that the patient and/or his partner can perform the procedure properly.[23] Autonomic dysreflexia is a risk for any method of sperm retrieval in patients with a level of injury T6 and above.[27] Briefly, autonomic dysreflexia is a potentially life-threatening medical complication that can occur in patients injured at or above T6. Autonomic dysreflexia is an uninhibited sympathetic reflex response of the nervous system to an irritating stimulus below the level of injury. Symptoms of autonomic dysreflexia include hypertension, bradycardia, sweating, chills, and headache. In some cases, autonomic dysreflexia can lead to dangerously high blood pressure levels, and this complication can lead to stroke, seizure, or even death. Autonomic dysreflexia symptoms can be well managed or prevented by oral administration of nifedipine.[27]

PVS may be attempted using any of a number of commercially available devices sold over the counter as wand massagers. One of the most effective commercially available vibrators is the Ferti Care (Multicept, Denmark), engineered specifically for inducing ejaculation in men with SCI (Figure 77.5). The advantage of this vibrator is its ability to deliver high-amplitude stimulation i.e., 2.5 mm excursions of the vibrating head, at a frequency of 90–100 Hz. These stimulus parameters were found to be most effective for ejaculatory success in men with SCI.[28]

If a patient is unable to ejaculate with a high amplitude vibrator, then auxiliary methods may be employed to facilitate ejaculation with PVS, such as application of two vibrators (Figure 77.6),[29] use of abdominal electrical stimulation in addition to PVS (Figure 77.7),[30] or oral administration of Viagra prior to PVS.[31] It is advisable to collect sperm via PVS because total motile sperm yields are highest with PVS

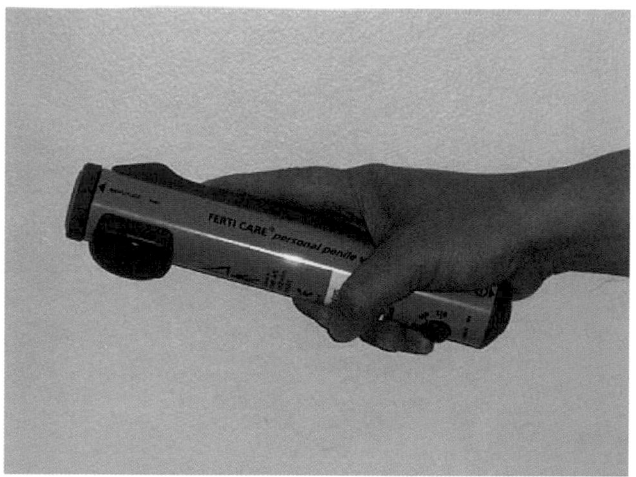

Figure 77.5
The Ferti Care vibrator, pictured here, was engineered specifically for ejaculation of men with SCI.

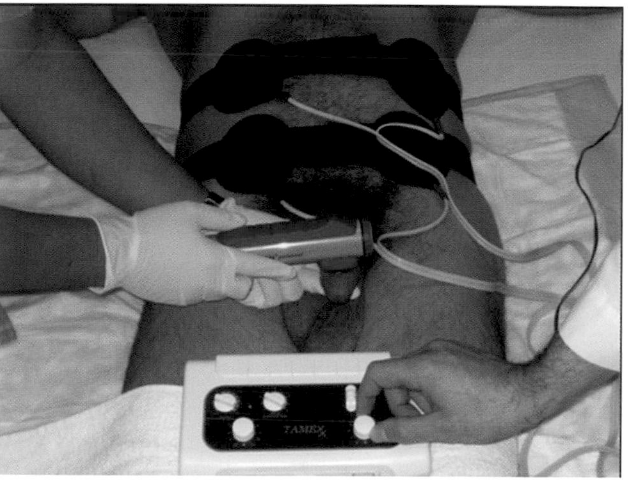

Figure 77.7
PVS, in combination with abdominal electrical stimulation using a commercially-available device, has been shown to be successful in some men who do not respond to PVS alone.

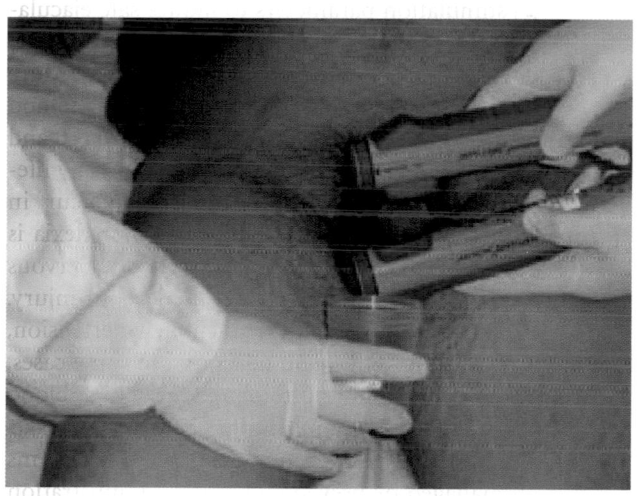

Figure 77.6
Individuals who cannot respond to PVS with one vibrator may respond to PVS with two vibrators.

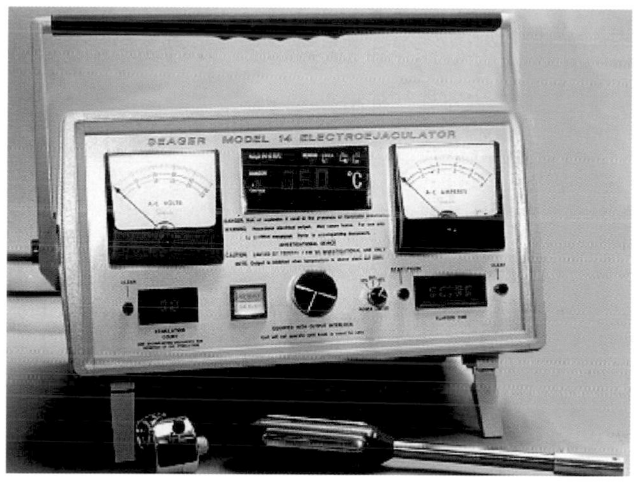

Figure 77.8
Electroejaculation is a method to retrieve semen when PVS fails.

compared to EEJ, surgical sperm retrieval, or prostate massage.[32,33] Higher yields of total motile sperm allow for the use of a wider range of assisted reproductive technologies.[34,35]

Electroejaculation

Individuals who cannot respond to PVS are often referred for EEJ (Figure 77.8). EEJ is performed with the patient in the lateral decubitus position (Figure 77.9). A probe is placed in the rectum, and electrodes on the probe are oriented anteriorly toward the prostate and seminal vesicles. Current delivered through the probe stimulates nerves that lead to emission of semen.

The method of EEJ was first developed in the 1930s for use in veterinary medicine,[36] and modified in the 1980s for use in humans.[37,38] Prior to the development of the high-amplitude vibrator in the mid-1990s, EEJ was the most common method of semen retrieval in men with SCI due to its higher success rate compared to PVS. Currently, EEJ is recommended for those individuals who fail to achieve semen retrieval via PVS because, compared to PVS, EEJ is more invasive, preferred less by patients, and results in a lower yield of total motile sperm in the antegrade fraction.[32,33]

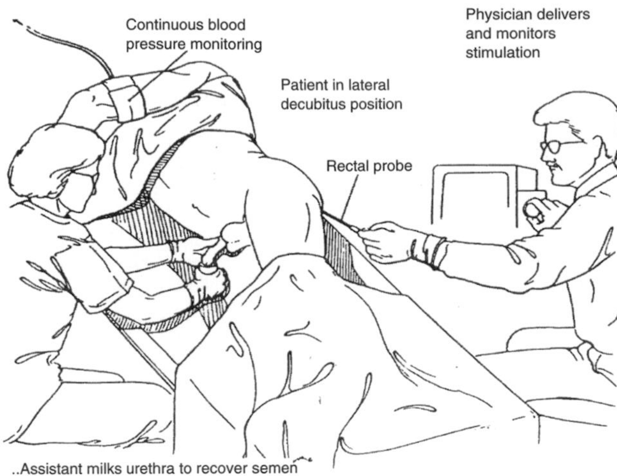

Figure 77.9
Electroejaculation must be performed by a specially trained physician. Electroejaculation is effective in retrieving semen in 95% of men with SCI.

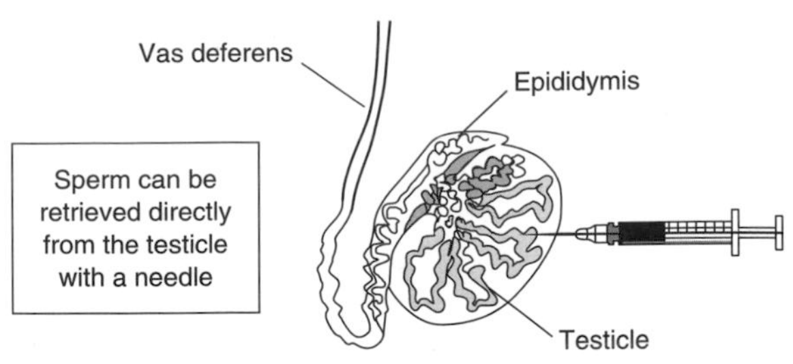

Figure 77.10
Sperm may be surgically removed from men with SCI. Use of surgical sperm retrieval in men with SCI is controversial.

Prostate massage

Prostate massage has been used to collect semen from men with SCI for use in insemination.[39,40] The physician inserts a gloved finger into the patient's rectum and massages the seminal vesicles and prostate. In a recent report, prostatic massage was used in 10 patients, resulting in two pregnancies (20% pregnancy rate).[41] It is not clear when this method is indicated in men with SCI. Some practitioners may not have PVS or EEJ equipment, and in these cases, prostate massage may be useful. The rationale for doing prostate massage is that sperm are stored in the ampulla of the vas deferens and, in men with SCI, are sequestered in the seminal vesicles as well.[42] The practitioner, therefore, attempts to mechanically push the sperm out through the ejaculatory ductal system.

Surgical sperm retrieval

Surgical sperm retrieval is a method of retrieving sperm from reproductive tissue (Figure 77.10). A variety of techniques may be used, including testicular sperm extraction (TESE), testicular sperm aspiration (TESA), microsurgical epididymal sperm aspiration (MESA), percutaneous epididymal sperm aspiration (PESA), and aspiration of sperm from the vas deferens.[43–49] Unlike the methods discussed previously, these methods were not developed to treat anejaculation. Instead, these methods were originally developed to retrieve sperm from men without SCI who were azoospermic, i.e., men who had no sperm in their ejaculate.

The application of surgical sperm retrieval to men with SCI is controversial. A recent survey [25] indicates that some practitioners are using surgical sperm retrieval as the first option of treatment for anejaculation in men with SCI. The primary reasons given by these practitioners for not offering PVS or EEJ were a lack of equipment and/or lack of training in these techniques.[25] It is unclear why practitioners are not being trained in the techniques of PVS and EEJ. One possible reason is that anejaculatory men with SCI represent only a small fraction of the male infertile population, whereas azoospermic men represent a much larger proportion of male infertile patients. Thus, physicians may possess the necessary equipment for, and become adept at, performing the procedures that are appropriate for the majority of their client population. Ejaculation success rates and pregnancy success rates indicate that PVS, EEJ, and interuterine insemination (IUI) warrant consideration in centers not currently offering these options for couples with SCI male partners.

Semen quality in men with spinal cord injury

With the advent of PVS and EEJ, data have accumulated on semen quality in men with spinal cord injury. The majority of these men have a distinct semen profile characterized by normal total sperm numbers but abnormally low sperm motility.[24,50–52] Furthermore, the sperm from men with SCI are 'fragile', i.e., they lose motility and viability faster than sperm from noninjured controls.[53]

Semen profiles of men with SCI are not related to lifestyle

Historically, there had been no precedent for understanding the cause of abnormal semen quality in men with SCI. Initial investigations tended to focus on lifestyle factors such as elevated scrotal temperature from sitting in a wheelchair,[54] infrequency of ejaculation,[55] methods of bladder management,[56] and methods of assisted ejaculation[32] as

Table 77.1 *Comparison of temperatures between subjects with SCI and control subjects*

	Room temperature (°C)	Oral temperature (°C)	Scrotal temperature (°C)	Difference between oral and scrotal temperature (°C)
Mean ± standard error of the mean				
SCI	22.6 ± 0.23	37.0 ± 0.06	35.4 ± 0.09	1.6 ± 0.09
Control	20.2 ± 0.18	37.0 ± 0.07	35.7 ± 0.16	1.3 ± 0.17

Scrotal temperature was not elevated in men with spinal cord injury. Group means were compared by analysis of variance. Adapted from Brackett et al.[54]

Table 77.2 *Comparison of semen quality by method of ejaculation*

	Masturbation: SCI men $n = 15$	PVS: SCI men $n = 106$	EEJ: SCI men $n = 90$	Controls: $n = 56$
Count / cc × 10^6	114.1 ± 24.6***	104.5 ± 8.1***	65.0 ± 7.7*	84.7 ± 6.2
% Motile sperm	29.0 ± 4.7**,***	26.0 ± 1.7**,***	14.8 ± 1.4*,**	63.6 ± 2.5*

SCI, spinal cord injured; PVS, penile vibratory stimulation; EEJ, electroejaculation *Significantly different from masturbation in SCI men. **Significantly different from controls; ***Significantly different from EEJ. Means were compared by analysis of variance. Adapted from Brackett et al.[60]

the cause for low sperm motility. Studies showed that such factors could not entirely account for the problem. For example, scrotal temperature was similar in injured and noninjured men (Table 77.1),[54] frequent ejaculation did not improve low sperm motility,[52,55,57–59] and sperm motility remained subnormal despite some improvements by the method of bladder management[56] and of assisted ejaculation (Table 77.2).[32,33]

Semen was obtained by PVS from 90 men with SCI, and by EEJ from 106 men with SCI. Parameters of sperm obtained by these two methods were compared to sperm parameters obtained by masturbation in 56 normal control subjects. The results showed that, although sperm motility was higher when obtained by PVS versus EEJ, sperm motility was significantly lower than that of normal control subjects. A minority of men with SCI can ejaculate by masturbation and 15 such men were recruited as additional controls. As is shown in Table 77.2, sperm motility obtained by masturbation in men with SCI was significantly lower than that obtained by masturbation in able-bodied men, and similar to that obtained by PVS of men with SCI. *The results of this study indicate that method of ejaculation alone cannot account for the pathophysiologic condition of low sperm motility in men with SCI.*[60]

With lifestyle factors apparently not the cause of abnormal sperm parameters in men with SCI, attention then turned to secondary physiologic factors as possible mechanisms for this condition. Again, this line of investigation yielded negative results. For example, there was no correlation between low sperm motility and level of injury, time post-injury, or age of subject.[52,61] Low sperm motility was also not related to hormone levels[62,63] or urinary tract infections.[56]

Accessory gland function is abnormal in men with SCI

In humans, semen is composed of fluids primarily from the seminal vesicles and prostate gland. Examination of semen from men with SCI shows numerous abnormalities in addition to abnormal sperm parameters. For example, 27% of men with SCI have brown-colored semen which does not become normally colored with repeated ejaculations.[64] The brown color is not simply hematospermia, but instead, indicates a dysfunction of the seminal vesicles.[64] Additional evidence of seminal vesicle dysfunction is the finding that men with SCI show an abnormal pattern of transport and storage of sperm in the seminal vesicles.[42]

In addition to dysfunction of the seminal vesicles in men with SCI, there is also evidence of prostate gland dysfunction in these men. Prostate-specific antigen (PSA) was higher in the blood, but lower in the semen of men with SCI compared to healthy, age-matched control subjects (Figure 77.11).[65] This pattern of PSA expression indicates a secretory dysfunction of the prostate gland in men with SCI.

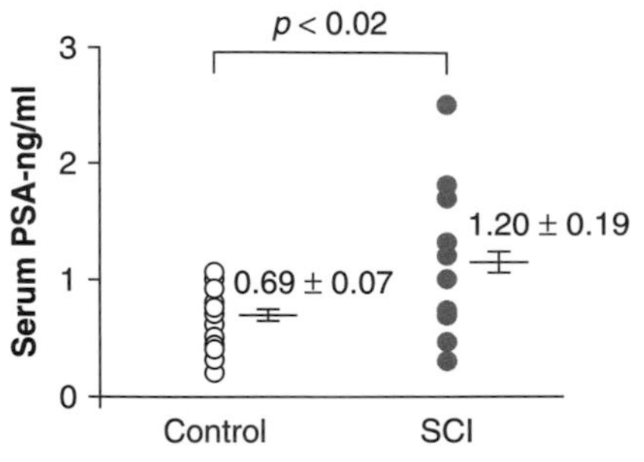

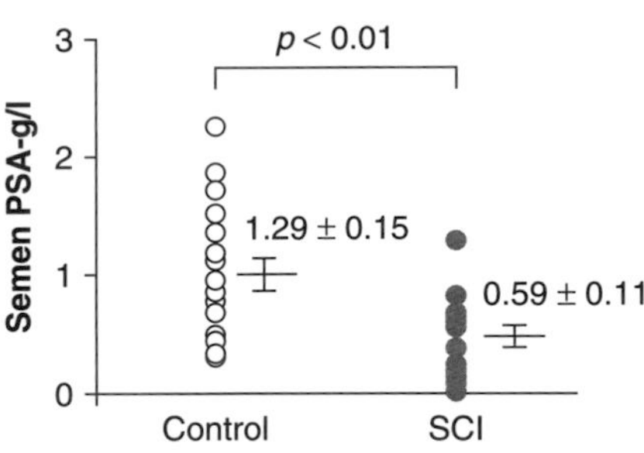

Figure 77.11
The prostate gland is dysfunctional in men with SCI as evidenced by higher concentrations of prostate-specific antigen (PSA) in the blood and lower concentrations of PSA in the semen of men with SCI compared to control subjects. Adapted from Lynne et al.[65]

Additional evidence of accessory gland dysfunction in men with SCI is found in studies showing abnormal concentrations of various biochemical substances in the semen of men with SCI versus compared to able-bodied subjects. For example, compared to able-bodied men, men with SCI have higher concentrations of platelet-acting factor acetylhydrolase (PAFah),[66] reactive oxygen species,[67–69] and somatostatin (in patients with lesions at or above T6).[70] Conversely, the semen of men with SCI has lower levels of fructose, albumin, glutamic oxaloacetic transaminase, alkaline phosphatase,[71] and transforming growth factor (TGF)-β1 compared to the semen of able-bodied men.[72]

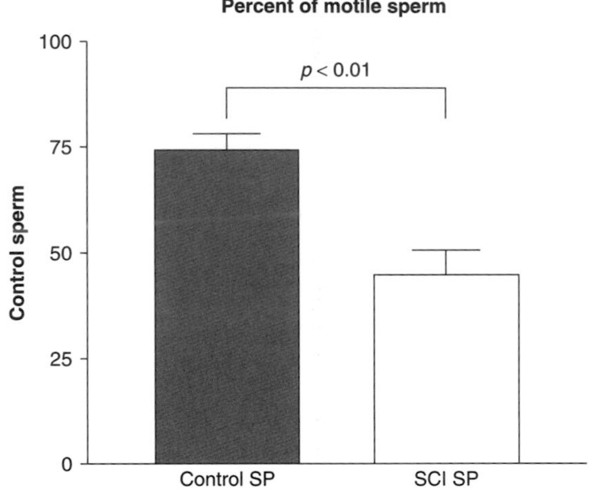

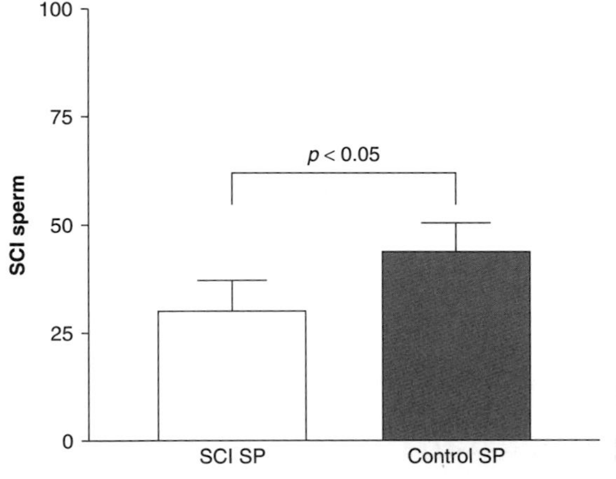

Figure 77.12
Seminal plasma (SP) from men with SCI inhibited sperm motility of nonSCI men, indicating that seminal plasma contributes to low sperm motility in men with SCI. Adapted from Brackett et al.[73]

Seminal plasma from men with SCI is toxic

Evidence of abnormal accessory gland function in men with SCI led to studies investigating the role of the seminal plasma as a contributing factor to the abnormal sperm parameters found in these men. The studies showed that the seminal plasma of men with SCI is toxic to normal sperm. For example, when seminal plasma of men with SCI was mixed with sperm from normospermic men, a rapid and profound impairment to normal sperm motility occurred (Figure 77.12).[73] Furthermore, sperm unexposed to the seminal plasma (i.e., aspirated from the vas deferens) had significantly higher motility than sperm in the ejaculate of these men (Figure 77.13).[74] These findings introduced the concept of an abnormal seminal plasma environment as a cause of impaired sperm motility in men with SCI.

Men with SCI have leukocytospermia

One of the most pronounced abnormalities in men with SCI is leukocytospermia, which is an abnormally high concentration of white blood cells in the semen (Figure 77.14).[75–77] Leukocytospermia has been studied in non-SCI men, especially with respect to its relationship with genitourinary tract infections and infertility.[56] These studies have established that cellular elements, in general, may be related to abnormal sperm parameters,[78–81] but the sperm–leukocyte interaction is not clearly understood.[80,82] Low sperm motility in men with SCI does not seem to be caused simply by local infection of the genitourinary tract. In these men, treatment of genitourinary infections with antibiotics does not result in improved sperm motility.[56]

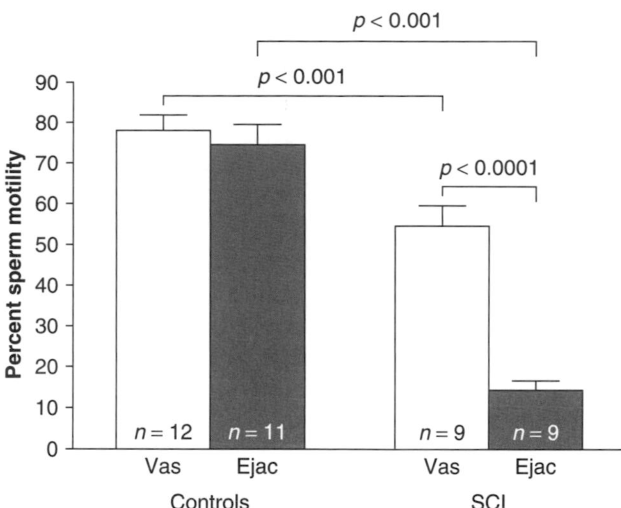

Figure 77.13
In each of 12 men with SCI, sperm motility was 2–13 times higher when obtained from the vas deferens than from the ejaculate. The net result was that mean sperm motility was significantly higher when obtained from the vas deferens versus the ejaculate (two bars on the right side of the graph). In contrast, in control subjects there was little difference in sperm motility between the two sites (two bars on left side of graph). *This study provided definitive evidence that seminal plasma is a major contributor to low sperm motility in men with spinal cord injury.*[74] The individual data clearly showed that in each SCI subject, sperm motility was much higher in the vas deferens than in the ejaculate. Although the vas aspirated sperm from these men generally had lower motility than that of controls, suggesting that some epididymal or testicular factor may also have a role in decreasing sperm motility, the major decrease in motility was obviously due to contact with the seminal plasma. These results represented a major step toward understanding the source of poor sperm motility in men with spinal cord injury. Adapted from Brackett et al.[74]

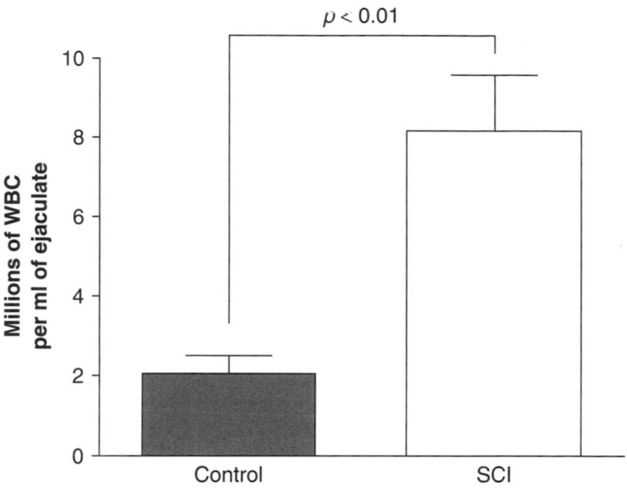

Figure 77.14
Most men with SCI have abnormally high concentrations of white blood cells (WBC) in their semen. This condition is termed leukocytospermia. Adapted from Basu et al.[75]

Men with SCI have immune abnormalities

There is ample experimental evidence that individuals with SCI suffer from immune regulatory dysfunction.[63,83–85] Typically, their circulating lymphocytes demonstrate suppressed responses to challenges that stimulate cell division (standard mitogen challenges), have reduced ratios of specific white blood cells, show reduced natural killer (NK) cell responses, and altered response to exercise challenges. The conclusion of these studies is that autonomic nervous system dysfunction results in alterations of the normal operations of the immune response, possibly via the interruption of sympathetic innervation of the lymphatics and spleen, the normal hypothalamic–pituitary–adrenal axis, or normal neurologic feedback from the periphery on these systems. The relationship of these findings to any disease state is unclear. In examining the semen of men with SCI during routine semen analysis, nearly all have an elevated number of white blood cells.[75] Flow cytometric analysis of the semen of these men has shown the presence of large numbers of activated T-lymphocytes,[75] which are known to secrete cytotoxic cytokines.[86] It is well known that activated T-lymphocytes can exert a damaging effect on other cells by cytotoxic cytokines.[86–89]

Cytokines contribute to low sperm motility in men with SCI

Cytokines play an important role in the function of the immune system.[86] Elevated concentrations of cytokines can be harmful to sperm.[90–92] It is possible that the activated T-lymphocytes observed in semen of men with SCI are secreting cytokines which impair sperm motility. It is hypothesized that semen cytokine concentrations are abnormal in men with SCI. Basu et al[72] measured levels of 10 cytokines in the seminal plasma of men with SCI versus age-matched, healthy, non-SCI control subjects. The results showed that, compared to control subjects, concentrations of 5 of the 10 cytokines were elevated in the seminal plasma of men with SCI.[72] Further, interfering with the actions of specific cytokines, by addition of monoclonal antibodies directly to the semen, improved sperm motility in men with SCI.[93] *This treatment represented the first intervention that significantly improved sperm motility in men with SCI.*

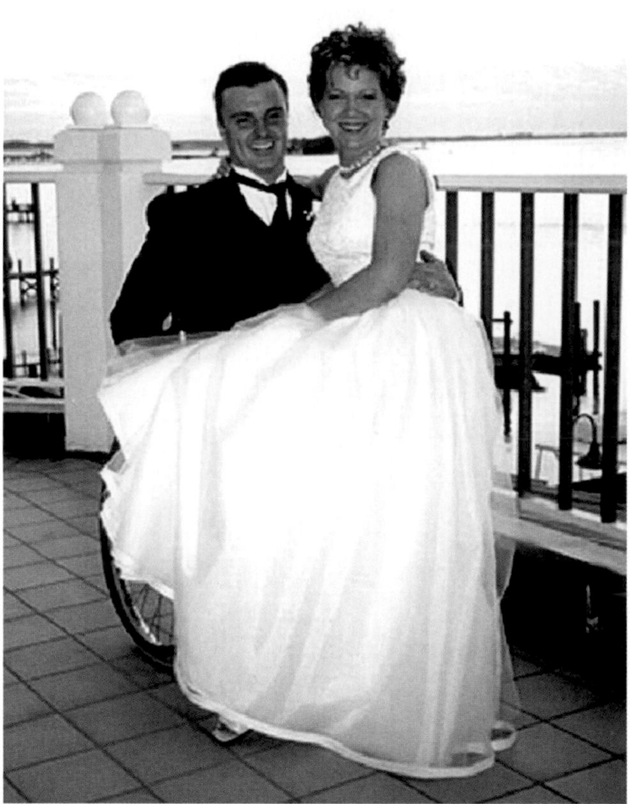

Figure 77.15
Many options are available to assist conception in couples with SCI male partners.

Reproductive options for couples with SCI male partners

Intravaginal insemination at home

The majority of men with SCI cannot ejaculate during sexual intercourse, and require some form of technical or medical assistance to father a child. With improvements in rehabilitation law and medicine, men with SCI have become increasingly integrated into society. Marriage and children are important to these men (Figure 77.15).

The least invasive and least expensive of the assisted reproductive options is intravaginal insemination, sometimes called 'in-home insemination'. It is advisable for couples to be evaluated in a clinic prior to attempting intravaginal insemination at home. The clinic should evaluate the male partner to determine the optimal method for safe and effective ejaculation at home. This evaluation should assess the male partner with SCI for risk of, and management of, autonomic dysreflexia. The evaluation should also determine the optimal method of inducing ejaculation, such as use of one vibrator,[23] two vibrators,[29] abdominal electrical stimulation plus PVS,[30] or oral medications, such as Viagra, prior to PVS.[31] The clinic should also evaluate the semen quality of the male partner with SCI. While minimum numbers of total motile sperm have not been established for successful pregnancy using intravaginally inseminated sperm from men with SCI, the clinic should discuss guidelines regarding the number of intravaginal insemination cycles that will be attempted prior to choosing more advanced methods of assisted conception.

The female partner should be evaluated for the absence of any tubal or uterine pathology and for the presence of normal ovulatory cycles. She should also be counseled regarding methods of ovulation prediction at home. Insemination should occur at the time of ovulation. If the male partner with SCI cannot ejaculate during intercourse, the couple may collect his semen by PVS into a clean specimen cup. The semen is then drawn into the barrel of a syringe. The semen is delivered by inserting the syringe deep into the vagina. Some clinics advise the female to remain recumbent for 15–30 minutes following insemination, to allow gravity to help keep the semen in the vagina, however there are no data to indicate whether this recumbence increases the probability of pregnancy.

There are reports in the literature of the successful use of intravaginal insemination to achieve pregnancy in couples with a male partner with SCI (see Table 77.3). Sonksen et al[94] reported a 25% pregnancy rate per couple for 16 couples undergoing PVS and vaginal self-insemination. Basal body temperature was used to predict ovulation timing and multiple ovulation cycles were required within a period of 2 years. Löchner-Ernst et al[95] reported a total of 60 pregnancies in 35 couples with male partners with SCI. Of these, 37 pregnancies occurred in 22 couples who performed semen collection and insemination at home, and 23 pregnancies occurred in 13 couples after intravaginal insemination in the clinic, but the study did not provide details on the proportion of couples that achieved pregnancy. Additionally, the study did not provide details about the ovulation cycles needed for this outcome, such as the number of cycles, or whether the female partner took fertility drugs to produce multiple eggs per cycle.

Nehra et al[96] reported pregnancies in 5 out of 8 couples (63% pregnancy rate) following PVS and the use of intravaginal or cervical self-insemination during multiple ovulation cycles. Dahlberg et al[97] reported 12 pregnancies in 8 couples after PVS and intravaginal insemination during multiple cycles using luteinizing hormone kits for timing of ovulation. Couples attempted intravaginal insemination at home approximately 6 times before going on to more advanced assisted reproductive technologies. Elliott[15] reported 28 infants born to 31 couples, with almost half of the couples conceiving at home using PVS.[15]

Table 77.3 *Summary of studies using intravaginal insemination in couples with male partners with SCI*

Author	Couples (*n*)	Cycles (*n*)	Pregnancies (*n*)
Sonksen et al 1997[94]	16	ND	4
Löchner-Ernst et al 1997[95]	35	ND	60
Nehra et al 1996[96]	8	ND	5
Dahlberg et al 1995[97]	8	≤48*	12
Elliott 2003[15]	31	ND	14*
Rutkowski et al 1999[98]	17	45	6
Hultling et al 1997[99]	19	ND	8

For each study, the total number of couples, the total number of attempts at pregnancy (cycles), and the total number of pregnancies are summerized. (*n*), number; ND, no data; *data estimated from information in study.

Table 77.4 *Summary of studies using intrauterine insemination in couples with male partners with SCI*

Author	Couples (*n*)	Cycles (*n*)	Pregnancies (*n*)	Medications used in study
Sonksen, et al 1997[94]	4	17	3	CC/hCG
Nehra et al 1996[96]	13	25	5	None/CC/hMG
Dahlberg, et al 1995[97]	15	≤90*	9	CC/hMG
Ohl et al 2001[100]	87	479	41	CC/hMG/hCG/LA
Pryor et al 2001[105]	10	19	6	CC/hCG
Rutkowski et al 1999[98]		5	10	3 ND
Taylor et al 1999[39]	14	92	11	ND
Chung et al 1996[62]	10	50	5	CC/hCG
Heruti et al 2001[103]	15	33	4	ND

For each study, the total number of couples, the total number of attempts at pregnancy (cycles), and the total number of pregnancies are summarized. Medications used in the study are listed. Some women had multiple cycles with different medications. (*n*), number; CC, clomiphene citrate; hCG, human chorionic gonadotropin; hMG, human menopausal gonadotropin; LA, leuprolide acetate; ND, no data; *data estimated from information provided in study.

Rutkowski et al[98] retrospectively reviewed outcomes of infertility management in their male patients with SCI. The clinic used PVS or EEJ as the semen retrieval technique. Intravaginal insemination was attempted in 17 couples. A total of 6 pregnancies was achieved in 45 cycles. Five of these pregnancies occurred in 23 cycles of PVS (22% pregnancy rate per cycle), and one pregnancy occurred in 22 cycles of EEJ (5% pregnancy rate per cycle).

Hultling et al[99] reported on 19 couples who tried PVS and intravaginal insemination at home; 8 of the 19 couples (42%) conceived.

Intrauterine insemination

Intrauterine insemination (IUI) has been used to achieve pregnancy in couples with an SCI male partner (see Table 77.4). IUI involves collecting semen from the SCI male partner and processing it in a laboratory to separate the sperm from the semen, and to isolate the motile from the nonmotile sperm. In men with SCI, semen to be used in IUI is usually collected by PVS or EEJ. The processed sperm is placed inside the uterus of the woman (Figure 77.16). IUI can be performed during unstimulated cycles

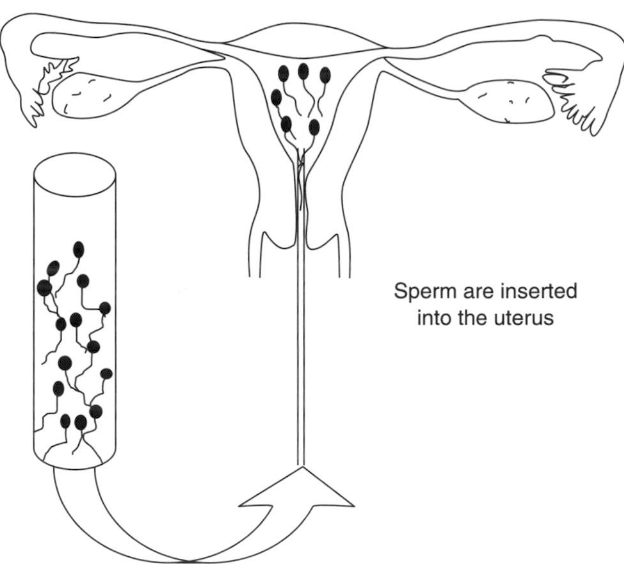

Figure 77.16
Intrauterine insemination has been used successfully to achieve pregnancy in couples with SCI male partners.

where no fertility drugs are prescribed to the woman or during stimulated cycles where fertility drugs are prescribed to stimulate the production of eggs and/or to stimulate ovulation.

Sonksen et al[94] reported the results of 17 IUI cycles in 4 couples. The women received medications to stimulate ovulation in 14 of the 17 cycles. PVS and EEJ were used as semen retrieval methods. Median total sperm count was 65 million (range 100 thousand to 480 million) with a median motility of 13% (range 1% to 60%). Three pregnancies occurred in 2 of the 4 couples (i.e., 1 couple had 2 pregnancies) for a 50% pregnancy rate per couple, and a 17.6% pregnancy rate per cycle.

Nehra et al[96] reported no pregnancies in 11 natural (no fertility drugs) cycles of IUI, but achieved 5 pregnancies in 13 couples after 25 cycles of IUI in which medications were administered to stimulate ovulation. Dahlberg et al[97] reported 9 pregnancies in 15 couples where IUI was tried for 4–6 cycles (≤ 90 cycles).

Ohl et al[100] studied 121 consecutive couples who used EEJ in combination with assisted reproductive technology in the treatment of anejaculatory infertility. For those couples that did not conceive within 3–6 cycles of IUI, gamete intrafallopian transfer (GIFT) or *in vitro* fertilization (IVF) procedures were recommended. Eighty-seven of the 121 couples had male partners with SCI. In 479 cycles of EEJ with IUI in these couples, 41 pregnancies were obtained. This outcome represents an 8.6% pregnancy rate per cycle and 32.2% pregnancy rate per couple.

Ohl et al[100] concluded that the type of fertility drug used to stimulate egg production and/or ovulation, and the method of monitoring and timing of insemination, did not affect IUI cycle fecundity. No multiple gestations were observed with natural cycle/IUI procedures. In comparing ranges of motile sperm counts and IUI cycle fecundity, the authors suggested that patients with counts of <4 million total motile sperm should proceed directly to high-level assisted reproductive technologies, since below this threshold the pregnancy rate per cycle decreased sharply to 1.1%. Based on a cost-effectiveness comparison of IUI and IVF, they recommended that couples should attempt 3–6 cycles of IUI before proceeding to IVF. When inseminated total motile sperm counts were greater than 40 million, the pregnancy rate per cycle was 17.6%. They concluded that an IUI program can be successful and cost-effective in men with SCI.

Some studies discussed whether semen specimens were obtained by antegrade (out the tip of the penis) or retrograde (into the bladder) ejaculation. Men with SCI often experience retrograde ejaculation due to dis-coordination between the external urinary sphincter and the bladder neck, which, in normal circumstances, ensures that the ejaculate flows forcefully out the end of the urethra. Pryor et al[101] reviewed outcomes in 10 couples undergoing IUI. Ejaculates were obtained by PVS in 2 patients and by EEJ in 9 patients. Retrograde samples with <5 million motile sperm were not used if the antegrade sample had >5 million motile sperm. Six pregnancies were achieved in 10 couples after 19 cycles of IUI when the women received human chorionic gonadotropin (hCG) to stimulate ovulation. No pregnancies occurred in 19 unstimulated cycles of IUI in 5 couples. Also, no pregnancies in the same 5 couples when the women received a combination of clomiphene citrate (CC) plus hCG to stimulate ovulation. Pryor's study, like Ohl's,[100] underlined the vital role that semen quality plays in the chances for pregnancy, and the importance of semen preparation techniques which isolate the most motile sperm for insemination. This study again emphasized the consideration of cost in assisted fertility procedures and also suggested that initial conception attempts should be made by IUI if adequate numbers of motile sperm are available.

Rutkowski et al[98] reviewed pregnancy results with IUI. In 5 couples who had EEJ and IUI, 3 pregnancies were achieved during 10 cycles. This outcome represents a 30% pregnancy rate per cycle, which was an improvement over the 13% pregnancy rate per cycle obtained with intravaginal insemination. The authors emphasized that conventional insemination techniques such as IUI will remain an important option in couples with SCI male partners, particularly in healthcare systems where IVF procedures such as intracytoplasmic sperm injection (ICSI) are beyond the financial reach of many couples.

Taylor et al[39] studied 19 couples with an anejaculatory male partner with SCI. Semen was obtained with PVS, PVS plus prostate massage, or EEJ. Assisted reproduction treatments offered were IUI, GIFT, and ICSI. Patients with motile sperm were first offered IUI. The pregnancy rate per cycle for IUI was 12% (11 pregnancies out of 92 cycles). Of the 14 couples treated with IUI, 6 achieved at least 1 pregnancy (42.9%). The authors suggested that sperm numbers within the normal range with at least 10% good progressive motility can be used for timed IUI with washed concentrated sperm, a procedure they characterize as 'relatively inexpensive and minimally invasive'.

Chung et al[102] reported their experience with EEJ combined with IUI or IVF. Female partners received clomiphene citrate 50 mg/day (days 3–7) during IUI cycles to improve pregnancy rates. EEJ was performed on the day of insemination and both antegrade and retrograde specimens were processed by swim-up technique. A total of 50 IUIs was performed in 10 couples, resulting in 5 pregnancies in 3 couples, with 2 couples conceiving twice. Pregnancy thus occurred in 30% of the couples and in 10% of the IUI cycles. One couple failed to conceive after 8 cycles of IUI, but successfully delivered twins after IVF.

Heruti et al[103] studied 15 couples with SCI male partners who underwent assisted reproductive technology. Semen was collected by EEJ in all patients. Four pregnancies were achieved after 33 cycles of IUI for a pregnancy rate per couple of 28.6%.

In vitro insemination/ intracytoplasmic sperm injection

Advanced assisted reproductive technologies are available when fertilization is not possible or not indicated by intravaginal insemination or IUI. IVF is a procedure where sperm from the man are placed in a laboratory dish with ova retrieved from the woman. The sperm–ova mixture is then placed in an incubator for up to 5 days. Sperm are allowed to fertilize the ova. Embryos that develop to the highest quality blastocyst stage are then placed into the uterus of the woman. Transfer of high-quality blastocysts is associated with higher pregnancy rates compared to transfer of poorly formed blastocysts.[104] This method whereby sperm are allowed to fertilize ova is termed 'conventional IVF' (Figure 77.17).

When the number of motile sperm is too low for conventional IVF, the method of ICSI is often used to achieve fertilization. ICSI is a procedure in which a single sperm is injected directly into the ovum (Figure 77.18). IVF and ICSI have been used to achieve pregnancy in couples with SCI male partners (Table 77.5). Hultling et al[99] reported a longitudinal descriptive study on the benefit of IVF in cases of anejaculatory infertility due to SCI, and the results achieved by ICSI. Sperm were retrieved through PVS or EEJ. If sperm quality was judged to be sufficient, conventional IVF was

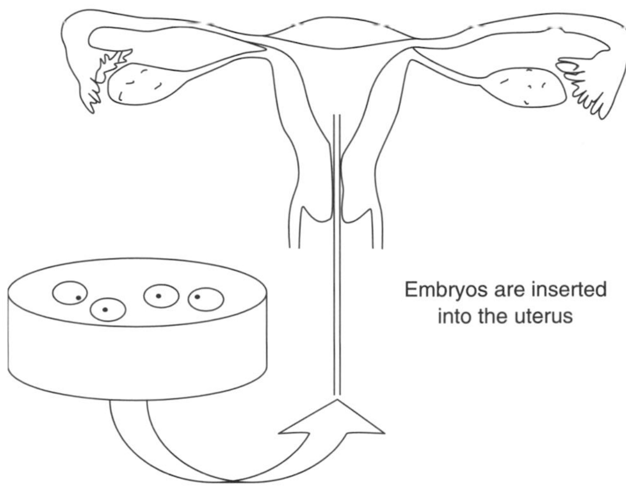

Figure 77.17
Example of conventional IVF in which sperm and ova are mixed together in a lab dish. Sperm are allowed to fertilize the ova. Well-developed embryos are transferred to the uterus.

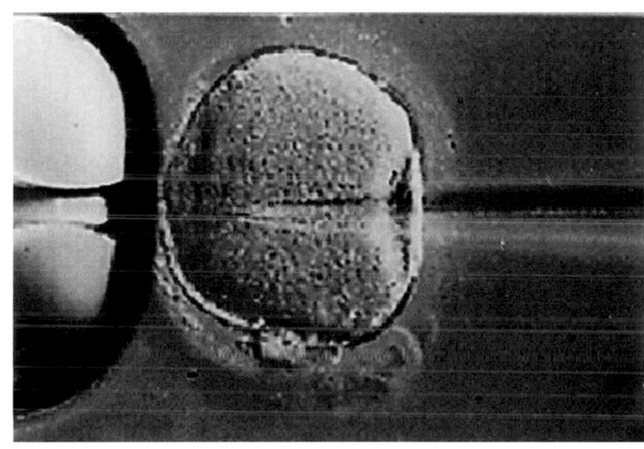

Figure 77.18
Intracytoplasmic sperm injection is a method of injecting sperm directly into an ovum. This method is used to increase the chance of fertilization.

performed. If sperm quality was very poor, ICSI was performed. Twenty-five couples underwent 52 cycles. Total sperm counts ranged from 0.01 to 978 million. Although the fertilization rate improved from 30% with conventional IVF to 88% with ICSI, there was no difference in pregnancy rate between the two methods. A total of 16 clinical pregnancies was established leading to 11 deliveries, for a pregnancy rate of 56% per couple.

Heruti et al[103] reported 18 pregnancies after 68 cycles of IVF/ICSI in 20 couples. Sonsken et al[94] reported 3 pregnancies in 10 cycles of IVF/ICSI in 8 couples. Brinsden et al[105] reported on the treatment of 35 couples with a male

Table 77.5 *Summary of studies using in couples with male partners with SCI*

Author, Year	Couples (*n*)	Cycles (*n*)	Pregnancies (*n*)	Medications used in study
Hultling et al 1997[99]	25	52	18	GnRH/hMG/FSH/hCG
Heruti et al 2001[103]	20	68	15	ND
Sonksen et al 1997[94]	8	10	3	GnRH/hMG/hCG
Brindten et al 1997[103]	35	85	18	GnRH/hMG/FSH
Shieh et al 2003[106]	9	11	9	GnRH/hMG/FSH
Löchner-Ernst, et al 1997[95]	11	ND	13	ND
Nehra et al 1996[96]	12	15	6	LA/hMG/FSH/hCG
Dahlberg et al 1995[97]	9	14	4	CC/hMG
Rutkowski et al 1999[98]	21		42	8 ND
Taylor et al 1999[39]	15	40	12	ND

For each study, the total number of couples, the total number of attempts at pregnancy (cycles), and the total number of pregnancies are summarized. Medications used in the study are listed. Some women had multiple cycles with different medications. (*n*), number; GnRH, gonadotropin releasing hormone agonist; hMG, human menopausal gonadotropin; hCG, human chorionic gonadotropin; ND, no data; LA, leuprolide acetate; FSH, follicle stimulating hormone; CC, clomiphene citrate.

partner with SCI. Sperm was obtained by EEJ. Eighteen clinical pregnancies were obtained in 85 cycles of IVF. The pregnancy rate per treatment cycle was 18/85 = 21.2%. The pregnancy rate per couple was 18/35 = 51.4%.

Shieh et al[106] reported on 9 couples undergoing 11 cycles of ICSI. Nine pregnancies were achieved (1 pregnancy per couple). Seven of the couples achieved pregnancy in 8 cycles of EEJ and ICSI. One couple achieved pregnancy in 2 cycles of PVS and ICSI, and one couple achieved pregnancy with donor sperm + ICSI.

Löchner-Ernst et al[95] reported on 13 pregnancies (2 sets of twins) in 11 couples using IVF and ICSI. Semen was obtained by PVS or surgical sperm retrieval. Nehra et al[96] reported pregnancy rates in 12 couples. GIFT was performed in 5 couples, and 4 achieved pregnancy in 8 cycles, for a 50% pregnancy rate per cycle and 80% pregnancy rate per couple. ICSI was performed in 7 couples, resulting in 2 pregnancies in 7 cycles for a 29% pregnancy rate per cycle, and a 29% pregnancy rate per couple.

Dahlberg et al[97] reported on pregnancy outcomes in 9 couples. Four couples had 6 cycles of IVF with sperm obtained by PVS or EEJ. Two pregnancies were achieved by this method. Two pregnancies were also achieved in five couples who had 8 cycles of IVF with sperm obtained from the vas deferens. Taylor et al[39] achieved 12 pregnancies in 15 couples undergoing 40 cycles of GIFT or ICSI. Six of 7 couples achieved 7 pregnancies (2 pregnancies in one couple) in 18 cycles of GIFT. Three of 8 couples achieved 5 pregnancies (3 pregnancies in one couple) in 22 cycles of ICSI.

Although definitive studies have not yet been performed, pregnancy outcomes using sperm from men with SCI seem to be similar to those using sperm from non-SCI patients with male factor infertility. Similar pregnancy rates are found between the two groups for IUI, conventional IVF, and ICSI.[94,106,107] Although there are some studies showing impaired sperm function in men with SCI,[51,108] these functional impairments apparently do not lower pregnancy rates in couples. These findings may reflect the increasing ability of laboratory-assisted reproductive technologies to overcome all forms of male infertility.[109,110]

Selection of ART approach

Recent improvements in the treatment of male factor infertility *in general* have led to a problem for couples with SCI male partners *in particular*. The ejaculates of many of these men are not being examined as a source of sperm for assisted reproductive technology (ART) procedures. Instead, sperm are being retrieved directly from their testes or epididymes as a first line of treatment for anejaculation. This development has resulted in many centers recommending ICSI as a first line of treatment for assisted conception to couples with an SCI male partner. For many such couples, the cost of ICSI is prohibitive. ICSI is currently the most invasive of the available ART options.

The risks to the female partner and the incidence of multiple gestations are significantly higher with IVF compared to IUI procedures.[111] If ICSI is the only treatment option offered to couples, many will not attempt biologic parenthood. This outcome will impede rather than encourage progress in treatment of infertility in these couples.

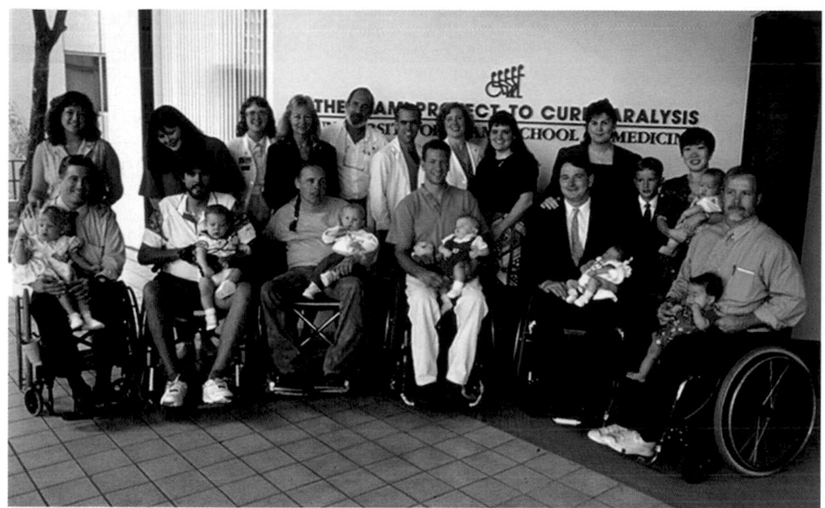

Figure 77.19
Photo of the first 7 babies born at the Miami Project to Cure Paralysis Male Fertility Program, including one set of twins (far right). All of these couples met and got married after the man's injury. One man (second from right) had a child from a previous marriage prior to his SCI. To date, over 150 babies have been born with the help of this program.

Studies have shown that semen may be easily obtained by PVS or EEJ in 95% of men with SCI. Centers cite lack of familiarity, training, or equipment as the primary reasons for not offering these procedures.[25] It is understandable that centers may not want to invest a large sum of money to purchase electroejaculation equipment for use in a small number of cases. The majority of SCI patients, however, can ejaculate easily with a low-cost vibrator.

Kafetsoulis et al[25] showed that: (1) the majority of men with SCI have reasonable yields of total motile sperm in their ejaculates, and (2) IUI has been successfully used to achieve pregnancy in these couples. It is recommended that centers continue (or begin) to examine semen as a source of sperm and consider IUI as a treatment option for assisted conception in couples with SCI male partners.

Summary

Young men comprise the overwhelming majority of individuals with spinal cord injury. Fertility is severely impaired in men with SCI due to erectile dysfunction, ejaculatory dysfunction, and semen abnormalities. The same treatments that are effective for erectile dysfunction in the general population are effective for treatment of erectile dysfunction in the SCI population. These treatments include oral PDE-5 inhibitors, intracavernous or intra-urethral injections of alprostadil, vacuum erection devices, and penile implants. Similarly, the same treatments that are effective to assist conception in couples with non-SCI male-factor patients are effective in assisting conception in SCI male-factor patients. These treatments include IUI, IVF, and ICSI.

The most apparent differences in male-factor symptoms between SCI and non-SCI patients are the high occurrences of anejaculation and atypical semen profiles in men with SCI. Methods are available to assist ejaculation in men with SCI. These treatments include PVS and EEJ. The use of surgical sperm retrieval as the first line of treatment for anejaculation in men with SCI is currently controversial.

Most men with SCI have a unique semen profile characterized by normal sperm concentration, but abnormally low sperm motility and viability. Abnormal accessory gland function, possibly due to dis-innervation of the prostate gland and seminal vesicles, may lead to abnormalities in the seminal plasma which contribute to this condition. Despite abnormal sperm parameters, pregnancy outcomes using sperm from men with SCI seem to be similar to pregnancy outcomes using sperm from non-SCI men. Future studies in the field of infertility in men with SCI should focus on improving natural ejaculation, and improving semen quality in these men.

References

1. National Spinal Cord Injury Center. Spinal cord injury. Facts and figures at a glance. J Spinal Cord Med 2005; 28: 379–80.
2. O'Connor P. Incidence and patterns of spinal cord injury in Australia. Accid Anal Prevent 2002; 34: 405–15.
3. Kuptniratsaikul V. Epidemiology of spinal cord injuries: a study in the Spinal Unit, Siriraj Hospital, Thailand, 1997–2000. J Med Assoc Thailand 2003; 86: 1116–21.
4. Mena Quinones PO, Nassal M, Al Bader KI, Al Muraikhi AE, Al Kahlout SR. Traumatic spinal cord injury in Qatar: an epidemiological study. Mid E J Emerg Med 2002; 1: 1–5.
5. Kondakov EN, Simonova IA, Poliakov IV. The epidemiology of injuries to the spine and spinal cord in Saint Petersburg, Russia, Zhurnal Voprosy Neirokhirurgii Imeni N-N-Burdenko 2002; 2: 50–3.
6. Exner G, Meinecke FW. Trends in the treatment of patients with spinal cord lesions seen within a period of 20 years in German centers. Spinal Cord 1997; 35: 415–9.
7. Pickett GE, Campos-Benitez M, Keller JL, Duggal N. Epidemiology of traumatic spinal cord injury in Canada. Spine 2006; 31: 799–805.
8. Polinder S, Meerding WJ, Mulder S, Petridou E, van Beeck E. Assessing the burden of injury in six European countries. Bull World Health Org 2007; 85: 27–34.

9. Farooque M, Suo Z, Arnold PM et al. Gender-related differences in recovery of locomotor function after spinal cord injury in mice. Spinal Cord 2006; 44: 182–7.
10. Sipski ML, Jackson AB, Gomez-Marin O, Estores I, Stein A. Effects of gender on neurologic and functional recovery after spinal cord injury. Arch Phys Med Rehab 2004; 85: 1826–36.
11. Kolettis PN, Lambert MC, Hammond KR et al. Fertility outcomes after electroejaculation in men with spinal cord injury. Fertil Steril 2002; 78: 429–31.
12. Sipski ML. The impact of spinal cord injury on female sexuality, menstruation and pregnancy: a review of the literature. J Am Paraplegic Soc 1991; 14: 122–6.
13. Anderson KD. Targeting recovery: priorities of the spinal cord-injured population, J Neurotrauma 2004; 21: 1371–83.
14. White MJ, Rintala DH, Hart KA, Young ME, Fuhrer MJ. Sexual activities, concerns, and interests of men with spinal cord injury. Am J Phys Med Rehab 1992; 71: 225–31.
15. Elliott S. Sexual dysfunction and infertility in men with spinal cord disorders. In: Lin V, ed. Spinal Cord Medicine: Principles and Practice. New York: Demos Medical Publishing, 2003: 349–65.
16. Padma-Nathan H, Giuliano F. Oral drug therapy for erectile dysfunction. Urol Clin North Am 2001; 28: 321–34.
17. Sanchez RA, Vidal J, Jauregui ML et al. Efficacy, safety and predictive factors of therapeutic success with sildenafil for erectile dysfunction in patients with different spinal cord injuries. Spinal Cord 2001; 39: 637–43.
18. Derry FA, Dinsmore WW, Fraser M et al. Efficacy and safety of oral sildenafil (Viagra) in men with erectile dysfunction caused by spinal cord injury. Neurology 1998; 51: 1629–33.
19. Giuliano F, Rubio-Aurioles E, Kennelly M et al. Efficacy and safety of vardenafil in men with erectile dysfunction caused by spinal cord injury. Neurology 2006; 66: 210–6.
20. Brown DJ, Hill ST, Baker HW. Male fertility and sexual function after spinal cord injury. Prog Brain Res 2006; 152: 427–39.
21. Brackett NL, Ferrell SM, Aballa TC et al. An analysis of 653 trials of penile vibratory stimulation on men with spinal cord injury. J Urol 1998; 159: 1931–4.
22. DeForge D, Blackmer J, Garritty C et al. Fertility following spinal cord injury: a systematic review. Spinal Cord 2005; 43: 693–703.
23. Brackett NL. Semen retrieval by penile vibratory stimulation in men with spinal cord injury. Hum Reprod Update 1999; 5: 216–22.
24. Sonksen J, Ohl DA. Penile vibratory stimulation and electroejaculation in the treatment of ejaculatory dysfunction. Int J Androl 2002; 25: 324–32.
25. Kafetsoulis A, Brackett NL, Ibrahim E, Attia GR, Lynne CM. Current trends in the treatment of infertility in men with spinal cord injury. Fertil Steril 2006; 86: 781–9.
26. Elliott S, Krassioukov A. Malignant autonomic dysreflexia in spinal cord injured men. Spinal Cord 2006; 44: 386–92.
27. Sheel AW, Krassioukov AV, Inglis JT, Elliott SL. Autonomic dysreflexia during sperm retrieval in spinal cord injury: influence of lesion level and sildenafil citrate. J Appl Physiol 2005; 99: 53–8.
28. Sonksen J, Biering-Sorensen F, Kristensen JK. Ejaculation induced by penile vibratory stimulation in men with spinal cord injuries. The importance of the vibratory amplitude. Paraplegia 1994; 32: 651–60.
29. Brackett NL, Kafetsoulis A, Ibrahim E, Aballa TC, Lynne CM. Application of 2 vibrators salvages ejaculatory failures to 1 vibrator during penile vibratory stimulation in men with spinal cord injuries. J Urol 2007; 177: 660–3.
30. Kafetsoulis A, Ibrahim E, Aballa TC et al. Abdominal electrical stimulation rescues failures to penile vibratory stimulation in men with spinal cord injury: a report of two cases. Urology 2006; 68: 204–11.
31. Giuliano F, Rubio-Aurioles E, Kennelly M et al. Efficacy and safety of vardenafil in men with erectile dysfunction caused by spinal cord injury. Neurology 2006; 66: 210–6.
32. Brackett NL, Padron OF, Lynne CM. Semen quality of spinal cord injured men is better when obtained by vibratory stimulation versus electroejaculation. J Urol 1997; 157: 151–7.
33. Ohl DA, Sonksen J, Menge AC, McCabe M, Keller LM. Electroejaculation versus vibratory stimulation in spinal cord injured men: sperm quality and patient preference. J Urol 1997; 157: 2147–9.
34. Wainer R, Albert M, Dorion A et al. Influence of the number of motile spermatozoa inseminated and of their morphology on the success of intrauterine insemination. Hum Reprod 2004; 19: 2060–5.
35. van der WL, Naaktgeboren N, Verburg H, Dieben S, Helmerhorst FM. Conventional in vitro fertilization versus intracytoplasmic sperm injection in patients with borderline semen: a randomized study using sibling oocytes. Fertil Steril 2006; 85: 395–400.
36. Gunn RMC. Fertility in sheep: artificial production of seminal ejaculation and the characteristics of the spermatozoa contained therein. Aust Commonwealth Council Sci Ind Res 1936; 94: 1–5.
37. Brindley GS. Electroejaculation and the fertility of paraplegic men. Sexual Disabil 1980; 3: 223–9.
38. Halstead LS, Ver Voot S, Seager SW. Rectal probe electrostimulation in the treatment of anejaculatory spinal cord injured men. Paraplegia 1987; 25: 120–9.
39. Taylor Z, Molloy D, Hill V, Harrison K. Contribution of the assisted reproductive technologies to fertility in males suffering spinal cord injury. Aus NZ J Obstet Gynaecol 1999; 39: 84–7.
40. Marina S, Marina F, Alcolea R et al. Triplet pregnancy achieved through intracytoplasmic sperm injection with spermatozoa obtained by prostatic massage of a paraplegic patient: case report. Hum Reprod 1999; 14: 1546–8.
41. Engin-Uml Stün Y, Korkmaz C, Duru NK, Baser I. Comparison of three sperm retrieval techniques in spinal cord-injured men: pregnancy outcome. Gynecol Endocrinol 2006; 22: 252–5.
42. Ohl DA, Menge A, Jarow J. Seminal vesicle aspiration in spinal cord injured men: insight into poor semen quality. J Urol 1999; 162: 2048–51.
43. Craft I, Tsirigotis M. Simplified recovery, preparation and cryopreservation of testicular spermatozoa. Hum Reprod 1995; 10: 1623–6.
44. Tsirigotis M, Pelekanos M, Beski S et al. Cumulative experience of percutaneous epididymal sperm aspiration (PESA) with intracytoplasmic sperm injection. J Assist Reprod Genet 1996; 13: 315–9.
45. Haberle M, Scheurer P, Muhlebach P et al. Intracytoplasmic sperm injection (ICSI) with testicular sperm extraction (TESE) in non-obstructive azoospermia – two case reports. Andrologia 1996; 28(Suppl 1): 87–8.
46. Kahraman S, Ozgur S, Alatas C et al. High implantation and pregnancy rates with testicular sperm extraction and intracytoplasmic sperm injection in obstructive and non-obstructive azoospermia. Hum Reprod 1996; 11: 673–6.
47. Craft I, Tsirigotis M, Courtauld E, Farrer-Brown G. Testicular needle aspiration as an alternative to biopsy for the assessment of spermatogenesis. Hum Reprod 1997; 12: 1483–7.
48. Westlander G, Hamberger L, Hanson C et al. Diagnostic epididymal and testicular sperm recovery and genetic aspects in azoospermic men. Hum Reprod 1999; 14: 118–22.
49. Chiang H, Liu C, Tzeng C, Wei H. No-scalpel vasal sperm aspiration and in vitro fertilization for the treatment of anejaculation. Urology 2000; 55: 918–21.
50. Linsenmeyer TA. Male infertility following spinal cord injury. J Am Paraplegic Soc 1991; 14: 116–21.
51. Denil J, Ohl DA, Menge AC, Keller LM, McCabe M. Functional characteristics of sperm obtained by electroejaculation. J Urol 1992; 147: 69–72.
52. Brackett NL, Nash MS, Lynne CM. Male fertility following spinal cord injury: facts and fiction. Phys Ther 1996; 76: 1221–31.

53. Brackett NL, Santa-Cruz C, Lynne CM. Sperm from spinal cord injured men lose motility faster than sperm from normal men: the effect is exacerbated at body compared to room temperature. J Urol 1997; 157: 2150–3.
54. Brackett NL, Lynne CM, Weizman MS, Bloch WE, Padron OF. Scrotal and oral temperatures are not related to semen quality or serum gonadotropin levels in spinal cord-injured men. J Androl 1994; 15: 614–9.
55. Laessoe L, Sonksen J, Bagi P et al. Effects of ejaculation by penile vibratory stimulation on bladder reflex activity in a spinal cord injured man. J Urol 2001; 166: 627.
56. Ohl DA, Denil J, Fitzgerald-Shelton K et al. Fertility of spinal cord injured males: effect of genitourinary infection and bladder management on results of electroejaculation. J Am Paraplegic Soc 1992; 15: 53–9.
57. Siosteen A, Forssman L, Steen Y, Sullivan L, Wickstrom I. Quality of semen after repeated ejaculation treatment in spinal cord injury men. Paraplegia 1990; 28: 96–104.
58. Hamid R, Patki P, Bywater H, Shah PJ, Craggs MD. Effects of repeated ejaculations on semen characteristics following spinal cord injury. Spinal Cord 2006; 44: 369–73.
59. Das S, Dodd S, Soni BM et al. Does repeated electro-ejaculation improve sperm quality in spinal cord injured men? Spinal Cord 2006; 44: 753–6.
60. Brackett NL, Lynne CM. The method of assisted ejaculation affects the outcome of semen quality studies in men with spinal cord injury: a review. Neurorehab 2000; 15: 89–100.
61. Brackett NL, Ferrell SM, Aballa TC, Amador MJ, Lynne CM. Semen quality in spinal cord injured men: does it progressively decline post-injury? Arch Phys Med Rehab 1998; 79: 625–8.
62. Brackett NL, Lynne CM, Weizman MS, Bloch WE, Abae M. Endocrine profiles and semen quality of spinal cord injured men. J Urol 1994; 151: 114–9.
63. Naderi AR, Safarinejad MR. Endocrine profiles and semen quality in spinal cord injured men. Clin Endocrinol 2003; 58: 177–84.
64. Wieder JA, Lynne CM, Ferrell SM, Aballa TC, Brackett NL. Brown-colored semen in men with spinal cord injury. J Androl 1999, 20: 594–600.
65. Lynne CM, Aballa TC, Wang TJ et al. Serum and seminal plasma prostate specific antigen (PSA) levels are different in young spinal cord injured men compared to normal controls. J Urol 1999; 162: 89–91.
66. Zhu J, Brackett NL, Aballa TC et al. High seminal platelet-activating factor acetylhydrolase activity in men with spinal cord injury. J Androl 2006; 27: 429–33.
67. Padron OF, Brackett NL, Sharma RK et al. Seminal reactive oxygen species and sperm motility and morphology in men with spinal cord injury. Fertil Steril 1997; 67: 1115–20.
68. de Lamirande E, Leduc BE, Iwasaki A, Hassouna M, Gagnon C. Increased reactive oxygen species formation in semen of patients with spinal cord injury. Fertil Steril 1995; 63: 637–42.
69. Rajasekaran M, Hellstrom WJ, Sparks RL, Sikka SC. Sperm-damaging effects of electric current: possible role of free radicals. Reprod Toxicol 1994; 8: 427–32.
70. Odum L, Sonksen J, Biering-Sorensen F. Seminal somatostatin in men with spinal cord injury. Paraplegia 1995; 33: 374–6.
71. Hirsch IH, Jeyendran RS, Sedor J, Rosecrans RR, Staas WE. Biochemical analysis of electroejaculates in spinal cord injured men: comparison to normal ejaculates. J Urol 1991; 145: 73–6.
72. Basu S, Aballa TC, Ferrell SM, Lynne CM, Brackett NL. Inflammatory cytokine concentrations are elevated in seminal plasma of men with spinal cord injuries. J Androl 2004; 25: 250–4.
73. Brackett NL, Davi RC, Padron OF, Lynne CM. Seminal plasma of spinal cord injured men inhibits sperm motility of normal men. J Urol 1996; 155: 1632–5.
74. Brackett NL, Lynne CM, Aballa TC, Ferrell SM. Sperm motility from the vas deferens of spinal cord injured men is higher than from the ejaculate. J Urol 2000; 164: 712–5.
75. Basu S, Lynne CM, Ruiz P et al. Cytofluorographic identification of activated T-cell subpopulations in the semen of men with spinal cord injuries. J Androl 2002; 23: 551–6.
76. Aird IA, Vince GS, Bates MD, Johnson PM, Lewis-Jones ID. Leukocytes in semen from men with spinal cord injuries. Fertil Steril 1999; 72: 97–103.
77. Trabulsi EJ, Shupp-Byrne D, Sedor J, Hirsh IH. Leukocyte subtypes in electroejaculates of spinal cord injured men. Arch Phys Med Rehab 2002; 83: 31–3.
78. Diemer T, Huwe P, Ludwig M, Hauck EW, Weidner W. Urogenital infection and sperm motility. Andrologia 2003; 35: 283–7.
79. Omu AE, Al-Qattan F, Al-Abdul-Hadi FM, Tunde Fatinikun M, Fernandes S. Seminal immune response in infertile men with leukocytospermia: effect on antioxidant activity. Eur J Ob/Gyn Reprod Biol 1999; 86: 195–202.
80. Maegawa M, Kamada M, Irahara M et al. A repertoire of cytokines in human seminal plasma. J Reprod Immunol 2002; 54: 33–42.
81. Henkel R, Schill WB. Sperm separation in patients with urogenital infections. Andrologia 1998; 30: 91–7.
82. Rossi A, Aitken R. Interactions between leucocytes and the male reproductive system. The unanswered questions. In: Ivell and Holstein, ed. The Fate of the Male Germ Cell. New York: Plenum Press, 1997: 245–52.
83. Cruse JM, Lewis RE, Dilioglou S et al. Review of immune function, healing of pressure ulcers, and nutritional status in patients with spinal cord injury. J Spinal Cord Med 2000; 23: 129–35.
84. Popovich PG, Jones TB. Manipulating neuroinflammatory reactions in the injured spinal cord: back to basics. Trends Pharmacol Sci 2003; 24: 13–7.
85. Kawashima N, Nakazawa K, Ishii N, Akai M, Yano H. Potential impact of orthotic gait exercise on natural killer cell activities in thoracic level of spinal cord-injured patients. Spinal Cord 2004; 42: 420–4.
86. Parham P. The Immune System. New York: Garland Science, 2005.
87. Hoek JB, Pastorino JG. Cellular signaling mechanisms in alchol-induced liver damage. Sem Liver Disease 2004; 24: 257–72.
88. Yamaoka J, Kabashima K, Kawanishi M, Toda KMY. Cytotoxicity of IFN-gamma and TNF-alpha for vascular endothelial cell is mediated by nitric oxide. Biochem Biophys Res Commun 2002; 291: 780–6.
89. van Soeren MH, Diehl-Jones WL, Maykut RJ, Haddara WM. Pathophysiology and implications for treatment of acute respiratory distress syndrome. AACN Clin Issues 2000; 11: 179–97.
90. Kocak I, Yenisey C, Dundar M, Okyay P, Serter M. Relationship between seminal plasma interleukin-6 and tumor necrosis factor alpha levels with semen parameters in fertile and infertile men. Urol Res 2002; 30: 263–7.
91. Eggert-Kruse W, Boit R, Rohr G et al. Relationship of seminal plasma interleukin (IL)-8 and IL-6 with semen quality. Hum Reprod 2001; 16: 517–28.
92. Sikka SC, Champion HC, Bivalacqua TJ et al. Role of genitourinary inflammation in infertility: synergistic effect of lipopolysaccharide and interferon-gamma on human spermatozoa. Int J Androl 2001; 24: 136–41.
93. Cohen DR, Basu S, Randall JM et al. Sperm motility in men with spinal cord injuries is enhanced by inactivating cytokines in the seminal plasma. J Androl 2004; 25: 922–5.
94. Sonksen J, Sommer P, Biering-Sorensen F et al. Pregnancy after assisted ejaculation procedures in men with spinal cord injury. Arch Phys Med Rehab 1997; 78: 1059–61.
95. Löchner-Ernst D, Mandalka B, Kramer G, Stohrer M. Conservative and surgical semen retrieval in patients with spinal cord injury. Spinal Cord 1997; 35: 463–8.
96. Nehra A, Werner M, Bastuba, Title C, Oates R. Vibratory stimulation and rectal probe electroejaculation as therapy for patients with spinal cord injury: semen parameters and pregnancy rates. J Urol 1996; 155: 554–9.

97. Dahlberg A, Ruutu M, Hovatta O. Pregnancy results from a vibrator application, electroejaculation, and a vas aspiration programme in spinal-cord injured men. Hum Reprod 1995; 10: 2305–7.
98. Rutkowski SB, Geraghty TJ, Hagen DL et al. A comprehensive approach to the management of male infertility following spinal cord injury. Spinal Cord 1999; 37: 508–14.
99. Hultling C, Rosenlund B, Levi R et al. Assisted ejaculation and in-vitro fertilization in the treatment of infertile spinal cord-injured men: the role of intracytoplasmic sperm injection. Hum Reprod 1997; 12: 499–502.
100. Ohl DA, Wolf LJ, Menge AC et al. Electroejaculation and assisted reproductive technologies in the treatment of anejaculatory infertility. Fertil Steril 2001; 76: 1249–55.
101. Pryor JL, Kuneck PH, Blatz SM et al. Delayed timing of intrauterine insemination results in a significantly improved pregnancy rate in female partners of quadriplegic men. Fertil Steril 2001; 76: 1130–5.
102. Chung PH, Verkauf BS, Eichberg RD et al. Electroejaculation and assisted reproductive techniques for anejaculatory infertility. Obstet Gynecol 1996; 87: 22–6.
103. Heruti RJ, Katz H, Menashe Y et al. Treatment of male infertility due to spinal cord injury using rectal probe electroejaculation: the Israeli experience. Spinal Cord 2001; 39: 168–75.
104. Balaban B, Urman B, Sertac A et al. Blastocyst quality affects the success of blastocyst-stage embryo transfer. Fertil Steril 2000; 74: 282–7.
105. Brinsden PR, Avery SM, Marcus S, Macnamee MC. Transrectal electroejaculation combined with in-vitro fertilization: effective treatment of anejaculatory infertility due to spinal cord injury. Hum Reprod 1997; 12: 2687–92.
106. Shieh JY, Chen SU, Wang YH et al. A protocol of electroejaculation and systematic assisted reproductive technology achieved high efficiency and efficacy for pregnancy for anejaculatory men with spinal cord injury. Arch Phys Med Rehab 2003; 84: 535–40.
107. Brackett NL, Abae M, Padron OF, Lynne CM. Treatment by assisted conception of severe male factor infertility due to spinal cord injury or other neurological impairment. J Assist Reprod Genet 1995; 12: 210–6.
108. Buch JP, Zorn BH. Evaluation and treatment of infertility in spinal cord injured men through rectal probe electroejaculation. J Urol 1993; 149: 1350–4.
109. Maduro MR, Lamb DJ. Understanding new genetics of male infertility. J Urol 2002; 168: 2197–205.
110. Isidori A, Latini M, Romanelli F. Treatment of male infertility. Contraception 2005; 72: 314–8.
111. Winston RM, Hardy K. Are we ignoring potential dangers of in vitro fertilization and related treatments? Nat Cell Biol 2002; 4(Suppl): S14–8.

78

Pregnancy in spinal cord injury

Carlotte Kiekens

Introduction

In Western countries, spinal cord injury (SCI) is a relatively rare condition with an incidence varying between 1 and 4 per 100 000 inhabitants per year. Eighty percent of the subjects are male.[1] The mean age at onset being the early thirties, sexuality and fertility issues are relevant, but literature concerning these topics in women is scarce. However, motherhood is an important issue for the quality of life of these disabled women and their motivation to carry on with their lives after such a devastating event.

Concerning female fertility issues such as pregnancy rates, live births, and complications or obstetric management following SCI, only case reports and opinion articles are available and a systematic review by De Forge et al in 2005 was restricted to male fertility post SCI.[2]

Menstruation, fertility, and contraception

Menarche has been reported to occur normally in girls who have been injured as preadolescents. When an SCI is sustained after menarche, it is usually followed by an episode of amenorrhea. On average, women resume menses after 3 to 6 months, with 50% of the women presenting menses at 6 months and 90% of the women by one year post-injury. At that moment fertility status returns to the premorbid status.[3–5] The same pattern of regularity or irregularity then usually appears and the level and completeness of the lesion do not seem to influence the menstrual cycle.[5] However, a multicenter survey in 472 women, published by Jackson and Wadley in 1999, showed that menstrual cramping is less frequent after SCI, which is in contrast to an increase in premenstrual syndrome. Exacerbation of autonomic symptoms occurs at particular times in the cycle. These spinal cord injured women had fewer gynecologic check-ups, mammographies, and PAP smears post-injury. Menopause was induced by SCI, immediately or within 12 months, in 14% of the subjects, but except for an increase in mood disorders, menopausal symptoms were fairly comparable in women with or without an SCI.[3] The use of oral contraceptives may be contraindicated because of the challenged cardiovascular status and increased risk of deep venous thrombosis. Especially in women who smoke or are over 35 years of age, the risks are increased.[6] Due to the sensory loss, intrauterine devices (IUDs) can be dangerous in case of urogenital infection or other complications.[4] Condoms can be used and offer the additional benefit of protection from sexually transmitted disease.[7]

Pregnancy

Pregnancy rate is lower in women with an SCI. This does not seem to be due to fertility problems but rather to secondary factors such as decreased sexual activity, decreased involvement in relationships, not wanting children, or perceived difficulty in caring for the children.[4]

Different problems can occur during pregnancy and a regular follow-up by a multidisciplinary team is mandatory. This team should at least be composed of the general practitioner, a gynecologist, and a physician specialized in physical medicine and rehabilitation. Ideally also the urologist, anesthesiologist, physical therapist, occupational therapist, and midwife are involved. Where possible, it is optimal to give preconceptual counseling. This counseling comprises an evaluation of the medication scheme of the mother in order to avoid teratogenous effects on the fetus. Women with SCI due to spina bifida should take folic acid in a dose of 4 mg daily.[8] Psychologic aspects can be discussed in preparation of pregnancy, particularly in women who might not be able to care independently for their baby. A renal/urologic and pulmonary assessment is appropriate.

The following information is mainly based on the review on pregnancy and SCI published in 1996 by Baker and Cardenas,[9] and the data reported respectively by Charlifue et al in 1992[4] and Jackson and Wadley in 1999.[3] During pregnancy, weight gain can decrease mobility and independence for activities of daily living (ADL, e.g. transfers and wheelchair propulsion). Extra help as well as technical aids sometimes need to be provided, as can be the case for tetraplegic mothers for the care of the baby. Due to sensory loss, fetal movements might not be perceived. In that case the mother should be taught to feel these movements by palpating the abdominal wall. Bladder management is often disturbed: incontinence increases and more frequent intermittent catheterization may be necessary. As the presence of asymptomatic bacteriuria and urinary tract infections increases, it is important to insure sufficient fluid intake and to minimize residual volumes in order to avoid pyelonephritis, which might induce preterm labour and delivery. Indwelling or suprapubic catheters are contraindicated and frequent surveillance cultures are advised. Some suggest to switch from 'clean' to 'sterile' intermittent catheterization, for example using a self-contained 'touchless' catheter and bag.[5] Due to a decrease in gastric motility during pregnancy, bowel management requires prevention of constipation with, again, sufficient fluid (and fiber) intake and, if necessary, mild laxatives.

The pregnant woman with SCI often shows anemia and fatigue, water retention, and edema of the lower extremities. Augmented spasticity and pain have also been described. These factors, together with the decreased mobility, can cause decubitus ulcers. The risk for thromboembolism increases and compression stockings as well as LMWH (low molecular weight heparin) administration from the 4th month on until the end of the postpartum period are recommended. In high thoracic and cervical lesions, respiratory capacity is challenged during pregnancy, requiring adapted respiratory rehabilitation. Spasticity can be exacerbated during pregnancy, but oral baclofen can have side-effects for the fetus. Roberts et al reported on two cases where an intrathecal baclofenpump (ITB) was implanted before or during pregnancy, and one case where intrathecal baclofen was administered via an external catheter with good tolerance and good effect on spasticity.[10]

The most important and dangerous complication during pregnancy (and delivery) is autonomic dysreflexia.[11] This is a syndrome characterized by a sudden exaggerated reflex increase in blood pressure known as an important and possibly life-threatening complication, for the mother as well as the baby. It is reported to occur in 48 to 85% of all SCI patients with an SCI at T6 or above, but isolated cases in patients with SCI as low as T8 have been reported. Any stimulus below the lesion that enters the spinal cord through intact peripheral nerves, such as a distended bladder or bowel, a urinary tract infection, a pressure sore, or labor, can trigger the orthosympathetic nervous system (segments T1–T5) and induce an uncontrolled increase in blood pressure due to the lack of inhibitory descending tracts. The symptoms are those of an infralesional vasoconstriction with supralesional vasodilatation. General symptoms are systemic hypertension, compensatory bradycardia, and anxiety. Above the lesion we notice pounding headache, flushing, sweating, and, if the lesion is higher than T1, mydriasis. Below the lesion the patient presents mainly cool extremities and piloerection. Possible complications include retinal, subarachnoidal or intracerebral hemorrhage, myocardial infarction, seizure, and death. During pregnancy differential diagnosis has to be made with pre-eclampsia, of which the treatment is different.[6] Prevention of autonomic dysreflexia by avoiding irritations, such as a full bladder or bowel, infection, constipation or skin ulcers, is absolutely mandatory. When treating autonomic dysreflexia, antihypertensive agents with rapid action and short duration are preferred (mostly nifedipine or captopril), but hypotension should be avoided as this is more poorly tolerated by the fetus then acute hypertension.

Labor and delivery

Labor and delivery depend on the level of the lesion. The uterus is innervated by the segments T10–L1. Women presenting lesions lower than L1 have preservation of uterine sensibility. Women with a lesion in T10–L1, may present insufficient labor. When the lesion is situated in L1 or above, the onset of labor may not be perceived due to the sensory impairment. As is the case during pregnancy, women with lesions at T6 or higher present a risk for autonomic dysreflexia.

Different authors report an increase in preterm labor and delivery. Labor indicators differ greatly following SCI and can be pain above the level of injury, abnormal pain, ruptured membranes (which can be confused with urinary incontinence), significantly increased spasticity (usually of the legs or the abdomen), respiratory changes, symptoms of autonomic dysreflexia, and increased bladder spasms.[3,4] Some women report normal labor sensation but others do not experience any type of labor sensation, depending on the level and completeness of the lesion. Unattended delivery should be avoided in patients who are unable to sense contractions reliably. Therefore, cervical examinations once or twice weekly are recommended after 28 weeks, and hospitalization after 36 weeks or earlier if labor begins or the cervix dilates or is effaced.[6] The patient should be taught uterine palpation techniques and home uterine activity monitoring could be beneficial. Labor duration does not differ significantly even though the clinical perception of labor may be present only at advanced labor and not at latent labor.[9]

During labor and delivery, rigorous prevention of pressure ulcers is of extreme importance, and a special support, regular changes in position, and skin examination are mandatory. Frequent bladder emptying by intermittent or continuous catheterization will prevent overdistention of the bladder, which is important as an (over)distended bladder can induce autonomic dysreflexia.

In the series published by Charlifue et al, 53% of the women had vaginal deliveries without forceps, 22% with forceps assistance, and 25% were cesarean deliveries. Of the cesarean deliveries, 5 were done by physician choice, 2 to deliver transverse lying twins, 2 for autonomic dysreflexia during delivery, 1 because of placenta previa, and 1 because of prolonged labor.[4] Cross et al reported cesarean section in 43% of the patients for the following reasons: breech presentation, transverse presentation, lack of progress, onset of labor one day post-spinal fusion, and a mother's request to have tubal ligation.[6] Finally, Pereira described rates of spontaneous vaginal delivery in 37% of SCI women, assisted vaginal delivery in 31%, and cesarean delivery in 32%.[8]

If autonomic dysreflexia can occur, this means in all women with a lesion at or above T6, then an epidural anesthesia and continuous blood pressure monitoring are necessary. To avoid skin breakdown at the episiotomy site, the use of nonabsorbable sutures has been recommended.[5]

There are some specificities concerning women presenting a cauda equina syndrome.[12] Women who preserved an ability for walking often lose this at the end of the pregnancy. Sensibility of the internal genital organs is preserved, meaning that fetal movements as well as onset of labor will be perceived, so early hospitalization is usually not necessary in this group of patients. The abdominal muscles will help to expel the baby. However, the risk of perineal distention or even rupture is increased due to hypotonia of the pelvic floor and the cicatrization of episiotomy can be problematic. A cesarean section might be indicated in order to protect the fragile pelvic floor.

Postpartum and breastfeeding

During the postpartum period the risk for thromboembolic disease remains increased. Patients should be assessed for bladder distention and bladder management has to be adapted. Bowel management also still requires extra attention.[8,9] In case of impaired balance or upper limb function, extra help needs to be organized for the care of the baby. This may require some psychologic adaptation of the mother. Technical aids, and tips and tricks can be given by the occupational therapist.

Breastfeeding is possible even though milk production might be decreased in lesions above T6 due to decreased nipple sensation. In neurologically intact mothers infant suckling activates tactile receptors in the breast. This signal is carried via afferent nerves in the T4–6 dorsal roots to the spinal cord and then to neurons in the hypothalamus (Figure 78.1), which release oxytocin in the bloodstream, triggering milk ejection from the breast.[13] Cowley reported on three tetraplegic women maintaining breastfeeding for an extended period (12 to 54 weeks). One of them used mental imaging and relaxation techniques and another needed oxytocin nasal spray to facilitate the let-down reflex. In Charlifue's series of 29 women who breastfed their infants, only 4 were reported to have insufficient milk.[4] Halbert drew attention to the fact that additional support with breastfeeding aids, such as pillows to support the baby or adapted nursing bras with easy opening and closing, might be necessary.[14]

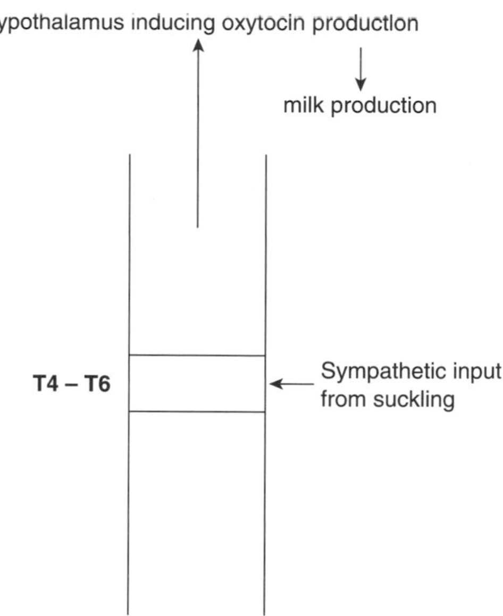

Figure 78.1
Under normal conditions the sympathetic input from suckling enters the spinal cord at the level of T4–T6 and from there travels up to the hypothalamus, which in turn induces oxytocin production and increases milk production. In lesions at or above T6 this normal pathway is partially or completely interrupted, which can result in a decrease of milk production.

Motherhood

Literature on the impact of SCI on mothering is very scarce. In 1994 a paper was published on 26 mothers with SCI with 47 children.[15] No women felt that their family roles and the relationships between family members differed from those of other families. Neither did they have the impression that their children were unable to participate in regular activities because of their SCI. The 10 children who were able to fill out the questionnaire did not perceive their mothers as different from other mothers because of their SCI. Fathers did not report that they felt that they had more responsibilities than partners of able-bodied women. In some other studies very few problems were reported by mothers with SCI. One woman noted that she had problems going on field trips. Another woman, though, stated that having a child actually provided a motivation to stay healthy.[5]

In 2002 Alexander et al published a randomized controlled trial of mothers with SCI and their children, matched to able-bodied mothers and their children on key demographic variables.[16] Eighty-eight mothers, 46 of their partners, and 31 of their children participated. In this study SCI did not appear to affect their children adversely in terms of individual adjustment, attitudes towards their parents, self-esteem, gender roles, and family functioning. Moreover, SCI mothers saw their children as being less rigid and more comfortable in adjusting to novel situations in their environment. SCI mothers did not show more stress than the able-bodied mothers, even if they were more likely to report feeling a lack of emotional and active support from their partners in the area of child management. Partners of SCI mothers, however, seemed to enjoy more satisfying relationships with their children. Just the presence of maternal SCI does not predict difficulties in children's psychologic adjustment, nor does it lead to problems in areas of parenting satisfaction, parenting stress, marital adjustment, or family functioning.

Summary

Spinal cord injury is a relatively rare condition and mainly strikes men. Literature on pregnancy in SCI is very scarce and consists mainly of case reports and opinion articles. However, motherhood is an important topic for women with SCI. After an episode of amenorrhea, fertility returns to the premorbid status. Contraception should be prescribed if necessary, taking into account the specific risks of each method. Pregancy rates are lower in women with SCI. During pregnancy appropriate multidisciplinary follow-up is mandatory. The most dangerous complication is autonomic dysreflexia, which can occur in patients with a lesion at T6 or above. Other potential complications are bladder and bowel problems, pressure sores, anemia and fatigue, increased spasticity or pain, decreased respiratory capacity, and thromboembolic events. Extra monitoring is advised from the 28th week and hospitalization at 36 weeks in order to prevent preterm delivery. Delivery depends on the level of the lesion, the innervation of the uterus being autonomic and situated in T10–L1. Even though spontaneous vaginal delivery is often possible there is an increased percentage of assisted vaginal delivery or cesarean delivery. In patients presenting a lesion at T6 or above, continuous monitoring of blood pressure and epidural anesthesia is necessary during delivery because of the risk for autonomic dysreflexia. Breastfeeding is recommended because of its beneficial effects for the mother as well as the baby. In patients with a lesion above T6, the hypothalamus reaction to suckling-inducing oxytocin production might be decreased, with insufficient milk production as a consequence. With some extra care though, most of the women succeed in breastfeeding. The presence of maternal SCI does not seem to predispose for psychologic adjustment problems in their children, nor does it lead to decreased parenting satisfaction or family functioning.

Pregnancy and motherhood are certainly possible for women with SCI, but multidisciplinary follow-up with prevention of possible complications during pregnancy, labor, and delivery is mandatory.

References

1. DeVivo M, Epidemiology of traumatic spinal cord injury. In: Kirshblum S, Campagnolo DI, De Lisa JA, eds. Spinal Cord Medicine. Lippincott Williams & Wilkins, 2002: 69–81.
2. DeForge D, Blackmer J, Garritty et al. Fertility following spinal cord injury: a systematic review. Spinal Cord 2005; 43: 693–703.
3. Jackson AB, Wadley V. A multicenter study of women's self-reported reproductive health after spinal cord injury. Arch Phys Med Rehabil 1999; 80: 1420–8.
4. Charlifue SW, Gerhart KA, Menter RR et al. Sexual issues of women with spinal cord injuries. Paraplegia 1992; 30: 192–9.
5. Linsenmeyer TA. Sexual function and infertility following spinal cord injury. Phys Med Rehab Clin N Am 2000; 11: 141–56.
6. Cross LL, Meythaler JM, Tuel SM, Cross AL. Pregnancy, labor and delivery post spinal cord injury. Paraplegia 1992; 30: 890–902.
7. Sipski ML. Spinal cord injury and sexual function: an educational model. In: Sipski ML, Alexander CJ, eds. Sexual Function in People with Disability and Chronic Illness. Aspen Publishers, Inc. Gaitherburg, MD. 1997: 149–76.
8. Pereira L. Obstetric management of the patient with spinal cord injury. Obstetr Gynaecol Survey 2003; 58: 678–86.
9. Baker ER, Cardenas DD. Pregnancy in spinal cord injured women. Arch Phys Med Rehab 1996; 77: 501–7.
10. Roberts AG, Graves CR, Konrad PE et al. Intrathecal baclofenpump implantation during pregnancy. Neurology 2003; 61: 1156–7.
11. Campagnolo DI, Merli GJ. Autonomic and cardiovascular complications of spinal cord injury. In : Kirshblum S, Campagnolo DI, De Lisa JA, eds. Spinal Cord Medicine. Lippincott Williams & Wilkins, 2002: 123–34.
12. Perrouin-Verbe B, Labat JJ. Sexualité et procréation des syndromes de la queue de cheval. In: Costa P, Lopez S, Pélissier J, eds, Sexualité, Fertilité et Handicap. Masson, 1996: 81–8.
13. Cowley KC. Psychogenic and pharmacological induction of the letdown reflex can facilitate breastfeeding by tetraplegic women: a report of 3 cases. Arch Phys Med Rehab 2005; 86: 1261–4.
14. Halbert LA. Breastfeeding in the woman with a compromised nervous system. J Hum Lact 1998; 14: 327–31.
15. Westgren N, Levi R. Motherhood after traumatic spinal cord injury. Paraplegia 1994; 32: 517–23.
16. Alexander CJ, Hwang K, Sipski M. Mothers with spinal cord injuries: impact on marital, family, and children's adjustment, Arch Phys Med Rehab 2002; 83: 24–30.

Part XI

Prognosis and follow-up

79

Evolution and follow-up of lower urinary tract dysfunction in spinal cord injury patients

Jean-Jacques Labat and Brigitte Perrouin-Verbe

Introduction

Neurologic lesions can disrupt bladder-sphincter functioning and its central neurologic control. Consequently, these problems can alter the quality of life by inducing incontinence and even threatening the upper urinary tract, particularly of spinal cord injury (SCI) patients. For a long time, urinary complications have been the leading cause of death in SCI. Today, this is not the case. Better knowledge of the evolution and prognostic factors of neurologic bladder has enabled the development of pertinent follow-up strategies, screening for risky situations, and taking account of aging urinary systems as well as aging SCI patients themselves. Neuro-urologic assessment is never definitive. The evolution of therapeutic methods will permit new, more adequate treatments for use tomorrow.

Background

In 1927, Harvey Cushing observed that 80% of SCI patients died within weeks after the trauma because of infections, urinary catheters and bedsores. The mortality rate during the acute phase has evolved over the years due to improved care management. It dropped from 60–80% during World War II to 30% in the 1960s and 6% in the 1980s.[1]

The decrease in mortality of urinary origin is partly responsible for this survival gain. In SCI patients who survived World War II and the Korean war,[2] deaths from urinary causes were estimated to be 43%. Then they declined with time, with the rate not exceeding 10% in the 1980s and 1990s.[3] In 50 years of follow-up, the risk of death attributed to urinary factors has diminished by half in each successive decade.[4]

This favorable evolution in terms of mortality is also seen for morbidity, with preventive measures tending to replace hospitalization for urologic complications. The leading cause of rehospitalization, reported at 1-, 5-, 10-, 15-, and 20-year follow-ups, was disease of the genitourinary system, including urinary tract infections.[5] At present, 43% of rehospitalizations are for urinary reasons (the leading cause of rehospitalization),[6] but in most cases they are more for a check-up than for care. The average length of hospitalization is 7.9 days, with a median length of 3 days. These figures thus confirm that there has been a progression from care to prevention, showing the importance of bladder-sphincter follow-up.

Prognostic factors in upper urinary tract changes

Follow-up objectives

There are many neuro-bladder classifications, but they do not enable prognostic assessment because, even if they do identify the dysfunction type, they do not estimate the balance of urodynamic forces present. The classical criteria of bladder disequilibrium, which are postvoid residual urine, urinary infection, vesicoureteral reflux, ureterohydronephrosis, lithiasis, and incontinence, reflect the deterioration when they occur, but they do not have good prognostic value. The follow-up objectives are thus to solve the problems encountered by SCI patients with lower urinary tract dysfunction, this means improving urinary continence, restricting of infections, facilitating micturition, while preserving patient autonomy. It is equally important to strive for an equilibrated bladder today without any risks for tomorrow, that is, to protect the upper urinary tract apparatus. This equilibrium is not a constant but a daily balance that cannot be considered as unchanging.

The role of elevated intravesical pressure during the storage phase

In 1981, MacGuire et al[7] brilliantly illuminated the harmful role of elevated intravesical pressures in SCI patients. When bladder leak-point pressure (BLPP) is lower than or equal to 40 cmH_2O, there is no vesicoureteral reflux and only 10% of dilatation on intravenous pyelography (IVP). When BLPP is more than 40 cmH_2O, we find 61% of reflux and 81% of upper urinary tract dilatation.

We have confirmed these data in a retrospective study of 200 myelomeningocele patients,[8] followed for a period of 3 to 17 years (average 9.02 years). The prognostic value of BLPP is demonstrated by the study of survival curves testing the rate of upper urinary tract degradation according to its dilatation and the BLPP: if BLPP rises during the follow-up, the probability of an undilated upper urinary tract at 12 years post-trauma is no more than 20%, while it is 86% if BLPP stays low; a patient with BLPP exceeding 40 cmH_2O has 7 times more risk of upper urinary tract damage than someone with stable BLPP.

SCI patients show a correlation between vesicoureteral reflux and elevated intravesical pressure:[9] when bladder pressure exceeds 60 cmH_2O, 22% have reflux, but when the pressure is normal, reflux occurs in only 5%. In detrusor hyperreflexia, we find upper urinary tract alteration in 16% and a normal upper urinary tract in 84%, corresponding to patients whose BLPP is 115 cmH_2O and 72 cmH_2O respectively, on average.[10] Similarly, in detrusor areflexia, the upper urinary tract is altered in 18% and normal in 82%. The corresponding BLPP values are 58 cmH_2O and 24 cmH_2O, respectively.

BLPP is thus an essential prognostic factor with a particularly bad significance when it exceeds 40 cmH_2O.

The physiopathology of upper urinary tract damage

Bladder hyperpressure, either related to detrusor hyperreflexia (SCI patients with prolonged and strong amplitude bladder contractions) or to poor bladder compliance of detrusor areflexia (particularly in myelomeningocele), will have a dual effect: hydrodynamic perturbations and morphologic changes. Bladder hyperpressure will alter urethral flow, as the latter occurs at low pressure; in the beginning, the ureter compensates by an increased amplitude and frequency of contractions; then, above 40 cmH_2O, statis presents with dilatation (or even vesicoureteral reflux). The situation will deteriorate rapidly if the duration of exposure to high pressure is prolonged. This upper urinary tract alteration is initially reversible by continuous catheterization or by restoring detrusor pressure to an acceptable level.

Detrusor hyperpressure can be the consequence but, above all, the cause of bladder wall deformities (trabeculae, diverticula); these may some times affect the watertightness of the vesicoureteral junction and induce vesicoureteral reflux. They will facilitate the development of infectious sites, increasing hyperreflectivity. Collagen will seep progressively into and accumulate between smooth muscle fibers which become rarified. These structural changes may have variable repercussions. When the bladder is active, they induce a decrease of detrusor contractility and lead to a new pressure equilibrium, a veritable homeostasis phenomenon aimed at protecting the upper urinary tract. More deformed bladders are not always the most poorly tolerated by the upper urinary tract level. The collagen excess also favors irreversible detrusor fibrosis, particularly in inactive or congenital neurobladders. This fibrosis, which thickens the detrusor wall, contributes to stenosis of the lower ureter and hydronephrosis. After bladder wall lesions are definitively installed, treatment of hyperreflexia cannot stop the vesicoureteral reflux.

The context and antecedents

Age at onset

Children

In childhood-acquired paraplegia, the prognosis of lower urinary tract dysfunction is relatively good compared to paraplegia occurring during adulthood.[11] In the long-term (6–30 years), 10.4% of childhood paraplegics[12] will incur Bricker's syndrome, which has a lower rate than for adults in the same reference period (1960s–1980s).

The elderly

Spinal cord lesions in the elderly mean complications. Rehabilitation failure is common because of difficulties in adapting to the new situation, a lower urinary tract altered by age (prostate hyperplasia, cystocele, sphincter failure) with slower reflexes, and detrusor hypoactivity. These elements explain the frequency of surgical procedures in men and the use of indwelling cathethers. When the lesion occurs after age 60 years, 50% have an indwelling cathether, and 50% of men undergo a de-obstruction procedure. Traditional rehabilitation often fails.[13] The prognosis for old people is, therefore, linked more to personal factors than to the neuro-urologic situation itself.

Gender

Studies published a few years ago show that women are less exposed than men to urologic complications. In 1983, 99%

of 200 SCI women who survived the initial phase retained a normal IVP for the following 20 years;[14] the woman/man complication rate was 1 for 4.4; 1 woman died of renal failure for every 19 men. This difference has not been seen in recent years. In 1992, the urologic complication rate with time was not significantly different between men and women, and renal failure was no higher in women with an indwelling catheter than in men with a condom catheter.[15]

The drainage method significantly influences the complication rate, and the harmful role of indwelling catheters can be found here compared to reflex voiding or intermittent catheterization. This was very significant in a population of 70 SCI women followed for 11–13 years.[16] It raises questions as to better choices of treatment, given the absence of urine collectors for women.

The neurologic lesion

In a study by Gerridzen et al[10] of 140 SCI patients, of whom 62% were tetraplegic and 38% paraplegic, somewhat surprisingly, 51% of paraplegics had detrusor hyperreflexia versus 49% who presented with detrusor areflexia. Among the tetraplegics, 86% had detrusor hyperreflexia and 14% bladder areflexia. Eight years after the lesion, alterations of the upper urinary tract were twice as frequent among tetraplegics, as 17% of them had a damaged upper urinary tract versus 8% of paraplegics.

The incidence of reflux is higher in complete than in incomplete SCI,[17] but the frequency is identical in paraplegics and tetraplegics. It is probable that the perception of an equivalent of a micturition need limits the risk of increased intravesical pressure because the patient can urinate sooner.

Drainage method

In the initial stage

The complication rate in the initial period after the trauma is closely linked to the bladder drainage method, with particularly high risks of damage from indwelling catheters:[18] acute pyelonephritis, purulent cystitis, paraurethral abscess, ureteral fistula, urethral strictures, and severe hematuric cystitis.

In the long term

In a very large study of 316 exclusively male SCI patients, Weld[19] examined the influence of drainage methods on urologic complications. One hundred and fourteen patients had an indwelling catheter (changed every month), 92 practiced proper intermittent catheterization, 74 voided spontaneously (defined as reflex voidings with postvoid residual urine volume less than 100 ml and voiding pressure less than 40 cmH_2O), and 36 carried a suprapubic catheter. Three hundred and ninety-eight urologic complications occurred in 126 patients. The complications were more frequent in patients with continuous bladder drainage since, 53.5% of these cases had 236 of the complications (61 patients), 4.4% of suprapubic catheter patients had 48 complications (16 patients), 32.4% of patients who voided spontaneously had 57 complications (24 patients), and 27.2% of intermittent catheterization patients had 57 complications (25 patients).

Tetraplegic cases

The independence of tetraplegics is more or less limited, and so the choice of their micturition mode is necessarily influenced by voiding autonomy. Among 73 SCI patients of more than 20 years' duration,[20] 32 had an indwelling catheter, and 41 another mode of micturition (reflex voiding, sphincterotomy, intermittent catheterization): there was no difference between the two groups for creatinine level, but the indwelling catheter group had a higher rate of hydronephrosis and renal atrophy. Alternatively to indwelling catheters, suprapubic catheters seemed to be a good drainage method since 34 of 61 tetraplegics used this mode for an average of 8.6 years (for 27 intermittent catheterizations, the average was 9.9 years), and no upper urinary tract deterioration was observed in any of these groups.[21] However, we noted a much higher frequency of lithiasis in the suprapubic catheter group, and more frequent urinary infections with intermittent catheterization.

Intermittent catheterization seems to be the safest method for SCI patients in terms of urologic complications. In contrast, indwelling catheters appear to incur the highest rate of complications, particularly in the long term.

Urinary infection

Symptomatic infections

The elements that indicate urinary infections in SCI patients sometimes clearly appear with fever and shivering, smelly urine, or hematuria, but are most often subtle: intense renal or bladder pain, urinary leakage or micturition changes, increased spasticity, lethargy, general malaise, and discomfort.

Asymptomatic infections

It is extremely difficult to find a consensus concerning the criteria of asymptomatic urinary infection in SCI patients and, above all, to see them applied, even if only to clinical studies. Nevertheless, criteria have been defined in a

National Institute on Disability and Rehabilitation Research Consensus Statement[22] according to the micturtion mode and can be viewed as extremely rigorous: bacteriuria exceeding 10^2/ml in intermittent catheterization patients, greater than 10^4/ml in patients with a condom catheter, and no matter what the concentration is when patients have an indwelling catheter. The banality of asymptomatic infections is such that they may be neglected most of the time.

Universally accepted risk factors

The risk factors of urinary infections have been classified universally by Cardenas and Hooton:[23] bladder distention, vesicoureteral reflux, elevated intravesical pressure, postvoid residual urine volume, stones, lower bladder outlet obstruction, decreased immunity, pregnancy, repeated urethral traumas, anatomic anomalies of the urinary tract, perineum hygiene, and presence of an indwelling or suprapubic catheter. We must also consider some of the more subjective elements, including possible behavioral risks as well as psychologic factors: degree of patient comprehension, inactivity, self-esteem, social acceptance. Finally, intermittent catheterization is a source of increased infections only when it is done for tetraplegics by nontrained persons (in this case, with infection risk even higher than with indwelling catheters).

Infectious complications

Epididymitis was found in 16.1% of patients, and pyelonephritis in 3.5%. Ninety-four percent of patients had been treated at least once for lower urinary tract infection. Indwelling catheters are the main cause of infectious complications: pyelonephritis and especially epididymitis. Intermittent catheterization leads to less epididymitis than reflex voiding.[18]

Renal function

All bladder drainage methods may preserve the upper urinary tract, but continuous drainage is a risk factor for upper urinary tract damage and renal failure. With continuous bladder drainage, 18.6% of patients undergo upper urinary tract changes. This rate is 7.8% with reflex voiding, and 6.5% with intermittent catheterization.[24] If death (from all causes) is twice as frequent in the continuous drainage group, it is not necessarily significant, because patients in this group are older.

Among the associated factors, patient age and lesion duration are correlated with higher blood creatinine, lower creatinine clearance, and frequent proteinuria. Vesicoureteral reflux is correlated with renal function damage and radiologic anomalies of the upper urinary tract. Blood creatinine levels alone seem not to be a very sensitive factor in early deterioration of the upper urinary tract compared with proteinuria, creatinine clearance, and upper urinary tract imaging.

The two most sensitive methods of screening for renal function deterioration are creatinine clearance and isotopic scintigraphy. Blood creatinine declines with age and body mass reduction; hence, it can remain normal despite decreasing glomerular filtration, and is not sensitive enough. Measurement of endogenous creatinine clearance is acceptable, but poses a problem of 24-hour urine collection in SCI patients. Isotopic clearance (Tc DTPA) seems to be the best method of examination.

Renal scintigraphy represents the most sensitive screening procedure for renal function changes. Effective renal plasma flow (ERPF) decreases by 4.5 ml per year in the 10 years following spinal cord lesion.[25] The factors associated with declining ERPF are age, female sex, renal or bladder lithiasis, tetraplegia, frequent shivering, and fever episodes, but there is no relationship with lesion age or bacteriuria, and no link with lesion severity.

Radiology

Urethral complications

Urethral stricture has been noted in 11.7% of patients, and periurethral abscess in 2.8%.[18] Indwelling catheters cause many urethral strictures, and intermittent catheters two times less, but significantly more than suprapubic catheters or reflex micturition.

Lithiasis

Upper urinary tract lithiasis has been found in 35.1% of patients,[18] and lower urinary tract lithiasis in 14.6%. Indwelling catheters lead to significantly more lithiasis complications of the upper urinary tract and bladder than intermittent catheterization and spontaneous micturition. Recurrent urinary tract infections, indwelling catheters, vesicoureteral reflux, and immobilization hypercalcuria are a few of the major risk factors for the development of urolithiasis among spinal cord injury patients.[26] Temporal evolution shows that lithiasis risk is always present[26] – 3.1% at 5 years, 5.1% at 10 years, 6% at 15 years, and 10.8% at 20 years – but with significant variations according to the voiding method: suprapubic and indwelling catheters represent a high risk while intermittent catheterization has a negligible risk. In men who cannot use intermittent catheterization, or when the bladder cannot empty spontaneously, suprapubic cystostomy is better than urethral catheterization to avoid renal stone formation.[27]

Upper urinary tract changes

Vesicoureteral reflux has been found in 15.8% of patients, and upper urinary tract alteration in 26.3%.[18] Intermittent catheterization and reflex micturition are accompanied by significantly less reflux than indwelling or suprapubic catheters. Injuries between T10 and L2 involve the sympathetic nervous system; patients with such injuries often exhibit vesicoureteral reflux in the early stage of spinal cord injury.

Urodynamics

Postvoid residual urine

Contrary to what we have always thought, even if postvoid residual urine volume is a sign of bladder-sphincter dysfunction, it is not a prognostic factor. The upper urinary tract can deteriorate without any residual volume; the bladder may work to avoid residual urine volume, but this exhausts the urinary system in the long term. In 1977, 38% of dilatation was found 2 to 6 years after SCI in the absence of residual volume.[28] However, major, chronic postvoid urine volume can be tolerated perfectly for years, especially in hypoactive bladders with high compliance.

The prognosis is thus not linked to postvoid residual volume, but depends on urodynamic balance. Postvoid urine volume is a sign of obstruction because it is also a function of adaptation to detrusor contraction. It is as much the consequence of primary insufficient detrusor contraction or decompensation as obstruction. It can be particularly dangerous if there is an associated compliance deficit, or if there are prolonged dyssynergic contractions, as the bladder is then subjected permanently to high pressures.

Bladder reflectivity and contractility

The complication rate of upper urinary tract damage is clearly higher in patients with reflex micturition (32%) compared to patients who void spontaneously (0%) or who have an inactive detrusor or a detrusor inactivated by anticholinergics (7%).[29] All hyperreflexias are not dangerous in the same way: they will be more hazardous if the contractions are strong, prolonged, and frequent; otherwise, they may just manifest as a brief peak of hyperpressure but much less harmful than hyperpressure of the filling phase. In paraplegics, there is a correlation between high intravesical pressure and reflux, with 22% of reflux occurring when intravesical pressure is greater than 60 cmH_2O versus 5% when it is lower than this value.[30]

Dyssynergia

Detrusor-sphincter dyssynergia

Bladder hyperreflexia is harmful in SCI patients because it is associated with bladder-sphincter dyssynergia. In suprasacral lesions,[31] 7.4% of patients have no dyssynergia, 80.3% have intermittent dyssynergia, and 12.3% have continuous dyssynergia. Complete spinal cord lesion is usually accompanied by continuous dyssynergia, while intermittent dyssynergia is seen only with incomplete lesion. Dyssynergia is associated with complete lesions, with high intravesical pressure, and with upper urinary tract complications. These associations are more pronounced in continuous dyssynergia than in intermittent dyssynergia. The proportion of patients suffering from a particular type of bladder-sphincter dyssynergia has not changed with time.

These parameters are, in fact, correlated. Indeed, dyssynergia is responsible for high intravesical pressures which are themselves a source of risk for the upper urinary tract. On the other hand, what value should be given to this classification of detrusor-sphincter dyssynergia in case of anticholinergic treatment, since the latter does not alter the type of dyssynergia although it modifies the other risk factors (decreased intravesical pressure)? Under these conditions, would it be worthwhile to distinguish the different types of dyssynergia or to evaluate the pressures that they engender?

Compliance

Measurement of compliance deficiency seems less significant than BLPP, but explores high pressures in the same way during the filling phase and their danger. In contrast, flaccid and compliant bladders do not develop any changes of the bladder wall and upper urinary tract; this may be the case for cauda equina syndrome after disc herniation.

Evaluation of compliance is difficult in SCI patients because of hyperreflexia, and studies are rare. Hypocompliant bladders are seldom found in SCI patients.[32] In the population with initially normal compliance (higher than 20%), the upper urinary tract remains normal 3 years later in 78% of cases, but when initial compliance is low (17%), we find only 23% with a normal upper urinary tract after this time period.[33]

A threshold of 12.5 ml/cmH_2O significantly indicates the presence of various upper urinary tract complications: vesicoureteral reflux, upper urinary tract distention, pyelonephritis, and upper urinary tract lithiasis.[34] In suprasacral lesions (complete and incomplete), bladder hypocompliance is more frequent in patients with continuous drainage than in those who use intermittent catheterization. Whatever the drainage method, low compliance is more frequent in sacral lesions than in suprasacral lesions, and in complete than in incomplete lesions. Regression curve analysis shows that compliance is more often altered with time in the continuous drainage group than in the reflex micturition and intermittent catheterization groups. The risk of altered compliance with indwelling catheters increases by 23% every 5 years.

The evolution of bladder compliance thus appears to be a fundamental element of surveillance for all neurologic bladders.

Cytology and cystoscopy

The risk of bladder tumor is high in aging SCI patients and notably in those with indwelling catheters (over 8 years) or bladder lithiasis.[35] Groah et al[36] examined 3670 SCI patients by cystoscopy and showed that the risk of bladder cancer with SCI using an indwelling catheter is 77 per 100 000 person-years. This corresponds to an age- and gender-adjusted standardized morbidity ratio of 25.4 when compared with the general population. After adjusting for age at injury, gender, level and severity of SCI, history of bladder calculi, and smoking, those using solely indwelling catheters had a risk of bladder cancer 4.9 times than those using nonindwelling methods. However, the incidence of invasive bladder cancer in the European population appears to be lower than that reported in other series.[37] Gross hematuria in individuals with SCI warrants aggressive assessment for bladder cancer.[38] These findings suggest a screening by annual cystoscopy after 8 years of indwelling catheter use in the at-risk patient group (lithiasis, repeated infections, etc.). The BTA (bladder tumor antigen) stat, survivin assay, and urine cytology were unable to predict bladder cancer cases in patients with SCI.[39] Cystoscopy, therefore, remains the gold standard for bladder cancer surveillance in patients with SCI.

Longitudinal follow-up

Patient compliance in follow-up

Clinical practice demonstrates the importance of some elements that are difficult to quantify. Patient compliance in follow-up is one of these parameters. The three most significant elements when complications occur are ignorance of follow-up importance, lack of confidence in their general practioner, and examination cost.[40] The other significant elements are living far from services, transport difficulties, and length of time since the accident.

It is common for SCI individuals to change their bladder-emptying method over time. At least 10 years after a traumatic spinal cord injury the use of clean intermittent catheterization (CIC) rose from 11% at the initial discharge to 36% at the time of follow-up. The use of suprapubic tapping fell from 57 to 31% in the same period, while the use of the Credé maneuver rose from 5 to 19%. During follow-up, 46% changed the bladder-emptying method. The results showed the following trends in change of method: a high proportion of discontinuation in normal bladder emptying, suprapubic tapping, and abdominal pressure, and a high proportion of continuation when using CIC.[41,42]

Delayed complications

Radiologically, 63% of SCI patients have bladder anomalies – wall deformities, lithiasis, upper urinary tract changes – that appear in 3/4 of cases in the first year, especially in patients who had an indwelling catheter for a prolonged initial period (more than 8 weeks). In contrast, new radiologic anomalies occur in only 1% of cases after 10 years.[43] Upper urinary tract complications (23.7% of 105 SCI patients)[44] can present at any time of follow-up, between 1 month and 34 years, with an average of 10.4 years. Forty-four percent of reflux appears during the first 2 years, and 23% during the 2 following years, with the rates decreasing regularly with time.[16] Thus, the first years after the trauma are the most dangerous.

If we compare drainage methods,[18] we find that the complication rate increases in the indwelling catheter group 5 years after the trauma, and after 15 years in patients with suprapubic catheters, with no significant changes in time for the two other groups (intermittent catheterization and spontaneous micturition) which, therefore, remain safe methods for the long term.

Patients at risk

It is possible to define SCI populations at higher risk of urinary complications.

Tetraplegic patients have a higher risk

They have a higher risk because they frequently have bladder hyperreflexia and because they do not take any anticholinergics to facilitate spontaneous micturition in a condom catheter.

Paraplegic patients have a relative decrease in risk

The decreased risk in paraplegics is linked to a lower frequency of hyperreflexia with high pressures because these patients are treated with intermittent catheterization and anticholinergics. In this group, the only deterioration occurs in patients not taking anticholinergics.

Men have more risks than women

The caricatural difference of a few years ago is subsiding, thanks to progress made in the follow-up of SCI patients.

Surveillance will be especially close as intravesical pressures are high

In hyperreflexia, dyssynergia is responsible for type 3 high pressures. This is characteristic of complete lesions. In areflexia, low compliance of the peripheral bladder is the source of the high pressures. In all cases, it is important to suspect compliance <20 and to avoid compliance <12.5.

Micturition mode

Patients with an indwelling catheter in the initial phase and in the long term present more complications. The suprapubic catheter is a better method, except for the risk of intravesical lithiasis. It is preferable to use anticholinergics in association with intermittent catheterization than to urinate in a reflex way.

Lesion duration

Surveillance should be close in the first 2 years. Complications may occur later (after 5 years of an indwelling catheter and after 15 years of a suprapubic catheter). In patients without an indwelling or suprapubic catheter, the situation may remain stable for over 15 years. Cystoscopy is necessary in patients with an indwelling catheter for over 8 years or for those with augmentation ileocystoplasty.

Patient profile

It is important to pay attention to loss of follow-up in patients who live far away and who have a great deal of trust in their general practitioner. It is important to inform patients of the necessity of regular and specialized follow-up.

Conclusion: follow-up proposals

SCI patient follow-up is based on clinical care and systematic check-ups.[45] The clinical elements that lead patients to consultation are generally linked to infectious complications or to changes in continence. The search for an irritative cause is part of the check-up: eschar, fecaloma, ingrown nail, prolapse. The paraclinical elements derive from an appreciation of post-micturition residual volume, from biologic examinations that explore renal function (creatinine clearance annually), imaging (urinary ultrasound with abdomen X-rays, computer tomography without and with injection), and urodynamics (cystometry, urethral pressure measurements). All these parameters do not possess the same value, as some screen for certain complications (imaging), while others try to prevent them (urodynamics).

However, there is a lack of consensus in the specific methods used for surveillance of the urinary system.[46] The follow-up of SCI patients should be adapted to the clinical situation. Nevertheless, we can still try to respect standard procedures that will be adapted in terms of the data collected during these check-ups and risky situations.

In the first 2 years, the patient should be followed up clinically, urodynamically, and echographically every 6 months. In the subsequent 5 years, follow-up will be annual.[47] In the following 8 years, follow-up should be every 2 years, with clinical, echographic, and urodynamic assessment indications to be discussed in terms of each situation. After 15 years, clinical and echographic follow-up every 2–5 years may be enough if the patient urinates in a reflex way or by intermittent catheterization.

Certainly, the presentation of risk factors (particularly elevated intravesical pressures) and urinary complications will lead to changes in follow-up and treatment plans.

References

1. Hartkopp A, Bronnum-Hansen H, Seidenschnur AM, Biering-Sorensen F. Survival and cause of death after traumatic spinal cord injury. A long-term epidemiological survey from Denmark. Spinal Cord 1997; 35: 76–85.
2. Hackler RH. A 25 years prospective mortality study in a spinal cord injured patient: comparison with the long term living paraplegic. J Urol 1977; 117: 486–8.
3. Whiteneck GG, Charlifue SW, Frankel HL et al. Mortality, morbidity, and psychosocial outcomes of persons spinal cord injured more than 20 years ago. Paraplegia 1992; 30: 617–30.
4. Frankel HL, Coll JR, Charlifue SW et al. Long-term survival in spinal cord injury: a fifty year investigation. Spinal Cord 1998; 36: 266–74.
5. Cardenas DD, Hoffman JM, Kirshblum S, McKinley W. Etiology and incidence of rehospitalization after traumatic spinal cord injury: a multicenter analysis. Arch Phys Med Rehabil 2004; 85: 1757–63.
6. Vaidyanathan S, Soni BM, Gopalan L et al. A view of the readmissions of patients with tetraplegia to the Regional Injuries Centre,

Southport, United Kingdom, between January 1994 and December 1995. Spinal Cord 1998; 36: 838–46.
7. McGuire EJ, Woodside JR, Borden TA, Weiss RM. Prognostic value of urodynamic testing in myelodysplastic patients. J Urol 1981; 126: 205–9.
8. Bouchot O, Labat JJ, Glemain P, Buzelin JM. Les facteurs du pronostic urinaire des myélo-méningocèles. J Urol (Paris) 1988; 94: 145–51.
9. Anderson RU. Urologic complications in spinal cord injured patients. Urology 1988; 32(Suppl): 31–2.
10. Gerridzen RG, Thijssen AM, Dehoux E. Risk factors for upper tract deterioration in chronic spinal cord injury patients. J Urol 1992; 147: 416–18.
11. Fanciullacci F, Zanollo A, Sandri S, Catanzaro F. The neuropathic bladder in children with spinal cord injury. Paraplegia 1988; 26: 83–6.
12. Lacert P, Picard A, Richard F, Bourgeois-Gavardin T. Résultats à long terme de la rééducation urinaire au cours des paraplégies acquises de l'enfant. Ann Urol 1982; 16: 44–6.
13. Madersbacher H, Oberwalder M. The elderly para and tetraplegic: special aspects of urologic care. Paraplegia 1987; 25: 318–23.
14. Watson N. Spinal cord injury in the female. Paraplegia 1983; 21: 143–8.
15. Jackson AB, DeVivo M. Urological long term follow-up in women with spinal cord injuries. Arch Phys Med Rehabil 1992; 73: 1029–35.
16. Bennet CJ, Young MN, Adkins RH, Diaz F. Comparison of bladder management complication outcomes in female spinal cord injury patients. J Urol 1995; 153: 1458–60.
17. Lamid S. Long term follow-up of spinal cord injury patients with vesicoureteral reflux. Paraplegia 1988; 26: 27–34.
18. Zermann D, Wunderlich H, Derry F, Schroder S, Schubert J. Audit of early bladder management complications after spinal cord injury in first treating hospitals. Eur Urol 2000; 37: 156–60.
19. Weld JK. Effect of bladder management on urological complications in spinal cord injured patients. J Urol 2000; 163: 768–72.
20.. Chao R, Clowers D, Mayo ME. Fate of upper urinary tracts in patients with indwelling catheters after spinal cord injury. Urology 1993; 42: 259–62.
21. Mitsui T, Minami K, Furuno T, Morita H, Koyanagi T. Is suprapubic cystostomy an optimal urinary management in high quadriplegics? A comparative study of suprapubic cystostomy and clean intermittent catheterisation. Eur Urol 2000; 38: 434–8.
22. National Institute on Disability and Rehabilitation Research Consensus Statement. January 27–29, 1992. The prevention and management of urinary tract infections among people with spinal cord injuries. J Am Paraplegia Soc 1992; 15: 194–204.
23. Cardenas DD, Hooton TM. Urinary tract infection in persons with spinal cord injury. Arch Phys Med Rehabil 1995; 76: 272–80.
24. Weld KJ. Influences on renal function in chronic spinal cord injured patients. J Urol 2000; 164: 1490–3.
25. McKinley WO, Jackson AB, Cardenas DD, DeVivo MJ. Long term medical complications after traumatic spinal cord injury: a regional model systems analysis. Arch Phys Med Rehabil 1999; 80: 1402–10.
26. Ost MC, Lee BR. Urolithiasis in patients with spinal cord injuries: risk factors, management, and outcomes. Curr Opin Urol 2006; 16: 93–9.
27. Ku JH, Jung TY, Lee JK, Park WH, Shim HB. Risk factors for urinary stone formation in men with spinal cord injury: a 17-year follow-up study. BJU Int 2006; 97: 790–3.
28. Stover SL, Lloyd LK, Nepomuceno CS, Gale LL. Intermittent catheterization: follow-up. Paraplegia 1977; 15: 38–46.
29. Killorin W, Gray M, Bennett JK, Green BG. The value of urodynamics and bladder management in predicting upper urinary tract complications in male spinal cord injury patients. Paraplegia 1992; 30: 437–41.
30. Arnold EP, Cowan IA. Clinical significance of ureteric diameter on intravenous urography after spinal cord injury. Br J Urol 1988; 62: 131–5.
31. Weld JK. Clinical significance of detrusor sphincter dyssynergia type in patients with post-traumatic spinal cord injury. Urology 2000; 56: 565–9.
32. Ruutu M. Cystometrographic patterns in predicting bladder function after spinal cord injury. Paraplegia 1985; 23: 243–52.
33. Hackler RH, Hall MK, Zampieri TA. Bladder hypocompliance in the spinal cord injury population. J Urol 1989; 141: 1390–3.
34. Weld JK. Differences in bladder compliance with time and associations of bladder management with compliance in spinal cord injured patients. J Urol 2000; 163: 1228–33.
35. Stonehill WH, Goldman HB, Dmochowski RR. Risk factors for bladder tumors in spinal cord injury patients. J Urol 1996; 155: 1248–50.
36. Groah SL, Weitzenkamp DA, Lammertse DP et al. Excess risk of bladder cancer in spinal cord injury: evidence for an association between indwelling catheter use and bladder cancer. Arch Phys Med Rehab 2002; 83: 346–51.
37. Subramonian K, Cartwright RA, Harnden P, Harrison SC. Bladder cancer in patients with spinal cord injuries. BJU Int 2004; 93: 739–43.
38. Hess MJ, Zhan EH, Foo DK, Yalla SV. Bladder cancer in patients with spinal cord injury. J Spinal Cord Med 2003; 26: 335–8.
39. Davies B, Chen JJ, McMurry T et al. Efficacy of BTA stat, cytology, and survivin in bladder cancer surveillance over 5 years in patients with spinal cord injury. Urology 2005; 66: 908–11.
40. Canupp KC, Waites KB, DeVivo MJ, Richards JS. Predicting compliance with annual follow-up evaluations in persons with spinal cord injury. Spinal Cord 1997; 35: 314–19.
41. Hansen RB, Biering-Sorensen F, Kristensen JK. Bladder emptying over a period of 10–45 years after a traumatic spinal cord injury. Spinal Cord 2004; 42: 631–7.
42. Drake MJ, Cortina-Borja M, Savic G, Charlifue SW, Gardner BP. Prospective evaluation of urological effects of aging in chronic spinal cord injury by method of bladder management. Neurourol Urodyn 2005; 24: 111–16.
43. Gupta S, Chawla JC. Review of urinary tract abnormalities in 100 patients with spinal cord paralysis. Paraplegia 1994; 32: 531–9.
44. Van Kerrebroeck PE, Koldewijn EL, Scherpenhuizen S, Debruyne FM. The morbidity due to lower urinary tract function in spinal cord injury patients. Paraplegia 1993; 31: 320–9.
45. Ruffion A, de Sèze M, Denys P, Perrouin-Verbe B, Chartier-Kastler E. Care of neurogenic bladder in spinal cord injured patients and patients with myelomeningocele: review of the literature and therapeutic recommendations. Pelv Perineol 2006; 1: 304–23.
46. Razdan S, Leboeuf L, Meinbach DS, Weinstein D, Gousse AE. Current practice patterns in the urologic surveillance and management of patients with spinal cord injury. Urology 2003; 61: 893–6.
47. Nosseir M, Hinkel A, Pannek J. Clinical usefulness of urodynamic assessment for maintenance of bladder function in patients with spinal cord injury. Neurourol Urodyn 2007: 228–33.

80

Neurogenic bladder surveillance in children

Lysanne Campeau and Jacques Corcos

Introduction

Most neurogenic bladder in children is secondary to neural tube congenital defects.[1] These include myelomeningocele and sacral agenesis, both of which can be detected at birth (Figure 80.1). Other defects encountered are occult dysraphisms, whose diagnoses are more subtle due to the absence of median lumbosacral cutaneous anomalies. Acquired neurogenic bladder can affect all levels of the spinal cord, being secondary to spinal trauma or cord compression of a mass.

The vesical pressures considerably influence the follow-up of these vesical dysfunctions. It is uncommon to encounter structural or functional injury to the upper tract system with low pressure neurogenic bladders.[2] These patients may then be followed less frequently (every 24 months in our practice). On the other hand, patients with an overactive neurogenic bladder face a higher risk of renal deterioration requiring a closer follow-up (every 3 to 12 months according to the case). This surveillance follows detrusor-sphincter dysfunction changes, but is also aimed at assessing the efficacy of several pharmacologic and surgical treatments (anticholinergics, botulinum toxin injections, bladder augmentation, artificial sphincter, etc.).

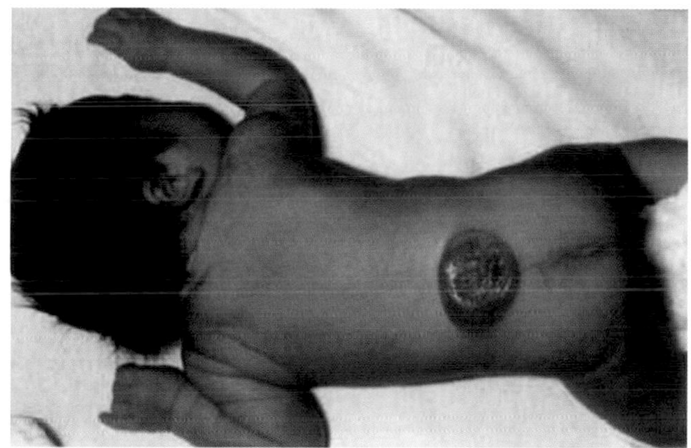

Figure 80.1
Cutaneous manifestations of spina bifida.

The natural evolution of neurogenic bladders

Neurogenic bladders have a wide spectrum of progression towards renal deterioration (defining vital prognosis) and urinary incontinence (defining functional prognosis). The surveillance of these often handicapped patients intends to minimize as much as possible both of these complications, thereby improving the patient's prognosis and quality of life.

Storing dysfunction and detrusor-sphincter incoordination cause an increased workload on the bladder and progressively worsening detrusor hypertrophy. This structural anomaly brings about a decreased bladder compliance, which degenerates to a high-pressure storage system and incontinence. The neurogenic bladder dysfunction weakens the efficacy of the intravesical ureter antireflux mechanism, and along with detrusor high pressures produce a vesicoureteral reflux. This reflux disturbs renal function and can lead to renal failure alone or in combination with recurrent infections.[3]

Neurogenic bladder surveillance strives for slowing down or stopping the natural progression towards incontinence and renal failure. This surveillance is based on 10 essential elements that can establish the child's functional and vital prognosis. Alone or combined, these elements gather sufficient information to decide on the optimal timing of therapeutic interventions. These elements are described in the following sections.

Clinical history

A detailed clinical history evaluates the *severity* of the neurologic and functional urologic condition along with their impact on the child's quality of life. The questions asked at the initial assessment represent an important reference and baseline status to which will be compared subsequent evaluations. The questionnaire directed to the child or his caregivers starts with an elaborate layout of his *neurologic* and *neurourologic* impairment, his evaluations, and response to previous or ongoing treatments. Other impairments, past medical and surgical history, and allergies complete the initial history taking.

The history thereafter will be focused on the child's urinary symptoms: frequency of voiding episodes (spontaneously or self-catheterization), type of urinary jet (normal, intermittent, drops, etc.), need to strain to urinate (often detected with observation of the 'patient squatting'), presence of urgency, presence and type of incontinence, and control measures (no protection, pads, diapers, etc.). All these elements are usually difficult to gather from the child himself as he might minimize his symptoms, or from the parents as they might not have observed him. A frequency volume chart may become very useful to confirm these symptoms, but is quite difficult to obtain from the pediatric population. This chart objectively measures the voiding function and its changes observed after treatments.[4] When the child requires self-catheterization, the history should reveal difficulties or concerns with this process. If these catheterizations are performed with difficulty, the technique (detailed steps, catheter type, lubricant type, etc.) and catheterized access (Mitrofanoff, urethra, or other) should be verified.

Recent changes in urinary symptoms are important hints in the detection of the neurologic condition evolution. For example, the appearance of an overactive bladder with urinary leakage, or of a hydronephrosis, can represent the first clinical symptoms of a progressive spinal process such as a syringomyelia or a tethered cord, which should prompt the clinician to carry out a magnetic resonance imaging of the spinal cord.

Finally, the enquiry should include possible fecal elimination troubles, such as fecal incontinence, constipation, and rectal tenesmus, along with the different nutritional adjustments or medications to treat them. It is often warranted to guide the child's daily treatment of constipation that may affect the voiding function or worsen the risk of urinary tract infections. It is of great importance for the questionnaire to address the evolution of *urinary tract infections* because they can cause deterioration of the detrusor muscle and the renal function. The history should determine the frequency and symptoms associated as well as the presence of fever, which is often a sign of concomitant pyelonephritis.[5]

Quality of life evaluation

The evaluation and surveillance of a child with a neurogenic bladder should take into account the patient's and parent's perception of the condition and treatment outcome. There is, however, no validated questionnaire to evaluate in a standardized fashion the quality of life of a child suffering from a neurogenic bladder. However, simple and focused questions can allow the clinician to estimate the negative impact the voiding and fecal function may have on the quality of life of the patient and his caregivers. For the teenage patient, the evaluation should address sexual function and expectations towards sexual relationships, and paternity or maternity. These legitimate expectations may require specialized consultations in sexology, gynecology, or urology.

Physical exam

The abdominal and external genitalia physical exam should be performed at the initial assessment, but repeated on subsequent assessments if clinically pertinent (presence of a costo-vertebral angle tenderness, a full bladder, or other tenderness, etc.). If possible, the observation of the child voiding can be very informative in terms of urinary flow, presence of intermittent flow, or need to strain, although these elements will later be objectified during the urodynamic evaluation.

Urine analysis and culture

A routine urine analysis is a crude but good indicator of renal injury. Urine cultures are done only in the presence of symptoms (pain, fever, or changes of voiding pattern).[6] Asymptomatic bacteriuria should not be systematically treated in children using self-catheterization.

Serum creatinine

Biologic serum testing of creatinine concentration and creatinine excretion rate can give an approximate calculation of the renal function.

Postvoid residual measurement

If the child voids spontaneously, the postvoid residual volume can establish a complete or partial emptying ability. There is no a normal value for residual volume, but the expected value should be zero based on a normal child's voiding pattern. In a context of a patient suffering from a neurologic condition, the postvoid residual value

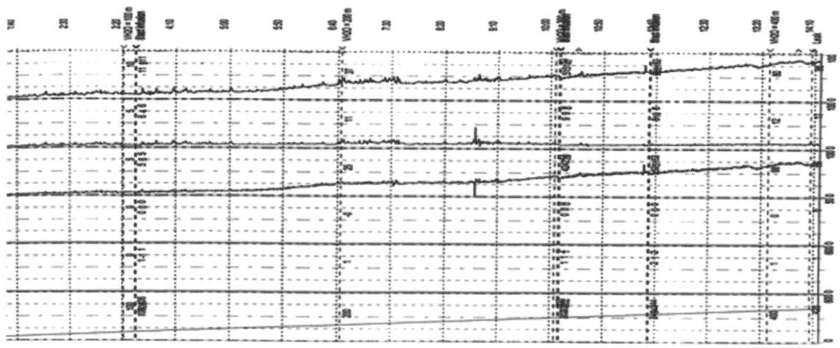

Figure 80.2
Cystometrogram of a child with myelomeningocele showing loss of detrusor compliance leading to a lower "safe" bladder capacity (at detrusor pressure < 40 cmH_2O) despite a close to normal cystometric bladder capacity.

interpretation needs a correlation with the clinical context and elements of the history such as the presence of incontinence, urgency, urinary tract infection, etc. For example, a small asymptomatic residual volume may be ignored. This measurement can be carried out in a child using self-catheterization to confirm the efficacy of the technique.

Urodynamic evaluation

The urodynamic evaluation in a young child is achieved by active participation of the physician along with good cooperation and relaxation from the child, often requiring the parent's presence during the exam, or occasionally sedation via suppositories or injections. The urodynamic study is crucial at all steps of the diagnosis and surveillance. A more frequent study is indicated in patients at risk of structural damage (recurrent urinary tract infections, newly diagnosed hydronephrosis) or in patients who are refractory to conservative treatments (Figure 80.2). The timing of the first urodynamic study and the frequency of the following studies vary from one patient to another. In general, the first evaluation is performed at 3–4 years old and repeated every year after. Any new neurologic or urologic event (recurrent urinary tract infections) or new treatment calls for a repeat study.[7]

Ultrasound

The surveillance involves the prevention of upper urinary tract anatomic changes. A renal ultrasound evaluates in a noninvasive fashion the size and growth of the kidneys along with the presence of hydronephrosis or nephrolithiasis (Figure 80.3). This study does not, however, predict renal function nor determine the presence and the degree of an obstruction or vesicoureteral reflux.[8]

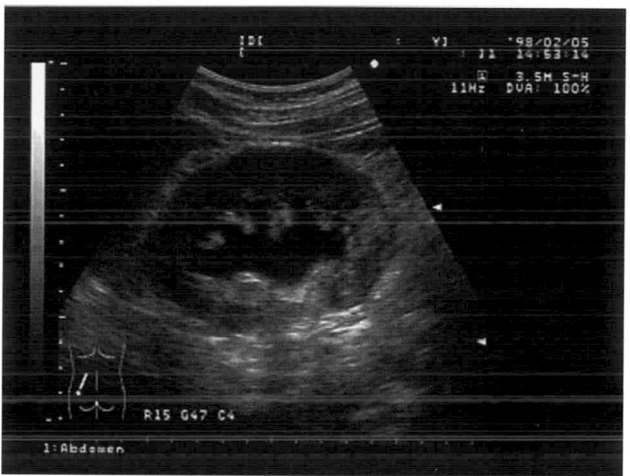

Figure 80.3
Ultrasound of renal hydronephrosis.

Retrograde cystography

The cystography can be nuclear or radiographic, alone or within a video-urodynamic exam. The contrast agent instilled in the bladder in a retrograde fashion via a urethral catheter allows a precise visualization of the bladder contour and a crude evaluation of bladder capacity. A neurogenic bladder often demonstrates a characteristic shape with a verticalization of its long axis and/or a thickened wall (Figure 80.4). In a severe state, it can have a 'Christmas tree' appearance with its trabeculations and diverticula.[3] In addition, the filling of the bladder to its maximal capacity can reveal a passive or low-pressure reflux or an active reflux during voiding.[5] Finally, the voiding cystography is the only exam that can confirm the results of a vesicoureteral reflux.

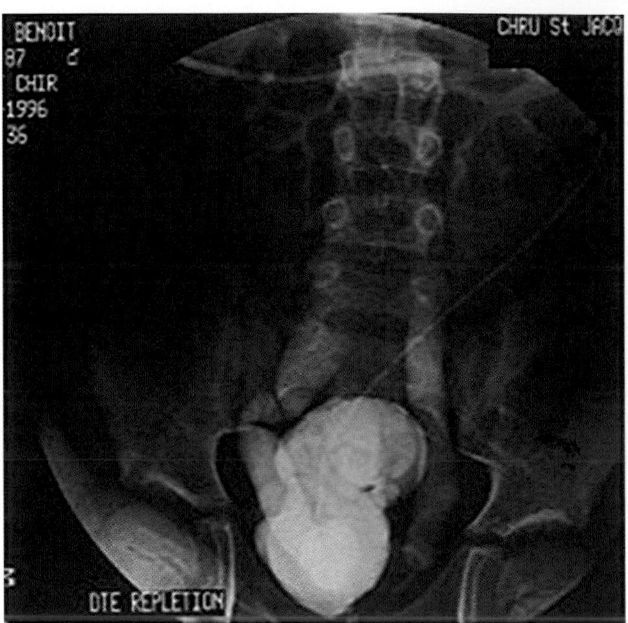

Figure 80.4
Cystography of a neurogenic bladder with vesico-ureteral reflux.

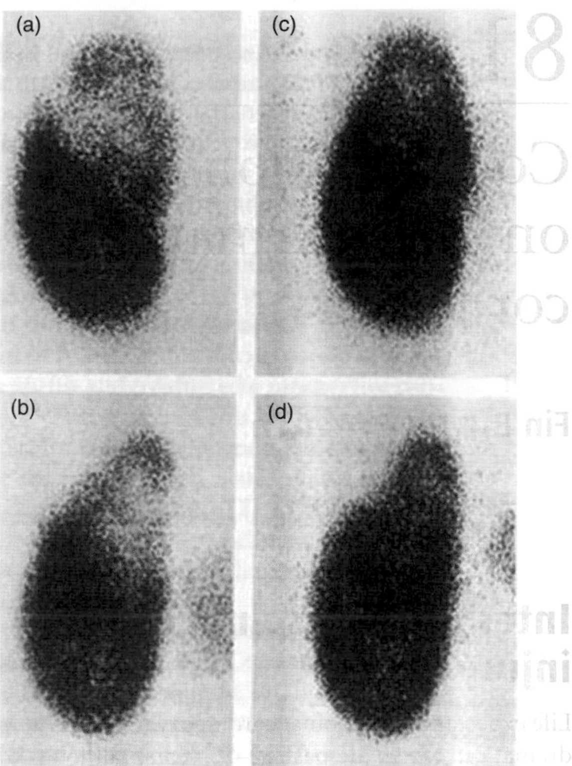

Figure 80.5
DMSA study of left renal scar in a five year-old child. (a) Posterior view; (b) Posterior oblique view.

Nuclear renal scan

This exam of low invasiveness and low radiographic dose is used more liberally in the pediatric population. A functional and anatomic nuclear study is recommended if there is a suspicion of pyelonephritic renal scars or hydronephrosis secondary to reflux or obstruction (Figure 80.5). The nuclear renal scan not only delineates the morphology and location of the kidneys, but also determines the differential renal function, the glomerular filtration rate, and degree of obstruction.

Conclusion

The careful surveillance of pediatric patients with neurogenic bladder anticipates renal and bladder function deterioration. It also facilitates assessment of the impact of pharmacologic and surgical treatments. It is of the greatest importance to establish and apply these surveillance modalities, because the main neurologic and orthopedic condition can undergo a clinically silent progression and thereby cause a deterioration in kidney and bladder function. Thus a basic annual surveillance including all or most of the proposed elements is the minimum required in children with a neurogenic bladder. Any symptom or treatment change should prompt a more frequent follow-up.

References

1. Aslan AR, Kogan BA. Conservative management in neurogenic bladder dysfunction. Current Opinion in Urology 2002; 12: 473–77.
2. Fowler CJ, O'Malley KJ. Investigation and Management of Neurogenic Bladder Dysfunction. Journal of Neurologic and Neurosurgical Psychiatry 2003; 74; 27–31.
3. Guys JM, Camerlo A, Hery G. Vessies neurologiques de l'enfant: Approche diagnostique et therapeutique. Annales d'urologie – EMC Urologie 2006; 40: 15–27.
4. Bankhead RW, Kropp BP, Cheng EY. Evaluation and Treatment of Children with Neurogenic Bladders. Journal of Child Neurology 2000; 15(3): 141–9.
5. Corcos J, Schick E. Textbook of the Neurogenic Bladder (Adults and Children). London, Martin Dunitz (eds) 2004: p. 361.
6. Elliot SP, Villar R, Duncan B. Bacteriuria Management and Urological Evaluation of Patients with Spina Bifida and Neurogenic Bladder: A Multicenter Survey. Journal of Urology 2005; 173: 217–20.
7. Tarcan T, Bauer S, Olmedo E et al. Long-term follow up of newborns with myelodysplasia and normal urodynamic findings: is follow-up necessary? J Urol 2001; 165: 564–7.
8. Blok BFM, Karsenty G, Corcos J. Urological surveillance and management of patients with neurogenic bladder: results of a survey among practicing urologists in Canada. Can J Urol 2006; 13(5): 3034–8.
9. Del Gado R, Perrone L, Del Gaizo D et al. Renal size and function in patients with neuropathic bladder due to myelomeningocele: the role of growth hormone. J Urol 2003; 170(5): 1960–1.

81

Considerations on the international data set on lower urinary tract function following spinal cord injury

Fin Biering-Sørensen

International spinal cord injury data set

Life expectancy after spinal cord injury (SCI) has increased dramatically over the past 60–70 years,[1] although within the last three decades research has shown the absence of a substantial decline in mortality after the first 2 years post-injury.[2] The life expectancy of people with SCI is still below that of the general population.[3–7] The causes of death in SCI have changed from being primarily due to urinary tract disease to increasingly due to cardiovascular disease and respiratory complications,[3–5,8] thus becoming similar to the causes of death in the general population. Improved early medical care, specialized rehabilitation, and regular follow-up visits have contributed to this development.

Because of the increasing prevalence of individuals living with SCI, after a traumatic as well as nontraumatic spinal cord lesion there is an increasing need for data pertaining to SCI. To facilitate comparisons regarding injuries, treatments, and outcomes between patients, centers, and countries, such data should be in the form of common international data sets collected on individuals with SCI.[9]

Many countries have established SCI databases. It is becoming increasingly important to have comparable data so that the services affecting worldwide outcome of SCI can be assessed and compared. For those countries or centers seeking to develop or upgrade an SCI database, the ability to learn from the experience of others is critical.

After a one-day workshop on 2 May 2002 in Vancouver, British Columbia, Canada, before the combined annual scientific meeting between the American Spinal Injury Association (ASIA) and the International Spinal Cord Society (ISCoS), it was decided to establish a partnership for developing international data sets for SCI. There was a consensus that guidelines for the recommended minimal number of data elements could provide a lowest common denominator and be the start of a common language among SCI centers. The aim was to assist centers to develop new SCI databases, enable researchers to be more consistent and effective in the design and publication of clinical research studies through the use of international data sets, and thus to facilitate comparison between SCI populations worldwide.[9]

It is also hoped that internationally recognized and endorsed data sets can build on the experience and positive momentum of the worldwide dissemination of the ASIA and now ASIA/ISCoS International Standards for Neurological Classification of SCI.[10] To obtain this kind of success, it is important that the data sets are simple and perceived relevant to the clinicians so they will use them. In addition, it is imperative that these data sets can be both easily retrieved and available for use for no cost and without any specific restrictions other than those protecting the privacy of the individuals whose information resides in subsequent registries based on the data sets.

International Classification of Functioning, Disability, and Health

In 2001, the World Health Organization endorsed the International Classification of Functioning, Disability, and Health (ICF).[11] Since the ICF is an internationally accepted classification of the consequences of disease, it is considered to be a useful conceptual framework for data sets related to the consequences of SCI.

In this classification scheme, disability is an umbrella term for any or all of the following:

- impairment of body function or structure
- limitation in activities
- restriction in participation.

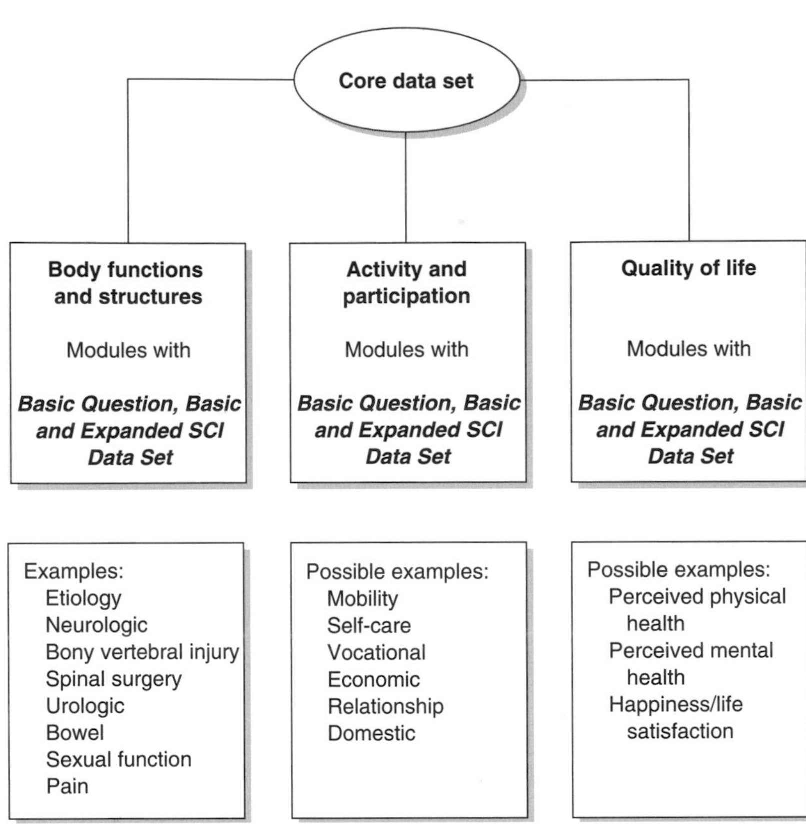

Figure 81.1
General structure of the International Spinal Cord Injury Data Sets.

Environmental factors make up the physical, social, and attitudinal environment in which people live and conduct their lives. These are either barriers to or facilitators of the person's functioning.

With more than 1400 categories, the ICF classification can serve as a reference but is not applicable in clinical practice. Tools such as *ICF Core Sets* are needed to make the ICF useful, and such an ICF Core Set for SCI will be developed alongside the International SCI Data Sets.[12]

Structure and terminology for the International SCI Data Sets

The overall framework for the International SCI Data Sets is illustrated in Figure 81.1.

Core Data Set

The Core Data Set was the first one to be developed.[13] The purpose of the Core Data Set is to standardize the collection and reporting of a minimal amount of information necessary to evaluate and compare results of published studies. At minimum, published studies should include information on the gender and age of the study population at the time of injury, the current age of the study population if different from age at injury, the length of time elapsed after injury when data are being collected, the calendar time frame during which the study was conducted, the causes of spinal cord lesion, and the neurologic status of the study population according to the International Standards for Neurological Classification of SCI.[10] In addition, studies of health services and rehabilitation outcomes should also contain information on the total number of days hospitalized, whether a bony vertebral injury or associated injury was present, whether spinal surgery was performed, whether the patient was ventilator-dependent, and the place of discharge from inpatient care. These data are included in the Core Data Set and are recommended to be included as a descriptive table in most publications including individuals with SCI. Inclusion of more detailed information will depend on the research topic. This information should be provided in either table or text format for the overall study population and for each study group. It is extremely important that data be collected in a uniform manner. The Core Data Set is available at www.iscos.org.uk, and www.asia-spinalinjury.org, including training cases.

Basic Question

This is a question, which, with an affirmative answer, implies that it is possible to go on to one or more specific data set(s) with more detailed information on the particular topic. There will not be such questions for all data sets.

Examples of Basic Questions:

- Bony vertebral injury: Yes/No/Unknown (from the Core Data Set), if Yes → Bony vertebral injury Basic SCI Data Set.
- Spinal surgery: Yes/No/Unknown (from the Core Data Set), if Yes → Spinal surgery Basic SCI Data Set.
- Etiology of lesion: Sports/Assault/Transport/Fall/Other traumatic/Nontraumatic (from the Core Data Set), if traumatic → Etiology module (SCI version of International Classification of External Causes of Injury (ICECI (http://www.iceci.org/)[14]).
- Pain: Have you had any pain during the last 7 days including today: Yes/No, if Yes → Pain Basic SCI Data Set.

Module

A Module may consist of Basic and Expanded SCI Data Sets, and other data (e.g. specific scoring systems), which are appropriate for the particular module.

Possible examples of Modules:

Urologic module:

- Lower Urinary Tract Function Basic SCI Data Set
- Lower Urinary Tract Function Expanded SCI Data Set
- Urodynamic Basic SCI Data Set
- Urodynamic Expanded SCI Data Set
- Urinary tract imagine Basic SCI Data Set
- Urinary tract imagine Expanded SCI Data Set.

Pain module:

- Pain Basic SCI Data Set
- Pain Expanded SCI Data Set
- Pain scoring.

Basic SCI Data Set

This is the minimal number of data elements, including the possible Basic Question, which together should be collected in daily clinical practice for a particular topic. This means that the various Basic SCI Data Sets in the future may be the basis for a structured record in centers worldwide caring for persons with SCI.

Examples of Basic SCI Data Sets:

- Bony vertebral injury Basic SCI Data Set
- Spinal surgery Basic SCI Data Set
- Lower Urinary Tract Function Basic SCI Data Set
- Bowel Basic SCI Data Set
- Pain Basic SCI Data Set
- Urodynamic Basic SCI Data Set
- Urinary tract imagine Basic SCI Data Set.

Expanded SCI Data Set

This is a more detailed data set, which may be used as optional for a topic, but may be recommended for specific research studies within the particular area.

Examples of possible Expanded SCI Data Sets:

- Lower urinary tract function Expanded SCI Data Set
- Bowel Expanded SCI Data Set
- Pain Expanded SCI Data Set
- Urodynamic Expanded SCI Data Set
- ICECI (International Classification of External Causes of Injury) for SCI.[14]

In summary, each module may consist of a basic question, a two-level data set: the basic SCI data set and the expanded SCI data set, and eventually other data sets.

International SCI Data Set developments

For development of further Data Sets, the Executive Committee for the International SCI Standards and Data Sets creates topic-specific expert working groups. The establishment of working groups in the various areas is done in cooperation with relevant international societies and organizations working with the respective topics.

Initially, priority has been given to the development of Basic Questions and Data Sets within the following areas:

- bony vertebral injury
- spinal surgery
- nontraumatic spinal cord lesions
- etiology/prevention, based on the WHO International Classification of External Causes of Injury (http://www.iceci.org/)
- urology
- bowel
- sexual function
- pain
- activity, participation, and well-being.

For each data set a syllabus including definitions, coding schemes, and instructions on how to collect each data item is developed.

Organization

The Executive Committee for the International Spinal Cord Injury Standards and Data Sets is a steering committee for the specific working groups created for the development of specific topic Modules and Data Sets. International organizations and societies within the fields of spinal cord injury, neurosurgery, orthopedic surgery, rehabilitation, and others are being invited to appoint members to join the review process for the creation and evaluation of the best possible International SCI Data Set.

Process for approval of International SCI Data Sets

A process for approval of the data sets has been established following the points below:

1. The particular SCI Data Set working group itself finalizes the data set.
2. The Executive Committee of the International SCI Standards and Data Sets reviews the data set.
3. Comments from the Committee are discussed in the particular SCI Data Set working group and a response is made and possible adjustments of the Data Set performed.
4. ISCoS Scientific Committee and ASIA Board review the data set.
5. Comments from the Committee/Board are discussed in the particular SCI Data Set working group and a response is made and possible adjustments of the Data Set performed.
6. Relevant and interested (international) organizations, societies, and persons review the data set.
7. Comments are discussed in the particular SCI Data Set working group and responses are made and possible adjustments of the Data Set performed.
8. ISCoS Scientific Committee, Council, and ASIA Board review the data set for final approval.
9. ISCoS and ASIA general meetings have the data set for final approval.
10. Endorsement of the data set by relevant (international) organizations and societies.

Data Set presentation

As soon as a new International SCI Data Set is developed in this iterative manner, consensus has been obtained, and the final draft has been approved together with an appropriate training program, the information will be disseminated at meetings, and published in international journals and through the web sites of ISCoS (www.iscos.org.uk), and ASIA (www.asia-spinalinjury.org).

Training programs

For each developed Data Set, training cases will be created and made accessible through the ISCoS and ASIA web sites, from which the data guidelines will be freely available. The training cases should preferable precede download of the particular Data Set. This training will provide examples on how to code the data set and will give a minimal introduction to those using the data sets in their own environment.

International SCI Urologic Data Set Working Group

Due to the central role of urologic issues for most individuals with spinal cord lesions, this topic was given early high priority for establishing a working group to develop SCI data sets in this area. The working group was established after consultation with the International Continence Society (ICS), European Association of Urology (EAU), ISCoS, ASIA, and representatives of the American Urologic Association. A group was then created, consisting of Michael Craggs, representing the EAU, Michael Kennelly, representing ASIA, Erik Schick, representing ICS, Jean-Jacques Wyndaele, representing ISCoS, and Fin Biering-Sørensen representing The Executive Committee of the International Spinal Cord Injury Standards and Data Sets ASIA/ISCoS (chair).

An example: Lower Urinary Tract Function Basic SCI Data Set

The purpose of the Lower Urinary Tract (LUT) Function Basic SCI Data Set for individuals with SCI is to standardize the collection and reporting of a minimal amount of information on the lower urinary tract in daily practice. This will also make it possible to evaluate and compare results from various published studies. The data in the LUT Function Basic SCI Data Set should be seen in connection with data in the Core Data Set.

A spinal cord lesion may be of traumatic or nontraumatic etiology. All lesions to the spinal cord, conus medullaris, and cauda equina are included in the context of the LUT Function Basic SCI Data Set. As for all data sets, it is extremely important that data be collected in a uniform manner. For this reason, each variable and each response category within each variable have been specifically defined in a way that is designed to promote the collection and reporting of comparable minimal data. Use of a standard format is essential for combining data from multiple investigators and locations. Various formats and coding schemes may be equally effective and could be used in individual studies or by agreement of the collaborating investigators.

This collection of data on lower urinary tract function may be carried out at any time after the spinal cord lesion. Follow-up of persons with spinal cord lesions should, as advised, be at least every 1–2 years,[15] and for these follow-up visits the LUT Function Basic SCI Data Set will provide a helpful screening.

The complete LUT Function Basic SCI Data Set including comments may be downloaded from www.iscos.org.uk and www.asia-spinalinjury.org, including training cases. As far as possible, definitions approved by the ICS are applied.[16] The data in the LUT Function Basic SCI Data Set should be seen in connection with data in the Core Data Set.[13]

The data elements included in the International LUT Function Basic SCI Data Set are described briefly below:

Date of data collection: YYYYMMDD

The date of data collection is imperative to be able to identify the data collected in relation to other data collected on the same individual at various time points. In addition, the date is likewise important to enable calculation of the time interval from the date of birth (age), and the time interval from the date of the lesion, i.e. time since spinal cord lesion.

Urinary tract impairment unrelated to spinal cord lesion:
❑ No ❑ Yes, specify________ ❑ Unknown

Urinary tract impairment unrelated to spinal cord lesion is stated to enable evaluation of the LUT function in an individual with spinal cord lesion.

Awareness of the need to empty the bladder:
❑ No ❑ Yes ❑ Not applicable ❑ Not known

Awareness of the need to empty the bladder is meant as any kind of bladder sensation as defined by ICS.[16] 'Not applicable' is to be used when the individual with a spinal cord lesion has, e.g, an unclamped indwelling catheter or noncontinent urinary diversion.

Bladder-emptying:	Main	Supplementary
Normal voiding		
Bladder reflex triggering		
Voluntary (tapping, scratching, anal stretch, etc.)	❑	❑
Involuntary	❑	❑
Bladder expression		
Straining (abdominal straining, Valsalva's manoeuvre)	❑	❑
External compression (Credé manoeuvre)	❑	❑
Intermittent catheterisation		
Self-catheterisation	❑	❑
Catheterisation by attendant	❑	❑
Indwelling catheter		
Transurethral	❑	❑
Suprapubic	❑	❑
Sacral anterior root stimulation	❑	❑
Non-continent urinary diversion/ostomy	❑	❑

Other method, specify______________
❑ Unknown

This variable documents the method(s) used by the spinal cord lesioned individual to empty the bladder on the date of collecting the data. For each method of bladder emptying it should be stated whether this is a main or a supplementary method. Two main and more supplementary methods may be indicated (adopted from (17)). Definitions in general are in accordance with ICS (16).

Average number of voluntary bladder emptying per day during the last week ____________

This number refers to the number of voluntary bladder emptying irrespective of the method.

Any involuntary urine leakage (incontinence) within the last three months:
❑ No ❑ Yes, average daily
❑ Yes, average weekly
❑ Yes, average monthly
❑ Not applicable ❑ Unknown

Urinary incontinence is defined by ICS (16) as the complaint of any involuntary leakage of urine. In each specific circumstance the urinary incontinence should be further described by specifying relevant factors such as type, frequency, severity, precipitating factors, social impact, effect on hygiene and quality of life, etc. (16). In the Basic SCI Data Set a simple indication of severity and collection of urine is given only. Bladder reflex triggering including into a collection system, e.g. condom catheter may be voluntary and thus not considered as incontinence. But, if the condom or ostomy bag fall off and the individual complains of incontinence then it should be recorded as Yes. No incontinence within the last three months implies no leakage of urine outside the urinary tract or a closed urinary collection system. Instances of leakage less than monthly is considered as "no" unless the individual with spinal cord lesion does consider it a problem, and then it is to be coded as "monthly". Not applicable may be used when the spinal cord lesioned individual has for instance a non-continent urinary diversion.

Collecting appliances for urinary incontinence:

❑ No ❑ Yes, condom catheter/sheath
❑ Yes, diaper/pad
❑ Yes, ostomy bag
❑ Yes, other, specify ______________

❑ Unknown

Collecting appliances are any externally applied aids to avoid urinary leakage, or devices for collection of urine. Regular use of one or more collecting appliances is to be recorded. Individuals with spinal cord lesions that use such appliances less than once a month, "for the sake of safety", and have no more than exceptional episodes of leakage during a year should be excluded (adapted from (17)).

Any drugs for the urinary tract within the last year:
❑ No
❑ Yes, bladder relaxant drugs (anticholinergics, tricyclic antidepressant, etc.)
❑ Yes, sphincter/bladder neck relaxant drugs (alpha adrenergic blockers, etc.)
❑ Yes, antibiotics/antiseptics:
❑ For treatment of urinary tract infection
❑ For prophylactic reasons

Yes, other, specify________________

❑ Unknown

This variable documents use of any drugs, systemic or intravesical, for the urinary tract.
This does not include treatment with injections into the detrusor or sphincter.

Surgical procedures on the urinary tract:
❑ No ❑ Yes, supra-pubic catheter insertion, date last performed YYYYMMDD
❑ Yes, bladder stone removal, date last performed YYYYMMDD
❑ Yes, upper urinary tract stone removal, date last performed YYYYMMDD
❑ Yes, bladder augmentation, date last performed YYYYMMDD
❑ Yes, sphincterotomy/urethral stent, date last performed YYYYMMDD
❑ Yes, botulinum toxin injection, date last performed YYYYMMDD
❑ Yes, artificial sphincter, date last performed YYYYMMDD
❑ Yes, ileovesicostomy, date last performed YYYYMMDD
❑ Yes, ileoureterostomy, date last performed YYYYMMDD
❑ Yes, content catheterizable values, date last performed YYYYMMDD
❑ Yes, sacral anterior root stimulator, date performed YYYYMMDD
❑ Yes, other, specify________________, date performed YYYYMMDD

❑ Unknown

This variable documents any surgical procedures on the urinary tract up to the date of collecting the data. If more procedures of the same kind have been performed, only the last one is documented with date of performance. Bladder stone or upper urinary tract stone removal includes any type of removal, including via endoscopy, extracorporal shock wave lithotripsy (ESWL), or open lithotomy.

Any change in urinary symptoms within the last year:
❑ No ❑ Yes ❑ Unknown

LUT symptoms are, according to ICS, the subjective indicator of a disease or change in conditions as perceived by the individual with a spinal cord lesion, attendant, or partner, and may lead him/her to seek help from healthcare professionals.[16] Symptoms may either be volunteered or described during the interview with the individual with a spinal cord lesion. They may be qualitative as well as quantitative, e.g. change in frequency, urgency, nocturia, incontinence, hesitancy, slow stream, etc. Many individuals with spinal cord lesion and bacteriuria have no associated signs or symptoms. Chills and fever are often considered to be signs of acute pyelonephritis; however, these signs do not confirm an infection in the upper urinary tract.[18] Still, chills and fever may be the only symptoms in persons with spinal cord lesion and pyelonephritis, bacteremia, upper tract obstruction by calculi, renal abscesses, and periphrenic abscess. Other suspicious signs and symptoms may include increased sweating, abdominal discomfort, costovertebral angle pain or tenderness, and increased muscle spasticity.[18] Cloudy and malodorous urine and changes in urine pH may be signs of urinary tract infection, but can also occur with colonization, changes of bacterial organisms, and various food intakes. Increased spontaneous voiding or larger residual urine including acute urinary retention may be seen with acute infection.[18]

Summary

It is extremely important that the LUT Function Basic SCI Data Set be collected in a uniform manner. For this reason, each variable and each response category within each variable have been specifically defined in a way that is designed to promote the collection and reporting of comparable minimal data.

Before using the LUT Function Basic SCI Data Set, individuals should review each training case at www.iscos.org.uk and www.asia-spinalinjury.org, complete a sample data collection form, and compare it with the correct results that are also posted. Generally speaking, International SCI Data Sets and Standards are imperative for the continuous improvement of examination, treatment, rehabilitation, and prevention of SCI in the future. Regarding prevention, the Data Sets may, depending on the topic, be of importance both in primary prevention (ICECI[14]) and in secondary and tertiary prevention regarding relapse of disease and occurrence of possible complications, if screening with the Data Sets can pinpoint areas of special concern for the particular individual.

When considering breakthrough studies it is unlikely that one center alone will be able to recruit enough participants. Therefore, standardized international data sets like the LUT Function Basic SCI Data Set are necessary for the many multicenter trials and investigations which will take place in the years to come.

Acknowledgment

Coloplast A/S, Denmark, have supported the work on this Lower Urinary Tract Function Basic SCI Data Set with an unconditional grant. We are grateful for comments and suggestions received from Susan Charlifue, Volker Dietz, Brigitte Schurch, and Lawrence C Vogel.

References

1. Kemp BJ, Adkins RH, Thompson L. Aging with a spinal cord injury: what recent research shows. Top Spinal Cord Inj Rehab 2004; 10: 175–97.
2. Strauss DJ, Devivo MJ, Paculdo DR, Shavelle RM. Trends in life expectancy after spinal cord injury. Arch Phys Med Rehab 2006; 87: 1079–85.
3. Frankel HL, Coll JR, Charlifue SW et al. Long term survival in spinal cord injury: a fifty year investigation. Spinal Cord 1998; 36: 266–74.
4. Hartkopp A, Brønnum-Hansen H, Seidenschnur A-M, Biering-Sørensen F. Survival and cause of death after traumatic spinal cord injury. A long-term epidemiological survey from Denmark. Spinal Cord 1997; 35: 78–85.
5. DeVivo MJ, Krause JS, Lammertse DP. Recent trends in mortality and causes of death among persons with spinal cord injury. Arch Phys Med Rehab 1999; 80: 1411–19.
6. Krause JS, DeVivo MJ, Jackson AB. Health status, community integration, and economic risk factors for mortality after spinal cord injury. Arch Phys Med Rehab 2004; 85: 1764–73.
7. O'Connor PJ. Survival after spinal cord injury in Australia. Arch Phys Med Rehab 2005; 86: 37–47.
8. Soden R, Walsh J, Middleton JW et al. Causes of death after spinal cord injury. Spinal Cord 2000; 38: 604–10.
9. Biering-Sørensen F, Charlifue S, DeVivo M et al. International Spinal Cord Injury Data Sets. Spinal Cord 2006; 44: 530–4.
10. Marino RJ, Barros T, Biering-Sorensen F et al. International standards for neurological classification of spinal cord injury. J Spinal Cord Med 2003; 26(Suppl 1): S50–6.
11. World Health Organization. International Classification of Functioning. Disability and Health. Geneva: WHO; 2001.
12. Biering-Sørensen F, Scheuringer M, Baumberger M et al. Developing core sets for persons with spinal cord injuries based on the International Classification of Functioning, Disability and Health as a way to specify functioning. Spinal Cord 2006; 44: 541–6.
13. DeVivo M, Biering-Sørensen F, Charlifue S et al. International Spinal Cord Injury Core Data Set. Spinal Cord 2006; 44: 535–40.
14. World Health Organisation: International Classification of External Causes of Injury (ICECI). Available from: http://www.iceci.org/
15. Stöhrer M, Castro-Diaz D, Chartier-Kastler E et al. Guidelines on Neurogenic Lower Urinary Tract Dysfunction. European Association of Urology 2006.
16. Abrams P, Cardozo L, Fall M et al. The Standardisation of Terminology of Lower Urinary Tract Function: Report from the Standardisation Sub-committee of the International Continence Society. Neurourol Urodyn 2002; 21: 167–78.
17. Levi R, Ertzgaard P. The Swedish Spinal Cord Injury Council 1998. Quality indicators in spinal cord injury care: A Swedish collaboration project. Scand J Rehab Med 1998; (Suppl 38): 1–80.
18. Stover SL, Lloyd K, Waites KB et al. Review article. Urinary tract infection in spinal cord injury. Arch Phys Med Rehab 1989; 70: 47–54.

Part XII

Ethical considerations

82

Ethical considerations in neurogenic lower urinary tract dysfunction

Jocelyne Tessier

Why bioethics?

Following the medical scandals that resulted from Nazi experimentation held during World War II and that led to the Nuremberg Code[1] and article by Beecher[2] published in the *New England Journal of Medicine* exposing medical research aberrations, the bioethics movement evolved during the second half of the 20th century. However, even though this seems strange to many doctors, bioethics has always been part of medical practice at various levels. An example dating back to the beginning of medicine is the Hippocratic Oath,[3] which delimits medical practice including doctors' conduct per se to the end result of administered treatments.

The contribution of philosophy and law helped develop this new discipline with regard to both theory and language. Bioethics often seems closed to practitioners, who nevertheless unknowingly use it on a daily basis! Each decision made concerning a patient is an ethics act. One often realizes the involvement of bioethics only when confronted with problem cases, such as the absence of adequate resources to perform intermittent catheterization on a quadriplegic patient with numerous complications involving an indwelling catheter.

Neurogenic bladder treatment does not imply ethical issues specific to this area. However, the very nature of the breach of the patient's physical integrity has a greater chance of forcing the attending physician to deal with problems regarding quality of life and autonomy, for instance, than the treatment of a common urinary tract infection. The purpose of this chapter is to introduce bioethics basic concepts and suggest a method for solving ethical problems.

Values and ethical conflicts

Even though they belong to a given community, each member of such a group believes in his or her own value system. These values influence them with regard to the life choices that they must make, especially when dealing with medical treatment having considerable impact of their lives. Here is a list of the values mentioned most often.

Autonomy

This is the most important value. It is at the heart of the bioethics movement in the United States; it goes against paternalism. It refers to a person's self-determination in as much as a person cannot be governed by another one since all persons are equal. From this value comes the free and informed consent, the right to the truth, the refusal of treatment, and the need for a legal representative in case of incompetence.

Self-determination may be limited by society through laws, for instance, or by other ethical values, such as the respect for life or justice.

Respect for life

This value sanctions the fundamental importance of human life. This explains why it is an integral part of many religions (Judaeo-Christian, Buddhism, etc.) and numerous Acts that prohibit murder, assisted suicide, etc. Without this value, human society would be in peril. Must life be respected in all circumstances? For vitalists, this is a nonquestion since life must be protected at all costs. For others, quality of life is an important element in the equation when a decision regarding treatment must be made.[4] The quality of human life is therefore valued over the sole biologic life. This type of reasoning is often the basis for decisions on the cessation of treatment, such as artificial nutrition or breathing termination, or no resuscitation.

Quality of life

This value is not easily defined. Some have tried to quantify it,[5,6] but the experience has proven to be difficult and potentially discriminatory for certain categories of people. What is a good quality of life for an elderly man or a severely handicapped person? It is probably inappropriate to compare the lives of different individuals, but more relevant to compare what the life of one individual was to what it could be.

Justice

This is a value which is difficult to define, since the viewpoints that address it vary. It is involved, notably, in the accessibility to care, exploitation of vulnerable populations for research, discrimination, and resource allocation. The principle of justice is often invoked when resources are scarce. For instance, among all the candidates for a kidney transplant, who must be chosen? The one who is most deserving socially? The one who has greatest chance of recovery? The one whose name was written on the list first? The one who has the greatest life expectancy?

Beneficence

This principle requires that we act for the patient's good. Some authors make it such an obligation for physicians that it even justifies compromising the doctor's personal comfort or financial situation.[7] For others, this principle must be carefully considered as it has paternalistic overtones (I know what is good for you). Nevertheless, embedded in a value system, beneficence can only contribute to the humanism of physicians.

Nonmaleficence

This is the *primum non nocere* (first, do no harm) of the Hippocratic tradition. This value is closely linked to beneficence, since we cannot be satisfied with not harming alone. It often comes up in discussions about life-prolonging medical treatment, futility of treatment, dignity, etc.

When these values go against the attending physician's values, an ethical conflict ensues. It is then possible to ethically define the nature of the conflict. For instance, a patient's refusal to undergo treatment that is recognized and suited to his or her medical condition brings into play the patient's autonomy and the physician's obligation to beneficence.

1. Facts
   - Clinical facts
     - Current disease, co-existing diseases
     - Higher mental functions
     - Diagnostic, prognosis
   - Psychosocial facts
     - Social history
     - Family dynamics
     - Patient's will
     - Reactions of the patient and his or her family to the situation
   - Reactions of the healthcare team
   - Identification of the question
2. Spontaneous option
   - Intuitive solution that does not need to be shared with the group
3. Identification of the values
   - Patient's values
     - Moral values
     - Religious values
   - Values of the family or membership group
   - Values of the healthcare providers
     - Personal values (moral, religious)
     - Professional values
4. Identification of the problem or moral dilemma
   - Determination of the values at stake
   - Identification of the conflicting values that create ethical dilemmas
5. Alternatives
   - Enumeration of all possible options with related normative and legal aspects (including step-by-step solutions)
   - Probable consequences of each alternative
   - Values underlying each option
   - Argumentation on the eventual priority to be established
6. Consideration of the spontaneous option
   - Intuitive solution that does not need to be shared with the group
7. Decision (advice)
   - Recommendations
   - Justification

Figure 82.1
Analytical grid for ethics cases

Decision-making

In most cases of ethical conflicts, the decision is made quickly and usually proves to be the best option among several alternatives. Experience and evaluation of various data pertaining to the patient and his or her disease are part of the decision-making process, which initially appears to be largely intuitive. However, what seems intuitive is more the fruit of a methodology that has been extensively discussed in the literature.[8]

The problem-solving method used in bioethics is closely related to that used in medicine. It entails a series of steps that lead to a global understanding of the situation, followed by the drafting of a list of possible solutions. Constraints and particularities are then included to eliminate a certain number of solutions and achieve a final decision supported by valid arguments. In bioethics, there are numerous decision-making models[9,10] that are helpful to structure the decision-making process in cases of ethical conflicts that seem more difficult to address. The use of these models allows for a global vision of the problematic situation, which usually extends beyond the medical framework. The accuracy and completeness of the facts, the degree of medical certainty, and the amount of creativity in the solutions considered are all assets useful to achieve an adequate decision based on ethical arguments.

Irrespective of the method used, there is a clear advantage to examining the problem in a group since the analysis of the problem and the solutions considered are enriched by the contributions of the various participants. As an example, the Crowe and Durand[9] analytical grid is presented in Figure 82.1. Interestingly, step 2 consists in stating the solution that comes to mind spontaneously during the summary analysis of the problem and step 6 is to modify that solution following the detailed analysis of the problem.

Conclusion

Bioethics is here to stay. Whatever the area of practice, a physician should gradually familiarize him- or herself with the language and method of the discipline that he or she is already practicing intuitively. The use of ethical analytical grids that structure the decision-making process can only promote this learning.

References

1. http://www.frsq.gouv.qc.ca/fr/ethique/pdfs_ethique/nuremberg_f. pdf.
2. Beecher HK. Ethics and clinical research. N Engl J Med 1966; 274: 1354–60.
3. http://www.cmq.org/CmsPages/PageCmsSimpleSplit.aspx?PageID=05aa9276-c26a-4528-aab1-105fe58a800c.
4. Keyserlingk EW, Le caractère sacré de la vie ou la qualité de la vie: du point de vue de l'éthique, de la médecine et du droit. Document published by the LRCC, Ottawa, 1979.
5. Fagot-Largeault A. Réflexions sur la notion de qualité de vie. Jurisprud Arch 1991; 36: 135–54.
6. Williams A. The value of QALYs. Health Soc Serv J 1985: 3.
7. Pellegrino E, Thomasma DC. For the patient's good. In: The Restoration of Beneficence in Health Care. New York: Oxford University Press, 1988: 27.
8. Drane JF. Theory and practice in medical ethical decision-making. In: Clinical Bioethics. Sheed & Ward, Kansas City, 1994: 38–9.
9. Durand G. Introduction à la Bioéthique. (Fides, Montreal 1999), 437–4.
10. Richard Martin A clinical model for decision-making. J Med Ethics 1978; 4: 200–6.

Part XIII

Reports and guidelines

83

Reports and guidelines in relation to neurogenic bladder dysfunction: a selection

Erik Schick

In the Appendices of the first edition of this textbook, in 2004, we reproduced four documents, terminology reports and guidelines, in relation to neurogenic bladder dysfunction. Since then several other reports have been published and the existing ones updated. It became apparent that these documents are rapidly changing and become outdated. As almost all of them are available on the Web, it seems to be more useful to establish a repertoire of these websites where all of them can be consulted in their most recent, updated version, instead of reproducing some of them *in extenso* in this book.

The reader will find herein a collection of these websites with their electronic addresses, the name and composition of the groups who developed them and the bibliographic reference when they were published.

1 Evidence-based medicine overview of the main steps for developing and grading guideline recommendations

The Agency for Health Care Policy and Research (AHCPR), a US government agency, has used specified evidence levels to justify recommendations for the investigation and treatment of a variety of conditions. The Oxford Centre for Evidence Based Medicine has produced a widely accepted adaptation of the work of the AHCPR. It seems to be highly desirable that Guidelines follow this accepted grading system supported by explicit levels of evidence. Even if not strictly related to the topic of this book, we find that this important document has its place in the repertoire of different reports and guidelines in relation to neurogenic bladder dysfunction.

Authors: Bob Phillips, Dave Sachett, Doug Badenoch, Sharon Straus, Brian Haynes, and Martin Dawes.

Website: http://www.cebm.net/levels_of_evidence.asp#levels
http://www.cebm.net/levels_of_evidence.asp#notes

Printed version: Recently, fundamental principles of evidence based clinical practice have been outlined using examples from the literature and practice of urology. (Scales CD Jr, Premingr GM, Keitz SA, Dahm P. Evidence based clinical practice: a primer for urologists. J Urol 2007; 178: 775–82.)

2 The standardization of terminology of lower urinary tract function: Report from the standardization subcommittee of the International Continence Society (ICS)

This report is one of the first which gained wide acceptance within the urologic community and which deals with the standardization of the terminology used in clinical practice and research. It was published for the first time 20 years ago and underwent an extensive revision in 2002. It is certainly the most frequently quoted report of its kind in the urologic literature.

Authors: Paul Abrams, Linda Cardozo, Magnus Fall, Derek Griffiths, Peter Rosier, Ulf Ulmsten, Philip van Kerrebroeck, Arne Victor, and Alan Wein.

Website: www.icsoffice.org

Printed version: Neurourology and Urodynamics 2002; 21: 167–78.

3 The standardization of terminology in neurogenic lower urinary tract dysfunction with suggestions for diagnostic procedures

This report of a subcommittee of the International Continence Society was first published in 1999 and has not been revised since then. It represents not simply an effort to standardize terminology in the neurogenic bladder patient, but also contains some suggestions for diagnostic procedures, including clinical assessment, investigations, comments on clinical value and classification of urodynamic investigations, as well as supplemental investigations.

Website: www.icsoffice.org

Authors: Manfred Stöhrer, Mark Goepel, Atsuo Kondo, Guus Kramer, Helmut Madersbacher, Richard Millard, Alain Rossier and Jean-Jacques Wyndaele.

Printed version: Neurourology and Urodynamics 1999; 18: 139–58.

4 The standardization of terminology and assessment of functional characteristics of intestinal urinary reservoirs

This report deals with the terminology of surgical procedures, patient assessment, procedures related to the evaluation of urine storage and evacuation of an intestinal urinary reservoir, as well as a proposed classification of the storage function in an intestinal urinary reservoir.

Website: www.icsoffice.org

Authors: Joachim W Thüroff, Anders Mattiasson, Jens Thorup Anderson, Hans Hedlund, Frank Hinman Jr, Markus Hochenfellner, Wiking Mansson, Anthony B Mundy, Randall G Rowland and Kenneth Steven.

Printed version: Neurourology and Urodynamics 1996; 15: 499–511.

5 Good urodynamic practice: uroflowmetry, filling cystometry, and pressure–flow studies

Urodynamics is the cornerstone in the investigation, the elaboration of an appropriate treatment plan, and a meaningful follow-up of patients with neurogenic bladder dysfunction. It represents the first report of the International Continence Society on the development of comprehensive guidelines for good urodynamic practice for the measurement, quality control, and documentation of urodynamic investigations. It deals with the three most frequently performed urodynamic examinations, i.e. uroflowmetry, filling cystometry, and pressure–flow studies.

Website: www.icsoffice.org

Authors: Werner Schafer, Paul Abrams, Limin Liao, Anders Mattiasson, Francesco Pesce, Anders Spangberg, Arthur M Sterling, Norman R Zinner, and Philip van Kerrebroeck

Printed version: Neurourology and Urodynamics 2002; 21: 261–74.

6 Guidelines on neurogenic lower urinary tract dysfunction

The European Association of Urology put together a working party to provide information on the incidence, definitions, diagnosis, therapy, quality of life issues, and follow-up of patients with neurogenic bladder dysfunction that will be useful for clinical practitioners. It has a broader spectrum than the ICS report on the same subject and represents a state of the art reference for all clinicians. Each section is followed by an important reference list. The most recent update was published in 2006.

Website: www.uroweb.org

Authors: Manfred Stöhrer, David Castro-Diaz, Emmanuel Chartier-Kastler, Guus Kramer, Anders Mattiasson, and Jean-Jacques Wyndaele.

Printed version: European Association of Urology Guidelines, Anheim, European Association of Urology, 2007.

7 The standardization of terminology of lower urinary tract function in children and adolescents

This report from the Standardization Committee of the International Children's Continence Society (ICCS) focuses on voiding function and dysfunction in childhood and during adolescence. Symptoms are followed by investigational tools, signs, conditions, and treatment parameters, but in no way does the report tell researchers and clinicians what to do, only what words to use. The document also contains a number of appendices, including encopresis and functional fecal incontinence, an alphabetic list of commonly used terms defined in the ICCS terminology, urodynamic instruments in children, and maximum voided volume formula.

Website: www.i-c-c-s.org

Authors: Tryggve Nevéus, Alexander von Gontard, Piet Hoebeke, Kelm Hjälmås, Stuart Bauer, Wendy Bower, Troels Munch Jørgensen, Søren Rittig, Johan Vande Walle, Chung-Kwong Yeung, and Jens Christian Djurhuus.

Printed version: Journal of Urology 2006, 176: 314–24.

8 International urodynamic basic spinal cord injury data set

A detailed description of this data set can be found in Chapter 81 of this textbook.

Websites: www.iscos.org.uk
www.asia-spinalinjury.org

Authors: Fin Biering-Sørensen, Michael Craggs, Michael Kennelly, Erik Schick and Jean-Jacques Wyndaele.

Printed version: Spinal Cord 2008; 46: 325–30.

Index